Hepatology
A Textbook of Liver Disease

VOLUME II

DAVID ZAKIM, MD
Professor of Medicine Emeritus
Cornell University Medical College
New York, New York

THOMAS D. BOYER, MD
John J. Lee Professor of Medicine
Director, Liver Research Institute
University of Arizona
Tucson, Arizona

FOURTH EDITION

with 556 *illustrations and* 186 *color plates*

SAUNDERS
An Imprint of Elsevier Science
Philadelphia London New York St. Louis Sydney Toronto

SAUNDERS
An Imprint of Elsevier Science

The Curtis Center
Independence Square West
Philadelphia, Pennsylvania 19106

HEPATOLOGY 0-7216-9051-3

NOTICE

Hepatology is an ever-changing field. Standard safety precautions must be followed, but as new research and clinical experience broaden our knowledge, changes in treatment and drug therapy may become necessary or appropriate. Readers are advised to check the most current product information provided by the manufacturer of each drug to be administered to verify the recommended dose, the method and duration of administration, and contraindications. It is the responsibility of the licensed prescriber, relying on experience and knowledge of the patient, to determine dosages and the best treatment for each individual patient. Neither the publisher nor the editor assumes any liability for any injury and/or damage to persons or property arising from this publication.

Library of Congress Cataloging-in-Publication Data

Hepatology / [edited by] David Zakim, Thomas D. Boyer.—4th ed.
p. ; cm.
Includes bibliographical references and index.
ISBN 0-7216-9051-3 (alk. paper)
1. Liver—Diseases. I. Zakim, David. II. Boyer, Thomas D.
[DNLM: 1. Liver Diseases. WI 700 H5292 2002]
RC845.H46 2002
616.3′62—dc21 2002021749

Acquisitions Editor: Sue Hodgson
Developmental Editor: Jennifer Shreiner
Publishing Services Manager: Pat Joiner
Project Manager: Rachel E. Dowell
Book Design Manager: Gail Morey Hudson
Cover Art: Jayne Jones

GW/MVY

Printed in the United States of America

Last digit is the print number: 9 8 7 6 5 4 3 2 1

Hepatology

To the memory of our parents:
Sam and Ruth Zakim
and
Clayton and Agellah Boyer

Contributors

Gary A. Abrams, MD
Assistant Professor of Medicine
Division of Gastroenterology and Hepatology,
Medical Director, GI/Hepatology Inpatient Service
University of Alabama at Birmingham
Birmingham, Alabama

Helmut Albrecht, MD
Associate Professor of Medicine
Division of Infectious Diseases
Emory University;
Director, Infectious Diseases Clinics,
Director, ID Clinical Research Unit
Emory University Hospitals and Emory Healthcare
Atlanta, Georgia

Karl E. Anderson, MD
Professor, Departments of Preventative Medicine & Community Health, Internal Medicine, and Pharmacology & Toxicology,
Active Member of the Medical Staff
University of Texas Medical Branch
Galveston, Texas

Miguel R. Arguedas, MD, MPH
Assistant Professor of Medicine
University of Alabama at Birmingham
Birmingham, Alabama

Vicente Arroyo, MD
Professor of Medicine
Medical School, University of Barcelona;
Director, Institute of Digestive Disease
Hospital Clinic
Barcelona, Spain

Veronica A. Arteaga, MD, BS
Doctor of Medicine, Department of Surgery
Cedars-Sinai Medical Center
Los Angeles, California;
Clinical Researcher
New England Hepatobiliary Disease Center
Dartmouth-Hitchcock Medical Center
Lebanon, New Hampshire

Bruce R. Bacon, MD
James F. King, MD, Endowed Chair in Gastroenterology
Professor of Internal Medicine,
Director, Division of Gastroenterology & Hepatology
Saint Louis University School of Medicine
St. Louis, Missouri

Norman H. Bell, MD
Distinguished University Professor of Medicine
Medical University of South Carolina
Charleston, South Carolina

Marina Berenguer, MD
Hospital Universitario Lafe Servicio de Medicina Digestiva
Valencia, Spain

D. Montgomery Bissell, MD
Professor of Medicine,
Director, Division of Gastroenterology
University of California;
Attending Physician, University of California Hospitals
San Francisco General Hospital Medical Center
San Francisco, California

Thomas D. Boyer, MD
John J. Lee Professor of Medicine
Director, Liver Research Institute
University of Arizona
Tucson, Arizona

Mary T. Brophy, MD, MPH
Assistant Professor of Medicine
Boston University School of Medicine;
Staff Hematologist/Oncologist, VA Boston Health Care System
Boston, Massachusetts

Naga Chalasani, MD
Assistant Professor of Medicine
Division of Gastroenterology & Hepatology
Indiana University School of Medicine
Indianapolis, Indiana

David E. Cohen, MD, PhD
Associate Professor of Medicine and Biochemistry
Marion Bessin Liver Research Center
Albert Einstein College of Medicine;
Attending Physician, Montefiore Medical Center
Jacobi Medical Center
Bronx, New York

Arthur J.L. Cooper, PhD, DSc
Professor of Medicine
Weill Medical College of Cornell University at
Burke Medical Research Institute
White Plains, New York

John R. Craig, MD, PhD
Associate Clinical Professor
University of Southern California School of Medicine
Los Angeles, California;
Director of Laboratory, St. Luke Medical Center
Pasadena, California;
Medical Director, Oncology Services, St. Jude Medical Center
Fullerton, California

James M. Crawford, MD, PhD
Professor and Chair, Department of Pathology, Immunology, &
Laboratory Medicine
University of Florida College of Medicine
Gainesville, Florida

Oscar W. Cummings, MD
Associate Professor of Pathology, Department of Pathology
Indiana University School of Medicine
Indianapolis, Indiana

Albert J. Czaja, MD
Professor of Medicine, Mayo Medical School;
Consultant, Gastroenterology and Hepatology, Mayo Clinic
Rochester, Minnesota

Lawrence J. Dahm, PhD
Manager, Drug Safety Evaluation, Pfizer, Inc.
Global Research and Development
Groton, Connecticut

Valeer J. Desmet, MD, PhD
Emeritus Professor of Pathology and Histology
University of Leuven Medical School
Leuven, Belgium

Daniel Deykin, BA, MD
Professor of Medicine and Public Health
Boston University School of Medicine and Public Health
Boston, Massachusetts

Carlos A. DiazGranados, MD
Infectious Diseases Fellow, Division of Infectious Diseases
Emory University School of Medicine
Atlanta, Georgia

David D. Douglas, MD
Assistant Professor of Medicine, Mayo Medical School
Rochester, Minnesota;
Medical Director, Liver Transplantation, Mayo Clinic Hospital
Phoenix, Arizona

Wayne A. Duffus, MD, PhD
Infectious Diseases Fellow, Division of Infectious Diseases
Emory University School of Medicine
Atlanta, Georgia

Michael B. Fallon, MD
Associate Professor of Medicine,
Director, Section of Hepatology
University of Alabama at Birmingham;
Chief, Gastroenterology and Hepatology
Birmingham Veterans Administration Medical Center
Birmingham, Alabama

Louis D. Fiore, MD, MPH
Assistant Professor of Medicine and Public Health
Boston University School of Medicine and Public Health;
Acting Chief, Oncology Section, Medical Service
VA Boston Health Care System
Boston, Massachusetts

Lawrence S. Friedman, MD
Professor of Medicine, Harvard Medical School;
Physician, Gastrointestinal Unit,
Chief, Walter Bauer Firm (Medical Services)
Massachusetts General Hospital
Boston, Massachusetts

Hans Fromm, MD
Professor of Medicine, Dartmouth Medical School;
Director, New England Hepatobiliary Disease Center
Section of Gastroenterology
Dartmouth-Hitchcock Medical Center
Lebanon, New Hampshire

Toyomi Fukushima, MD, MPH
Director of Digestive Diseases
Tokyo Adventist Hospital (Tokyo Eisei Byoin)
Tokyo, Japan

G. Gerken, MD
Professor of Medicine,
Director, Department of Gastroenterology and Hepatology
University of Essen
Essen, Germany

Fayez K. Ghishan, MD
Professor and Head, Department of Pediatrics
University of Arizona Health Sciences Center;
Director, Steele Memorial Children's Research Center
Tucson, Arizona

Rajbir K. Gill, PhD
Assistant Professor of Medicine
Medical University of South Carolina
Charleston, South Carolina

Pere Ginès, MD
Associate Professor of Medicine, Department of Medicine
University of Barcelona School of Medicine;
Consultant in Hepatology, Liver Unit
Institute for Digestive Diseases, Hospital Clinic
Barcelona, Spain

Jonathan D. Gitlin, MD
Helene B. Roberson Professor of Pediatrics
Washington University School of Medicine
St. Louis, Missouri

Steve Goldschmid, MD
Associate Professor of Clinical Medicine
University of Arizona Health Sciences Center;
Director, GI Lab, University Medical Center
Tucson, Arizona

Hartmut M. Hanauske-Abel, MD, PhD
Assistant Professor of Pediatrics and Obstetrics,
Gynecology, and Women's Health,
Head, Section on Matrix Biology, New Jersey Medical School
Newark, New Jersey

Theo Heller, MB, BCh
Clinical Associate, Liver Diseases Section
National Institute of Health
Bethesda, Maryland

J. Michael Henderson, MD
Chairman, Department of General Surgery
The Cleveland Clinic Foundation
Cleveland, Ohio

Bruce W. Hollis, PhD
Professor of Medicine, Medical University of South Carolina
Charleston, South Carolina

Jay H. Hoofnagle, MD
Director, Division of Digestive Disease and Nutrition
National Institute of Diabetes and Digestive and
Kidney Diseases
National Institutes of Health
Bethesda, Maryland

John G. Hunter, MD
Professor & Chairman, Department of Surgery
Oregon Health & Science University
Portland, Oregon

Peter L.M. Jansen, MD, PhD
Professor of Gastroenterology, University of Groningen;
Head, Department of Gastroenterology and Hepatology
University Hospital Groningen
Groningen, The Netherlands

David L. Jaye, MD
Instructor, Department of Pathology and Laboratory Medicine
Emory University School of Medicine
Atlanta, Georgia

Dean P. Jones, PhD
Professor of Medicine, Emory University
Atlanta, Georgia

Jerry Kaplan, PhD
Professor, Department of Pathology,
Assistant Vice President for Health Sciences for Basic Science,
Associate Dean for Health Sciences Research
University of Utah
Salt Lake City, Utah

Emmet B. Keeffe, MD
Professor of Medicine
Stanford University School of Medicine;
Chief of Hepatology, Co-Director, Liver Transplant Program
Stanford University Medical Center
Stanford, California

Raymond S. Koff, MD
Professor of Medicine
University of Massachusetts Medical School;
Hepatologist, Division of Gastroenterology
UMass Memorial Health Care
Worcester, Massachusetts

Douglas R. LaBrecque, MD
Professor of Internal Medicine,
Director, Liver Service
University of Iowa College of Medicine;
Professor of Internal Medicine,
Director, Liver Service
University of Iowa Hospitals and Clinics
Iowa City Veterans Administration Hospital
Iowa City, Iowa

Jay H. Lefkowitch, MD
Professor of Clinical Pathology
Columbia University College of Physicians and Surgeons;
Attending Physician in Pathology
Columbia-Presbyterian Medical Center
New York, New York

Michael J. Levy, MD
Senior Associate Consultant, Mayo Clinic
Rochester, Minnesota

Keith D. Lindor, MD
Professor of Medicine, Mayo Medical School;
Chair, Division of Gastroenterology and Hepatology
Mayo Clinic
Rochester, Minnesota

Sagar Lonial, MD
Assistant Professor
Bone Marrow and Stem Cell Transplant Center
Winship Cancer Institute, Emory University
Atlanta, Georgia

Jacquelyn J. Maher, MD
Associate Professor of Medicine
University of California, San Francisco;
Director, Liver Center Laboratory
San Francisco General Hospital
San Francisco, California

Paul Martin, MD
Professor of Medicine, UCLA School of Medicine;
Medical Director, Liver Transplantation
Cedars Sinai Medical Center
Los Angeles, California

Enrique J. Martinez, MD, FACP
Assistant Professor, Division Digestive Diseases,
Medical Director, Liver Transplant Program
Emory University
Atlanta, Georgia

Samer G. Mattar, MD
Clinical Instructor, Endosurgery, Emory University
Atlanta, Georgia

Karl-Hermann Meyer zum Büschenfelde, MD, PhD, DrHC, FRCP
Emeritus, First Department of Internal Medicine
Johannes Gutenberg University Mainz
Mainz, Germany

Esteban Mezey, MD
Professor of Medicine
Johns Hopkins University School of Medicine
Baltimore, Maryland

J. Paul Miller, BM, BCh, MSc, DPhil, FRCP
Honorary Lecturer, University of Manchester;
Consultant Gastroenterologist
South Manchester University Hospitals
Manchester, United Kingdom

Darius Moradpour, MD
Assistant Professor of Medicine, University of Freiberg;
Staff Physician, Department of Medicine II
University Hospital Freiburg
Freiburg, Germany

Michael Müller, PhD
Professor of Nutrition, Metabolism, and Genomics, Division of Human Nutrition and Epidemiology
University of Wageningen
Wageningen, The Netherlands

Santiago J. Muñoz, MD
Associate Professor of Medicine
Director, Center for Liver Disease,
Head, Division of Hepatology
Albert Einstein Medical Center, Jefferson Medical College
Philadelphia, Pennsylvania

Satheesh Nair, MD
Clinical Assistant Professor of Medicine, Tulane University;
Medical Director, Liver Transplantation
Ochsner Clinic Foundation
New Orleans, Louisiana

Amin A. Nanji, MD, FRCPC, FRCPath
Professor, Department of Pathology, University of Hong Kong;
Senior Consultant, Clinical Biochemistry
Queen Mary Hospital
Hong Kong

Robert P. Perrillo, MD
Clinical Professor of Medicine
Tulane University School of Medicine;
Director, Section of Gastroenterology and Hepatology
Ochsner Clinic Foundation
New Orleans, Louisiana

Jorge Rakela, MD
Professor of Medicine, Mayo Medical School
Rochester, Minnesota;
Chair, Division Transplantation Medicine
Mayo Clinic Scottsdale
Scottsdale, Arizona

Davendra Ramkumar, MB, BS
Assistant Professor, University of Iowa Health Care;
Assistant Professor, University of Iowa
Iowa City, Iowa

Juan Rodés, MD
Professor of Medicine, University of Barcelona;
Research Director, Hospital Clinic
Barcelona, Spain

Tania A. Roskans, MD, PhD
Professor of Pathology, University of Leuven Medical School;
Staff Member, Department of Pathology
University Hospital Leuven
Leuven, Belgium

A. Catharine Ross, PhD
Professor of Medicine, Department of Nutritional Science
College of Health and Human Development
Pennsylvania State University
University Park, Pennsylvania

Jayanta Roy Chowdhury, MD, MRCP
Professor of Medicine and Molecular Genetics
Albert Einstein College of Medicine
Bronx, New York

Namita Roy Chowdhury, PhD
Professor of Medicine and Molecular Genetics
Albert Einstein College of Medicine
Bronx, New York

Eduardo Ruchelli, MD
Assistant Professor of Pathology & Laboratory Medicine
University of Pennsylvania School of Medicine;
Associate Pathologist, Children's Hospital of Philadelphia
Philadelphia, Pennsylvania

Arun J. Sanyal, MBBS, MD
Professor of Medicine, Pharmacology
Chairman, Division of Gastroenterology, Hepatology, and Nutrition
Virginia Commonwealth University
Richmond, Virginia

Romil Saxena, MD, FRCPath
Assistant Professor
Department of Pathology & Laboratory Medicine
Indiana University School of Medicine
Indianapolis, Indiana

Shobha Sharma, MD
Assistant Professor of Pathology, Emory University Hospital
Atlanta, Georgia

Jerry L. Spivak, MD
Professor of Medicine and Oncology
Johns Hopkins University School of Medicine;
Active Staff, Johns Hopkins Hospital
Baltimore, Maryland

Charles A. Staley, MD
Associate Professor of Surgery
Emory University School of Medicine
Atlanta, Georgia

R. Todd Stravitz, MD, BS
Associate Professor of Medicine, Section of Hepatology, Division of Gastroenterology
Virginia Commonwealth University;
Attending Physician, Medical College of Virginia Hospitals
H.H. McGuire Veterans Affairs Hospital
Richmond, Virginia

Michael B. Streiff, MD
Assistant Professor of Medicine, Division of Hematology
Johns Hopkins School of Medicine
Baltimore, Maryland

Jayant A. Talwalkar, MD, MPH
Instructor of Medicine, Mayo Medical School;
Senior Associate Consultant
Division of Gastroenterology and Hepatology
Mayo Foundation
Rochester, Minnesota

Rebecca A. Taub, MD
Professor of Genetics
University of Pennsylvania School of Medicine
Philadelphia, Pennsylvania

Anthony S. Tavill, MD, FACP, FRCP
Professor of Medicine and Nutrition
Case Western Reserve University at MetroHealth Medical Center
Cleveland, Ohio

Rebecca W. Van Dyke, MD
Professor of Medicine, University of Michigan Medical School;
Attending Physician, University of Michigan Hospitals;
Staff Physician, Ann Arbor Veterans Hospital
Ann Arbor, Michigan

Anthony Van Ho, MD
Hematology/Oncology Fellow
Department of Internal Medicine, Division of Hematology/Oncology, University of Utah
Salt Lake City, Utah

Donald A. Vessey, PhD
Professor of Biochemistry (Medicine)
University of California San Francisco;
Career Scientist
Department of Veterans' Affairs Medical Center
San Francisco, California

John M. Vierling, MD
Professor of Medicine
University of California Los Angeles School of Medicine;
Director of Hepatology,
Medical Director of Multi-Organ Transplantation
Cedars-Sinai Medical Center
Los Angeles, California

Edmund K. Waller, MD, PhD
Associate Professor of Hematology/Oncology
Winship Cancer Institute
Emory University School of Medicine;
Director, Bone Marrow and Stem Cell Transplant Center
Emory University Hospital
Atlanta, Georgia

Jack R. Wands, MD
Professor of Medicine, Brown Medical School;
Director, Division of Gastroenterology,
Director, Liver Research Center
Rhode Island Hospital and the Miriam Hospital
Providence, Rhode Island

Walter H. Watson, PhD
Professor of Medicine, Department of Biochemistry
Emory University School of Medicine
Atlanta, Georgia

Karin Weissenborn, MD
Professor of Neurology,
Consultant, Medizinische Hochschule Hannover
Hannover, Germany

C. Mel Wilcox, MD
Professor of Medicine
Director, Division of Gastroenterology and Hepatology
University of Alabama at Birmingham
Birmingham, Alabama

C.L. Witzleben, BS, MD
Emeritus Professor of Pathology
University of Pennsylvania Medical School;
Emeritus Pathologist-in-Chief
Children's Hospital of Philadelphia
Philadelphia, Pennsylvania

Teresa L. Wright, MD
Professor of Medicine, University of California San Francisco;
Chief, Gastroenterology Section
Veterans Administration Medical Center
San Francisco, California

Mahmoud M. Yousfi, MD
Gastroenterology & Hepatology Fellow, Mayo Clinic
Scottsdale, Arizona

Andy S. Yu, MD
Assistant Professor of Medicine
Division of Gastroenterology and Hepatology
Stanford University School of Medicine;
Attending Physician, Liver Transplant Program
Stanford University Medical Center,
Stanford, California;
Attending Physician, Liver Transplant Program
Palo Alto VA Medical Center
Palo Alto, California

David Zakim, MD
Professor of Medicine Emeritus
Cornell University Medical College
New York, New York

Thomas R. Ziegler, MD
Associate Professor of Medicine
Divisions of Endocrinology/Metabolism and Digestive Diseases
Emory University School of Medicine
Atlanta, Georgia

Stephen D. Zucker, MD
Assistant Professor of Medicine
Director, Gastroenterology Training Program, Division of Digestive Diseases
University of Cincinnati
Cincinnati, Ohio

Preface

Four editions of *Hepatology* in 20 years validate the extent to which clinically useful information has grown in the field of hepatology. In addition, we believe that *Hepatology* (and texts like it) is a more significant resource today than when the first edition appeared. Thus while a burgeoning knowledge base about disease makes it increasingly satisfying to practice medicine, it also makes it increasingly difficult to use new information effectively and provide patients the full benefits of up-to-date clinical thinking. Modern information technology has not changed the manner in which doctors acquire new concepts and facts, assimilate these with old knowledge and experience, and then apply new ideas in clinical settings. Reading remains the best way to achieve these goals. But while reading is more important than ever because of the quickening pace of medical science, students of medicine at all levels know there is "too much" to read.

A key purpose of the fourth edition of *Hepatology* is to reduce this problem to a manageable level. *Hepatology* is thus a series of essays, each of which evaluates and synthesizes data in hundreds to thousands of primary references to generate a clinically useful body of knowledge that applies to a relatively narrow aspect of medicine in the author's field of expertise. Every chapter is intended to keep the reader current in that particular facet of liver disease. Given the pace of medical science and the overwhelming burden of staying current, the discipline imposed by a page limit for *Hepatology* is appropriate. The range of topics is intended to cover what we believe needs to be known. No completely new topics have been added to the fourth edition. But to extend discussion in established areas of liver disease that increasingly are amenable to therapeutic intervention, we have dropped some chapters from prior editions. We have combined basic science and clinical aspects of gallstone formation and copper metabolism to save space. As compared with prior editions, hepatitis B virus and hepatitis C virus are treated separately in the fourth edition. There are two new chapters on other viral liver diseases. The basic science and clinical aspects of alcoholic liver disease are no longer combined but are now discussed in separate chapters, to enhance focus on the clinical problem. Most important perhaps is that to keep the material fresh, about half of the fourth edition is written by authors who did not contribute to prior editions.

David Zakim

Thomas D. Boyer

Acknowledgments

A large textbook is a cooperative effort for which only some contributors receive public acknowledgment. Those behind the scenes are as important, however, as the people whose names appear on the spine of the book and at the chapter headings. We are deeply indebted, in this regard, to Jennifer Shreiner and Rachel E. Dowell, who deserve most of the credit for producing this edition in a timely manner. Jennifer Shreiner provided inestimable assistance in helping us organize the book and recruit authors. Always with good humor and patience, she kept us moving forward so that we could keep the schedule to which we were committed. She ran interference with authors to keep manuscripts flowing from them to us to the compositors. Rachel Dowell was equally important on the production side. Jennifer and Rachel also helped to resolve problems gracefully when they arose with figures and equation style to get us the quality of text we wanted. We thank Sue Hodgson, acquisition editor at Elsevier, for the exciting cover design of the fourth edition, which breaks dramatically with the staid appearance of previous editions. Its execution was the work of the art department at Elsevier. And besides these key people, many others at W.B. Saunders, Harcourt, and Elsevier, whose names we don't know, converted the idea of this book to a reality.

Last but not least, we acknowledge the patience, indulgence, and support of our families through the gestation of this book.

Color Plate Index

Contents

VOLUME I
NORMAL LIVER FUNCTION AND SYSTEMIC EFFECTS OF LIVER DYSFUNCTION

VOLUME II
ETIOLOGIES, CLINICAL FEATURES, DIAGNOSIS, AND TREATMENT OF SPECIFIC LIVER DISEASES

Hepatology

SECTION

IV A

Toxic Injury to the Liver and Associated Diseases

CHAPTER

26

Mechanisms of Chemically Induced Liver Disease

Walter H. Watson, PhD, Lawrence J. Dahm, PhD, and Dean P. Jones, PhD

CLASSIFICATION OF CHEMICALLY INDUCED LIVER INJURY

Liver injury can be caused by therapeutically useful drugs and by foreign chemicals, which are often termed xenobiotic agents. These toxic compounds are classified into two broad categories: agents that cause intrinsic toxicity, and those that cause idiosyncratic toxicity.[1,2] Hepatotoxic agents in the former group produce a dose-related, reproducible lesion in all exposed individuals after a predictable latent period. Additionally, the lesion is reproducible in animals, which serve as models to study the mechanism of injury. Hepatotoxic agents in the idiosyncratic group produce lesions with a variable, non-dose-related injury. The temporal relationship from administration of the agent to the onset of liver injury is variable, and only a small fraction of individuals exposed to the agent are affected. In addition, the lesions often are not reproducible in experimental animals. Consequently, there is a better understanding of mechanisms involved in intrinsic toxicity although in some cases idiosyncratic reactions have been attributed to host-specific, immune-mediated injury and specific alterations in biotransformation pathways.[3]

Attention has focused on the hepatocyte as a direct target for hepatotoxic agents because it makes up such a substantial portion of the liver and is most active in biotransformation of drugs and xenobiotic agents to toxic metabolites. However, injury to the liver also involves non-parenchymal cells such as Kupffer cells, endothelial cells, pit cells, and other cells lining the hepatic sinusoids and bile ducts. The type of injury induced by a specific hepatotoxicant may be classified as necrotic, cholestatic, steatotic, or a mixed lesion. Necrotic lesions may be focal or diffuse, and the nature of the lesion can tell us something about the mechanism of injury. Cholestasis results from the cessation of bile flow through the ductular network. Many clinically relevant drugs (e.g., chlorpromazine, erythromycin estolate, contraceptive steroids) cause cholestasis in a low percentage of the human population. Additional information on the mechanisms of cholestatic liver injury has been obtained with model compounds such as alpha-naphthylisothiocyanate (ANIT) in laboratory animals.[4] Steatosis, or fatty liver, is observed after intoxication with carbon tetrachloride (CCl_4), ethionine, puromycin, tetracycline, and other compounds. Many hepatotoxicants cause mixed lesions, such as necrosis and steatosis (e.g., CCl_4) or necrosis and cholestasis (e.g., ANIT) (see Chap. 27 for discussions of individual drugs).

In this chapter, we focus on mechanisms of chemically induced hepatocellular death and we do not consider mechanisms of cholestasis or steatosis. Also, the mechanisms by which chronic toxicant exposure leads to fibrosis and cirrhosis will not be discussed. In our approach, we have classified hepatotoxicants into the general pathways by which they elicit injury (Table 26-1), recognizing that more than one pathway may be involved for specific toxic agents. This classification is not comprehensive; however, it conveniently categorizes the most common pathways leading to irreversible hepatocellular injury. Further, within each pathway, we consider the most widely held mechanisms of hepatocellular death. In our discussion, we briefly address topics considered elsewhere in this book (e.g., hepatic biotransformation). In instances where there may be overlap, the reader should refer to those chapters for additional details (see Chap. 8).

Distinctions Between Apoptosis and Necrosis in Hepatocytes

Considerable progress has been made during the past decade in understanding the mechanisms of cell death. Previously, necrosis was considered to be synonymous with cell death. Necrosis is a morphologic term referring to tissue changes during injury that are characterized by cellular and organellar swelling and membranal lysis with release of cytoplasmic contents. After such changes, outlines of cells are often indistinct and the cells themselves have an amorphous or coarsely granular appearance. Detailed morphologic studies of pathologic and normal tissues revealed a distinct morphology of cell death, originally termed "shrinkage necrosis,"[5] and now termed "apoptosis."[6] In apoptosis, typical changes include cell shrinkage, organellar compaction, nuclear condensation, deoxyribonucleic acid (DNA) fragmentation into oligonucleosomal lengths, fragmentation of cells into smaller "apoptotic bodies," and appearance of

TABLE 26-1
General Pathways Leading to Hepatocellular Injury

Pathway	Examples
Bioactivation to electrophiles	Acetaminophen, bromobenzene
Bioactivation to free radicals	CCl_4, halothane, ethanol
Redox cycling	Quinones (menadione, Adriamycin)
Failure of energy supply	Cyanide, rotenone
Immune mechanisms	
Cell-mediated or humoral	Halothane, tienilic acid
Kupffer cell activation	Endotoxin, CCl_4, allyl alcohol, 1,2-dichlorobenzene
Neutrophil activation	α-Naphthylisothiocyanate

CCl_4, Carbon tetrachloride.

phagocytotic signals on the cell surface.[7] Apoptotic cells are rapidly removed by phagocytosis.

Mechanistic studies show that apoptosis generally involves activation of a family of highly conserved enzymes, termed caspases, which function to cleave specific target sequences, resulting in characteristic morphology and leading to cell elimination by phagocytosis.[8] Activation occurs through plasma membrane-associated death receptor activation of caspase 8,[9] through mitochondria-mediated activation of caspase 9,[10] and through endoplasmic reticulum activation of caspase 12.[11] Chemicals that alter expression and function of the death receptor components, disrupt mitochondrial function, or disrupt the secretory pathway therefore can be expected to activate apoptosis (Figure 26-1). In addition, disruption of the cell cycle and inhibition of proteosomes also activate apoptosis. Thus many agents previously thought to kill cells by disruption of critical homeostatic processes are now believed to do so by activation of apoptosis.

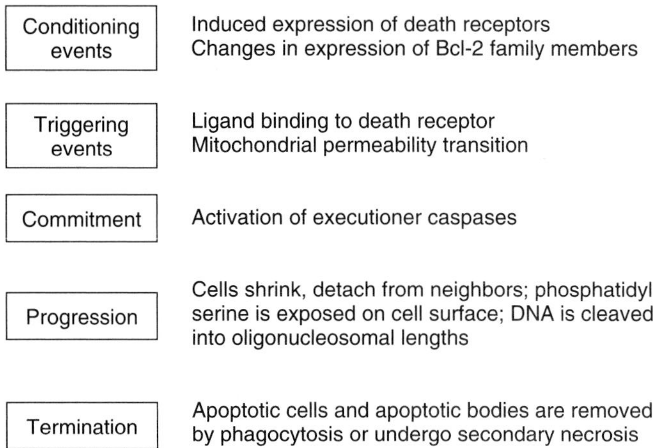

Figure 26-1 Stages of apoptosis.

True distinction between necrosis and apoptosis as causative mechanisms in liver toxicity may not be possible. Apoptotic cells undergo secondary necrosis if there are inadequate phagocytic cells to remove the apoptotic cells. Thus, when large fields of contiguous cells undergo apoptosis, the region is likely to have a necrotic appearance as a result of deficient phagocytosis. Alternatively, if high doses of toxicant disrupt ionic homeostasis and, at the same time, activate the caspase cascade, the cells may swell and lyse even though they have characteristics of apoptosis.

The intrinsic hepatotoxicity of many chemicals has a necrotic appearance. However, many chemicals result in increased apoptotic cells when given at doses lower than those causing necrosis. This difference can often be reconciled because of mitochondrial involvement. Disruption of only a fraction of mitochondria can result in sufficient cytochrome c release to activate the caspase 9/caspase 3 pathway without disrupting cellular energetics. Under these conditions, cells maintain osmotic regulation and undergo apoptosis. However, with greater disruption of mitochondria, cellular energetics are impaired, osmotic regulation is lost, and cells undergo swelling and lysis. Because of this, the mechanisms involved in activation of caspases or loss of osmotic regulation appear to be key to understanding chemically induced liver disease.

BIOACTIVATION OF XENOBIOTIC AGENTS TO ELECTROPHILES

Lipophilic compounds are not readily removed by the kidneys and must be converted to more water-soluble derivatives. Although this occurs to some extent in many organs, the liver is the primary organ for biotransformation of xenobiotic agents and also for many endogenously produced lipophilic compounds (e.g., bile acids, bile pigments). During biotransformation, lipophilic compounds are converted to more water-soluble derivatives by phase I and phase II drug-metabolizing enzymes (see Chap. 8). Phase I reactions involve oxidation, reduction, and hydrolysis (e.g., esterases, amidases) of the parent molecule; phase II reactions serve as conjugation reactions to add endogenous substrates (e.g., glucuronic acid, sulfate, glutathione [GSH]) to phase I metabolites or to reactive groups on the parent molecule. Many of the phase I enzymes are in the endoplasmic reticulum, the membrane fraction that is isolated as small vesicles termed microsomes. These phase I enzymes include a superfamily of enzymes collectively known as cytochrome

P450 (CYP) and the microsomal flavin-containing monooxygenase system that is especially important in humans for biotransformation of sulfur-containing chemicals. Phase II enzymes may be microsomal, cytosolic (i.e., soluble in cell cytoplasm), or mitochondrial and are composed of GSH S-transferases, glucuronosyltransferases, sulfotransferases, *N*-acetyltransferases, and enzymes catalyzing methylation and amino acid conjugation.

The mixed-function oxidases include CYP, a heme-containing protein that oxidizes xenobiotic compounds, and an associated flavin-containing enzyme, nicotinamide adenine dinucleotide phosphate (NADPH):cytochrome P450 reductase. The enzymes have a hydrophobic binding site where lipophilic compounds can bind in association with the heme site for oxygen (O_2) binding and activation. The enzymes often have very broad and overlapping substrate specificities and can catalyze different chemical reactions. The latter can occur because the reaction proceeds through an activated oxygen intermediate that is reactive with different functional groups.

Molecular biologic approaches have shown the existence of 481 CYP genes in eukaryotes and prokaryotes.[8,12] These have been classified into 74 major families on the basis of amino acid sequence identity. By definition, CYPs with more than a 40 percent sequence identity are included in the same family, which is designated by an Arabic number. Those with greater than 55 percent similarity are included in the same subfamily and designated by a capital letter. Individual CYP genes then are assigned an arbitrary number. Mammals express 14 of the 74 families of CYP genes, and these 14 families are made up of 26 mammalian subfamilies. It is not yet known whether expression of specific forms is associated with the risk of chemically induced liver injury in humans, but this is suggested by animal and clinical studies.[13]

Both phase I and phase II reactions may result in chemical detoxification, meaning that biotransformation results in less toxic metabolites. However, some compounds are not toxic to liver in the parent form but are bioactivated to reactive species. One of the more common mechanisms of bioactivation involves conversion to compounds with electron-seeking properties (i.e., electrophiles). In most cases, these electrophiles are the result of phase I metabolism by CYP-dependent reactions. Epoxides, which have the general structure,

```
        O
       / \
R—CH——CH—R
```

are an important class of toxic electrophiles. Bromobenzene and aflatoxin B1 are metabolized by hepatic mixed-function oxidases to the epoxide intermediates bromobenzene-3,4-oxide[14,15] and aflatoxin B1-8,9-oxide,[16] respectively. Other electrophilic species include alkyl and aryl halides; carbonium and diazonium ion intermediates; aldehydes; esters; alpha, beta-unsaturated carbon compounds; and compounds containing doubly bound nitrogen (e.g., isothiocyanates, isocyanates, quinazolines).[17] Phase II metabolism also may result ultimately in toxic electrophiles, exemplified by toxic GSH S-conjugates, glucuronides, and sulfates;[18,19] these metabolites may be toxic to liver and to extrahepatic organs.

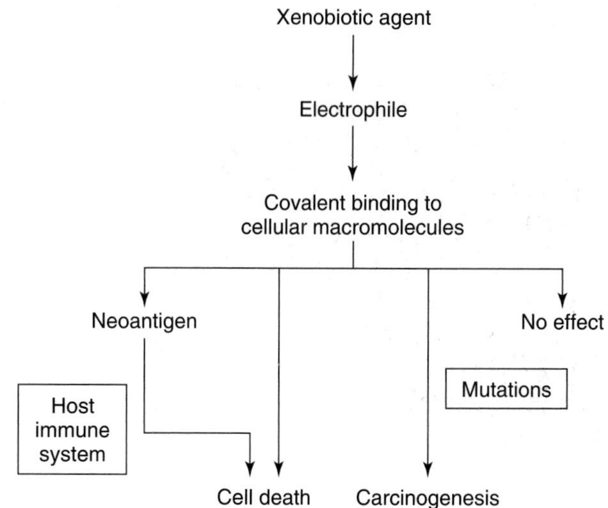

Figure 26-2 Cellular response after covalent binding of electrophile. Note that the electrophile may be formed via phase I or phase II metabolism.

Covalent Binding of Reactive Electrophiles

One of the first documented mechanisms of liver injury involves binding of reactive electrophiles to cellular macromolecules that contain nucleophilic centers (e.g., protein thiols). Covalent binding can lead to hepatocellular death if critical macromolecules necessary for cell survival are targeted. In principle, this could involve any macromolecule, but most evidence suggests that the chemical reactivity and physical properties of the toxicant result in reaction with specific macromolecules or sites.[20] Toxicity can result when a critical component is inhibited or activated to a level that disrupts cellular homeostasis. For instance, earlier research showed that calcium transport systems in the plasma membrane[21] and endoplasmic reticulum[22,23] contain oxidizable cysteine thiol groups that are critical for function. More recent studies show that molecular chaperones, proteolytic systems, and transcription factors are susceptible to redox modifications.[24-26] DNA may be a target of electrophiles, in which case the lesion may cause acute hepatocellular cell death or lead to carcinogenicity (Figure 26-2). The epoxide of aflatoxin B1 formed during hepatic biotransformation binds guanine residues at the N-7 position in DNA, which ultimately results in hepatocarcinogenesis.[16,27] Covalent modification of proteins can result in the formation of a neoantigen against which an immune response can be mounted (see Figure 26-2 and the following sections). Metabolites of halothane and tienilic acid, a diuretic that was withdrawn from the U.S. market in 1980, may cause liver injury by this type of idiosyncratic mechanism.[3,28]

Although covalent binding of reactive electrophiles is certain to be responsible for injury caused by some toxicants, the evidence implicating covalent binding and cell death is often indirect, relying upon experimental measures known to enhance or diminish chemically induced hepatocellular injury. The rationale is that covalently bound electrophiles (e.g., to hepatocellular protein) should increase after treatments that enhance toxicity of the parent compound and decrease after treatments that prevent injury if covalent binding is indeed involved in cell death. Current methods using proteomic techniques provide hope that specific protein targets can be identified and used as the basis for interventions to avoid chemical induced injury.

Role of Glutathione in Chemical Detoxification of Reactive Electrophiles

GSH is a major low-molecular-weight thiol compound that makes up more than 90 percent of the acid-soluble thiol pool in hepatocytes and accounts for about 30 percent of the total thiol groups in the liver.[29] Its disulfide form, glutathione disulfide (GSSG), makes up less than 5 percent of the total cellular glutathione pool, but is increased under certain pathophysiologic conditions such as oxidative stress (see the following section). In the liver, glutathione serves many important functions, including detoxification of peroxides and electrophiles, maintenance of protein thiols in a reduced state, serving as a non-toxic storage form of cysteine, synthesis of leukotrienes and prostaglandins, and reduction of ribonucleotides to deoxyribonucleotides.[29] Glutathione is synthesized in all cells in two adenosine triphosphate (ATP)-dependent reactions within the cytoplasm. The first step is rate-limiting and is catalyzed by gamma-glutamylcysteine synthetase; in this reaction, cysteine and glutamate are converted to gamma-glutamylcysteine. The enzyme is feedback-inhibited by glutathione, which provides a mechanism for regulating glutathione concentrations. However, expression of this enzyme in cells is variable, and glutathione concentrations can vary considerably in different proliferative states. The second enzyme is glutathione synthetase, which adds a glycine residue to yield glutathione. The liver, unlike most other tissues, can convert methionine to cysteine in the cystathionine pathway and therefore can use methionine to support synthesis of glutathione.[30]

Glutathione is compartmentalized within hepatocytes. Glutathione levels in cytoplasm are about 4 to 8 mM and compose 85 to 90 percent of total cellular glutathione; the remaining 10 to 15 percent has been attributed to a mitochondrial pool.[31,32] Because GSH synthetic enzymes are present in the cytoplasm and not in mitochondria, mitochondria probably accumulate GSH via transport from cytoplasm.[33] Under conditions in which cytosolic GSH is depleted, there is release of mitochondrial GSH to cytoplasm,[32] indicating that there is bidirectional flux of GSH between these compartments. GSH and GSSG in the lumen of the endoplasmic reticulum have been suggested to function in the introduction of disulfide bonds in newly synthesized proteins.[34] Other studies also have shown the existence of a separate nuclear GSH pool,[35,36] the functions of which are not completely understood.

Of most relevance to chemical toxicity, GSH is involved in detoxification of electrophiles. The thiol group of GSH is a nucleophilic center that undergoes *S*-conjugation with electrophiles; in most cases, this leads to detoxification. Many electrophiles form GSH *S*-conjugates non-enzymatically to some extent, which is a function of charge localization of both electrophile and nucleophile.[37] Chemicals having a high charge density are said to be "hard," whereas those having a low charge density, such as GSH, are termed "soft." Generally, chemicals of like charge density react non-enzymatically, whereas those of differing densities require catalysis. Assuming favorable charge densities, the capacity of GSH to form GSH *S*-conjugates non-enzymatically is determined by two factors—the concentration of GSH and pH. Given that the pKa for the ionization of the thiol in GSH is 9.2,[38] formation of the ionized and reactive species (i.e., thiolate anion, GS-) is favored at alkaline pH. Thus, non-enzymatic generation of GSH *S*-conjugates is favored at alkaline pH.

Hepatocytes and other cells do not rely on non-enzymatic conjugation of electrophiles; instead, they contain enzymes termed GSH *S*-transferases that catalyze *S*-conjugation of GSH to electrophiles. Four major classes of cytosolic GSH *S*-transferases (i.e., alpha, mu, pi, delta) and one microsomal enzyme have been characterized in mammalian tissues.[39] The cytosolic GSH *S*-transferases have been studied in the most detail and have been shown to be a multi-gene family of enzymes. Each cytosolic GSH *S*-transferase is composed of two subunits (i.e., dimers); a discrete gene codes for each subunit, only subunits of the same class form dimers, and dimers may contain identical subunits (homodimers) or different subunits (heterodimers). The cytosolic enzymes are expressed to various extents in different tissues and are important in detoxification of several groups of xenobiotic agents including polycyclic aromatic hydrocarbons, aflatoxins, aromatic amines, and alkylating agents.[40] The liver is most active in GSH-dependent detoxification of electrophiles, and human liver is particularly rich in GSH *S*-transferases of the alpha class; in other species such as rat, the mu class of GHS S-transferases also is abundant in liver.

Factors Affecting GSH-Dependent Detoxification of Electrophiles in Liver

Generation of large quantities of electrophiles in the liver ultimately will deplete cellular GSH pools, resulting in enhanced covalent binding to critical macromolecules and cell death. Because GSH and the GSH *S*-transferases play such an integral role in detoxification of electrophilic species in the liver, physiologic or pathophysiologic conditions that either decrease or elevate levels or activities in the liver would be expected to affect chemical detoxification in the appropriate direction. Experimentally, this has been demonstrated for a variety of electrophiles. For example, depletion of hepatocellular GSH exacerbates hepatotoxicity associated with electrophiles, including metabolites of acetaminophen[41] and bromobenzene.[15] Depletion of GSH can be accomplished by prior treatment with another electrophile such as diethylmaleate or inhibition of GSH synthesis with buthionine sulfoximine. In addition to chemical treatment, certain physiologic states may reduce hepatic GSH content. Fasting for 1 or 2 days decreases hepatic GSH content by 30 to 50 percent,[42] and enhances the liver injury caused by many electrophilic agents. Animal studies also have revealed a diurnal variation in hepatic GSH stores of about 25 to 30 percent,[43] with higher levels at night and early morning when the animals have eaten. Thus, the injury caused by a given hepatotoxicant may be influenced by the time of day of exposure as a result of the availability of GSH for detoxification.

Maintenance or augmentation of cellular GSH levels can prevent the hepatotoxicity caused by electrophiles. This can be accomplished chemically by treatment with certain anti-oxidants such as butylated hydroxyanisole, by supplying cysteine for GSH synthesis via the cysteine pro drugs *N*-acetylcysteine or oxothiazolidine-4-carboxylate, or by administering GSH esters.[44] *N*-acetylcysteine elevates and maintains hepatic GSH stores and serves as a clinical treatment against the hepatotoxicity caused by acetaminophen overdose.[45]

The activities and isoenzymatic forms of GSH *S*-transferases also are important in detoxification of electrophiles in the liver. These enzymes have relatively slow enzymatic turnover rates but are extremely abundant in the cytoplasm of hepatic parenchymal cells; they comprise about 10 percent of hepatic cytosolic protein.[46] Some isoforms have a high binding capacity for lipophilic compounds, and this property may allow short-term sequestration of reactive or lipophilic compounds that is protective independent of the enzyme activity.

Similar to the CYPs, the GSH *S*-transferases have relatively broad and overlapping substrate specificities. Of significance, exposure to certain drugs, environmental chemicals, and dietary components increases the activities of hepatic GSH *S*-transferases by inducing increased synthesis of the enzymes. Because many inducers have the same effect on some of the CYPs, such induction can enhance clearance of compounds but not necessarily have any effect on their toxicity, especially those requiring bioactivation to a toxic metabolite. In this case, induction will result both in greater bioactivation by CYP and in enhanced detoxication of the reactive metabolite by GSH *S*-transferases. Recent studies with dietary inducers contained in cruciferous vegetables show that these agents induce GSH *S*-transferases and other protective phase II enzymes without having a significant effect on the CYPs.[47-50] These results are particularly exciting because they suggest that increased intake of foods containing these agents may provide a simple and effective means to prevent toxicity and cancer caused by toxicants.

Role of Bioactivation and Covalent Binding in Acetaminophen Hepatotoxicity

Acetaminophen (*N*-acetyl-p-aminophenol) is a widely used analgesic that is without deleterious side effects when used in therapeutic doses. In overdose, however, it can result in severe hepatocellular necrosis around the central vein (i.e., centrilobular necrosis).[51] Evidence indicates that bioactivation of acetaminophen to an electrophilic species plays a pivotal role in the hepatocellular injury. Under therapeutic conditions, acetaminophen is sulfated and glucuronidated in detoxification pathways; it undergoes immediate phase II metabolism because the parent compound is already hydroxylated. These pathways are saturated in overdosage, and a significant portion of acetaminophen is biotransformed by hepatic CYP to the electrophilic intermediate *N*-acetyl-p-benzoquinoneimine (NAPQI) (Figure 26-3).[52] In humans, CYP2E1 and 1A2 account for a large fraction of this conversion.[53] At low rates of production, NAPQI is detoxified by *S*-conjugation with GSH; however, at higher rates of NAPQI production, hepatocellular GSH pools are depleted and extensive covalent binding to cellular macromolecules occurs.[54,55]

Considerable effort has been expended in trying to identify the specific targets of acetaminophen hepatotoxicity. This has been approached conceptually in two ways: by trying to identify systems that lose function early in the process and by trying to identify proteins that are specifically modified. The logic of the former approach is that energy-producing systems (mitochondria and the glycolytic pathway) and ion-transporting ATPases are critical to cellular homeostasis and that their failure often contributes to cell death. Ultrastructural and functional studies have shown that mitochondria are an early target in the hepatocellular necrosis caused by acetaminophen (Figure 26-4).[56-59] Regarding the second approach, acetaminophen treatment does result in extensive covalent binding to mitochondrial, microsomal, and cytosolic proteins in hepatocytes. The identification of

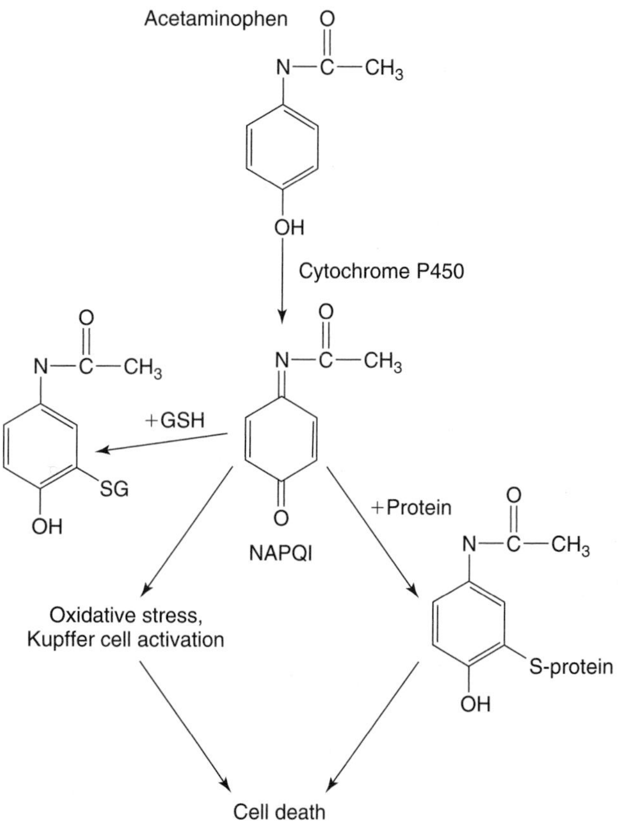

Figure 26-3 Proposed mechanisms for acetaminophen-induced hepatotoxicity. *NAPQI, N*-acetyl-p-benzoquinoneimine; *GSH,* glutathione.

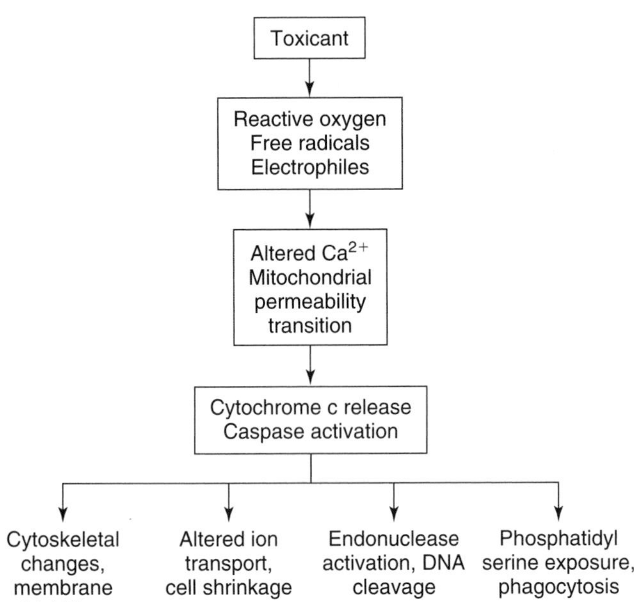

Figure 26-4 Central role of mitochondria in chemically induced apoptosis.

specific NAPQI targets has been aided by developing immunologic methods to detect and localize the protein-bound adducts. Acetaminophen metabolites form adducts to hepatic proteins in the cytosol, microsomes, mitochondria, nuclei, and plasma membranes.[28] Arylation of a 58-kDa cytosolic protein on cysteinyl residues correlates very well with the extent of hepatocellular necrosis after various experimental manipulations to enhance or ameliorate the injury in mice. This protein has been identified as a selenium-binding protein, the function of which has not been established.[60,61] A similar 58-kDa hepatic protein was targeted in a human acetaminophen overdosage.[62] Thus the 58-kDa cytosolic protein may be a critical target in acetaminophen hepatotoxicity.

Some chemical treatments alter acetaminophen hepatotoxicity without affecting covalent binding,[63-66] suggesting that other mechanisms also may be involved in the pathogenesis of liver cell injury. For example, NAPQI is a good oxidant in biologic systems and causes extensive oxidation of soluble and protein thiols and of adenine nucleotides.[65,67,68] Also, recent evidence suggests that Kupffer cell activation is a prerequisite for the toxicity of acetaminophen.[69]

BIOACTIVATION OF XENOBIOTIC AGENTS TO FREE RADICALS

The hepatic mixed-function oxidase system can metabolize xenobiotic agents to free radicals, which are chemically reactive species containing an unpaired electron. They can be formed by CYP by three different mechanisms: a one-electron oxidation to form a cation radical ($R \rightarrow \bullet R^+ + e^-$), a one-electron reduction to yield an anion radical ($R + e^- \rightarrow \bullet R^-$), or a homolytic bond scission to yield a neutral radical ($R\text{-}R \rightarrow \bullet R + \bullet R$).[70] Hepatotoxicants of occupational, environmental and clinical interest are bioactivated in liver to free radical species. CCl_4 will be discussed briefly later, although this is only one representative of a large number of halogenated hydrocarbons that can be activated in a similar manner. In addition to free radicals of the parent compound, reactive oxygen radicals such as the hydroxyl radical ($\bullet OH$) may be generated during pathophysiologic conditions. These conditions include redox cycling of xenobiotic agents, activation of the respiratory burst in host phagocytic cells, and exposure to ionizing radiation. Whether free radicals are oxygen-centered (e.g., $\bullet OH$) or carbon-centered as in the case of certain radicals generated from CCl_4, they may initiate events (e.g., covalent binding, oxidative stress, lipid peroxidation) that have been linked to the pathogenesis of lethal cell injury. The free radical nitric oxide ($NO\bullet$) is an important signaling agent in biologic systems and can contribute to oxidative injury via reaction with superoxide anion radical ($\bullet O_2^-$) to generate peroxynitrite.[71-73]

Additionally, changes in reactive oxygen intermediates may contribute to pathogenesis without directly causing cell death. For instance, transcription factors *Fos* and *Jun* of the activator protein-1 (AP-I) complex contain a critical cysteine thiol that is under redox regulation and must be reduced for DNA binding and transcriptional activation.[74] Several other transcription factors have been shown to be sensitive to changes in redox state.[26] Thus even though the following text focuses on oxidative stress as a mechanism leading to acute necrosis, pathologic processes also can occur as a consequence of sublethal modulation of cellular redox state.

All of the classes of cellular macromolecules can be targets of free radical–induced liver injury. As discussed previously regarding covalent modification, proteins are most often considered the critical targets in acute necrosis. However when free radicals are generated, lipid peroxidation can be a critical event in the pathogenesis of injury because it amplifies free radical–induced injury. Free radicals also damage DNA, and efficient repair systems normally function to minimize these alterations.

Free Radical–induced Lipid Peroxidation

Lipid peroxidation of organelle membranes (e.g., plasma membrane, endoplasmic reticulum) is initiated by both carbon-centered and oxygen-centered radicals and is thought to be a primary mechanism by which free radicals cause death to hepatocytes and other cells. Lipid peroxidation decreases membrane fluidity and is associated with inactivation of membrane-bound receptors and enzymes, increased permeability of membranes, and generation of toxic degradation products of lipid peroxidation.[75,76] The manner in which free radicals cause lipid peroxidation is shown in Figure 26-5. Upon generation (e.g., after biotransformation of the parent molecule by hepatic mixed-function oxidases) a free radical can abstract hydrogen from a methylene carbon of polyunsaturated fatty acids of membranal lipids, leaving a lipid radical. After rearrangement reactions in the lipid radical to form a species containing conjugated double bonds (i.e., conjugated diene), a lipid peroxy radical can be formed in the presence of O_2. This radical, in turn, can abstract

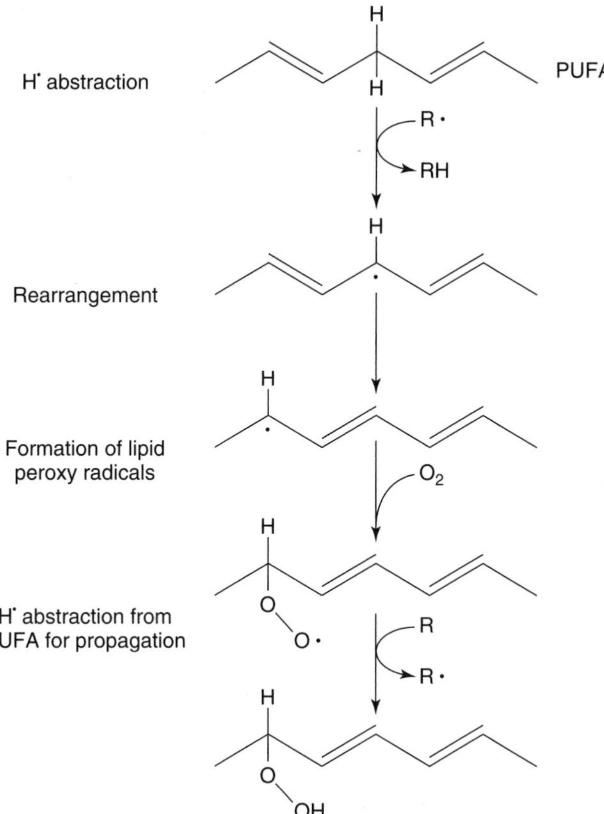

Figure 26-5 Chemistry of lipid peroxidation. *PUFA,* Polyunsaturated fatty acid; *R-,* lipid radical.

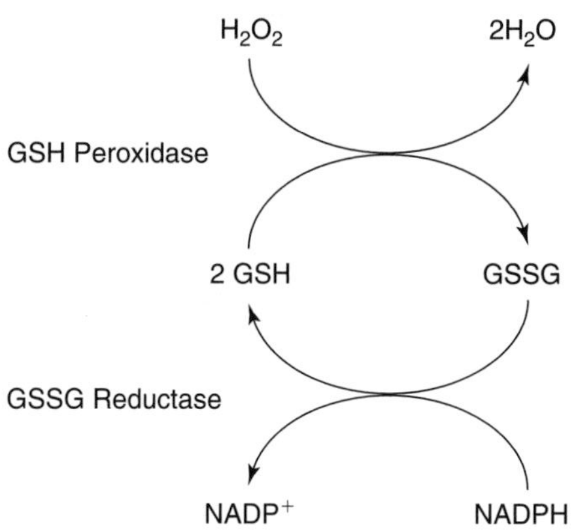

Figure 26-6 Glutathione redox cycle. *GSH,* Glutathione; *GSSG,* glutathione disulfide; *NADP+,* nicotinamide adenine dinucleotide phosphate; *NADPH,* nicotinamide adenine dinucleotide phosphate (reduced form).

hydrogen from another polyunsaturated fatty acid molecule to yield the lipid hydroperoxide and another lipid radical. In this way, there is propagation of the original event, and it is estimated that 4 to 10 propagation steps occur per initiation.[77] Additionally, lipid hydroperoxides can react with metal ions or with metalloproteins to generate alkoxyl radicals as well as lipid peroxy radicals,[76,77] both of which can initiate lipid peroxidation. Thus these 4 to 10 propagation steps can be amplified an additional fourfold to tenfold. This vicious cycle of free radical reactions is halted by disproportionation and termination reactions in which stable non-radical species are produced. It is rather ironic that many of these termination reactions (e.g., lipid radical lipid radical interaction) are thought to alter membrane structure and fluidity and participate in the injury caused by lipid peroxidation.[75]

Role of GSH in Free Radical–induced Lipid Peroxidation

GSH plays a central role in protection against lipid peroxidation through enzyme-catalyzed reactions and through non-enzymatic reduction of other anti-oxidants (vitamins C and E). GSH is required for degradation of lipid hydroperoxides and other hydroperoxides in reactions catalyzed by the selenium-dependent GSH peroxidase (Figure 26-6 and Table 26-2). Detoxication of lipid hydroperoxides by selenium-dependent GSH peroxidase requires an additional step compared to hydrogen peroxide (H_2O_2); lipid hydroperoxides are associated with phospholipid and are not accessible to the cytosolic enzyme as compared to the freely diffusible H_2O_2. Thus, the fatty acid hydroperoxide must be released first from the bulk lipid by the action of phospholipase A2.[78,79] A separate selenium-dependent "phospholipid hydroperoxide GSH peroxidase" that directly detoxifies phospholipid hydroperoxides without a requirement for phospholipase A2 has been characterized.[80,81] A selenium-independent GSH peroxidase, which has been ascribed to GSH *S*-transferases of the alpha class,[82] also detoxifies lipid hydroperoxides; it, like the selenium-dependent GSH peroxidase, requires release of the fatty acid peroxide from the membrane. The selenium-independent form also is active in detoxification of cumene hydroperoxide and nucleic acid hydroperoxides.[83]

GSH also can play an important role in protection against free radical processes by interfering with propagation reactions. GSH may terminate lipid peroxidation reactions by donating an electron to a free radical (R•) to form RH and a thiyl radical (GS•).[84] Additionally, GSH is involved in regeneration of α-tocopherol (vitamin E) from the α-tocopheroxy radicals,[85] which is formed after donation of an electron to a lipid radical. GSH is a good reductant for dehydroascorbate[86,87] and therefore can maintain the ascorbate pool during oxidative stress. Ascorbate is an efficient reductant for alkoxy radicals (RO•) and reduces the α-tocopheroxy radical form of vitamin E back to vitamin E.[88] Vitamin E appears to be the most important chain terminator for lipid peroxidation, reducing both carbon-centered (R•) and peroxyradicals (ROO•). Thus the two major free radical terminators, ascorbate and α-tocopherol, are either directly or indirectly preserved by GSH.

Finally, GSH detoxifies toxic degradation products of lipid hydroperoxides, most notably the 4-hydroxyalkenals (e.g., 4-hydroxynonenal) via *S*-conjugation. 4-Hydroxynonenal is an extremely toxic product of lipid peroxidation, with submicromolar concentrations causing genotoxic lesions to cultured rat hepatocytes.[89] Its conjugation with GSH is catalyzed by a specific form of

TABLE 26-2

Cellular Anti-oxidant Enzyme Systems that Degrade Reactive Oxygen Species

Enzyme	Distribution	Reaction
Superoxide dismutase	Cytoplasm, mitochondria	$2O_2^{\cdot} + 2H+ \rightarrow H_2O_2 + O_2$
Catalase	Peroxisomes	$H_2O_2 \rightarrow H_2O + O_2$
GSH peroxidases	Cytoplasm, mitochondria	$2GSH + H_2O_2 \rightarrow GSSG + 2H_2O$
		$2GSH + ROOH \rightarrow GSSG + ROH + H_2O$

GSH, Glutathione.

glutathione S-transferase,[90,91] suggesting that this reaction may be fundamentally important in the prevention of free radical-mediated liver injury.

Lipid Peroxidation as a Mechanism of Lethal Cell Injury

Lipid peroxidation has been studied with methods that measure the process at different stages, which include loss of unsaturated fatty acids, measurement of primary peroxidation products (e.g., malondialdehyde), and measurement of secondary carbonyls (e.g., 4-hydroxynonenal) and hydrocarbon gases (e.g., ethane).[92] For studies in vitro with hepatocytes, levels of malondialdehyde, thiobarbituric acid-reactive substances, and conjugated dienes have been used most commonly to assess lipid peroxidation. Malondialdehyde is a degradation product of lipid hydroperoxides; it can be measured specifically or as thiobarbituric acid-reactive substance, of which it is a major component. Conjugated dienes are a conjugated series of double bonds formed in the polyunsaturated fatty acid molecule after initiation and rearrangement reactions (see Figure 26-5). For studies in vivo, measurement of ethane or pentane, which are derived from n-3 and n-6 fatty acids, respectively, in the expired gases is a common marker of lipid peroxidation. Other markers associated with lipid peroxidation, including vitamin E loss, protein thiol loss, and carbonyl formation, also provide useful ways to assess lipid peroxidation in some systems.

In considering lipid peroxidation as a mechanism of cell death, several criteria must be met. First, lipid peroxidation must be measurable after intoxication with an agent that generates free radicals. Regarding markers of lipid peroxidation, one must consider their specificity, particularly in tissue samples, to ensure that they are actually detecting free radical-induced lipid peroxidation. An additional concern is that lipid peroxidation is measured in the tissue actually undergoing injury. This is not so much of a problem for studies in vitro or in perfused organs, but for studies in vivo it is difficult to attribute elevations of expired ethane or pentane to a specific site of lipid peroxidation in the body. Second, lipid peroxidation must precede cell death. This is a particularly important point given that different markers of lipid peroxidation all may be elevated after intoxication but may show different time courses.[93] If these are only a consequence of degradation of dead cells, then they provide only a measure of injury and no information concerning mechanisms or treatments. Third, lipid peroxidation and injury should be increased or decreased by experimental measures that decrease or increase anti-oxidant defenses, respectively.

Although there is agreement that lipid peroxidation does occur after generation of free radicals in the liver, some investigators have questioned its role in causing lethal hepatocellular injury. Tribble and colleagues[94] have reviewed the literature on chemically induced lipid peroxidation in the liver and have concluded that lipid peroxidation, per se, probably does not play a causal role in hepatocellular death. However, when it does occur, it may be an important determinant of the extent of injury because of its capacity to amplify free radical injury. Tribble and colleagues based their conclusions primarily on the ambiguous results obtained with free radical scavengers and clear examples of dissociation of lipid peroxidation from cell lethality. They support the view that lipid peroxidation contributes to the pathogenesis of cell injury by tying up GSH and GSH peroxidases required in the detoxification of other peroxides (e.g., H_2O_2) that also may be present. An additional proposal is that lipid peroxidation contributes to the pathogenesis of free radical-mediated liver injury by generating toxic degradation products. These aldehyde products, typified by the 4-hydroxyalkenals, react with soluble and protein thiols, inactivate a variety of enzymes, and bind to DNA to produce genotoxicity.[89] Thus lipid peroxidation may not be required for the lethal cell injury caused by free radicals but may serve to exacerbate it.

Lipid Peroxidation and CCl_4-induced Liver Injury

CCl_4 is hepatotoxic, causing a centrilobular necrosis and associated fatty liver. Caspase 3 is activated and released into the plasma with a time course suggesting initial activation of apoptosis followed by secondary necrosis.[95] In addition, CCl_4 is nephrotoxic and a suspected carcinogen. Even though occupational and environmental poisonings resulting from CCl_4 are relatively rare today, CCl_4 has been one of the most intensively studied hepatotoxicants to date and provides a relevant model for other halogenated hydrocarbons that are widely used.[96] A primary event in the pathogenesis is the reductive dehalogenation of CCl_4 to the trichloromethyl free radical ($\bullet CCl_3$) by hepatic mixed function oxidases (Figure 26-7). $\bullet CCl_3$ can abstract hydrogen from polyunsaturated fatty acids to initiate lipid peroxidation. Alternatively, in

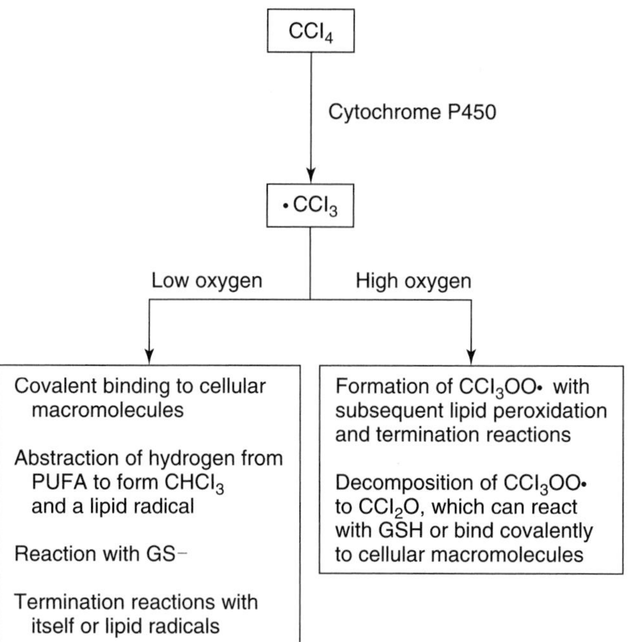

Figure 26-7 Metabolism of carbon tetrachloride in liver. *PUFA,* Polyunsaturated fatty acid; *GSH,* glutathione; *GS−*, glutathione thiolate anion.

the presence of oxygen, it forms the more reactive trichloromethylperoxy free radical ($CCl_3OO\bullet$), which also can participate in lipid peroxidation, or it decomposes to phosgene (CCl_2O) (Figure 26-7).

The lipid peroxidation in liver associated with CCl_4 exposure occurs early in the pathogenesis of the injury and has been viewed as a critical event because it is also associated with reductions of enzyme activity in the endoplasmic reticulum, fatty acid transport, and protein synthesis.[75] Treatments that either increase or decrease CCl_4 hepatotoxicity in vivo and in vitro affect the extent of lipid peroxidation in the manner expected to support a role for lipid peroxidation in the pathogenesis of injury. For instance, treatment of animals with inducers of hepatic mixed-function oxidases (e.g., phenobarbital) augments production of free radicals and lipid peroxidation and exacerbates hepatotoxicity.[97-99] Conversely, treatment with inhibitors of mixed-function oxidases, such as SKF-525A, decreases the extent of lipid peroxidation and injury as determined by microsomal dysfunction in vitro and lethality in vivo.[97,100,101] Although these observations and others support a role for lipid peroxidation in CCl_4-induced hepatocellular injury, some experimental treatments show dissociation between lipid peroxidation and hepatocellular lethality. For example, the anti-oxidant *N,N′*-diphenyl-p-phenylenediamine prevents hepatocellular injury caused by CCl_4 but does not prevent lipid peroxidation.[102-104] Similarly, vitamin E protects against the hepatocellular injury in vivo[105] but does not affect the production of certain markers of lipid peroxidation (i.e., lipid peroxides and malondialdehyde) in microsomal lipids.[104,106] Thus, even though lipid peroxidation is typically associated with CCl_4 intoxication, this appears to be more of a symptom than a causal process in CCl_4 hepatotoxicity.

In contrast, CCl_4-induced free radical processes appear to cause an early inactivation of Ca^{2+}-sequestering capacity of endoplasmic reticulum.[107,108] Elevation of cellular Ca^{2+} establishes conditions for activation of the mitochondrial permeability transition with associated cytochrome c release and caspase activation (see Figure 26-4).

Other mechanisms have been proposed to explain the hepatotoxicity caused by CCl_4. Aldehyde products of lipid hydroperoxide degradation, such as 4-hydroxynonenal, are toxic to hepatocytes and have been considered "toxic second messengers." In many instances, 4-hydroxynonenal and other 4-hydroxyalkenals mimic the toxicities caused by CCl_4, including mitochondrial dysfunction; inhibition of protein, RNA, and DNA synthesis; decreased triglyceride secretion; loss of CYPs and Ca^{2+} sequestering activity; and cell death.[109] Additionally, after CCl_4 treatment, 4-hydroxyalkenals are generated at levels high enough to account for these toxicities. However, their involvement in CCl_4 hepatotoxicity has been questioned primarily on the basis of two arguments. First, the toxic aldehydes *S*-conjugate with GSH[90,91] and would be expected to deplete cellular GSH pools. Hepatocellular GSH levels, however, are unchanged or decreased only slightly by CCl_4.[110,111] Second, the aldehydes are sufficiently reactive to raise questions about their ability to diffuse to targets of injury that are far removed from the sites of aldehyde generation. Thus, 4-hydroxyalkenals may be responsible for some of the cellular manifestations of injury but probably are not required for CCl_4-induced hepatocellular death.

Another particularly interesting mechanism to explain CCl_4 hepatotoxicity is that the agent activates Kupffer cells, which are phagocytic cells lining the hepatic sinusoids, to release products toxic to hepatocytes. Evidence supporting such a mechanism comes largely from agents that either enhance[112] or inhibit[113] Kupffer cell function. See the following section for further discussion on phagocytic cell–mediated liver injury. Continuing research on mechanisms of CCl_4 hepatotoxicity surely will yield additional details of its mechanism of all injury.

REDOX CYCLING XENOBIOTIC AGENTS

Redox cycling refers to a pathway whereby a compound undergoes a series of one-electron reductions and oxidations. These reactions are coupled to generation of toxic oxygen species, which are thought to trigger a series of events ultimately leading to cell death. Isolated or cultured hepatocytes, perfused livers, and in vivo models have been used to study the hepatotoxicity associated with redox cycling compounds; however, these agents usually cause toxicity to other organ systems when administered in vivo. Examples are the lung injury associated with paraquat[114] and the cardiotoxicity caused by Adriamycin.[115] The relative insensitivity of liver parenchyma may be explained at least in part by the large capacity of the liver to detoxify reactive oxygen species.

A variety of flavoproteins catalyze one-electron reductions. In the presence of oxygen, the reduced product can spontaneously oxidize back to the parent compound, and this oxidation is coupled to the reduction of molecular oxygen to $\bullet O_2^-$. $\bullet O_2^-$ may cause lipid peroxidation or trigger other events leading to lethal cell injury.[76,116] Additionally, it may be metabolized to, or used in the generation of, other toxic oxygen species. The first case is exemplified by the degradation of $\bullet O_2^-$ to H_2O_2 (Table 26-2), which may be catalyzed by a Cu/Zn form of superoxide dismutase in cytoplasm or an Mn form in mitochondria.[117] H_2O_2, which also is toxic to hepatocytes and other cells, is degraded primarily by GSH peroxidases[118] (see Table 26-2 and Figure 26-6). As indicated previously, these consist of a selenium-dependent form localized to cytoplasm and mitochondria, a selenium-independent form identified as GSH *S*-transferases of the alpha class,[82] and a selenium-dependent phospholipid hydroperoxide GSH peroxidase.[80,81] In addition, there is evidence for a nicotinamide adenine dinucleotide-dependent pathway in the liver that uses ascorbate to detoxify organic peroxides,[119,120] although its role in H_2O_2 degradation is not clear. Hepatocytes also contain catalase to degrade H_2O_2; however, it is commonly believed that its role in H_2O_2 detoxification is limited, owing to its localization in peroxisomes and its high Km for H_2O_2.[118]

$\bullet O_2^-$ and H_2O_2 probably cause lethal cell injury to hepatocytes through formation of •OH by the iron-catalyzed Haber Weiss reaction (i.e., Fenton reaction) as shown in the equations following. •OH is very reactive and may initiate lipid peroxidation or bind to critical cellular

$$\begin{array}{c} \bullet O_2^- + Fe^{3+} \rightarrow O_2 + Fe^{2+} \\ Fe^{2+} + H_2O_2 \rightarrow Fe^{3+} + -OH + \bullet OH \\ \hline \bullet O_2^- + H_2O_2 \rightarrow -OH + \bullet OH + O_2 \end{array}$$

targets within close proximity to sites of generation. These reactions ultimately will quench •OH but may initiate events leading to irreversible cell injury. Fortunately, hepatocytes and other cells contain "free radical scavengers" such as ascorbate, which donate an electron and become a free radical themselves before being reduced back to the parent compound.

NADPH supply for reduction of peroxides often becomes limiting in oxidative stress.[119,121] GSSG formed during detoxification of H_2O_2 via GSH peroxidases cannot be reduced back to GSH by GSSG reductase because the latter enzyme has a requirement for NADPH (see Figure 26-6). Consequently, cellular GSH pools are depleted while GSSG levels increase, and GSSG is released from the cell. Studies in isolated perfused rat livers and in vivo show that GSSG is released across the sinusoidal membrane into the vasculature[122,123] in a process that is faster than in other organ systems. Thus, elevations of plasma GSSG (i.e., for studies in vivo) or in the vascular perfusate (i.e., for perfused liver studies) have been suggested to provide a measure of oxidative stress in the liver.

Redox Cycling of Menadione and Hepatocellular Injury

Menadione (2-methyl-1,4-naphthoquinone; vitamin K_3) is a quinone compound that undergoes redox cycling. In hepatocytes and other cells, it can undergo a two-electron reduction to the hydroquinone in a reaction catalyzed by quinone reductase, a cytosolic enzyme also known as DT-diaphorase (Figure 26-8). This 2-electron reduction is considered a detoxification reaction because the hydroquinone can be conjugated by sulfotransferases or uridine diphosphate glucuronosyltransferases. Furthermore, DT-diaphorase knock-out mice are more sensitive to the hepatotoxicity of menadione.[124] Menadione also undergoes one-electron reductions to the semiquinone free radical, which is catalyzed by many flavoenzymes including NADPH:cytochrome P450 reductase.[70] This free radical can undergo another one-electron reduction to the hydroquinone. Alternatively, in the presence of oxygen, the semiquinone free radical can be oxidized back to menadione with the liberation of $\bullet O_2^-$ from O_2. Redox cycling of menadione generates large amounts of $\bullet O_2^-$ and other reactive oxygen species, such as H_2O_2 and •OH, by the mechanisms described previously.

The oxidative stress caused by redox cycling of menadione leads to irreversible cell injury via a complex interplay between oxidation of soluble thiols (e.g., GSH) and protein thiols, causing a sustained rise in Ca^{2+} that is critical to activation of mitochondria-mediated apoptosis. Oxidation of critical protein thiols decreases microsomal Ca^{2+} sequestering capacity[22,23] and plasma membrane extrusion of Ca^{2+} from cells.[21] Oxidation of soluble

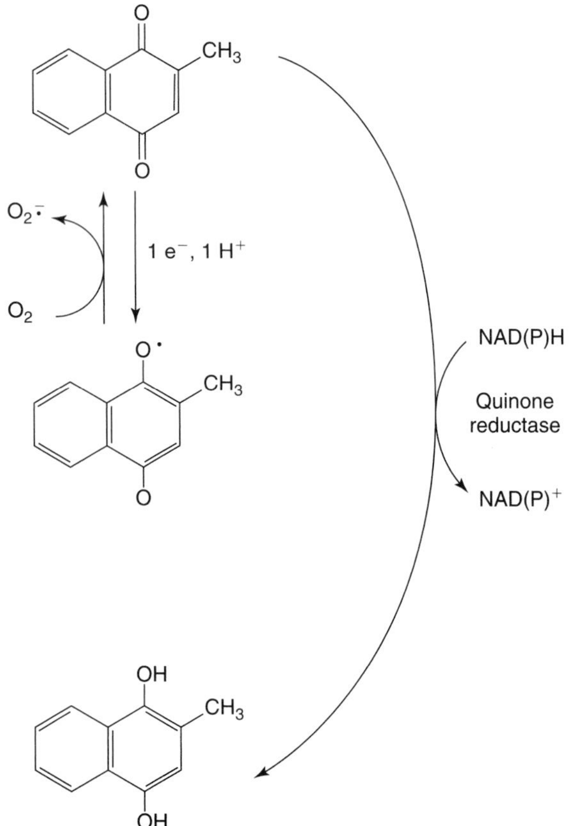

Figure 26-8 Redox cycling of menadione. *NAD+,* Nicotinamide adenine dinucleotide; *NADH,* nicotinamide adenine dinucleotide (reduced form); *NADP+,* nicotinamide adenine dinucleotide phosphate; *NADPH,* nicotinamide adenine dinucleotide phosphate (reduced form).

thiols precedes this and is a contributing factor in inhibition of the microsomal Ca^{2+} pump because GSH keeps the protein thiols in a reduced and functional form. In the presence of elevated Ca^{2+}, mitochondria load Ca^{2+}, and this loading sets conditions appropriate for activation of the mitochondrial permeability transition.[125]

The permeability transition (PT) occurs in response to opening of a high-conductance channel in the mitochondrial inner membrane.[125] Ordinarily, the inner membrane is highly impermeable to solutes. However in the presence of matrix Ca^{2+}, certain agents trigger the opening of the high conductance PT pore. The prevailing interpretation is that the PT pore is a protein complex containing adenine nucleotide translocase (ANT, inner membrane), voltage-dependent anion channel (VDAC, outer membrane), cyclophilin D (associated with ANT), and peripheral benzodiazepine receptor (associated with VDAC). Sensitivity to oxidants and thiol reagents, especially arsenicals, indicates that the PT pore contains thiols, probably vicinal thiols, which control opening. Thus, in the presence of elevated Ca^{2+}, oxidants trigger opening of the PT pore, with resulting swelling and release of cytochrome c[126] and other proapoptotic components.[127,128] Cytochrome c binds an assembly protein, ApaF-1, that allows recruitment and activation successively of procaspase 9 and procaspase 3.[129]

FAILURE OF ENERGY METABOLISM

Hepatocytes require a nearly continuous supply of energy in the form of ATP; decreased ATP supply may lead to cell injury by indirect or direct mechanisms. GSH synthesis is ATP-dependent. Thus chemical detoxification and repair of injury place increased demands on the cell for ATP; if these are not met, cell death may ensue. On the other hand toxicants that act as mitochondrial poisons (e.g., cyanide) or conditions that impair O_2 supply (e.g., hypoxia) act directly to decrease the energy supply to the cell.

Generation of free radicals from halogenated hydrocarbons by CYP is increased under the reductive conditions of hypoxia,[130,131] and hypoxic cells are more sensitive to oxidative injury.[132] Supply of NADPH is limited because of use of glucose 6-phosphate by glycolysis instead of the pentose phosphate pathway. There is, in addition, a decrease in glucose 6-phosphate dehydrogenase and GSH peroxidase activities.[133] Hypoxia and oxidant chemicals induce the mitochondrial permeability transition in liver cells in vitro, causing uncoupling of oxidative phosphorylation and further ATP depletion.[134] Thus hypoxia and other conditions that induce the mitochondrial permeability transition may impair cellular energetics and produce a situation in which the liver is more vulnerable to chemically induced injury.

IMMUNE MECHANISMS IN CHEMICALLY INDUCED LIVER INJURY

Hypersensitivity or Allergic Reactions

Because this issue is covered in Chapters 37 and 38 it will be discussed only briefly here. Many clinically relevant agents in the "idiosyncratic" liver injury group are thought to cause toxicity via hypersensitivity or allergic reactions. As reviewed by Pohl,[3] the liver injury caused by these agents usually occurs after repeated exposures and is often dose-independent. When the drug is removed, the injury subsides; however, upon rechallenge the liver injury is manifested again. One mechanism for these idiosyncratic reactions appears to involve activation of T lymphocytes (cell-mediated immune response), which are targeted to the liver. The second mechanism involves a humoral immune response in which specific antibodies are directed toward the liver. Although drugs causing these idiosyncratic reactions usually do so by one or the other mechanism, both may be involved. Whichever case operates, sensitized T lymphocytes or specific antibodies are directed toward chemically modified hepatic macromolecules (e.g., from covalently bound metabolite, termed neoantigens), or against normal liver macromolecules (i.e., autoantigens).

Halothane is an anesthetic that produces hepatitis in an idiosyncratic manner. Halothane is oxidized by CYP to a trifluoroacetylhalide that forms covalent adducts with microsomal proteins.[28] These neoantigens are present in all patients exposed to halothane, but only those individuals that develop halothane hepatitis produce autoantibodies against these proteins.[135]

Role of Phagocytic Cells in Liver Injury

Phagocytic cells, including monocytes, macrophages, and polymorphonuclear leukocytes (PMNs), have the capacity to produce and release a variety of cytotoxic agents such as reactive oxygen and nitrogen species, proinflammatory cytokines, bioactive lipids, and hydrolytic enzymes.[136] Normally, this arsenal is directed toward an invading pathogen, but occasionally host tissue can be injured. The liver injury produced by several hepatotoxins is dependent, at least in part, on the recruitment and activation of PMNs and macrophages.

Several approaches have been used to establish that phagocytic cells can injure hepatic parenchymal cells. Co-culture studies between PMNs and hepatocytes showed that PMNs activated with phorbol ester,[137-139] dead bacteria,[140] the oligopeptide *N*-formyl-methionyl-leucyl-phenylalanine,[139] and opsonized zymosan[141] caused hepatocellular injury as indicated by release of transaminases from hepatocytes. Further, the mechanism appeared to relate to release of proteases and not reactive oxygen species. Similar co-culture experiments between Kupffer cells and hepatocytes have shown that upon activation, Kupffer cells release products injurious to hepatocytes.[142] Studies with isolated perfused rat livers showed that activated PMNs caused elevated transaminases in perfusate and histologic lesions when compared to perfusions with unactivated PMNs.[143] A combination of superoxide dismutase and catalase afforded protection from injury, suggesting that reactive oxygen species released by the PMNs could injure hepatic parenchyma.

Studies in vivo also have implicated phagocytic cells in liver injury. Some investigators have depleted animals of circulating PMNs with polyclonal antibodies[144,145] to show that PMN depletion protected against chemically induced liver injury. Others have shown protection with antibodies to PMN adherence molecules (i.e., CD 11b/CD18),[146,147] which are normally expressed by PMNs and required for extravasation of PMNs through endothelium. Other in vivo studies have demonstrated the involvement of Kupffer cells, the resident macrophages of the liver. Gadolinium chloride, a Kupffer cell toxicant, protects the liver from the toxicity of acetaminophen,[148] CCl_4,[113] ethanol (see Chap. 30), dichlorobenzene,[149] allyl alcohol,[150] and endotoxin (bacterial lipopolysaccharide).[151]

There continue to be growing interest and awareness that phagocytic cells mediate liver injury under a variety of pathophysiologic conditions. For this discussion, it is perhaps most pertinent to consider the role of phagocytic cells in chemically induced liver injury. The endotoxin models are perhaps the most well-characterized models of liver injury. In one model, intravenous administration of killed *Corynebacterium parvum* to rats results in mobilization of macrophages to the liver, and treatment with endotoxin 6 days later causes extensive hepatocellular necrosis.[152,153] Inhibition of macrophage function with gadolinium chloride treatment decreases the extent of hepatic necrosis as determined by histopathology and serum alanine aminotransferase activity,[154] indicating that Kupffer cells may play a causal role in the injury. Macrophages isolated from the livers of treated rats are primed for oxygen radical release,[155,156] showing that they respond to stimuli with a greater oxidative burst (i.e., more $\bullet O_2^-$) than cells from untreated rats. $\bullet O_2^-$ or products derived from it appear to be involved in the pathogenesis because administration of superoxide dismutase before endotoxin reduces the hepatotoxicity. Other factors released by hepatic Kupffer cells also may be involved in the liver injury. TNF-α levels are elevated in this model,[154] and it is known that TNF-α can induce apoptosis via a receptor-mediated pathway.[9] In another well-established model, galactosamine, rather than *C. parvum*, is used to sensitize the liver to endotoxin. Endotoxin alone causes PMN sequestration in the hepatic sinusoids, but no liver injury. However, coadministration of galactosamine causes the PMNs to transmigrate from the sinusoids and attack the hepatocytes.[157] In this model, release of TNF-α as well as leukotriene D_4 (LTD_4) by Kupffer cells is involved in the pathogenesis.[158,159] They also show that Kupffer cells release factors that are chemotactic for PMNs, that up-regulate PMN adhesion molecules, and that prime PMNs for oxygen radical release.[160] Thus there appears to be a complex interplay between Kupffer cells/infiltrating macrophages and PMNs in endotoxin-induced liver injury (Figure 26-9).

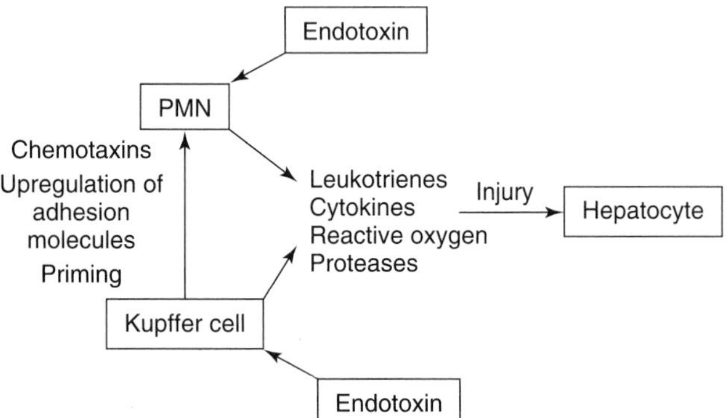

Figure 26-9 Phagocytic cell involvement in endotoxin-induced liver injury.

CONCLUDING COMMENT

The rapidly developing knowledge about the mechanisms of apoptosis dramatically changed the perception of how chemicals induce hepatic injury. In the past, injury was considered to be due to failure of critical cell machinery, especially that controlling Ca^{2+} homeostasis. Now, however, attention has shifted to mechanisms of apoptosis, which is executed by a proteolytic cascade that is activated by specific signaling involving death receptors or disruption of mitochondria, endoplasmic reticulum, and nuclei. Central features of chemically induced liver injury remain the same, but death is now viewed to occur through targeted cleavage of specific proteins rather than generalized failure. Bioactivation of organic compounds to reactive electrophiles occurs prominently in the liver because of high concentrations of enzyme systems designed to aid in the elimination of foreign compounds. Electrophilic agents covalently modify macromolecules, disrupting normal functions, including protein-protein interactions and protein degradation by proteosomes. Oxidants alter expression of death receptor machinery, enhancing death-receptor mediated apoptosis, and target the mitochondrial membrane permeability transition pore, triggering mitochondria-mediated apoptosis. Protection against reactive electrophiles and oxidants occurs through systems that depend upon GSH, and maintenance of glutathione provides a central approach for protection against chemically induced liver injury.

References

1. Klatskin G: Toxic and drug-induced hepatitis. In Schiff L, ed: Diseases of the liver, ed 3. Philadelphia, Lippincott, 1969:498-601.
2. Zimmerman HJ: The adverse effects of drugs and other chemicals on the liver. New York, Appleton-Century-Crofts, 1978:464-476.
3. Pohl LR: Drug-induced allergic hepatitis. Semin Liv Dis 10:305, 1990.
4. Plaa GL, Priestly BG: Intrahepatic cholestasis induced by drugs and chemicals. Pharmacol Rev 28:207, 1977.
5. Kerr JF: Shrinkage necrosis: a distinct mode of cellular death. J Pathol 105:13, 1971.
6. Kerr JF, Wyllie AH, Currie AR: Apoptosis: a basic biological phenomenon with wide-ranging implications in tissue kinetics. Br J Cancer 26:239, 1972.
7. Arends MJ, Wyllie AH: Apoptosis: mechanisms and roles in pathology. Int Rev Exp Pathol 32:223, 1991.
8. Samali A, Zhivotovsky B, Jones D, et al: Apoptosis: cell death defined by caspase activation. Cell Death Differ 6:495, 1999.
9. Ashkenazi A, Dixit VM: Death receptors: signaling and modulation. Science 281:1305, 1998.
10. Li P, Nijhawan D, Budihardjo I, et al: Cytochrome c and dATP-dependent formation of Apaf-1/caspase 9 complex initiates an apoptotic protease cascade. Cell 91:479, 1997.
11. Nakagawa T, Zhu H, Morishima N, et al: Caspase-12 mediates endoplasmic-reticulum-specific apoptosis and cytotoxicity by amyloid-beta. Nature 403:98, 2000.

12. Nelson DR, Koymans L, Kamataki T, et al: P450 superfamily: Update on new sequences, gene mapping, accession numbers, and nomenclature. Pharmacogenetics 6:1, 1996.
13. Lin JH, Lu AYH: Interindividual variability in inhibition and induction of cytochrome P450 enzymes. Annu Rev Pharmacol Toxicol 41:535, 2001.
14. Brodie BB, Reid WD, Cho AK, et al: Possible mechanism of liver necrosis caused by aromatic organic compounds. Proc Natl Acad Sci U S A 68:160, 1971.
15. Jollow DJ, Mitchell JR, Zampaglione N, et al: Bromobenzene-induced liver necrosis. Protective role of glutathione and evidence for 3,4-bromobenzene oxide as the hepatotoxic metabolite. Pharmacology 11:151, 1974.
16. Garner RC, Martin CN: Fungal toxins, aflatoxins and nucleic acids. In Grover PL, ed: Chemical Carcinogens and DNA, vol I. Boca Raton, Fla., CRC, 1979:187-225.
17. Douglas KT: Reactivity of glutathione in model systems for glutathione S-transferases and related enzymes. In Sies H, Ketterer B, eds: Glutathione conjugation. Mechanisms and biological significance. London, Academic, 1988:1-41.
18. Monks TJ, Lau SS: Reactive intermediates and their toxicological significance. Toxicology 52:1, 1988.
19. Anders MW, Lash L, Dekant W, et al: Biosynthesis and biotransformation of glutathione S-conjugates to toxic metabolites. Crit Rev Toxicol 18:311, 1988.
20. Miller EC, Miller JA: Mechanisms of chemical carcinogenesis: nature of proximate carcinogens and interactions with macromolecules. Pharmacol Rev 18:805, 1966.
21. Nicotera P, Moore M, Mirabelli F, et al: Inhibition of hepatocyte plasma membrane Ca2+-ATPase activity by menadione and its restoration by thiols. FEBS Lett 181:149, 1985.
22. Jones DP, Thor H, Smith MT, et al: Inhibition of ATP-dependent microsomal Ca2+ sequestration during oxidative stress and its prevention by glutathione. J Biol Chem 258:6390, 1983.
23. Thor H, Hartzell P, Svensson SA, et al: On the role of thiol groups in the inhibition of liver microsomal Ca2+ sequestration by toxic agents. Biochem Pharmacol 34:3717, 1985.
24. Freeman ML, Borrelli MJ, Meredith MJ, Lepock JR: On the path to the heat shock response: destabilization and formation of partially folded protein intermediates, a consequence of protein thiol modification. Free Radic Biol Med 26:737, 1999.
25. Ueda S, Nakamura H, Masutani H, et al: Redox regulation of caspase-3(-like) protease activity: regulatory roles of thioredoxinand cytochrome c. J Immunol 161:6689, 1998.
26. Moran LK, Gutteridge JM, Quinlan GJ: Thiols in cellular redox signaling and control. Curr Med Chem 8:763, 2001.
27. Essigman JM, Croy RG, Nadzan AM, et al: Structural identification of the major DNA adduct formed by aflatoxin BI in vivo. Proc Natl Acad Sci U S A 74:1870, 1977.
28. Pumford NR, Halmes NC: Protein targets of xenobiotic reactive intermediates. Annu Rev Pharmacol Toxicol 37:91, 1997.
29. Deleve LD, Kaplowitz N: Importance and regulation of hepatic glutathione. Semin Liv Dis 10:251, 1990.
30. Beatty PW, Reed DJ: Involvement of the cystathionine pathway in the biosynthesis of glutathione by isolated rat hepatocytes. Arch Biochem Biophys 204:80, 1980.
31. Wahllander A, Soboll S, Sies H: Hepatic mitochondrial and cytosolic glutathione content and the subcellular distribution of GSH S-transferases. FEBS Lett 97:138, 1979.
32. Meredith MJ, Reed DJ: Status of the mitochondrial pool of glutathione in the isolated hepatocyte. J Biol Chem 257:3747, 1982.
33. Griffith OW, Meister A: Origin and turnover of mitochondrial glutathione in the isolated hepatocyte. Proc Natl Acad Sci U S A 82:4668, 1977.
34. Hwang C, Sinskey AJ, Lodish HF: Oxidized redox state of glutathione in the endoplasmic reticulum. Science 257:1496, 1992.
35. Bellomo G, Vairetti M, Stivala L, et al: Demonstration of nuclear compartmentalization of glutathione in hepatocytes. Proc Natl Acad Sci U S A 89:4412, 1992.
36. Jevtovic-Todorovic V, Guenthner TM: Depletion of a discrete nuclear glutathione pool by oxidative stress, but not by buthionine sulfoximine. Biochem Pharmacol 44:1383, 1992.
37. Coles B: Effects of modifying structure on electrophile reactions with biological nucleophiles. Drug Metab Rev 15:1307, 1985.
38. Kosower NS, Kosower EM: The glutathione status of cells. Int Rev Cytol 54:109, 1978.
39. Mannervik B, Awasthi YC, Board PG, et al: Nomenclature for human glutathione transferases. Biochem J 282:305, 1992.
40. Coles B, Ketterer B: The role glutathione and glutathione transferases in chemical carcinogenesis. Crit Rev Biochem Mol Biol 25:47, 1990.
41. Mitchell JR, Jollow DJ, Potter WZ, et al: Acetaminophen-induced hepatic necrosis. IV. Protective role of glutathione. J Pharmacol Exp Ther 187:211, 1973.
42. Reed DJ: Cellular defense mechanisms against reactive metabolites. In Anders MW, ed: Bioactivation of foreign compounds. Orlando, Fla., Academic, 1985:71-108.
43. Beck LV, Rieks VD, Duncan B: Diurnal variation in mouse and rat liver sulfhydryl. Proc Soc Exp Biol Med 97:224, 1958.
44. Meister A: Selective modification of glutathione metabolism. Science 220:472, 1983.
45. Prescott LF, Critchley JAJH: The treatment of acetaminophen poisoning. Annu Rev Pharmacol Toxicol 23:87, 1983.
46. Kaplowitz N: Physiological significance of glutathione S-transferases. Am J Physiol 239:G439, 1980.
47. Prochaska HJ, Santamaria AB, Talalay P: Rapid detection of inducers of enzymes that protect against carcinogens. Proc Natl Acad Sci U S A 89:2394, 1992.
48. Zhang Y, Talalay P, Cho CO, et al: A major inducer of anticarcinogenic protective enzymes from broccoli: Isolation and elucidation of structure. Proc Natl Acad Sci U S A 89:2399, 1992.
49. Dinkova-Kostova AT, Talalay P: Persuasive evidence that quinone reductase type 1 (DT diaphorase) protects cells against the toxicity of electrophiles and reactive forms of oxygen. Free Radic Biol Med 29:231, 2000.
50. Kensler TW, Curphey TJ, Maciutenko Y, et al: Chemoprotection by organosulfur inducers of phase 2 enzymes: dithiolethiones and dithiins. Drug Metabol Drug Interact 17:3, 2000.
51. McClain CJ, Price S, Barve S, et al: Acetaminophen hepatotoxicity: an update. Curr Gastroenterol Rep 1:42, 1999.
52. Dahlin DC, Miwa GT, Lu A, et al: N-acetyl-p-benzoquinone imine: A cytochrome P450-mediated oxidation product of acetaminophen. Proc Natl Acad Sci U S A 81:1327, 1984.
53. Raucy JL, Lasker JM, Lieber CS, et al: Acetaminophen activation by human liver cytochromes P45011E1 and P4501A2. Arch Biochem Biophys 271:270, 1989.
54. Jollow DJ, Mitchell JR, Potter WZ, et al: Acetaminophen-induced hepatic necrosis. II. Role of covalent binding in vivo. J Pharmacol Exp Ther 187:195, 1973.
55. Potter WZ, Thorgeirsson SS, Jollow DJ, et al: Acetaminophen-induced hepatic necrosis. V. Correlation of hepatic necrosis, covalent binding and glutathione depletion in hamsters. Pharmacology 12:129, 1974.
56. Walker RM, Racz WJ, McElligott TF: Acetaminophen-induced hepatotoxicity in mice. Lab Invest 42:181, 1980.
57. Placke ME, Ginsberg GL, Wyard DS, et al: Ultrastructural changes during acute acetaminophen-induced hepatotoxicity in the mouse: A time and dose study. Toxicol Pathol 15:431, 1987.
58. Myers LL, Beierschmitt WP, Khairallah EA, et al: Acetaminophen-induced inhibition of hepatic mitochondrial respiration in mice. Toxicol Appl Pharmacol 93:378, 1988.
59. Burcham PC, Harman AW: Mitochondrial dysfunction in paracetamol hepatotoxicity: in vitro studies in isolated mouse hepatocytes. Toxicol Lett 50:37, 1990.
60. Bartolone JB, Birge RB, Bulera SJ, et al: Purification, antibody production, and partial amino acid sequence of the 58-kDa acetaminophen-binding liver proteins. Toxicol Appl Pharmacol 113:19–29, 1992.
61. Pumford NR, Martin BM, Hinson JA: A metabolite of acetaminophen covalently binds to the 56 kDa selenium binding protein. Biochem Biophys Res Commun 182:1348, 1992.
62. Birge RB, Bartolone JB, Emeigh-Hart SG, et al: Acetaminophen hepatotoxicity: correspondence of selective protein arylation in human and mouse liver in vitro, in culture, and in vivo. Toxicol Appl Pharmacol 105:472, 1990.
63. Labadarios D, Davis M, Portmann B, et al: Paracetamol-induced hepatic necrosis in the mouse: relationship between covalent binding, hepatic glutathione depletion and the protective effect of α-mercaptopropionylglycine. Biochem Pharmacol 26:31, 1977.
64. Devalia JL, Ogilvie RC, McLean AEM: Dissociation of cell death from covalent binding of paracetamol by flavones in a hepatocyte system. Biochem Pharmacol 31:3745, 1982.

65. Albano E, Rundgren M, Harvison P, et al: Mechanisms of N-acetyl-p-benzoquinone imine cytotoxicity. Mol Pharmacol 28:306, 1985.
66. Tee LBG, Boobis AR, Huggett AC, et al: Reversal of acetaminophen toxicity in isolated hamster hepatocytes by dithiothreitol. Toxicol Appl Pharmacol 83:294, 1986.
67. Moore M, Thor H, Moore G, et al: The toxicity of acetaminophen and N-acetyl-p-benzoquinone imine in isolated hepatocytes is associated with thiol depletion and increased cytosolic Ca2+. J Biol Chem 260:13035, 1985.
68. Coles B, Wilson I, Wardman P: The spontaneous and enzymatic reaction of N-acetyl-p-benzoquinoneimine with glutathione: a stopped-flow kinetic study. Arch Biochem Biophys 264:253, 1988.
69. Michael SL, Pumford NR, Mayeux PR, et al: Pretreatment of mice with macrophage inactivators decreases acetaminophen hepatotoxicity and the formation of reactive oxygen and nitrogen species. Hepatology 30:186, 1999.
70. Anders MW: Bioactivation mechanisms and hepatocellular damage. In Arias IM, Jakoby WB, Popper H, et al, eds: The liver: biology and pathobiology, ed 2. New York, Raven, 1988:389-400.
71. Beckman JS, Beckman TW, Chen J, et al: Apparent hydroxyl radical production by peroxynitrite: Implications for endothelial injury from nitric oxide and superoxide. Proc Natl Acad Sci U S A 87:1620, 1990.
72. Radi R, Beckman JS, Bush KM, et al: Peroxynitrite-induced membrane lipid peroxidation: The cytotoxic potential of superoxide and nitric oxide. Arch Biochem Biophys 288:481, 1991.
73. Beckman JS, Crow JP: Pathological implications of nitric oxide, superoxide and peroxynitrite formation. Biochem Soc Trans 21:330, 1993.
74. Abate C, Patel L, Rauscher FS III, et al: Redox regulation of Fos and Jun DNA-binding activity in vitro. Science 249:1157, 1990.
75. Recknagel RO, Glende EA Jr, Dolak JA, et al: Mechanisms of carbon tetrachloride toxicity. Pharmacol Ther 43:139, 1989.
76. Halliwell B, Chirico S: Lipid peroxidation: its mechanism, measurement, and significance. Am J Clin Nutr 57(suppl):715S, 1993.
77. Sevanian A, Hochstein P: Mechanisms and consequences of lipid peroxidation in biological systems. Annu Rev Nutr 5:365, 1985.
78. van Kuijk FJGM, Handelman GJ, Dratz EA: Consecutive action of phospholipase A2 and glutathione peroxidase is required for reduction of phospholipid hydroperoxides and provides a convenient method to determine peroxide values in membranes. Free Radic Biol Med 1:421, 1986.
79. van Kuijk FJGM, Sevanian A, Handelman GJ, et al: A new role for phospholipase A2: protection of membranes from lipid peroxidation damage. Trends Biochem Sci 12:31, 1987.
80. Ursini F, Maiorino M, Gregolin C: The selenoenzyme phospholipid hydroperoxide glutathione peroxidase. Biochim Biophys Acta 839:62, 1985.
81. Ursini F, Bindoli A: The role of selenium peroxidases in the protection against damage of membranes. Chem Phys Lipids 44:255, 1987.
82. Prohaska JR, Ganther HE: Glutathione peroxidase activity of glutathione-S-transferases purified from rat liver. Biochem Biophys Res Commun 76:437, 1977.
83. Ketterer B, Meyer DJ, Dark AG: Soluble glutathione transferase isozymes. In Sies H, Ketterer B, eds: Glutathione conjugation. Mechanisms and biological significance, London, Academic, 1988:73-135.
84. Wardman P: Conjugation and oxidation of glutathione via thiyl free radicals. In Sies H, Ketterer B, eds: Glutathione conjugation. Mechanisms and biological significance, London, Academic, 1988:43-72.
85. McCay PB, Brueggeman G, Lai EK, et al: Evidence that alpha-tocopherol functions cyclically to quench free radicals in hepatic microsomes. Requirement for glutathione and a heat-labile factor. Ann N Y Acad Sci 570:32, 1989.
86. Wells WW, Xu DP, Yang Y, et al: Mammalian thioltransferase (glutaredoxin) and protein disulfide isomerase have dehydroascorbate reductase activity. J Biol Chem 265:15361, 1990.
87. Meister A: Glutathione, ascorbate and cellular protection. Cancer Res (suppl) 54:1969s, 1994.
88. McCay PB: Vitamin E: interactions with free radicals and ascorbate. Annu Rev Nutr 5:323, 1985.
89. Esterbauer H, Schaur RJ, Zollner H: Chemistry and biochemistry of 4-hydroxynonenal, malonaldehyde and related aldehydes. Free Radic Biol Med 11:81, 1991.
90. Jensson H, Guthenberg C, Alin P, et al: Rat glutathione transferase 8-8, an enzyme efficiently detoxifying 4-hydroxyalk-2-enals. FEBS Lett 203:207, 1986.
91. Danielson UH, Esterbauer H, Mannervik B: Structure-activity relationships of 4-hydroxyalkenals in the conjugation catalysed by mammalian glutathione transferases. Biochem J 247:707, 1987.
92. Gutteridge JMC, Halliwell B: The measurement and mechanism of lipid peroxidation in biological systems. Trends Biochem Sci 15:129, 1990.
93. Smith MT, Thor H, Hartzell P, et al: The measurement of lipid peroxidation in isolated hepatocytes. Biochem Pharmacol 31:19, 1982.
94. Tribble DL, Aw TY, Jones DP: The pathophysiological significance of lipid peroxidation in oxidative cell injury. Hepatology 7:377, 1987.
95. Sun F, Hamagawa E, Tsutsui C, et al. Evaluation of oxidative stress during apoptosis and necrosis caused by carbon tetrachloride in rat liver. Biochim Biophys Acta 1535:186, 2001.
96. Plaa GL: Chlorinated methanes and liver injury: highlights of the past 50 years. Pharmacol Toxicol 40:43, 2000.
97. Rao KS, Glenda EA Jr, Recknagel RO: Effect of drug pretreatment on carbon tetrachloride-induced lipid peroxidation in rat liver microsomal lipids. Exp Mol Pathol 12:324, 1970.
98. Garner RC, McClean AEM: Increased susceptibility to carbon tetrachloride poisoning in the rat after pretreatment with oral phenobarbitone. Biochem Pharmacol 18:645, 1969.
99. Riely CA, Cohen G, Lieberman M: Ethane evolution: a new index of lipid peroxidation. Science 183:208, 1974.
100. Marchand C, McLean S, Plaa GL, et al: Protection by 2-diethylaminoethyl-2,2-diphenylvalerate hydrochloride against carbon tetrachloride hepatotoxicity. A possible mechanism of action. Biochem Pharmacol 20:869, 1971.
101. Recknagel RO, Glende EA Jr: Carbon tetrachloride hepatotoxicity: an example of lethal cleavage. Crit Rev Toxicol 2:263, 1973.
102. Comporti M, Benedetti A, Casini A: Carbon tetrachloride-induced liver alterations in rats pretreated with N,N′-diphenyl-p-phenylenediamine. Biochem Pharmacol 23:421, 1974.
103. Torrielli MV, Ugazio G, Gabriel L, et al: Time course of protection by N,N′-diphenyl-p-phenylenediamine (DPPD) against carbon tetrachloride hepatotoxicity. Agents Actions 4:383, 1974.
104. deFerreyra EC, Castro JA, Diaz-Gornez MI, et al: Diverse effects of antioxidants on carbon tetrachloride hepatotoxicity. Toxicol Appl Pharmacol 32:504, 1975.
105. Hove EL: Interrelation between α-tocopherol and protein metabolism. III. The protective effect of vitamin E and certain nitrogenous compounds against CCl_4 poisoning in rats. Arch Biochem 17:467, 1948.
106. Green J, Bunyan J, Cawthome MA, et al: Vitamin E and hepatotoxic agents. 1. Carbon tetrachloride and lipid peroxidation in the rat. Br J Nutr 23:297, 1969.
107. Moore L, Davenport GR, Landon EJ: Calcium uptake of a rat liver microsomal subcellular fraction in response to in vivo administration of carbon tetrachloride. J Biol Chem 251:1197, 1976.
108. Long RM, Moore L: Elevated cytosolic calcium in rat hepatocytes exposed to carbon tetrachloride. J Pharmacol Exp Ther 238:186, 1986.
109. Comporti M: Three models of free radical-induced cell injury. Chem Biol Interact 72:1, 1989.
110. Harris RN, Anders MW: Effect of fasting, diethyl maleate, and alcohols on carbon tetrachloride-induced hepatotoxicity. Toxicol Appl Pharmacol 56:191, 1980.
111. Pohl LR, Branchflower RV, Highet RJ, et al: The formation of diglutathionyl dithiocarbonate as a metabolite of chloroform, bromotrichloromethane and carbon tetrachloride. Drug Metab Dispos 9:334, 1981.
112. Nolan JP: Intestinal endotoxins as mediators of hepatic injury: an idea whose time has come again. Hepatology 10:887, 1989.
113. Edwards MJ, Keller BJ, Kauffman FC, et al: The involvement of Kupffer cells in carbon tetrachloride toxicity. Toxicol Appl Pharmacol 119:275, 1993.
114. Bus JS, Aust SD, Gibson JE: Lipid peroxidation: a possible mechanism for paraquat toxicity. Res Commun Chem Pathol Pharmacol 11:31, 1975.
115. Myers CE, McGuire WP, Liss RH, et al: Adriamycin: the role of lipid peroxidation in cardiac toxicity and tumor response. Science 197:165, 1977.

116. Poli G, Albano E, Dianzani MU: The role of lipid peroxidation in liver damage. Chem Phys Lipids 45:117, 1987.
117. Fridovich I: Superoxide radical: an endogenous toxicant. Annu Rev Pharmacol Toxicol 23:239, 1983.
118. Jones DP, Ekiow L, Thor H, et al: Metabolism of hydrogen peroxide in isolated hepatocytes. Relative contributions of catalase and glutathione peroxidase in decomposition of endogenously generated H_2O_2. Arch Biochem Biophys 210:505, 1981.
119. Kowalski DP, Aw TY, Park Y, et al: Postanoxic oxidative injury in rat hepatocytes: lactate-dependent protection against tert-butylhydroperoxide. Free Radic Biol Med 12:205, 1992.
120. Jones DP: NADH-, ascorbate-dependent peroxidase activity in rat liver microsomes. Toxicologist 12:76, 1992.
121. Tribble DL, Jones DP: Oxygen dependence of oxidative stress. Rate of NADPH supply for maintaining the GSH pool during hypoxia. Biochem Pharmacol 39:729, 1990.
122. Sies H, Wahlländer A, Waydhas C, et al: Functions of intracellular glutathione in hepatic hydroperoxide and drug metabolism and the role of extracellular glutathione. Adv Enzyme Regul 18:303, 1980.
123. Adams JD, Lauterburg BH, Mitchell JR: Plasma glutathione and glutathione disulfide in the rat: Regulation and response to oxidative stress. J Pharmacol Exp Ther 227:749, 1983.
124. Radjenirane V, Joseph P, Lee YH, et al: Disruption of the DT-diaphorase (NQO1) gene in mice leads to increased menadione toxicity. J Biol Chem 273:7382, 1998.
125. Bernardi P: Mitochondrial transport of cations: channels, exchangers, and permeability transition. Physiol Rev 79:1127, 1999.
126. Yang J, Liu X, Bhalla K, et al: Prevention of apoptosis by Bcl-2: release of cytochrome c from mitochondria blocked. Science 275:1129, 1997.
127. Susin SA, Lorenzo HK, Zamzami N, et al: Molecular characterization of mitochondrial apoptosis-inducing factor. Nature 397:441, 1999.
128. Li LY, Luo X, Wang X: Endonuclease G is an apoptotic DNase when released from mitochondria. Nature 412:95, 2001.
129. Li P, Nijhawan D, Budihardjo I, et al: Cytochrome c and dATP-dependent formation of Apaf-1/caspase-9 complex initiates an apoptotic protease cascade. Cell 91:479, 1997.
130. Cousins MJ, Sharp LH, Gourlay GK, et al: Hepatotoxicity and halothane metabolism in an animal model with application for human toxicity. Anaesth Intensive Care 7:9, 1979.
131. Strubelt O, Breining H: Influence of hypoxia on the hepatotoxic effects of carbon tetrachloride, paracetamol, allyl alcohol, bromobenzene and thioacetamide. Toxicol Lett 6:109, 1980.
132. Tribble DL, Jones DP, Edmondson DE: Effect of hypoxia on tert-butylhydroperoxide-induced oxidative injury in hepatocytes. Mol Pharmacol 34:413, 1988.
133. Shan X, Aw TY, Smith ER, et al: Effect of chronic hypoxia on detoxification enzymes in rat liver. Biochem Pharmacol 43:2421, 1992.
134. Lemasters JJ, Nieminen AL, Qian T, et al: The mitochondrial permeability transition in toxic, hypoxic and reperfusion injury. Mol Cell Biochem 174:159, 1997.
135. Losser M, Payen D: Mechanisms of liver damage. Sem Liver Dis 16:357, 1996.
136. Laskin DL, Laskin JD: Role of macrophages and inflammatory mediators in chemically induced toxicity. Toxicology 160:111, 2001.
137. Guigui B, Rosenbaum J, Preaux AM, et al: Toxicity of phorbol myristate acetate-stimulated polymorphonuclear neutrophils against rat hepatocytes. Demonstration and mechanism. Lab Invest 59:831, 1988.
138. Harbrecht BG, Billiar TR, Curran RD, et al: Hepatocyte injury by activated neutrophils in vitro is mediated by proteases. Ann Surg 218:120, 1993.
139. Ganey PE, Bailie MB, VanCise S, et al: Activated neutrophils from rat injured isolated hepatocytes. Lab Invest 70:53, 1994.
140. Holman JM, Saba TM: Hepatocyte injury during post-operative sepsis: activated neutrophils as potential mediators. J Leukoc Biol 43:193, 1988.
141. Mavier P, Preaux AM, Guigui B, et al: In vitro toxicity of polymorphonuclear neutrophils to rat hepatocytes: evidence for a proteinase-mediated mechanism. Hepatology 8:254, 1988.
142. Kobayashi S, Clemens MG: Kupffer cell exacerbation of hepatocyte hypoxia/reoxygenation injury. Circ Shock 37:245, 1992.
143. Dahm LJ, Schultze AE, Roth RA: Activated neutrophils injure the isolated, perfused rat liver by an oxygen radical-dependent mechanism. Am J Pathol 139:1009, 1991.
144. Dahm LJ, Schultze AE, Roth RA: An antibody to rat neutrophils attenuates α-naphthylisothiocyanate-induced liver injury. J Pharmacol Exp Ther 256:412, 1991.
145. Hewett JA, Schultze AE, VanCise S, et al: Neutrophil depletion protects against liver injury from bacterial endotoxin. Lab Invest 66:347, 1992.
146. Vedder NB, Fouty BW, Winn RK, et al: Role of neutrophils in generalized reperfusion injury with resuscitation from shock. Surgery 106:509, 1989.
147. Jaeschke H, Farhood A, Smith CW: Neutrophil-induced liver cell injury in endotoxin shock is a GDI lb/CD18-dependent mechanism. Am J Physiol 261:G1051, 1991.
148. Laskin DL, Gardner CR, Price VF, Jollow DJ: Modulation of macrophage functioning abrogates the acute hepatotoxicity of acetaminophen. Hepatology 21:1045, 1995.
149. Gunawardhana L, Mobley SA, Sipes IG: Modulation of 1,2-dichlorobenzene hepatotoxicity in the Fischer-344 rat by a scavenger of superoxide anions and an inhibitor of Kupffer cells. Toxicol Appl Pharmacol 119:205, 1993.
150. Przybocki JM, Reuhl KR, Thurman RG, et al: Involvement of nonparenchymal cells in oxygen-dependent hepatic injury by allyl alcohol. Toxicol Appl Pharmacol 115:57, 1992.
151. Sarphie TG, D'Souza NB, Deaciuc IV: Kupffer cell inactivation prevents lipopolysaccharide-induced structural changes in the rat liver sinusoid: an electron-microscopic study. Hepatology 23:788, 1996.
152. Ferluga J, Allison AL: Role of mononuclear infiltrating cells in pathogenesis of hepatitis. Lancet 2:610, 1978.
153. Arthur MJP, Bentley IS, Tanner AR, et al: Oxygen-derived free radicals promote hepatic injury in the rat. Gastroenterology 89:1114, 1985.
154. Arai M, Mochida S, Ohno A, et al: Sinusoidal endothelial cell damage by activated macrophages in rat liver necrosis. Gastroenterology 104:1466, 1993.
155. Arthur MJP, Kowolski-Saunders P, Wright R: Corynebacterium parvum-elicited hepatic macrophages demonstrate enhanced respiratory burst activity compared to resident Kupffer cells in the rat. Gastroenterology 91:174, 1986.
156. Arthur MJP, Kowolski-Saunders P, Wright R: Effect of endotoxin on release of reactive oxygen intermediates by rat hepatic macrophages. Gastroenterology 95:1588, 1988.
157. Lawson JA, Fisher MA, Simmons CA, et al: Parenchymal cell apoptosis as a signal for sinusoidal sequestration and transendothelial migration of neutrophils in murine models of endotoxin and Fas-antibody-induced liver injury. Hepatology 28:761, 1998.
158. Tiegs G, Wendel A: Leukotriene-mediated liver injury. Biochem Pharmacol 37:2569, 1988.
159. Tiegs G, Wolter M, Wendel A: Tumor necrosis factor is a terminal mediator in galactosamine/endotoxin-induced hepatitis in mice. Biochem Pharmacol 38:627, 1989.
160. Doi F, Goya T, Torisu M: Potential role of hepatic macrophages in neutrophil-mediated liver injury in rats with sepsis. Hepatology 17:1086, 1993.

C H A P T E R

27

Drug-induced Liver Disease and Environmental Toxins

Davendra Ramkumar, MB, BS, and Douglas R. LaBrecque, MD

The liver has a central role in the metabolic hierarchy of the human body (see Chaps. 3, 4, 5, and 8). It serves as the primary regulator of the contents of blood plasma, processing a vast array of chemicals supplied by the portal vein and hepatic artery. In addition to foodstuffs absorbed in the intestines that are necessary for growth, development and homeostasis, and the numerous by-products of normal metabolism, the liver is faced with an ever-increasing number of chemicals that are either intentionally—in the case of therapeutic drugs—or unintentionally—in the case of industrial and environmental exposures, introduced into the body. How the liver deals with an individual substance depends on a variety of factors. The final outcome is not always predictable. Some drugs and chemicals will be toxic to the liver despite its impressive metabolic capacity and flexibility. Others may be metabolized to toxic chemicals that subsequently damage the liver. Genetic aberrations and competition for particular elements of the metabolic machinery by different drugs and chemicals may produce unique interactions that ultimately result in hepatotoxicity.

Since the advent of the industrial age, a bewildering number of new chemicals have been synthesized and their number continues to grow exponentially. A total of 35,969,051 chemical substances had been registered with the Chemical Abstracts Service of the American Chemical Society as of January 28, 2002. They included 19,221,161 organic and inorganic substances and 16,747,880 sequences. The list grows by over 4000 each day, with 6,310,378 added in 1999 and 2000 alone. More than 3 million are available commercially. The Food and Drug Administration (FDA) lists more than 10,000 approved drug products in addition to 3000 substances that are added to foods in the United States. This is only a partial list of food additives because federal law allows some ingredients to be added under a "generally recognized as safe" category that does not require evaluation by the FDA. One must also recognize that 99.99 percent of the pesticides we ingest are natural ones, produced by plants to protect themselves from insects and other predators. Approximately 10,000 such natural pesticides have been identified and are generally present in much higher concentrations in the food we eat than synthetic pesticides.[1,2] Cooking food generates thousands of additional chemicals (more than 1000 have been identified in a cup of coffee alone). Considered in the context of the entire spectrum of liver disease, it is a logical assumption that the morbidity and mortality caused by drug and chemical hepatotoxicity will increase exponentially in the future. Whereas understanding of the somewhat finite number of infectious, autoimmune, and hereditary metabolic liver diseases is improving and translating into better management, recognition of hepatotoxicity resulting from one of the almost infinite number of new chemicals requires de novo evaluation to determine mechanisms of injury and management. Thus drug- and other chemical-induced liver injuries provide a challenging problem for physicians and health agencies and the pharmaceutical industry.

The clinical, biochemical, and histologic abnormalities caused by drugs and toxins may mimic virtually any liver disease. Often the diagnosis is one of exclusion. Moreover, severity may vary from subclinical or slowly progressive disease to fulminant hepatic failure. The reported incidence of drug-induced liver disease is often skewed based on how the cases are defined. Clinical judgment is probably the most frequent method used to identify a hepatotoxin. In an attempt to eliminate the inherent subjectivity of this process of decision-making, different methods seeking to improve the reliability of causality assessment have been developed. These vary in complexity and, as noted in a recent comparison between two clinical scales applied to the same patients, do not always agree.[3] Overestimation can occur as a result of using too sensitive a test to define disease (e.g., minimally abnormal liver enzymes or transient abnormality with reversion to normal). Conversely, liver tests may be normal in slowly progressive damage, as with the use of methotrexate, and underreporting may result. Case reports in the literature tend to concentrate on unique, severe, or fatal outcomes. The overall incidence of environmental and industrial toxin-induced liver injury is likely underestimated. Many cases are not recognized because they were never suspected, not properly investigated, or simply not reported.

EPIDEMIOLOGY

Chemical hepatotoxicity can occur in many settings. Commonly it is a result of the ingestion of drugs for medicinal purposes. These may be accepted, government regulated and approved medicines or folk remedies, herbal compounds, or others that do not require government regulation. An example of the latter is the ingestion of "bush tea" made from the *Senecio* species that can result in veno-occlusive disease (VOD) if taken in sufficient quantities. Other substances may be taken with suicidal intent, such as ingestion of acetaminophen or paraquat. Worldwide, the most common hepatotoxic agent is ethanol. In other situations the toxic agent may be accidentally or unknowingly ingested, as can occur when aflatoxin-contaminated grain is consumed. In the workplace, exposure to hepatotoxic agents may occur routinely. Chemicals may not be recognized as toxic to the liver, or when adequate precautions may not be taken against well-known toxic agents. Exposure also may be accidental. An increasing problem is exposure to chemicals that pollute the environment, such as herbicides and pesticides.

Estimates of the actual incidence of chemical-induced hepatotoxicity must be interpreted with several caveats in mind. In the case of pharmaceuticals, much of the data on toxicity are based on clinical experience with the drug in phase IV trials in the postmarketing setting. These trials usually involve a healthier subset of patients in the median range of the age spectrum as opposed to the young and the elderly, who have a statistically greater chance of developing toxicity. Selection is such that comorbid conditions and concurrent medication intake are at a minimum. The trials may not last long enough for the toxicity to become manifest in the case of drugs whose toxicity depends on a cumulative effect. These trials are designed to test efficacy first and foremost and may not be sensitive enough to detect subtle evidence of toxicity. Dose-dependent effects are usually well described in such trials but the total number of patients is usually not sufficient to recognize the rarer idiosyncratic reactions that occur in subjects predisposed by reason of immune or metabolic factors. For drugs and chemicals that have been in use for some time, individual or grouped case reports are usually the medium through which further information about a substance's toxicity is gleaned. These reports often concentrate on new and unusual effects or more serious problems that result in significant morbidity and mortality. Known drug reactions often are not reported. Because there is no incentive to report these cases, clinicians may find it difficult to justify taking the time to properly evaluate cases and submit their findings for peer review. It is estimated that fewer than 10 percent of adverse drug reactions caused by already approved drugs are reported to the FDA by physicians caring for affected patients. These data are not useful in estimating overall incidence. In addition, patients may not report an adverse event. They may feel sick and simply stop taking the drug or avoid the perceived toxic chemical. In addition, with mild toxicity, patients may not complain. Therefore the effect is not suspected and subsequently not recognized. Conversely, the effect may be recognized, but its etiology may be ascribed to other factors (i.e., misdiagnosis). Despite all of these limitations, serious drug-induced liver injury is the number one reason for withdrawal of drugs from the market.

The incidence of drug toxicity as the cause of fulminant liver failure is well described. In the United States one recent series estimated this to be about 20 percent.[4] The Acute Liver Failure Study Group found that, between 1998 and 2000, 52 percent of all cases of acute liver failure in the United States were due to drug-induced liver injury. In the United Kingdom the incidence was reported to be 60 percent to 70 percent. The offending agent is most often acetaminophen. Studies attempting to quantify the overall occurrence of liver toxicity resulting from drugs are uncommon. In the Boston Collaborative Drug Surveillance Program 66,995 medical and surgical inpatients were evaluated.[5] Twenty cases of drug-induced toxicity, of which 14 cases were probable and seven were definite, were found. Possible cases were not included, therefore these figures may be an underestimation. Eleven of the cases received the drugs in question during hospitalization, and nine were taking the medications before being hospitalized. The overall frequency was 1:3350 cases. An earlier study had reported 15 in 23,600 or a frequency of 1:1573 cases.[6] A review of adverse drug reactions in psychiatric hospitals found 31 probable and definite cases (7.6 percent) of increased transaminases in a total of 406 intensively monitored patients. Thirty-nine cases (0.8 percent) were spontaneously reported in 5096 patients monitored less intensively. The Danish Committee on Adverse Drug Reactions reported on 1100 cases of hepatic toxicity from 1978 to 1987.[7] The causality assessment between drug intake and hepatic injury was definite in 57 (5.2 percent) cases, probable in 989 (89.9 percent), possible in 50 (4.5 percent), and unclassifiable in 4 (0.4 percent). Hepatic injuries accounted for 6 percent of all adverse drug reactions reported, including 14.7 percent of the lethal adverse drug reactions. The major categories of drug effect were 47.2 percent acute cytotoxic, 26.9 percent elevated transaminases, and 16.2 percent acute cholestasis. In 4.7 percent of cases the hepatic injury was lethal and 1.3 percent of cases had chronic manifestations. Halothane accounted for 25 percent of all cases with a trend toward decreasing incidence over the duration of the observations. Next to halothane, sulfasalazine was the drug most often suspected. A similar report by the Committee on the Safety of Medicines in the United Kingdom indicated that hepatotoxicity as a manifestation of adverse drug reactions occurred in 3.5 percent of 1600 cases reported in the course of 1 year. Of these, 7 percent were fatal. Cholestasis and hepatitis occurred with greatest frequency and the drugs most commonly implicated were halothane, antibiotics, and oral contraceptives.

Within the last 20 years, several new methods have been developed to improve vigilance. In the United Kingdom the Prescription Event Monitoring System has been instituted. The identity of patients prescribed a particular drug and their physicians are identified from National Health Service prescriptions. A personalized questionnaire is mailed to each physician on the first anniversary of the initial prescription requesting information about any events their patients may have experienced since commencing the drug.[8] To date more than 65 studies have been completed and information regarding jaundice with erythromycin use,[9] liver test abnormalities with meloxicam use,[10] and liver toxicity with itraconazole use[11] have been published. Another method involves the use of medical record linkage, in which large databases of administrative and clinical data can be linked and information about medication use and hepatotoxicity extrapolated. To date this has been used to study hepatotoxicity from phenothiazines, cimetidine[12,13] and non-steroidal anti-inflammatory drugs (NSAIDs),[14,15] among others. Because of the large number of patients reviewed, the chances of detecting rare drug effects are improved.

CAUSALITY ASSESSMENT

A significant problem in the study of adverse effects of drugs and chemicals on the liver (and other organs) is that of causality assessment. The latter term refers to the process whereby the likelihood of the diagnosis of chemical-induced liver disease is determined. This process of deduction involves analysis of the relevant data and should include an assessment of the temporal relationship, clinical features, laboratory data, histologic data if available, and what is currently known about the chemical in question. From a statistical standpoint the most scientifically sound approach is to use Bayes theorem. Using this technique, an attempt is made to estimate the overall probability of a particular adverse event occurring to a particular individual in a particular situation (posterior probability), given the probability of this event occurring in a group of individuals similarly exposed (prior probability). Individual and situational details considered include the subject's clinical history, temporal relationships, histologic pattern of injury, resolution with discontinuation of the agent, and whether rechallenge with the agent resulted in the adverse event recurring. These details are used to develop a likelihood ratio; the product of this ratio and the prior probability is a measure of the posterior probability. The major problems that limit the application of Bayes theorem in practice are that it is time-consuming, and data needed to compute the likelihood ratio, e.g., background incidence, are often unavailable.

Most causality assessment is done using causality schemes. Subjectivity can result in significant intra- and interobserver variations when the same person or different people analyze a case of presumed chemical-induced hepatotoxicity.[16] To obviate this problem various algorithms and schemes have been developed.[16] Evidence that is weighed at the nodal points of these schemas includes the specificity of the clinicopathologic pattern, the temporal relationship between the onset and resolution of the adverse event and the intake and discontinuation of the agent being considered, and the exclusion of other potential causes. Based on the degree of certainty of a causal interaction between intake of a chemical and hepatic injury, different terms are used to describe the strength of the relationship. A relationship termed *definite* is usually supported by a specific clinicopathologic pattern, a strong temporal correlation, including a positive rechallenge, and exclusion of all other potential causes. Weaker relationships are termed *probable* or *possible* in descending order of strength; these terms are used when the required evidence is equivocal. The advantages of this approach are that it should allow more consistency in the evaluation of individual cases and different cases are more likely to be evaluated in the same way. This, in theory, should lead to better communication between groups evaluating the same problem. This is not always the case and critics argue that enough subjectivity is allowed in some of these processes to significantly alter the outcomes.[17] Different causality assessment schemes do not always agree. A recent study used two such scales to look at the same clinical data and demonstrated a low (18 percent) absolute agreement. A possible explanation was that too much was left to interpretation and judgment in one of the scales.[3]

Problems notwithstanding, many pharmaceutical firms, national monitoring committees, and drug regulatory boards require standardization. An international consensus meeting—The Council for International Organization of Medical Sciences (CIOMS)—proposed a series of standard designations of drug-induced liver disorders and criteria of causality assessment. These are summarized in Table 27-1[18] and provide useful guidance in evaluating causality. An attempt to produce a score predictive

TABLE 27-1

Summary of the CIOMS Consensus Meeting on Criteria for Drug-induced Liver Disorders[18]

Designations of Drug-induced Liver Disorders on the Basis of Liver-Test Abnormalities

1. When liver biopsy or autopsy has been performed, the lesion should be named according to the histologic findings (e.g., cirrhosis, chronic liver disease, hepatic necrosis, hepatitis).
2. In the absence of histology data such terms as *hepatitis, hepatic necrosis, chronic liver disease,* or *cirrhosis* should not be used in reporting. The preferred term is *liver injury.* The signs and symptoms of liver injury (asthenia, abdominal pain, nausea, vomiting, pruritus, and jaundice) are not specific enough to ascertain a liver disorder. Confirmation of liver injury is based on results of biochemical tests of the liver. The term *liver tests* should be used instead of *liver function tests.*
   A. Liver injury
      The term *liver injury* should be used if there is an increase of more than twice the upper limit of normal (2N) in ALT or CB, or a combined increase in AST, ALP, and TB, provided one of them is above 2N. No other biochemical test is specific to liver disorder.

Continued

TABLE 27-1

Summary of the CIOMS Consensus Meeting on Criteria for Drug-induced Liver Disorders[18]—cont'd

- Liver injury is designated *hepatocellular* when there an increase of more than 2N in ALT alone or $R \geq 5$ (where R [ratio] is serum activity of ALT/serum activity of ALP). Each activity is expressed as a multiple of N. Both should be measured simultaneously at the time of recognition of liver injury
- Liver injury is designated *cholestatic* when there is an increase of more than 2N in ALP alone or $R \leq 2$
- Liver injury is designated *mixed* when both ALT (above 2N) and ALP are increased, and $2 < R < 5$. R is of greatest value in patients with jaundice. R may vary during the course of the liver injury
- Acute liver injury is considered present when these increases have lasted less than 3 months
- Chronic liver injury is considered present when the increases have lasted more than 3 months. It should be distinguished from chronic liver disease, which may be used only on the basis of histologic findings
- The term *severe liver injury* is used in the presence of (in order of increasing severity):
  - Jaundice
  - Prothrombin time greater than 1.5 of control or prothrombin levels < 50% of normal
  - Hepatic encephalopathy
- *Fulminant liver injury* is the term used to designate rapid (days to weeks) development of hepatic encephalopathy and severe coagulation disorders

B. Abnormalities of liver tests
- Isolated increase, even more than 2N, in AST, ALP, or TB should be considered only a biochemical abnormality and not necessarily a sign of liver injury
- When the increase in ALT, AST, ALP, or TB is between N and 2N the term *abnormality of liver tests* should be used, not *liver injury*

Causality Assessment of Drug-induced Liver Injury: Acute Hepatocellular Liver Injury

1. Time to apparent onset of action

	Suggestive	COMPATIBLE		INCOMPATIBLE	
	from onset of drug administration	**From onset of drug administration**	**From cessation of drug administration**	**From onset of drug administration**	**From cessation of drug administration**
Initial treatment	5-90 days	<5 or >90 days	≤15 days	Drug taken after the onset of action	>15 days except for slowly metabolized drugs
Subsequent treatment	1-15 days	>15 days	≤15 days		

2. Course of the reaction

A. After cessation of the administration of the drug:
- The course is very suggestive if there is a decrease of ALT ≥ 50% of the excess over the upper limit of normal within 8 days and no additional elevation of ALT within a month. The course is suggestive if the decrease of ALT ≥ 50% occurs within 30 days
- The course is not suggestive (i.e, against a causal role for the drug), if the variations in level of ALT are different from above
- The course is inconclusive if there is no information regarding liver tests

B. If the drug is continued:
- The course is always inconclusive as regards causality assessment (i.e, no reliable conclusion can be drawn)

3. In case of re-administration of the drug
- The response is positive if there is at least a doubling of ALT irrespective of date, duration, or combination with other uninterrupted drugs
- The response is negative if the increase is less than N, provided the drug has been given in the same dose, for the same duration, and with the same combined drugs as for the first administration
- The response is not interpretable under other conditions

4. Information to be collected to permit the most accurate assessment of causality
- Information about the patient: age, sex, underlying disease or condition, weight, height.

A. Important risk factors in the development of drug-induced liver injury
- Use of one or more other drugs at the same time as the suspect drug, with accurate record of dates and times of administration
- Use of alcohol (amount, regularity, duration)

5. Information or results of investigations to exclude non-drug-related causes of liver injury
- Alcohol-induced injury, which is suggested when the ratio of AST/ALT ≥ 2
- IgM anti-HBc, which indicates recent infection by HBV

TABLE 27-1

Summary of the CIOMS Consensus Meeting on Criteria for Drug-induced Liver Disorders[18]—cont'd

- IgM anti-HAV, which indicates recent infection by HAV
- Non-A, non-B hepatitis: anti-HCV antibody (which may be present only after 1 or 2 months—sometimes 4 months—after the acute phase of liver injury), or circumstantial evidence, including administration of blood or blood products between 2 and 6 months previously, or recent travel to areas where hepatitis is endemic*
- Ultrasonography of the liver and biliary tract to exclude cholelithiasis and biliary tract abnormalities
- Episode of recent acute hypotension
- Results of tests to determine recent infection by CMV or EBV (optional)

Causality Assessment of Drug-induced Liver Injury: Acute Cholestatic or Mixed Liver Injury

1. Time to apparent onset of the reaction

		COMPATIBLE		INCOMPATIBLE	
	Suggestive from onset of drug administration	From onset of drug administration	From cessation of drug administration	From onset of drug administration	From cessation of drug administration
Initial treatment	5-90 days	<5 or >90 days	≤1 month	Drug taken after the onset of action	>1 month
Subsequent treatment	1-90 days	>90 days	≤1 month		

2. Course of the reaction
   A. After cessation of the drug:
      - The course is suggestive if reduction of at least 50% of the excess above the upper limit of normal of ALP or TB occurs within 6 months
      - The course is compatible if this reduction is <50% within 6 months
      - The course is inconclusive if the levels are stable or increase
   B. If the drug is continued:
      - The course is always inconclusive as regards causality assessment (i.e, no reliable conclusion can be drawn)
3. Re-administration
   - The response to re-administration is positive if there is at least a doubling of the ALP irrespective of date, duration, or combination with other uninterrupted drugs
   - The response to re-administration is negative if the increase is lower than N and if the drug has been given in the same dose, for the same duration, and with the same combined drugs as for the first administration
   - The response is not interpretable under other conditions
4. Information to be collected to allow the most accurate measurement of causality
   - Information on the patient: age, sex, weight, height, and underlying disease or condition
   A. Important risk factors in the development of drug-induced liver injury:
      - Use of concomitant drugs, with accurate record of date and times of administration
      - Use of alcohol (amount, regularity, duration)
      - Pregnancy
5. Information or investigations to exclude non-drug-related causes of liver injury
   - Ultrasonography of the liver and biliary tract to exclude cholelithiasis and biliary tract abnormalities
   - History of alcohol-induced injury, which is suggested when the ratio of AST/ALT is ≥2
   - IgM anti-HBc, which indicates recent infection by HBV
   - IgM anti-HAV, which indicates recent infection by HAV
   - Non-A, non-B hepatitis: anti-HCV antibody (which may be present only after 1 or 2 months—sometimes 4 months—after acute phase of liver injury), or circumstantial evidence, including administration of blood or blood products between 2 and 6 months previously, or recent travel to areas where hepatitis is endemic.*

CIOMS, Council for International Organization of Medical Sciences; *ALT,* alanine aminotransferase; *CB,* conjugated bilirubin; *AST,* aspartate aminotransferase; *ALP,* alkaline phosphatase; *TB,* total bilirubin; *IgM,* immunoglobulin M; *anti-HBc,* antibody against hepatitis B core antigen; *HBV,* hepatitis B virus; *anti-HAV,* antibody against hepatitis A virus; *HAV,* hepatitis A virus; *HCV,* hepatitis C virus; *CMV,* cytomegalovirus; *EBV,* Epstein-Barr virus.

*Author note: PCR for HCV virus should be positive within days of infection and is recommended if diagnosis is unclear. HCV-PCR was not included in the CIOMS criteria, which were developed before the routine availability of HCV-PCR.

of causality was published using the CIOMS criteria in 1993.[19] Ultimately, the physician must always be alert to the possibility of drug toxicity, have a low threshold of suspicion, and promptly discontinue any suspect drug. Neil Kaplowitz stated the maxim succinctly: "Suspicion is more important than proof."[17]

MECHANISMS OF INJURY

Chemicals that can induce damage in the liver often do so in a predictable manner that is usually dose-dependent and readily reproducible in animals and man. Others will induce damage in only a few individuals, and the damage is usually not dose-dependent. The former drug toxicities are frequently termed *predictable* and the latter *unpredictable*. The terms *idiosyncratic* and, less accurately, *allergic* are sometimes substituted for unpredictable. Agents that produce predictable toxicity tend to produce liver cell toxicity that affects a particular zone of the liver lobule, producing characteristic histologic changes. Unpredictable or idiosyncratic toxins can produce hepatic damage when they are present in concentrations that are therapeutic, in the case of medications, or at least not harmful to the majority of people exposed to similar concentrations, in the case of other chemicals. The mechanism of toxicity with idiosyncratic hepatotoxins is usually immunogenic or the result of defective. In immunogenic types of reactions there may be systemic features of an immune response such as fever, arthralgias, myalgias, skin rash, eosinophilia, or a serum sickness-type syndrome. In some instances the development of specific antibodies has been identified. These features suggest the development of an allergic reaction to the drug or an intermediate metabolite (e.g., a drug-enzyme complex). As more is learned about the enzyme systems present in the liver, their individual functions, and the metabolic pathways for individual chemicals, explanations for many of the non-allergic unpredictable drug reactions are being suggested (e.g., genetically defective sulfoxidation) in the setting of normal hydroxylation enhances the likelihood of chlorpromazine-induced jaundice[20]; genetically impaired epoxide hydrolase activity may lead to phenytoin hepatotoxicity due to impaired detoxification of a toxic epoxide intermediate.[21]

Rarely, substances are toxic in their de novo state. White phosphorus is a good example.[22] For the most part, however, most substances that are ingested are metabolized, and in some cases toxic intermediates or toxic end-products are created. Chemicals may be processed in the gut by gastric, intestinal, or bacterial enzymes to form the toxic product that reaches the liver via the portal circulation. Examples include the conversion of cycasin to methylazoxymethanol by intestinal bacteria[23] and activation of the carcinogenic dialkylnitrosamines in intestinal epithelial cells[24] (although in this latter example, activation also occurs via the cytochrome P450 system in the liver[25]). The most common scenario, however, occurs when the liver processes the chemical to produce toxic intermediates, which in turn produce hepatotoxicity. Although other tissues and organs in the body possess complex metabolic machinery to deal with alien substances, none are nearly as extensive or able to deal with as wide an array of chemicals as the liver. This is due to the strategic location of the liver, such that most of what is ingested must pass through the liver before entering the systemic circulation. From an evolutionary standpoint, the development of such a versatile enzyme system would seem to be an important requirement for improved survival. In addition to the vulnerability to hepatotoxicity by reason of its location and metabolic capacity, the liver's risk of injury is increased further in some instances because the toxic agents concentrate in the liver secondary to (presumed) binding to proteins. Drugs that are excreted in bile may produce toxic effects related to disruption of the ultrastructure and function of this complex drainage system. Drugs that undergo enterohepatic circulation may be more likely to cause hepatotoxicity because of prolonged exposure (if the drug or its metabolites are intrinsically toxic).

Often a precise categorization of the drug toxicity is not possible; however, the frequency and latency of such occurrences are generally helpful. Thus as noted previously, direct or predictable toxicities occur in a high percentage of those exposed after a short latent period. Immune-mediated reactions are infrequent and have a longer latency period (4 to 6 weeks), whereas metabolic idiosyncrasy is suggested by a variable but delayed latent period and low frequency.

THE DRUG-METABOLIZING ENZYMES OF THE LIVER AND THEIR ROLE IN TOXICITY

Biotransformation of non-polar substances to polar or water-soluble products that can be excreted in either bile or urine occurs in two phases. Phase I metabolism provides the compound with polar groups, preparing it for conjugation by phase II enzymes. The primary enzyme system involved in phase I reactions is the mixed-function oxidase system that uses the cytochromes P450, which are substrate- and oxygen-binding enzymes. The flavin monooxygenase system also catalyzes phase I reactions. These enzymes are primarily located in the smooth endoplasmic reticulum. These catalyze mainly oxidation and to a lesser extent reduction and hydrolysis reactions. In phase II the polar group created in phase I is conjugated to glucuronic acid, glycine, glutamine, ornithine, arginine, taurine, sulfates, glutathione, acetyl coenzyme A (CoA), or water. The phase II enzymes are primarily located in the cytosol. Phase I reactions may result in the production of reactive species that can cause hepatotoxicity, and as a consequence are sometimes referred to as the toxification phase. Phase II has been called the detoxifying phase because its products are generally non-toxic, polar substances that are readily excreted.

Cytochrome P450 consists of many isoforms that are grouped into families and subfamilies. Molecular-genetic techniques have established the gene sequences of the various isoforms of cytochrome P450 isoenzymes. A total of 27 gene families responsible for the variety of human cytochrome P450 enzymes had been identified by 1996.[26]

Of these the CYP1, CYP2, and CYP3 families are considered to be the most important in the hepatic metabolism of drugs, with a lesser role from the CYP4 family.[25]

Cytochrome P450 enzymes consist of two major protein components—a hemoprotein containing iron and a flavoprotein portion—which is responsible for the transfer of electrons from nicotinamide adenine dinucleotide phosphate (NADP) to the cytochrome P450 substrate complex. The binding site for drugs on the cytochrome P450 molecule is located in close proximity to a heme iron. This iron molecule, which initially is in the ferric form (Fe^{+3}), is reduced to the ferrous form (Fe^{+2}) by transfer of an electron from NADP via NADP reductase. The heme iron is then oxidized back to Fe^{+3} with concomitant insertion of an oxygen molecule into the substrate. A second oxygen molecule is then used to form water. If an oxygen radical is added to the parent drug, a reactive molecule is formed that may be highly toxic. The possible outcomes from phase I metabolism are illustrated in Figure 27-1 (phase I).

Different isoforms are specific for different substrates but, as alluded to, some substrates share the same isoform. When there is competition for a particular isoform of cytochrome P450 by two different chemicals, hepatotoxicity can result if one of the chemicals is intrinsically toxic and has a narrow therapeutic index. Liver damage occurs as a result of accumulation of this drug if the other chemical possesses a higher affinity for the P450 enzyme.

In response to some lipophilic substances individual isoforms of P450 may undergo induction whereby the substance up-regulates the production of the messenger ribonucleic acid (mRNA) endoplasmic reticulum. This results in more efficient metabolism and elimination of the inducing agent; however, this can also result in toxicity if another substance is ingested that is metabolized by the same isoform to produce a toxic metabolite. The rate of toxin production may exceed detoxification capacity as a result of the increased enzyme activity.

Other factors that can affect drug metabolism include decreased availability of the enzymes secondary to decreased synthesis and increased destruction or inactivation and suboptimal function as a result of an altered immediate milieu (e.g., secondary to hypoxia). Inhibition of enzyme activity by other drugs or chemicals can lead to toxic accumulation of a drug because of decreased clearance of the parent drug or toxicity because of failure to clear a toxic metabolite.

DETERMINANTS OF INDIVIDUAL SUSCEPTIBILITY TO HEPATOTOXICITY

Hepatotoxicity becomes manifest when a susceptible individual is exposed to a potentially toxic substance. The degree of toxicity is dependent on individual characteristics of the drug and how it is normally metabolized in addition to factors that might serve to make an individual more susceptible. Host determinants of toxicity include age, sex, and other endocrine factors; co-existing systemic or liver disease; nutritional status; the effects of other drugs, including alcohol; and genetic factors.

The effect of age on susceptibility to hepatotoxicity mirrors the effect of age on metabolism. For substances that require metabolic activation to produce a toxic species, immaturity of the metabolic machinery may lead to resistance to toxicity. On the other hand, immaturity may lead to worse toxicity from substances that are intrinsically toxic or are activated to toxic species and

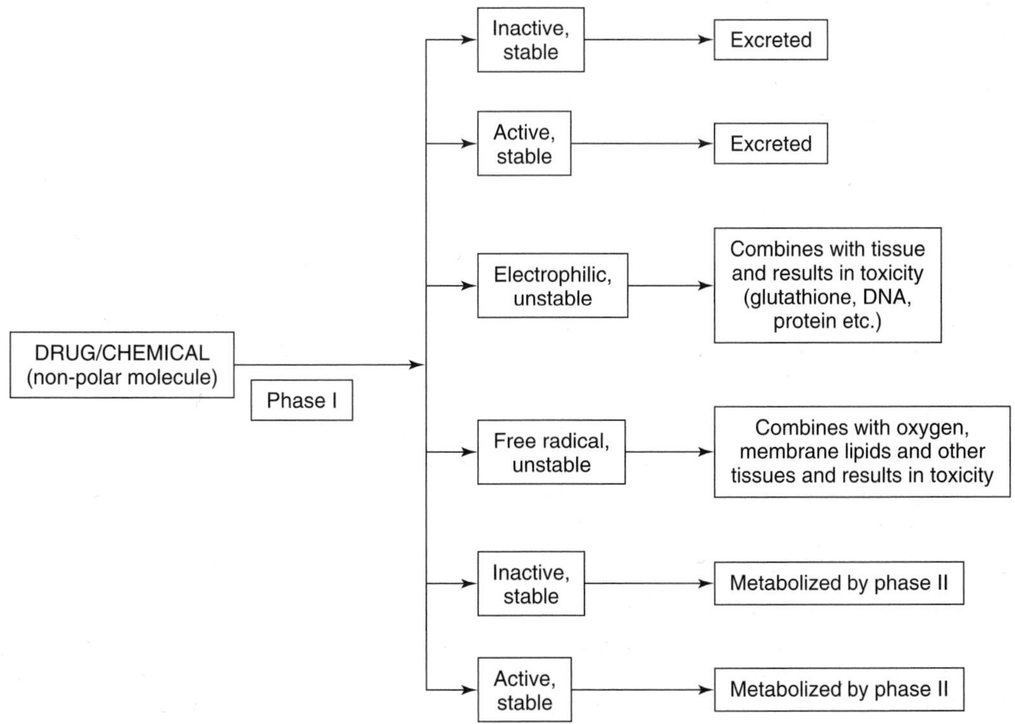

Figure 27-1 Phase I reactions.

depend on the liver for detoxification. Children and individuals younger than 20 years old are less susceptible to isoniazid,[27] with an increasing incidence of toxicity in older individuals. Similarly, children are less susceptible to hepatic injury related to the use of acetaminophen,[28] chlorpromazine, halothane, and erythromycin estolate. However, children and people younger than 20 years are more susceptible than older individuals to injury from valproate.[29] The elderly may be more susceptible to hepatotoxicity because of a reduction in the activity of the mixed-function oxidase (MFO) system, induction or inhibition of enzyme systems related to the ingestion of multiple medications, reduced volumes of distribution, reduced hepatic blood flow and mass, reduced renal clearance, prolonged half-lives, and reduced regenerating capacity of the liver.[30]

Limited data suggest that there are minor gender-related differences in susceptibility to hepatotoxicity. Women appear to be more susceptible to tetracycline-induced hepatotoxicity than men. This becomes more pronounced during pregnancy.[31] In addition, females seem to be more susceptible to developing hepatotoxicity to halothane, chlorpromazine, methyldopa, ticrynafen, and diclofenac.[32] Women are clearly more susceptible to the development of hepatic adenomas, especially in association with the use of estrogen in the form of oral contraceptive pills. The reasons for these differences are not clear, but hormonal influences on the immune system and on enzyme induction may be important. There are a few instances in which the male gender is more susceptible to hepatotoxicity. In the post-renal transplantation setting men are more prone to develop VOD, nodular regenerative hyperplasia, and non-occlusive portal hypertension with the use of azathioprine.[33]

Although well-documented in animal models, disorders of the endocrine system—including diabetes mellitus, hypothyroidism, and hyperthyroidism—and disorders of the hypothalamic-pituitary-adrenal axis have not been conclusively established as important factors in the causation of chemical-induced hepatotoxicity. Given their known effects on metabolism, they are likely to be important, however. Hypo- and hyperthyroidism result in decreased and increased susceptibility to carbon tetrachloride, respectively. This is thought to be related to down-regulation and up-regulation of the MFO system in the respective conditions.[34] Similarly, glucocorticoid excess may be protective in the setting of an immune-mediated adverse response. On the other hand, it may result in enhanced toxicity by causing increased accumulation of a lipophilic toxin. Changes in body temperature and hepatic blood flow may also be important variables that can be affected by endocrine factors.

The importance of nutritional status in the pathogenesis of hepatotoxicity is controversial. It was formerly thought that protein malnutrition enhanced the effect of all hepatotoxins. This notion has been shown to be somewhat inaccurate in recent years. Protein deficiency has been shown to decrease the activity of the MFO system. For toxins—such as carbon tetrachloride—that require metabolic activation, this will lead to a decreased susceptibility. Dimethylnitrosamine, which also requires metabolic activation to exert its hepatotoxic and carcinogenic effects, causes fewer problems in individuals on a low-protein diet. On the other hand, for agents such as aflatoxin that require detoxification to decrease their toxic potency, protein malnutrition may be deleterious. In addition, hypoalbuminemia—whether nutritional or from other causes (e.g., protein losing enteropathy or protein losses in burn victims and the nephrotic syndrome)—may result in increased toxicity of substances that are predominantly protein-bound (e.g., aspirin). Obesity is associated with an increased incidence of halothane-induced toxicity. This has been assumed to occur because of a prolonged storage of halothane in adipose tissue, although in a rat model of obesity there is increased activity of components of the MFO system that produce the toxic metabolites of halothane. Another nutritional factor that may affect the degree of toxicity of some substances is fasting, which reduces levels of glutathione that are protective against damage (e.g., in acetaminophen toxicity).[35] Individual components of the diet, apart from protein and carbohydrate, including ascorbic acid, tocopherol, essential fatty acids, zinc, selenium, and other vitamins and minerals can also affect drug metabolism.

Pre-existing diseases may affect the injury by some hepatotoxins. Acquired immunodeficiency syndrome (AIDS) has been associated with increased toxicity of sulfamethoxazole-trimethoprim, dapsone, and oxacillin.[36-38] Individuals with certain rheumatologic disorders, including systemic lupus erythematosus (SLE) and juvenile rheumatoid arthritis, appear to be more susceptible to salicylate-induced liver injury.[38]

Pre-existing liver disease may cause enhanced hepatotoxicity to a select few drugs. Methotrexate toxicity appears to be more pronounced in patients with pre-existing liver disease.[39] Concurrent therapy with medicines or exposure to other foreign chemical compounds may increase susceptibility for various reasons, some of which were discussed under "Mechanisms of Injury." Patients taking multiple drugs are more likely to develop hepatotoxicity.[40] These effects are likely the result of the effects of metabolism of one agent on another. In this regard, chemicals can interact in many different ways. If the same MFO enzyme processes them both, intrinsically toxic substances may accumulate; if they are competing for the same detoxification pathway (phase II), toxic intermediates may accumulate. Enzyme induction by one substance may result in increased metabolism with the potential for accumulation of a toxic intermediate of the other chemical. In some cases concurrent therapy enhances toxicity, whereas with other combinations some protection against hepatotoxicity seems to be afforded. Isoniazid is less toxic when administered alone than when administered with other agents (e.g., rifampin,[41] ethanol). Hepatotoxicity of valproic acid appears to be enhanced by simultaneous treatment with other anti-convulsants such as phenytoin. Alcohol ingestion increases the toxicity of acetaminophen and carbon tetrachloride.[42]

Genetic polymorphisms that result in increased susceptibility to hepatic injury are increasingly recognized as the cause of many idiosyncratic, non-immune-related cases of hepatotoxicity. Some examples are listed in Table 27-2 and will be discussed further in the following sections.

TABLE 27-2
Susceptibility to Drug Hepatotoxicity

Host factor	Increased susceptibility
Age	
• Infancy	Isoniazid, NSAIDs
• Older age groups	Valproic acid
Sex	
• Female	Halothane, isoniazid, zidovudine
• Male	Amoxicillin-clavulanate
Race	
• African	Isoniazid
• Asian	Isoniazid
Renal insufficiency	NSAIDs, methotrexate
Hypoalbuminemia	Aspirin, methotrexate
Pre-existing liver disease	Isoniazid, methotrexate, acetaminophen
Obesity	Halothane, methotrexate
HIV/AIDS	Oxacillin, trimethoprim-sulfamethoxazole
Other drugs	
• Alcohol	Acetaminophen, NSAIDs, methotrexate
• Isoniazid	Acetaminophen
• Anti-convulsants	Acetaminophen, valproic acid
• Rifampin	Isoniazid
Genetic polymorphisms/defects	
• Slow acetylators	Isoniazid
• P450 2D6 (debrisoquine 4-hydroxylase)	Perhexiline maleate
• Urea cycle	Valproic acid
• Mitochondrial beta-oxidation	Valproic acid, aspirin
• UDP glucuronosyl transferase	Acetaminophen

NSAIDs, Non-steroidal anti-inflammatory drugs; *HIV,* human immunodeficiency virus; *AIDS,* acquired immunodeficiency virus; *UDP,* uridine diphosphate.

CLINICOPATHOLOGIC SPECTRUM OF DRUG HEPATOTOXICITY

Drugs and other chemicals can mimic virtually any recognized liver disorder, both clinically and histologically. Many agents produce a characteristic histologic pattern that forms the basis for one classification of drug-induced liver damage. Table 27-3 outlines the various patterns that can occur with representative examples. The patterns listed are by no means mutually exclusive. Some chemicals may cause one type of injury, but with significant individual variation in severity of damage (e.g., halothane,[43] whose effects can range from mild asymptomatic disease to fatal hepatic failure with corresponding minimally abnormal histology to massive hepatocellular necrosis). Other substances can cause a variety of injury patterns, depending on a number of factors such as dose and duration of treatment. For instance, methotrexate can produce damage ranging from liver test abnormalities with no histologic change to varying degrees of steatosis, hepatitis, and fibrosis. The presence of underlying liver disease can sometimes confuse the picture. Probably the most common scenario that occurs in practice is the need to differentiate the effects of alcohol intake and those resulting from the chemical in question. These observations all underscore the basic tenet that liver biopsies need to be interpreted in the context of the entire clinicopathologic circumstance. This includes clinical features, history of drug or chemical exposure, laboratory tests including biochemistries and serologies, and findings on imaging studies. The pathologist must be provided with all the relevant information if he or she is to make an accurate interpretation of the biopsy.

Acute Hepatocellular Injury

Acute hepatocellular or cytotoxic injury is manifested by necrosis and apoptosis of hepatic parenchymal cells. Necrosis refers to disintegration of the hepatocyte, initiated by direct damage to the plasma membrane and resulting in debris.[44] Apoptosis, on the other hand, refers to lethal cell injury, which mimics programmed cell death. These include cell shrinkage, clumping of the nuclear chromatin, nuclear shrinkage, nuclear fragmentation (karyorrhexis), and cytoplasmic blebs. The condensed hepatocytes are referred to as acidophil or apoptotic bodies. Inflammation is rare in the setting of acute hepatocellular injury. Cells that are damaged but not dead may accumulate lipid droplets (steatosis). Minor drug effects may be suggested by the appearance of "induced hepatocytes," which appear pale on hematoxylin and eosin staining because of the presence of large amounts of smooth endoplasmic reticulum. Hepatocellular injury is usually suggested by an elevation of the hepatocellular enzymes: alanine aminotransferase (ALT), which is

TABLE 27-3

Liver Injury Patterns Resulting from Drugs

Category	Examples
Altered liver tests without histologic liver disease	
Microsomal enzyme induction	Phenytoin, warfarin, phenobarbital
Hyperbilirubinemia	Rifampin, novobiocin, flavaspidic acid
Acute hepatocellular injury	
Zonal	
Zone 1	Phosphorus, ferrous sulfate, allyl formate
Zone 2	Beryllium
Zone 3	Acetaminophen, carbon tetrachloride, mushroom poisoning, halothane
Non-zonal	
Massive necrosis	Halothane, valproic acid, non-steroidal anti-inflammatory drugs
Bridging necrosis	Isoniazid, alpha-methyldopa
Focal necrosis	Cloxacillin, isoniazid, halothane
Chronic parenchymal injury	
Chronic active hepatitis	Alpha-methyldopa, nitrofurantoin, dantrolene, minocycline
Fibrosis and cirrhosis	Methotrexate, hypervitaminosis A
Fatty liver	
Microvesicular	Tetracycline, valproic acid, didanosine
Macrovesicular	Alcohol, methotrexate, corticosteroids, asparaginase
Phospholipidosis/pseudoalcoholic	Amiodarone, perhexiline maleate, sulfamethoxazole-trimethoprim
Granulomatous reactions	Hydralazine, allopurinol, carbamazepine, phenylbutazone, dapsone
Acute cholestasis	
With hepatitis	Chlorpromazine, amoxicillin-clavulanate, erythromycin estolate, piroxicam
Without hepatitis/ductal injury	Oral contraceptive steroids, anabolic steroids
Chronic cholestasis	
Sclerosing cholangitis	Intraarterial floxuridine, formalin treatment of hydatid cysts
Vanishing bile ducts	Chlorpromazine, flucloxacillin, prochlorperazine, ajmaline, amitriptyline
Vascular lesions	
Hepatic vein thrombosis	Oral contraceptive steroids, total parenteral nutrition
Veno-occlusive disease	Pyrrolizidine alkaloids, oncotherapy, azathioprine
Portal vein thrombosis	Oral contraceptive steroids
Non-cirrhotic portal hypertension	Vinyl chloride, hypervitaminosis A, azathioprine
Peliosis hepatis	Anabolic steroids, oral contraceptives steroids, Thorotrast
Nodular regenerative hyperplasia	Azathioprine, 6-thioguanine
Sinusoidal dilation	Oral contraceptive steroids
Prolapse of hepatocytes into the central veins	Anabolic steroids
Hepatoportal sclerosis	Arsenic, azathioprine
Hepatic tumors	
Adenomas	Oral contraceptive steroids, anabolic steroids
Nodular transformation	Oral contraceptive steroids, anabolic steroids, aniline-rapeseed oil, oncotherapy
Hepatocellular carcinoma	Oral contraceptive steroids, anabolic steroids, thorotrast
Angiosarcoma	Inorganic arsenic, thorotrast, vinyl chloride
Cholangiocarcinoma	Thorotrast
Pigment deposition	
Lipofuscin	Phenothiazine, phenacetin, aminopyrine, cascara
Hemosiderin	Alcoholism, iron overload syndromes, toxic porphyrias
Thorotrast	Thorotrast
Gold	Gold compounds used in the treatment of arthritis
Titanium	Drug abuse, occupational exposure
Anthracite	Miners

specific for the liver, and aspartate aminotransferase (AST), which is less specific.

Hepatocellular necrosis may occur in a zonal or non-zonal manner. Zone I (periportal) refers to the areas most peripheral to the central veins, zone 3 (centrolobular or perivenular) to the area immediately around the central veins, and zone 2 to the area intermediate to zones 1 and 3. There may be overlaps (e.g., extensive zone 3 necrosis may encroach on zone 2). In general, predictable reactions are zonal, whereas unpredictable or idiosyncratic reactions tend to be non-zonal. Zone 3 necrosis occurs with acetaminophen, halothane, carbon tetrachloride, chloroform, and mushroom poisoning resulting from *Amanita phalloides.* Zone 1 necrosis occurs with ferrous sulfate, white phosphorus, cocaine and allyl alcohol, and esters. Isolated zone 2 necrosis is rare, and this zone tends to be involved mainly as extensions from zone 1 and 3. Beryllium is an example of a substance that produces isolated zone 2 necrosis. The zonality of necrosis may be related to the mechanism of injury. The location of the isoforms of cytochrome P450 that convert individual substances to their toxic metabolites may be a major factor. In addition to this, the higher oxygen tension in zone 1, resulting from its proximity to the hepatic arteriole, is thought to promote the conversion of allyl alcohol and esters to their toxic metabolites. Also, the concentrations of chemicals may vary in a zonal manner, as can the cellular content of protective species such as glutathione. Zonal necrosis may either progress to fulminant hepatic failure or heal with discontinuation of the drugs or chemicals. Healing tends to occur without extensive scarring and the hepatic architecture is maintained. There is no chronic variant of this damage.

Massive (panacinar), bridging, and focal (spotty) necrosis are forms of non-zonal necrosis that tend to be manifestations of idiosyncratic hepatotoxicity. Massive necrosis is typified by diffuse cell death throughout the hepatic lobule. This can usually be differentiated from extensive zone 3 necrosis because the latter tends to spare a thin rim of hepatocytes in the periportal area and the liver architecture is generally maintained. In addition to diffuse necrosis and degeneration with collapse of the liver architecture, evidence of regeneration and bile duct proliferation may be seen. At the extreme, massive necrosis can result in fulminant hepatic failure. With healing, postnecrotic nodular scarring and cirrhosis may ensue but most cases of fulminant hepatic failure that recover do so with no residual scarring. Drugs that can induce this reaction include halothane, isoniazid, valproic acid, and phenytoin. In focal necrosis there are single or small groups of necrotic hepatocytes that display ballooning degeneration and evidence of apoptosis. There may be a mononuclear cell infiltrate in the portal triads and Kupffer cells, laden with the scavenged remnants of degenerated cells. With healing, ceroid-laden macrophages may be noted.

Chronic Parenchymal Injury

Chronic Hepatitis

Chronic hepatitis can be a manifestation of the hepatotoxicity caused by certain drugs. The primary importance of this observation is that the clinical and histologic picture is difficult to distinguish from chronic viral hepatitis. It may also mimic autoimmune hepatitis in which severe liver damage with prominent plasma cell infiltration may be present. These similarities are often used as a means to classify these types of drug reactions (Table 27-4).

TABLE 27-4
Drugs Causing Chronic Hepatitis

Autoimmune-like	Dantrolene
	Diclofenac
	Hydralazine
	Methyldopa
	Nitrofurantoin
	Oxyphenisatin
	Phenytoin
	Propyluracil
	Tienilic acid
	Sulfonamides
Chronic viral hepatitis-like	Amiodarone
	Aspirin
	Halothane
	Isoniazid
	Ethanol
	Etretinate

Autoimmune hepatitis-like manifestations may also include striking titers of anti-nuclear antibodies (ANA) or anti–smooth muscle antibodies (ASMA). Examples of drugs that can cause this reaction include dantrolene, diclofenac, methyldopa, nitrofurantoin, oxyphenisatin, phenytoin, propyluracil, and tienilic acid.

The literature regarding a chronic hepatitis–like picture published before the advent of reliable testing for hepatitis C has to be interpreted carefully because some of these cases were likely chronic viral hepatitis C. Examples of drugs that cause this type of hepatotoxicity include isoniazid and halothane.

In many cases chronic hepatitis is not recognized as a manifestation of hepatotoxicity, resulting in continued exposure to the agent with serious consequences. The course after discontinuation is variable. Usually there is prompt and complete reversal of the hepatic lesion (e.g., aspirin- and acetaminophen-induced chronic hepatitis). In other cases, especially when the hepatitis is in an advanced state or the drug had been continued after the onset of symptoms, resolution may be slow and progress to a fatal outcome (e.g., isoniazid).

Steatosis

Lipid droplets within the cytoplasm of hepatocytes are a common expression of hepatotoxicity for many chemicals. The droplets are composed primarily of triglycerides, with phospholipids less commonly accounting for the droplets seen with some drugs or chemicals. Although the distribution of lipid-laden hepatocytes tends not to follow a zonal distribution for most instances of toxicity, there are a few exceptions. Some agents lead primarily to a zone 3 distribution of fat (e.g., tetracycline, ethanol). Others lead to zone 1 distribution (e.g., white phosphorus, ethionine). It is presumed that the accumulation of lipids occurs as a result of impaired cellular metabolism of fatty acids. Although steatosis is a physical manifestation of disturbances in the metabolic machinery of the hepatocyte, it does not imply that this is the mediator of cell injury. It is likely that lipid droplets are one of many aberrations in cellular metabolism. Hence the degree of cellular dysfunction seen for a given extent of steatosis is variable.

With deposition of triglycerides, two patterns are described. In the more common macrovesicular form the droplets are large, effectively fill the hepatocyte and displace the nucleus to the periphery, giving the hepatocyte the appearance of an adipose cell. This type of steatosis is encountered most commonly in metabolic disorders such as obesity, diabetes mellitus, malnutrition, and jejunoileal bypass. Chemicals that can cause this pattern of toxicity include ethanol, corticosteroids, and methotrexate. When present in isolation, this type of steatosis is rarely associated with significant abnormalities in liver function. However, as in the case of alcoholic steatosis, it can be associated with polymorphonuclear leukocyte infiltration (alcoholic hepatitis), Mallory bodies (hyaline degeneration), cholestasis, and fibrosis, which can be associated with varying degrees of liver dysfunction. When these manifestations occur in the absence of alcohol, the condition is referred to as pseudoalcoholic liver disease or non-alcoholic steatohepatitis (NASH) and can be seen with amiodarone, nifedipine, and perhexiline maleate toxicity. There are a few situations in which a seemingly pure expression of macrovesicular steatosis has led to significant liver dysfunction or liver failure (e.g., zidovudine, the anti–human immunodeficiency virus [HIV] medication, which is associated with fatal lactic acidosis resulting from mitochondrial malfunction).

In microvesicular steatosis the lipid droplets are smaller and distributed evenly throughout the cytoplasm, with the nucleus maintaining its central location. The aberrations in lipid metabolism in microvescicular steatosis, involve impaired mitochondrial oxidation of fatty acids. As a consequence, microvesicular steatosis is more likely to be associated with significant liver dysfunction despite a liver that appears to have minimal histologic injury. Manifestations include elevated ammonia, ALT, and AST levels; coagulopathy; hepatic encephalopathy; and death as a consequence of liver failure. This pattern of injury is less common than the macrovesicular variety and can be seen in the setting of fatty liver of pregnancy, Reye's syndrome, and inborn errors of fatty acid metabolism. Chemicals that can mimic this pattern include valproic acid, tetracycline, and hypoglycin, a toxin found in unripe ackee, a tropical fruit.

Although macrovesicular and microvesicular steatosis can occur exclusively, often a combination of the two is recognized. The classic example of this is ethanol toxicity. Here the predominant form of steatosis tends to be macrovesicular, but varying degrees of microvesicular steatosis can be observed. The administration of large doses of vitamin A can lead to the focal deposition of lipids in hepatic stellate (Ito) cells. This can progress to fibrosis and cirrhosis.[45-47] Phospholipid accumulation can occur as a manifestation of chemical-induced toxicity. The agents that can produce this pattern of injury include the anti-dysrhythmic amiodarone[48] and the antianginal perhexiline maleate,[49] which are discussed further in their respective subsections.

Inflammatory and Granulomatous Reactions

Inflammatory responses can be secondaary to hepatocellular injury and necrosis or they can be induced directly by a toxin. Liver damage in this instance can be secondary to inflammation. In general, the degree of inflammatory infiltrate in toxin hepatocellular injury or necrosis tends to be less severe than that seen with similar degrees of liver dysfunction in viral-induced hepatitis. However, the distinction between chemical- and viral-induced hepatitis cannot always be made with reasonable certainty, which leads to controversy in assessing the actual incidence of chemical-induced toxicity and complicates management of individual cases. When drugs and chemicals with intrinsic hepatotoxicity result in hepatocellular injury or necrosis, the inflammatory infiltrate is usually a variable infiltrate consisting primarily of polymorphonuclear leukocytes and less commonly of eosinophils. The inflammatory cells are usually distributed around necrotic cells, which may be in a zonal distribution, and close to the portal areas. A marked portal inflammatory infiltrate may mimic that seen with infectious mononucleosis, cytomegalovirus infections, and hepatitis A and hepatitis C. Many chemicals can give this picture, including phenytoin, carbamazepine, allopurinol, and dapsone.

Non-caseating granulomas may result from exposure to some chemicals. The granulomas are composed of epithelioid histiocytes, giant cells, and other inflammatory cells such as eosinophils and lymphocytes. They are thought to arise from a hypersensitivity reaction to the drug (i.e., they tend to be associated with idiosyncratic-type reactions). The finding of increased numbers of eosinophils in a biopsy bolsters this theory. Increased eosinophils in numbers of sinusoids suggest peripheral eosinophilia. If sought, granulomas may be found in other organs as well. Some examples of drugs associated with this effect include quinidine, sulfonamides, sulfonylurea derivatives, allopurinol, halothane, and hydralazine. In addition, chronic occupational exposure to metals such as copper and beryllium can cause this histologic finding. In this setting other etiologies for non-caseating granulomas such as sarcoidosis, fungal and Q fever infections, and foreign material must be ruled out before the finding can be ascribed to a chemical.

Cholestasis

Cholestasis is defined as impairment of bile flow. Clinically, this may be associated with scleral icterus, jaundice, dark urine, pale stools, and pruritus. Biochemically, this is manifested by elevations in the serum bilirubin, which may be primarily conjugated, unconjugated, or a mixture of the two depending on the site of impairment. Other biochemical abnormalities include elevated alkaline phosphatase (ALP) and gamma-glutamyl transferase (GGT). Histologically, cholestasis is characterized by retained bile, as manifested by bile plugs or casts in the bile canaliculi. Cholestatic injury may occur in a seemingly pure form with no parenchymal damage evident or it may be accompanied by parenchymal injury. Several subtypes of injury have been described.

In pure or bland cholestasis, which is also referred to as canalicular cholestasis, ALT is normal or minimally elevated and histologically there is no evidence of hepatocellular damage or inflammation. Bile casts are evident. The prototypical drugs that cause this picture are anabolic and contraceptive steroids. Recovery from this type of injury is usually prompt and complete after discontinuation of the offending agent.

In cholestatic hepatitis, which is also referred to as hepatocanalicular, hypersensitivity, or cholangiolitic cholestasis, there is evidence of hepatocellular necrosis (acidophil bodies) and portal and lobular inflammation in addition to the cholestasis. Clinically, patients tend to experience systemic symptoms in addition to the symptoms of cholestasis. These include fever, rash, and arthralgias. Significant elevations of ALT and AST occur with the typical biochemical changes of cholestasis. The injury that occurs with chlorpromazine and erythromycin estolate typifies cholestatic hepatitis. Recovery is usual with withdrawal of the offending agent, although in instances of more severe ductular injury (i.e., ductopenic cholestasis), the disease may follow a prolonged course. Jaundice tends to be more severe and systemic symptoms such as fever, malaise, and abdominal pain may occur, often raising the question of bacterial ascending cholangitis. Flucloxacillin can cause cholestasis with bile duct injury that can progress to the more chronic form of cholestasis, referred to as *vanishing bile duct syndrome.*

Chronic cholestasis in the setting of chemical exposure is defined as persistent liver abnormalities for more than 3 months after exposure (and withdrawal) of the agent. Vanishing bile duct syndrome is a form of chronic cholestasis that results from the destruction of small intrahepatic bile ducts. The clinical presentation and laboratory abnormalities mirror those seen with primary biliary cirrhosis, with the exception that anti-mitochondrial antibodies are absent. Although jaundice may be present early in the clinical course after exposure to the drug or chemical, this may disappear. Subsequent clinical and laboratory features may include pruritus, xanthelasma, and hypercholesterolemia. The liver biopsy is notable for the absence or paucity of intralobular bile ducts and portal fibrosis. In addition to flucloxacillin, anti-psychotics including chlorpromazine, haloperidol, and carbamazepine have been implicated in causing this syndrome (Table 27-5). Environmental toxins such as alpha-naphthylisothiocyanate and 4,4′-diaminodiphenylmethane may also result in vanishing duct syndrome. The latter agent is a hardener used in the plastics industry and caused the epidemic of jaundice in Epping, Essex, Great Britain (i.e., Epping jaundice), when a batch of flour became contaminated with this chemical.[50,51]

Another form of chronic cholestasis is sclerosing cholangitis. This is also referred to as biliary sclerosis or cholangiosclerotic (septal) cholestasis. Histologically and at endoscopic retrograde cholangiography, this condition is identical to primary sclerosing cholangitis and can be produced by intraarterial infusion of the anti-neoplastic agent 5-fluorodeoxyuridine. Presumably, biliary strictures result from ischemic injury to the large intra- and extrahepatic bile ducts caused by disruption of their fragile blood supply by chemical arteritis. Other agents that can cause sclerosing cholangitis include 2 percent formaldehyde and 20 percent sodium chloride when they are injected into lesions in hydatid disease. These agents presumably directly injure adjacent bile ducts.

TABLE 27-5

Drugs and Environmental Toxins Implicated in the Causation of Vanishing Bile Duct Syndrome

Drugs
Ajmaline
Carbamazepine
Chlorpromazepine
Chlorpropamide
Co-trimoxazole
Cyproheptadine
Flucloxacillin
Haloperidol
Thiabendazole
Tolbutamide
Tricyclic anti-depressants
Environmental Toxins
4,4′-diaminodiphenylmethane
Alpha-naphthylisothiocyanate

Vascular Disorders

The primary target of a drug- or toxin-induced liver injury can be one or more of the components of the hepatic vasculature. Examples of this type of injury include hepatic vein thrombosis, VOD, portal vein thrombosis, non-cirrhotic portal hypertension, peliosis hepatis, nodular regenerative hyperplasia, sinusoidal dilation, or prolapse of hepatocytes into the central veins and hepatoportal sclerosis.

Hepatic vein thrombosis refers to occlusion of a large hepatic vein as occurs in Budd-Chiari syndrome. Drugs that cause this thrombosis are thought to promote a procoagulant state. Oral contraceptive agents (primarily estrogens) have been strongly linked to the occurrence of hepatic vein thrombosis.

In drug- or toxin-induced VOD the agent causes endothelial damage, which in turn causes secondary thrombosis. Examples of causative chemicals include the pyrrolidizine alkaloids such as those found in the plant genera *Senecio* and *Crotalaria.* These plants are used to make "bush tea" in various parts of the world. Other examples are azathioprine, 6-mercaptopurine, and several alkylating agents that are used in cancer chemotherapy. The characteristic lesion is zone 3 congestion with hemorrhage into the hepatic cell plates and hepatocyte necrosis. Clinically, the patient may have an acute, subacute, or chronic syndrome of hepatic dysfunction with hepatosplenomegaly, ascites, and other complications of cirrhosis and portal hypertension. As a drug- or chemical-induced complication, portal vein thrombosis is rare. It tends to occur in the setting of increased coagulation tendencies that occur with use of the sex steroids.

Non-cirrhotic portal hypertension can result from the stimulation of perisinusoidal fibrosis. Prototypical examples include exposure to the industrial chemical vinyl chloride (monomer form), the anti-metabolite immunosuppressive azathioprine, and the radiocontrast agent thorium dioxide. The clinical features are those of the complications of portal hypertension. Hepatoportal sclerosis, histologically characterized by the presence of primarily portal fibrosis and focal occlusive lesions in medium-sized intrahepatic veins, is seen rarely with the use of azathioprine. In addition, it occurs with inorganic arsenic poisoning, thorium dioxide, oral contraceptives, methotrexate, and vitamin A.

In peliosis hepatis the toxic agent presumably targets the sinusoidal endothelial cell. This results in destruction of the sinusoids with development of blood-filled lakes or lacunae and associated hepatic cell atrophy. When the lacunae are in close proximity to the liver capsule, they may rupture with catastrophic consequences. When unrecognized or unsuspected the condition may progress to hepatic failure. The drugs or chemicals associated with this complication include anabolic steroids, danazol, diethylstilbestrol, tamoxifen, estrogens, glucocorticoids, thorium dioxide, hypervitaminosis A, and a variety of anti-neoplastic agents. Sinusoidal dilation may represent a mild or early form of peliosis hepatis, which was originally described in areas of hepatic parenchyma close to hepatocellular carcinoma and other hepatic neoplasms. Zone 1 dilation is also seen in patients taking oral contraceptives. Clinical features are rare and include asymptomatic hepatomegaly.

Nodular regenerative hyperplasia is thought to result from obliterative portal venopathy. In many circles it is considered to result from disordered hepatocyte growth or regeneration. It has been described in a variety of disorders including rheumatoid arthritis, diabetes mellitus, lymphoma, inflammatory bowel disease, and after renal transplantation. Grossly, the liver appears cirrhotic; histologically multiple nodules that are not clearly separated from the adjacent hepatic parenchyma by fibrosis are seen. The adjacent parenchyma is compressed. It has been described in association with the use of anabolic and contraceptive steroids, corticosteroids, anti-convulsants, azathioprine, and a few anti-neoplastic drugs. Prolapse of hepatocytes into the central veins has been described with the use of anabolic steroids and is a rare finding.

Hepatic Tumors

Hepatocellular adenomas are benign tumors. They occur primarily in women of childbearing age who use oral contraceptives containing estrogens. Anabolic steroids are rarely associated with this tumor. Histologically, although the parenchymal cells may be indistinguishable from normal hepatocytes, this tumor generally lacks the characteristic cellular components that make up the normal liver. Kupffer cells are usually absent, as are bile ducts, portal veins, and hepatic veins. "Free-floating" hepatic arterioles with no other associated portal structures are a common finding. Some of these tumors may have malignant potential. These lesions may come to attention because of abdominal pain associated with intralesional hemorrhage or rupture but are most often detected during the evaluation of hepatomegaly or unrelated abdominal pain. Focal nodular hyperplasia is a benign proliferative lesion in which all of the cellular components of the liver are represented. It is regarded as a hamartoma produced by a congenital vascular malformation. Pathologically, it is characterized by a central fibrous scar with septae radiating to the periphery that contain numerous bile ductules. The lesion simulates a picture of focal cirrhosis. It is usually found incidentally and has been weakly associated with oral contraceptive use. Rather, oral contraceptives may stimulate growth and increased vascularity, which may in turn give rise to the development of symptoms. Hepatocellular carcinoma, a malignant tumor of hepatocytes, has been associated with the use of oral contraceptives and anabolic steroids. The tumors tend to be well-differentiated and may be of the fibrolamellar variety. Aflatoxin, an environmental carcinogen produced by a fungus, can also cause hepatocellular carcinoma. Aflatoxin, thorium dioxide, and sex steroids have also been implicated in the genesis of cholangiocarcinoma, although a causal relationship is not well established. Angiosarcoma of the liver has been observed in people occupationally exposed to the vinyl chloride monomer. Other drugs or toxins that may be associated with this tumor include thorium dioxide, long-term exposure to inorganic arsenic, patients with psoriasis using Fowler's solution, and androgens. The prognosis is usually poor in patients with this diagnosis.

Pigment Deposition

Lipofuscin shows up as a brown pigment on hematoxylin eosin staining. It is lysosomal in origin and tends to accumulate with aging. It has minimal clinical significance. Some exogenous chemicals can lead to enhanced deposition. These include phenothiazine, phenacetin, aminopyrine, some anti-convulsants, and cascara. Hemosiderin deposits are a nonspecific finding for the most part. When there is hepatocyte death, Kupffer cells engulf and process the remains, a byproduct of which is hemosiderin. Some exposures tend to be associated with more prominent deposition. These include the secondary iron overload seen with alcoholism, especially in the setting of porphyria cutanea tarda, and after exposure to the industrial chemical hexachlorobenzene. The other setting in which there is excessive hemosiderin deposition is hemolysis caused by a drug or chemical. With breakdown of the heme, hemosiderin accumulates in Kupffer cell. Bilirubin may be seen in association with intrahepatic cholestasis. This tends to be more prominent in zone 3. Copper deposits occurring as a consequence of chemical toxicity are rare and may be seen in the setting of a primary biliary cirrhosis-like syndrome that can occur with chlorpromazine. Any cause of prolonged cholestasis can lead to copper deposition. Some drugs and chemicals may themselves be deposited in the liver. Usually this is an incidental finding and has little clinical significance apart from indicating prior exposure. Examples include gold compounds, thorium dioxide, and titanium.

DIAGNOSIS OF CHEMICAL-INDUCED LIVER INJURY

When patients present liver dysfunction or abnormal liver tests, it often requires a high index of suspicion to recognize that this may be the result of exposure to a medication or an environmental toxin. The patient may be a healthy outpatient using one or two medications that were commenced recently or who is exposed to a known environmental toxin. When there are no other risk factors for chronic liver disease the diagnosis is usually easy to make in this setting. Alternatively, the patient may be critically ill and currently in the medical intensive care unit after a prolonged hospital course, during which multiple medications were commenced and various organ failures and infections have further complicated the issue. Determining the actual cause of the liver dysfunction and narrowing the list of suspected drugs is a significant clinical challenge.

The major goals of the clinical evaluation of patients with suspected chemical-induced liver dysfunction are to recognize that this is indeed what is occurring by establishing that there are sufficient criteria to assign a causal relationship to a particular agent. At the same time other causes of acute and chronic liver diseases must be ruled out because, as alluded to previously, chemically induced liver disease can mimic almost all known liver diseases. Information regarding the severity of the liver dysfunction should also be gathered.

Important details to establish in the patient's history include all therapeutic agents used recently and some time ago. The temporal relationship between onset or cessation of the medications and symptoms or laboratory abnormalities should be established. In addition to documenting prescription medications, a list of over-the-counter and herbal remedies and details of their use should be compiled. The patient's symptoms should be categorized. Pruritus and, to a lesser extent, jaundice suggest cholestasis. Confusion, alterations in the sleep-wake cycle, ascites, and evidence of coagulopathy all suggest more advanced or severe liver dysfunction.

Other conditions that could account for the presenting clinical scenario need to be ruled out. These would include risk factors for viral hepatitis and a family history of chronic liver disease such as hemochromatosis, α_1-antitrypsin deficiency, and Wilson's disease. A personal or family history of autoimmune conditions may be suggestive of autoimmune liver disease. A concomitant history of inflammatory bowel disease may suggest primary sclerosing cholangitis. Conditions that result in elevated right-sided venous pressure suggest that hepatic congestion could be contributing to clinical and laboratory abnormalities. The social history should delve into details of alcohol and recreational drug use. The occupational and travel history may suggest an etiology and should be obtained routinely.

The finding of fever or a rash, supported by peripheral eosinophilia, may suggest a drug hypersensitivity reaction. Features that attest to the severity and extent of the impaired liver function such as asterixis, confusion, or the presence of pedal edema or ascites should be sought.

Laboratory tests serve mainly to establish details of extent and severity and exclude other causes of liver disease. The pattern of liver test abnormalities may suggest the type of liver injury and based on previously reported patterns of illness suggest a particular offending agent. There are a few specific tests that identify a small number of adverse drug reactions—including anti-mitochondrial antibody type 6 for iproniazid, ASMA for clometacin, liver-kidney microsomal antibody type 2 for tienilic acid, anti-liver microsomal antibody for dihydralazine, and anti-mitochondrial antibody type 2 for halothane.

Specific syndromes that may be seen with different drugs will be described in the sections dealing with individual drugs and drug categories. Because many drugs that cause idiosyncratic hepatotoxicity may do so via an immune-mediated process, other methods of in vitro diagnosis have been devised. An example is lymphoblastic transformation after challenge with the chemical in question. These tests in general lack specificity and sensitivity and for now remain experimental. In general, drug levels are not important because most drug reactions are not dose-dependent. Exceptions to this rule are acetaminophen and salicylate. Levels of these two drugs provide prognostic information and guidelines for drawing up a plan of therapy.

Liver biopsy is indicated in instances where the diagnosis remains unclear, despite discontinuation of the suspected drug. Liver biopsy is also indicated when clinical and laboratory features suggest advanced liver dysfunction, raising the possibility that emergent liver transplantation may be necessary. Histologic features that suggest a drug or chemical etiology include a zonal distribution of necrosis, microvesicular fatty change, eosinophilic infiltration, destructive bile duct lesions, granulomas, bland cholestasis, and vascular lesions such as peliosis hepatis and VOD.

The initial section of this chapter provided a discourse on causality assessment. This is of critical importance in establishing the diagnosis. This may be straightforward in some instances—as when only one drug is involved with clinical, laboratory, and liver biopsy findings consistent with previously reported reactions caused by the agent in question and resolution after withdrawal of the agent. The situation becomes more complicated when several drugs are in use, baseline information is not known, and the patient has multiple other medical problems that are ongoing. Rechallenge provides one of the strongest lines of evidence that can causally link a chemical to hepatotoxicity. In most clinical settings this is done inadvertently and, barring occurrence of a severe reaction, provides very useful information. If the initial reaction was mild, there are no suitable drug alternatives, and the potential benefits of the drug in question outweigh the risk of a deliberate rechallenge, this may be undertaken with the understanding that significant morbidity and possible mortality may occur. Reference texts on drug hepatotoxicity should be consulted for guidelines before performing deliberate rechallenge. As noted in the previous section, when considering causality "suspicion is more important than proof."[52]

MANAGEMENT

Early recognition is of utmost importance in the management of chemical-induced hepatotoxicity. In this regard, anticipation and proactively seeking evidence for hepatotoxicity in patients who are on medications or are exposed to known hepatotoxins in the work environment are critical. Even when a substance is not known to cause hepatotoxicity, a high index of suspicion needs to be maintained, especially if the temporal relations are appropriate. Another preventive method is avoidance of potentially hepatotoxic drugs in patients who have risk factors for hepatotoxicity. Examples include avoidance of halothane use in patients with a family history of halothane toxicity, avoidance of aspirin in children with febrile illnesses (to prevent Reye's syndrome), and the avoidance of methotrexate in patients with pre-existing liver disease, especially in the setting of alcohol use. In the future it may become possible to profile a person's metabolic capability, especially by determining the make-up of their MFO system. Thus predictions based on known information about the way various chemicals are metabolized can be used to determine which substances will be more likely to cause hepatotoxicity in a given individual. These substances can then be avoided, and alternatives with more suitable metabolic profiles chosen instead.

After a diagnosis of hepatotoxicity is made, the most important step is to discontinue the offending agent. Appropriate supportive care needs to be given based on the type of liver injury or degree of dysfunction. This would include treatment of encephalopathy and ascites in the case of liver failure, in addition to the appropriate work-up for urgent liver transplantation, and treatment of pruritus in severe cholestasis. Supplementation with fat-soluble vitamins is also an integral part of management.

Specific drug treatment is limited in toxicity related to the use of acetaminophen. Although immunosuppressive medications, including corticosteroids, were used primarily for acute hepatitis type of hepatotoxicity, their efficacy for the most part has not been proven. There are a few settings in which the use of corticosteroids may be considered, including the granulomatous hepatitis that can occur with allopurinol- and diclofenac-induced hepatitis. Use in these situations is reasonable if there has been no improvement, or if actual worsening of the toxicity occurs, despite passage of a reasonable interval since the discontinuation of the offending agent.

ANALGESIC, ANTI-INFLAMMATORY, AND MUSCLE RELAXANT DRUGS

Acetaminophen

Historical Perspective

Acetaminophen was first synthesized in the latter part of the nineteenth century, but its clinical utility was not discovered until the 1950s[53] when it was recognized as the active metabolite of phenacetin and acetanilide. At that time its anti-pyretic and analgesic properties were appreciated. It became readily available as an over-the-counter medication in the 1960s. It distinguished itself as being effective as an analgesic and an anti-pyretic without the gastrointestinal side effects of aspirin and the NSAIDs. At therapeutic doses, there are few if any side effects. However, in 1966 two cases were reported in which fatality occurred as a result of large overdose.[54] Additional cases were documented in the late 1960s and early 1970s. Beginning in the early 1970s, initially in Great Britain and subsequently in the United States, acetaminophen became a popular method for attempted suicide. The incidence of this method of attempted suicide has remained high and continues to account for a large fraction of cases of fulminant liver failure.[4,55,56] From data collected from 13 hospitals in the United States in a 2-year period, it was estimated that acetaminophen accounted for 20 percent of all liver transplants for fulminant liver failure.[4] In 1999 approximately 108,000 instances of toxicity in roughly 90,000 individuals, presumed to be caused by acetaminophen, were reported to the Toxic Exposure Surveillance Program of the American Association of Poison Control Centers.[57] Of these, about 61,000 instances were related to the ingestion of acetaminophen alone; about 47,000 represented intake of preparations of acetaminophen in combination with other agents (the most common of which were narcotic agents). A total of 42,254 instances of ingestion were intentional (i.e., with suicidal intent); 62,322 were unintentional; 177 deaths were reported.

Today, acetaminophen is widely available as an over-the-counter medication. In addition, it can be found in various combinations, most notably with narcotic analgesics and aspirin. The ease of acetaminophen availability and the addictive potential of its narcotic combination forms both serve to promote an increased incidence of hepatotoxicity.

The mechanisms of acetaminophen injury were elucidated primarily in the early 1970s. This in turn led to the development and clinical use of hepatoprotective antidotes, of which N-acetylcysteine proved to be the most acceptable. Acetaminophen hepatotoxicity is therefore well understood in no small part because of the frequency of its occurrence. It is unique in that it stands alone as a model of drug-induced hepatotoxicity in which the concepts of drug metabolism and toxicity have translated to pathogenesis and management.

Metabolism and Mechanism of Hepatotoxicity of Acetaminophen

The metabolic pathways and mechanisms of toxicity have been worked out in detail over the past three decades and are well detailed in the literature (Figure 27-2).[58,59] It has been established that acetaminophen must undergo metabolism for hepatotoxicity to occur.

At low doses acetaminophen undergoes conjugation with glucuronic acid or sulphate mediated by the enzymes glucuronyl transferase and sulfotransferase, respectively. These conjugates are water-soluble and readily excreted in the urine. Only small amounts are metabolized by the cytochrome P450 2E1 enzyme (primarily), with smaller contributions from other isoenzymes of the MFO system. This converts the parent compound into the toxic intermediate N-acetyl-p-semiquinone imine (NAPSQI) and subsequently N-acetyl-p-benzoquinone imine (NAPQI). These are highly reactive electrophiles and powerful oxidants. They usually are eliminated first by conjugation of NAPQI with reduced glutathione and subsequent conversion to cysteine and N-acetylcysteine derivatives, which are then excreted in the urine as mercapturic acid.

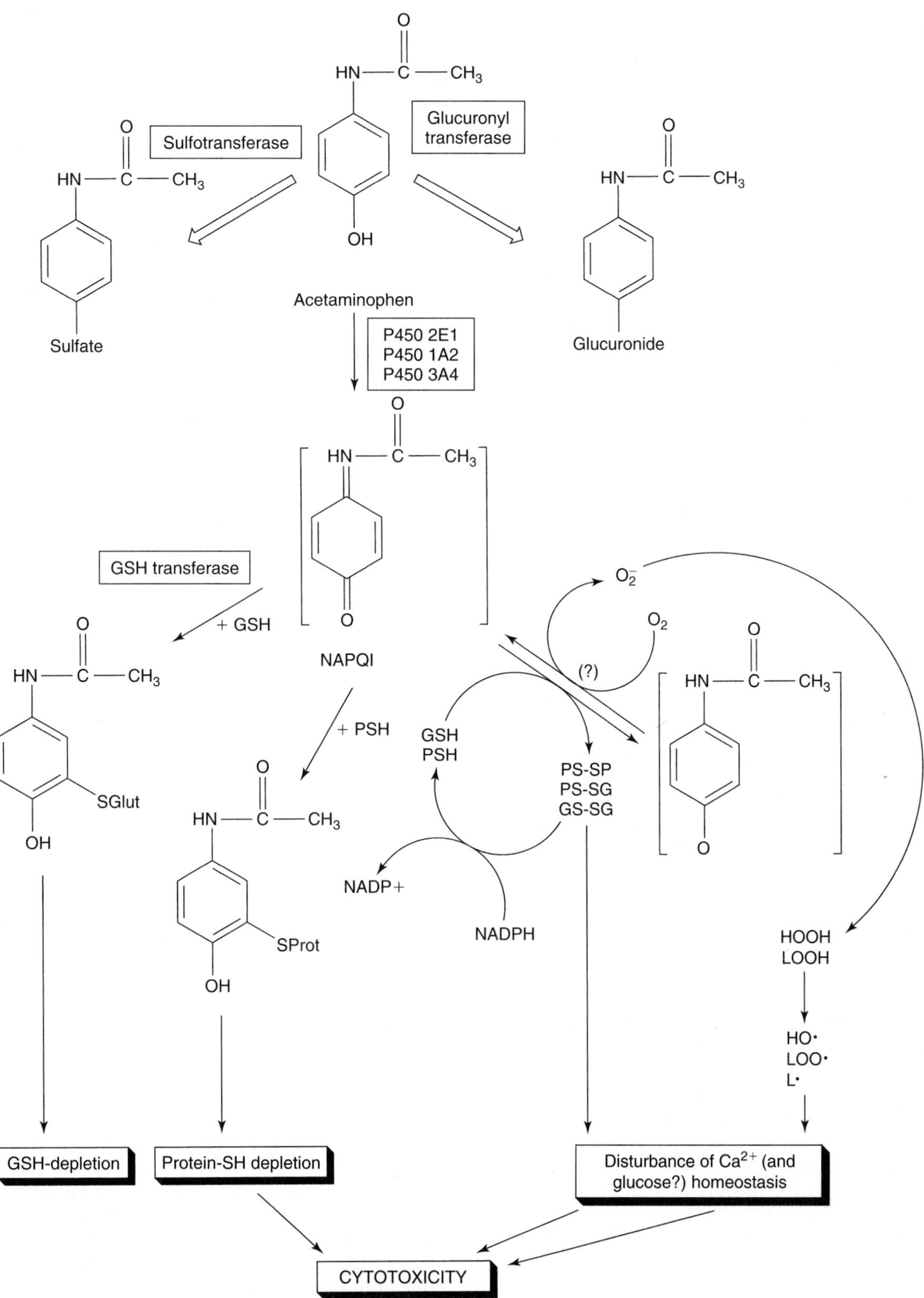

Figure 27-2 Mechanisms of cell injury by acetaminophen. (From Vermeulen NP, Bessems JG, Van de Straat R: Molecular aspects of paracetamol-induced hepatotoxicity and its mechanism-based prevention. Drug Metab Rev 24:367, 1992.)

At higher doses of acetaminophen the initial step in its metabolism—the conjugation with glucuronic acid or sulfate—becomes rapidly saturated. Conjugation is likely limited by depletion of stores in the liver of inorganic sulfate[60] and glucuronic acid.[61] This leaves a larger fraction of the parent compound to be oxidized by cytochrome P450 2E1, 1A2, and 3A4 isoenzymes and results in larger quantities of toxic intermediates (e.g., NAPQI). As noted previously, the elimination of this intermediate requires conjugation with reduced glutathione. Further, it has been established that hepatotoxicity caused by acetaminophen only occurs when there is extensive depletion of glutathione. With higher doses of ingested acetaminophen, the hepatic stores of glutathione become depleted and the rate of synthesis is insufficient to keep up with the demands produced by the toxic intermediates. These reactive species then proceed to inflict both structural and functional disruption on the hepatocyte. This damage appears to occur as a result of two processes, both of which are dependent on the highly electrophilic and oxidative nature of NAPQI. The processes are (1) covalent binding of NAPSQI and NAPQI to various macromolecules in the cell, especially proteins, which are essential for homeostasis, and (2) the production of oxidative stress within the hepatocyte. The latter mechanism involves oxidation of protein and non-protein thiols and lipid peroxidation. The relative importance of these two processes for hepatotoxicity has been the subject of debate. Covalent binding occurs primarily with the sulfhydryl groups of the cysteine moieties of proteins. This binding of NAPQI tends to occur primarily to proteins in the plasma and mitochondrial membranes,[62] although a 58-kd protein in the cytosol is also a target.[63] Studies have documented a correlation between the extent of covalent binding and the histologic and biochemical (level of ALT) extent of liver injury.[64] However, there is evidence that suggests that covalent adduct formation is not the only process that results in hepatotoxicity. The drugs that are most effective in the treatment of acetaminophen toxicity—N-acetylcysteine, cimetidine, and anti-oxidants—do so without significantly affecting the degree of covalent adduct formation.[58,59] In addition, other studies have suggested that there is no or little relationship between covalent binding and hepatotoxicity.[59] This observation has been supported by a few in vitro studies that instead support a major role of oxidative stress and disruption of calcium homeostasis as playing a more central role in injury.[65] However, there are many variables in the clinical setting that cannot be controlled for in vitro. Conversely, NADQI, acting on protein and non-protein thiols (S-thiolation) and pyridine nucleotides, especially in the mitochondria, causes oxidative stress.[58,59] Lipid peroxidation has also been observed but appears to be a consequence of cell death, not a cause of it.[66] Although there are many elegant in vitro models demonstrating the importance of oxidative stress in the hepatotoxicity caused by acetaminophen, its role is more difficult to validate in animal studies.[67]

Disruption of cellular calcium homeostasis appears to be the key event preceding and likely causing cell death. Calcium levels go up precipitously at this stage. This may occur as a result of oxidation of critical thiol groups in the Ca^{2+} adenosine triphosphatase (ATPase) in the plasma membrane—this being the key means by which the cell actively extrudes calcium.[68] Covalent adduct formation has also been associated with inhibition of Ca^{2+} transport.[67] With the increase in intracellular, and thus intranuclear and intramitochondrial Ca^{2+}, there is activation of various Ca^{2+}-dependent proteases, phospholipases, and endonucleases. These produce the terminal damage that results in cell death.[58] Although an inflammatory infiltrate is not a typical histologic finding, cell death will attract the attention of the immune system; white blood cells invading the damaged areas may promote further hepatocyte injury and death by the release of reactive oxygen species.

In addition to the dose, the risk factors for acetaminophen toxicity are summarized in Table 27-6. Hepatotoxicity occurs when the rate of formation of toxic intermediates exceeds the liver's ability to effectively detoxify them by conjugation with glutathione. These risk factors affect the levels of NAPQI by effects on the rates of production or detoxification. Higher doses of drug increase the formation of NAPQI by saturating the conjugating capacity of the liver to detoxify the parent compound. This leaves a larger fraction of the drug available for metabolism by the P450 system of mixed function oxidases. This of course leads to increased formation of NAPQI. The amount taken is not always available, and when it is may be unreliable based on the state of consciousness and motives of the subject and whether of not vomiting occurred. Even when it is reliable, however, it does not always predict outcome because there is variability in the way acetaminophen is metabolized. The rates of glucuronidation and sulfation and the rates of oxidation may vary from individual to individual.[69] A more reliable index of dose is the level of acetaminophen in the serum, making this an important risk factor.

Infants and children are less susceptible to acetaminophen toxicity. This may be related to changes in liver metabolism that occur with age.[70] Greater conjugation ability coupled with reduced formation of NAPQI is presumably the reason for this finding. Women are more likely to present with acetaminophen toxicity than men because they use this as a method of suicide more often. However, when men present, they tend to have more significant hepatotoxicity. This may be related to the higher prevalence of alcoholism in men and the ingestion of higher doses.[55]

Chronic excessive intake of alcohol has been widely recognized as a risk factor for hepatotoxicity.[55,58,59,71,72] Alcoholics are more susceptible to hepatotoxicity and have a poorer prognosis. Alcohol induces the activity of the mixed-function oxidases (primarily P450 2E1) that are responsible for the synthesis of the toxic species NAPQI. Other factors that may contribute to the poorer outcomes include late presentation[55] and depletion of hepatic glutathione resulting from poor nutrition and the direct effect of the metabolism of ethanol.[73] Acute alcohol intoxication can paradoxically have a protective effect in that alcohol competes with acetaminophen for P450 2E1 and thus reduces the formation of NAPQI.[55,58,74]

TABLE 27-6
Factors Affecting Hepatotoxicity as a Result of Acetaminophen

Factor	Effect
Dose	Suicidally intended single dose >10 g in 95% of cases In cases of therapeutic misadventure, the dose is within that accepted as non-toxic (<6 g) in 60% of cases Death unlikely unless >20 g taken The toxic dose in children is usually >150 mg/kg
Sex	Higher incidence of ingestion with suicidal intent in women The prognosis tends to be worse in men
Age	Children are resistant to hepatotoxicity, presumably related to decreased production of NAPQI and greater conjugation
Acetaminophen blood level	Taken within 24 hours, but more so in the period between the 4 and 16 hours after ingestion, remains the best predictor of hepatic injury
Time of presentation	With early presentation (<12 hours after ingestion), hepatotoxicity can be prevented with antidote Most deaths are among late presenters Prognosis is altered only if treatment is instituted early
Hepatic-reduced glutathione stores	Reduced glutathione reacts with NAPQI, detoxifying it Depletion of stores of reduced glutathione reduces detoxifying ability The hepatic stores must fall below 15% before hepatocyte cell death occurs
Nutritional status	Fasting decreases glucuronidation, leading to increased production of NAPQI Fasting may also decrease the hepatic stores of reduced glutathione Obesity may lead to increased toxicity by increasing the activity of P450 2E1, and thus enhance formation of NAPQI
Genetic	Hereditary deficiency of UDP-glucuronosyl transferase in Gilbert's syndrome may increase the risk of hepatotoxicity by decreasing conjugation of the parent compound
Concomitant alcohol and other drugs	Alcohol induces P450 2E1 and, to a lesser extent, 3A4. This leads to enhanced production of NAPQI Alcohol also decreases glutathione stores, probably related to poor nutrition Isoniazid can enhance the activity of P450 2E1 Phenytoin, phenobarbital, and carbamazepine induce 3A4, among other isoforms Zidovudine presumably decreases glucuronidation Cimetidine inhibits P450-mediated metabolism and thus reduces the formation of NAPQI

NAPQI, N-acetyl-p-benzoquinone imine.

Concomitant use of other medications may also affect the metabolism of acetaminophen and thus alter the risk for developing hepatotoxicity. These effects are mediated primarily by the P450 system of enzymes. Anti-convulsants, including phenobarbital, carbamazepine, and phenytoin, and the anti-tuberculosis agent isoniazid[75] all induce the activity of the essential P450 isoenzymes and thus increase the formation of NAPQI. On the other hand, inhibitors of these enzymes confer protective effects. Other agents that reduce hepatotoxicity are described in the following section under the heading "Treatment."

Clinical and Laboratory Findings

Patients present with either an obvious history of ingesting a large single dose of acetaminophen or, in the case of therapeutic misadventure, having taken therapeutic doses at intervals more frequently than approved, often in the presence of other risk factors (e.g., alcohol use). During the first 12 to 24 hours after ingestion of a single large dose, there may be a phase characterized by diaphoresis, nausea, and vomiting. Concurrent sedation in this setting usually indicates that there was co-ingestion of other substances such as alcohol or narcotic agents. These symptoms usually subside and are followed by a so-called latent phase in which there are no clinical or laboratory features. This may last a further 24 to 48 hours, during which time there is a progressive build-up of toxic intermediates and the commencement of hepatic injury that is not as yet clinically or biochemically manifest.

The latent phase ends 72 to 96 hours after ingestion. Acute hepatocellular necrosis is now overt and results in clinical features. These include anorexia, malaise, nausea, vomiting, abdominal pain, and, in more severe cases, progressive jaundice, a tender liver that is often clinically reduced in size, and other manifestations of fulminant liver failure including hepatic encephalopathy and neurologic changes associated with cerebral edema. In this phase of acute injury the serum aminotransferase levels increase dramatically. In alcoholics the serum AST may be disproportionately higher.[71] Levels several hundredfold greater than normal are not unusual.[76] There are variable increases in the serum bilirubin and the prothrombin time. Other hepatocellular proteins including ferritin and glutathione transferases are elevated in the serum. In the acute phase of toxicity the serum ALP and GGT are not elevated (an elevation in the latter may be seen with chronic alcohol ingestion or by induction by anti-convulsants). Elevation in these latter two enzymes tends to occur in the recovery phase when active regeneration is occurring. With more severe toxicity, metabolic acidosis with hypokalemia and hypoglycemia may ensue.[77] Renal failure secondary to acute tubular necrosis may further complicate the clinical course.[74,78] Myocardial toxicity can also occur. Ultrasound or computed tomography (CT) of the liver may reveal a reduction in the size of the liver.

The outcome after the phase of acute injury is complete clinical and histologic recovery in most instances. The symptoms resolve, although there may be transient pruritus. This occurs secondary to the cholestasis that develops during healing. In cases of fulminant liver failure in which liver transplant is not performed, death occurs in 4 to 18 days after ingestion. Prognostic factors for a poor outcome are listed in Table 27-7. Risk is predicted by plotting the serum acetaminophen level against the time of presentation on a semi-logarithmic scale (Figure 27-3).

Hepatotoxic reaction as a therapeutic misadventure usually occurs in subjects taking the drug with therapeutic intent. Many of these patients take therapeutic doses, but over a short period. Sixty percent of the cases take less than 6 g per day, whereas 40 percent take more than 6 g per day. It is estimated that 65 percent imbibe more than 60 g of alcohol per day.[53] The chronic alcohol intake results in induction of the MFO system, resulting in increased levels of NAPQI, and reduced glutathione levels. The reduced glutathione levels occur as a result of malnutrition and fasting as well as inhibitory effects on its synthesis. The typical scenario is the development of pain resulting from another illness. This leads to the escalating intake of acetaminophen. A key that suggests that this is the cause for liver dysfunction in an alcoholic is that the serum AST tends to be elevated out of proportion to the ALT and to a greater degree than would be expected from pure alcoholic liver disease. Metabolic acidosis may also be evident.[79]

Acetaminophen Toxicity Associated with the Treatment of Febrile Infants

There are several reports of acetaminophen toxicity in febrile infants.[53] In most of the reported cases the doses have been excessive. Elevated aminotransferase levels and zone 3 necrosis characterize these cases. Contributing risk factors may include fasting with resultant depletion of reduced glutathione versus other factors yet to be defined.

Histology

Maximal injury is localized in zone 3 of the liver lobule, with massive hepatic necrosis seen in more severe toxicity. There is minimal inflammatory response. Sinusoids of zone 3 are often congested and dilated. The location of maximal injury matches that of the enzymes responsible

TABLE 27-7

Prognostic Factors in Acetaminophen Hepatotoxicity

Factor
Acetaminophen serum level: Based on the level at presentation, can define possible (20%-30% risk) versus probable (60% risk) mortality
Age: Children in general have a better prognosis
Alcohol ingestion: Worsens prognosis for the reasons described in the text
Severity of liver failure • Prothrombin time > 100 seconds • Grade III-IV encephalopathy • Cerebral edema • Serum bilirubin > 200 μmol/L • Hypoglycemia
Co-existing renal failure
Metabolic acidosis (pH < 7.3)
Long interval between ingestion and treatment

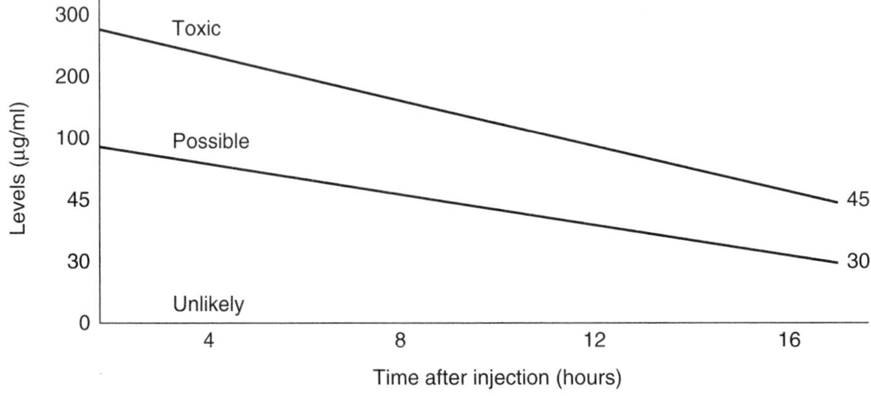

Figure 27-3 Likelihood of liver damage based on acetaminophen level and time after ingestion.

for the production of NAPQI.[53] With recovery, there is complete normalization of the liver histology. There are reports of a chronic form of toxicity seen in subjects taking 2 to 6 g daily for several months to years.[80,81] The histologic changes include low-grade zone 3 necrosis, a chronic inflammatory infiltrate, and fibrosis. In the cases reported there was complete recovery of the liver after cessation of acetaminophen. These cases were reported before the advent of proper testing for hepatitis C, a fact that should be taken into account when considering the reports.

Diagnosis

In obtaining a history from a patient after an acute ingestion it is important to document the time of ingestion, how many tablets were ingested, and the formulation of the tablets. Whether vomiting has occurred and the content of the vomitus must be established. Because the history is often unreliable, objective data such as a report from a knowledgeable third party or pill counts should be performed. Other ingested medications also need to be documented. This is especially important in the case of prescription analgesics, many of which contain acetaminophen in combination with a narcotic. The medication list should be reviewed to exclude drugs that can enhance the hepatotoxicity of acetaminophen. Details of alcohol usage and state of fasting should be elicited. The physical exam tends not to be very helpful early on because it is frequently normal.

The serum acetaminophen level should be determined as quickly as possible. The level should then be plotted on a nomogram that correlates the likelihood of liver damage with the acetaminophen level during the first 24 hours after ingestion. Various nomograms have been developed. Figure 27-3 is a composite created from several nomograms (i.e., Rumack-Mattews, Prescott, and Vale nomograms).[53,76,82,83]

The differential diagnoses of acetaminophen hepatotoxicity are the conditions that cause acute hepatocellular destruction. These include acute viral hepatitis, other forms of drug-induced hepatotoxicity, acute alcoholic hepatitis, and, rarely, autoimmune liver disease. Even if other conditions are suspected, after acetaminophen toxicity is considered a possibility, treatment should be instituted pending confirmation of the diagnosis.

Liver biopsy is rarely required for the management of patients with acetaminophen toxicity. However, in confusing cases, and in situations where emergent liver transplantation is being considered, liver biopsy to look for the typical pattern of acetaminophen-induced damage and to determine the extent of damage should be performed. Because of severe coagulopathy, a transjugular approach is often required.

Treatment

The primary objectives of treatment are to institute measures to prevent further absorption of acetaminophen in cases that present early enough for this to make a difference, to stimulate hepatic synthesis of reduced glutathione to minimize the hepatotoxicity of NAPQI, and, in patients in whom significant damage has already occurred, to provide adequate supportive care to allow recovery or liver transplantation. In patients who present early (within 1 to 3 hours of ingestion), a naso- or orogastric tube should be used to lavage the stomach. Activated charcoal also should be used in an effort to bind drug in the gut lumen.

For the purpose of preventing hepatotoxicity from an overdose of acetaminophen, N-acetylcysteine is the drug of choice and, as alluded to previously, should be administered without delay. This agent has been used extensively since the 1970s and is safe and effective if used within 16 hours of ingestion.[84-88] In the United States N-acetylcysteine is available only in an oral form. In Europe and in many other countries the drug is administered intravenously. When used intravenously, there is precise delivery of the calculated dose. With oral administration, primarily because of the unpleasant taste and smell of the drug, vomiting is frequent (53 percent) and delivery of the dose is not always assured.[88] Otherwise, the major side effects of oral drug used orally are rash and diarrhea. Use of a nasogastric tube or anti-emetic drugs may be necessary. One of the primary concerns with administration of N-acetylcysteine via the intravenous route is the increased incidence of anaphylactoid reactions. These occur with a frequency of 0.2 percent to 20.8 percent.[88] Manifestations may include flushing, rash, tachycardia, angioedema, nausea, vomiting, hypotension, anaphylaxis, and bronchospasm. The incidence is higher with larger doses and presumably is related to the higher serum levels achieved by using the intravenous route. Pretreatment with an anti-histamine may be prudent.

The effectiveness of N-acetylcysteine as an antidote depends on stimulating hepatic production of reduced glutathione. This in turn conjugates NAPQI, and the resultant harmless, water-soluble conjugate is eventually excreted in the urine. To be effective, N-acetylcysteine must be administered at the time of maximal production of NAPQI. This corresponds to the first 12 to 16 hours after ingestion. In the study by Prescott and associates[85] the incidence of significant hepatic damage after early administration (less than 10 hours) of intravenous N-acetylcysteine was estimated at 1.6 percent as compared with 52.6 percent for late administration (more than 10 hours) or 58 percent for no administration. Significant liver damage was defined as ALT > 1000 I.U. The numbers of deaths within each group were 0, 2, and 3, respectively. In the national multi-center study reported by Smilkstein and colleagues in which oral N-acetylcysteine was used, there was severe liver damage in 6 percent of patients treated within 6 hours of ingestion as opposed to 35 percent in those treated between 10 and 24 hours after ingestion. Subsequent studies have demonstrated that, even though the reduction in morbidity is not as striking as when N-acetylcysteine is administered early, administration after 10 or more hours still appears to be beneficial.[89] The improved outcomes are thought to be related to beneficial effects of N-acetylcysteine on the hepatic microcirculation.

The drug is used when the serum acetaminophen level (taken 4 or more hours after ingestion) indicates that the patient is at risk for liver toxicity (probable or possible) based on the nomogram in Figure 27-3. However, regardless of whether a serum level can be obtained expeditiously or not, if there is convincing evidence that the patient ingested a significant amount of acetaminophen (more than 7 g), the drug should be started immediately on an empiric basis, pending the determination of the acetaminophen level. The threshold for institution of treatment should be low in those with other risk factors for acetaminophen hepatotoxicity (see Table 27-6). If the level of acetaminophen is high, N-acetylcysteine can be continued; on the other hand, if the level indicates that the patient is at minimal risk drug can be stopped. In current treatment regimens the initial or loading dose of oral N-acetylcysteine is usually calculated as 140 mg/kg of body weight. Subsequent doses are 70 mg/kg and are administered every 4 hours for a total of 17 doses.[76] Intravenous regimens are variable. Some use a similar dosing and interval schedule as for oral administration. The study by Prescott and colleagues used a loading dose of 150 mg/kg in 200 ml of 5 percent dextrose water, to be infused over 15 minutes, followed by 50 mg/kg in 500 ml over 4 hours, followed by 100 mg/kg in 1 L administered over the following 20 hours. The intravenous preparation is not approved for use in the United States, but the sterile liquid form of the inhalational preparation has been used intravenously when the patient is unable to keep the oral preparation down because of continued vomiting.

Methionine works by a similar mechanism as N-acetylcysteine. It may be used in patients who are clearly allergic to N-acetylcysteine, as can occur in patients with a history of multiple suicide attempts using acetaminophen, who were treated with N-acetylcysteine in the past. Methionine is administered orally, and nausea and vomiting are common.[90] The recommendation is a 2.5 g loading dose and 2.5 g every 4 hours up to a total of 10 g.

Another possible approach to treating acetaminophen hepatotoxicity would be to attempt to reduce the formation of NAPQI by competitively inhibiting cytochrome P450-mediated production. In animal models of acetaminophen toxicity cimetidine has shown promise.[91] The presumed mechanism is inhibition of cytochrome P450, although this is not known with certainty.[92] Although anecdotal reports suggest some benefit in humans,[93,94] there is little objective evidence that cimetidine has benefit. In a prospective study the outcome in 61 patients treated with N-acetylcysteine alone was compared with that obtained with treatment with both N-acetylcysteine and cimetidine in 44 patients.[95] The cimetidine was administered after 8 hours of ingestion and the dose was 300 mg every 6 hours. There was no appreciable difference between the two groups. The effect of larger doses or continuous infusion is unknown.

NSAIDS

Aspirin (Acetylsalicylic Acid)

Aspirin first became available for use in the late 1800s as an anti-pyretic. Although it has been used extensively since as an anti-pyretic, anti-inflammatory, analgesic, and, most recently, as an anti-platelet agent, its ability to cause hepatotoxicity was first recognized in the early 1970s.[96] The primary risk factor for aspirin-induced hepatotoxicity appears to be the dose of the drug and, as a consequence, the serum salicylate levels.[97] Most patients with hepatotoxicity as evidenced by elevated aminotransferase levels are taking 2 to 6 g of aspirin daily and have serum levels of salicylates exceeding 15 mg/dl (usually more than 25 mg/dl), although toxicity has been seen at levels as low as 10 mg/dl.[96] Predisposing conditions have been suggested as being risk factors as well. These include having the connective tissue disorders rheumatoid arthritis, SLE, and juvenile rheumatoid arthritis. However, the increased incidence in this subgroup is probably in large part explained by the higher doses used in treating these conditions rather than an intrinsic susceptibility, although the cytokine milieu in systemic inflammatory diseases may predispose to hepatotoxicity.[98] The same explanations are likely for the increased incidence seen in cases of rheumatic fever. In patients who develop Reye's syndrome aspirin intake appears to be one of—probably the most common—triggers for the development of the characteristic features, namely a microvesicular hepatic steatosis and acute encephalopathy. This occurs in the setting of a febrile illness in children, most commonly induced by a viral infection. The underlying predisposing condition is as yet unclear, but may involve congenital mitochondrial enzyme defects or deficiencies, the effect of which is exacerbated by the use of aspirin.[97,99] In experimental animals, salicylic acid inhibits mitochondrial beta-oxidation of long chain fatty acids[100] and up to one third of children who develop Reye's syndrome have inborn errors of metabolism in this very pathway.[101] The incidence of Reye's syndrome is decreasing, mirroring the decline in use of aspirin for childhood viral illnesses.[97]

Mechanism

In this dose-dependent type of hepatotoxicity the mechanism is likely related to an intrinsic ability to injure the hepatocyte. Based on the ultrastructural histology, the site of injury appears to be the mitochondrion. Other mechanisms that have been postulated include lipid peroxidation, hydroxyl radical scavenging, and injury to the hepatocyte membrane.[97]

Clinical Features and Laboratory Findings

Apart from the features of the disease condition necessitating the use of aspirin, findings are minimal. Tender hepatomegaly may occur. Liver injury is most often recognized by finding elevated serum AST and ALT levels, and, less commonly, ammonia and bilirubin levels. Up to 50 percent of individuals with serum levels of salicylate greater than 15 mg/dl have elevated AST and ALT.[96] Acute liver failure, characterized by coagulation abnormalities and hepatic encephalopathy, is rare.[102]

Histology

The classic histologic description of liver injury from aspirin is a non-specific focal hepatitis. Ballooning degeneration that is more prominent in zone 3 is a typical finding. Hepatocyte necrosis is also seen, and inflammatory cell infiltration is minimal. Steatosis is unusual in the hepatotoxicity associated with high doses of aspirin. However, in Reye's syndrome microvesicular steatosis is the hallmark. There is no conclusive evidence that aspirin can cause chronic hepatitis.

Management

Aspirin overdose is managed by discontinuation of the drug, with supportive care in the rare individual who has severe hepatotoxicity. If aspirin is absolutely essential in the individual's management, restarting at a lower dose after the liver tests have returned to normal may be attempted. Close monitoring of the liver tests in this rechallenge is necessary.

Prognosis

Aspirin hepatotoxicity is rapidly reversible when the drug is discontinued. Case fatalities are very rare but have been reported.[103]

Other NSAIDs

NSAIDs as a class of analgesics are important causative agents of hepatotoxicity. Although the incidence of hepatotoxicity differs for different agents, the overall incidence of overt dysfunction is low (less than 0.1 percent).[97] However, because of the large number of people who use NSAIDs on a regular basis (it is estimated that there are 20 million such subjects in the United States) the actual number of cases that occur is ultimately substantial.[97] There are no large series reported in the United States that can be used to glean the actual incidence of hepatotoxicity caused by NSAIDs. It is estimated, from Medicaid billing data, that acute hepatitis, probably related to NSAID use, results in about 2.2 hospitalizations per 100,000 people.[104] In a retrospective Canadian study looking at 228,392 adult patients who contributed 645,456 person years, the age- and sex-matched risk ratio for hospitalization for acute liver injury related to NSAID use was 1.7, or about 5 episodes per 100 000 patient years.[105] Risk factors for developing hepatotoxicity from NSAIDs include advanced age, renal insufficiency, multiple drug use, and high doses.[106] As noted, the different NSAIDs have different propensities to cause hepatotoxicity. Benoxaprofen proved to be an agent that caused liver injury with a high incidence and fatalities, prompting its withdrawal from medical use. Other agents have minimal potential for hepatotoxicity. NSAIDs that are capable of causing hepatotoxicity are listed in Table 27-8. The most common mechanism of injury appears to be idiosyncratic, probably as a result of metabolic abnormalities, and the most common type of injury appears to be hepatocellular injury. Cross-reactivity between different classes of NSAIDs may occur.[107]

Salicylates Other than Aspirin

Diflunisal (Dolobid). This is a difluorophenyl derivative of salicylic acid that has been reported to cause a cholestatic and mixed hepatocellular type injury.[108,109]

Benorilate. This is an acetaminophen ester of acetylsalicylic acid. Reported toxicity usually has the characteristics of acetaminophen toxicity.[110] The drug itself has very little use clinically.

ACETIC ACID DERIVATIVES

Indomethacin (Indocin)

This is probably the most used NSAID in this particular category. It is an indole derivative of acetic acid. There are relatively few reports of indomethacin-related hepatic injury as compared with other organ toxicities caused by this drug.[97,111] In one series, although indomethacin accounted for relatively fewer instances of hepatotoxicity (compared with other NSAIDS), the incidence of fatalities was higher.[111] Case fatalities have been reported.[111-113] Children may be more susceptible to severe injury and, as such, the drug is not recommended for use in the pediatric age group.[97]

Mechanism

Based on the few case reports available, the mechanism of toxicity appears to be metabolic idiosyncrasy.

Clinical Features

Features are usually non-specific with laboratory values suggesting hepatocellular injury and much less often a mixture with cholestasis.

Histology

Massive hepatocellular necrosis, primarily located centrally,[112] is typical. Microvesicular steatosis and cholestasis may occur.

Management

Discontinuation of the drug and supportive measures should be instituted.

Prognosis

A good outcome is expected with early detection and withdrawal. However, case fatalities have been reported.

Sulindac (Clinoril)

Sulindac is also an indole derivative of acetic acid and therefore has some structural similarities to in-

TABLE 27-8
Non-steroidal Anti-inflammatory Drugs

Class/agent	Type of injury	Proposed mechanism
Salicylates		
Aspirin	Hepatocellular	Toxic
Diflunisal	Cholestatic	Idiosyncratic-metabolic
Benorilate	Hepatocellular	Toxic
Salicylates	Hepatocellular	Toxic
Acetic Acid Derivatives		
Amfenac	Hepatocellular	Idiosyncratic-metabolic
Clometacin	Hepatocellular	Idiosyncratic-metabolic
Diclofenac	Hepatocellular	Idiosyncratic-metabolic
Etodolac	Hepatocellular	Idiosyncratic
Fenclofenac	Hepatocellular	Idiosyncratic-metabolic
Fenclofenamic acid	Hepatocellular	Idiosyncratic-metabolic
Fenclozic acid	Cholestatic	Idiosyncratic-metabolic
Fentiazac	Hepatocellular	Idiosyncratic-metabolic
Indomethacin	Hepatocellular	Idiosyncratic
Isoxepac	Hepatocellular	Idiosyncratic-metabolic
Nabumetone	Cholestatic	Idiosyncratic
Sulindac	Cholestatic	Idiosyncratic-immune
Tolmetin	Hepatocellular	Idiosyncratic
Propionic Acid Derivatives		
Benoxaprofen	Cholestatic	Idiosyncratic-metabolic
Carpofen	Hepatocellular	Idiosyncratic-metabolic
Fenbufen	Hepatocellular	Idiosyncratic-metabolic
Fenoprofen	Hepatocellular/cholestatic	Idiosyncratic
Flurbiprofen	Hepatocellular	Idiosyncratic-metabolic
Ibufenac	Hepatocellular	Idiosyncratic-metabolic
Ibuprofen	Hepatocellular	Idiosyncratic-metabolic
Ketoprofen	Hepatocellular	Idiosyncratic-immune
Naprosyn	Hepatocellular/cholestatic	Idiosyncratic-immune
Oxaprozin	Hepatocellular	Idiosyncratic-immune
Pirprofen	Hepatocellular	Idiosyncratic-metabolic
Fenamates		
Cinchophen	Hepatocellular	Idiosyncratic-metabolic
Glafenine	Hepatocellular	Idiosyncratic-metabolic
Meclofenamic acid	Hepatocellular	Idiosyncratic-metabolic
Mefenamic acid	Hepatocellular	Idiosyncratic-metabolic
Niflumic acid	Hepatocellular	Idiosyncratic-immune
Tolfenamic acid	Hepatocellular	Idiosyncratic-metabolic
Oxicams		
Droxicam	Hepatocellular/cholestatic	Idiosyncratic
Isoxicam	Cholestatic	Idiosyncratic-metabolic
Piroxicam	Hepatocellular/cholestatic	Idiosyncratic
Sudoxicam	Hepatocellular	Idiosyncratic-metabolic

domethacin. There are many reported cases of hepatotoxicity related to this drug, which is a potent analgesic and has relatively fewer gastrointestinal side effects compared with other NSAIDs. However, it is still considered one of the most likely NSAIDs to produce hepatic injury.[97] In an analysis of 91 cases reported to the FDA the ratio of females to males was 3:5.[114]

Mechanism

Based on the reported cases, the mechanism for most cases appeared to be a generalized hypersensitivity reaction (immune mediated), which included liver involvement. Metabolic idiosyncrasy may account for a minor subset.[114]

Clinical Features and Laboratory Findings

Patients present with features of a hypersensitivity reaction including fever, skin rash, pruritus, and tender hepatomegaly. Stevens-Johnson syndrome may occur. The onset is usually within 4 weeks of starting the drug.[115-117] Jaundice may occur in about two thirds of cases.[114] Laboratory tests often reveal significant hepatocellular damage. Eosinophilia tends to be more common when the pattern of injury is cholestatic than when it is primarily hepatocellular.[114] Pancreatitis may occur in some cases.[118]

Histology

Cholestasis is prominent in most cases, with only about 25 percent showing hepatocellular injury.[114]

Management

Withdrawal of the drug and supportive treatment.

Prognosis

Five percent (4 cases of 91) of patients with sulindac-associated jaundice died.[119] Although the cause of death in most cases was attributable to systemic hypersensitivity, death from liver failure secondary to massive hepatocellular necrosis can occur.[114] Rechallenge with the drug may result in the reappearance of the hypersensitivity reaction after only a few doses.[116]

Diclofenac (Voltaren)

Diclofenac is a phenylacetic acid derivative that has been in use for some time. Although the most common manifestation of hepatotoxicity is asymptomatic elevations in the liver tests, there are numerous reports in the literature of significant hepatotoxicity and even fatalities attributable to use of this drug.[120,121] It is estimated that 1 to 5 of 100,000 individuals have significant hepatotoxicity, and the onset is anywhere from 3 weeks to 12 months from commencing the drug.[120,121] Elderly women with osteoarthritis seem to be more susceptible to liver injury.[120]

Mechanism

Data from the reported cases suggest that the cause in most cases is immunologic idiosyncrasy. However, metabolic idiosyncrasy has seemed to be the more logical explanation in other cases.

Clinical Features and Laboratory Abnormalities

Symptoms are non-specific in most cases, with nausea, vomiting, abdominal discomfort, and jaundice being hallmarks of more severe hepatitis. Rash and fever occur in a minority of cases. The liver test abnormalities favor hepatocellular damage. In rare cases the ANA titers may be elevated and care should be taken to rule out autoimmune chronic hepatitis.[121,122]

Histology

Zone 3 or spotty acute hepatocellular necrosis is the most common finding. Other features may include granulomas, cholestasis, hepatic eosinophilia, and chronic hepatitis.

Management

Overdose is managed through withdrawal of the agent and supportive care.

Prognosis

With early withdrawal, prognosis is good, even with severe hepatitis.

Clometacine (Dupéran)

This drug is an isomer of indomethacin. It is an effective analgesic that is used primarily in European countries,[97] where most of the case reports of hepatotoxicity have originated. There appears to be a female preponderance,[123,124] and although there is a wide age range, it is more likely to affect elderly women after a latency period of approximately 6 months.[97] The higher incidence in the older age group may reflect increased exposure or, on the other hand, may lend support to the theory that the drug induces chronic hepatitis, similar to that seen with autoimmune hepatitis.

Mechanism

The mechanism is presumed to be immunologic idiosyncrasy (drug allergy), although intrinsic toxicity has also been implicated in cases of overdose.

Clinical Features and Laboratory Findings

Jaundice, fatigue, and weight loss were the most common symptoms in one series.[124] Less common were edema, ascites, and palmar erythema. Laboratory studies may reveal eosinophilia, thrombocytopenia, and mild renal insufficiency (interstitial nephritis). The liver tests show a pattern more consistent with hepatocellular injury in 75 percent of cases and predominantly cholestasis in 25 percent. There is usually hypergammaglobulinemia. ANAs and ASMAs are present in about 60 percent of cases.[123,124]

Histology

Chronic hepatitis with centrolobular necrosis is common. Increased fibrosis and cirrhosis are not uncommon.[123,124] Granulomatous hepatitis and cholestatic hepatitis have also been reported.[97]

Management

Management is withdrawal of the drug and supportive care.

Prognosis

In most instances there is resolution after withdrawal of the drug. In a series of 30 patients hepatitis was directly implicated in the death of 3 patients. Chronic hepatitis may progress to cirrhosis in some cases.[124]

Other Acetic Acid Derivatives

- Amfenac (Fenazox) can cause abnormal liver tests; however, no cases of significant hepatotoxicity have been reported. The pattern and scenarios of enzyme elevation suggest that the process is primarily hepatocellular and caused by metabolic idiosyncrasy.
- Etodolac (Lodine) can cause borderline elevations in liver tests in up to 15 percent of patients. However, meaningful elevations (more than 3 times the upper limit of normal) occur in fewer than 1 percent of patients (based on the product information). There is one case report of a 67-year-old woman succumbing to fulminant liver failure after taking etodolac for about 4 months.[125] The liver histology at autopsy showed submassive bridging necrosis, early fibrosis, and microvesicular steatosis. Overall, the incidence of significant hepatotoxicity appears to be low and the recommendation for management of cases of mild elevations in liver tests is to discontinue the drug if there is a persistent or increasing trend or if there is any other clinical evidence of liver dysfunction. The presumed mechanism of injury is metabolic idiosyncrasy.
- Tolmetin (Tolectin) is a pyrrol acetic acid derivative that has a low incidence of hepatotoxicity. Cases of jaundice and microvesicular steatosis have been recognized.[97]
- Nabumetone (Relafen) is an acetic acid derivative that has diminished ability to inhibit cyclo-oxygenase 2. It can cause minor elevations in liver tests (hepatocellular). Hyperbilirubinemia has been observed.[97]
- Isoxepac, fenclofenac (Flenac), fenclofenamic acid, fenclozic acid, fentiazac (Fentiazac), and ketorolac (Toradol, Acular) are other acetic acid derivatives that are no longer in clinical use or have a low incidence of significant hepatotoxicity.

PROPIONIC ACID DERIVATIVES

Benoxaprofen (Oraflex)

Benoxaprofen was abruptly withdrawn from clinical use shortly after its introduction because of several reports of fatalities resulting from hepatorenal toxicity, especially in elderly female patients.[126] Onset occurred within 1 to 12 months of initiating therapy.[97] Other reported adverse reactions included photosensitization of the skin, Stevens-Johnson syndrome, and gastrointestinal toxicity.[97]

Mechanism

The exact mechanism is unknown. Although toxicity (not hepatotoxicity) was associated with fatality in overdose,[127] the cause of death in most cases was not related to overdose, suggesting that the method of toxicity is idiosyncratic. The weight of evidence suggests that the mechanism is metabolic idiosyncrasy.[97] The reason for the striking cholestasis may relate to occlusion of the bile canaliculi by deposition of the conjugated metabolites of the parent compound. These accumulate because of impaired metabolism as result of age-related changes in the MFO system. Systemic and renal toxicity secondary to elevated serum levels of either the parent compound or its metabolites is probably the main determinant of poor outcomes[97] rather than liver failure.

Clinical and Laboratory Features

Progressive painless jaundice was the typical manifestation of hepatotoxicity with elevation of the bilirubin and ALP, with less striking increases in the hepatocellular enzymes.[97]

Histology

Histology of benoxaprofen is cholestasis with minimal hepatocellular necrosis.

Management

This drug is no longer in clinical use.

Ibuprofen (Motrin)

Despite its widespread use, there are relatively few case reports of significant hepatotoxicity.[97,128,129] It is a derivative of ibufenac. This latter agent was withdrawn from clinical use after it was noted that up to 30 percent of patients taking therapeutic doses had elevated aminotransferases and 5 percent developed jaundice.[130] Several deaths were reported with use of ibufenac.

Mechanism

The mechanism of hepatotoxicity from ibuprofen is presumed to be idiosyncratic. Some cases suggest immunologic idiosyncrasy with a hypersensitivity type of reaction being characteristic.[97] There is one reported case fatality. The affected patient developed microvesicular steatosis, suggesting that metabolic idiosyncrasy may sometimes play a role.[131] A further report of acute intoxication in the setting of an overdose of ibuprofen suggests a role for intrinsic toxicity (albeit minor, as the degree of injury noted was minimal).[132] There is one case series that reported an apparent interaction of ibuprofen in patients with chronic hepatitis C, wherein the transaminase levels were quite elevated while the patients were taking ibuprofen, but decreased while they were off the drug.[133]

Clinical Features and Laboratory Tests

Tests are those of systemic hypersensitivity. Laboratory tests usually indicate a hepatocellular-type injury, although cholestasis may be the predominant feature in some cases. There is one case report in which treatment with ibuprofen resulted in vanishing bile duct syndrome.[134]

Management

Discontinue the drug and provide supportive treatment.

Prognosis

Prognosis is good. There is a risk of cross-reaction with diclofenac.[120]

Naproxen (Naprosyn, Naprelan, Anaprox DS)

This propionic acid derivative has rarely been implicated in instances of hepatotoxicity.[97,135] Although the mechanism of toxicity is not clearly defined, it is likely idiosyncratic. Fever and hepatic eosinophilia in some reports suggest that hypersensitivity plays a role at least in some cases.[97] Clinical presentations have included hepatocellular jaundice, cholestatic jaundice, and a case with fulminant hepatic failure.[97]

Pirprofen

This agent, in addition to causing abnormal liver tests, can have more serious outcomes. There are cases reported in the literature of fulminant liver failure and at least five patients who have had fatal outcomes.[136,137] The cases presented within 6 weeks to 9 months after commencing the drug. Clinical features included anorexia, nausea, and jaundice. The absence of hypersensitivity manifestations and the presence of centrolobular necrosis with microvesicular steatosis suggest that the mechanism is metabolic idiosyncrasy.[136]

Other Propionic Acid Derivatives

Carpofen, fenbufen, fenoprofen, flurbiprofen, ketoprofen, oxaprozin, and suprofen are the other NSAIDs of note in this category. There are no reports of significant toxicity caused by carprofen, flurbiprofen, and suprofen beyond abnormal liver tests. Fenbufen has been documented to cause elevated liver tests in a significant fraction of patients, presumably by an idiosyncratic reaction.[138] Although ketoprofen has been used fairly extensively, there are relatively few reports of toxicity. One case of fulminant hepatitis was associated with pancreatitis and renal insufficiency. Other cases of acute hepatitis and jaundice have been reported related to its use.[139,140] The incidence of hepatotoxicity of oxaprozin is also low, but a few cases of significant toxicity have been reported.[141]

Fenamates

Cinchophen was once used extensively for the treatment of arthritis and gout. However, because of its propensity for hepatocellular injury, it is now rarely used. The mechanism of injury in most cases was probably metabolic idiosyncrasy.

Glafenine is similar in structure to cinchophen, and as with cinchophen, is no longer in clinical use because of significant hepatotoxicity. Reported deaths from liver failure were mediated by metabolic idiosyncrasy.

Meclofenamic Acid, Mefenamic Acid, Niflumic Acid, and Tolfenamic Acid

These agents appear to be relatively devoid of hepatic side effects, with few reports of significant toxicity.

Oxicams

Piroxicam (Feldene)

Piroxicam is a carboxamide derivative. There have been a number of cases of severe hepatic necrosis fatalities from massive or submassive necrosis and cholestatic jaundice reported in the literature.[97] Patients older than age 60 seem to be most susceptible. The presumed mechanism is immunologic idiosyncrasy. Some cases were reported to have co-existing renal insufficiency.[142]

Sudoxicam

Sudoxicam is similar in structure to, and actually preceded, piroxicam. However, it was withdrawn from clinical use because of excessive hepatotoxicity.

Isoxicam

This is a relatively new drug. There is a single case report of hepatotoxicity, which appeared to be mediated by immunologic idiosyncrasy.[143]

Droxicam

All of the reports and letters regarding hepatotoxicity caused by this drug are from Spain.[144-150] The pattern of injury most commonly described is acute cholestatic hepatitis that is correlated temporally with the commencement of droxicam. The mechanism seems to be idiosyncratic, and some of the reports suggest that toxicity may be immune-mediated.[147] There is one report of chronic autoimmune hepatitis after one episode of hepatotoxicity.[144]

Pyrazolone Derivatives

Phenylbutazone (Butazolidin)

Phenylbutazone was formerly used for the treatment of rheumatoid arthritis and related disorders. At present its use is restricted to veterinary medicine.[97] It was withdrawn from clinical use because of an unacceptably high rate of side effects. Numerous instances of hepatotoxicity have been reported. The preponderance of evidence suggests that the mechanism of injury in most cases was immunologic idiosyncrasy. Toxicity became manifest within 1 to 6 weeks of commencing the drug. In many cases the classic findings of fever, rash, peripheral, and hepatic eosinophilia and granulomas in the liver would suggest a hypersensitivity reaction. Intrinsic toxicity was a probable mechanism in children receiving an overdose of the drug.[151] The predominant type of injury was hepatocellular with prominent cholestasis in a smaller fraction.[97,151] There are no specific interventions to minimize toxicity, and treatment is supportive. The prognosis apparently depended on the morphologic form of injury. The patients with granulomas and prominent cholestasis fared much better than those with predominantly severe hepatocellular necrosis.[97,151]

Aminophenazone, Feprazone, and Oxyphenbutazone

There are few reports, if any, of hepatotoxicity caused by these drugs. The mechanism of injury in these cases seems to be immunologic idiosyncrasy.

Celecoxib

This sulfonamide derivative belongs to a new class of NSAIDs that are selective cyclo-oxygenase 2 inhibitors and that have a reduced incidence of gastrointestinal side effects. Celecoxib is indicated for the treatment of rheumatoid arthritis and osteoarthritis. In analyses of data from trials to evaluate the safety and efficacy of the drug in patients with arthritis, it was found that the incidence of hepatic side effects was much lower with celecoxib as compared with other NSAIDs.[152,153] These data notwithstanding, there are two reports of hypersensitivity-type liver injury occurring, one of which was reminiscent of sulfonamide-type hepatotoxicity.[154,155]

Other Anti-rheumatic Agents

Allopurinol

Allopurinol is widely used to treat gout and hyperuricemia in the setting of cancer chemotherapy. Since its introduction in the 1960s it has been associated with various side effects, most of which are mild and include diarrhea, skin rash, and headache.[156] Significant hepatotoxicity is a rare event. In those few reported cases there seems to be a preponderance of men, although this is probably because gout is more common in men. Patients taking thiazide diuretics and those with renal insufficiency seem to be more susceptible, and there is one case report of possible potentiation by tamoxifen.[157,158]

Mechanism. The mechanism appears to be by immunologic idiosyncrasy, although the reasons for potentiation by thiazides and renal insufficiency are unexplained by this theory. These latter features suggest that the drug levels (or the levels of a metabolite) may have some intrinsic toxicity.

Clinical Features and Laboratory Abnormalities. The onset of toxicity is within 1 to 5 weeks of commencing the drug. Fevers, skin rash, and leukocytosis with eosinophilia are all features that support a hypersensitivity-type reaction.[156] Liver tests indicate hepatocellular injury and elevation of the cholestatic indices.

Histology. Granulomas are common; these are present within the parenchyma as well as in the portal tracts. A case with fibrin-ring granulomas that are typical of Q-fever has been described.[159] Hepatocellular necrosis, primarily in zone 3 (centrolobular), is characteristic. Other findings may include steatosis and infiltration of the parenchyma with neutrophils and eosinophils.[156]

Management. Overdose is managed by withdrawal of the agent and supportive care. Corticosteroids do not seem to have any benefit.[156]

Prognosis. Prognosis is good in most cases after withdrawal of the drug. In patients who died from allopurinol toxicity the cause of death was not usually liver failure (i.e., it is usually the result of a severe systemic reaction), although liver failure has occurred.[156]

Methotrexate

This is a derivative of aminopterin and is a folate antagonist that inhibits dihydrofolate reductase, which causes arrest of rapidly dividing cells in the S-phase of the cell cycle. This property has been used in the treatment of leukemias and, more recently, as a disease-modifying agent in various chronic inflammatory conditions including psoriasis, rheumatoid arthritis, and chronic idiopathic inflammatory bowel disease, among others. Hepatotoxicity has been recognized as a potential major adverse reaction that can occur with long-term use. Case reports describing cirrhosis as a result of methotrexate use first appeared in the 1960s.[160]

Mechanism

The pathogenesis is poorly understood. It has been hypothesized that methotrexate can activate hepatic stellate (Ito) cells, which leads to increased collagen deposition. Others speculate that the drug itself, and its metabolites (polyglutamates), may accumulate, leading to prolonged folate inhibition with resultant impairment of nucleotide and methionine synthesis that in turn lead to hepatocyte injury.[160] Patients with underlying preexisting liver disease seem to be more susceptible to toxicity.[161]

Clinical Features and Laboratory Abnormalities

The factors associated with increased risk of methotrexate toxicity are listed in Table 27-9.

Acute symptoms are rare. With advanced toxicity and cirrhosis, clinical features will reflect these changes and are therefore nonspecific. Minor elevations in liver tests may occur in a significant number (20 percent to 48 percent) of patients taking methotrexate, but this does not necessarily imply significant toxicity.[162] Conversely, liver tests may be normal in the setting of severe fibrosis. With advanced disease, the laboratory findings will reflect the findings associated with cirrhosis and its complications.

Histology

In 1982 the Psoriasis Task Force (Roenigk and colleagues) devised a classification scheme for the liver biopsy findings in methotrexate hepatotoxicity. A revised version is shown in Table 27-10. This is probably the most popular classification scheme, although its main drawback is its subjective nature. Ultrastructural changes precede microscopic changes and include deposition of fibrous tissue in the space of Disse and an increase in the size and number of hepatic stellate (Ito) cells in the perisinusoidal space.[160] Microscopic changes include macrovesicular steatosis; nuclear variability; infiltration with chronic inflammatory cells; focal liver cell necrosis; fibrosis in the perivenular, pericellular, and portal regions; and eventually cirrhosis. Of significance, many of these findings may be a result of other underlying conditions, many of which have been identified as being risk factors for hepatotoxicity.

TABLE 27-9
Risk Factors for Methotrexate Hepatotoxicity

Association	Factor
Strong association	Previous heavy alcohol use
	Pre-existing liver disease
	Daily dosing of methotrexate
Probable association	Duration of treatment with methotrexate > 2 years
	Cumulative dose > 1500 mg
	Prior treatment with arsenicals
	Obesity with diabetes mellitus
Possible association	Maximum weekly dose > 25 mg
	Obesity alone
	Diabetes mellitus alone
	Heterozygous α_1-antitrypsin deficiency
	Felty's syndrome
	Prior treatment with vitamin A
	Concurrent NSAID use
	Concurrent cyclosporine use
	Concurrent PUVA therapy
Negative association	Concurrent folate supplementation
	Concurrent hydroxychloroquine use
No association	Gender
	HLA phenotype
	Extent of psoriasis
	Duration of rheumatoid arthritis
	Corticosteroid therapy

From West SG: Methotrexate hepatotoxicity. Rheum Dis Clin North Am 23:883, 1997.
NSAID, Non-steroidal anti-inflammatory drug; *PUVA,* psoralen plus ultraviolet A; *HLA,* human leukocyte antigen.

Management

There is no antidote for methotrexate. Patients with cirrhosis have required transplantation. Prevention of significant toxicity requires close monitoring of patients on long-term methotrexate. In cases where a pre-existing liver disease is strongly suspected, a baseline liver biopsy should be performed. Thereafter, liver tests should be followed every 4 to 8 weeks for as long as the patient is on methotrexate. Subjects should avoid alcohol and should be placed on folic acid supplements. Patients with diabetes mellitus should be strictly controlled and obese patients strongly advised to lose weight. Patients with no history of liver disease, but who develop abnormal liver tests early after starting methotrexate (within a few months), should have a liver biopsy before continuing with further treatment. Otherwise, when the patient has received a predetermined cumulative dose (the American College of Rheumatology recommends after 1.5 g initially and thereafter every 1 to 1.5 g), liver biopsies should be performed. If the Roenigk classification is used, the findings of Grade IIIb or Grade IV fibrosis are grounds to discontinue the drug.

Prognosis

Prognosis is good with early detection and cessation of methotrexate.

Gold Salts

Gold salts are an old method of treating refractory rheumatoid arthritis. They are still used in difficult cases, although much less frequently. Use of gold salts is associ-

TABLE 27-10
Roenigk Classification of Methotrexate Toxicity

	Fatty infiltration	Nuclear variability	Portal inflammation and necrosis	Fibrosis
Grade I	Mild or none	Mild or none	Mild or none	None
Grade II	Moderate to severe	Moderate to severe	Moderate to severe	None
Grade IIIa	May or may not be present	May or may not be present	May or may not be present	Mild
Grade IIIb	May or may not be present	May or may not be present	May or may not be present	Moderate to severe
Grade IV	May or may not be present	May or may not be present	May or may not be present	Cirrhosis

ated with a 30 percent to 40 percent chance of toxicity, most of which consists of mucocutaneous reactions, with others involving the kidney and bone marrow.[163] Nonetheless, hepatotoxicity resulting from the use of gold is a recognized problem, but many of the cases reported in the literature had liver disease that may have been due to viral hepatitis rather than true toxicity. Two forms of injury are described: a relatively non-inflammatory cholestatic form that occurs within a few weeks of starting the drug[164] and a hepatocellular form that appears to be dose-dependent.[163,165]

Mechanism

Many of the cases of cholestatic injury have features that are in keeping with immunologic-type of idiosyncratic reaction. These include onset within 1 to 4 weeks of commencing the drug, the presence of fever, skin rash, eosinophilia, and elevated immunoglobulin E levels.[163] In the cumulative, dose-dependent hepatocellular form of injury the mechanism appears to be intrinsic toxicity.[163,165]

Clinical Features and Laboratory Findings

Features of a hypersensitivity reaction are present with the cholestatic-type injury. Conversely, hepatotoxicity tends to occur after a cumulative dose of 1.1 to 2.5 g in the hepatocellular-type injury, and clinical and laboratory features reflect the degree of hepatic dysfunction. Case fatalities have been described with the latter type of injury.[166,167]

Histology

In the cholestatic-type injury there is canalicular cholestasis with minimal hepatocellular injury. Conversely, in the predominantly hepatocellular type of injury, there is massive or submassive hepatocellular necrosis, with a mixed inflammatory infiltrate (likely reactive to the primary injury). At an ultrastructural level there are increased gold deposits in lysosomes (so-called autosomes) that are characteristically dense and needle-shaped.[165]

Management

Management of gold salts overdose consists of withdrawal of the agent and supportive care. There is a single case report of a cholestatic injury with concomitant pure red cell aplasia that seemed to respond to prednisone and N-acetylcysteine. This has not been substantiated and may be coincidental.[168]

Prognosis

In the cholestatic-type injury complete recovery occurs in a timely fashion. In the hepatocellular type of injury without liver failure, recovery and regeneration of the liver is a slow process that takes months. To prevent this latter type of injury, monitoring similar to that done with methotrexate seems to be a prudent measure in management of patients on chronic gold therapy.

Opiate Analgesics

Dextropropoxyphene (Propoxyphene, Darvon)

Dextropropoxyphene is an opiate analgesic often available in combination with aspirin or acetaminophen. It is a well-recognized cause of hepatotoxicity, with several reports in the literature suggesting a typical scenario. Hepatotoxicity related to dextropropoxyphene use is probably underdiagnosed because of its similarity in presentation to large duct obstruction.[169]

Mechanism. The mechanism is unknown, but it is not dose-related, and based on the lack of evidence of immune features, it is presumed to be metabolic idiosyncrasy.

Clinical Features and Laboratory Findings. Although some reports suggest that the reaction is more common in women,[170] both men and women with the age range inclusive of young adults and the elderly can be affected. Jaundice, upper abdominal pain, nausea, vomiting, and various constitutional symptoms including fever, chills, and malaise are the typical presenting symptoms, often leading to the incorrect diagnosis of ascending cholangitis.[169,170] Laboratory features usually suggest primarily hepatocellular damage initially, with subsequent elevation in bilirubin levels.[170]

Histology. Histologic changes typically consist of centrolobular cholestasis, portal tract inflammation, and bile duct abnormalities, all features reminiscent of large bile duct obstruction.[169]

Management. Discontinue the agent.

Prognosis. There is resolution of the clinical and laboratory features within weeks, and certainly within 3 months after discontinuation of the drug. Recurrence has been described with rechallenge.[170]

Buprenorphine

This is a narcotic that is used as a substitution drug in the treatment of heroin addicts. It is known to affect mitochondrial function in animals.[171] When used in therapeutic doses, usually sublingually, the concentrations that enter the general circulation should not be high enough to cause toxicity. However, some addicts have used the agent intravenously. In a setting in which mitochondrial dysfunction may already exist, as in patients with hepatitis C or patients using other drugs that affect mitochondrial function, hepatotoxicity may occur.[172] Hepatocellular-type injury with significant elevations in the ALT and AST may be seen.[172] More severe disease may be associated with jaundice. The toxicity seems easily reversed with discontinuation of intravenous use, and in keeping with the metabolic idiosyncrasy theory of mechanism, cases rechallenged with sublingual (low-dose) buprenorphine do not seem to have recurrent toxicity.[172]

Muscle Relaxants

Dantrolene Sodium

Dantrolene sodium is a hydantoin derivative that is a long-acting skeletal muscle relaxant. The drug is used to control muscle spasticity in patients with various neurologic disorders. In one series of 1044 patients 19 (1.8 percent) developed hepatotoxicity when monitored for at least 60 days, and 3 died presumably as a result of the toxicity, although this was not stated explicitly.[173] The patients in this series, plus an additional 31 cases reported to the FDA, were reviewed and were all older than age 30 and on the drug for at least 2 months. Most of the reactions were seen between 1 and 6 months of therapy. Higher daily doses (more than 300 mg per day) were associated with a higher incidence of toxicity and fatality. A case fatality rate of 28 percent was reported.[173] Other reports have not substantiated the dose relationship, with toxicity noted with lower doses.[174]

Mechanism. The reaction is idiosyncratic, with most of the features suggesting a metabolic mechanism.[173,174]

Clinical Features and Laboratory Findings. In a significant number of cases the hepatotoxicity is asymptomatic[173,174] and there may be extensive liver damage with minimal symptoms.[174] Otherwise the symptoms are non-specific and reminiscent of those seen with acute or chronic hepatitis—anorexia, malaise, lethargy, and jaundice.[174] Laboratory findings suggest a mixture of hepatocellular injury and cholestasis.

Histology. Chronic hepatitis was the most common finding in one series. Other patterns noted were varying degrees of necrosis, acute hepatocellular injury, and varying degrees of non-specific portal inflammation.[173]

Management. Management consists of discontinuing the agent.

Prognosis. There is a high case fatality rate, as noted. Monitoring for liver test abnormalities and early cessation of the drug seem prudent.

Chlorzoxazone

This muscle relaxant has both a local and central effect in producing its effects. There have been several reports of hepatotoxicity.[175,176] The injury appears to be hepatocellular, but beyond this, there is minimal information to infer a mechanism of toxicity.

HERBS AND BOTANICALS

Although herbs and botanical products have been a mainstay in the treatment of medical conditions worldwide for centuries, they are marketed in the United States as nutritional supplements that boost organ health and strengthen the immune system. Because these products are not marketed as drugs, they do not come under the purview of the FDA and are not subject to the rigorous testing for efficacy, side effects, and uniformity of composition that therapeutic drugs must pass before they are approved for clinical use. Their use is ubiquitous and often not reported to physicians. Some $5.4 billion was spent on botanicals alone in 1997.[177] Although the characteristics of toxicity for a few of these products have been well characterized, for most this remains to be realized. Confounding factors in this process include that many users simply stop using the substance when an ill effect is perceived. In addition, because of the lack of standardization in the preparation and distribution of these substances, the preparation ingested is often impure, and may contain other chemicals. Storage is often improper, and decomposition may lead to the production of toxic species. Often, when patients present with a clinical picture suggesting hepatic injury, they will not volunteer details about their use of over-the-counter drugs or herbal remedies—this information must be specifically sought.[178]

Pyrrolizidine Alkaloids

Toxicity related to these substances, found in more than 350 species of plants, has been well recognized for some time.[178] Toxicity often results from the ingestion of herbal teas containing pyrrolidizines,[178] and is endemic in areas such as Africa where the use of such teas is routine. Species include *Senecio, Crotalaria, Heliotropium,* and *Symphytum.* The major manifestation of liver disease is VOD. This may occur acutely, subacutely, or as a chronic form of liver injury. *Crotalaria* and *Senecio* were the species of plants that caused VOD in Jamaican children in the 1950s.[178] A species of *Senecio* is found in an herb, gordolobo yerba, which is used to make an antitussive tea by Mexican-Americans in Arizona and was the cause of the first reported case of pyrrolizidine toxicity described in the United States of America.[179]

Mechanism

Toxicity is dose-dependent when it occurs, suggesting intrinsic toxicity, possibly caused by metabolic idiosyncrasy. Large doses, ingested over a short period, cause acute disease, whereas smaller doses ingested regularly over a long period cause chronic disease. It is presumed that the pyrrolizidine alkaloid undergoes biotransformation to more toxic metabolites by the MFO system of enzymes. These metabolites may be alkylating agents that in turn mediate the toxic effects.[178]

Clinical Features and Laboratory Findings

In acute VOD abdominal pain associated with distension, ascites, edema, and hepatomegaly commonly occur. The transaminases and bilirubin, primarily conjugated, are usually markedly elevated. In the less acute forms of toxicity the pain and the degree of elevation of the transaminases may not be as spectacular, but the features are otherwise similar.

Histology

Histologic features are typical for VOD, namely nonthrombotic occlusion of the terminal hepatic venules, with central congestion of the sinusoids and centrolobular hepatic necrosis. In the less acute forms there is central fibrosis that leads to bridging between perivenular spaces and, ultimately, cirrhosis.

Management

Discontinuing the agent and supportive care are appropriate. There is no specific antidote.

Prognosis

From 15 percent to 20 percent of acute pyrrolizidine alkaloid toxicity is fatal. Fifty percent recover completely. A significant subfraction of the remainder have a chronic course that culminates in decompensated cirrhosis in about 15 percent.[178]

Chaparral

The leaves of this evergreen desert shrub are used to make teas, salves, or capsules for a variety of ailments including skin conditions, to retard aging, and to facilitate weight loss. It is also thought to have anti-microbial properties. The active ingredient is thought to be nordihydroguaiaretic acid, which is a potent inhibitor of the cyclo-oxygenase and lipoxygenase pathways. Hepatotoxicity as a result of chaparral use is a well-recognized complication.[180,181]

Mechanism of injury

The mechanism of injury is not known, but it is thought to be mediated by the active ingredient nordihydroguaiaretic acid.

Clinical Features and Laboratory Findings

Symptoms of hepatitis, with malaise and jaundice, are common. This occurs anywhere from 3 to 52 weeks after ingestion and resolves in 1 to 17 weeks after discontinuation.[181] The serum aminotransferases and bilirubin are markedly elevated.[180]

Histology

Histology ranges from mild cholangitis and cholestasis to frank hepatocellular necrosis.

Management

Overdose is managed by discontinuing the agent and supportive care.

Prognosis

Patients have progressed to fulminant hepatic failure and cirrhosis requiring liver transplantation.[180] Most patients have complete recovery.

Germander (*Labiatae* Family)

The blossoms of this plant have been used to prepare teas, tablets, and liquors that have been used for relieving fever, abdominal ailments, as a treatment for obesity, as a choleretic, and as an antiseptic.[178] It was used extensively in France in the mid- and late 1980s for treatment of obesity, and it was during this period that the hepatotoxic potential was fully realized,[178] leading to the drug being banned from sale.

Mechanism of Toxicity

The extract from germander is composed of several compounds, including glycosides, flavonoids, and neoclerodane diterperoids. The latter chemicals are thought to be oxidized by the cytochrome P450 mixed-function oxidases to reactive species that are similar to aflatoxins. These, in turn, bind covalently to proteins, leading to depletion of glutathione and protein thiols and subsequent cytoskeletal and plasma membrane disruption.[182,183] Dietary factors may be involved; rats fed with sulfur amino acid–deficient diets appear to be more susceptible to injury.[182] Because the doses used are small, toxicity is not seen universally. Some subjects may be more susceptible by reason of metabolic idiosyncrasy. Others have suggested that an immunoallergic response may be responsible for the findings in some cases, with the target antigen being epoxide hydrolase.[184]

Clinical and Laboratory Features

Most reported patients are middle-aged women, and liver injury was documented on average after 2 months of therapy.[185,186] Non-specific symptoms of acute hepatitis with jaundice and asthenia are common. Marked elevations in the serum aminotransferase and bilirubin levels are seen.[186,187] Cases of chronic cryptogenic cirrhosis have been reported in which the clinical and laboratory evidence of damage were insidious.[188]

Histology

Centrolobular necrosis and portal lymphoplasmacytic infiltrates are seen.

Management

Overdose is managed by discontinuing the agent and with supportive care.

Prognosis

Most cases resolve completely within 2 to 6 months of discontinuation of the agent.

Pennyroyal *(Hedeoma pulegioides, Mentha pulegium)*

These herbs are used to make squaw mint oil and contain pulegone and other monoterpenes found in the mint species.[178] Various preparations are used as abortifacients and to induce menses. In addition they are used to rid household pets of fleas.

Mechanism

Oxidized metabolites of pugelone, metabolized by the cytochrome P450 enzymes, are responsible for the toxicity of these agents. Menthofuran, one of these metabolites, has been shown to bind covalently to various cellular proteins leading to, among other effects, glutathione depletion.[189]

Clinical Features

Clinical features occurred mostly in young women who were using the agent as an abortifacient.[190] Gastrointestinal upset and central nervous system effects, including seizures, develop within 1 to 2 hours of ingestion. Larger doses are associated with more symptoms and 15 ml or more was ingested in fatal cases.[190] Laboratory evidence of hepatocellular injury and renal insufficiency is found within 24 hours of ingestion.

Histology

Centrolobular necrosis is typical.

Management

Management of overdose consists of supportive care. There is one reported patient who had been receiving small doses of the agent, and immediately before presentation took a larger dose (15 ml). N-acetylcysteine was promptly administered and hepatocellular necrosis did not develop.

Prognosis

In the review alluded to previously, 3 of 18 patients died. In those who survived there were no signs of residual liver injury.[190]

Atractylis gummifera and *Callilepsis laureola*

Atractylis gummifera, or glue thistle, has been used as an herbal remedy for various purposes including as an emetic, purgative, diuretic, and anti-pyretic. The gum-like substance secreted by the plant is also used by children as chewing gum. Its hepatotoxic potential is well documented.

Mechanism

Potassium atractylate and gummiferin are two components of the gum that are implicated in its toxicity. They inhibit oxidative phosphorylation and steps in the Krebs' cycle.[178]

Clinical and Laboratory Features

The subjects are usually young children. They present within 24 hours of ingestion with headache, abdominal pain, and vomiting.[178,191] Hepatocellular enzyme elevations are marked. Later, severe hypoglycemia and renal failure ensue.

Histology

Centrolobular and panlobular hepatocellular necrosis are typical histologic findings.

Management

Overdose management consists of supportive care, with close monitoring for hypoglycemia.

Prognosis

Many case fatalities have been reported.

Callilepsis laureola has active ingredients similar to *Atractylis gummifera* and, as such, a similar type of hepatotoxicity may occur.

Jin Bu Huan

Jin bu huan is an herbal remedy extracted from *Lycopodium serratum.* It is a traditional Chinese treatment for insomnia and is also an analgesic. There seem to be distinct syndromes of toxicity: in children acute ingestion leads to life-threatening neurologic and cardiovascular manifestations. Chronic ingestion by adults is associated with hepatitis.

Mechanism

The mechanism of jin bu huan toxicity is not well characterized. Based on the case reports, there is evidence suggestive of immune-related idiosyncrasy, including fever and peripheral and hepatic eosinophilia. Other reports have noted the presence of microvesicular steatosis, the etiology of which is more in keeping with a metabolic idiosyncrasy.[192]

Clinical and Laboratory Features

Acute hepatitis occurred after a mean of 20 weeks (range, 7 to 52 weeks) of jin bu huan ingestion and resolved in six patients within a mean of 8 weeks (range, 2 to 30 weeks).[192] Clinical features included fever, fatigue, nausea, pruritus, abdominal pain, and signs of jaundice and hepatomegaly.[192,193] The laboratory features support a hepatitis like picture.

Histology

Both acute and chronic types of hepatitis, the latter with varying degrees of fibrosis, have been described. As alluded to previously, microvesicular steatosis has also been seen.[192,194,195]

Management and Prognosis

Management is supportive. There is complete resolution in most cases with cessation of the agent. Reducing the dose of the agent has led to resolution of the biochemical changes. Recurrent hepatitis has been described with rechallenge.[192]

Mushroom Poisoning

Most episodes of mushroom poisoning are caused by ingestion of members of the *Amanita* species. Several members of this species, and in particular *Aphalloides*, have an appearance that is very similar to that of edible, non-poisonous mushrooms, which accounts for most of the episodes of poisoning seen.

Mechanism

Amatoxin and phalloidin are the toxins that mediate hepatotoxicity. Phalloidin leads to polymerization of F-actin and G-actin, which in turn causes disruption of the hepatocyte cell membrane.[178] Amatoxin, which is heat-stable and resistant to gastric acidity, inhibits RNA polymerase II, which leads to impaired mRNA synthesis; ultimately, protein synthesis is impaired. This leads to cell necrosis in tissues that have high rates of protein synthesis, such as the liver. The amatoxins are readily absorbed by the intestines, excreted in bile, and subject to enterohepatic circulation, making them ideal hepatotoxins. The dose of toxin per mushroom is variable in different species and within species by season, region, and local conditions, but in general 15 to 20 mushrooms can supply a lethal dose.[178]

Clinical and Laboratory Features

In less severe cases the presenting symptoms are crampy abdominal pain, nausea, vomiting, and watery diarrhea. With ingestion of toxic doses, the first 6 to 24 hours may be devoid of symptoms. In the ensuing 12 to 24 hours severe gastrointestinal upset is the hallmark. This is usually followed by a second latent period. Then, within 48 to 96 hours of ingestion, abnormal liver tests become evident with marked elevations of the aminotransferases, coagulopathy, and jaundice.[178] When liver failure occurs, it is usually fully manifest by the sixth to sixteenth day postingestion. Renal failure and pancreatitis are also common occurrences.

Histology

Varying degrees of hepatocellular necrosis are evident, depending on the severity of the toxicity. Zone 3 (centrilobular) is the primary location of these changes. Steatosis is also common.[196]

Management

The amount of mushrooms ingested provides good prognostic information and should be carefully appraised and documented. Induction of emesis, administration of activated charcoal, and other measures to reduce residual material in the gut should be performed if the patient presents in the appropriate time frame. Supportive measures, including maintaining fluid and electrolyte balance, should be provided. There is no proven role for hemodialysis or charcoal hemoperfusion. Treatment with silymarin, an extract from milk thistle (*Silybum marianum)*, seems to improve outcomes especially when started early, but may be beneficial even after 48 hours.[196,197] High doses of penicillin G also seem to help, possibly by increasing renal excretion by competitive inhibition of resorption.[178,196] Close communication with a poison control center and a liver transplant center should be maintained at all times.

Prognosis

The case fatality rate with ingestion of a potentially toxic dose of mushrooms is high. In the past this was quoted to be as high as 30 percent to 50 percent. More recently, the rates are more in the region of 20 percent to 30 percent.[178] When fulminant hepatic failure occurs, liver transplantation is the treatment of choice. There are reports of chronic liver disease in patients with severe acute episodes of toxicity.[198]

Aflatoxins

Aflatoxins are the metabolites of the fungus *Aspergillus flavus*. This fungus is found commonly in foods, primarily grains and nuts, which are stored for prolonged periods under hot, humid conditions. This is a significant problem in less-developed countries within the boundaries of the tropical latitudes.

Mechanism

Aflatoxin B_1 is the most common aflatoxin contaminant and has been found to be the most hepatotoxic and hepatocarcinogenic.[178] Since the recognition of their hepatotoxic potential initially in poultry and other animals in 1960, aflatoxins have been implicated in the genesis of various forms of liver injury. Acute fatty liver[199] and toxic hepatitis[200] are some of the more acute variants of presentation, whereas cirrhosis and, most importantly, hepatocellular carcinoma are more chronic manifestations. Acute presentations are very rare. Risk factors as inferred from animal studies include malnutrition, young age, alcohol ingestion, protein-deficient diets, and high doses and a long duration of intake of aflatoxins. Some investigators have proposed that concurrent hepatitis B infection provides a synergistic effect on the risk of hepatocellular carcinoma.[201]

Mechanism of Injury

Aflatoxins are metabolized to reactive species by the liver microsomal enzymes. These metabolites bind to guanine residues on deoxyribonucleic acid (DNA). This in turn leads to impairment in the function of RNA polymerase and subsequent inhibition of nuclear RNA formation.[178,202] This process explains many of the acute findings. In many of the cases of hepatocellular carcinoma that are thought to be related to aflatoxin exposure, there is a mutation at codon 249 of the p53 tumor suppressor gene.[178,201,203]

Clinical Features

Acute toxicity in humans is not clearly described. The clinical and laboratory features of hepatocellular carcinoma are described elsewhere (see Chaps. 44 and 45).

Histology

Microvesicular steatosis reminiscent of Reye's syndrome may be seen.[199] There are no specific histologic features of the hepatocellular carcinoma.

Kava (Piper methysticum)

Products containing the herb kava have been marketed to relieve stress, anxiety, tension, insomnia, and premenstrual syndrome. Sales exceeded $30 million in the United States in 2001 as reported by the American Botanical Council.[203a] Recently, Switzerland banned products containing kava, and Germany proposed to do the same when concerns arose about possible liver toxicity. Six cases of liver failure and approximately 25 reports of liver toxicity in Switzerland and Germany led to the ban. On December 19, 2001, the FDA issued a letter to health care professionals asking them to determine whether patients with liver toxicity might have been using kava-containing dietary supplements. Such reporting of side effects resulting from dietary supplements is mandatory in Europe, but voluntary in the United States.

Other Herbs and Botanicals

Direct drug effects and interactions of herbs and botanicals continue to be uncovered as the metabolic effects of these agents become better understood. Two popular agents, *Echinacea* species and St. John's Wort, affect cytochrome P450 3A4. *Echinacea* inhibits CYP3A4 whereas St. John's wort induces CYP3A4. These herbs must be used with caution in patients taking drugs metabolized by CYP3A4 (e.g, cyclosporine, indinavir).

ANESTHETIC AGENTS

It is often difficult to ascribe a causal relationship between hepatotoxicity and the use of anesthetic agents because one of the key requirements in causality assessment is elimination of other potential confounding factors. In the setting of surgery this cannot always be accomplished with reasonable certainty. Other variables that may account for liver dysfunction or injury include liver hypoperfusion that may be related to anesthesia-associated decrease in splanchnic blood flow or to excessive blood loss. In addition, the level of oxygenation of the blood flowing through the liver may have an influence on the way the liver metabolizes halogenated hydrocarbons such as halothane and other related haloalkanes.

The role of halogenated anesthetics in causing hepatotoxicity was validated in a unique report of an anesthesiologist who had had repeated exposures to halothane and had suffered recurrent and progressive liver disease. The recurrences were documented with detailed clinical, biochemical, and histologic findings.[204] It should be noted that with the administration of currently available halogenated hydrocarbon anesthetic agents, the incidence of hepatotoxicity is very low. Ethyl ether, nitrous oxide, and cyclopropane do not appear to be directly injurious to the liver.

Halothane

This is a commonly used anesthetic and produces two distinct syndromes of toxicity. By far the more common of the two is a mild subclinical alteration of the liver tests. The other is a rare but often fatal acute hepatitis.[205-208]

Incidence

The mild form of halothane-induced hepatotoxicity has an incidence of one in four patients.[208] The incidence of the more severe form ranges from 1 in 10,000 to 1 in 35,000 patients undergoing anesthesia; in those undergoing repeated anesthesia, the incidence may approach 7 in 10,000.[206,207,209] A recent review of incidence suggested that the rates were lower than they had been in the past.[210] Most of the patients (10 of 15) had had prior exposures to halothane and many (6 of 10) had unrecognized evidence of hepatotoxicity after the initial exposure. The prognosis of this often-fatal hepatotoxicity is favorably altered by liver transplantation if this can be accomplished in time.[210] The risk of significant hepatotoxicity appears to be higher in female and obese patients.[209] The risk is significantly lower in children and young adults when compared with older individuals.[211]

Mechanism

Hepatic hypoxia may be important in some episodes of toxicity because it is known that most inhaled anesthetics have the potential to decrease hepatic blood flow from both the portal and hepatic arterial sources. In addition, halothane is a potent myocardial depressant that can reduce hepatic oxygen delivery further by decreasing the mean arterial blood pressure.[209] This appears to be an important mechanism in some animal models, but the actual importance in humans is unclear.

As noted, there are two distinct forms of hepatotoxicity associated with exposure to halothane. In the milder forms a metabolic etiology has been proposed based on findings in animal models.[208] Halothane is metabolized primarily by the liver. This metabolism is catalyzed by the CYP2B and CYP2E1 of cytochrome P450 MFO system.[212] In conditions of normal oxygen tension, oxidation is favored. Conversely, in conditions of low oxygen tension reductive metabolism predominates. Both pathways can result in the production of reactive species, which can lead to dysfunction by covalent binding to various molecules, including proteins, and by lipid peroxidation.[206,208]

In the severe form of hepatotoxicity the finding that many of the patients have had prior exposure to halothane and that many exhibit systemic features such as delayed onset of fever, rash, arthralgias, eosinophilia, circulating immune complexes, and autoantibodies to normal tissue components has suggested that this disorder is immunologically mediated. This is supported by various studies.[213-219]

Immune sensitization to halothane-induced antigens is only seen in the setting of halothane hepatitis. It is not seen in patients exposed to halothane who do not develop hepatitis or in those with viral hepatitis who have recently undergone anesthesia with halothane.[208,218] The immune reaction does not seem to be directed against the drug itself; rather, it appears that sensitization occurs as a result of injury and not vice versa.

Many elegant studies have been performed in attempts to elucidate the sequence of events that lead to hepatotoxicity. The halothane-induced antigens are expressed on hepatocytes from livers of rabbits, rats, and mice exposed to halothane; on isolated hepatocytes exposed to halothane in vitro; and liver biopsies from halothane-anesthetized humans.[206,208] Two distinct groups of halothane-induced antigens have been characterized. One group comprises peripherally located membrane proteins and the other comprises integral membrane proteins.[206] The antigens themselves appear to be polypeptides covalently bound to trifluoroacetylated derivatives of halothane.[206,208] Presumably, halothane undergoes metabolism by the cytochrome P450 MFO system of enzymes to produce trifuoroacetylated reactive species that covalently bind to various proteins.[206,208,209] These proteins include endoplasmin Erp99,[220] Erp72,[221] calreticulin,[222] microsomal carboxylesterase,[223,224] cytochrome P450 2E1,[225] and protein disulfide isomerase,[226] among others.[208] These are all peripheral membrane proteins that are abundant and normally reside within the lumen of the endoplasmic reticulum. The adducts are thought to form within this organelle and ultimately are expressed on the plasma membranes of hepatocytes by membrane flow from the endoplasmic reticulum via the secretory pathway.[208] These adducts are found in virtually all halothane-exposed patients and animals; however, they are only recognized as antigens by antibodies found in the sera of patients with severe forms of halothane hepatitis.[208] The trifluoroacetylated proteins expressed on the cell membranes of hepatocytes are recognized as foreign and an immune response is directed against them, resulting in hepatocellular necrosis. The antigens are formed with a half-life of 6 hours and are long-lived.[208] Antibodies specific to halothane-induced antigens are found in up to 70 percent of sera from patients with halothane hepatitis.[206,208] These can be detected by immunoblotting. An additional immunologic mechanism that has been postulated is the generation of autoantibodies (i.e, antibodies to non-trifluoroacetylated epitopes expressed on the same proteins). It is thought that these arise because of loss of T-cell tolerance resulting from the trifluoroacetylation of the same proteins at other sites. These antibodies have been detected in up to 90 percent of patients with halothane hepatitis.[208]

The reason why only a select subfraction of individuals develop halothane hepatotoxicity and others do not is unclear. The initial metabolism to produce trifluoroacetylated species by the cytochrome CYP2E1 is universal. However, there may be individual variations in the levels of the isoenzyme and thus the amount of antigen generated, in the way the antigen is presented to the immune system, in the way the antigen is recognized, or there may be variations in immunologic tolerance.[208] Other factors that may be significant include variations in dose; intra- or postoperative hypoxemia; impairment in splanchnic, hepatic, or lobular blood flow; and concomitant drug administration (and the effect such drugs may have on the expression of the cytochrome isoenzymes). Familial susceptibility factors related to the metabolism of halothane have also been suggested.[227] As is the case with many other diseases in which an immune response is triggered, there is always the possibility that the immune response seen occurs as a result of liver injury and not vice versa.

In summary there are a number of different mechanisms by which liver damage can occur. There is evidence to support many in both animal and human studies. Within an individual, and in the setting of surgery, there are a multitude of potentially interrelating variables that can affect the outcome with respect to hepatotoxicity, and there appears to be interplay between both metabolic and, ultimately, immunologic mechanisms that result in what is eventually seen clinically. This is summarized in Figure 27-4.

Clinical Features and Laboratory Findings

In the milder forms of hepatotoxicity there are usually no symptoms and the presentation is purely subclinical and is manifest only by elevations in the AST and ALT. Symptoms and signs of more severe halothane hepatotoxicity most often appear several days to up to 2 to 3 weeks after exposure.[228] This interval is reduced to a few days when there has been prior exposure to halothane,[229] lending credence to the theory of immunologic idiosyncrasy. The clinical onset often begins with fever and other non-specific signs and symptoms of hepatotoxicity including anorexia, nausea, jaundice, myalgias, and tender hepatomegaly. In more severe cases this is followed by signs of liver failure, including ascites, encephalopathy, and coagulopathy. Laboratory abnormalities in severe cases are notable for marked elevations in the serum aminotransferase levels. With more severe cases, there are increases in the serum bilirubin, ammonia, and prothrombin time.

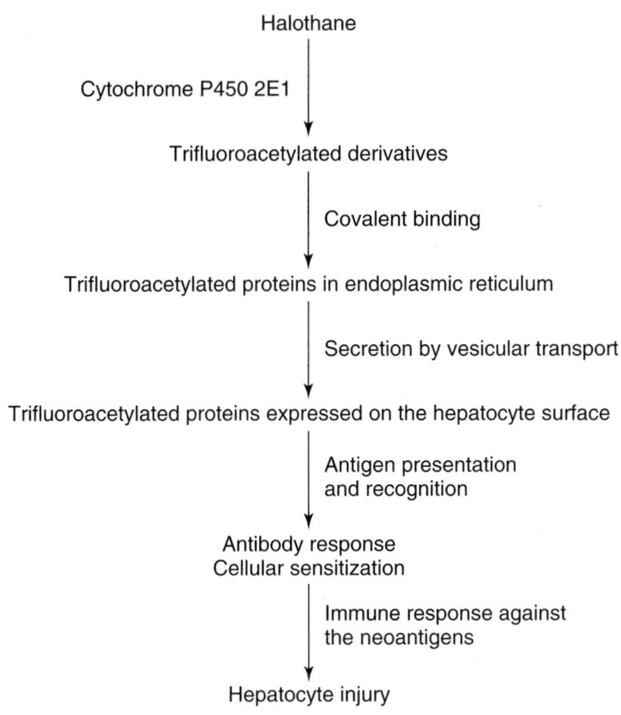

Figure 27-4 Scheme of the possible mechanism of halothane-induced hepatotoxicity based on the available evidence.

Histology

The findings are reminiscent of those seen in cases of severe viral hepatitis. There is focal to massive necrosis depending on the severity, with the centrolobular zones being more affected. In general, evidence of inflammation is sparse. Rarer findings include eosinophilic infiltration and granuloma formation.

Management

The non-specific nature of the clinical, laboratory, and histologic findings caused by halothane hepatitis makes it essential to rule out other causes of liver disease, especially viral hepatitis, medication, or alcohol-induced causes. Other differential diagnoses in the postoperative setting include sepsis, bile duct obstruction, postoperative intrahepatic cholestasis, and hemolysis. Prevention is an important tenet in management. Any patient with a prior history of liver dysfunction thought to be due to halothane, regardless of the severity, should not receive the drug again. Care should be taken to limit the dose of the drug administered, minimize surgical blood loss, and prevent excessive or inadequate oxygenation. In established hepatotoxicity supportive management with evaluation for liver transplantation should be carried out as necessary.

Of note, there is potential cross-reactivity with respect to hepatotoxicity.[230] Most of the reported cases are of hepatotoxicity related to the use of enflurane in patients previously exposed to halothane, although there are reports of cross-reactivity with isoflurane and methoxyflurane as well.[230,231] In a rat model it has been shown that the degree to which protein acetylation occurs is greatest with halothane; this is followed by enflurane, isoflurane, and desflurane, in descending order.[219] This suggests that there may be some similarity in the mechanism of toxicity, which may help explain the differences seen in the incidence of hepatotoxicity and provide a rational explanation for cross-reactivity.

Prognosis

As noted previously, the prognosis is poor in severe cases; however, mortality rates may be improved with liver transplantation.

Methoxyflurane

This inhalation agent causes a type of hepatitis very similar to that caused by halothane. The agent is commonly used in obstetric cases, and some of the case reports have been related to use in these settings.[232] Cases of hepatotoxicity have also been seen in the setting of long-term use of subanesthetic doses.[233] The clinical presentation, laboratory findings, and histology are similar to those seen for halothane hepatotoxicity, and presumably the mechanism of toxicity is the same. Methoxyflurane is metabolized to a greater extent than halothane (50 percent versus 20 percent) and, as such, its potential for causing hepatotoxicity by the presumed mechanism described may be greater. The prognosis in severe cases is poor with a reported mortality of 58 percent.[234] Cross-reactivity with halothane has been described.[235] Methoxyflurane has also been noted to cause nephrotoxicity, which may occur with or without hepatotoxicity.[236] The acute renal failure that occurs appears to be due to renal tubular damage caused by the effects of the fluoride release that occurs with methoxyflurane metabolism.[208]

Enflurane

Enflurane is also a halogenated inhalation anesthetic, and there are many reported cases of hepatotoxicity that are similar in clinical presentation, laboratory abnormalities, and histologic findings to those seen with halothane; the incidence, however, is lower.[208,237] Enflurane is metabolized to a lesser extent than halothane (2 percent to 4 percent as opposed to 20 percent) and this may provide an explanation for this disparity. The mechanism of toxicity is presumed to be the same as for halothane. Reactive species are produced by metabolism via the P450 2E1 isoenzyme. There is evidence in support of the generation of neoantigens by covalent binding and subsequent sensitization of the immune system.[208,219] There are also reports of cross-sensitization between enflurane and halothane.[219,238]

Isoflurane

Although this was questioned initially,[239] there is more convincing evidence now available to suggest that hepatitis and fatalities occur with the use of isoflurane.[240-246]

Overall, however, this appears to be rare. Isoflurane is minimally metabolized, causes a lesser reduction in hepatic blood flow and oxygenation, and is a less effective inducer of heat shock proteins (targets for acetylation and subsequent neoantigen formation) than halothane.[219,247,248] The clinical, laboratory, and histologic features are similar to those of halothane-induced hepatotoxicity and presumably occur by similar mechanisms, although the targets of the immune system may be different.[242] Cross-reactivity with halothane has also been described.[231 249]

Desflurane

This is a newer halogenated inhalation anesthetic agent. It appears to be safe from the point of view of causing hepatotoxicity. There is one case report of possible hepatotoxicity related to its use.[250] Experience is as yet too limited to gauge its true hepatotoxic potential.

Sevoflurane

Sevoflurane is also a newer halogenated inhalation anesthetic agent. It can be metabolized by the cytochrome P450 system of enzymes, but its hepatotoxic potential seems to be minimal.[251] However, there are a few case reports of possible hepatotoxicity, including a likely cross-reactivity with enflurane.[252,253] Experience is as yet too limited to gauge its true hepatotoxic potential.

ANTI-CONVULSANTS

Anti-convulsants are important in the pathogenesis of hepatotoxicity from a number of standpoints. They are potentially hepatotoxic in their own right, but in addition, they are inducers of enzymes that are important in the biotransformation of other drugs. If these drugs are used, they may increase the risk of toxicity from other agents, as in the case of acetaminophen.[254,255] The commonly used anti-convulsants are all known to produce hepatotoxicity and include the hydantoin derivatives such as phenytoin, valproic acid, carbamazepine, and phenobarbital. The toxicities of many of the newer agents are not as well defined but should become more obvious with further use.

Hydantoin Derivatives

Phenytoin

Liver dysfunction has been documented in the setting of long-term use by abnormal liver tests[256] and structural changes.[257-259] Some of these changes may be related to enzyme induction and are not considered to be important clinically. Phenytoin routinely induces a several-fold increase in GGT activity. When this is an isolated finding, it is of no consequence, except in alerting the clinician to the increased potential for drug interactions. A type of chronic hepatitis has been described as well, although this appears to be rare.[260] Acute liver injury is well-documented,[261-266] and prompt recognition and management are critical to the patient's survival.

Mechanism. As alluded to previously, abnormal liver tests, primarily elevations in the GGT and ALP, that may be seen with chronic use may simply represent enzyme induction. The acute cases of hepatic injury appear to be mediated primarily by immunologic mechanisms. Several different lines of evidence support this finding. Clinically, the time between commencing the drug and the onset of hepatotoxicity is remarkably consistent, occurring between 1 and 8 weeks.[267] The clinical features of rash, fever, and lymphadenopathy also support an immune mechanism. Peripheral eosinophilia and eosinophilic infiltrates in liver biopsies and the occasional occurrence of granulomas suggest an immunologic mechanism. Rechallenge almost always leads to prompt recurrence of these findings.[264,268] Lymphoblastic transformation studies in patients recovering from phenytoin toxicity and the demonstration of antibodies against the drug also support a hypersensitivity scenario.[269] There is evidence to support some degree of genetic predisposition to phenytoin hepatotoxicity.[270,271] Phenytoin is metabolized to a dihydrodiol derivative with an arene oxide as an intermediate.[270] This intermediate can covalently bind to sulfhydryl groups and other reducing groups on proteins and other molecules. This binding may in itself produce hepatotoxicity much in the way acetaminophen does, or alternatively the resultant compound may serve as a hapten that induces an immunologic response. The genetic defect in susceptible individuals appears to be a defect in an epoxide hydrolase that detoxifies the arene oxide intermediate.[270] In summary, there are many intriguing possibilities as to the pathogenesis of acute phenytoin hepatotoxicity. The initiating mechanism may vary and genetic predisposition may be an important factor in this regard, but the final manifestations seem to be a result of a hypersensitivity reaction.

Clinical and Laboratory Findings. The onset of hepatotoxicity usually occurs within the first 8 weeks.[268] Fewer than 1 percent of individuals are affected. Symptoms include fever, rash, lymphadenopathy, hepatomegaly, anorexia, and myalgias or arthralgias.[268] The clinical presentation may be confused with infectious mononucleosis or acute viral hepatitis. Physical findings may include tender hepatomegaly, jaundice, and splenomegaly. Rarely, severe hypersensitivity such as that seen with Stevens-Johnson syndrome and toxic epidermal necrolysis is seen.[272,273] The laboratory abnormalities include elevations in peripheral eosinophils, serum aminotransferases, lactic dehydrogenase, ALP, bilirubin, and prothrombin time. The pattern of liver test abnormalities suggests a hepatocellular type of injury. Atypical lymphocytes may be seen on review of the peripheral smear. Agranulocytosis has been reported.[274] Other unusual presentations have included renal dysfunction, rhabdomyolysis, and pseudolymphoma.[267,275] In severe cases signs of progressive liver failure such as encephalopathy ensue, portending a poor prognosis. Often in this setting the pattern of liver injury suggested by the liver tests is poor synthetic function and severe cholestasis.

Histology. A picture reminiscent of acute viral hepatitis characterizes most cases. There is severe hepatocellular damage, primarily in a centrolobular location. A marked inflammatory response is present, with the number of eosinophils being disproportionately increased. Atypical lymphocytes may be seen in the hepatic sinusoids. Granulomatous changes may also be seen.[276]

Management. Immediate cessation of phenytoin is warranted. Otherwise, treatment is largely supportive. Corticosteroids have been employed in a number of instances,[266,277] but there is no convincing evidence that survival or the course of the hepatic lesion is altered in any significant way.[272,278,279]

Prognosis. Early detection and cessation of drug are important, as reversal with no residual disease is the rule. As noted, rechallenge may result in prompt recurrence, often with fatal consequences. If there is any suspicion that phenytoin was possibly the cause of a prior episode of hepatotoxicity, rechallenge should not be attempted. In severe cases, many examples of which are reported in the literature, deaths from hepatic failure may occur. These may have manifestations of Stevens-Johnson syndrome.

Carbamazepine

As with phenytoin, carbamazepine is an aromatic anticonvulsant. This drug is also well documented to cause hepatotoxicity. Although the exact incidence is not known, such injuries may be more common than thought because of misdiagnosis.[280-288] This drug is also instrumental in unleashing the hepatotoxic potential of other drugs by virtue of its enzyme-induction capabilities; interactions with isoniazid, methyldopa, and ritonavir, among others, have been reported.[289-292] There is a case report of possible transient carbamazepine hepatotoxicity developing in a neonate who was exposed prenatally and through breast milk after birth.[293]

Mechanism. Carbamezapine is processed by the cytochrome P450 system to form an arene oxide that is probably detoxified by epoxide hydrolase. It is presumed, based on the similarity of the clinical, laboratory, and histologic findings, that the mechanism of injury is immune related as in the case of phenytoin. The arene (epoxide) intermediate is likely the key substrate in the sequence of reactions. There are reports of tremendous elevations in the serum transaminases with acute administration of high doses of the drug[294]; this suggests that intrinsic toxicity may also occur.

Clinical and Laboratory Findings. Clinical manifestations of hepatotoxicity appear within 1 and 8 weeks of commencing the drug. Fever, rash, lymphadenopathy, and eosinophilia feature prominently. Although the severe exfoliative picture that occurs with phenytoin is less common, it does occur.[286] A case with associated cutaneous pseudolymphoma has been reported.[295] The pattern of injury as revealed by laboratory tests may suggest primarily hepatocellular, cholestatic, or mixed types of injury.

Histology. Histology is variable, with some cases showing changes consistent with predominantly hepatocellular necrosis and inflammation and others showing a more cholestatic picture. Granulomatous changes may also be seen.[281,282,296,297] These latter changes are more commonly in the setting of cholangitis or cholestasis. Cholangitis may lead to vanishing bile duct syndrome.[298]

Management. Management involves withdrawal of the agent and supportive care.

Prognosis. The occurrence of severe reactions with fatalities appears to be much less frequent with carbamazepine than with phenytoin.

Valproic Acid

This drug differs from phenytoin and carbamazepine in structure. It is a branched medium-chain-length fatty acid that is used in the treatment of petit mal epilepsy. As with phenytoin and carbamazepine, however, it is a well-established cause of hepatotoxicity. It commonly causes slight (less than twofold), transient increases in serum transaminases in as many as 44 percent of cases.[299] Elevations occur after 10 to 12 weeks of treatment and appear to be in part dose-related.[300] The exact incidence of overt liver injury is unknown. Children and infants appear to be more susceptible.[301-303] Similarly, case fatalities are highest in the young.[303] Many of the affected children are mentally retarded and the increased incidence in these children is likely a reflection of the increased susceptibility to seizure disorders in this subgroup rather than a risk factor per se. Polytherapy, especially with phenytoin and phenobarbital, appears to increase the risk of hepatotoxicity. Genetic factors may also play a role in susceptibility; there are reports of a familial tendency to developing hepatotoxicity.[304] Based on the proposed mechanisms of injury, it is conceivable that inborn errors of metabolism could play a role in the development of toxicity.[305-307] High serum levels of valproic acid represent an additional risk factor. The risk of hepatotoxicity appears to be highest (1:500) in infants between 0 and 2 years of age who are receiving valproate as part of polytherapy.[301]

Mechanism. There is no clear dose relationship to toxicity, implying that the mechanism of toxicity is not direct. The low incidence and lack of clinical and laboratory evidence in support of an immunologic mechanism suggest that metabolic idiosyncrasy is the primary mediator of toxicity. This is supported by the fact that microvesicular steatosis is the major histologic feature and the time lag to toxicity, often occurring months after commencement of the drug, is too long in most instances to postulate an immune mechanism. Studies have suggested that valproic acid or its metabolites significantly impair mitochondrial oxidation of long-chain fatty acids. In addition, use of valproic acid is associated with decreases in hepatocellular acetyl CoA and serum levels of β-hydroxybutyrate and ketones and impaired urea synthesis and gluconeogenesis.[308-312] The exact mechanism that results in toxicity is not known. The site of primary injury appears to be the mitochondrion. Along with the uncoupling of oxidative phosphorylation, there are various ultrastructural changes that support this notion.[313,314]

One theory suggests that one of the metabolites of valproate metabolism may be the primary mediator of toxicity. Ordinarily, valproate is inactivated by glucuronidation or beta oxidation. Smaller amounts undergo metabolism by the cytochrome P450 system. That toxicity seems to be enhanced by concurrent treatment with phenytoin and phenobarbital suggests that induction of these enzymes may play a role in the production of a toxic intermediate.[309] One of these metabolites, 4-en-valproic acid, is a likely candidate. In vitro studies on cultured hepatocytes suggest that this compound is very toxic.[315] It also induces microvesicular hepatic steatosis in vivo in the rat model.[309] There are reports that levels of 4-en-valproic acid are elevated in cases of toxicity but tend to be low in treated patients with no evidence of hepatotoxicity.[316] High serum levels of 4-en-valproic acid also seem to correlate with some of the risk factors including young age, high serum valproic acid levels, and polypharmacy.[317] In addition, 4-en-valproic acid is a known inhibitor of beta oxidation of fatty acids. It appears to do this by formation of CoA esters,[309,310] that deplete CoA. 4-En-valproic acid also inhibits its own disposal by inhibiting the P450 enzymes and fatty acid beta oxidation.[318] 4-En-valproic acid is similar in structure to hypoglycin A, the agent found in ackee fruit that causes Jamaican vomiting sickness.[310] Another compound with which 4-en-valproic acid shares structural similarities is 4-pentanoic acid, the agent that induces microvesicular steatosis in the rat model of Reye's syndrome. There are cases in which classic toxicity has occurred but levels of 4-en-valproic acid were not elevated.[319]

In summary, the weight of evidence supports the theory that certain predisposing conditions—including the induction of isoenzymes of the cytochrome P450 system—allow the increased formation of toxic intermediates such as 4-en-valproic acid. These intermediates sequestor CoA and impair fatty acid beta oxidation among other processes, resulting in the physical manifestation of microvesicular steatosis. Liver dysfunction and failure ultimately result from pervasive mitochondrial dysfunction.

Clinical and Laboratory Abnormalities. Symptoms may occur anywhere from a few weeks to as long as 2 years after commencing therapy with valproic acid. The majority of cases become manifest between the first and fourth months of therapy.[320] There is often a characteristic course that commences with a prodrome typified by drowsiness, malaise, weakness, and facial edema. There is often loss of seizure control. Fever may be present. Later, anorexia, nausea, vomiting, and weight loss occur and, with progression, symptoms and signs of liver insufficiency and ultimately failure with jaundice, ascites, coagulopathy, and hepatic encephalopathy. The serum transaminases and bilirubin tend to be moderately elevated and there is usually significant prolongation of the prothrombin time and hypofibrinogenemia. Other indices of synthetic function, including serum albumin, are decreased. In advanced cases hypoglycemia and metabolic acidosis may be seen. Elevated serum ammonia with hepatic encephalopathy and ataxia may occur with or without enzymatic evidence of significant hepatotoxicity.[321-323]

In cases that resemble Reye's syndrome there is usually rapid progression, with anorexia, nausea, vomiting, and lethargy followed by fever and the neurologic consequences of cerebral edema. The serum AST and ammonia may be significantly elevated in this setting.[304,324,325] Other complications may include pancreatitis,[326] alopecia, and renal insufficiency.[327]

Histology. As noted, the primary histologic feature is microvesicular steatosis, which is most prominent in zones 2 and 3. Accompanying this is hepatocellular necrosis also occurring in zones 2 and 3. These findings are reminiscent of those seen in Reye's syndrome. However, differences include the presence of bile ductular injury and the degree of necrosis seen tends to be more striking.[328] Congestion and hemorrhage around the central veins may be noted, and there are reports of VOD occurring.[320,328]

Management. Prevention of hepatotoxicity can be attempted by avoiding polytherapy with other anticonvulsants, avoiding excessively high doses, and monitoring liver tests and serum valproate levels, especially during the first 6 months of treatment.[303] Whenever possible, the drug should be avoided in infants younger than 2 years old. Because mild liver test abnormalities are common with valproic acid use, this has to be followed closely after appropriate dose reductions. The drug should be stopped if there is no improvement, worsening of the liver test abnormalities, or if symptoms of anorexia, lethargy, nausea, or vomiting develop. The drug should also be avoided in patients with a known metabolic disorder that can increase the susceptibility to hepatotoxicity, such as ornithine carbamoyl transferase or other urea cycle enzyme deficiency or carnitine deficiency. The drug should also be avoided in cases of known abnormalities in fatty acid metabolism.

Prognosis. With early recognition, withdrawal of the agent and supportive management are sufficient to result in reversal in some cases, although with advanced toxicity, the case-fatality rates are high.[320] Successful treatment with liver transplantation has been described.[329]

Progabide

This anti-convulsant has seen use in Europe, but has not been used in the United States. Abnormal liver tests with use have been noted[330] and one case of severe hepatic failure developing after 4 weeks of use has been reported in the literature.[331] The findings in this case were in keeping with an immune-related mechanism.

Felbamate

This is a relatively new anti-convulsant that has the potential to cause hepatotoxicity. Released for use in the United States in 1993, its use has been curtailed significantly since its potential for causing idiosyncratic aplastic anemia and hepatotoxicity was recognized.[332] Cases of fulminant liver failure have been reported. The risk of hepatotoxicity approximates that seen with valproic acid.[332] Likewise, the susceptibility to hepatotoxicity seems to be increased by concomitant treatment with other anti-convulsants.[333] The mechanism of toxicity is unclear, but appears to involve metabolic idiosyncrasy. A metabolic scheme involving the formation of a reactive aldehyde metabolite from a one of the primary metabolites, a monocarbamate, has been proposed.[334]

ANTI-MICROBIAL AGENTS

Penicillins

Ampicillin

This penicillin is associated with very rare occurrences of hepatotoxicity.[335] In the reported cases the mechanism was probably immunologic idiosyncrasy. There is a case report of Stevens-Johnson syndrome that may have been due to either ampicillin or cephalexin.[336] Another case of chronic cholestasis with paucity of bile ducts and Stevens-Johnson syndrome has been reported.[337]

Amoxicillin and Amoxicillin-Clavulanic Acid

By itself, amoxicillin is a rare cause of hepatotoxicity. There is a recent report of a hypersensitivity type of reaction that presented 3 weeks after a course of amoxicillin with clinical and biochemical manifestations of acute cholestasis. Histology was consistent with acute cholestasis.[338]

Much more common are reports of hepatotoxicity with the amoxicillin-clavulanic acid combination.[339-345] The addition of this β-lactamase inhibitor apparently increases this adverse effect. The frequency of jaundice is estimated to be in about 1:80,000 to 1:100,000 cases.[346,347] Male sex, advanced age, and prolonged treatment may increase the risk of toxicity.[348]

Mechanism. Based on the onset of toxicity within 3 to 6 weeks of starting drug and the occurrence of rash, fever, and other manifestations of a systemic hypersensitivity, the presumed mechanism is immunologic idiosyncrasy.[348] Subtypes of the haplotype human leukocyte antigen (HLA)-DRB1 appear to confer an increased risk of hepatotoxicity.[346,349]

Clinical Manifestations and Laboratory Features. Jaundice is present in almost all cases of amoxicillin toxicity. This may be accompanied by pruritus.[346,347] Other symptoms of cholestasis are also seen. There is often marked elevation in the serum bilirubin and the ALP may be elevated twofold to sevenfold. Serum aminotransferases may be elevated twofold to tenfold.[347]

Histology. The most common injury pattern displays a combination of hepatocellular and cholestatic features. There is perivenular bile stasis, accompanying reactive ceroid-laden macrophages, and portal inflammation with focal injury to interlobular bile ducts.[346] Necrosis is minimal. Granulomatous changes may be seen.[350]

Management. Management is supportive.

Prognosis. Complete recovery occurs within 1 to 4 months after discontinuation of treatment in most cases.[348] The jaundice resolves within 1 to 8 weeks and complete resolution occurs within 16 weeks.[347] Some cases may resolve in a delayed manner. Others may be more severe but complete recovery is usual.[346] Case fatalities are rare, but may occur in the frail and elderly.[346]

Ticarcillin

Ticarcillin by itself is not known to be hepatotoxic. However, in combination with clavulanic acid, it can cause hepatotoxicity similar to amoxicillin-clavulanic acid combinations.

Oxacillin

Oxacillin is a semi-synthetic, penicillinase-resistant penicillin. There have been reports of the development of hepatotoxicity with this agent, especially in the setting of treating staphylococcal infections using high doses intravenously.[351-354] Patients infected with HIV may be more susceptible to oxacillin hepatitis; 80 percent of HIV-positive patients compared with 45 percent of HIV-negative patients develop reversible aminotransferase elevations during treatment with this antibiotic.

Mechanism. That high doses are a frequent coinciding event in patients who develop oxacillin toxicity suggests that the mechanism may be intrinsic toxicity. The time course to the onset of toxicity, often in the range of a week, and lack of clinical evidence to support a systemic hypersensitivity lend support to this theory. However, some patients have been noted to have peripheral eosinophilia,[355] which is more suggestive of a hypersensitivity reaction.[356] The exact mechanism of injury remains unclear.

Clinical and Laboratory Features. After about 1 week (2 to 21 days[356]) of high-dose intravenous therapy with oxacillin, the patient may develop anorexia, nausea, vomiting, and occasionally fever. Many patients are asymptomatic.[351,355] There may be right upper quadrant discomfort and hepatomegaly. The laboratory picture supports a primarily hepatocellular type of injury with serum aminotransferases in the 1000-second range and minimal elevations in the serum bilirubin or ALP.[351]

Histology. In the few patients in whom liver biopsies have been performed, a non-specific hepatitic pattern of injury was noted.

Management. Patients on high-dose oxacillin therapy should have frequent assessments of their liver tests. Immediate withdrawal of the agent and substitution of an alternate penicillinase-resistant penicillin or another antibiotic based on sensitivity assay is warranted.

Prognosis. Complete reversal occurs with withdrawal. The reaction can recur with rechallenge and there is a report of possible cross-reactivity with nafcillin.[357]

Carbenicillin

A clinical, laboratory, and histologic syndrome similar to that encountered with oxacillin can occur with carbenicillin. Rechallenge can lead to recurrence.[358,359]

Flucloxacillin

This is a useful penicillin in the treatment of gram-positive infections. It is known to cause cholestatic hepatitis. The risk, based on a case-controlled study, is estimated to be 7.6 per 100,000 users.[360] Another study reported a similar risk (1 in 15,000).[361] Increasing age (older than 55 years) and prolonged intake (longer than 14 days) are particular risk factors.[361]

Mechanism. The exact mechanism of toxicity is unknown. There are a few clinical indicators to support immunologic idiosyncrasy as the cause. In addition to the time course of onset related to exposure to the drug, the findings of lymphocyte sensitization[362] and tissue eosinophilia[363] in a few cases lend support to this as the likely mechanism. Based on the pattern of injury, the target of the immune response appears to be the biliary epithelium.

Clinical and Laboratory Findings. The onset of symptoms occurs 1 to 3 weeks after initiation of therapy with the drug.[361,364] The usual presenting symptoms are jaundice and pruritus.[361] Laboratory abnormalities suggest a primary cholestatic process. Serum bilirubin and ALP are markedly elevated. Serum aminotransferase levels are elevated to a lesser extent. Although resolution is the most common outcome, some cases may be prolonged and permanent; irreversible damage may result.[365]

Histology. Liver pathology shows centrizonal bile stasis with portal tract inflammation and variable loss of bile ducts.[361] Tissue eosinophilia may be observed.[363] Degenerative changes in the bile duct epithelium may lead to marked bile duct depletion and are correlated with a prolonged recovery period.[365] Secondary biliary cirrhosis may result.

Management. Prevention is an important tenet in management. Hepatotoxicity has been widely reported in Sweden and Australia, but is relatively rare in the United States. This is thought to be primarily related to inappropriate use of the antibiotic; attention to this may be important in reducing the overall incidence of the problem.[361,366] When cholestatic hepatitis does occur, treatment is supportive with appropriate management of pruritus and other problems as they arise.

Prognosis. As noted, most cases resolve completely with supportive therapy. Fatal outcomes have been described, though uncommonly.[361]

Cephalosporins

Hepatotoxicity appears to be an extremely rare occurrence with the use of cephalosporins.[367,368] Given the frequency with which drugs from this class are used, it is safe to assume that the mechanism of toxicity is idiosyncratic. A report of two cases suggests that a hypersensitivity mechanism may play a role in at least some cases.[367] However, reports are so rare, it is conceivable that in some cases metabolic idiosyncrasy may play a role as well.

Erythromycin

This macrolide antibiotic is a well-established cause of cholestatic reactions. The molecule is a large lactone ring with amino and neutral sugars attached by glycosidic bonds. Different preparations have different propensities for hepatotoxicity. Erythromycin estolate is the most commonly hepatotoxic. The other preparations, namely propionate, ethylsuccinate, and stearate, can cause hepatotoxicity, but do so less frequently; cross-reactivity can occur.[369-371] Troleandomycin is a related macrolide that is also a known cause of cholestatic hepatitis. The frequency with which hepatotoxicity occurs has been estimated at 3.6 per 100,000 adult users of all forms of erythromycin, and 2.5 per 100,000 for non-estolate users.[372,373] Children appear to be less susceptible than adults.[374]

Mechanism. The preponderance of evidence supports an immunologic mechanism of injury. There is no apparent dose relationship. The detection of serum antibodies against erythromycin in a patient previously sensitized and subsequently re-exposed to the drug, who developed cholestatic hepatitis, supports immunologic idiosyncrasy.[375] It is known that erythromycin and troleandomycin can induce cytochrome P450 isoenzymes. These isozymes actively demethylate and oxidize macrolides into nitrosoalkanes, which are thought to be reactive intermediates. The reactive intermediates can deplete glutathione and bind to sulfhydryl groups of cysteine in various intracellular proteins, leading to hepatocellular dysfunction. This may be the explanation for the commonly seen elevation in liver tests with use of these drugs. Further, with hepatic cell necrosis, there may be release into the circulation of plasma membrane proteins altered by the covalent binding of metabolites. Such modified liver antigens may be recognized as foreign and may trigger, in an exceptional subject, an immunoallergic type of clinical hepatitis.[376] Other lines of evidence, including disruption of intracellular calcium homeostasis,[377] support a role for direct toxicity.[377,378]

Clinical and Laboratory Features. Symptoms develop between a few days and 3 to 4 weeks after initial intake.[379] With re-exposure, the reaction is characteristically prompt,[370,371] with the development of symptoms often occurring after a single dose. The clinical syndrome may resemble acute cholecystitis or ascending cholangitis, and in some situations, patients presenting with erythromycin-induced hepatotoxicity have been subjected to surgery. Severe right upper quadrant pain associated with fever, anorexia, nausea, and vomiting may precede jaundice and pruritus, thus mimicking ascending cholangitis.[374,379] Hepatotoxicity from these drugs has even been known to cause a false-positive technetium-99m diisopropyl iminodiacetic acid study.[380] Hepatomegaly with hepatic tenderness may be appreciated on physical examination. The laboratory findings may show a mixed picture initially with evidence to support both hepatocellular and cholestatic types of injury, but with time tend more toward a cholestatic pattern. Peripheral eosinophilia may be seen.

Histology. Centrolobular distributed cholestasis and a portal inflammatory cell infiltrate are common. The infiltrate may contain relatively large numbers of eosinophils. Foci of hepatocellular necrosis and acidophil bodies may be seen in the centrolobular areas.

Management. Management is supportive.

Prognosis. After withdrawal (if the patient is still taking the drug) there is spontaneous resolution in most cases. Fatalities have been reported.[381] As noted, readministration of the same or a different preparation of erythromycin may be associated with a prompt and florid reaction.

Fluoroquinolones

Although gastrointestinal events such as nausea and vomiting are the most common adverse effects, mild hepatic reactions are a class effect, usually presenting as mild increases in transaminase levels without clinical symptoms.[382] For norfloxacin, this is estimated to occur in about 0.1 percent of patients receiving the antibiotic. Cases of more severe hepatotoxicity have been described.[383-386] In one of these cases presentation occurred within 12 days of commencing the drug, the serum transaminase levels were markedly elevated, and biopsy was notable for moderate fatty change.[384] This suggests metabolic idiosyncrasy. Another case was notable for eosinophilic necrotizing granulomatous hepatitis,[385] which is more in keeping with a hypersensitivity reaction. Support for an immune-related mechanism is provided by detection of autoantibodies that may form as a result of protein modification by either the quinolone itself or one of its metabolites.[387]

Ciprofloxacin appears to be less likely to cause significant hepatotoxicity, although cases of severe hepatotoxicity and one fatality, occurring within 3 weeks of exposure and with biopsy findings of severe hepatocellular necrosis, have been described.[388,389]

Trovafloxacin has been reported to cause an acute hepatitis that appears to result from immunologic idiosyncrasy.[390-392] The lack of a dose relationship and the presence of tissue and peripheral eosinophilia support this explanation. One case was notable for severe centrolobular necrosis that probably resulted in a veno-occlusive-like presentation with hepatosplenomegaly and ascites.[391]

Tetracyclines

Tetracycline

Tetracycline a relatively old antibiotic that has long been recognized to cause hepatotoxicity, producing a characteristic histologic pattern of microvesicular steatosis.[393-396] It was initially recognized when the drug was used in high doses intravenously. However, it is now well established that hepatotoxicity can also occur with oral administration. High doses and associated high serum levels of the drug are definite risk factors. Women and, in particular, pregnant women, appear to be at high risk for the development of hepatic toxicity with tetracycline use. Children seem to be less susceptible. Renal insufficiency is important from the standpoint of drug excretion. With renal impairment, very high serum levels can result, increasing the risk of toxicity.

Mechanism. Toxicity is dependent on high serum levels and is reproducible.[394,395] Large doses, intravenous administration, and reduced excretion secondary to renal insufficiency can all facilitate the development of high serum levels. Microvesicular steatosis is the principal histologic finding. These features, combined with the paucity of findings suggestive of an ongoing immunologic process, imply that the mechanism of injury is intrinsic toxicity of the drug or one of its metabolites. Studies have established that there is impaired secretion of triglycerides from the liver.[395] Within the hepatocyte, tetracycline appears to accumulate in the mitochondria.[397] Impaired mitochondrial beta oxidation of fatty acids appears to play a role in the pathogenesis of the liver damage.[398,399] The physiologic decline in fatty acid oxidation in late pregnancy may account for the increased susceptibility to tetracycline hepatotoxicity in this group of patients.[400] Tetracycline is also known to impair protein synthesis.[401] Impaired production of the apoprotein of very low-density lipoproteins may lead to decreased egress of triglycerides from the liver.

Clinical and Laboratory Features. Symptoms usually commence within 3 to 7 days of initiating the drug. The syndrome resembles viral hepatitis in its presentation, with non-specific complaints including malaise, anorexia, nausea, vomiting, and upper abdominal discomfort. The discomfort is usually in the right upper quadrant, and the liver may be enlarged and tender. Occasionally pain typical of pancreatitis may occur because this can be a complication. Fever may also be present. With progressive injury, jaundice and features suggestive of liver failure, including encephalopathy, ascites, and complications of coagulopathy, ensue. Laboratory tests reveal moderate elevations in the serum aminotransferase levels and the AST is usually higher that the ALT (indicative of mitochondrial injury). Moderate hyperbilirubinemia is present. With advanced injury, azotemia, metabolic acidosis, hypoglycemia, and a prolonged prothrombin time occur.

Histology. As noted, microvesicular steatosis is marked with the nuclei remaining in a central location within the cell. The pattern is reminiscent of that in Reye's syndrome, fatty liver of pregnancy, hypoglycin toxicity (Jamaican vomiting sickness or ackee poisoning), and valproic acid toxicity. In severe cases the distribution is panlobular. In milder cases zone 1 may be spared. There is minimal inflammation. This finding is characteristic enough; its detection in a patient who develops liver dysfunction while taking tetracycline is strong evidence that tetracycline hepatotoxicity is the culprit. This is in contradistinction to the non-specific findings that are observed in most drug reactions.

Management. Intravenous doses and high doses of the drug in general should be avoided. The drug is contraindicated in pregnancy and should be used very judiciously in patients with renal insufficiency. Discontinuation of the agent and supportive care are otherwise the pillars of care in those who develop hepatotoxicity.

Prognosis. Jaundice is an unfavorable sign and patients who develop this should be monitored closely for acute liver failure and evaluated expeditiously for possible liver transplantation.

Other Tetracyclines

Other tetracyclines such as oxytetracycline, chlortetracycline, minocycline,[402] and demeclocycline can all lead to dose-related microvesicular steatosis. Doxycycline presumably could also cause steatosis, although this has not been reported. In addition to steatosis, minocycline has also been reported to cause a hepatitis that has many features of a hypersensitivity reaction and in other cases, an autoimmune type of hepatitis.[403-410] The hypersensitivity type of reaction appears after a few weeks of use, whereas the lupus-like syndrome may appear in women after a year or more of use (usually for treatment of acne).[407] In the latter cases the histologic picture is chronic hepatitis, and autoimmune serologies including ANA and anti–double-stranded DNA antibody may be positive. Treatment is cessation of the agent and supportive care. Some patients with an autoimmune type of presentation follow a chronic course, and it is unclear whether the drug is causative or merely unmasks a tendency to develop chronic autoimmune hepatitis.

Sulfonamides

Sulfonamides were the first anti-bacterial agents introduced for clinical use in the 1930s. They are well recognized as a cause of acute hepatitis. Hepatotoxicity with features suggestive of hypersensitivity was recognized early. Sulfa drugs that have been implicated include sulfanilamide,[411,412] sulfadimethoxine,[413,414] Azulfidine, sulfamethoxazole, sulfones, sulfamethizole, and sulfamethoxypyridizine. With the sulfonamides that are in current use, the risk of a hypersensitivity reaction appears to be lower that with the older drugs in this class. Co-trimoxazole, a combination of sulfamethoxazole and trimethoprim, has been appreciated as a cause of hepatocellular injury.[415,416] A case fatality occurred after a small dose and presumably represented a rechallenge subsequent to a prior immune sensitization.[416] Patients with AIDS seem to be more susceptible to hypersensitivity reactions.[36] In one series of patients being treated for *Pneumocystis carinii* only 5 of 37 patients started on trimethoprim-sulfamethoxazole were able to complete treatment and, in 19 patients, treatment was changed because of adverse reactions that included rash, fever, neutropenia, thrombocytopenia, and transaminase elevations.[36]

Clinical and Laboratory Features

These are typical for a hypersensitivity type of reaction. Onset occurs within 5 to 14 days of starting the drug. Fever, rash, lymphadenopathy, and eosinophilia are typical, but not universally seen. The liver tests reflect a mixed hepatocellular and cholestatic injury.[417]

Histology

Cholestasis, varying degrees of hepatocellular necrosis, bile duct injury, and a portal tract infiltrate that may contain eosinophils are the usual findings on biopsy.[417]

Management

Early recognition and discontinuation of therapy are the basic steps.

Prognosis

Prognosis is generally good, although fatalities can occur with rechallenge.[416]

Other types of hepatotoxic reactions that have been reported to occur with sulfonamides include granulomatous hepatitis[418] and chronic hepatitis.[419]

Nitrofurantoin

Nitrofurantoin is a known cause of chronic hepatitis.[420] Cases of cholestatic hepatitis and pure cholestasis[421] have also been described; these tend to have a more acute presentation. The drug is used commonly for prophylactic therapy in cases of recurrent urinary tract infections, and this may in part be the reason for the reported higher incidence of hepatotoxicity in women.[422]

Mechanism of Injury

In acute cholestasis, the relatively short interval (about 6 weeks) between first exposure and manifestations of hepatotoxicity and the presence of fever, rash, and eosinophilia, all suggest that the mechanism of injury is hypersensitivity reaction to the drug or one of its metabolites.

With chronic hepatitis induced by nitrofurantoin, the features are reminiscent of those seen in chronic autoimmune hepatitis. The patients have usually been taking the drug for more than 6 months. An autoimmune process is supported by ANA and ASMA in a large proportion of cases.[423] Cell-mediated mechanisms may also play a role.[424]

Clinical Features and Laboratory Abnormalities

In the acute hypersensitivity reaction the onset of clinical manifestations of hepatotoxicity occurs within 6 weeks of commencing the drug. In addition to the features of hypersensitivity noted previously, jaundice is common. The laboratory abnormalities reflect a cholestatic injury with elevations in the serum bilirubin, ALP, and GGT and minimal elevations in the hepatocellular enzymes. In the more chronic form of hepatotoxicity the patients have usually been taking the drug for a longer period and there is elevation of the serum transaminase and gamma globulin levels. As noted, the autoimmune serologies may be positive. Cirrhosis may ensue, with its corresponding clinical complications.[422,425-428] Pulmonary toxicity (fibrosis) may be seen concomitantly in some chronic cases.[429]

Histology

In the acute presentation of toxicity, cholestasis is the predominant feature, along with other features of a hypersensitivity reaction. Granulomatous hepatitis has been noted.[430] In the chronic form of toxicity a chronic hepatitis with various degrees of hepatic necrosis and cirrhosis may be seen.[428]

Management

Withdrawal of the agent and supportive treatment are indicated. There does not seem to be a role for the use of corticosteroids in the chronic form despite the similarities to chronic autoimmune hepatitis.

Prognosis

Case fatalities have been reported in several series. This is usually in the setting of end-stage liver disease as a result of cirrhosis but in rare cases in elderly women fulminant liver failure may occur.[422,431] In most cases, however, with timely detection and early withdrawal there is complete reversal in both types of toxicity. Rechallenge with nitrofurantoin may result in severe reactions and should not be attempted.[432] Cross-reactivity has also been noted with other furan derivatives (e.g, furosemide, furazolidone).[433]

ANTI-FUNGAL AGENTS

Griseofulvin

This anti-fungal agent may cause a cholestatic reaction in humans.[434] It may also trigger acute intermittent porphyria.[435] Overall, hepatotoxicity is rare.

Amphotericin

Hepatotoxicity with this agent is rare. However, cases of possible reactions have been described.[436]

Ketoconazole

Of the anti-fungals, this commonly used drug has been well documented as a causative agent of hepatotoxicity. The spectrum of effects ranges from mild reversible changes in liver tests to fulminant liver failure resulting in death or liver transplantation. The incidence of significant, symptomatic reactions is estimated to be about 1 in 2000 to 1 in 15,000 cases.[437,438] In one series the mean age of occurrence was 57 years. It is seen predominantly in women.[437-439] The onset is between 11 and 168 days after the start of therapy, with an average of 61 days. There does not seem to be any clear dose relationship.

Mechanism

With the paucity of clinical and laboratory evidence supporting a hypersensitivity type of reaction, metabolic idiosyncrasy seems to be the most plausible explanation in most cases. Although ketoconazole is extensively metabolized by hepatic microsomal enzymes, the nature, route of formation, and toxicity of suspected metabolites are largely unknown.[440] N-diacetyl ketoconazole is one of the initial metabolites and is thought to undergo metabolism by the MFO system to form a potentially cytotoxic dialdehyde.[441,442]

Clinical Features and Laboratory Tests

These include anorexia, malaise, nausea, and vomiting in up to one third of cases.[437] Rash and eosinophilia are rare. Laboratory tests in approximately 60 percent of cases are in keeping with a hepatocellular type of process. The majority of the remainder demonstrates a mixed picture, with a few demonstrating a primarily cholestatic pattern.[437-439]

Histology

A predominantly hepatocellular pattern was seen in about 60 percent of patients with variable degrees of centrolobular necrosis and mild to moderate bridging.[438] In the other 40 percent of cases cholestasis predominated.[439] In fatal cases autopsy has shown massive hepatocellular necrosis.[437]

Management and Prognosis

Withdrawal of the agent results in complete reversal in most cases. In clinically evident toxicity, the mortality rate is probably about 3 percent to 5 percent.[439] Fatalities occur more often if the drug is continued despite the clinical manifestations of toxicity.[439] The drug should be avoided in patients with underlying liver disease and a point could be made for routine monitoring of liver tests for evidence of toxicity.

Other Azoles

Fluconazole

This is a relatively new but commonly used anti-fungal agent that appears to be much less hepatotoxic than ketoconazole.[443] It is excreted primarily by renal mechanisms. It has been noted to cause a hepatocellular type of injury that is dose dependent.[444,445] A case of near-fatal hepatotoxicity was described in the setting of high serum levels that occurred as a result of amphotericin.[446,447] In patients with AIDS there may be clinical or laboratory evidence of a mixed hepatocellular and cholestatic injury, with microscopic evidence of mitochondrial aberrations in patients taking fluconazole for extended periods.[448] Toxicity is reversed with withdrawal of therapy. Phenytoin hepatotoxicity has been induced by concomitant treatment with fluconazole resulting from inhibition of cytochrome P450 with resulting increases in phenytoin levels. Similar problems are common post-transplant with cyclosporine, FK506, and other drugs that require P450 metabolism (e.g, warfarin, theophylline).[449]

Miconazole, itraconazole, and clotrimazole[450-452] can all cause elevations in liver tests. Itraconazole has been noted to cause hepatotoxicity in the treatment of and prophylaxis against fungal infections in patients with AIDS.[453,454]

ANTI-PARASITIC AGENTS

Fansidar (Pyrimethamine and Sulfadoxine)

This agent, used in the treatment of malaria, has been implicated in instances of hepatic injury.[411,412,455-457] The mechanism appears to be hypersensitivity, and presumably the sulfa component is the inciting stimulus, although pyrimethamine used independently can cause hepatotoxicity.

Amodiaquine

This drug was used as prophylaxis against and treatment of malaria. It has been implicated as a cause of hepatotoxicity[458-460] and hematologic reactions.[446,461] Hepatotoxicity ranges from mild, completely reversible elevations in the aminotransferases to severe cholestasis and fulminant hepatitis. The mechanism appears to be metabolic idiosyncrasy, with bioactivation of amodiaquine by cytochrome P450 to a reactive metabolite that conjugates with glutathione and protein.[462] Amodiaquine is no longer used.

Sodium Stibogluconate

This drug is a mainstay in the treatment of leishmaniasis. It has been noted to cause a hepatocellular pattern of liver injury and it is recommended that liver tests be followed closely in those on therapy with this agent.[463,464]

Albendazole

This anti-helminthic agent causes elevated aminotransferase levels in a large fraction of patients treated long term (10 of 12 patients in one series).[465-468] The drug is known to partially inhibit microsomal enzyme function but it induces its own metabolism, which may be pivotal in the pathogenesis of hepatotoxicity. Close monitoring of liver tests is recommended.[465]

Thiabendazole

This agent has been implicated as the cause of severe intrahepatic cholestatic jaundice in patients who have undergone long-term therapy.[469] It appears to cause biliary ductular injury that may be immunoallergic in origin and may result in vanishing bile duct syndrome.[470] The occurrence of sicca syndrome in one case led to the postulation of a common antigen in the ductular systems of the affected organs. Cases that have progressed to cirrhosis and transplantation have been described.[470,471]

Hycanthone

This agent was a mainstay in the treatment of schistosomiasis. It has been discontinued from clinical use because of its hepatotoxic potential. The injury appeared to be due to inherent hepatotoxicity of the agent and was dose-related, with laboratory tests revealing a hepatocellular pattern of injury. Histology showed toxic hepatitis and in some instances massive hepatocellular necrosis.[472,473] Cases of fulminant hepatic failure resulting in death have been reported.[474]

ANTI-TUBERCULOSIS AGENTS

Isoniazid

Isoniazid has been prescribed since the early 1950s for the treatment of active and latent tuberculosis and as prophylaxis for subjects who were exposed to proven cases. Despite its extensive use, it was not until the early 1970s, some 20 years after its introduction, that its hepatotoxic potential was first recognized. Over the ensuing years the range of clinical presentations, laboratory and histologic findings, and possible mechanisms of pathogenesis have been described.

Two types of hepatic reaction can occur. The more common effect is seen in 10 percent to 20 percent of all recipients of isoniazid.[475,476] It develops within the first few months of isoniazid use and tends to be asymptomatic and mild. It appears to occur less often in children than in adults.[477,478] In most cases the reaction subsides even if the drug is continued.

In about 1 percent of patients taking the drug, a more severe hepatotoxic reaction may occur. This tends to be clinically overt and often resembles an episode of acute hepatitis.[476] There is a striking age dependency, with the reaction being very uncommon in subjects less than 20 years old, whereas an incidence approaching 2 percent is seen in patients 50 years or older.[479,480] Other subgroups that appear to be at increased risk for this type of hepatotoxic reaction include those who chronically imbibe excessive amounts of alcohol[480] and those undergoing concomitant therapy with other anti-tuberculosis drugs, especially rifampicin[481,482] and pyrazinamide.[483,484] The reaction appears to be more severe, and this may translate into higher mortality rates, in black American women[475] although actual incidence does not appear to be affected by gender. The severity appears to be greater at higher doses.[485] The severity of the toxicity also appears to be enhanced in carriers of chronic hepatitis B.[486] Patients with AIDS may be at higher risk for developing toxicity.[487] Malnutrition may play a role in the reported higher incidence seen in third-world countries.[488] It was initially believed that people with a fast acetylator phenotype were at increased risk of developing hepatotoxicity.[489] There are now good data supporting the converse (i.e, a higher incidence in slow acetylators).[490]

Mechanism

The weight of evidence supports the theory that isoniazid or one of its metabolites is a chemical toxin that produces the hepatotoxicity. In support of this there is minimal evidence, clinical or otherwise, to support a hypersensitivity type of reaction. The toxicity appears to be dose-related,[485] and animal experiments clearly show that metabolism of isoniazid leads to the formation of a potent hepatotoxin.[491,492] The initial step in inactivation of isoniazid is acetylation to form acetylisoniazid. This latter compound appears to be harmless, but after hydrolysis, acetylhydrazine and isonicotinic acid result. Isonicotinic acid also appears to be harmless. However, acetylhydrazine, after undergoing cytochrome P450–mediated oxidation, forms toxic intermediates. This oxidation may be enhanced in patients taking rifampin concomitantly because this induces cytochrome P450 enzymes. The toxic intermediates are thought to produce their damaging effects by acylating or alkylating macromolecules within the liver cells.[491,493,494] The actual toxic intermediates and the mechanism by which they cause liver cell injury or cell death have not been identified. This may involve an immune mechanism related to the formation of neo-antigens resulting from covalent binding.

The relationship of acetylator status to hepatotoxicity has been extensively studied, but its role in individual cases continues to be poorly defined. It would seem logical that fast acetylators would be more at risk of developing hepatotoxicity because this would allow the generation of higher concentrations of acetylisoniazid, which in turn undergoes hydrolysis to form acetylhydrazine that is oxidized to the toxic intermediates. This view was initially supported by a few studies.[476,489] Subsequent work has failed to show a greater susceptibility in fast acetylators compared with slow acetylators.[495–498] In fact, some studies have suggested that slow acetylators may be more at risk.[490,499] A possible explanation for this phenomenon is the observation that in fast acetylators, not only is the parent compound acetylated at an enhanced rate, but the precursor of the toxic intermediates, acetylhydrazine, is also acetylated to the harmless diacetylhydrazine.[494,500] This is excreted in the urine, thus removing substrate for the harmful oxidation reaction mediated by the cytochrome P450 system. However, an additional observation confuses the issue further; the potentially "protective" acetylation of acetylhydrazine to form diacetylhydrazine is inhibited by isoniazid itself[501] and the rate of this reaction proceeds five times slower than acetylation of isoniazid. Therefore it would be expected that for a given dose of isoniazid acetylhydrazine would accumulate in slow acetylators and predispose to hepatotoxicity.

Another potential pathway for the development of hepatotoxicity is hydrolysis of isoniazid to produce hydrazine and isonicotinic acid. Hydrazine is known to be directly hepatotoxic and this hydrolysis is enhanced in alcoholics.[502] Rifampicin also seems to enhance this process, which may be the explanation for why co-treatment with the two drugs enhances isoniazid hepatotoxicity. This mechanism of disposal seems to be more important in slow acetylators and may explain the increased incidence of toxicity seen in this subgroup of patients in some studies.

Clinical and Laboratory Features

In the mild form of hepatotoxicity, patients are usually asymptomatic. If the liver tests are followed, a transient mild elevation of the AST and ALT is seen within the first few months of therapy. This usually resolves completely over time. In the more severe but less common form of hepatotoxicity, clinical and laboratory findings become evident in the first few months in about half of the cases. Other patients may not manifest toxicity until they have received up to 12 months of therapy.[476] These latter patients, who display a delayed onset of toxicity, and those in whom the drug is continued after the onset of symptoms seem to fare the worst.[476,503,504] As noted previously, toxicity resembles viral hepatitis including its spectrum of severity. Toxicity typically presents as a flu-like syndrome with anorexia, nausea, vomiting, and fatigue, with variable degrees of right upper quadrant pain. In more severe cases jaundice and symptoms and signs of acute liver failure may supersede. Physical findings include fever, jaundice, tender hepatomegaly, and in severe cases encephalopathy, evidence of coagulopathy, and ascites. Findings that are typical of hypersensitivity reactions, such as rash and arthritis, are rare.

Laboratory tests reflect a hepatocellular process, with predominantly elevated AST and ALT. There is a variable increase in the ALP, bilirubin, and prothrombin time.

Histology

Histology mimics the spectrum seen with viral hepatitis and ranges from acute hepatitis with ballooning degeneration and acidophil bodies, with or without bridging necrosis, to massive or submassive necrosis. In more subacute or chronic courses the histology is similar to that seen in chronic viral hepatitis. With a chronic smoldering course, macronodular cirrhosis may result.

Management

Management consists of withdrawing the agent and providing supportive care. If fulminant liver failure occurs, liver transplant evaluation should proceed.

Prognosis

The mild changes in liver enzymes that occur in 10 percent to 20 percent of patients taking isoniazid, as noted previously, usually do not progress and may actually resolve with time. This would seem to make surveillance of liver enzymes of all patients taking isoniazid of limited importance. The counterpoint to this argument is that such a protocol may prevent the early detection and prevention of the potentially more severe hepatotoxicity that can occur, especially because this syndrome may present as fulminant liver failure. Observations in large series of patients being treated with isoniazid have led to the recommendation that aminotransferase levels be followed in patients older than age 35 years (e.g, every 4 weeks); if the levels exceed fourfold normal and are persistent, continued treatment should be reevaluated. This approach seems to reduce the incidence of severe liver injury.[505] Enzymes should always be checked and the drug stopped in patients who develop symptomatic hepatitis. In patients with overt hepatotoxicity the case fatality rates have been estimated to be about 10 percent (or about 4.2 per 100,000 people beginning therapy).[475,506,507] Middle-aged black women seem to fare worse.[475] This is usually a result of fulminant liver failure. In most other cases there is clinical and biochemical resolution in 1 to 2 months. As noted previously, a more protracted course mimicking chronic viral hepatitis may ensue and result in cirrhosis.[475,506]

Rifampin

Rifampin belongs to a group of chemicals referred to as rifamycins and is produced by *Streptomyces mediterranei.* It is one of the drugs used to treat mycobacterial tuberculosis and non-tuberculous mycobacteria. It is also effective in the treatment of pruritus. The administration of rifampin may exacerbate hyperbilirubinemia (in patients with preexisting liver disease) because the drug impairs the uptake of bilirubin and bile acids by the hepatocyte. It is a potent inducer of the cytochrome P450 system and, as such, decreases its own elimination half-life. In addition, this effect may enhance the toxicity of other drugs, most notably isoniazid, with which it is often used.[482] In fact, hepatotoxicity is seen more often when rifampin is used concomitantly with isoniazid than when either drug is used separately.[482,495] Synergism is also noted in children, in whom isoniazid hepatotoxicity is rare.[508] This is especially so when the drugs are used to treat tuberculous meningitis in children.[509,510] In these patients other potentiating factors include the use of higher doses of the drugs, malnutrition, and concomitant therapy with cytochrome P450-inducing anti-convulsant medications.

The mechanism of this increase in toxicity likely involves rifampin's ability to induce the microsomal enzymes and thus increase the production of oxidized metabolites of isoniazid. When isoniazid and rifampin are taken together, the incidence of hepatotoxicity appears to be higher in slow acetylators than in fast acetylators.[509] As noted in the discourse on isoniazid, acetylhydrazine tends to accumulate in slow acetylators. This latter compound is the substrate for cytochrome P450 production of reactive species that mediate toxicity. In addition rifampin induces direct hydrolysis of isoniazid to produce hydrazine, a known hepatotoxin. This is especially a problem in slow acetylators. In addition to its effect on bilirubin uptake and the increase in hepatotoxicity noted with isoniazid, rifampin has the potential to cause its own hepatitis-like drug reaction.[482,511] The exact incidence of this is unclear because most reported cases were in patients taking more than one agent[482,511,512] or in patients with underlying liver disease.[513]

In instances of hepatitis ascribed to rifampin in one series the onset appeared to be sooner than that of isoniazid, and the histology was remarkable for a paucity of inflammatory cells.[511]

Para-aminosalicylic acid

This drug is used rarely as an anti-tuberculosis agent. It is known to cause hepatitis in which clinical features and laboratory findings suggest an immunologically (hypersensitivity) mediated reaction (i.e, a drug allergy). These include fever, rash, lymphadenopathy, jaundice, and eosinophilia.

ANTI-VIRAL AGENTS

Zidovudine

This agent is a thymidine analog that is used to treat HIV infections. There were initial reports of reversible liver test abnormalities[514] and cholestatic jaundice[515] with zidovudine. More recent reports have centered on the potentially fatal occurrence of marked hepatic steatosis associated with severe lactic acidosis.[516-520] This probably represents a class effect of the nucleoside analogs because similar changes have been noted with the use of stavudine, didanosine (ddI), and zalcitabine.[521-524]

Clinical and Laboratory Findings

Affected patients presenting tend to be obese females, although some reports describe the findings in predominantly male patients.[525] On presentation they often complain of flu-like symptoms including mild fever, myalgias, anorexia, nausea, vomiting, and diarrhea. Most have been receiving the drug for several months when lactic acidosis is discovered.[525] Tender hepatomegaly may be detected on physical examination. A low-grade fever, tachypnea, and tachycardia are often found. Laboratory features include an anion-gap metabolic acidosis with elevated serum lactate levels (lactic acid levels higher than 5 mmol/L). The lactic acidosis is of the aerobic type (not resulting from tissue hypoxia) (i.e, type B). There is moderate elevation in the aminotransferases, and minimal changes if any in the serum ALP or bilirubin levels.[519]

Mechanism

The mechanism is likely to be metabolic idiosyncrasy. At an ultrastructural level, severe aberrations in the mitochondria are noted.[525,526] The mechanism of action of the drug (i.e, its ability to substitute as a nucleoside) results in inhibition of HIV reverse transcriptase. Presumably it inhibits the γ-DNA polymerase necessary for mitochondrial replication. Blocks in the citric acid cycle lead to low ATP/ADP and increased NADH/NAD ratios that in turn lead to increased lactate production and acidosis.[519] Zidovudine has been shown to directly inhibit NADP-linked respiration as well.[519]

Histology

Histology reveals massive steatosis that microscopically is a mixture of macrovesicular and microvesicular inclusions.[519,525] There is otherwise minimal distortion of the liver architecture and minimal inflammation. There are, as noted previously, ultrastructural changes that include lipid inclusions, prominent endoplasmic reticulum, increased density of the inner mitochondrial membrane, and enlarged mitochondria containing paracrystalline inclusions and dense bodies.[525]

Management

Withdrawal of the agent and supportive treatment, including attempts to correct severe acidosis, are standard management protocols.

Prognosis

The majority of reports in the literature suggest that the mortality rate is about 50 percent to 60 percent.[516,518,519,527-529] There are a few reports of a milder syndrome with better outcomes.[525] There are no apparent long-term sequelae in those who recover.

ddI, Stavudine, and Zalcitabine

Although not described as often as with zidovudine, these three nucleoside analogs also appear to cause lactic acidosis.[521,522,530-534] ddI has been reported to cause Mallory bodies,[535] and a case of hepatitis has been described.[536] Its toxicity may be enhanced in patients receiving concomitant ribavirin therapy.[537-539]

Ribavirin

Ribavirin is a nucleoside analog that has been used for many years as an inhalational agent in the treatment of respiratory syncytial virus infection in infants and young children. More recently, an oral preparation has been used in combination with interferon-α to treat hepatitis C. Nucleoside analogs are inhibitors of reverse transcriptase. A common feature of such compounds is the inhibition of mitochondrial DNA synthesis by blocking DNA polymerase.[540] The resultant deficiency of oxidative phosphorylation is a key factor in the development of lipodystrophy, neuropathy, pancreatitis, lactic acidemia, and liver toxicity.[541] Recently, five cases of hepatic toxicity in patients co-infected with the hepatitis C virus (HCV) and HIV were reported after patients were started on interferon-α plus ribavirin therapy.[542,543] All five had been on long-term, highly active anti-retroviral therapy (HAART). The patients presented with weakness, weight loss, and clinical or biochemical signs of liver disease and pancreatitis. These changes became evident after 4 to 6 months of therapy. At least one patient developed ascites. Laboratory studies revealed elevated amylase, lipase, γ-glutamyl transferase, and ALP levels. Lactic acidemia was a common thread in these patients. Liver biopsies showed significant micro- and macrovesicular steatosis. It is hypothesized that the combined effects of ribavirin and HAART on the mitochondria,[542] along with the potentiation of other nucleoside activities resulting from ribavirin's promotion of nucleoside phosphorylation,[537,543,544] may act synergistically to increase mitochondrial toxicity.[538,539,545-547] HCV and HIV infections alone have also been noted to induce mitochondrial disruption.[548] More such toxicities are reportedly being seen in the clinical trials evaluating hepatitis C therapy in patients with HCV and HIV co-infection. For now it is recommended that patients on long-term HAART therapy have markers of mitochondrial and pancreatic toxicity, including lactic acid amylase, and lipase, monitored closely if they are placed on ribavirin therapy. Toxicity appears to be a particular concern in patients with cirrhosis, who have limited hepatic reserve.

Fialuridine

Fialuridine is also a nucleoside analog, and it was evaluated for the treatment of chronic hepatitis B. It was withdrawn from development because it caused steatosis and mitochondrial dysfunction, leading to several cases of fatal lactic acidosis and liver failure.[549-551] The cumulative dose appears to be important, and in in vitro studies,[551] incorporation of the drug into the mitochondrial DNA correlated with mitochondrial dysfunction and steatosis. This may explain the finding of toxicity beginning months after stopping the agent.

Indinavir (and Other Protease Inhibitors)

Indinavir is an anti-HIV agent of the protease inhibitor class. There are several reports of hepatitis occurring as a result of its use.[552-554] The mechanism is unclear. There is a report of nelfinavir causing acute hepatitis with cholestatic features in two patients.[555] There are reports suggesting that ritonavir may have hepatotoxic potential.[556-558] This is probably enhanced by co-treatment with other drugs. There is a report of acute hepatitis in a patient who was also being treated with saquinavir.[557] A case of lactic acidosis similar to that described in patients taking nucleoside analogs seemed to have been precipitated by ritonavir (although the patient was also taking stavudine and lamivudine).[558]

ANTI-NEOPLASTIC AND IMMUNOSUPPPRESSIVE AGENTS

Medical treatment of cancer evolved rapidly in the last three decades, and the number of drugs available as options to treat malignant neoplasms is ever-increasing (Table 27-11). Although this leads to improved survival and quality of life overall, toxicity for various organ systems including the liver can result, and knowledge of such toxicities can lead to early recognition and the institution of corrective measures.

Causality assessment of hepatotoxicity in the setting of cancer chemotherapy is often difficult. There are several reasons for this.

1. Abnormal liver tests may result from metastasis or infiltration of the liver parenchyma or biliary tree by tumor. A Budd-Chiari-like picture may resemble VOD and may occur as a result of the procoagulant state caused by many tumors.

TABLE 27-11

Hepatotoxic Manifestations of Anti-neoplastic Agents

Manifestation of hepatotoxicity	Agent
Veno-occlusive disease	Mitomycin
	6-Thioguanine
	Azathioprine
	Cytarabine
	Dacarbazine
	Indicine-N-oxide
	Daunorubicin
	Combination chemotherapy
	Radiation therapy plus
	Cyclophosphamide
	Busulfan
	Carmustine
	Mitomycin C
	Other regimens
Hepatocellular necrosis	Common
	Mithramycin
	L-Asparaginase
	Streptozocin
	Methotrexate (high dose)
	Rare
	Nitrosoureas
	6-Thioguanines
	Cytarabine
	Adriamycin
	5-Fluorouracil
	Cyclophosphamide
	Etoposide
	Vinca alkaloids
Hepatic steatosis	L-asparaginase
	Actinomycin-D
	Mitomycin C
	Bleomycin
	Methotrexate
Cholestasis	6-Mercaptopurine
	Azathioprine
	Busulfan
	Amsacrine
Fibrosis	Methotrexate
	Azathioprine
Sclerosing cholangitis	Floxuridine
Peliosis hepatitis	Androgens
	Hydroxyprogesterone
	Azathioprine
	Hydroxyurea
	Tamoxifen
Nodular regenerative hyperplasia	Azathioprine
	6-Thioguanine
	Androgens
	Estrogens
Hepatic neoplasms	Estrogens
	Androgens
	Methotrexate

2. Immune suppression may result in sepsis and shock with its attendant cytokine-induced effects on the liver, such as cholestasis. Occasionally, the liver itself may be opportunistically infected or transfusion may result in viral hepatitis.
3. Multiple drugs are often used in overlapping schedules, making it difficult to establish temporal correlation.
4. Different modalities of treatment (i.e, non-chemotherapy treatment) may lead to hepatotoxicity. Examples include the direct effects of radiation and graft-versus-host disease in patients undergoing bone marrow or stem cell transplants.
5. Drugs that have minimal hepatotoxic potential when used alone may produce severe liver disease when used in combination with other chemotherapeutic agents or with radiation therapy.
6. Barring the availability of skilled services to perform high-risk transjugular liver biopsies, liver biopsy is often contraindicated because of thrombocytopenia and coagulation abnormalities caused by treatment.
7. Toxicity in other organ systems may result in abnormal liver tests (e.g, Adriamycin-induced cardiac failure may result in hepatic congestion and its resultant liver test abnormalities).

ANTI-METABOLITES

See the section on anti-inflammatory agents for information on methotrexate.

6-Mercaptopurine and Azathioprine

As with methotrexate, these agents probably see more widespread use as immunosuppressive agents in the treatment of chronic inflammatory disorders and in the post-transplant setting than as anti-neoplastic agents. Azathioprine is a derivative of 6-mercaptopurine (6-MP) and appears to be less hepatotoxic than its parent compound.

6-MP has been in use for the last 60 years. It is a thiopurine analog of the natural purine bases. Its potential to cause hepatotoxicity is well recognized. Cholestatic liver injury appears to be the most common manifestation of this toxicity and may occur in 6 percent to 40 percent of recipients,[559-561] although many of these observations were made at a time when chronic hepatitis C was not a recognized entity. The effect appears to be dose-dependent. Doses exceeding 2.5 mg/kg have the highest likelihood of toxicity.[560,562,563] The latent period between commencement of drug and onset of toxicity is anywhere from 1 to 18 months. Adults appear to be more susceptible to injury than children.[564]

Mechanism

6-MP is metabolized extensively in the liver. Whether this has any bearing on its hepatotoxic potential is not known. The mechanism of toxicity appears to be intrinsic. Evidence in support of this conclusion includes the paucity of evidence that would suggest a hypersensitivity-mechanism (i.e, the long lag time before the onset of symptoms and lack of hypersensitivity features such as rash and eosinophilia). Other supporting facts include the relatively high incidence and dose dependence.

Clinical and Laboratory Features

Jaundice and pruritus are the main presenting symptoms. The laboratory studies reflect a mixed hepatocellular and cholestatic injury with moderate elevations in AST, ALT, ALP, and serum bilirubin.[562,563]

Histology

This is also a mixed picture, with features of both cholestasis and hepatocellular necrosis.

Management

Management consists of discontinuating of the agent.

Prognosis

Cases of fatal hepatic necrosis, in the setting of continued use despite evidence of toxicity, have been described.[563] Rechallenge has led to recurrent hepatotoxicity in some cases.[563]

Azathioprine, as noted, has a lesser tendency to cause hepatotoxicity. This fact notwithstanding, the spectrum of hepatotoxicity is wider than that seen with 6-MP. In addition to the cholestatic injury seen with 6-MP,[565,566] other patterns have been recognized. Predominant cholestasis, with evidence of a hypersensitivity reaction, has been recognized.[567] The converse (i.e, primarily hepatocellular type of injury) has been seen in other settings, especially in post-renal transplant patients.[568]

More recently, several other lesions with a common pathogenesis—in that they involve an insult to the vascular endothelium—have been appreciated. These conditions include striking sinusoidal dilation,[569] peliosis hepatis in 12 patients,[570] nodular regenerative hyperplasia,[571,572] hepatoportal sclerosis,[571] and VOD.[573-575] These observations were all made in the post-renal transplant setting and, in one series, the incidence of VOD was estimated to be 2.5 percent.[575] The onset of VOD occurs from 2 months to as long as 9 months after transplant. There is a male preponderance. In one series co-infection with a hepatatrophic virus was questioned as a probable contributing factor in the pathogenesis of VOD.[575] Clinically, signs of portal hypertension with minimal elevations of the liver tests in a non-specific pattern are noted. Portal hypertension may progress, which may have an effect on future morbidity and mortality.[575] The hepatotoxicity appears to be primarily an idiosyncratic reaction, although azathioprine is converted to 6-MP in vivo and direct toxicity may also play a role. Also, as alluded to previously, patients may display features of a hypersensitivity reaction in some instances of toxicity. Histology is usually classic for VOD or the other pathologies described. The tenets of management involve early detection, which is often difficult given the insidious nature of onset and progression, and withdrawal of the drug. This has led to reversal, and in one instance, recurrence with rechallenge.[576]

6-Thioguanine

6-Thioguanine is also a purine analog, used primarily in the treatment of acute and chronic leukemia. As with azathioprine, this agent also appears to result in endothelial dysfunction leading to manifestations of VOD, nodular regenerative hyperplasia, and hepatoportal sclerosis.[560,577,578] In one study the incidence of portal hypertension in patients with chronic myeloid leukemia who were treated with busulfan alone or busulfan with 6-thioguanine was determined. In the latter group 18 of 675 patients compared with none in the busulfan alone group developed portal hypertension. Histologically, idiopathic portal hypertension with minimal morphologic abnormalities or nodular regenerative hyperplasia was the major finding; three patients developed cirrhosis and its attendant complications.[577] Other studies have described VOD in patients treated with 6-thioguanine and cytosine arabinoside.[579,580]

5-Fluorouracil

5-Fluorouracil (5-FU) is used in the treatment of malignancies of the digestive system, breast, and ovary. It is a pyrimidine-base analog. It is metabolized by the liver and has little hepatotoxicity when used orally.

A derivative of 5-FU, floxuridine, is administered by continuous intravenous infusion or directly into the hepatic artery for treatment of hepatic metastasis from colon cancer.[581,582] This leads to higher remission rates and improved survival, but at the cost of increased hepatic injury. Damage appears to be more common with direct hepatic artery infusions,[560] which cause a chemical hepatitis in more than half of the cases.[583] Liver tenderness and elevation in the AST, ALT, ALP, and bilirubin characterize the reaction. In a smaller subset of patients sclerosing cholangitis may develop.[583-586] This is usually heralded by the onset of jaundice and marked elevations in the ALP. In one study of intra-arterial infusion 35 of 35 patients had a predominantly cholestatic pattern of liver tests. Seven patients receiving intra-arterial therapy were studied with cholangiography, which, in all cases, demonstrated sclerosis of the intrahepatic or extrahepatic bile ducts. In addition, liver biopsies showed cholestasis and pericholangitis with minimal hepatocytic damage. It was suggested that biliary sclerosis is probably more common than the often-described chemical hepatitis.[583] Chemical hepatitis usually resolves after therapy is complete or is discontinued. Fatal cirrhosis has been reported to result from the more serious sclerosing cholangitis.[587] Cases with sclerosing cholangitis are managed on their merit, with endoscopic retrograde cholangiopancreatography (ERCP) and stenting versus surgical therapy if complications develop or are impending. The biliary tree is highly dependent on the hepatic arterial supply for oxygenation and delivery of nutrients, and presumably damage or dysfunction of the arteries caused by the chemotherapeutic agent leads to the biliary sclerosis.

Cytosine Arabinoside

Cytosine arabinoside is also a pyrimidine analog. Hepatotoxicity appears to be dose-related and ranges from mild increases in the AST, ALT, and ALP to more significant elevations with frank cholestatic jaundice.[588-591] These changes are usually reversible.

L-Asparaginase

This is an enzyme that catalyses the hydrolysis of L-asparagine to aspartic acid and ammonia. Because leukemic cells cannot produce L-asparagine, whereas the normal cell can, L-asparaginase is used to treat acute lymphocytic leukemia and T-cell lymphoblastic lymphoma. Abnormal liver tests have been reported in up to 75 percent of recipients.[592]

Mechanism

Hypersensitivity type of reactions, especially after repeated doses, are common and have been reported in 43 percent of recipients, although anaphylactic-like reactions only occur in about 10 percent of recipients.[593,594] Steatosis, a finding more typical of a metabolic aberration, is common, occurring in 50 percent to 90 percent of recipients.[595] This is likely a result of impaired protein synthesis at the mitochondrial level. Given the frequency of its occurrence, liver injury is likely to be a direct toxic effect of the drug itself (rather than metabolic idiosyncrasy).

Clinical and Laboratory Findings

The clinical features of reactions to L-asparaginase usually develop within 1 hour after administration and include pruritus, dyspnea, urticaria, swelling at the injection site, angioedema, rash, abdominal pain, laryngospasm, nasal stuffiness, bronchospasm, and hypotension.[593] The liver test abnormalities include modestly elevated AST, ALT, bilirubin, and ALP. The serum albumin and several other proteins that are synthesized by the liver are decreased. These proteins include factors I, II, VII, IX, and X; ceruloplasmin; haptoglobin; transferrin; and lipoproteins.[592] Coagulopathy may be a prominent feature. Elevated ammonia levels may occur (in keeping with the mechanism of action).

Histology

The most prominent histologic finding is microvesicular steatosis.[595]

Management

In cases of significant toxicity, it is necessary to stop the drug. However, abnormal liver tests are common and it is often difficult to differentiate hepatotoxicity from other toxic effects of the drug.

Prognosis

Fatal outcomes can occur. A less immunogenic form of the drug (pegaspargase) has been developed and reportedly is less likely to result in hypersensitivity reactions.[593]

Mithramycin (Plicamycin)

This is an antibiotic that can intercalate into DNA and thus inhibit RNA synthesis. In addition to its use as an anti-cancer agent, it is sometimes used in the treatment of hypercalcemia and Paget's disease. Direct hepatotoxicity is the likely mechanism because abnormal liver tests occur in almost all patients treated.[596,597] Hepatocellular enzymes may be quite elevated, and the level correlates with dose. Depression of coagulation factor production and thrombocytopenia may result in a bleeding diathesis. Hepatocellular necrosis (zone 3) and steatosis have been observed.[597] The lower doses used to treat hypercalcemia and Paget's disease are reportedly associated with less frequent hepatotoxicity.[560]

Adriamycin (Doxorubicin)

Adriamycin is also an antibiotic. It has rarely been implicated as the cause of hepatic injury. In six cases of acute lymphoblastic leukemia it was thought to have caused acute or chronic hepatitis.[598] It has also been postulated that Adriamycin potentiates the hepatotoxicity of 6-MP.[599] It may increase the incidence of radiation-induced injury when used before radiation therapy.[600] Adriamycin can produce cardiomyopathy that can result in congestive heart failure (CHF). The resultant liver congestion can sometimes be misleading but reverses with appropriate treatment of the CHF.

Dactinomycin (Actinomycin D)

This antibiotic has been used for many years without much evidence of hepatotoxicity. A few cases of severe hepatic injury have been described when the agent is used alone or with vincristine.[601-603] Cases of VOD have also been described, especially in the setting of concomitant irradiation for treatment of Wilms' tumor.[604-607]

Cyclosporin A

This peptide is extracted from *Tolypocladium inflatum*. It is used primarily as an immune suppressant in transplant medicine and has a narrow therapeutic window. It has been reported to cause a mild, dose-dependent cholestatic injury,[608,609] with a frequency of 4 percent to 86 percent.[609]

Mechanism

The mechanism is unclear. There is experimental evidence that a dose-dependent decrease occurs in both bile flow and secretion of bile solute in the presence of cyclosporine; this may be secondary to inhibition of vesicular transport in the liver.[610]

Clinical and Laboratory Features

In many patients cyclosporin A toxicity is subclinical.[608,609] The liver tests reveal a mild, often transient increase in ALP levels, occasionally accompanied by slight elevations in serum bilirubin and aminotransferase levels.[609] Cyclosporine levels tend to be on the high side of the therapeutic range.[608]

Histology

Histology is not well documented.

Management

Dose reduction is recommended. In the settings in which this drug is used there are often multiple other potential causes of liver dysfunction (e.g, infection); confounding conditions should therefore be ruled out, especially graft rejection. Lliver biopsy may be helpful.

Prognosis

It appears that hepatotoxicity is of little prognostic significance. Nephrotoxicity and neurotoxicity are more important from this standpoint.

Vinca Alkaloids

These alkaloids are derived from the periwinkle plant. Their anti-tumor effects are dependent on their ability to disrupt cellular microtubule function.

Vincristine appears to increase liver toxicity when used with radiation therapy.[560] Rarely it may result in a mild increase in aminotransferase levels outside of the setting of radiation.[611] Otherwise, these agents do not appear to be significant hepatotoxins.

Etoposide (VP-16)

Also an alkaloid, etoposide is a derivative of podophyllotoxin. The drug disrupts the formation of the mitotic spindle. Acute hepatocellular necrosis has been reported.[612] In combination with ifosfamide severe hepatotoxicity has been described.[613]

ALKYLATING AGENTS

Cyclophosphamide

This alkylating agent is a commonly used anti-cancer drug in regimens for leukemia, lymphoma, and solid tumors. It is also used in the treatment of a few chronic inflammatory conditions such as Wegener's granulomatosis and SLE. It is metabolized to its active form by the cytochrome P450 system. The alkylating species usually are formed only in cells with high turnover rates. However, hepatotoxicity may result from a metabolic idiosyncrasy in some individuals who form toxic amounts of these species in the hepatocytes. Hepatotoxicity appears to be a rare complication of therapy. There are case reports in the literature of hepatocellular necrosis that were possibly related to the use of cyclophosphamide.[614] In patients with collagen vascular diseases cyclophosphamide has rarely caused hepatic injury, including mild hepatitis to massive hepatocellular necrosis.[615] A convincing case of toxicity with resolution after withdrawal and recurrence on rechallenge was seen in a patient with SLE. There was jaundice and marked elevation in the ALT.[616] There are increasing reports of VOD in patients undergoing bone marrow transplant who receive a conditioning regimen containing cyclophosphamide and busulfan.[617-620] There is a report of VOD in the non-transplant setting related to the use of cyclophosphamide.[621]

Busulfan

Busulfan appears to be a contributing factor in the causation of VOD, as described previously.

Ifosfamide

A cholestatic injury has been reported when this agent is used in combination with etoposide (VP-16).[613]

Chlorambucil

This drug rarely causes hepatotoxicity. There is a recent report of an acute cholestatic hepatitis with the use of this drug. Older, sparse reports focus more on a hepatocellular injury.[622]

Nitrosoureas (Carmustine [BCNU], Lomustine, Semustine, Streptozocin)

These compounds can all cause what appears to be reversible hepatic dysfunction, with jaundice and an elevated AST in up to 25 percent of cases. Higher doses have been noted to increase the AST in up to 40 percent of patients.[623,624] With high doses of BCNU, fatal hepatic necrosis can occur.[623] Pericholangitis and intrahepatic cholestasis accompany mild hepatic necrosis in most cases. Recent animal studies provide evidence that lipoperoxidation and alterations in the anti-oxidant system may significantly contribute to BCNU-induced hepatotoxicity, and some anti-oxidant agents may be of benefit in reducing the incidence of cholestasis.[625]

Dacarbazine

This also is an alkylating agent, used primarily to treat malignant melanoma and some lymphomas. Recent case reports implicate this drug in the causation of acute hepatocellular necrosis secondary to VOD.[626-628] This seems to occur within a few days of the second dose of the drug, and eosinophilia may be a feature, raising the possibility of an immunologically mediated process. Massive elevations in the AST and ALT occur, and histology is consistent with VOD. There tends to be minimal inflammatory infiltration.[626] Management is supportive. It has been recommended that if eosinophilia develops after the first dose of dacarbazine, subsequent doses should be avoided.[626]

BIOLOGIC RESPONSE MODULATORS

Interferons

These agents are used in the treatment of chronic viral hepatitis (C and B), some solid tumors (e.g, Kaposi's sarcomas in patients with HIV disease), melanoma, and certain leukemias. Hepatotoxicity is extremely rare with the low percutaneous doses used to treat hepatitis. However, a few cases that probably represent induction of autoimmune hepatitis by interferon-induced enhancement of the immune system have been described.[629] In addition, it has been our experience that a small subset of patients being treated for chronic hepatitis C often has mild elevations in AST and ALT, despite good virologic responses. This corrects at the end of the treatment course when the interferon is withdrawn, suggesting that interferon-α has a role to play in its pathogenesis. Interferon is not recommended in patients with decompensated cirrhosis. The incidence of liver enzyme abnormalities seems somewhat more common with the pegylated interferons. Three percent of patients receiving 1.5 mg/kg pegylated interferon α-2b plus 800 mg ribavirin developed ALT elevations greater than two times, but less than five times, baseline.[630] Transaminase elevations are frequent with systemic administration. Sixty percent of melanoma patients have an increase in AST (2 percent, ALT). In Kaposi's sarcoma the incidence of AST and ALT elevations rises from 10 percent with 30 million units twice per week to 40 percent and 15 percent respectively with 35 million units per day.[630a] Bilirubin, ALP, and LDH elevations often occur in conjunction with transaminase increases.[631] Rare cases of jaundice and hepatic failure have been reported with interferon α-2b.[631] Interferon α-2a was associated with elevations in AST (77 percent), ALP (48 percent), and bilirubin (31 percent) in a large series of cancer patients.[632]

Tumor Necrosis Factor

This is a biologic agent that is produced in response to several types of injury such as alcoholic liver disease and chronic inflammatory bowel disease. It has been implicated in the pathogenesis of cholestasis,[633] and therefore it is not surprising that it has been found to cause profound cholestasis when it is used as treatment in advanced colorectal cancer.[634]

Interleukin-2

Interleukin-2 (IL-2) immunotherapy is associated with the development of profound reversible cholestasis and hyperbilirubinemia in a large subfraction of patients (up to 85 percent of treated patients).[635-638] There is evidence to suggest that this reversible cholestasis is a direct result of IL-2-dependent reduced excretion of bile.[635] Clinical features include jaundice, right upper quadrant pain and tenderness, nausea, pruritus, and hepatomegaly. The administration of total parenteral nutrition has been noted to reduce the incidence of this phenomenon.[636]

DRUGS USED IN THE TREATMENT OF CARDIOVASCULAR DISEASES

Antihypertensive and Diuretic Agents

Alpha-methyldopa

Alpha-methyldopa has been used to treat hypertension since 1960. Hepatotoxicity was described soon after its release, and case reports of toxicity have continued to this day. It is not used as often as it previously was in the Western world, but it continues to be a common drug in third-world countries because of its relatively low cost. Because it is considered to be relatively safe in pregnancy, it remains popular in the treatment of hypertension during pregnancy. Even in this latter setting there are case reports, albeit rare, of hepatotoxicity.[639-641] There is an array of different presentations, but the majority of cases fall into two main categories: acute hepatocellular injury[642,643] and chronic hepatitis.[643-646] Other, less-common manifestations include acute granulomatous hepatitis,[647,648] cholestatic disease,[643,649] fatty liver,[650] and acute massive or submassive necrosis.[651,652]

Asymptomatic elevations in liver tests occur in 10 percent to 30 percent of all recipients.[644] The incidence of clinically significant hepatotoxicity is less clear. But methyldopa accounted for 10 percent of all drug-induced hepatotoxicity reported to the Swedish Adverse Drug Reaction Committee in a 10-year period.[653] Females are affected three times as often as males. The incidence appears to be increased in patients in their 50s and 60s. There are reports of multiple cases within a single family, suggesting possible genetic determinants.[654,655] Preexisting liver disease does not appear to be a risk factor in the development of toxicity, although the drug should be avoided in such patients because of the potential for diagnostic confusion and further deterioration of liver function, should hepatotoxicity develop.

Mechanism. The mechanism of toxicity has not been elucidated entirely and may be different in the acute and chronic diseases. Toxicity appears to be independent of dose. Multiple autoimmune phenomena, including positive lupus erythematosis (LE) cell preparations, positive Coombs' test, hemolytic anemia, hypergammaglobulinemia, elevated titers of ANA and ASMA, and recurrence with rechallenge all suggest that an immune mechanism is playing a role. These features are common and the chronic hepatitis syndrome that can occur most resembles the findings in autoimmune hepatitis. Methyldopa has been found to inhibit T-suppressor cell function and this may allow unregulated B-cell production of antibodies.[656,657] This is unlikely to be the only pathogenetic mechanism, however. Classic findings of hypersensitivity reactions, such as eosinophilia, are rare. In addition, experimental data have accumulated to suggest that methyldopa is metabolized by the cytochrome P450 system to form a reactive species that can covalently bind to proteins. This product is believed to be a semiquinone or quinone formed by oxidation of methyldopa.[658,659] Presumably, covalent binding of these reactive species to plasma membrane proteins forms neo-antigens that are detected by the immune system. This is supported by the finding that antibodies in the sera from patients with methyldopa-induced liver disease only bind to rabbit hepatocyte membranes after treatment with both methyldopa and a cytochrome P450-inducing agent.[660] Thus it appears that both metabolic idiosyncrasy and autoimmune phenomena contribute to the pathogenesis of methyldopa-induced toxicity.

Clinical Features

Acute Hepatitis. Methyldopa-induced acute hepatitis resembles acute viral hepatitis in its presentation. Anorexia, chills, headache, nausea, and fever usually precede jaundice, occurring within 1 to 20 weeks after starting the drug.[642] Other symptoms include right upper quadrant pain, dark urine, and pale stools. In patients with cholestasis, pruritus may occur.[661] As noted previously, rash, lymphadenopathy, and eosinophilia are rare. The laboratory features are similar to those in acute viral hepatitis. There is marked elevation in serum AST and ALT, often greater than 1000 U/L, with moderate elevations in the ALP. Bilirubin is low at the outset, but increases later. Other common findings include a Coombs'-positive hemolytic anemia and positive ANA and ASMA.[642] Fulminant hepatic failure can occur.[662]

Chronic Hepatitis. This tends to present after a longer period of drug intake, usually after 6 months.[654] It resembles chronic autoimmune hepatitis in its clinical and laboratory features.

Histology

Acute Hepatitis. Methydopa-induced acute hepatitis resembles acute viral hepatitis. There are inflammatory infiltrates, mainly lymphocytes and neutrophils, primarily located in the portal and periportal zones. Hepatocellular degeneration, acidophil bodies, and areas of necrosis that may bridge portal areas are seen.[644,661]

Chronic Hepatitis. The inflammatory response tends to be more intense, with plasma cells, lymphocytes, and occasionally eosinophils being present.[661] Steatosis and variable degrees of necrosis are seen.[650,652] Fibrous tissue, ranging from thickening of intralobular septa to macronodular cirrhosis may be found.

Management. Patients should be counseled regarding premonitory symptoms. Evaluation for hepatotoxicity should be performed for unexplained fever or other symptoms or signs of hepatitis. There is a high incidence of mild elevations in the liver tests. Because of this, there does not appear to be too much benefit in monitoring liver tests in all patients. The drug should be discontinued if abnormalities are discovered. There is no evidence to suggest that the use of corticosteroids in either the acute or chronic autoimmune-like scenarios is beneficial.

Prognosis. With early detection and withdrawal most patients do well. However, case fatalities and progression to cirrhosis are well described.[651,661] Recurrences can be prompt or delayed, and fatalities can occur.[644,661]

Angiotensin-converting Enzyme Inhibitors

They have been implicated in the causation of cholestatic hepatitis, although a mixed hepatocellular cholestatic picture and predominant hepatocellular reactions have also been reported. Captopril has been the culprit in many of these cases.[663-669] The frequent presence of fever, rash, and eosinophilia and the relative rarity of the condition suggest a hypersensitivity reaction,[667] although this is not entirely clear. Another potential mechanism may involve modulation of eicosanoid metabolism by inhibition of kininase II and subsequent increased hepatic bradykinin activity.[670] This latter substance may induce cholestasis. Yet another contributor to the pathogenesis of hepatotoxicity may be metabolism by the cytochrome P450 enzymes to reactive species that may cause either direct or immune-mediated toxicity.[671]

The onset is usually within 1 to 20 weeks of initiating the drug.[663] Histology usually reveals marked cholestasis with variable degrees of hepatocellular injury. Discontinuation of the drug results in slow resolution over 1 week to 6 months.[663] Hepatic failure and death can occur if this condition is unrecognized.[663]

- Enalapril has similarly been implicated in causing cholestatic and occasionally mixed and hepatocellular hepatic injury.[670,672-675] The drug is structurally similar to captopril and there are reports of cross-reactivity.[676]
- Lisinopril has been implicated in one case of fulminant hepatic failure.[677] Other studies have also reported chronic hepatitis.[678,679]
- Fosinopril has recently been reported to have produced a case of severe, prolonged cholestasis.[680]

Hydralazine and Dihydralazine

These agents can cause hepatocellular,[681-684] cholestatic,[685] and granulomatous[686] injury and acute cholangitis[687]—all of which appear to be reversible. As with methyldopa, this drug is favored in pregnancy, and cases of hepatotoxicity have been reported in this setting.[688] There is a 3:1 female to male ratio[689] of patients reported to have experienced hepatotoxicity.

Mechanism

The sera of patients with hepatocellular type of injury contain anti-liver microsomal antibodies that are directed against cytochrome P450 1A2.[690-692] It appears that these drugs are metabolized by this enzyme into highly reactive species that in turn bind to the enzyme itself, thus creating a neo-antigen to which antibodies subsequently develop. This results in an autoimmune hepatitis-like injury. This theory therefore invokes roles by both metabolic and immune idiosyncrasies in the pathogenesis of hepatotoxicity. Acetylator status in the equilibrium between toxication and detoxication pathways has not been clearly defined.

Clinical and Laboratory Features

The interval between initiation of the drug and onset of hepatotoxicity is usually a few days to several weeks, although months or years[684] may have elapsed. In the hepatocellular-type injury, which appears to be the most common manifestation, there is marked elevation of the AST and ALT. Fever, rash, and eosinophilia may occur. Evidence of more severe liver dysfunction such as coagulopathy and encephalopathy may ensue in some cases.

Histology

Histology shows variable degrees of necrosis in a zone 3 distribution.

Management

Management consists of withdrawing the agent. There does not appear to be a role for corticosteroids.

Prognosis

Reversal of injury after cessation of the drugs is almost the rule. There are few reported fatal cases.[693]

Tienilic Acid (Ticrynafen)

Tienilic acid is a uricosuric diuretic that is no longer in clinical use.[694] A large number of cases of hepatocellular injury, including acute and chronic hepatitis and cirrhosis,[695] were reported with its use and led to its withdrawal. The syndrome of hepatotoxicity was similar to acute viral hepatitis. An immunoallergic mechanism of toxicity was postulated, as the sera of patients who developed this injury contained anti-liver kidney antibodies directed against cytochrome P450 2C9, the isoenzyme that catalyzed the 5-hydroxylation of this compound.[691,696,697]

Furosemide

Although no convincing cases of human toxicity have been reported,[698] there are experimental models in mice linking hepatotoxicity to the conversion of the parent compound to a toxic intermediate by the cytochrome P450 system.[699,700]

Thiazide Diuretics

Rare cases of hepatotoxicity have been reported. The mechanism is unclear, but probably involves a hypersensitivity reaction.[701,702]

ANTI-ARRHYTHMIC AGENTS

Quinidine

Quinidine is one of the older anti-arrhythmic agents. Beginning in the late 1960s, case reports of hepatotoxicity were reported. In one series the incidence was estimated to be as high as 6 percent.[703] One of the more consistent characteristic findings was presentation with fever[704] occurring within 1 to 2 weeks of starting treatment. Other clinical and laboratory features include the development of a rash, diarrhea, nausea, elevated aminotransferase levels, milder increases in ALP and bilirubin, and occasional eosinophilia and thrombocytopenia.[704,705] These resolve rapidly with discontinuation of the drug, but promptly recur with rechallenge.[704] Histology is variable and may include a granulomatous hepatitis,[703,706,707] and hepatocellular injury evidenced by degeneration and focal necrosis.[708] The relatively short period between initiation and the development of toxicity, many of the clinical features including fever and rash, and prompt recurrence with rechallenge all suggest that this manifestation of hepatotoxicity is a hypersensitivity reaction to the drug.[704]

Ajmaline

This quinidine-related anti-arrhythmic agent is an alkaloid derived from the root of *Rauwolfia serpentina*. Neither it nor its congener prajmaline are available for use in the United States. Experience in Europe suggests that this agent can cause an acute cholestatic injury most commonly and chronic cholestasis[709] and hepatocellular injury[710] less commonly. The onset of clinical evidence of hepatotoxicity is usually within 4 weeks of commencing the agent. Fever, chills, right upper quadrant pain, jaundice, and pruritus are typical symptoms. The presentation may mimic ascending cholangitis, secondary to choledocholithiasis.[709] Eosinophilia is common. Liver tests are consistent with cholestasis with markedly elevated ALP, GGT, and bilirubin, and lesser elevations in the aminotransferases. Thrombocytopenia and acute renal failure have been described.[711] The short duration from exposure to the development of hepatotoxicity, recurrence with rechallenge,[712,713] and the clinical and laboratory features suggest that a hypersensitivity reaction is the most likely pathogenesis.[714] Histology reveals centrolobular cholestasis, mild hepatocyte lesions, and portal inflammation.[713] Electron microscopy disclosed dilation of the endoplasmic reticulum with disorganization of the hepatocyte microfilament network. Biliary canaliculi were enlarged with absent or blunted microvilli.[715] Resolution may be slow after discontinuation of the agent, taking anywhere from 6 to 24 months,[709] but appears to be complete in most cases.[716] Persistent cholestasis 5 years after an acute episode has been described.[717]

Amiodarone

Amiodarone is an iodinated benzofuran derivative that is used to treat patients with recurrent or refractory ventricular tachyarrhythmias. It has some structural similarities to perhexiline maleate and produces a similar type of hepatotoxicity. Amiodarone causes mild, asymptomatic elevations of the aminotransferase levels in 15 percent to 82 percent of patients taking the drug.[718-723] In a prospective study 23 percent of patients developed abnormal liver tests.[723] In many of these cases, values returned to normal during treatment.[724] Clinically significant liver disease, which mimics alcoholic hepatitis, only occurs in a small subset of these patients (0.6 percent to 3 percent).[723-728] Other rarer manifestations of hepatotoxicity include Reye's syndrome,[729,730] acute hepatitis,[728,731-734] and cholestatic injury.[725,735,736]

Mechanism

Amiodarone is amphiphilic (has both polar and non-polar moieties); as a result, it possesses the ability to cause phospholipidosis. It shares this tendency with a number of other drugs, most notably perhexiline maleate and diethylaminoethoxyhexestrol. *Phospholipidosis* is the term used to describe the finding on electron microscopy of lysosomes engorged with phospholipids. These appear as striking accumulations of concentric whorled membranous arrays (myeloid figures) in lysosomes, similar to those seen in Niemann-Pick and Tay-Sachs diseases.[737] The amphipathic nature of amiodarone leads to its entrapment in lysosomes,[738] where it binds phospholipids. In addition, it inhibits phospholipases, leading to further build-up of phospholipids. The development of phospholipidosis is therefore a property of the drug and it will develop in all users given time. It is not necessarily associated with clinical hepatotoxicity.

In patients who develop clinically significant liver disease (0.6 percent to 3 percent of patients) the histology is reminiscent of alcoholic hepatitis, with steatosis (which is usually a mixture of macro- and microvesicular), focal neutrophil infiltration, perinuclear (Mallory's) hyaline, and centrizonal fibrosis. This is often referred to as pseudoalcoholic liver disease (PSALD). The mechanism by which this occurs is unclear. Amiodarone inhibits both mitochondrial beta oxidation of fatty acids and oxidative phosphorylation in animal models.[307,739] The role of cumulative doses of the drug remains controversial.[720,740] Higher serum levels of the drug and its major metabolite, desethylamiodarone, have been implicated.[732-734] In the early acute hepatitis after intravenous loading of the drug polysorbate 80, a surfactant present in the vehicle, has been suggested to be the cause of the hepatotoxic reaction.[734] Another potential source of toxicity is the propensity of amiodarone and its metabolite desethylamiodarone to inhibit various enzymes in the cytochrome P450 system, thereby altering the metabolism of various other drugs.[741,742]

Clinical and Laboratory Features

The majority of patients with phospholipidosis are asymptomatic. Symptoms of toxicity (resulting from phospholipidosis or otherwise) in other organs, including the lung, peripheral nerves, the thyroid, and the heart, may predominate. In patients who develop clinically significant hepatotoxicity, the latent period varies from 1 month to several years. When serious hepatotoxicity has occurred, liver disease developed insidiously and asymptomatically, with mild to moderate elevations in the aminotransferases and mild elevation in the ALP levels. Jaundice is unusual; weight loss is common. The most common physical finding is hepatomegaly. In those who progress to cirrhosis, clinical evidence of this may be present.[743] With significant phospholipidosis the liver may appear radiopaque on plain x-rays because of the increased iodine content. It also may have an increased density on CT scanning.[744,745] After withdrawal, the drug may take a long time to be completely eliminated from the body.[727] This may prolong idiosyncratic toxicity.[736]

Histology

The findings of phospholipidosis and PSALD were described previously. Early PSALD shows changes typical of alcoholic steatohepatitis.[746] When PSALD progresses to cirrhosis, it is micronodular, as in alcoholic cirrhosis.[737] The presence of granular cells has been noted in patients with the early acute form of hepatitis.[747,748]

Management

When significant liver disease develops, withdrawal of the agent is the logical next step. However, this is not always a simple decision because the patient's life span may be limited mainly by their underlying heart disease. Discontinuation of this potent anti-arrhythmic, which may be the only effective therapy for the patient's condition, may hasten their demise.[749] Ex vivo studies in cultured human cells suggest that vitamin E may be beneficial in the prevention of the phospholipidosis.[750,751]

Prognosis

Improvement in the hepatotoxicity may occur after withdrawal.[719,726] Fatalities as a result of continuing therapy[752] and after intravenous loading[733] have been reported. However, prognosis is complicated by co-morbid conditions and other issues in these often very ill patients.

Perhexiline Maleate

This anti-anginal agent is not available for use in the United States. It is of interest in that, as with amiodarone, it can cause phospholipidosis and PSALD. These two drugs share the chemical property of being cationic amphipathic molecules, which accumulate in lysosomes. There is a high incidence (up to 50 percent) of elevated aminotransferase levels in patients taking this drug.[753-755] The incidence of significant liver disease is probably similar to that with amiodarone.[754] Hepatotoxicity appears to depend on several factors, including plasma levels,[755] duration of intake,[756] and genetic susceptibility.[757,758] The latter is thought to be important because an inherited deficiency of cytochrome P450 2D6, the enzyme responsible for hydroxylation of perhexiline,[758] has been found in some affected patients. Weight loss is a prominent feature. The clinical and laboratory findings and the histologic abnormalities are similar to those caused by amiodarone.

Aprindine

This is a long-acting anti-arrhythmic agent. Hepatotoxicity has been noticed with its use.[759] The injury appears to be a mixture of hepatocellular, cholestatic, and mixed reactions.[760-762] Reports of onset within 3 weeks of initiation, resolution after withdrawal, and prompt recurrence with rechallenge suggest an idiosyncratic reaction with an immune basis,[762] although the mechanism remains largely unknown.

Calcium Channel Blockers

Nifedipine is a dihydropyridine calcium channel blocker. It is reported to cause a syndrome of acute liver injury.[763-765] The features of this reaction, including onset within a few days to weeks of initiation of the drug and clinical features such as fever and eosinophilia, suggest a hypersensitivity reaction. Lymphocyte sensitization tests bear this out.[766] Histology shows a portal inflammatory cell infiltrate that contains eosinophils.[764] Reversal occurs with withdrawal. A case of alcoholic hepatitis-like liver injury, with steatohepatitis and Mallory bodies, has been reported.[767]

There are a few reports of acute hepatic injury including granulomatous hepatitis that may occur with the use of diltiazem.[768-770] The presentation usually suggests an immune-mediated injury.

Verapamil is a phenylalkylamine calcium channel blocker. It has been implicated in a few instances of hepatotoxicity,[771-775] usually shortly after commencing the drug. The injury is primarily hepatocellular and, in a few instances, cholestatic.[773] The mechanism is presumed to be an idiosyncratic immune reaction,[776] although this is not known with certainty.

Procainamide

Although the more significant toxicity of this drug is SLE, it has been reported to cause an acute hepatocellular or cholestatic injury,[777-779] with features most suggestive of an immune-mediated injury, although other factors may be involved. Granulomas may be seen on histology.[778]

β-Adrenergic Blocking Agents

Labetalol

This agent is a selective α_1- and a non-selective β-adrenergic receptor antagonist. It is a relatively new beta blocker, and several instances of hepatotoxicity have been reported.[780-785] In a review of the cases presented to the FDA, 9 of 11 were women, with a median onset of 60 days after starting drug.[782] In five cases in which histology was obtained, hepatocellular necrosis was seen in four and chronic active hepatitis in one.[782] There were 3 deaths in the 11 cases. Nine of eleven cases resolved with discontinuation of the agent and one case recurred with rechallenge. The mechanism of injury remains unclear. There is minimal evidence to support an immune-mediated mechanism. One of the enantiomers of labetalol, dilevalol, is a known cause of hepatotoxicity. A hypersensitivity mechanism has been proposed to account for this observation based on the finding of lymphocyte sensitization in a patient who developed hepatotoxicity.[785]

Metoprolol

This drug is a β_1-adrenergic receptor antagonist. It is metabolized by cytochrome P450 2D6, and as a consequence it accumulates in subjects who are P450 2D6-deficient (so-called poor debrisoquine metabolizer phenotype). This fact was thought to play a role in the pathogenesis of the very rarely seen hepatotoxicity,[786] but this has not been borne out.[787] The presentation is one of acute hepatitis and recurrence with rechallenge has been seen in one case.[787]

HYPOLIPIDEMIC AGENTS

Fibrate Hypolipidemic Agents

Clofibrate can cause mildly abnormal aminotransferase levels.[788,789] This may be seen in about 10 percent of users, although concurrent creatine phosphokinase levels may be indicative of muscle damage that can also cause increases in AST.[788] There are rare reports of clinically significant hepatotoxicity including cholestasis, hepatitis, and granulomatous changes.[790-792] The fibrate hypolipidemics are known peroxisome proliferators and may cause mitochondrial damage by stimulating formation of reactive oxygen species, which eventually contribute to cell death.[793] These drugs have also been found to induce hepatocarcinogenesis in rodents,[793] but there is no evidence of carcinogenesis in humans. The drugs in this class are all lithogenic,[794] and complications related to the formation of cholesterol gallstones may occur. Cross-reactivity in the causation of hepatotoxicity has been observed between clofibrate and fenofibrate.[792]

Fenofibrate and gemfibrozil have also been implicated in episodes of cholestasis and hepatitis.[795,796]

3-Hydroxy-3-Methylglutaryl-CoA Reductase Inhibitors

The drugs in this class include atorvastatin, cerivastatin, fluvastatin, lovastatin, pravastatin, and simvastatin. Dose-related minor and reversible elevations of liver enzymes are commonly encountered (4 percent to 5 percent for simvastatin and pravastatin[797]). Serious hepatotoxic reactions are rare, but have been reported increasingly in recent years. Simvastatin has been reported to cause hepatitis, which may have predominant cholestatic features.[798-800] These presumably result from an immune idiosyncrasy.[799] Acute cholestatic hepatitis has also been reported with pravastatin[801] and with atorvastatin.[802,803] Lovastatin causes cholestatic and non-cholestatic hepatitis.[804-807] In one case, histology revealed centrolobular necrosis, centrolobular cholestasis, and infiltrates with mononuclear and polymorphonuclear cells, including eosinophils.[806] There are no reports of clinically significant hepatotoxicity with cerivastatin or fluvastin.

Niacin/Nicotinic Acid

This agent is the oldest drug used in the treatment of dyslipidemias. It has beneficial effects on low-density lipoprotein cholesterol, high-density lipoprotein cholesterol, triglycerides, and lipoprotein(a), all of which lead to a lower risk for coronary artery disease.[808] The major factor limiting widespread use has been a high incidence of side effects, including flushing and gastrointestinal discomfort. Minor elevations in serum ALT levels may accompany use.[808-811] A sustained-release preparation was developed primarily to counter flushing. Studies have shown that clinically significant hepatotoxicity (hepatitis) seems to be more common with this form of the drug than with immediate-release (crystalline) preparations.[809-811] Abnormal liver tests and clinical hepatotoxicity increase with higher doses. With crystalline niacin this is usually in excess of 4 to 5 g daily.[810] The doses that induce significant hepatotoxicity are lower for the sustained-release form of the drug.[810]

Clinical and Laboratory Features

The interval between initiation of the drug and the development of clinical hepatotoxicity is variable and in one series of patients on sustained-release niacin, symptoms developed 2 days to 7 weeks after initiation. This interval has been said to be shorter in general for sustained-release niacin than the crystalline form,[810] which tends to develop after several months of use. Clinical and laboratory presentations are usually consistent with an acute hepatitis. Unusual presentations include focal fatty infiltration and coagulopathy.[812]

Mechanism

The mechanism of toxicity is unclear. It is dose-dependent. Other factors that may contribute to the development of toxicity include alcohol use, preexisting liver disease, and concurrent oral sulfonylurea therapy.[813] Genetic factors may play a role as well; in one series, identical twin brothers and two sisters developed hepatotoxicity with sustained-release niacin.[811] There may be differences in the mechanism of toxicity for sustained-release as opposed to crystalline preparations. Patients switched from the latter preparation (on which they had no hepatotoxicity) to a sustained-release preparation developed hepatotoxicity within 2 days.[814] In support of this is the observation that patients who develop hepatotoxicity with sustained-release niacin did not have evidence of recurrent hepatocellular damage when rechallenged with crystalline niacin.[815] It has been proposed that hepatotoxicity reflects the high demand for methyl groups imposed by niacin catabolism, leading to a reduction in hepatic levels of S-adenosylmethionine.[816] The exact mechanism of injury is unknown.

Management

Management consists of withdrawal of the agent. It has been proposed that methyl group donors such as betaine may protect against hepatotoxicity.[816]

Prognosis

Reversal of injury follows discontinuation of the drug. Acute liver failure has been reported in a patient taking low-dose sustained-release niacin.[817]

Heparin

Abnormal liver tests have been reported with the use of heparin and with low-molecular weight heparin.[818-820] These are reversible with discontinuation. In a case of liver injury thought to be due to low-molecular weight heparin, serum complement 3 activity was reduced, and on histology there was ballooning degeneration with scattered foci of hepatocyte necrosis, suggesting complement-mediated hepatocellular damage.[819] A cholestatic reaction has also been described.[821]

Coumarin Derivatives

There are several reports of hepatitis resulting from the use of phenprocoumon, an oral anti-coagulant used in Europe.[822-825] The reports suggest immune idiosyncrasy as the cause.

HORMONES

Estrogens

Both natural and synthetic estrogens affect the structure and function of the liver in several important ways. In addition to their effects on intermediary metabolism estrogens appear to cause several pathologic/hepatotoxic effects. These include the following:

1. Cholestasis
2. Predisposition to cholesterol gallstone formation
3. Predisposition to hepatic tumors
4. Predisposition to Budd-Chiari syndrome
5. Predisposition to vascular tumors

Estrogen-induced Cholestasis

Estrogen has long been recognized as a cause of hepatotoxicity in man and animals.[826,827] Cholestasis of pregnancy was recognized to be due to estrogens in the late 1950s.[828-830] After the introduction of oral contraceptive pills (OCPs) in the early 1960s, reports of jaundice resulting from OCPs began to appear. It was recognized that the cholestasis of pregnancy and that of OCP use were fundamentally the result of the same pathophysiologic process, a metabolic idiosyncrasy in which estrogens impaired bile secretion. A wide variation in individual susceptibility and response to this particular impairment has been recognized. The incidence of cholestasis related to OCP use appears to be higher in Chile and Scandinavia (1:4000 as opposed to 1:10,000 elsewhere).[831-834] In Chile women of Araucanian ancestry appear to be more susceptible to cholestasis of pregnancy and to OCP-induced cholestasis.[833] Women with Dubin-Johnson syndrome and a history of cholestasis of pregnancy seem to be more susceptible to OCP-induced cholestasis.[828,835]

Mechanism. OCPs are used extensively, yet only a small fraction of users develop cholestasis. Explanations must take this and its dose dependence and genetic or ethnic predisposition into account. Estrogen and its metabolites have a number of different effects on the liver. Many of these may have some bearing on the pathogenesis of cholestasis. Estrogens interfere with the secretion of bromosulphthalein (BSP) into bile.[836] The structure of the estrogen molecule may have some bearing on its ability to produce cholestasis. One group found that oxygen in the C3 position led to greater inhibition of BSP secretion into bile.[837,838] Subsequent studies have shown that D-ring glucuronides are more likely to cause dose-dependent cholestasis and inhibition of bile flow than are A-ring glucuronides or D-ring glucuronides with A-ring sulfation.[839,840] An interesting observation in support of these experimental findings is that women with cholestasis of pregnancy have a relative decrease in A-ring glucuronides and an increase in D-ring glucuronides.[841] Sulfation of the A-ring may be an important step in decreasing the cholestatic potential of the D-ring glucuronides, and a decrease (e.g, resulting from a decrease in sulfate supply or an enzyme deficiency) may predispose individuals to cholestasis. This remains unproven.

The mechanism by which estrogen or its metabolites cause cholestasis is unclear. There is evidence to suggest that these steroid hormones can directly alter the physical properties and function of the hepatocyte membrane. Estrogens increase the cholesterol ester content of the membrane by increasing cholesterol uptake and increasing lecithin-cholesterol acyltransferase activity.[842,843] The increased content of cholesterol esters leads to an increase in membrane fluidity and impaired Na^+/K^+-ATPase activity.[843,844] These effects can be reversed by the non-ionic detergent Triton WR-1339.[845] Estrogen-induced changes in the hepatic plasma membranes are localized predominantly to the basolateral (sinusoidal) surfaces of the cell, and the decrease in the membrane fluidity and decrease in activity of the Na^+/K^+-ATPase are therefore observed on the sinusoidal surface rather than on the canalicular surface.[845] Whether these changes are important in pathogenesis remains to be elucidated. The observation that spironolactone also decreases membrane fluidity and the activity of Na^+/K^+-ATPase, but actually increases bile flow as opposed to estrogens, argues against this being the sole or major factor in the pathogenesis of cholestasis.[846] It has been suggested that cholestasis induced by estrogen metabolites is a result of impaired bile acid transport. However, it appears that bile acids and estrogen glucuronides are transported into the hepatocyte by different carrier systems so that the cholestasis induced by the estrogen D-ring glucuronides cannot be explained by an inhibition of bile acid uptake.[847] The bile salt sodium taurocholate has been shown in experiments in vitro to prevent estrogen D-ring glucuronide-induced cholestasis.[848] The reason for this is not known. S-adenosyl-L-methionine, a methyl donor, has been observed to suppress the cholestatic effect of ethynylestradiol in animal studies. This is thought to result from conversion of ethynylestradiol into its methyl-derivatives.[849] S-adenosyl-L-methionine has been found in one study to improve pruritus and to decrease serum bilirubin and bile salts in women with cholestasis of pregnancy.[850] This was not confirmed in a subsequent placebo-controlled study,[851] and S-adenosyl-L-methionine is therefore not of therapeutic importance.

In summary, estrogen has many effects on the liver that can potentially lead to cholestasis. Given the fact that pregnancy-induced cholestasis and OCP-induced cholestasis rarely occur, the possibility of a genetic susceptibility factor has to be considered. Population-based linkage disequilibrium screening suggests that there may be a novel cholestasis-associated gene located on chromosome 2. Whatever this abnormality is, it probably allows the increased formation of a metabolite of estrogen, such as the D-ring glucuronides. This in turn, by mechanisms yet to be clearly defined, decreases bile acid–independent bile flow and causes cholestasis.

Clinical and Laboratory Features. Cholestasis usually appears within the first few months of OCP use. Jaundice, pruritus, pale stools, and dark urine are the typical findings. Constitutional symptoms such as malaise and fatigue may occur, but are rare. Fever, rash, arthralgia, and other evidence of an immunoallergic reaction are notably absent. On physical exam, jaundice and scleral icterus are found. Spider angiomata may be prominent. Hepatomegaly is rare. Unconjugated hyperbilirubinemia is the typical laboratory finding. Mild elevations in the serum ALP and aminotransferases may occur. Prothrombin time is normal.

Histology. The typical descriptor used is bland cholestasis. There is canalicular and hepatocellular bile accumulation, with minimal other findings. There tends to be little or no inflammation or evidence of hepatocellular necrosis. The cholestasis tends to be more pronounced in the perivenular regions of the hepatic lobule. Ultrastructural changes include dilation of the smooth endoplasmic reticulum and abnormally shaped mitochondria containing paracrystalline material.[852]

Management. Discontinuation of the agent leads to reversal in about 2 months in almost all cases. Testing to rule out chronic biliary diseases such as primary biliary cirrhosis should be pursued if normalization does not occur after a reasonable time.

Prognosis. Prognosis is good for complete reversal with discontinuation. Patients with OCP-induced cholestasis may be at increased risk for the development of pregnancy-induced cholestasis (discussed in another section).

Predisposition to Gallstones

The predisposition to gallstones is described in detail elsewhere in this textbook (see Chap. 59). There is convincing evidence that the incidence of gallstones is higher in users of OCPs and in postmenopausal women on hormone replacement therapy.[853-857] This may be a result of decreased gallbladder contractility[858,859] or increased saturation of the bile by cholesterol.[860,861] The latter effect appears to be reversed by S-adenosyl-L-methionine.[862] The primary importance of the association between gallstones and estrogen use is that cholelithiasis should be considered in patients on estrogen therapy who present with jaundice.

Predisposition to Hepatic Tumors

Hepatic tumors are described in greater detail elsewhere in this textbook (see Chap. 45) and in the introductory section of this chapter. The relationship between hepatic tumors and estrogens was first suggested in the early 1970s.[863] Since then many reports of hepatic tumors related to the use of estrogen preparations have been made. The tumors that have been associated with estrogen use include hepatic adenomas, focal nodular hyperplasia, hepatocellular carcinoma—including the fibrolamellar variant of hepatocellular carcinoma—and hemangioendotheliomas. They usually develop after long-term use of these agents.

Predisposition to Budd-Chiari Syndrome and Other Vascular Tumors

The use of estrogen preparations has long been reported[864] to be an etiologic factor in the pathogenesis of Budd-Chiari syndrome (see Chap. 53). Many cases have been reported.[865-872] In the more recent reports many of the patients, in addition to using oral contraceptives, were found to also have one of the various relatively newly discovered coagulation defects that predispose to intravascular clotting.[869] These include the factor V Leiden mutation, prothrombin gene mutation, and inherited deficiencies of protein C, protein S, and anti-thrombin. It is therefore important that an evaluation for these disorders be performed in all patients on estrogen preparations who are diagnosed with Budd-Chiari syndrome. Other vascular syndromes that have been described in association with estrogen use include peliosis hepatis,[873,874] hepatic infarction,[874,875] and unilobular hepatic vein obstruction.[876]

Tamoxifen

Tamoxifen is an estrogen receptor antagonist with partial agonist activity. It has become the treatment of choice for estrogen receptor–positive breast cancer. Cases with intrahepatic cholestasis have been described.[877] More recently, however, many case reports of NASH, which can progress to cirrhosis, have been reported.[878-884] In one study 40 of 104 patients developed steatosis (by CT imaging) within the first 2 years of using tamoxifen.[882] Of these 40, 21 had abnormal transaminases, and 6 of 7 patients with imaging evidence of steatosis who underwent liver biopsy had NASH.[882] A case of submassive necrosis has been described.[884]

Androgens and Anabolic Steroids

These drugs are used legitimately for medical treatment of aplastic anemia, male impotence, female transsexualism, and other conditions. They are also used illicitly by body builders and other athletes for muscle enhancement.[885] Adverse effects are therefore seen more commonly than one would otherwise expect, although the incidence is much less than that seen with estrogen-based drugs.

A bland cholestasis similar to that seen with the use of estrogen-based preparations and in the cholestasis of pregnancy can occur, usually after short-term use. Hepatic tumors and vascular lesions may occur after use for longer durations.[886,887]

Cholestasis

As is the case with estrogens, the cholestasis caused by anabolic steroids such as methyltestosterone is believed to be due to an intrinsic hepatotoxic effect, possibly mediated by metabolic idiosyncrasy.

Mechanism. Cholestasis is seen far more commonly with synthetic androgens such as methyltestosterone and norethandrolone. These have alpha substitutions at the 17-carbon (D-ring), as opposed to testosterone and its esters, which do not have the alpha substitution, and rarely if ever cause cholestasis.[888] The 7alpha-alkylated steroids seem to be implicated most often in hepatotoxicity (cholestasis and tumors). As with estrogens, the exact mechanism of cholestasis is incompletely understood.

Clinical and Laboratory Features. Features are similar to those seen with estrogens. Occasionally severe cholestasis may occur.[889]

Histology. Hisotology is similar to that described for estrogens.

Management. Resolution with withdrawal of the drug is the rule. However, some cases may take a long time, and an anecdotal report suggests that treatment with ursodeoxycholic acid may lead to improvement.[890]

Peliosis Hepatis

This unusual condition, as described earlier, is characterized by blood-filled spaces within the hepatic parenchyma that may or may not be lined with sinusoidal endothelium. It has been associated with the chronic administration of anabolic steroids.[891-899]

Clinical Features. Many cases of peliosis hepatis are asymptomatic or may have hepatomegaly; others are found incidentally at autopsy. Clinically they may manifest as liver failure.[899] Rarely they may present with evidence of an intraperitoneal bleed.[891]

Mechanism. Based on the histologic appearance, it has been suggested that the primary process may be hepatocyte hyperplasia, (perhaps caused by the anabolic effect of methyltestosterone) that causes nodules and tumors and formation of cysts through mechanical obstruction of hepatic veins.[900] Obstruction of the hepatic veins may occur as a result of accumulation of hepatocytes between the endothelium and the supporting collagen of the hepatic veins.[900] However, the exact mechanism is unknown.

Prognosis. If peliosis hepatis is diagnosed antemortem, withdrawal of toxic drug has led to reversal of this lesion.[899]

Hepatic Tumors

Tumors that can develop include hepatic adenomas, hepatocellular carcinoma, and hepatic angiosarcoma.[901-907] The pathogenesis (which is presumably the same for estrogens) probably involves cell proliferation induced by these hormones with resultant increased sensitivity to subthreshold doses of carcinogens and enhanced clonal expansion of preneoplastic cells.

ORAL HYPOGLYCEMICS

Oral hypoglycemics have been used for more than 40 years in the treatment of diabetes mellitus. They have an excellent record of safety. Sulfonylureas were the first class of compounds to be developed and, although infrequent, hepatic injury has been seen.[908] With the sulfonylureas cholestasis has been the principal manifestation of injury, with hepatocellular-type injury being less common. One sulfonylurea, metahexamide, was removed from the market because of hepatotoxicity.[908] There is some uncertainty as to the role of sulfonylureas in some case reports because a rechallenge was not associated with a recurrence of jaundice in several patients.[909] Other agents used to treat diabetes also rarely cause liver injury.[908] This situation changed with the development of a peroxisome proliferator-activator receptor agonist (PPAR-gamma), however.

PPAR-gamma Receptor Agonists (Troglitazone)

PPAR-gamma receptor agonists are a new type of oral agent used for treating diabetes mellitus. The drug is thought to act by increasing peripheral insulin sensitivity. The first of this type of drug to be developed was troglitazone (Rezulin). During clinical trials, 2 percent of patients developed elevated liver tests and some developed jaundice.[910] After release of the drug there were numerous reports of severe hepatic injury and some deaths, leading to withdrawal of the drug, first in England and then in the United States.

Patients present with evidence of liver dysfunction about 4 to 10 months after the start of treatment with troglitazone.[911-914] They may present with jaundice or symptoms of acute hepatitis. Most of the reported cases occurred in women. Patients were frequently taking other diabetes medications as well.

Mechanism

The mechanism by which troglitazone causes liver injury is unknown. Given the lack of other features of an immune-mediated injury and the infrequency of the event, it is most likely due to a metabolic idiosyncrasy.

Laboratory Findings

Liver tests are abnormal, with elevated serum aminotransferase (hundreds to less than 2000 IU/liter) and ALP levels. Serum bilirubin levels may be quite high (more than 20 mg/dl) in some cases. In more severe cases a significant coagulopathy may develop as well as other features of hepatic failure.

Histology

The liver biopsy shows submassive hepatic necrosis with cholestasis. Portal areas contain a mild infiltrate of chronic inflammatory cells.

Management

Troglitazone has been withdrawn from the market in the United States but may be found in other countries. Patients taking troglitazone should be switched to another medication. If there is evidence of liver injury, the drug should be discontinued immediately.

Prognosis

Troglitazone caused severe hepatic injury in many patients, leading to death or liver transplantation in a few. If the injury resolves with discontinuation of the drug, complete recovery is expected. However, long-term follow-up of these patients is lacking, so it remains unclear whether the liver returns completely to normal.

Other PPAR-gamma Agonists

Other PPAR-gamma agonists that have been developed for the treatment of diabetes mellitus are rosiglitazone (Avandia) and pioglitazone. The frequency of liver injury from these two newer agents appears to be significantly less than with troglitazone. However, liver injury and fatal liver failure have been reported with rosiglitazone.[915] Because of the risk of liver injury the manufacturer recommends monitoring of AST and ALT levels every 2 months during the first 12 months of therapy. If the aminotransferase levels increase to more than three times the upper limit of normal the drug should be discontinued.

References

1. Ames BN, Profet M, Gold LS: Nature's chemicals and synthetic chemicals: comparative toxicology. Proc Natl Acad Sci U S A 87:7782, 1990.
2. Ames BN, Profet M, Gold LS: Dietary pesticides (99.99% all natural). Proc Natl Acad Sci U S A 87:7777, 1990.
3. Lucena MI, Camargo R, Andrade RJ, et al: Comparison of two clinical scales for causality assessment in hepatotoxicity. Hepatology 33:123, 2001.
4. Schiodt FV, Atillasoy E, Shakil AO, et al: Etiology and prognosis for 295 patients with acute liver failure. Gastroenterology 112:A1376, 1997.
5. Jick H, Walker AM, Porter J: Drug-induced liver disease. J Clin Pharmacol 21:359, 1981.
6. Bjorneboe M, Iversen O, Olsen S: Infective hepatitis and toxic jaundice in a municipal hospital during a five-year period. Incidence and prognosis. Acta Med Scand 182:491, 1967.
7. Friis H, Andreasen PB: Drug-induced hepatic injury: an analysis of 1100 cases reported to the Danish Committee on Adverse Drug Reactions between 1978 and 1987. J Intern Med 232:133, 1992.
8. Rawson NS, Pearce GL, Inman WH: Prescription-event monitoring: methodology and recent progress. J Clin Epidemiol 43:509, 1990.
9. Inman WH, Rawson NS: Erythromycin estolate and jaundice. BMJ 286:1954, 1983.
10. Jick SS: The risk of gastrointestinal bleed, myocardial infarction, and newly diagnosed hypertension in users of meloxicam, diclofenac, naproxen, and piroxicam. Pharmacotherapy 20:741, 2000.
11. Haria M, Bryson HM, Goa KL: Itraconazole. A reappraisal of its pharmacological properties and therapeutic use in the management of superficial fungal infections. Drugs 51:585, 1996.

12. Garcia Rodriguez LA, Wallander MA, Stricker BH: The risk of acute liver injury associated with cimetidine and other acid-suppressing anti-ulcer drugs. Br J Clin Pharmacol 43:183, 1997.
13. Jones JK, Van de Carr SW, Zimmerman H, et al: Hepatotoxicity associated with phenothiazines. Psychopharmacol Bull 19:24, 1983.
14. Garcia Rodriguez LA, Williams R, Derby LE, et al: Acute liver injury associated with nonsteroidal anti-inflammatory drugs and the role of risk factors. Arch Intern Med 154:311, 1994.
15. Jick H, Derby LE, Garcia Rodriguez LA, et al: Nonsteroidal antiinflammatory drugs and certain rare, serious adverse events: a cohort study. Pharmacotherapy 13:212, 1993.
16. Stricker BHCH: Drug-induced Hepatic Injury, ed 2. Amsterdam, Elsevier, 1992.
17. Hutchinson TA, Lane CA: Assessing methods for causality assessment of suspected adverse drug reactions. J Clin Epidemiol 42:5, 1989.
18. Standardization of definitions and criteria of causality assessment of adverse drug reactions. Drug-induced liver disorders: report of an international consensus meeting. Int J Clin Pharmacol Ther Toxicol 28:317, 1990.
19. Danan G, Benichou C, Flahault A: [Score of suspected drug-induced acute liver disorders. Presentation of an evaluation sheet]. Gastroenterol Clin Biol 17:H22, 1993.
20. Watson RG, Olomu A, Clements D, et al: A proposed mechanism for chlorpromazine jaundice—defective hepatic phoxidation combined with rapid hydroxylation. J Hepatol 7:72, 1988.
21. Spielberg SP: In vitro assessment of pharmacogenetic susceptibility to toxic drug abolites in humans. Federation Proc 43:2308, 1984.
22. Warnet JM, Claude JR, Truhaut R: [Experimental biological toxicology of white sphorus]. Eur J Toxicol Hyg Environ 6:57, 1973 (review).
23. Laqueur GL, Spatz M: Toxicology of cycasin. Cancer Res 28:2262, 1968 (review).
24. Asahina S, Friedman MA, Arnold E, et al: Acute synergistic toxicity and hepatic necrosis following oral inistration of sodium nitrite and secondary amines to mice. Cancer Res 31:1201, 1971.
25. Loeppky RN, Li YE: Nitrosamine activation and detoxication through free radicals and their ived cations. IARC Sci Publ 105:375, 1991.
26. Wrighton SA, VandenBranden M, Ring BJ: The human drug metabolizing cytochromes P450. J Pharmacokinet Biopharm 24:461, 1996.
27. Comstock GW, Edwards PQ: The competing risks of tuberculosis and hepatitis for young adult tuberculin reactors. Am Rev Respir Dis 111:572, 1975.
28. Rhumack RH, Mathew H: Acetaminophen and toxicity. Pediatrics 55:871, 1975.
29. Zimmmerman HJ, Ishak KG: Valproate-induced hepatic injury: analysis of 23 fatal cases. Hepatology 2:592, 1982.
30. Rikans LE: Influence of aging on chemically induced hepatotoxicity: role of age-related changes in metabolism. Drug Metab Rev 20:87, 1989.
31. Davis J: Liver damage due to tetracycline and its relationship to pregnancy. In Meyler PH, ed: Drug-induced Diseases. Amsterdam, Excerpta Medica Foundation, 1968:103.
32. Zimmerman HJ: Hepatoxicity ed 2. Philadelphia, Lippincott Williams & Wilkins, 1999.
33. Liano F, Moreno A, Matesanz R: Veno-occlusive disease of the liver in renal transplantation: is azathioprine the cause? Nephron 51:501, 1989.
34. Calvert DN, Brody TM: The effects of thyroid function upon carbon tetrachloride hepatoxicity. J Pharmacol Exp Ther 134:30, 1961.
35. Lauterburg BH Velez ME: Glutathione deficiency in alcoholics: risk factor for paracetamol hepatotoxicity. Gut 29:1153, 1988.
36. Gordin FM, Simon GL, Wofsy CB, et al: Adverse reactions to trimethoprim-sulfamethoxazole in patients with the acquired immunodeficiency syndrome. Ann Intern Med 100:495, 1984.
37. Leoung GS, Mills J, Hopewell PC, et al: Dapsone-trimethoprim for *Pneumocystis carinii* pneumonia in acquired immune deficiency syndrome. Ann Intern Med 105:45, 1986.
38. Zimmerman HJ: Effects of aspirin and acetaminophen on the liver. Arch Intern Med 141:333, 1981.
39. Lewis JH, Schiff EF: Methotrexate-induced chronic liver injury: guidelines for detection and prevention. Am J Gastroenterol 88:1337, 1988.
40. Sotoniemi E, Hokkanen O, Keipeinen WJ: Hepatic injury and multiple drug treatment. Ann Clin Res 3:200, 1971.
41. Cohen CD, Sayed AR, Kirsh RE: Hepatic complications of antituberculous therapy revisited. S Afr Med J 63:138, 1983.
42. Zimmerman HJ: Effects of alcohol on other hepatotoxins. Alcohol: Clin Exp Res 10:3, 1986 (review).
43. Benjamin SE, Goodman ZD, Ishak KG, et al: The morphologic spectrum of halothane-induced hepatic injury. Hepatology 5:1163, 1985.
44. Rosser BG, Gores GJ: Liver cell necrosis: cell mechanisms and clinical implications. Gastroenterology 108:252, 1995.
45. Bioulac-Sage P, Quinton A, Saric J, et al: Chance discovery of hepatic fibrosis in patient with asymptomatic hypervitaminosis A. Arch Pathol Lab Med 112:505, 1988.
46. Guarascio P, Portmann B, Visco G, Williams R: Liver damage with reversible vitamin A intoxication: demonstration of Ito cells. J Clin Pathol 36:769, 1983.
47. Babb R, Kieraldo JH: Cirrhosis due to hypervitaminosis A. West Med J 128:244, 1978.
48. Guigui B Perrot S, Berry JP et al: Amiodarone induced hepatic phospholipoidosis. A morphological alteration independent of pseudo-alcoholic liver disease. Hepatology 8:1063, 1988.
49. Roberts RK, Cohn D, Petroff V, Senevirante B: Liver disease induced by perhexiline maleate. Med J Aust 2:553, 1981.
50. Kopelman H: The Epping jaundice after two years. Postgrad Med J44:78, 1968.
51. Kopelman H, Robertson MH, Sanders PG, et al: The Epping jaundice. BMJ 5486:514, 1966.
52. Kaplowitz N: Causality assessment versus guilt-by-association in drug hepatotoxicity. Hepatology 33:308, 2001.
53. HJZimmerman: Acetaminophen hepatotoxicity. Clin Liver Dis 2:523, 1998.
54. Davidson DG Eastham WN: Acute liver necrosis following overdose of paracetamol. BMJ 2:497, 1966.
55. Brotodihardjo AE, Batey RG, Farrell P, et al: Hepatotoxicity from paracetamol self poisoning in Western Sydney: a continuing challenge. Med J Aust 157:382, 1992.
56. Makin AJWendon J, Wiliams R: A 7 year experience of severe acetaminophen-induced hepatotoxicity (1987-1993). Gastroenterology 109:1907, 1995.
57. Litovitz TL, et al: 1999 AAPCC Annual Report. Am J Emerg Med 18:560, 2000.
58. Nelson SD: Molecular mechanisms of the hepatotoxicity caused by acetaminophen. Semin Liver Dis 10:267, 1990.
59. Vermeulen NP, Bessems JG, Van de Straat R: Molecular aspects of paracetamol-induced hepatotoxicity and its mechanism-based treatment. Drug Metab Rev 24:367, 1992.
60. Clements JA, Critchley JAJ, Prescott LF: The role of sulphate conjugation in the metabolism and disposition of oral and intravenous paracetamol in man. Br J Clin Pharm 18:481, 1984.
61. Hjelle JJ: Hepatic UDP-glucuronic acid regulation during acetaminophen biotransformation in rats. Pharmacol Exp Ther 237:750, 1986.
62. Pumford NR, Roberts DW, Benson RW, Hinson JA: Immunochemical quantitation of 3-(cystein-S-yl) acetaminophen protein adducts insubcellular fractions in a hepatotoxic dose of acetaminophen. Biochem Pharmacol 40:573, 1990.
63. Bartolone JB, Birge RB, Bulera SJ, et al: Purification, antibody production and partial amino acid sequence of the 58-kDa acetaminophen-binding proteins. Toxicol Appl Pharmacol 113:19, 1992.
64. Jollow DJ, Mitchell JR, Potter WZ, et al: Acetaminophen induced hepatic hecrosis. Role of covalent binding in-vitro. J Pharm Ther 187:195, 1973.
65. Gerson RJ, Casini A, Gilfor D, et al: Oxygen mediated cell injury in the killing of cultured hepatocytes by acetaminophen. Biochem Biophys Res Commun 126:1127, 1985.
66. Kamiyama T, Sato C, Liu J, et al: Role of lipid perioxidation in acetaminophen-induced hepatotoxicity: comparison with carbon tetrachloride. Toxicol Lett 77:7, 1993.
67. Smith CV, Mitchell JR: Acetaminophen toxicity in vivo is not accompanied by oxidant stress. Biochem Biophys Res Commun 133:329, 1985.
68. Moore M, Thor H, Moore G, et al: The toxicity of acetaminophen and N-acetyl-p-benzoquinone imine in isolated hepatocytes is associated with thiol depletion and increased cytosolic Ca^{2+}. J Biol Chem 260:13035, 1985.

69. Critchley JA, Nimmo GR, Gregson CA, et al: Inter-subject and ethnic differences in paracetamol metabolism. Br JClin Pharm 22:649, 1986.
70. Miller RP, Roberts RJ, Fischer LJ: Acetaminophen elimination kinetics in neonates, children and adults. Clin Pharmacol Ther 19:284, 1976.
71. Johnston SC, Pelletier LL: Enhanced hepatotoxicity of acetaminophen in the alcoholic patient. Medicine 76:185, 1997.
72. Leist MH, Gluskin LE, Payne JA: Enhanced toxicity of acetaminophen in alcoholics: report of thre cases. J Clin Gastroenterol 7:55, 1985.
73. Lauterberg BH, Velez ME: Glutathione deficiency in alcoholics: risk factor for paracetamol hepatotoxicity. Gut 29:1153, 1988.
74. Thomas SHL: Paracetamol (acetaminophen) poisoning. Pharmacol Ther 60:91, 1993.
75. Murphy R, Swartz R, Watkins PB: Severe acetaminophen toxicity in a patient receiving isoniazid. Ann Intern Med 113:799, 1990.
76. Rumack BH: Acetaminophen overdose. Am J Med 75(suppl):104, 1983.
77. Meredith TJ, Prescott LF, Vale JA: Why do patients still die from paracetamol poisoning? BMJ 293:345, 1986.
78. Jones AF, Vale JA: Paracetamol poisoning of the kidney. J Clin Pharmacol Ther 18:5, 1993.
79. Schiodt FV, Rochling FA, Casey DL: Acetaminophen toxicity in an urban county hospital. N Engl J Med 337:1112, 1997.
80. Barker JD Jr, de Carle DJ, Anuras S: Chronic excessive acetaminophen use and liver damage. Ann Intern Med 87:299, 1977.
81. Bonokowsky HL, Mudge GH, McMurtry RJ: Chronic hepatic inflammation and fibrosis due to low doses of paracetamol. Lancet 1:1016, 1978.
82. Prescott LF: Paracetamol overdosage: pharmacological considerations and clinical management. Drugs 25:290, 1983.
83. Vale JA, Meredith TJ, Goulding R: Treatment of acetaminophen poisoning: the use of oral methionone. Arch Intern Med 141:394, 1981.
84. Piperno E, Berssenbruegge DA: Reversal of experimental paracetamol toxicosis with N-acetylcysteine. Lancet 2:738, 1976.
85. Prescott LF, Illingsworth RN, Critchley JAJH, et al: Intravenous N-acetylcysteine: the treatment of choice for paracetamol poisoning. BMJ 2:1097, 1979.
86. Smilkstein MJ, Knapp GL, Kulig KW, et al: Efficacy of oral N-acetylcysteine in the treatment of acetaminophen toxicity. Analysis of the national multicenter study. N Engl J Med 319:1577, 1988.
87. Rumack BH, Peterson RG, Koch GC, et al: Acetaminophen overdosage: 622 cases with evaluation of oral N-acetylcysteine treatment. Arch Intern Med 141:380, 1981.
88. Yip L, Dart RC, Hurlbut KM: Intravenous administration of N-acetylcysteine. Crit Care Med 26:40, 1998.
89. Harrison PM, Keays R, Bray GP, et al: Improved outcome of paracetamol induced fulminant hepatic failure by late administration of acetylcysteine. Lancet 335:1572, 1990.
90. Prescott LF, Critchley JAJH: The treatment of acetaminophen poisoning. Ann Rev Pharm Toxicol 23:87, 1983.
91. Speeg KV: Potential use of cimetidine for treatment of acetaminophen overdose. Pharmacotherapy 7:125s, 1987.
92. Kaufenberg AJ, Shererd MF: Role of cimetidine in the treatment of acetaminophen poisoning. Am J Health Syst Pharmacol 55:1516, 1998.
93. Rolband GC, Marcuard SP: Cimetidine in the treatment of acetaminophen overdose. J Clin Gastroenterol 13:79, 1991.
94. Jackson JE: Cimetidine protects against acetaminophen toxicity. Life Sci 5:31, 1982.
95. Burkhart KK, Janco N, Kulig KW, et al: Cimetidine as adjunctive treatment for acetaminophen poisoning. Human Exp Toxicol 14:299, 1995.
96. Zimmermann HJ: Effects of aspirin and acetaminophen on the liver. Arch Intern Med 141:333, 1981.
97. Lewis JH: NSAID induced hepatotoxicity. Clin Liver Dis 2:543, 1998.
98. Seaman WE, Plotz PH: Effect of aspirin on liver tests in patients with RA and SLE and in normal volunteers. Arthr Rheum 19:155, 1976.
99. Martens ME, Chang CH, Lee CP: Reye's syndrome: mitochondrial swelling and calcium release induced by Reye's plasma, allantoin, and salicylate. Arch Biochem Biophys 244:773, 1986.
100. Deschamps D, Fisch C, Fromenty B, et al: Inhibition by salicylic acid of the activation of and thus oxidation of long chain fatty acids. Possible role in the development of Reye's symdrome. J Pharmacol Exp Ther 259:694, 1991.
101. Glascow JFT, Moore R: Reye's syndrome 30 years on. BMJ 307:950, 193.
102. Ulshen MH, Grand RJ, Crain JD, et al: Hepatotoxicity with encephalopathy associated with aspirin therapy in rheumatoid arthritis. J Pediatr 93:1034, 1978.
103. Scully RE, Galdabini JJ, McNeely BU: Case records of the Massachusetts General Hospital: case 23-1977. N Engl J Med 296:1337, 1977.
104. Carson JL, Strom BL, Duff A, et al: Safety of nonsteroidal anti-inflammatory drugs with respect to acute liver disease. Arch Intern Med 153:1331, 1993.
105. Garcia Rodriguez LA, Perez Gutthann S, Walker AM, et al: The role of non-steroidal anti-inflammatory drugs in acute liver injury (erratum appears in BMJ 305(6859):920, 1992). BMJ 305(6858):865, 1992.
106. Bush TM, Shlotzhauer TL, Imai K: Nonsteroidal anti-inflammatory drugs. Proposed guidelines for monitoring toxicity. West J Med 155:39, 1991.
107. Adebajo AO, Eastmond CJ: Hepatotoxicity to several nonsteroidal anti-inflammatory drugs with diclofenac induced histological changes. Clin Rheumatol 11:120, 1992.
108. Cook DJ, Achong MR, Murphy FR: Three cases of difliunisal hypersensitivity. Can Med Assoc J 138:1029, 1988.
109. Warren NS: Diflunisal induced cholestatic jaundice. BMJ 2:736, 1978.
110. Symon DN, Gray ES, Mammer OJ, et al: Fatal paracetamol poisoning from benorylate therapy in a child with cystic fibrosis. Lancet 2:1153, 1982.
111. Cuthbert MF: Adverse reactions to nonsteroidal anti-inflammatory drugs. Curr Med Res Opin 2:12, 1974.
112. Kelsey WM, Scharyj M: Fatal hepatitis probably due to indomethacin. JAMA 199:154, 1967.
113. Jacobs JS: Sudden death in arthritic children treated with large doses of indomethacin. JAMA 199:923, 1967.
114. Tarazi E, Harter JG, Zimmermann HJ, et al: Sulindac-associated hepatic injury. Analysis of 91 cases reported to the FDA. Gastroenterology 104:569, 1992.
115. McIndoe GAJ, Menzies KW, Reddy J: Sulindac (Clinoril) and cholestatic jaundice. N Z Med J 94:430, 1981.
116. Dhand AK, LaBrecque DR, Metzger J: Sulindac (Clinoril) hepatitis. Gastroenterology 80:585, 1981.
117. Whittaker SJ, Amar JN, Wanless IR, et al: Sulindac hepatotoxicity. Gut 23:875, 1982.
118. Klein SM, Muhammad AK: Hepatitis, toxic epidermal necrolysis and pancreatitis in association with sulindac therapy. J Rheumatol 10:1983, 1983.
119. Terazi E, Harter JG, Zimmermann HJ, et al: Sulindac-associated hepatic injury. Analysis of 91 cases reported to the FDA. Gastroenterology 104:569, 1992.
120. Banks AT, Ishak KG, Zimmermann HJ, et al: Diclofenac-associated hepatotoxicity: analysis of 180 cases reported to the Food and Drug Administration. Hepatology 22:820, 1995.
121. Bhogaraju A, Nazeer S, Al-Baghdadi Y, et al: Diclofenac associated hepatitis. South Med J 92:711, 1999.
122. Scully LJ, Clark D, Barr RJ: Diclofenac induced hepatitis: 3 cases with features of autoimmune chronic active hepatitis. Dig Dis Sci 38:744, 1993.
123. Islam S, Mekhloufi F, Paul JM, et al: Characteristics of clometacin-induced hepatitis with special reference to the presence of anti-actin cable antibodies. Autoimmunity 2:213, 1989.
124. Pariente EA, Hamoud A, Goldfain D, et al: Hepatitis caused by clometacin (Duperan). Retrospective study of 30 cases. A model for autoimmune drug-induced hepatitis. Gastroenterol Clin Biol 13:769, 1989.
125. Mabee CL, Mabee SW, Baker PB, et al: Fulminant hepatic failure associated with etodolac use. Am J Gastroenterol 90:659, 1995.
126. Taggart HM, Alderdice JM: Fatal cholestatic jaundice in elderly patients taking benoxaprofen. BMJ 284:1372, 1982.
127. Fancourt GJ, Adams H, Walls J, et al: Fatal self-poisoning with benoxaprofen. Human Toxicol 3:517, 1984.
128. Cuthbert MF: Adverse reactions to non-steroidal antirheumatic drugs. Curr Med Res Opin 2:600, 1974.
129. Friis H, Andreasen PB: Drug-induced hepatic injury: an analysis of 1100 cases reported to the Danish Committee on Adverse Drug Reactions between 1978 and 1987. J Int Med 232:95, 1992.

130. Thompson M, Stephenson P, Percy JS: Ibufenac in the treatment of arthritis. Ann Rheum Dis 23:397, 1964.
131. Bravo JF, Jacobson MP, Mertens BF: Fatty liver and pleural effusions associated with ibuprofen therapy. J Pediatr 90:651, 1977.
132. Lee CY, Finkler A: Acute intoxication due to ibuprofen overdose. Arch Path Lab Med 110:747, 1986.
133. Riley TR, Smith JP: Ibuprofen-induced hepatotoxicity in patients with chronic hepatitis C: a case series. Am J Gastroenterol 93:1563, 1998.
134. Alam I, Ferrel LD, Bass NB: Vanishing bile duct syndrome associated with ibuprofen use. Am J Gastroenterol 91:1626, 1996.
135. Victorino RMM, Silveira JCB, Baptista A, et al: Jaundice associated with naprosyn. Postgrad Med 56:368, 1980.
136. Depla AC, Vermeersch PH, van Gorp LH, et al: Fatal acute liver failure associated with pirprofen. Report of a case and a review of the literature. Neth J Med 37:32, 1990.
137. Danan G, Trunet P, Bernuau J: Pirprofen-induced fulminant hepatitis. Gastroenterology 89:210, 1985.
138. Becker A, Hoffmeister RT: Fenbufen, a new non-steroidal antiinflammatory agent in rheumatoid arthritis, its efficacy and toxicity. J Int Med Res 8:333, 1980.
139. Flamenbaum M, Abergel A, Marcato N, et al: Regressive fulminant hepatitis, acute pancreatitis and renal insufficiency after taking ketoprofen. Gastroenterol Clin Biol 22:975, 1998.
140. Nores JM, Rambaud S, Remy JM: Acute hepatitis due to ketoprofen. Clin Rheum 10:215, 1991.
141. Kethu SR, Rukkannagari S, Lansford CL: Oxaprozin-induced symptomatic hepatotoxicity. Ann Pharmacother 33:942, 1999.
142. Marsepoil T, Levesque P, Agard D, et al: [Hepatonephritis caused by piroxicam]. Gastroenterol Clin Biol 11(10):712, 1987.
143. Ollagnon HO, Perpoint B, Decousus H, et al: Hepatitis induced by isoxicam. Hepatogastroenterology 33(3):109, 1986.
144. Perez-Aguilar F, Berenguer M, Ramirez-Palanca JJ, et al: [Chronic autoimmune hepatitis following cholestatic hepatitis caused by droxicam]. Med Clin 106(12):460, 1996.
145. Berenguer M, Perez-Aguilar F, Gisbert C, et al: [Droxicam-induced toxic hepatitis]. Rev Esp Enferm Dig 88(1):49, 1996.
146. Ferrer A, Buenestado J, Rene JM, et al: [Acute cholestatic hepatitis caused by droxicam]. Atencion Prim 14(1):583, 1994.
147. Garcia Gonzalez M, Sanroman AL, Herrero C, et al: [Droxicam-induced hepatitis. Description of 3 new cases and review of the literature]. Rev Clin Esp 194(3):170, 1994.
148. Omar M, Mediavilla-Garcia JD, Corrales Torres AJ, et al: [Droxicam-induced hepatitis: a report of 2 cases]. Rev Esp Enferm Dig 84(4):277, 1993
149. Morillas Arino J, Sanchez de la Fuente MF, Garcia-Cano Lizcano J, et al: [Hepatotoxicity induced by droxicam: presentation of 4 cases]. Rev Esp Enferm Dig 83(3):197, 1993.
150. Primo J, Hinojosa J, Moles JR: [Hepatitis caused by droxicam]. Rev Esp Enferm Dig 83(2):138, 1993
151. Benjamin SB, Ishak KG, Zimmermann HJ, et al: Phenylbutazone liver injury: a clinical pathologic survey of 23 cases and review of the literature. Hepatology 1:255, 1981.
152. Maddrey WC, Maurath CJ, Verburg KM, et al: The hepatic safety and tolerability of the novel cyclooxygenase-2 inhibitor celecoxib (erratum appears in Am J Ther 7(5):341, 2000). Am J Ther 7(3):153, 2000.
153. Silverstein FE, Faich G, Goldstein JL, et al: Gastrointestinal toxicity with celecoxib vs nonsteroidal anti-inflammatory drugs for osteoarthritis and rheumatoid arthritis: the CLASS study: a randomized controlled trial. Celecoxib Long-term Arthritis Safety Study (see comments). JAMA 284(10):1247, 2000.
154. Carrillo-Jimenez R, Nurnberger M: Celecoxib-induced acute pancreatitis and hepatitis: a case report. Arch Intern Med 160(4):553, 2000.
155. Galan MV, Gordon SC, Silverman AL: Celecoxib-induced cholestatic hepatitis. Ann Intern Med 134(3):254, 2001.
156. Al-Kawas FH, Seeff LB, Berendson RA, et al: Allopurinol hepatotoxicity. Ann Intern Med 95:588, 1981.
157. Shah KA, Levin J, Rosen N, et al: Allopurinol toxicity potentiated by tamoxifen. N Y State Med J 82:1745, 1982.
158. Chawla SK, Patel HD, Parrino GR, et al: Allopurinol hepatotoxicity. Arthr Rheum 20:1546, 1977.
159. Vanderstigel M, Zafrani ES, Lejonc JL, et al: Allopurinol hypersensitivity syndrome as a cause of fibrin-ring granulomas. Gastroenterology 90:188, 1986.
160. West SG: Methotrexate hepatotoxicity. Rheum Dis Clin North Am 23:883, 1997.
161. Bridges SL, Alarcon GS, Koopman WJ: Methotrexate-induced liver abnormalities in rheumatoid arthritis. J Rheumatol 16:1180, 1989.
162. Rau R, Karger T, Herborn G, et al: Liver biopsy findings in patients with rheumatoid arthritis undergoing treatment with methotrexate. J Rheumatol 16:489, 1989.
163. te Boekhorst PA, Barrera P, Laan RF, et al: Hepatotoxicity of parenteral gold therapy in rheumatoid arthritis: a case report and review of the literature. Clin Exp Rheumatol 17:359, 1999.
164. Howrie CL, Gartner JC Jr: Gold-induced hepatotoxicity: case report and review of the literature. J Rheumatol 9:727, 1982.
165. Fleischner GM, Morecki R, Hanaichi T, et al: Light- and electron-microscopical study of a case of gold salt-induced hepatotoxicity. Hepatology 14:422, 1991.
166. Watkins PB, Schade R, Mills AS, et al: Fatal hepatic necrosis associated with parenteral gold therapy. Dig Dis Sci 33:1025, 1988.
167. Van Linthoudt D, Buss W, Beyner F, et al: [Fatal hepatic necrosis due to a treatment course of rheumatoid arthritis with gold salts]. Schweiz Med Wochenschr J Suisse Med 121:1099, 1991.
168. Hansen RM, Varma RR, Hanson GA: Gold induced hepatitis and pure red cell aplasia. Complete recovery after corticosteroid and N-acetylcysteine therapy. J Rheumatol 18:1251, 1991.
169. Rosenberg WM, Ryley NG, Trowell JM, et al: Dextropropoxyphene induced hepatotoxicity: a report of nine cases. J Hepatol 19:470, 1993.
170. Bassendine MF, Woodhouse KW, Bennett M, et al: Dextropropoxyphene induced hepatotoxicity mimicking biliary tract disease. Gut 27:444, 1986.
171. Berson A, Fau D, Fornacciari R, et al: Mechanisms for experimental buprenorphine hepatotoxicity: major role of mitochondrial dysfunction versus metabolic activation. J Hepatol 34:261, 2001.
172. Berson A, Gervais A, Cazals D, et al: Hepatitis after intravenous buprenorphine misuse in heroin addicts. J Hepatol 34:346, 2001.
173. Utili R, Boitnott JK, Zimmerman HJ: Dantrolene-associated hepatic injury. Incidence and character. Gastroenterology 72:610, 1977.
174. Wilkinson SP, Portmann B, Williams R: Hepatitis from dantrolene sodium. Gut 20:33, 1979.
175. Kronenberg A, Krahenbuhl S, Zimmermann A, et al: [Severe hepatocellular damage after administration of paracetamol and chlorzoxazone in therapeutic dosage]. Schweiz Rundschau Med Praxis 87:1356, 1998.
176. Chlorzoxazone hepatotoxicity. Med Lett Drugs Ther 38:46, 1996.
177. Eisenberg CM, Davis RB, Ettner SL, et al: Trends in alternative medicine use in the United States, 1990-1997: results of a follow-up national survey. JAMA 280:1569, 1998.
178. Schiano TD: Liver injury from herbs and other botanicals. Clin Liver Dis 2:607, 1998.
179. Stillman AS, Huxtable R, Consroe P, et al: Hepatic veno-occlusive disease due to pyrrolizidine (*Senecio*) poisoning in Arizona. Gastroenterology 73:349, 1977.
180. Gordon CW, Rosenthal G, Hart J, et al: Chaparral ingestion. The broadening spectrum of liver injury caused by herbal medications. JAMA 273:489, 1995.
181. Sheikh NM, Philen RM, Love LA: Chaparral-associated hepatotoxicity. Arch Intern Med 157:913, 1997.
182. Lekehal M, Pessayre D, Lereau JM, et al: Hepatotoxicity of the herbal medicine germander: metabolic activation of its furano diterpenoids by cytochrome P450 3A depletes cytoskeleton-associated protein thiols and forms plasma membrane blebs in rat hepatocytes. Hepatology 24:212, 1996.
183. Kouzi SA, McMurtry RJ, Nelson SC: Hepatotoxicity of germander (Teucrium chamaedrys L.) and one of its constituent neoclerodane diterpenes teucrin A in the mouse. Chem Res Toxicol 7:850, 1994.
184. De Berardinis V, Moulis C, Maurice M, et al: Human microsomal epoxide hydrolase is the target of germander-induced autoantibodies on the surface of human hepatocytes. Mol Pharmacol 58:542, 2000.
185. Pauwels A, Thierman-Duffaud D, Azanowsky JM, et al: [Acute hepatitis caused by wild germander. Hepatotoxicity of herbal remedies. Two cases]. Gastroenterol Clin Biol 16:92, 1992.
186. Larrey D, Vial T, Pauwels A, et al: Hepatitis after germander (Teucrium chamaedrys) administration: another instance of herbal medicine hepatotoxicity. Ann Intern Med 117:129, 1992.
187. Laliberte L, Villeneuve JP: Hepatitis after the use of germander, a herbal remedy. CMAJ154:1689, 1996.

188. Dao T, Peytier A, Galateau F, et al: [Chronic cirrhogenic hepatitis induced by germander]. Gastroenterol Clin Biol 17:609, 1993.
189. Thomassen D, Slattery JT, Nelson SC: Menthofuran-dependent and independent aspects of pulegone hepatotoxicity: roles of glutathione. J Pharmacol Exp Ther 253:567, 1990.
190. Anderson IB, Mullen WH, Meeker JE, et al: Pennyroyal toxicity: measurement of toxic metabolite levels in two cases and review of the literature. Ann Intern Med 124:726, 1996.
191. Georgiou M, Sianidou L, Hatzis T, et al: Hepatotoxicity due to Atractylis gummifera. Clin Toxicol 26:487, 1988.
192. Woolf GM, Petrovic LM, Rojter SE, et al: Acute hepatitis associated with the Chinese herbal product jin bu huan. Ann Intern Med 121:729, 1994.
193. Kaptchuk TJ: Acute hepatitis associated with jin bu huan. Ann Intern Med 122:636, 1995.
194. Horowitz RS, Feldhaus K, Dart RC, et al: The clinical spectrum of Jin Bu Huan toxicity. Arch Intern Med 156:899, 1996.
195. Picciotto A, Campo N, Brizzolara R, et al: Chronic hepatitis induced by Jin Bu Huan. J Hepatol 28:165, 1998.
196. Parish RC, Doering PL: Treatment of Amanita mushroom poisoning: a review. Vet Human Toxicol 28:318, 1986.
197. Hruby K, Csomos G, Fuhrmann M, et al: Chemotherapy of Amanita phalloides poisoning with intravenous silibinin. Human Toxicol 2:183, 1983.
198. Bartoloni St Omer F, Giannini A, Botti P, et al: Amanita poisoning: a clinical-histopathological study of 64 cases of intoxication. Hepatogastroenterology 32:229, 1985.
199. Becroft CM, Webster CR: Aflatoxins and Reye's disease. BMJ 4:117, 1972.
200. Krishnamachari KA, Bhat RV, Nagarajan V, et al: Hepatitis due to aflatoxicosis. An outbreak in Western India. Lancet 1:1061, 1975.
201. Katiyar S, Dash BC, Thakur V, et al: p53 tumor suppressor gene in patients with hepatocellular cancer in India. Cancer 88:1565, 2000.
202. Pong RS, Wogan GS: Time course and dose response characteristics of aflatoxin B1 effects on rat liver RNA polymerase and ultrastructure. Cancer Res 30:299, 1970.
203. Hsu IC, Metcalf RA, Sun T, et al: Mutational hotspot in the p53 gene in human hepatocellular carcinomas. Nature 350:427, 1991.
203a. USA Today, December 31, 2001-January 1, 2002:1.
204. Klatskin G, Kimberg DV: Recurrent hepatitis attributable to halothane sensitation in an anesthetist. N Engl J Med 275:515, 1969.
205. Brown BR Jr: Hepatotoxicity of halogenated inhalation anesthetics. Contemp Anesth Pract 4:171, 1981.
206. Elliott RH, Strunin L: Hepatotoxicity of volatile anaesthetics. Br J Anaesth 70:339, 1993.
207. Ray DC, Drummond GB: Halothane hepatitis. Br J Anaesth 67:84, 1991.
208. Kenna JG, Jones RM: The organ toxicity of inhaled anesthetics. Anesth Analg 81:S51, 1995.
209. Holt C, Csete M, Martin P: Hepatotoxicity of anesthetics and other central nervous system drugs. Gastroenterol Clin North Am 24:853, 1995.
210. Lo SK, Wendon J, Mieli-Vergani G, et al: Halothane-induced acute liver failure: continuing occurrence and use of liver transplantation. Eur J Gastroenterol Hepatol 10:635, 1998.
211. Wark H: Halothane metabolism in children. Br J Anaes 64:474, 1990.
212. Gruenke LD, Konopka K, Koop DR, et al: Characterization of halothane oxidation by hepatic microsomes and P-450 using a gas chromatographic mass spectrometric assay. JPharmacol Exp Ther 246:454, 1988.
213. Paronetto F, Popper H: Lymphocyte stimulation induced by halothane in patients with hepatitis following exposure to halothane. N Engl J Med 283:277, 1970.
214. Williams BD, White N, Amlot PL, et al: Circulating immune complexes after repeated halothane anesthesia. BMJ 2:159, 1977.
215. Price CD, Gibbs AR, Williams WJ: Halothane macrophage migration inhibition factor test in halothane-associated hepatitis. J Clin Pathol 30:312, 1977.
216. Satoh H, Fukada Y, Anderson DK, et al: Immunological mechanism of halothane-induced hepatotoxicity: immunolohistochemical evidence of trifluoroacetylated hepatocytes. J Pharmacol Exp Ther 233:857, 1985.
217. Vergani D, Tsantoulas D, Eddleston ALWF, et al: Sensitation of halothane-altered liver components in severe hepatic necrosis after halothane anesthesia. Lancet 2:801, 1978.
218. Neuberger J, Kenna JG: Halothane-hepatitis: a model of imune mediated drug hepatotoxicity. Clin Sci 72:263, 1987.
219. Njoku D, Laster MJ, Gong CH, et al: Biotransformation of halothane, enflurane, isoflurane, and desflurane to trifluoroacetylated liver proteins: association between protein acylation and hepatic injury. Anesth Analg 84:173, 1997.
220. Thomassen D, Martin BM, Martin JL, et al: The role of stress protein in the development of a drug-induced allergic response. Eur J Pharmacol 183:1138, 1989.
221. Pumford NR, Martin BM, Thomassen C: Serum antibodies from halothane hepatitis patients react with the rat endoplasmic reticulum protein ERp72. Chem Res Toxicol 6:609, 1993.
222. Butler LE, Thomassen D, Martin JL, et al: The calcium binding protein calreticulin is covalently modified in rat liver by a reactive metabolite of the inhalational anesthetic halothane. Chem Res Toxicol 5:406, 1992.
223. Satoh H, Martin BM, Schulick AH, et al: Human anti-endoplasmic reticulum antibodies in sera of patients with halothane induced hepatitis are directed against a trifluoroacetylated carboxylesterase. Proc Natl Acad Sci U S A 86:322, 1989.
224. Smith GCM, Kenna JG, Harrison DJ, et al: Autoantibodies to hepatic microsomal carboxylesterase in halothane hepatitis. Lancet 342:963, 1993.
225. Kenna JG: Immunological allergic drug-induced hepatitis: lessons from halothane. J Hepatol 26:5, 1997.
226. Martin JL, Kenna JG, Martin BM, et al: Halothane hepatitis patients have antibodies that react with protein disulfide isomerase. Hepatology 18:858, 1993.
227. Farrell G, Prendergast D, Murray M: Halothane hepatitis: detection of a constitutional susceptibility factor. N Engl J Med 313:1310, 1985.
228. Neuberger J, Williams R: Halothane anesthesia and liver damage. BMJ 289:1136, 1984.
229. Inman WHW, Mushin WW: Jaundice after repeated exposure to halothane: a further analysis of reports to the Committee on Safety of Medicines. BMJ 2:817, 1978.
230. Mikatti NE, Healy TE: Hepatic injury associated with halogenated anaesthetics: cross-sensitization and its clinical implications. Eur J Anaes 14:7, 1997.
231. Hasan F: Isoflurane hepatotoxicity in a patient with a previous history of halothane-induced hepatitis. Hepatogastroenterology 45:518, 1998.
232. Delia JE, Maxson WS, Breen JL: Methoxyflurane hepatitis: two cases following obstetric analgesia. Int J Gynaecol Obstet 21:89, 1983.
233. Okuno T, Takeda M, Horishi M, et al: Hepatitis due to repeated inhalation of methoxyflurane in subanaesthetic concentrations. Can Anaes Soc J 32:53, 1985.
234. Joshi PH, Conn HO: The syndrome of methoxyflurane associated hepatitis. Ann Intern Med 80:395, 1974.
235. Judson JA, De Jongh HJ, Walmsley JB: Possible cross-sensitivity between halothane and methoxyflurane: report of a case. Anesthesiology 35:527, 1971.
236. Blettery B, Foissac-Durand J, Michiels R, et al: [Renal tubular necrosis and cytolytic hepatitis following repeated anaesthetic inhalation of methoxyflurane]. Eur J Toxicol 5:257, 1972.
237. Reeves M: Acute hepatitis following enflurane anaesthesia. Anaes Inten Care 25:80, 1997.
238. Sigurdsson J, Hreidarsson AB, Thjodleifsson B: Enflurane hepatitis. A report of a case with a previous history of halothane hepatitis. Acta Anaesthesiol Scand 29:495, 1985.
239. Stoelting RK, Blitt CD, Cohen PJ, et al: Hepatic dysfunction after isoflurane anesthesia. Anesth Analg 66:147, 1987.
240. Carrigan TW, Straughen WJ: A report of hepatic necrosis and death following isoflurane anesthesia. Anesthesiology 67:581, 1987.
241. Cherng CH, Ho ST, Chen CF, et al: [Acute hepatitis in an uremic patient following isoflurane anesthesia]. Ma Zui Xue Za Zhi Anaesthesiol Sinica 26:239, 1988.
242. Martin JL, Keegan MT, Vasdev GM, et al: Fatal hepatitis associated with isoflurane exposure and CYP2A6 autoantibodies. Anesthesiology 95:551, 2001.
243. Scheider CM, Klygis LM, Tsang TK, et al: Hepatic dysfunction after repeated isoflurane administration. J Clin Gastroenterol 17:168, 1993.

244. Turner GB, O'Rourke D, Scott GO, et al: Fatal hepatotoxicity after re-exposure to isoflurane: a case report and review of the literature. Eur J Gastroenterol Hepatol 12:955, 2000.
245. Webster JA: Acute hepatitis after isoflurane anesthesia. CMAJ135: 1343, 1986.
246. Weitz J, Kienle P, Bohrer H, et al: Fatal hepatic necrosis after isoflurane anaesthesia. Anaesthesia 52:892, 1997.
247. Gelman S, Rimerman V, Fowler KC, et al: The effect of halothane, isoflurane, and blood loss on hepatotoxicity and hepatic oxygen availability in phenobarbital-pretreated hypoxic rats. Anesth Analg 63:965, 1984.
248. Yamasaki A, Takahashi T, Suzuki T, et al: Differential effects of isoflurane and halothane on the induction of heat shock proteins. Biochem Pharmacol 62:375, 2001.
249. Gunaratnam NT, Benson J, Gandolfi AJ, et al: Suspected isoflurane hepatitis in an obese patient with a history of halothane hepatitis. Anesthesiology 83:1361, 1995.
250. Martin JL, Plevak CJ, Flannery KD, et al: Hepatotoxicity after desflurane anesthesia. Anesthesiology 83:1125, 1995.
251. Ghantous HN, Fernando J, Gandolfi AJ, et al: Sevoflurane is biotransformed by guinea pig liver slices but causes minimal cytotoxicity. Anesth Analg 75:436, 1992.
252. Shichinohe Y, Masuda Y, Takahashi H, et al: [A case of postoperative hepatic injury after sevoflurane anesthesia]. Masui 41:1802, 1992.
253. Ogawa M, Doi K, Mitsufuji T, et al: [Drug induced hepatitis following sevoflurane anesthesia in a child]. Masui 40:1542, 1991.
254. Bray GP, Harrison PM, O'Grady JG, et al: Long-term anticonvulsant therapy worsens outcome in paracetamol-induced fulminant failure. Hum Exp Toxicol 11:265, 1992.
255. Brackett CC, Bloch JC: Phenytoin as a possible cause of acetaminophen hepatotoxicity: case report and review of the literature. Pharmacotherapy 20:229, 2000.
256. Bush-Andreasen J, Lyngbye J, Trolle E: Abnormalities in liver function tests during long-term diphenylhydantoin therapy in epileptic putpatients. Acta Med Scand 194:261, 1973.
257. Aiges HW, Daum F, Olson M, et al: The effects of phenobarbital and diphenylhydantoin on liver function and morphology. J Pediatr 97:22, 1980.
258. Pamperl H, Gradner W, Fridrich L, et al: Influence of long-term anticonvulsant therapy on liver ultrastructure in man. Liver 4:294, 1984.
259. Jezequel AM, Librari ML, Mosca P, et al: Changes induced on human liver by long-term anticonvulsant therapy. Liver 4:307, 1984.
260. Roy AK, Mahoney HC, Levine RA: Phenytoin-induced chronic hepatitis. Dig Dis Sci 38:740, 1993.
261. Harinasula U, Zimmerman HJ: Diphenylhydantoin sodium hepatitis. JAMA 203:1015, 1968.
262. Brown M, Schubert T: Phenytoin hypersensitivity hepatitis and mononucleosis syndrome. J Clin Gastroenterol 8:469, 1986.
263. Carro JA, Senior J, Rubio CE, et al: Phenytoin induced fatal hepatic injury. Bol Asoc Med P R 81:359, 1989.
264. Prosser TR, Lander RC: Phenytoin-induced hypersensitivity reactions. Clin Pharm 6:728, 1987.
265. Lee TJ, Carney CN, Lapis JL, et al: Diphenylhydantoin-induced hepatic necrosis. A case study. Gastroenterology 70:422, 1976.
266. Fonseca JC, Azulay CR, Rozembau I, et al: [Hypersensitivity syndrome caused by phenytoins and phenobarbital]. Med Cutanea Ibero-Latino-Am 12:187, 1984.
267. Mullick FG, Ishak KG: Hepatic injury associated with diphenylhydantoin therapy. A clinicopathologic study of 20 cases. Am J Clin Pathol 74:442, 1980.
268. Smythe MA, Umstead GS: Phenytoin hepatotoxicity: a review of the literature. Dicp Ann Pharmac 23:13, 1989.
269. Kleckner HB, Yakulis V, Heller P: Severe hypersensitivity to diphenylhydantoin with circulating antibodies to the drug. Ann Int Med 83:522, 1975.
270. Spielberg SP, Gordon GB, Blake CA, et al: Predisposition to phenytoin hepatotoxicity assessed in vitro. N Engl J Med 305:722, 1981.
271. Gennis MA, Glazko AJ: Familial occurrence of hypersensitivity to phenytoin. Am J Med 91:631, 1991.
272. Sherertz EF, Jegasothy BV, Lazarus GS: Phenytoin hypersensitivity reaction presenting with toxic epidermal necrolysis and severe hepatitis. Report of a patient treated with corticosteroid "pulse therapy." J Am Acad Dermat 12:178, 1985.
273. Conger LA Jr, Grabski WJ: Dilantin hypersensitivity reaction. Cutis 57:223, 1996.
274. Kakar A, Byotra SP: Phenytoin induced severe agranulocytosis and hepatitis. J Assoc Physicians India 47:644, 1999.
275. Korman LB, Olson MJ: Phenytoin-induced hepatitis, rhabdomyolysis, and renal dysfunction. Clin Pharm 8:514, 1989.
276. Cook IF, Shilkin KB, Reed WC: Phenytoin induced granulomatous hepatitis. Aust N Z J Med 11:539, 1981.
277. Howard PA, Engen PL, Dunn MI: Phenytoin hypersensitivity syndrome: a case report. Dicp Ann Pharmac 25:929, 1991.
278. Lisker-Melman M, Hoofnagle JH: Phenytoin hepatotoxicity masked by corticosteroids. Arch Intern Med 149:1196, 1989.
279. Powers NG, Carson SH: Idiosyncratic reactions to phenytoin. Clin Pediatr 26:120, 1987.
280. Haukeland JW, Jahnsen J, Raknerud N: [Carbamazepine-induced hepatitis]. Tidsskr Nor Laegeforen 120:2875, 2000.
281. Levy M, Goodman MW, Van Dyne BJ, et al: Granulomatous hepatitis secondary to carbamazepine. Ann Intern Med 95:64, 1981.
282. Mitchell MC, Boitnott JK, Arregui A, et al: Granulomatous hepatitis associated with carbamazepine therapy. Am J Med 71:733, 1981.
283. Hopen G, Nesthus I, Laerum OC: Fatal carbamazepine-associated hepatitis. Report of two cases. Acta Med Scand 210:333, 1981.
284. Soffer EE, Taylor RJ, Bertram PD, et al: Carbamazepine-induced liver injury. South Med J 76:681, 1983.
285. Ponte CC: Carbamazepine-induced thrombocytopenia, rash, and hepatic dysfunction. Drug Intel Clin Pharm 17:642, 1983.
286. Davion T, Capron JP, Andrejak M, et al: [Acute hepatitis due to carbamazepine (Tegretol). Study of a case and review of the literature]. Gastroenterol Clin Biol 8:52, 1984.
287. Morales-Diaz M, Pinilla-Roa E, Ruiz I: Suspected carbamazepine-induced hepatotoxicity. Pharmacotherapy 19:252, 1999.
288. Queyrel V, Catteau B, Michon-Pasturel U, et al: [DRESS (Drug Rash with Eosinophilia and Systemic Symptoms) syndrome after sulfasalazine and carmazepine: report of two cases]. Rev Med Intern 22:582, 2001.
289. Berkowitz FE, Henderson SL, Fajman N, et al: Acute liver failure caused by isoniazid in a child receiving carbamazepine. Int J Tuberc Lung Dis 2:603, 1998.
290. Barbare JC, Lallement PY, Vorhauer W, et al: [Hepatotoxicity of isoniazid: influence of carbamazepine?]. Gastroenterol Clin Biol 10:523, 1986.
291. Kato Y, Fujii T, Mizoguchi N, et al: Potential interaction between ritonavir and carbamazepine. Pharmacotherapy 20:851, 2000.
292. Orozco Lopez P, Roman Martinez J, Sorribes Puelles R, et al: [Carbamazepine and methyldopa: a hepatotoxic combination?]. Med Clin 81:40, 1983.
293. Frey B, Schubiger G, Musy JP: Transient cholestatic hepatitis in a neonate associated with carbamazepine exposure during pregnancy and breast-feeding. Eur J Pediatr 150:136, 1990.
294. Luke CR, Rocci ML, Schaible CH, et al: Acute hepatotoxicity after excessively high doses of carbamazepine on two occasions. Pharmacotherapy 6:108, 1986.
295. Nathan CL, Belsito CV: Carbamazepine-induced pseudolymphoma with CD-30 positive cells. J Am Acad Dermatol 38:806, 1998.
296. Levander HG: Granulomatous hepatitis in a patient receiving carbamazepine. Acta Med Scand 208:333, 1980.
297. Noguerado A, Isasia T, Martinez MC, et al: [Granulomatous hepatitis caused by carbamazepine]. Rev Clin Espan 181:116, 1987.
298. Forbes GM, Jeffrey GP, Shilkin KB, et al: Carbamazepine hepatotoxicity: another cause of the vanishing bile duct syndrome. Gastroenterology 102:1385, 1992.
299. Brown TR: Valproic acid. N Engl J Med 302:661, 1980.
300. Coulter DL, Wu H, Allen RJ: Valproic acid therapy in childhood epilepsy. JAMA 244:785, 1980.
301. Dreifuss FE, Santilli N, Langer CH, et al: Valproic acid hepatic fatalities: a retrospective review. Neurology 37:379, 1987.
302. Bryant AE, Dreifuss FE: Valproic acid hepatic fatalities. U.S. experience since 1986. Neurology 46:465, 1996.
303. Konig SA, Siemes H, Blaker F, et al: Severe hepatotoxicity during valproate therapy: an update and report of eight new fatalities. Epilepsia 35:1005, 1994.
304. Powell-Jackson PR, Tredger JM, Williams R: Hepatotoxicity to sodium valproate: a review. Gut 25:673, 1984.

305. Appleton RE, Farrell K, Applegarth CA, et al: The high incidence of valproate hepatotoxicity in infants may relate to familial metabolic defects. Can J Neurologic Sci 17:145, 1990.
306. Zafrani ES, Berthelot P: Sodium valproate in the induction of unusual hepatotoxicity. Hepatology 2:648, 1982.
307. Fromenty B, Pessayre C: Inhibition of mitochondrial beta-oxidation as a mechanism of hepatotoxicity. Pharmacol Ther 67:101, 1995.
308. Turnbull CM, Bone AJ, Bartlett K, et al: The effects of valproate on intermediary metabolism in isolated rat hepatocytes and intact rats. Biochem Pharmacol 32:1887, 1983.
309. Kesterson JW, Granneman GR, Machinist JM: The hepatotoxicity of valproic acid and its metabolites in rats. I. Toxicologic, biochemical and histopathologic studies. Hepatology 4:1143, 1984.
310. Granneman GR, Wang SI, Kesterson JW, et al: The hepatotoxicity of valproic acid and its metabolites in rats. II. Intermediary and valproic acid metabolism. Hepatology 4:1153, 1984.
311. Turnbull CM, Dick CJ, Wilson L, et al: Valproate causes metabolic disturbance in normal man. J Neurol Neurosurg Psychiatry 49:405, 1986.
312. Strolin Benedetti M, Rumigny JF, Dostert P: [Mechanisms of action and biochemical toxicology of valproic acid]. Encephale 10:177, 1984.
313. Jimenez-Rodriguezvila M, Caro-Paton A, Duenas-Laita A, et al: Histological, ultrastructural and mitochondrial oxidative phosphorylation studies in liver of rats chronically treated with oral valproic acid. J Hepatol 1:453, 1985.
314. Jezequel AM, Bonazzi P, Novelli G, et al: Early structural and functional changes in liver of rats treated with a single dose of valproic acid. Hepatology 4:1159, 1984.
315. Kingsley E, Gray P, Tolman KG, et al: The toxicity of metabolites of sodium valproate in cultured hepatocytes. J Clin Pharmacol 23:178, 1983.
316. Kochen W, Schneider A, Ritz A: Abnormal metabolism of valproic acid in fatal hepatic failure. Eur J Pediatr 141:30, 1983.
317. Kondo T, Kaneko S, Otani K, et al: Associations between risk factors for valproate hepatotoxicity and altered valproate metabolism. Epilepsia 33:172, 1992.
318. Rettie AE, Rettenmeier AW, Howald WN, et al: Cytochrome P-450-catalyzed formation of 4-en-VPA, a toxic metabolite of valproic acid. Science 235:890, 1987.
319. McLaughlin CB, Eadie MJ, Parker-Scott SL, et al: Valproate metabolism during valproate-associated hepatotoxicity in a surviving adult patient. Epilepsy Res 41:259, 2000.
320. Zimmerman HJ, Ishak KG: Valproate induced hepatic injury. Analysis of 23 fatal cases. Hepatology 2:591, 1982.
321. Rawat S, Borkowski WJ, Swick HM: Valproic acid and secondary hyperammonemia. Neurology 31:1173, 1981.
322. Ratnaike RN, Schapel GJ, Purdie G, et al: Hyperammonaemia and hepatotoxicity during chronic valproate therapy: enhancement by combination with other antiepileptic drugs. Br J Clin Pharmacol 22:100, 1986.
323. Kane RE, Kotagel S, Bacon BR, et al: Valproate use associated with persistent hyperammonemia and mitochondrial injury in a child with Down's syndrome. J Pediatr Gastroenterol Nutr 14:223, 1992.
324. Young RSK, Bergman I, Gang DL, et al: Fatal Reye-like syndrome associated with valproic acid. Ann Neurol 7:389, 1980 (letter).
325. Klein M, Wendt U: [Reye-like syndrome following valproate therapy in an adult]. Psychiatrie Neurol Medizin Psychol 40:353, 1988.
326. Binek J, Hany A, Heer M: Valproic-acid-induced pancreatitis. Case report and review of the literature. J Clin Gastroenterol 13:690, 1991.
327. Dickinson RG, Bassett ML, Searle J, et al: Valproate hepatotoxicity: a review and report of two instances in adults. Clin Exp Neurol 21:79, 1985.
328. Suchy FJ, Balistreri WF, Buchino JJ, et al: Acute hepatic failure associated with the use of sodium valproate. N Engl J Med 300:962, 1979.
329. Bell EA, Shaefer MS, Markin RS, et al: Treatment of valproic acid-associated hepatic failure with orthotopic liver transplantation. Ann Pharmacother 26:18, 1992.
330. de Pasquet EG, Scaramelli A, de Caceres MP, et al: Double-blind, placebo-controlled, cross-over trial of progabide as add-on therapy in epileptic patients. Epilepsia 32:133, 1991.
331. Munoz SJ, Fariello R, Maddrey WC: Submassive hepatic necrosis associated with the use of progabide: a GABA receptor agonist. Dig Dis Sci 33:375, 1988.
332. Pellock JM: Felbamate. Epilepsia 40:S57, 1999.
333. Pellock JM: Felbamate in epilepsy therapy: evaluating the risks. Drug Safety 21:225, 1999.
334. Kapetanovic IM, Torchin CD, Thompson CD, et al: Potentially reactive cyclic carbamate metabolite of the antiepileptic drug felbamate produced by human liver tissue in vitro. Drug Metabol Disp 26:1089, 1998.
335. Beard K, Belic L, Aselton P, et al: Outpatient drug-induced parenchymal liver disease requiring hospitalization. J Clin Pharmacol 26:633, 1986.
336. McArthur JE, Dyment PG: Stevens-Johnson syndrome with hepatitis following therapy with ampicillin and cephalexin. N Z Med J 81:390, 1975.
337. Cavanzo FJ, Garcia CF, Botera RC: Chronic cholestasis, paucity of bile ducts and the Stevens-Johnson syndrome. Gastroenterology 9:854, 1990.
338. Bolzan H, Spatola J, Castelletto R, et al: [Intrahepatic cholestasis induced by amoxicillin alone]. Gastroenterol Hepatol 23:237, 2000.
339. Alexander P, Roskams T, Van Steenbergen W, et al: Intrahepatic cholestasis induced by amoxicillin/clavulanic acid (Augmentin): a report on two cases. Acta Clin Belg 46:327, 1991.
340. Belknap MK, McClelland KJ: Cholestatic hepatitis associated with amoxicillin-clavulanate. Wis Med J 92:241, 1993.
341. Beurton I, Germanese JC, Becker MC, et al: [Acute hepatitis and destructive cholangitis probably induced by amoxicillin-clavulanic acid combination]. Gastroenterol Clin Biol 23:1097, 1999.
342. Bralet MP, Zafrani ES: [Hepatitis caused by the amoxicillin-clavulanic acid combination. An example of drug-induced biliary hepatotoxicity]. Ann Pathol 16:425, 1996.
343. Bustamante Balen M, Perez Aguilar F, Rayon Martin M, et al: [Cholestatic hepatitis caused by amoxycillin-clavulanic acid. Report of a new case]. Gastroenterol Hepatol 20:187, 1997.
344. Ersoz G, Karasu Z, Yildiz C, et al: Severe toxic hepatitis associated with amoxycillin and clavulanic acid. J Clin Pharm Ther 26:225, 2001.
345. Gresser U: Amoxicillin-clavulanic acid therapy may be associated with severe side effects—review of the literature. Eur J Med Res 6:139, 2001.
346. O'Donohue J, Oien KA, Donaldson P, et al: Co-amoxiclav jaundice: clinical and histological features and HLA class II association. Gut 47:717, 2000.
347. Larrey D, Vial T, Micaleff A, et al: Hepatitis associated with amoxycillin-clavulanic acid combination: report of 15 cases. Gut 33:368, 1992.
348. Mari JY, Guy C, Beyens MN, et al: [Delayed drug-induced hepatic injury. Evoking the role of amoxicillin-clavulinic acid combination]. Therapie 55:699, 2000.
349. Hautekeete ML, Horsmans Y, Van Waeyenberge C, et al: HLA association of amoxicillin-clavulanate–induced hepatitis. Gastroenterology 117:1181, 1999.
350. Silvain C, Fort E, Levillain P, et al: Granulomatous hepatitis due to combination of amoxicillin and clavulanic acid. Dig Dis Sci 37:150, 1992.
351. Pollock AA, Berger SA, Simberkoff MS, et al: Hepatitis associated with high-dose oxacillin therapy. Arch Intern Med 138:915, 1978.
352. Bruckstein AH, Attia AA: Oxacillin hepatitis. Two patients with liver biopsy, and review of the literature. Am J Med 64:519, 1978.
353. Goldstein LI, Granoff M, Waisman J: Hepatic injury due to oxacillin administration. Am J Gastroenterol 70:171, 1978.
354. Halloran TJ, Clague MC: Hepatitis associated with high-dose oxacillin therapy. Arch Intern Med 139:376, 1979.
355. Olans RN, Weiner LB: Reversible oxacillin hepatotoxicity. J Pediatr 89:835, 1976.
356. Onorato IM, Axelrod JL: Hepatitis from intravenous high-dose oxacillin therapy: findings in an adult inpatient population. Ann Intern Med 89:497, 1978.
357. Miller WI, Souney PF, Chang JT: Hepatic dysfunction following nafcillin and cephalothin therapy in a patient with a history of oxacillin hepatitis. Clin Pharm 2:465, 1983.
358. Wilson FM, Belamaric J, Lauter CB, et al: Anicteric carbenicillin hepatitis. Eight episodes in four patients. JAMA 232:818, 1975.
359. Gump CW: Elevated SGOT levels after carbenicillin. N Engl J Med 282:1489, 1970.
360. Derby LE, Jick H, Henry CA, et al: Cholestatic hepatitis associated with flucloxacillin. Med J Aust 158:596, 1993.

361. Devereaux BM, Crawford CH, Purcell P, et al: Flucloxacillin associated cholestatic hepatitis. An Australian and Swedish epidemic? Eur J Clin Pharmacol 49:81, 1995.
362. Victorino RM, Maria V. A, Correia AP, et al: Floxacillin-induced cholestatic hepatitis with evidence of lymphocyte sensitization. Arch Intern Med 147:987, 1987.
363. Miros M, Kerlin P, Walker N, et al: Flucloxacillin induced delayed cholestatic hepatitis. Aust N Z J Med 20:251, 1990.
364. Koek GH, Stricker BH, Blok AP, et al: Flucloxacillin-associated hepatic injury. Liver 14:225, 1994.
365. Turner IB, Eckstein RP, Riley JW, et al: Prolonged hepatic cholestasis after flucloxacillin therapy. Med J Aust 151:701, 1989.
366. Roughead EE, Gilbert AL, Primrose JG: Improving drug use: a case study of events which led to changes in use of flucloxacillin in Australia. Soc Sci Med 48:845, 1999.
367. Eggleston SM, Belandres MM: Jaundice associated with cephalosporin therapy. Drug Intell Clin Pharm 19:553, 1985.
368. Ammann R, Neftel K, Hardmeier T, et al: Cephalosporin-induced cholestatic jaundice. Lancet 2:336, 1982.
369. Horn S, Aglas F, Horina JH: Cholestasis and liver cell damage due to hypersensitivity to erythromycin stearate—recurrence following therapy with erythromycin succinate. Wien Klin Wochenschr 111:76, 1999.
370. Keeffe EB, Reis TC, Berland JE: Hepatotoxicity to both erythromycin estolate and erythromycin ethylsuccinate. Dig Dis Sci 27:701, 1982.
371. Luherne JY, Pariente EA, Maitre F: [Crossed hepatotoxicity of erythromycin propionate and troleandomycin?] Gastroenterol Clin Biol 12:869, 1988.
372. Derby LE, Jick H, Henry CA, et al: Erythromycin-associated cholestatic hepatitis. Med J Aust 158:600, 1993.
373. Carson JL, Strom BL, Duff A, et al: Acute liver disease associated with erythromycins, sulfonamides, and tetracyclines. Ann Intern Med 119:576, 1993.
374. Braun P: Hepatotoxicity of erythromycin. J Infect Dis 118:300, 1973.
375. Gomez-Lechon MJ, Carrasquer J, Berenguer J, et al: Evidence of antibodies to erythromycin in serum of a patient following an episode of acute drug-induced hepatitis. Clin Exp Allergy 26:590, 1996.
376. Pessayre D, Larrey D, Funck-Brentano C, et al: Drug interactions and hepatitis produced by some macrolide antibiotics. J Antimicrob Chemother 16:181, 1985.
377. Richelmi P, Baldi C, Manzo L, et al: Erythromycin estolate impairs the mitochondrial and microsomal calcium homeostasis: correlation with hepatotoxicity. Arch Toxicol 7:298, 1984.
378. Sorensen EM, Acosta C: Erythromycin estolate-induced toxicity in cultured rat hepatocytes. Toxicol Lett 27:73, 1985.
379. Braun P: Hepatotoxicity of erythromycin. J Infect Dis 119:300, 1969.
380. Swayne LC, Kolc J: Erythromycin hepatotoxicity. A rare cause of a false-positive technetium-99m DISIDA study. Clin Nuclear Med 11:10, 1986.
381. Gholson CF, Warren GH: Fulminant hepatic failure associated with intravenous erythromycin lactobionate. Arch Intern Med 150:215, 1990.
382. Ball P, Mandell L, Niki Y, et al: Comparative tolerability of the newer fluoroquinolone antibacterials. Drug Safety 21:407, 1999.
383. Davoren P, Mainstone K: Norfloxacin-induced hepatitis. Med J Aust 159:423, 1993.
384. Lopez-Navidad A, Domingo P, Cadafalch J, et al: Norfloxacin-induced hepatotoxicity. J Hepatol 11:277, 1990.
385. Bjornsson E, Olsson R, Remotti H: Norfloxacin-induced eosinophilic necrotizing granulomatous hepatitis. Am J Gastroenterol 95:3662, 2000.
386. Romero-Gomez M, Suarez Garcia E, Fernandez MC: Norfloxacin-induced acute cholestatic hepatitis in a patient with alcoholic liver cirrhosis. Am J Gastroenterol 94:2324, 1999.
387. Gauffre A, Mircheva J, Glotz D, et al: Autoantibodies against a kidney–liver protein associated with quinolone-induced acute interstitial nephritis or hepatitis. Nephrol Dial Transplant 12:1961, 1997.
388. Villeneuve JP, Davies C, Cote J: Suspected ciprofloxacin-induced hepatotoxicity. Ann Pharmacother 29:257, 1995.
389. Grassmick BK, Lehr VT, Sundareson AS: Fulminant hepatic failure possibly related to ciprofloxacin. Ann Pharmacother 26:636, 1992.
390. Chen HJ, Bloch KJ, Maclean JA: Acute eosinophilic hepatitis from trovafloxacin. N Engl J Med 342:359, 2000.
391. Lazarczyk CA, Goldstein NS, Gordon SC: Ovafloxacin hepatotoxicity. Dig Dis Sci 46:925, 2001.
392. Lucena MI, Andrade RJ, Rodrigo L, et al: Trovafloxacin-induced acute hepatitis. Clin Infect Dis 30:400, 2000.
393. Dowling HF, Lepper LH: Hepatic reactions to tetracycline. JAMA 188:307, 1964.
394. Whalley PJ, Adams RJ, Combes B: Tetracycline toxicity in pregnancy. JAMA 189:357, 1964.
395. Hansen CH, Pearson LH, Schenker S, et al: Impaired secretion of triglycerides by the liver: a cause of tetracycline induced fatty liver. Proc Soc Exp Biol Med 128:143, 1968.
396. Horwitz ST, Marymont H Jr: Fatal liver disease during pregnancy associated with tetracycline therapy. Obstet Gynecol 23:826, 1964.
397. DuBuy HG, Showacre JL: Selective localization of tetracycline in the mitochondria of living cells. Science 133:196, 1961.
398. Zussman WV: Hepatic alterations following experimental tetracycline toxicity. Anat Rec 162:301, 1968.
399. Labbe G, Fromenty B, Freneaux E, et al: Effect of various tetracycline derivatives on the in vitro and in vivo beta-oxidation of fatty acids, egress of triglycerides from the liver, accumulation of hepatic triglycerides, and mortality in mice. Biochem Pharmacol 41:638, 1991.
400. Grimbert S, Fromenthy B, Fisch C, et al: Decreased mitochondrial oxidation of fatty acids in pregnant mice: possible relevance to the development of acute fatty liver of pregnancy. Hepatology 17:628, 1993.
401. Hoyumpa AM, Greene HL, Dunn GD, et al: Fatty liver: biochemical and clinical considerations. Am J Dig Dis 20:1142, 1968.
402. Boudreaux JP, Hayes CH, Mizrahi S, et al: Fulminant hepatic failure, hepatorenal syndrome, and necrotizing pancreatitis after minocycline hepatotoxicity. Transplant Proc 25:1873, 1993.
403. Eichenfield AH: Minocycline and autoimmunity. Curr Opin Pediatr 11:447, 1999.
404. Goldstein NS, Bayati N, Silverman AL, et al: Minocycline as a cause of drug-induced autoimmune hepatitis. Report of four cases and comparison with autoimmune hepatitis. Am J Clin Pathol 114:591, 2000.
405. Bhat G, Jordan J Jr, Sokalski S, et al: Minocycline-induced hepatitis with autoimmune features and neutropenia. J Clin Gastroenterol 27:74, 1998.
406. Castex F, Canva-Delcambre V, Maunoury V, et al: [Acute hepatitis induced by minocycline]. Gastroenterol Clin Biol 19:640, 1995.
407. Lawrenson RA, Seaman HE, Sundstrom A, et al: Liver damage associated with minocycline use in acne: a systematic review of the published literature and pharmacovigilance data. Drug Safety 23:333, 2000.
408. Malcolm A, Heap TR, Eckstein RP, et al: Minocycline-induced liver injury. Am J Gastroenterol 91:1641, 1996.
409. Nietsch HH, Libman BS, Pansze TW, et al: Minocycline-induced hepatitis. Am J Gastroenterol 95:2993, 2000.
410. Pointud P: Minocycline related lupus. J Rheumatol 24:1851, 1997.
411. Wejstal R, Lindberg J, Malmvall BE, et al: Liver damage associated with fansidar. Lancet 1:854, 1986.
412. Lazar HP, Murphy RL, Phair JP: Fansidar and hepatic granulomas. Ann Intern Med 102:722, 1985.
413. Kaufman SF: A rare complication of sulfadimethoxine (Madribon) therapy. Calif Med 107:344, 1967.
414. Espiritu CR, Kim TS, Levine RA: Granulomatous hepatitis associated with sulfadimethoxine hypersensitivity. JAMA 202:985, 1967.
415. Colucci CF, Lo Cicero M: Letter: hepatic necrosis and trimethoprim-sulfamethoxazole. JAMA 233:952, 1975.
416. Ransohoff CF, Jacobs G: Terminal hepatic failure following a small dose of sulfamethoxazole-trimethoprim. Gastroenterology 80:816, 1981.
417. Fries J, Siraganian R: Sulfonamide hepatitis: case due to sulfamethoxazole and sulfisoxazole. N Engl J Med 274:95, 1966.
418. Rigberg LA, Robinson MJ, Espiritu CR: Chlorpropamide-induced granulomas. A probable hypersensitivity reaction in liver and bone marrow. JAMA 235:409, 1976.
419. Tonder M, Nordoy A: Sulfonamide-induced chronic liver disease. Scand J Gastroenterol 9:93, 1974.
420. Young TL, Achkar E, Tuthill R, et al: Chronic active hepatitis induced by nitrofurantoin. Cleve Clin Q J 52:253, 1985.

421. Berry WR, Warren GH, Reichen J: Nitrofurantoin-induced cholestatic hepatitis from cow's milk in a teenaged boy. West J Med 140:278, 1984.
422. Dam-Larsen S, Kromann-Andersen H: [Hepatic toxicity of nitrofurantoin. Cases reported to the Center for Monitoring Adverse Drug Reactions 1968-1998]. Ugeskr Laeger 161:6650, 1999.
423. Stricker BCCH, Blok APR, Claas FHJ, et al: Hepatic injury associated with the use of nitrofurans: a clinicopathological study of 52 reported cases. Hepatology 8:599, 1988.
424. Kelly BD, Heneghan MA, Bennani F, et al: Nitrofurantoin-induced hepatotoxicity mediated by CD8+ T cells. Am J Gastroenterol 93:819, 1998.
425. Klemola H, Penttila O, Runeberg L, et al: Anicteric liver damage during nitrofurantoin medication. Scand J Gastroenterol 10:501, 1975.
426. Fagrell B, Strandberg I, Wengle B: A nitrofurantoin-induced disorder simulating chronic active hepatitis. A case report. Acta Med Scand 199:237, 1976.
427. Burger HC, Meiring JL, Nel PJ: [Chronic active hepatitis caused by nitrofurantoin: a case report]. S Afr Med J 67:125, 1985.
428. Sharp JR, Ishak KG, Zimmerman HJ: Chronic active hepatitis and severe hepatic necrosis associated with nitrofurantoin. Ann Intern Med 92:14, 1980.
429. Reinhart HH, Reinhart E, Korlipara P, et al: Combined nitrofurantoin toxicity to liver and lung. Gastroenterology 102:1396, 1992.
430. Strohscheer H, Wegener HH: [Nitrofurantoin-induced granulomatous hepatitis]. MMW - Munchener Medizinische Wochenschrift 119:1535, 1977.
431. Edoute Y, Karmon Y, Roguin A, et al: Fatal liver necrosis associated with the use of nitrofurantoin. Israel Med Assoc J 3:382, 2001.
432. Paiva LA, Wright PJ, Koff RS: Long-term hepatic memory for hypersensitivity to nitrofurantoin. Am J Gastroenterol 87:891, 1992.
433. Engel JJ, Vogt TR, Wilson CE: Cholestatic hepatitis after administration of furan derivatives. Arch Intern Med 135:733, 1975.
434. Chiprut RO, Viteri A, Jamroz C, et al: Intrahepatic cholestasis after griseofulvin administration. Gastroenterology 70:1141, 1976.
435. Bickers CR: Environmental and drug factors in hepatic porphyria. Acta Derm Venereol Suppl 100:29, 1982.
436. Gill J, Sprenger HR, Ralph ED, et al: Hepatotoxicity possibly caused by amphotericin B. Ann Pharmacother 33:683, 1999.
437. Lewis JH, Zimmerman HJ, Benson GD, et al: Hepatic injury associated with ketoconazole therapy. Analysis of 33 cases. Gastroenterology 86:503, 1984.
438. Stricker BH, Blok AP, Bronkhorst FB, et al: Ketoconazole-associated hepatic injury. A clinicopathological study of 55 cases. J Hepatol 3:399, 1986.
439. Lake-Bakaar G, Scheuer PJ, Sherlock S: Hepatic reactions associated with ketoconazole in the United Kingdom. BMJ 294:419, 1987.
440. Rodriguez RJ, Acosta D Jr: Metabolism of ketoconazole and deacetylated ketoconazole by rat hepatic microsomes and flavin-containing monooxygenases. Drug Metab Disp 25:772, 1997.
441. Rodriguez RJ, Acosta C: N-deacetyl ketoconazole-induced hepatotoxicity in a primary culture system of rat hepatocytes. Toxicology 117:123, 1997.
442. Rodriguez RJ, Proteau PJ, Marquez BL, et al: Flavin-containing monooxygenase-mediated metabolism of N-deacetyl ketoconazole by rat hepatic microsomes. Drug Metab Disp 27:880, 1999.
443. Trujillo MA, Galgiani JN, Sampliner RE: Evaluation of hepatic injury arising during fluconazole therapy. Arch Intern Med 154:102, 1994.
444. Bronstein JA, Gros P, Hernandez E, et al: Fatal acute hepatic necrosis due to dose-dependent fluconazole hepatotoxicity. Clin Infect Dis 25:1266, 1997.
445. Wells C, Lever AM: Dose-dependent fluconazole hepatotoxicity proven on biopsy and rechallenge. J Infect 24:111, 1992.
446. Woodtli W, Vonmoos P, Siegrist P, et al: [Amodiaquine-induced hepatitis with leukopenia]. Schweiz Med Wochenschr 116:966, 1986.
447. Crerar-Gilbert A, Boots R, Fraenkel D, et al: Survival following fulminant hepatic failure from fluconazole induced hepatitis. Anaesth Intensive Care 27:650, 1999.
448. Guillaume MP, De Prez C, Cogan E: Subacute mitochondrial liver disease in a patient with AIDS: possible relationship to prolonged fluconazole administration. Am J Gastroenterol 91:165, 1996.
449. Cadle RM, Zenon GJ 3rd, Rodriguez-Barradas MC, et al: Fluconazole-induced symptomatic phenytoin toxicity. Ann Pharmacother 28:191, 1994.
450. Clerig Arnau U, Garcia Rodriguez J, Perez Lidon G, et al: [Cholestatic hepatitis secondary to clotrimazole]. Med Clin 98:757, 1992.
451. Gallardo-Quesada S, Luelmo-Aguilar J, Guanyabens-Calvet C: Hepatotoxicity associated with itraconazole. Int J Dermatol 34:589, 1995.
452. Hann SK, Kim JB, Im S, et al: Itraconazole-induced acute hepatitis. Br J Dermatol 129:500, 1993.
453. Chotmongkol V, Sukeepaisarncharoen W: Maintenance therapy with itraconazole after treatment of cryptococcal meningitis in the acquired immunodeficiency syndrome. J Med Assoc Thai 80:767, 1997.
454. Hecht FM, Wheat J, Korzun AH, et al: Itraconazole maintenance treatment for histoplasmosis in AIDS: a prospective, multicenter trial. J Acquir Immune Defic Syndr 16:100, 1997.
455. Gersch K, Broker HJ, Morl H, et al: [Drug-induced hepatitis caused by Fansidar]. Schweiz Med Wochenschr 117:1544, 1987.
456. Meier P, Schmid M, Staubli M: [Acute hepatitis following administration of fansidar]. Schweiz Med Wochenschr 120:221, 1990.
457. Okazaki Y, Watanabe N, Uchiyama J, et al: [A case of hypersensitivity type of liver injury induced by pyrimetamine and sulfadoxin (Fansidar)]. Nippon Shokakibyo Gakkai Zasshi 94:129, 1997.
458. Larrey D, Castot A, Pessayre D, et al: Amodiaquine-induced hepatitis. A report of seven cases. Ann Intern Med 104:801, 1986.
459. Bernuau J, Larrey D, Campillo B, et al: Amodiaquine-induced fulminant hepatitis. J Hepatol 6:109, 1988.
460. Raymond JM, Dumas F, Baldit C, et al: Fatal acute hepatitis due to amodiaquine. J Clin Gastroenterol 11:602, 1989.
461. Sturchler D, Schar M, Gyr N: Leucopenia and abnormal liver function in travellers on malaria chemoprophylaxis. J Trop Med Hyg 90:239, 1987.
462. Jewell H, Maggs JL, Harrison AC, et al: Role of hepatic metabolism in the bioactivation and detoxication of amodiaquine. Xenobiotica 25:199, 1995.
463. Hepburn NC, Siddique I, Howie AF, et al: Hepatotoxicity of sodium stibogluconate therapy for Am cutaneous leishmaniasis. Trans R Soc Trop Med Hyg 88:453, 1994.
464. Hepburn NC, Siddique I, Howie AF, et al: Hepatotoxicity of sodium stibogluconate in leishmaniasis. Lancet 342:238, 1993.
465. Steiger U, Cotting J, Reichen J: Albendazole treatment of echinococcosis in humans: effects on microsomal metabolism and drug tolerance. Clin Pharmacol Ther 47:347, 1990.
466. Morris CL, Smith PG: Albendazole in hydatid disease—hepatocellular toxicity. Trans R Soc Trop Med Hyg 81:343, 1987.
467. el-Mufti M, Kamag A, Ibrahim H, et al: Albendazole therapy of hydatid disease: 2-year follow-up of 40 cases. Ann Trop Med Parasitol 87:241, 1993.
468. Choudhuri G, Prasad RN: Jaundice due to albendazole. Indian J Gastroenterol 7:245, 1988.
469. Jalota R, Freston JW: Severe intrahepatic cholestasis due to thiabendazole. Am J Trop Med Hyg 23:676, 1974.
470. Skandrani K, Richardet JP, Duvoux C, et al: [Hepatic transplantation for severe ductopenia related to ingestion of thiabendazole]. Gastroenterol Clin Biol 21:623, 1997.
471. Roy MA, Nugent FW, Aretz HT: Micronodular cirrhosis after thiabendazole. Dig Dis Sci 34:938, 1989.
472. Cohen C: Liver pathology in hycanthone hepatitis. Gastroenterology 75:103, 1978.
473. Shekhar KC: Schistosomiasis drug therapy and treatment considerations. Drugs 42:379, 1991.
474. Stolte JB: [Letter: 3 deaths following administration of hycanthone (Etrenol)]. Ned Tijdschr Geneeskd 120:795, 1976.
475. Black M, Mitchell JR, Zimmerman HJ, et al: Isoniazid-associated hepatitis in 114 patients. Gastroenterology 69:289, 1975.
476. Mitchell JR, Zimmerman HJ, Ishak KG, et al: Isoniazid liver injury: clinical spectrum, pathology, and probable pathogenesis. Ann Intern Med 84:181, 1976.
477. Beaudry PH, Brickman HF, Wise MB, et al: Liver enzyme disturbances during isoniazid chemoprophylaxis in children. Am Rev Respir Dis 110:581, 1974.
478. Litt IF, Cohen MI, McNamara H: Isoniazid hepatitis in adolescents. J Pediatr 89:133, 1976.
479. Stein MT, Liang C: Clinical hepatotoxicity of isoniazid in children. Pediatrics 64:499, 1979.
480. Kopanoff CE, Snider CE Jr, Caras GJ: Isoniazid-related hepatitis: a U.S. Public Health Service cooperative surveillance study. Am Rev Respir Dis 117:991, 1978.

481. Lees AW, Allan GW, Smith J, et al: Toxicity from rifampicin plus isoniazid and rifampicin plus ethambutol therapy. Tubercle 52:182, 1971.
482. Pessayre D, Bentata M, Degott C, et al: Isoniazid-rifampin fulminant hepatitis. A possible consequence of the enhancement of isoniazid hepatotoxicity by enzyme induction. Gastroenterology 72:284, 1977.
483. Durand F, Jebrak G, Pessayre D, et al: Hepatotoxicity of antitubercular treatments. Rationale for monitoring liver status. Drug Safety 15:394, 1996.
484. Anonymous. From the Centers for Disease Control and Prevention. Update: Fatal and severe liver injuries associated with rifampin and pyrazinamide for latent tuberculosis infection, and revisions in American Thoracic Society/CDC recommendations—United States, 2001. JAMA 286:1445, 2001.
485. Altman C, Biour M, Grange JC: [Hepatic toxicity of antitubercular agents. Role of different drugs. 199 cases]. Presse Med 22:1212, 1993.
486. Wu JC, Lee SD, Yeh PF, et al: Isoniazid-rifampin-induced hepatitis in hepatitis B carriers. Gastroenterology 98:502, 1990.
487. Ozick LA, Jacob L, Comer GM, et al: Hepatotoxicity from isoniazid and rifampin in inner-city AIDS patients. Am J Gastroenterol 90:1978, 1995.
488. Krishnaswamy K, Prasad CE, Murthy KJ: Hepatic dysfunction in undernourished patients receiving isoniazid and rifampicin. Trop Geogr Med 43:156, 1991.
489. Mitchell JR, Thorgeirsson UP, Black M, et al: Increased incidence of isoniazid hepatitis in rapid acetylators: possible relation to hydrazine metabolites. Clin Pharmacol Ther 18:70, 1975.
490. Sarma GR, Immanuel C, Kailasam S, et al: Rifampin-induced release of hydrazine from isoniazid. A possible cause of hepatitis during treatment of tuberculosis with regimens containing isoniazid and rifampin. Am Rev Respir Dis 133:1072, 1986.
491. Nelson SD, Mitchell JR, Timbrell JA, et al: Isoniazid and iproniazid: activation of metabolites to toxic intermediates in man and rat. Science 193:901, 1976.
492. Mitchell JR, Snodgrass WR, Gillette JR: The role of biotransformation in chemical-induced liver injury. Environ Health Perspect 15:27, 1976.
493. Lauterburg BH, Smith CV, Todd EL, et al: Oxidation of hydrazine metabolites formed from isoniazid. Clin Pharmacol Ther 38:566, 1985.
494. Lauterburg BH, Smith CV, Todd EL, et al: Pharmacokinetics of the toxic hydrazine metabolites formed from isoniazid in humans. Pharmacol Exp Ther 235:566, 1985.
495. Gronhagen-Riska C, Hellstrom PE, Froseth B: Predisposing factors in hepatitis induced by isoniazid-rifampin treatment of tuberculosis. Am Rev Respir Dis 118:461, 1978.
496. Snider CE Jr, Caras GJ: Isoniazid-associated hepatitis deaths: a review of available information. Am Rev Respir Dis 145:494, 1992.
497. Ellard GA, Mitchison CA, Girling CJ, et al: The hepatic toxicity of isoniazid among rapid and slow acetylators of the drug. Am Rev Respir Dis 118:628, 1978.
498. Jordan TJ, Lewit EM, Reichman LB: Isoniazid preventive therapy for tuberculosis. Decision analysis considering ethnicity and gender. Am Rev Respir Dis 144:1357, 1991.
499. Dickinson CS, Bailey W. C, Hirschowitz BI, et al: Risk factors for isoniazid (NIH)-induced liver dysfunction. J Clin Gastroenterol 3:271, 1981.
500. Timbrell JA, Wright JM, Baillie TA: Monoacetylhydrazine as a metabolite of isoniazid in man. Clin Pharmacol Ther 22:602, 1977.
501. Peretti E, Karlaganis G, Lauterburg BH: Acetylation of acetylhydrazine, the toxic metabolite of isoniazid, in humans. Inhibition by concomitant administration of isoniazid. J Pharmacol Exp Ther 243:686, 1987.
502. Gent WL, Seifart HI, Parkin CP, et al: Factors in hydrazine formation from isoniazid by paediatric and adult tuberculosis patients. Eur J Clin Pharmacol 43:131, 1992.
503. Comstock GW: New data on preventive treatment with isoniazid. Ann Intern Med 98:663, 1983.
504. Maddrey WC, Boitnott JK: Isoniazid hepatitis. Ann Intern Med 79:1, 1973.
505. Bailey WC, Byrd RB, Glassroth JL, et al: Preventive treatment of tuberculosis. Chest 87:128S, 1985.
506. Garibaldi RA, Drusin RE, Ferebee SH, et al: Isoniazid-associated hepatitis. Report of an outbreak. Am Rev Respir Dis 106:357, 1972.
507. Millard PS, Wilcosky TC, Reade-Christopher SJ, et al: Isoniazid-related fatal hepatitis. West J Med 164:486, 1996.
508. Thulasimany M: Increased incidence of hepatitis induced by isoniazid-rifampin combination in children. J Pediatr 100:174, 1982.
509. Parthasarathy R, Sarma GR, Janardhanam B, et al: Hepatic toxicity in South Indian patients during treatment of tuberculosis with short-course regimens containing isoniazid, rifampicin and pyrazinamide. Tubercle 67:99, 1986.
510. O'Brien RJ, Long MW, Cross FS, et al: Hepatotoxicity from isoniazid and rifampin among children treated for tuberculosis. Pediatrics 72:491, 1983.
511. Scheuer PJ, Summerfield JA, Lal S, et al: Rifampicin hepatitis. A clinical and histological study. Lancet 1:421, 1974.
512. Most JA, Markle GB: A nearly fatal hepatotoxic reaction to rifampin after halothane anesthesia. Am J Surg 127:593, 1974.
513. Bachs L, Pares A, Elena M, et al: Effects of long term administration of rifampin in primary biliary cirrhosis. Gastroenterology 102:2077, 1992.
514. Melamed AJ, Muller RJ, Gold JW, et al: Possible zidovudine-induced hepatotoxicity. JAMA 258:2063, 1987.
515. Dubin G, Braffman MN: Zidovudine-induced hepatotoxicity. Ann Intern Med 110:85, 1989.
516. Sundar K, Suarez M, Banogon PE, et al: Zidovudine-induced fatal lactic acidosis and hepatic failure in patients with acquired immunodeficiency syndrome: report of two patients and review of the literature. Crit Care Med 25:1425, 1997.
517. Olano JP, Borucki MJ, Wen JW, et al: Massive hepatic steatosis and lactic acidosis in a patient with AIDS who was receiving zidovudine. Clin Infect Dis 21:973, 1995.
518. Freiman JP, Helfert KE, Hamrell MR, et al: Hepatomegaly with severe steatosis in HIV-seropositive patients. AIDS 7:379, 1993.
519. Acosta BS, Grimsley EW: Zidovudine-associated type B lactic acidosis and hepatic steatosis in an HIV-infected patient. South Med J 92:421, 1999.
520. Stein DS: A new syndrome of hepatomegaly with severe steatosis in HIV-seropositive patients. AIDS Clin Care 6:1721, 1994.
521. Miller KD, Cameron M, Wood LV, et al: Lactic acidosis and hepatic steatosis associated with use of stavudine: report of four cases. Ann Intern Med 133:192, 2000.
522. Mokrzycki MH, Harris C, May H, et al: Lactic acidosis associated with stavudine administration: a report of five cases. Clin Infect Dis 30:198, 2000.
523. Carr A, Morey A, Mallon P, et al: Fatal portal hypertension, liver failure, and mitochondrial dysfunction after HIV-1 nucleoside analogue-induced hepatitis and lactic acidaemia. Lancet 357:1412, 2001.
524. Henry K, Acosta EP, Jochimsen E: Hepatotoxicity and rash associated with zidovudine and zalcitabine chemoprophylaxis. Ann Intern Med 124:855, 1996.
525. Lonergan JT, Behling C, Pfander H, et al: Hyperlactatemia and hepatic abnormalities in 10 human immunodeficiency virus-infected patients receiving nucleoside analogue combination regimens. Clin Infect Dis 31:162, 2000.
526. Chariot P, Drogou I, de Lacroix-Szmania I, et al: Zidovudine-induced mitochondrial disorder with massive liver steatosis, myopathy, lactic acidosis, and mitochondrial DNA depletion. J Hepatol 30:156, 1999.
527. Lenzo NP, Garas BA, French MA: Hepatic steatosis and lactic acidosis associated with stavudine treatment in an HIV patient: a case report. AIDS 11:1294, 1997.
528. Fouty B, Frerman F, Reves R: Riboflavin to treat nucleoside analogue-induced lactic acidosis. Lancet 352:291, 1998.
529. Brinkman K: Editorial response: hyperlactatemia and hepatic steatosis as features of mitochondrial toxicity of nucleoside analogue reverse transcriptase inhibitors. Clin Infect Dis 31:167, 2000.
530. Bleeker-Rovers CP, Kadir SW, van Leusen R, et al: Hepatic steatosis and lactic acidosis caused by stavudine in an HIV-infected patient. Neth J Med 57:190, 2000.
531. Brivet FG, Nion I, Megarbane B, et al: Fatal lactic acidosis and liver steatosis associated with didanosine and stavudine treatment: a respiratory chain dysfunction? J Hepatol 32:364, 2000 (letter; comment).
532. Ellozy S, Massen R, Chao L, et al: Antiretroviral-induced hepatic steatosis and lactic acidosis: case report and review of the literature. Am Surg 67:680, 2001.

533. Bissuel F, Bruneel F, Habersetzer F, et al: Fulminant hepatitis with severe lactate acidosis in HIV-infected patients on didanosine therapy. J Intern Med 235:367, 1994.
534. Lai KK, Gang CL, Zawacki JK, et al: Fulminant hepatic failure associated with 2′,3′-dideoxyinosine (ddI). Ann Intern Med 115:283, 1991.
535. Hu B, French SW: 2′,3′-Dideoxyinosine-induced Mallory bodies in patients with HIV. Am J Clin Pathol 108:280, 1997.
536. Ware AJ, Berggren RA, Taylor WE: Didanosine-induced hepatitis. Am J Gastroenterol 95:2141, 2000.
537. Hartman NR, Ahluwalia GS, Cooney CA, et al: Inhibitors of IMP dehydrogenase stimulate the phosphorylation of the anti-human immunodeficiency virus nucleosides 2′,3′-dideoxyadenosine and 2′,3′-dideoxyinosine. Mol Pharmacol 40:118, 1991.
538. Balzarini J, Lee CK, Herdewijn P, et al: Mechanism of the potentiating effect of ribavirin on the activity of 2′,3′-dideoxyinosine against human immunodeficiency virus. J Biol Chem 266:21509, 1991.
539. Harvie P, Omar RF, Dusserre N, et al: Ribavirin potentiates the efficacy and toxicity of 2′,3′- dideoxyinosine in the murine acquired immunodeficiency syndrome model. J Pharmacol Exp Ther 279:1009, 1996.
540. Brinkman K, Smeitink JA, Romijn JA, et al: Mitochondrial toxicity induced by nucleoside-analogue reverse-transcriptase inhibitors is a key factor in the pathogenesis of antiretroviral-therapy-related lipodystrophy. Lancet 354:1112, 1999.
541. Carr A, Miller J, Law M, et al: A syndrome of lipoatrophy, lactic acidaemia and liver dysfunction associated with HIV nucleoside analogue therapy: contribution to protease inhibitor-related lipodystrophy syndrome. AIDS 14:F25, 2000.
542. Lafeuillade A, Hittinger G, Chadapaud S: Increased mitochondrial toxicity with ribavirin in HIV/HCV coinfection. Lancet 357:280, 2001.
543. Salmon-Ceron D, Chauvelot-Moachon L, Abad S, et al: Mitochondrial toxic effects and ribavirin. Lancet 357:1803, 2001.
544. Kakuda TN, Brinkman K: Mitochondrial toxic effects and ribavirin. Lancet 357:1802, 2001.
545. Allen LB, Quenelle CC, Westbrook L, et al: In vitro and in vivo enhancement of ddI activity against Rauscher murine leukemia virus by ribavirin. Antiviral Res 27:317, 1995.
546. Japour AJ, Lertora JJ, Meehan PM, et al: A phase-I study of the safety, pharmacokinetics, and antiviral activity of combination didanosine and ribavirin in patients with HIV-1 disease. AIDS Clin Trials Group 231 Protocol Team. J Acq Immune Defic Syndr 13:235, 1996.
547. Brinkman K, Kakuda TN: Mitochondrial toxicity of nucleoside analogue reverse transcriptase inhibitors: a looming obstacle for long-term antiretroviral therapy? Opin Infect Dis 12:5, 2000.
548. Genini D, Sheeter D, Rought S, et al: HIV induces lymphocyte apoptosis by a p53-initiated, mitochondrial-mediated mechanism. FASEB J 15:5, 2001.
549. Kleiner CE, Gaffey MJ, Sallie R, et al: Histopathologic changes associated with fialuridine hepatotoxicity. Mod Pathol 10:192, 1997.
550. McKenzie R, Fried MW, Sallie R, et al: Hepatic failure and lactic acidosis due to fialuridine (FIAU), an investigational nucleoside analogue for chronic hepatitis B. N Engl J Med 333:1099, 1995.
551. Cui L, Yoon S, Schinazi RF, et al: Cellular and molecular events leading to mitochondrial toxicity of 1-(2-deoxy-2-fluoro-1-beta-D-arabinofuranosyl)-5-iodouracil in human liver cells. J Clin Invest 95:555, 1995.
552. Brau N, Leaf HL, Wieczorek RL, et al: Severe hepatitis in three AIDS patients treated with indinavir. Lancet 349:924, 1997.
553. Vergis E, Paterson CL, Singh N: Indinavir-associated hepatitis in patients with advanced HIV infection. Int J STD AIDS 9:53, 1998.
554. Matsuda J, Gohchi K: Severe hepatitis in patients with AIDS and haemophilia B treated with indinavir. Lancet 350:364, 1997.
555. Trape M, Barnosky S: Nelfinavir in expanded postexposure prophylaxis causing acute hepatitis with cholestatic features: two case reports. Infect Contr Hosp Epidemiol 22:333, 2001.
556. Cozza KL, Swanton EJ, Humphreys CW: Hepatotoxicity with combination of valproic acid, ritonavir, and nevirapine: a case report. Psychosomatics 41:452, 2000.
557. Vandercam B, Moreau M, Horsmans C, et al: Acute hepatitis in a patient treated with saquinavir and ritonavir: absence of cross-toxicity with indinavir. Infection 26:313, 1998.
558. Picard O, Rosmorduc O, Cabane J: Hepatotoxicity associated with ritonavir. Ann Intern Med 129:670, 1998.
559. Zimmermann HJ: Oncotherapeutic and immunesuppresive agents. In Zimmerman HJ, ed: Hepatotoxicity, ed 2. Lippincott, Williams and Wilkins, 1999:687.
560. Perry MC: Chemotherapeutic agents and hepatotoxicity. Semin Oncol 19:551, 1992.
561. McDonald GB, Tirumali N: Intestinal and liver toxicity of antineoplastic drugs. West J Med 140:250, 1984.
562. Shorey J, Schenker S, Suki WN, et al: Hepatotoxicity of mercaptopurine. Arch Intern Med 122:54, 1968.
563. Einhorn M, Davidshohn I: Hepatotoxicity of 6-mercaptopurine. JAMA 188:802, 1964.
564. Topley JM, Benson J, Squier MV, et al: Hepatotoxicity in the treatment of acute lymphoblastic leukaemia. Med Pediatr Oncol 7:393, 1979.
565. Greaves MW, Dawber R: Azathioprine in psoriasis. BMJ 2:237, 1970.
566. Horsmans Y, Rahier J, Geubel AP :Reversible cholestasis with bile duct injury following azathioprine therapy. A case report. Liver 11:89, 1991.
567. Knowles SR, Gupta AK, Shear NH, et al: Azathioprine hypersensitivity-like reactions—a case report and a review of the literature. Clin Exp Dermatol 20:353, 1995.
568. Malekzadeh MH, Grushkin CM, Wright HT, Jr, et al: Hepatic dysfunction after renal transplantation in children. J Pediatr 81:279, 1972.
569. Gerlag PG, van Hooff JP: Hepatic sinusoidal dilatation with portal hypertension during azathioprine treatment: a cause of chronic liver disease after kidney transplantation. Transplant Proc 19:3699, 1987.
570. Degott C, Rueff B, Kreis H, et al: Peliosis hepatis in recipients of renal transplants. Gut 19:748, 1978.
571. Mion F, Napoleon B, Berger F, et al: Azathioprine induced liver disease: nodular regenerative hyperplasia of the liver and perivenous fibrosis in a patient treated for multiple sclerosis. Gut 32:715, 1991.
572. Watanabe A, Obata T, Nagashima H, et al: Nonicteric liver damage with a gamma-glutamyl transpeptidase level of 5,609 units/l in a renal-transplant recipient receiving azathioprine. Acta Med Okayama 38:533, 1984.
573. Haboubi NY, Ali HH, Whitwell HL, et al: Role of endothelial cell injury in the spectrum of azathioprine-induced liver disease after renal transplant: light microscopy and ultrastructural observations. Am J Gastroenterol 83:256, 1988.
574. Marubbio AT, Danielson B: Hepatic veno-occlusive disease in a renal transplant patient receiving azathioprine. Gastroenterology 69:739, 1975.
575. Liano F, Moreno A, Matesanz R, et al: Veno-occlusive hepatic disease of the liver in renal transplantation: is azathioprine the cause? Nephron 51:509, 1989.
576. Sterneck M, Wiesner R, Ascher N, et al: Azathioprine hepatotoxicity after liver transplantation. Hepatology 14:806, 1991.
577. Shepherd PC, Fooks J, Gray R, et al: Thioguanine used in maintenance therapy of chronic myeloid leukaemia causes non-cirrhotic portal hypertension. Results from MRC CMLIITrial comparing busulphan with busulphan and thioguanine. Br J Haematol 79:185, 1991.
578. Shepherd P, Harrison CJ: Idiopathic portal hypertension associated with cytotoxic drugs. J Clin Pathol 43:206, 1990.
579. Satti MB, Weinbren K, Gordon-Smith EC: 6-thioguanine as a cause of toxic veno-occlusive disease of the liver. J Clin Pathol 35:1086, 1982.
580. Griner PF, Elbadawi A, Packman CH: Veno-occlusive disease of the liver after chemotherapy of acute leukemia. Report of two cases. Ann Intern Med 85:578, 1976.
581. Ambiru S, Miyazaki M, Ito H, et al: [Intraportal infusion of 5-FU and lipiodol-aclarubicin after hepatic resection for colorectal liver metastasis]. Nippon Geka Gakkai Zasshi 96:145, 1995.
582. Klotz HP, Weder W, Largiader F: Local and systemic toxicity of intra-hepato-arterial chemotherapy for treatment of unresectable liver metastases of colorectal cancer with 5-fluorouracil and high dose leucovorin. Helv Chir Acta 60:283, 1993.
583. Hohn D, Melnick J, Stagg R, et al: Biliary sclerosis in patients receiving hepatic arterial infusions of floxuridine. J Clin Oncol 3:98, 1985.

584. Bolton JS, Bowen JC: Biliary sclerosis associated with hepatic artery infusion of floxuridine. Surgery 99:119, 1986.
585. Remick SC, Benson AB 3rd, Weese JL, et al: Phase I trial of hepatic artery infusion of 5-iodo-2′-deoxyuridine and 5-fluorouracil in patients with advanced hepatic malignancy: biochemically based combination chemotherapy. Cancer Res 49:6437, 1989.
586. Rougier P, Laplanche A, Huguier M, et al: Hepatic arterial infusion of floxuridine in patients with liver metastases from colorectal carcinoma: long-term results of a prospective randomized trial. J Clin Oncol 10:1112, 1992.
587. Pettavel J, Gardiol D, Bergier N, et al: Fatal liver cirrhosis associated with long-term arterial infusion of floxuridine. Lancet 2:1162, 1986.
588. Faggioli P, De Paschale M, Tocci A, et al: Acute hepatic toxicity during cyclic chemotherapy in non Hodgkin's lymphoma. Haematologica 82:38, 1997.
589. Goodell B, Leventhal B, Henderson E: Cytosine arabinoside in acute granulocytic leukemia. Clin Pharmacol Ther 12:599, 1971.
590. Traggis CG, Dohlwitz A, Das L, et al: Cytosine arabinoside in acute leukemia of childhood. Cancer 28:815, 1971.
591. Herzig RH, Wolff SN, Lazarus HM, et al: High-dose cytosine arabinoside therapy for refractory leukemia. Blood 62:361, 1983.
592. Haskell CM, Canellos GP, Leventhal BG, et al: L-asparaginase: therapeutic and toxic effects in patients with neoplastic disease. N Engl J Med 281:1028, 1969.
593. Shanholtz C: Acute life-threatening toxicity of cancer treatment. Crit Care Clin 17:483, 2001.
594. Weiss RB: Hypersensitivity reactions to cancer chemotherapeutic agents. Ann Intern Med 94:66, 1981.
595. Biggs JC, Chesterman CN, Holliday J: L-asparaginase—clinical experience in leukaemia, lymphoma and carcinoma. Aust N Z J Med 1:1, 1971.
596. Ansfield FJ: Clin studies with mithramycin. Oncology 23:283, 1969.
597. Kennedy BJ: Metabolic and toxic effects of mithramycin during tumor therapy. Am J Med 49:494, 1970.
598. Aviles A, Herrera J, Ramos E, et al: Hepatic injury during doxorubicin therapy. Arch Pathol Lab Med 108:912, 1984.
599. Minow RA, Stern MH, Casey JH, et al: Clinico-pathologic correlation of liver damage in patients treated with 6-mercaptopurine and Adriamycin. Cancer 38:1524, 1976.
600. Kun LE, Camitta BM: Hepatopathy following irradiation and Adriamycin. Cancer 42:81, 1978.
601. Pritchard J, Raine J, Wallendszus K: Hepatotoxicity of actinomycin-C. Lancet 1:168, 1989.
602. D'Angio GJ: Hepatotoxicity with actinomycin C. Lancet 2:104, 1987.
603. Jayabose S, Shende A, Lanzkowsky P: Hepatotoxicity of chemotherapy following nephrectomy and radiation therapy for right-sided Wilms tumor. J Pediatr 88:898, 1976.
604. Czauderna P, Katski K, Kowalczyk J, et al: Venoocclusive liver disease (VOD) as a complication of Wilms' tumour management in the series of consecutive 206 patients. Eur J Pediatr Surg 10:300, 2000.
605. Hazar V, Kutluk T, Akyuz C, et al: Veno-occlusive disease-like hepatotoxicity in two children receiving chemotherapy for Wilms' tumor and clear cell sarcoma of kidney. Pediatr Hematol Oncol 15:85, 1998.
606. Bisogno G, de Kraker J, Weirich A, et al: Veno-occlusive disease of the liver in children treated for Wilms tumor. Med Pediatr Oncol 29:245, 1997.
607. Flentje M, Weirich A, Potter R, et al: Hepatotoxicity in irradiated nephroblastoma patients during postoperative treatment according to SIOP9/GPOH. Radiother Oncol 31:222, 1994.
608. Lorber MI, Van Buren CT, Flechner SM, et al: Hepatobiliary and pancreatic complications of cyclosporine therapy in 466 renal transplant recipients. Transplantation 43:35, 1987.
609. Kassianides C, Nussenblatt R, Palestine AG, et al: Liver injury from cyclosporine A. Dig Dis Sci 35:693, 1990.
610. Roman ID, Monte MJ, Gonzalez-Buitrago JM, et al: Inhibition of hepatocytary vesicular transport by cyclosporin A in the rat: relationship with cholestasis and hyperbilirubinemia. Hepatology 12:83, 1990.
611. el Saghir NS, Hawkins KA: Hepatotoxicity following vincristine therapy. Cancer 54:2006, 1984.
612. Tran A, Housset C, Boboc B, et al: Etoposide (VP 16-213) induced hepatitis. Report of three cases following standard-dose treatments. J Hepatol 12:36, 1991.
613. Paschke R, Worst P, Brust J, et al: [Hepatotoxicity with etoposide-ifosfamide combination therapy]. Onkologie 11:273, 1988.
614. Menard CB, Gisselbrecht C, Marty M, et al: Antineoplastic agents and the liver. Gastroenterology 78:142, 1980.
615. Cleland BC, Pokorny CS: Cyclophosphamide related hepatotoxicity. Aust N Z J Med 23:408, 1993.
616. Bacon AM, Rosenberg SA: Cyclophosphamide hepatotoxicity in a patient with systemic lupus erythematosus. Ann Intern Med 97:62, 1982.
617. Umeda K, Lin Y. W, Watanabe K, et al: [Hematopoietic stem cell transplantation with busulfanthiotepa-cyclophosphamide conditioning for pediatric patients with high-risk acute lymphoblastic leukemia]. Rinsho Ketsueki 42:685, 2001.
618. Andersson BS, Gajewski J, Donato M, et al: Allogeneic stem cell transplantation (BMT) for AML and MDS following i.v. busulfan and cyclophosphamide (i.v. BuCy). Bone Marrow Transplant 25:S35, 2000.
619. Worth L, Tran H, Petropoulos D, et al: Hematopoietic stem cell transplantation for childhood myeloid malignancies after high-dose thiotepa, busulfan and cyclophosphamide. Bone Marrow Transplant 24:947, 1999.
620. Lee JL, Gooley T, Bensinger W, et al: Veno-occlusive disease of the liver after busulfan, melphalan, and thiotepa conditioning therapy: incidence, risk factors, and outcome. Biol Blood Marrow Transplant 5:306, 1999.
621. Modzelewski JR, Jr, Daeschner C, Joshi VV, et al: Veno-occlusive disease of the liver induced by low-dose cyclophosphamide. Mod Pathol 7:967, 1994.
622. Pichon N, Debette-Gratien M, Cessot F, et al: [Acute cholestatic hepatitis due to chlorambucil]. Gastroenterol Clin Biol 25:202, 2001.
623. Phillips GL, Fay JW, Herzig GP, et al: Intensive 1,3-bis(2-chloroethyl)-1-nitrosourea (BCNU), NSC #4366650 and cryopreserved autologous marrow transplantation for refractory cancer. A phase I-II study. Cancer 52:1792, 1983.
624. Lokich JJ, Drum CE, Kaplan W: Hepatic toxicity of nitrosourea analogues. Clin Pharmacol Ther 16:363, 1974.
625. Girgin F, Tuzun S, Demir A, et al: Cytoprotective effects of trimetazidine in carmustine cholestasis. Exp Toxicol Pathol 51:326, 1999.
626. Quinio P, Bouche O, Lambolais C, et al: Fatal hepatic toxicity of DTIC: a new case. Inten Care Med 23:1099, 1997.
627. Voigt H, Caselitz J, Janner M: [Veno-occlusive syndrome with acute liver dystrophy following decarbazine therapy of malignant melanoma (author's transl)]. Klin Wochenschr 59:229, 1981.
628. Asbury RF, Rosenthal SN, Descalzi ME, et al: Hepatic veno-occlusive disease due to DTIC. Cancer 45:2670, 1980.
629. Vial T, Descotes J: Clin toxicity of the interferons. Drug Safety 10:115, 1994.
630. Manns MP, McHutchison JG, Gordon SC, et al: Peginterferon alfa-2b plus ribavirin compared with interferon alfa-2b plus ribavirin for initial treatment of chronic hepatitis C: a randomised trial. Lancet 358:958, 2001.
630a. Prod Info: (R) A, interferon alfa 2-b, recombinent, Schoring Corp., Kenilworth, NJ, USA (revised 2/2001).
631. Quesada JR, Talpaz M, Rios A, et al: Clinical toxicity of interferons in cancer patients: a review. J Clin Oncol 4:234, 1986.
632. Jones GJ, Itri LM: Safety and tolerance of recombinant interferon alfa-2a (Roferon-A) in cancer patients. Cancer 57:1709, 1986.
633. Whiting JF, Green RM, Rosenbluth AB, et al: Tumor necrosis factor-alpha decreases hepatocyte bile salt uptake and mediates endotoxin-induced cholestasis. Hepatology 22:1273, 1995.
634. Kemeny N, Childs B, Larchian W, et al: A phase II trial of recombinant tumor necrosis factor in patients with advanced colorectal carcinoma. Cancer 66:659, 1990.
635. Fisher B, Keenan AM, Garra BS, et al: Interleukin-2 induces profound reversible cholestasis: a detailed analysis in treated cancer patients. J Clin Oncol 7:1852, 1989.
636. Samlowski WE, Wiebke G, McMurry M, et al: Effects of total parenteral nutrition (TPN) during high-dose interleukin-2 treatment for metastatic cancer. J Immunother 21:65, 1998.
637. Haga Y, Sakamoto K, Egami H, et al: Changes in production of interleukin-1 and interleukin-2 associated with obstructive jaundice and biliary drainage in patients with gastrointestinal cancer. Surgery 106:842, 1989.
638. Hoffman M, Mittelman A, Dworkin B, et al: Severe intrahepatic cholestasis in patients treated with recombinant interleukin-2 and

lymphokine-activated killer cells. J Cancer Res Clin Oncol 115:175, 1989.
639. Smith GN, Piercy WN: Methyldopa hepatotoxicity in pregnancy: a case report. Am J Obstet Gynecol 172:222, 1995.
640. Thomas LA, Cardwell MS: Acute reactive hepatitis in pregnancy induced by alpha-methyldopa. Obstet Gynecol 90:658, 1997.
641. Picaud A, Walter P, de Preville G, et al: [Fatal toxic hepatitis in pregnancy. A discussion of the role of methyldopa]. J Gynecol Obstet Biol Reprod 19:192, 1990.
642. Rodman JS, Deutsch CJ, Gutman SI: Methyldopa hepatitis. A report of six cases and review of the literature. Am J Med 60:941, 1976.
643. Toghill PJ, Smith PG, Benton P, et al: Proceedings: Liver damage in patients taking methyldopa. Gut 15:342, 1974.
644. Hoyumpa AM Jr, Connell AM: Methyldopa hepatitis. Report of three cases. Am J Dig Dis 18:213, 1973.
645. Goldstein GB, Lam KC, Mistilis SP: Drug-induced active chronic hepatitis. Am J Dig Dis 18:177, 1973.
646. Seeff LB: Drug-induced chronic liver disease, with emphasis on chronic active hepatitis. Semin Liver Dis 1:104, 1981.
647. Seeverens H, de Bruin CC, Jordans JG: Myocarditis and methyldopa. Acta Med Scand 211:233, 1982.
648. Bezahler GH: Fatal methyldopa-associated granulomatous hepatitis and myocarditis. Am J Med Sci 283:41, 1982.
649. Moses A, Zahger C, Amir G: Cholestatic liver injury after prolonged exposure to methyldopa. Digestion 42:57, 1989.
650. Arranto AJ, Sotaniemi EA: Histologic follow-up of alpha-methyldopa-induced liver injury. Scand J Gastroenterol 16:865, 1981.
651. Thomas E, Bhuta S, Rosenthal WS: Methyldopa-induced liver injury. Rapid progression to fatal postnecrotic cirrhosis. Arch Pathol Lab Med 100:132, 1976.
652. Schweitzer IL, Peters RL: Acute submassive hepatic necrosis due to methyldopa. A case demonstrating possible initiation of chronic liver disease. Gastroenterology 66:1203, 1974.
653. Furhoff AK: Adverse reactions with methyldopa—a decade's reports. Acta Med Scand 203:425, 1978.
654. Sotaniemi EA, Hokkanen OT, Ahokas JT, et al: Hepatic injury and drug metabolism in patients with alpha-methyldopa-induced liver damage. Eur J Clin Pharmacol 12:429, 1977.
655. Granlien M, Ostergaard Kristensen HP: [Methyldopa hepatitis in 2 sisters]. Ugeskrift Laeger 140:978, 1978.
656. Delpre G, Grinblat J, Kadish U, et al: Case report. Immunological studies in a case of hepatitis following methyldopa administration. Am J Med Sci 277:207, 1979.
657. Kirtland HH 3rd, Mohler CN, Horwitz CA: Methyldopa inhibition of suppressor-lymphocyte function: a proposed cause of autoimmune hemolytic anemia. N Engl J Med 302:825, 1980.
658. Dybing E, Nelson SD, Mitchell JR, et al: Oxidation of alpha-methyldopa and other catechols by cytochrome P-450-generated superoxide anion: possible mechanism of methyldopa hepatitis. Mol Pharmacol 12:911, 1976.
659. Dybing E, Nelson SC: Metabolic activation of methyldopa and other catechols. Arch Toxicol Suppl 1:117, 1978.
660. Neuberger J, Kenna JG, Nouri Aria K, et al: Antibody mediated hepatocyte injury in methyl dopa induced hepatotoxicity. Gut 26:1233, 1985.
661. Toghill PJ, Smith PG, Benton P, et al: Methyldopa liver damage. BMJ 3:545, 1974.
662. Puppala AR, Steinheber FU: Fulminant hepatic failure associated with methyldopa. Am J Gastroenterol 68:578, 1977.
663. Crantock L, Prentice R, Powell L: Cholestatic jaundice associated with captopril therapy. J Gastroenterol Hepatol 6:528, 1991.
664. Hagley MT: Captopril-induced cholestatic jaundice. South Med J 84:100, 1991.
665. Hagley MT, Hulisz CT, Burns CM: Hepatotoxicity associated with angiotensin-converting enzyme inhibitors. Ann Pharmacother 27:228, 1993.
666. Parker WA: Captopril-induced cholestatic jaundice. Drug Intell Clin Pharm 18:234, 1984.
667. Rahmat J, Gelfand RL, Gelfand MC, et al: Captopril-associated cholestatic jaundice. Ann Intern Med 102:56, 1985.
668. Schattner A, Kozak N, Friedman J: Captopril-induced jaundice: report of 2 cases and a review of 13 additional reports in the literature. Am J Med Sci 322:236, 2001.
669. Vandenburg M, Parfrey P, Wright P, et al: Hepatitis associated with captopril treatment. Br J Clin Pharmacol 11:105, 1981.
670. Todd P, Levison C, Farthing MJ: Enalapril-related cholestatic jaundice. J Royal Soc Med 83:271, 1990.
671. Jurima-Romet M, Huang HS: Comparative cytotoxicity of angiotensin-converting enzyme inhibitors in cultured rat hepatocytes. Biochem Pharmacol 46:2163, 1993.
672. Valle R, Carrascosa M, Cillero L, et al: Enalapril-induced hepatotoxicity. Ann Pharmacother 27:1405, 1993.
673. Jeserich M, Ihling C, Allgaier HP, et al: Acute liver failure due to enalapril. Herz 25:689, 2000.
674. Hurlimann R, Binek J, Oehlschlegel C, et al: [Enalapril (Reniten)-associated toxic hepatitis]. Schweiz Med Wochenschr 124:1276, 1994.
675. Lunel F, Grippon P, Cadranel JF, et al: [Acute hepatitis after taking enalapril maleate (Renitec)]. Gastroenterol Clin Biol 11:174, 1987.
676. Hagley MT, Benak RL, Hulisz CT: Suspected cross-reactivity of enalapril- and captopril-induced hepatotoxicity. Ann Pharmacother 26:780, 1992.
677. Larrey D, Babany G, Bernuau J, et al: Fulminant hepatitis after lisinopril administration. Gastroenterology 99:1832, 1990.
678. Lindgren A, Olsson R: [Liver damage following antihypertensive therapy. A case report of hepatitis induced by lisinopril and a review]. Lakartidningen 90:1557, 1993.
679. Droste HT, de Vries RA: Chronic hepatitis caused by lisinopril. Neth J Med 46:95, 1995.
680. Nunes AC, Amaro P, Mac as F, et al: Fosinopril-induced prolonged cholestatic jaundice and pruritus: first case report. Eur J Gastroenterol Hepatol 13:279, 2001.
681. Bartoli E, Massarelli G, Solinas A, et al: Acute hepatitis with bridging necrosis due to hydralazine intake. Report of a case. Arch Intern Med 139:698, 1979.
682. Forster HS: Hepatitis from hydralazine. N Engl J Med 302:1362, 1980.
683. Itoh S, Ichinoe A, Tsukada Y, et al: Hydralazine-induced hepatitis. Hepatogastroenterology 28:13, 1981.
684. Itoh S, Yamaba Y, Ichinoe A, et al: Hydralazine-induced liver injury. Dig Dis Sci 25:884, 1980.
685. Shaefer MS, Markin RS, Wood RP, et al: Hydralazine-induced cholestatic jaundice following liver transplantation. Transplantation 47:203, 1989.
686. Rice C, Burdick CO: Granulomatous hepatitis from hydralazine therapy. Arch Intern Med 143:1077, 1983.
687. Myers JL, Augur NA Jr: Hydralazine-induced cholangitis. Gastroenterology 87:1185, 1984.
688. Hod M, Friedman S, Schoenfeld A, et al: Hydralazine-induced hepatitis in pregnancy. Int J Fertil 31:352, 1986.
689. Roschlau G, Baumgarten R, Fengler JC: [Dihydralazine hepatitis. Morphologic and clinical criteria for diagnosis]. Zentralblatt Allgemeine Pathol Anat 136:127, 1990.
690. Beaune P, Bourdi M, Belloc C, et al: Immunotoxicology and expression of human cytochrome P450 in microorganisms. Toxicology 82:53, 1993.
691. Beaune PH, Lecoeur S, Bourdi M, et al: Anti-cytochrome P450 autoantibodies in drug-induced disease. Eur J Haematol 60:89, 1996.
692. Boitier E, Beaune P: Cytochromes P450 as targets to autoantibodies in immune mediated diseases. Mol Aspects Med 20:84, 1999.
693. Machnik G, Bergert A, Justus J, et al: [Drug-induced hepatitis after dihydralazine treatment with fatal consequences]. Zentralblatt Allgemeine Pathol Anat 134:167, 1988.
694. Manier JW, Chang WW, Kirchner JP, et al: Hepatotoxicity associated with ticrynafen—a uricosuric diuretic. Am J Gastroenterol 77:401, 1982.
695. Pariente EA, Andre C, Zafrani ES, et al: [Tienilic acid can induce acute hepatitis, chronic hepatitis and cirrhosis. A report of three cases (author's transl)]. Gastroenterol Clin Biol 5:567, 1981.
696. Neuberger J, Williams R: Immune mechanisms in tienilic acid associated hepatotoxicity. Gut 30:515, 1989.
697. Lecoeur S, Andre C, Beaune PH: Tienilic acid-induced autoimmune hepatitis: anti-liver and-kidney microsomal type 2 autoantibodies recognize a three-site conformational epitope on cytochrome P4502C9. Mol Pharmacol 50:326, 1996.
698. Mousson C, Justrabo E, Tanter Y, et al: [Acute granulomatous interstitial nephritis and hepatitis caused by drugs. Possible role of an allopurinol-furosemide combination]. Nephrologie 7:199, 1986.

699. Mitchell JR, Nelson WL, Potter WZ, et al: Metabolic activation of furosemide to a chemically reactive, hepatotoxic metabolite. J Pharmacol Exp Ther 199:41, 1976.
700. Walker RM, McElligott TF: Furosemide induced hepatotoxicity. J Pathol 135:301, 1981.
701. Weisburst M, Self T, Peace R, et al: Jaundice and rash associated with the use of phenobarbital and hydrochlorothiazide. South Med J 69:126, 1976.
702. Hourmand-Ollivier I, Dargere S, Cohen D, et al: [Fatal subfulminant hepatitis probably due to the combination benazepril-hydrochlorothiazide (Briazide)]. Gastroenterol Clin Biol 24:464, 2000.
703. Geltner D, Chajek T, Rubinger D, et al: Quinidine hypersensitivity and liver involvement. A survey of 32 patients. Gastroenterology 70:650, 1976.
704. Knobler H, Levij IS, Gavish D, et al: Quinidine-induced hepatitis. A common and reversible hypersensitivity reaction. Arch Intern Med 146:526, 1986.
705. Guharoy SR, Shahin J, Levin S: Quinidine-induced hepatotoxicity revisited. Vet Human Toxicol 33:613, 1991.
706. Bramlet CA, Posalaky Z, Olson R: Granulomatous hepatitis as a manifestation of quinidine hypersensitivity. Arch Intern Med 140:395, 1980.
707. Chajek T, Lehrer B, Geltner D, et al: Quinidine-induced granulomatous hepatitis. Ann Intern Med 81:774, 1974.
708. Pariente EA, Maitre F, Marchand JP: [Hepatitis caused by quinidine. Study of a case and review of the literature]. Gastroenterol Clin Biol 10:255, 1986.
709. Larrey D, Pessayre D, Duhamel G, et al: Prolonged cholestasis after ajmaline-induced acute hepatitis. J Hepatol 2:81, 1986.
710. Dossing M, Andreasen PB: Drug-induced liver disease in Denmark. An analysis of 572 cases of hepatotoxicity reported to the Danish Board of Adverse Reactions to Drugs. Scand J Gastroenterol 17:205, 1982.
711. Faller JP, Simon G, Rodier L, et al: [Anuria, cholestatic jaundice, thrombocytopenia, hemolysis. Immunoallergic complication due to ajmaline]. Ann Med Intern 136:386, 1985.
712. Henning H, Vogel HM, Ihlenfeld J, et al: [Liver damage due to N-propyl-ajmalin bitartrate (NPAB)]. Zeitschr Gastroenterol 13:501, 1975.
713. Pariente EA, Pessayre D, Bentata-Pessayre M, et al: [Hepatitis due to ajmaline. Report of cases and review of the literature]. Gastroenterol Clin Biol 4:240, 1980.
714. Rotmensch HH, Liron M, Yust I, et al: Cholestatic jaundice: an immune response to prajmalium bitartrate. Postgrad Med J 56:738, 1980.
715. Monges B, Monges G, Salducci J: [Ajmaline-induced hepatitis. A case report with ultrastructural study]. Gastroenterol Clin Biol 7:540, 1983.
716. Borsch G, Schmidt G, Hopmann G, et al: Prajmaliumbitartrate-associated liver damage. Report on seven further cases with follow-up for two to five years. Klin Wochenschr 62:998, 1984.
717. Chammartin F, Levillain P, Silvain C, et al: [Prolonged hepatitis due to ajmaline—description of a case and review of the literature]. Schweiz Rundschau Med Praxis 78:582, 1989.
718. Anastasiou-Nana MI, Anderson JL, Nanas JN, et al: High incidence of clinical and subclinical toxicity associated with amiodarone treatment of refractory tachyarrhythmias. Can J Cardiol 2:138, 1986.
719. Elving LD, Hoefnagels WH, Van Haelst UJ, et al: Amiodarone hepatotoxicity. Neth J Med 29:303, 1986.
720. Flaharty KK, Chase SL, Yaghsezian HM, et al: Hepatotoxicity associated with amiodarone therapy. Pharmacotherapy 9:39, 1989.
721. Guccione P, Paul T, Garson A Jr: Long-term follow-up of amiodarone therapy in the young: continued efficacy, unimpaired growth, moderate side effects. J Am Coll Cardiol 15:1118, 1990.
722. Lahoti S, Lee WM: Hepatotoxicity of anticholesterol, cardiovascular, and endocrine drugs and hormonal agents. Gastroenterol Clin North Am 24:907, 1995.
723. Lewis JH, Ranard RC, Caruso A, et al: Amiodarone hepatotoxicity: prevalence and clinicopathologic correlations among 104 patients. Hepatology 9:679, 1989.
724. Rigas B: The evolving spectrum of amiodarone hepatotoxicity. Hepatology 10:116, 1989.
725. Morse RM, Valenzuela GA, Greenwald TP, et al: Amiodarone-induced liver toxicity. Ann Intern Med 109:838, 1988.
726. Rigas B, Rosenfeld LE, Barwick KW, et al: Amiodarone hepatotoxicity. A clinicopathologic study of five patients. Ann Intern Med 104:348, 1986.
727. Simon JB, Manley PN, Brien JF, et al: Amiodarone hepatotoxicity simulating alcoholic liver disease. N Engl J Med 311:167, 1984.
728. Pye M, Northcote RJ, Cobbe SM: Acute hepatitis after parenteral amiodarone administration. Br Heart J 59:690, 1988.
729. Jones CB, Mullick FG, Hoofnagle JH, et al: Reye's syndrome-like illness in a patient receiving amiodarone. Am J Gastroenterol 83:967, 1988.
730. Yagupsky P, Gazala E, Sofer S, et al: Fatal hepatic failure and encephalopathy associated with amiodarone therapy. J Pediatr 107:967, 1985.
731. Lupon-Roses J, Simo-Canonge R, Lu-Cortez L, et al: Probable early acute hepatitis with parenteral amiodarone. Clin Cardiol 9:223, 1986.
732. Morelli S, Guido V, De Marzio P, et al: Early hepatitis during intravenous amiodarone administration. Cardiology 78:291, 1991.
733. Kalantzis N, Gabriel P, Mouzas J, et al: Acute amiodarone-induced hepatitis. Hepatogastroenterology 38:71, 1991.
734. Rhodes A, Eastwood JB, Smith SA: Early acute hepatitis with parenteral amiodarone: a toxic effect of the vehicle? Gut 34:565, 1993.
735. Rumessen JJ: Hepatotoxicity of amiodarone. Acta Med Scand 219:235, 1986.
736. Chang CC, Petrelli M, Tomashefski JF Jr, et al: Severe intrahepatic cholestasis caused by amiodarone toxicity after withdrawal of the drug: a case report and review of the literature. Arch Pathol Lab Med 123:251, 1999.
737. Guigui B, Perrot S, Berry JP, et al: Amiodarone-induced hepatic phospholipidosis: a morphological alteration independent of pseudoalcoholic liver disease. Hepatology 8:1063, 1988.
738. Joshi U. M, Rao P, Kodavanti S, et al: Fluorescence studies on binding of amphiphilic drugs to isolated lamellar bodies: relevance to phospholipidosis. Biochim Biophys Acta 1004:309, 1989.
739. Berson A, De Beco V, Letteron P, et al: Steatohepatitis-inducing drugs cause mitochondrial dysfunction and lipid peroxidation in rat hepatocytes. Gastroenterology 114:764, 1998.
740. Babany G, Mallat A, Zafrani ES, et al: Chronic liver disease after low daily doses of amiodarone. Report of three cases. J Hepatol 3:228, 1986.
741. Ohyama K, Nakajima M, Suzuki M, et al: Inhibitory effects of amiodarone and its N-deethylated metabolite on human cytochrome P450 activities: prediction of in vivo drug interactions. Br J Clin Pharmacol 49:244, 2000.
742. Marcus FI: Drug interactions with amiodarone. Am Heart J 106:924, 1983.
743. Bach N, Schultz BL, Cohen LB, et al: Amiodarone hepatotoxicity: progression from steatosis to cirrhosis. Mt Sinai J Med 56:293, 1989.
744. Goldman IS, Winkler ML, Raper SE, et al: Increased hepatic density and phospholipidosis due to amiodarone. AJR Am J Roentgenol 144:541, 1985.
745. Jones W. P, Shin MS, Stanley RJ, et al: Dense liver in a 72-year-old woman with congestive heart failure. Investig Radiol 20:911, 1985.
746. Lewis JH, Mullick F, Ishak KG, et al: Histopathologic analysis of suspected amiodarone hepatotoxicity. Human Pathol 21:59, 1990.
747. Jain D, Bowlus CL, Anderson JM, et al: Granular cells as a marker of early amiodarone hepatotoxicity. J Clin Gastroenterol 31:241, 2000.
748. Shepherd NA, Dawson AM, Crocker PR, et al: Granular cells as a marker of early amiodarone hepatotoxicity: a pathological and analytical study. J Clin Pathol 40:418, 1987.
749. Dean PJ, Groshart KD, Porterfield JG, et al: Amiodarone-associated pulmonary toxicity. A clinical and pathologic study of eleven cases. Am J Clin Pathol 87:7, 1987.
750. Honegger UE, Scuntaro I, Wiesmann UN: Vitamin E reduces accumulation of amiodarone and desethylamiodarone and inhibits phospholipidosis in cultured human cells. Biochem Pharmacol 49:1741, 1995.
751. Scuntaro I, Kientsch U, Wiesmann UN, et al: Inhibition by vitamin E of drug accumulation and of phospholipidosis induced by desipramine and other cationic amphiphilic drugs in human cultured cells. Br J Pharmacol 119:829, 1996.

752. Gilinsky NH, Briscoe GW, Kuo CS: Fatal amiodarone hepatoxicity. Am J Gastroenterol 83:161, 1988.
753. Pessayre D, Bichara M, Degott C, et al: Perhexiline maleate-induced cirrhosis. Gastroenterology 76:170, 1979.
754. Poupon R, Rosensztajn L, Prudhomme de Saint-Maur P, et al: Perhexiline maleate-associated hepatic injury prevalence and characteristics. Digestion 20:145, 1980.
755. Garson W. P, Gulin RC, Phear CN: Proceedings: clinical experience with perhexiline maleate in forty-six patients with angina. Postgraduate Med J 49(suppl):90, 1973.
756. Bertrand L, Baldet P, Blanc F, et al: [Cirrhogenic hepatitis due to perhexiline maleate: general review based upon one new case with ultrastructural study (author's translation)]. Ann Intern Med 129:565, 1978.
757. Dawes P, Moulder C: Perhexiline hepatitis and HLA-B8. Lancet 2:109, 1982.
758. Morgan MY, Reshef R, Shah RR, et al: Impaired oxidation of debrisoquine in patients with perhexiline liver injury. Gut 25:1057, 1984.
759. Danilo P Jr: Aprindine. Am Heart J 97:119, 1979.
760. Brandes JW, Schmitz-Moormann P, Lehmann FG, et al: [Jaundice after aprindin (author's translation)]. Deutsche Med Wochenschr 101:111, 1976.
761. Elewaut A, Van Durme JP, Goethals L, et al: Aprindine-induced liver injury. Acta Gastroenterol Belg 40:236, 1977.
762. Herlong HF, Reid PR, Boitnott JK, et al: Aprindine hepatitis. Ann Intern Med 89:359, 1978.
763. Abramson M, Littlejohn GO: Hepatic reactions to nifedipine. Med J Aust 142:47, 1985.
764. Shaw CR, Misan GM, Johnson RCL Nifedipine hepatitis. Aust N Z J Med 17:447, 1987.
765. Sawaya GF, Robertson PA: Hepatotoxicity with the administration of nifedipine for treatment of preterm labor. Am J Obstet Gynecol 167:512, 1992.
766. Davidson AR: Lymphocyte sensitisation in nifedipine-induced hepatitis. BMJ 281:1354, 1980.
767. Babany G, Uzzan F, Larrey D, et al: Alcoholic-like liver lesions induced by nifedipine. J Hepatol 9:252, 1989.
768. Sarachek NS, London RL, Matulewicz TJ: Diltiazem and granulomatous hepatitis. Gastroenterology 88:1260, 1985.
769. Toft E, Vyberg M, Therkelsen K: Diltiazem-induced granulomatous hepatitis. Histopathology 18:474, 1991.
770. Traverse JH, Swenson LJ, McBride JW: Acute hepatic injury after treatment with diltiazem. Am Heart J 127:1636, 1994.
771. Brodsky SJ, Cutler SS, Weiner CA, et al: Hepatotoxicity due to treatment with verapamil. Ann Intern Med 94:490, 1981.
772. Guarascio P, D'Amato C, Sette P, et al: Liver damage from verapamil. BMJ 288:362, 1984.
773. Burgunder JM, Abernethy CR, Lauterburg BH: Liver injury due to verapamil. Hepatogastroenterol 35:169, 1988.
774. Nash CT, Feer TC: Hepatic injury possibly induced by verapamil. JAMA 249:395, 1983.
775. Stern EH, Pitchon R, King BD, et al: Possible hepatitis from verapamil. N Engl J Med 306:612, 1982.
776. Hare CL, Horowitz JC: Verapamil hepatotoxicity: a hypersensitivity reaction. Am Heart J 111:610, 1986.
777. Worman HJ, Ip JH, Winters SL, et al: Hypersensitivity reaction associated with acute hepatic dysfunction following a single intravenous dose of procainamide. J Intern Med 232:361, 1992.
778. Rotmensch HH, Yust I, Siegman-Igra Y, et al: Granulomatous hepatitis: a hypersensitivity response to procainamide. Ann Intern Med 89:646, 1978.
779. Farber HI: Fever, vomiting, and liver dysfunction with procainamide therapy. Postgrad Med 56:155, 1974.
780. Anonymous. Labetalol hepatotoxicity. Ann Intern Med 114:341, 1991.
781. Chon EM, Middleton RK: Labetalol hepatotoxicity. Ann Pharmacother 26:344, 1992.
782. Clark JA, Zimmerman HJ, Tanner LA: Labetalol hepatotoxicity. Ann Intern Med 113:210, 1990.
783. Stronkhorst A, Bosma A, van Leeuwen CJ: A case of labetalol-induced hepatitis. Neth J Med 40:200, 1992.
784. Thiele CL: Labetalol hepatotoxicity. Am J Med 87:361, 1989.
785. Maria VA, Victorino RM: Hypersensitivity immune reaction as a mechanism for dilevalol-associated hepatitis. Ann Pharmacother 26:924, 1992.
786. Lennard MS: Metoprolol-induced hepatitis: is the rate of oxidation related to drug-induced hepatotoxicity? Hepatology 9:163, 1989.
787. Larrey D, Henrion J, Heller F, et al: Metoprolol-induced hepatitis: rechallenge and drug oxidation phenotyping. Ann Intern Med 108:67, 1988.
788. Smith AF, Macfie WG, Oliver MF: Clofibrate, serum enzymes, and muscle pain. BMJ 2:86, 1970.
789. Vester JW, Sunder JH, Aarons JH, et al: Long-term monitoring during clofibrate therapy. Clin Pharmacol Ther 11:689, 1970.
790. Jacobs WH: Intrahepatic cholestasis following the use of Atromid-S. Am J Gastroenterol 66:69, 1976.
791. Pierce EH, Chesler CL: Possible association of granulomatous hepatitis with clofibrate therapy. N Engl J Med 299:314, 1978.
792. Migneco G, Mascarella A, La Ferla A, et al: [Clofibrate hepatitis. A case report]. Minerva Med 77:799, 1986.
793. Qu B, Li QT, Wong KP, et al: Mechanism of clofibrate hepatotoxicity: mitochondrial damage and oxidative stress in hepatocytes. Free Radic Biol Med 31:659, 2001.
794. Sirtori CR, Calabresi L, Werba JP, et al: Tolerability of fibric acids. Comparative data and biochemical bases. Pharmacol Res 26:243, 1992.
795. Bustamante Balen M, Plume Gimeno G, Bau Gonzalez I, et al: [Acute hepatitis caused by gemfibrozil]. Gastroenterol Hepatol 21:419, 1998.
796. Lepicard A, Mallat A, Zafrani ES, et al: [Chronic lesion of the interlobular bile ducts induced by fenofibrate]. Gastroenterol Clin Biol 18:1033, 1994.
797. Ballare M, Campanini M, Airoldi G, et al: Hepatotoxicity of hydroxy-methyl-glutaryl-coenzyme A reductase inhibitors. Minerva Gastroenterol Dietol 38:41, 1992.
798. Roblin X, Becot F, Piquemal A, et al: [Simvastatin-induced hepatitis]. Gastroenterol Clin Biol 16:101, 1992.
799. Ballare M, Campanini M, Catania E, et al: Acute cholestatic hepatitis during simvastatin administration. Recenti Prog Med 82:233, 1991.
800. Feydy P, Bogomoletz WV: [A case of hepatitis caused by simvastatin]. Gastroenterol Clin Biol 15:94, 1991.
801. Hartleb M, Rymarczyk G, Januszewski K: Acute cholestatic hepatitis associated with pravastatin. Am J Gastroenterol 94:1388, 1999.
802. Nakad A, Bataille L, Hamoir V, et al: Atorvastatin-induced acute hepatitis with absence of cross-toxicity with simvastatin. Lancet 353:1763, 1999.
803. Jimenez-Alonso J, Osorio JM, Gutierrez-Cabello F, et al: Atorvastatin-induced cholestatic hepatitis in a young woman with systemic lupus erythematosus. Grupo Lupus Virgen de las Nieves. Arch Intern Med 159:1811, 1999.
804. Raveh D, Arnon R, Israeli A, et al: Lovastatin-induced hepatitis. Israel J Med Sci 28:101, 1992.
805. Gavilan Carrasco JC, Bermudez Recio F, Salgado Ordonez F, et al: [Hepatitis due to lovastatin]. Med Clin 107:557, 1996.
806. Grimbert S, Pessayre D, Degott C, et al: Acute hepatitis induced by HMG-CoA reductase inhibitor, lovastatin. Dig Dis Sci 39:2032, 1994.
807. Bruguera M, Joya P, Rodes J: [Hepatitis associated with treatment with lovastatin. Presentation of 2 cases]. Gastroenterol Hepatol 21:127, 1998.
808. Knopp RH: Clin profiles of plain versus sustained-release niacin (Niaspan) and the physiologic rationale for nighttime dosing. Am J Cardiol 82:24U, 1998.
809. McKenney JM, Proctor JD, Harris S, et al: A comparison of the efficacy and toxic effects of sustained- vs immediate-release niacin in hypercholesterolemic patients. JAMA 271:672, 1994.
810. Etchason JA, Miller TD, Squires RW, et al: Niacin-induced hepatitis: a potential side effect with low-dose time-release niacin. Mayo Clin Proc 66:23, 1991.
811. Henkin Y, Oberman A, Hurst CC, et al: Niacin revisited: clinical observations on an important but underutilized drug. Am J Med 91:239, 1991.
812. Coppola A, Brady PG, Nord HJ: Niacin-induced hepatotoxicity: unusual presentations. South Med J 87:30, 1994.
813. Gray CR, Morgan T, Chretien SD, et al: Efficacy and safety of controlled-release niacin in dyslipoproteinemic veterans. Ann Intern Med 121:252, 1994.
814. Dalton TA, Berry RS: Hepatotoxicity associated with sustained-release niacin. Am J Med 93:102, 1992.
815. Henkin Y, Johnson KC, Segrest JP: Rechallenge with crystalline niacin after drug-induced hepatitis from sustained-release niacin. JAMA 264:241, 1990.

816. McCarty MF: Co-administration of equimolar doses of betaine may alleviate the hepatotoxic risk associated with niacin therapy. Med Hypoth 55:189, 2000.
817. Hodis HN: Acute hepatic failure associated with the use of low-dose sustained-release niacin. JAMA 264:181, 1990.
818. Carlson MK, Gleason PP, Sen S: Elevation of hepatic transaminases after enoxaparin use: case report and review of unfractionated and low-molecular-weight heparin-induced hepatotoxicity. Pharmacotherapy 21:108, 2001.
819. Hui CK, Yuen MF, Ng IO, et al: Low molecular weight heparin-induced liver toxicity. J Clin Pharmacol 41:691, 2001.
820. AL-Mekhaizeem KA, Sherker AH: Heparin-induced hepatotoxicity. Can J Gastroenterol 15:527, 2001.
821. Manfredini R, Boari B, Regoli F, et al: Cholestatic liver reaction and heparin therapy. Arch Intern Med 160:3166, 2000.
822. Weber T, Hinterreiter M, Knoflach P: [Phenprocoumon-associated necrotizing hepatitis]. Deutsche Med Wochenschr 126:1060, 2001.
823. Bux-Gewehr I, Zotz RB, Scharf RE: Phenprocoumon-induced hepatitis in a patient with a combined hereditary hemostatic disorder. Thromb Haemost 83:799, 2000.
824. Ehrenforth S, Schenk JF, Scharrer I: Liver damage induced by coumarin anticoagulants. Semin Thromb Hemost 25:79, 1999.
825. Hohler T, Schnutgen M, Helmreich-Becker I, et al: Drug-induced hepatitis: a rare complication of oral anticoagulants. J Hepatol 21:447, 1994.
826. Coe JE, Ishak KG, Ross MJ: Diethylstilbestrol-induced jaundice in the Chinese and Armenian hamster. Hepatology 3:489, 1983.
827. Adlercreutz H, Tenhunen R: Some aspects of the interaction between natural and synthetic female sex hormones and the liver. Am J Med 49:630, 1970.
828. Kreek MJ, Weser E, Sleisenger MH, et al: Idiopathic cholestasis of pregnancy. The response to challenge with the synthetic estrogen, ethinyl estradiol. N Engl J Med 277:1391, 1967.
829. Kreek MJ, Sleisenger MH, Jeffries GH: Recurrent cholestatic jaundice of pregnancy with demonstrated estrogen sensitivity. Am J Med 43:795, 1967.
830. Kreek MJ: Female sex steroids and cholestasis. Semin Liver Dis 7:8, 1987.
831. Orellana-Alcalde JM, Dominguez JP: Jaundice and oral contraceptive drugs. Lancet 2:1279, 1966.
832. Metreau JM, Dhumeaux C, Berthelot P: Oral contraceptives and the liver. Digestion 7:318, 1972.
833. Reyes H, Gonzalez MC, Ribalta J, et al: Prevalence of intrahepatic cholestasis of pregnancy in Chile. Ann Intern Med 88:487, 1978.
834. Dalen E, Westerholm B: Occurrence of hepatic impairment in women jaundiced by oral contraceptives and in their mothers and sisters. Acta Med Scand 195:459, 1974.
835. Lindberg MC: Hepatobiliary complications of oral contraceptives. J Gen Intern Med 7:199, 1992.
836. Mueller MN, Kappas A: Estrogen pharmacology. I. Influence of estradiol and estriol on hepatic disposal of sulfobromophthalein (BSP) in man. J Clin Invest 43:1905, 1964.
837. Gallagher TF, Mueller MN, Kappas A: Estrogen pharmacology. IV. Studies of the structural basis for estrogen-induced impairment of liver function. Medicine 45:471, 1966.
838. Gallagher TF, Mueller MN, Kappas A: Studies on the mechanism and structural specificity of the estrogen effect on BSP metabolism. Trans Assoc Am Phys 78:187, 1965.
839. Meyers M, Slikker W, Pascoe G, et al: Characterization of cholestasis induced by estradiol-17 beta-D-glucuronide in the rat. J Pharmacol Exp Ther 214:87, 1980.
840. Vore M: Estrogen cholestasis. Membranes, metabolites, or receptors? Gastroenterology 93:643, 1987.
841. Adlercreutz H, Tikkanen MJ, Wichmann K, et al: Recurrent jaundice in pregnancy. IV. Quantitative determination of urinary and biliary estrogens, including studies in pruritus gravidarum. J Clin Endocrinol Metab 38:51, 1974.
842. Davis RA, Kern F, Showalter R, et al: Alterations of hepatic Na^+,K^+-atpase and bile flow by estrogen: effects on liver surface membrane lipid structure and function. Proc Natl Acad Sci U S A 75:4130, 1978.
843. Simon FR, Gonzalez M, Sutherland E, et al: Reversal of ethinyl estradiol-induced bile secretory failure with Triton WR-1339. J Clin Invest 65:851, 1980.
844. Scharschmidt BF, Keeffe EB, Vessey CA, et al: In vitro effect of bile salts on rat liver plasma membrane, lipid fluidity, and ATPase activity. Hepatology 1:137, 1981.
845. Rosario J, Sutherland E, Zaccaro L, et al: Ethinylestradiol administration selectively alters liver sinusoidal membrane lipid fluidity and protein composition. Biochemistry 27:3939, 1988.
846. Smith CJ, Gordon ER: Role of liver plasma membrane fluidity in the pathogenesis of estrogen-induced cholestasis. J Lab Clin Med 112:679, 1988.
847. Brock W. J, Durham S, Vore M: Characterization of the interaction between estrogen metabolites and taurocholate for uptake into isolated hepatocytes. Lack of correlation between cholestasis and inhibition of taurocholate uptake. J Steroid Biochem 20:1181, 1984.
848. Adinolfi LE, Utili R, Gaeta GB, et al: Cholestasis induced by estradiol-17 beta-D-glucuronide: mechanisms and prevention by sodium taurocholate. Hepatology 4:30, 1984.
849. Stramentinoli G, Di Padova C, Gualano M, et al: Ethynylestradiol-induced impairment of bile secretion in the rat: protective effects of S-adenosyl-L-methionine and its implication in estrogen metabolism. Gastroenterology 80:154, 1981.
850. Frezza M, Pozzato G, Chiesa L, et al: Reversal of intrahepatic cholestasis of pregnancy in women after high dose S-adenosyl-L-methionine administration. Hepatology 4:274, 1984.
851. Ribalta J, Reyes H, Gonzalez MC, et al: S-adenosyl-L-methionine in the treatment of patients with intrahepatic cholestasis of pregnancy: a randomized, double-blind, placebo-controlled study with negative results. Hepatology 13:1084, 1991.
852. Perez V, Gorosdisch S, De Martire J, et al: Oral contraceptives: long-term use produces fine structural changes in liver mitochondria. Science 165:805, 1969.
853. Uhler ML, Marks JW, Judd HL: Estrogen replacement therapy and gallbladder disease in postmenopausal women. Menopause 7:162, 2000.
854. Jorgensen T: Estrogen use and gallstone disease. Am J Public Health 79:654, 1989.
855. Scragg RK, McMichael AJ, Seamark RF: Oral contraceptives, pregnancy, and endogenous oestrogen in gall stone disease—a case-control study. BMJ 288:1795, 1984.
856. Weiss GN, Weiss EB: Hormonal therapy and cholelithiasis. Int Surg 61:472, 1976.
857. Hammond CB, Maxson WS: Estrogen replacement therapy. Clin Obstet Gynecol 29:407, 1986.
858. Keane P, Colwell D, Baer HP, et al: Effects of age, gender and female sex hormones upon contractility of the human gallbladder in vitro. Surg Gynecol Obstet 163:555, 1986.
859. Messa C, Maselli MA, Cavallini A, et al: Sex steroid hormone receptors and human gallbladder motility in vitro. Digestion 46:214, 1990.
860. Everson GT, McKinley C, Kern F Jr: Mechanisms of gallstone formation in women. Effects of exogenous estrogen (Premarin) and dietary cholesterol on hepatic lipid metabolism. J Clin Invest 87:237, 1991.
861. Chen A, Huminer C: The role of estrogen receptors in the development of gallstones and gallbladder cancer. Med Hypoth 36:259, 1991.
862. Frezza M, Tritapepe R, Pozzato G, et al: Prevention of S-adenosylmethionine of estrogen-induced hepatobiliary toxicity in susceptible women. Am J Gastroenterol 83:1098, 1988.
863. Baum JK, Bookstein JJ, Holtz F, et al: Possible association between benign hepatomas and oral contraceptives. Lancet 2:926, 1973.
864. Ecker JA, McKittrick JE, Failing RM: Thrombosis of the hepatic veins. "The Budd-Chiari syndrome"—a possible link between oral contraceptives and thrombosis formation. Am J Gastroenterol 45:429, 1966.
865. Rothwell-Jackson RL: Budd-Chiari syndrome after oral contraceptives. BMJ 1:252, 1968.
866. Clubb AW, Giles C: Budd-Chiari syndrome after oral contraceptives. BMJ 1:252, 1968.
867. Krass I: Budd-Chiari syndrome after oral contraceptives. BMJ 1:708, 1968.
868. Grayson MJ, Reilly MC: Budd-Chiari syndrome after oral contraceptives. BMJ1:512, 1968.
869. Janssen HL, Meinardi JR, Vleggaar FP, et al: Factor V Leiden mutation, prothrombin gene mutation, and deficiencies in coagulation inhibitors associated with Budd-Chiari syndrome and portal vein thrombosis: results of a case-control study. Blood 96:2364, 2000.

870. Minnema MC, Janssen HL, Niermeijer P, et al: Budd-Chiari syndrome: combination of genetic defects and the use of oral contraceptives leading to hypercoagulability. J Hepatol 33:509, 2000.
871. Simsek S, Verheesen RV, Haagsma EB, et al: Subacute Budd-Chiari syndrome associated with polycythemia vera and factor V Leiden mutation. Neth J Med 57:62, 2000.
872. Hines C Jr, Mitchell WT Jr: Hepatic vein thrombosis in a woman taking oral contraceptives: a case report. Jthe Louisiana State Med Society. 129:189, 1977.
873. Schonberg LA: Peliosis hepatis and oral contraceptives. A case report. J Reproductive Medicine. 27:753, 1982.
874. Takiff H, Brems JJ, Pockros PJ, et al: Focal hemorrhagic necrosis of the liver. A rare cause of hemoperitoneum. Dig Dis Sci 37:1910, 1992.
875. Jacobs MB: Hepatic infarction related to oral contraceptive use. Arch Intern Med 144:642, 1984.
876. Saint-Marc Girardin MF, Zafrani ES, Prigent A, et al: Unilobar small hepatic vein obstruction: possible role of progestogen given as oral contraceptive. Gastroenterology 84:630, 1983.
877. Riippa P, Kauppila A, Sundstrom H, et al: Hepatic impairment during simultaneous administration of medroxyprogesterone acetate and tamoxifen in the treatment of endometrial and ovarian carcinoma. Anticancer Res 4:109, 1984.
878. Pratt CS, Knox TA, Erban J: Tamoxifen-induced steatohepatitis. Ann Intern Med 123:236, 1995.
879. Pinto HC, Baptista A, Camilo ME, et al: Tamoxifen-associated steatohepatitis—report of three cases. J Hepatol 23:95, 1995.
880. Van Hoof M, Rahier J, Horsmans Y: Tamoxifen-induced steatohepatitis. Ann Intern Med 124:855, 1996.
881. Cai Q, Bensen M, Greene R, et al: Tamoxifen-induced transient multifocal hepatic fatty infiltration. Am J Gastroenterol 95:277, 2000.
882. Murata Y, Ogawa Y, Saibara T, et al: Unrecognized hepatic steatosis and non-alcoholic steatohepatitis in adjuvant tamoxifen for breast cancer patients. Oncol Rep 7:1299, 2000.
883. Dray X, Tainturier MH, De La Lande P, et al: [Cirrhosis with non alcoholic steatohepatitis: role of tamoxifen]. Gastroenterol Clin Biol 24:1122, 2000.
884. Storen EC, Hay JE, Kaur J, et al: Tamoxifen-induced submassive hepatic necrosis. Cancer J 6:58, 2000.
885. Johnson FL: The association of oral androgenic-anabolic steroids and life-threatening disease. Med Sci Sports 7:284, 1975.
886. Dourakis SP, Tolis G: Sex hormonal preparations and the liver. Eur J Contraception Reprod Health Care 3:7, 1998.
887. Gelfand MM, Wiita B: Androgen and estrogen-androgen hormone replacement therapy: a review of the safety literature, 1941 to 1996. Clin Ther 19:383, 1997.
888. Westaby D, Ogle SJ, Paradinas FJ, et al: Liver damage from longterm methyltestosterone. Lancet 2:262, 1977.
889. Gurakar A, Caraceni P, Fagiuoli S, et al: Androgenic/anabolic steroid-induced intrahepatic cholestasis: a review with four additional case reports. J Oklahoma State Med Assoc 87:399, 1994.
890. Mork H, al-Taie O, Klinge O, et al: [Successful therapy of persistent androgen-induced cholestasis with ursodeoxycholic acid]. Zeitschrift fur Gastroenterologie 35:1087, 1997.
891. Hirose H, Ohishi A, Nakamura H, et al: Fatal splenic rupture in anabolic steroid-induced peliosis in a patient with myelodysplastic syndrome. Br J Haematol 78:128, 1991.
892. Cabasso A: Peliosis hepatis in a young adult bodybuilder. Med Sci Sports Exercise 26:2, 1994.
893. Yap I, Yeoh KG, Wee A, et al: Peliosis hepatis: a case report. Ann Acad Med Singapore. 22:381, 1993.
894. Kuhbock J, Radaszkiewicz T, Walek H: (Peliosis hepatis, complicating treatment with anabolic steroids [author's translation]). Medizin Klin 70:1602, 1975.
895. Leblay R, Brissot P, leCalve J, et al: (Peliosis hepatis after treatment with androgens. A recent case). Nouvelle Presse Med 7:1026, 1978.
896. Karasawa T, Shikata T, Smith RC: Peliosis hepatis. Report of nine cases. Acta Pathol Jpn 29:457, 1979.
897. Nuzzo JL, Manz HJ, Maxted WC: Peliosis hepatis after long-term androgen therapy. Urology 25:518, 1985.
898. Chopra S, Edelstein A, Koff RS, et al: Peliosis hepatis in hematologic disease. Report of two cases. JAMA 240:1153, 1978.
899. Nadell J, Kosek J: Peliosis hepatis. Twelve cases associated with oral androgen therapy. Arch Pathol Lab Med 101:405, 1977.
900. Paradinas FJ, Bull TB, Westaby D, et al: Hyperplasia and prolapse of hepatocytes into hepatic veins during longterm methyltestosterone therapy: possible relationships of these changes to the development of peliosis hepatis and liver tumours. Histopathology 1:225, 1977.
901. Watanabe S, Cui Y, Tanae A, et al: Follow-up study of children with precocious puberty treated with cyproterone acetate. Ad Hoc Committee for CPAJ Epidemiology 7:173, 1997.
902. Gleeson D, Newbould MJ, Taylor P, et al: Androgen associated hepatocellular carcinoma with an aggressive course. Gut 32:1084, 1991.
903. Grange JD, Guechot J, Legendre C, et al: Liver adenoma and focal nodular hyperplasia in a man with high endogenous sex steroids. Gastroenterology 93:1409, 1987.
904. Johnson FL, Lerner KG, Siegel M, et al: Association of androgenic-anabolic steroid therapy with development of hepatocellular carcinoma. Lancet 2:1273, 1972.
905. Nakao A, Sakagami K, Nakata Y, et al: Multiple hepatic adenomas caused by long-term administration of androgenic steroids for aplastic anemia in association with familial adenomatous polyposis. J Gastroenterol 35:557, 2000.
906. Balazs M: Primary hepatocellular tumours during long-term androgenic steroid therapy. A light and electron microscopic study of 11 cases with emphasis on microvasculature of the tumours. Acta Morphol Hungarica 39:201, 1991.
907. Sale GE, Lerner KG: Multiple tumors after androgen therapy. Arch Pathol Lab Med 101:600, 1977.
908. Zimmermann HJ: Hepatotoxicity, ed 2. Philadelphia, Lippincott Williams and Wilkins, 1999:575.
909. Van Thiel D, De Belle R, Mellow M, et al: Tolazamide hepatotoxicity. A case report. Gastroenterology 67:506, 1974.
910. Watkins PB, Whitcomb RW: Hepatic dysfunction associated with troglitazone. N Engl J Med 338:916, 1998 (letter).
911. Li H, Heller DS, Leevy Cb, et al: Troglitazone-induced fulminant hepatitis. Report of a case with autopsy findings. J Diabetes Complications 14:175, 2000.
912. Malik AH, Prasad P, Saboorian M, et al: Hepatic injury due to troglitazone. Dig Dis Sci 45:210, 2000.
913. Menon KV, Angulo P, Lindor KC: Severe cholestatic hepatitis from troglitazone in a patient with nonalcoholic steatohepatitis and diabetes mellitus. Am J Gastroenterol 96:1631, 2001.
914. Gitlin N, Julie N, Spurr C, et al: Two cases of severe clinical and histologic hepatotoxicity associated with troglitazone. Ann Intern Med 12:36, 1998.
915. McMorran M, Vu C: Rosiglitazone (Avandia): hepatic, cardiac and hematological reactions. Can Med Assoc J165:82, 2001.

C H A P T E R

28

Preoperative and Postoperative Hepatic Dysfunctions

Enrique J. Martinez, MD, FACP, and Thomas D. Boyer, MD

INTRODUCTION

The liver is the major site for the metabolism of many drugs and is responsible for the synthesis of most serum proteins and the removal of endogenous toxins. Therefore postoperative liver dysfunction may slow the recovery of a patient who has undergone surgery. Because of the liver's role in drug metabolism it is susceptible to injury by a variety of xenobiotics. Alterations in hepatic blood flow also may affect liver function, especially in the patient with underlying chronic liver disease. Therefore it is not unexpected that abnormalities of liver tests are noted frequently in patients after surgery.[1] However, clinical jaundice is rare (less than 1 percent) in patients with normal livers, and its development should prompt a thorough evaluation of its cause. Before reviewing the causes of postoperative liver dysfunction in this chapter, there will be a brief discussion of the evaluation of the patient with abnormal liver tests found during preoperative testing. If the surgery is critical to the patient, the presence of preoperative liver dysfunction should have no effect on the decision to operate. However, if the surgery is elective, the finding of abnormal liver tests preoperatively should prompt an evaluation as to their cause, and an estimate of liver function should be made.

PREOPERATIVE LIVER DYSFUNCTION

The frequency of unsuspected liver disease is approximately 1 in 700 of otherwise healthy surgical candidates, making this a common clinical problem.[2,3] Of most concern to surgeons and anesthesiologists are elevations of the serum aspartate aminotransferase (AST), alanine aminotransferase (ALT), and bilirubin and disorders of coagulation. Elevations of alkaline phosphatase or gamma glutamyltranspeptidase are of little clinical significance and should not prompt an evaluation unless associated with other clinical findings (see Chap. 23). The significance of a low serum albumin is difficult to interpret because of the multiple causes of a fall in the concentration of this protein (see Chap. 23). It is useful to combine patients with preoperative liver dysfunction into three groups: (1) asymptomatic with normal physical examination; (2) symptomatic; and (3) physical and biochemical findings of chronic liver disease.

Asymptomatic patients with a normal physical examination and abnormal liver tests (increased AST/ALT) are encountered frequently, raising concerns that they have underlying liver disease that may increase the risk of surgery. The abnormal liver tests most likely reflect a subacute or chronic form of liver injury resulting from viral hepatitis, drugs or alcohol, or fatty liver. We lack information as to whether this group of patients is at any increased risk from surgery, but it is the authors' opinion that if the serum bilirubin, albumin, and clotting tests are normal and the increase in aminotransferases mild (twofold to fivefold), there is little if any increase in surgical risk. Deciding to perform surgery and ensuring its successful completion in this type of patient should not be an end to the evaluation of the liver disease. After surgery the liver tests need to be monitored; if persistently abnormal, a thorough evaluation should be performed.

Greater increases in aminotransferases are more problematic only because they suggest more significant hepatic injury. Anesthetic agents may adversely affect hepatic function because of decreases in splanchnic blood flow and thereby oxygen delivery to the liver.[4,5] Early studies suggested that this may be a real clinical concern when an increase in operative mortality was observed in patients with acute hepatitis.[6-8] However, in other studies no increase in mortality has been found when surgery was performed in patients with coincidental acute viral hepatitis.[9-11] All of these studies suffer from being anecdotal and reporting on small numbers of patients. In addition many patients were jaundiced, suggesting the presence of significant liver injury. Despite these uncertainties, if the surgery is elective, a delay in the operation is the most conservative approach. Liver tests should be performed 2 to 3 weeks later, and if the abnormalities persist for several months, the patient should be evaluated completely. If it is decided to perform an elective operation when AST/ALT is elevated more than fivefold but normal albumin, prothrombin time, and bilirubin exist, the risk to the patient probably remains quite small. However, if the liver tests worsen postoperatively, defining whether the surgery or the initial illness is at fault will be difficult. Because there is no evidence that the presence of liver disease increases the risk of developing anesthetic-induced hepatitis[12] (see Chap. 27), there is no need to alter the choice of anesthetic agent used for the surgery.

Isolated elevations in the serum bilirubin usually are due to Gilbert's syndrome (see Chap. 9); this syndrome does not increase the risk of surgery. If the elevations of bilirubin are seen in association with elevations of AST/ALT or alkaline phosphatase, the cause of the liver injury needs to be determined before any elective surgery is performed. Isolated prolongation of the prothrombin time is an unusual manifestation of liver disease but suggests the presence of cirrhosis or a severe acute or subacute injury.

The symptomatic patient with elevated liver tests is of greater concern when elective surgery is planned. The presence of symptoms (nausea, vomiting) in association with elevated liver tests suggests that the patient is developing an acute illness that may worsen before it improves. Therefore if the patient is subjected to surgery and the liver tests worsen, it will be very difficult to determine whether the patient is suffering from a preexisting condition or a complication of surgery (i.e., halothane hepatitis). In addition, there is uncertainty as to whether or not acute viral hepatitis increases the risk of surgery[7-11]; therefore, elective surgery should be postponed until the hepatitis has resolved.

A special subset of the symptomatic patient is represented by patients with markedly elevated transaminases. This group is varied as to cause of these elevations and range from ischemia or cardiac dysfunction, drugs, liver trauma, cancer metastases to liver, and rhabdomyolysis. A recent review demonstrated that the overall mortality of patients with serum AST greater than 3000 was 55 percent and that ischemic hepatitis patients had a 75 percent mortality compared to 33 percent for all other causes. This group should clearly be excluded from consideration for any elective surgery.[13]

The presence of clinical (i.e., splenomegaly, spiders, palmar erythema, or ascites) and biochemical (i.e., low albumin or prolonged prothrombin time) evidence of chronic liver disease is of greatest concern when planning elective surgery. The risk of the surgery is determined by how well the liver is functioning[14] and the presence or absence of symptoms. For example, patients with chronic hepatitis appear to have an increased surgical risk if they are symptomatic.[14,15] Elective surgery in patients with evidence of chronic liver disease should be delayed until the cause of the liver disease is determined and the severity of the injury is fully assessed.

The most common cause of chronic liver disease in the Western world is alcoholism. Alcoholic liver disease can manifest as fatty liver, alcoholic hepatitis. cirrhosis, or a combination of the above (see Chap. 30). The risk of surgery in the patient with fatty liver appears to be small.[14] Surgical studies would suggest that it is not uncommon to find unsuspected cirrhosis in obese patients at the time of bariatric surgery. In a recent report of 125 patients with cirrhosis detected at surgery, the authors were able to proceed with their planned bariatric surgery in 74 percent of patients; the result was no intraoperative deaths and only a 4 percent mortality rate.[16] Alcoholic hepatitis can be present as an asymptomatic illness or be associated with jaundice and liver failure. Elective surgery in a patient with decompensated liver disease resulting from any cause is ill advised. Even in patients with better preserved liver function, elective surgery in patients with acute symptomatic alcoholic hepatitis is associated with increased morbidity and mortality and should not be performed.[14,17] The effect of asymptomatic alcoholic hepatitis on surgical mortality has been studied best in patients undergoing portal-systemic shunt surgery. The presence of large amounts of alcoholic hyalin in a liver biopsy specimen indicated a high likelihood of mortality in some series.[18,19] In another series the 1-year survival of patients after the insertion of a portal-systemic shunt was 70 percent to 74 percent in the absence of alcoholic hyalin and only 10 percent in those with alcoholic hyalin in a liver biopsy.[20] In contrast, other investigators have found no correlation between the presence of alcoholic hyalin and survival.[21-23] Despite these uncertainties, performance of elective surgery in a patient with alcoholic hepatitis should be avoided. It is very difficult, however, to determine whether an alcoholic patient has fatty liver or a more serious lesion (i.e., alcoholic hepatitis) based on liver test results alone. Therefore the most conservative approach in a chronic alcoholic patient who requires elective surgery and who has abnormal liver tests is either a liver biopsy to define the nature of the liver injury or a period of abstinence (2 to 3 months) to allow the acute injury to resolve preceding surgery.

There is little question that the presence of cirrhosis increases the risk of surgery, especially if it is an intraabdominal operation. Published mortality rates vary from 5 to 67 percent and morbidity rates from 7 to 39 percent.[14] These differences in survival reflect the variability in the clinical state of the patients reported in the different studies. The risk of surgery is defined best by the clinical severity of the cirrhosis (i.e., Child's classification).[14,24-26] Patients with good hepatic function, no ascites, and a good nutritional state (Child's A) do well with surgery, whereas those with jaundice, low serum albumin, ascites, and muscle wasting have a high operative mortality and postoperative morbidity. The presence of umbilical hernias is reported to be as high as 42 percent if ascites is present versus 10 percent if no ascites is present.[26] In cases of spontaneous rupture of these umbilical hernias, supportive care is associated with a 50 percent mortality versus a 14 percent mortality with repair, but repair may be associated with wound dehiscence or peritonitis in a patient with cirrhotic ascites.[27-29] Postoperative decreases in ascites either with medical management or with a transjugular intrahepatic portosystemic shunt decreases the recurrence of umbilical hernias postrepair.[29] Groin hernia repair in cirrhotics appears to be less affected by ascites, with reports of 8 percent recurrence versus 60 percent for umbilical hernias in similar patients with ascites.[30] Elective surgery can be performed in patients with decompensated liver disease but the surgeon must have experience in the management of this type of patient to minimize the risks of surgery.

A difficult problem that faces many surgeons is performing a cholecystectomy in a patient with cirrhosis. Mortality rates of 7.5 percent to 25.5 percent and morbidity rates of 4.8 percent to 25 percent have been reported.[31] In addition, many patients require transfusions—especially if they have decompensated liver disease.[31] A subtotal cholecystectomy used to be suggested for patients with cirrhosis and portal hypertension.[32] Previously, open cholecystectomy had been recommended for patients with cirrhosis, but recent studies would suggest that in Child's A-B patients, elective laparoscopic cholecystectomy is preferred because of less bleeding, fewer wound infections, and decreased lengths of stay compared with open cholecystectomy.[33-38] The complications rates after urgent cholecystectomy are significantly higher (36 percent) as compared to elective laparoscopic cholecystectomy in cirrhotics (16 percent), suggesting that if possible, stabilization of the patient with medical management followed by elective surgery would be preferred.[38] Given the high rates of mortality and morbidity in patients with advanced cirrhosis undergoing cholecystectomy and the increased difficulty associated with liver transplantation in patients with a previous cholecystectomy, the authors believe that the presence of recurrent cholecystitis in a patient with advanced liver disease should be considered an indication for liver transplantation while conservative management is being performed. Percutaneous cholecystostomy tubes may be attempted but may be difficult to perform in patients with significant ascites.

TABLE 28-1
Causes of Postoperative Liver Dysfunction

Hepatitis-like
Drugs
Anesthetic needs
Ischemia
Cardiac
Shock (non-cardiac)
Iatrogenic (ligation hepatic artery)
Viral hepatitis
Cholestasis
Benign postoperative cholestasis
Sepsis
Drugs
Antibiotics, anti-emetics
Bile duct injury
Choledocholithiasis/pancreatitis
Cholecystitis

POSTOPERATIVE LIVER DYSFUNCTION

Table 28-1 lists the most common causes of liver dysfunction and jaundice in postoperative patients. In a recent review of surgical complications in cirrhotics, the 30-day mortality rate was reported to be 11.6 percent, with a 30.1 percent perioperative complication rate.[39] The causes of this mortality rate are separated into two large groups but many patients have a mixed picture, which increases the difficulty in making a correct diagnosis.

Anesthetic-induced Liver Injury

Anesthetic-induced hepatitis is of most concern because of a high incidence of hepatic failure; it is discussed in detail in Chapter 27. Liver injury resulting from any of the currently used anesthetics is rare. By 1985 more than 500 cases of halothane hepatitis had been reported; however, the estimated frequency of hepatitis resulting from halothane is 1 in 10,000 operations.[12,40] The putative toxin is a metabolic product of halothane; therefore, other halogenated anesthetic agents that are less extensively metabolized than halothane have an even lower incidence of hepatotoxicity.[12,40] Published mortality rates vary from 10 percent to 80 percent, with rates of 10 percent to 30 percent being most representative.[40]

The development of symptoms (fever or jaundice) is seen 7 to 14 days after a single exposure and 5 to 7 days after multiple exposures to halothane. Fever is the most common symptom of halothane-induced hepatitis and may be present in the absence of jaundice. Laboratory tests show a marked increase (greater than tenfold above normal) in serum levels of aminotransferases. Patients with severe injury may have a rise in serum bilirubin and prolongation of the prothrombin time. Many, however, have only a rise in aminotransferases without clinical icterus and therefore the injury may be missed unless laboratory tests are obtained in patients with postoperative fever.[40-42] Eosinophilia and renal insufficiency also may be present.[40-42] The other halogenated anesthetics also cause a hepatitis-like injury with clinical features that are similar to those seen with halothane hepatitis.

Ischemic Hepatitis

Surgery is commonly performed in patients with cardiac disease, and if they develop congestive heart failure, they may develop ischemic hepatitis. Ischemic hepatitis is marked by a rapid rise in serum levels of AST, ALT, and lactate dehydrogenase (LDH). The levels frequently are greater than tenfold above normal and in severe cases may be associated with jaundice and prolongation of the prothrombin time.[43] In contrast to halothane hepatitis, elevation in liver tests can be seen any time after surgery and is not associated with fever or eosinophilia. In addition, the liver tests tend to return rapidly to normal (elevations last 3 to 11 days).[43] Non-cardiogenic shock liver is seen in association with hypotensive episodes (resulting from bleeding or sepsis) and also is marked by a rapid rise and fall in serum levels of AST and ALT. When comparing all causes of massive elevations of AST (more than 3000 U/L), ischemic hepatitis can be found to be associated with a mortality rate of 75 percent versus 33 percent for all other causes combined.[44] Accidental or deliberate ligation of the hepatic artery or its branches may result in hepatic ischemia and necrosis associated with a rise in serum levels of AST and ALT.[45] When accidental ligation of the hepatic artery occurs, it is usually during cholecystectomy and should be suspected in a patient who develops a rise in serum levels of AST and ALT after that operation.

Acute Viral Hepatitis

The development of acute viral hepatitis in the postoperative period is rare if patients are shown to have normal liver tests preceding the surgery. If the patient does develop acute viral hepatitis, a gradual rise in the serum levels of AST and ALT will be observed with or without other systemic symptoms (see Chap. 23). Of note, the serum levels of LDH are only slightly increased relative to the degree of elevation of the AST and ALT; hence, measurement of the serum LDH is a useful test for separating ischemic and drug-induced hepatitis from viral hepatitis. The appropriate tests for the diagnosis of acute viral hepatitis are discussed in Chapters 31-33.

Drug-induced Hepatitis

There are a large number of drugs that may cause an acute hepatitis-like injury and these are discussed in detail in Chapter 27. Acetaminophen is a direct hepatotoxin and is used commonly in the postoperative patient. Toxicity from acetaminophen is generally observed when more than 7.5 g is ingested as a single dose.[46] More recently, however, it has become apparent that therapeutic doses of acetaminophen ingested by alcoholics may be associated with significant hepatic injury.[47] In addition, the toxic metabolite of acetaminophen is formed by P450 2E1; this enzyme is susceptible to induction by a number of drugs, including alcohol.[46] The co-administration of an inducing agent may increase the generation of the toxic metabolite of acetaminophen and cause toxicity with ingestion of therapeutic doses (3 to 4 g per day) of the drug. Therefore if a patient develops an increase in serum levels of AST/ALT postoperatively, the amount of acetaminophen taken by the patient should be determined. Most hepatitis-like drug reactions are idiosyncratic and can be due to a variety of agents, as discussed in Chapter 27. An important fact in the differential diagnosis of postoperative liver dysfunction is that most idiosyncratic drug reactions develop after at least 2 weeks of therapy. Therefore the development of abnormal liver tests within 2 weeks of surgery is unlikely to be due to drugs started after the operation. In addition, drugs taken for more than 12 months preceding the surgery are unlikely causes of postoperative liver dysfunction.

Benign Postoperative Cholestasis

The development of jaundice postoperatively is observed in less than 1 percent of patients undergoing major surgery. Patients with preexisting liver or cardiovascular disease and who suffer trauma have a significantly higher incidence of jaundice.[1] The cause of the jaundice is multi-factorial and includes anesthetic-induced reduction in liver function because of decreased hepatic blood flow, increased pigment load from hematomas and transfused blood, and impaired bile formation secondary to bacterial sepsis.[1,48-52] The breakdown of 50 ml of blood yields 250 mg of bilirubin, which can be easily handled by the normal liver but leads to a rapid rise in serum bilirubin in patients with impaired liver function.[1] A fall in liver blood flow is observed with almost all general anesthetics, which may lead to a decline in liver function, especially in patients with underlying liver disease.[4,5,14] If the patient has suffered an episode of hypotension, it will affect hepatocyte function and predispose the patient to the development of cholestasis.[1] Last, endotoxemia reduces bile flow, and intra-abdominal sepsis is frequently associated with abnormal liver tests and jaundice.[48,51]

Benign postoperative cholestasis develops most commonly within the first 10 days after surgery. Cholestasis is observed most frequently in patients with sepsis, after cardiovascular surgery, and after prolonged operations during which and after the patient received multiple transfusions.[48-51] Although an increase in serum bilirubin is common and may reach levels of 40 mg/dl, it is not universal. Serum levels of alkaline phosphatase are frequently elevated, whereas AST and ALT levels are normal or only mildly elevated (less than fivefold). Serum albumin levels may be normal or reduced slightly and the prothrombin time is usually normal. Liver biopsy shows cholestasis and variable degrees of fat.[1,50]

The condition is referred to as benign because if the patient recovers from the surgery and any associated complications, the cholestasis resolves. However, patients developing postoperative cholestasis have a significant mortality. Patients with serum bilirubin levels of greater than 6 have a 46 percent mortality if they have suffered abdominal trauma and a 86 percent mortality if they have intra-abdominal sepsis.[52] These latter groups of patients frequently die with the syndrome termed *multiple organ system failure*, and worsening liver function is seen in association with renal failure and acute respiratory distress syndrome.[37,53] The liver plays a passive role in multiple organ system failure in that acute liver failure (encephalopathy with a coagulopathy) is not the cause of death.

Bile Duct Obstruction

A common concern is the development of extrahepatic bile duct obstruction in the postoperative patient who becomes icteric. Coincidental choledocholithiasis after surgery is rare. A far more common occurrence is bile duct injury after biliary tract or gastric surgery. Bile duct injury after laparoscopic cholecystectomy is an increasingly common problem and frequently goes unrecognized during the cholecystectomy.[53,55] The patient develops clinical jaundice with or without signs of cholangitis days to weeks after the initial surgery. Diagnosis is made by endoscopic retrograde cholangiopancreatography or transhepatic cholangiography (see Chap. 61). Postoperative pancreatitis also may cause bile duct obstruction because of edema of the head of the pancreas. The diagnosis is made by finding an elevated serum level of amylase and a computed tomography scan of the abdomen showing edema of the pancreas and bile duct dilation. The jaundice resolves as the patient recovers from the pancreatitis.[56] In the postoperative jaundiced patient who has not undergone biliary or gastric surgery and who does not have evidence of pancreatitis, biliary tract disease is uncommon and other causes of jaundice should be considered initially. Acute cholecystitis (calculous or acalculous) may occur postoperatively and can be asso-

TABLE 28-2
Differential Diagnosis of Postoperative Liver Dysfunction

Disorder	Type of surgery	Fever	Onset postoperatively	ALT U/L	AP
Halothane hepatitis	No relationship	Common	2-15 days	>500	sl ↑
Viral hepatitis	No relationship	Uncommon	>3 weeks	>500	sl ↑
Benign postoperative jaundice	Major surgery with sepsis	Common	<7 days	sl ↑	↑↑
Shock	No relationship (cardiac disease)	Uncommon	1-4 days	>500	sl ↑ (↑LDH)
Bile duct injury	Biliary tract and stomach	Common	Days-weeks	200-300	↑↑

ALT, Alanine aminotransferase; *AP,* alkaline phosphatase; *Sl,* slight; *LDH,* lactate dehydrogenase; ↑, increase; ↑↑, greater increase.

ciated with abnormal liver tests and clinical jaundice.[57] The presence of right upper quadrant abdominal pain and fever suggests the diagnosis, with the ultrasound findings of pericholecystic fluid, thickening of the gallbladder wall, and perhaps stones supporting the clinical suspicion.[58] Gangrene, perforation, and empyema of the gallbladder are common in the postoperative patient and associated with a high mortality.[57]

Abnormal liver tests are observed frequently in patients receiving total parenteral nutrition (TPN), which is discussed in detail in Chapter 57. Fatty liver with mild elevations of the serum aminotransferases and alkaline phosphatase is observed commonly.[59] Less common but of greater concern, especially in children, is the development of jaundice. The abnormal liver tests develop days to weeks after the institution of therapy.[59] The liver biopsy findings are non-specific and the diagnosis is one of excluding the other causes of postoperative hepatic dysfunction. The cause of the disorder remains poorly understood.

Evaluation of the Patient with Postoperative Liver Dysfunction

If the patient is within the first 2 weeks of surgery and has a hepatitis-like injury, anesthetic-related hepatitis or ischemic hepatitis is of major concern (Table 28-2). Injury by a direct hepatotoxin such as acetaminophen should also be considered. The development of cholestasis in the immediate postoperative period in a patient who has undergone biliary or gastric surgery suggests bile duct injury. If the patient has undergone major cardiac or abdominal surgery and is infected or has received multiple blood transfusions, benign postoperative cholestasis should be the initial diagnosis. If the abnormal liver tests develop more than 2 weeks after surgery, drug- or TPN-induced liver injury should be considered, as should bile duct injury if gallbladder surgery had been performed. Postoperative cholecystitis is associated with abdominal pain and fever, which are unusual features of the other types of injury, and abdominal ultrasonography should be performed in this situation. Hepatitis C should be considered in the transfused patient who develops elevated AST/ALT levels more than 3 weeks after exposure to blood products. Antibody tests may be negative during the acute illness and identification of viral ribonucleic acid in the serum by polymerase chain reaction may be required (see Chap. 33). Tests for acute hepatitis A and B are usually not necessary because they infrequently cause post-transfusion hepatitis.

References

1. LaMont JT: Postoperative jaundice. Surg Clin North Am 54:637, 1974.
2. Schemel WH: Unexpected hepatic dysfunction found by multiple laboratory screening. Anesth Analg (Cleve) 55:810, 1976.
3. Wataneeyawech M, Kelly KA Jr: Hepatic diseases unsuspected before surgery. NY State J Med 75:1278, 1975.
4. Ngai SH: Effects of anesthetics on various organs. N Engl J Med 302:564, 1980.
5. Cooperman LH: Effects of anesthesia on the splanchnic circulation. Br J Anaesth 44:967, 1972.
6. Harville DD, Summerskill WHJ: Surgery in acute hepatitis. JAMA 184:257, 1963.
7. Powell-Jackson P, Greenway B, Williams R: Adverse effects of exploratory laparotomy in patients with unsuspected liver disease. Br J Surg 69:449, 1982.
8. Shaldon S, Sherlock S: Virus hepatitis with features of prolonged bile retention. BMJ 2:734, 1957.
9. Hardy KJ, Hughes ESR: Laparotomy in viral hepatitis. Med J Aust 1:710, 1968.
10. Strauss AA, Strauss SF, Schwartz AH, et al: Decompression by drainage of the common bile duct in subacute and chronic jaundice: a report of 73 cases with hepatitis or concomitant biliary duct infection as cause. Am J Surg 97:137, 1959.
11. Bourke JB, Cannon P, Ritchie HD: Laparotomy for jaundice. Lancet ii:521, 1967.
12. Farrell GC: Postoperative hepatic dysfunction. In Zakim D, Boyer TD, eds: Hepatology: A Textbook of Liver Disease, ed 2, Philadelphia, WB Saunders, 1990:869.
13. Johnson RD, O'Connor ML, Kerr RM: Extreme serum elevations of aspartate aminotransferase. Am J Gastro 90:1244, 1995.
14. Friedman LS, Maddrey WC: Surgery in the patient with liver disease. Med Clin North Am 71:453, 1987.
15. Hargrove MD: Chronic active hepatitis possible adverse effect of exploratory laparotomy. Surgery 68:771, 1970.
16. Brolin RE: Unsuspected cirrhosis discovered during elective obesity operations. Arch Surg 133:84, 1998.
17. Greenwood SM, Leffler CT, Minkowitz S: The increased mortality rate of open liver biopsy in alcoholic hepatitis. Surg Gynecol Obstet 134:600, 1972.
18. Mikkelsen W: Therapeutic portacaval shunt. Preliminary data on controlled trial. Arch Surg 108:302. 1974.
19. Pande N, Resnick R, Yee W, et al: Cirrhotic portal hypertension: morbidity of continued alcoholism. Gastroenterology 74:64, 1978.
20. Eckhauser F, Appelman H, O'Leary T, et al: Hepatic pathology as a determinant of prognosis after portal decompression. Am J Surg 139:105, 1980.
21. Kanel G, Kaplan M, Zawacki I, et al: Survival in patients with postnecrotic cirrhosis and Laennec's cirrhosis undergoing therapeutic portacaval shunt. Gastroenterology 73:679, 1977.

22. Bell RH, Miyai K, Orloff MJ: Outcome in cirrhotic patients with acute alcoholic hepatitis after emergency portacaval shunt for bleeding esophageal varices. Am J Surg 147:78, 1984.
23. Reichle R, Fahmy W, Golsorkhi M: Prospective comparative clinical trial with distal splenorenal and mesocaval shunts. Am J Surg 137:13, 1979.
24. Garrison RN, Cryer HM, Howard DA, et al: Clarification of risk factors for abdominal operations in patients with hepatic cirrhosis. Ann Surg 199:648, 1984.
25. Brown MW, Burk RF: Development of intractable ascites following upper abdominal surgery in patients with cirrhosis. Am J Med 80:879, 1986.
26. Chapman CB, Snell AM, Rowntree LG: Decompensated portal cirrhosis. Report on one hundred and twelve cases. Clinical features of the ascitic stage of cirrhosis of the liver. JAMA 97:237, 1981
27. Leonetti JP, Aranha GV, Wilkinson WA, et al: Umbilical herniorrhaphy in cirrhotic patients. Arch Surg 119:442, 1984.
28. Yonemoto RH, Davidson CS: Herniorrhaphy in cirrhosis of the liver with ascites. N Engl J Med 255:733, 1956.
29. Maniatis AG, Hunt CM: Therapy for spontaneous umbilical hernia rupture. Am J Gastro 90:310, 1995.
30. Hurst RD: Management of groin hernias in patients with ascites. Ann Surg 216:696, 1992.
31. Bloch RS, Allaben RD, Wait AJ: Cholecystectomy in patients with cirrhosis. Arch Surg 120:669, 1985.
32. Bornman PC, Terblanche I: Subtotal cholecystectomy: for the difficult gallbladder in portal hypertension and cholecystitis. Surgery 98:1, 1985.
33. Yerdel MA, Tsuge H, Mimura H, et al: Laparoscopic cholecystectomy in cirrhotic patients: expanding indications. Surg Laparosc Endosc 3:180, 1993.
34. Yerdel MA: Laparoscopic versus open cholecystectomy in cirrhotic patients: a prospective study. Surg Laparosc Endosc 7:483, 1997.
35. Sleeman D: Laparoscopic cholecystectomy in cirrhotic patients. J Am Coll Surg 187:400, 1998.
36. Gopalswamy N: Risks of intra-abdominal nonshunt surgery in cirrhotics. Dig Dis 16:225, 1998.
37. D'Alburquerque LA: Laparoscopic cholecystectomy in cirrhotic patients. Surg Laparosc Endosc 5:272, 1995.
38. Friel CM: Laparoscopic cholecystectomy in patients with hepatic cirrhosis: a five-year experience. J Gastrointest Surg 3:286, 1999.
39. Ziser A, Plevak DJ, Weisner RH, et al: Morbidity and mortality in cirrhotic patients undergoing anesthesia and surgery. Anesthesiology 90:42, 1999.
40. Farrell GC: Liver disease due to anaesthetic agents. In Farrell GC, ed: Drug-Induced Liver Disease. Edinburgh, Churchill Livingstone, 1994:389.
41. Touloukian J, Kaplowitz N: Halothane-induced hepatic disease. Semin Liver Dis 1:134, 1981.
42. Cousins MJ, Plummer JL, Hall PM: Risk factors for halothane hepatitis. Aust NZ J Surg 59:5, 1989.
43. Gibson PR, Dudley FJ: Ischemic hepatitis clinical features, diagnosis and prognosis. Aust NZ I Med 14:822, 1984.
44. Johnson RD, O'Connor ML, Kerr RM: Extreme serum elevations of aspartate aminotransferase. Am J Gastro 90:1244, 1995.
45. Brittain RS, Marchioro TL, Hermann G, et al: Accidental hepatic artery ligation in humans. Am J Surg 107:822, 1964.
46. Farrell GC: Paracetamol-induced hepatotoxicity In Farrell GC, ed: Drug-Induced Liver Disease. Edinburgh, Churchill Livingstone, 1994:205.
47. Kumar S, Rex DK: Failure of physicians to recognize acetaminophen hepatotoxicity in chronic alcoholics. Ann Intern Med 151:1189, 1991.
48. Gottlieb JE, Menashe PI, Cruz E: Gastrointestinal complications in critically ill patients: the intensivists' overview. Am J Gastroenterol 81:227, 1986.
49. LaMont JT, Isselbacher KJ: Postoperative jaundice. N Engl J Med 288:305, 1974.
50. Schmid M, Hefti ML, Gattiker R, et al: Benign postoperative intrahepatic cholestasis. N Engl J Med 272:545, 1965.
51. Kantrowitz PA, Jones WA, Greenberger NJ, Isselbacher KJ: Severe postoperative hyperbilirubinemia simulating obstructive jaundice. N Engl J Med 276:591, 1967.
52. Boekhorst T, Urlus M, Doesburg W, et al: Etiologic factors of jaundice in severely ill patients. A retrospective study in patients admitted to an intensive care unit with severe trauma or with septic intra-abdominal complications following surgery and without evidence of bile duct obstruction. J Hepatol 7:111, 1988.
53. Waxman K: Postoperative multiple organ failure. Crit Care Clin 3:429, 1987.
54. Moossa AR, Easter DW, Van Sonnenberg E, et al: Laparoscopic injuries to the bile duct. A cause for concern. Ann Surg 215:203, 1992.
55. Davidoff AM, Pappas TN, Murran EA, et al: Mechanisms of major biliary injury during laparoscopic cholecystectomy. Ann Surg 215:196, 1992.
56. Thompson JS, Bragg LE, Hodgson PE, Rikkers LF: Postoperative pancreatitis. Surg Gynecol Obstet 167:377, 1988.
57. Frazee RC, Nagorney DM, Mucha P: Acute acalculous cholecystitis. Mayo Clin Proc 64:163, 1989.
58. Becker CD, Burckhardt B, Terrier F: Ultrasound in postoperative acalculous cholecystitis. Gastrointest Radiol 11:47, 1986.
59. Baker AL, Rosenberg IH: Hepatic complications of total parenteral nutrition. Am J Med 82:489, 1987.

CHAPTER

29

Alcoholic Liver Disease

Amin A. Nanji, MD, FRCPC, FRCPath

Alcohol abuse costs the United States more than $116 billion per year, of which about 12 percent is for direct costs of medical care.[1,2] Alcohol accounts for about 100,000 deaths per year in the United States.[3] A study of middle-aged men in Malmö, Sweden, over nearly 6 years in the early 1980s showed that premature deaths caused by alcoholism were as frequent as deaths resulting from cancer or coronary artery disease.[4] Nineteen percent of the deaths resulting from alcoholism could be attributed to cirrhosis. The basic reason for this large epidemic of alcohol-related disease is that ethanol is an effective drug in relieving anxiety, depression, and the pressures of modern society. The easy availability of ethanol and the social acceptability of ethanol consumption are advertised widely and aggressively. About $1.2 billion is spent to advertise alcohol consumption as manly, facilitating sociability, leading to wealth and prestige, and enhancing romantic settings.[5] The industry promotes "responsible drinking" in its advertising. Yet it is known that the incidence of alcohol abuse increases rapidly as per capita consumption increases and that the amount of alcohol drunk per event increases as frequency of drinking increases.[6,7] The public seems unaware that chronic use of ethanol in the absence of addiction can lead to serious medical illness, the development of adverse social consequences, or both.

Consumption of ethanol is widespread; about three quarters of the population of the United States use it. The incidence of alcoholism in the United States is approximately 7 percent. In some states, such as California, it exceeds 10 percent. In 1992, 7.41 percent of adults in the United States met the criteria for alcohol dependence or abuse.[8] Alcohol abuse and dependence rates were higher for men (11 percent) than for women (4.08 percent) and higher for non-blacks than for blacks (non-black males 11.33 percent, females 4.25 percent; black males 8.25 percent, females 2.88 percent). Despite these differences blacks have a higher rate of cirrhosis than non-blacks. We are confronted, therefore, with a public health and social problem of enormous proportions—that is, a group of alcohol-related diseases that are completely preventable. The discussion in this chapter is limited to the impact of ethanol consumption on the incidence of hepatic disease and the possible causal relationship between ethanol use and liver disease. The clinical manifestations, the course of ethanol-associated liver disease, and the management of these complications of ethanol abuse are discussed in Chap. 30.

Prevention (or treatment or both) of alcoholism is a problem for which we have no certain answers. Nor does there seem to be strong public resolve in this respect.[9] It is clear that we will have to continue to manage the medical complications of alcoholism and to improve the usefulness of therapy. With regard to liver disease, we need to devise therapies that diminish the impact of ethanol on hepatic function. To do so depends on an understanding of the mechanisms by which ethanol ingestion leads to liver disease and whether ethanol per se is the cause of liver disease or whether ethanol abuse, environmental factors, and genetic predisposition act in concert to produce liver disease. Answers to these questions may be sought via experiments in animals aimed at elucidating the biochemical effects of ethanol metabolism and through studies of the natural history of ethanol-induced liver disease in patients. We hence devote a large portion of this chapter to a consideration of the biochemical basis for the hepatotoxicity of ethanol and to studies in experimental animals of ethanol-induced liver disease.

RELATIONSHIP BETWEEN ETHANOL CONSUMPTION AND THE INCIDENCE OF LIVER DISEASE

The concept of ethanol as a substance producing irreversible damage to the liver rests primarily on the clinicopathologic observation that cirrhosis with a fairly typical histologic appearance (see Chap. 30) occurs in patients consuming large amounts of ethanol. Ethanol can be shown to have a variety of toxic effects on livers in otherwise normal animals, including normal men and women (Table 29-1), but whether any of these changes are cirrhogenic is debatable. Moreover, the animal models for ethanol-induced cirrhosis are not satisfactory (see the following section) and may indeed not apply to humans. Hence it is important to keep in mind that epidemiologic evidence, not biochemical studies of the toxicity of ethanol, leads us to conclude that ethanol ingestion is an important factor in the genesis of cirrhosis; as for example, cirrhosis at autopsy is several-fold more frequent in alcoholics than in non-alcoholics.[10-12] Data on consumption reveal a positive correlation between average per capita ingestion of ethanol and the frequency of cirrhosis found postmortem (Figure 29-1) and show that decreases in the availability of ethanol-containing beverages are associated with declines in deaths resulting from cirrhosis (Figure 29-2). These relationships are strengthened by the separate observation that the incidence of alcohol abuse increases with per capita consumption of alcohol.[6]

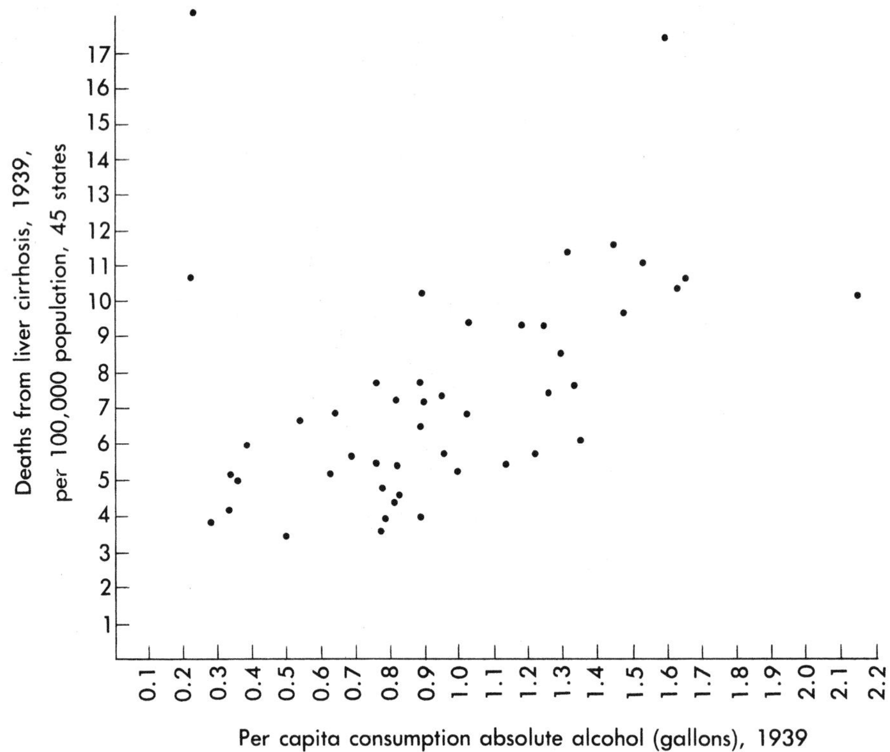

Figure 29-1 The relationship of death from cirrhosis of the liver per 100,000 1939 population of 45 states of the United States to the 1939 per capita consumption of absolute alcohol in the same states. (From Jollife N, Jellinek EM: Q J Stud Alcohol 2:544, 1941.)

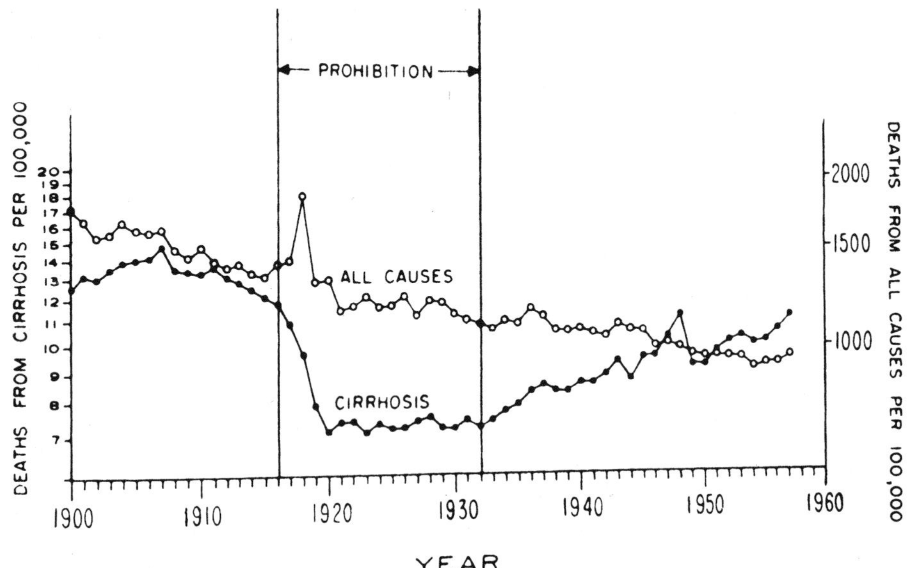

Figure 29-2 Cirrhosis mortality in the United States between 1900 and 1957 compared with death from all causes per 100,000. (From Martini GA, Bode CH. In Engel A, Larsson T, eds: Alcoholic Cirrhosis and Other Toxic Hepatopathias. Stockholm, Nordiska Bokhandelns Förlag, 1970:315.)

After the repeal of prohibition the United States in 1933, the mortality rate from chronic liver disease and cirrhosis gradually increased until it peaked in 1973 at 15.0 deaths per 100,000 population. Since 1973 this rate has steadily decreased and, by 1988, it had dropped to 9.1 deaths per 100,000 population.[13,14] This decrease in cirrhosis mortality is consistent with the reported decrease in per capita consumption of ethanol. Similar phenomena have been reported in Canada and Europe, thus documenting the link between per capita consumption of alcohol and mortality rates from cirrhosis.

Given the epidemiologic data indicating that ethanol causes liver disease (although the mechanism of its toxic effects remains to be elucidated), the next logical question is, How much ethanol induces clinically significant liver disease? Lelbach, in Germany, studied in retrospect the relationship between consumption of ethanol and the incidence of liver disease by correlating consumption with histologic evidence of disease.[15,16] Not surprisingly, he found that the amount ingested and duration of intake were important factors in the induction of alcohol-associated liver disease. The incidence of biopsy-proven alcoholic hepatitis, cirrhosis, or both increased as consumption increased, and cirrhosis was most frequent in the subgroup of alcoholics who had drunk the most for the longest times (Figure 29-3). On the other hand, no level or duration of consumption was associated uniformly with the appearance of clinically significant liver disease. Lelbach's patients had the highest incidence of cirrhosis of any group of alcoholic patients reported in the literature. Cirrhosis of the liver was present in 40 percent to 50 percent of the alcoholic subgroup consuming the largest amount of ethanol for the longest time, but 60 percent of patients consuming as much as 200 g per day of ethanol (for a 70-kg man or woman) for as long as 10 years had normal liver biopsies or uncomplicated fatty livers. To put this level of ethanol intake into perspective, note that it is only slightly less than the maximum amount metabolized in 24 hours by a 70-kg adult.

Lelbach's data suggest that there is no threshold level of ethanol intake at which the risk of liver disease occurs abruptly, but that the relationship between risk and level of consumption is a smooth function. If there were a threshold level, in fact, this probably could not be discerned.[6] The dose-response curves (i.e., risk of liver disease as a function of intake), however, are different for men and women. Risk increases faster for women for relatively low levels of consumption.[17] In addition, the

TABLE 29-1

Some Ways Ethanol Ingestion Can Directly or Indirectly Stress Liver Cell Function

Disorganizes the Lipid Portion of Cell Membranes, Leading to Adaptive Changes in Their Composition

Increased fluidity and permeability of membranes
Impaired assembly of glycoproteins into membranes
Impaired secretion of glycoproteins
Impaired binding and internalization of large ligands
Formation of abnormal mitochondria
Impairment of transport of small ligands
Impairment of membrane-bound enzymes
Adaptive changes in lipid composition, leading to increased lipid peroxidation
Abnormal display of antigens on the plasma membrane

Alters the Capacity of Liver Cells to Cope With Environmental Toxins

Induces xenobiotic metabolizing enzymes
Directly inhibits xenobiotic metabolizing enzymes
Induces deficiency in mechanisms protecting against injury resulting from reactive metabolites
Enhances the toxicity of oxygen

Oxidation of Ethanol Produces Acetaldehyde, a Toxic and Reactive Intermediate

Inhibits export of proteins from the liver
Modifies hepatic protein synthesis in fasted animals
Alters the metabolism of co-factors essential for enzymic activity—pyridoxine, folate, choline, zinc, vitamin E
Alters the oxidation-reduction potential of the liver cell
Induces malnutrition

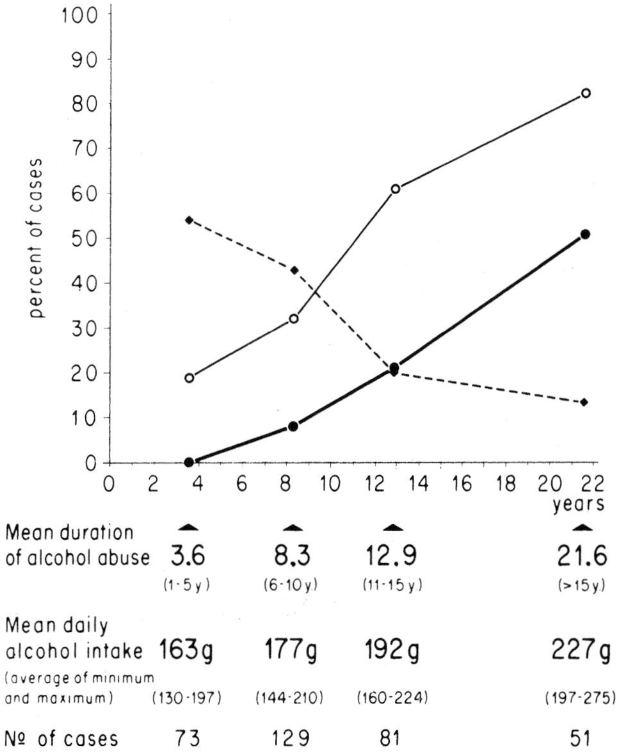

Figure 29-3 Relative frequency of cirrhosis and precirrhotic lesions and its relation to the volume of alcohol abuse among 334 drinkers. (From Lelbach WK: Cirrhosis in the alcoholic and its relation to the volume of alcohol abuse. Ann N Y Acad Sci 285:85, 1975.)

course of liver disease appears to be accelerated in women.[18-20] Fortunately, the incidence of alcoholism in women is about one sixth that in men.[21]

The incidence of cirrhosis in the hospitalized patients studied by Lelbach was about 50 percent for the group of patients drinking the largest amounts of ethanol for 20 years. Estimates of cirrhosis in the overall alcoholic population range from 8 percent to about 15 percent.[22-27] There are several possible causes for this discrepancy. The populations in Lelbach's studies were self-selected, in that the patients admitted themselves to the hospital for detoxification. All studies of hospitalized patients may suffer from the same uncertainty: Do the patients in hospitals accurately reflect the larger group in the population using ethanol? On the other hand, the documentation of ethanol intake is far better in Lelbach's work than in other published surveys for the overall incidence of liver disease in abusers of alcohol. (More recent surveys of the incidence of alcoholism and cirrhosis in several areas of the world can be found in Chapters 5 to 10 of reference 28.) Whatever the exact incidence of liver disease in alcoholics, it is clear that some abusers of ethanol are resistant to its deleterious effects on the liver. Perhaps ethanol abuse that leads to cirrhosis requires malnutrition, a specific type of predisposed host, or the presence of factors not yet described. To give perspective to the complexity of this problem and to provide a basic level of background information for understanding of controversies in the literature, we review the metabolism of ethanol and the posited hepatotoxic effects of ethanol.

OXIDATIVE METABOLISM OF ETHANOL

Ninety percent to ninety-five percent of ingested ethanol is metabolized in the body to acetaldehyde and then to acetate.[29] The remainder is excreted intact via the lungs and kidneys and in sweat. Because oxidation in the liver accounts for nearly all ethanol metabolism (small amounts are oxidized in kidneys, muscles, intestines, and lungs), the study of ethanol metabolism has focused on oxidation by enzyme systems in this organ.

Ethanol oxidation is catalyzed by enzymes within the cytosolic compartment of the liver cell and by enzymes that are attached to the endoplasmic reticulum. The former system is quantitatively more significant compared with the latter.[30-33] Nevertheless, there is a great deal of interest in the oxidation of ethanol by membrane-bound enzymes.

Oxidation of Ethanol by the Combined Activity of Alcohol Dehydrogenases and Aldehyde Dehydrogenases

Reactions [1] and [2] describe the predominant pathways for the oxidation of ethanol. Reaction [1], which is reversible, is catalyzed by alcohol dehydrogenase (ADH). Reaction [2] is catalyzed by aldehyde dehydrogenases.

$$\underset{\text{Ethanol}}{C_2H_5OH} + NAD^+ \leftrightarrow \underset{\text{Acetaldehyde}}{CH_3CHO} + NADH + H^+ \quad [1]$$

$$\underset{\text{Acetaldehyde}}{C_2H_4O} + NAD^+ \rightarrow \underset{\text{Acetate}}{CH_3COOH} + NADH + H^+ \quad [2]$$

Alcohol Dehydrogenases

ADHs are non-specific enzymes broadly distributed throughout nature. These enzymes have a wide variety of endogenous and exogenous substrates[34-38] and catalyze the oxidations of alcohols to the corresponding aldehydes and ketones. ADHs catalyze the oxidation of several physiologic intermediates, for example, glycerol to glyceraldehyde, retinol to retinal, and steroid alcohols to aldehydes.

Multiple molecular forms of human liver ADH have been described. All are dimeric molecules with subunits of 40 Kd that contain zinc. Currently, more than 20 different isoenzymes encoded by seven gene loci are known. They are grouped into five classes of enzymes (Table 29-2).[35,37]

The class I enzymes correspond to what is regarded usually as the common liver ADHs. These isoenzymes are

TABLE 29-2
Human Alcohol Dehydrogenases

Class	Gene locus	Allele	Subunit	Tissue distribution
I	ADH_1	ADH1	α_1	Liver
I	ADH_2	ADH2*1	β_1	Liver, lung
I		ADH2*2	β_2	
I		ADH2*3	β_3	
I	ADH_3	ADH3*1	γ_1	Liver, stomach
I		ADH3*2	γ_2	
II	ADH_4	ADH4	π	Liver, cornea, kidney, lung
				All tissues
III	ADH_5	ADH5	χ	Liver, stomach, skin, cornea
IV	ADH_7	ADHΔ	δ	
			μ	Liver, stomach
IV		ADHμ	?	
V	ADH_6	ADH6		

ADH, Alcohol dehydrogenase.

formed by random dimeric association of any of the three types of polypeptide subunits, α, β, and γ. These subunits are encoded by three separate gene loci, designated ADH_1, ADH_2, and ADH_3, respectively.[39] Class I ADH enzymes have a high affinity for ethanol with a Michaelis constant (K_m) of approximately 0.1 to 1.0 mm (4.6 mg/dl). They are sensitive to inhibition by pyrazole.[40]

Humans express one class II ADH, designated π-ADH.[41] It is detected principally in the liver with minor activity in the intestine. The π-ADH has a K_m for ethanol of about 34 mm (156 mg/dl) and is less sensitive to inhibition by 4-methylpyrazole than are class I enzymes. At low concentrations of ethanol, the activity of π-ADH is less than 10 percent of that of class I ADHs, but π-ADH could be important for oxidation of ethanol at high concentrations of substrate.

Class III ADHs consist of the χ-isoenzyme, which has very low affinity for ethanol ($K_m > 1$ M).[42] This isoform of ADH is not inhibited by 4-methylpyrazole. Only long-chain alcohols such as 1-pentanol and aromatic alcohols are oxidized efficiently by χ-ADH. Class III ADH functions normally in vivo as a glutathione-dependent, formaldehyde dehydrogenase.

Class IV ADHs consist of ADHσ and ADHμ, which are expressed predominantly in the stomach.[43,44] These types of ADH have characteristics similar to those of class II enzymes (e.g., a high K_m for ethanol [41 mm]). The ADH6 gene of a class V ADH has been cloned.[45] This gene encodes a subunit with about 60 percent homology to the other classes of ADH. It is expressed in liver and stomach and has a K_m for ethanol of about 28 mm (129 mg/dl). The importance of this enzyme in ethanol oxidation is unknown at present.

As shown in Table 29-2 ADH isoenzymes have tissue-specific expression. Although most studies in rats show a prevalent perivenular distribution of ADH in the liver,[46,47] others have found either no particular anatomic distribution[48,49] or a periportal distribution.[50] These discrepancies reflect differences in techniques used to measured zonal activities. In humans there is a continuous increase in ADH activity from the perivenous to periportal regions. Immunohistochemical analysis shows a perivenous distribution of ADH even in cirrhotic livers.[51] A temporal sequence of expression of class I ADH isoenzymes in the liver has been described for liver (ADH1-ADH2-ADH3).[53] ADH activity is higher in women than in men.[52]

Distribution of the different ADH alleles in various racial groups has been studied extensively in attempts to correlate frequencies of alleles with known variations in ethanol elimination rates, susceptibility to alcoholism, and incidence of liver disease in alcoholics.[35,37] Class I ADH genes show polymorphism, which may be important in this regard.[35] Allelic variants at the ADH_2 (β subunit) and ADH_3 (γ subunit) locus are known, but no polymorphisms have been reported at the ADH_1 (α subunit) locus.[35] The three known polymorphic alleles at the ADH_2 locus are designated ADH_2^1, ADH_2^2, and ADH_2^3. These encode the ADH-β1, ADH-β2, and ADH-β3 subunits, respectively. ADH-β1 is predominant in white and black populations; ADH-β2 is predominant in Asia with a frequency of 85 percent in Japanese populations; and ADH-β3 appears in 25 percent of the black population. With respect to polymorphism of ADH3, ADH_3^1 encodes γ_1 and ADH_3^2 encodes γ_2 subunits. The two γ alleles appear with roughly equal frequencies in white populations, but γ_1 predominates in the Japanese, Chinese, and black populations.

As alluded to previously, there are substantial differences in catalysis between the various isoenzymes of ADH; these differences explain the variations in oxidation rates of ethanol (Table 29-3).[35] Isoenzymes with γ, α, β, and π subunits efficiently oxidize ethanol in that order. χ-ADH is efficient only for oxidizing long-chain alcohols.[54] Hence only isoenzymes with the α, β, γ, π, and σ subunits exhibit high activity with concentrations of ethanol that are close to pharmacologic or near-physiologic levels in liver (22 mm or 100 mg/dl).

The association between polymorphisms of ADH and the occurrence of alcoholic liver disease (ALD) has been the focus of many studies. Day and associates found a disproportionately high frequency of ADH_3^1 in alcoholic cirrhosis.[55] ADH_2^2 and ADH_3^1 were less prevalent than other genotypes in Chinese alcoholics.[56] Poupon and colleagues[57] found no correlation between alleles at the ADH_3 locus and the occurrence of cirrhosis in

TABLE 29-3

Steady-state Kinetic Constants of Homodimeric ADH Isoenzymes

	ISOENZYMES						
	CLASS I				CLASS II		
	$\alpha\alpha$	$\beta_1\beta_1$	$\beta_2\beta_2$	$\beta_3\beta_3$	$\gamma_1\gamma_1$	$\gamma_2\gamma_2$	$\pi\pi$
K_m ethanol (mm)	4.2	0.049	0.94	36.0	1.0	0.63*	34.5
K_m acetaldehyde (mm)	4.3	0.1	0.2	3.4	0.3	0.2	30.5
K_m NAD (μm)	13.3	7.4	180	710	7.9	8.7	14.5
K_m NADH (μm)	11.3	6.4	105	260	7.0	—	2.5
V_{max} (U/mg)	0.6	0.23	8.6	7.9	2.2	0.87	0.5

V_{max}, Maximum velocity.

alcoholics. One of the problems with these studies is the small number of patients evaluated. Possibly, allelic variation at more than one of the above loci alters the risk of alcoholics developing liver disease. Further studies with larger numbers of patients will be necessary to resolve this question.

There is considerable homology between the α, β, and γ peptides of the class I enzymes but not between subunits in different classes. Enzymes of different classes differ extensively in substrate specificities. For example, ethylene glycol and methanol are metabolized only by class I enzymes. Ethanol is not metabolized by the class III enzyme and, as mentioned, ethanol is a relatively poor substrate for all the isoforms of ADH, indicating that these enzymes have other biologic functions.[58-61]

Note in Table 29-3 that polymorphisms in class I ADHs can have large effects on capacity for ethanol metabolism. Rates of metabolism of ethanol in vivo in people with an atypical enzyme, such as $\beta_2\beta_2$, are only slightly greater, however, than in the "normal" population.[62] The basis for this discordance between the activity of alcohol dehydrogenase and rates of utilization of ethanol in vivo is discussed in the following section.

Aldehyde Dehydrogenases

Mammalian tissues contain several aldehyde dehydrogenases that catalyze Reaction [2]. More than 90 percent of the acetaldehyde generated from ethanol is oxidized further to acetate by aldehyde dehydrogenases (ALDHs).[38] As with the ADHs, the ALDHs display broad substrate specificity. Also, ALDHs are present in most cells in the body, with the highest activity in liver. The ALDH family of isoenzymes has been grouped into three classes according to their catalytic and structural characteristics and subcellular localization.[63] Only the class 1 and 2 isoenzymes (E1 and E2), which are encoded by $ALDH_1$ and $ALDH_2$ loci, respectively, are thought to be involved in oxidation of acetaldehyde.

$ALDH_1$ is the high-K_m isoenzyme for acetaldehyde (30 μm) and is expressed constitutively in cytosol. It is NAD^+-dependent. $ALDH_2$ has a low K_m for acetaldehyde (3 μm) and catalyzes most acetaldehyde oxidation in the liver. It is expressed constitutively, is present exclusively in mitochondria, and is NAD^+-dependent. $ALDH_2$ in rat liver is more concentrated in periportal than in perivenous cells.[49] Inhibition of mitochondrial $ALDH_2$ increases acetaldehyde levels, and mutations in $ALDH_2$ are associated with elevated levels of acetaldehyde and the alcohol-induced flush reaction.[37] In humans, unlike in experimental animals, small amounts of acetaldehyde are oxidized by both mitochondrial and cytosolic ALDH. Larger amounts seem to be oxidized mainly by mitochondrial ALDH.[63,64]

Electrophoretic methods indicate that there are polymorphisms for both $ALDH_1$ and $ALDH_2$. $ALDH_1$ variants occur with low frequency, however. The most important ALDH variant, clinically, is $ALDH_{22}$, which is detected in about 50 percent of Japanese and Chinese.[66] It is referred to as the "deficient" phenotype because affected people have very low acetaldehyde-oxidizing activity. The inactivity is a result of substitution of lysine for glutamine in $ALDH_2$.[67] Also, individuals who are $ALDH_2$-deficient by phenotype and $ALDH_2^1/ALDH_2^2$ or $ALDH_2^2/ALDH_2^2$ by genotype have lower elimination rates for ethanol than those with active ALDH.[68]

The alcohol "flushing" reaction is believed to be due to the $ALDH_2$-deficient phenotype and associated increases in levels of acetaldehyde.[69] The attenuation of flushing by histamine antagonists and non-steroidal anti-inflammatory agents supports a role for acetaldehyde-mediated release of vasoactive substances by mast cells in the flushing reaction.[37] For obvious reasons, individuals with the $ALDH_2^2$ isoform are less likely to be heavy drinkers than people with a normal capacity for oxidizing acetaldehyde. Liver fibrosis is less common in alcoholics who are heterozygotes for the $ALDH_2^2$ isoenzyme.[70]

Although flushing and occurrence of the $ALDH_2^2$ genotype have often been used interchangeably, the relationship between flushing and genotype is not always true, even in Asians.[71] The confusion surrounding various aspects of alcohol-induced flushing, within the various ethnic groups, warrants a systematic examination of these groups that incorporates genotypic information.[71]

Deficiency of $ALDH_2$ can be detected with reasonable ease. The enzyme is present normally in hair roots, for example.[72] Moreover, individuals who lack $ALDH_2$ are sensitive (i.e., develop erythema) to patch testing with ethanol because the enzyme also is absent from their skin.[73,74] The sensitivity of these patients to patch testing with ethanol can be blocked by prior treatment of the skin with inhibitors of alcohol dehydrogenase.[75] Results from the patch test depend on the oxidation of ethanol to acetaldehyde, which then accumulates in and irritates the skin.

Microsomal Ethanol-oxidizing System and Cytochrome P450 2E1

Chronic ethanol consumption is associated in rats and humans with proliferation of hepatic endoplasmic reticulum. This observation led to the hypothesis that liver endoplasmic reticulum could be a site for a distinct and adaptive system of ethanol oxidation.[76-78] Subsequently, such a system was demonstrated in vitro and named the microsomal ethanol oxidizing system (MEOS).[79,80] MEOS has a relatively high K_m for ethanol (8 to 10 mm) compared with 0.2 to 2.0 mm for ADH. Therefore ADH accounts normally for the bulk of ethanol oxidation at low levels of alcohol in blood. At higher levels of alcohol or after chronic use of alcohol, MEOS becomes more significant, quantitatively, for the oxidation of ethanol.[81]

The properties of MEOS—that is, co-factor requirements and response to inhibitors—suggested that it was a cytochrome P450-dependent monooxygenase.[81,82] This has been confirmed. It has been shown also that chronic consumption of ethanol induces a unique P450.[82] An ethanol-inducible form of P450 (LM 3a), purified from rabbit liver microsomes, catalyzed ethanol oxidation at rates much higher than rates for other P450 isoenzymes.[83,84] Similar results were obtained with cytochrome P450j, a major hepatic P450 isoenzyme purified from ethanol- or isoniazid-treated rats.[85-87] There is also evidence that a P450j-like enzyme is present in humans.[88,89] In the new nomenclature for cytochromes P450 it was proposed that the ethanol-inducible form be designated P450 IIE1 or CYP 2E1.[90] The term *MEOS* refers to the overall capacity of microsomes for oxidizing ethanol in that cytochrome P450 isoenzymes other than IIE1 also contribute to oxidation of ethanol.

CYP 2E1 has its highest expression in the liver. The expression of the enzyme, both constitutively and after administration of ethanol, is restricted to the centrilobular (perivenous) region particularly to the three or four layers of hepatocytes most proximal to the central vein.[91,92] The regio-selective nature for expression of CYP 2E1 is of obvious interest because ethanol causes selective damage to the centrolobular region. Using immunofluorescence CYP 2E1 is identified to be distributed uniformly across the entire surface of the hepatocyte plasma membrane.[93] The exact significance of CYP 2E1 in hepatocyte plasma membranes is unknown.

The molecular basis for induction of CYP 2E1 by ethanol remains controversial. Proposed mechanisms in ethanol-fed animals and humans include increased 2E1 messenger ribonucleic acid (mRNA) secondary to transcriptional activation, stabilization of mRNA, enhanced synthesis of the enzyme, or decreased degradation.[94] Notably, the mechanism of induction appears to differ with the treatment given and species examined.[94] In general, ethanol administration to rats is not associated with an increase in hepatic CYP 2E1 transcripts unless extremely high concentrations of ethanol are achieved. This rules out transcriptional activation of the 2E1 gene or stabilization of 2E1 mRNA in rats at moderate doses of ethanol. A post-translational mechanism, namely a decrease in degradation of 2E1 because ethanol stabilizes the enzyme, has been proposed by a number of investigators.[95-98] Thus CYP 2E1-specific substrates protect the enzyme from degradation in hepatocytes. Acetone prolongs the half-life in vivo in rat liver by eliminating the fast phase component associated with normal degradation of the enzyme.[95]

Although stabilization of enzyme is a generally recognized mechanism for induction of CYP 2E1 by ethanol, elevations of mRNA have been described in rats receiving ethanol via continuous intragastric infusion.[99-101] Blood ethanol levels were cyclical in nature in these experiments and ranged between 10 and 500 mg/dl. A two-step induction of CYP 2E1 by ethanol was proposed. At ethanol levels less than 300 mg/dl the increase in hepatic CYP 2E1 content was not accompanied by an increase in mRNA for CYP 2E1. At levels above 300 mg/dl a marked elevation of CYP 2E1 mRNA occurred via transcription of the CYP 2E1 gene. Other species in which induction was associated with increases in CYP 2E1 mRNA are hamsters[102] and man.[103] Using in situ hybridization with a human CYP 2E1 complementary deoxyribonucleic acid (cDNA) probe, the distribution of CYP 2E1 transcripts in liver tissue was primarily perivenular in non-drinking subjects. A threefold increase in CYP 2E1 transcripts occurred in subjects who were drinking actively.[103] A strong correlation between the content of CYP 2E1 mRNA and enzyme protein suggested that CYP 2E1 expression in human livers was linked closely to translation of mRNA. The enhancement of CYP 2E1 message and protein was seen only in alcoholic subjects who had consumed alcohol within the previous 36 hours. It was not observed in patients who had been abstinent for at least 96 hours. These findings are consistent with the high turnover rate reported for CYP 2E1.[94,95] Not all investigators have found a correlation, however, between concentrations of mRNA and levels of CYP 2E1 in human liver.[104]

CYP 2E1 and Lipid Peroxidation

Interest in CYP 2E1 extends beyond the oxidation of ethanol because the enzyme possesses high oxidase activity. CYP 2E1 is the most efficient isoenzyme of P450 in the initiation of nicotinamide adenine dinucleotide phosphate (NADPH)–dependent peroxidation of fatty acids.[105-107] It can initiate lipid peroxidation of membrane lipids in the presence of small amounts of non-heme iron.[108] Inhibitors of CYP 2E1 have been used to evaluate the importance of induction of CYP 2E1 as a mechanism for ethanol-dependent lipid peroxidation.

Diallylsulfone, a metabolite of diallyl sulfide (DAS), inhibits CYP 2E1.[109] When used chronically, DAS inhibits the rate of transcription of CYP 2E1.[110] When DAS (an ingredient of onion and garlic) was administered to ethanol-fed rats, the activity of CYP 2E1 decreased, lipid peroxidation decreased, and liver pathology was ameliorated.[111] An interesting observation in these studies was that inhibition of CYP 2E1 by DAS was accompanied by increases in CYP 2E1 in periportal cells.[112] This shift in the hepatic distribution of CYP 2E1 was accompanied by a shift in the localization of fatty change from the perivenous to periportal region. Chlormethiazole, an inhibitor of CYP 2E1 gene transcription, also reduced the level of CYP 2E1 and lipid peroxidation when administered to ethanol-fed rats.[113] Inhibition of CYP 2E1 also significantly decreased concentrations of hydroxyethyl free radicals,[114] which bind covalently to microsomal proteins[115] and elicit an immune response to the modified protein.[116,117] Studies showing concomitant inhibition of CYP 2E1 and a reduction in the severity of lipid peroxidation and liver pathology support the idea that induction of CYP 2E1 and lipid peroxidation are contributors to ALD. The use of electron spin resonance spectroscopy also has demonstrated that hydroxylethyl radicals are generated during ethanol metabolism by CYP 2E1.[118] Formation of hydroxyethyl radicals is associated with formation of lipid peroxides and development of liver injury.[119] Furthermore, hydroxyethyl radicals alkylate liver proteins, leading to induction of specific antibodies in experimental animals and alcoholics.[120,121]

CYP 2E1 also oxidizes acetaldehyde.[122] Acetaldehyde binds to CYP 2E1 and other microsomal proteins and forms adducts.[123] By metabolizing both ethanol and its primary oxidation product acetaldehyde, CYP 2E1 leads to the formation of both acetaldehyde protein adducts and serum protein adducts with the products of lipid peroxidation (e.g., malondialdehyde and 4-hydroxynonenal).[124]

Nutrient Regulation of CYP 2E1

The expression of CYP 2E1 is influenced by hormonal and nutritional factors.[102] Starvation of rats increases the amount of CYP 2E1 and its corresponding mRNA.[125,126] Starvation exerts a pronounced synergistic effect on the induction of CYP 2E1 by ethanol.[127] Indeed, ethanol in combination with a low-carbohydrate diet causes a tenfold induction of CYP 2E1 in the liver.[127]

The effect of the type of dietary fat on induction of CYP 2E1 by ethanol has received a great deal of recent attention.[128-135] The level of CYP 2E1 induction is regulated by the type of dietary fat in the absence of ethanol. Dietary corn oil, in rats for example, increased the level of CYP 2E1 twofold compared with a fat-free diet,[129] and rats fed corn oil or menhaden oil had higher levels of CYP 2E1 in liver as compared to rats fed lard or olive oil.[130] The effect of the type of dietary fat influenced levels of CYP 2E1 in ethanol-fed rats. The combination of corn oil and ethanol caused a much higher level of induction of CYP 2E1 than saturated fat and ethanol.[131,132] The induction of CYP 2E1 occurred before the development of pathologic changes. Thus induction of CYP 2E1 appears important in the pathogenesis of alcoholic liver injury and not a consequence of injury.[132]

Using the intragastric feeding model (see section on Animal Models of Alcoholic Liver Injury), a threefold higher level of CYP 2E1 was seen in rats fed fish oil plus ethanol as compared with corn oil plus ethanol. And, the higher level of CYP 2E1-induction was accompanied by enhanced lipid peroxidation and more severe liver pathology in rats fed fish oil plus ethanol.[134] A significant correlation between the amount of CYP 2E1, NADPH-dependent lipid peroxidation, and severity of pathology has been confirmed.[135]

Induction of other P450s that may contribute to enhanced MEOS in ethanol-fed rats includes the phenobarbital-inducible cytochrome P450. Coordinate induction of both CYP 2B1 and CYP 2E1 has been seen using the Lieber-DeCarli feeding regimen[128] or the intragastric feeding model.[132] The contribution of CYP 2B1 induction to ethanol-induced liver pathology is unknown.

Cytochrome P450 2E1 and Non-alcoholic Steatohepatitis

Non-alcoholic steatohepatitis (NASH) and ALD have similar pathologic features. NASH is considered a progressive disease that leads to cirrhosis in 25 percent of affected patients.[136] One similarity between NASH and alcoholic steatohepatitis (ASH) is induction of CYP 2E1 in both.[137] A connection between induction of CYP 2E1 and NASH was first suggested in studies of rats fed a methionine-choline-deficient (MCD) diet.[138] These rats developed steatosis and hepatic inflammation accompanied by up-regulation of catalytically active CYP 2E1. CYP 2E1 was also induced in humans with NASH.[139] Studies in mice fed the MCD diet showed that the activity of CYP 2E1 accounted for more than 90 percent of NADPH-dependent lipid peroxidation in hepatic microsomes.[140] Further studies of NASH in mice lacking CYP 2E1 showed induction of alternate microsomal enzymes that promote lipid peroxidation and steatohepatitis. The activity of CYP 4A10 accounted for more than half of the microsomal lipid peroxidation in vitro in CYP 2E1-deficient mice. CYP 2E1 -/- mice also develop alcoholic liver injury.[141] An abundance of data suggests that the catalytic activity of CYP 2E1 is highly significant for developing ASH and NASH.[142] Further work is needed to clarify the significance of other initiators of oxidative stress in livers with ASH or NASH.[143]

Catalase

Reaction [3], which describes MEOS-catalyzed oxidation of ethanol, also could describe the oxidation of ethanol by catalase, an enzyme bound to microsomes.

$$C_2H_5OH + O_2 + NADPH + H^+ \rightarrow CH_3CHO + NADP^+ + 2H_2O \qquad [3]$$

Catalase catalyzes Reaction [4].[144]

$$H_2O_2 + C_2H_5OH \rightarrow CH_3CHO + 2H_2O \qquad [4]$$

Hydrogen peroxide (H_2O_2) in this reaction is generated by flavoprotein oxidase enzymes—Reaction [5]—which are plentiful in microsomes.

$$NADPH + H^+ + O_2 \xrightarrow[\text{oxidase}]{\text{Flavoprotein}} H_2O_2 + NADP^+ \qquad [5]$$

Addition of Reactions [4] and [5] yields the stoichiometry of Reaction [3]. The direct participation of cytochrome P450 in Reaction [3] cannot be inferred, therefore, on the basis of the stoichiometry of the oxidation of ethanol catalyzed by microsomes. The carbon monoxide-induced inhibition of microsomal-catalyzed oxidation of ethanol also does not validate catalysis by cytochrome P450 in the metabolism of ethanol because cytochrome P450 can generate H_2O_2, according to Reaction [5].

The oxidation of ethanol by microsomes is inhibited by specific inhibitors of catalase, or by removing catalase from microsomes,[145-150] but catalase and P450s do not account completely for all the oxidation of ethanol by microsomes.[151-158] NADPH-cytochrome *c* reductase produces •OH (hydroxide radical) from H_2O_2,[153-155] and •OH oxidizes alcohols non-enzymatically (Reaction [6]).

$$\bullet OH + \text{ethanol} \rightarrow \text{acetaldehyde} \qquad [6]$$

Oxidation of ethanol by catalase, by •OH, or by cytochrome P450-mediated reactions can be dissected out because each reaction can be inhibited selectively. Note, however, that the stoichiometry of all three reactions for microsomal-catalyzed oxidation of ethanol is identical.

It has been proposed that the contribution of catalase to ethanol oxidation in vivo is enhanced by fatty acids.[159] In perfused livers from fasted rats, for example, rates of H_2O_2 production were increased significantly, from 10 to about 80 μmol/g per hour, by the addition of fatty acid-albumin complexes (palmitate and oleate). The explanation for this is that the peroxisomal beta oxidation of fatty acids (see Chap. 3) generates H_2O_2. One potentially confounding and interesting aspect of the problem is that NADH produced from alcohol dehydrogenase-dependent metabolism of alcohol in the cytosol inhibits production of H_2O_2.[160,161] This interaction represents a potentially important mechanism for regulation of ethanol oxidation. In the alcohol dehydrogenase-negative (ADH^-) deermouse catalase is the predominant pathway for alcohol metabolism; in the ADH^+ deermouse, about 50 percent of alcohol metabolism is catalyzed by catalase at low blood levels of ethanol (<50 mg/dl). Catalase-dependent metabolism predominates at higher blood levels of alcohol.[162] The exact relevance of this observation to other mammalian species and humans is unknown but it suggests that catalase is important in the metabolism of ethanol. Nevertheless, some investigators have failed to confirm that catalase activity and peroxisomal beta oxidation of fatty acids are important for ethanol metabolism.[160,163]

Chronic feeding of ethanol to rats increases rates of beta oxidation of fatty acids in peroxisomes in the pericentral regions of the liver.[164] Because H_2O_2 produced in this reaction is a precursor of a number of oxygen-derived free radicals,[165] it is reasonable to postulate that elevated rates of peroxisomal, beta oxidation of fatty acids could contribute to the pericentral toxicity of ethanol.

Non-oxidative Pathways for the Metabolism of Ethanol

A non-oxidative pathway for ethanol metabolism was identified first in rabbit hearts. It was demonstrated that ethanol reacted with long-chain fatty acids to form ethyl esters.[166] This reaction has been documented in human hearts. The enzyme catalyzing the reaction has been purified.[167,168] The esterification reaction is unusual in that there is a direct esterification of fatty acids with ethanol. By contrast, all esterification reactions of fatty acids with glycerol (but not cholesterol) require formation of the acyl co-enzyme A (CoA) derivative, which depends on cleavage of adenosine triphosphate (ATP) to adenosine monophosphate (AMP) and inorganic pyrophosphate. Esterification of fatty acids with ethanol occurs independently of CoA and ATP. Because ethyl esters accumulate in tissue, it was proposed that their formation accounted for the known deleterious effects of ethanol on myocardial metabolism and contractility.[169,170]

In humans the pancreas and liver have by far the largest enzymatic capacity for esterifying ethanol with long-chain fatty acids.[171] The esters are present in above-normal amounts in a variety of tissues from alcoholics who have no ethanol in the blood at the time of death[171]; they are found in greater amounts in organs of patients dying while intoxicated. And, levels of fatty acid ethyl esters (FAEE) in plasma correlate with levels of alcohol.[172] Although it has been proposed that the ethyl esters could have a deleterious effect on tissue and could account for the toxic effects of ethanol, no data as yet connect the presence of the esters with pathogenic events in vivo.

Studies of cytotoxic treatment of isolated organelles with FAEE in non-physiologic vehicles, such as emulsions, show detrimental effects.[173,174] Also, in vitro studies using intact cells and low-density lipoproteins (LDL) as a carrier for FAEE show that FAEE was incorporated into Hep G2 cells with a resultant decrease in cell proliferation and protein synthesis.[175] The concentrations of FAEE used in this last study were 250-fold to 300-fold higher than levels in intoxicated individuals (16 ± 3 μmol/L with about 2.5 μmol/L being present in LDL).[176]

Gastric Alcohol Dehydrogenase and First-pass Metabolism

Studies in rats and humans show that intravenous administration of a low dose of ethanol results in higher concentrations of ethanol in blood than does oral administration.[177,178] Theoretically, this first-pass metabolism (FPM) of oral ethanol could occur in the stomach, intestine, or liver. And the concept that the stomach makes a significant contribution to FPM is now widely accepted. That is, gastric metabolism of ethanol defines the difference between the quantity of alcohol reaching the systemic circulation after ethanol is given intravenously or orally.[177-181]

Multiple isoforms of ADH occur in the mucus-producing epithelial cells that line the gastric mucosa.[182,183] Total enzyme is abundant and is the most important system for metabolism of ethanol in the gastric mucosa.[184] The isoenzymes in stomach include the class I ADH isoenzymes, a class III or χ-ADH, and a σ-ADH (40 mmol/L).[185] Although this isoform has a high K_m for ethanol, the σ-ADH is efficient for oxidation of ethanol at concentrations in the stomach after ingestion of ethanol.[186] The importance of gastric ADH in FPM is supported by observations that FPM disappears when enteral ethanol bypasses the stomach[177] and by clinical associations between the magnitude of FPM and variation of ADH activity in the stomach.[180,187] Decreased FPM in women and alcoholics correlates with decreased gastric ADH on endoscopic biopsy of gastric mucosa.[180,187] Some H_2 receptor antagonists that inhibit gastric ADH appear to decrease the effect,[188] but this finding has not been confirmed by all investigators.[189] The discrepancies may be related to choice of experimental subjects and whether individuals were fasting at the time of ethanol ingestion.[184]

There are opposing views for the significance of the stomach in the FPM of ethanol.[190,191] These arguments are based on the established fact that the maximal capacity of the liver to metabolize ethanol is much greater than that of gastric mucosa.[190] The alternative hypothesis is that the varying saturation of liver metabolism by ethanol accounts for the reported observations concerning FPM. Even at concentrations of 40 mmol/L of ethanol, the gastric enzyme is at only half its maximal activity; therefore, very high concentrations of ethanol are required for significant metabolism of ethanol by gastric ADH. A further argument against a dominant role for gastric ADH in FPM is that the absence of gastric ADH in Asians does not lead to a higher blood ethanol in response to ingested ethanol.[192] However, high rates for alcohol metabolism in these individuals could be due to hepatic isoenzymes of ADH not found in the Caucasian population.[193] The controversy regarding the role of the stomach in FPM is far from settled, but the balance of available evidence today favors the idea that the stomach makes a significant contribution.

Factors Determining the Rate of Oxidation of Ethanol by Alcohol Dehydrogenase

It is generally true that the rate of elimination of ethanol is zero order (constant) so long as the concentration of ethanol in vivo is higher than 50 mg/100 ml blood. This statement is not exactly correct. The rate of ethanol metabolism in humans increases at very high concentrations in blood because metabolism catalyzed by the class II type of ADH becomes increasingly larger at high concentrations of ethanol.[194] In fact, at high concentrations of ethanol (200 mg/100 ml) the elimination rate, as a result of metabolism, was nearly twice as great as at 50 mg/100 ml.[195] Moreover, this high rate was sustained until blood levels of ethanol fell to 25 mg/ml. The basis for this last effect is unclear. The high rates of ethanol metabolism at high concentrations of ethanol are observed in alcoholics and controls.[195,196]

One can make a reasonable estimate of the rate of ethanol metabolism in an average, well-fed individual who is not a chronic user of large amounts of ethanol. The rate is about 100 mg ethanol/hour/kg body weight for as long as the plasma concentration of ethanol exceeds 50 mg/100 ml. There can be considerable variability, however. Nutritional state, genetic polymorphism, and previous intake of ethanol influence rate of metabolism (see the following section).

The rate of oxidation of ethanol depends on the amount of alcohol dehydrogenase and the constraints under which it functions in the intact hepatocyte. It is uncertain whether the latter or former limits metabolism in vivo. Reaction [1] is reversible, but levels of acetaldehyde in tissue and blood remain low as compared with those for ethanol during the metabolism of ethanol. In vivo, therefore, there is no tendency for Reaction [1] to come to equilibrium or reverse. On the other hand, the NADH produced in Reaction [1] is not as easily reoxidized to NAD^+ as the acetaldehyde is disposed of.

Oxidation of ethanol alters the ratio of NAD^+ to NADH in the hepatocyte. The reduced form of the nucleotide (i.e., NADH) accumulates at the expense of the oxidized form. It appears that the rate of reoxidation of NADH, not the amount of alcohol dehydrogenase, limits the metabolism of ethanol in an intact animal.[30,31,197-200] Direct observations in humans tend to confirm this idea. Thus as previously mentioned, the rates of oxidation of ethanol in individuals with ADH_2 are only slightly faster than in the "normal" population.[33] We review briefly the reactions accounting for the reoxidation of NADH in hepatocytes.

Alcohol dehydrogenase is in the cytoplasm of the cell. NADH can be reoxidized to NAD^+ in this compartment according to the scheme in Reaction [7]. However, the amount of substrates in these systems is limited as compared with the amount of ethanol usually ingested. Reactions such as those in [7] hence cannot support the oxidation of ethanol. Instead, NADH produced by Reaction [1] must be transferred to the mitochondria to be oxidized by the electron-transport system. NADH and NAD^+ do not cross the inner membrane of the mitochondria, however (see Chap. 3). The hydrogen and electrons abstracted from ethanol and transferred to NAD^+ in Reaction [1] are shuttled across the inner mitochondrial membrane attached to carrier molecules, as depicted in Figure 29-4. The carrier systems for hydrogen and electrons, the malate-aspartate and α-glycerophosphate cycles, are the two most important such systems in liver.[201,202]

Once inside the mitochondria, the reduced carriers are oxidized, thereby passing the hydrogen and electrons derived from ethanol to the components of the electron-transport chain. The energy of the oxidation-reduction reactions comprising the electron-transport system is conserved as ATP, which is why ethanol is a food yielding 7.1 calories/g on complete oxidation to CO_2.

The coupling of the oxidation of ethanol to the synthesis of ATP limits the rate at which ethanol can be oxidized because the rate of synthesis of ATP is regulated carefully: synthesis equals utilization. The rate of flow of electrons through the electron-transport system and hence the rate of oxidation of NADH and glycerol-1-P are constrained in normal tissue by the rate at which the cell uses ATP. The rate of this last process may determine the maximal rate of ethanol oxidation in fed animals. For example, uncouplers of oxidative phosphorylation, which allow the electron-transport system to function independently of a supply of ADP, enhance the rate of metabolism of ethanol.[171,195,197] Fructose increases the rate of oxidation of ethanol by intact animals[202-204] because it increases the concentration of ADP in the cell (Reaction [7]).

$$\text{Fructose} + \text{ATP} \xrightarrow{\text{Fructokinase}} \text{fructose-1-P} + \text{ADP} \qquad [7]$$

In addition, direct oxidation of NADH is coupled to reduction of fructose to sorbitol.

Calculations of the elimination rate for ethanol, based on the amounts and catalytic constants for alcohol dehydrogenases, predict with good accuracy actual rates of elimination, in humans and rats, whether fed or fasted.[205-208] These data are posited to support the idea that the amounts of the dehydrogenases determine the elimination rate for ethanol. On the other hand, although the rate of oxidation of ethanol is thought to be increased in people who use it on a chronic basis as compared with rates in those who consume it sporadically,[31,198,209-211] more recent studies suggest that the rate of oxidation does not increase with chronic consumption.[195]

Fasting diminishes the rate of oxidation of ethanol compared with the fed state.[199,212] This is associated with a decrease in total ADH in the liver, but no change in the amount per gram of liver.[110] The best evidence available is compatible with the idea that the rate of ethanol oxidation in fasted rats is limited by the activity of the shuttle systems for transporting reducing equivalents from the cytoplasm to the mitochondria. Treatment of fasted rats with agents that enhance the maximum capacity of either of the shuttle systems in Figure 29-4 increases the rate of oxidation of ethanol. The same treatments are without effect on the rate of oxidation of ethanol when administered to fed rats.[199,212]

Diets deficient in protein, when fed to rats and alcoholic patients, decrease the alcohol and aldehyde dehydrogenases in liver.[212-217] The decrease in activity of the latter enzyme is no greater than for alcohol dehydrogenase in protein-restricted rats. Whether levels of alcohol

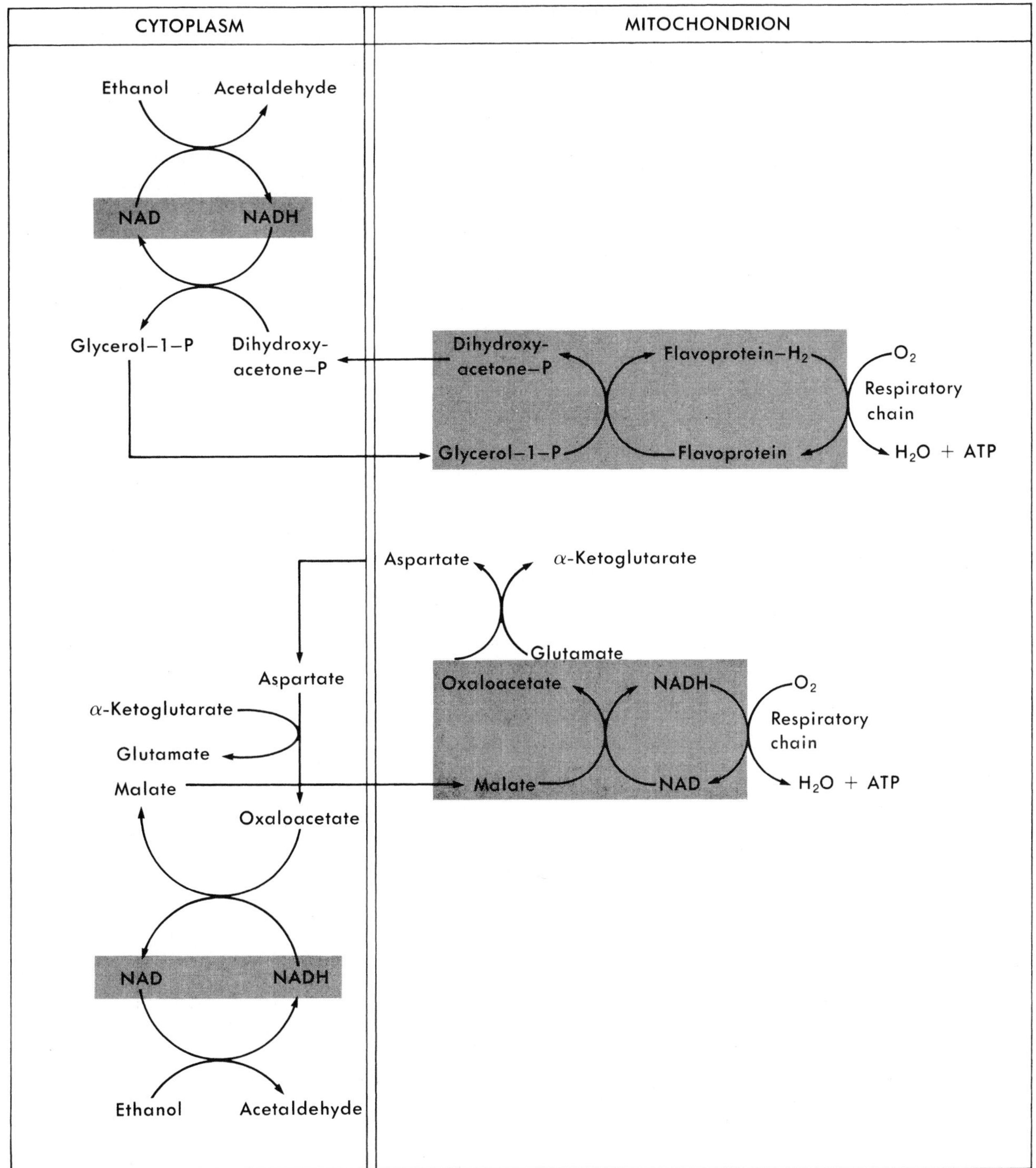

Figure 29-4 Shuttle systems for transporting electrons and hydrogen from cytoplasm to the mitochondrial respiratory chain.

dehydrogenase limit the metabolism of ethanol in vivo in protein-deficient animals or whether the activity of the shuttle systems does, as in fasting, is unstudied.

Metabolism of Acetaldehyde

Acetaldehyde levels in peripheral venous blood are at the level of detectability (approximately 2 μm) after oral administration of ethanol to non-alcoholics.[218] Earlier data for levels of acetaldehyde in human blood, which reported higher values,[217,219-222] were probably incorrect because of methodologic problems in quenching the production of acetaldehyde in blood.[218,223,224]

Only about 1 percent of acetaldehyde produced in the liver from Reaction [2] leaves the liver.[219,225] In addition, red blood cells (RBCs) oxidize acetaldehyde.[218,226,227]

These two factors account for the low levels of acetaldehyde in peripheral blood in normal people. But levels of acetaldehyde in blood are higher in alcoholics with liver disease and in alcoholics without evident liver disease than in non-alcoholic subjects given identical test doses of ethanol by any route (Figure 29-5).[228-232] The basis for this difference in levels of acetaldehyde in the blood of alcoholics compared with non-alcoholics is probably reduced levels of aldehyde dehydrogenases in liver and RBCs of alcoholics.[228-232] Thus rates of ethanol oxidation are equal in controls and alcoholics, so accumulation of acetaldehyde in alcoholics must reflect slower than normal rates of metabolism of acetaldehyde. Moreover, it has been found that the cytosolic isoform of aldehyde dehydrogenase in liver is reduced in alcoholics as compared with non-alcoholics.[230-232] Whether or not the mitochondrial form of the enzyme is also reduced is not clear.[229] The reduction of ALDH persists after abstention in some alcoholics,[231] but in others the abnormality disappears with abstention.[224] Whether these results are due to the presence and the extent of irreversible liver disease in some alcoholics has not been examined. Interestingly, the isoform of ALDH in RBCs is the same as the isoform reduced in cytosol from livers of alcoholics, and the activity of this enzyme in RBCs is decreased in alcoholics.[227] The activity of this same ALDH is decreased in liver in some patients with a variety of liver diseases that are not the result of alcohol,[228] but levels of ALDH in RBCs have not been reported in this subset of patients. Patients with liver disease not resulting from alcohol have slightly greater concentrations of acetaldehyde in peripheral blood after administration of a test dose of ethanol as compared with controls.

As mentioned previously, the mitochondrial form of ALDH is believed to be the only form of the enzyme in liver that catalyzes the oxidation of significant amounts of acetaldehyde. On the other hand, if, as claimed, alcoholic liver disease causes a selective reduction in a cytosolic ALDH and a decrease in rates of oxidation of acetaldehyde, then it is quite likely that cytosolic ALDH metabolizes significant amounts of acetaldehyde in normal liver.

The compromised metabolism of acetaldehyde in alcoholics may lead to its metabolism by a non-oxidative pathway. Evidence has been presented that 2,3-butanedione accumulates in serum after ingestion of ethanol and that levels are higher in alcoholics than in non-alcoholics.[233] The likely pathway for the synthesis of this compound is a condensation between hydroxyethylthiamine pyrophosphate (bound to the pyruvate dehydrogenase complex) and acetaldehyde to produce acetoin. The latter is reduced by NADH to 2,3-butanediol.

There is a positive correlation between the hepatic concentrations of ethanol and acetaldehyde. It is noteworthy, however, that the concentration of acetaldehyde is quite low compared with that of ethanol, even at high levels of the latter.[219,220,222,223] The liver thus oxidizes acetaldehyde at a rate almost equal to its production. There are many uncertainties as to how this is accomplished. We say this because, as mentioned previously, reoxidation of the NADH produced in Reaction [2] is effected by the enzymes of the mitochondrial electron-transport system, which may control the rate of Reaction [1] in the fed state by limiting the rate of reoxidation of the NADH. Yet oxidation of acetaldehyde keeps pace under almost all conditions with the rate of oxidation of ethanol. There appears to be a mechanism by which oxidation of acetaldehyde takes precedence over that of ethanol to ensure that acetaldehyde does not accumulate.

The rate of metabolism of acetaldehyde by liver mitochondria from rats fed ethanol on a chronic basis is slower than that by liver mitochondria from untreated rats,[234] suggesting that chronic exposure to ethanol may interfere with the oxidation of acetaldehyde in vivo. However, measurement of ALDH activity in mitochon-

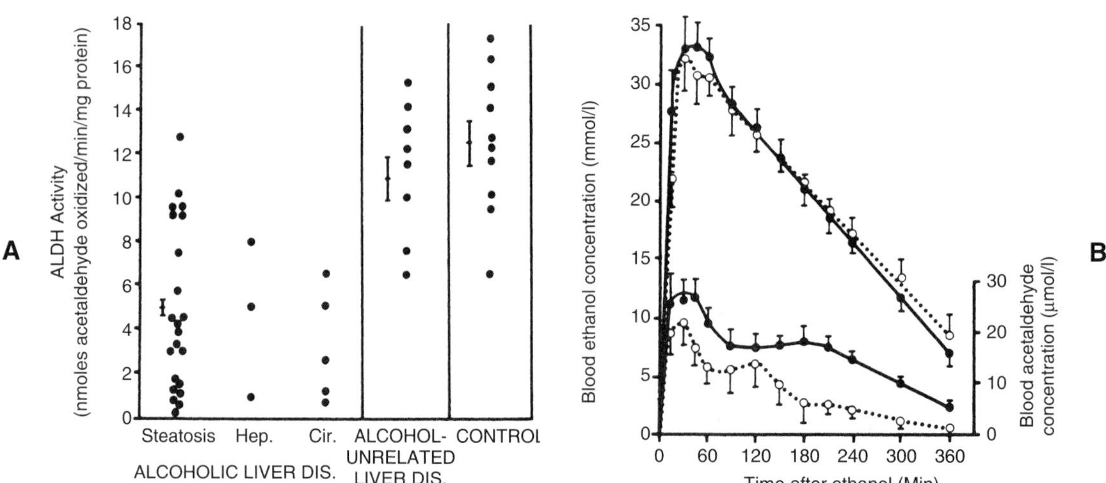

Figure 29-5 **A,** Activities of acetaldehyde dehydrogenase in liver biopsies from indicated groups of patients. **B,** Concentrations of ethanol and acetaldehyde (lower part of figure) in alcoholics (•) or controls (○) after a test dose of ethanol. (From Palmer KR, Jenkins WJ: Impaired acetaldehyde oxidation in alcoholics. Gut 23:729, 1982.)

dria from ethanol-treated rats demonstrates that the rats' deficient metabolism of this intermediate is not the result of a reduction in the amount of this enzyme but reflects a more complicated injury to mitochondrial function.[234]

Diet affects the metabolism of acetaldehyde. Levels of acetaldehyde are greater in rats fed diets containing low levels of protein,[215-217] but the relationship between levels of dietary protein and plasma levels of acetaldehyde after administration of a standard dose of ethanol is complex. The relationship is biphasic with regard to the amount of protein in the diet.[235] Also, after prolonged feeding of protein-deficient diets, levels of acetaldehyde in plasma are normal after administration of ethanol. After challenge of rats with ethanol, the concentration of acetaldehyde in liver is also affected by the amount of protein in the diet. As for the concentration of acetaldehyde in plasma, there is a biphasic response to levels of protein in the diet, but hepatic concentrations of acetaldehyde in response to ethanol administration do not become abnormal with persistent feeding of protein-deficient diets.[235] None of these effects of dietary protein can be explained on the basis of variable effects on the amounts of ADH and ALDH in liver.[215-217] Nor are there any data in this respect for humans. Nevertheless, any manipulation that alters the concentration of a potentially toxic agent deserves scrutiny. Of note for its potential application to humans is that starvation of rats markedly decreases plasma levels of acetaldehyde compared with rats fed normal or protein-restricted diets.[217] We note, however, that starvation also decreases the elimination rate for ethanol. The effect of starvation on levels of acetaldehyde in liver is unknown.

METABOLIC CONSEQUENCES OF ETHANOL INGESTION

We would like to know whether ethanol itself, independent of other factors, leads inexorably to liver disease. If this represents the true relationship between ethanol intake and liver disease, then from a strictly analytic view, therapeutic efforts have to be directed toward persuading patients to cease abuse of ethanol, and toward altering the metabolism of ethanol or its metabolic consequences or both. If, on the other hand, the hepatotoxicity of ethanol depends on interactions with factors in the environment, the problem of ameliorating the deleterious effects of ethanol, at least with respect to hepatic function, might be easier to achieve.

Theories abound as to the manner in which ethanol ingestion directly produces liver disease. Most of these are based on observations of the effects of ethanol on the biochemistry and morphology of liver in experimental animals. These studies are important because they extend our opportunity to modify the effects of ethanol beyond what can be done in patients. Nevertheless, a great deal remains to be learned from observation of patients. As we try to emphasize in the following sections, for example, answers have not been sought to several direct, simple questions about the natural history of liver disease in the alcoholic.

TOXIC EFFECTS OF ETHANOL AND ETHANOL OXIDATION

Acetaldehyde

Acetaldehyde has several important pharmacologic and chemical effects. It is a vasoactive substance.[236,237] Infusion in humans leads to a prompt flushing reaction on the trunk, especially the face. More serious symptoms are dyspnea and a sense of anxiety. A vascular reaction to acetaldehyde usually is not seen in individuals ingesting ethanol because the concentration of acetaldehyde in blood is too low to produce one.

The unpleasantness of the side effects of acetaldehyde has been used therapeutically to encourage abusers of ethanol to abstain. The approach used is to administer an inhibitor of ALDH. Disulfiram (Antabuse) is the agent used for this purpose.[238,239]

$$(C_2H_5)_2-N-\overset{\overset{\displaystyle S}{|}}{C}-S-S-\overset{\overset{\displaystyle S}{|}}{C}-N(C_2H_5)_2$$

Disulfiram

The best evidence indicates that disulfiram forms a disulfide link with a thiol group of ALDH, thereby inhibiting it.[240] Maximum inhibition occurs between 16 and 40 hours after administration, and the effect of a single dose persists for several days because the binding of disulfiram to ALDH is irreversible.[241] Also, the drug has a long half-life in the body.[242] Disulfiram-induced inhibition of ALDH is overcome only when new molecules of enzyme are synthesized. Experiments in vivo suggest that disulfiram does not have a uniform inhibitory effect on different isoenzymes of ALDH. The mitochondrial isoenzyme with a high affinity for acetaldehyde seems to be the form most sensitive to inhibition,[243] although the cytosolic forms in rat also are inhibited by disulfiram.[244] The symptoms experienced by a patient ingesting ethanol while under treatment with disulfiram are compatible with the idea that they are caused by acetaldehyde alone. In fact, acetaldehyde, when infused into patients who have previously experienced the ethanol-disulfiram reaction, evokes a response that is perceived by these patients as identical to it.

Disulfiram is not the only drug alleged to interfere with the metabolism of acetaldehyde. Pargyline and reserpine are inhibitors of ALDH.[245,246] Disulfiram-ethanol–like reactions have been reported to occur after ingestion of ethanol by patients being treated with sulfonylureas, phenylbutazone, metronidazole, and chemically related compounds.[237,246-252] However, the interactions between these drugs and ethanol have not been evaluated carefully in patients in all instances. Metronidazole has no demonstrable effect on the metabolism of acetaldehyde. Sulfonylureas in combination with ethanol produce symptoms of acetaldehyde toxicity only at large doses of the former. Studies of this last entity indicate that naloxone prevents flushing in response to the combination of ethanol and chlorpropamide.[252,253] In addition, the flush in these patients can be evoked by infusion of met-enkephalin. Ethanol-induced flushing in patients receiving chlorpropamide thus may have nothing to do with accumulation of acetaldehyde and appears instead to be a dominantly inherited trait in association with diabetes.[252,253] Hence the clinical significance of the reported disulfiram-ethanol-like interactions between ethanol and other drugs remains clouded. By contrast, it is established that the edible mushroom *Coprinus atramentarius* produces a disulfiram-ethanol-like reaction when ingested with ethanol.

In addition to exogenous ethanol, there are other endogenous sources of acetaldehyde such as deoxypentosephosphate aldolases,[254] pyruvate dehydrogenase,[255] and phosphorylphosphoethanolamine phosphorylase.[256] Cleavage of threonine to acetaldehyde and glycine by threonine reductase[257] and production of ethanol and acetaldehyde by microbial metabolism of sugars[258] are other potential sources of acetaldehyde.

Acetaldehyde can affect the functions of many tissues but its most important effects occur in the liver. It has been suggested that acetaldehyde is a key factor in the hepatic injury caused by ethanol.[259-261] Acetaldehyde binds covalently to proteins, lipids, and DNA[262,263] to form stable and unstable adducts, which damage key functions of the cell. Also, adducts between normal cellular proteins and acetaldehyde can be "neoantigens" and stimulate immune response and immune-mediated injury.[261,264] Finally, acetaldehyde can promote oxidative stress by reacting with and depleting cellular glutathione (GSH).[265]

Acetaldehyde binds covalently to soluble enzymes,[266] hemoglobin,[267] albumin,[268] microsomal membrane proteins including cytochrome P450 2E1,[269,270] cytoskeletal proteins,[271] and calmodulin.[272] Reaction occurs between acetaldehyde and the ϵ-amino group of lysine. Unstable adducts, which are Schiff bases, are intermediates in formation of stable adducts.[273] Adduct formation with different lysine residues in a given protein may be modified depending on the concentration of acetaldehyde.[273] Amino acids other than lysine, which are sites for interaction with acetaldehyde, include valine, tyrosine, and cysteine.[263] The competition between acetaldehyde and pyridoxal phosphate for protein binding may account for increased degradation of pyridoxal phosphate in alcohol-induced deficiency of vitamin B_6.[263]

Although the covalent binding of acetaldehyde to hepatic proteins is well established, its precise importance in causing liver injury remains to be clarified. One possibility by which adducts could cause toxicity involves the altered biologic properties of modified proteins. For example, the ethanol-induced impairment of hepatic protein synthesis (see Chap. 5) is prevented by pyrazole (an alcohol dehydrogenase inhibitor)[274] and enhanced by pretreating the animals with cyanamide (an ADH inhibitor).[275] A possible site rendered defective by ethanol ingestion, probably related to acetaldehyde toxicity, is the hepatic microtubular system.[276] Tubulin, when modified covalently by acetaldehyde, in vitro, does not polymerize to form microtubules.[271,277] Because microtubules promote the intracellular transport and secretion of proteins, long-term administration of alcohol delays the secretion of proteins and causes their retention in liver.[278] The high susceptibility of collagen to form adducts with acetaldehyde may be the cause of increased production of collagen in alcoholic liver disease.[279] Additionally, acetaldehyde per se is a potent stimulant of collagen synthesis in isolated systems.[280,281] The formation of collagen-acetaldehyde adducts may impair collagen degradation and promote fibrosis in this way, too.[280,281]

Protein-acetaldehyde adducts are detected predominantly in the perivenous zone of rat liver.[282] An acetaldehyde-protein adduct, with reactivity to antibodies to collagen and susceptibility to collagenase, is present in the hepatic cytosol of patients with alcoholic liver disease.[279] The association between this adduct and liver inflammation suggests that the adduct may contribute to hepatic injury in alcoholics. The acetaldehyde-collagen adducts occur in areas of active fibrogenesis, and their presence on initial biopsy correlates with progression of liver fibrosis.[263] In the ethanol-fed micropig a similar association of the location of acetaldehyde-collagen adducts and deposition of collagen in the perivenous region[284] is further evidence for a link between adduct formation and liver fibrosis.[285,286]

The demonstration that acetaldehyde adducts elicit an immune response, which may be directed against liver cells in alcoholics, suggests an immune mechanism in the pathogenesis of alcoholic liver injury.[287] An increase in circulating antibodies that react against acetaldehyde adducts has been described in the sera of patients with alcoholic liver disease and in animals fed ethanol.[287,288] Support for the idea that acetaldehyde-protein adducts promote an immune-mediated liver injury comes from studies showing that lesions similar to alcoholic hepatitis can be induced in ethanol-fed guinea pigs previously immunized with acetaldehyde-protein adducts.[289] Koskinas and co-workers also showed that circulating antibodies from patients with alcoholic liver disease recognize adducts between acetaldehyde and liver proteins,[290] that the circulating antibodies are of the immunoglobulin (Ig)A type, and that they specifically recognize a 200-Kd cytosolic protein adduct, which they speculated to be a procollagen conjugate. The high incidence of anti-adduct IgA in alcoholics has been confirmed, as have increased levels of other classes of immunoglobulins with specificity directed to acetaldehyde-protein adducts.[291] Titers of IgA are higher, however, in patients with alcoholic liver disease as compared with levels in heavy drinkers without liver disease. Titers of immunoglobulin-modified proteins correlated with the clinical and laboratory indices of liver disease severity. The observed IgA response, also reported by others,[292] is significant because increased levels of IgA in serum and deposition of IgA in the liver are characteristic of alcoholic liver disease.[293,294] Spleen cells modified by treatment with acetaldehyde generate a cytotoxic T-cell response, which can cause liver cell damage.[295] In addition to acetaldehyde derived from oxidation of ethanol, aldehydic products of lipid peroxidation, such as malondialdehyde (MDA) and 4-hydroxynonenal (HNE), form Schiff base adducts with proteins.[296] MDA is a highly reactive dialdehyde originating from non-enzymatic lipid peroxidation of unsaturated fatty acid.[297] The free-radical mediated oxidation of long-chain polyunsaturated fatty acids leads to the production of HNE, which reacts with sulfhydryl groups of protein.[297] Protein

TABLE 29-4

Reactive Compounds from Ethanol Metabolism that Form Adducts in Alcoholics

Metabolite	Key target protest	Possible functional consequence
Acetaldehyde	Tubulin	Altered microtubule function with impairment of protein secretion
	Ketosteroid	Interference with bile acid synthesis
Acetaldehyde, malondialdehyde	Collagen	Fibrogenesis
Acetaldehyde, malondialdehyde (malondialdehyde-acetaldehyde), hydroxyethyl radical 4-hydroxynonenal	Several (e.g., CYP 2E1)	Stimulation of immunologic response to adduct leading to liver injury

Modified from Niemela O: Aldehyde-protein adducts in the liver as a result of ethanol-induced oxidative stress. Front Biosci 4:506-513, 1999.

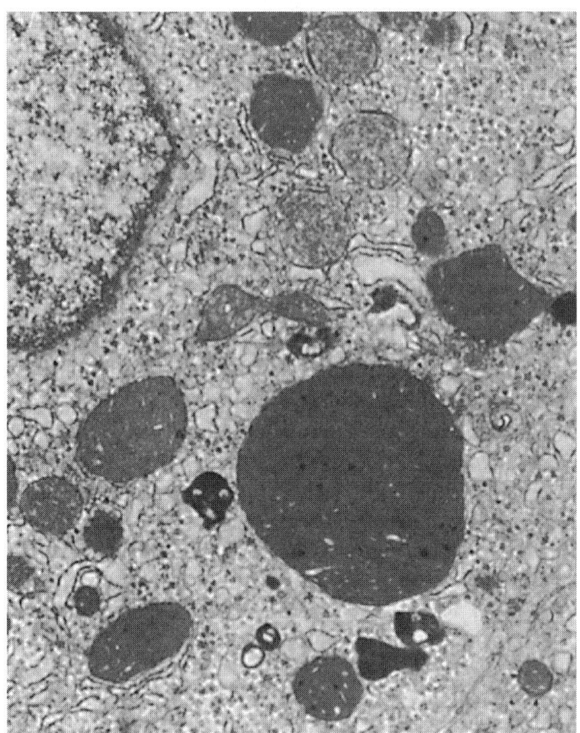

Figure 29-6 Electron micrograph of enlarged "megamitochondria" in rat liver after administration of ethanol. A nucleus is in the upper left-hand corner. Magnification ×32,300. (Courtesy of Dr. Sam French.)

adducts of both MDA and HNE occur in livers of animals fed ethanol[298,299] and in patients with ALD.[300]

A final possible mechanism of acetaldehyde toxicity is via production of free radicals (see the following section). Other products of ethanol metabolism are also capable of forming adducts with proteins (Table 29-4).

Effects of Ethanol on the Structure and Function of Hepatic Mitochondria

One of the earliest manifestations of ethanol consumption is a change in the structure of hepatic mitochondria.[301-303] The mitochondria are often enlarged and misshapen, appearing either as swollen or elongated structures, with the cristae either disrupted or without normal organization (Figure 29-6). These morphologic and histochemical changes in experimental animals and alcoholic patients have been interpreted as evidence that mitochondrial abnormalities are important in the pathogenesis of ALD.[304] This interpretation has been challenged.[305-307] Nevertheless, current concepts maintain that mitochondrial dysfunction contributes to cellular injury by one of two processes: failure of oxidative phosphorylation with loss of synthesis of ATP or a change in membrane permeability that leads to cell injury independent of ATP depletion.

Liver mitochondria isolated from animals fed ethanol for prolonged periods show numerous defects in the electron-transport chain and oxidative phosphorylation (Figure 29-7; see Chap. 3). In general, respiration in the presence of ADP (state 3 respiration) with NADH-linked substrates or fatty acids is decreased in coupled mitochondria from rats fed ethanol for 3 weeks.[308] With longer intervals of feeding, succinate-driven, state 3 respiration and respiration through the cytochrome oxidase pathway is decreased.[309,310] This depression in the rate of state 3 respirations, which is about 20 percent to 45 percent lower in mitochondria from ethanol-fed rats versus controls, demonstrates that chronic consumption of ethanol decreases the rate at which hepatic mitochondria synthesize ATP.[11]

State 4 respiration is the rate of respiration in the absence of ADP and is a measure of the functional viability of mitochondria. An increase in state 4 respiration indicates that mitochondria have a lesser ability to conserve the proton gradient generated by electron transport and therefore are less well coupled.[311] Significant increases in state 4 respiration are observed after extended periods of ethanol consumption, although the changes are less dramatic than for state 3 respiration.[309,312] State 4 respiration through cytochrome oxidase is significantly depressed. The significant degree of change in state 3 respiration and the lack of uncoupling indicated by the relatively constant state 4 respiration indicate that the *rate* of ATP synthesis is affected more by ethanol administration than is the *efficiency* of ATP synthesis.[311] This has been verified in several studies in which the rate of ATP synthesis was depressed more dramatically than the P/O ratio, which measures the efficiency of ATP synthesis.[310,313]

IMPAIRED OXYGEN UTILIZATION BY LIVER MITOCHONDRIA (CHRONIC ETHANOL-FED BABOONS)

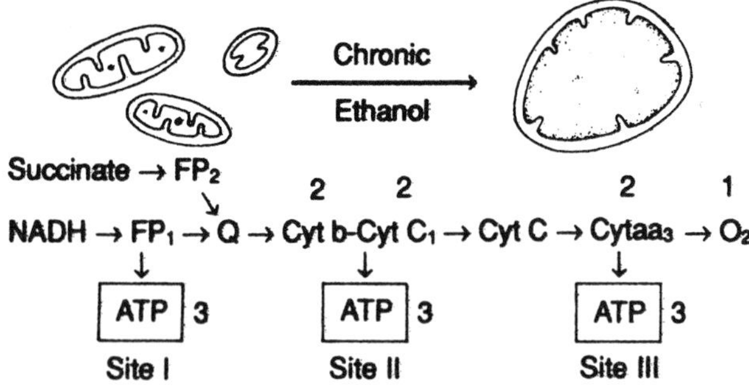

↑ Mitochondrial Redox State NADH ↑
NAD ↓
↓ Fatty Acid and Acetaldehyde Oxidation
1 ↓ Cytochrome Oxidase
2 ↓ Cytochrome aa3, b and C + C1
↓ Respiratory Control
3 ↓ Oxidative Phosphorylation (Site I, II and III)
↓ Oxygen Extraction at High Alcohol Levels
↓ Glutamate Dehydrogenase (GD)
↓ Succinate-Cytochome c Reductase

Figure 29-7 Evidence for ethanol-induced mitochondrial "injury." (From Palmer TN, ed: Alcoholism: A Molecular Perspective. New York, Plenum, 1991:57.)

The rate of substrate oxidation in mitochondria is controlled by several components of the oxidative phosphorylation system. The most consistent ethanol-induced alteration is a 50 percent to 70 percent decrease in the activity and heme content of cytochrome oxidase.[314,315] Other components showing a lesser decrease include cytochrome b and some of the iron-sulfur centers associated with the NADH-ubiquinone reductase portion of the electron-transport chain. The additional depression in the rate of ATP synthesis that cannot be attributed to alterations in the electron transport system per se is associated with alterations in ATP synthase activity.[311] The enzyme ATP synthase is composed of two principal domains, an extramembranous catalytic domain, F_1, and a membrane-embedded proton-translocating domain, F_0.[316] The source of energy for ATP synthesis is the transmembrane electrochemical potential of protons. The two assays normally used to measure the catalytic capacity of ATP synthase are its adenosine triphosphatase (ATPase) and ATP-inorganic phosphorus (Pi) exchange activities. The ethanol-dependent lesion, believed to be responsible for the altered activity of ATP synthase, is located in the F_0 moiety of the enzyme complex.[317,318] A decrease in the synthesis of two mitochondrial-encoded polypeptides of ATP synthase (subunits 6 and 8) is responsible for the loss of ATPase activity. Another important property of the ATP synthase that is altered by ethanol consumption is sensitivity to oligomycin,[316] which binds to the F_0 subunits of ATP synthase and inhibits both ATPase and ATP synthetic activities. Ethanol consumption lowers the oligomycin sensitivity of ATP synthase and renders it less tightly attached to the inner membrane and therefore makes the enzyme less active.[318] The effects of chronic ethanol intake on energy conservation processes in liver mitochondria are summarized in Table 29-5.[319]

TABLE 29-5

Effect of Chronic Ethanol Intake on Energy Conservation Processes in the Liver Mitochondria

Processes Decreased by Chronic Alcohol Intake
30%-50% depression of state 3 respiration with NAD-linked substrates
10%-15% decrease of state 4 respiratory activity
ATP-Pi exchange
Iron-sulfur clusters N-2, N-3, and N-4 of NADH dehydrogenase
Cytochrome aa_3
Cytochrome b
Activity of oligomycin-sensitive F_0-F_1 ATPase
Processes Not Affected by Chronic Alcohol Intake
Cytochromes C and C_1
Proton permeability
Succinate dehydrogenase
Iron-sulfur clusters N-1a, N-1b of NADH dehydrogenase and S1, S-3 of succinate hydrogenase
Oligomycin-insensitive F_1 ATPase
Adenine nucleotide translocator
Proton motive force

Modified from Hoek JB: Mitochondrial energy metabolism in chronic alcoholism. Curr Top Bioenergetics 17:197, 1994.

Hepatic glycogen stores also modify rates of ATP depletion during inhibition of oxidative phosphorylation by supplying glucose for generation of ATP from glycolysis.[320] ATP depletion rapidly ensues after depletion of glycogen stores. In ethanol-fed rats and in human alcoholics liver glycogen stores are depleted, particularly in the centrolobular areas.[321]

The second factor, other than ATP depletion, associated with mitochondrial dysfunction is changes in mitochondrial permeability.[322] Under normal circumstances, the inner mitochondrial membrane is impermeant to solutes that move across the inner membrane only via specific transport mechanisms (see Chap. 3). Cell injury appears to be coupled to changes in the permeability of the inner membrane, referred to as the mitochondrial membrane permeability transition (MMPT).[323] The MMPT initiates a collapse of ion gradients across the mitochondrial membrane, causing mitochondrial dysfunction. Mitochondrial contents "leak" into the cytoplasm, and cytoplasmic components gain access into the mitochondrial matrix. Mitochondrial swelling, which occurs as a morphologic manifestation of this form of mitochondrial injury,[324] is also a feature of alcoholic liver injury.[306,307] Factors that are operative in the pathogenesis of alcoholic liver injury, such as lipid peroxidation and fatty acid accumulation, also result in MMPT.[324] The interaction between ATP depletion and MMPT in alcoholic liver injury requires further work to clarify their individual contributions to cell injury. It appears, however, that the ethanol-dependent decrease in the rate of ATP synthesis is multi-factorial and reflects changes in the activities of enzymes such as cytochrome oxidase, NADH-quinone reductase, and ATP synthase and changes in permeability of the inner membrane of the mitochondrion.

An increased prevalence of maternally transmitted deletions of mitochondrial DNA (mt DNA) occurs in alcoholics.[325,326] All deletions are flanked by short or long tandem repeats.[326] These deletions are particularly frequent in alcoholics with microvesicular steatosis, a lesion thought to be due to impaired beta oxidation. Although most damaged mt DNA is repaired without causing deletions, repeated episodes of damage and repair eventually may cause deletions of mt DNA. In support of this hypothesis alcoholic binges in mice cause extensive degradation of mt DNA,[327] possibly because of increased peroxidation of mitochondrial lipids and increased levels of carbonyls in mitochondrial proteins. Depletion of mt DNA is prevented completely by 4-methylpyrazole, which inhibits alcohol dehydrogenase and cytochrome P450 2E1.

The Physical Effects of Ethanol on Membranes

The effects of ethanol on mitochondrial function, and indeed, its effects on other organelles of the hepatocyte usually are considered to be consequences of the metabolism of ethanol. However, the best known effect of ethanol—the capacity to induce narcosis—is related to its physical properties, not to metabolism. Thus ethanol, as with other lipid-soluble chemicals, is a membrane-active agent.

Many enzymes that are embedded within membranes of cells are sensitive to the chemical and physical properties of the lipid components of the membrane.[328-331] The functions of these integral membrane-bound enzymes can be regulated to some extent by changes within the lipid portions of biologic membranes. This is not surprising, because the function of a protein depends on its conformation, which in turn depends on environmental conditions, and the membrane lipids are a significant part of the proximate environment of membrane-bound proteins.[332,333]

Phospholipids are amphipathic molecules. They contain a polar region and a hydrophobic region. The former is the so-called head group of the phospholipid molecule and can be one of several different possible groups, for example, phosphocholine or phosphoethanolamine. The hydrophobic region of a phospholipid consists of the long hydrocarbon chains attached, usually via ester linkages, to the 1 and 2 positions of the glycerol backbone of the molecule. These chains are at least 14 carbons long in humans. The hydrocarbon chains can be unsaturated to a

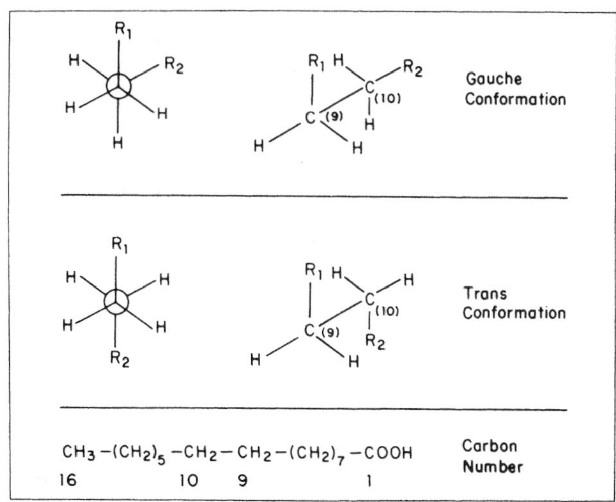

Figure 29-8 Effect of rotation about C—C— bonds on conformation in fatty acids. The schematic is for rotation about the $C_9—C_{10}$ bond, but identical possibilities for conformation exist for all —C—C— bonds in the fatty acid. (From Zakim D: Interface between membrane biology and clinical medicine. Am J Med 80:645, 1986.)

variable extent. Typical of naturally occurring phospholipids is the presence of an unsaturated chain at position 2 and a saturated chain at position 1. Given the number of possible fatty acids (hydrocarbon region) that can be esterified with glycerol and the number of possible polar groups, there are hundreds of different species of phospholipids within the membranes of higher animals.

The phospholipids organize with each other to maximize the interaction of the hydrocarbon—or acyl tail—region of one molecule with the hydrocarbon regions of another. This arrangement excludes water from interacting with the non-polar portions of the molecule and maximizes interactions between the polar regions and water. These thermodynamic requirements can be satisfied in a variety of ways, depending primarily on the structure of the polar region but also on the state of hydration of the polar groups and on the ionic strength and pH of the aqueous phase. Under in vivo conditions, including the natural abundance of phospholipids of different classes, the phospholipids organize as bilayers.

The manner in which phospholipids pack together seems to be their most important characteristic for modulating the function of enzymes embedded within phospholipid bilayers. The term *fluidity* has been used to describe and quantitate one important aspect of packing. The concept of fluidity is simple and can be understood in the following way. When the hydrocarbon chain of a phospholipid is fully saturated, there is free rotation around all of its carbon-carbon bonds. All positions of rotation are not equally probable, however, because of mutual repulsion between bulky groups when these are close to each other (Figure 29-8). This familiar idea predicts that the most favorable conformation of the carbon-carbon bonds occurs when the bulky groups are trans. The least favorable position obviously is for the bulky groups—the proximal and distal regions of the hydrocarbon chain—to be cis or partially eclipsed. Thus the most likely conformation of the acyl chains is with all carbon-carbon bonds as trans, as depicted in Figure 29-9. The acyl chains have maximal length in this configuration. More important, the cross-sectional area is minimal when all carbon-carbon bonds are trans. The energy barrier between trans and partially eclipsed, or gauche, conformations for each carbon-carbon bond is relatively low; the barrier is crossed easily at room temperature. Hence there is a constant "wiggling" of the acyl chains of phospholipids as different carbon-carbon bonds rotate from trans to gauche separately and together. Gauche configurations about a carbon-carbon bond have a kink in the chain. Figure 29-9 shows that acyl chains containing a kink have a larger cross-sectional area than chains in the all-trans state. This effect on cross-sectional area is not important when we consider only a single molecule of phospholipid, but it is important in a bilayer in which there are thousands of phospholipid molecules. The packing together of many phospholipids makes it less likely that a carbon-carbon bond will rotate spontaneously from trans to gauche because introducing a kink in an otherwise all-trans chain increases the volume of the chain. The kink occurs only when the environment provides a sufficient volume to accommodate the kinked chain. So when phospholipids pack together, the creation of a kink in one acyl chain requires that surrounding chains be pushed aside. The extent to which trans-gauche changes occur therefore depends on the tightness of packing of the acyl chains, which in turn depends on van der Waals interactions. These interactions between two acyl chains are quite small, but the total energy of attraction becomes quite large when there are millions of chains limiting the wiggling of neighboring chains. The organization is cooperative because close approximation of chains maximizes van der Waals energies. As these increase, wiggling is diminished. This in turn diminishes the volume occupied by a single chain, which increases van der Waals energies. Hence the normal tendency for free rotation about the carbon-carbon bonds in a single acyl chain attached to an isolated molecule of phospholipid is constrained severely when there is an array of acyl chains. This constraint leads to high viscosities or low fluidities within the bilayer of a membrane. The tightness of packing can be disturbed in many ways: by unsaturated fatty acids, by introducing bulky detergent molecules, by substituting phosphocholine for phosphoethanolamine, and so forth. Cholesterol has complex effects. It increases fluidity when added to a highly viscous (non-fluid) membrane but decreases fluidity when added to a highly fluid membrane.

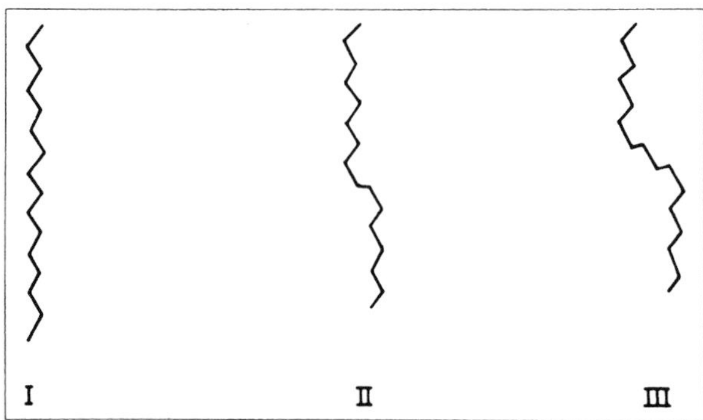

Figure 29-9 Extended views of conformational isomers of palmitate. (From Zakim D: Interface between membrane biology and clinical medicine. Am J Med 80:645, 1986.)

Ethanol in vitro generally enhances the fluidity of biologic membranes.[334] Large amounts of ethanol (and other short-chain alcohols) can cause the basic bilayer structure to break down.[335,336] These effects probably are not important in vivo. On the other hand, after chronic administration of ethanol, ethanol in vitro does not increase the "fluidity" of membranes from ethanol-treated animals to as great an extent as it increases fluidity of membranes from control animals.[337-342] Resistance to the membrane-active effects of ethanol, as defined by its effect on fluidity, can be attributed to an adaptive change in the lipid composition of the membrane.[339,341,343-347]

This tolerance to ethanol is not associated with a change in the composition of the main phospholipid classes of the membrane, however. There are changes in the acyl composition of specific phospholipids,[348] and especially of the phosphatidylinositols (PI).[349] The major adaptive response in rat liver microsomal PI to chronic administration of ethanol is a decrease in the percent of arachidonic acid that is compensated partially by increases in oleic and eicosatrienoic acids.

Microsomal membranes from rats fed ethanol chronically are also resistant to hydrolysis by exogenous phospholipase A_2,[350] which is believed to reflect changes in the composition of fatty acids of phosphatidylserines. In mitochondrial membranes tolerance is associated with about a 25 percent decrease in the linoleyl content of cardiolipin, the predominant anionic phospholipid in the inner membrane.[351] After discontinuing ethanol-containing diets, there is an accompanying loss of the ability of cardiolipin to confer tolerance to reconstituted phospholipid bilayers.[348,352] Because the loss of tolerance occurs more rapidly than the recovery of the acyl composition of normal cardiolipin, it is unlikely that changes in fatty acid composition are sufficient to explain all the phenomena.

The development of membrane tolerance after chronic ingestion of ethanol has been hypothesized to contribute to mitochondrial dysfunction.[353] For example, cardiolipin alters the function of mitochondrial membranes and some enzymes affected by ethanol treatment. Some but not all cardiolipin-dependent enzyme changes in mitochondria are affected by chronic treatment with ethanol; however, recovery of mitochondrial enzyme function takes longer than the recovery of membrane tolerance. Therefore factors besides membrane tolerance must be important for ethanol-induced mitochondrial dysfunction.[353]

The apparent adaptation of membranes is almost certainly not the result of metabolism of ethanol but of its physical properties. For example, exposure to ethanol leads to adaptive changes in the lipid compositions of membranes from *Escherichia coli* and *Tetrahymena* species, neither of which oxidizes ethanol.[354-356]

The physical interactions between ethanol and membranes in vitro are associated with acute changes in ATPase and several other enzyme activities,[346,347,357,358] decreased transport of amino acids[330,331] and bile acids,[361] and an increased permeability of membranes to Na^+.[361] Chronic administration of ethanol has been reported to enhance the solubility of halogenated anesthetics in liver membranes.[362] There appears to be an unusual limitation of glucose transport across hepatocyte plasma membranes during acute withdrawal after chronic administration of ethanol to rats.[363] In addition, administration of ethanol seems to interfere with the flow of glycoproteins from the Golgi to plasma membranes.[364] Interference by ethanol of secretion of liver glycoproteins could be one of the consequences of this effect because mechanisms for the secretion of proteins and the assembly of proteins into membranes have many similarities.[364] The reported decrease in the number of glucagon receptors on hepatocyte plasma membranes[365] and reduced binding and internalization of asialoglycoproteins[366,367] in rats fed alcohol on a chronic basis may be a reflection of an ethanol-induced abnormality in the "trafficking" of proteins to plasma membranes.[364] The effects of ethanol on membrane structure and function also may contribute to putative abnormalities of immune function in the alcoholic with liver disease (see the following section).

The most dramatic effects of chronic consumption of ethanol on membranes are on the morphology of mitochondria,[368-370] but whether the "giant" mitochondria induced by ethanol (see Figure 29-6) are unable to sustain the viability of hepatocytes is unclear. In addition, the morphologic changes of mitochondria in liver specimens from alcoholic patients are not specific. They are seen in specimens from obese patients and diabetics and increase as a function of the patient's age (see ref. 371).

As mentioned previously, studies with mitochondria in vitro indicate that ingestion of ethanol inhibits the respiration of intact hepatocytes secondary to decreased amounts of respiratory enzymes and inhibition of the coupled oxidation of several mitochondrial substrates. Various experiments with perfused liver, liver slices, and intact animals show, however, that chronic ingestion of ethanol increases mitochondrial respiration in intact hepatocytes.[209,372-374] Oxygen consumption by liver is increased, compared with controls, by chronic ingestion of ethanol in the preparations described. There is evidence, too, that hepatic synthesis and utilization of ATP are increased by ingestion of ethanol (this evidence is discussed in the section Effects of Ethanol on Hepatic Consumption of O_2). It therefore seems that the behavior of mitochondria in vitro does not correlate well with their function in intact cells. Nevertheless, it would be unwise to dismiss as biochemical curiosities the effects of ethanol on the function of hepatic mitochondria. First, careful scrutiny of the literature dealing with the toxic effects of ethanol on cells leads one to conclude that derangement of mitochondrial function is one type of injury that is well established experimentally and that would diminish the viability of hepatocytes. Second, ethanol ingestion clearly has the capacity to alter the function of mitochondria in some environments. The biochemical functions of mitochondria from ethanol treated rats deteriorate rapidly under the stress of isolation, for example.[347]

PROTECTIVE EFFECT OF POLYENYLPHOSPHATIDYLCHOLINE IN ALCOHOLIC LIVER INJURY

Soybean polyenylphosphatidylcholine (PPC) is a mixture of 94 percent to 96 percent polyunsaturated phosphatidylcholines, about half of which is dilinoleoylphatadylcholine (DLPC).[375] In contrast to mammalian phospholipids, this plant phospholipid contains unsaturated fatty acids in both the 1 and 2 positions of the glycerol backbone, which confers high bioavailability.

PPC has been shown to have protective effects on several pathophysiologic events relevant to alcohol-induced liver injury. PPC was originally shown to protect against liver fibrosis and cirrhosis in the baboon.[375,376] Subsequent studies showed that PPC also decreases hepatic stellate cell activation, prevents the acetaldehyde-induced increase in collagen accumulation in hepatic stellate cells in culture,[377] and attenuates the hepatic fibrosis caused by carbon tetrachloride and heterologous albumin in rats.[378] The exact mechanism by which PPC protects against hepatic fibrosis remains unresolved but reduced lipid peroxidation and increased collagenase activity are possible mechanisms.

In addition to its anti-fibrogenic effects, PPC also protects against earlier changes induced by alcohol consumption. For example, PPC leads to attenuation of alcoholic fatty liver in rats.[379] The mechanism for the preventive effect of PPC on fatty liver is correction of the ethanol-induced impairment in hepatic oxidation of fatty acids in mitochondria. In particular, the ethanol-induced inhibition of mitochondrial oxidation of palmitoyl-L-carnitine and depression of cytochrome oxidase activity are corrected by PPC. PPC also protects against oxidative stress generated through CYP 2E1 induction[380] and restores glutathione levels.[381]

DLPC, the main component of PPC, also modulates the lipopolysaccharide (LPS)-induced activation of Kupffer cells.[382] DLPC decreases the LPS induced release of tumor necrosis factor alpha (TNFα) but increases the production of interleukin (IL)-1β by Kupffer cells. It is hypothesized that the increased production of IL-1β by DLPC is potentially protective against TNFα-induced hepatotoxicity.[383]

Effects of Ethanol on Hepatic Consumption of O_2

There is a well-known lobular gradient of O_2 tension between portal and central vein cells. Hepatic levels of O_2 are low compared with those in other tissues because 75 percent of hepatic blood flow comes from the venous system rather than the arterial system. It is interesting in this context that the centrolobular cells, which under normal conditions receive blood with the lowest concentration of O_2, are the ones principally affected in patients with alcoholic hepatitis. It has been proposed that chronic ingestion of ethanol increases the consumption of O_2 by human liver to the point that centrolobular cells become anoxic.[384-388] This leads to cell death, the morphologic constellation of central hyaline necrosis, and the clinical syndrome of alcoholic hepatitis. This hypothesis has been tested in rats by feeding ethanol chronically and then exposing the test animals to lower-than-normal O_2

tension in inspired air.[388] Rats treated in this way develop extensive centrolobular necrosis. Animals not exposed to ethanol before breathing air with a diminished content of O_2 do not develop hepatic necrosis. Clearly, ethanol can sensitize the liver to the noxious effects of low levels of inspired O_2.

To assess the validity of the hypoxic theory in man, hepatic venous O_2 tensions have been measured in alcoholics with liver pathology. Some studies reveal a strong association between alcoholic liver injury and reduced O_2 tension in the hepatic vein,[389,390] a result compatible with the idea that centrolobular hepatocytes were close to a state of anoxia after chronic use of ethanol. Others find normal hepatic venous O_2 concentration, determined as O_2 saturation or O_2 tension.[391] Unfortunately, many of the studies in patients were conducted in the withdrawal state, which makes interpretation of the data difficult. For example, effects on hepatic O_2 during the withdrawal state disappear or are reduced when alcohol is present in the blood.[392,393] Under withdrawal conditions, a hyperadrenergic state can contribute to the "hypermetabolic" state and increased O_2 utilization.[394] Increases in O_2 utilization secondary to ethanol administration can be offset partially by increases in splanchnic blood flow.[395,396]

In ethanol-fed rats with minimal liver injury an enhanced hepatic consumption of O_2 is adequately compensated by a concomitant increase in hepatic blood flow and O_2 delivery.[395] In rats exhibiting centrolobular necrosis the increment in O_2 delivery is too small to compensate for the increase in O_2 consumption.[397] These uncoordinated changes in hepatic O_2 metabolism lead to increased O_2 extraction by liver of ethanol-fed rats and a reduction in the O_2 content of hepatic venous blood. Further support for the hypoxia hypothesis is provided by studies using the anti-thyroid drug, propylthiouracil (PTU). The use of PTU is based on the assumption that the drug reduces hepatic O_2 demand during administration of ethanol.[398] PTU, in vitro, prevents the ethanol-induced increase in liver O_2 consumption.[399,400] In vivo PTU administration to rats suppressed hepatic hypermetabolism after the long-term administration of ethanol.[401]

One of the postulated mechanisms for increased O_2 consumption in rats chronically fed ethanol that exhibit centrolobular necrosis is induction of MEOS, which uses 50 percent more O_2 to oxidize ethanol to acetate versus the alcohol dehydrogenase pathway.[402] Thus induction of MEOS by ethanol could increase O_2 consumption by the liver. Interestingly, a high-fat diet induces MEOS and potentiates centrolobular necrosis in the alcohol-fed rat.[403-405]

Another mechanism leading to hepatic hypoxia, suggested by administration of an acute dose of ethanol to baboons fed ethanol chronically, is defective O_2 utilization.[406] Impaired utilization of O_2 in this setting is associated with a striking accumulation of reducing equivalents, especially in the mitochondria. On the other hand, inhibition of xanthine oxidase by allopurinol protects the liver against damage by hypoxia, which indicates the complexity of attributing causes to general types of effects.[407]

Based on the hypothesis that a hypermetabolic state and hypoxia are important in the genesis of ALD and the prevention of the putative hypermetabolic state by propylthiouracil,[404] clinical studies were conducted to test the efficacy of PTU in alcoholic hepatitis. In the first of three studies the effect of propylthiouracil (300 mg/day for 30 days) on the rate of recovery was evaluated.[408] Those patients who had milder disease and received PTU showed more rapid improvement that those receiving placebo; there was no difference in the patients' short-term survival. A study by a second group of investigators failed to show any benefit of therapy.[409] The most recent study investigated the effect of long-term use of PTU on the clinical course of ALD.[410] PTU reduced mortality from 0.25 percent in the placebo group to 0.13 percent in the treated group. This positive effect was seen only in patients with severe disease because the death rate in those with mild disease was so low as to prevent a meaningful comparison. The patients who benefited most from PTU had the lowest consumption of alcohol (based on the alcohol concentration in a morning urine). Heavy drinkers were not protected by the drug. Although the high attrition rate weakens any conclusions regarding long-term effects, it is interesting that a beneficial effect of PTU was observed in specific subgroups of patients. There has been little subsequent interest in PTU, however, and caution is recommended in the use of this agent pending further studies.

Energy Metabolism in ALD

The metabolism of adenine nucleotides in the liver of alcohol-fed animals has been studied as a mechanism linking hypoxia with alcohol-induced liver injury.[411,412] Although a number of reports show decreased levels of ATP in liver of animals fed ethanol chronically,[413,414] the levels of ATP in these studies have been measured after an overnight fast. Most metabolic changes induced by acute or chronic ingestion of ethanol are reversed by abstinence from ethanol.[411,413] Using the intragastric feeding model, Miyamoto and French measured levels of ATP in liver at high levels of blood alcohol.[415] In rats fed a high-fat, low-protein diet plus ethanol (to match the diet of malnourished human alcoholics[416,417]) levels of ATP and the total adenylate pool decreased as compared with controls. Levels of AMP and ADP were not changed by ethanol feeding. Thus the decrease in total adenylate pool was due to the decrease in ATP. Levels of ATP decreased over the first 2 months of feeding alcohol and then remained constant at 35 percent lower than levels of ATP in control animals.

The same investigators also studied the effect of hypoxia and hyperoxia on hepatic levels of ATP in ethanol-fed and control rats using the same long-term intragastric feeding model.[415] Hypoxia resulted in a decrease in hepatic levels of ATP in both ethanol-fed and control rats, but the magnitude of the decrease was significantly greater in the ethanol-fed group. When the same ethanol-fed rats inhaled 100 percent O_2 for 3 minutes, reversal of ATP to normal levels was accompanied by reciprocal changes in ADP and AMP. Spach and colleagues, using hepatocytes from ethanol-fed and control rats, suggested that the energy state of liver cells from ethanol-fed rats is influenced more by O_2 tension than is the case in liver cells from control animals.[418] They hypothesized that depletion of substrate by ethanol could explain the much more dramatic decrease in energy state in response to hypoxia in rats fed ethanol chronically. These investigators also emphasized the importance of measuring the energy state of livers from ethanol and control animals under normal conditions of oxygenation. In their review of previously published reports (Table 29-6),[413-415,419,420] which indicate that chronic consumption of ethanol decreases the energy state of the liver, they concluded that the O_2 supply to the liver was terminated before the liver tissue was excised and frozen. When livers are freeze-clamped while perfused by the animal's blood, no significant decrease in energy state is seen in ethanol-fed rats.[418]

To overcome the breakdown of ATP during sampling and preparation of tissue, phosphorus-31 (^{31}P) nuclear magnetic resonance (NMR) spectroscopy was used to study hepatic energy metabolism in response to ethanol.[421-423] Results with this non-invasive technique corroborated with the results using chemical measurements of adenine nucleotides after excision of samples.[424] Over a 6-month period the ratio of Pi/ATP in ethanol-fed rats was significantly increased during the first 3 to 5 weeks of ethanol feeding. This is the time frame in which livers, in this feeding model, begin to show fatty change. Levels of ADP measured by high-pressure liquid chromatography remain relatively constant in this model.[425] Hence changes in the ratio Pi/ATP would be related inversely to the phosphorylation potential, that is, ATP/ADP $\times$ Pi. A progressive increase in the ratio Pi/ATP continued up to the twenty-fourth week of ethanol feeding. There was no correlation, however, between changes in ATP and liver pathology.

Clinical studies evaluating changes in energy metabolism by ^{31}P NMR have shown that some changes in man are similar to those seen in the intragastric feeding model in rats.[426] First, the ratio phosphomonoesters (PME)/ATP was increased in patients with alcoholic hepatitis. No increase was seen in cirrhotic patients, who had been abstinent from alcohol for 6 months, or in patients with fatty liver and abstinent for at least 72 hours. These findings reflect that the energy state may be a consequence of ethanol feeding per se and not a result of pathologic change. In patients with minimal liver injury recent drinking was associated with elevations in the ratios phosphodiesters (PDE)/ATP and PME/ATP.[427] After abstinence from alcohol the ratio PME/ATP decreased promptly toward normal whereas the PDE/ATP took longer to normalize. A strong correlation between the ratio PME/ATP and scores of liver pathology was seen in alcoholic hepatitis[426]; an increase in the ratio was seen also in patients with alcoholic cirrhosis.[427] The elevation of PME is caused by an accumulation of phosphoryl ethanolamine. Not all studies have shown relative changes in ^{31}P metabolites in patients with ALD,[428] although absolute decreases in concentrations of all ^{31}P metabolites have been observed in both alcoholic hepatitis and cirrhosis. Differences between studies may reflect the fasted/fed status before ^{31}P NMR measurements and the period of abstinence from alcohol.

The mechanism for a low hepatic energy state during chronic ethanol intake remains unclear. Possibilities include a reduction in synthesis of ATP by depressed adenosine transferase activity[433]; dysfunction of the mitochondrial respiratory chain[429-432]; and an increase in utilization of ATP secondary to an activated sodium pump.[414] When ATP depletion is mediated by oxidant stress the predominant mechanism involved is activation of the DNA repair enzyme, poly-ADP-ribose polymerase, which consumes NAD and interferes in this way with ATP metabolism.[433] The relationship between depletion of ATP in liver and hepatocellular damage secondary to alcohol ingestion is unclear. Although the firm relationship between ATP depletion and cell injury is not always clear, several cell functions are altered profoundly by depletion of ATP. Increased cell permeability[434] and substantial alterations in the cytoskeleton,[435] together with disruptions in glucose and phosphate transport,[433,436] may be important for disordered cell function.

VASOCONSRTICTOR/VASODILATOR IMBALANCE IN ALCOHOLIC INJURY

One of the hypotheses forwarded for the reduced supply of O_2 to liver of ethanol-fed animals is a vasoconstrictive effect of ethanol on the perisinusoidal vessels.[437,438] This effect, in contrast to the vasodilatory effect of ethanol, is seen at high concentrations of ethanol. Of the various agents that cause vasoconstriction, endothelin (ET) has been shown recently to be responsible in part for

TABLE 29-6

Summary of Measurements of the Effect of Chronic Ethanol Consumption on Rat Liver ATP Concentration

ATP CONCENTRATION (μMOL/G WET WEIGHT LIVER)			
Liquid diet control	Ethanol-fed	Tissue fixation procedure (manipulation before extraction)	Reference
2.44 ± 0.14	1.42 ± 0.07	Animal killed; lobe excised and frozen in liquid nitrogen	375
2.43 ± 0.27	1.70 ± 0.20	Animal killed; section excised and frozen in liquid nitrogen	376
2.56 ± 0.58	1.86 ± 0.45	Animal anesthetized; liver biopsy section frozen in liquid nitrogen	377
2.62 ± 0.13	1.37 ± 0.08	Animal killed; section excised and frozen or frozen in situ	381
1.4 ± 0.1	0.9 ± 0.1	Animal anesthetized; liver excised and frozen in liquid nitrogen	382

From Spach PI, Herbert JS, Cunningham CC: The interaction between chronic ethanol consumption and oxygen fusion influencing the energy state of rat liver. Biochim Biophys Acta 1056:40, 1991.

ethanol-induced perturbations of the hepatic microcirculation.[439] The effect of ET, mediated by ethanol, would be additive to those of thromboxanes and isoprostanes (see section on dietary fats and alcoholic liver disease).

ETs are a family of three peptides (i.e., ET-1, ET-2, and ET-3) with potent and characteristically sustained vasoconstrictor and vasopressor effects.[402,403] Two distinct receptors for ET have been cloned. The ET_A receptor is preferentially activated by ET and is the main receptor subtype causing vasoconstriction; the ET_B receptor is activated equally by all three isoforms of ET. It is present on the luminal surface of endothelial cells.[442] ET-1 is a potent vasoconstrictive peptide that predominates in the vascular endothelium. ET-1 has a half-life in serum of about 2 minutes. It is thought to have predominantly local effects.[443,444] Despite the short half-life the pressor effects of ET-1 are long-lasting, persisting for as long as 1 hour after administration to humans.[444] The potency and duration of the vasopressor effects of ET have led to speculation that they reflect generation of eicosanoids, such as the products cyclooxygenase and lipoxygenase enzymes, which regulate vascular tone, coagulation, and inflammation.[445,446] ET-1 stimulates production of platelet activating factor (PAF) by rat Kupffer cells.[447] PAF exerts profound effects on the liver,[448] for example, vasoconstriction, chemotaxis, degranulation of leukocytes, and production of arachidonic acid and eicosanoids by Kupffer cells.[449,450] There is now both experimental and clinical evidence for involvement of ET in liver disease.[451,452]

ET-1 is synthesized and released from non-parenchymal hepatic cells in response to mediators such as endotoxin and transforming growth factor beta (TGF-β). ET-1 also is released during hypoxia. All these factors can cause vasoconstriction and cell injury mediated through the effects of ET. Additionally, ethanol is a direct stimulus for release of ET-1 from endothelial cells. When rats are infused intragastrically with ethanol increased levels of ET are seen only in rats that develop liver injury.[453]

The idea that sinusoidal constriction occurs in response to ET is controversial. Several groups have reported that Ito cells contract in response to ET.[454,455] Others have shown little contractility in freshly isolated Ito cells from normal rats, but that cells from cirrhotic rats are highly contractile in response to ET-1.[456,457] Infusion of ET into the portal vein of rats reveals extreme heterogeneity of responses of the liver circulation to ET.[458] Constriction of the sinusoids predominates at low doses of ET-1, whereas at higher doses sinusoidal dilation occurred. These effects are mediated probably by receptors designated ET_A, which are expressed on Ito cells in hepatic sinusoids.[456] Thus sites of sinusoidal constriction colocalize with the sites of Ito cells based on fluorescence of vitamin A in the isolated perfused rat liver.[459] Endothelial cells and Kupffer cells express only receptors designated ET_B.[456] Infusion of ET to achieve physiologic concentrations in sinusoids decreases oxygenation of the liver in association with vasoconstriction of sinusoids.[460]

There is evidence that the increase in blood flow at low concentrations of ethanol is a compensatory mechanism for the ethanol-induced increase in hepatic consumption of O_2.[461,462] One mediator of an ethanol-dependent increase in hepatic blood flow is prostacyclin (see section on dietary fats and ALD). Another possible mediator is the potent vasodilator nitric oxide (NO). NO is synthesized from L-arginine by nitric oxide synthase (NOS),[463-465] which is expressed constitutively in the vascular endothelium and regulates vasomotor tone. NOS also is inducible in vascular endothelium, macrophages, smooth muscle cells, and hepatocytes in response to inflammatory cytokines and endotoxin.[463-465] Ethanol-fed rats that develop pathologic liver injury have decreased production of NO by non-parenchymal cells and a compensatory increase in production of NO by hepatocytes.[466] Inhibition of NO production, using an inhibitor of NOS, exacerbates liver injury in ethanol-fed rats; supplementation with arginine is protective against liver injury.[466] Factors determining whether NO reduces or enhances toxicity are poorly understood, however.[467] The protective or toxic effect of an increase in production of NO by hepatocytes may depend on the biochemical milieu in the liver. NO produced by hepatocytes could de-energize mitochondria and lead to hepatocyte damage.[468] Alternatively, NO could combine with superoxide to form strong oxidizing agents such as peroxynitrite,[469] which in the presence of depleted anti-oxidant reserves (see the following section) can lead to cell damage.[470]

Impairment of NO production by non-parenchymal cells of liver in alcohol-fed rats has many possible deleterious consequences. NO inhibits platelet aggregation.[471] Thus decreased concentrations of NO favor adhesion and aggregation of platelets with consequent release of vasoconstrictor mediators. These would exacerbate a reduced supply of O_2 to the liver. Decreased concentrations of NO also are associated with increased adhesion of leukocytes to postcapillary venules, thereby promoting recruitment of leukocytes.[472] In addition to modulating blood flow and O_2 supply, there is evidence that NO can be an anti-oxidant.[473] Inhibition of NO production in vivo, enhances production of superoxide by the liver.[474] And, NO acts synergistically with prostacyclin to prevent endotoxin-mediated liver injury.[475]

One of the effects of NO relevant to vasoconstrictor-vasodilator imbalance is that NO terminates ET-1 signaling by displacing ET-1 from receptors and by interfering with postreceptor mobilization of calcium.[476] This "crosstalk" between NO and ET could account for alterations in blood flow and O_2 supply to the liver after ethanol administration.

The mechanisms contributing to the ethanol-induced decrease in NO production by non-parenchymal hepatic cells are unknown. Possible inhibitors of NO production include lipid peroxides, TNFα and TGF-β.[477-479] TNFα, which is increased in alcoholic hepatitis, enhances degradation of NOS.[478] TGF-β suppresses induction of NOS by decreasing the stability and translation of the enzyme mRNA and by increasing degradation of the enzyme itself.[479]

THE EFFECTS OF ETHANOL ON THE METABOLISM OF FATTY ACIDS

Ethanol-induced Fatty Liver

The central role of the liver in the metabolism of fatty acids and a pathogenetic discussion of fatty liver are presented in detail in Chap. 3. A general scheme of the circulation of fatty acids between peripheral tissues and liver is depicted in Figure 29-10. The amount of fatty acids in the liver depends on the balance between the processes of delivery and removal. The former are de novo synthesis in the liver and release from adipose tissue. The latter are oxidation of fatty acids and their resecretion as very low-density lipoproteins (VLDL). Ingestion of ethanol alters the rates of all these processes.[480]

Many mechanisms have been proposed as a basis for alcohol-induced fatty liver but it is not clear which is the most important.[481] Also, the basis for fatty liver appears to change with the stage of disease.[481]

Mechanisms of Ethanol-induced Fatty Liver: Increased Supply of Substrate

The two principal substrates for synthesis of triacylglycerol (TAG) are glycerol-3-phosphate (3-GP) and free (nonesterified) fatty acids.[482] Hepatic levels of 3-GP are increased after ethanol ingestion secondary to an increase in the ratio of NADH to NAD^+ in the liver, which drives the equilibrium of Reaction [8] to the right.[483]

$$\text{Dihydroxyacetone P} + \text{NADH} + H^+ \rightarrow \text{glycerol-3-P} + NAD^+ \quad \textbf{[8]}$$

A consequence of increasing concentrations of 3-GP is enhanced rates of esterification of fatty acids.[484] The significance of a shift in the equilibrium of [8] for the pathogenesis of alcoholic fatty liver and control of TAG synthesis has been questioned, however, because increased synthesis of triglycerides, in association with alcohol ingestion, can be independent of an altered hepatic redox state and the concentration of 3-GP in the liver.[485,486]

Of perhaps greater importance in the pathogenesis of alcoholic fatty liver is the increased levels of free fatty acids in blood.[487] Fatty acids that accumulate in the liver originate from dietary fatty acids rather than from endogenous sources.[488] Large amounts of ethanol enhance the lipolytic rate in adipose tissue because of direct stimulatory effects on the adrenal and pituitary-adrenal axis.[489,490] Fatty acids released from adipose tissue are then taken up by the liver. Several studies using isolated hepatocytes have shown that the rate of synthesis of TAG depends on the extracellular concentration of free fatty acids.[485,491,492] Moreover, chronic consumption of ethanol inhibits oxidation of fatty acids in liver. The activity of carnitine palmitoyl transferase (CPT) I, which is located in the outer half of the inner mitochondrial membrane, controls the entry of acyl-CoAs into the mitochondria before β-oxidation.[493,494] This activity is decreased by alcohol consumption. And, because the activity of CPT determines, at least in part, the partitioning of fatty acids between oxidation and esterification,[495,496] inhibition tends to increase esterification of fatty acids (Figure 29-11). Another factor contributing to inhibition of fatty acid oxidation in mitochondria is the increase in NADH generated by ethanol oxidation. Prolonged ethanol administration to rats causes profound alterations in the zonation pattern of the different fatty acid synthetic and oxidative pathways.[497] Ethanol administration abolishes the zonal asymmetry of the lipogenic process, and inverts the acinar distribution of fatty acid oxidation (i.e., the rates of fatty acid oxidation and CPT 1 activity are higher in perivenous than in portal hepatocytes).

Stimulation of esterification due to a specific effect of alcohol on phosphatidate phosphohydrolase (PAP) has received some recent attention.[498] Hepatocytes contain two distinct forms of PAP: a "metabolic" form present in

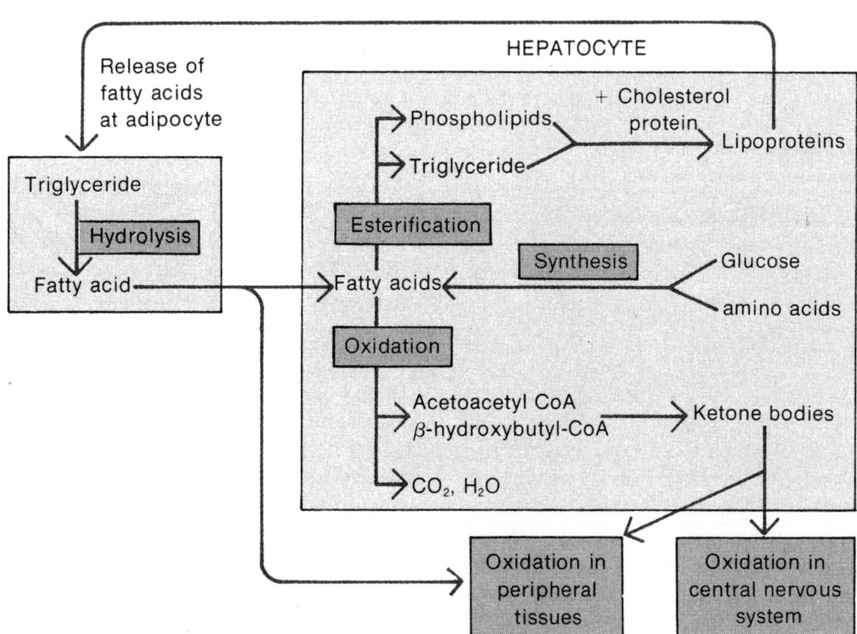

Figure 29-10 The flow of fatty acids between liver and adipose tissue. (From Zakim D: The pathophysiology of liver disease. In Smith LH Jr, Thier SO, eds: International Textbook of Medicine, vol 1. Pathophysiology, ed 2. Philadelphia, WB Saunders Co, 1985:1267.)

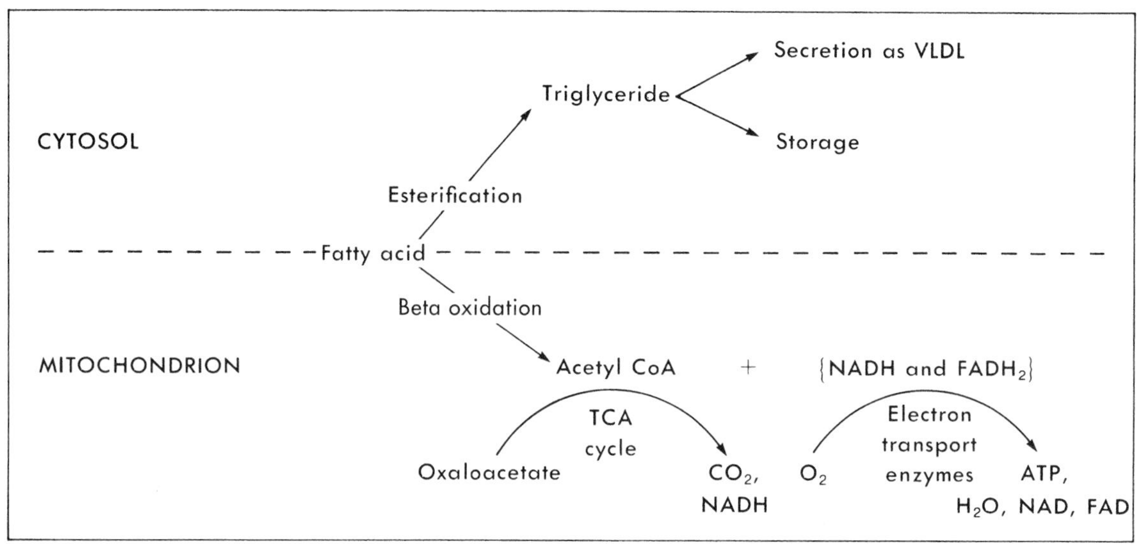

Figure 29-11 Disposition of fatty acids between esterification and oxidation. In ethanol-fed animals the block in oxidation of fatty acids is at the entry site into the TCA cycle, that is, the oxidation of acetyl CoA lost to carbon dioxide. Ethanol also stimulates esterification of fatty acids. *TCA,* Tricarboxylic acid; *CoA,* co-enzyme A.

the cytosol and microsomes, sensitive to inhibition by N-ethylmaleimide (NEM) and involved in triglyceride synthesis, and a physically distinct "cell-signaling" form located predominantly in the plasma membrane and insensitive to inhibition by NEM.[499,500] Physiologically relevant concentrations of fatty acids (0.15-0.30 mm) cause a concentration-dependent translocation of PAP from a metabolically inactive site in the cytosol to the membranes of the endoplasmic reticulum, where the enzyme can participate in synthesis of glycerolipids.[501] Alcohol feeding to baboons[502] and hamsters[503] demonstrates increased cytosolic and microsomal PAP activity in the early stages of fatty liver. A single large dose of ethanol also stimulates hepatic PAP activity.[504] Measurements of NEM-sensitive and NEM-insensitive PAP activities in needle biopsy specimens of liver from patients with severe steatosis show increased activity of the NEM-sensitive form of PAP (which catalyzes the rate-limiting step in triglyceride synthesis).[505] It is hypothesized that alcohol-stimulated increases of PAP activity are due to hormonal effects, particularly an increase in glucocorticoids and glucagon relative to insulin.[506]

Increased Uptake of Fatty Acids

An increased uptake of hepatic fatty acids from plasma is a central mechanism involved in alcoholic fatty liver. Uptake of fatty acids by the liver occurs through both simple diffusion[507] and a carrier-mediated process.[508] Fatty acids bind to a hepatic cytosolic fatty acid binding protein (L-FABP). L-FABP has an important role not only in the uptake and transport of fatty acids but also facilitates cholesterol and triglyceride synthesis and activates some enzymes involved in fatty acid metabolism.[508] Chronic ethanol administration produces a striking increase in levels of L-FABP in the livers of male rats.[509] This increase is hypothesized to prevent an increase in the levels of fatty acids in the cytosol, thereby preventing liver cell damage. Ethanol administration to female rats, in some but not all studies, produces a smaller increase in hepatic L-FABP compared to males[510,511]; this smaller increase results in a lesser ability to bind potentially toxic fatty acids and might account, in part, for increased vulnerability of females to alcohol-induced liver injury.[512,513]

Inhibition of Fatty Acid Oxidation

Inhibition of fatty acid oxidation by ethanol has been demonstrated in vitro,[514,515] in perfused rat liver,[516] and in vivo in man and experimental animals.[517] The block in oxidation of fatty acids is not at entry to or within the beta oxidation cycle but in the oxidation of the acetyl CoA produced by beta oxidation (Figure 29-11).[518,519] The simplest explanation for these observations is that ethanol increases the ratio of NADH to NAD^+. This suppresses both the beta oxidation spiral and the tricarboxylic acid (TCA) cycle, which completes the oxidation of fatty acid–derived acetyl-CoA to CO_2.[516] The inhibitory effect of the redox shift on the TCA cycle is further compounded by the alcohol-derived increase in the concentration of acetyl CoA.[514]

Studies in human liver showing persistence of a defect in CO_2 production from fatty acids after a period of abstinence suggest that mechanisms other than the redox change or competitive substrate oxidation may be important.[520] Derangements in the organization and function of liver mitochondria, after ethanol administration, might contribute to non-redox-related defects in beta oxidation.

Increased Endogenous Synthesis of Fatty Acids

The majority of fatty acids that accumulate in the liver originate from dietary sources.[488] There is controversy about the effect of ethanol on hepatic fatty acid synthesis in alcohol-fed rats.[521,522] Early studies reported an increase in fatty acid synthesis attributed to an increase in the NADPH:NADP ratio in rats fed ethanol. Other experimental observations have not confirmed these earlier findings,[523,524] and the biochemical explanations for them are now known to be invalid. One study even showed a decrease in endogenous fatty acid synthesis secondary to feedback inhibition by the accumulated triglyceride.[524]

Decreased Export of Triglycerides

The normal fate of hepatic triglycerides is incorporation into VLDL followed by secretion into sinusoidal blood. Under normal conditions the rates of these two processes are sufficient to keep triglycerides in the liver at low levels. When the triglyceride load increases because of increased synthesis of fatty acids, increased mobilization of fatty acids from adipocytes, or decreased oxidation, the rates of synthesis and secretion of VLDL also increase. Alcohol, however, inhibits the secretion of VLDL[525] after chronic ethanol ingestion but not after acute administration.[526] The defect in VLDL secretion has been localized to the Golgi in that VLDL-like particles accumulate in the Golgi apparatus in both rats and humans after ethanol intake.[527,528] One proposed mechanism for a defect in secretion of VLDL is the formation of adducts between tubulin and acetaldehyde, which prevents polymerization of tubulin to form microtubules.[529] The selective blockade of VLDL secretion in perivenous hepatocytes may contribute to fatty infiltration in the perivenular area.[497]

Ethanol-induced fatty liver is a toxic effect of ethanol that occurs independently of nutritional deficiency. It has been suggested repeatedly that the fatty liver is a harbinger of more serious liver disease and that the fatty liver is a natural event on the path to cirrhosis. In a large prospective study of men with alcohol-related steatosis the severity of steatosis on initial liver biopsy predicted the development of cirrhosis on a subsequent biopsy 10 years later, independent of the level of continuing alcohol intake.[492] Both animals and patients with alcohol-induced fatty liver show evidence of increased collagen synthesis and turnover.[493,494]

Adaptation to Fatty Acid Overload

Peroxisome proliferation-activated receptors (PPAR) are members of the nuclear receptor family of transactivating factors that mediate the pleiotropic hepatic response to xenobiotics that cause proliferation of peroxisomes.[533,534] Long chain fatty acids and their metabolites are important physiologic ligands of PPAR. PPAR-responsive genes include key enzymes of the mitochondrial and extramitochondrial pathways of fatty acid oxidation and cytosolic L-FABP.[535] A mechanism common to many diseases associated with fatty acid overload is impairment of mitochondrial fatty acid oxidation.[536] PPAR-α is the predominant isoform of PPAR in liver.[533] PPAR-α is believed to be a sensor of fatty acid overload and an effector of the adaptive gene response to this state. Under conditions of fatty acid overload fatty acids are directed toward synthesis of triglyceride and extramitochondrial oxidation in peroxisomes and endoplasmic reticulum. In the latter ω-oxidation of the acyl chain initiates the formation of dicarboxylic fatty acids primarily through the P450 4A subfamily of cytochrome P450 enzyme.[537] Alcohol induces CYP 4A expression in rats with formation of ω and ω-1 oxidized metabolites.[538,539] Although key to adaptation to fatty acid overload, the increase in peroxisomal and microsomal oxidation of fatty acid produces metabolites that also are potentially toxic.[540]

By histochemistry and in-situ hybridization, expression of peroxisomal fatty acyl CoA oxidase and CYP 4A1 is greater in the centrolobular region of the liver.[541] The expression of L-FABP is predominantly in the periportal and midzonal regions.[542] Thus greater formation of toxic metabolites together with reduced fatty acid buffering capacity could contribute to the predominant centrolobular damage in ALD.[543] In studies in which the expression of PPAR-α and PPAR-α–regulated genes was measured in rats fed alcohol and a high-fat diet, induction of PPAR-α and CYP 4A1 was associated with the lack of appropriate induction of L-FABP and peroxisomal fatty acyl CoA oxidase in the animals with liver injury.[544]

Role of Microsomal Triglyceride Transfer Protein

Microsomal triglyceride transfer protein (MTP) is required for the secretion of apo B–containing lipoprotein from hepatocytes.[545] MTP is located within the lumen of the endoplasmic reticulum and transfers both neutral and polar lipids but transfer is most efficient with neutral lipids (triglycerides and cholesterol esters). Studies in liver-specific *mtp* knockout mice show that MTP is essential for transferring the bulk of triglycerides into the lumen of the endoplasmic reticulum for assembly of VLDL, and is required for the secretion of apo B-100 from the liver.[546] Histologic studies of the liver in the knockout mice reveal marked steatosis. Exposure of Hep G2 cells to low concentrations of ethanol (between 0.01 percent and 0.1 percent) significantly decreases levels of MTP mRNA, activity of MTP, and rates of secretion of apo B.[547] Studies in vivo of rats confirm that ethanol ingestion leads to decreased hepatic MTP mRNA.[535] Mice with heterozygous MTP deficiency and levels of MTP comparable to those in alcohol-fed mice have diminished rates of secretion of apo B from liver and modest increases in liver triglycerides.[548]

Role of Kupffer Cells in Hepatic Fat Accumulation

Experimental evidence suggests that Kupffer cells may be involved in the accumulation of fat in hepatocytes of ethanol-fed rats.[549] When ethanol-fed rats are administered gadolinium chloride, an agent that inactivates Kupffer cells,[550] or non-absorbable antibiotics that decrease levels of gut-derived endotoxin, fat accumulation in that liver is diminished considerably. These results suggest that endotoxin is a likely stimulus for the Kupffer cell–mediated increase in hepatic triglyceride storage. The postulated mechanism for the endotoxin-mediated fatty liver is that endotoxin causes an increase in intracellular calcium in Kupffer cells, which results in an increase in prostaglandin (PG)E_2 production.[551] PGE_2 acting on EP_2/EP_4 receptors increases intracellular cyclic AMP, which in turn increases triglyceride accumulation in hepatocytes.[552]

Alcohol and Hepatic Fatty Acid Composition

The most consistent finding with respect to changes in composition is a decrease in arachidonic acid (AA) (20:4 n-6).[553-556] In some studies this decrease is accompanied by an increase in linoleic acid (LA) (18:2 n-6),[557] although this is not a constant finding.[558] There are a number of possible interpretations of the alteration in the ratio of LA:AA, such as selective uptake of LA and selective utilization of AA, but a commonly held view is that these changes indicate a reduced conversion of LA to AA.[559]

Direct evidence for this has been obtained by measurements of hepatic Δ6 desaturase and Δ5 desaturase (Figure 29-12). The Δ6 desaturase converts both LA and α-linolenic acid (18:3 n-3) to γ-linolenic acid (18:3 n-6) and 18:4 n-4. After chain elongation Δ5 desaturase converts dihomo-γ-linolenic acid (20:3 n-6) to AA and 20:4 n-3 to eicosapentaenoic acid (20:5 n-3). Ethanol inhibits both of these enzymes.[560-562]

In rat studies a uniform decrease in three desaturases (Δ6, Δ5, and Δ9) has been reported with ethanol feeding.[560,561] This general effect on desaturases could reflect suppression of the microsomal electron transport system or CoA ligase by ethanol because the electron transport system and ligase are common components in all three desaturases. The effect of ethanol on activities of Δ5 and Δ6 desaturases varies in different strains of rats, which may explain why ethanol administration has apparently inconsistent effects on liver fatty acid composition in different animals.[563] Also, activities of Δ6 and Δ5 desaturases but not of Δ9 desaturase decrease in a pig model of alcoholism.[564] This result suggests that ethanol affects desaturase activities directly and not via an effect on components common to all three desaturases.

In keeping with the lack of an ethanol effect on Δ9 desaturase in pigs, oleic acid (18:1 n-9) concentrations are increased in liver cell membranes after ethanol feeding.[565] Δ9 Desaturase is influenced more significantly by dietary lipids than are Δ6 and Δ5 desaturases.[566] Thus alterations in oleate may reflect dietary availability rather a specific effect of ethanol.

In studies using intragastric feeding of ethanol to rats there is a reduction in long-chain polyunsaturated fatty acids in animals fed corn oil and ethanol.[509] Feeding saturated fat (medium-chain triglycerides), which protects the liver from ethanol-induced injury,[567] increases rather than decreases concentrations of AA. In both groups, there is a significant correlation ($P < .01$) between the percentage changes in AA and oleic acid, suggesting that the change in oleic acid is a specific response to a

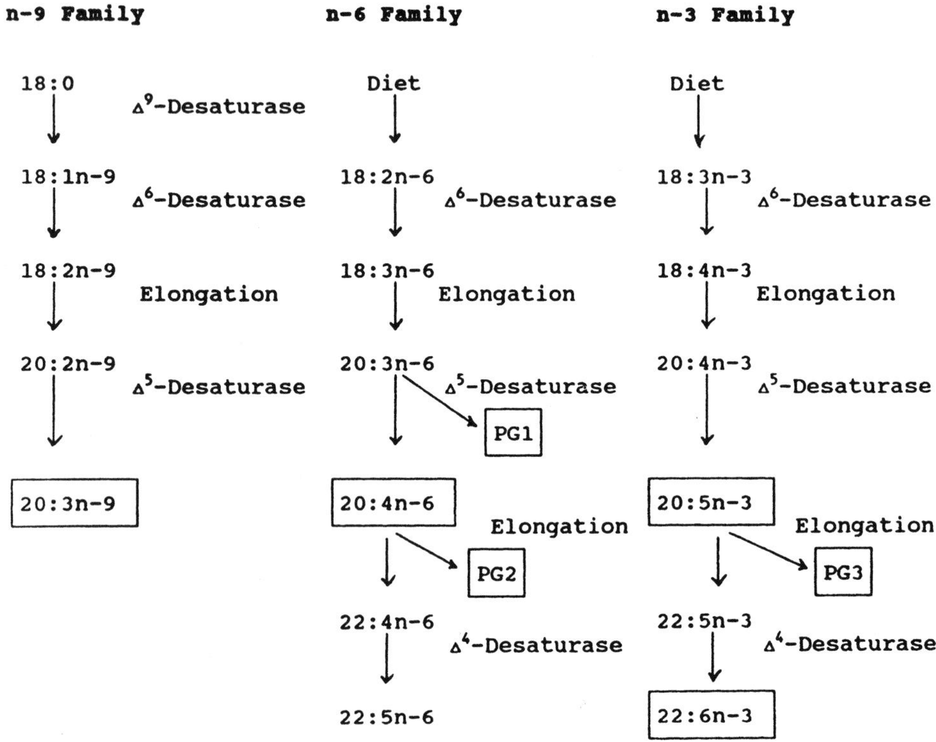

Figure 29-12 The fatty acids enclosed in boxes represent the major polyunsaturated fatty acids that are found in membranes. Three of the fatty acids give rise to prostaglandins, and these conversions are represented by PG enclosed in boxes. Ethanol has been shown to have an effect on all of the desaturases except the Δ^4-desaturase. (From Reitz RC: Dietary fatty acids and alcohol: effects on cellular membranes. Alcohol Alcohol 28:59, 1993.)

change in AA. The change in microsomal fatty acid composition in rats fed saturated fat and ethanol may be related to the hepatoprotective effect of this diet. This hypothesis is supported by observations that a diet low in linoleic acid prevents the fatty acid changes seen with ethanol feeding and protects against the increase in mitochondrial fragility caused by ethanol ingestion.[568] In rats fed fish oil and ethanol a significant decrease occurs in concentrations of palmitic acid (16:0), whereas 18:2 n-6 increases.[569] In contrast to the decrease in 20:4 n-6 seen in rats fed corn oil–ethanol diets, an increase in 20:4 n-6 occurs in rats fed ethanol with fish oil. The exact significance of the differences between these two groups is unknown.

Varying the percentage of calories derived from fat also affects the fatty acid composition of liver organelles in a dose-dependent manner.[570,571] In male rats a high-fat diet (34.2 percent of calories) and ethanol caused a decrease in concentrations of 16:0, 20:4 n-6, and 22:6 n-3, and an increase in concentrations of 18:1 n-9 and 18:2 n-6.[572] A low-fat diet (4.6 percent of calories) led only to an increase in the concentration of 18:2 n-6 and a decrease in the concentration of 20:4 n-6. In females only the levels of 16:0 and 18:0 were affected by alcohol, and the amount of dietary fat had no effect. Fractionation of mitochondrial phospholipids showed that the major alterations were in phosphatidylcholines with less significant changes in other classes of phospholipids.[556]

Enzymes—excluding desaturases—that may be responsible for ethanol-induced alterations in the fatty acid composition of various hepatic phospholipids include phospholipase A_2 and the acyl CoA:phospholipid acyltransferases.[573] The interaction between these two groups of enzymes is largely responsible for the incorporation of polyunsaturated fatty acids (containing three or more double bonds) during the process of phospholipid synthesis. A role for CYP 2E1 in the pathogenesis of ethanol-induced changes in liver fatty acid composition also has been suggested.[574] Increased formation of diene conjugates and the level of CYP 2E1 in ethanol-fed rats correlated in one study with the decrease in arachidonic acid in liver microsomes.[573] This suggests a role for CYP 2E1–induced lipid peroxidation in the selective utilization of 20:4. When CYP 2E1 induction is inhibited in ethanol-fed rats there is partial amelioration of the decrease of arachidonic acid in microsomes, lipid peroxidation, and severity of fatty liver.[574] A strong negative correlation that is seen between activity of CYP 2E1 and the ratio of 20:4/18:2 indicates the importance of CYP 2E1 in the differential oxidation of these fatty acids. CYP 2E1 may be important in the oxidation of arachidonic acid by the liver to form two monohydroxylated eicosatetraenoic acids (HETEs).[575,576] The 19(s)-HETE formed in this reaction has vascular reactivity and stimulates the Na^+/K^+-ATPase pump. Na^+K^+-ATPase activity is increased in red cells and liver membranes of ethanol-fed rats.[577,578] Selective utilization of arachidonic acid secondary to ethanol feeding also may explain the increased production of arachidonic acid metabolites such as thromboxane B_2 and leukotriene B_4.[579]

Role of Dietary Fat in Ethanol-induced Liver Injury

There is considerable evidence that the amount of fat in the diet is a key determinant of the lesions in ALD. Initial studies in rats fed the Lieber-DeCarli diet showed a steatogenic effect of dietary fat in ALD and that dietary fatty acids were an important source of the lipids accumulating in the liver of ethanol-fed animals.[580] More recent data, using continuous intragastric feeding of ethanol, confirm the role of dietary fat in ALD.[581-583] When fat constituted 5 percent of the calories, focal necrosis and severe steatosis were induced in centrolobular areas of livers of rats.[581] When the experiments were repeated using the same diet but a fat content of 25 percent of total calories, more than half of the rats developed centrolobular fibrosis resembling that in baboon and man.[582] The rate of development of fatty liver also was related to the fat content of the diet.[584]

The importance of dietary fat in ALD is also supported by epidemiologic correlations, which suggest that susceptibility to alcohol is related to different types of dietary fat.[585,586] Interestingly, mortality from cirrhosis in different populations correlates with the per capita consumption of pork.[585] No correlation was seen between mortality rates from cirrhosis and per capita consumption of total fat or beef, but pork fat has more linoleic acid than beef fat and the position of the unsaturated fatty acids is different in lard and beef tallow. Additionally, when the deviation from expected mortality from cirrhosis was correlated with dietary intake of saturated fat, cholesterol, and unsaturated fat in 17 different countries, saturated fat was relatively protective against the development of ALD.

Rats fed ethanol and tallow (beef fat) develop none of the features of ALD. Animals fed ethanol and lard develop minimal to moderate ALD, and animals fed ethanol and corn oil develop severe ALD.[587] In each of these instances the percent of calories derived from fat in the diet was the same. Because the degree of histopathologic abnormality in liver correlated with the amount of linoleic acid in the diet, it was postulated that this feature of the diet accounted for differences in the incidence of ALD in the tallow-, lard-, and corn oil–fed groups and therefore that linoleic acid was essential in the pathogenesis of ALD. To test this hypothesis, rats were fed ethanol plus tallow or 2.5 percent linoleic acid.[588] The rats supplemented with linoleic acid showed all the features of ALD, confirming the importance of linoleic acid in the pathogenesis of experimental alcoholic liver injury.[588]

The importance of polyunsaturated fatty acids rather than linoleic acid alone also was demonstrated. More severe liver injury is produced by feeding fish oil and ethanol versus corn oil and ethanol.[589,590] In particular, the degree of necrosis and inflammation was more severe in the rats fed fish oil and ethanol. Two mechanisms for the relationship between dietary fats and alcoholic liver injury have been investigated in some detail. These are the metabolism of eicosanoids and the effect of different dietary fats on induction of CYP 2E1.

The chemistry of the eicosanoid biosynthetic pathway is well known.[591,592] PGs are formed by the oxidative cyclization of the central 5 carbons within the 20-carbon polyunsaturated fatty acids. Cyclooxygenase (Cox or PGH synthase) is the key regulatory enzyme for this pathway, in which arachidonic acid is converted to PGG_2 and PGH_2. PGH_2 is converted subsequently to a variety of eicosanoids (e.g., PGE_2, PGF_2, $PFG_2\alpha$, prostacyclin, and thromboxane [Tx]A_2), depending on the downstream enzymatic machinery present in a particular cell type.

There are two different isoforms of Cox, designated Cox-1 and Cox-2.[593-596] Cox-1 is the constitutive isoform that is present in most tissues; it mediates the synthesis of PGs required for normal physiologic functions. Cox-2 is not detectable in most normal tissues but is induced by cytokines and growth factors. It is the major isoform in inflammatory cells.[593-596] Other differences between Cox-1 and Cox-2 include utilization of different pools of arachidonic acid substrate. Endogenous arachidonic acid is a substrate for Cox-2 but not for Cox-1. The latter isoform appears to require exogenous substrate.[597] The importance of endogenous arachidonic acid as a substrate for Cox-2–dependent synthesis of prostanoids is highlighted by demonstration of synergy between proinflammatory mediators and induction of Cox-2 in vivo.[598] Thus production of eicosanoids was highest when phospholipase A_2–mediated production of arachidonic acid was greatest. This observation is relevant to the observed association between induction of Cox-2, production of eicosanoids, and increased activity of phospholipase A_2 in livers of rats with inflammatory liver injury (reviewed in refs. 599, 600, and 601). The difference in utilization of arachidonic acid by the Cox isoforms could explain why linoleic acid (a precursor of arachidonic acid) is necessary for alcohol-induced liver injury[602] and why ethanol decreases the concentration of endogenous arachidonic acid in rats that develop liver injury but not in rats protected against liver damage.[603]

Cox-2 and Hepatic Inflammation

Chronic inflammatory changes are a hallmark of alcoholic hepatitis.[599,600] Inflammation increases the synthesis of prostanoids as a result, in part, of upregulation of Cox-2.[593-595] Consistent with this prevailing opinion, mRNA and Cox-2 protein are generally undetectable in liver and most other normal tissues but increase in inflamed tissues along with strong enhancement of prostanoid production.[594]

Perhaps the most pivotal observation linking Cox-2 to hepatocellular injury is the study of Dinchuk and colleagues in Cox-2–deficient mice.[604] Cox-2–deficient mice and controls were sensitized to TNF-α–induced hepatocellular toxicity with D-galactosamine. Levels of TNF-α increased in response to endotoxin to similar extents in control and Cox-2–deficient mice. There was extensive hepatocyte necrosis in control animals whereas injury was mild or absent in the Cox-2–deficient mice. These results clearly indicate that macrophage priming for LPS-induced TNF-α production was normal in Cox-2–deficient mice. The absence of hepatocellular injury in this group underscores the importance of Cox-2 and TNFα in hepatocellular injury.

Of the inflammatory mediators that induce Cox2, endotoxin and TNFα[600] are the most relevant to alcoholic liver injury. Endotoxemia occurs in clinical and experimental ALD.[606-609] Levels of endotoxin in rats correlate with the severity of liver pathology.[609] Similarly, increased levels of TNFα are seen in clinical and experimental ALD.[600] Endotoxin induces TNFα and Cox-2. Selective inhibition of Cox-2 inhibits many of the endotoxin-related responses in vivo and in macrophages.[594] Lipid peroxidation[605] is also important for alcoholic liver injury.

Reactive O_2 intermediates and lipid hydroperoxides regulate expression of Cox-2 in vitro.[610-612] Lipid hydroperoxides also activate Cox; in addition to their effects on the amounts and activities of Cox isoform, lipid peroxides activate phospholipase A_2 activity to provide increased arachidonic acid as substrate for Cox. Thus a small increase in the level of hydroperoxides in cells can cause dramatic increases in Cox activity, resulting in an explosive production of prostanoids.[610] Studies of alveolar macrophages showed that the synthesis of Cox-2 in response to endotoxin was regulated by oxidant tone[610] and that initiation of Cox-2 activity required considerably lower levels of hydroperoxides than did Cox-1. This differential regulation would allow prostanoid synthesis by Cox-2 to proceed at levels of hydroperoxides in cells too low to stimulate Cox-1.

In the intragastrically fed rat increased levels of Cox-2 are seen in rats showing evidence of necroinflammatory injury,[613] as are increased levels of TNFα, endotoxin, and lipid peroxidation. The highest levels of Cox-2 are detected in the Kupffer cells. Interestingly, TNFα and Cox-2 are co-expressed in Kupffer cells in ethanol-fed rats with evidence of necroinflammatory changes.

The importance of TNFα and Cox-2 in promoting liver injury is further suggested by studies in female rats.[614] Male and female rats fed fish oil and dextrose have increased expression of TNFα mRNA. However, only female rats have enhanced expression of Cox-2. And female but not male rats have evidence of liver injury when fed fish oil and dextrose.

The relationship between oxidative stress, Cox-2, and fibrosis is supported by in vitro experiments that link CYP 2E1–dependent oxidative stress, induction of Cox-2, and activation of collagen gene expression.[615] The results of this study suggest that induction of CYP 2E1 activity generates oxidative stress, which leads to increased Cox-2 activity and collagen production.

Eicosanoids produced by the activity of Cox-1 protect against liver injury. A protective role for Cox-1 as a "housekeeping" gene and for generation of cytoprotective prostanoids is suggested by a number of studies.[618-620] Cox-1 products (PGE_2) and prostacyclin are lower in rats with pathologic changes after alcohol administration.[616,617] Increased Cox-1 expression in the vascular bed of liver occurs concomitantly with increased synthesis of prostacyclin.[618] Decreased expression of Cox-1 occurs in Kupffer cells of ethanol-fed rats; this decrease can explain decreased production of prostacyclin and PGE_2 in liver injury.[609-621]

In rats fed corn oil plus ethanol, which causes ALD, the progression of liver injury was accompanied by a decline in production of PGE_2 and an increase in production of leukotriene B and TxB_2 by non-parenchymal liver cells.[622] The best correlate of liver pathology was the ratio in plasma of TxB_2:PGE_2.[623] In addition to changes in TxB_2 and PGE_2 the levels of 6 ketoprostaglandin $F_1\alpha$ in plasma and in non-parenchymal cells decreased before development of liver injury.[624] The question arises as to why, with continued alcohol feeding, the ratio of eicosanoids shifts away from prostacyclin and PGE_2 to TxB_2. There is evidence to suggest that the level of lipid peroxides in cells has a profound effect on the enzymes of the arachidonic acid cascade,[625] such as prostaglandin endoperoxide synthase, which catalyzes the conversion of arachidonic acid to PGH_2, and prostacyclin synthase, which catalyzes conversion of PGH_2 to PGI_2.[626] There is also evidence that vitamin E affects eicosanoid metabolism via changes in lipid peroxidation by the states of activation of enzymes involved in the synthesis of eicosanoids.[627] Ethanol feeding increases levels of lipid peroxides and decreases levels of vitamin E in plasma and liver.[628,629] It is not surprising then that concentrations of eicosanoids are altered in a manner that increases synthesis of thromboxane and decreases synthesis of prostacyclin.[630]

The mechanism by which thromboxanes cause liver injury is unknown. TxA_2 was described originally as a potent vasoconstrictor and agent of platelet aggregation.[631] Vasoconstriction may lead to hypoxia (see previous), and platelet aggregation releases secretory products that cause cell injury.[632] Additionally, TxB_2 causes bleb formation in isolated hepatocytes,[633] which is a consequence of toxic or ischemic cell injury.[634] TxA_2 also may promote inflammation; thromboxanes mediate diapedesis by activation of neutrophil adhesion receptors interacting with basally expressed intercellular adhesion molecules (ICAM)-1.[635] Besides causing cell injury, thromboxanes can contribute to the long-term effects of alcohol such as fibrosis.[636,637] In the kidney, for example, thromboxanes increase cell-associated laminin, fibronectin, and collagen,[638] partly by stimulation of TGF-β that in turn stimulates synthesis of cell matrix proteins.[639]

The increase in TxA_2 cannot explain the enhanced severity of liver injury in rats fed fish oil and ethanol because fish oil reduces production of thromboxane by a variety of cells.[640,644] One possible explanation for the enhancement of alcoholic liver injury by fish oil, however, is the formation of 8-isoprostanes. Recently, Morrow and associates found a series of PG-like compounds with potent biologic activity.[642,643] These compounds are produced in vivo in humans and experimental animals as products of free radical catalyzed peroxidation of unsaturated fatty acids. The formation of these compounds occurs independently of the catalytic activity of the cyclooxygenase enzymes. In the case of arachidonic acid the formation of these PG-like compounds proceeds through intermediates composed of four positional peroxyl radical isomers of arachidonic acid, which undergo endocyclization to yield bicyclic endoperoxide PGG_2-like compounds. These are reduced to PGF_2-like compounds. In a study of the effect of CCl_4 on formation of 8-isoprostane in liver and plasma the induction of 8-isoprostane was linked to lipid peroxidation rather than hepatic necrosis.[642] Also, a reduction in levels of 8-isoprostane was seen in the presence of an inhibitor of cytochrome P450, implicating these enzymes in the formation of 8-isoprostanes. When 8-isoprostane levels were measured in rats fed different dietary fats plus ethanol, the highest levels were seen in rats fed fish oil and ethanol.[644] As mentioned previously, the highest levels of CYP 2E1 are seen in rats fed fish oil and ethanol.[589] These animals have the highest levels of 8-isoprostane.

The biologic activities of 8-isoprostanes are believed to be mediated by interaction with Tx receptors.[645] Thus 8-isoprostanes can act via the same receptor as TxA_2, and possibly via a separate isoprostane receptor.[646] The activation of these receptors causes vasoconstriction and activation of phospholipase C.[647] These effects are abolished by treating with antagonists of the Tx receptor. The formation of Tx and isoprostanes and their relationship to alcoholic liver injury are shown in Figure 29-13.

The effect of ethanol and different dietary fats on induction of CYP 2E1 has been studied in some detail. As stated earlier, lower levels of induction are found in rats fed saturated fat and ethanol compared with rats fed corn oil and ethanol.[648,649] The level of induction of CYP 2E1 correlates with the decline in microsomal arachidonic acid, which in turn correlates with the formation of conjugated dienes.[650] Although it cannot be determined conclusively that lipid peroxidation is related directly to induction of CYP 2E1 or is part of a more generalized process, the data support the former hypothesis. A correlation between activation of phospholipases A and C and a decline in microsomal levels of arachidonic acid and induction of CYP 2E1 suggests that these processes are interlinked and that phospholipase-catalyzed generation of arachidonic acid leads to conversion of this fatty acid to lipid peroxides. The level of induction of CYP 2E1 is threefold higher in rats fed fish oil and ethanol as compared with rats fed corn oil and ethanol.[589] A significant correlation is obtained between levels of CYP 2E1 and conjugated dienes. This supports a role for CYP 2E1–mediated lipid peroxidation in ALD and provides an additional explanation for the varying severity of liver injury in rats fed different dietary fats plus ethanol.

The observation that saturated fatty acids protect against alcoholic liver injury has been used as a strategy to treat established alcoholic liver injury. When rats fed fish oil and ethanol were treated with palm oil and dextrose, significant decreases in the severity of fatty liver, necrosis, and inflammation were observed.[651] In rats fed fish oil and dextrose no significant improvement in pathology was seen. These differences in liver pathology could be explained, in part, by differences in lipid peroxidation, composition of liver fatty acids, and activity of CYP 2E1. Higher levels of polyunsaturated fatty acids in the groups fed fish oil were accompanied by an increased index of peroxidation in liver tissue. The protective effect of palm oil and dextrose was replicated by medium-chain triglycerides and dextrose.[652]

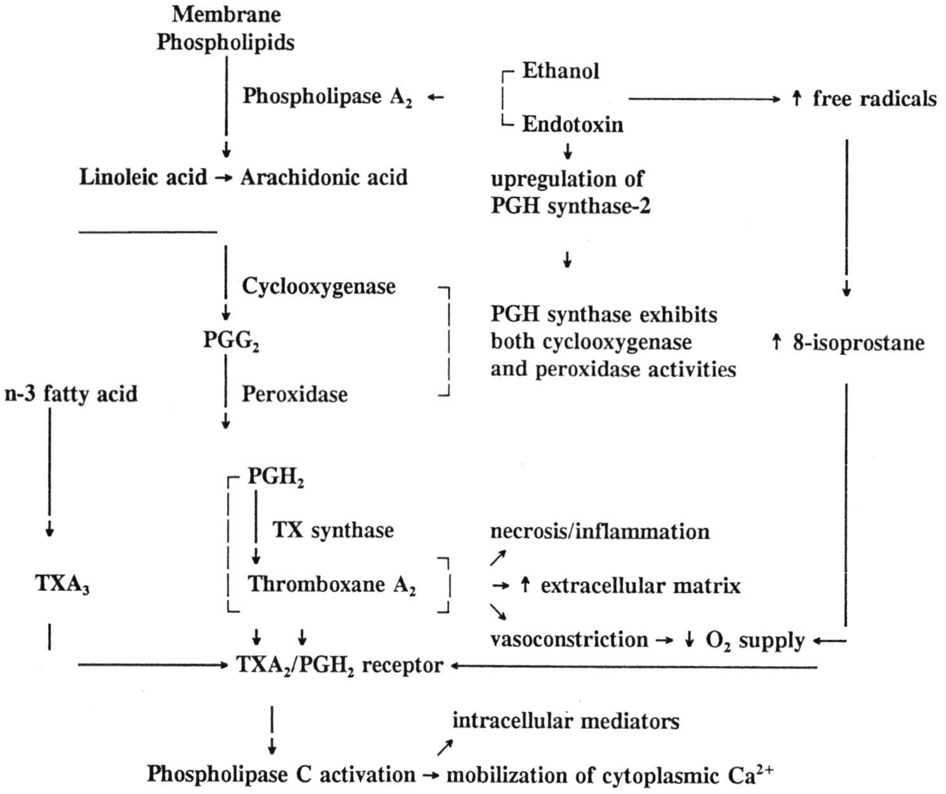

Membrane Phospholipids
Phospholipase A_2 ←
Ethanol
Endotoxin
↑ free radicals
Linoleic acid → Arachidonic acid
upregulation of PGH synthase-2
Cyclooxygenase
PGG_2
Peroxidase
PGH synthase exhibits both cyclooxygenase and peroxidase activities
↑ 8-isoprostane
n-3 fatty acid
PGH_2
TX synthase
Thromboxane A_2
TXA_3
necrosis/inflammation
→ ↑ extracellular matrix
vasoconstriction → ↓ O_2 supply ←
TXA_2/PGH_2 receptor
intracellular mediators
Phospholipase C activation → mobilization of cytoplasmic Ca^{2+}

Figure 29-13 Arachidonic acid release from membrane phospholipids can result in formation of either thromboxanes or isoprostanes. Both can act through the same TXA_2/PGH_2 receptor. *TxA_2*, Thromboxane A_2; *PGH_2*, prostaglandin H_2.

Another lipid-based therapy of potential benefit in ALD that affects collagen production and degradation is polyunsaturated lecithin (PUL).[653] Baboons fed PUL did not show progression beyond the stage of perivenular fibrosis. PUL selectively prevented acetaldehyde-induced accumulation of collagen in lipocytes in culture. Other lipids—for example, a saturated phospholipid, a monounsaturated lipid, or linoleate—had no effect. PUL also increased collagenase activity in vitro. The protection afforded against alcohol-induced fibrosis by PUL was reproduced by the same amount of phosphatidylcholine given in a purified extract consisting of 94 percent to 96 percent phosphatidylcholine.[654,655] The phosphatidylcholines given exogenously consisted of several species, but mainly of dilinoleoylphosphatidylcholine and palmitoyl-linoleoylphosphatidylcholine. Only dilinoleoylphosphatidylcholine duplicated the effect of PUL on collagenase. It is believed to be the active agent in the protective effect of phosphatidylcholine against the development of fibrosis and cirrhosis.[654] Part of this protective effect may be due to restoration of an alcohol-induced decrease in the activity of phosphatidylethanolamine-N-methyltransferase,[656] which is important for the synthesis of phosphatidylcholines.[655] Regardless of the mechanism, the possible protective effect of selected phosphatidylcholines against fibrosis and cirrhosis in humans has potential value.

Effects of Ethanol Oxidation on Synthesis of Glucose

The most significant interaction between the metabolism of ethanol and glucose synthesis is that the former process inhibits the hepatic synthesis of glucose.[657-660] Ethanol does not alter the rate of hydrolysis of glycogen to glucose in a controlled setting, so inhibition of gluconeogenesis in response to ethanol is important clinically only in individuals who have no hepatic glycogen. A normal man or woman essentially is depleted of hepatic glycogen after about 48 hours of fasting. Normal subjects or alcoholics with and without liver disease may become hypoglycemic if they ingest ethanol at a time when they lack hepatic glycogen. This is a direct effect of ethanol on the liver and can be understood on the basis of the ethanol-induced shifts in the oxidation-reduction potential of the cytoplasmic compartment of the liver cell (Figure 29-14). (Chap. 3 describes hepatic gluconeogenesis.)

The increase in the ratio of NADH:NAD^+ during oxidation of ethanol shifts several oxidation-reduction couples to the reduced substrate: for example, oxaloacetate is reduced to malate, dihydroxyacetone-P is reduced to glycerol-1-P (Reaction [2]), and pyruvate is reduced to lactate. These intermediates are precursors of glucose. The ethanol-induced effect on levels of NADH thereby shunts intermediates of the gluconeogenic pathway away from the synthesis of glucose. A more important effect is that ox-

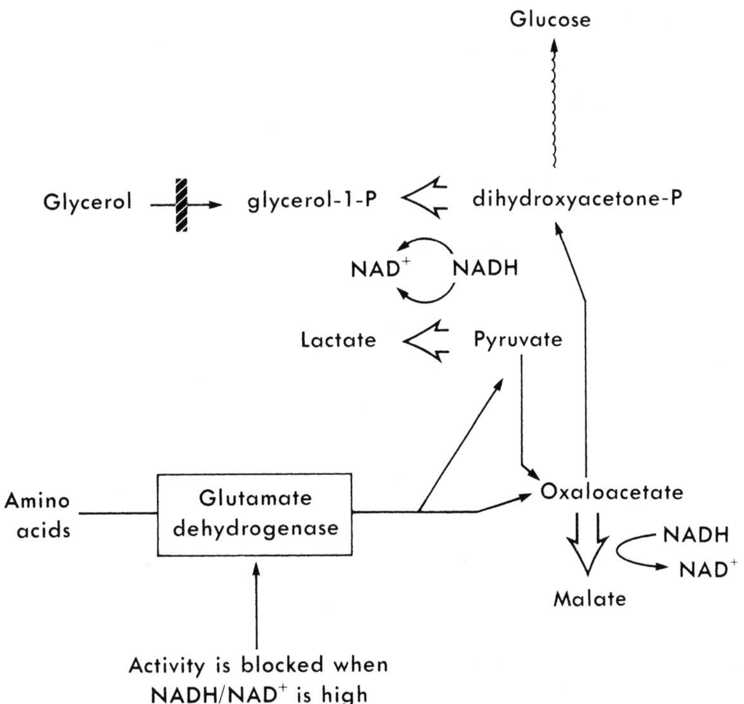

Figure 29-14 Effects of ethanol on synthesis of glucose. Ethanol blocks the flow of carbon to glucose by alteration in the ratios of lactate to pyruvate, dihydroxyacetone-P to glycerol-1-P, and oxaloacetate to malate secondary to increasing the ratio of NADH to NAD^+. Ethanol also leads to functional inhibition of glutamate dehydrogenase.

idation of ethanol interferes with the entry of carbon into the gluconeogenic pathway. This also is a consequence of the high NADH:NAD^+ ratio, which inhibits glutamate dehydrogenase (see the discussion of gluconeogenesis in Chap. 3).[661,662] Glutamate dehydrogenase is an important enzyme in the synthesis of glucose because it allows continued recycling of α-ketoglutarate in aminotransferase reactions, which provides for a continuous flow of carbon from amino acids to glucose. It has been found, too, that ethanol ingestion is associated with a reduction in the hepatic activity of two important gluconeogenic enzymes: pyruvate carboxylase and fructose-1,6-diphosphatase.[663] Measurement of the concentrations of gluconeogenic substrates in hepatocytes of fasted rats given ethanol suggests, however, that any changes in the activities of these two enzymes are less important than inhibition of the entry of substrates into the gluconeogenic pathway.[664] In addition to the alterations in intracellular processes mentioned previously, ethanol inhibits gluconeogenesis at two other sites.[665] Uptake of lactate, glycerol, and alanine by the liver is depressed in the presence of elevated blood ethanol levels. Furthermore, ethanol lowers circulating levels of alanine by inhibiting its release from muscle.

The effects of ethanol on gluconeogenesis are self-limited. Inhibition of gluconeogenesis is present only so long as the NADH:NAD^+ ratio is above normal. As soon as all administered ethanol is metabolized and NADH is reoxidized to NAD^+, the flow of substrate into and through the gluconeogenic pathway resumes. We want to stress, however, that ethanol-induced hypoglycemia can have serious clinical consequences requiring diagnosis and treatment with glucose. One should not delay administration of glucose while waiting for the ethanol to be metabolized completely. It also is important that certain individuals are at high risk for development of ethanol-induced hypoglycemia: patients who are malnourished or thyrotoxic, those consuming high-protein diets with limited carbohydrates, and children.[666] Ethanol-induced hypoglycemia in children has a 25 percent fatality rate.[666] The combination of ethanol and administration of insulin has produced severe hypoglycemia.[667] By contrast, obese patients and patients taking glucocorticoids are resistant to the hypoglycemic effects of ethanol.

Ethanol slightly decreases peripheral utilization of glucose.[668] In addition to direct interactions between the metabolism of ethanol and the synthesis of glucose, ethanol appears to influence the metabolism of glucose via effects on the endocrine system. Ethanol, when ingested by chronic users, interferes with the pituitary-adrenal axis, so that ethanol in this setting can limit the normal endocrine response to hypoglycemia,[669] potentiating the effects of ethanol on rates of gluconeogenesis and delaying recovery. Prior administration of ethanol enhances the response of the pancreatic cells to selected stimulators of insulin secretion. Ethanol, for example, potentiates arginine-induced but not glucagon-induced secretion of insulin by the pancreas.[670,671]

Hypoglycemia presumed secondary to ingestion of ethanol has been reported to occur in well-fed individuals who were exercising vigorously in the cold.[670,672] The mechanism of this phenomenon is unclear. Exercise, of course, potentiates utilization of glucose. In the presence of hepatic glycogen, however, we would not expect hypoglycemia to ensue. It has been suggested, therefore, that ethanol ingestion may impede glycogenolysis. This point has not been documented and is difficult to accept in view of published studies of normal volunteers. It has also been reported that reactive hypoglycemia is potentiated by ethanol ingestion.[673,674] Controlled studies in humans indicate that the combined intake of ethanol and a large sugar load may enhance insulin release.[658,674] The timing of ethanol administration relative to glucose ingestion seems critical for duplicating this result.[674,675]

Ethanol administration also causes alterations in glucose transporters. Glucose is transported into parenchymal cells by facilitated transport.[676-678] Within the family of glucose transporters detected so far the low-affinity type of glucose transporter in liver (GLUT 2) carries out the symmetric transport of glucose. The glucose transporter (designated GLUT 1) facilitates unidirectional transport of glucose into cells. GLUT 1 is localized to hepatocytes of the first row of cells around the terminal hepatic venule.[679] Cells with GLUT 1 as their glucose transporter are not well endowed for gluconeogenesis. Ethanol administration to rats, in amounts that cause liver injury, depletes liver glycogen, decreases expression of GLUT 2, and increases centrolobular expression of GLUT 1.[680] Unidirectional transport by GLUT 1 allows GLUT 1 to enhance inward transport of glucose when intracellular demand for glucose is high, for example, during endotoxemia, hypoxia, or increased oxidative stress.[681] Increased expression of GLUT 1 may provide energy to replenish ATP reduced by ethanol administration.

ETHANOL AND OXIDATIVE STRESS

The carbon adjacent to the double bond, especially in a polyunsaturated fatty acid, is highly susceptible to attack by free radicals (R•), which extract a proton, leaving behind a free radical form of the acyl chain (Reaction [9]).[682-688]

$$\text{LIPID-H} + \text{R}\bullet \rightarrow \text{LIPID}\bullet + \text{RH} \qquad [9]$$

O_2 can react with the lipid radical (Reaction [10]) to produce a peroxyradical that can react further with another unsaturated acyl chain (Reaction [11]) to produce

$$\text{LIPID}\bullet + O_2 \rightarrow \text{LIPID-}O_2 \qquad [10]$$

$$\text{LIPID-}O_2\bullet + \text{LIPID-H} \rightarrow \text{LIPID-OOH} + \text{LIPID}\bullet \qquad [11]$$

a lipid peroxide and a new lipid radical. The lipid peroxide can react further with Fe^{2+} and other transition metals to produce new free radicals (Reactions [12] and [13]).

$$\text{Lipid-OOH} + Fe^{2+} \rightarrow Fe^{3+} + OH^- + \text{Lipid-O}\bullet \qquad [12]$$

$$\text{Lipid-OOH} + Fe^{3+} \rightarrow \text{Lipid-}O_2 + H^+ + Fe^{2+} \qquad [13]$$

This chain of radical formation obviously can cause extensive alterations in the lipid regions of membranes. In addition, the free radicals generated in the membrane can react with several functional groups in proteins, thereby altering the function of enzymes. The products of metabolism of the acyl peroxides—for example, reactive aldehyde—also will react with proteins and DNA, causing damage to the cell.[689-692]

The metabolism of many direct hepatotoxins is associated with generation of free radicals and peroxidation of membrane lipids (see Chaps. 26 and 27). Whether or not this kind of mechanism is critical for the initiation of hepatotoxicity is the subject of controversy,[689-692] but there is a fair amount of evidence to indicate that peroxidation of lipids at least contributes to the overall hepatotoxicity of many agents. Prior treatment with antioxidants diminishes the hepatotoxicity of carbon tetrachloride, for example.[693]

Normal metabolism within the liver cell also gives rise constantly to toxic forms of O_2.[683,684,694,695] The superoxide anion of O_2 ($O_2^-\bullet$) is the most abundant of these. It is produced by a variety of flavin dehydrogenase enzymes and by cytochrome P450 (see Figure 29-14) (see Chap. 8).[684,685,694,695] The does not seem to be directly toxic, but it reacts with H_2O_2 to produce hydroxyl free radicals (•OH) (Reaction [14]).

$$O_2\bullet + H_2O_2 \rightarrow O_2 + OH^- + \bullet OH \qquad [14]$$

Reaction [14] requires a catalyst in vivo, which probably is a form of Fe^{3+}.[153] The H_2O_2 for Reaction [14] can be produced by many flavoprotein oxidases (Reaction [5]). The hydroxyl radical (•OH) is the proximate, toxic form of O_2.

The superoxide anion is detoxified by the enzyme superoxide dismutase (Reaction [15]), which is distributed widely in tissues.[684-688]

$$2\,O_2^-\bullet + 2\,H^+ \rightarrow H_2O_2 + O_2 \qquad [15]$$

H_2O_2 produced in other reactions is detoxified by catalase and glutathione peroxidase (Reaction [16]).[6]

$$\text{ROOH} + \text{GSH} \rightarrow \text{ROH} + \text{GSSG} + H_2O \qquad [16]$$

Oxidant-antioxidant Imbalance in ALD

A significant body of evidence supports increased production of reactive O_2 intermediates in alcohol-induced liver injury.[697,698] Enhanced ethanol-dependent lipid peroxidation has been confirmed by many but not all investigators.[699-701] A number of possible reasons may account for observed discrepancies (Table 29-7).[702]

The possible mechanisms by which ethanol promotes oxidative stress and sources of free radicals in the liver are listed in Table 29-8. Currently the main candidates for oxidative stress generated by ethanol metabolism include superoxide, a dioxygen molecule with an additional electron, H_2O_2, hydroxyl radical (•OH), and alcohol-derived free radical (hydroxyethyl radical). Acetaldehyde also can generate free radicals when oxidized by xanthine oxidase.[703]

TABLE 29-7

Variables that May Account for the Controversies Regarding the Role of Free Radicals and Lipid Peroxidation in Ethanol-induced Liver Injury

Variable	Comments
Acute versus chronic	Lipid peroxidation occurs more readily during acute rather than chronic administration of ethanol
	Dose of alcohol varies
Nature of diet	Use of liquid diets of variable composition
	Use of ethanol in drinking water
Controls	Chow-fed or controls pair-fed dextrose
Nutritional state of animal	Fed versus starved
	Duration of ethanol administration
Parameter assayed	TBARS, conjugated dienes, alkanes, fatty acid composition, free radicals, chemiluminescence, and DNA cleavage
	Presence of iron or buffers to remove endogenous iron
Organelle assayed	Whole liver homogenate, isolated microsomes or mitochondrial fractions
Presence/absence of pathologic changes (e.g., fatty liver, inflammation)	Contribution by lipids and inflammatory cells to generation of reactive oxygen intermediates

Modified from Cederbaum AI: Introduction: role of lipid peroxidation and oxidative stress in alcohol toxicity. Free Radic Biol Med 7:537, 1989.
TBARS, Thiobarbituric acid reacting substances; *DNA*, deoxyribonucleic acid.

TABLE 29-8

Possible Mechanisms by which Ethanol Promotes Oxidative Stress and Sources of Free Radicals

Organelle	Enzyme Substrate	Free Radical
Microsomes	Cytochrome P450 2E1	$O_2^-\bullet$ (superoxide)
		$\bullet CHOHCH_3$ (1-hydroxyethyl)
		$\bullet CH_2CH_2OH$ (2-hydroxyethyl)
		$CH_3CH_2O\bullet$ (ethoxy)
	Cytochrome P450 reductase	$O_2^-\bullet$
	Membrane lipids	Lipid-derived (probably involves CYP 2E1)
Mitochondria	Respiratory chain	H_2O_2, $O_2^-\bullet$
Peroxisomes	Peroxisomal beta oxidation	H_2O_2
Cytosol	Xanthine oxidase	$O_2^-\bullet$, H_2O_2
	Aldehyde oxidase	$O_2^-\bullet$, H_2O_2
Nuclei	NADPH and NADH-cytochrome c reductase	$O_2^-\bullet$

Importance of Microsomes

In the presence of NADPH, microsomes from ethanol-fed rats generate increased amounts of reactive intermediates of O_2.[704,705] Increases of a lesser magnitude occur with NADH as the reductant.[706] In the presence of transition metals, especially iron (see also subsection on iron), microsomes catalyze the production of potent oxidizing species that initiate lipid peroxidation.[707] Microsomes isolated from livers of rats treated chronically with ethanol generate $O_2^-\bullet$ and H_2O_2 at elevated rates compared with pair-fed controls.[704,708] In the presence of iron, microsomes from ethanol-treated rats are more reactive in generating •OH and in catalyzing lipid peroxidation.[707] Another free radical, the α-hydroxyethyl radical, is derived from the one-electron oxidation of ethanol in microsomes.[709]

Most reactive O_2 produced in microsomes from ethanol-fed rats appears to be generated through the cytochrome P450 system (Figure 29-15).[710] Using a DNA-strand cleavage assay for detection of hydroxyl radicals, the increased generation of •OH in the presence of NADPH and NADH was found to be due, at least in part, to induction of CYP.[711] The DNA-strand cleavage assay also showed that NADH supported microsomal production of reactive species of O_2, although not as effectively as NADPH. This observation is important in view of the reduction of the NAD^+/NADH redox state during oxidation of ethanol by alcohol dehydrogenase. Because generation of •OH radical was inhibited by catalase and superoxide dismutase, H_2O_2 and O_2 are probably important in the overall reaction. Induction of CYP 2E1 leading to increased production of O_2 radicals is also supported by studies showing that the increase in lipid per-

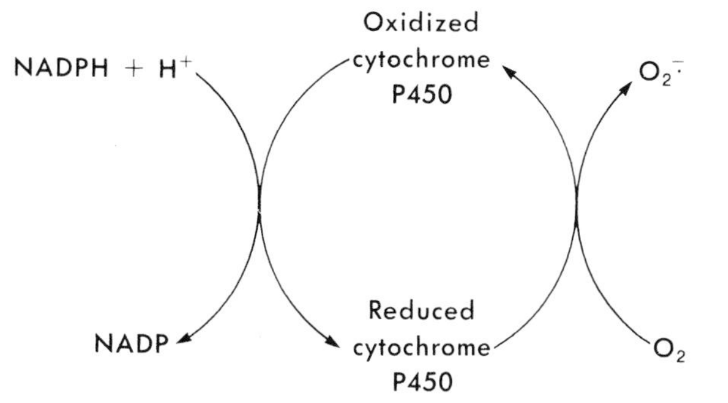

NADPH + H+
Oxidized cytochrome P450
O_2^{-}
NADP
Reduced cytochrome P450
O_2

Figure 29-15 The generation of a toxic oxygen radical.

oxidation can be blocked by anti-P450 2E1 IgG[620] and other inhibitors of CYP 2E1[712] (see Chap. 8). A prominent role for CYP 2E1 does not exclude, however, the contribution of the peroxidase activities of other forms of P450.[713]

Hydroxyl radicals can be generated in microsomes by NADPH cytochrome P450 reductase. This flavoenzyme produces superoxide, which can generate •OH through an iron-catalyzed, Haber-Weiss reaction.[714] Enhanced reductase activity has been described after chronic intake of ethanol.[715] The exact nature of the iron derivative active in vivo remains to be determined. However, stimulation of •OH production is observed readily in the presence of ferric complexes such as ferric-EDTA. This is more difficult to study in the presence of physiologic ferric chelates such as ferric-ATP, ferric-citrate, or ferric-histidine. With the DNA-strand cleavage assay concentrations of ferric-histidine as low as 0.5 μm were catalytically more reactive in the NADPH-dependent reaction compared with NADH.[711] Because NADPH is the preferred co-factor for donating electrons to cytochrome P450 (at least for the first electron), the increased effectiveness of NADPH, compared with NADH, is not surprising.

The spin-trapping method is useful for studying mechanisms of free radical formation in alcohol-fed animals. The principle of spin-trapping is reaction of a highly reactive radical with a spin-trapping agent to form a secondary, more stable radical referred to as a "spin adduct." Electroparamagnetic resonance studies are then with the relatively long-lived spin adduct to characterize the free radical intermediates with which the "trap" reacted. Spin-trapping experiments demonstrate that hepatic microsomes metabolize ethanol to the 1-hydroxyethyl radical in a reaction that requires NADPH.[709,716,717] The formation of 1-hydroxyethyl radical increases with the concentration of ethanol added to microsomes, and the production of this radical is greater in ethanol-fed rats as compared with controls and is highly sensitive to agents that chelate iron. Inhibition of radical formation from ethanol by chelators of iron and inhibitors of catalase suggests that some ethanol radicals might be generated through a hydroxyl radical intermediate or by another, highly reactive, iron-oxygen complex. The chemical nature of iron-containing oxidants is unknown, but the ferryl ion has been suggested as one intermediate.[718] Thus it appears that at least two pathways generate 1-hydroxyethyl radicals from ethanol. One involves •OH radicals in a Fenton-type reaction from endogenously formed H_2O_2. The other is cytochrome P450–mediated.[717] Formation of hydroxyethyl radical has been assessed in the intragastric feeding model using spin trapping in vitro and immunohistochemical staining for hydroxyethyl radicals bound covalently to microsomal protein.[719] A sevenfold increase in radical formation occurred in ethanol-fed rats compared with controls. When induction of CYP 2EI by ethanol was inhibited by treatment with diallylsulfide or phenyethylisothiocyanate, there was a marked reduction in the generation of hydroxyethyl radicals.[720] Furthermore, a significant correlation was observed between the content of CYP 2E1 in liver microsomes of ethanol-fed and inhibitor-treated groups and capacity for generating hydroxyethyl radicals. A similar correlation between content of CYP 2E1 and degree of spin-trapping of hydroxyethyl radical was also seen in human liver microsomes.[720] Destruction of Kupffer cells with gadolinium chloride reduced formation of hydroxyethyl radical in ethanol-fed rats.[721] The exact role of the Kupffer cell in generation of hydroxyethyl radical is unknown, and little is known about whether gadolinium chloride affects the function of liver microsomes. The significance of CYP 2E1 for generating hydroxyethyl radicals in humans was investigated in alcoholics by measuring oxidation of chlorox-azone (measure of CYP 2E1 activity in vivo).[722] IgG-reactive hydroxyl radical-protein adducts were detected only in alcoholics with increased CYP 2E1 activity; adducts were absent in patients with normal CYP 2E1 activity.

The mechanism by which hydroxyethyl radicals contributes to liver injury is unclear. Chemically generated hydroxyethyl radicals react with glutathione, ascorbic acid, and α-tocopherol[723] and hence are likely to deplete anti-oxidants in liver.

Caution should be exercised in interpreting results from spin-trapping studies. 5,5-Dimethylpyroline-N-oxide interacts with Fe^{3+} to produce a signal that is indistinguishable from that of the •OH radical adduct[724]; α-(4-pyridyl 1-oxide)-N-t-butylnitrone) interacts with Fe^{3+} to yield 1-hydroxyethyl radicals that are not necessarily part of the biologic system under study.[725] The concentration of phosphate buffer used in the spin-trapping experiments also markedly influences the rates of free radical formation in microsomes isolated from ethanol-fed rats.[726]

Importance of Mitochondria

Generation of superoxide radicals results from the activity of the mitochondrial respiratory chain. The presence of several electron carriers and membranes rich in polyunsaturated fatty acids makes this organelle highly susceptible to attack by free radicals. Because mitochondria contain an active superoxide dismutase, they can generate hydrogen peroxide that can be metabolized by mitochondrial glutathione peroxidase. However, in the presence of iron, a portion of the H_2O_2 can generate free radicals. These may damage mitochondrial structure and function.

Production of superoxide by liver mitochondria is increased after an acute load of ethanol.[727] Increased generation of superoxide does not adversely affect the mitochondrial electron transport chain, however. Chronic ethanol consumption, on the other hand, results in decreased production of both superoxide[728] and H_2O_2 by mitochondria.[729] It thus appears that liver mitochondria cannot be implicated as a major source of free radicals after chronic feeding of ethanol.

Short-term treatment of hepatocytes with ethanol decreases the mitochondrial membrane potential and increases mitochondrial permeability.[730] The mitochondrial changes in ethanol-exposed hepatocytes correlate with decreased mitochondrial glutathione levels. Decreased mitochondrial glutathione enhances apoptosis and DNA fragmentation in hepatocytes exposed to ethanol.[731] In alcohol-induced fatty liver, mitochondria exhibit ultrastructural abnormalities, including swelling and disruption of the inner membrane.[732] These anatomic abnormalities correlate with biochemical abnormalities, which include inhibition of mitochondrial respiration, increased mitochondrial oxidants, depletion of mitochondrial glutathione, and DNA deletions.[730] These abnormalities enhance hepatocyte cell death in response to TNFα; normal hepatocytes are resistant to TNFα.[733] The exact molecular mechanisms by which ethanol contributes to enhance vulnerability of hepatocytes to TNFα is unknown.

Importance of Peroxisomes

Catalase plays a minor role in alcohol metabolism in the absence of fatty acids (see also discussion of catalase in section on ethanol oxidation).[734] Oxidation of ethanol can be stimulated significantly by the addition of fatty acids, however; the magnitude of the stimulation is dependent on the chain length of the fatty acid.[735] It may be hypothesized, therefore, that a portion of the H_2O_2 produced inside the peroxisomes during beta oxidation of fatty acids contributes in the presence of iron to the generation of toxic free radicals.

Because chronic treatment with ethanol increases the lipid content in pericentral regions of the liver, elevated substrate supply for peroxisomal beta oxidation could enhance production of H_2O_2 and cause oxidative stress leading to hepatocellular damage. In a study in which tissue cylinders were isolated from pericentral and periportal regions of the liver, generation of H_2O_2 was approximately four times higher in the pericentral region compared with the periportal region.[736] This increase was due at least in part to elevated rates of peroxisomal beta oxidation of fatty acids. Acyl CoA oxidase activity was increased significantly only in the pericentral regions of the liver from ethanol-treated rats. Elevated levels of lipid in the pericentral regions, resulting from ethanol treatment, also contribute by providing substrate for peroxisomal beta oxidation. Thus higher rates of H_2O_2 generation in pericentral areas most likely occur because of increased availability of fatty acid substrate and elevated acyl CoA oxidase activity. In a study in which total liver rather than different regions was examined, acyl CoA oxidase was not affected by chronic administration of ethanol.[737]

Cytosol

The possibility that acetaldehyde contributes to an ethanol-induced increase in free radical generation is based on studies demonstrating that acetaldehyde increases the production of alkanes,[738,739] anti-oxidant-sensitive respiration[740] in perfused rat liver, and lipid peroxidation in isolated hepatocytes.[741] Administration of acetaldehyde to rats increases hepatic lipid peroxidation and decreases hepatic GSH.[742] Inhibition of lipid peroxidation by 4-methylpyrazole, an inhibitor of alcohol dehydrogenase, also provides evidence for a role for acetaldehyde in ethanol-induced lipid peroxidation.[743] It should be noted, however, that the specificity of alkyl pyrazoles as inhibitors of alcohol dehydrogenase has been questioned. Inhibition of cytochrome P450[744] and the catalase-H_2O_2 complex[745] by 4-methylpyrazole and its metabolites has been demonstrated. Furthermore, inhibition of fatty acyl CoA synthase by 4-methylpyrazole reduces the availability of H_2O_2 for catalase-dependent ethanol metabolism and for free radical generation.[746]

The best-characterized cytosolic oxidase that produces toxic species of O_2 is the xanthine oxidase–xanthine dehydrogenase system. In mammalian tissues xanthine oxidase exists as an NAD-dependent dehydrogenase (xanthine dehydrogenase, XDH) that can be converted into an oxidase form (xanthine oxidase, XO). The activity of XDH, which does not produce superoxide normally, prevails over that of XO in the liver.[747,748] Acute and repeated exposure to ethanol favors the conversion of XDH to XO.[749-751] This effect of ethanol may be related to hypoxia, which converts XDH to XO,[747] and to inhibition of XDH activity by an increase in the NADH/NAD ratio.[748] XO produces superoxide with acetaldehyde as a substrate.[752,753] This reaction has been considered to be a possible source of free radicals during exposure to ethanol.[749,750] However, unrealistically high concentrations of acetaldehyde are needed, and the in vitro systems lack ADH activity.[752,754] Concentrations of acetaldehyde in liver after ethanol administration (0.1 to 0.2 mm)[755] are extremely low compared with the concentration required for half-maximal velocity of XO (K_m greater than 30 mm) with acetaldehyde as substrate.[756] Cyanamide, an inhibitor of ALDH, reduced lipid peroxidation despite increased hepatic levels of acetaldehyde.[757] The investigators concluded that acetaldehyde was not a substrate for free radical production by XO in vivo. Their proposed mechanism for generation of free radicals by xanthine oxidase required inhibition of XDH by NADH (generated by ethanol metabolism) and the provision of breakdown products of purine metabolism (hypoxanthine and xanthine) as substrates for XO. An increase in purine degradation leading to increased concentration of substrates for free radical formation,[758] together with the higher activity of ADH[759,760] and xanthine oxidase[761] in the centrolobular area of the liver, would support lipid peroxidation as a mechanism leading to centrolobular liver injury.

Besides XO, another closely related molybdo-flavo enzyme (aldehyde oxidase) with a low K_m for acetaldehyde (1 mm) should be considered as a source of free radicals.[762] Tungstate, which inhibits both aldehyde oxidase and XO, reduces lipid peroxidation to a greater extent in rat hepatocytes than does allopurinol, which inhibits XO only.[763]

Liver Anti-oxidant Enzymes

The first line of defense against O_2 radicals is cytochrome oxidase and comparable enzymes that carry out the reduction of O_2 intermediates to water. The second line of defense is enzymes that remove the intermediates of dioxygen reduction. These enzymes include catalase, superoxide dismutase (SOD), and enzymes of the glutathione redox cycle, which are the primary intracellular, anti-oxidant defense mechanisms to cope with increased oxidant stress. They eliminate $O_2^-\bullet$ and hydroperoxides that can oxidize cellular substrates.

Catalase is a 240,000-MW tetrameric hemoprotein that catalyzes the decomposition of H_2O_2 to water. Catalase has appreciable reductive activity only for small molecules such as H_2O_2 and methyl or ethyl hydroperoxides. It does not metabolize large molecular peroxides, as for example, the lipid hydroperoxide products of lipid peroxidation.[764] Catalase is highly compartmentalized in mammalian cells; in hepatocytes, peroxisomes exhibit the highest catalase activity although activity is found also in microsomes and cytosol.[764]

The key enzyme for reduction of hydroperoxides is glutathione peroxidase (GSH-P_x), which is a 85,000-Kd tetrametric protein with four atoms of selenium bound as selenocysteine.[765,766] GSH-P_x requires glutathione as co-substrate and uses organic hydroperoxides (reaction [16]) as preferred substrates over H_2O_2 (reaction [17]).

$$2GSH + H_2O_2 \xrightarrow{\text{GSH-Pzx}} GSSG + 2H_2O \qquad [17]$$

GSH-P_x is bound tightly to GSH reductase, predominantly in the cytosol.

Two classes of SODs occur in eukaryotes.[767] Mn-containing SODs are present primarily in the mitochondrial matrix but are found in the cytosol as well. CuZnSOD is present mainly in the cytosol, but is found also in the nucleus. These two different forms of SOD promote the same biochemical reaction: the dismutation of the superoxide anion to H_2O_2 and O_2. Hydrogen peroxide is removed by hydroperoxidases such as GSH-P_x.

The effect of ethanol on the activity of anti-oxidant enzymes in the liver is dependent on whether ethanol is given acutely or chronically. Acute administration of ethanol decreases the activity of catalase, which precedes the decrease in CuZnSOD activity.[768,769] This is likely to be related to the effect of superoxide in inactivating catalase[770] and hydrogen peroxide in inactivating CuZnSOD.[771] GSH-P_x activity is not altered by acute treatment with ethanol.[772] In rats fed alcohol chronically, decreased activities of catalase and CuZnSOD[773,774] are observed. In the pig model for alcoholism a decrease in GSH-P_x and CuZnSOD but an increase in MnSOD activities is seen.[775,776] These results have been interpreted to mean that a compromised anti-oxidant defense system leads to increased oxidative damage in alcoholic liver injury. We note, however, that significant pathologic liver injury was not present in any of the animal models studied.

In an attempt to study the regulation of the various anti-oxidant enzymes in relationship to liver pathology and lipid peroxidation, mRNA levels of catalase, GSH-P_x, and MnSOD were studied in different dietary models for intragastric feeding of ethanol. The highest levels of mRNA for catalase and GSH-P_x occurred in animals with the most severe liver injury, and levels of H_2O_2 and conjugated dienes correlated with the increase in catalase and GSH-P_x mRNA.[777] These observations are consistent with an ethanol-induced increase in both production of H_2O_2 and catalase activity in rat liver.[778] The increases in mRNAs for anti-oxidant enzymes are probably a compensatory response to enhanced oxidative stress.

A decrease in MnSOD mRNA was seen only in rats exhibiting pathologic liver injury. Although the mechanism leading to a decrease in MnSOD mRNA is unknown, it could be extremely important in view of the known relationship between MnSOD and cytotoxicity of TNF.[779-781] Cells expressing increased mRNA for MnSOD are resistant to TNF cytotoxicity, for example, whereas cells with lower expression of MnSOD are extremely sensitive to TNF.[779-781] Cytotoxicity of TNF can be mediated through induction of oxidative radicals such as $O_2^-\bullet$, H_2O_2, and $\bullet OH$.[782] TNF is important in clinical and experimental ALD.[783-785] The association of low levels of MnSOD mRNA and enhanced cytotoxicity mediated by TNF provides an additional explanation for the importance of mitochondrial injury in ALD. The decrease in MnSOD mRNA and increase in TNF are seen after 1 month of ethanol feeding and can explain why mitochondrial abnormalities are among the earliest lesions during administration of ethanol.[786] The increase in GSH-P_x and catalase may protect the cell against injury and delay the onset of pathologic alterations. Increased hepatic cytosolic glutathione-S-transferase activity (GST) has been reported to be associated with chronic ethanol feeding.[787,788] GST shares the characteristic of inducibility with the microsomal drug-metabolizing enzymes.[789] An ethanol-induced increase in GST activity in the perivenous region coincides with the induction of CYP 2E1 in the same region,[790] suggesting that the increase in GST could reflect an attempt by the cells to adapt to increased production of reactive products secondary to induction of CYP 2E1.

No single defect in hepatic anti-oxidant enzyme defense is seen consistently in ethanol-fed animals.

GSH

GSH is the most abundant non-protein thiol in cells. It is crucial in anti-oxidant defense and detoxification of xenobiotics.[791-793] In most cells the intracellular concentration of GSH is maintained in the range between 0.5 and 10 mm, and less than 5 percent of GSH is in the oxidized state. In hepatocytes cytosolic GSH accounts for 90 percent of total GSH, with the remainder in mitochondria. Mitochondrial GSH is derived from the cytosol by way of a mitochondrial transporter.[794-796] The cellular level of GSH is determined by a balance of its rates of synthesis and utilization by conjugation and loss by export from the cell. Synthesis of GSH from its constituent amino acids requires two ATP steps: (1) formation of γ-glutamylcysteine from glutamate and cysteine and (2) formation of GSH from γ-glutamylcysteine and glycine.[797] The rate of GSH synthesis is determined by the availability of cysteine and the activity of the rate-limiting enzyme, γ-glutamylcysteine synthase (GCS).

A decrease in the level of GSH is one of the most constant changes in liver anti-oxidants induced by an acute load of ethanol.[798-800] The mechanisms responsible for the decrease are probably multi-factorial because the decline in GSH can be prevented by the administration of an iron chelator such as desferrioxamine or by a non-steroidal anti-inflammatory drug such as piroxicam.[801]

There is little agreement, however, on the effects of chronic administration of ethanol on hepatic GSH content. Some investigators report no change[802]; others have found GSH either decreased[803] or increased.[804] In models in which levels of GSH decrease, there is increased sinusoidal efflux and not biliary secretion[805]; efflux of GSH from hepatocytes of ethanol-fed rats is greater than for controls because of a decrease in K_m for transport of GSH.[805] Decrease in concentration of GSH, secondary to ethanol ingestion, is not caused by a limitation on enzymatic capacity for resynthesis. The activity of γ-glutamylcysteine synthetase, which is the rate-limiting enzymatic step in synthesis of GSH, is affected minimally by ethanol, as is the transsulfuration pathway.[806] However, hepatic GCS activity is increased in the rats fed ethanol intragastrically.[807] This increased GCS activity is due mainly to the increase in level of the heavy subunit of GCS.[807] On the other hand, there is diminished availability of precursors to maintain synthesis of GSH, for example, decreased synthesis of serine, after administration of ethanol.[808]

Using the Lieber-DeCarli model a 40 percent to 50 percent decrease in mitochondrial GSH has been observed in isolated hepatocytes and in vivo.[809] Using the intragastric feeding model a progressive decrease was seen in mitochondrial GSH (39 percent decrease at 3 weeks, 61 percent at 6 weeks, and 85 percent at 16 weeks). In contrast, modest decreases (28 percent to 39 percent) in cytosolic GSH occurred when concentrations were expressed per gram of liver.[810] Depletion of mitochondrial GSH is more severe in perivenous than periportal cells in ethanol-fed rats, and the degree of depletion correlates with the decrease in levels of ATP and mitochondrial membrane potential.[811]

The change in mitochondrial GSH is an important contributor to liver injury after chronic feeding of ethanol.[805,809] GSH in mitochondria is a key component for protecting the cell against the reactive metabolites of O_2 that are generated in the electron transport chain.[806] Because mitochondria do not contain catalase (the only exception being heart mitochondria), the GSH redox system is the only mitochondrial defense for metabolism of reactive O_2.[809] It is not surprising that decreasing concentrations of GSH in mitochondria precede the loss of mitochondrial function and histologic evidence of liver injury. Raising the concentration of GSH in the cytosol of hepatocytes of ethanol-fed rats does not yield a significant increase in mitochondrial GSH, however.[809,811] Glutathione ethylester, a more permeable form of GSH, increases mitochondrial GSH, but its potential toxicity may limit its usefulness.[812]

S-Adenosyl-L-Methionine

Methionine adenosyl transferase (MAT) is an essential enzyme that catalyzes the only reaction that generates S-adenosylmethionine (SAM). SAM is the principal methyl donor and precursor for polyamine synthesis.[813] In mammals two genes—MAT 1A and MAT 2A—encode for two homologous MAT catalytic subunits α1 and α2.[814] MAT 1A is expressed only in the liver. Rats fed ethanol intragastrically show induction of mRNA of both isoforms of MAT.[710c] However, only the protein level of the non-liver-specific MAT is increased. S-adenosyl-L-methionine (adomet) is the principal methylating agent in transmethylation reactions of proteins and nucleic acids. Biosynthesis of phosphatidylcholine uses methionine, through its activated form of adomet, to sequentially methylate membrane-bound phosphatidylethanolamine. [816] Adomet also is important in the synthesis of polyamines and provides a source of cysteine for synthesis of GSH. Ethanol feeding increases the hepatic activities of enzymes involved in methionine catabolism, specifically Adomet synthase and cystathionine synthase, and decreases methionine synthase.[817] These changes impair conservation of methionine by committing it to the catabolic and transsulfuration pathways. Ethanol administration is associated with decreased hepatic levels of adomet in the rat,[818] baboon,[819] and man.[820]

Depletion of GSH or adomet by ethanol is reversed by administration of adomet in the baboon[819] and human alcoholics.[821] In addition to causing deficiency of GSH, adomet deficiency enhances the vulnerability of rats to TNF-mediated hepatotoxicity.[822] Compared with methionine administration, adomet has the advantage of bypassing the ethanol-induced deficit in synthesis of adomet from methionine. In rats, decreased formation of methionine through the N^5-tetrahydrofolate pathway after long-term consumption of alcohol is compensated for by an adaptive increase in the activity of betaine-homocysteine methyltransferase, which uses betaine as a methylating agent to help maintain hepatic levels of methionine and adomet.[823] Even though the rat can produce sufficient betaine to meet its normal requirements via oxidation of choline, this amount of betaine is apparently inadequate to maintain levels of adomet during administration of ethanol; feeding betaine generates a level of adomet that is sufficient to protect against alcohol-induced fatty infiltration in the rat.[824] Adomet supplementation in the baboon has no effect on ethanol-induced steatosis. The differences are likely to be species-related. Administration of adomet to ethanol-fed rats causes significant increases in concentrations of GSH in cytosol and mitochondria in both perivenous and periportal cells.[825] Adomet, in addition to being a precursor of GSH in the rat, restores and stabilizes ethanol-induced abnormalities in the physical properties of membranes.

Role of Iron in the Generation of Free Radicals in the Liver of Ethanol-fed Rats

Clinical experience suggests a synergistic hepatotoxic effect between alcohol and iron overload.[826-828] Hepatic iron overload is observed in about 30 percent of alcoholics.[828] To explain increased iron storage in livers of alcoholics, attention has focused on transferrin. Several groups report increased concentrations of abnormal transferrin molecules, i.e., molecules with a reduced content of sialic acid in the serum of alcoholics.[824-831] Studies in vivo with asialotransferrin from humans or rats show an increased uptake of iron by rat liver from iron bound to asialotransferrin as compared with transferrin.[832,833] Short-term exposure of freshly isolated rat hepatocytes to ethanol depresses uptake of iron from transferrin[834,835] by an effect mediated through ADH-catalyzed metabolism of alcohol. Long-term exposure of hepatocytes to ethanol depresses hepatocyte uptake of iron from asialotransferrin and transferrin.[836,837] In contrast to these studies in vitro Rouach and associates found a significant increase in uptake of radiolabeled iron by the liver in rats given an acute ethanol load.[838] These investigators proposed that either a modification of transferrin structure by endothelial cells or a reduction in the amount of iron associated with transferrin, produced by NADH during oxidation of ethanol, was responsible for enhanced uptake of iron, and that one of these effects was necessary before the iron could be taken up by the liver.

One facet of disordered iron metabolism in alcoholics is a contribution of iron-mediated lipid peroxidation to alcoholic liver injury. The mechanistic connection between ethanol and toxicity of iron is that iron catalyzes the formation of free radicals and thereby can enhance the oxidative stress on liver cells resulting from ethanol alone. The synergistic effect of ethanol and iron on liver injury was studied in patients with hereditary hemochromatosis who also abused alcohol.[839] Protein adducts with MDA and hydroxynonenal were localized to zone 1 hepatocytes in patients with hemochromatosis and followed the distribution of storage iron. As expected, the aldehyde adducts were found in zone 3 in alcohol abusers. In patients with hemochromatosis who abused alcohol the adducts were more abundant and panlobular in distribution.

Iron within the liver (see Chap. 14) is found in several biochemical forms such as ferritin, hemosiderin, and heme, and in the putative "intracellular low-molecular weight" chelate pool.[840,841] Although the identity of this intracellular low-molecular weight iron is not firmly established, iron apparently is bound to weak chelators, for example, AMP and ATP. Iron in this form catalyzes formation of hydroxyl radical. An important factor is the influence of ethanol on the distribution of iron in the liver.[842]

There is no consistency in results from experiments to determine the effects of acute administration of ethanol on the concentration of non-heme iron in liver.[843-845] Chronic feeding of ethanol has been shown generally, however, to increase the non-heme iron in liver in rodents.[846-848] An increase in non-heme iron also has been shown to occur in the presence of ischemia,[849,850] which may contribute to ALD.[851] Moreover, a proposed mechanism for the increase in the pool of non-heme iron during hypoxia is via formation of reducing equivalents, which mobilize iron from ferritin.[852] Of note is that oxidation of ethanol via alcohol dehydrogenase and MEOS generates reducing equivalents.[851] Another molecule mobilizing iron from ferritin is superoxide,[853,854] and superoxide-induced mobilization of iron is enhanced by hypoxia.[855] But there is evidence for[856] and against[857,858] a role for superoxide in releasing iron from ferritin.

Further support for the role of iron in alcoholic liver injury comes from studies to prevent liver injury with chelators of iron. An oral iron chelator, 1,2 dimethyl-3-hydroxypyrid-4-one, reduced free iron in liver, lipid peroxidation, and accumulation of fat in rats fed ethanol chronically.[848] In contrast, a parenterally administered chelator (hydroxyethylstarch-deferoxamine) enhanced lipid peroxidation and the severity of liver injury in rats fed ethanol chronically.[859] Perhaps desferrioxamine forms radicals itself that enhance liver injury.[860-862] Another mechanism by which iron may play a key role in alcoholic liver injury is through formation of lipid neutrophil chemoattractants.[863] The formation of these chemoattractants involves oxyradicals. The generation of these chemoattractants is inhibited by •OH scavengers but enhanced when rat liver cytosol is deficient in GSH.[864] Chemoattractant production is virtually undetectable when the iron chelator desferrioxamine is added to cultures of iron-loaded cells.[863]

Vitamin E

Vitamin E is a general term that refers to different tocopherols and tocotrienols.[865,866] Alpha-tocopherol (α-Toc) is the biologically most active form of vitamin E and is a major anti-oxidant in cell membranes. α-Toc is viewed as the "last line of defense" against peroxidation of membrane lipids. α-Toc, by donating a hydrogen atom, acts as a chain reaction terminator and functions as a scavenger of free radicals. In addition to its anti-oxidant function, vitamin E influences the cellular response to oxidative stress through modulation of signal-transduction pathways.[866] Several investigators have shown a reduction in levels of α-Toc in plasma and liver after ethanol feeding.[867-869] The responsible mechanisms are unclear, but include decreased intestinal absorption, impaired uptake of lipoproteins by hepatocytes, increased mobilization of tocopherol from the liver, and increased conversion of α-Toc to α-tocopherol quinone.[867] In the intragastric feeding model of alcoholic injury in the rat the decrease in γ-TOC was greater than the decrease in α-Toc, in both liver and plasma.[870] The levels of α-Toc in liver correlated inversely with the levels of conjugated dienes and thiobarbituric acid reactive substances, suggesting an interconnection between these parameters.[870]

Based on the effect of ethanol on vitamin E, it seems reasonable to propose that addition of vitamin E to the diet will block lipid peroxidation and prevent liver injury. Few studies have addressed, however, whether supplementation with vitamin E reduces liver injury in ethanol-fed rats. Vitamin E supplementation (172 IU of vitamin E/kg diet) has normalized α-Toc levels in ethanol-fed rats.[871] However, no measurements of lipid peroxidation were made.[871] In ethanol-fed rats given extremely high doses of α-Toc acetate (1200 times the normal dietary intake), the high hepatic levels of α-Toc were accompanied by decreased peroxidation of lipids but not by decreased severity of injury.[872] Possibly, α-Toc acetate was not incorporated into intracellular membranes but remained in plasma membranes.[873] Thus Lamb and co-workers,[874] using an in vitro model of ethanol-dependent injury to liver cells, showed that cell viability was improved by supplementation with vitamin E phosphate as compared with cells exposed to α-Toc acetate. These investigators proposed that the phosphate ester of vitamin E partitioned into the phospholipid bilayers of intracellular membranes. There is also evidence that α-Toc acetate does not accumulate at critical sites of cell injury. Vitamin E succinate inhibits lipid peroxidation more effectively as compared with α-Toc acetate because it accumulates at a unique and critical mitochondrial site.[875] Vitamin E administered as a component in liposomes accumulated in Kupffer cells[876] and protected against carbon tetrachloride–induced hepatotoxicity. Thus accumulation of vitamin E at critical sites in liver organelles, such as mitochondria and in Kupffer cells, may be important for a cytoprotective effect in alcoholic liver injury.

Effect of Ethanol on Protein Metabolism in the Liver

Acute ethanol administration inhibits protein synthesis in vitro in isolated hepatocytes,[877] in perfused livers,[878] and in rat liver in vivo.[879] In humans intravenous infusion of ethanol reduces excretion of nitrogen.[880] The isocaloric replacement of glucose and lipids with ethanol in the diet of normal[881] or alcoholic subjects[882,883] results in negative nitrogen balance and weight loss, despite adequate provision of amino acids in the diet.[884] Ethanol, in amounts consumed during social drinking, decreases the rate of oxidation of leucine and fractional secretory rates of hepatic proteins, albumin, and fibrinogen.[885]

A direct toxic effect of ethanol on protein trafficking in the liver has been demonstrated in vitro and in vivo.[886-888] As early as 1 week after ethanol administration to rats, receptor-mediated endocytosis of asialoglycoproteins is altered.[888] The hepatic uptake of asialoglycoproteins from serum depends on a galactose- specific receptor on the hepatocyte plasma membrane.[889] The receptor binds circulating asialoglycoproteins; the receptor-ligand complexes are then internalized by way of a coated pit-vesicle pathway. The ligand is usually transported to lysosomes for degradation, and the receptor is recycled back to the plasma membrane where it is reinserted.[890,891] Binding, internalization, degradation, receptor-ligand dissociation, and receptor recycling are all impaired in hepatocytes isolated from ethanol-fed animals, and especially in the perivenular region of the liver,[892-894] the site at which ethanol exerts its major toxic effects. Decreased recycling of extracellular matrix receptors has been suggested as one cause of the perturbations of interactions between the hepatocyte and the extracellular matrix in ethanol-fed rats.[893] Ethanol administration also results in hepatic accumulation of protein.[895,896] Decreased proteolysis in lysosomes is considered the responsible primary factor for this accumulation of protein.[897] In turn, decreased levels of proteases within hepatic lysosomes may be due to either decreased synthesis or perturbed trafficking.[898] Ethanol increases protein oxidation in the liver and slows the rate of protein catabolism. Oxidized proteins accumulate in liver because of decreased proteolysis related specifically to multi-catalytic alkaline proteases.[899,900] Degradation of protein substrates by the multi-catalytic protease depends on prior covalent attachment of ubiquitin, which marks a protein for degradation.[901] The 20S proteosome expresses at least three distinct peptidase activities (i.e., chymotrypsin-like [ChT-L], trypsin-like [T-L], and peptidylglutamyl peptide hydrolase). Voluntary ethanol feeding has no effect on the three peptidase activities of the proteosome.[902] In contrast, intragastric ethanol administration for 4 or 8 weeks causes a significant decline in the specific activities of ChT-L and T-L of the multi-catalytic enzyme.[902,903] The decrease in the peptidase activities is probably a result of partial inactivation of the holoenzyme. Oxidative stress generated through cytochrome P450 2E1 is a likely cause of the inhibition of proteolysis of oxidized protein because inhibitors of cytochrome P450 2E1 ameliorate the decline in the peptidase activities.[903]

Effects of Ethanol on Synthesis of Protein by the Liver

Some hepatotoxins are known to be inhibitors of hepatic protein synthesis, and a casual interpretation of this association suggests that the two phenomena are linked. Whether they are or not remains to be determined. Thus inhibiting the synthesis of a given protein will have an impact on the survival of a cell only when that protein is essential for the cell's life. We do not know which cellular proteins are essential for survival of liver cells, although we could make reasonable guesses. We do know, on the other hand, that the liver must have adaptive mechanisms for maintaining its critically important proteins. These mechanisms ensure survival of hepatocytes when conditions for maximal synthesis of proteins are not met—during severe malnutrition, for example. Data relating the toxicity of an agent to an effect on protein synthesis hence must be interpreted cautiously. Finally, although ethanol does inhibit the synthesis of some proteins, this effect is not general. Ethanol, for example, induces the synthesis of xenobiotic-metabolizing enzymes (see the following section on drug metabolism).[904-906]

Effects of Ethanol on Hepatic Detoxification of Xenobiotics

It is clear from the preceding discussion of lipid peroxidation that administration of ethanol will influence the toxicity of xenobiotics simply because ethanol will alter the stress placed on systems that normally protect against liver damage caused by free radicals. In addition, ethanol will alter the metabolism of drugs directly (Table 29-9). Several lines of evidence indicate that this is an important problem for study and one that has more relevance to problems of disease in humans than many other lines of alcohol-related research.

Effects on P450

In humans and experimental animals there is induction of a specific form of P450 that catalyzes, at relatively high rates, the oxidation of ethanol, isoniazid, aniline, acetaminophen, carbon tetrachloride, and several nitrosamines (see Chap. 8).[907-913] This specific form of P450 in humans is designated P450 HL_j.[911] Although it is clear that the P450 HL_j form is increased in humans in response to ethanol, other forms also may be induced. Induction of P450s by ethanol is not limited to the liver,[912,913] which is important medically because the likely connection between alcoholism and the increased incidence of cancer of the head, neck, and colorectal regions in alcoholics is induction by ethanol of cytochrome P450s that metabolize nitrosamines (and perhaps other agents) to proximate carcinogens.[914-917]

Induction of P450 probably is the mechanism by which ethanol enhances the hepatotoxicity of CCl_4 and contributes to the toxicity of acetaminophen (see the following section) and cocaine.[918] In experimental animals, for example, prior treatment with a single dose of ethanol sensitizes the animal to the hepatotoxic effects of CCl_4. The interaction is greatest when the time between administrations of ethanol and CCl_4 is about 18 hours; it is independent of the metabolism of ethanol.[918-923] The ethanol-induced potentiation of toxicity is not limited to CCl_4 but extends to other halogenated hydrocarbons (including halothane), which are also metabolized by the P450 system.[918] The clinical correlate of enhanced toxicity caused by CCl_4 in ethanol-fed animals is that fatal CCl_4 poisoning in people occurs almost exclusively in alcoholics—that is, poisoning is almost never fatal in the non-alcoholic patient.[918] The significance of induction of P450 for acetaminophen-induced hepatotoxicity is more complex than for CCl_4 and is discussed at the end of this section.

TABLE 29-9

Mechanisms by which Ethanol Can Modify the Metabolism of Xenobiotics

Selective induction of specific types of P450
Competitive inhibition of P450
Selective induction of glucuronosyltransferases
Decreased production of UDP-glucuronic acid
Stimulation of acetylation by increasing the hepatic concentration of acetyl CoA

UDP, Uridine diphosphate.

Glucuronosyltransferase and Other Conjugating Reactions

Ethanol appears to be an inducer of this family of enzymes, which also are located in the endoplasmic reticulum of the liver and which represent the most important pathway for detoxification of xenobiotics by conjugation (see Chap. 8). It is not proved, however, that prior administration of ethanol increases the amounts of any type of this enzyme. What is known is that glucuronidating activity, measured with many but not all substrates, is greater in liver microsomes from ethanol-fed rats than in microsomes from controls.[919-922] However, if ethanol is being metabolized, it interferes with glucuronidation in intact animals by decreasing the hepatic concentration of uridine diphosphate-glucuronic acid, probably as a result of the ethanol-induced increase in the ratio of NADH/NAD.[920,923,924]

Ethanol metabolism inhibits sulfation in association with decreases in the hepatic concentration of 3′phosphoadenosine-5′phosphosulfate, which is the sulfodonor in this detoxification reaction.[924] Chronic feeding of ethanol does not depress sulfotransferase activities. On an acute basis ethanol would also be expected to decrease conjugation with GSH because of its effects on the concentration of this intermediate. The effects on conjugation with GSH in chronically treated animals are uncertain, however, because concentrations of GSH are decreased in mitochondria but normal in liver cytosol in these animals.[925] On the other hand, fasting per se leads to a decrease in total hepatic GSH.[926] In the clinical setting, therefore, the effects of chronic intake of alcohol on conjugation with GSH could be mediated by the influence of alcohol on nutrition.

Ethanol stimulates acetylation reactions because its metabolism increases concentrations of acetyl CoA in liver (Reaction [2]).[918,927,928] Whether this effect has toxicologic significance—for example, whether increased rates of acetylation contribute to the increased hepatotoxicity of isoniazid in the alcoholic—is unstudied.

Alcohol and the Hepatotoxicity of Acetaminophen

Figure 29-16 depicts the major pathways for metabolism of acetaminophen (see Chaps. 8 and 26). Ethanol should enhance the hepatotoxicity of acetaminophen because it induces the type of P450 that metabolizes acetaminophen to reactive metabolites, it interferes with glucuronidation and sulfation, and at least acutely decreases the hepatic concentration of GSH.

However, ethanol and acetaminophen compete for the same P450, so in the presence of ethanol, metabolism of acetaminophen could be limited. Nevertheless, it is clear that ethanol augments the hepatotoxicity of acetaminophen in small laboratory animals.[918,929,931] The important clinical question is whether ethanol enhances the hepatotoxicity of therapeutic doses of acetaminophen. The answer seems to be yes.[932-934] Several reports have shown that relatively large but therapeutic doses of acetaminophen cause acute hepatotoxicity and death in alcoholics.[932-934] But, in contrast to these data in people, chronic administration of ethanol did not augment the hepatotoxicity of therapeutic amounts of acetaminophen given to baboons.[935] Obviously, we cannot be certain of the significance of these discrepant results in humans and baboons. But it is worthwhile to point out that the environment and dietary intake of the baboons were controlled,[935] whereas those for the patients were not.[932-934] The lesson from comparing the data in patients and experimental animals may be that the true hepatotoxicity of ethanol is much harder to demonstrate in the controlled experiment than in the world of clinical medicine because the hepatotoxicity of ethanol is determined to a considerable degree by undefined factors in a patient's environment and not simply by the intake of ethanol. We will return to this idea in the sections following on animal models and ethanol-nutrient interactions.

Alcohol, Vitamin A, and the Hepatotoxicity of Vitamin A

Vitamin A is not a xenobiotic, but it is hepatotoxic, and its hepatotoxicity is potentiated by ethanol (see Chap. 6). In hypervitaminosis A in rats there is a release of protease from liver lysosomes with swelling of rat liver mitochondria.[936] These phenomena reflect that excessive amounts of vitamin A decrease the stability of biologic membranes.[937,938] Because of interactions between the hydroxyl of retinol and the phosphates in the polar region of the membrane, α-retinol, a biologically inactive analog of vitamin A, has lytic effects on membranes almost identical to those of retinol. Hence the observed surface-active effects of retinol on membranes are not necessarily related to the physiologic action of this vitamin. It is possible also to produce the clinical manifestations of hypervitaminosis A in animals by administering large amounts of all-trans-retinoic acid.[939,940] The 13-cis-retinoic acid has no toxicity.[940]

The recommended daily intake of vitamin A by an adult is 5000 IU per day. Intakes several-fold (>40,000 IU/day) greater than this level, when prolonged for years, may lead to a chronic form of liver disease.[941-948] The amount of vitamin A ingested determines the interval between onset of excess intake and clinical manifestations of liver disease. Indeed, acute vitamin A intoxication occurs after massive intake. This has been reported to occur after ingestion of livers from animals whose livers contain enormous stores of vitamin A, such as fish and the polar bear. The more common cause of intoxication, however, is intake of vitamin A as a medication.

About half the patients with vitamin A intoxication have hepatomegaly and splenomegaly. Some of these patients have cirrhosis, with an elevated wedged hepatic vein pressure and ascites. The morphologic characteristics of the liver are variable in these patients. Changes range from non-specific degeneration to fibrosis to cirrhosis. There may be sclerosis of portal and central veins as well as perisinusoidal fibrosis. The latter changes undoubtedly lead to the associated portal hypertension and ascites. In addition, storage of excess vitamin A in Kupffer cells leads to their swelling, and this may be an additional factor producing sinusoidal hypertension. Dilated vitamin A storage cells are seen typically in liver biopsy specimens from affected patients. Laboratory abnormalities in chronic vitamin A intoxication are not specific. Jaundice, when present, usually is mild.

It is important to appreciate that excess vitamin A causes liver disease that is potentially curable.

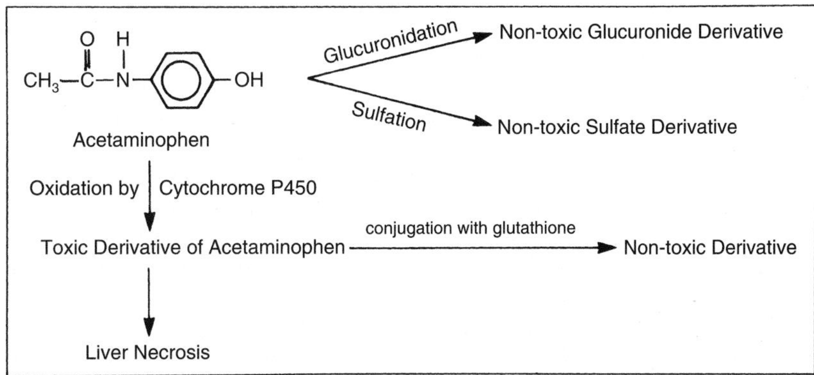

Figure 29-16 Metabolic pathways for the disposition of acetaminophen. Conjugation with glucuronic acid and sulfate is preferred to oxidation by P450; however, interference with the former pathways, and especially with glucuronidation, forces more substrate into the oxidative pathway, which produces toxic intermediates. (From Zakim D: Interface between membrane biology and clinical medicine. Am J Med 80:645, 1986.)

Discontinuation of exposure to excess vitamin A leads in many instances to complete recovery. This is not true, however, for patients in whom the disease has progressed to a cirrhotic stage; the manifestations of vitamin A-induced liver disease can persist in these patients. Nevertheless, it is reasonable to expect that removal of excess vitamin A from the diets of these patients will ameliorate some features of their disease. In addition to liver disease, vitamin A excess causes systemic signs and symptoms—for example, fever, night sweats, anemia, leukopenia, proteinuria, pruritus, loss of head and body hair, and bone pain and tenderness.

Hepatic storage capacity for vitamin A and serum levels of vitamin A-retinol-binding protein are decreased in cirrhotic as well as in many non-cirrhotic forms of liver disease.[949] These changes can account for night blindness in patients with liver disease. In addition, zinc deficiency in cirrhosis can interfere with the metabolism of vitamin A in the retina (alcohol dehydrogenases contain zinc), which can cause night blindness even in the vitamin A-repleted patient.

Chronic ethanol intake reduces the level of retinoids in liver in the rat, baboon, and man.[950-952] This effect occurs in the absence of pathologic changes, but the extent of the decrease from normal increases as patients progress from fatty liver to alcoholic hepatitis to cirrhosis. By contrast, the level of retinol in serum is constant despite progressive reduction in levels of retinoids in liver.[952] Associated with the decrease in total retinoids is a relative increase in retinyl oleate and a relative decrease in retinyl palmitate.[953,954] The status of zinc in experimental animals modulates ethanol-induced changes in the metabolism of vitamin A.[843] Deficiency of zinc diminishes the effect of ethanol on decreasing stores of vitamin A in liver and in epithelial tissues.[955]

The ethanol-induced reduction in hepatic vitamin A is not explained by malnutrition, malabsorption, or reduced uptake via chylomicron remnants. Ethanol administration appears instead to enhance metabolism of retinoic acid (RA) and retinol by microsomal enzymes.[956-960] Increased catabolism of RA to 4-oxo-RA and 4-hydroxy RA after ethanol administration is thought to be a cytochrome P450-dependent process. Cytochrome P450 2E1-catalyzed metabolism is a major pathway for degradation of RA.[961] Studies in vitro with specific inhibitors of CYP 2E1 inhibited RA catabolism by about 75 percent. Nonspecific inhibitors of cytochrome P450 also blocked RA catabolism, suggesting that other CYP 450s contribute to ethanol-induced catabolism of RA. Additionally, there is impaired conversion of carotenoids to retinoids administered to normal subjects.[962] Whereas carotenoid levels correlate with retinoid levels in patients with alcoholic liver cirrhosis,[963] the ratio of hepatic α- and β-carotene to retinoids is abnormally elevated, suggesting impaired conversion.[962] Ethanol feeding also delays the clearance of β-carotene from plasma, resulting in increased β-carotene in liver with a relative lack of a corresponding rise in hepatic retinoids.[964]

A relationship between vitamin A depletion, Ito cell activation, and hepatic fibrosis has been proposed by a number of investigators.[965-967] One possible link between these processes is the up-regulation of RA receptors (RARs) in ethanol-fed mice and rats.[968,969] Up-regulation of RAR-β is seen in ethanol-fed rats that develop severe liver injury.[969] RA, acting via the RARs, can both down-regulate the expression of collagenase and metalloproteinase genes and induce expression of laminin.[970,971] Thus modulation of RAR-β by products of retinoic acid metabolism can modulate genes for components of the extracellular matrix. The increase in expression of RAR-β in ethanol-fed rats may also explain why vitamin A supplementation enhances liver toxicity in these rats.[972] Because RAR-β receptors are ligand-activated, administration of vitamin A or RA is expected to further increase the changes induced by ethanol. Retinoids also modulate the immune functions of macrophages and lymphocytes.[973,974] RA deficiency in hepatic macrophages from ethanol-fed rats leads to increased TNFα synthesis.[975] RA destabilizes TNFα mRNA; therefore, diminished RA would increase TNFα mRNA stability.[975] Studies in rats fed ethanol intragastrically support the inverse relationship between endogenous RA levels and TNFα mRNA stability and the notion that diminished RA signaling may be a causal factor for sustained up-regulation of TNFα expression by hepatic macrophages in alcoholic liver injury.[975]

Some investigators have recommended vitamin A supplementation of alcoholics and patients with chronic liver disease as preventive and curative therapy, but monitoring of serum vitamin A is necessary to limit the risk of toxicity.[976] As noted previously, the recommended daily intake of vitamin A by an adult is 5000 IU per day; intakes several-fold (>40,000 IU/day) greater than this level, when prolonged for years, may lead to a chronic form of liver disease.[941-948,977,978] Vitamin A toxicity is not common in healthy adults given "moderate" supplemental vitamin A, but it is suggested that doses of vitamin A considered safe in healthy adults cause toxicity when consumed by alcoholics. Non-toxic amounts of vitamin A (about 200 U/day or about fivefold greater than amounts usually fed to rats) fed in combination with ethanol are associated with necrosis, inflammation, and fibrosis in rat liver.[972] This interaction between vitamin A and ethanol has not been confirmed by all investigators.[979]

When β-carotene, a precursor of vitamin A, is given to baboons in high doses, the ethanol-induced depletion of total retinoids is not corrected.[964] This is not surprising in view of the ethanol-induced impairment in the conversion of carotenoids to retinoids. In fact, in the baboons fed alcohol with β-carotene, multiple ultrastructural lesions appear, including degenerated mitochondria. Whether the results seen in baboons can be extrapolated to humans deserves further study because, in other primates, similarities and differences with humans with respect to carotene metabolism have been described.[980] Because of the toxicity of β-carotene in baboons, studies were carried out in ethanol-fed rats to determine whether the toxicity was due to the beadlets used as a carrier for β-carotene.[981] Potentiation of hepatic mitochondrial changes, similar to those in baboons, occurred in ethanol-fed rats supplemented with β-carotene in beadlets.[981] Contrary to expectation, β-carotene did not alleviate, but rather potentiated, increases in markers of hepatic lipid peroxidation.

Attempts to correct hepatic depletion of vitamin A in animals fed alcohol were not successful and had deleterious effects on liver mitochondria. The mechanisms for these deleterious effects remain to be determined. The safe amounts of β-carotenoids or retinoids in alcohol abusers is not known; however, maintaining physiologic concentrations of retinoids is potentially important because retinoid deficiency is a factor in the pathogenesis of liver fibrosis.[982] β-Carotene, in the presence of heavy alcohol consumption, must be used with caution.

Immunologic Reactions in Alcoholic Liver Injury

There has been long-term speculation that alcohol-associated liver disease is due in part to immune attack on the liver.[983-987] The proposed mechanisms that could lead to liver disease on this basis are summarized in Table 29-10 (see Chap. 37).

Interactions between CD4 and CD8 lymphocytes and class I and class II major histocompatibility complex (MHC) molecules mediate antigen-dependent cell injury. The liver antigen that is the target of T cells is unknown. However, to postulate the importance of immunologic reactions, one has to demonstrate the presence of modified antigens or neoantigens in hepatocytes or on the liver cell plasma membrane.[988] Several studies show that such antigens are indeed present in ALD. They include adducts between normal proteins and acetaldehyde and hydroxyethyl radicals, which can elicit the response of cytotoxic T lymphocytes.[989]

Cytoxic lymphocytes exert their activity by adhering to target cells. The cell surface antigens important in this process are ICAMs. Thus induction of ICAM-1 mediates adhesion of lymphocytes,[990] and its expression is increased in sinusoidal lining cells and hepatocytes in alcoholic hepatitis.[991] Increased plasma levels of circulating ICAM-1 also are seen in alcoholic cirrhosis.[992]

The demonstration that lymphocytes are present in the livers of alcoholic patients[993] and that these lymphocytes may be activated and liberate chemotactic factors for neutrophils[994] has stimulated investigations to better characterize the lymphocytes in the liver. T lymphocytes, mainly CD8, are the predominant cells in the livers of alcoholics; they also bear the DR marker, which indicates cell activation. CD3 cells expressing $CD4^+$ or $CD8^+$ surface molecules are also increased.[969,984] Efficient lysis of target cells by $CD8^+$ cytotoxic lymphocytes requires that target cells carry class I HLA antigens in addition to specific antigens. In the Veterans Administration cooperative study $CD4^+$ and $CD8^+$ cells were found in large numbers at the interface between necrotic and fibrotic areas, infrequent B cells correlated with portal inflammation, and natural killer cells were absent.[995] The correlation of $CD8^+$ and class II MHC molecules with Mallory bodies suggested an antigenic role for this protein in alcoholic hepatitis. These observations suggest that T-cell-mediated injury may perpetuate ALD through autoimmune mechanisms.[996] Natural killer cells are absent in the liver of patients with ALD, suggesting that they are not important for liver injury.

It has long been known that IgA, IgM, and IgG are elevated in blood of chronic alcoholics, and continuous staining of sinusoids with IgA has been shown repeatedly in patients with ALD.[997,998] Staining with IgA does not correlate with severity of liver disease. It is observed also in patients with fatty liver only. The pathogenetic significance of sinusoidal deposition of IgA is not established, but may be related to the release of TNF by monocytes in alcoholic patients.[999] Because deposition of IgA is seen infrequently in other types of liver disease, it probably represents a specific effect of ethanol on the liver.

TABLE 29-10

Evidence for Derangement of the Immune System in Patients with ALD

Humoral Factors
- Increased levels of IgA and other immunoglobulins
- IgA deposition along liver sinusoids
- Presence of circulating antibodies: anti-nuclear and anti-smooth muscle antibodies
- Antibodies to liver cell membrane, liver-specific protein, and asialoglycoprotein
- Antibodies to protein changed by reaction with acetaldehyde, malondialdehyde, hydroxynonenal, and hydroxyethyl radicals ("neoantigens")
- Antibodies to alcoholic hyalin

Cell-mediated Factors
- Transformation of T cells by acetaldehyde or alcoholic hyalin, producing cytotoxic lymphocytes
- Increased reactivity of T and B cells
- Alcohol promotes expression of MHC class I antigens
- Alcohol and acetaldehyde increase expression of class II (DR) histocompatibility antigens on blood mononuclear cells

Role of Cytokines in Modulating Immune Function
- Reduced proliferative response of T cells to IL-2
- Increased levels of TNF, IL-1, and IL-6
- Blockage of cytokine receptors on macrophages

Other Factors
- Co-existing malnutrition, which affects immune function
- Co-existing viral infections (e.g., hepatitis B and C)

ALCOHOL AND THE CYTOSKELETON

The cytoskeleton has critical significance for the structure and function of the hepatocyte. The hepatocyte cytoskeleton is composed of three major types of filaments: microfilaments consisting of F actin, the intermediate filaments consisting of subunits of cytokeratin, and the microtubules consisting of polymerized tubulin. Many diseases of the liver, the most prominent example being alcoholic hepatitis, are associated with changes in the cytoskeletal network.[1000,1001]

The first indications that microtubules in the liver were affected by ethanol were the observations that ethanol feeding improved the yield of isolated Golgi vesicles from rat liver and that ethanol dramatically increased the number of VLDL particles found in the Golgi apparatus.[1002] The latter effect is similar to that of colchicine, which is an anti-microtubule agent.[1003] Ethanol, as with colchicine, also inhibits the secretion of hepatic proteins,[1004,1005] and the effects of ethanol and colchicine are additive.[1006] The defect in secretion is believed to reflect a decrease in polymerized tubulin. A decrease in tubulin occurs in both experimental and human ALD.[1007,1008] The net effect of the retention of export proteins and fat is the enlargement and ballooning of hepatocytes in rats and man.

Normal liver parenchymal cells from adults have a fairly simple cytokeratin (CK) composition.[1009,1010] They express only one CK pair: CK 8 (a type II CK, MW 52 Kd) and CK 18 (a type I CK, MW 45 Kd). The corresponding CKs in the rat and mouse are sometimes referred to as CK A (MW 55 Kd) and CK D (MW 49 Kd). The cytoskeletal preparations from control hepatocytes show the major cytokeratin proteins: 55 Kd (CK 8), 52 Kd (possibly a degradation product of CK 55), and 49 Kd (CK 18). In ethanol-treated hepatocytes, CK 55 Kd is extensively phosphorylated; CK 52 Kd and CK 49 Kd also show enhanced phosphorylation in this setting.[1011] Phosphorylation of intermediate filaments may lead to their disassembly, thereby altering membrane traffic and secretory functions.

A pathologic phenomenon, in which hepatocyte cytokeratins are altered, is manifested on light microscopy as balloon cell degeneration with or without Mallory bodies.[1012] One of the hallmarks of ALD is the disappearance of the cytokeratin cytoskeleton and the focal aggregation of these filaments to form "alcoholic hyalin" or Mallory bodies in groups of liver cells associated with inflammation and scarring.[1012-1015] The Mallory body, a cytoplasmic inclusion found in swollen, irregularly shaped hepatocytes, stains positively for ubiquitin, for CK 18, and sometimes for CK 7 and 19, but rarely for CK 8.[1011] Hepatocytes not containing Mallory bodies also may stain for CK 7 and CK 19. It is unlikely, however, that this finding (i.e., hepatocytes immunoreactive for these "bile duct types" of CKs) is indicative that Mallory bodies will develop.[1011]

Mallory bodies contain high concentrations of ϵ-(γ-glutamyl)-lysine dipeptides, suggesting increased transglutaminase activity as a mechanism for cross-linking of cytokeratins.[1016] Other changes described in the filaments of Mallory bodies are phosphorylation[1011] and polyubiquitinization.[1017,1018] Ubiquitin is a common component in various types of inclusion bodies derived from intermediate filaments.[1019] It is produced in response to stress, and the ATP-dependent formation of ubiquitin-protein conjugates is a signal for the selective degradation of abnormal proteins.[1019] High molecular weight cytokeratins, a result of covalent cross-linking of normal cytokeratins, also are found in Mallory bodies.[1020,1021] Mallory bodies in hepatocyte cultures incorporate [^{35}S]-methionine at a faster rate than normal intermediate filaments in the same cell, suggesting that Mallory bodies are incorporating cytokeratin monomers at an accelerated rate.[1022] Also, CK 8, CK 18, and actin exhibit modifications in phosphorylation.[1023] Recently, the induction of Mallory bodies has been associated with expression of heat shock proteins (HSP).[1024] In the intragastric feeding model of alcoholism an increase in HSP70 mRNA correlated with severity of liver injury and lipid peroxidation.[1025] The levels of HSP70 protein were no different in ethanol-fed and control groups, however, which suggests that binding of HSP70 protein to damaged proteins decreased the concentration of "free" HSP70 protein and that this, in turn, stimulated synthesis of HSP70 mRNA.

It is unclear whether the derangement of the network of intermediate filaments in ALD is caused directly by ethanol or by its metabolites. Vitamin A deficiency may be a factor triggering aggregation of cytokeratin filaments and formation of Mallory bodies,[1026] which in combination with other unknown factors may determine the histologic severity in ALD. An increased frequency of CK inclusions is found in alcoholic patients with fatty liver, hepatitis, bridging fibrosis, and cirrhosis.[1027] The frequency of CK inclusions increases significantly with the dose of ethanol ingested, and distinct Mallory bodies are found mostly in patients with daily alcohol intakes exceeding 160 g. Clearly chronic heavy alcohol abuse is a prerequisite for forming Mallory bodies.

Although our knowledge of the morphologic, biochemical, and immunologic composition of hepatic cytoskeletal components in livers from normal and alcoholic livers has increased dramatically, the precise mechanisms responsible for the derangements in ALD remain to be elucidated.

EFFECTS OF ALCOHOL ON NON-PARENCHYMAL CELLS AND ASSOCIATED FACTORS

An interesting facet of the history of research on ALD was the idea first proposed by Rojkind that the effects of this disease could be ameliorated by preventing the fibrosis that accompanies it.[1028-1030] Work on this idea began before an appreciation of the full significance of the matrix of the liver for the function and development of liver cells and the importance of factors (cytokines) provoked by the inflammatory response in stimulating fibrogenesis. Recently, there has been an explosion of knowledge about cytokine-mediated inflammation and how, in addition to fibrogenesis, these mediators may be involved in pathogenetic mechanisms of liver diseases. These areas are reviewed in detail in Chapters 12 and 13. Although it is not clear as yet how this work will affect our ideas about the genesis of liver disease or the treatment of ALD, there is a reason to be hopeful. For example, therapy in the future could be directed at the selective interdiction of inflammatory signals that incite cells in the liver to increase the synthesis of collagen, or it could be directed at preventing synthesis of collagen before its secretion from cells.[1031,1032] Indeed, data show that a prostaglandin inhibited the generation of fibrous tissue in rats fed a cirrhogenic diet (deficient in choline and protein).[1031]

Alcohol and Kupffer Cells

Kupffer cells are important in host defense mechanisms because they phagocytize blood-borne particles such as bacteria.[1033,1034] Kupffer cells also produce mediators of inflammation and liver function, which include cytokines, prostanoids, and O_2 free radicals.[1035-1039] Alcohol ingestion, acute or chronic, modifies the homeostatic responses of the Kupffer cell by altering the membrane surface and secretory mechanisms of this cell. Alcohol acutely stimulates and chronically inhibits Kupffer cell responses to agonists. The inhibition of Kupffer cell function—for example, secretion of TNF—may be dose-related.

Infusion of colloidal carbon into the isolated, perfused rat liver stimulates glycogenolysis.[1040] Because colloidal carbon is cleared by non-parenchymal cells, it is likely that active, phagocytizing Kupffer cells signal hepatocytes to produce glucose by mobilizing glycogen reserves, possibly to support the increased metabolic demands of the Kupffer cells. When livers from fed rats are perfused with ethanol, ethanol induces the effect of colloidal carbon on glucose production.[1041] Methylpyrazole, an inhibitor of alcohol dehydrogenase, does not abolish this effect. So it is not the result of the oxidation of ethanol. On the other hand, this response to ethanol is blocked by the cyclooxygenase inhibitor, indomethacin,[1041] and attenuated by adrenergic blockade.[1042] Other effects of ethanol on Kupffer cells are the down-regulation of superoxide and the production and inhibition of secretion of TNF.

High levels of alcohol depress, and low levels stimulate, the Kupffer cell response to endotoxin.[1043,1044] It is believed that part of these effects are mediated by calcium, which is the major second messenger in the activation of Kupffer cells.[917] Voltage-dependent calcium channels are involved in the mechanism of TNF production and phagocytosis by Kupffer cells.[1045] Short-term treatment with ethanol inactivates these channels, which suppresses Kupffer cell function.[1046] Activation of Kupffer cells after chronic exposure to alcohol reflects that treatment with ethanol makes it easier to open calcium channels in Kupffer cells, and thereby activate the cells.[1047]

Basal uptake of O_2 increases about 2 to 3 hours after treatment with ethanol.[1048] This phenomenon is termed *swift increase in alcohol metabolism* (SIAM).[1048-1050] Inactivation of Kupffer cells by gadolinium chloride blocks the increases in respiration and ethanol metabolism that characterize SIAM.[1050] In the intragastric feeding model, rates of ethanol elimination are normally elevated twofold to threefold in rats exposed to ethanol for 2 to 4 weeks.[1051] But when Kupffer cells are inactivated by gadolinium chloride, these enhanced rates of ethanol metabolism and consumption of O_2 are prevented.[1052] The severity of pathologic liver injury also is reduced significantly.[1052] Inactivation of Kupffer cells prevents conversion of xanthine dehydrogenase to xanthine oxidase and subsequent generation of free radicals during hypoxia of these cells.[1053]

Hepatic Stellate (Ito) Cells and Ethanol-induced Fibrosis

Liver scarring occurs when the normal balance of collagen formation and breakdown is altered to favor formation.[1054-1055] The biochemical composition of hepatic extracellular matrix in alcoholic fibrosis is similar to that in cirrhosis of other etiologies (see Chap. 12). The major constituent of abnormal connective tissue is collagen with fibrillar collagens (types I and III) predominating.[1055] With progression of fibrosis there is a disproportionate increase in type I collagen. This process takes place in the space of Disse located between the liver cell and endothelial cells lining the sinusoids. Perisinusoidal and pericellular scarring occurs first in the centrolobular zone in ALD and then extends to connect adjacent central veins and portal tracts.[1056] Focal intralobular scarring in areas of inflammation and necrosis also occurs.[1057] When these processes reach the periportal zone, adjacent hepatocytes undergo a phenotypic switch to form bile ductules (bile ductular metaplasia). The process of periportal scarring extends to form fibrous connections between adjacent portal tracts and central veins to alter the liver architecture permanently (portal cirrhosis).

Despite the early controversy over the primary source of extracellular matrix in liver fibrosis, there is compelling evidence to implicate Ito cells (e.g., fat-storing cells, hepatic lipocytes, stellate cells) as the ultimate source of collagen.[1058-1060] Thus Ito cells maintain the normal structural scaffolding of collagen (extracellular matrix) of the liver sinusoid. Scarring results when Ito cells are activated in response to cytokines, growth factors, products of necrotic hepatocytes, and lipid peroxides derived from inflammatory cells or Kupffer cells.[1061,1062] Activation of Ito cells is demonstrable in the scars and sinusoids of livers in rats developing pathologic injury.[1063] Similarly, activation of Ito cells is seen within the scars in the livers of patients with alcoholic hepatitis.[1064] Even though Ito cells are activated diffusely in liver injury, scarring is localized. This implies that local factors—for example, hepatocyte necrosis and inflammation—are necessary for scar formation. In a long-term, serial, morphometric study in alcohol-fed rats, Ito cell activation was accompanied by or preceded by morphologic evidence of liver injury.[1063] Activation of Ito cells seems to be a late event in the course of ALD in that activation is significant only in the presence of scar tissue.

The significance of acetaldehyde for the activation of Ito cells is controversial. Many investigators have shown that acetaldehyde in vitro increases production of collagen by Ito cells and increases gene transcription of procollagen and fibronectin,[1065,1066] but the interpretation of these studies depends on the conditions used in cell culture. Results may not extend to the situation in vivo.[1067] Acetaldehyde at pharmacologic concentrations stimulates production of collagen only 1.6 times the control levels in fibroblasts and myofibroblasts.[1068] Shiratori and co-workers could not induce collagen synthesis in lipocytes with 200 μm acetaldehyde,[1069] which is a level substantially above those in vivo. These observations cast doubt on the relevance of acetaldehyde-initiated fibrosis in ALD. Acetaldehyde, however, may be a secondary stimulus to fibrogenesis after an initiating event has occurred.[1070]

Ito cells isolated from rat livers in the early stages of alcoholic liver injury proliferate rapidly and have decreased amounts of vitamin A. A later stage of activation is myofibroblastic in nature, with increased expression of the genes for collagen, TGF-β1, and smooth muscle α actin.[1061,1071] Vitamin A depletion in hepatic stellate cells appears to be an early effect of chronic ethanol intake but does not predict cellular activation. Activation is more closely related to a reduction in cellular levels of retinol-binding protein.[1072] Increased production of TGF-β1 by Kupffer cells, which enhances expression of the collagen gene in Ito cells, is thought to be an important mediator of cellular events between early and late activation.[1061,1073] TNFα stimulates DNA synthesis in Ito cells.[1074] It also works synergistically with TGF-β1 to stimulate synthesis of fibronectin by cultured Ito cells.[1075] IL-6 stimulates expression of the collagen gene in Ito cells.[1076] Among these cytokines TGF-β is considered the most potent in stimulating matrix gene expression.

The pathogenetic importance of lipid peroxidation in fibrogenesis, in alcohol-fed animals, has received recent attention.[1062] There are significant correlations between indices of lipid peroxidation and hepatic levels of hydroxyproline.[1077] Also, malondialdehyde and 4-hydroxynonenal stimulate collagen synthesis by Ito cells in vitro.[1078,1079] These results support the idea that lipid peroxidation contributes to alcoholic liver fibrosis. Moreover, dietary iron stimulates lipid peroxidation and alcohol-induced fibrosis.[1080]

Role of Endothelial Cells in ALD

The importance of the endothelium in alcohol-induced liver injury was first suggested by observations of the capillarization of the hepatic sinusoid in patients with alcoholic cirrhosis.[1081] Major features of this process include a reduction in endothelial fenestrae, development of a subendothelial basal lamina, collagenosis of the space of Disse, and diffuse interstitial fibrosis. Similar findings have been described in the rat model for ALD.[1082] An early feature of alcoholic liver injury in rats chronically fed ethanol is arrest of endothelial cells at the G_1/S phase of the cell cycle. The extent of this arrest correlates with the severity of pathologic injury.[1083]

One of the main functions of sinusoidal endothelial cells is the continuous exchange of compounds between the liver parenchyma and the blood stream.[1084] One of these compounds, hyaluronic acid, has been used as a marker of endothelial cell dysfunction in a variety of liver diseases.[1085-1087] In humans high levels of hyaluronic acid are associated with capillarization of the sinusoids.[1088] And, in ethanol-fed rats levels of hyaluronic acid in blood correlate with the number of endothelial cells arrested at G_1/S.[1089] Capillarization is thought to occur in response to mediators released by Kupffer cells in response to stimulation by endotoxin.[1090,1091] An increased concentration of hyaluronic acid in plasma and decreased uptake by sinusoidal endothelial cells after administration of endotoxin and ethanol are abolished by gadolinium chloride, which, as noted, selectively suppresses Kupffer cell function.[1091]

Endotoxin and ALD

Endotoxins are lipopolysaccharide components of the outer cell wall of most gram-negative bacteria.[1092-1094] They consist of a lipid component called lipid A linked to a complex polysaccharide (Figure 29-17). The polysaccharide is divided into two regions: a core polysaccharide that is largely conserved among gram-negative bacteria and an outer region that shows great variability between bacterial species. This outer polysaccharide is known as the O-antigen or O-specific polysaccharide. When bacteria multiply, but also when they die and lyse, endotoxin is set free from the surface.

The gram-negative flora of the terminal ileum and large intestine form a large reservoir of endotoxins. Nolan and co-workers suggest that endotoxins do not cross the gut as passively permeable solutes but are transported actively.[1095] Thus absorption of endotoxin from the gut with portal endotoxemia is a normal physiologic process, and liver is the major site for removal of gut-derived endotoxin from the circulation. Accumulating evidence from a number of sources shows that endotoxin is taken up almost exclusively by the Kupffer cell, where it is internalized and subsequently modified.[1096,1097] In patients with portosystemic shunting inefficient clearance of endotoxin can lead to systemic endotoxemia.[1098]

Endotoxin is necessary for the development of a variety of experimentally induced liver diseases, both chronic and acute.[1099-1106] Broitman and associates[1099] demonstrated, for example, that endotoxin was necessary for the development of choline-deficiency cirrhosis in rats. Adult rats fed a choline-deficient diet were protected from development of cirrhosis (but not hepatic steatosis) by addition of neomycin to their drinking water; addition of endotoxin (6 mg percent) to the neomycin-containing drinking water overcame the protection afforded by the antibiotic. The presence of endotoxin also is required for the acute liver toxicity associated with exposure to CCl_4 and D-galactosamine.[1099-1101] Impairment of the clearance of circulating endotoxins from peripheral circulation has been shown in CCl_4-induced liver disease; pretreatment with the anti-endotoxin polymyxin B protected animals from CCl_4 toxicity.[1102] However, gentamicin, which does not interact with endotoxin, had no protective effect.[1103]

Resection of the small bowel and colon eliminates the normal flora as a source of endotoxin and protects rabbits from D-galactosamine hepatotoxicity,[1104] which is mediated by depletion of uridine nucleotides and impairs macromolecular synthesis.[1105] D-Galactosamine also may impair hepatic metabolism of endotoxins in the portal vein. The concept that hepatotoxin sensitivity correlates with endotoxin sensitivity was demonstrated with endotoxin-resistant mice (strain C3H/HeJ) and the histocompatible, endotoxin-sensitive strain C3H/HeN. Unlike the HeN strain, HeJ mice are resistant to D-galactosamine–associated hepatitis.[1106] But adoptive transfer of macrophages from sensitive to lethally irradiated endotoxin-resistant strains transferred both endotoxin and D-galactosamine sensitivity.[1106] These results suggest that the active cell in D-galactosamine–associated endotoxin toxicity is a macrophage and most probably the Kupffer cell. Moreover, the interaction between endotoxin and D-galactosamine appears to be mediated by exquisite sensitivity to cytokines.[1107] Mice treated with D-galactosamine become sensitive to submicrogram quantities of TNF, one of the products of endotoxin-sensitized macrophages.[1108]

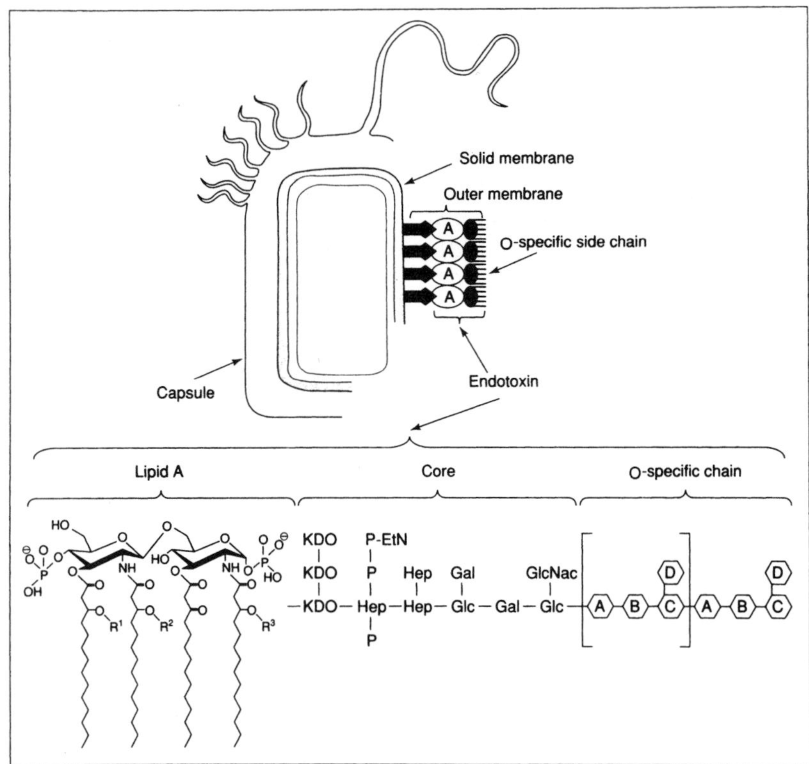

Figure 29-17 Structure of bacterial wall and endotoxin molecule. The endotoxin molecule is a lipopolysaccharide found in the outer membrane of most pathogenic gram-negative bacteria. This diagram illustrates the three distinct domains of this molecule: a lipid, referred to as lipid A; a core sugar; and an outer sugar known as the O-specific side chain. (From Quezado ZMN, Banks SM, Natanson C: New strategies for combating sepsis. Trends Biotech 13:56, 1995.)

Endotoxin also is an essential component in the pathogenesis of murine hepatitis induced by frog virus 3. This virus is lethal to Kupffer cells.[1109] Prior colectomy of mice protects against the fatal effects of the virus.[1110] The direct role of endotoxin in frog virus 3 hepatitis also was shown by inoculation of colectomized mice with 1 percent of a lethal dose of endotoxin plus the virus, which negated the protective effects of colectomy.[1109] Germ-free or C3H/HeJ mice are resistant to the virus, and pretreatment of mice with polymyxin B significantly ameliorated the effects of viral infection as reflected by decreased levels of serum alanine aminotransferase and decreased mortality.[1111]

Considerable evidence supports the hypothesis that endotoxin(s) are involved in alcohol-dependent liver injury. Plasma levels of endotoxin are increased after acute ingestion of ethanol and in patients with ALD.[1112,1113] Increased plasma levels of endotoxin have been described in the intragastric feeding model for ALD.[1114,1115] Endotoxin levels begin to increase within 2 weeks of ethanol administration, and increase nearly fivefold to sixfold in plasma by 8 weeks.[1114] A significant correlation is observed in this model between severity of liver injury and levels of endotoxin in plasma, but the mechanism by which alcohol induces endotoxemia is unknown. The possibilities include a reduction in the capacity of Kupffer cells to detoxify endotoxin,[1116] an increase in the permeability of mucous membranes to endotoxin,[1117,1118] and an increase in the gram-negative bacterial flora of the jejunum, which would provide a reservoir for increased production of endotoxin.[1119] Ethanol, in vitro, increases the permeability of the small intestine to endotoxin and to other molecules, such as polyvinyl pyrolidomacromolecules.[1118,1119]

Further support for the hypothesis that endotoxin (derived from intestinal bacteria) is a contributory factor in alcohol-induced liver injury comes from studies in which blockage of endotoxin production ameliorates liver injury. There is a marked decrease in circulating levels of endotoxin, accompanied by a virtual absence of pathologic changes in the liver,[1120] in rats fed ethanol with lactobacillus GG (a strain of lactobacillus resistant to effects of gastric acid). Lactobacillus GG suppresses the growth of a broad spectrum of gram-negative bacteria, probably by elaborating low-molecular weight substances with antibiotic activity.[1121,1122] As mentioned previously, intestinal sterilization with polymyxin B or neomycin results in a significant reduction in levels of endotoxin in ethanol-fed rats[1123] accompanied by an improvement in the severity of pathology and hepatic hypoxia.

The principles of endotoxin-induced damage to tissue are fairly well understood. Endotoxin, through its lipid A component, interacts with a number of cell types, including Kupffer and endothelial cells. Endotoxins, however, are not toxic because they kill cells or inhibit their functions. Endotoxin stimulates Kupffer cells to produce bioactive lipids, reactive species of O_2, and peptides such as TNF, IL-1, IL-6, IL-8, and IL-10. These mediators, acting independently or in sequence, can be hepatotoxic directly or recruit neutrophils or other inflammatory cells that potentiate liver injury.[1124,1125]

Multiple mammalian receptors for endotoxin have been identified over the last decade. Of these receptors, two glycoproteins are clearly implicated in the molecular and cellular basis of the interaction between endotoxin and macrophages.[1126,1127] The first, lipopolysaccharide-binding protein (LBP), present in normal serum, recognizes and binds LPS with high affinity through its lipid A moiety.[1128,1129] LPS-LBP complexes then activate cells through the second glycoprotein, membrane-bound CD14 (mCD14), to produce inflammatory mediators.[1127,1130,1131] An important role for CD14 is suggested by studies in which transfection of human CD14 into 70Z/3 B cells (normally CD14 negative) increases sensitivity to LPS in the presence of LBP by 10,000-fold compared with 70Z/3 control, non-transfected cells.[1132] Second, several reports have shown CD14 to be critical to the response of macrophages to low concentrations of LPS in the presence of LBP.[1133-1135] Furthermore, CD14 transgenic mice are extremely sensitive to the toxic effects of LPS,[1136] whereas CD14 knockout mice are much less sensitive.[1137]

LBP and CD14 mRNA levels were evaluated in rats fed ethanol intragastrically.[1138] The highest levels of LBP and CD14 mRNAs were found in rats that demonstrated the presence of necrosis and inflammation. Expression of CD14 mRNA was restricted to Kupffer cells and LBP expression to hepatocytes. Although there is little doubt that CD14 binds LPS and initiates signal transduction, CD14 is not by itself capable of initiating a transmembrane activation signal. CD14 lacks a transmembrane domain and therefore has no intrinsic signaling capabilities.[1139] Also, LPS receptor antagonists inhibit the effects of LPS at concentrations that are too low to block LPS binding to CD14.[1140] These observations have led many to postulate that the LPS/CD14 complexes interact with a transmembrane receptor that is responsible for ligand specificity and signal transduction.[1141,1142] Recently, members of the Toll receptor family have been implicated in LPS signaling.[1143] Toll, a type I transmembrane receptor, exhibits homology to the intracellular portion of the IL-1 receptor. A family of Toll-like receptors (TLRs) has been described and two members, TLR2 and TLR4, have been identified as LPS-signaling receptors.[1144-1147] Recently Su and co-workers showed that in Kupffer cells, TLR4 signaling occurred downstream of LBP and CD14.[1148] In keeping with the proposed view that LPS does not directly bind to TLR4, it has been proposed that TLR4 acts as a "sensor," responding to alterations in membrane structure resulting from CD14-mediated LPS internalization.[1149] Studies in the rat intragastric feeding model show increased levels of TLR4 expression in rats exhibiting pathologic liver injury.[1149a] Alterations in membrane structure by alcohol and polyunsaturated fatty acids could, in part, explain up-regulation of Toll 4 in this model. Further support for a role for both CD14 and TLR4 is provided in studies that show that both CD14-deficient[1150] and TLR4-deficient[1151] mice are protected against alcoholic liver injury.

Role of Nuclear Factor-Kappa B

Nuclear factor-kappa B (NF-κB) is a ubiquitous transcription factor that is implicated in the activation of many genes, several of which are involved in alcoholic liver injury.[1152,1153] In unstimulated cells NF-κB is a heterodimeric complex that is sequestered in the cytoplasm by its interaction with the IκB family of inhibitors. When cells are stimulated, IκB is phosphorylated and NF-κB is released; NF-κB then translocates to the nucleus, where it binds to specific sequences in the promoter region of target genes.[1152,1153] Endotoxemia and oxidative stress cause liver injury via NF-κB. Activation of NF-κB occurs in experimental alcoholic liver injury in association with endotoxemia, lipid peroxidation, and liver injury.[1154] In rats fed alcohol intragastrically nuclear translocation of NF-κB is associated with necroinflammatory changes in ethanol-fed rats.[1154] Activation of NF-κB in these rats was secondary to proteolytic degradation of IκBα. Monocytes from patients with alcoholic hepatitis display greater NF-κB activity than monocytes from control subjects.[1155] But activation of NF-κB in patients with alcoholic hepatitis differs from effects after acute exposure to ethanol. For example, acute exposure to ethanol inhibits LPS-induced activation of NF-κB and production of TNFα by rat Kupffer cells.[1156] Acute ethanol ingestion by humans suppresses endotoxin-induced activation of NF-κB and production of TNFα by peripheral blood mononuclear cells.[1157]

Although NF-κB is an attractive therapeutic target for inflammatory liver injury, inhibition of NF-κB can initiate fulminant liver injury and hepatocyte apoptosis.[1158] Thus NF-κB can be hepato-protective. P65 knockout mice die in utero of massive apoptosis in liver; macrophages from these knockout mice are extremely sensitive to killing by TNFα.[1159]

Despite elevated levels of endotoxin in plasma of patients with alcoholic cirrhosis, systemic reactions are absent in most patients. This phenomenon has been attributed to down-regulation of secretion of proinflammatory cytokines. The mechanisms of tolerance to endotoxemia in ALD are poorly understood. In one study of patients with alcoholic cirrhosis and endotoxemia tolerance to endotoxin was associated with increased levels of anti-inflammatory cytokines (IL-10 and IL-receptor antagonist) and reduced levels of TNF receptors in plasma.[1160]

Cytokines and Alcoholic Liver Injury

Many of the features of ALD are associated with the acute phase response, which includes fever, malaise, anorexia, and leukocytosis.[1161,1162] Many of these features also occur after injecting experimental animals with cytokines (Table 29-11).[1163]

Several models of alcohol-related liver injury have been linked to increased production of cytokines. Rats fed ethanol chronically, for instance, are more susceptible to endotoxin-mediated liver injury.[1164,1165] Furthermore, ethanol-fed rats exposed to lipopolysaccharide have

TABLE 29-11

Biologic Effects of Cytokines and Similarities in Clinical and Laboratory Findings in ALD

Fever	Increased acute phase proteins
Anorexia	Collagen deposition
Neutrophilia	Increased liver triglycerides
Muscle catabolism	Hypermetabolic state

higher levels of TNF as compared with controls.[1166] On the basis of these and other experiments[1167,1168] it can be concluded that high concentrations of TNFα in serum, as found in ethanol-fed, LPS-injected rats, are associated with liver injury; that feeding ethanol and injection of LPS are necessary for significant liver injury to occur; and that the increase in TNFα is due to increased synthesis. Isolation of non-parenchymal cells shows that Kupffer cells are responsible for the increased synthesis of TNFα.[1168]

Using the intragastric feeding model, mRNA for TNFα was increased in rats with pathologic liver injury; mRNA for TNFα was not present in the absence of liver injury.[1169] In the same model Kupffer cells isolated from ethanol-fed rats had increased spontaneous and LPS-stimulated secretion of TNF as compared with cells from control rats.[1170] Compelling data for the significance of TNFα come from TNF-receptor knockout mice (TNR-R1 mice) and use of anti-TNF antibodies to prevent alcoholic liver injury. After 4 weeks of continuous ethanol exposure, liver injury did not occur in the TNR-R1 knockout mice but was present in wild-type mice or TNF-R2 knockout mice.[1171] These results are consistent with the idea that the p55 (R1) receptor promotes inflammatory changes in response to endotoxin.[1172] Furthermore, mice lacking TNF-R1 are resistant to challenge with endotoxin,[1173] and alcohol-induced liver injury is blocked by antibodies to TNFα.[1174] Analysis of TNFα promoter polymorphisms in humans showed an association between alcohol-induced steatohepatitis and an allele that upregulated expression of TNF.[1175] Increased production of TNFα occurs in vitro in monocytes from patients with alcoholic hepatitis.[1176] Several laboratories also have demonstrated increased TNF activity in patients with ALD. Felver and associates showed that concentrations of TNF were increased in patients with alcoholic hepatitis.[1177] During a 2-year follow-up period the patients who died had elevated concentrations of TNF. Surviving patients did not have increased concentrations of TNF. Bird and colleagues also demonstrated significantly increased concentrations of TNF in patients with severe alcoholic hepatitis,[1178] although many of the patients in this study had documented infections.

IL-8 is another cytokine of importance in ALD. Rat hepatocytes, when exposed to ethanol, release a chemotactic factor whose activity is abolished by anti-serum against rat IL-8.[1179] IL-8 causes neutrophilia and enhances the release of lysosomal enzymes and expression of adhesion molecules on granulocytes.[1180] Levels of IL-8 are increased in patients with alcoholic hepatitis and in alcohol-dependent patients without liver injury.[1181] Furthermore, tissue levels of IL-8 correlate with neutrophil infiltration.[1182] Thus the accumulation and activation of neutrophils by IL-8 may contribute to liver injury in alcoholics.

Measurements of serum IL-1, using the thymocyte proliferation assay, have shown increased levels in patients with alcoholic hepatitis.[1183,1184] Monocytes from patients with ALD also secrete more IL-1 in response to LPS than monocytes from controls.[1185]

Levels of IL-6, a cytokine responsible for much of the hepatic acute phase response,[1186] are increased in the serum of patients with ALD.[1187,1188] In patients with alcoholic hepatitis concentrations of IL-6 in plasma correlate with biochemical and clinical features of the disease.[1188] A decrease in levels of IL-6 correlates with clinical improvement. The pathogenetic mechanisms leading to increased production of cytokines in ALD are not completely understood. Likely stimuli for production of cytokines by macrophages and other types of cells in the liver are endotoxin,[1189] prostanoids,[1190] and GSH.[1191]

Endotoxin, in addition to increasing production of TNFα mRNA, enhances the responsiveness of hepatocytes to TNF by enhancing the binding of TNFα to plasma membranes.[1192] The diminished production of PGE_2 seen in experimental and clinical ALD may lead to impaired regulation of cytokine production.[1190] GSH is an important regulator of TNFα production or release. In summary, the depletion of GSH in alcohol-fed animals could augment release of TNF.[1190]

The correlation between production of cytokines and severity of disease in patients with ALD makes it clear that cytokines are important factors in alcohol-induced injury to the liver.

ALCOHOL AND LIVER REGENERATION

Alcohol is one of the few liver toxins that causes injury without inducing a compensatory proliferative response in surviving hepatocytes. Data from a number of laboratories indicate that ethanol inhibits the regenerative capacity of the liver.[1193] Thus alcohol may induce liver injury not only by directly injuring the liver but also by impairing the regenerative response to injury. There are a number of possible regenerative pathways that could be interrupted by ethanol.

Role of TNFα

Liver regeneration after partial hepatectomy is significantly delayed in germ-free, athymic, and LPS-resistant mice, which have limited ability to release cytokines in response to endotoxin.[1194,1195] Several groups subsequently demonstrated that TNFα was, at least in part, responsible for the compensatory hepatic regenerative response to toxin-induced liver injury.[1196-1198] Treatment of rats with anti-TNF antibody significantly inhibits the posthepatectomy increase in ^{3}H-thymidine incorporation into hepatic DNA.[1199] Anti-TNF antibodies have a similar effect in retarding regeneration of liver cells in ethanol-fed rats.[1200] Furthermore, the amount of TNF required to achieve a proliferative response in ethanol-fed rats is greater compared with pair-fed control animals.[1201]

Because TNF is believed to be an important mediator of inflammatory changes in ALD, additional work is necessary to define whether antagonizing the effects of TNF will have therapeutic benefit.

Other cytokines such IL-1 and IL-6 are also important in the regenerative response.[1201] For example, the postpartial-hepatectomy increase in IL-6 levels is attenuated in TNF R-1 null transgenic mice.[1201]

Mitogenic Factors

Little is known about the mechanisms that operate within the regenerating liver to coordinate the production of mitogenic factors (see Chap. 2). Evidence is accumulating that hepatic stellate cells (see Chap. 13), the principal source of liver extracellular matrix, also produce mitogens during liver regeneration.[1202] Stellate cells are a rich source of hepatocyte growth factor, for example, which is a potent hepatic mitogen. Hepatic stellate cells also are targets for injury-related cytokines. Under certain circumstances TNFα stimulates stellate cells to produce mitogenic factors.[1193] The effect of alcohol consumption on the production of mitogens and comitogens by stellate cells has not been adequately studied.

Effect of Light Ethanol Consumption

Although heavy alcohol consumption has a detrimental effect on hepatic regenerative activity, there are limited data on the effects of light, daily ethanol consumption. A recent study indicates that light ethanol consumption enhances hepatic regenerative activity after partial hepatectomy in rats.[1203] The mechanisms for the beneficial effects of light ethanol consumption on hepatic regeneration are unknown, but depolarization of hepatic membrane potentials and reduced p53 levels may contribute.[1203]

APOPTOSIS AND ALD

"Acidophilic bodies" in ALD represent instances of apoptosis.[1204] In humans ALD markers of apoptosis are expressed in hepatocytes with Mallory bodies, suggesting that hepatocytes containing Mallory bodies are eliminated at least in part by apoptosis.[1205] In experimental animals chronic alcohol administration significantly increases the percentage of apoptotic hepatocytes.[1206] For example, in normal rat liver, apoptosis is localized to the first two rows of hepatocytes around the central vein[1207]; in ethanol-fed animals, apoptosis extends to several rows.[1208,1209] In rats fed ethanol intragastrically the greatest degree of apoptosis is observed in rats exhibiting the worst liver injury.[1210]

Mechanisms Involved in Apoptosis in ALD

Cytochrome P450 2E1

As pointed out previously, induction of cytochrome P450 2E1 and the formation of reactive O_2 intermediates and lipid peroxides appears to be one of the mechanisms for ethanol-induced hepatotoxicity.[1211] To establish a link between CYP 2E1, unsaturated fatty acids, lipid peroxidation, and cell injury, Hep G2 cells were transduced with human CYP 2E1 cDNA and exposed to arachidonic acid.[1212] Enhanced lipid peroxidation was associated with cytotoxicity that was apoptotic in nature. A variety of anti-oxidants including α-tocopherol acetate and Trolox prevented apoptosis. 4-Methyl pyrazole, which is an inhibitor of CYP 2E1, also prevented cellular damage, indicating that ethanol toxicity required active CYP 2E1.

Oxidative Stress. In addition to CYP 2E1, iron overload is a major cause of free radical formation in ALD. Hepatic iron overload is seen in about 30 percent of alcoholics[1213] and iron accumulation in rats is associated with increased apoptosis of hepatocytes.[1214] Chronic ethanol exposure also selectively decreases the mitochondrial pool of GSH.[1215] This depletion sensitizes the hepatocytes in ethanol-fed rats to the cytotoxic effects of TNFα.[1216,1217] GSH is also cytoprotective against apoptosis mediated by oxidative stress-mediated during acute ethanol intoxication.[1218] Finally, oxidant stress also upregulates Fas ligand mRNA in liver cells[1219] (see the following section on Fas and Fas ligand).

Fas and Fas-Ligand (Fas-L). Fas (also called CD95 or Apo 1) and Fas-L are important in apoptosis .[1220,1221] There is accumulating evidence that the Fas-Fas-L interaction contributes to the pathogenesis of many liver diseases, including ALD.[1222] Fas and Fas L are up-regulated in patients with alcoholic hepatitis.[1223] Fas L, in addition to being present on inflammatory cells, was also up-regulated in hepatocytes. These findings suggest that hepatocytes might mediate their own death by paracrine or autocrine mechanisms.[1224]

TNF and TNF Receptors. TNF has different activities depending on the cell type and metabolic milieu of the cell. TNF can induce apoptosis or necrosis, stimulate proliferation, or be cytoprotective.[1225,1226] TNF rarely triggers apoptosis unless protein synthesis is blocked.[1225] As discussed previously, increased levels of TNF occur in patients with ALD and in rats with ethanol-induced liver injury. The effect of TNF on cells is mediated by binding to two cell surface receptors, TNF receptors 1 (p55) and 2 (p75).[1226,1227] In patients with alcoholic hepatitis strong cytoplasmic staining for both receptors is seen.[1228] Similar results are seen in experimental animals.[1227] Upon binding of TNF, TNF R1 trimerizes, which induces association of the receptor's death domains and activates caspases and apoptosis. Hepatocytes are rich in TNFα receptors, rendering them susceptible to TNFα–induced injury.[1220] Binding of TNF to its receptor also leads to activation of NF-κB, which paradoxically contributes to preventing TNFα–induced cell death.[1229]

Mitochondria. At least three general mechanisms are thought to be important in relation to mitochondria and apoptosis.[1230] These are (1) disruption of the electron transport chain, oxidative phosphosphorylation, and ATP generation; (2) release of proteins such as cytochrome C that trigger activation of the caspase family of proteases; and (3) alteration of cellular-reduction oxidation (redox) potential. Many of these mitochondrial abnormalities are present after alcohol administration (see section on Mitochondria). A consequence of many apoptotic stimuli is the collapse of the mitochondrial inner membrane potential indicating the opening of the mitochondrial permeability transition pore.[1231] Opening of this pore leads to volume dysregulation and swelling and uncoupling of mitochondria that, if unrestrained, can lead to apoptosis or necrosis.

ANIMAL MODELS OF ALCOHOLIC LIVER INJURY

The variation in animal models used in the study of ALD reflects the formidable task of developing a suitable experimental model that exactly replicates the human prototype. Each model emphasizes one or more features seen in humans. In this way each model makes a contribution to some aspect of our understanding of the pathogenesis of ALD.[1233]

Many studies involving alcoholic liver injury in animal models do not include an assessment of liver pathology. This is unfortunate because investigation of experimental ALD should employ designs that allow correlation between pathogenetic factors and particular types of liver injury. In a recent review of the pathology of ALD in humans French and co-workers[1232] highlighted the following features:

1. Moderate elevation of serum aspartate aminotransferase and alanine aminotransferase with aspartate aminotransferase greater than alanine aminotransferase
2. Cholestasis
3. Fatty liver
4. Ballooning degeneration of hepatocytes with loss of immunostaining for cytokeratin
5. Formation of Mallory bodies
6. Bile ductular metaplasia of hepatocytes at the limiting plate
7. Proliferation of periportal Ito cells, transformation, and fibrosis
8. Perivenular proliferation of Ito cells, transformation, and fibrosis
9. Megamitochondria
10. Acinar inflammation
11. Apoptosis
12. Spotty necrosis
13. Zonal necrosis
14. Cirrhosis

These features should be evaluated as markers of alcohol-associated liver injury in experimental models. The features of ALD that have been reported in the various animal models are summarized in Table 29-12. Mammalian models of ALD include the rat, mouse, miniature pig, guinea pig, hamster, ferret, and various primates.

Rat Models

The first major obstacle to development of a model for ALD was the natural aversion of animals to alcohol. This was overcome by Lieber and DeCarli by incorporating ethanol into a liquid diet.[1234,1235] This regimen ensured that rats received diet and ethanol in amounts sufficient to induce fatty liver after 1 month of feeding. The severity of the fatty change was dependent on the percent of calories from fat.[1236] When 10 percent of calories were derived from fat, there was a doubling in the amount of liver fat stores; increasing the fat content to 45 percent of total calories increased fat stores sevenfold.

The liquid diet has been criticized as not being nutritionally adequate and not supporting optimal growth in rats.[1237] Rodents decrease their overall food intake when ethanol is introduced in the liquid diet. This factor is controlled by pair-feeding each control animal with amounts of the liquid diet equal to those ingested by the corresponding alcohol-treated littermate.[1238] Under these conditions, numerous dietary ingredients become suboptimal. However, supplementation of the liquid diet with minerals and vitamins fails to prevent alcohol-induced fatty liver.[1239]

The role of a decreased carbohydrate supply in the liquid diet has been suggested as one cause of the hepatic effects attributed in ethanol.[1240,1241] This issue had been anticipated and was addressed previously when ethanol was used not only as isocaloric replacement for carbohydrate but also as a substitute for fat, to assure identical carbohydrate content in the alcohol-containing and control diets.[1235] Under these conditions ethanol-fed animals developed fatty liver, which was not seen in the pair-fed controls. This result incriminated alcohol and not reduced carbohydrates as a pathogenetic factor. Energy restriction itself had no ill effects in the content of hepatic fat. Other studies show, however, that decreased intake of carbohydrate, in ethanol-fed rats, increases the severity of fatty liver.[1242,1243] It can be concluded, nevertheless, that the use of the Lieber-DeCarli alcohol liquid diet in the rat provides a useful model for studying alcohol-induced fatty liver. But advanced stages of alcoholic liver injury, such as necrosis, inflammation, and fibrosis, are not seen with this diet. Other models of ALD, such as the intragastric tube feeding method, must be used to study these effects of alcohol.

The development of the intragastric tube feeding of ethanol and liquid diet by continuous infusion grew out of the idea that sustained high levels of alcohol in blood were necessary for the induction of progressive liver injury. In the intragastric cannula model, ethanol and liquid diet are delivered simultaneously so that both the amount of alcohol and diet can be varied independently.[1244-1246] Chronic ethanol feeding, via intragastric infusion at a constant rate (10 to 14 g/kg/day), causes a cyclic oscillation in the blood and urinary alcohol levels.[1247] Ethanol levels peak at approximately 500 mg/dl and then fall to about 100 mg/dl. It has been suggested that fluctuations in the activities of alcohol dehydrogenase and cytochrome P450 2E1 (CYP 2E1) drive the cyclic fluctuations of alcohol.[1248] CYP 2E1 inhibitors fail to explain a role for CYP 2E1 as a cause for the oscillations.[1249] It was, however, noticed that the rate of O_2 consumption and body temperature, peaked at the nadir of the blood alcohol cycle.[1250] To further characterize the mechanisms involved in the cycle-induced alterations in ethanol, body temperature, and O_2 consumption, French and colleagues evaluated the role of endotoxin, cytokines, and the hypothalamic-pituitary-thyroid axis.[1251] The ethanol cycling was not related to endotoxin or cytokine levels but required an intact hypothalamic-pituitary-thyroid axis. Thyroid hormone levels correlated positively with the rate of O_2 consumption, and administration of propylthiouracil

TABLE 29-12

Models of ALD in Experimental Animals

Animal	Fatty liver	Alcoholic hepatitis	Cirrhosis	Ductular metaplasia	MB	Centrolobular fibrosis	Balloon cells	Apoptosis	Elevated AST/ALT	Chole-stasis	Megamito-chondria	Inflam-mation	Spotty necrosis	Zonal necrosis	Duration of feeding	Reference
Rabbit	X		X										X		10 mo-5yrs	1070
Rabbit[a]	X		X	X										X	93-244 days	1071
Dog[b]	X		X	X		X				X		X			106 days	1072
Dog[c]	X	X			X	X		X	X	X	X	X	X	X	10-18 mo	1073
Rat[d]	X														1 mo	1074
Rat[e]	X											X	X		12 wk	1075
Rat[f]	X						X						X		12 wk	1076
Rat[d]	X		X*			X		X	X			X	X	X	4 mo	1077
Baboon[d]	X	X	X		X	X	X		X	X	X	X		X	8-22 mo	1057
Baboon[d]	X						X		X	X	X	X			18 mo-5 yrs	1063
Micropig[d]	X					X									12 mo	1065
Mouse[d]	X														4-10 wk	1078
Guinea pig[d]	X														8 wk	1079

Modified fron French SW, Morimoto M, Tsukamoto H: Animal models of alcohol associated liver injury. In Hall P, ed: Alcoholic Liver Disease: Pathology and Pathogenesis. London, Edward Arnold, 1995:279.

MB, Mallory bodies; *AST*, aspartate aminotransferase; *ALT*, alanine aminotransferase; *X*, indicates presence of a pathologic entity.

*When ethanol-high fat diet is supplemented with carbonyl-iron.

[a]The diet was high in protein (40% calories) high in fat (48%), contained lecithin (3.8%) and vitamin supplements. Cirrhosis was formed by portal-portal bridging fibrosis. Arch Pathol 30:165, 1940.

[b]A diet high in lean meat alternating with a high lard content was given with alcohol via stomach tube.

[c]Alcohol was fed with a beef diet through a gastric fistula 5 days a week for 10-18 months. The diet was enriched with choline.

[d]See text.

[e]Addition of 4-methylpyrazole to the diet resulted in high blood alcohol levels (260-350 mg/dl). After 12 weeks of treatment, fatty liver, spotty necrosis, granulocytic and lymphocytic infiltrates were observed.

[f]Administration of pyrazole and alcohol with a high-fat diet produces balloon degeneration and necrosis of hepatocytes in the centrolobular area.

or ablating the pituitary gland eliminated the cycling of body temperature and alcohol levels. The authors concluded that the signal that initiates the reversal of the increasing levels of alcohol in blood is the decrease in body temperature that in turn stimulates the cold-sensitive neurons in the hypothalamus to activate the pituitary-thyroid axis.[1251] Also of note is that the greatest degree of liver injury occurred at the time the alcohol levels were at their lowest.

The combination of a low-fat (5 percent of calories) diet (with adequate carbohydrates) and alcohol fed by continuous intragastric infusion induces fatty liver, focal necrosis, and inflammation in the liver.[1252] When the dietary fat is increased to 25 percent of calories, advanced liver injury ensues, including liver fibrosis.[1253] A further increase in the fat content to 35 percent has no additional effect on centrolobular necrosis or fibrosis.[1254] When a diet marginal in protein, vitamins, and choline is fed with ethanol together with a high-fat diet, liver damage becomes more severe, especially centrolobular fibrosis.[1255] Pericellular fibrosis also is seen and bridging fibrosis is prominent. When young rats (approximately 200 g) are fed via the intragastric route, the calorie content of the diet and ethanol has to be increased by about 50 percent to sustain growth and high levels of alcohol in blood.[1256] The liver injury in these rats is more severe; focal centrolobular fibrosis occurs as early as 1 month after the start of feeding. When 0.25 percent weight in volume of carbonyl iron was infused intragastrically with ethanol and a high-fat diet for 16 weeks, diffuse central-central bridging fibrosis was evident in most rats and micronodular cirrhosis developed in 2 of 10 animals.[1257] The iron-potentiated, alcohol-induced liver fibrogenesis was associated closely with diffuse, intense immunostaining for adducts containing epitopes of malondialdehyde and 4-hydroxynonenal.

Primate Models

The *Macaca mulatta* monkey (Rhesus) develops fatty liver, fibrosis, and cirrhosis when fed ethanol plus a high-fat, low-protein, low-choline diet, and the diet is given by lavage three times a week.[1258] Cirrhosis is seen in animals fed the same diet without ethanol, however, because choline deficiency alone induces cirrhosis in the Rhesus monkey.[1259] Moreover, feeding alcohol and a nutritious diet led to no significant liver pathology.[1260] Even when monkeys *(Macaca radiatas)* were fed the Lieber-DeCarli liquid diet and ethanol for 4 years, only fatty liver and megamitochondria were observed.[1261]

In a series of studies Lieber and associates described an alcoholic hepatitis-like lesion and cirrhosis in baboons fed ethanol and liquid diet.[1262-1265] Cirrhosis developed in only one third of the animals and was preceded by perivenular fibrosis at the stage of fatty liver.[1266] The baboon model has been successful in the laboratory of Lieber and associates, but studies of baboons in other laboratories have not resulted in cirrhosis.[1267,1268] In a study by Ainley and co-workers, for example, chronic feeding of ethanol did not cause hepatic fibrosis or cirrhosis even though six of the baboons were fed ethanol for periods ranging from 36 to 60 months.[1268] The ethanol intake of 25 g/kg/day in these experiments was far higher than what baboons can metabolize and higher than the dose of 4.5 to 8.3 g/kg/day used by Lieber and associates.[1263] Blood ethanol levels in both studies were remarkably similar, but the animals in the Lieber study failed to gain weight, whereas in the study by Ainley and co-workers, the weight gain was similar to that in controls.[1268] This has led to questions as to whether deficiency of specific nutrients is important in the pathogenesis of fibrosis and cirrhosis in the baboon model. To rule out choline deficiency, Lieber and associates fed baboons an ethanol-containing diet supplemented with choline.[1265] This failed to prevent cirrhosis. On the other hand, supplementation of the diet with polyunsaturated phosphatidylcholine prevented cirrhosis,[1269] suggesting that choline supplemented in this way prevented liver injury. The reasons for the inability of various investigators to replicate the findings of Lieber and associates remain unknown.

Pig Model

The requirement for a diet high in polyunsaturated fats plus alcohol to induce significant liver pathology has been demonstrated in the miniature pig. When the pig is fed a diet containing 10 percent of calories as protein, 25 percent as carbohydrate, 5 percent as fat, and 4 g ethanol/kg (60 percent of calories) for up to 11 months, the animals gain no weight and exhibit increases in serum aminotransferases, but not changes in liver histology.[1270] Even when fat was increased to 12 percent of calories and the feeding extended to 20 months, there were no pathologic changes.[1271] When the dietary fat component was increased to 33 percent of calories, significant fatty liver was observed.[1272]

Other Small Animal Models

Other animal models that have been used include the mouse, ferret, guinea pig, and hamster.[1273,1274] Some animals such as the guinea pig show fatty change on administration of ethanol. In other models such as the ferret toxic changes in bone marrow complicate the interpretation of results and limit the duration of feeding. Major requirements for an animal model that produces ethanol-induced pathology resembling human ALD include maintaining a high level of alcohol in the blood, feeding a diet rich in polyunsaturated fatty acids that has a high content of fat and little carbohydrate, and maintaining a pair-feeding regimen to allow for adequate comparison.[1273] The intragastric feeding model developed by Tsukamoto and French[1244-1246] satisfies all of these requirements.

INTERACTIONS BETWEEN ETHANOL AND CHOLINE

Rats

The toxic effects of ethanol described to date establish conditions under which nutritional deficiency leads to cirrhosis and vice versa, but the toxic effects of ethanol per se (e.g., accumulation of fat, megamitochondria, lipid peroxidation) do not cause liver disease in experimental animals. Precisely what toxic effects of ethanol interact with dietary deficiency (or in fact with what dietary deficiency) to produce cirrhosis remain to be elucidated. It is known, however, that choline deficiency per se will cause cirrhosis in the rat when combined with protein deficiency[1285] and that ethanol increases the choline requirement of the rat.[1286-1289]

The rat synthesizes choline-containing phosphatides (Figure 29-18), but the rate of synthesis does not appear to be sufficient for meeting all the animal's needs. Choline hence is an essential dietary ingredient for the rat. Deficiency is associated almost immediately with an inability of the animal's liver to secrete VLDL. Fatty liver ensues. Fibrous tissue develops in the liver of the choline-deficient rat, and depending on the amount of dietary protein, the liver eventually becomes cirrhotic. There is no evidence of hepatitis during the development of cirrhosis, and the molecular events leading to cirrhosis in the choline-deficient rat are completely unknown. Nevertheless, given the importance of phosphatidylcholine for the structural and functional integrity of the plasma and intracellular membranes (in which it comprises two thirds of the phospholipids) of the hepatocyte and its role in maintaining the activities of some enzymes that are integral components of these membranes, it is not difficult to propose mechanisms by which choline deficiency can interfere with the viability of liver cells.

Choline deficiency is not sufficient for production of cirrhosis in the rat; the cirrhogenic potential of choline deficiency can be modulated. Cirrhosis is prevented by administration of non-absorbable antibiotics to choline-deficient rats.[1290] Fatty liver persists in these animals. Diets containing large amounts of protein also block the cirrhogenic effect of choline deficiency, so that choline deficiency leads to cirrhosis in the rat only when combined with a diet low in protein. Interestingly, the accumulation of fat in the livers of choline-deficient rats fed a high-protein diet is greater than that in animals fed a choline-deficient, low-protein diet. Thus a high-protein diet does not correct choline deficiency but alters the hepatic response to it. Choline deficiency, therefore, is only one of the factors involved in the genesis of cirrhosis in the choline-deficient rat.

Secondary malnutrition occurs in rats fed ethanol on a chronic basis. As mentioned previously, animals fed ethanol do not gain weight as rapidly as controls ingesting the same quantity of calories,[1291] and these animals display evidence of multiple vitamin deficiencies despite a nutritionally adequate diet.[1292,1293] What is clear, therefore, is that minimal daily requirements for nutrients determined for normal animals (humans probably included) do not apply to animals consuming large amounts of ethanol. One simple reason for this is the effect of ethanol on absorption of nutrients in the gut (Table 29-13).[1294-1298] Finally, the amounts of carbohydrate and fat fed along with ethanol have a profound effect on the genesis of cirrhosis and fibrosis in rat liver. As alluded to previously, fibrosis does not occur if ethanol is substituted for fat instead of for sugar.[1299,1300] The usual diets used to induce cirrhosis in the rat substitute ethanol for carbohydrates.

There are many reasons why ethanol ingestion could alter the minimal daily requirements for choline and other nutrients. As mentioned, ethanol ingestion increases the utilization of choline in the rat.[1286-1289] It also has important effects on the metabolism of folate, which can interact with the enzyme systems synthesizing choline. As shown in Figure 29-19, adequate stores of folate are important for synthesis of choline. Also, choline can serve as a source of $—CH_3$ groups for synthesis of methionine, thereby circumventing an ethanol-induced block of folate-mediated methyl transfer reactions.[1301]

Sorting out the significant interactions between ethanol and the metabolism of nutrients obviously will be an enormously difficult task. These complexities probably explain why a fixed choline supplement that prevents ethanol-induced fibrosis in monkeys[1302,1303] does not do so in baboons.[1304] The idea that ethanol per se is not toxic for baboons is underlined too by the observa-

TABLE 29-13

Reversible Intestinal Abnormalities in Alcoholics Without Liver Disease

Malabsorption of folic acid, thiamine, fat, nitrogen B_{12}, and B_2
Decreased output of HCO_3, amylase, lipase, and chymotrypsin in response to secretin

HCO_3, Bicarbonate.

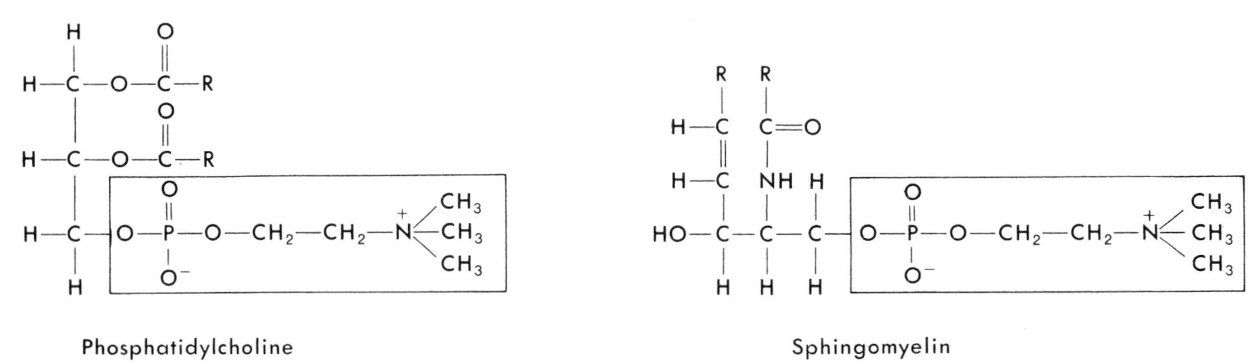

Phosphatidylcholine

Sphingomyelin

Figure 29-18 Choline-containing phosphatides.

tion that hepatic fibrosis develops in only one third of baboons fed ethanol. Two thirds of the animals fed ethanol plus a diet of questionable nutritional adequacy are able to compensate for the toxic effects of ethanol. This is not unlike the situation in humans. However, there is no good evidence that baboons ever develop alcoholic hepatitis.

Relevant Experimental Data in Humans

There has been no long-term prospective study of the incidence of liver disease in alcoholic individuals. There are, however, well-controlled studies of the effects of ethanol when administered to patients recovering from alcoholic hepatitis.[1305-1309] In one such study the patients all had decompensated alcoholic cirrhosis.[1305] After it was clear that the patients were able to eat, they were given large oral doses of ethanol. Patients consumed approximately 3000 calories each day, of which one third were derived from ethanol. The amount of ethanol ingested was sufficient in these patients to exceed their capacity to metabolize it completely within 24 hours. As liver function improved and the metabolic rate for ethanol increased, more ethanol was added to the diet. Liver function tests for the patients treated in this manner are shown in Figure 29-20. Data for a patient with acute sclerosing hyaline necrosis are shown in Figure 29-21. Clinical observations of the progress of the patients in this study indicated continued improvement over the course of the experiment. Patients with decompensated, alcohol-induced liver disease recovered from their disease even while ingesting large amounts of ethanol as long as they also were consuming nutritionally adequate diets. The best available data from controlled investigations in humans indicate, therefore, that the response of humans to ethanol is similar to that of rats and primates. The data in humans imply that ethanol abuse is not the only factor essential for producing cirrhosis in the alcoholic, because, given an "adequate" diet, humans adapt to the hepatotoxic effects of ethanol. These results thus do not fit with the idea that ethanol is a direct hepatotoxin.

The idea that liver disease in the alcoholic is secondary to the malnutrition seen so frequently in this group, rather than to their alcohol intake per se, is an old one. This view has never been accepted as fact because malnutrition, defined as protein and calorie deprivation, does not cause irreversible liver disease in humans. During World War II, for example, the incidence of cirrhosis did not increase in those areas in which starvation was present. Similarly, children who have kwashiorkor or marasmus do not develop cirrhosis. And, because malnutrition cannot be shown to cause cirrhosis in humans (it does in rats and primates), it has been difficult to accept the concept that malnutrition in the alcoholic causes cirrhosis.

Documentation that ethanol itself had deleterious effects on the function of the liver, causing, for example, fatty liver, abnormalities of endoplasmic reticulum, and swollen mitochondria, seemed to rationalize the idea that ethanol per se was the cause of cirrhosis in alcoholics and that diet was unimportant. However, advances in biochemistry have taught us that most clinical diseases are the end result of concerted effects, each of which may not cause clinical abnormality when acting alone. This is appreciated most easily in disease states secondary to inborn errors of metabolism. Patients lacking the hepatic form of fructose-1-P aldolase, for example, become ill after eating fructose, but are well as long as they avoid it.[1310] Clinical disease, therefore, is not caused by either fructose

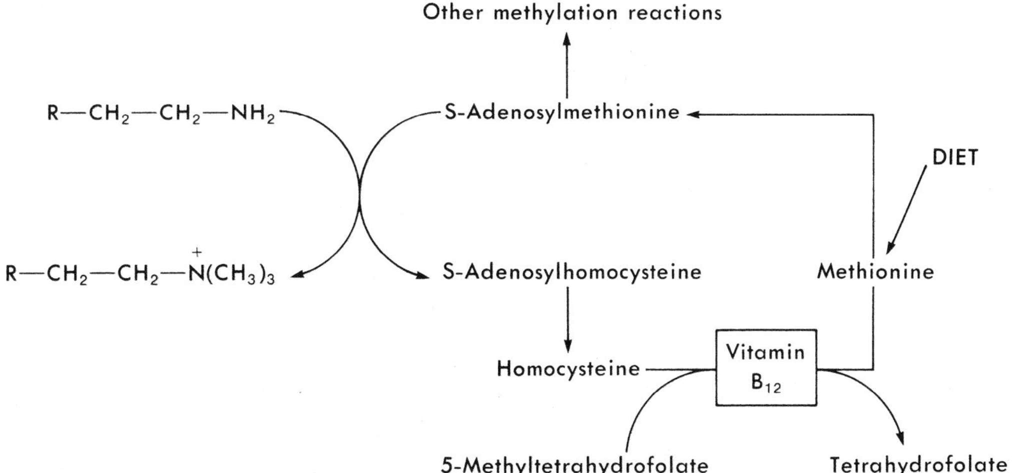

Figure 29-19 The synthesis of choline and its dependence on vitamin B_{12} and folate. R-CH_2-CH_2-NH_2 represents phosphatidyl ethanolamine, which is methylated three times to form phosphatidylcholine. Three moles of *S*-adenosylmethionine are required for synthesis of each mole of phosphatidylcholine. Regeneration of *S*-adenosylmethionine can be effected with dietary methionine or by synthesis of methionine from homocysteine. The latter conversion requires 5-methyltetrahydrofolate as a methyl group donor and vitamin B_{12} as co-factor. The scheme shows how choline- and methionine-deficient diets might induce folate deficiency by draining folate (the folate trap hypothesis) from DNA synthesis. *DNA,* Deoxyribonucleic acid.

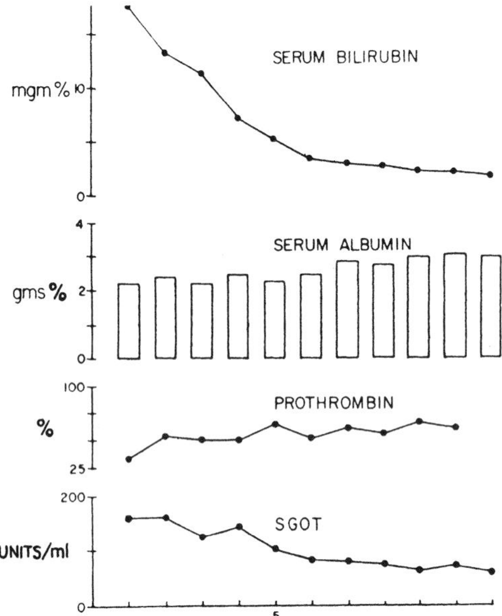

Figure 29-20 Composite results of laboratory tests performed on 10 patients with alcoholic hepatitis who were given alcohol. Alcohol intake was increased to match an increasing alcohol metabolic rate. (From Reynolds TB, Redeker AG, Kuzma OT: Role of alcohol in pathogenesis of alcoholic cirrhosis. In McIntyre NM, Sherlock S, eds: Therapeutic Agents and the Liver. Oxford, Blackwell, 1965:131.)

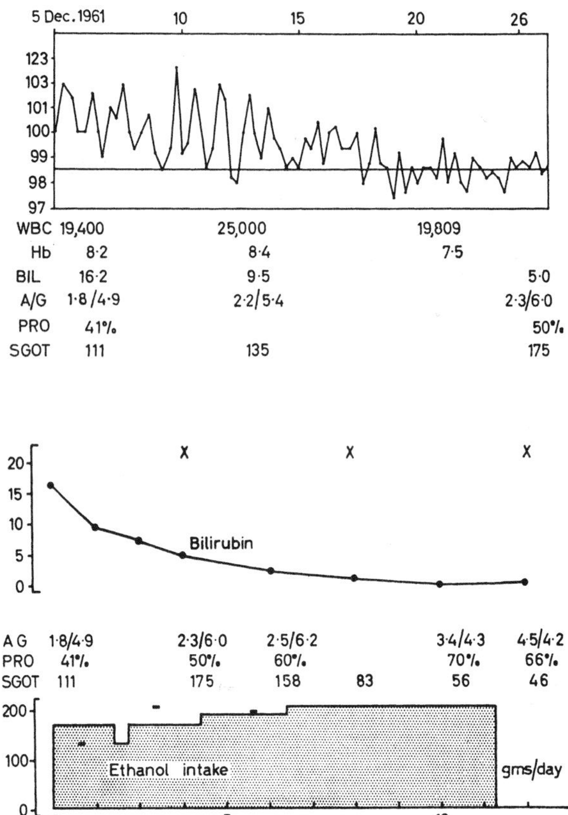

Figure 29-21 The top part of this figure reflects the clinical course of a patient with acute sclerosing hyaline necrosis. The two bottom sections are the results of laboratory tests of the patient. The small bars associated with the ethanol intake chart represent estimations of the alcohol metabolic rate. (From Reynolds TB, Redeker AG, Kuzma OT: Role of alcohol in pathogenesis of alcoholic cirrhosis. In McIntyre NM, Sherlock S, eds: Therapeutic Agents and the Liver. Oxford, Blackwell, 1965:131.)

or deficiency of fructose-1-P adolase, but by both acting in concert. Another example that is more relevant to disease in the alcoholic is the importance of ethanol and thiamine deficiency for producing Wernicke-Korsakoff syndrome. This disease is seen predominantly in malnourished alcoholics. Interestingly, however, those patients who develop Wernicke-Korsakoff psychosis, in addition to being alcoholics and thiamine-deficient because of their alcoholism, have an apparently greater than normal requirement for thiamine because of a genetic abnormality. The affinity of transketolase from these patients for its co-factor thiamine-PP is abnormally low,[1311,1312] which explains why only a minority of malnourished alcoholics develop Wernicke-Korsakoff syndrome. With regard to the problem of ethanol-induced liver disease, some proponents seem to argue that malnutrition in the alcoholic is the causal factor; others argue that ethanol causes liver disease regardless of diet. Neither of these views is supported by experiments.

Nutritional Status of Alcoholics

Not all alcoholics are malnourished, nor do all alcoholics have liver disease. On the other hand, data in the literature show that most alcoholics with liver disease are malnourished, on the basis of weight loss, specific evidence of malnutrition, or both.[1313-1331] This is true because ethanol interferes with intestinal absorption of nutrients (see Table 29-13) and it diminishes appetite for nonethanolic calories, which can lead to further deficiencies in absorptive function. It is mentioned often that dietary histories of alcoholics fail to show diminished intake of protein in those with liver disease, yet objective studies of these same patients show repeatedly that abstention from alcohol and ingestion of a normal diet in a controlled setting correct many abnormalities considered to reflect protein deficiency: weight gain, gain of muscle mass, correction of defective pancreatic secretion, and return of skin sensitivity to foreign antigens. Moreover, surveys of nutritional status in alcoholics consistently show that objective evidence of malnutrition is more prevalent in alcoholics with liver disease than in alcoholics without liver disease. Alcoholic patients with liver disease weigh less than they ideally should; alcoholics without liver disease are in excess of ideal body weight. Evidence of gross malnutrition is almost always present in patients with ALD and must be considered a significant and probably critical feature of their disease.

We should not assume that liver disease in the alcoholic patient, when it occurs, is continuously progressive. Clinical experience indicates that the intake of alcohol of a given patient with acute liver disease is not invariant. Instead, the history reveals quite frequently that admission to the hospital with acute decompensated liver disease was preceded by increasing intake of ethanol superimposed on a history of chronic alcoholism. Correlation of dietary intake with indices of liver function and without regard for the possible dynamic interactions between ethanol, diet, and hepatic function may give a skewed picture of the interrelations among these factors. Another problem that could confound studies of the relationship between ethanol, diet, and cirrhosis is that ethanol may interact not only with the diet but also with a genetic predisposition. That some malnourished alcoholics escape the problems of alcoholic hepatitis or cirrhosis is not evidence that malnutrition is not the critical pathogenic mechanism in those alcoholics that develop liver disease. Observations of the effects of ethanol in primates emphasize this idea.

Liver Disease in Patients Who Are Obese

An exceedingly interesting lesion is observed frequently (about 5 percent to 10 percent of the time) in patients who are morbidly obese.[1332-1337] Liver biopsy specimens from these patients are strikingly similar to those from patients with alcohol-associated liver disease. The frequency of the hepatic abnormalities increases to as much as 50 percent in patients who have had jejunoileal bypass procedures for control of their obesity.[1332-1340] The jejunoileal bypass gives rise to several potential problems for the liver of the treated patient who is deficient in essential nutrients, has a blind intestinal loop, and has abnormal hepatotoxic bile acids in serum.[1339-1342] The combination of these effects, especially the malnutrition, may account for the high incidence of severe hepatic lesions in patients who have had jejunoileal bypass procedures. In a few instances the hepatic lesions found after bypass surgery have responded to intravenous hyperalimentation.[1342-1344] We do not know why this lesion is present in obese patients, but neither do we know very much about the nutrient balance in such patients. Of interest is that being overweight potentiates the metabolic effects of ethanol, leading to cirrhosis even in the absence of alcoholic hepatitis.[1345] There is an important correlation between obesity, insulin resistance, and non alcoholic steatohepatitis (NASH).[1346] The common denominator for ALD and NASH appears to be fatty liver. Factors discussed already in the context of ALD and fatty liver are likely to bear on the etiology of NASH in patients with obesity and/or insulin resistance.

Increased Susceptibility of Women to ALD

Women develop alcohol-induced liver injury more rapidly than men[1347-1349]; liver injury progresses faster in women with alcoholic hepatitis, even after cessation or reduced drinking.[1350,1351] The reasons for this increased sensitivity to alcohol remain uncertain. Women have a higher blood alcohol level than men for a similar intake of ethanol,[1350] which is believed to reflect differences in body size, amount of body fat, and a lesser first-pass effect.[1352,1353]

The intragastric feeding model has helped to elucidate mechanisms leading to enhanced susceptibility of females to alcoholic liver injury.[1354] Levels of endotoxin are higher in female than in male rats fed alcohol. Because estrogens increase the permeability of gut to endotoxin in rats fed ethanol,[1355] greater permeability of female gut to endotoxin could account for higher levels after feeding alcohol to females versus males. Moreover, the effects of endotoxin on liver are mediated, in part, through the estrogen-responsive CD14 receptor of Kupffer cells.[1356] Pharmacologic doses of estrogen increase CD14 expression on Kupffer cells in rats. Levels of CD14 mRNA are greater in female rats compared to male rats fed ethanol.[1357] Ovariectomized rats show decreased severity of liver injury after feeding ethanol.[1355] Levels of lipid peroxides are significantly higher in female versus male liver after feeding ethanol, but levels of cytochrome P450 2E1, a major contributor to oxidative stress, are similar in male and female rats fed ethanol.[1358]

As mentioned previously, NF-κB is a possible link between endotoxemia, lipid peroxidation, and ethanol-induced liver injury. Levels of NF-κB are increased in female rats fed ethanol compared with male rats,[1147] as are expression of two NF-κB responsive genes (e.g., TNFα, Cox-2).[1358] These data support the concept that higher levels of endotoxin and oxidative stress in female as compared with male rats activate proinflammatory genes via NF-κB to promote greater liver injury in female rats.[1357-1359] Estrogen, which increases lipopolysaccharide binding-protein, also sensitizes Kupffer cells to LPS.[1360] Another mechanism by which estrogen might enhance the toxicity of endotoxin in vivo is lowered levels of lipoproteins, which would impair pathways neutralizing endotoxin.[1361]

In the ethanol-fed micropig the generation of protein-aldehyde adducts is associated with sex-steroid-dependent induction of several cytochrome P450s.[1362] Castrated animals show higher levels of CYP 2A than do non-castrated micropigs.

There are important gender differences in the effects of alcohol on hepatic lipid metabolism. Alcohol consumption inhibits mitochondrial beta oxidation of fatty acids,[1362] while inducing CYP 2E1 and CYP 4A1. The latter enzymes catalyze omega oxidation (hydroxylation at the terminal carbon of the fatty acid) and omega1 oxidation (hydroxylation at the penultimate carbon) of fatty acids, respectively.[1364] Further oxidation of these intermediates generates dicarboxylic acid (for reaction at the terminal carbon) or oxo-carboxylic acids (for reaction at the penultimate carbon). These products are less toxic than the parent compounds. The dicarboxylic acids generated during ethanol oxidation initiate transcription of proteins (e.g., cytosolic fatty acid binding protein) involved in fatty acid disposition.[1365] Chronic administration of alcohol increases omega oxidation more effectively in males than in female rats.[1366] The net effect of alcohol on beta and omega oxidation is greater accumulation of deleterious monocarboxylic acids in females versus male rats.[1367] Similar gender differences occur in humans.[1368] The lesser degree of the compensatory response in women could promote a greater accumulation of toxic fatty acids in their livers.

References

1. Harwood HJ, Napcitano DM, Kristiansen PL, et al: Economic costs to society of alcohol and drug abuse and mental illness: 1980. Research Triangle Institute: Report submitted to the Alcohol, Drug Abuse, and Mental Health Administration, Rockville, MD, 1984.
2. Boar°d of Trustees Report: Alcohol. Advertising, counter advertising and depiction in the public media. JAMA 256:1485, 1986.
3. West LJ, ed: Alcoholism and Related Problems: Issues for the American Public. Englewood Cliffs, NJ, Prentice Hall, 1984.

4. Trell E, Kristenson H, Petersson B: A risk factor approach to alcohol related disease. Alcohol Alcohol 20:333, 1985.
5. Breed W, DeFoe JR: Themes in magazine alcohol advertisements: a critique. J Drug Issues 9:511, 1979.
6. Skog OJ: The wetness of drinking cultures: a key variable in the epidemiology of alcoholic liver disease. Acta Med Scand (suppl) 703:157, 1985.
7. Cohalan D: Epidemiology: alcohol use in American Society. In Gomberg EL, White HR, Carpenter JD, eds: Alcohol Science and Society Revisited. Ann Arbor, University of Michigan Press, 1982:96-98.
8. Fuller RK, Allen JP, Litten RZ: Diagnosis and management of alcohol problems. Clin Liver Dis 2:649-660, 1998.
9. Kendell RE: Alcoholism: medical or political problem? BMJ 1:367, 1979.
10. Gorwitz K, Bahn A, Warthen FJ, et al: Some epidemiological data on alcoholism in Maryland. Q J Stud Alcohol 31:423, 1970.
11. Schmidt W, DeLint J: Causes of death of alcoholics. Q J Stud Alcohol 33:171, 1972.
12. Lelbach WK: Quantitative aspects of drinking in alcoholic liver cirrhosis. In Israel Y, Khanna J, Kalant H, eds: Alcoholic Liver Pathology. Toronto, Addiction Research Foundation, 1975.
13. Grant BF, DeBakey S, Zobek TS: Liver cirrhosis mortality in the United States, 1973-1988. NIAAA Surveillance Report No. 18. DHHS Publ. No. (ADM) 281-89-0001. Washington DC, Section of Documents, US Government Printing Office, 1991.
14. Mann RE, Smart RG, Aglin L, Adlaf EM: Reductions in cirrhosis deaths in the United States: associations with per capita consumption and AA membership. J Stud Alcohol 52:361, 1991.
15. Lelbach WK: Cirrhosis in the alcoholic and its relation to the volume of alcohol abuse. Ann N Y Acad Sci 285:85, 1975.
16. Lelbach WK: Epidemiology of alcoholic liver disease. Prog Liver Dis 5:494, 1976.
17. Tuyns AJ, Pequignot G: Greater risk of ascitic cirrhosis in females in relation to alcohol consumption. Int J Epidem 13:53, 1984.
18. Spain DM: Portal cirrhosis of the liver: a review of 250 necropsies with reference to sex differences. Am J Clin Pathol 15:215, 1945.
19. Krasner N, Davis M, Portmann B, et al: Changing pattern of alcoholic liver disease in Great Britain: relation to sex and signs of autoimmunity. BMJ 1:1487, 1977.
20. Morgan MY, Sherlock S: Sex-related differences among 100 patients with alcoholic liver disease. BMJ 1:939, 1977.
21. Robins LN, Helzer JE, Weissman MM, et al: Lifetime prevalence of specific psychiatric disorders in three sites. Arch Gen Psychiatr 41:949, 1984.
22. Jolliffe N, Jellinek EM: Vitamin deficiencies and liver cirrhosis in alcoholism. VII. Cirrhosis of the liver. Q J Stud Alcohol 2:544, 1941.
23. Popham RE: The Jellinek alcoholism estimation formula and its application to Canadian data. Q J Stud Alcohol 17:559, 1956.
24. Klatskin G: Alcohol and its relation to liver damage. Gastroenterology 41:443, 1961.
25. Steiner PE: World problem in the cirrhotic diseases of the liver. Their incidence, frequency, types and etiology. Trop Geogr Med 16:175, 1964.
26. Bhathol PS, Wilkinson P, Clifton S, et al: The spectrum of liver disease in alcoholism. Aust NZ J Med 5:49, 1975.
27. Saunders JB, Williams R: The genetics of alcoholism: is there an inherited susceptibility to alcohol-related problems? Alcohol Alcohol 3:189, 1983.
28. Hall PA, ed: Alcoholic Liver Disease Pathobiology, Epidemiology and Clinical Aspects. New York, John Wiley & Sons, 1985.
29. Lundquist F: The metabolism of ethanol. In Israel Y, Mardonec J, eds: Biological Basis of Alcoholism. New York, John Wiley and Sons, 1971:1.
30. Williamson JR, Tischler M: Ethanol metabolism in perfused liver and isolated hepatocytes with associated methodologies. In Majchrowicz E, Noble EP, eds: Biochemistry and Pharmacology of Ethanol. New York, Plenum, 1979:167.
31. Hawkins RD, Kalant H: The metabolism of ethanol and its metabolic effects. Pharmacol Rev 24:67, 1972.
32. Roach MD, Khan M, Knapp M, et al: Ethanol metabolism in vivo and the role of hepatic microsomal ethanol oxidation. Q J Stud Alcohol 33:751, 1972.
33. Lieber CS: Metabolism of ethanol. In Lieber CS, ed: Metabolic Aspects of Alcoholism. Baltimore, University Park Press, 1977:1.
34. Chambers GK: The genetics of human alcohol metabolism. Gen Pharmacol 21:267, 1990.
35. Bosron WF, Ehring T, Li TK: Genetic factors in alcohol metabolism and alcoholism. Semin Liver Dis 13:126, 1993.
36. Lumeng L, Crabb DW: Genetic aspects and risk factors in alcoholism and alcoholic liver disease. Gastroenterology 107:572, 1994.
37. Arnon R, Esposti D, Zern MA: Molecular biologic aspects of alcohol-induced liver disease. Alcohol Clin Exp Res 19:247, 1995.
38. Yoshida A, Hsu LC, Yasunami M: Genetics of human alcohol-metabolizing enzymes. Prog Nucl Acid Res 40:255, 1991.
39. Agarwal DP, Goedde HW: Pharmacogenetics of alcohol dehydrogenase. Pharmacol Ther 45:69, 1990.
40. Agarwal DP, Goedde HW: Enzymology of alcohol degradation. In Goedde HW, Agarwal DP, eds: Alcoholism: Biomedical and Genetic Aspects. New York, Pergamon Press, 1990.
41. Bosron WF, Li TK: Genetic polymorphism of human liver alcohol and aldehyde dehydrogenases and their relationship to alcohol metabolism and alcoholism. Hepatology 6:502, 1986.
42. Julia P, Boleda MD, Farres J, Pares X: Mammalian alcohol dehydrogenase: characteristics of class III isozymes. Alcohol Alcohol (suppl 1): 169, 1987.
43. Moreno A, Pares X: Purification and characterization of a new alcohol dehydrogenase from human stomach. J Biol Chem 266:1128, 1991.
44. Yin SJ, Wang MF, Liao CS, et al: Identification of a human stomach alcohol dehydrogenase with distinctive kinetic properties. Biochem Int 22:829, 1990.
45. Yasunami M, Chen CS, Yoshida A: A human alcohol dehydrogenase gene (ADH_6) encoding an additional class of isozyme. Proc Natl Acad Sci U S A 88:7610, 1991.
46. Yamauchi M, Potter J, Mezey E: Lobular distribution of alcohol dehydrogenase in the rat liver. Hepatology 8:243, 1988.
47. Kato S, Ishii H, Yamashita S, et al: Histochemical and immunohistochemical evidence for hepatic zone 3 distribution of alcohol dehydrogenase in rats. Hepatology 12:66, 1990.
48. Vaananen H, Salspuro M, Lindros K: The effect of chronic ethanol ingestion on ethanol metabolizing enzymes in isolated periportal and perivenous rat hepatocytes. Hepatology 5:862, 1984.
49. Chen L, Sidner RA, Lumeng L: Distribution of alcohol dehydrogenase and low K_m form of aldehyde dehydrogenase in isolated perivenous and portal hepatocytes in rats. Alcohol Clin Exp Res 16:23, 1992.
50. Greenberger N, Cohen RB, Isselbacher KJ: The effect of chronic alcohol administration on liver alcohol dehydrogenase activity in the rat. Lab Invest 14:264, 1965.
51. Sokal EM, Collette C, Buts JP: Continuous increase of alcohol dehydrogenase activity along the liver plate in normal and cirrhotic human livers. Hepatology 17:202, 1993.
52. Maly IP, Sasse D: Intraacinar profiles of alcohol dehydrogenase and aldehyde dehydrogenase activities in human liver. Gastroenterology 101:1716, 1991.
53. Van Ooij C, Snyder RC, Paeper BW, Duester G: Temporal expression of the human alcohol dehydrogenase gene family correlates with differential promoter activation by hepatocyte nuclear factor 1, CCAA/enhancer binding protein alpha, liver activator protein and D-element binding protein. Mol Cell Biol 12:3023, 1992.
54. Burnell JC, Bosron WF: Genetic polymorphism of human liver alcohol dehydrogenase and kinetic properties of the isoenzymes. In Crow KE, Batt RD, eds: Human Metabolism of Alcohol, Vol. II. Boca Raton, FL, CRC Press, 1989:65.
55. Day CP, Bashir R, James OFW, et al: Investigation of the role of polymorphisms at the alcohol and aldehyde dehydrogenase loci in genetic predisposition to alcohol-related end-organ damage. Hepatology 14:798, 1991.
56. Thomasson HR, Edenberg HJ, Crabb DW, et al: Alcohol and aldehyde dehydrogenase genotypes and alcoholism in Chinese men. Am J Hum Genet 48:677, 1991.
57. Poupon RE, Nalpas B, Coutelle C, et al: Polymorphisms of alcohol dehydrogenase, alcohol and aldehyde dehydrogenase activities: implications in alcoholic cirrhosis in white patients. Hepatology 15:1017, 1992.
58. Vallee BL, Bazzone TJ: Isoenzymes of human liver alcohol dehydrogenase. Curr Topics Biol Med Res 8:219, 1983.

59. Vallee BL: A novel approach to human ethanol metabolism: isoenzymes of alcohol dehydrogenases. Proc Cong Eur Brew Conv 20:65, 1985.
60. Wagner FW, Burger AR, Vallee BL: Kinetic properties of human liver alcohol dehydrogenase: oxidation of alcohols by class I isoenzymes. Biochemistry 22:1857, 1983.
61. Ditlow CD, Holmquist B, Morelock M, et al: Physical and enzymatic properties of a class II alcohol dehydrogenase isoenzyme of human liver: π ADH. Biochemistry 23:6363, 1984.
62. Von Wartburg JP, Schürch PM: Atypical liver alcohol dehydrogenase. Ann N Y Acad Sci 151:936, 1968.
63. Anonymous: Nomenclature of mammalian aldehyde dehydrogenases. Prog Clin Biol Res 290:xix, 1989.
64. Tsutsumi M, Takada A, Takase S, Sugata K: Hepatic aldehyde dehydrogenase isoenzymes: differences with respect to species. Alcohol 5:33, 1988.
65. Meier-Tackmann D, Korencke GC, Agarwal DP, Goedde HW: Human liver aldehyde dehydrogenase: subcellular distribution in alcoholics and non-alcoholics. Alcohol 5:73, 1988.
66. Goedde HW, Agarwal DP, Fritze G, et al: Distribution of ADH_2 and $ALDH_2$ genotypes in different populations. Hum Genet 88:344, 1992.
67. Yoshida A, Huang IY, Ikawa M: Molecular abnormality of an inactive aldehyde dehydrogenase variant commonly found in Orientals. Proc Natl Acad Sci U S A 81:258, 1984.
68. Thomasson HR, Crabb DW, Edenberg HJ, Li TK: Alcohol and aldehyde dehydrogenase polymorphisms and alcoholism. Behav Genet 23:131, 1993.
69. Crabb DW, Dipple KM, Thomasson HR: Alcohol sensitivity, alcohol metabolism, risk of alcoholism and role of alcohol and aldehyde dehydrogenase enzymes. J Lab Clin Med 122:234, 1993.
70. Enomoto N, Takase S, Takada N, Takada A: Alcoholic liver disease in heterozygotes of mutant and normal aldehyde dehydrogenase-2 genes. Hepatology 13:1071, 1991.
71. Chao HM: Alcohol and the mystique of flushing. Alcohol Clin Exp Res 19:104, 1995.
72. Harada S, Agarwal DP, Goedde HW: Isoenzyme variations in acetaldehyde dehydrogenase (EC 1.2.1.3) in human tissues. Hum Genet 44:181, 1978.
73. Wilhin JK, Fortner G: Cutaneous vascular sensitivity to lower aliphatic alcohols and aldehydes in Orientals. Alcoholism 9:522, 1985.
74. Higuchi S, Muramatsu T, Saito M, et al: Ethanol patch test for low K_m aldehyde dehydrogenase deficiency. Lancet i:629, 1987 (letter).
75. Ikawa M, Impraim CC, Wang G, et al: Isolation and characterization of aldehyde dehydrogenase isoenzymes from usual and atypical human livers. J Biol Chem 258:6282, 1983.
76. Iseri OA, Gottlieb LS, Lieber CS: The ultrastructure of ethanol-induced fatty liver. Fed Proc 23:579, 1964.
77. Iseri OA, Lieber CS, Gottlieb LS: The ultrastructure of fatty liver induced by prolonged ethanol ingestion. Am J Pathol 48:535, 1966.
78. Lane BP, Lieber CS: Ultrastructural alterations in human following ingestion of ethanol with adequate diets. Am J Pathol 49:593, 1966.
79. Lieber CS, DeCarli LM: Hepatic microsomal enzymes in man and rat: induction and inhibition by ethanol. Science 162:167, 1968.
80. Lieber CS, DeCarli LM: Hepatic microsomal ethanol oxidizing system: in vitro characteristics and adaptive properties in vivo. J Biol Chem 245:2505, 1970.
81. Lieber CS: The microsomal ethanol oxidizing system. Biochem Soc Trans 16:232, 1988.
82. Ohnishi K, Lieber CS: Reconstitution of the microsomal ethanol oxidizing system (MEOS): qualitative and quantitative changes of cytochrome P450 after chronic ethanol consumption. J Biol Chem 252:7124, 1977.
83. Koop DR, Morgan ET, Tarr GE, Coon MJ: Purification and characterization of a unique isoenzyme of cytochrome P450 from liver microsomes of ethanol treated rabbits. J Biol Chem 257:8472, 1982.
84. Morgan ET, Koop DR, Coon MJ: Catalytic activity of cytochrome P-450 isoenzyme 3a isolated from liver microsomes of ethanol-treated rabbits. J Biol Chem 257:13951, 1982.
85. Ryan DE, Ramanathan L, Iida S, et al: Characterization of a major form of rat hepatic microsomal cytochrome P450 induced by isoniazid. J Biol Chem 260:6385, 1985.
86. Patten CJ, Ning SM, Lu AYH, Yang CS: Acetone-inducible cytochrome P450: purification, catalytic activity and interaction with cytochrome b5. Arch Biochem Biophys 251:629, 1986.
87. Johannson I, Ekstrom G, Schotte B, et al: Ethanol-, fasting- and acetone inducible cytochromes P-450 in rat liver: regulation and characteristics of enzymes belonging to the IIB and IIE gene subfamilies. Biochemistry 27:1925, 1988.
88. Wrighton SA, Thomas PE, Ryan DE, Levin W: Purification and characterization of ethanol-inducible human hepatic cytochrome HLj. Arch Biochem Biophys 258:292, 1987.
89. Lasker JM, Paucy J, Kubota S, et al: Purification and characterization of human liver cytochrome-P450-ALC. Biochem Biophys Res Commun 148:232, 1988.
90. Gonzalez FJ, Guengerich FP, Gulsalus IC, et al: The P450 superfamily: update on new sequences, gene mapping and recommended nomenclature. DNA Cell Biol 10:1, 1991.
91. Ingelman-Sundberg M, Johannson I, Pentilla K, et al: Centrilobular expression of ethanol-inducible cytochrome P450 (IIE1) in rat liver. Biochem Biophys Res Commun 157:55, 1988.
92. Tsutsumi M, Lasker JM, Shimizu M, et al: The intralobular distribution of ethanol-inducible P450 IIE1 in rat and human liver. Hepatology 10:437, 1989.
93. Wu D, Cederbaum AI: Presence of functionally active cytochrome P-450 IIE1 in the plasma membrane of rat hepatocytes. Hepatology 15:515, 1992.
94. Koop DR, Tierney DJ: Multiple mechanisms in the regulation of ethanol-inducible cytochrome P450 IIE1. Bioessays 12:429, 1990.
95. Song BJ, Veech RL, Park SS, et al: Inducible of rat hepatic N-dinitrosodimethylamine dimethylase by acetone is due to protein stabilization. J Biol Chem 264:3568, 1989.
96. Eliasson E, Johannson I, Ingelman-Sundberg M: Ligand-dependent maintenance of ethanol-inducible cytochrome P-450 in primary hepatocyte cultures. Biochem Biophys Res Commun 150:436, 1988.
97. Ronis MJJ, Ingelman-Sundberg M: Acetone-dependent regulation of cytochrome-P450j (IIE1) and P-450b (IIB1) in rat liver. Xenobiotica 19:1161, 1989.
98. Eliasson E, Johansson I, Ingelman-Sundberg M: Substrate, hormone and cAMP-regulated cytochrome P450 degradation. Proc Natl Acad Sci U S A 87:3225, 1990.
99. Badger TM, Huang J, Ronis M, Lumpkin CK: Induction of cytochrome P450 2E1 during chronic ethanol exposure occurs via transcription of the CYP 2E1 gene when blood alcohol concentrations are high. Biochem Biophys Res Commun 190:780, 1993.
100. Ronis MJJ, Huang J, Crouch J, et al: Cytochrome P450 2E1 induction during chronic ethanol exposure occurs by a two-step mechanism associated with blood alcohol concentrations in rats. J Pharmacol Exp Ther 264:944, 1993.
101. Badger TJ, Ronis MJJ, Ingelman-Sundberg M, Hakkak R: Pulsatile blood alcohol and CYP 2E1 induction during chronic alcohol infusions in rats. Alcohol 10:453, 1993.
102. Kubota S, Lasker JM, Lieber CS: Molecular regulation of ethanol-inducible cytochrome P450 IIE1 in hamsters. Biochem Biophys Res Commun 150:304, 1988.
103. Takahashi T, Lasker JM, Rosman AS, Lieber CS: Induction of cytochrome P450 2E1 in the human liver by ethanol is caused by a corresponding increase in encoding messenger RNA. Hepatology 17:236, 1993.
104. Wrighton SA, Thomas PE, Molowa DT, et al: Characterization of ethanol-inducible human liver N-nitrosodimethylamine dimethylase. Biochemistry 25:6731, 1986.
105. Ingelman-Sundberg M, Johansson I, Terelius Y, et al: Ethanol-inducible CYP 2E1: toxicological importance and regulation by nutrients. In Parke DV, Ioannides C, Walker R, Smith-Gordon, eds: Food, Nutrition and Chemical Toxicology. Amsterdam, Netherlands, Elsevier Science, 1992:149.
106. Ingelman-Sundberg M, Johannson I: Mechanisms of hydroxyl radical formation and ethanol oxidation by ethanol-inducible and other forms of rabbit liver microsomal cytochrome P450. J Biol Chem 259:6447, 1984.
107. Ekstrom G, Ingelman-Sundberg M: Rat liver microsomal NADPH-supported oxidase activity and lipid peroxidation dependent on ethanol-inducible cytochrome P450 (P-450 IIE1). Biochem Pharmacol 38:1313, 1989.
108. Castillo T, Koop DR, Kamimura S, et al: Role of cytochrome P450 2E1 in ethanol-, carbon tetrachloride- and iron-dependent microsomal lipid peroxidation. Hepatology 16:992, 1992.

109. Brady JF, Wang MH, Hong JY, et al: Modulation of rat hepatic microsomal monooxygenase enzymes and cytotoxicity by diallylsulfide. Toxicol Appl Pharmacol 108:342, 1991.
110. Kwak MK, Kim SG, Kwak JY, et al: Inhibition of cytochrome P450 2E1 expression by organosulfur compounds allylsulfide, allylmercaptan and allylmethylsulfide in rats. Biochem Pharmacol 47:531, 1994.
111. Morimoto M, Hagbjork AL, Nanji AA, et al: Role of cytochrome P450 2E1 in alcoholic liver disease pathogenesis. Alcohol 10:459, 1993.
112. Morimoto M, Hagbjork AL, Wan YY, et al: Modulation of experimental alcohol-induced liver disease by cytochrome P450 2E1 inhibitors. Hepatology 21:1610, 1995.
113. Hu Y, Mishin V, Johansson I, et al: Chlormethiazole as an efficient inhibitor of cytochrome P450 2E1 expression in rat liver. J Pharmacol Exp Ther 269:1286, 1994.
114. Albano E, Clot P, Morimato M, et al: Role of cytochrome P4502E1-dependent formation of hydroxyethyl free radical in the development of liver damage in rats intragastrically fed with ethanol. Hepatology 23:155, 1996.
115. Albano E, Parola M, Comoglio A, Dianzani MU: Evidence for the covalent binding of hydroxyethyl radicals to rat liver microsomal proteins. Alcohol Alcohol 28:453, 1993.
116. Moncada C, Torres V, Vargese E, et al: Ethanol derived immunoreactive species formed by free radical mechanisms. Mol Pharmacol 46:786, 1994.
117. Clot P, Bellomo G, Tabone M, et al: Detection of antibodies against proteins modified by hydroxyethyl free radicals in patients with alcoholic cirrhosis. Gastroenterology 108:201, 1995.
118. Albano E, French SW, Ingelman-Sundberg M: Hydroxyethyl radicals in ethanol hepatotoxicity. Front Biosci 4:533-540, 1999.
119. Albano E, Clot P, Morimoto M, et al: Role of cytochrome P4502E1-dependent formation of hydroxyethyl free radical in the development of liver damage in rats intragastrically fed with ethanol. Hepatology 23:155-163, 1996.
120. Dupont I, Lucas D, Clot P, et al: Cytochrome P4502E1 inducibility and hydroxyethyl radical formation among alcoholics. J Hepatol 28:564-571, 1998.
121. Clot P, Albano E, Eliasson E. et al: Cytochrome P4502E1 hydroxyethyl radical adducts as the major antigen in autoantibody formation among alcoholics. Gastroenterology 111:206-216, 1996.
122. Terelius Y, Norsten-Hoog C, Cronholm T, Ingelman-Sundberg M: Acetaldehyde as a substrate for ethanol-inducible cytochrome P450 (CYP 2E1). Biochem Biophys Res Commun 179:689, 1991.
123. Lucas D, Lambouef Y, Blanquat GD, Menez JF: Ethanol-inducible cytochrome P450 activity and increase in acetaldehyde bound to microsomes after chronic administration of acetaldehyde or ethanol. Alcohol Alcohol 25:395, 1990.
124. French SW, Wong K, Jui L, et al: Effect of ethanol on cytochrome P450 2E1 (CYP 2E1); lipid peroxidation and serum protein adduct formation in relation to liver pathology pathogenesis. Exp Mol Pathol 58:61, 1993.
125. Hong J, Pan J, Gonzalez FJ, et al: The induction of a specific form of cytochrome P450 (P-450j) by fasting. Biochem Biophys Res Commun 142:1077, 1987.
126. Porter TD, Khani SC, Coon MJ: Induction and tissue-specific expression of rabbit cytochrome P450 IIE1 and IIE2 genes. Mol Pharmacol 36:61, 1989.
127. Johannson I, Ekstrom G, Scholte B, et al: Ethanol-, fasting- and acetone-inducible cytochromes P450 in rat liver: regulation and characteristics of enzymes belonging to the IIB and IIE gene subfamilies. Biochemistry 27:1925, 1988.
128. Lieber CS, Lasker JM, DeCarli LM, et al: Role of acetone, dietary fat and total energy intake in induction of hepatic microsomal ethanol oxidizing system. J Pharmacol Exp Ther 247:791, 1988.
129. Yoo JH, Hong JY, Ning SM, Yang CS: Roles of dietary corn oil in the regulation of cytochromes P450 and glutathione-S-transferases in rat liver. J Nutr 120:1718, 1990.
130. Yoo JH, Ning SM, Pantuck CB, et al: Regulation of hepatic microsomal cytochrome P450 2E1 level by dietary lipids and carbohydrates in rats. J Nutr 121:959, 1991.
131. Takahashi H, Johansson I, French SW, Ingelman-Sundberg M: Effects of dietary fat composition on activities of the microsomal ethanol-inducible cytochrome P450 (CYP 2E1) in the liver of rats chronically fed ethanol. Pharmacol Toxicol 70:347, 1992.
132. Nanji AA, Zhao S, Lamb RG, et al: Changes in cytochromes P-450 2E1, 2B1 and 4A and phospholipases A and C in the intragastric feeding rat model for alcoholic liver disease: relationship to dietary fats and pathologic liver injury. Alcohol Clin Exp Res 18:902, 1994.
133. French SW: Nutrition in the pathogenesis of alcoholic liver disease. Alcohol Alcohol 28:97, 1993.
134. Nanji AA, Zhao S, Sadrzadeh SMH, et al: Markedly enhanced cytochrome P450 2E1 induction and lipid peroxidation is associated with severe liver injury in fish oil-ethanol-fed rats. Alcohol Clin Exp Res 18:1280, 1994.
135. Morimoto M, Zern MA, Hagbjork AL, et al: Fish oil, alcohol, and liver pathology: role of cytochrome P450 2E1. Proc Soc Exp Biol Med 207:197, 1994.
136. Matteonic CA, Younossi AM, Gramlich T, et al: Non-alcoholic fatty liver disease: a spectrum of clinical and pathological severity. Gastroenterology 116:1413-1419, 1999.
137. Robertson G, Leclerq I, Farrell GC: Non-alcoholic steatosis and steatohepatitis-cytochrome P450 enzymes and oxidative stress. Am J Physiol Gatrointest Liver Physiol 281:G1136-G1139, 2001.
138. Weltman MD, Farrell GC, Liddle C: Increased hepatocyte CYP2E1 expression in a rat nutritional model of hepatic steatosis with inflammation. Gastroenterology 111:1645-1653, 1996.
139. Weltman MD, Farrell GC, Hall P, et al: Hepatic cytochrome P450 2E1 is increased in patients with nonalcoholic steatohepatitis. Hepatology 27:128-133, 1998.
140. Leclercq IA, Farrell GC, Field J, et al: CYP2E1 and CYP4A as microsomal catalysts of lipid peroxides in murine nonalcoholic steatohepatitis. J Clin Invest 105:1067-1075, 2000.
141. Kono H, Bradford BU, Yin M, et al: CYP2E1 is not involved in early alcohol-induced liver injury. Am J Physiol 277:G1259-1267, 1999.
142. Lieber CS: Microsomal ethanol-oxidizing system (MEOS): the first 30 years. Alcohol Clin Exp Res 23:991-1007, 1999.
143. Maher J: The CYP2E1 knockout delivers another punch: first ASH, now NASH. Hepatology 33:311-312, 2001.
144. Keilin D, Hartree ER: Properties of catalase. Catalysis of coupled oxidation of alcohol. Biochem J 39:293, 1945.
145. Isselbacher KJ, Carter EA: Ethanol oxidation by liver microsomes: evidence against a separate and distinct enzyme system. Biochem Biophys Res Commun 39:530, 1970.
146. Thurman RG, Ley HG, Scholz R: Hepatic microsomal ethanol oxidation: hydrogen peroxide formation and the role of catalase. Eur J Biochem 25:420, 1972.
147. Vatsis KP, Schulman MP: Absence of ethanol metabolism in acatalatic hepatic microsomes that oxidize drugs. Biochem Biophys Res Commun 52:588, 1973.
148. Oshino N, Oshino R, Chance B: The characteristics of 'peroxidatic' reaction of catalase in ethanol oxidation. Biochem J 131:555, 1973.
149. Ohnishi K, Lieber CS: Reconstitution of the microsomal ethanol-oxidizing system. J Biol Chem 252:7124, 1977.
150. Miwa GT, Levin W, Thomas PE, et al: The direct oxidation of ethanol by a catalase- and alcohol dehydrogenase-free reconstituted system containing cytochrome P-450. Arch Biochem Biophys 137:464, 1978.
151. Teschke R, Hasumura Y, Lieber CS: Hepatic microsomal ethanol-oxidizing system: solubilization; isolation, and characterization. Arch Biochem Biophys 163:404, 1974.
152. Teschke R, Hasamura Y, Lieber CS: Hepatic microsomal alcohol oxidizing system: affinity for methanol, ethanol, propanol and butanol. J Biol Chem 250:7397, 1975.
153. Fong KL, McCay PB, Poyer JL, et al: Evidence that peroxidation of lysosomal membranes is initiated by hydroxyl free radicals produced during flavin enzyme activity. J Biol Chem 248:7792, 1973.
154. Dorfman LM, Adams GE: Reactivity of the Hydroxyl Radical in Aqueous Solutions. NSRRS, National Bureau of Standards, Washington, DC, 1992:46.
155. Cederbaum AI, Dicker E, Cohen G: Effect of hydroxyl radical scavengers on microsomal oxidation of alcohols and on associated microsomal reactions. Biochemistry 17:3058, 1978.
156. Krikun G, Lieber CS, Cederbaum AI: Increased microsomal oxidation of ethanol by cytochrome P-450 and hydroxyl radical-dependent pathways after chronic ethanol consumption. Biochem Pharmacol 33:3309, 1984.
157. Krikun G, Cederbaum AI: Evaluation of microsomal pathways of oxidation of alcohols and hydroxyl radical scavenging agents

with carbon monoxide and cobalt protoporphyrin IX. Biochem Pharmacol 34:2929, 1985.
158. Feierman DE, Cederbaum AI: Inhibition of microsomal oxidation of ethanol by pyrazole and 4-methylpyrazole in vitro. Biochem J 239:671, 1986.
159. Handler JA, Thurman RG: Catalase-dependent ethanol oxidation in perfused rat liver. Requirement for fatty acid-stimulated H_2O_2 production by peroxisomes. Eur J Biochem 176:477, 1988.
160. Inatomi N, Kato S, Ito D, Lieber CS: Role of peroxisomal fatty acid beta-oxidation in ethanol metabolism. Biochem Biophys Res Commun 163:418, 1989.
161. Handler JA, Thurman RG: Redox interactions between catalase and alcohol dehydrogenase pathways of ethanol metabolism in perfused rat liver. J Biol Chem 265:1510, 1990.
162. Bradford UB, Seed CB, Handler JA, et al: Evidence that catalase is a major pathway of ethanol oxidation in vivo: dose-response studies in deer mice using methanol as a selective substrate. Arch Biochem Biophys 303:172, 1993.
163. Kato S, Alderman J, Lieber CS: Respective roles of the microsomal ethanol oxidizing system (MEOS) and catalase in ethanol metabolism by deermice lacking alcohol dehydrogenase. Arch Biochem Biophys 254:586, 1987.
164. Misra UK, Bradford UB, Handler JA, Thurman RG: Chronic ethanol treatment induces H_2O_2 production selectively in pericentral regions of the liver lobule. Alcohol Clin Exp Res 16:839, 1992.
165. Imlay JA, Linn DS: DNA damage and oxygen radical toxicity. Science 240:1302, 1988.
166. Lange LG, Bergman SR, Sobel BE: Identification of fatty acid ethyl esters as products of rabbit myocardial ethanol metabolism. J Biol Chem 256:12968, 1981.
167. Lange LG, Sobel BE: Myocardial metabolites of ethanol. Circ Res 52:479, 1983.
168. Mogelson S, Lange LG: Non-oxidative ethanol metabolism in rabbit myocardium: purification to homogeneity of fatty acyl ethyl ester synthase. Biochemistry 23:4075, 1984.
169. Ryan TJ, Kororenidis G, Moschoz CB, et al: The acute metabolic and hemodynamic responses of the left ventricle to ethanol. J Clin Invest 45:270, 1966.
170. Lange LG, Sobel BE: Mitochondrial dysfunction induced by fatty acid ethyl esters, myocardial metabolites of ethanol. J Clin Invest 72:724, 1983.
171. Laposata EA, Lange LG: Presence of non-oxidative ethanol metabolism in human organs commonly damaged by ethanol abuse. Science 231:497, 1986.
172. Doyle KM, Rind DA, Al-Soliki S, et al: Fatty acid ethyl esters are present in serum after ethanol ingestion. J Lipid Res 35:428-437, 1994.
173. Lange LG, Sobel BE: Mitochondrial dysfunction induced by fatty acid ethyl esters, myocardial metabolites of ethanol. J Clin Invest 72:724, 1983.
174. Haber PS, Wilson JS, Apte MV, Pirola RC: Fatty acid ethyl esters increase rat pancreatic lysosomal fragility. J Lab Clin Med 121:759, 1993.
175. Szczepiorkowski ZM, Dickersin GR, Laposata M: Fatty acid ethyl esters decrease human hepatoblastoma cell proliferation and protein synthesis. Gastroenterology 108:515, 1995.
176. Spector AA: Fatty acid ethyl esters: insight or intoxication. Gastroenterology 108:605, 1995.
177. Cabelleria J, Baraona E, Lieber CS: The contribution of the stomach to ethanol oxidation in the rat. Life Sci 41:1021, 1987.
178. Julkunen RJK, DiPadova C, Lieber CS: First pass metabolism of ethanol—a gastrointestinal barrier against the systemic toxicity of ethanol. Life Sci 37:567, 1985.
179. Julkunen RJK, Tannenbaum L, Baraona E, Lieber CS: First pass metabolism of ethanol: an important determinant of blood levels after alcohol consumption. Alcohol 2:437, 1985.
180. DiPadova C, Worner TM, Julkunen RJK, Lieber CS: Effects of fasting and chronic alcohol consumption on the first-pass metabolism of ethanol. Gastroenterology 92:1169, 1987.
181. Caballeria J, Frezza M, Hernandez-Munoz R, et al: Gastric origin of first pass metabolism in humans: effects of gastrectomy. Gastroenterology 97:1205, 1989.
182. Pestalozzi DM, Buhler R, vonWartburg JP, Hess M: Immunohistochemical localization of alcohol dehydrogenase in the human gastrointestinal tract. Gastroenterology 85:1011, 1983.
183. Maly JP, Arnold M, Krieger K, et al: The intramucosal distribution of gastric alcohol dehydrogenase and aldehyde dehydrogenase activity in rats. Histochemistry 98:311, 1992.
184. Gentry RT, Baraona E, Lieber CS: Agonist: gastric first pass metabolism of alcohol. J Lab Clin Med 123:21, 1994.
185. Moreno A, Pares X: Purification and characterization of a new alcohol dehydrogenase from human stomach. J Biol Chem 266:1128, 1991.
186. Halsted CH, Robles EA, Mezey E: Distribution of ethanol in the human gastrointestinal tract. Am J Clin Nutr 26:831, 1973.
187. Frezza M, DePadova C, Pozzato G, et al: High blood alcohol levels in women. The role of decreased gastric alcohol dehydrogenase activity and first-pass metabolism. N Engl J Med 322:95, 1990.
188. Cabelleria J, Baraona E, Rodamilans M, Lieber CS: Effects of cimetidine on gastric alcohol dehydrogenase activity and blood ethanol levels. Gastroenterology 96:388, 1989.
189. Raulman JP, Notar-Francesco V, Rafiello R, Strauss E: Histamine-2-receptor antagonists do not alter serum ethanol levels in fed non-alcoholic men. Ann Intern Med 118:489, 1993.
190. Levitt MD: Antagonist: the case against first-pass metabolism of ethanol in the stomach. J Lab Clin Med 123:28, 1994.
191. Smith T, DeMaster E, Furne J, et al: First-pass gastric mucosal metabolism of ethanol is negligible in the rat. J Clin Invest 89:1802, 1992.
192. Baraona E, Yokoyama A, Ishii H, et al: Lack of alcohol dehydrogenase isoenzyme activities in the stomach of Japanese subjects. Life Sci 49:1929, 1991.
193. Gentry RT, Baraona E, Lieber CS: Rebuttal to antagonist. J Lab Clin Med 123:32, 1994.
194. Li TK, Bosron WF, Dafeldecker WP, et al: Isolation of π-alcohol dehydrogenase of human liver: is it a determinant of alcoholism? Proc Natl Acad Sci U S A 74:4378, 1977.
195. Keiding S, Christian NJ, Damgaard SE, et al: Ethanol metabolism in heavy drinkers after massive and moderate alcohol intake. Biochem Pharm 32:3097, 1983.
196. Korsten MA, Matsuzaki S, Feinman L, et al: High blood acetaldehyde levels after ethanol administration. N Engl J Med 292:386, 1975.
197. Israel Y, Khanna JM, Lin J: Effect of 2,4 dinitrophenol on the rate of ethanol elimination in the rat in vivo. Biochem J 120:447, 1970.
198. Videla L, Israel Y: Factors that modify the metabolism of ethanol in rat liver and adaptive changes produced by its chronic administration. Biochem J 118:275, 1970.
199. Meijer AJ, Von Woerkon G, Williamson JR, et al: Rate limiting factors in the oxidation of ethanol by isolated rat liver cells. Biochem J 150:205, 1975.
200. Bucher T, Klingenberg M: Wege des Wasserstoffe in der Lebendigen Organisation. Angew Chem 70:552, 1958.
201. Klingenberg M, Bucher T: Glycerin 1-P und Flugmuskelmitochondrien. Biochem Z 334:1, 1961.
202. Grunnet N, Quistorff B, Thieden HID: Rate limiting factors in ethanol oxidation by isolated rat liver parenchymal cells. Effect of ethanol concentration on fructose, pyruvate, and pyrazole. Eur J Biochem 40:275, 1973.
203. Thurman RG, Ji S, Lemasters JJ: Lobular oxygen gradient: a possible role in alcohol-induced hepatotoxicity. In Thurman RG, Kauffman FC, Jungerman K, eds: Regulation of Hepatic Metabolism. New York, Plenum, 1986:293.
204. Scholz R, Wohl H: Mechanism of the stimulatory effect of fructose on ethanol oxidation in perfused rat liver. Eur J Biochem 63:449, 1976.
205. Bosron WF, Li TK: Genetic polymorphism of human liver alcohol and dehydrogenases, and their relationship to alcohol metabolism and alcoholism. Hepatology 6:502, 1986.
206. Lumeng L, Bosron WF, Li TK: Quantitative correlation of ethanol elimination rates in vivo with liver alcohol dehydrogenase activities in fed, fasted and food restricted rats. Biochem Pharm 28:1547, 1979.
207. Wilson JS, Korsten MA, Lieber CS: The combined effects of protein deficiency and chronic ethanol administration on rat ethanol metabolism. Hepatology 6:823, 1986.
208. Crabb DW, Bosron WF, Li TK: Steady state kinetic properties of purified rat liver alcohol dehydrogenase: application to predicting alcohol elimination rates in vivo. Arch Biochem Biophys 224:299, 1983.

209. Videla L, Bernstein J, Israel Y: Metabolic alterations produced in the liver by chronic ethanol administration. Increased oxidative capacity. Biochem J 134:507, 1973.
210. Hawkins RD, Kalant H, Khanna JM: Effect of chronic intake of ethanol on rate of ethanol metabolism. Can J Physiol Pharmacol 44:241, 1966.
211. Mendelson JH, Mello NK: Metabolism of ^{14}C ethanol and behavioral adaptation of alcoholics during experimentally induced intoxication. Trans Am Neurol Assoc 89:133, 1964.
212. Cederbaum AI, Dicker E, Rubin E: Transfer and reoxidation of reducing equivalents as the rate limiting steps in the oxidation of ethanol by liver cells isolated from fed and fasted rats. Arch Biochem Biophys 183:638, 1977.
213. Kerner E, Westerfeld WW: Effect of diet on rate of alcohol oxidation by the liver. Proc Soc Exp Biol Med 83:530, 1953.
214. Bode C: Factors influencing ethanol metabolism in man. In Thurman RG, Yonetani T, Williamson JR, et al, eds: Alcohol and Aldehyde Metabolizing Systems, vol 1. New York, Academic Press, 1974:457.
215. Lindros KO, Pekkanen L, Kiovula T: Effect of low protein diet on acetaldehyde metabolism in rats. Acta Pharmacol Toxicol 40:134, 1977.
216. Lindros KO, Pekkanen L, Koivula T: Enzymatic and metabolic modification of hepatic ethanol and acetaldehyde oxidation by the dietary protein level. Biochem Pharmacol 28:2313, 1979.
217. Lindros KO: Regulatory factor in hepatic acetaldehyde metabolism during ethanol oxidation. In Lindros KO, Eriksson CJP, eds: The Role of Acetaldehyde in the Actions of Ethanol. The Finnish Foundation for Alcohol Studies 23:67, 1975.
218. Nuutinen HU, Salaspuro MP, Valle M, et al: Blood acetaldehyde concentration gradient between hepatic and antecubital venous blood in ethanol-intoxicated alcoholics and controls. Eur J Clin Invest 14:306, 1984.
219. Weiner H: Acetaldehyde metabolism. In Majchrowicz F, Noble EP, eds: Biochemistry and Pharmacology of Ethanol. New York, Plenum, 1979:125.
220. Tank AW, Weiner H, Thurman JA: Enzymology and subcellular localization of aldehyde oxidation in rat liver. Oxidation of 3,4-dihydroxyphenylacetaldehyde derived from dopamine to 3,4-dihydroxyphenylacetic acid. Biochem Pharmacol 30:2365, 1981.
221. Corrall RJ, Havre P, Margolis J, et al: Subcellular site of acetaldehyde oxidation in rat liver. Biochem Pharmacol 25:17, 1976.
222. Eriksson CJP, Sippel HW: The distribution and metabolism of acetaldehyde in rats during ethanol oxidation. I. The distribution of acetaldehyde in liver, brain, blood and breath. Biochem Pharmacol 26:241, 1977.
223. Eriksson CJP, Hilboni ME, Sovijarvi ARA: Difficulties in measuring human blood acetaldehyde concentration during ethanol intoxication. In Begleiter H, ed: Biological Effects of Alcohol. New York, Plenum, 1979.
224. Truitt EB Jr: Blood acetaldehyde levels after alcohol consumption by alcoholic and non-alcoholic subjects. In Biological Aspects of Alcohol, Advances in Mental Science, vol 3. Austin, University of Texas Press, 1971:212.
225. Weiner H: Aldehyde dehydrogenase: mechanism of action and possible physiological roles. In Majchrowicz E, Noble EP, eds: Biochemistry and Pharmacology of Ethanol. New York, Plenum, 1979:107.
226. Agarwal DP, Tobar-Rojas L, Meier-Taikman D, et al: Human erythrocyte aldehyde dehydrogenase: a biochemical marker of alcoholism? Alcohol Clin Exp Res 6:426, 1982.
227. Matthewson K, Record CO: Erythrocyte aldehyde dehydrogenase activity in alcoholic subjects and its value as a marker for hepatic aldehyde dehydrogenase in subjects with and without liver disease. Clin Sci 70:295, 1986.
228. Matthewson K, Al Mardini H, Bartlett K, et al: Impaired acetaldehyde metabolism in patients with nonalcoholic liver disorders. Gut 27:756, 1986.
229. Palmer KR, Jenkins WJ: Impaired acetaldehyde oxidation in alcoholics. Gut 23:729, 1982.
230. Jenkins WJ, Peter TJ: Selectively reduced hepatic acetaldehyde dehydrogenase in alcoholics. Lancet i:629, 1980.
231. Thomas M, Halsall S, Peters TJ: Role of hepatic acetaldehyde dehydrogenase in alcoholism: demonstration of a persisting reduction of cytosolic activity in abstaining patients. Lancet ii:1057, 1982.
232. Jenkins WJ, Cakebread K, Palmer KR: Effect of alcohol consumption on hepatic aldehyde dehydrogenase activity in alcoholic patients. Lancet i:1048, 1984.
233. Rutstein DD, Nickerson RJ, Vernon AA, et al: 2,3-butanediol: an unusual metabolite in the serum of seriously alcoholic men during acute intoxication. Lancet ii:534, 1983.
234. Hasumura Y, Teschke R, Lieber CS: Characteristics of acetaldehyde oxidation in rat liver mitochondria. J Biol Chem 251:4903, 1976.
235. Lindros KO, Pekkanen L, Koivula T: Biphasic influence of dietary protein levels on ethanol-derived acetaldehyde concentrations. Acta Pharmacol Toxicol 43:409, 1978.
236. Asmussen E, Hald J, Larsen V: The pharmacological action of acetaldehyde on the human organism. Acta Pharmacol Toxicol 4:311, 1948.
237. Truitt EJ Jr, Walsh MJ: The role of acetaldehyde in the actions of ethanol. In Kissin B, Begleiter HB, eds: The Biology of Alcoholism, vol 1. New York, Plenum, 1971:161.
238. Faiman M: Biochemical pharmacology of disulfuram. In Majchrowicz E, Noble EP, eds: Biochemistry and Pharmacology of Ethanol. New York, Plenum, 1979.
239. Haley TJ: Disulfiram (tetraethylthioperoxydicarbonic diamide): a reappraisal of its toxicity and therapeutic applications. Drug Metab Rev 9:319, 1979.
240. Sanny CG, Weiner H: Inactivation of horse liver mitochondrial aldehyde dehydrogenase by disulfuram. Evidence that disulfiram is not an active-site-directed reagent. Biochem J 242:499, 1987.
241. Lundwall L, Baekeland F: Disulfiram treatment of alcoholism. J Nerv Ment Dis 153:381, 1971.
242. Ritchie JM: The aliphatic alcohols. In Goodman LS, Gilman A, eds: The Pharmacological Basis of Therapeutics, ed 4. New York, Macmillan, 1970:135.
243. Berger D, Weiner J: In vivo interactions of chloral hydrate and disulfiram with the metabolism of catecholamines. In Galanter M, ed: Currents in Alcoholism. New York, Grune and Stratton, 1977:231.
244. Hellstrom-Lindahl E, Weiner H: Effects of disulfuram on oxidation of benzaldehyde and acetaldehyde in rat liver. Biochem Pharm 34:1529, 1985.
245. Cohen G, Heikkila RE, Allis B, et al: Destruction of sympathetic nerve terminals by 6-hydroxydopamine: protection by 1-phenyl-3-(2 thiazolyl)-2-thiourea, diethyl *d-l*-thiocarbamate, methimazole, cysteamine, ethanol and n-butanol. J Pharmacol Exp Ther 199:336, 1976.
246. Lebsack ME, Peterson DR, Collins AC, et al: Preferential inhibition of the low K_m aldehyde dehydrogenase activity by pargyline. Biochem Pharmacol 26:1151, 1977.
247. Kitson TM: The disulfiram-ethanol reaction. J Stud Alcohol 38:96, 1977.
248. Bonfiglio G, Donadio G: Results of the clinical testing of a new drug "metronidazole" in the treatment of chronic alcoholism. Br J Addiction 62:249, 1967.
249. Truitt EB, Duritz G, Morgan AM, et al: Disulfiramlike actions produced by hypoglycemic sulfonylurea compounds. Q J Stud Alcohol 23:197, 1962.
250. Reeves DS, Davies AJ: Antabuse effect with cephalosporins. Lancet 2:540, 1980.
251. Kalant H, LeBlanc AE, Guttman M, et al: Metabolic and pharmacologic interaction of ethanol and metronidazole in the rat. Can J Physiol Pharmacol 50:476, 1972.
252. Leslie RDG, Pyke DA: Chlorpropamide-alcohol flushing: a dominantly inherited trait associated with diabetes. BMJ 2:1519, 1978.
253. Leslie RDG, Pyke DA, Stubbs WA: Sensitivity to encephalin as a cause of non-insulin-dependent diabetes. Lancet 1:341, 1979.
254. Lionetti FJ, Fortier NL, Jedziniak JA: Acetaldehyde, product of deoxynucleoside metabolism in human erythrocyte ghosts. Proc Soc Exp Biol Med 116:1080, 1964.
255. McManus IR, Brotsky E, Olson RE: The origin of ethanol in mammalian tissues. J Biol Chem 241:349, 1966.
256. Fleshood HL, Pitot HC: The metabolism of O-phosphoryl ethanolamine in animal tissues. J Biol Chem 245:4414, 1970.
257. Bird MI, Nunn PB: Metabolic homeostasis of L-threonine in normally fed rat. Biochem J 214:687, 1983.
258. Baraona E, Julkunen R, Tannenbaum L, Lieber CS: Role of intestinal bacterial overgrowth on ethanol production and metabolism in rats. Gastroenterology 90:103, 1986.

259. Sorrell MF, Tuma DJ: Hypothesis: alcoholic liver injury and the covalent binding of acetaldehyde. Alcohol Clin Exp Res 9:306, 1985.
260. Barry RE, McGivan JD: Acetaldehyde alone may initiate hepatocellular damage in acute alcoholic liver disease. Gut 26:1065, 1985.
261. Lauterberg BH, Bilzer M: Mechanisms of acetaldehyde hepatotoxicity. J Hepatol 7:384, 1988.
262. Lumeng L, Lin RC: Protein-acetaldehyde adducts as biochemical markers of alcohol consumption. In Litten R, Allen J, eds: Measuring Alcohol Consumption. Humana Press, 1992:161.
263. Lin RC, Lumeng L: Alcohol and hepatic protein modification. In Watson RR, ed: Drug and Alcohol Abuse Reviews, vol 2. Liver Pathology and Alcohol. Totowa, NJ, Humana Press, 1991:221.
264. Bloor JH, Mapoles JE, Simon FR: Alcoholic liver disease: new concepts of pathogenesis and treatment. Adv Intern Med 39:49, 1994.
265. Sorrell MF, Tuma DJ: The functional implications of acetaldehyde binding to cell constituents. Ann N Y Acad Sci 492:50, 1987.
266. Mauch TJ, Donohue TM, Zetterman RK, et al: Covalent binding of acetaldehyde selectively inhibits the catalytic activity of lysine-dependent enzymes. Hepatology 6:263, 1986.
267. San George RC, Hoberman HD: Reaction of acetaldehyde with hemoglobin. J Biol Chem 261:6811, 1986.
268. Tuma DJ, Donohue TM, Medina VA, et al: Enhancement of acetaldehyde-protein adduct formation by L-ascorbate. Arch Biochem Biophys 234:377, 1984.
269. Nomura F, Lieber CS: Binding of acetaldehyde to rat liver microsomes: enhancement after chronic ethanol consumption. Biochem Biophys Res Commun 100:131, 1981.
270. Behrens UJ, Hoerner M, Lasker JM, Lieber CS: Formation of acetaldehyde adducts with ethanol-inducible P450IIE1 in vivo. Biochem Biophys Res Commun 154:584, 1988.
271. Tuma DJ, Smith SL, Sorrell MF: Acetaldehyde and microtubules. Ann N Y Acad Sci 625:786, 1991.
272. Jennett RB, Saffari-Fard A, Sorrell MF, et al: Increased covalent binding of acetaldehyde to calmodulin in the presence of calcium. Life Sci 24:281, 1989.
273. Tuma DJ, Hoffmann T, Sorrell MF: The chemistry of acetaldehyde-protein adducts. Alcohol Alcoholism Suppl 1:271, 1991.
274. Volentine GD, Tuma DJ, Sorrell MF: Acute effects of ethanol on hepatic glycoprotein secretion in the rat in vivo. Gastroenterology 84:225, 1984.
275. Volentine GD, Oglen KA, Kortje DK, et al: Role of acetaldehyde in ethanol-induced impairment of hepatic glycoprotein secretion in the rat in vivo. Hepatology 7:490, 1987.
276. Jennett RB, Tuma DJ, Sorrell MF: Effects of acetaldehyde on hepatic proteins. Prog Liver Dis 9:325, 1990.
277. Smith SL, Jennett RB, Sorrell MF, et al: Acetaldehyde substoichiometrically inhibits bovine neurotubulin polymerization. J Clin Invest 84:337, 1989.
278. Baraona E, Leo MA, Borowsky SA, Lieber CS: Pathogenesis of alcohol-induced accumulation of protein in the liver. J Clin Invest 60:546, 1977.
279. Svegliatia-Baroni G, Baraona E, Rosman AS, Lieber CS: Collagen-acetaldehyde adducts in alcoholic and non-alcoholic liver disease. Hepatology 20:111, 1994.
280. Moshage H, Casini A, Lieber CS: Acetaldehyde selectively stimulates collagen production in cultured rat liver fat-storing cells but not in hepatocytes. Hepatology 12:511, 1990.
281. Casini A, Cunningham M, Rojkind M, Lieber CS: Acetaldehyde increases procollagen type I and fibronectin gene transcription in cultured rat fat storing cells through a protein synthesis-dependent mechanism. Hepatology 13:758, 1991.
282. Lin RC, Zhou FC, Fillenworth MJ, Lumeng L: Zonal distribution of protein acetaldehyde adducts in the liver of rats fed alcohol for long periods. Hepatology 18:864, 1993.
283. Holstege A, Bedossa P, Poynard T, et al: Acetaldehyde-modified epitopes in liver biopsy specimens of alcoholic and non-alcoholic patients: localization and association with progression of liver fibrosis. Hepatology 19:367, 1994.
284. Halsted CH, Villanueva J, Chandler CJ, et al: Centrilobular distribution of acetaldehyde and collagen in the ethanol-fed micropig. Hepatology 18:954, 1993.
285. Niemela O, Juvonen T, Parkilla S: Immunohistochemical demonstration of acetaldehyde-modified epitopes in human liver after alcohol consumption. J Clin Invest 87:1367, 1990.
286. Niemela O, Parkilla S, Yla-Herttuala S, et al: Covalent protein adducts in the liver as a result of ethanol metabolism and lipid peroxidation. Lab Invest 70:537, 1994.
287. Israel Y, Hurwitz E, Niemela O, Arnon R: Monoclonal and polyclonal antibodies against acetaldehyde-containing epitopes in acetaldehyde-protein adducts. Proc Natl Acad Sci U S A 83:7923, 1986.
288. Tuma DJ, Klassen LW: Immune response to acetaldehyde-protein adducts: role in alcoholic liver disease. Gastroenterology 103:1969, 1992.
289. Yokoyama H, Ishii H, Nagata S, et al: Experimental hepatitis induced by ethanol after immunization with acetaldehyde adducts. Hepatology 17:14, 1993.
290. Koskinas J, Kenna JG, Bird GL, et al: Immunoglobulin A antibody to a 200-kilodalton cytosolic acetaldehyde adduct in alcoholic hepatitis. Gastroenterology 103:1860, 1992.
291. Viitala K, Israel Y, Blake JE, Niemela O: Serum IgA, IgG, and IgM antibodies directed against acetaldehyde-derived epitopes: relationship to liver disease severity and alcohol consumption. Hepatology 25:1418-1424, 1997.
292. Worrall S, DeJersey J, Shanley BC, Wilce PA: Antibodies against acetaldehyde-modified epitopes: an elevated IgA response in alcoholics. Eur J Clin Invest 21:90, 1991.
293. Swerdlow MD, Chowdury LN: IgA deposition in liver in alcoholic liver disease. Arch Pathol Lab Med 108:416, 1984.
294. Van de Wiel A, vanHattum J, Schurman HJ, Kater L: Immunoglobulin A in the diagnosis of alcoholic liver disease. Gastroenterology 94:457, 1988.
295. Terbayashi H, Kolber MA: The generation of cytotoxic T lymphocytes against acetaldehyde-modified syngeneic cells. Alcohol Clin Exp Res 14:893, 1990.
296. Niemela O: Aldehyde-protein adducts in the liver as a result of ethanol-induced oxidative stress. Front Biosci 4:506-513, 1999.
297. Esterbauer H, Schaur JR, Zollner H: Chemistry and biochemistry of 4-hydroxynonenal, malonaldehyde and related aldehydes. Free Radic Biol Med 11:81-128, 1991.
298. French SW, Wong K, Jui L, et al: Effect of ethanol on cytochrome P450 2E1, lipid peroxidation, and serum protein adduct formation in relation to liver pathology pathogenesis. Exp Mol Pathol. 58:61-75, 1993.
299. Niemela O, Parkkila S, Passanen M, et al: Early alcoholic liver injury: formation of protein adducts with acetaldehyde and lipid peroxidation products, and expression of CYP2E1 and CYP3A. Alcohol Clin Exp Res. 22:2118-2124, 1998.
300. Ohhira M, Ohtake T, Matsumoto A, et al: Immunohistochemical detection of 4-hydroxy-2-nonenal-modified-protein adducts in human alcoholic liver diseases. Alcohol Clin Exp Res. 22:1455-1459, 1998.
301. French SW: Succinic dehydrogenase histochemical "shift" in hepatic lobular distribution induced by ethanol. Lab Invest 13:1051, 1964.
302. French SW: Fragility of liver mitochondria in ethanol-fed rats. Gastroenterology 54:1106, 1968.
303. Koch OR, Roatta LL, Bolanas LP, et al: Ultrastructural and biochemical aspects of liver mitochondria during recovery from ethanol-induced alterations. Am J Pathol 90:325, 1973.
304. Bruguera M, Bertman A, Bombi JA, et al: Giant mitochondria in hepatocytes. A diagnostic hint for alcoholic liver disease. Gastroenterology 73:1383, 1977.
305. Jenkins WJ, Peters TJ: Mitochondrial enzyme activities in liver biopsies from patients with alcoholic liver disease. Gut 19:341-344, 1978.
306. French SW: Role of mitochondrial damage in alcoholic liver disease. In Majchrowicz E, Noble EP, eds: Biochemistry and Pharmacology of Ethanol, vol I. New York, Plenum, 1979:409.
307. French SW, Ruebner BH, Mezey E, et al: Effect of chronic ethanol feeding on hepatic mitochondria in the monkey. Hepatology 3:34, 1983.
308. Cederbaum AI, Rubin E: Molecular injury to mitochondria produced by ethanol and acetaldehyde. Fed Proc 34:2045, 1975.
309. Spach PI, Cunningham CC: Control of state 3 respiration in liver mitochondria from rats subjected to chronic ethanol consumption. Biochim Biophys Acta 894:460, 1987.
310. Thayer WS, Rubin E: Molecular alterations in the respiratory chain of rat liver after chronic ethanol consumption. J Biol Chem 256:6090, 1981.

311. Cunningham CC, Coleman WB, Spack PI: The effects of chronic ethanol consumption on hepatic mitochondrial energy metabolism. Alcohol Alcohol 25:127, 1990.
312. Cunningham CC, Kouri DL, Beeker KR, Spach PI: Comparison of effects of long term ethanol consumption on the heart and liver of the rat. Alcohol Clin Exp Res 13:58, 1989.
313. Cederbaum AI, Lieber CS, Beattie DS, Rubin E: Effect of chronic ethanol ingestion or fatty acid oxidation by hepatic mitochondria. J Biol Chem 250:5122, 1975.
314. Bernstein JD, Penniall R: Effects of chronic ethanol treatment upon rat liver mitochondria. Biochem Pharmacol 27:2337, 1978.
315. Schilling RJ, Reitz RC: A mechanism for ethanol-induced damage to liver mitochondrial structure and function. Biochim Biophys Acta 603:266, 1980.
316. Hatefi Y: ATP synthesis in the mitochondria. Eur J Biochem 218:759, 1993.
317. Cunningham CC, Coleman WB, Spach PI: Chronic alcoholism and the mitochondrial FoF_1-ATP synthase. Methods in Toxicology 2:354, 1993.
318. Coleman WB, Cahill A, Ivestger P, Cunningham CC: Differential effects of ethanol consumption on synthesis of cytoplasmic and mitochondrial encoded subunits of the ATP synthase. Alcohol Clin Exp Res 18:947, 1994.
319. Hoek JB: Mitochondrial energy metabolism in chronic alcoholism. Curr Top Bioenergetics 17:197, 1994.
320. Annundi I, King J, Owen DA, et al: Fructose prevents hypoxic cell death in the liver. Am J Physiol 253:G390, 1987.
321. Nanji AA, Fogt F, Griniuviene B: Alteration in glucose transporter proteins in alcoholic liver disease in the rat. Am J Pathol 146:329, 1995.
322. Rosser BG, Gores GJ: Liver cell necrosis: cellular mechanisms and clinical implications. Gastroenterology 108:252, 1995.
323. Pastorino JG, Snyder JW, Serroni A, et al: Cyclosporine and carnitine prevent anoxic death of cultured hepatocytes by inhibiting the mitochondrial permeability transition. J Biol Chem 268: 13791, 1993.
324. Gunter TE, Pfeiffer DR: Mechanisms by which mitochondria transport calcium. Am J Physiol 258:C755, 1990.
325. Mansouri A, Fromety B, Berson A, et al: Multiple hepatic mitochondrial DNA deletions suggest premature oxidative aging in alcoholic patients. J Hepatol 27:96-102, 1997.
326. Fromenty B, Grimbert S, Mansouri A, et al: Hepatic mitochondrial DNA deletion in alcoholics: association with microvesicular steatosis. Gastroenterology. 108:193-200, 1995.
327. Mansouri A, Gaou I, Kerguence C, et al: An alcoholic binge causes massive degradation of hepatic mitochondrial DNA in mice. Gastroenterology. 117:181-190, 1999.
328. Zakim D, Vessey DA: The effects of lipid-protein interactions on the kinetic parameter of microsomal UDP-glucuronyltransferase. In Martonosi A, ed: The Enzymes of Biological Membranes, vol 2. New York, Plenum, 1976:443.
329. Vessey DA, Zakim D: Membrane fluidity and the regulation of membrane-bound enzymes. Horizons Biochem Biophys 1:139, 1975.
330. Quinn PJ: The Molecular Biology of Cell Membranes. London, Macmillan, 1976.
331. Martonosi A, ed: The Enzymes of Biological Membranes, vol. 4. Electron Transport Systems and Receptors. New York, Plenum Press, 1976.
332. Zakim D: Interface between membrane biology and clinical medicine. Am J Med 80:645, 1986.
333. Sandermann H: Regulation of membrane enzymes by lipids. Biochim Biophys Acta 515:209, 1978.
334. Chin JH, Goldstein DB: Effects of low concentrates of ethanol on the fluidity of spin-labeled erythrocyte and brain membranes. Mol Pharmacol 13:435, 1977.
335. Rowe ES: Lipid chain length and temperature dependence of ethanol-phosphatidylcholine interactions. Biochemistry 22:3299, 1983.
336. Herold LL, Rowe ES, Khalifah RG: ^{13}C-NMR and spectrophotometric studies of alcohol-lipid interactions. Chem Phys Lipids 43:215, 1987.
337. Chin JH, Goldstein DB: Drug tolerance in biomembranes: a spin-label study of the effects of ethanol. Science 196:684, 1977.
338. Johnson DA, Friedman HJ, Cooke R, et al: Adaptation of brain lipid bilayers to ethanol induced fluidization. Biochem Pharmacol 29:1673, 1980.
339. Johnson DA, Lee NM, Cooke R, et al: Ethanol-induced fluidization of brain lipid bilayers: required presence of cholesterol in membranes for expression of tolerance. Mol Pharmacol 15:739, 1979.
340. Goldstein DB: The effects of drugs on membrane fluidity. Ann Rev Pharmacol Toxicol 24:43, 1984.
341. Taraschi TF, Ellingson JS, Wu A, et al: Membrane tolerance to ethanol is rapidly lost after withdrawal: a model for studies of membrane adaptation. Proc Natl Acad Sci U S A 83:3669, 1986.
342. Rottenberg H: Membrane solubility of ethanol in chronic alcoholism. The effect of ethanol feeding and its withdrawal on the protection by alcohol of rat red blood cells from hypotonic hemolysis. Biochim Biophys Acta 855:211, 1986.
343. French SW, Ihrig TJ, Morin RJ: Lipid composition of RBC ghosts, liver mitochondria and microsomes of ethanol-fed rats. Q J Stud Alcohol 31:801, 1970.
344. Thompson JA, Reitz RC: Studies on the acute and chronic effects of ethanol ingestion on choline oxidation. Ann N Y Acad Sci 273:194, 1976.
345. Hosein EA, Hofmann I, Linder E: Ethanol and Mg^{2-}-stimulated ATPase. Arch Biochem Biophys 183:64, 1977.
346. Hosein EA, Lee H, Hofmann I: The influence of chronic ethanol feeding to rats on liver mitochondrial membrane structure and function. Can J Biochem 58:1147, 1980.
347. Spach PI, Parce JW, Cunningham CC: Effect of chronic ethanol administration on energy metabolism and phospholipase A_2 activity in rat liver. Biochem J 178:23, 1979.
348. Taraschi TF, Ellingson JS, Janes N, Rubin E: The role of anionic phospholipids in membrane adaptation to ethanol. Alcohol Alcohol 26(suppl 1):241, 1991.
349. Taraschi TF, Ellingson JS, Wu A, et al: Phosphotidylinositol from ethanol-fed rats confers membrane tolerance to ethanol. Proc Natl Acad Sci U S A 83:9398, 1986.
350. Stubbs CD, Kisielewski AE, Rubin E: Chronic ethanol ingestion modifies liver microsomal phosphatidylserine inducing resistance to hydrolysis by phospholipase A2. Biochim Biophys Acta 1070:349, 1991.
351. Ellingson JS, Taraschi TF, Wu A, et al: Cardiolipin from ethanol-fed rats confers tolerance to ethanol in liver mitochondrial membranes. Proc Natl Acad Sci U S A 85:3353, 1988.
352. Taraschi TF, Ellingson JS, Wu-Sun A, Rubin E: Rats withdrawn from ethanol rapidly re-acquire membrane tolerance after resumption of ethanol feeding. Biochim Biophys Acta 1021:51, 1990.
353. Hoek JB: Mitochondrial energy metabolism in chronic alcoholism. Curr Top Bioenergetics 17:197, 1994.
354. Buthke TM, Ingram LO: Mechanism of ethanol-induced changes in lipid composition of *Escherichia coli:* inhibition of saturated fatty acid synthesis in vivo. Biochemistry 17:637, 1978.
355. Berger B, Carty CE, Ingram LO: Alcohol-induced changes in the phospholipid molecular species of *Escherichia coli.* J Bacteriol 142:1040, 1980.
356. Nandini-Kishove SG, Mattox SM, Martin CE, et al: Membrane changes during growth of Tetrahymena in the presence of ethanol. Biochim Biophys Acta 551:315, 1979.
357. Swann AC: Free fatty acids and (Na^+,K^+)-ATPase: effects of cation regulation, enzyme conformation, and interactions with ethanol. Arch Biochem Biophys 233:354, 1984.
358. Dreiling CE, Schilling RJ, Reitz RC: Effects of chronic ethanol ingestion on the activity of rat liver mitochondrial 2′,3′-cyclic nucleotide 3′-phosphohydrolase. Biochim Biophys Acta 640:121, 1981.
359. Dorio RJ, Hock JB, Rubin E: Ethanol treatment selectively decreases neutral amino acid transport in cultured hepatocytes. J Biol Chem 259:11430, 1984.
360. O'Neill B, Weber F, Honig D, et al: Ethanol selectively affects Na^+ gradient-dependent intestinal transport systems. FEBS Lett 194:183, 1986.
361. Mills PR, Meier PJ, Smith DJ, et al: The effect of changes in the fluid state of rat liver plasma membrane on the transport of taurocholate. Hepatology 1:61, 1987.
362. Fassoulaki A, Eger EI II: Alcohol increases in solubility of anesthetics in the liver. Br J Anaesth 58:551, 1986.

363. Kosenko EA, Kaminsky YG: Limitation in glucose penetration from the liver into blood and other metabolic symptoms of ethanol withdrawal in rats. FEBS Lett 200:210, 1986.
364. Tuma DJ, Mailliard ME, Casey CA, et al: Ethanol-induced alterations of plasma membrane assembly in the liver. Biochim Biophys Acta 856:5171, 1986.
365. Lee H, Hosein EA: Chronic alcohol feeding and its withdrawal on the structure and function of the rat liver plasma membrane: a study with ^{125}I-labelled glucagon binding as a metabolic probe. Can J Physiol Pharmacol 60:1171, 1982.
366. Sharma RJ, Grant DA: A differential effect between the acute and chronic administration of ethanol on the endocytotic rate constant, k_e, for the internalization of asialoglycoproteins by hepatocytes. Biochim Biophys Acta 862:199, 1986.
367. Casey CA, Kragskow SL, Sorrell MF, et al: Chronic ethanol administration impairs the binding and endocytosis of asialo-orosomucoid in isolated hepatocytes. J Biol Chem 262:2704, 1987.
368. Kiessling K-H, Lindgren L, Strandberg B, et al: Electron microscopic study of liver mitochondria from human alcoholics. Acta Med Scand 85:413, 1964.
369. Uchida T, Kronborg I, Peters RL: Giant mitochondria in alcoholic liver disease—their identification, frequency and pathologic significance. Liver 4:29, 1984.
370. Stewart RV, Dincsoy HP: The significance of giant mitochondria in liver biopsies as observed by light microscopy. Am J Clin Pathol 78:293, 1982.
371. French SW: Role of mitochondrial damage in alcoholic liver disease. In Majchrowicz E, Noble EP, eds: Biochemistry and Pharmacology of Ethanol. New York, Plenum, 1979:409.
372. Israel Y, Videla L, Videla-Fernandez V, et al: Effects of chronic ethanol treatment and thyroxine administration on ethanol metabolism and liver oxidative capacity. J Pharmacol Exp Ther 192:565, 1975.
373. Thurman RG, McKenna WR, McCaffrey TB: Pathways responsible for the adaptive increase in ethanol utilization following chronic treatment with ethanol: inhibition studies with hemoglobin-free perfused rat liver. Mol Pharmacol 12:156, 1956.
374. Kessler BJ, Liebler JB, Bronfin GJ, et al: Hepatic blood flow and splanchnic oxygen consumption in alcoholic fatty liver. J Clin Invest 33:1338, 1954.
375. Lieber CS, Robins SJ, Li J et al: Phosphatidylcholine protects against fibrosis and cirrhosis in the baboon. Gastroenterology 106:152-159,1994.
376. Lieber CS, DeCarli LM, Mak KM, et al: Attenuation of alcohol-induced hepatic fibrosis by polyunsaturated lecithin. Hepatology 12:1390-1398, 1990.
377. Poniachik J, Baraona E, Zhao, J, Lieber CS: Dilinoleoylphosphatidylcholine decreases hepatic stellate cell activation. J Lab Clin Med 133:342-348, 1999.
378. Ma X, Zhoa J, Lieber CS: Polyenylphosphatidylcholine attenuates non-alcoholic hepatic fibrosis and accelerates its regression. J Hepatol 24:604-613, 1996.
379. Navder KP, Baraona E, Lieber CS: Polyenylphosphatidylcholine attenuates alcohol-induced fatty liver and hyperlipemia in rats. J Nutr 127:1800-1806, 1997.
380. Aleynik MK, Leo MA, Aleynik SI, Lieber CS: Polyenylphosphatidylcholine opposes the increase of cytochrome P-4502E1 by ethanol and corrects its iron-induced decrease. Alcohol Clin Exp Res 23:96-100, 1999.
381. Aleynik SI, Leo MA, Aleynik MK, Lieber CS: Polyenylphosphatidylcholine protects against alcohol but not iron-induced oxidative stress in the liver. Alcohol Clin Exp Res. 24:196-206, 2000.
382. Oneta CM, Mak KM, Lieber CS: Dilinoleoylphosphatidylcholine selectively modulates lipopolysaccharide-induced Kupffer cell activation. J Lab Clin Med 134:466-470, 1999.
383. Bohlinger I, Leist M, Barsig J, et al: Interleukin-1 and nitric oxide protect against tumor necrosis factor-alpha induced liver injury through distinct pathways. Hepatology 22:1829-1837, 1995.
384. Videla L, Bernstein J, Israel Y: Metabolic alterations produced in the liver by chronic ethanol administration: changes related to energetic parameters of the cell. Biochem J 134:515, 1973.
385. Israel Y, Videla L, Bernstein J: Liver hypermetabolic state after chronic ethanol consumption. Hormonal inter-relations and pathogenic implications. Fed Proc 34:2052, 1975.
386. Israel Y, Kalant H, Orrego H, et al: Experimental alcohol induced hepatic necrosis: suppression by propylthiouracil. Proc Natl Acad Sci U S A 72:1137, 1975.
387. Orrego H, Kalant H, Israel Y: Effect of short-term therapy with propylthiouracil in patients with alcoholic liver disease. Gastroenterology 76:105, 1979.
388. French SW, Benson NC, Sun PS: Centrilobular liver necrosis induced by hypoxia in chronic ethanol-fed rats. Hepatology 4:912, 1984.
389. Itrruriage H, Ugarte H, Israel Y: Hepatic vein oxygenation, liver blood flow and the rate of ethanol metabolism in recently abstinent alcoholic patients. Eur J Clin Invest 10:211, 1980.
390. Hayashi N, Nakamura A, Kurokawa K, et al: Oxygen supply to the liver in patients with alcoholic liver disease assessed by oxygen reflectance spectrophotometry. Gastroenterology 88:881, 1985.
391. Bendtsen F, Henriksen JH, Widding A, et al: Hepatic venous oxygen content in alcoholic cirrhosis and non-cirrhotic alcoholic liver disease. Liver 7:176, 1987.
392. Shaw S, Heller E, Friedman H, et al: Increased hepatic oxygenation following ethanol administration in the baboon. Proc Soc Exp Biol Med 156:509, 1977.
393. Sato N, Kamada T, Kawano S, et al: Effect of acute and chronic ethanol consumption on hepatic tissue oxygen tension in rats. Pharmacol Biochem Behav 18:443, 1983.
394. Linnoila M, Mefford I, Nutt D, Adinoff B: Alcohol withdrawal and noradrenergic function. Ann Intern Med 107:875, 1987.
395. Bredfeldt JE, Riley EM, Groszmann RJ: Compensatory mechanisms in response to an elevated hepatic oxygen consumption in chronically ethanol-fed rats. Am J Physiol 248:G507, 1985.
396. McKaigney JP, Carmichael FJ, Saldivia V, et al: Role of ethanol metabolism in the ethanol-induced increase in splanchnic circulation. Am J Physiol 250:G519, 1986.
397. Tsukamoto H, Xi XP: Incomplete compensation of enhanced hepatic oxygen consumption in rats with alcoholic centrilobular necrosis. Hepatology 9:302, 1989.
398. Israel Y, Kalant H, Orrego H, et al: Experimental alcohol-induced hepatic necrosis: suppression by propylthiouracil. Proc Natl Acad Sci U S A 72:1137, 1975.
399. Rachamin G, Okuno F, Israel Y: Inhibitory effect of propylthiouracil on the development of metabolic tolerance to ethanol. Biochem Pharmacol 34:2377, 1985.
400. Yuki T, Israel Y, Thurman RG: The swift increase in alcohol metabolism: inhibition by propylthiouracil. Biochem Pharmacol 31:2403, 1982.
401. Carmichael FJ, Orrego H, Saldivia V, Israel Y: Effect of propylthiouracil on the ethanol-induced increase in liver oxygen consumption in awake rats. Hepatology 18:415, 1993.
402. Pirola RC, Lieber CS: The energy costs of the metabolism of drugs including ethanol. Pharmacology 7:185, 1972.
403. Tsukamoto H, Towner SJ, Ciofalo LM, et al: Ethanol-induced liver fibrosis in rats fed high fat diet. Hepatology 6:814, 1986.
404. Tsukamoto H, French SW, Benson N, et al: Severe and progressive steatosis and focal necrosis in rat liver induced by continuous intragastric infusion of ethanol and low fat diet. Hepatology 5:224, 1985.
405. French SW: Biochemistry of alcoholic liver disease. CRC Crit Rev Clin Lab Sci 29:83, 1992.
406. Lieber CS, Baraona E, Hernandez-Munoz R, et al: Impaired oxygen utilization—a new mechanism for the hepatotoxicity of ethanol in sub-human primates. J Clin Invest 83:1682, 1989.
407. Younes M, Strubelt O: Enhancement of hypoxic liver damage by ethanol. Involvement of xanthine oxidase and the role of glycolysis. Biochem Pharmacol 36:2973, 1987.
408. Orrego H, Kalant H, Israel Y, et al: Effect of short-term therapy with propylthiouracil (PTU) in patients with alcoholic liver disease. Gastroenterology 76:105, 1979.
409. Halle P, Pare P, Kaptein E, et al: Double-blind controlled trial of propylthiouracil in patients with severe acute alcoholic hepatitis. Gastroenterology 82:925, 1982.
410. Orrego H, Blake JE, Blendis LM, et al: Long-term treatment of alcoholic liver disease with propylthiouracil. N Engl J Med 317:1421, 1987.
411. French SW: Effect of acute and chronic ethanol ingestion on rat liver ATP. Proc Soc Exp Biol Med 121:681, 1966.

412. Ammonn HPT, Estler CJ: Influence of acute and chronic administration of alcohol on carbohydrate breakdown and energy metabolism in the liver. Nature 216:158, 1967.
413. Gordon ER: Mitochondrial functions in an ethanol-induced fatty liver. J Biol Chem 248:8271, 1973.
414. Bernstein J, Videla L, Israel Y: Metabolic alterations produced in the liver by chronic ethanol administration. Biochem J 134:515, 1973.
415. Miyamoto K, French SW: Hepatic adenine nucleotide metabolism measured in vivo in rats fed ethanol and a high fat-low protein diet. Hepatology 8:53, 1988.
416. Mitchell MC, Herlong HF: Alcohol and nutrition: caloric value, bioenergetics and relationship to liver damage. Ann Rev Nutr 6:457, 1986.
417. Mezey E: Liver disease and protein needs. Ann Rev Nutr 2:21, 1982.
418. Spach PI, Herbert JS, Cunningham CC: The interaction between chronic ethanol consumption and oxygen tension in influencing the energy state of rat liver. Biochim Biophys Acta 1056:40, 1991.
419. Gordon E: ATP metabolism in an ethanol-induced fatty liver. Biochem Pharmacol 26:1229, 1977.
420. Gillam E, Ward L: Cellular energy charge in the heart and liver of the rat. The effects of ethanol and acetaldehyde. Int J Biochem 18:1031, 1986.
421. Desmoulin F, Canioni P, Crotte C, et al: Hepatic metabolism during acute ethanol administration: a phosphorus-31-nuclear magnetic resonance study on the perfused rat liver under normoxic or hypoxic conditions. Hepatology 7:315, 1987.
422. Cunningham CC, Malloy CR, Radda GK: Effect of fasting and acute ethanol administration on the energy state in vivo liver as measured by ^{31}P-NMR spectroscopy. Biochim Biophys Acta 885:12, 1986.
423. Helzberg JH, Brown MS, Smith DJ, et al: Metabolic state of the rat liver with ethanol: comparison of in vivo 31-phosphorus nuclear magnetic resonance spectroscopy with freeze clamp assessment. Hepatology 7:83, 1987.
424. Willson RA: ^{31}Phosphorus nuclear magnetic resonance spectroscopy: what does it tell us about alcohol-induced liver disease. Hepatology 12:1246, 1990.
425. Takahashi H, Geoffrion Y, Butler KW, French SW: In vivo hepatic energy metabolism during the progression of alcoholic liver disease: a noninvasive ^{31}P nuclear magnetic resonance study in rats. Hepatology 11:65, 1990.
426. Angus PW, Dixon RM, Rajagopalan B, et al: A study of patients with alcoholic liver disease by ^{31}P nuclear magnetic resonance spectroscopy. Clin Sci 78:33, 1990.
427. Menon DK, Harris M, Sargentoni J, et al: In vivo hepatic magnetic resonance spectroscopy in chronic alcohol abusers. Gastroenterology 108:776, 1995.
428. Meyerhoff DJ, Boska MD, Thomas AM, Weiner MW: Alcoholic liver disease: quantitative image-guided ^{31}P MR spectroscopy. Radiology 173:343, 1989.
429. Thayer WS, Rubin E: Effects of chronic ethanol intake on oxidative phosphorylation in rat liver submitochondrial particles. J Biol Chem 254:7717, 1979.
430. Schilling RJ, Reitz RC: A mechanism for ethanol-induced damage to liver mitochondrial structure and function. Biochim Biophys Acta 603:266, 1980.
431. Bottenus RE, Spach PI, Filus F, Cunningham CC: Effect of chronic ethanol consumption on energy-linked processes associated with oxidative-phosphorylation: proton translocation and ATP-Pi exchange. Biochem Biophys Res Commun 105:1368, 1982.
432. Arai M, Leo M, Naakano M, et al: Biochemical and morphological alterations of baboon hepatic mitochondria after chronic ethanol consumption. Hepatology 4:165, 1984.
433. Andreoli SP: ATP depletion and cell injury: what is the relationship. J Lab Clin Med 122:232, 1993.
434. Mandel LJ, Bacallao R, Zamphigi R: Uncoupling of the molecular "fence" and paracellular "gate" functions in epithelial tight junctions. Nature 361:552, 1993.
435. Molitoris BA: Ischemia-induced loss of epithelial polarity: potential role of the actin cytoskeleton. Am J Physiol 260:F769, 1991.
436. Li HY, Dai LJ, Quamme GA: Effect of chemical hypoxia on intracellular ATP and cytosolic Mg^{2+} levels. J Lab Clin Med 122:260, 1993.
437. Hijioka T, Sato N, Mastumara T, et al: Ethanol-induced disturbance of hepatic microcirculation and hepatic hypoxia. Biochem Pharmacol 41:1551, 1991.
438. Oshita M, Sato N, Yoshihara H, et al: Ethanol-induced vasoconstriction causes focal hepatocellular injury in the isolated perfused rat liver. Hepatology 16:1007, 1992.
439. Oshita M, Takei Y, Kawano H, et al: Roles of endothelin-1 and nitric oxide in the mechanism for ethanol-induced vasoconstriction in rat liver. J Clin Invest 91:1337, 1993.
440. Haynes WG, Webb DJ: The endothelin family of peptides: local hormones with diverse roles in health and disease. Clin Sci 84:485, 1993.
441. Marsen TA, Schramek H, Dunn MJ: Renal actions of endothelin-1: linking cellular signalling pathways to kidney disease. Kidney Int 45:336, 1994.
442. Rubanyi GM, Polokoff MA: Endothelins: molecular biology, biochemistry, pharmacology, physiology and pathophysiology. Pharmacol Rev 46:325, 1994.
443. Angaard E, Galton S, Rae G, et al: The fate of radioiodinated endothelin 1 and endothelin 3 in the rat. J Cardiovasc Pharmacol 13(suppl 5):S46, 1989.
444. Kiowski W, Luscher TF, Linder L, Buhler FR: Endothelin-1 induced vasoconstriction in humans. Reversal by calcium channel blockade but not by nitrovasodilators or endothelium-derived relaxing factor. Circulation 83:469, 1991.
445. Millul V, Lagente V, Gillardeux O, et al: Activation of guinea pig alveolar macrophages by endothelin-1. J Cardiovasc Pharmacol 17(suppl 7):S233, 1991.
446. Hollenberg SM, Tong W, Shelhamer JH, et al: Eicosanoid production by human aortic endothelial cells in response to endothelin. Am J Physiol 267:H2290, 1994.
447. Mustafa SB, Gandhi CR, Harvey SAK, Olson MS: Endothelin stimulates platelet-activating factor synthesis in cultured rat Kupffer cells. Hepatology 21:545, 1995.
448. Zhou W, Chao W, Levine BA, Olson MS: Role of platelet-activating factor in hepatic responses after bile duct ligation in rats. Am J Physiol 263:G587, 1992.
449. Chao W, Liu WL, DeBuysere M, et al: Identification of receptors for platelet-activating factor in rat Kupffer cells. J Biol Chem 264:13591, 1989.
450. Buxton DG, Fisher RA, Hanahan DJ, Olson MS: Platelet-activating factor-mediated vasoconstriction and glycogenolysis in perfused rat liver. J Biol Chem 261:644, 1986.
451. Goto M, Takei Y, Kawano S, et al: Endothelin-1 is involved in the pathogenesis of ischemia-reperfusion liver injury by hepatic microcirculatory disturbances. Hepatology 19:675, 1994.
452. Moore K, Wendon J, Frazer M, et al: Plasma endothelin immunoreactivity in liver disease and the hepatorenal syndrome. N Engl J Med 327:1774, 1992.
453. Nanji AA, Khwaja S, Khettry U, Sadrzadeh SMH: Plasma endothelin levels in chronic ethanol-fed rats: relationship to pathologic liver injury. Life Sci 54:423, 1994.
454. Pinzani M, Failli P, Ruocco C, et al: Fat-storing cells as liver-specific pericytes: spatial dynamics of agonist-stimulated intracellular calcium transients. J Clin Invest 90:642, 1992.
455. Sakamoto M, Ueno T, Kin M, et al: Ito cell contraction in response to endothelin-1 and substance P. Hepatology 18:978, 1993.
456. Housset C, Rockey DC, Bissell DM: Endothelin receptor in rat liver: lipocytes as a contractile target for endothelin 1. Proc Natl Acad Sci U S A 90:9266, 1993.
457. Rockey DC, Housset CN, Friedman SL: Activation-dependent contractility of rat hepatic lipocytes in culture and in vivo. J Clin Invest 92:1795, 1993.
458. Bauer M, Zhang JX, Bauer I, Clemens MG: ET-1 induced alteration of hepatic microcirculation: sinusoidal and extrasinusoidal sites of action. Am J Physiol 267:G143, 1994.
459. Zhang JX, Pegoli W Jr, Clemens MG: Endothelin-1 induces direct constriction of hepatic sinusoids. Am J Physiol 266:G624, 1994.
460. Okumura S, Takei Y, Kawano S, et al: Vasoactive effect of endothelin-1 on rat liver in vivo. Hepatology 19:155, 1994.
461. Mendeloff A: Effects of intravenous infusions of ethanol upon estimated hepatic blood flow in man. J Clin Invest 33:1298, 1954.
462. Bredfelt JE, Riley EM, Groszmann RJ: Compensatory mechanisms in response to an elevated hepatic oxygen consumption in chronically ethanol-fed rats. Am J Physiol 248:G507, 1985.
463. Stamler JS, Singel DJ, Loscalzo J: Biochemistry of nitric oxide and its redox-activated forms. Science 258:1898, 1992.
464. Moncada S, Palmer RMJ, Higg EA: Nitric oxide: physiology, pathophysiology and pharmacology. Pharmacol Rev 43:109, 1991.

465. Moncada S, Higgs EA: The L-arginine-nitric oxide pathway. N Engl J Med 329:2002, 1993.
466. Nanji AA, Greenberg SS, Tahan SR, et al: Nitric oxide production in experimental alcoholic liver disease in the rat: role in protection from injury. Gastroenterology 109:899, 1995.
467. Billiar TR: The delicate balance of nitric oxide and superoxide in liver pathway. Gastroenterology 108:603, 1995.
468. Richter C, Gogvadze V, Schlapbach R, et al: Nitric oxide kills hepatocytes by mobilizing mitochondrial calcium. Biochem Biophys Res Commun 205:1143, 1994.
469. Radi R, Beckman JS, Bush KM, Freeman BA: Peroxynitrite-induced membrane lipid peroxidation: the cytotoxic potential of superoxide and nitric oxide. Arch Biochem Biophys 288:481, 1991.
470. Garcia Ruiz C, Morales A, Ballesta A, et al: Effect of chronic ethanol feeding on glutathione and functional integrity of mitochondria in periportal and perivenous hepatocytes. J Clin Invest 94:193, 1994.
471. Radomski MW, Palmer RMJ, Moncada S: An arginine/nitric oxide pathway present in human platelets regulates aggregation. Proc Natl Acad Sci U S A 87:5193, 1990.
472. Kubes P, Suzuki M, Granger DN: Nitric oxide: an endogenous modulator of leukocyte adhesion. Proc Natl Acad Sci U S A 88:4651, 1991.
473. Cooke JP, Tsao PS: Cytoprotective effects of nitric oxide. Circulation 88:2451, 1993.
474. Bautista AP, Spitzer JJ: Inhibition of nitric oxide formation in-vivo enhances superoxide release by perfused rat liver. Am J Physiol 266:G783, 1994.
475. Harbrecht BG, Stadler J, Demetris AJ, et al: Nitric oxide and prostaglandins interact to prevent hepatic damage during murine endotoxemia. Am J Physiol 266:G1004, 1994.
476. Goligorsky MS, Tsukahara H, Magazine H, et al: Termination of endothelin signaling: role of nitric oxide. J Cell Physiol 158:485, 1994.
477. Ignarro LJ: Endothelium-derived nitric oxide: action and properties. FASEB J 3:31, 1989.
478. Toshizumi M, Perella MA, Burnett JC, Lee ME: Tumor necrosis factor downregulates an endothelial nitric oxide synthase mRNA by shortening its half life. Circ Res 73:205, 1993.
479. Vodovotz Y, Bogdan C, Paik J, et al: Mechanisms of suppression of macrophage nitric oxide release by transforming growth factor β. J Exp Med 178:605, 1993.
480. Baraona E, Lieber CS: Effects of ethanol on lipid metabolism. J Lipid Res 20:289, 1979.
481. Day CP, Yeaman SJ: The biochemistry of alcohol-induced fatty liver. Biochim Biophys Acta 1215:33, 1994.
482. Nikkila EA, Ojala K: Role of hepatic c-d glycerophosphate and triglyceride synthesis in the production of fatty liver by ethanol. Proc Soc Exp Biol Med 113:814.
483. Zakim D: Effect of ethanol on hepatic acyl-coenzyme a metabolism. Arch Biochem Biophys 111:253, 1965.
484. Ylikahri RH: Ethanol-induced changes in hepatic α-glycerophosphate and triglyceride concentrations in normal and thyroxine treated rats. Metabolism 19:1036, 1970.
485. Stals HH, Mannaerts GP, DeClercq PE: Factors influencing triacylglycerol synthesis in permeabilized rat hepatocytes. Biochem J 283:719, 1992.
486. Ryle CR, Chakraborty J, Thomson AD: The effect of methylene blue on the hepatocellular redox state and liver lipid content during chronic ethanol feeding in the rat. Biochem J 232:877, 1985.
487. Mavrelis PG, Ammon HV, Gleysteen JJ, et al: Hepatic free fatty acids in alcoholic liver disease and morbid obesity. Hepatology 3:226, 1983.
488. Lieber CS, Spritz N, DeCarli LM: Role of dietary, adipose and endogenously synthesized fatty acids in the pathogenesis of the alcoholic fatty liver. J Clin Invest 45:51, 1966.
489. Klingman GI, McGoodall C: Urinary epinephrine and levarterenol excretion during alcohol intoxication in dogs. J Pharmacol Exp Ther 121:313, 1957.
490. Forbec JC, Duncan GM: The effects of acute ethanol intoxication on the adrenal glands of rats and guinea pigs. Q J Stud Alcohol 12:355, 1951.
491. Ontko JA: Metabolism of free fatty acids in isolated liver cells. J Biol Chem 247:1788, 1972.
492. Ide T, Ontko JA: Increased secretion of very low density lipoprotein triglyceride following inhibition of long chain fatty acid oxidation in isolated rat liver. J Biol Chem 256:10247, 1981.
493. Guzman M, Castro J, Maquedano A: Ethanol feeding to rats reversibly decreases hepatic carnitine palmitoyl transferase activity and increases enzyme sensitivity to malonyl-coA. Biochem Biophys Res Commun 149:443, 1987.
494. Guzman M, Castro J: Alterations in the regulatory properties of hepatic fatty acid oxidation and carnitine palmitoyl transferase I activity after ethanol feeding and withdrawal. Alcohol Clin Exp Res 14:472, 1990.
495. Zammit VA: Mechanism of regulation of partition of fatty acids between oxidation and esterification in the liver. Prog Lipid Res 23:39, 1984.
496. Zammit VA: Carnitine acyltransferases in the physiologic setting: the liver. Biochem Soc Trans 14:679, 1986.
497. Guzman M, Castro J: Zonal heterogeneity of the effects of chronic ethanol feeding on hepatic fatty acid metabolism. Hepatology 12:1098, 1990.
498. Simpson KJ, Venkatesan S, Peters TJ, et al: Hepatic phosphatidate phosphohydrolase activity in acute and chronic alcohol-fed rats. Biochem Soc Trans 17:1115, 1989.
499. Jamal Z, Martin A, Gomez-Munoz A, Brindley DN: Plasma membrane fractions from rat liver contain a phosphatidate phosphohydrolase distinct from that in endoplasmic reticulum and cytosol. J Biol Chem 266:2988, 1991.
500. Day CP, Yeaman SJ: Physical evidence for the presence of two forms of phosphatidate phosphohydrolase in rat liver. Biochim Biophys Acta 1127:87, 1992.
501. Brindley DN: Intracellular translocation of phosphatidate phosphohydrolase and its possible role in the control of glycerolipid synthesis. Prog Lipid Res 23:115, 1984.
502. Savolainen MJ, Baraona E, Pikkarainen P, Lieber CS: Hepatic triacylglycerol synthesizing activity during progression of alcoholic liver injury in the baboon. J Lipid Res 25:813, 1984.
503. Lamb RG, Wood CK, Fallon HJ: The effect of acute and chronic ethanol intake on hepatic glycerolipid synthesis in the hamster. J Clin Invest 63:14, 1979.
504. Savolainen MJ: Stimulation of hepatic phosphatidate phosphohydrolase activity by a single dose of ethanol. Biochem Biophys Res Commun 75:511, 1977.
505. Day CP, James OFW, Brown AJM, et al: The activity of the metabolic form of hepatic phosphatidate phosphohydrolase correlates with the severity of alcoholic fatty liver in human beings. Hepatology 18:832, 1993.
506. Pittner RA, Fears R, Brindley DN: Interactions of insulin, glucagon and dexamethasone in controlling the activity of glycerol phosphate acyltransferase and the activity and subcellular distribution of phosphatidate phosphohydrolase in cultured rat hepatocytes. Biochem J 230:525, 1985.
507. Ferraresi-Filho O, Ferraresi ML, Costantin J, et al: Transport and metabolism of palmitate in the rat liver. Net flux and unidirectional fluxes across the cell membrane. Biochim Biophys Acta 1103:239, 1992.
508. Glatz JFC, Van der Vusse GJ: Cellular fatty acid-binding proteins: current concepts and future directions. Mol Cell Biochem 98:237, 1990.
509. Pignon JP, Bailey NC, Baraona E, Lieber CS: Fatty acid-binding protein: a major contributor to the ethanol-induced increase in liver cytosolic proteins in the rat. Hepatology 7:865, 1987.
510. Sherchuk O, Baraona E, Ma XL, et al: Gender differences in the response of hepatic fatty acids and cytosolic fatty acid-binding capacity to alcohol consumption in rats. Proc Soc Exp Biol Med 198:584, 1991.
511. Wantanabe S, Wakatsuki Y, Yoshioka H, et al: Biochemical and histochemical studies of liver fatty acid binding protein in alcohol-treated rats. J Clin Biochem Nutr 14:171, 1993.
512. Morgan MY, Sherlock S: Sex-differences among 100 patients with alcoholic liver disease. BMJ 1:939, 1977.
513. Nakamura S, Takezawa Y, Sato T, et al: Alcoholic liver disease in women. Tohoku J Exp Med 129:351, 1979.
514. Ontko JA: Effects of ethanol on the metabolism of free fatty acids in isolated liver cells. J Lipid Res 14:78, 1973.
515. Gordienko AD: The effect of hepatoprotectors on the functional activity of rat hepatocyte mitochondria in in vitro and in vivo systems. Eskp Klin Farmacol 55:18, 1992.
516. Williamson JR, Scholz R, Browning ET, et al: Metabolic effects of ethanol in perfused rat liver. J Biol Chem 244:5044, 1969.
517. Grunnet N, Kondrup J, Dich J: Effect of ethanol or lipid metabolism in cultured hepatocytes. Biochem J 228:673-681, 1985.

518. Toth A, Lieber CS, Cederbaum AI, et al: Effects of ethanol and diet on fatty acid oxidation by hepatic mitochondria. Gastroenterology 64:198, 1973.
519. Zakim D, Green J: Quantitative importance of reduced fatty acid oxidations in the pathogenesis of ethanol-fatty liver. Proc Soc Exp Biol Med 27:138, 1963.
520. Leung NWY, Peters TJ: Palmitic acid oxidation and incorporation into triglyceride by needle liver biopsy specimens from control subjects and patients with alcoholic liver disease. Clin Sci 71:253, 1986.
521. Lieber CS, Schmid R: The effect of ethanol on fatty acid metabolism: stimulation of hepatic fatty acid synthesis in vitro. J Clin Invest 40:394, 1961.
522. Reboucas G, Isselbacher K: Studies on the pathogenesis of the ethanol-induced fatty liver: synthesis and oxidation of fatty acids by the liver. J Clin Invest 40:1355, 1961.
523. Kim CL, Leo MA, Lowe N, Lieber CS: Effects of vitamin A and ethanol on liver plasma membrane fluidity. Hepatology 8:735, 1988.
524. Venkatesan S, Ward RJ, Peters TJ: Fatty acid synthesis and triacylglycerol accumulation in rat liver after chronic ethanol consumption. Clin Sci 73:159, 1987.
525. Venkatesan S, Ward RJ, Peters TJ: Effect of chronic ethanol feeding on the hepatic secretion of very-low-density lipoproteins. Biochim Biophys Acta 960:61, 1988.
526. Zakim D, Alexander D, Slesinger MH: The effect of ethanol on hepatic secretion of triglycerides into plasma. J Clin Invest 44:1115, 1965.
527. Cairns SR, Peters TJ: Isolation of micro- and macro-droplet fractions of needle biopsy specimens of human liver and determination of subcellular distribution of the accumulating liver lipids in alcoholic fatty liver. Clin Sci 67:337, 1984.
528. Venkatesan S, Cooper PJ, Simpson KJ: Morphometric and biochemical evidence for inhibited very low density lipoprotein secretion in chronic low-fat alcohol-fed rats. Biochem Soc Trans 17:1117, 1989.
529. Jennett RB, Sorrell MF, Saffari-Ward A, et al: Preferential covalent binding of acetaldehyde to the α-chain of purified rat liver tubulin. Hepatology 9:57, 1989.
530. Sorensen TIA, Orholm M, Bentsen KD, et al: Lancet 2:241, 1984.
531. Fernman G, Lieber CS, Feiman L, Lieber CS: Hepatic collagen metabolism: effect of alcohol consumption in rats and baboons. Science 176:795, 1972.
532. Mezey E, Potter JJ, Maddrey WC: Hepatic collagen turnover in alcoholic liver disease. Gastroenterology 67:815, 1974.
533. Kersten S, Dasvergne B, Wahli W: Roles of PPARs in health and disease. Nature 405:421-424, 2000.
534. Vumecg J, Latruffe N: Medical significance of peroxisome proliferator-activated receptors. Lancet 354:141-148, 1999.
535. Bass NM: Interaction of fatty acid-binding protein (FABP) with peroxisomal proliferator-activated receptor (PPARα): evidence for FABP modulation of the gene response to fatty acid overload. In Van der Hoek(de): Frontiers in Bioactive Lipids. New York, Plenum Press, 1996:67-72.
536. Fromenty B, Pessayre D: Inhibition of mitochondrial beta-oxidation as a mechanism of hepatotoxicity. Pharmacol Ther 67:101-154, 1995.
537. Gibson GG: Co-induction of cytochrome P450 IVA and peroxisome proliferation: a causal or casual relationship. Xenobiotica 22:1101-1109, 1992.
538. Amet Y, Adas F, Nanji AA: Fatty acid omega and (omega-1) hydroxylation in experimental alcoholic liver disease: relationship to different dietary fatty acids. Alcohol Clin Exp Res 22:1493-1500, 1998.
539. Ma XL, Baraona E, Lieber CS: Alcohol consumption enhances fatty acid omega-oxidation, with a greater increase in male than in female rats. Hepatology 18:1247-1253, 1993.
540. Kaikaus RM, Chan WK, Lysenko N, et al: Induction of peroxisomal fatty acid beta-oxidation and liver fatty acid-binding protein by peroxisome proliferators. Mediation via the cytochrome P-450IVA1 omega-hydroxylase pathway. J Biol Chem 268:9593-9603, 1993.
541. Bell DR, Bars RG, Elcombe CR: Differential tissue-specific expression and induction of cytochrome P450IVA1 and acyl-CoA oxidase. Eur J Biochem 206:979-986, 1992.
542. Bass NM: Cellular binding proteins for fatty acids and retinoids: similar or specialized functions. Mol Cell Biochem 123:191-202, 1993.
543. Bass NM, Appel R, Goetzl EJ, et al: Peroxisome proliferator-activated receptor α-mediated gene expression and adaptation to fatty acid overload in alcoholic liver disease. Alcohol Clin Exp Res 22:749, 1998.
544. Nanji AA, Dannenberg AJ, Bass NM: Dietary fat composition influences cell injury in experimental alcoholic liver disease and has divergent effects on the expression of liver fatty acid binding protein and enzymes of extramitochondrial fatty acid oxidation. Gastroenterology 10 A1274, 1996.
545. Gordon DA: Recent advances in elucidating the role of the microsomal triglyceride transfer protein in apolipoprotein B lipoprotein assembly. Curr Opin Lipidol 8:131-137, 1997.
546. Raabe M, Veniant M, Sullivan MT, et al: Analysis of the role of microsomal triglyceride transfer protein in the liver of tissue-specific knockout mice. J Clin Invest 103:1287-1298, 1999.
547. Lin MC, Li JJ, Wang EJ, et al: Ethanol down-regulates the transcription of microsomal triglyceride transfer protein gene. FASEB J 11:1145-1152, 1997.
548. Leung GK, Veniant MM, Kim SK, et al: A deficiency of microsomal triglyceride transfer protein reduces apolipoprotein B secretion. J Biol Chem 275:7515-7520, 2000.
549. Kapadia C: Alcoholic steatosis: the Kupffer cell a villain? Gastroenterology 120:581-582, 2001.
550. Adachi Y, Bradford BU, Gao W, et al: Inactivation of Kupffers cells prevents early alcohol-induced liver injury. Hepatology 20:453-460, 1994.
551. Kawada N, Mizoguchi K, Kobayashi T, et al: Calcium-dependent prostaglandin biosynthesis by LPS-stimulated rat Kupffer cells. Prostaglandins Leukot Essent Fatty Acids. 47:209-214, 1992.
552. Enomoto N, Ikejima K, Yamashina S, et al: Kupffer cell-derived prostaglandin E_2 is involved in alcohol-induced fat accumulation in rat liver. Am J Physiol 279:G100-106. 2000.
553. French SW, Ihrig TJ, Morin RJ: Lipid composition of RBC, liver mitochondria and microsomes of ethanol-fed rats. J Stud Alcohol 31:810, 1970.
554. Alling C, Aspenstrom G, Dencker SJ, Svennerhold L: Essential fatty acids in chronic alcoholism. Acta Med Scand Suppl 631:1, 1979.
555. Cairns SR, Peters TJ: Biochemical analysis of hepatic lipid in alcoholic and diabetic subjects. Clin Sci 65:645, 1983.
556. Cunningham CC, Filus B, Bottenus RE, Spach RI: Effect of ethanol consumption on the phospholipid composition of rat liver microsomes and mitochondria. Biochim Biophys Acta 797:320, 1982.
557. Rietz RC: The effects of ethanol on lipid metabolism. Prog Lipid Res 18:87, 1978.
558. Cunnane SC, McAdoo KR, Horrobin DF: Long-term ethanol consumption in the hamster: effects on tissue lipids, fatty acids and erythrocyte hemolysis. Ann Nutr Metab 31:265, 1987.
559. Horrobin DF: Essential fatty acids, prostaglandins and alcoholism: an overview. Alcohol Clin Exp Res 11:2, 1987.
560. Nervi AM, Peluffo RO, Brenner RR: Effect of ethanol administration on fatty acid desaturation. Lipids 15:263, 1980.
561. Wang DL, Reitz RC: Ethanol ingestion and polyunsaturated fatty acids effects on the acyl CoA desaturases. Alcohol Clin Exp Res 7:220, 1983.
562. Reitz RC: Relationship of the acyl CoA desaturases to certain membrane fatty acid changes induced by ethanol consumption. Proc West Pharmacol Soc 27:247, 1984.
563. DeAntueno RJ, Elliot M, Horrobin DF: Liver $\Delta 5$ and $\Delta 6$ desaturase activity differs among laboratory rat strains. Lipids 29:327, 1994.
564. Nakamura MT, Tang AB, Villanueva J, et al: Selective reduction of $\Delta 6$ and $\Delta 5$ desaturase activities but not $\Delta 9$ desaturase in micropigs chronically fed ethanol. J Clin Invest 93:450, 1994.
565. Reitz RC: Dietary fatty acids and alcohol: effects on cellular membranes. Alcohol Alcohol 28:59, 1993.
566. Oshino N, Sato R: The dietary control of the microsomal stearyl-CoA desaturation enzyme system in rat liver desaturation enzyme system. Arch Biochem Biophys 149:369, 1972.
567. Nanji AA, Sadrzadeh SMH, Dannenberg AJ: Liver microsomal fatty acid composition in ethanol-fed rats: effect of different dietary fats and relationship to liver injury. Alcohol Clin Res 18:1024, 1994.
568. French SW, Sheinbaum A, Morin RJ: Effect of ethanol and fat free diet on hepatic mitochondrial fragility and fatty acid composition. Proc Soc Exp Biol Med 130:781, 1969.

569. Nanji AA, Zhao S, Sadrzadeh SMH, et al: Markedly enhanced cytochrome P450 2E1 induction and lipid peroxidation is associated with severe liver injury in fish oil-ethanol fed rats. Alcohol Clin Exp Res 18:1280, 1994.
570. Reitz RC: Dietary fatty acids and alcohol: effects on cellular membranes. Alcohol Alcohol 28:59, 1993.
571. Thompson JA, Reitz RC: Effects of ethanol ingestion and dietary fat levels on mitochondrial lipids in male and female rats. Lipids 13:540, 1978.
572. Reitz RC: Effects of dietary fatty acids and alcohol on the fatty acid composition in cellular membranes. In Watson RR, Watzl B, eds: Nutrition and Alcohol. Boca Raton, CRC Press, 1992:191.
573. Nanji AA, Lamb RG, Sadrzadeh SMH, et al: Changes in microsomal phospholipases and arachidonic acid in experimental alcoholic liver injury: relationship to cytochrome P450 2E1 induction and conjugated diene formation. Alcohol Clin Exp Res 17:598, 1993.
574. Morimoto M, Reitz RC, Morin RJ, et al: Fatty acid composition of hepatic lipids in rats fed ethanol and high fat diet intragastrically: effect of CYP 2E1 inhibitors. J Nutr 125:2953-2964, 1995.
575. Laetham RM, Balazy M, Falck JR, et al: Formation of 19(S)-and 18(R)-hydroxyeicosatetraenoic acids by alcohol-inducible cytochrome P450 2E1. J Biol Chem 268:12912, 1993.
576. Rifkind AB, Lee C, Chang TKH: Arachidonic acid metabolism by human cytochrome P450s 2C8, 2C9, 2E1 and 1A2. Arch Biochem Biophys 320:380, 1995.
577. Israel Y, Kalant H, LeBlanc E, et al: Changes in cation transport and (Na^+K^+)-activated adenosine triphosphatase produced by chronic administration of ethanol. J Pharmacol Exp Ther 174:330, 1970.
578. Sadrzadeh SMH, Price P, Nanji AA: Ethanol-induced changes in membrane ATPases: inhibition by iron chelation. Biochem Pharmacol 47:745, 1994.
579. Nanji AA, Khettry U, Sadrzadeh SMH, Yamanaka T: Severity of liver injury in experimental alcoholic liver disease: correlation with plasma endotoxin, prostaglandin E_2, leukotriene B_4 and thromboxane B2. Am J Pathol 142:367, 1993.
580. Lieber CS, DeCarli LM: Quantitative relationship between amount of dietary fat and severity of alcoholic fatty liver. Am J Clin Nutr 23:474, 1970.
581. Tsukamoto H, French SW, Benson N, et al: Severe and progressive steatosis and focal necrosis in rat liver induced by continuous intragastric infusion of ethanol and low fat diet. Hepatology 5:224, 1985.
582. Tsukamoto H, Towner SJ, Ciofalo LM, French SW: Ethanol-induced liver fibrosis in rats fed high fat diet. Hepatology 6:814, 1986.
583. French SW, Miyamoto K, Tsukamoto H: Ethanol-induced hepatic fibrosis in the rat: role of amount of dietary fat. Alcohol Clin Exp Res 10:13S, 1986.
584. Nanji AA, Tsukamoto H, French SW: Relationship between fatty liver and subsequent development of necrosis, inflammation, and fibrosis in experimental alcoholic liver disease. Exp Mol Pathol 51:141, 1989.
585. Nanji AA, French SW: Relationship between pork consumption and cirrhosis. Lancet 1:681, 1985.
586. Nanji AA, French SW: Dietary factors and alcoholic cirrhosis. Alcohol Clin Exp Res 10:271, 1986.
587. Nanji AA, Mendenhall CL, French SW: Beef fat prevents alcoholic liver disease in the rat. Alcohol Clin Exp Res 13:15, 1989.
588. Nanji AA, French SW: Dietary linoleic acid is required for development of experimentally induced alcoholic liver injury. Life Sci 44:223, 1989.
589. Nanji AA, Zhao S, Sadrzadeh SMH, et al: Markedly enhanced cytochrome P450 2E1 induction and lipid peroxidation is associated with severe liver injury in fish oil-ethanol-fed rats. Alcohol Clin Exp Res 18:1280, 1994.
590. French SW: Nutrition in the pathogenesis of alcoholic liver disease. Alcohol Alcohol 28:97, 1993.
591. Kaminski DL: Arachidonic acid metabolites in hepatobiliary physiology and disease. Gastroenterology 97:781-792, 1989.
592. Eberhart CE, DuBois RN: Eicosanoids and the gastrointestinal tract. Gastroenterology 109:285-301, 1995.
593. DuBois RN, Abramson SB, Grofford L, et al: Cyclooxygenases in biology and disease. FASEB J 12:1063-1073, 1998.
594. Mitchell JA, Larkin S, Williams TJ: Cyclooxygenase-2 regulation and relevance to inflammation. Biochem Pharmacol 50:1535-1542, 1995.
595. Herschmann HR: Prostaglandin synthetase-2. Biochem Biophys Acta 1299:125-140, 1996.
596. Needleman P, Isakson PC: The discovery and function of COX-2. J Rheumatol 24:6-8, 1997.
597. Nakatsugi S, Sugimoto N, Furukawa M: Effects of non-steroidal anti inflammatory drugs on prostaglandin E_2 production by cyclooxygenase-2 from endogenous and exogenous arachidonic acid in rat peritoneal macrophages stimulated with lipopolysaccharide. Prostoglandins Leukot Essent Fatty Acids 55:451-457, 1996.
598. Hamilton LC, Mitchell JA, Tomlinson AM, Warner TD: Synergy between cyclooxygenase-2 induction and arachidonic acid supply in vivo: Consequences for non-steroidal drug efficacy FASEB J 13:245-251, 1999.
599. Nanji AA, Zakim D: Alcoholic liver disease. In Zakim D, Boyer TD (eds): Hepatology: A Textbook of Liver Disease, ed. 3. Philadelphia, WB Saunders, 1996:891-962.
600. Hill DB, Deauciuc IV, Nanji AA, McClain CJ: Mechanisms of hepatic injury in alcoholic liver disease. Clin Liver Dis 2:703-722, 1998.
601. Nanji AA, Lamb RG, Sadrzadeh SMH, et al: Changes in microsomal phospholipases and arachidonic acid in experimental alcoholic liver injury: relationship to cytochrome P450 2E1 induction and conjugated diene formation. Alcohol Clin Exp Res 17:595-603, 1993.
602. Nanji AA, French SW: Dietary linoleic acid is required for development of experimentally-induced alcoholic liver disease. Life Sci 44:223-227, 1989.
603. Nanji AA, Sadrzadeh SMH, Dannenberg AJ: Liver microsomal fatty acid composition in ethanol-fed rats: effect of different dietary fats and relationship to liver injury. Alcohol Clin Exp Res 18:1024-1028, 1994.
604. Dinchuk JE, Car BD, Focht RJ, et al: Renal abnormalities and an altered inflammatory response in mice backing cyclooxygenese II. Nature 378:406-409, 1995.
605. Cederbaum AI: Role of lipid peroxidation and oxidative stress in alcohol toxicity. Free Radic Biol Med 7:537-539, 1989.
606. Bode C, Kugler V. Bode JC: Endotoxemia in patients with alcoholic and non-alcoholic cirrhosis and in patients with no evidence of chronic liver disease following acute alcohol excess. J Hepatol 4:8-13, 1987.
607. Fukai H, Brauner B, Bode JC, Bode C: Plasma endotoxin concentrations in patients with alcoholic and non-alcoholic liver disease: re-evaluation with improved chromogenic assay. Hepatology 12:162-168, 1991.
608. Thurman RG, Bradford BU, Iimuro Y, et al: The role of gut-derived bacterial toxins and free radicals in alcohol-induced liver injury. J Gastroenterol Hepatol 13(suppl):S39-S50, 1998.
609. Nanji AA, Khettry U, Sadrzadeh SMH, Yamanaka T: Severity of liver injury in experimental alcoholic liver disease: correlation with plasma endotoxin, prostaglandin E_2, leukotriene B_4 and thromboxane B2. Am J Pathol 142:367-373, 1993.
610. Hempel SL, Monick MM, Yano BT, Hunninghake GV: Synthesis of prostaglandin H synthase-2 by human alveolar macrophage in response to lipopolysaccharide is inhibited by decreased cell oxidant tone. J Biol Chem 269:32979-32984, 1994.
611. Kulmacz RJ, Wang LH: Comparison of hydroperoxide initiator requirements for the cyclooxygenase activities of prostaglandin H synthase-1 and -2. J Biol Chem 270:24019-24023, 1995.
612. Feng L, Xia Y, Garcia GE, et al: Involvement of reactive oxygen intermediates in cyclooxygenase-2 expression induced by interleukin-1, tumor necrosis factor-α and lipopolysaccharide. J Clin Invest 95:1669-1675, 1995.
613. Nanji AA, Miao L, Thomas P, et al: Enhanced cyclooxygenase-2 gene expression in alcoholic liver disease in the rat. Gastroenterology 112: 943-951, 1997.
614. Nanji AA, Fotouhinia M, Miao L, et al: Enhanced severity of alcoholic liver injury in female rats. Hepatology 26:272A, 1997.
615. Nieto N, Greenwel P, Friedman SL, et al: Ethanol and arachidonic acid increase $\alpha 2$(I) collagen expression in rat hepatic stellate cells overexpressing CYP 2E1: role of H_2O_2 and cyclooxygenase 2. J Biol Chem 275:20136-20145, 2000.
616. Nanji AA, Khettry U, Sadrzadeh SMH, Yamanaka T: Severity of liver injury in experimental alcoholic liver disease: correlation with plasma endotoxin, prostaglandin E_2 leukotriene B_4 and thromboxane B_2. Am J Pathol 142:367-373, 1993.

617. Nanji AA, Sadrzadeh SMH, Thomas P, Yamanaka T: Eiscosanoid profile and evidence for endotoxin tolerance in chronic ethanol-fed rats. Life Sci 55:611-620, 1994.
618. Hou MC, Cahill PA, Zhang S, et al: Enhanced cyclooxygenase-1 expression within the superior mesenteric artery portal hypertensive rats: role in the hyperdynamic circulation. Hepatology 27:20-27, 1998.
619. Jun SS, Chen Z, Pace MC, Shaul PW: Estrogen upregulates cyclooxgenase-1 gene expression in ovine fetal pulmonary artery endothelium. J Clin Invest 102:176-183, 1998.
620. Wu KK: Regulation of prostaglandin H 1 synthase gene expression. Adv Exp Biol Med 400A:121-126, 1997.
621. Nanji AA, Sadrzadeh SMH, Thomas P, Yamanaka T: Eicosanoid profile and evidence for endotoxin tolerance in chronic ethanol-fed rats. Life Sci 55:611-619, 1994.
622. Nanji AA, Sadrzadeh SMH, Thomas P, Yamanaka T: Eicosanoid profile and evidence for endotoxin tolerance in chronic ethanol-fed rats. Life Sci 55:611, 1994.
623. Nanji AA, Khettry U, Sadrzadeh SMH, Yamanaka T: Severity of liver injury in experimental alcoholic liver disease: correlation with plasma endotoxin, prostaglandin E_2, leukotriene B_4 and thromboxane B_2. Am J Pathol 142:367, 1993.
624. Nanji AA, Khwaja S, Sadrzadeh SMH: Decreased prostacyclin production by liver non-parenchymal cells precedes liver injury in experimental alcoholic liver disease. Life Sci 54:455, 1994.
625. Warso MA, Lands WEM: Lipid peroxidation in relation to prostacyclin and thromboxane physiology and pathophysiology. Br Med Bull 39:277, 1983.
626. Hecker M, Ullrich V: On the mechanism of prostacyclin and thromboxane A_2 biosynthesis. J Biol Chem 264:141, 1989.
627. Chan AC: Vitamin E and the arachidonic acid cascade. In Mino M, ed: Vitamin E—Its Usefulness in Health and Curing Disease. Japan Sci Soc Press, Tokyo, 1993:197.
628. Sadrzadeh SMH, Nanji AA, Price PL, Meydani M: The effect of chronic ethanol feeding on serum and liver alpha and gamma tocopherol levels in normal and vitamin E deficient rats. Biochem Pharmacol 47:2005, 1994.
629. Kawase T, Kato S, Lieber CS: Lipid peroxidation and antioxidant defense systems in rat liver after chronic ethanol feeding. Hepatology 10:815, 1989.
630. Nanji AA, Khwaja S, Sadrzadeh SMH: Eicosanoid production in experimental alcoholic liver disease is related to vitamin E levels and lipid peroxidation. Mol Cell Biochem 140:85, 1994.
631. Smith WL: Prostanoid biosynthesis and mechanisms of action. Am J Physiol 263:F181, 1992.
632. Schror K, Braun M: Platelets as a source of vasoactive mediators. Stroke 21(suppl IV):32, 1990.
633. Horton AA, Wood JM: Prevention of thromboxane B_2 induced hepatocyte plasma membrane bleb formation by certain prostaglandins and a proteinase inhibitor. Biochim Biophys Acta 1022:319, 1990.
634. Gores GJ, Herman B, LeMasters JJ: Plasma membrane bleb formation and rupture: a common feature of hepatocellular injury. Hepatology 11:690, 1990.
635. Goldman G, Welbourn R, Klausner JM, et al: Thromboxane mediates diapedesis after ischemia by activation of neutrophil adhesion receptors interacting with basally expressed ICAM-1. Circ Res 68:1013, 1991.
636. Kohan DE: Eicosanoids: potential regulators of extracellular matrix formation in the kidney. J Lab Clin Med 120:4, 1992.
637. Bruggeman LA, Pellicoro JA, Horigan EA, Klotman PE: Thromboxane and prostacyclin differentially regulate murine extracellular matrix gene expression. Kidney Int 43:1219, 1993.
638. DeRubertis FR, Craven PA: Eicosanoids in the pathogenesis of functional and structural alterations in the kidney in diabetes. Am J Kidney Dis 22:727, 1993.
639. Negrete H, Studer RK, Craven PA, DeRubertis FR: Role for transforming growth factor β in thromboxane-induced increases in mesangial cell fibronectin synthesis. Diabetes 44:335, 1995.
640. Lands WEM: Biochemistry and physiology of n-3 fatty acids. FASEB J 6:2530, 1992.
641. Ferreti A, Judd JT, Taylor PR, et al: Ingestion of marine oil reduces excretion of 11-dehydrothromboxane B_2, an index of intravascular production of thromboxane A2. Prostaglandins Leukot Essent Fatty Acids 48:305, 1993.
642. Morrow JD, Awad JA, Kato T, et al: Formation of novel non-cyclooxygenase-derived prostanoids (F2-isoprostanes) in carbon tetrachloride hepatotoxicity. J Clin Invest 90:2502, 1992.
643. Morrow JD, Awad JA, Boss HJ, et al: Non-cyclooxygenase-derived prostanoids (F2-isoprostanes) are formed in situ on phospholipids. Proc Natl Acad Sci U S A 89:10721, 1992.
644. Nanji AA, Khwaja S, Tahan SR, Sadrzadeh SMH: Plasma levels of a novel non-cyclooxygenase-derived prostanoid (8-isoprostane) correlate with severity of liver injury in experimental alcoholic liver disease. J Pharmacol Exp Ther 269:1280, 1994.
645. Takahashi K, Nammour TK, Fukunaga M, et al: Glomerular actions of a free radical-generated novel prostaglandin, 8-epi-prostaglandin $F_{2\alpha}$ in the rat: evidence for interaction with thromboxane A_2 receptors. J Clin Invest 90:136, 1992.
646. Fukunaga M, Makuta N, Roberts LJ, et al: Evidence for the existence of F_2-isoprostane receptors on rat vascular smooth muscle cells. Am J Physiol 264:C1619, 1993.
647. Fukunaga M, Takahashi K, Badr KF: Vascular smooth muscle actions and interactions of 8-isoprostaglandin F_2 and an E_2 isoprostane. Biochem Biophys Res Commun 195:507, 1993.
648. Takahashi H, Johansson I, French SW, et al: Effects of dietary fat composition on activities of the microsomal ethanol oxidizing system and ethanol-inducible cytochrome P450 (CYP 2E1) in the liver of rats chronically fed ethanol. Pharmacol Toxicol 70:347, 1992.
649. Nanji AA, Zhao S, Lamb RG, et al: Changes in cytochrome P450, 2E1, 2B1 and 4A and phospholipases A and C in the intragastric feeding rat model for alcoholic liver disease: relationship to dietary fats and pathologic liver injury. Alcohol Clin Exp Res 18:902, 1994.
650. Nanji AA, Zhao S, Lamb RG, et al: Changes in microsomal phospholipases and arachidonic acid in experimental alcoholic liver injury: relationship to cytochrome P450 2E1 induction and conjugated diene formation. Alcohol Clin Exp Res 17:598, 1993.
651. Nanji AA, Sadrzadeh SMH, Yang EK, et al: Dietary saturated fatty acids: a novel treatment for alcoholic liver disease. Gastroenterology 109:547, 1995.
652. Nanji AA, Sadrzadeh SMH, Yang EK, et al: Medium chain triglycerides and vitamin E are effective in treating alcoholic liver injury. Gastroenterology 108:A1131, 1995.
653. Lieber CS, DeCarli LM, Mak KM, et al: Attenuation of alcohol-induced hepatic fibrosis by polyunsaturated lecithin. Hepatology 12:1390, 1990.
654. Lieber CS, Robins SJ, Li J, et al: Phosphatidylcholine protects against fibrosis and cirrhosis in the baboon. Gastroenterology 106:152, 1994.
655. Duce AM, Ortiz P, Cabrero C, Mato IM: S-adenosyl-L-methionine synthetase and phospholipid methyltransferase are inhibited in human cirrhosis. Hepatology:65, 1988.
656. Lieber CS, Robins SJ, Leo MA: Hepatic phosphatidylethanolamine methyltransferase activity is decreased by ethanol and increased by phosphatidylcholine. Alcohol Clin Exp Res 18:592, 1994.
657. Field JB, Williams HE, Mortimore GE, et al: Studies on the mechanism of ethanol-induced hypoglycemia. J Clin Invest 42:497, 1963.
658. Freinkel N, Singer DL, Arky RA, et al: Alcohol hypoglycemia. I. Carbohydrate metabolism of patients with clinical alcohol hypoglycemia and the experimental reproduction of the syndrome with pure ethanol. J Clin Invest 42:1112, 1963.
659. Forsander OA, Raiha N, Salasporo M, et al: Influence of ethanol on the liver metabolism of fed and starved rats. Biochem J 94:259, 1965.
660. Madison LL, Lochner A, Wolff J: Ethanol-induced hypoglycemia. Diabetes 16:252, 1967.
661. Frieden C: Glutamic dehydrogenase. III. The order of substrate addition in the enzymatic reaction. J Biol Chem 234:2891, 1959.
662. Ideo G, DeFranchis R, Del Ninno ED, et al: Decrease of rat liver glutamate dehydrogenase after chronic administration of ethanol. Enzymologia 43:245, 1972.
663. Stifel FB, Greene HL, Lufkin EG, et al: Acute effects of oral and intravenous ethanol on rat hepatic enzyme activities. Biochim Biophys Acta 428:633, 1976.
664. Zakim D: The effect of ethanol on the concentration of gluconeogenic intermediates in rat liver. Proc Soc Exp Biol Med 129:393, 1968.

665. Arky RA: Hypoglycemia associated with liver disease and ethanol. Endocrinol Metab Clin North Am 18:75, 1989.
666. Madison LL: Ethanol induced hypoglycemia. Adv Metab Dis 3:85, 1968.
667. Kreisberg RA, Siegal AM, Owen WC: Glucose-lactate interrelationships: effect of ethanol. J Clin Invest 50:175, 1971.
668. Arky RA, Veverbrants E, Abramson EA: Irreversible hypoglycemia: a complication of alcohol and insulin. JAMA 206:575, 1968.
669. Chalmers RJ, Bennie EH, Johnson RH, et al: The growth hormone response to insulin induced hypoglycemia in alcoholics. Psychol Med 7:607, 1977.
670. Kuhl C, Anderson O: Glucose- and tolbutamide-mediated insulin response after pure infusion with ethanol. Diabetes 23:821, 1974.
671. Gohen S: A review of hypoglycemia and alcoholism with and without liver disease. Ann N Y Acad Sci 273:338, 1976.
672. Haight JSJ, Keatinge WR: Failure of thermoregulation in the cold during hypoglycemia induced by exercise and alcohol. J Physiol 229:87, 1973.
673. O'Keefe SJD, Marks V: Lunchtime gin and tonic: a cause of reactive hypoglycemia. Lancet 1:1286, 1977.
674. Metz R, Berger S, Mako M: Potentiation of the plasma insulin response to glucose by prior administration of alcohol. Diabetes 18:517, 1969.
675. Singh SP, Patel DG: Effects of ethanol on carbohydrate metabolism. I. Influence on oral glucose tolerance test. Metabolism 25:239, 1976.
676. Mueckler M: Facilitative glucose transporters. Eur J Biochem 219:713, 1994.
677. Could GW, Holman GD: The glucose transporter family: structure, function and tissue specific expression. Biochem J 295:329, 1993.
678. Bell GI, Burant CF, Takeda G, Gould GW: Structure and function of mammalian facilitative sugar transporters. J Biol Chem 268:19161, 1993.
679. Tal M, Scheider DL, Thorens B, Lodish HF: Restricted expression of the erythroid/brain glucose transporter isoform to perivenous hepatocytes in rats: modulation by glucose. J Clin Invest 86:986, 1990.
680. Nanji AA, Fogt F, Griniuviene B: Alterations in glucose transporter proteins in alcoholic liver disease in the rat. Am J Pathol 146:329, 1995.
681. Loike JD, Cao L, Brett J, et al: Hypoxia induces glucose transporter expression in endothelial cells. Am J Physiol 263:C326, 1992.
682. Porter NA, Caldwell SE, Mills KA: Mechanisms of free radical oxidation of unsaturated lipids. Lipids 30:277, 1995.
683. Bulkley GB: Free radicals and other reactive oxygen metabolites. Surgery 113:479, 1993.
684. Aust SD, Chignell CF, Bray TM, et al: Free radicals in toxicology. Toxicol Appl Pharmacol 120:168, 1993.
685. North JA, Spector AA, Buettner GR: Cell fatty acid composition affects free radical formation during lipid peroxidation. Am J Physiol 267:c177, 1994.
686. Kehrer JP: Free radicals as mediators of tissue injury and disease. Crit Rev Toxicol 23:21, 1993.
687. Gardner HW: Oxygen radical chemistry of polyunsaturated fatty acids. Free Rad Biol Med 7:65, 1989.
688. Dargel HW: Lipid peroxidation—a common pathogenetic mechanism. Exp Toxic Pathol 14:169, 1992.
689. Dix TA, Aikens J: Mechanisms and biologic relevance of lipid peroxidation initiation. Chem Res Toxicol 6:2, 1993.
690. Shigenega MK, Hagen TM, Ames BN: Oxidative damage and mitochondrial decay in aging. Proc Natl Acad Sci U S A 91:10771, 1994.
691. Poli G, Albano E, Dianzani HU: The role of lipid peroxidation in liver damage. Chem Phys Lipids 45:117, 1987.
692. Ungemach FR: Pathobiological mechanisms of hepatocellular damage following lipid peroxidation. Chem Phys Lipids 45:171, 1987.
693. Yao T, Esposti SD, Huang L, et al: Inhibition of carbon tetrachloride-induced liver injury by liposomes containing vitamin E. Am J Physiol 267:G476, 1994.
694. Mason RP: Free radical metabolites of foreign compounds and their toxicological significance. In Hodgson E, Bend JR, Philpot RM, eds: Review of Biochemical Toxicology. New York, Elsevier-North Holland, 1979:151.
695. McCoy PB, Poyer JL: Enzyme generated free radicals as initiators of lipid peroxidation in biological membranes. In Martonosi A, ed: The Enzymes of Biological Membranes, vol 4. New York, Plenum, 1976:239.
696. Sies H: Strategies of antioxidant defense. Eur J Biochem 215:213, 1993.
697. DiLuzio NR: Prevention of the acute ethanol-induced fatty liver by antioxidants. Physiologist 6:169, 1963.
698. DiLuzio NR, Hartman AD: Role of lipid peroxidation in the pathogenesis of ethanol-induced fatty liver. Fed Proc 26:1436, 1967.
699. Dianzani MU: Lipid peroxidation in ethanol poisoning: a critical re-consideration. Alcohol Alcohol 20:161, 1985.
700. Videla LA, Valenzuela LA: Alcohol ingestion, liver glutathione and lipoperoxidation. Life Sci 31:2395, 1985.
701. Bondy SC: Ethanol toxicity and oxidative stress. Toxicol Lett 63:231, 1992.
702. Cederbaum AI: Introduction: role of lipid peroxidation and oxidative stress in alcohol toxicity. Free Radic Biol Med 7:537, 1989.
703. Nordmann R, Ribiere C, Rouach H: Implication of free radical mechanisms in ethanol-induced cellular injury. Free Radic Biol Med 12:219, 1992.
704. Thurman RG: Induction of hepatic microsomal NADPH-dependent production of hydrogen peroxide by chronic prior treatment with ethanol. Mol Pharmacol 9:670, 1973.
705. Puntarulo SP, Cederbaum AI: Increased NADPH-dependent chemiluminescence by microsomes after chronic ethanol consumption. Arch Biochem Biophys 266:435, 1988.
706. Dicker E, Cederbaum AI: Increased NADH-dependent production of reactive oxygen intermediates by microsomes after chronic ethanol consumption. Arch Biochem Biophys 293:274, 1992.
707. Cederbaum AI: Oxygen radical generation by microsomes: role of iron and implications for alcohol metabolism and toxicity. Free Radic Biol Med 7:559, 1989.
708. Boveris A, Fraga CG, Varsavsky AI, Koch OR: Increased chemiluminescence and superoxide production in the livers of chronically ethanol-treated rats. Arch Biochem Biophys 227:534, 1983.
709. Reinke LA, Lai EK, DuBose CM, McCay PB: Reactive free radical generation in vivo in heart and liver of ethanol-fed rats: correlation with radical formation in vitro. Proc Natl Acad Sci U S A 84:9223, 1987.
710. Ekstrom G, Ingelman-Sundberg M: Rat liver microsomal NADPH-supported oxidase activity and lipid peroxidation dependent on ethanol-inducible cytochrome P450 (P450 IIE1). Biochem Pharmacol 38:2505, 1989.
711. Kukielka E, Cederbaum AI: DNA strand cleavage assay as a sensitive assay for the production of hydroxyl radicals by microsomes: role of cytochrome P450 2E1 in the increased activity after ethanol treatment. Biochem J 302:773, 1994.
712. Morimoto M, Hagbjork AL, Nanji AA, et al: Role of cytochrome P450 2E1 in alcoholic liver disease pathogenesis. Alcohol 10:459, 1993.
713. Albano E, Tomasi A, Persson JO, et al: Role of ethanol-inducible cytochrome P450 (P450 IIE1) in catalyzing the free radical activation of aliphatic alcoholics. Biochem Pharmacol 41:1895, 1991.
714. Ekstrom G, Cronholm T, Ingelman-Sundberg M: Hydroxyl-radical production and ethanol oxidation by liver microsomes isolated from ethanol treated rats. Biochem J 233:755, 1986.
715. Joly JG, Ishii H, Teschke R, et al: Effect of chronic alcohol feeding on the activities and submicrosomal distribution of reduced nicotinamide adenine dinucleotide phosphate-cytochrome P450 reductase and demethylase for aminopyrine and ethylmorphine. Biochem Pharmacol 22:1532, 1973.
716. Albano E, Tomasi A, Goria-Gatti L, Dianzani MU: Spin trapping of free radical species produced during the microsomal metabolism of ethanol. Chem Biol Inter 65:223, 1988.
717. McCay PB, Rau JM, Rienke LA: Hydroxyl radicals are generated by hepatic microsomes during NADPH oxidation: relationship to ethanol metabolism. Free Radic Res Commun 15:335, 1992.
718. Rienke LA, Rau JM, McCay PB: Characteristics of an oxidant formed during iron (II) antioxidation. Free Radic Biol Med 16:485, 1994.
719. Albano E, Clot P, Morimoto M, et al: Role of cytochrome P4502E1-dependent formation of hydroxyethyl free radical in the

development of liver damage in rats intragastrically fed with ethanol. Hepatology 23:155-163, 1996.
720. Albano E, French SW, Ingelman-Sundberg M: Hydroxyethyl radicals in ethanol hepatotoxicity. Front Biosci 4:533-540, 1999.
721. Knecht KT, Adachi Y, Bradford BU, et al: Free radical adducts in the bile of rats treated chronically with intragastric alcohol: inhibition by destruction of Kupffer cells. Mol Pharmacol 47:1028-1934, 1995.
722. Dupont I, Lucas D, Clot P, et al: Cytochrome P4502E1 inducibility and hydroxyethyl radical formation among alcoholics. J Hepatol 28:564-571, 1998.
723. Stoyanovsky DA, Wu D, Cederbaum AI: Interaction of 1-hydroxyethyl radical with glutathione, ascorbic acid and α-tocopherol. Free Radical Biol Med 24:132-138, 1998.
724. Makino K, Hagiwara T, Hagi A, et al: Cautionary note for DMPO spin trapping in the presence of iron ion. Biochem Biophys Res Commun 172:1073, 1990.
725. Rienke LA, Moore DR, Hague CM, McCay PB: Metabolism of ethanol to 1-hydroxyethyl radicals in rat liver microsomes: comparative studies with three spin trapping agents. Free Radic Res Commun 21:213, 1994.
726. Reinke LA, Moore DR, Rau JM, McCay PB: Inorganic phosphate promotes redox cycling of iron in liver microsomes: effects of free radical reactions. Arch Biochem Biophys 316:758, 1995.
727. Ribiere C, Sabourault D, Saffar C, Nordmann R: Mitochondrial generation of superoxide free radicals during acute ethanol intoxication in the rat. Alcohol Alcohol 1(suppl):241, 1987.
728. Ribiere C, Hininger I, Saffar-Boccara C, et al: Mitochondrial respiratory activity and superoxide radical generation in the liver, brain and heart after chronic ethanol intake. Biochem Pharmacol 47:1827, 1994.
729. Koch OR, Boveris A, Sirotzky S, et al: Biochemical lesion of liver mitochondria from rats after chronic alcohol consumption. Exp Mol Pathol 27:213, 1977.
730. Kurose I, Higuchi H, Kato S, et al: Oxidative stress on mitochondria and cell membrane of cultured rat hepatocytes and perfused liver exposed to ethanol. Gastroenterology 112:1331-1343, 1997.
731. Kurose I, Higuchi H, Miura S, et al: Oxidative stress-mediated apoptosis of hepatocytes exposed to acute ethanol intoxication. Hepatology 25:368-378, 1997.
732. Bruguera M, Bertran A, Bombi JA, Rodes J: Giant mitochondria in hepatocytes: a diagnostic hint for alcoholic liver disease. Gastroenterology 73:1383-1387, 1997.
733. Tilg H, Diehl M: Cytokines and alcoholic and non-alcoholic steatohepatitis. N Engl J Med. 343:1467-1476, 2000.
734. Oshino N, Jamieson D, Chance B: The properties of hydrogen peroxide production under hyperoxic and hypoxic conditions of perfused rat liver. Biochem J 146:53, 1975.
735. Handler JA, Thurman RG: Catalase-dependent ethanol oxidation in perfused rat liver: requirement for fatty acid stimulated H_2O_2 production by peroxisomes. Eur J Biochem 176:477, 1988.
736. Misra UK, Bradford BU, Handler JA, Thurman RG: Chronic ethanol treatment induces H_2O_2 production selectively in pericentral regions of the liver lobule. Alcohol Clin Exp Res 16:839, 1992.
737. Panchenko LF, Pirozhkov SV, Popova SV, Antonenkov VD: Effect of chronic ethanol treatment on peroxisomal acyl-coA oxidative activity and lipid peroxidation in rat liver and heart. Experientia 43:580, 1987.
738. Muller A, Sies H: Role of alcohol dehydrogenase activity and of acetaldehyde in ethanol-induced ethane and pentane production by isolated perfused rat liver. Biochem J 206:153, 1982.
739. Muller A, Sies H: Ethane release during metabolism of aldehydes and monoamines in perfused rat liver. Eur J Biochem 134:599, 1983.
740. Videla LA, Villena MI: Effect of ethanol, acetaldehyde, and acetate on the anti-oxidant sensitive respiration in the perfused rat liver: influence of fasting and diethylmaleate treatment. Alcohol 3:163, 1986.
741. Stege TE: Acetaldehyde-induced lipid peroxidation in isolated hepatocytes. Res Commun Chem Pathol Pharmacol 36:287, 1982.
742. Videla LA, Fernandez V, de Marinis A: Liver lipoperoxidative pressure and glutathione status following acetaldehyde and aliphatic alcohol pretreatment of rats. Biochem Biophys Res Commun 104:965, 1982.
743. Kera Y, Ohbora Y, Kumura S: The metabolism of acetaldehyde and not acetaldehyde itself is responsible for in-vivo ethanol-induced lipid peroxidation in rats. Biochem Pharmacol 37:3633, 1988.
744. Damgaard SE: The D(V/K) isotope effect of the cytochrome P450-mediated oxidation of ethanol and its biological applications. Eur J Biochem 125:593, 1982.
745. Feytmans E, Morales MN, Leighton F: Effect of pyrazole on rat liver catalase. Biochem Pharmacol 23:1293, 1974.
746. Bradford BU, Forman DT, Thurman RG: 4-Methylpyrazole inhibits fatty acyl coenzyme synthetase and diminishes catalase-dependent alcohol metabolism: has the contribution of alcohol dehydrogenase to alcohol metabolism been previously overestimated? Mol Pharmacol 43:115, 1993.
747. Engerson JD, McKelvey TG, Rhyne DB, et al: Conversion of xanthine dehydrogenase to oxidase in ischemic rat tissues. J Clin Invest 79:1564, 1987.
748. Della Corte E, Stirpe F: The regulation of xanthine oxidase. Biochem J 117:97, 1970.
749. Oei HHH, Zoganas HC, McCord JM, Schaffer SW: Role of acetaldehyde and xanthine oxidase in ethanol-induced oxidative stress. Res Commun Chem Pathol Pharmacol 51:195, 1986.
750. Sultatos LG: Effect of acute ethanol administration on the hepatic xanthine dehydrogenase/oxidase system in the rat. J Pharmacol Exp Ther 246:946, 1988.
751. Abbondanza A, Batteli MG, Soffritti M, Cessi C: Xanthine oxidase status in ethanol-intoxicated rat liver. Alcohol Clin Exp Res 13:841, 1989.
752. Kellogg EW, Fridovich I: Superoxide, hydrogen peroxide, and singlet oxygen in lipid peroxidation by a xanthine oxidase system. J Biol Chem 250:8812, 1975.
753. Fridovich I: Oxygen radicals from acetaldehyde. Free Radic Biol Med 7:557, 1989.
754. Shaw S, Jayatilleke E: Acetaldehyde-mediated hepatic lipid peroxidation: role of superoxide and ferritin. Biochem Biophys Res Commun 143:984, 1987.
755. Erikkson CJP: Ethanol and acetaldehyde metabolism in rat strains genetically selected for ethanol preference. Biochem Pharmacol 22:2283, 1973.
756. Fridovich I: The mechanism of the enzymatic oxidation of aldehydes. J Biol Chem 241:3126, 1966.
757. Kato S, Kawase T, Alderman J, et al: Role of xanthine oxidase in ethanol-induced lipid peroxidation in rats. Gastroenterology 98:203, 1990.
758. Purg JG, Fox IH: Ethanol-induced activation of adenine nucleotide turnover. Evidence for a role of acetate. J Clin Invest 74:936, 1984.
759. Buehler R, Hess M, von Wartburg JP: Immunohistochemical localization of human alcohol dehydrogenase in liver tissue, cultured fibroblasts and Hela cells. Am J Pathol 108:89, 1982.
760. Morrison GR, Brock FE: Quantitative measurement of alcohol dehydrogenase in the lobule of normal livers. J Lab Clin Med 70:116, 1967.
761. Chen L, Davis GJ, Lumeng L: Zonal distribution of xanthine oxidase in rat liver. (Abstract) Clin Res 39:537, 1989.
762. Rajagopalan KV, Handler P: Hepatic aldehyde oxidase III. The substrate binding site. J Biol Chem 239:2027, 1964.
763. Shaw S, Jayatilleke E: The role of aldehyde oxidase in ethanol-induced hepatic lipid peroxidation. Biochem J 268:579, 1990.
764. Yu BP: Cellular defenses against damage from reactive oxygen species. Physiol Rev 74:139, 1994.
765. Sies H: Strategies of antioxidant defense. Eur J Biochem 215:213, 1993.
766. Ichikawa I, Kiyama S, Yoshioka T: Renal antioxidant enzymes: their regulation and function. Kidney Int 45:1, 1994.
767. Fridovich I: Superoxide dismutases. J Biol Chem 264:7761, 1989.
768. Ribiere C, Sinaceur J, Sabourault D, Nordmann R: Hepatic catalase and superoxide dismutases after acute ethanol administration in rats. Alcohol 2:31, 1985.
769. Ribiere C, Sinaceur J, Nordmann J, Nordmann R: Discrepancy between the different subcellular activities of rat liver catalase and superoxide dismutases in response to acute ethanol administration. Alcohol Alcohol 20:13, 1985.
770. Kono Y, Fridovich I: Superoxide inhibits catalase. J Biol Chem 257:5751, 1982.

771. Sinet PM, Garber P: Inactivation of the human CuZn superoxide dismutase during exposure to O^{-}_2 and H_2O2. Arch Biochem Biophys 212:411, 1981.
772. Valenzuela A, Fernandez N, Fernandez V, et al: Effect of acute ethanol ingestion on lipoperoxidation and on the activity of the enzymes related to peroxide metabolism in rat liver. FEBS Lett 111:11, 1980.
773. DeMaster EG, Kaplan E, Chester E: The differential response of tissue catalase activity to chronic administration in the rat. Alcohol Clin Exp Res 5:45, 1981.
774. Schisler NJ, Singh SM: Effect of ethanol in vivo on enzymes which detoxify oxygen free radicals. Free Radic Biol Med 7:117, 1989.
775. Zindenberg-Cherr S, Halsted CH, Olin KL, et al: The effect of chronic alcohol ingestion on free radical defense in the miniature pig. J Nutr 120:213, 1990.
776. Zindenberg-Cherr S, Olin KL, Villanueva J, et al: Ethanol-induced changes in hepatic free radical defense mechanisms and fatty acid composition in the miniature pig. Hepatology 13:1185, 1991.
777. Nanji AA, Griniuviene B, Sadrzadeh SMH, et al: Effect of type of dietary fat and ethanol on antioxidant enzyme mRNA induction in rat liver. J Lipid Res 36:736, 1995.
778. Misra UK, Bradford BU, Handler JA, Thurman RG: Chronic ethanol treatment induces H_2O_2 production selectively in epicentral regions of the liver lobule. Alcohol Clin Exp Res 16:839, 1992.
779. Wong GHW, Elwell JH, Oberly LW, Goedell GV: Manganous superoxide dismutase is essential for cellular resistance to cytotoxicity of tumor necrosis factor. Cell 58:923, 1989.
780. Kizaki M, Sakashita A, Karmakar A, et al: Regulation of manganese superoxide dismutase and other antioxidant genes in normal and leukemic hematopoietic cells and their relationship to cytotoxicity by tumor necrosis factor. Blood 82:1142, 1993.
781. Hirose K, Longo DL, Oppenheim JJ, Matsushima K: Over expression of mitochondrial manganese superoxide dismutase promotes the survival of tumor cells exposed to interleukin 1, tumor necrosis factor, selected anti cancer drugs and ionizing radiation. FASEB J 7:361, 1993.
782. Zimmerman RJ, Chan A, Leadon SA: Oxidative damage in murine tumor cells treated in vitro by recombinant human tumor necrosis factor. Cancer Res 49:1644, 1989.
783. McClain CJ, Hill D, Schmidt J, Diehl AM: Cytokines and alcoholic liver disease. Semin Liver Dis 13:170, 1993.
784. McClain CJ, Cohen DA: Increased tumor necrosis factor production by monocytes in alcoholic hepatitis. Hepatology 9:349, 1989.
785. Nanji AA, Zhao S, Sadrzadeh SMH, Waxman DJ: Use of reverse transcription-polymerase chain reaction to evaluate in-vivo cytokine gene expression in rats fed ethanol for long periods. Hepatology 19:1483, 1994.
786. French SW: Role of mitochondrial damage in alcoholic liver disease. In Majchrowicz E, Noble EP, eds: Biochemistry and Pharmacology of Ethanol, vol 1. New York, Plenum, 1979: 409.
787. David RM, Nerland DE: Induction of mouse liver glutathione-S-transferase by ethanol. Biochem Pharmacol 32:2809, 1983.
788. Aykac C, Uysal M, Yalcin AS, et al: The effect of chronic ethanol ingestion on hepatic lipid peroxide, glutathione, glutathione peroxidase and glutathione transferase in rats. Toxicology 36:71, 1985.
789. Boyer TD: The glutathione-S-transferases: an update. Hepatology 9:486, 1989.
790. Hippel H, Pentilla KE, Lindros KO: Regioselective induction of liver glutathione transferase by ethanol and acetone. Pharmacol Toxicol 68:391, 1991.
791. Meister A, Anderson M: Glutathione. Ann Rev Biochem 52:711, 1983.
792. Fernandez-Checa JC, Lu S, Ookhtens M, et al: Regulation of hepatic GSH. In Tavaloni N, Berk P, eds: Hepatic Anion Transport and Bile Secretion: Physiology and Pathophysiology. New York, Raven Press, 1993:345.
793. Kaplowitz N, Aw TY, Ookhtens M: The regulation of hepatic glutathione. Ann Rev Pharmacol Toxicol 25:715, 1985.
794. Griffith OW, Meister A: Origin and turnover of mitochondrial glutathione. Proc Natl Acad Sci U S A 82:4668, 1985.
795. Martensson J, Lai CK, Meister A: High affinity transport of GSH is part of a multicomponent system essential for mitochondrial function. Proc Natl Acad Sci U S A 87:7185, 1990.
796. Kurosawa K, Hayashi N, Sato N, et al: Transport of GSH across mitochondrial membranes. Biochem Biophys Res Commun 167:367, 1991.
797. Lu SC: Regulation of hepatic glutathione synthesis. Semin Liver Dis. 18:331-343, 1998.
798. Videla LA, Valenzuela A: Alcohol ingestion, liver glutathione and lipoperoxidation: metabolic interrelationships and pathologic implications. Life Sci 31:2395, 1982.
799. Lauterburg BH, Davies S, Mitchell JR: Ethanol suppresses hepatic glutathione synthesis in rats in vivo. J Pharmacol Exp Ther 230:7, 1984.
800. Speisky H, MacDonald A, Giles G, et al: Increased loss and decreased synthesis of hepatic glutathione after acute ethanol administration. Biochem J 225:565, 1985.
801. De Pina MZ, Rocha-Hernandez AE, Balmori YS, et al: Restoration by piroxicam of liver glutathione levels decreased by acute ethanol intoxication. Life Sci 54:1433, 1994.
802. Callans DJ, Wacker LS, Mitchell MC: Effects of ethanol feeding and withdrawal on plasma glutathione elimination in the rat. Hepatology 7:496, 1987.
803. Fernandez-Checa JC, Ookhtens M, Kaplowitz N: Effect of chronic ethanol feeding on rat hepatocytic glutathione. Compartmentation, efflux and response to incubation with ethanol. J Clin Invest 80:57, 1987.
804. Yang CM, Carlson GP: Effects of ethanol on glutathione conjugation in rat liver and lung. Biochem Pharmacol 41:923, 1991.
805. Fernandez-Checa JC, Ookhtens M, Kaplowitz N: Effects of chronic ethanol feeding on rat hepatocytic glutathione: relationship to cytosolic glutathione to efflux and mitochondrial sequestration. J Clin Invest 83:1247, 1989.
806. Mitchell MC, Raiford DS, Mallat A: Effects of ethanol on glutathione metabolism. In: Watson RR, ed: Drug and Alcohol Abuse Reviews, vol 2. Totowa, NJ, Humana Press, 1991:169.
807. Lu SC, Huang ZZ, Yang JM, Tsukamoto H: Effect of ethanol and high-fat feeding on hepatic γ-glutamylcysteine synthetase subunit expression in the rat. Hepatology 30:209-214, 1999.
808. LaBaume LB, Merill DK, Clary GL: Effect of acute ethanol on serine biosynthesis in liver. Biochim Biophys Acta 256:569, 1987.
809. Fernandez-Checa JC, Garcia Ruiz MC, Ookhtens M, Kaplowitz N: Impaired uptake of glutathione by hepatic mitochondria from chronic ethanol-fed rats. J Clin Invest 87:397, 1991.
810. Hirano T, Kaplowitz N, Tsukamoto H, et al: Hepatic mitochondrial glutathione depletion and progression of experimental alcoholic liver disease in the rat. Hepatology 16:1423, 1992.
811. Garcia-Ruiz C, Morales A, Ballesta A, et al: Effect of chronic ethanol feeding on glutathione and functional integrity of mitochondria in periportal and perivenous hepatocytes. J Clin Invest 94:193, 1994.
812. Yang HD, Gattone VH, Martin LF, et al: The effect of glutathione content on renal function following warm ischemia. J Surg Res 46:633, 1989.
813. Mato JM, Alvarez L, Ortiz P, Pajares MA: S-adenosylmethionine synthesis: molecular mechanisms and clinical implications. Pharmacol Ther 73:265-280, 1997.
814. Katb M, Mudd SH. Mato JM, et al: Consensus nomenclature for the mammalian methionine adenosyltransferase genes and gene products. Trends Genet 13:51-52, 1997.
815. Lu SC, Huang ZZ, Yang H, et al: Changes in methionine adenosyltransferase and S-adenosylmethionine homeostasis in alcoholic rat liver. Am J Physiol Gastrointest Liver Physiol 279:G178-185, 2000.
816. Hirata J, Axelrod J: Phospholipid methylation and biological signal transduction. Science 209:1082, 1980.
817. Fonkelstein JD, Cello JP, Kyle WE: Ethanol-induced changes in methionine metabolism in rat liver. Biochem Biophys Res Commun 61:525, 1974.
818. Barak AJ, Beckenhauer HC, Tuma DJ, Badaksh S: Effects of prolonged ethanol feeding on methionine metabolism in rat liver. Biochem Cell Biol 65:230, 1987.
819. Lieber CS, Casini A, DeCarli LM, et al: S-adenosyl-L-methionine attenuates alcohol-induced liver injury in the baboon. Hepatology 11:165, 1990.

820. Duce AM, Ortiz P, Cabrero C, Mato JM: S-adenosyl-L-methionine synthetase and phospholipid methyltransferase are inhibited in human cirrhosis. Hepatology 8:65, 1988.
821. Vendemiale G, Altomare E, Trizio T, et al: Effects of oral S-adenosyl-L-methionine on hepatic glutathione in patients with liver disease. Scand J Gastroenterol 24:407, 1989.
822. Chawla R, Hill D, Watson B, et al: S-adenosylmethionine (Adomet) deficiency predisposes to TNF hepatotoxicity. Gastroenterology 108:1047A, 1995 (sbstract).
823. Barak AJ, Beckenhauer HC, Tuma DJ, Donohue TM: Adaptive increase in betaine-homocysteine methyltransferase activity maintains hepatic S-adenosylmethionine levels in ethanol-treated rats. IRCS Med Sci Biochem 12:866, 1984.
824. Barak AJ, Beckenhauer HC, Tuma DJ: S-adenosylmethionine generation and prevention of alcoholic fatty liver by betaine. Alcohol 11:501, 1994.
825. Garcia-Ruiz C, Morales A, Collell A, et al: Feeding S-adenosyl-L-methionine attenuates both ethanol-induced depletion of mitochondrial glutathione and mitochondrial dysfunction in periportal and perivenous hepatocytes. Hepatology 21:207, 1995.
826. Lundvall O, Weinfeld A, Lundin P: Iron stores in alcohol abusers. Acta Med Scand 185:259, 1969.
827. Powell LW: Normal human iron storage and its relation to ethanol consumption. Aust Ann Med 15:110, 1966.
828. Jacobovits A, Morgan MY, Sherlock S: Hepatic siderosis in alcoholics. Dig Dis Sci 24:305, 1979.
829. Stibler H, Borg S: Evidence of a reduced sialic acid content in serum transferrin in male alcoholics. Alcohol Clin Exp Res 5:545, 1981.
830. Vesterberg O, Petren S, Schmidt D: Increased concentrations of a transferrin variant after alcohol abuse. Clin Chim Acta 141:33, 1984.
831. Storey EL, Powell LW, Halliday JW: Use of chromatofocusing to detect a transferrin variant in serum of alcoholic subjects. Clin Chem 31:1543, 1985.
832. Rogoeczki E, Chindemi PA, Debanne MT: Transferrin glycans: a possible link between alcoholism and alcoholic siderosis. Alcohol Clin Exp Res 8:287, 1984.
833. Beguin Y, Bergamaschi G, Huebers H, Finch CA: The behavior of asialotransferrin-iron in the rat. Am J Hematol 29:204, 1988.
834. Beloqui O, Nunes RM, Blades B, et al: Depression of iron uptake from transferrin by isolated hepatocytes in the presence of ethanol is a pH-dependent consequence of ethanol metabolism. Alcohol Clin Exp Res 10:463, 1986.
835. Nunes RM, Beloqui O, Potter BJ, Berk PD: Iron uptake from transferrin by isolated hepatocytes: effect of ethanol. Biochem Biophys Res Commun 125:824, 1984.
836. Potter BJ, McHugh TA, Beloqui O: Iron uptake from transferrin and asialotransferrin by hepatocytes from chronically alcohol-fed rats. Alcohol Clin Exp Res 16:810, 1992.
837. Batey RG, Johnston R: Effect of alcohol, carbon tetrachloride, and choline deficiency on iron metabolism in the rat. Alcohol Clin Exp Res 17:931, 1993.
838. Rouach H, Houze P, Gentil M, et al: Effects of acute ethanol administration on the uptake of ^{59}Fe-labeled transferrin by rat liver and cerebellum. Biochem Pharmacol 47:1835, 1994.
839. Niemela O, Parkilla S, Britton RS, et al: Hepatic lipid peroxidation in hereditary hemochromatosis and alcoholic liver injury. J Lab Clin Med 133:451-460, 1999.
840. Badr MZ: Controversial role of intracellular iron in the mechanisms of chemically-induced hepatotoxicity. J Biochem Toxicol 9:25, 1994.
841. Bacon B, Tavill A: Role of the liver in normal iron metabolism. Semin Liver Dis 4:181, 1984.
842. Nordmann R, Ribiere C, Rouach H: Involvement of iron and iron-catalyzed free radical production in ethanol metabolism and toxicity. Enzyme 37:57, 1987.
843. Rouach H, Houze P, Orfanelli MT, et al: Effect of acute ethanol administration on the subcellular distribution of iron in rat liver and cerebellum. Biochem Pharmacol 39:1095, 1990.
844. Shaw S, Jayatilleke E, Lieber CS: Lipid peroxidation as a mechanism of alcoholic liver injury: role of iron mobilization and microsomal induction. Alcohol 5:135, 1988.
845. Valenzuela A, Fernandez V, Videla LA: Hepatic and biliary levels of glutathione and lipid peroxides following iron-overload in the rat: effects of simultaneous ethanol administration. Toxicol Appl Pharmacol 70:87, 1983.
846. Sanchez J, Casas M, Rama R: Effect of chronic ethanol administration on iron metabolism in the rat. Eur J Hematol 41:321, 1988.
847. Fairweather-Tait SJ, Southon S, Piper Z: The effect of alcoholic beverages on iron and zinc metabolism in the rat. Br J Nutr 60:209, 1988.
848. Sadrzadeh SMH, Nanji AA, Price PL: The oral iron-chelator, 1,2-dimethyl-3-hydroxypyrid-4-one reduces hepatic-free iron, lipid peroxidation and fat accumulation in chronically ethanol-fed rats. J Pharmacol Exp Ther 269:632, 1994.
849. Kirschner RE, Fantini GA: Role of iron and oxygen-derived free radicals in ischemia-reperfusion injury. J Am Coll Surg 179:103, 1994.
850. Robinson E, Hedlund B: Role of iron in ischemia and reperfusion. Circ Shock 27:367, 1989.
851. French SW: The mechanisms of organ injury in alcoholics: implications for therapy. Alcohol Alcohol 1(suppl):57, 1991.
852. Shaw S: Lipid peroxidation, iron mobilization and radical generation induced by alcohol. Free Radic Biol Med 7:541, 1989.
853. Biemond P, van Eijk HG, Swaak AJG, Koster FJ: Iron mobilization from ferritin by superoxide derived from stimulated polymorphonuclear leukocytes: possible mechanism in inflammation. J Clin Invest 73:1576, 1984.
854. Bolann BJ, Ulvik R: Release of iron from ferritin by xanthine oxidase: role of the superoxide radical. Biochem J 243:55, 1987.
855. Voogd A, Sluiter W, Van Eijk HG, Koster JF: Low molecular weight iron and the oxygen paradox in isolated rat hearts. J Clin Invest 90:2050, 1992.
856. Boyer RF, McCleary CJ: Superoxide ion as a primary reductant in ascorbate-mediated ferritin iron release. Free Radic Biol Med 3:389, 1987.
857. Bolånn BJ, Ulvik RJ: On the limited ability of superoxide to release iron from ferritin. Eur J Biochem 193:899, 1990.
858. Rerf DW: Ferritin as a source of iron for oxidative damage. Free Radic Biol Med 12:417, 1992.
859. Sadrzadeh SMH, Hallaway PE, Nanji AA: Macromolecular deferoxamine fails to protect against ethanol-induced hepatic injury. Hepatology 20:358A, 1994.
860. Davies MJ, Donkor R, Dunster CA, et al: Desferrioxamine (Desferal) and superoxide free radicals: formation of an enzyme-damaging nitroxide. Biochem J 246:7, 1987.
861. Morehouse KM, Flitter WD, Mason RP: The enzymatic oxidation of Desferal to a nitroxide free radical. FEBS Lett 222:246, 1987.
862. Braughler JM, Chase RL, Pregenzer JF: Stimulation and inhibition of iron-dependent lipid peroxidation by desferrioxamine. Biochem Biophys Res Commun 153:933, 1988.
863. Hultcrantz R, Bissell DM, Roll FJ: Iron mediates production of a neutrophil chemoattractant by rat hepatocytes metabolizing ethanol. J Clin Invest 87:45, 1991.
864. Neuschwander-Terri BA, Roll FJ: Chemotactic activity for human PMN generated during ethanol metabolism by rat hepatocytes: role of glutathione and glutathione peroxidase. Biochem Biophys Res Commun 167:1170, 1990.
865. Burton GW, Ingold KU: Vitamin E as an in vitro and in vivo antioxidant. Ann N Y Acad Sci 570:7, 1989.
866. Meydani M: Vitamin E. Lancet 345:170, 1995.
867. Kawase T, Kato S, Lieber CS: Lipid peroxidation and anti-oxidant defense systems in rat liver after chronic ethanol feeding. Hepatology 10:815, 1989.
868. Bjornboe GEA, Johnsen J, Bjornboe A, et al: Some aspects of antioxidant status in blood from alcoholics. Alcoholism 12:806, 1988.
869. Meydani M, Seitz H, Blumberg JB, Russell RM: Effect of chronic ethanol feeding on hepatic and extrahepatic distribution of vitamin E in rats. Alcohol Clin Exp Res 15:771, 1991.
870. Sadrzadeh SMH, Nanji AA, Price PL, Meydani M: Effect of chronic ethanol feeding on plasma and liver alpha and gamma tocopherol levels in normal and vitamin E deficient rats: relationship to lipid peroxidation. Biochem Pharmacol 47:2005, 1994.
871. Odeleye O, Eskelson CD, Mufti SI, Watson RR: Vitamin E attenuation of effects of chronic ethanol and cod liver oil consumption on rat liver lipid composition. Nutr Res 13:1253, 1993.

872. Sadrzadeh SMH, Meydani M, Nanji AA: High-dose vitamin E supplementation has no effect on ethanol-induced pathological liver injury. J Pharmacol Exp Ther 273:455, 1995.
873. Liebler DC: The role of metabolism on the antioxidant function of vitamin E. CRC Crit Rev Toxicol 23:147, 1993.
874. Lamb RG, Koch JC, Snyder JW, et al: An in-vitro model of ethanol-dependent liver cell injury. Hepatology 19:174, 1994.
875. Fariss MW: Oxygen toxicity: unique cytoprotective properties of vitamin E succinate in hepatocytes. Free Radic Biol Med 9:333, 1990.
876. Yao T, Esposti SD, Huang L, et al: Inhibition of carbon-tetrachloride-induced liver injury by liposomes containing vitamin E. Am J Physiol 267:G476, 1994.
877. Morland JA, Bessesen A, Svendsen L: Incorporation of labelled amino acids into proteins of isolated parenchymal and non-parenchymal rat liver cells in the absence and presence of ethanol. Biochim Biophys Acta 561:404, 1979.
878. Rothschild MA, Oratz M, Chrieber SS: Alcohol, amino acids, and albumin synthesis. Gastroenterology 67:1200, 1974.
879. Jejeebhoy KN, Phillips MJ, Bruce-Robertson A, et al: The acute effect of ethanol on albumin, fibrinogen and transferrin synthesis in the rat. Biochem J 126:1111, 1972.
880. Shelmet JJ, Reichcod GA, Skutches CL, et al: Ethanol causes acute inhibition of carbohydrate, fat, and protein oxidation and insulin resistance. J Clin Invest 81:1137, 1988.
881. McDonald JT, Margen S: Wine versus ethanol in human nutrition. I. Nitrogen and calorie balance. Am J Clin Nutr 29:1093, 1986.
882. Burnout D, Petermann M, Ugarte G, et al: Nitrogen economy in alcoholic patients without liver disease. Metab Clin Exp 36:651, 1987.
883. Reinus JF, Heymsfield SB, Wiskind R, et al: Ethanol: relative fuel value and metabolic effects in vivo. Metab Clin Exp Res 38:125, 1989.
884. Mitchell MC, Herlong HF: Alcohol and nutrition: caloric value, bioenergetics and relationship to liver damage. Ann Rev Nutr 6:457, 1986.
885. DeFio P, Volpi E, Lucidi P, et al: Ethanol impairs post-prandial hepatic protein metabolism. J Clin Invest 95:1472, 1995.
886. Casey CA, Kragskow SL, Sorrell MF, Tuma DJ: Chronic ethanol administration alters the binding and endocytosis of asialoorosomucoid in isolated hepatocytes. J Biol Chem 262:2704, 1987.
887. Tuma DJ, Maillard ME, Casey CA, et al: Ethanol-induced alterations in plasma membrane assembly in the liver. Biochim Biophys Acta 856:571, 1986.
888. Casey CA, Kragskow SL, Sorrell MF, Tuma DJ: Ethanol-induced impairments of receptor-mediated endocytosis of asialoorosomucoid in isolated rat hepatocytes: time course of impairments and recovery after ethanol administration. Alcohol Clin Exp Res 13:258, 1989.
889. Ashwell G, Harford J: Carbohydrate-specific receptors of the liver. Ann Rev Biochem 51:531, 1982.
890. Wall DA, Wilson G, Hubbard AL: The galactose-specific recognition system of mammalian liver: the route of ligand internalization in rat hepatocytes. Cell 21:79, 1980.
891. Tolleshaug H: Binding and internalization of asialoglycoproteins by isolated rat hepatocytes. Int J Biochem 13:45, 1981.
892. Casey CA, Kragskow SL, Sorrell MF, Tuma DJ: Zonal differences in ethanol-induced impairment in receptor mediated endocytosis of asialoglycoproteins in isolated rat hepatocytes. Hepatology 13:260, 1991.
893. Xu DS, Sorrell MF, Casey CA, Tuma DJ: Impaired attachment of hepatocytes to extracellular matrix components following chronic ethanol administration. Lab Invest 67:186, 1992.
894. Xu D, Sorrell MF, Casey CA, et al: Long-term ethanol feeding selectively impairs the attachment of rat perivenous hepatocytes to extracellular matrix substrates. Gastroenterology 106:473, 1994.
895. Baraona E, Leo MA, Borowsky SA, Lieber CS: Alcoholic hepatomegaly: accumulation of protein in the liver. Science 190:794, 1975.
896. Baraona E, Leo MA, Borowsky SA, Lieber CS: Pathogenesis of alcohol-induced accumulation of protein in the liver. J Clin Invest 60:546, 1977.
897. Donohue TM, McVicker DL, Kharbanda KK, et al: Alcohol Clin Exp Res 18:536, 1994.
898. Kharbanda KK, McVicker DL, Zetterman RK, Donohue TM: Effect of ethanol consumption on the proteolytic capacity and hydrolase activation of hepatic lysosomes. Hepatology 20:313A, 1994.
899. Baumeister W, Walz J, Zuhl F, Seemuller E: The proteasome: paradigm of a self-compartmentalizing protease. Cell 92:367-380, 1998.
900. Coux O, Tanaka K, Goldberg AL: Structure and functions of the 20S and 26S proteasomes. Annu Rev Biochem 65:801-847, 1996.
901. Mayer RJ, Arnold J, Lajos L, et al: Ubiquitin in health and disease. Biochim Biophys Acta 1089:141-157, 1991.
902. Donohue TM, Zetterman RR, Gouillon ZQ, French SW: Peptidase activities of the multicatalytic protease in rat liver after voluntary and intragastric ethanol administration. Hepatology 28:486-491, 1998.
903. Fataccioli V, Andraud E, Gentil M, et al: Effects of chronic ethanol administration on rat liver proteasome activities: relationship with oxidative stress. Hepatology 29:14-20, 1999.
904. Iseri OH, Lieber CS, Gottlieb LS: The ultrastructure of fatty liver induced by prolonged ethanol ingestion. Am J Pathol 48:535, 1966.
905. Rubin E, Hutterer F, Lieber CS: Ethanol increases hepatic smooth endoplasmic reticulum and drug metabolizing enzyme. Science 159:1469, 1968.
906. Joly J-G, Ishii H, Teschke R: Effect of chronic ethanol feeding on the activities and submicrosomal distribution of reduced nicotinamide adenine dinucleotide phosphate-cytochrome P-450 reductase and the demethylases for aminopyrine and ethylmorphine. Biochem Pharmacol 22:1532, 1983.
907. Koop DR, Nordblom GD, Coon MJ: Immunochemical evidence for a role of cytochrome P-450 in liver microsomal ethanol oxidation. Arch Biochem Biophys 235:228, 1984.
908. Koop DR, Crump BL, Nordblom GD, et al: Immunochemical evidence for induction of alcohol-oxidizing cytochrome P-450 of rabbit liver microsomes by diverse agents: ethanol, imidazole, trichloroethylene, acetone, pyrazole, and isoniazid. Proc Natl Acad Sci U S A 82:4065, 1985.
909. Park SS, Ko IY, Patten C, et al: Monoclonal antibodies to ethanol-induced cytochrome P-450 that inhibit aniline and nitrosamine metabolism. Biochem Pharmacol 35:2855, 1986.
910. Fujii H, Ohmachi T, Sagami I, et al: Liver microsomal drug metabolism in ethanol-treated hamsters. Biochem Pharmacol 34:3881, 1985.
911. Wrighton SA, Thomas PE, Mulowa DT, et al: Characterization of ethanol-inducible human liver N-nitrosodimethylamine demethylase. Biochemistry 25:6731, 1986.
912. Ueng T-H, Friedman FK, Miller H, et al: Studies on ethanol-inducible cytochrome P-450 in rabbit liver, lungs and kidneys. Biochem Pharmacol 36:2689, 1987.
913. Rush GF, Adler VL, Hook JB: The effect of ethanol administration on renal and hepatic mixed-function oxidases in the Fischer 344 rat. Toxicol Lett 12:265, 1982.
914. McCoy GD, Wynder EL: Etiological and preventative implications in alcohol carcinogenesis. Cancer Res 39:2844, 1979.
915. Pollack ES, Nomura ANY, Heilbrun LK, et al: Prospective study of alcohol consumption and cancer. N Engl J Med 310:617, 1984.
916. Porta EA, Markell N, Dorado RD: Chronic alcoholism enhances hepatocarcinogenicity of dimethylnitrosamine in rats fed a marginally methyl-deficient diet. Hepatology 5:1120, 1985.
917. Sohn OS, Fiala ES, Puz C, et al: Enhancement of rat liver microsomal metabolism of azoxymethane to methylazoxymethanol by chronic ethanol administration: similarity to the microsomal metabolism of N-nitrosodimethylamine. Cancer Res 47:3123, 1987.
918. Zimmermann HJ: Effects of alcohol on other hepatotoxins. Alcohol Clin Exp Res 10:3, 1986.
919. Finley BL, Ashley PJ, Neptune AG, et al: Substrate-selective induction of rabbit hepatic UDP-glucuronosyltransferases by ethanol and other xenobiotics. Biochem Pharmacol 35:2875, 1986.
920. Bodd E, Gadebolt G, Christensson PI, et al: Mechanisms behind the inhibitory effect of ethanol on the conjugation of morphine in rat hepatocytes. J Pharmacol Exp Ther 239:887, 1986.
921. Sieg A, Seitz HK: Increased production, hepatic conjugation, and biliary secretion of bilirubin in the rat after chronic ethanol consumption. Gastroenterology 93:261, 1987.

922. Sweeny DJ, Reinke LA: Effect of ethanol feeding on hepatic microsomal UDP-glucuronyltransferase activity. Biochem Pharmacol 36:1381, 1987.
923. Moldeus P, Anderson B, Norling AI: Interaction of ethanol oxidation with glucuronidation in isolated hepatocytes. Biochem Pharmacol 27:2583, 1978.
924. Reinke LA, Moyer MJ, Notley KA: Diminished rates of glucuronidation and sulfation in perfused rat liver after chronic ethanol administration. Biochem Pharmacol 35:439, 1986.
925. Fernandez-Checa JC, Ookhtens M, Klapowitz N: Effect of chronic ethanol feeding on rat hepatocytic glutathione. Compartmentation, efflux, and response to incubation with ethanol. J Clin Invest 80:57, 1987.
926. Price VF, Miller MG, Jollow DJ: Mechanisms of fasting-induced potentiation of acetaminophen hepatotoxicity in the rat. Biochem Pharmacol 36:427, 1987.
927. Olsen H, Morland J: Ethanol-induced increase in drug acetylation in man and isolated rat liver cells. BMJ 2:1260, 1978.
928. Olsen H: Interaction between drug acetylation and ethanol, acetate, pyruvate, citrate, and L-carnitine in isolated rat liver parenchymal cell. Acta Pharmacol Toxicol 50:67, 1982.
929. Strubelt U: Interactions between ethanol and other hepatotoxic agents. Biochem Pharmacol 29:1445, 1980.
930. Moldeus P, Andersson B, Norling A, et al: Effect of chronic ethanol administration on drug metabolism in isolated hepatocytes with emphasis on paracetamol activation. Biochem Pharmacol 29:1741, 1980.
931. Sato C, Matsuda Y, Lieber CS: Increased hepatotoxicity of acetaminophen after chronic ethanol consumption in the rat. Gastroenterology 80:140, 1981.
932. Licht H, Seeff LB, Zimmermann HJ: Apparent potentiation of acetaminophen hepatotoxicity by alcohol. Ann Intern Med 92:511, 1980.
933. Leist MH, Gluskin LE, Payne JA: Enhanced toxicity of acetaminophen in alcoholics: report of three cases. J Clin Gastroenterol 7:55, 1985.
934. Seeff LB, Cuccherini BA, Zimmermann HJ, et al: Acetaminophen hepatotoxicity in alcoholics. Ann Intern Med 104:399, 1986.
935. Altomare E, Leo MA, Sato C, et al: Interaction of ethanol with acetaminophen metabolism in the baboon. Biochem Pharmacol 33:2207, 1984.
936. Dingle JT, Lucy JA: Vitamin A carotenoids and cell function. Biol Rev Cambridge Philosophic Soc 40:422, 1965.
937. Lucy JA: Some possible roles for vitamin A in membranes: micelle formation and electron transfer. Am J Clin Nutr 22:1033, 1969.
938. Roels OA, Anderson OR, Lui NST, et al: Vitamin A and membranes. Am J Clin Nutr 22:1020, 1969.
939. Thompson JN, Pitt GAJ: Vitamin A acid and hypervitaminosis A. Nature 188:672, 1960.
940. Nettesheim P, Williams MI: The influence of vitamin A on the susceptibility of the rat lung to 3-methylcholanthrene. Int J Cancer 17:351, 1976.
941. Josephs HW: Hypervitaminosis A. Am J Dis Child 67:33, 1944.
942. Stimson WH: Vitamin A intoxication in adults: report of case with a summary of the literature. N Engl J Med 265:369, 1961.
943. Soler-Bicheva J, Joscia JL: Chronic hypervitaminosis A: report of a case in an adult. Arch Intern Med 112:462, 1963.
944. Lane BP: Hepatic microanatomy in hypervitaminosis A in man and rat. Am J Pathol 53:591, 1968.
945. Rubin E, Floorman AF, Degnan T, et al: Hepatic injury in chronic hypervitaminosis A. Am J Dis Child 119:132, 1970.
946. Muenter MD, Perry HO, Ludwig J: Chronic vitamin A intoxication in adults. Hepatic, neurologic and dermatologic complications. Am J Med 50:129, 1971.
947. Leo MA, Lieber CS: Hypervitaminosis A. Hepatology 8:412-417, 1988.
948. Russell RM, Boyer JL, Baghesi SA, et al: Hepatic injury from chronic hypervitaminosis A resulting in portal hypertension and ascites. N Engl J Med 291:435, 1974.
949. Popper H, Steigman F, Meyer KA, et al: Relation between hepatic and plasma concentrations of vitamin A in human beings. Arch Intern Med 72:439, 1943.
950. Sato M, Lieber CS: Hepatic vitamin A depletion after chronic ethanol consumption in baboons and rats. J Nutr 111:2015, 1981.
951. Leo MA, Lieber CS: Interaction of ethanol with vitamin A. Alcohol Clin Exp Res 7:15, 1983.
952. Leo MA, Lieber CS: Hepatic vitamin A depletion in alcoholic liver injury. N Engl J Med 307:597, 1982.
953. Rasmussen M, Blomhoff R, Helgerud P, et al: Retinol and retinyl esters in parenchymal and non-parenchymal rat liver cell fractions after long-term administration of ethanol. J Lipid Res 26:1112, 1985.
954. Bell H, Nilsson A, Norum KR, et al: Retinol and retinyl esters in patients with alcoholic liver disease. J Hepatol 8:26, 1989.
955. Mobarhan S, Leydan TJ, Friedman H, et al: Depletion of liver and esophageal epithelium vitamin A after chronic moderate ethanol consumption in rats: inverse relation to zinc nutriture. Hepatology 6:615, 1986.
956. Leo MA, Lieber CS: New pathway for retinol metabolism in liver microsomes. J Biol Chem 260:5228, 1985.
957. Leo MA, Iida S, Lieber CS: Retinoic acid metabolism by a system reconstituted with cytochrome P450. Arch Biochem Biophys 234:305, 1984.
958. Leo MA, Lasker JM, Raucy JL, et al: Metabolism of retinol and retinoic acid by human liver cytochrome P450 IIC8. Arch Biochem Biophys 269:305, 1989.
959. Martini R, Murray M: Participation of P450 3A enzymes in rat hepatic microsomal retinoic acid 4-hydroxylation. Arch Biochem Biophys 303:57, 1993.
960. Fiorella PD, Napoli JL: Microsomal retinoic acid metabolism. J Biol Chem 269:10538, 1994.
961. Liu C, Russell RM, Seitz HK, Wang XD: Ethanol enhances retinoic acid metabolism into polar metabolites in rat liver via induction of cytochrome P450 2E1. Gastroenterology 120:179-189, 2001.
962. Leo MA, Rosman AS, Lieber CS: Differential depletion of carotenoids and tocopherol in liver disease. Hepatology 17:977, 1993.
963. Schmitz HH, Poor CL, Wellman RB, Erdman JW: Concentrations of selected carotenoids and vitamin A in human liver, kidney and lung tissue. J Nutr 121:1613, 1991.
964. Leo MA, Kim CI, Lowe N, Lieber CS: Interaction of ethanol with β-carotene: delayed blood clearance and enhanced hepatotoxicity. Hepatology 15:883, 1992.
965. Ramadori G: The stellate cell (Ito-cell, fat-storing cell, lipocyte, perisinusoidal cell) of the liver. Virchows Arch B Cell Pathol 61:147, 1991.
966. Gressner AM: Perisinusoidal lipocytes and fibrogenesis. Gut 35:1331, 1994.
967. Yamane M, Tanaka Y, Marumo F, Sato C: Role of hepatic vitamin A and lipocyte distribution in experimental hepatic fibrosis. Liver 13:282, 1993.
968. Pallet V, Coustaut M, Naulet F, et al: Chronic ethanol administration enhances retinoic acid and triiodothyronine receptor expression in mouse liver. FEBS Lett 331:119, 1993.
969. Nanji AA, Yacoub LK, Tahan SR, et al: Relationship between severity of liver injury and retinoic acid receptor gene expression in experimental alcoholic liver disease. Alcohol Clin Exp Res 18:24A, 1994.
970. Lafyatis R, Kim SJ, Angel P, et al: Interleukin 1 stimulates and all-transretinoic acid inhibits collagenase gene expression through its 5′ activator protein-1 binding site. Mol Endocrinol 4:973, 1990.
971. Nicholson RC, Mader S, Nagpal S, et al: Negative regulation of the rat stromelysin gene promoter by retinoic acid is mediated by an AP-1 binding site. EMBO J 9:4443, 1990.
972. Leo MA, Lieber CS: Hepatic fibrosis after long-term administration of ethanol and moderate vitamin A supplementation in the rat. Hepatology 3:1, 1983.
973. Na SY, Kang BY, Chung SW, et al: Retinoids inhibit interleukin-12 production in macrophages through physical associations of retinoid X receptor and NF-kappa B. J Biol Chem 274:7674-7680, 1999.
974. Cantorna MT, Nashold FE, Chun, TY, et al: Vitamin A down-regulation of IFN-gamma synthesis in cloned mouse Th1 lymphocytes depends on the CD28 co-stimulatory pathway. J Immunol 156:2674-2679, 1996.
975. Motomura K, Ohata M, Satre M, Tsukamoto H: Destabilization of TNF-α mRNA by retinoic acid in hepatic macrophages: its implication in alcoholic liver disease. Am J Physiol Endocrinol Metab 281:E420, 2001.
976. Walt RP, Kemp CM, Lyness L, et al: Vitamin A treatment for night blindness in primary biliary cirrhosis. BMJ 288:1030, 1984.

977. Lane BP: Hepatic microanatomy in hypervitaminosis A in man and rat. Am J Pathol 53:591, 1968.
978. Muenter MD, Perry Ho, Ludwig J: Chronic vitamin A intoxication in adults. Hepatic, neurologic and dermatologic complications. Am J Med 50:129, 1971.
979. Bosma A, Seifert WF, Wilson JHP, et al: Chronic administration of ethanol with high vitamin A supplementation in a liquid diet to rats does not cause liver fibrosis. J Hepatol 13:240, 1991.
980. Snodderly DM, Russett MD, Land RI, Krinsky NI: Plasma carotenoids of monkeys (*Macacu fascicularis* and *Saimiri sciureus*) fed a non-purified diet. J Nutr 120:1663, 1990.
981. Leo MA, Aleynik SI, Aleynik MK, Lieber CS: β-Carotene beadlets potentiate hepatotoxicity of alcohol. Am J Clin Nutr 66:1461-1469, 1997.
982. Mezey E: Retinoids and alcoholic liver disease. Am J Clin Nutr 66:1301-1302, 1997.
983. Paronetto F: Immunologic reactions in alcoholic liver disease. Semin Liver Dis 13:183, 1993.
984. Paronetto F: Immunologic reactions in alcoholic liver disease. In Lieber CS, ed: Medical and Nutritional Complications of Alcoholism. New York, Plenum, 1992:283.
985. Zetterman R, Luisada-Opper A, Leevy C: Alcoholic hepatitis. Cell mediated immunologic response to alcoholic hyaline. Gastroenterology 70:382, 1976.
986. MacSween RNM, Anthony RS: Review: immune mechanisms in alcoholic liver disease. J Lab Clin Immunol 9:1, 1982.
987. Anonymous: Immunologic abnormalities in alcoholic liver disease. Lancet ii:605, 1983.
988. Niemela O, Juvonen T, Parkilla S: Immunohistochemical demonstration of acetaldehyde-modified epitopes in human liver after alcohol consumption. J Clin Invest 87:1367, 1991.
989. Terabayashi H, Kolber MA: The generation of cytotoxic T-lymphocytes against acetaldehyde-modified syngeneic cells. Alcohol Clin Exp Res 14:893, 1990.
990. Stoolman LM: Adhesion molecules controlling lymphocyte migration. Cell 56:907, 1989.
991. Burra P, Hubscher SG, Shaw J, et al: Is the intercellular adhesion molecule 1/leukocyte function associated antigen 1 pathway of leukocyte adhesion involved in tissue damage in alcoholic hepatitis? Gut 33:268, 1992.
992. Adams DH, Mainolfi E, Burra P, et al: Detection of circulating intercellular adhesion molecule-1 in chronic liver diseases. Hepatology 16:810, 1992.
993. French SW, Burbige EJ, Tarder G, et al: Lymphocyte sequestration by the liver in alcoholic hepatitis. Arch Pathol Lab Med 103:146, 1979.
994. Peters M, Liebman HA, Tong MJ, Tinberg HM: Alcoholic hepatitis: granulocyte chemotactic factor from Mallory body-stimulated human peripheral blood mononuclear cells. Clin Immunol Immunopathol 28:418, 1983.
995. Chedid A, Mendenhall CL, Moritz TE, et al: Cell-mediated hepatic injury in alcoholic liver disease. Gastroenterology 105:254, 1993.
996. Leevy CM, Leevy CB: Liver disease in the alcoholic. Gastroenterology 105:294, 1992.
997. Goldin RD, Cattle S, Boylston AW: IgA deposition in alcoholic liver disease. J Clin Pathol 39:1181, 1986.
998. Swerdlow MA, Chowdury LN: IgA subclasses in liver tissues in alcoholic liver disease. Am J Clin Pathol 80:283, 1983.
999. Deviere J, Vaerman JP, Content J, et al: IgA triggers tumor necrosis factor and secretion by monocytes: a study in normal subjects and patients with alcoholic cirrhosis. Hepatology 13:670, 1991.
1000. French SW, Okanue T, Swierenga SHH, Marceau N: The cytoskeleton of hepatocytes in health and disease. In Pathogenesis of Liver Disease, IAP Monograph No. 28. Baltimore, Williams & Wilkins, 1987:95.
1001. French SW: Cytoskeleton: intermediate filaments. In Arias IM, Boyer JL, Fausto N, et al, eds: The Liver: Biology and Pathobiology, ed 3. New York, Raven Press, 1994:33.
1002. Farguhar MG, Bergeron JJM, Palade GE: Cytochemistry of Golgi fractions prepared from rat liver. J Cell Biol 60:8, 1974.
1003. Stein O, Sanger L, Stein Y: Colchicine-induced inhibition of lipoprotein and protein secretion into the serum and lack of interference with secretion of biliary phospholipids and cholesterol by rat liver in vivo. J Cell Biol 62:90, 1974.
1004. Baraona E, Leo MA, Borowsky SA, Lieber CS: Pathogenesis of alcohol-induced accumulation of protein in the liver. J Clin Invest 60:546, 1977.
1005. Tuma DJ, Jennett RB, Sorrell MF: Effect of ethanol on the synthesis and secretion of hepatic secretory glycoproteins and albumin. Hepatology 1:590, 1981.
1006. French SW, Katsuma Y, Ray MB, Swierenga SHH: Cytoskeletal pathology induced by ethanol. Ann N Y Acad Sci 492:262, 1987.
1007. Matsuda Y, Baraona E, Salaspuro M, Lieber CS: Effects of ethanol on liver microtubules and Golgi apparatus. Possible role in altered hepatic secretion of plasma protein. Lab Invest 41:455, 1979.
1008. Okanoue T, Ongyoku O, Ohta M, et al: Effect of chronic ethanol treatment on cytoskeleton of rat hepatocytes. Acta Hepatol Japonica 25:210, 1984.
1009. Van Eyken P, Desmet VJ: Cytokeratins and the liver. Liver 13:113, 1993.
1010. Denk H, Lackinger E: Cytoskeleton in liver diseases. Semin Liver Dis 6:199, 1986.
1011. Kawahara H, Cadrin M, French SW: Ethanol-induced phosphorylation of cytokeratin in cultured hepatocytes. Life Sci 47:859, 1990.
1012. French SW, Nash J, Shitabata P, et al: Pathology of alcoholic liver disease. Semin Liver Dis 13:154, 1993.
1013. Worman HJ: Cellular intermediate filament networks and their derangement in alcoholic hepatitis. Alcohol Clin Exp Res 14:789, 1990.
1014. Jensen K, Gluud C: The Mallory body: morphological, clinical and experimental studies (part I of a literature survey). Hepatology 20:1061, 1994.
1015. Jensen K, Gluud C: The Mallory body: theories on development and pathologic significance (part 2 of a literature survey). Hepatology 20:1330, 1994.
1016. Zatloukal K, Fesus L, Denk H, et al: High amount of ϵ-(γ-glutamyl)-lysine cross-links in Mallory bodies. Lab Invest 66:774, 1992.
1017. Ohta M, Marceau N, Perry G, et al: Ubiquitin is present on cytokeratin intermediate filaments and Mallory bodies of hepatocytes. Lab Invest 59:848, 1988.
1018. Vyberg M, Leth P: Ubiquitin: an immunohistochemical marker of Mallory bodies and alcoholic liver disease. APMIS Suppl 23:46, 1991.
1019. Lowe J, Blanchard A, Morrell KA, et al: Ubiquitin is a common factor in intermediate filament inclusion bodies of diverse type in man including those of Parkinson's disease, Pick's disease, and Alzheimer's disease, as well as Rosenthal fibers in cerebellar astrocytomas, cytoplasmic bodies in muscle and Mallory bodies in alcoholic liver disease. J Pathol 155:9, 1988.
1020. Cadrin M, Marceau N, French SW: Cytokeratin of apparent high molecular weight in livers from griseofulvin-fed mice. J Hepatol 14:226, 1992.
1021. ZaHoukal K, Bock G, Rainer I, et al: High molecular weight components are main constituents of Mallory bodies isolated with a fluorescence activated cell sorter. Lab Invest 64:200, 1991.
1022. Kachi K, Cadrin M, French SW: Synthesis of Mallory body, intermediate filament and microfilament proteins in liver cell primary cultures. An electron microscopic autoradiography assay. Lab Invest 68:71, 1993.
1023. Cadrin M, McFarlane-Anderson N, Aasheim LH, et al: Modifications in cytokeratin and actin in cultured liver cells derived from griseofulvin-fed mice. Lab Invest 72:453, 1995.
1024. Yuan QX, Marceau N, French SW: Heat shock in vivo induces Mallory bodies in griseofulvin primed mouse liver. FASEB J 9:A425, 1995 (abstract).
1025. Nanji AA, Griniuviene B, Yacoub L, et al: Heat shock gene expression in alcoholic liver disease in the rat is related to severity of liver injury and lipid peroxidation. Proc Soc Exp Biol Med 210:12, 1995.
1026. Ray MB, Mendenhall CL, French SW, et al: Serum vitamin A deficiency and increased intrahepatic expression of cytokeratin antigen in alcoholic liver disease. Hepatology 8:1019, 1988.
1027. Savolainen VT, Laluk, Penttila A, et al: Cytokeratin inclusions in alcoholic liver disease and their relation to the amount of alcohol intake. Liver 14:281, 1994.
1028. Rojkind M, Dunn M: Hepatic fibrosis. Gastroenterology 76:849, 1979.

1029. Rojkind M, Kershenobick D: Effect of colchicine on collagen, albumin and transferrin synthesis by cirrhotic rat liver slices. Biochim Biophys Acta 378:415, 1975.
1030. Resnick R, Boitnolt J, Iber F, et al: Preliminary observations of *d*-penicillamine therapy in acute alcoholic liver disease. Digestion 11:257, 1974.
1031. Ruwart MJ, Rush BD, Snyder KF, et al: 16,16-dimethyl prostaglandin E_2 delays collagen formation in nutritional injury in the rat liver. Hepatology 8:61, 1988.
1032. Chojkier M, Brenner DA: Therapeutic strategies for hepatic fibrosis. Hepatology 8:176, 1988.
1033. McCuskey RS, McCuskey PA, Urbaschek R, Urbaschek B: Kupffer cell function in host defense. Rev Infect Dis 9:S619, 1987.
1034. Wardle EN: Kupffer cells and their function. Liver 7:63, 1987.
1035. Shiratori Y, Kawase T, Shiina S, et al: Modulation of hepatotoxicity by macrophages in the liver. Hepatology 8:815, 1988.
1036. Decker K: Biologically active products of stimulated liver macrophages (Kupffer cells). Eur J Biochem 192:245, 1990.
1037. Martinez F, Abril ER, Earnest DL, Watson RR: Ethanol and cytokine secretion. Alcohol 9:455, 1992.
1038. Yamada S, Mochida S, Ohno A, et al: Evidence for enhanced secretory function of hepatic macrophages after long term ethanol feeding in rats. Liver 11:220, 1991.
1039. Thiele DL: Tumor necrosis factor, the acute phase response and the pathogenesis of alcoholic liver disease. Hepatology 9:497, 1989.
1040. Cowper KB, Currin RT, Dawson TL, et al: A new method to monitor Kupffer cell function continuously in the perfused rat liver. Biochem J 266:141, 1990.
1041. D'Souza NB, Bagby GJ, Lang CH, et al: Ethanol alters the metabolic response of isolated, perfused rat liver to a phagocytic stimulus. Alcohol Clin Exp Res 17:147, 1993.
1042. Ohlakan A, Spolarics Z, Lang CH, Spitzer JJ: Adrenergic blockage attenuates endotoxin-induced hepatic glucose uptake. Circ Shock 39:74, 1993.
1043. Earnest DL, Sim W, Kirkpatrick DM, et al: Ethanol, acetaldehyde, and Kupffer cell function: potential role of Kupffer cells in alcohol-induced liver injury. In Seminara D, Watson RR, Pawlowski A, eds: Alcohol, Immunomodulation and AIDS; Progress in Clinical Biological Research, vol 325. New York, Alan R Liss, 1990:255.
1044. Basista MH, Gavaler J, Steiffenhofer A, et al: Effect of ethanol on Kupffer cell function. Alcohol Clin Exp Res 17:556, 1993.
1045. Hijioka T, Rosenberg RL, Lemasters JJ, Thurman RG: Kupffer cells contain voltage-dependent calcium channels. Mol Pharmacol 41:435, 1992.
1046. Hijioka T, Goto M, Lemasters JJ, Thurman RG: Effect of short-term ethanol treatment on voltage-dependent calcium channels in Kupffer cells. Hepatology 18:400, 1993.
1047. Goto M, Lemaster JJ, Thurman RG: Activation of voltage-dependent calcium channels in Kupffer cells by chronic treatment with alcohol in the rat. J Pharmacol Exp Ther 267:1264, 1993.
1048. Tuki T, Thurman RG: The swift increase in alcohol metabolism. Time course for increase in hepatic oxygen uptake and involvement of glycolysis. Biochem J 186:119, 1980.
1049. Thurman RG, Paschal DL, Wallace AT, et al: The swift increase in alcohol metabolism. Alcohol Clin Exp Res 6:316, 1982.
1050. Bradford BU, Misra UK, Thurman RG: Kupffer cells are required for the swift increase in alcohol metabolism. Res Commun Subst Abuse 14:1, 1993.
1051. Thurman RG, Bradford BU, Knecht KT, et al: Alcohol metabolism and its toxicity: role of Kupffer cells and free radicals. In Watson RR, ed: Drugs of Abuse and Immune Function. Boca Raton, FL, CRC Press, 1995:45.
1052. Adachi Y, Bradford BU, Gao W, et al: Inactivation of Kupffer cells prevents early alcohol-induced liver injury. Hepatology 20:453, 1994.
1053. Wiezorek JS, Brown DH, Kupperman DE, Brass CA: Rapid conversion to high xanthine oxidase activity in viable Kupffer cells during hypoxia. J Clin Invest 94:2224, 1994.
1054. Friedman SL: The cellular basis of fibrosis. N Engl J Med 328:1828, 1993.
1055. Maher JJ: Hepatic fibrosis caused by alcohol. Semin Liver Dis 10:66, 1990.
1056. French SW, Nash J, Shitabata P, et al: Pathology of alcoholic liver disease. Semin Liver Dis 13:154, 1993.
1057. Ray MB, Mendenhall CL, French SW, Gartside PS: Bile duct changes in alcoholic liver disease. Liver 13:36, 1993.
1058. Maher JJ, McGuire RF: Extracellular matrix gene expression increases preferentially in rat lipocytes and sinusoidal endothelial cells during hepatic fibrosis in vivo. J Clin Invest 86:1641, 1990.
1059. Milani S, Herbst H, Schuppan D, et al: Procollagen expression by non-parenchymal rat liver cells in experimental biliary cirrhosis. Gastroenterology 98:175, 1990.
1060. Nakatsukasa H, Nagy P, Evarts RP, et al: Cellular distribution of transforming growth factor $\beta 1$ and procollagen type I, III and IV transcripts in carbon tetrachloride-induced rat liver fibrosis. J Clin Invest 85:1833, 1990.
1061. Tsukamoto H: Activation of fat storing cells in alcoholic liver fibrosis: role of Kupffer cells and lipid peroxidation. In Surrentic, et al, eds. Falk Symposium No. 71, Fat-Storing Cells in Liver Fibrosis. Kluwer Academic Publishers, 1994:189.
1062. Tsukamoto H, Rippe R, Niemela O, Lin M: Role of oxidative stress in activation of Kupffer cells and Ito cells in liver fibrogenesis. J Gastroenterol Hepatol (in press).
1063. Takahashi H, Wong K, Nanji AA, et al: Effect of dietary fat on Ito cell activation by chronic ethanol intake: a long-term serial morphometric study on alcohol-fed and control rats. Alcohol Clin Exp Res 15:1060, 1991.
1064. French SW, Wong K, Nanji AA, et al: The role of the Ito cell in fibrogenesis in alcoholic liver disease. In Kuriyama K, Takada A, Ishii H, eds: Biomedical and Social Aspects of Alcohol and Alcoholism. Amsterdam, Elsevier, 1988:767.
1065. Casini A, Cunningham M, Rojkind M, Lieber CS: Acetaldehyde increases procollagen type I and fibronectin gene transcription in cultured rat fat-storing cells through a protein synthesis-dependent mechanism. Hepatology 13:758, 1991.
1066. Pares A, Potter JJ, Rennie L, Mezey E: Acetaldehyde activates the promoter of the mouse α_2 (I) collagen gene. Hepatology 19:498, 1994.
1067. Maher JJ, Zia S, Tzagarakis C: Acetaldehyde-induced stimulation of collagen synthesis and gene expression is dependent on conditions of cell culture: studies with rat lipocytes and fibroblasts. Alcohol Clin Exp Res 18:403, 1994.
1068. Brenner DA, Chojkier M: Acetaldehyde increases collagen transcription in cultured human fibroblasts. J Biol Chem 262:17690, 1987.
1069. Shiratori Y, Ichida T, Kawase T, Wisse E: Effect of acetaldehyde on collagen synthesis by fat storing cells isolated from rats treated with carbon tetrachloride. Liver 6:246, 1986.
1070. Friedman SL: Acetaldehyde and alcoholic fibrogenesis: fuel to the fire but not the spark. Hepatology 12:609, 1990.
1071. Tsukamoto H, Cheng S, Blaner WS: Fibroproliferative activation of Ito cells in experimental alcoholic liver fibrosis. Am J Physiol (in press).
1072. Tsukamoto H, Pham TV, Cheng S, Blaner WS: Effects of dietary fat on ethanol-induced hepatic stellate cell activation. Hepatology 22:226A, 1995.
1073. Matsuoka M, Zhang M, Tsukamoto H: Sensitization of hepatic lipocytes by high fat diet to stimulatory effects of Kupffer cell-derived factors: implication in alcoholic liver fibrogenesis. Hepatology 11:173, 1990.
1074. Matsuoka M, Pham NT, Tsukamoto H: Differential effects of interleukin 1α, tumor necrosis factor-α and transforming growth factor-$\beta 1$ on cell proliferation and collagen formation by cultured fat-storing cells. Liver 9:71, 1989.
1075. Bachem MG, Sell KM, Melchior R, et al: Tumor necrosis factor alpha (TNFα) and transforming growth factor $\beta 1$ (TGF$\beta 1$) stimulate fibronectin synthesis and the transdifferentiation of fat-storing cells in the rat liver into myofibroblasts. Virchows Archiv B Cell Pathol 63:123, 1993.
1076. Greenwel P, Rubin J, Schwartz M, et al: Liver fat-storing cell clones obtained from a CCl_4-cirrhotic rat are heterogeneous with regard to proliferation, expression of extracellular matrix components, interleukin 6 and connexin 43. Lab Invest 69:210, 1993.
1077. Kamimura S, Gaal K, Britton RS, et al: Increased 4-hydroxynonenal levels in experimental alcoholic liver disease: association of lipid peroxidation with liver fibrogenesis. Hepatology 16:448, 1992.

1078. Tsukamoto H, Kim CW, Luo ZZ, et al: Role of lipid peroxidation in vivo and in vitro models of liver fibrogenesis. Gastroenterology 104:A1012, 1993.
1079. Parola M, Pinzani M, Casini A, et al: Stimulation of lipid peroxidation or 4-hydroxynonenal treatment increases procollagen $\alpha 1$ (I) gene expression in human liver fat storing cells. Biochem Biophys Res Commun 194:1044, 1993.
1080. Tsukamoto H, Horne W, Kamimura S, et al: Experimental liver cirrhosis induced by alcohol and iron. J Clin Invest 96:620, 1995.
1081. Schafferer F, Popper H: Capillarization of hepatic sinusoids in man. Gastroenterology 44:239, 1963.
1082. Witte MH, Borgs P, Way DL, et al: Alcohol, hepatic sinusoidal microcirculation and chronic liver disease. Alcohol 9:473, 1992.
1083. Nanji AA, Tahan SR, Wei Y, et al: Hepatic sinusoidal endothelial cell G_1/S arrest correlates with severity of alcoholic liver injury in the rat. Gastroenterology 107:818, 1994.
1084. Smedsrod B, Pertoft H, Gustafson S, et al: Scavenger function of liver endothelial cells. Biochem J 266:313, 1990.
1085. Engstrom-Laurent A, Loof L, Nyberg A, et al: Increased serum levels of hyaluronate in liver disease. Hepatology 5:638, 1985.
1086. Frebourg T, Dalpech B, Bercoff E, et al: Serum hyaluronate in liver diseases: study by enzymoimmunological assay. Hepatology 6:392, 1986.
1087. Gibson PR, Fraser JRE, Brown TJ, et al: Hemodynamic and liver function predictors of serum hyaluronate in alcoholic liver disease. Hepatology 15:1054, 1992.
1088. Ueno T, Inuzuka S, Torimura T, et al: Serum hyaluronate reflects hepatic sinusoidal capillarization. Gastroenterology 105:475, 1993.
1089. Nanji AA, Tahan SR, Yacoub LK, et al: Plasma hyaluronic acid is a sensitive marker for endothelial dysfunction in the early stages of experimental alcoholic liver disease. Gastroenterology 108:A1131, 1995.
1090. Deauciuc IV, McDonough KH, Bagby GJ, et al: Alcohol consumption in rats potentiates the deleterious effect of gram-negative sepsis on hepatic hyaluronan uptake. Alcohol Clin Exp Res 17:1002, 1993.
1091. Deauciuc IV, Bagby GJ, Neissman MR, et al: Modulation of hepatic sinusoidal endothelial cell function by Kupffer cells: an example of intercellular communication in the liver. Hepatology 19:464, 1994.
1092. Reitschel ET, Kirikae T, Schade FU, et al: Bacterial endotoxin: molecular relationships of structure to activity and function. FASEB J 8:217, 1994.
1093. Fox ES, Broitman SA, Thomas P: Bacterial endotoxins and the liver. Lab Invest 63:733, 1990.
1094. Galanos C, Freudenberg MA: Bacterial endotoxins: biologic properties and mechanisms of action. Mediators Inflamm 2:S11, 1993.
1095. Nolan JP, Hare DK, McDevitt JJ, Ali MV: In vitro studies of endotoxin absorption. Gastroenterology 72:434, 1977.
1096. Fox ES, Thomas P, Broitman SA: Uptake and modification of an ^{125}I-lipopolysaccharide by isolated rat Kupffer cells. Hepatology 8:1550, 1988.
1097. Fox ES, Thomas P, Broitman SA: Comparative studies of endotoxin uptake by isolated rat Kupffer and peritoneal cells. Infect Immun 55:2962, 1987.
1098. Fox ES, Thomas P, Broitman SA: Hepatic mechanisms for clearance and detoxification of bacterial endotoxins. J Nutr Biochem 1:620, 1990.
1099. Broitman SA, Gottlieb LS, Zamcheck N: Influence of neomycin and ingested endotoxin in the pathogenesis of choline deficiency cirrhosis in the adult rat. J Exp Med 119:633, 1963.
1100. Nolan JP, Ali MV: Endotoxin and the liver. II. Effect of tolerance on carbon tetrachloride induced injury. J Med 4:28, 1973.
1101. Camera DS, Caruana JA, Schwartz KA, et al: D-Galactosamine liver injury: absorption of endotoxin and protective effect of small bowel and colon resection in rabbits. Proc Soc Exp Biol Med 172:255, 1983.
1102. Nolan JP, Leibowitz AI, Vladutiu AO: Influence of carbon tetrachloride on circulating endotoxin after exogenous administration of endotoxin in rats. Proc Soc Exp Biol Med 165:453, 1980.
1103. Nolan JP, Leibowitz AI: Endotoxin and the liver. III. Modification of acute carbon tetrachloride injury by polymyxin B and antiendotoxin. Gastroenterology 75:445, 1978.
1104. Galanos C, Freudenberg MA, Reutter W: Galactosamine-induced sensitization to the lethal effects of endotoxin. Proc Natl Acad Sci U S A 76:5939, 1979.
1105. Decker K, Keppler D: Galactosamine hepatitis: key role of the nucleotide deficiency period in the pathogenesis of cell injury and cell death. Rev Physiol Biochem Pharmacol 71:77, 1974.
1106. Freudenberg MA, Keppler D, Galanos C: Requirement for lipopolysaccharide responsive macrophages in galactosamine-induced sensitization to endotoxin. Infect Immun 51:891, 1986.
1107. Lehmann V, Freudenberg MA, Galanos C: Lethal toxicity of lipopolysaccharide and tumor necrosis factor in normal and D-galactosamine treated mice. J Exp Med 165:657, 1987.
1108. Old LJ: Tumor necrosis factor. Science 229:869, 1985.
1109. Gut JP, Schmitt S, Bingen A, et al: Protective effect of colectomy in frog virus 3 hepatitis of rats: possible role of endotoxin. J Infect Dis 146:594, 1982.
1110. Gut JP, Schmitt S, Bingen A, et al: Probable role of endogenous endotoxins in hepatocytolysis during murine hepatitis caused by frog virus 3. J Infect Dis 149:621, 1984.
1111. Kirn A, Gut JP, Gendrault JL: Interaction of viruses with sinusoidal cells. In Popper H, Schaffner F, eds: Progress in Liver Disease, vol VII. New York, Grune & Stratton, 1982:377.
1112. Bode C, Kugler V, Bode JC: Endotoxemia in patients with alcoholic and non-alcoholic cirrhosis and in subjects with no evidence of chronic liver disease following acute alcohol excess. J Hepatol 4:8, 1987.
1113. Fukui H, Brauner B, Bode JC, Bode C: Plasma endotoxin concentrations in patients with alcoholic and non-alcoholic liver disease: re-evaluation with an improved chromogenic assay. Hepatology 12:162, 1991.
1114. Nanji AA, Khettry U, Sadrzadeh SMH, Yamanaka T: Severity of liver injury in experimental alcoholic liver disease. Correlation with plasma endotoxin, prostaglandin E_2, leukotriene B_4 and thromboxane B2. Am J Pathol 142:367, 1993.
1115. Nanji AA, Sadrzadeh SMH, Thomas P, Yamanaka T: Eicosanoid profile and evidence for endotoxin tolerance in chronic ethanol-fed rats. Life Sci 55:611, 1994.
1116. Earnest DL, Sim WW, Smith TL, Eskelson CD: Ethanol, acetaldehyde and Kupffer cell function: potential role for Kupffer cells in alcohol induced liver injury. Prog Clin Biol Res 325:255, 1990.
1117. Bjarnason I, Ward K, Peters TJ: The leaky gut of alcoholism: possible route of entry for toxic compounds. Lancet I:179, 1984.
1118. Arai M: Effect of ethanol on intestinal uptake of endotoxin. Jpn J Gastroenterol 83:1060, 1986.
1119. Bode JC: Alcohol and the gastrointestinal tract. In Frick HP: Advances in Internal Medicine and Pediatrics. Heidelberg, Springer-Verlag, 1980:1.
1120. Nanji AA, Khettry U, Sadrzadeh SMH: Lactobacillus feeding reduces endotoxemia and severity of experimental alcoholic liver disease. Proc Soc Exp Biol Med 205:243, 1994.
1121. Goldin BR, Gorbach SL, Saxelin M, et al: Survival of lactobacillus species (strain GG) in human gastrointestinal tract. Dig Dis Sci 37:121, 1992.
1122. Silva M, Kacobus NV, Deneke C, Gorbach SL: Antimicrobial substance from a human lactobacillus strain. Antimicrob Agents Chemother 31:1231, 1987.
1123. Adachi Y, Moore LE, Bradford BU, et al: Antibiotics prevent liver injury in rats following long-term exposure to ethanol. Gastroenterology 108:218, 1995.
1124. Nolan JP, Camara DS: Intestinal endotoxins as cofactors in liver injury. Immun Invest 18:325, 1989.
1125. Nolan JP: Intestinal endotoxins as mediators of hepatic injury. An idea whose time has come again. Hepatology 10:887, 1989.
1126. Morrison DC, Ryan JL: Endotoxins and disease mechanisms. Annu Rev Med 38:417-432, 1987.
1127. Ulevitch RJ, Tobias PS: Receptor-dependent mechanisms of cell stimulation by bacterial endotoxin. Annu Rev Immunol 13:437-457, 1995.
1128. Schumann RR, Leong SR, Flaggs GW, et al: Structure and function of lipopolysaccharide binding protein. Science 249:1429-1431, 1990.
1129. Su GL, Simmons RL, Wang SC: Lipopolysaccharide binding protein participation in cellular activation by LPS. Crit Rev Immunol 15:201-214, 1995.

1130. Martin TR, Mongovin SM, Tobias PS, et al: The CD14 differentiation antigen mediates the development of endotoxin responsiveness during differentiation of mononuclear phagocytes. J Leukoc Biol 56:1-9, 1994.
1131. Wright SD, Ramos RA, Tobias PS, et al: CD14, a receptor for complexes of lipopolysaccharide (LPS) and LPS binding protein. Science 249:1431-1433, 1990.
1132. Lee JD, Kato K, Tobias PS, et al: Transfection of CD14 into 70Z/3 cells dramatically enhances the sensitivity to complexes of lipopolysaccharide (LPS) and LPS binding protein. J Exp Med 175:1697-1750, 1992.
1133. Dentener MA, Bazil V, Von Asmuth EJ, et al: Involvement of CD14 in lipopolysaccharide-induced tumor necrosis factor-alpha, IL-6 and IL-8 release by human monocytes and alveolar macrophages. J Immunol 150:2885-2891, 1993.
1134. Kielian TL, Blecha F: CD14 and other recognition molecules for lipopolysaccharide: a review. Immunopharmacology 29:187-205, 1995.
1135. Maliszewski CR: CD14 and immune response to lipopolysaccharide. Science 252:1321-1322, 1991.
1136. Ferrero E, Jiao D, Tsuberi BZ, et al: Transgenic mice expressing human CD14 are hypersensitive to lipopolysaccharide. Proc Natl Acad Sci U S A 90:2380-2384, 1993.
1137. Haziot A, Ferrero E, Lin XY, et al: CD14-deficient mice are exquisitely insensitive to the effects of LPS. Prog Clin Biol Res 392:349-351, 1995.
1138. Su GL, Rahemtulla A, Thomas P, et al: CD14 and lipopolysaccharide binding protein expression in a rat model of alcoholic liver disease. Am J Pathol 152:841-849, 1998.
1139. Fenton MJ, Golenbock DT: LPS-binding proteins and receptors. J Leukoc Biol 64:25-32, 1998.
1140. Kitchens RL, Munford RS: Enzymatically deacylated lipopolysaccharide (LPS) can antagonize LPS at multiple sites in the LPS recognition pathway. J Biol Chem 270:9904-9910, 1995.
1141. Ulevitch RJ, Tobias PS: Recognition of endotoxin by cells leading to transmembrane signaling. Curr Opin Immunol 6:125-130, 1994.
1142. Ingalls RR, Monks BG, Golenbock DT: Membrane expression of soluble endotoxin-binding proteins permits lipopolysaccharide signaling in Chinese hamster ovary fibroblasts independently of CD14. J Biol Chem 274:13993-13998, 1999.
1143. Rock FL, Hardiman G, Timans JC, et al: A family of human receptors structurally related to Drosophila Toll. Proc Natl Acad Sci U S A 95:588-593, 1998.
1144. Yang RB, Mark MR, Gray A, et al: Toll-like receptor-2 mediates lipopolysaccharide-induced cellular signalling. Nature 395:284-288, 1998.
1145. Hoshino K, Takeuchi O, Kawai T, et al: Cutting edge: Toll-like receptor 4 (TLR4)-deficient mice are hyporesponsive to lipopolysaccharide: evidence for TLR4 as the LPS gene product. J Immunol 162:3749-3752, 1999.
1146. Lien E, Means TK, Heine H, et al: Toll-like receptor 4 imparts ligand-specific recognition of bacterial lipopolysaccharide. J Clin Invest 105:497-504, 2000.
1147. Aderem A, Ulevitch RJ: Toll-like receptors in the induction of the innate immune response. Nature 406:782-787, 2000.
1148. Su GL, Klein RD, Aminlari A, et al: Kupffer cell activation by lipopolysaccharide in rats: role for lipopolysaccharide binding protein and toll-like receptor 4. Hepatology 31:932-936, 2000.
1149. Wright SD: Toll: a new piece in the puzzle of innate immunity. J Exp Med 189:605-609, 1999.
1149a. Su and Nanji: Unpublished observations.
1150. Yin M, Bradford BU, Wheeler MD, et al: Reduced early alcohol-induced liver injury in CD14-deficient mice. J Immunol 166: 4737-4742, 2000.
1151. Uesugi T, Froh M, Arteel GE, et al: Toll-like receptor 4 is involved in the mechanism of early alcohol-induced liver injury. Hepatology 34: 101-108, 2001.
1152. May MJ, Ghost S: Rel/NF-κB and IκB proteins: an overview. Semin Cancer Biol 8:63-73, 1997.
1153. Barnes PJ, Karin M: Nuclear factor-kappaB: a pivotal transcription factor in chronic inflammatory diseases. N Engl J Med 336:1066-1071, 1997.
1154. Nanji AA, Jokelainen K, Rahemtulla A, et al: Activation of nuclear factor kappa B and cytokine imbalance in experimental alcoholic liver disease in the rat. Hepatology 30:934-943, 1999.
1155. Hill DB, Barve S, Barve SJ, McClain CJ: Increased monocyte nuclear factor-kappaB activation and tumor necrosis factor production in alcoholic hepatitis. J Lab Clin Med 135:387-395, 2000.
1156. Fox ES, Cantrell CH, Leingang KA: Inhibition of the Kupffer cell inflammatory response by acute ethanol: NF-kappa B activation and subsequent cytokine production. Biochem Biophys Res Commun 225:134-140, 1996.
1157. Szabo G, Chavan S, Madrekar P, Catalano D: Acute alcohol consumption attenuates interleukin-8 (IL-8) and monocyte chemoattractant peptide-1 (MCP-1) induction in response to ex-vivo stimulation. J Clin Immunol 19:67-76, 1999.
1158. Bellas RE, FitzGerald MJ, Fauston, Sonenshein GE: Inhibition of NF-kappa B activity induces apoptosis in murine hepatocytes. Am J Pathol 151:891-896, 1997.
1159. Beg A, Baltimore D: An essential role for NF-κB in preventing TNF-α induced cell death. Science 274:782-784, 1998.
1160. Baehr V, Docke WD, Plauth M, et al: Mechanisms of endotoxin tolerance in alcoholic liver cirrhosis: role of interleukin 10, interleukin 1 receptor antagonist and soluble tumor necrosis factor receptors as well as effector cell desensitization. Gut 47:281-287, 2000.
1161. Mezey E: Alcoholic liver disease. Prog Liver Dis 7:555, 1982.
1162. French SW, Burridge EJ: Alcoholic hepatitis: clinical, morphologic, pathogenic and therapeutic aspects. Prog Liver Dis 6:557, 1979.
1163. McClain CJ, Barve S, Deauciuc I, et al: Cytokines in alcoholic liver disease. Semin Liver Dis 19: 205-219, 1999.
1164. Bhagwandeen BS, Apte M, Manwarring L, Dickeson J: Endotoxin-induced hepatic necrosis in rats on an alcohol diet. J Pathol 151:47, 1987.
1165. Arai M, Nakano S, Okuno F, et al: Endotoxin-induced hypercoagulability: a possible aggravating factor of alcoholic liver disease. Hepatology 9:846, 1989.
1166. Honchel R, Ray M, Marsano L, et al: Tumor necrosis factor in alcohol-enhanced endotoxin liver injury. Alcohol Clin Exp Res 16:665, 1992.
1167. Hansen J, Cherwitz DL, Allen JI: The role of tumor necrosis factor-α in acute endotoxin-induced hepatotoxicity in ethanol-fed rats. Hepatology 20:461, 1994.
1168. Hoffman R, Grewe M, Estler H, et al: Regulation of tumor necrosis factor-α mRNA synthesis and distribution of tumor necrosis factor-α-mRNA synthesizing cells in rat liver during experimental endotoxemia. J Hepatol 20:122, 1994.
1169. Nanji AA, Zhao S, Sadrzadeh SMH, Waxman DJ: Use of reverse transcription-polymerase chain reaction to evaluate in-vivo cytokine gene expression in rats fed ethanol for long periods. Hepatology 19:1483, 1994.
1170. Kamimura S, Tsukasmoto H: Cytokine gene expression of Kupffer cells in experimental alcoholic liver disease. Hepatology 21:1304, 1995.
1171. Yin M, Wheeler MD, Knon H, et al: Essential role of tumor necrosis factor alpha in alcohol-induced liver injury in mice. Gastroenterology 117:942-952, 1999.
1172. Amar S, Van Dyke TE, Eugster HP, et al: Tumor necrosis factor (TNF)-induced cutaneous necrosis is mediated by TNF receptor 1. J Inflamm 47:180-189, 1995.
1173. Acton RD, Dahlberg PS, Uknis ME, et al: Differential sensitivity to Escherichia coli infection in mice lacking tumor necrosis factor p55 or interleukin-1 p80 receptors. Arch Surg 131:1216-1221, 1996.
1174. Iimuro Y, Galluci RM, Luster MI, et al: Antibodies to tumor necrosis factor alfa attenuate hepatic necrosis and inflammation caused by chronic exposure to ethanol in the rat. Hepatology 26:1530-1537, 1997.
1175. Grove J, Daly AK, Bassendine M, Day C: Association of a tumor necrosis factor promoter polymorphism with susceptibility to alcoholic steatohepatitis. Hepatology 26:143-146, 1997.
1176. McClain CJ, Cohen DA: Increased tumor necrosis factor production by monocytes in alcoholic hepatitis. Hepatology 9:349, 1989.
1177. Felver ME, Mezey E, McGuire M, et al: Plasma tumor necrosis factor-α predicts decreased long term survival in severe alcoholic hepatitis. Alcohol Clin Exp Res 14:255-259, 1990.
1178. Bird GLA, Sheron N, Goka AKJ, et al: Increased plasma tumor necrosis factor in severe alcoholic hepatitis. Ann Intern Med 112:917, 1990.

1179. Shiratori Y, Takada H, Hikiba Y, et al: Production of chemotactic factor, interleukin 8, from hepatocytes exposed to ethanol. Hepatology 18:1477, 1993.
1180. Van Zee KJ, Fischer E, Hawes AS, et al: Effects of intravenous IL-8 administration on nonhuman primates. J Immunol 148:1746, 1992.
1181. Hill DB, Marsano LS, McClain CJ: Increased plasma interleukin-8 concentrations in alcoholic hepatitis. Hepatology 18:576, 1993.
1182. Sheron N, Bird G, Koskinas J, et al: Circulating and tissue levels of the neutrophil chemotaxin interleukin-8 are elevated in severe acute alcoholic hepatitis, and tissue levels correlate with neutrophil infiltration. Hepatology 18:41, 1993.
1183. McClain CJ, Cohen DA, Dinarello CA, et al: Serum interleukin-1 (IL-1) activity in alcoholic hepatitis. Life Sci 39:1479, 1986.
1184. Khoruts A, Stahnke L, McClain CJ, et al: Circulating tumor necrosis factor, interleukin 1 and interleukin 6 concentrations in chronic alcoholics. Hepatology 13:267, 1991.
1185. Deviere J, Content J, Denys C, et al: Excessive in-vitro bacterial polysaccharide induced production of monokine in cirrhosis. Hepatology 11:628, 1990.
1186. Kishimoto T: The biology of interleukin 6. Blood 74:1, 1989.
1187. Deviere J, Content J, Denys C, et al: High interleukin-6 serum levels and increased production by leukocytes in alcoholic liver cirrhosis. Clin Exp Immunol 77:221, 1989.
1188. Hill D, Marsano L, Cohen D, et al: Increased plasma interleukin 6 activity in alcoholic hepatitis. J Lab Clin Med 119:547, 1992.
1189. Ulich TR, Guo K, delCastillo J: Endotoxin-induced cytokine gene expression in vivo. I. Expression of tumor necrosis factor mRNA in visceral organs under physiologic conditions and during endotoxemia. Am J Pathol 134:11, 1989.
1190. McClain CJ, Hill DB, Schmidt J, Diehl AM: Cytokines and alcoholic liver disease. Semin Liver Dis 13:170, 1993.
1191. Peristeris P, Clark B, Gatti S, et al: N-acetylcysteine and glutathione as inhibitors of tumor necrosis factor production. Cell Immunol 140:390, 1992.
1192. Deauciuc IV, D'Souza NB, Bagby GJ, et al: Effect of acute alcohol administration on TNFα binding to neutrophils and isolated liver plasma membranes. Alcohol Clin Exp Res 16:533, 1992.
1193. Diehl AM: Alcohol and liver regeneration. Clin Liver Dis 2:723-738, 1998.
1194. Cornell RP: Gut-derived endotoxin elicits hepatotrophic factor secretion for liver regeneration. Am J Physiol 249:R551-562, 1985.
1195. Cornell RP, Lijequist BL, Bartizal KF: Depressed liver regeneration after partial hepatectomy of germ-free, athymic and lipopolysaccharide-resistant mice. Hepatology 11:916-922, 1990.
1196. Feingold KR, Barker ME, Jones AL, et al: Localization of tumor necrosis factor-stimulated DNA synthesis in the liver. Hepatology 13:773-779, 1991.
1197. Feingold KR, Soued M, Grunfeld C: Tumor necrosis factor stimulates DNA synthesis in the liver of intact rats. Biochem Biophys Res Commun 153:576-582, 1988.
1198. Mealy K, Wilmore DW: Tumour necrosis factor increases hepatic cell mass. Br J Surg 78:331-333, 1991.
1199. Akerman P, Cote P, Yang SQ, et al: Antibodies to tumor necrosis factor-alpha inhibit liver regeneration after partial hepatectomy. Am J Physiol 263:G579-585, 1992.
1200. Akerman P, Cote P, Yang SQ, et al: Long-term ethanol consumption alters the hepatic response to the regenerative effects of tumor necrosis factor-alpha. Hepatology 17:1066-1073, 1993.
1201. Yang SQ, Lin HZ, Yim M, et al: Effects of chronic ethanol consumption on cytokine regulation of liver regeneration. Am J Physiol 275:G696-704, 1998.
1202. Diehl AM, Rai R: Regulation of signal transduction during liver regeneration. FASEB J 10:215-227, 1996.
1203. Zhang M, Gong Y, Corbin I, et al: Light ethanol consumption enhances liver regeneration after partial hepatectomy in rats. Gastroenterology 119:1333-1339, 2000.
1204. French SW, Nash J, Shitabata P, et al: Pathology of alcoholic liver disease. Semin Liver Dis 13:154-169, 1993.
1205. Kawahara H, Matsuda Y, Takase S: Is apoptosis involved in alcoholic hepatitis? Alcohol 29(suppl 1):113-118, 1994.
1206. Goldin RD, Hunt NC, Clark J, et al: Apoptotic bodies in a murine model of alcoholic liver disease: reversibility of ethanol-induced changes. J Pathol 171:73-76, 1993.
1207. Benedetti A, Jezequel AM, Orlandi F: A quantitative evaluation of apoptotic bodies in rat liver. Liver 8:172-177, 1988.
1208. Benedetti A, Brunelli E, Risicato R, et al: Subcellular changes and apoptosis induced by ethanol in rat liver. J Hepatol 6:137-143, 1988.
1209. Benedetti A, Jezequel AM, Orlandi F: Preferential distribution of apoptotic bodies in acinar zone 3 of normal human and rat liver. J Hepatol 7:319-324, 1988.
1210. Yacoub LK, Fogt F, Nanji AA: Apoptosis and Bcl-2 protein expression in experimental alcoholic liver disease in the rat. Alcohol Clin Exp Res 19:854-859, 1995.
1211. Lieber CS: Cytochrome P4502E1: its physiological and pathological role. Physiol Rev 77:517-544, 1997.
1212. Chen Q, Galleano M, Cederbaum AI: Cytotoxicity and apoptosis produced by arachidonic acid in Hep G2 cells overexpressing human cytochrome P4502E1. J Biol Chem 272:14532-14541, 1997.
1213. Powell LW: The relationship between alcohol consumption and hepatic iron metabolism. Hepatology 2:9-14, 1981.
1214. Kato J, Kobune M, Kohgo Y, et al: Hepatic iron deprivation prevents spontaneous development of fulminant hepatitis and liver cancer in Long-Evans Cinnamon rats. J Clin Invest 98:923-923, 1996.
1215. Garcia Ruiz C, Morales A, Collel A, et al: Effect of chronic ethanol feeding on glutathione and functional integrity of mitochondria in periportal and perivenous rat hepatocytes. J Clin Invest 94:193-201, 1994.
1216. Hirano T, Kaplowitz N, Tsukamoto H, Kamimura S, et al: Hepatic mitochondrial glutathione depletion and progression of experimental alcoholic liver disease in rats. Hepatology 16:1423-1428, 1992.
1217. Colell A, Garcia-Ruiz C, Miranda M, et al: Selective glutathione depletion of mitochondria by ethanol sensitizes hepatocytes to tumor necrosis factor. Gastroenterology 115:1541-1551, 1998.
1218. Kurose J. Higuchi H, Miura S, et al: Oxidative-stress mediated apoptosis of hepatocytes exposed to acute ethanol intoxication. Hepatology 25:368-378, 1997.
1219. Hug H, Strand S, Grambihler A, et al: Reactive oxygen intermediates are involved in the induction of CD95 ligand mRNA expression by cytostatic drugs in hepatoma cells. J Biol Chem 272:28191-28193, 1997.
1220. Faubion W, Gores G: Death receptors in liver biology and pathobiology. Hepatology 29:1-4, 1999.
1221. Ashkenazi A, Dixit V: Death receptors: signaling and modulation. Science 281:1305-1308, 1998.
1222. Rust C, Gores GJ: Apoptosis and liver disease. Am J Med. 108:567-574, 2000.
1223. Galle PR, Hofmann WJ, Walczak H, et al: Involvement of the CD95 (APO-1/Fas) receptor and ligand in liver damage. J Exp Med 182:1223-1230, 1995.
1224. Mueller M, Scaffidi, Peters M, et al: Involvement of the CD95 system in alcohol-induced liver damage. Hepatology 26:270A, 1997 (abstract).
1225. Rath PC, Aggarwal BB: TNF-induced signaling in apoptosis. J Clin Immunol 19:350-364, 1999.
1226. Kuwano K, Hara N: Signal transduction pathways of apoptosis and inflammation induced by the tumor necrosis factor receptor family. Am J Respir Cell Mol Biol 22:147-149, 2000.
1227. Deaciuc IV, D'Souza NB, Spitzer JJ: Tumor necrosis factor-alpha cell-surface receptors of liver parenchymal and nonparenchymal cells during acute and chronic alcohol administration to rats. Alcohol Clin Exp Res 19:332-338, 1995.
1228. Spengler U, Zachoval R, Gallati H, et al: Serum levels and in situ expression of TNF-alpha and TNF-alpha binding proteins in inflammatory liver diseases. Cytokine 8:864-872, 1996.
1229. Barkett M, Gilmore TD: Control of apoptosis by Rel/NF-kappaB transcription factors. Oncogene 18:6910-6924, 1999.
1230. Green DR, Reed JC: Mitochondria and apoptosis. Science 281:1309-1312, 1998.
1231. Halestrap AP, Doran E, Gillespie JP, O'Toole A: Mitochondria and cell death. Biochem Soc Trans 28:170-177, 2000.
1232. French SW, Nash J, Shitabata P, et al: Pathology of alcoholic liver disease. Semin Liver Dis 13:154, 1993.
1233. Tsukamoto H: Animal models of alcoholic liver injury. Clin Liver Dis 2:739-752, 1998.
1234. Lieber CS, Jones DP, Mendelson J, DeCarli LM: Fatty liver, hyperlipemia and hyperuricemia produced by prolonged alcohol consumption despite adequate dietary intake. Trans Assoc Am Physicians 76:289, 1963.

1235. Lieber CS, Jones DP, DeCarli LM: Effects of prolonged ethanol intake. Production of fatty liver despite adequate diets. J Clin Invest 44:1009, 1965.
1236. Lieber CS, DeCarli LM: Quantitative relationship between the amount of dietary fat and severity of alcoholic fatty liver. Am J Clin Nutr 23:474, 1970.
1237. Rao GA, Larkin EC: Inadequate intake by growing rats of essential nutrients from liquid diets used for chronic alcohol consumption. Nutr Res 5:789, 1985.
1238. Lieber CS, DeCarli LM, Sorrell MF: Experimental models of ethanol administration. Hepatology 10:501, 1989.
1239. Lieber CS, DeCarli LM: Effects of mineral and vitamin supplementation on alcohol-induced fatty liver and microsomal induction. Alcohol Clin Exp Res 13:142, 1989.
1240. Rao GA, Riley DE, Larkin EC: Fatty liver caused by chronic alcohol ingestion is prevented by dietary supplementation with pyruvate or glycerol. Lipids 19:583, 1984.
1241. Yonekura I, Nakano M, Nakajima T, Sato A: Dietary carbohydrate intake as a modifying factor for the development of alcoholic fatty liver. Biochem Arch 5:41, 1989.
1242. Sankaran H, Larkin EC, Rao GA: Unsaturated fat and low energy intake induce whereas an increment in energy intake ameliorates fatty liver during prolonged alcohol consumption by rats. J Nutr 124:110, 1994.
1243. Yonekura K, Nakano M, Sato A: Effects of carbohydrate intake on the blood ethanol level and alcohol fatty liver damage in rats. J Hepatol 17:97, 1993.
1244. Tsukamoto H, Gaal K, French SW: Insights into the pathogenesis of alcoholic liver necrosis and fibrosis: status report. Hepatology 12:599, 1990.
1245. French SW, Miyamoto K, Ohta Y, Geoffrion Y: Pathogenesis of experimental alcoholic liver disease in the rat. Methods Achiev Exp Pathol 13:181, 1988.
1246. Tsukamoto H, Reidelberger RD, French SW, Largman C: Long-term cannulation model for blood sampling and intragastric infusion in the rat. Am J Physiol 247:R595, 1984.
1247. Tsukamoto H, French SW, Reidelberge RD, Largman C: Cyclical pattern of blood alcohol levels during continuous intragastric ethanol infusion in rats. Alcohol Clin Exp Res.9:31-37, 1985.
1248. Badger TM, Ronis MJ, Ingelman-Sundberg M, Hakkak R: Pulsatile blood alcohol and CYP2E1 induction during chronic alcohol infusions in rats. Alcohol 10:453-457, 1993.
1249. Badger TM, Ronis MJ, Ingelman-Sundberg M, Hakkak R: Inhibition of CYP2E1 activity does not abolish pulsatile urine alcohol concentrations during chronic alcohol infusions. Eur J Biochem 230:914-919, 1995.
1250. French SW, Li J, Yuan QX, et al: Pathogenesis of blood alcohol level 6-day cycle in the chronic alcohol feeding model. FASEB J 13:A738, 1999.
1251. Li J, Nguyen V, French BA, et al: Mechanism of the alcohol cyclic pattern: role of the hypothalamic-pituitary-thyroid axis. Am J Physiol Gastrointest Liver Physiol 279:G118-G125, 2000.
1252. Tsukamoto H, French SW, Benson N, et al: Severe and progressive steatosis and focal necrosis in rat liver induced by continuous intragastric infusion of ethanol and low fat diet. Hepatology 5:224, 1985.
1253. French SW, Miyamoto K, Tsukamoto H: Ethanol-induced hepatic fibrosis in the rat: role of the amount of dietary fat. Alcohol Clin Exp Res 10:13S, 1986.
1254. Tsukamoto H, Matsuoka M, French SW: Experimental models of hepatic fibrosis: a review. Semin Liver Dis 10:56, 1990.
1255. French SW, Miyamoto K, Wong K, et al: Role of the Ito cell in liver parenchymal fibrosis in rats fed alcohol and a high fat-low protein diet. Am J Pathol 132:73, 1988.
1256. Takahashi H, Wong K, Jui L, French SW: Effect of dietary fat on Ito cell activation by chronic ethanol intake: a long term serial morphometric study on alcohol-fed and control rats. Alcohol Clin Exp Res 15:1060, 1991.
1257. Tsukamoto H, Horne W, Kamimura S, et al: Experimental liver cirrhosis induced by alcohol and iron. J Clin Invest 96:620, 1995.
1258. Cueto J, Tajen N, Gilbert E, Currie RA: Experimental liver injury in the Rhesus monkey: I. Effects of a cirrhogenic diet and ethanol. Ann Surg 166:19, 1967.
1259. Ruebner BH, Moore J, Rutherford RB, et al: Nutritional cirrhosis in rhesus monkeys: electron microscopy and histochemistry. Exp Mol Pathol 11:53, 1969.
1260. Rogers AE, Fox JG, Murphy JC: Ethanol and diet interactions in male Rhesus monkeys. Drug Nutrient Interactions 1:3, 1981.
1261. French SW, Ruebner BH, Mezey E, et al: Effects of chronic ethanol feeding on hepatic mitochondria in the monkey. Hepatology 3:34, 1983.
1262. Rubin E, Lieber CS: Experimental alcoholic hepatitis: a new primate model. Science 182:712, 1973.
1263. Rubin E, Lieber CS: Fatty liver, alcoholic hepatitis and cirrhosis produced by alcohol in primates. N Engl J Med 290:128, 1974.
1264. Lieber CS, DeCarli LM: An experimental model of alcohol feeding and liver injury in the baboon. J Med Primatol 3:153, 1974.
1265. Lieber CS, DeCarli LM, Rubin E: Sequential production of fatty liver, hepatitis and cirrhosis in sub-human primates fed ethanol with adequate diets. Proc Natl Acad Sci U S A 72:437, 1975.
1266. Popper H, Lieber CS: Histogenesis of alcoholic fibrosis and cirrhosis in the baboon. Am J Pathol 98:695, 1980.
1267. Porto LC, Chevallier M, Grimaud JA: Morphometry of terminal hepatic veins. Follow up in chronically alcohol-fed baboons. Virchows Arch 414:299, 1988.
1268. Ainley CC, Senapati A, Brown IMH, et al: Is alcohol hepatotoxic in the baboon. J Hepatol 7:85, 1988.
1269. Lieber CS, Robins SJ, Li J, et al: Phosphatidylcholine protects against fibrosis and cirrhosis in the baboon. Gastroenterology 106:152, 1994.
1270. Zindenberg-Cherr S, Halstead CH, Olin KL, et al: The effect of chronic alcohol ingestion on free radical defense in the miniature pig. J Nutr 120:213, 1990.
1271. Zindenberg-Cherr S, Olin KL, Villanueva J, et al: Ethanol-induced changes in hepatic free radical defense mechanisms and fatty acid composition in the miniature pig. Hepatology 13:1185, 1991.
1272. Halsted CH, Villanueva J, Chandler CJ, et al: Centrilobular distribution of acetaldehyde and collagen in the ethanol-fed micropig. Hepatology 18:9549, 1993.
1273. French SW, Morimoto M, Tsukamoto H: Animal models of alcohol associated liver injury. In Hall P, ed: Alcoholic Liver Disease: Pathology and Pathogenesis. London, Edward Arnold, 1995:279.
1274. Goldin R: Rodent models of alcoholic liver disease. Int J Exp Pathol 75:1, 1994.
1275. Friedenwald J: The pathologic effects of alcohol on rabbits: an experimental study. JAMA 45:780, 1905.
1276. Connor CL: Some effects of chronic alcohol poisoning in rabbits. Arch Pathol 30:165, 1940.
1277. Connor CL, Chackoff IL: Production of cirrhosis in fatty liver with alcohol. Proc Soc Exp Biol Med 39:356, 1939.
1278. Chey WY, Losay S, Siplet H: Observations on hepatic histology and function in alcoholic dogs. Am J Dig Dis 16:825, 1971.
1279. Lieber CS, Jones DP, Mendelson J, DeCarli LM: Fatty liver, hyperlipemia and hyperuricemia produced by prolonged alcohol consumption despite adequate dietary intake. Trans Assoc Am Physicians 76:289, 1963.
1280. Lindros KO, Stowell L, Vaananen H, et al: Uninterrupted prolonged ethanol oxidation as a main pathogenetic factor of alcoholic liver damage: evidence from a new liquid diet animal model. Liver 3:79, 1983.
1281. Takada A, Matsuda Y, Takase S: Effects of dietary fat on alcohol-pyrazole hepatitis in rats: the pathogenic role of alcohol dehydrogenase pathway in alcohol-induced hepatic cell injury. Alcohol Clin Exp Res 10:403, 1986.
1282. Tsukamoto H, Towner SJ, Ciofalo LM, French SW: Ethanol-induced liver fibrosis in rats fed high-fat diet. Hepatology 6:814, 1986.
1283. Smith SM, Hoy HE: *Ad libitum* alcohol does not induce renal IgA deposition in mice. Alcohol Clin Exp Res 14:184, 1990.
1284. Yunice AA, Hsu JM, Fahmy A, Henry S: Ethanol-ascorbate interrelationship in acute and chronic alcoholism in the guinea pig. Proc Soc Exp Biol Med 177:262, 1984.
1285. Hartroft WS: The liver—nutritional guardian of the body. In Gall EA, Mostofi FK, eds: The Liver. Baltimore, Williams & Wilkins, 1973:131.
1286. Klatskin G, Krehl WA, Conn HO: Effect of alcohol on choline requirement: changes in rat's liver following prolonged ingestion of alcohol. J Exp Med 100:605, 1954.
1287. Fallon HJ, Gertman PM, Kemp ED: The effects of ethanol ingestion and choline deficiency on hepatic lecithin biosynthesis in the rat. Biochim Biophys Acta 187:94, 1969.

1288. Tuma DJ, Keefer RC, Beckenhauer HC, et al: Effect of ethanol on uptake of choline by the isolated perfused rat liver. Biochim Biophys Acta 218:141, 1970.
1289. Thompson JA, Reitz RC: Studies on the acute and chronic effects of ethanol ingestion on choline oxidation. Ann N Y Acad Sci 273:194, 1976.
1290. Rutenberg AM, Sonnenblick E, Koven E, et al: Role of intestinal bacteria in the development of dietary cirrhosis in rats. J Exp Med 106:1, 1957.
1291. Rao GA, Tsukamoto H, Larkin EC, et al: Nutritional inadequacy of diets for young growing rats used in models of chronic alcohol ingestion. Biochem Arch 1:97, 1985.
1292. Frank O, Baker H: Vitamin profile in rats fed starch and liquid ethanolic diets. Am J Clin Nutr 33:221, 1980.
1293. Rao GA, Larkin EC, Porta EA: Two decades of chronic alcoholism research with the misconception that liver damage occurred despite adequate nutrition. Biochem Arch 2:223, 1986.
1294. Mezey E: Intestinal function in chronic alcoholism. Ann N Y Acad Sci 252:215, 1975.
1295. Pinto J, Huang YA, Rivlin RS: Mechanisms underlying the differential effects of ethanol on the bioavailability of riboflavin and flavin adenine dinucleotide. J Clin Invest 79:1343, 1984.
1296. Mezey E, Potter JJ: Changes in exocrine pancreatic function produced by altered protein intake in drinking alcoholics. Johns Hopkins Med J 138:7, 1976.
1297. Roggin GM, Iber FL, Kater RMH, Tobon F: Malabsorption in the chronic alcoholic. Johns Hopkins Med J 125:321, 1969.
1298. Sarles H, Figarella C, Clemente F: The interaction of ethanol, dietary lipid and proteins on the pancreas. Digestion 4:13, 1971.
1299. Tsukamoto H, French SW, Benson N, et al: Severe and progressive steatosis and focal necrosis in rat liver induced by continuous intragastric ingestion of ethanol and low fat diet. Hepatology 5:224, 1985.
1300. Tsukamoto H, Towner SJ, Ciofalo LM, et al: Ethanol-induced liver fibrosis in rats fed high fat diet. Hepatology 6:814, 1986.
1301. Barak AJ, Beckewhauser HC, Tuma DJ, et al: Effects of prolonged ethanol feeding on methionine metabolism in rat liver. Biochem Cell Biol 65:230, 1987.
1302. Patek AJ Jr, Bowry S, Hayes KC: Cirrhosis of choline deficiency in rhesus monkey. Possible role of dietary cholesterol. Proc Soc Exp Biol Med 148:370, 1975.
1303. Mezey E, Potter JJ, French SW, et al: Effect of chronic ethanol feeding on hepatic collagen in the monkey. Hepatology 3:41, 1983.
1304. Lieber CS, Leo MA, Mak KM, et al: Choline fails to prevent liver fibrosis in ethanol-fed baboons but causes toxicity. Hepatology 5:561, 1985.
1305. Reynolds TB, Redeker AG, Kuzma OT: Role of alcohol in pathogenesis of alcoholic cirrhosis. In McIntyre NM, Sherlock S, eds: Therapeutic Agents and the Liver. Oxford, Blackwell, 1965:131.
1306. Patek AJ, Post J: Treatment of cirrhosis of the liver by a nutritious diet and supplements rich in vitamins. J Clin Invest 20:481, 1941.
1307. Volwiler W, Jones CM, Mallory TM: Criteria for the measurement of results of treatment in fatty cirrhosis. Gastroenterology 11:164, 1948.
1308. Summerskill WHJ, Wolfe SJ, Davidson CS: Response to alcohol in chronic alcoholics with liver disease. Lancet 1:335, 1957.
1309. Erenoglu E, Edreira JG, Patek AJ Jr: Observations on patients with Laennec's cirrhosis receiving alcohol while on controlled diets. Ann Intern Med 60:814, 1964.
1310. Froesch ER: Essential fructosuria, hereditary fructose intolerance, and fructose-1,6-diphosphatase deficiency. In Stanbury JB, Wyngaarden JB, Fredrickson DS, eds: The Metabolic Basis of Inherited Disease, ed 4. New York, McGraw-Hill, 1978:121.
1311. Blass JP, Gibson GE: Abnormality of thiamine-requiring enzyme in patients with Wernicke-Korsakoff syndrome. N Engl J Med 297:1367, 1977.
1312. Mukerjee AB, Svoronos S, Ghazanfari A, et al: An abnormality of transketolase in cultured fibroblasts from familial chronic alcoholic men and their male offspring. J Clin Invest 79:1039, 1987.
1313. Mitchell MC, Herlong HF: Alcohol and nutrition: caloric value, bioenergetics, and relationship to liver damage. Ann Rev Nutr 6:457, 1986.
1314. Mezey E: Liver disease and protein needs. Ann Rev Nutr 2:21, 1982.
1315. World MJ, Ryle PR, Thomson AD: Alcoholic malnutrition and the small intestine. Alcohol Alcohol 20:89, 1985.
1316. Mendenhall CL, Anderson S, Weesner RE, et al: Protein-calorie malnutrition associated with alcoholic hepatitis. Am J Med 76:211, 1984.
1317. Mills PR, Shenkin A, Anthony RS, et al: Assessment of nutritional status and in vivo immune response in alcohol liver disease. Am J Clin Nutr 38:849, 1983.
1318. Simko V, Connell AM, Banks B: Nutritional status in alcoholics with and without liver disease. Am J Clin Nutr 35:197, 1982.
1319. Hurt RD, Higgins JA, Nelson RA, et al: Nutritional status of alcoholics before and after admission to an alcoholism treatment unit. Am J Clin Nutr 34:386, 1981.
1320. Bunout D, Gattas V, Iturriaga H, et al: Nutritional status of alcoholic patients: its possible relationship to alcoholic liver disease. Am J Clin Nutr 38:469, 1983.
1321. Patek AJ Jr, Toth IG, Sanders GA, et al: Alcohol and dietary factors in cirrhosis. An epidemiologic study of 304 alcoholic patients. Arch Intern Med 135:1053, 1975.
1322. Small M, Longarini A, Zamcheck N: Disturbances of digestive physiology following acute drinking episodes in skid row alcoholics. Am J Med 27:575, 1959.
1323. Leevy CM, Baker N, Ten-Hove W, et al: B-complex vitamins in liver disease of the alcoholic. Am J Clin Nutr 16:399, 1965.
1324. Neville JN, Eagles JA, Samson G, et al: Nutritional status of alcoholics. Am J Clin Nutr 21:1329, 1968.
1325. Pekkanen L, Forsander O: Nutritional implications of alcoholism. Nutr Bull 4:91, 1977.
1326. Norton VP: Interrelationship of nutrition and voluntary alcohol consumption in experimental animals. Br J Addiction 72:205, 1977.
1327. Korsten MA, Lieber CS: Nutrition in the alcoholic. Med Clin North Am 63:963, 1979.
1328. McCullough AJ, Tavill AS: Disordered energy and protein metabolism in liver disease. Semin Liver Dis 11:265, 1991.
1329. Nompleggi DJ, Bonkovsky HL: Nutritional supplementation in chronic liver disease. Hepatology 19:518, 1994.
1330. Mendehall CL, Moritz TE, Roselle GA, et al: A study of oral nutritional support with oxandrolone in malnourished patients with alcoholic hepatitis: results of a Department of Veterans Affairs Cooperative Study. Hepatology 17:564, 1993.
1331. Mezey E: Interaction between alcohol and nutrition in the pathogenesis of alcoholic liver disease. Semin Liver Dis 13:210, 1993.
1332. Shibata HR, MacKenzie JR, Huary S-N: Morphological changes of the liver following small intestinal bypass for obesity. Arch Surg 103:229, 1971.
1333. Kern WH, Payne JH, Dewind IT: Hepatic changes after small intestinal bypass for morbid obesity. Am J Clin Pathol 61:763, 1974.
1334. Marrubbio AT, Buchwald H, Schwartz MZ, et al: Hepatic lesions of central pericellular fibrosis in morbid obesity, and after jejunoileal bypass. Am J Clin Pathol 66:684, 1976.
1335. Galambos J, Willis C: Relationship between 505 paired liver tests and biopsies in 242 obese patients. Gastroenterology 74:11191, 1978.
1336. Adler M, Schaffner F: Fatty liver, hepatitis and cirrhosis in obese patients. Am J Med 67:811, 1979.
1337. Zimmerman HJ, Ishak KG: Non-alcoholic steatohepatitis and other forms of pseudoalcoholic liver disease. In Hall P, ed: Alcoholic Liver Disease. London, Edward Arnold, 1995:175.
1338. Peters RL, Gay T, Reynolds TB: Post jejunoileal-bypass hepatic disease: its similarity to alcoholic hepatic disease. Am J Clin Pathol 63:318, 1975.
1339. Galambos JT: Jejunoileal bypass and nutritional liver injury. Arch Pathol Med 100:229, 1976.
1340. Iber FL, Cooper M: Jejunoileal bypass for the treatment of massive obesity. Prevalence, morbidity, and short- and long-term consequences. Am J Clin Nutr 30:4, 1977.
1341. Moxley RT, Pozefsky T, Lockwood DH: Protein nutrition and liver disease after jejunoileal bypass for morbid obesity. N Engl J Med 290:921, 1974.
1342. Campbell JM, Hunt TK, Karam JH, et al: Jejunoileal bypass as a treatment of morbid obesity. Arch Intern Med 135:602, 1977.
1343. Sherr HP, Nair PP, White JJ, et al: Bile acid metabolism and hepatic disease following small bowel bypass for obesity. Am J Clin Nutr 27:1369, 1974.

1344. Heimburger SL, Steiger E, Logerfo P, et al: Reversal of severe fatty hepatic infiltration after intestinal bypass for morbid obesity by calorie-free amino acid infusion. Am J Surg 129:1975.
1345. Naveau S, Giraud Y, Borotto E, et al: Overweight: risk factor of alcohol steatosis. Hepatology 22:241A, 1995.
1346. Angulo P: Nonalcoholic fatty liver disease. N Engl J Med 346:1221-1231, 2002.
1347. Nakamura S, Takezawa Y, Sato T, et al: Alcoholic liver disease in women. Tohoku J Exp Med 129:351-355, 1979.
1348. Loft S, Olesen K, Dossing M: Increased susceptibility to liver disease in relation to alcohol consumption in women. Scand J Gastroenterol 22:1251-1256, 1987.
1349. Pares A, Caballeria J, Brugueru M, et al: Histological cause of alcoholic hepatitis: Influence of abstinence, sex and extent of hepatic damage. J Hepatol 2:33-42, 1986.
1350. Krasner V, Davis M, Portmann B, Williams R: Changing pattern of alcoholic liver disease in Great Britain. Relation to sex and signs of autoimmunity. BMJ 1 (6075):1497-1500, 1977.
1351. Morbet VA, Branchi L, Meury V, Stalder GA: Long-term histological evaluation of the natural history and prognostic factors of alcoholic liver disease. J Hepatol 4:364-372, 1987.
1352. Ammon E, Schafer C, Hofmann V, Klotz V: Disposition and first-pass metabolism of ethanol in humans: Is it gastric or hepatic and does it depend on gender? Clin Pharmacol Ther 59:503-513, 1996.
1353. Gavaler JS, Dorin AM: Increased susceptibility of women to alcoholic liver disease: Antifactual or real? In Hall P (ed): Alcoholic Liver Disease Pathology and Pathogenesis, ed 2. London, Edward Arnold, 1995:123-137.
1354. Iimuro Y, Frankenberg MV, Arteel GE, et al: Female rats exhibit greater susceptibility to early alcohol-induced liver injury than males. Am J Physiol 272:G1186-1194, 1997.
1355. Yin M, Ikejima K, Wheeler MD, et al: Estrogen is involved in early alcohol-induced liver injury in a rat enteral feeding model. Hepatology 31:117-123, 2000.
1356. Wright SD, Ramos RA, Tobias PS, et al: CD14, a receptor for complexes of lipopolysaccharide (LPS) and LPS binding protein. Science 249:1431-1433, 1990.
1357. Kono H, Wheeler MD, Rusyn I, et al: Gender differences in early alcohol-induced liver injury: role of CD14, NF-κB and TNFα. Am J Physiol Gastrointest 278:G652-G661, 2000.
1358. Najji AA, Jokelainen K, Fotouhinia M, et al: Increased severity of alcoholic liver injury in female rats: role of oxidative stress, endotoxin and chemokines. Am J Physiol Gastrointest Liver Physio 281:G1348-G1356, 2002.
1359. Maher JJ: How does estrogen enhance endotoxin toxicity sensitivity? Let me count the ways. Hepatology 28:1720-1721, 1998.
1360. Ikejima K, Enomoto N, Iimuro Y, et al: Estrogen increases sensitivity of hepatic Kupffer cells to endotoxin. Am J Physiol 274:G669-676, 1998.
1361. Feingold KR, Funk JL, Moser AH, et al: Role for circulating lipoproteins in protection from endotoxin toxicity. Infect Immunol 63:2041-2046, 1995.
1362. Niemela O, Parkkila S, Psanen M, et al: Induction of cytochrome P450 enzymes and generation of protein-aldehyde adducts are associated with sex-dependent sensitivity to alcohol-induced liver disease in micropigs. Hepatology 30:1011-1017, 1999.
1363. Cedarbaum AI, Lieber CS, Beattie DS, Rubin E: Effect of chronic ethanol ingestion on fatty acid oxidation by mitochondria. J Biol Chem 250:5122-5129, 1975.
1364. Amet Y, Adas F, Nanji AA: Fatty acid omega and (omega-1)-hydroxylation in experimental alcoholic liver disease. Alcohol Clin Exp Res 22:1493-1500, 1998.
1365. Kalkaus RM, Chan WK, Ortiz de Montellano PR, Bass NM: Mechanisms of regulation of liver fatty acid binding protein. Mol Cell Biochem 123:93-100, 1993.
1366. Ma XL, Baraona E, Lieber CS: Alcohol consumption enhances fatty acid co-oxidation with greater increase in male than in female rats. Hepatology 18:1247-1253, 1993.
1367. Shevchuk O, Baraona E, Ma XL, et al: Gender differences in the response of hepatic fatty acids and cytosolic fatty acid-binding capacity to alcohol consumption in rats. Proc Soc Exp Biol Med 198:584-590, 1991.
1368. Ma X, Baraona E, Goozner BG, Lieber CS: Gender differences in medium-chain dicarboxylic aciduria in alcoholic men and women. Am J Med 106:70-75, 1999.

CHAPTER

30

Clinical Features and Management of Alcoholic Liver Disease and Non-alcoholic Steatohepatitis

Esteban Mezey, MD

ALCOHOLIC LIVER DISEASE

Alcoholic liver disease is defined by the development of three types of liver damage after chronic heavy alcohol consumption—namely, fatty liver, alcoholic hepatitis, and cirrhosis. These types of histologically detectable liver damage often overlap. Clinical features and laboratory tests frequently do not distinguish among these types of liver disease. There is a high prevalence of hepatitis C infection in alcoholic patients, and approximately 20 percent of alcoholic patients who have clinical and laboratory features compatible with alcoholic liver disease are found on liver biopsy to have pathology that suggests another cause of the liver disease. Hence liver biopsy is often necessary to arrive at a definitive cause of the liver disease, its activity, and its chronicity. Alcoholic hepatitis is generally regarded as a precursor of cirrhosis. Fatty liver without significant fibrosis is usually a benign reversible condition that disappears after abstinence from alcohol.

The quantity and length of ingestion of alcohol are principal factors in the development of alcoholic hepatitis and cirrhosis.[1] Women are more susceptible than men to hepatic damage. Intakes as low as 40 g for men and 20 g for women result in an increased risk of development of cirrhosis.[2] Twenty grams of ethanol approximates the amount of ethanol found in two beers, 2 ounces of whiskey, or 1 pint of wine. Only 10 percent to 20 percent of heavy drinkers develop alcoholic hepatitis or cirrhosis, indicating that other factors—either genetic, environmental, or nutritional—may contribute to the pathogenesis of this disease. Recent studies show that obesity of at least 10 years' duration in chronic alcoholic patients is a risk factor for steatosis, alcoholic hepatitis, and cirrhosis[3] and is associated with more severe histologic damage, in particular the presence of fibrosis in liver biopsies from patients with alcoholic hepatitis.[4] The pivotal factor in the therapy of alcoholic liver disease is prolonged abstinence from alcohol because abstinence by itself improves clinical state and survival. Nutritional supplementation in the malnourished patient and specific drug therapies for hospitalized patients with severe alcoholic hepatitis also have important roles in decreasing morbidity and improving survival. Liver transplantation is the ultimate successful therapy in patients with advanced inactive cirrhosis.

Fatty Liver

Fatty liver occurs commonly after the ingestion of moderate to large amounts of alcohol for even a short period of time. Severe fatty infiltration of the liver is associated with malaise, weakness, anorexia, nausea, abdominal discomfort, and tender hepatomegaly. Jaundice is present in about 15 percent of patients admitted to the hospital because of their symptoms. Fluid retention, portal hypertension with splenomegaly, and occasionally bleeding esophageal varices may occur in the most severe cases. Mild elevation of serum aspartate aminotransferase (AST) and serum alkaline phosphatase is common. Reduced serum albumin and elevated serum globulins are found in about 25 percent of patients. Ultrasonography is the most cost-effective method for detecting fatty infiltration of the liver. The fatty infiltration appears as increased parenchymal echogenicity ("bright liver") and is associated with attenuation of the ultrasound beam and decreased visualization of the portal and hepatic veins.[5] The overall sensitivity of ultrasound in this situation, however, is only 60 percent.[6] The sensitivity of ultrasound is related to the degree of fatty infiltration and increases to 80 percent to 90 percent when more than half of the hepatocytes in an imaged region contain macrovesicular fat. Fatty infiltration is usually diffuse but sometimes is very localized and may be present in only one well-defined area of the liver. Such localized fatty infiltration needs to be distinguished from space-occupying lesions.

Under light microscopy lipid accumulation in the alcoholic usually appears as large (macrovesicular) droplets that are more prominent in the centrolobular zones (Figure 30-1). Liver biopsy is usually not necessary for the diagnosis of fatty liver in patients with mild elevations of the serum aminotransferases (more than 2 times above normal) or alkaline phosphatase and normal serum bilirubin and in whom imaging techniques show a fatty liver. Liver biopsy, however, is indicated in symptomatic patients (i.e., with marked fatigue, who have more marked elevations of the liver enzymes for more than 6 months' duration, or with worsening symptoms or liver tests). In addition liver biopsy is indicated when there is any doubt of the diagnosis and to differentiate fatty liver from other types of alcoholic liver disease.

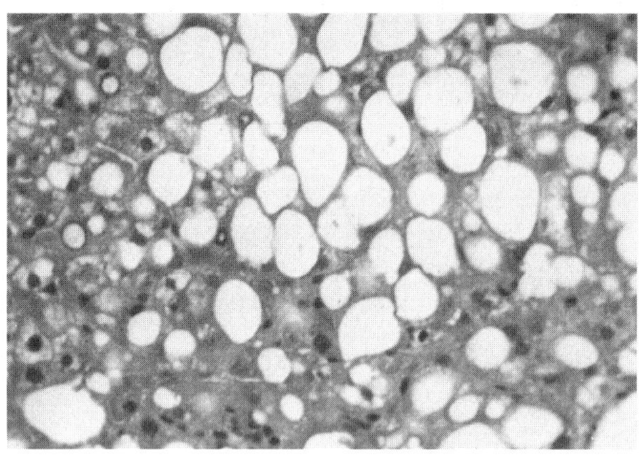

Figure 30-1 Macrovesicular and microvesicular steatosis (×63).

Treatment

The treatment of fatty liver consists of abstinence from alcohol and an adequate diet. Under this regimen the abnormal accumulation of fat disappears from the liver in 1 to 4 weeks. Bed rest is of no proven benefit. Androgenic steroids, which were found to increase the rate of lipid removal in some[7] but not other studies,[8] may be detrimental by producing cholestasis and are not indicated. Management of alcoholic patients with fatty liver often requires recognition and therapy of alcohol withdrawal. Preferred drugs for sedation in these patients are low doses of benzodiazepines. Multi-vitamins with folic acid are usually also provided because of the finding of frequent deficiencies in water-soluble vitamins in these patients.

Prognosis

Fatty liver in the alcoholic is usually a reversible condition; however, continued alcohol ingestion often leads to alcoholic hepatitis and cirrhosis. Dietary intake of fat and the development of fatty infiltration of the liver are important factors in the pathogenesis of alcoholic hepatitis and cirrhosis. Stellate cell activation was found on liver biopsies of patients with fatty liver with no evidence of alcoholic hepatitis or cirrhosis and the number of activated stellate cells correlated with the degree of steatosis.[9] The degree of fatty infiltration, the presence of Mallory bodies, and evidence of any pericellular or perivenular fibrosis on initial liver biopsy are all associated with an increased risk of developing cirrhosis.[10,11] Although the amount of dietary fat and its accumulation in the liver plays a role in alcohol-induced liver injury, the type of fat ingested may also be an important factor. In one study in France, dietary fat was higher in patients with alcoholic cirrhosis than in controls.[12] Comparison of dietary intake at similar per capita alcohol consumption in various countries indicated that a high intake of saturated fat was associated with a lower mortality from alcoholic cirrhosis. By contrast a high intake of unsaturated fat was associated with a higher mortality from cirrhosis.[13]

Alcoholic Hepatitis

Alcoholic hepatitis denotes the development of hepatocellular necrosis and inflammation occurring in chronic alcoholic patients. Alcoholic hepatitis is part of the spectrum of alcoholic liver disease that also includes fatty liver and cirrhosis. Alcoholic hepatitis often presents with acute symptoms but in most cases behaves as a chronic disease with progression to cirrhosis.[1] The mechanism that triggers the sudden development of alcoholic hepatitis in chronic alcoholics who have been drinking for many years remains a puzzle.

Clinical Presentation

The presenting symptoms in alcoholic hepatitis vary, but often include fatigue, anorexia, weight loss, jaundice, fever, and right upper quadrant abdominal pain. A very high fever can occur without evidence of sepsis. A few patients present for the first time with evidence of severe hepatocellular failure with ascites, hepatic encephalopathy, or gastrointestinal bleeding. Alcoholic hepatitis is a precursor of cirrhosis. The majority of patients presenting for the first time with alcoholic hepatitis who are biopsied already have evidence of significant fibrosis on liver biopsy and 50 percent already have cirrhosis.[14] Findings on physical examination often include low-grade fever, jaundice, parotid gland enlargement, spider angiomata, tender hepatomegaly, and sometimes splenomegaly and leg edema. Laboratory studies usually reveal anemia, macrocytosis, and leukocytosis. The cause of the anemia is multi-factorial and includes iron deficiency resulting from gastrointestinal bleeding, folate deficiency, hemolysis, and hypersplenism. Thrombocytopenia secondary to either ethanol-induced bone marrow suppression, folate deficiency, or hypersplenism may be present. Hypokalemia, hypophosphatemia, and hypomagnesemia are common. Hypokalemia and hypophosphatemia are major causes of muscle weakness. Hypomagnesemia can predispose the patient to seizures during alcohol withdrawal. The serum aminotransferases are moderately elevated, usually to less than 10 times above normal. Higher elevations of the aminotransferases indicate other types of liver injury such as viral hepatitis or acetaminophen toxicity. Characteristically, the serum AST is higher than the serum alanine aminotransferases (ALT). This is most likely related to pyridoxal 5′-phosphate (PLP) deficiency because it is a co-factor for the activity of aminotransferases and correction of PLP deficiency increases ALT with no change in AST. The serum glutamyl transpeptidase is also elevated, but it is of no value in the assessment of hepatocellular injury because it is often increased in alcoholics without significant liver injury as a result of microsomal enzyme induction by alcohol. Serum albumin is frequently depressed and prothrombin time prolonged. Cholestasis with striking elevation of serum alkaline phosphatase activity may occur and when associated with right upper quadrant pain, fever, and leukocytosis it may be confused with acute cholecystitis or extrahepatic biliary obstruction. Ideally, the diagnosis of alcoholic hepatitis should be confirmed by liver biopsy. The typical histologic picture of alcoholic hepatitis includes hepatocellular necrosis

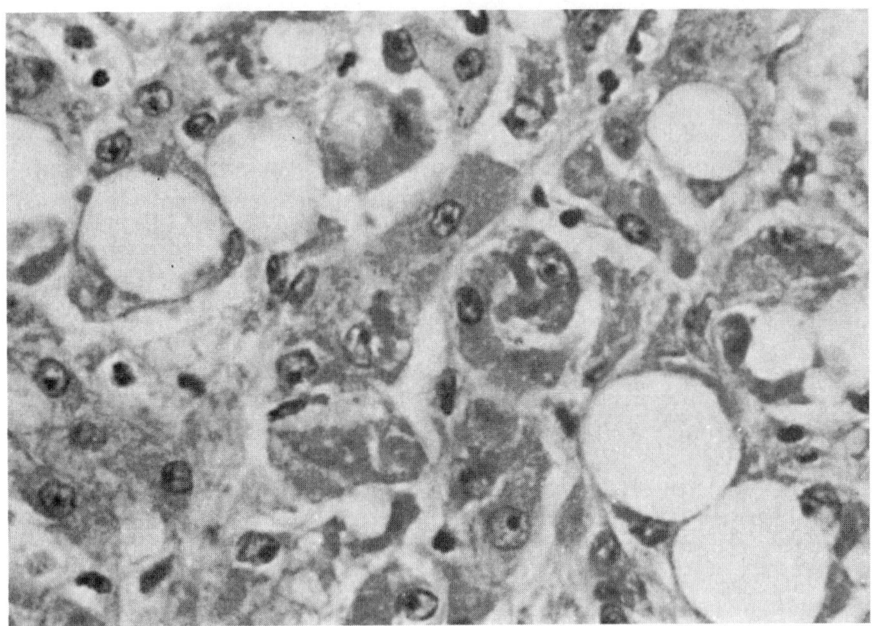

Figure 30-2 Mallory bodies and fatty changes in acute alcoholic hepatitis (×480).

and ballooning degeneration, alcoholic hyalin, and an inflammatory reaction with many polymorphonuclear leukocytes (Figure 30-2). Fatty infiltration is usually present. As noted previously, fibrosis is common and cirrhosis is often present. The pathologic findings in alcoholic hepatitis are most prominent in the centrolobular region. Fibrosis around the central veins can lead to obliteration and destruction of the hepatic vein branches (central hyalin sclerosis) (Figure 30-3). In many cases the diagnosis of alcoholic hepatitis is based on clinical data alone because a liver biopsy is not possible as a result of prolonged prothrombin time. Approximately 20 percent of patients with clinical and laboratory features compatible with alcoholic hepatitis are found on liver biopsy to have chronic hepatitis or other lesions such as granuloma.[15,16] Also complicating the diagnosis of alcoholic hepatitis is the high prevalence of antibodies to hepatitis C virus,[17] the concomitant use of illegal drugs, and the increased frequency of acquired immunodeficiency syndrome in chronic alcoholic patients.[18]

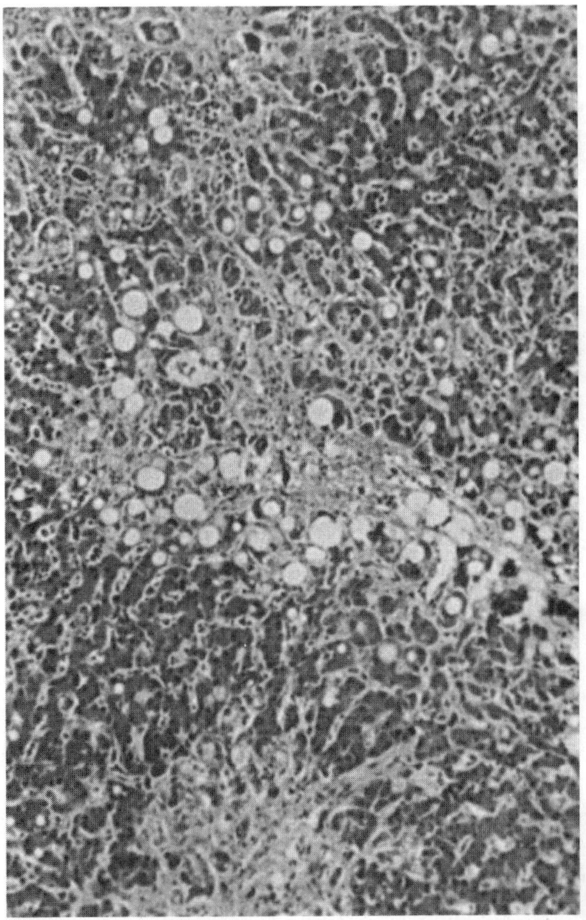

Figure 30-3 Chronic alcoholic liver disease manifested by sclerosing hyaline necrosis. Portal-central and intralobular fibrosis are pronounced (×75).

Differential Diagnosis

The diagnosis of viral hepatitis needs to be considered whenever serum aminotransferases are elevated more than 10 times above normal and when the AST is not higher than the ALT. The diagnosis of viral hepatitis is made by serologic measurements of viral hepatitis markers. In the case of hepatitis C the diagnosis requires the measurement of hepatitis C ribonucleic acid (RNA) because the antibody to hepatitis C may be falsely elevated in some patients with alcoholic hepatitis and hypergammaglobulinemia. Alcoholic patients presenting with very high elevations of serum aminotransferases should also be suspected of having superimposed acetaminophen hepatotoxicity. This diagnosis can be verified by a history of acetaminophen ingestion and high serum acetaminophen levels. Patients with acetaminophen hepatotoxicity often develop rapid worsening of prothrombin time. which is an unusual development in alcoholic hepatitis. Chronic alcohol ingestion increases the risk of developing acetaminophen hepatotoxicity because it enhances microsomal mixed function oxidase, which converts acetaminophen to its toxic metabolite and alcohol abuse decreases liver glutathione, which normally binds this toxic metabolite. Hence alcoholics may develop acetaminophen hepatotoxity after the ingestion of a dose of acetaminophen as low as 6 g (see Chap. 27).

Prognosis and Mortality

Patients with alcoholic hepatitis often worsen after admission to the hospital despite abstinence from alcohol, bed rest, and intake of an adequate diet.[19] The mortality rate in hospitalized patients varies from 4 percent to 40 percent in different series. Findings that correlate with poor prognosis are encephalopathy, depression of serum albumin, elevation of serum bilirubin above 20 mg/dl, and a prolonged prothrombin time (8 seconds or more above control) unresponsive to vitamin K administration.[19] The combination of elevated bilirubin and prolonged prothrombin time, which is the basis of the Maddrey's discriminant function of $4.6 \times$ (prothrombin time-control time [seconds] + bilirubin [mg/dl]) > 32, is a simple and very useful predictor of high mortality in patients with alcoholic hepatitis.[20] A combined clinical and laboratory index (CCLI) that correlates with prognosis in alcoholic liver disease has been developed.[21] The CCLI, which includes grading of seven clinical and five laboratory findings, has been useful in evaluating results of therapeutic clinical trials; however, it is cumbersome for routine evaluation of patients and less accurate because the assessment and grading of the clinical findings are subjective and influenced by observer variability. The Child-Turcotte classification and its Pugh modification originally developed to assess the ability of patients to tolerate shunt surgery are also good predictors of survival in patients with alcoholic cirrhosis.[22]

Long-term follow-up of patients with alcoholic hepatitis revealed that 38 percent of 61 patients who had no evidence of septum formation or cirrhosis on initial liver biopsy developed cirrhosis after a mean of 3.3 years.[14] Only 10 percent had complete resolution of their liver disease, whereas the remainder continued to have evidence of alcoholic hepatitis. The presence of alcoholic hepatitis on liver biopsy is associated with a worse long-term survival than the finding of inactive cirrhosis. The worst 5-year survival (46 percent) was in patients with alcoholic hepatitis superimposed on cirrhosis, and most of the deaths occurred in the first year after diagnosis.[23]

Treatment

Management of Alcohol Withdrawal. The initial management of patients with alcoholic liver disease often requires the recognition and therapy of alcohol withdrawal. Early symptoms of withdrawal are restlessness, anxiety, tremor, sweating, insomnia, and, occasionally, visual hallucinations. This is associated with an increased pulse rate and blood pressure and with dilation of the pupils. It can be followed by seizures or delirium tremens. The symptoms of alcohol withdrawal are sometimes difficult to distinguish from hepatic encephalopathy and both may co-exist. However, alcohol withdrawal is characterized by continuous symptoms of motor and autonomic hyperactivity and total insomnia, whereas in hepatic encephalopathy, the symptoms of hyperactivity and insomnia are usually transient, often occurring at night and alternating with episodes of somnolence during the day.

Delirium tremens, the most severe complication of alcohol withdrawal, usually occurs 2 to 3 days after the cessation of alcohol ingestion but may occur as late as 7 to 10 days. It is characterized by disorientation, confusion, hallucinations, agitation, marked autonomic activity, and, sometimes, seizures. The patient is usually febrile, with tachycardia, tachypnea, and diaphoresis, and has a flushed face and dilated pupils. The symptoms usually abate after 3 to 5 days. The most certain indication of the end of this syndrome is the occurrence of a deep sleep and of lucid intervals that increase in length. The mortality from delirium tremens has been reported to be as high as 30 percent.

Early alcohol withdrawal symptoms and their progression to seizures or to delirium tremens can be prevented by sedation. Preferred drugs for sedation in patients with liver disease are low doses of benzodiazepines such as oxazepam (Serax) or lorazepam (Ativan), which are metabolized and inactivated by glucuronidation, a pathway that is not affected by liver disease.[24] Oxazepam, 15 to 30 mg, or lorazepam, 0.5 to 1.0 mg, 3 times a day, is usually sufficient to control withdrawal symptoms without resulting in marked sedation. Patients with delirium tremens may need to be restrained initially while sedated with intravenous lorazepam 0.5 to 1.0 mg every 5 minutes until they are calm. Thereafter the restraints can be removed and subsequent doses of lorazepam can be individualized based on the lack of agitation. Benzodiazepines such as diazepam (Valium), which are initially metabolized to active forms by the mixed function oxidase system, should be avoided because the activity of this microsomal system can be increased by chronic alcohol ingestion or decreased in advanced liver disease. Management of alcohol withdrawal also requires attention to fluid and electrolyte replacement. This is given in accordance with what is estimated to be the daily requirements, taking into account the increased losses that occur with agitation, fever, and perspiration. In anorectic patients the fluids should provide a minimum of 1000 ml of 10 percent dextrose to prevent hypoglycemia and 1000 ml of normal saline. Thiamine, 100 mg intramuscularly, is administered to treat thiamine deficiency. Multi-vitamins, either intravenously or orally with folic acid 1 mg/day, are also provided because of the frequent deficiencies in water-soluble vitamins in these patients.

Nutritional Supplementation. The treatment of alcoholic hepatitis has consisted of abstinence from alcohol, bed rest, and intake of a normal 2500-calorie diet of normal protein content, provided there is no encephalopathy.

Replacement of nutrients and vitamins appears to be indicated because of the poor dietary intake, disturbed absorption and metabolism, and greater nutritional requirements induced by alcohol.[25] Furthermore, in the Veterans Administration Cooperative Study on Alcoholic Hepatitis, an association was found between the degree of protein-calorie malnutrition and the severity of illness and mortality.[26]

Patients with alcoholic hepatitis and malnutrition almost invariably have inadequate glycogen stores. Hence during fasting, their blood glucose is maintained by gluconeogenesis. A high demand for protein by gluconeogenesis and repair of liver injury results in enhanced release of amino acids from muscle that contributes to the muscle wasting often seen in these patients. It is therefore recommended that patients with alcoholic hepatitis who are unable to ingest a normal diet or who are subjected to prolonged periods of fasting be given continuous intravenous 10 percent dextrose (1-2 L per 24 hours) to maintain blood glucose.

Achievement of positive nitrogen balance by oral, enteric, or parenteral routes was an important determinant of survival in hospitalized patients with alcoholic hepatitis.[27] There was a 3.3 percent mortality in 30 patients who achieved a positive nitrogen balance compared with a 58 percent mortality in 19 patients who remained in negative nitrogen balance. An important effect of enteral formula feeding in malnourished patients with alcoholic liver disease is an increase in the digestibility and absorption of fat and protein. Controlled studies of the effects of enteral administration of nutrients have revealed improvement in nutritional parameters, clinical state, serum albumin, and liver function as measured by anti-pyrine clearance (Table 30-1).[28-30] There is no advantage in the administration of formulas enriched in branched chain amino acids over regular amino acids or casein hydrolysates. In one study encephalopathy improved after enteral administration of casein hydrolysates as a supplement to a hospital diet to achieve a mean protein intake of 103 g per day compared with a control group ingesting a mean of 50 g of dietary protein per day. Improved survival was demonstrated in only one small study in a group receiving 71 g of protein per day in the form of an enteral formula of amino acids enriched in branched chain amino acids compared with a control group ingesting a mean of 45 g of protein per day.[29] Controlled studies of parenteral amino acid supplementation in patients with alcoholic hepatitis also show improvement in nutritional parameters, clinical state, and serum albumin, bilirubin, prothrombin time, and liver function measured by galactose elimination capacity or aminopyrine clearance (Table 30-2). Parenteral amino acid supplementation for 1 month in patients with moderately severe biopsy-proven alcoholic hepatitis resulted in more rapid clinical improvement and greater resolution of fatty infiltration, but did not otherwise affect hepatic histology.[31] In patients with severe alcoholic hepatitis, Nasrallah and Galambos[35] showed that parenteral amino acid supplementation (70-85 g/day) resulted in greater clinical and laboratory improvement and increased survival. In a similar study of patients with severe alcoholic hepatitis by Mezey and colleagues[36] parenteral amino acid supplementation improved nutritional states and liver tests but did not affect 1-month hospital survival or 2-year follow-up survival. However, despite the lack of effect on survival, patients who had been treated with amino acids continued to have improvement in serum bilirubin, prothrombin time, retinol binding protein, and transferrin after discharge from the hospital. This delayed beneficial effect of amino acid therapy may be due to accelerated repair of hepatocellular damage.

Vitamin deficiencies are common in alcoholic liver disease. Low circulating levels of two or more water-soluble vitamins are found in approximately 40 percent of patients.[37] Folic acid is the vitamin most commonly found deficient, followed by thiamine, riboflavin, nicotinic acid, and pyridoxine. In most patients with mild to moderate alcoholic hepatitis, daily ingestion of a multivitamin preparation that contains folic acid (0.5 to 1.0 mg), thiamine (10-15 mg), and pyridoxine (2-4 mg) is sufficient to correct mild vitamin deficiencies or prevent their development. However, if the patient is unable to maintain an adequate oral intake or has severe vitamin deficiencies with clinical manifestations, much higher doses of the vitamins are indicated. Suggested daily doses are as follows: folic acid 1 to 5 mg; thiamine 50 to 100 mg; and pyridoxine 100 mg. Vitamin K_1 10 mg intramuscularly should always be administered as one dose

TABLE 30-1

Effect of Enteral Nutrition on Outcome in Alcoholic Hepatitis

References	Therapy	Patients (no.)	Duration of therapy (days)	Mean daily protein intake	Clinical improvement as compared to control	Mortality during therapy (%)
Mendenhall et al. (28)	BCAA (55 g/day)	34	30	98.3 g	Nutritional parameters only	17
	Control	18	30	81.3 g		21 (NS)
Cabre et al. (29)	AA + BCAA	16	23	71 g	Child's score	12
	Control	19	25	45 g	Albumin	47 (p = 0.02)
Kearns et al. (30)	Casein hydrolysate	16	11	1.5 g/kg	Encephalopathy Albumin	0
	Control	15	12	0.7 g/kg	Antipyrine elimination	13 (NS)

From Mezey E: Treatment of alcoholic liver disease. Semin Liver Dis 13:210-216, 1993.
BCAA, Branched chain amino acids; *NS,* not significant; *AA,* amino acids.

TABLE 30-2

Effect of Parenteral Nutritional Supplementation for 1 Month on Outcome in Alcoholic Hepatitis

References	Therapy	Patients (no.)	Mean protein intake (g/day)	Nitrogen balance (g/day)	Clinical and laboratory improvement as compared to control	Mortality (%)
Diehl et al. (31)	AA* (51.6 g/day)	5	138.6	10.5	More rapid improvement in composite clinical index‡	0
	Dextrose†	10	97.6	4.1		0
Bonkovsky et al. (32,33)	AA	9	125§	6.8§	Galactose clearance	
	Control	12	65	3.2		
Naveau et al. (34)	AA, dextrose/ Intralipid	20+	—	—	Bilirubin	5
	Control	20+	—	—		
Nasrallah and Galambos (35)	AA* (70-85 g/day)	17	—	—	Ascites, encephalopathy	0
	Control	18			Bilirubin, albumin	22 ($p < 0.02$)
Mezey et al. (36)	AA* (51.6 g/day) + dextrose	28	114.4	13.2	Bilirubin, AST‡ prothrombin time	21
	Dextrose	26	54.6	6.8	Aminopyrine clearance	19

From Mezey E: Treatment of alcoholic liver disease. Semin Liver Dis 13:210-216, 1993.
AA, Amino acids; *AST,* aspartate aminotransferase.
*FreAmine III, Kendall McGaw, Irvine, Calif.
†Patients with alcoholic cirrhosis.
‡Composite clinical index described by Orrego H, Israel Y, Blake JE, et al: Assessment of prognostic factors in alcoholic liver disease: toward a global quantitative expression of severity. Hepatology 3:896-905, 1983.
§Value approximated from figures in manuscript.

TABLE 30-3

Effect of Corticosteroids on Mortality in Patients with Severe Alcoholic Hepatitis

	MORTALITY/NUMBER STUDIED (%)		
References	Placebo	Corticosteroids	*p* value
Helman et al. (34)	6/17 (35)	1/20 (5)	NS
Encephalopathy subgroup	6/6 (100)	1/9 (11)	<.01
Maddrey et al. (19)	6/31 (19)	1/24 (4)	NS
DF > 93 subgroup*	6/8 (75)	1/7 (14)	<.05
Carithers et al. (20)	11/31 (35)	2/35 (6)	.006
Raymond et al. (35)	16/29 (55)	4/32 (12)	.001

From Mezey E: Treatment of alcoholic liver disease. Semin Liver Dis 13:210-216, 1993.
NS, Not significant; *DF,* discriminant function.
*DF = 4.6 × prothrombin time + serum bilirubin (mg/dl).

initially in all patients presenting with a prolonged prothrombin time. Any correction of the prothrombin time resulting from vitamin K deficiency will occur with one 10-mg dose of vitamin K_1; further daily administration of this vitamin is unnecessary. Some patients with alcoholic hepatitis require potassium, phosphorus, magnesium, or zinc replacement. Potassium can be replaced with oral solutions of 10 percent potassium chloride, which provides 40 mEq per ounce; alternatively, it can be given intravenously. Phosphorus deficiency, which can be a major cause of muscle weakness, is treated with Neutrophos tablets (K-phos neutral), which are given 4 times a day to provide a total daily dose of 1 g of phosphorus. Magnesium is replaced by intramuscular injection of 2 ml of a 50 percent solution of magnesium sulfate followed by daily ingestion of oral magnesium sulfate. Patients with evidence of poor wound healing or a low serum zinc level are given 200 mg of zinc sulfate daily.

Corticosteroids. Several randomized controlled studies investigated the benefit of corticosteroids in alcoholic hepatitis. In all these studies corticosteroids were given as 40 mg of prednisone or prednisolone or 32 mg of methylprednisolone per day for 4 to 6 weeks in the hospital.[1] This regimen did not increase survival when patients with varying severity of alcoholic hepatitis were considered together. However, corticosteroids increased survival in patients with severe illness manifested by encephalopathy or by very abnormal prothrombin times and bilirubin levels (Table 30-3). Patients presenting with infection or gastrointestinal bleeding were excluded from most of these trials. In the original controlled trial, the administration of prednisolone, 40 mg per day for 1 month, improved survival only in a subgroup of patients with hepatic encephalopathy.[38] Only one of nine patients on prednisolone died as compared with all six patients on placebo. In a subsequent study it was found that a discriminant function of 4.6 × prothrombin time (seconds) + bilirubin (mg/dl) > 93 predicted a high mortality and use of corticosteroids in this severely ill group of patients' improved survival.[19] It is important to note that vitamin K_1 was administered 24 hours before determination of the prothrombin time for use in the calculation of the discriminant function. In a multi-center study, it was demonstrated that methylprednisolone in a dose of 32 mg per day for 28 days improved survival in patients who were selected on the basis of the high discriminant function.[20] In a French study of patients with biopsy-proven alcoholic hepatitis with either spontaneous hepatic encephalopathy or a high discriminant function, prednisolone in a dose of 40 mg per day for 28 days resulted in improved 2-month survival.[39] The discriminant function in the last two studies[44,45] was modified to 4.6 × (prothrombin time of patient - control time [seconds] + bilirubin [mg/dl]) > 32 to reduce variability between different institutions. The corticosteroid therapy also was found to result in more rapid improvement in prothrombin time, bilirubin, albumin, and AST. Meta-analysis of 11 studies conducted between 1966 and 1989 comprising 562 patients, 45 percent of whom had encephalopathy, revealed that corticosteroids reduced mortality by 37 percent (95 percent confidence interval 20 percent to 50 percent).[40] Corticosteroids reduced mortality in the subgroup of patients with hepatic encephalopathy by 34 percent (95 percent confidence interval 15 percent to 48 percent), but not in those without encephalopathy. Also, the beneficial effect of corticosteroids was dependent on the exclusion of patients with acute gastrointestinal bleeding. Another meta-analysis of 10 studies also concluded that corticosteroids improved short-term survival.[41] There is no evidence that corticosteroids affect survival beyond 2 months after hospital discharge.

Complications of corticosteroid therapy have been minimal, consisting of hyperglycemia, infection occasionally with fungi, and pancreatitis in a few patients. The effect of corticosteroids in decreasing mortality in patients with hepatic encephalopathy in the initial controlled trial was associated with intake of more calories, suggesting that this was a factor in reducing mortality. However, in a subsequent study by the same group, prednisolone was again demonstrated to significantly improve survival in patients with alcoholic hepatitis and encephalopathy as compared to those receiving oral or intravenous nutrient supplements of at least 1600 calories/day.[42] Comparison of enteral feeding of a 2000-calorie daily diet containing 72 g of protein consisting of milk protein with added amino acids (31 percent branched chain amino acids) with prednisolone therapy for 28 days showed no difference in mortality between the two groups.[43] However, the deaths in the enteral feeding group occurred during the feeding, whereas those in the steroid group occurred in the immediate weeks after therapy and were mainly from infections.

Present recommendation is to treat patients with severe alcoholic hepatitis, defined by the presence of encephalopathy or the abnormal discriminant factor, with 40 mg of prednisolone (or 32 mg of methylprednisolone, which is the equivalent dose) for 1 month followed by tapering and discontinuation of the therapy in the following 2 to 4 weeks. Patients with evidence of infection or recent acute gastrointestinal bleeding do not qualify for this therapy.

Pentoxifylline. Pentoxifylline is a non-selective phosphodiesterase inhibitor, which has been shown to decrease tumor necrosis alpha (TNFα) production.[44] Elevations of TNFα correlate with severity of the disease and mortality in patients with alcoholic hepatitis.[45] In one randomized controlled study the administration of pentoxifylline to patients with severe alcoholic hepatitis, with Maddrey's discriminant function greater than 32, in a dose of 400 mg 3 times per day for 4 weeks, resulted in significant decreases in mortality and in the development of hepatorenal syndrome as compared to control patients on placebo.[46] The reduced mortality was mostly related to the decreased risk of developing the hepatorenal syndrome.

Propylthiouracil. The rationale for treatment of alcoholic hepatitis with propylthiouracil are animal experiments showing that it decreases an alcohol-induced hypermetabolic state and prevents centrolobular necrosis in rats exposed to low oxygen tensions.[47] In an initial study propylthiouracil in a dose of 300 mg per day for a maximum of 46 days resulted in a more rapid improvement in a CCLI reflecting common clinical findings and liver tests as compared to placebo.[21,48] In a subsequent study by the same group, propylthiouracil 300 mg per day given in cyclical periods of 3 months separated by 1-month intervals of placebo for a maximum of 2 years resulted in an improved survival as compared to placebo-treated patients.[49] The cumulative mortality was decreased to 13 percent in the patients receiving propylthiouracil compared with 25 percent in the placebo group. The therapy was most effective in increasing survival in individuals with more severe disease. Prolongations of the prothrombin time 3 seconds above control and decreases in hemoglobin levels to less than 90 percent below the lower limit of normal were found to be important prognostic factors. In patients with these severe abnormalities, propylthiouracil decreased mortality to 20 percent as compared with a mortality of 62 percent in the placebo group. Propylthiouracil did not increase survival in patients who continued to drink excessively as determined from high concentrations of alcohol in the urine. A confounding factor in the interpretation of the results of the study was a high dropout rate during follow-up. Propylthiouracil produced subclinical hypothyroidism as indicated by elevations of serum thyroid-stimulating hormone and decreases in serum thyroxine levels. No significant changes were observed in serum triiodothyronine levels. In another study administration of propylthiouracil for 6 weeks to patients with severe alcoholic hepatitis had no beneficial effect on morbidity or mortality.[50] Propylthiouracil is regarded as a potential therapeutic agent for alcoholic hepatitis. Its acceptance as a definitive therapeutic agent will require demonstration of a beneficial effect in additional large controlled clinical trials.

Anabolic Steroids. The administration of oxandrolone, 80 mg per day for 1 month, did not affect survival during this short-term administration but increased survival at 6 months in patients with moderate, but not severe, alcoholic hepatitis.[51] In a second study oxandrolone 80 mg per day for 1 month followed by 40 mg per day for 2 additional months together with branched chain amino acid supplements resulted again in an increase in survival at the 6 month follow-up point in a subgroup of patients with alcoholic hepatitis and moderate protein calorie malnutrition.[52] No such effect could be demonstrated in patients with mild or severe malnutrition. In another, smaller, study the combination of parenteral amino acids and oxandrolone for 21 days resulted in improvement in Child-Pugh score and antipyrine clearance as compared to standard hospital diet in patients with moderate to severe alcoholic hepatitis. Oxandrolone alone improved serum albumin and antipyrine clearance but to a lesser extent than when combined with parenteral nutrition. The beneficial delayed effect of oxandrolone on survival, found only in patients who present with moderate malnutrition, remains puzzling and requires further confirmation before its use can be recommended.

Insulin and Glucagon. The potential therapeutic use of insulin and glucagon in alcoholic hepatitis is based on observations that this combination of hormones accelerates hepatic regeneration after partial hepatectomy in experimental animals. A few initial studies showed improved survival after daily infusion of insulin and glucagon in patients with severe alcoholic hepatitis.[53] However, two other studies[54,55] in which insulin (30 IU) and glucagon (3 mg) in 250 to 500 ml of 5 percent dextrose were infused 12 hours each day for 3 weeks showed no benefit on clinical or biochemical parameters or in hospital survival or survival after 6 months of follow-up. Several patients developed significant hypoglycemia during the infusions. On the basis of the data available, insulin and glucagon infusions are not indicated in the therapy of alcoholic hepatitis, and may even be dangerous.

D-Penicillamine. D-penicillamine is known to reduce collagen synthesis by interference with cross-linking of collagen molecules. A 2-month controlled trial of 40 patients with alcoholic hepatitis treated with 1 g per day of D-penicillamine revealed no improvement in survival or liver tests.[56] However, hepatocellular injury and fibrosis appeared to be less in the biopsies of the treated patients as compared to the controls. In another study treatment with the same dose of D-penicillamine for 1 month did not improve liver histology.[57] An initially elevated hepatic proline hydroxylase activity, which catalyzes an early step in collagen synthesis, was further increased in four of five patients receiving placebo, but fell in all three receiving D-penicillamine.[58] It remains unknown whether therapy with D-penicillamine for a longer period will reduce hepatic fibrosis or alter survival.

Hepatoprotective Agents. Hepatoprotective agents such as (+)-cyanidanol-3, which are anti-oxidants and free radical scavengers, have not been found to have any consistent benefit in patients with alcoholic hepatitis or cirrhosis.[59] Recently in a large European cooperative study malotilate was found to marginally increase survival when given in a dose of 750 mg per day for 2 years; however, when given in a higher dose of 1500 mg per day it was of no benefit.[60]

Phosphatidylcholine. Phosphatidylcholine was shown to prevent the progression of early stages of pericentral and interstitial fibrosis to septal fibrosis and cirrhosis in alcohol-fed baboons.[61] A Veterans Administration Cooperative study is under way to test the usefulness of phosphatidylcholine in the prevention of fibrogenesis and cirrhosis in alcoholic liver disease.

Cirrhosis

Clinical Presentation

The clinical presentation of the patient with alcoholic cirrhosis is quite variable. Many of the patients are asymptomatic whereas others present with jaundice, ascites (see Chap. 22), bleeding varices (see Chap. 21), or hepatic encephalopathy (see Chap. 15). Laboratory tests also are quite variable. They may be normal in the patient who has stopped drinking for several months or they may reflect underlying alcoholic hepatitis (see previous section). Last, if the disease is advanced, hepatic insufficiency with low albumin and prolonged prothrombin times may be the principal laboratory abnormalities.

The diagnosis of alcoholic cirrhosis is based on a history of excessive alcohol intake (40-60 g/day in men, 20 g/day in women), negative serologies for the other causes of liver disease, and, if possible, a liver biopsy showing micronodular cirrhosis (Figure 30-4). If the patient has stopped drinking for several weeks to months, all the other histologic features of alcoholic liver disease (fat, alcoholic hyalin, polymorphonuclear infiltrate [PMNs]) may be lacking in the liver biopsy.

Treatment

Nutritional Supplementation. The treatment of uncomplicated cirrhosis consists of abstinence from alcohol, voluntary restriction of activity if the patient has weakness and fatigue, and a diet normal in protein (1 g/kg body weight/day) but low in salt. Therapy with oral or enteral formulas of casein hydrolysates or amino acids is indicated in anorectic malnourished patients or those intolerant of regular dietary protein and susceptible to encephalopathy. Oral and enteral administration of formulas providing 40 to 140 g protein/day improved nutritional status and serum albumin levels in patients with cirrhosis.[62] Oral administration of up to 80 g/day of branched chain amino acids improved nitrogen balance without causing encephalopathy in patients with cirrhosis.[63] Comparison of a casein-based supplement with branched chain amino acids revealed equal tolerance to intake of 60 to 70 g of daily protein without worsening

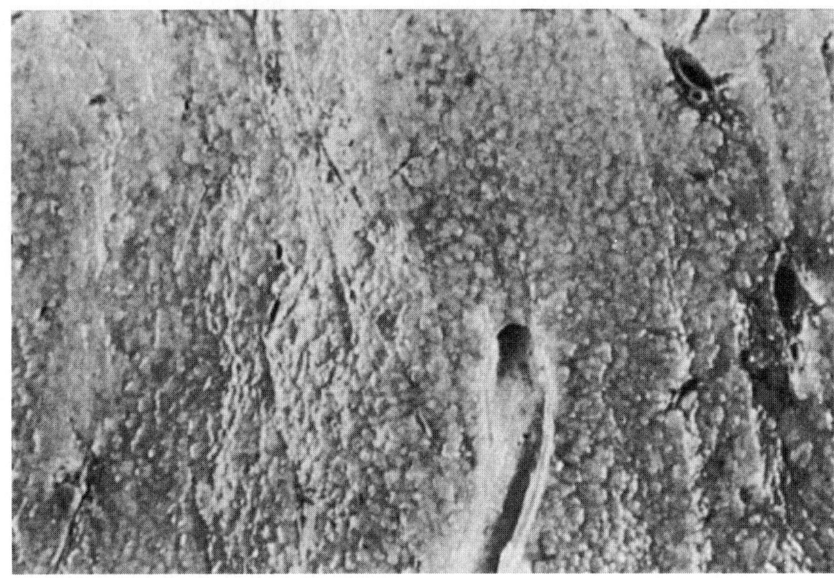

Figure 30-4 Micronodular cirrhosis. The regeneration nodules are small and uniform. The fibrosis that encircles them is delicate.

of mental status.[64] Multi-vitamins and folic acid, 1 mg/day, are given if the patient has evidence of vitamin deficiencies or is unable to achieve adequate dietary intake. Abstinence from alcohol improves long-term survival of patients with cirrhosis, with the exception of patients with advanced cirrhosis and portal hypertension.

Colchicine. Colchicine is a promising drug in the treatment of cirrhosis. It interferes with collagen synthesis by various mechanisms and it also increases collagenase production in vitro. Treatment with colchicine, 1 mg/day for 5 days per week, increased 5- to 10-year survival in patients with cirrhosis in one study.[65] Ten-year survivals were 56 percent in the group receiving colchicine compared with 30 percent in the placebo group. The results, however, are weakened by loss of follow-up in 20 percent of the patients and of poor compliance. Forty-one percent of the patients had alcoholic cirrhosis, 41 percent had posthepatic cirrhosis, and the remaining had cirrhosis of various causes. Histologic improvement was found in repeat liver biopsies of 9 of 30 patients on colchicine, but in none of 14 patients on placebo. In nine patients on colchicine who improved, the repeat liver biopsy showed fibrosis in seven and normal results in two. However, this result has to be interpreted with caution because of the known sampling variability of liver biopsies. In one study comparing the results from percutaneous liver biopsy immediately before autopsy to the findings at autopsy, cirrhosis was correctly diagnosed in only 80 percent of cases when only one specimen was taken at biopsy.[66] In another study colchicine therapy (1 mg per day) for 6 months in patients with alcoholic hepatitis and cirrhosis had no effect on survival or hepatic fibrosis.[67] Colchicine administration for 1 month did not alter survival in hospitalized patients with severe alcoholic hepatitis.[68] A large Veterans Administration cooperative trial is under way to obtain more definitive answers about the potential benefit of colchicine in alcoholic liver disease.

***S*-adenosylmethionine.** *S*-adenosylmethionine is known to increase depleted hepatic glutathione levels in experimental animals and in humans with alcoholic liver disease. Administration of *S*-adenosylmethionine in a dose of 1200 mg per day for 2 years to patients with alcoholic cirrhosis in a controlled trial resulted in a decreased mortality or delay in liver transplantation only in patients with Child's class A and B cirrhosis.[69]

Liver Transplantation. Liver transplantation is an important option in patients with alcoholic cirrhosis who have recognized their alcoholism and achieved sobriety in an alcoholism treatment program. Two-year survivals of 71 percent[70] and 73 percent[71] in two different studies of patients transplanted for alcoholic cirrhosis were similar to those found in patients with cirrhosis transplanted for other conditions. The rate of resumption of alcohol consumption during a 2-year follow-up period in the above two studies was 11.5 percent[70] and 15.1 percent.[71] Of importance was the finding that the resumption of alcohol consumption was 6.7 percent in the patients who had stopped drinking for more than 6 months before transplantation as compared to 43 percent in individuals who had been sober for less than 6 months before transplantation.[70] Patients transplanted for alcoholic hepatitis superimposed on cirrhosis had a survival similar to those transplanted for end-stage alcoholic cirrhosis.[72] However, resumption of alcoholic ingestion at 1 year after transplantation was 49 percent in those transplanted with alcoholic hepatitis as compared with 11 percent in those transplanted for cirrhosis alone. This difference presumably is due to lack of significant period of sobriety in patients with alcoholic hepatitis before transplantation. Patients transplanted for alcoholic liver disease who resumed alcoholic abuse are at risk of developing rapid recurrence of the disease. In 29 patients transplanted for alcoholic cirrhosis who resumed alcohol ingestion and were followed from 11 to 125 months (median 50 months), 3 (10 percent) developed alcoholic hepatitis, 8 (28 percent) centrolobular fibrosis, and 6 (23 percent) either bridging fibrosis or cirrhosis.[73] However, 5 of the latter 6 patients also had chronic hepatitis C. In another study three of six patients who returned to heavy alcohol ingestion after liver transplantation developed severe alcoholic hepatitis, causing their death at 9 months, 2.5 years, and 3.5 years after their transplant.[74] The results indicate that liver transplantation is an effective therapy for end-stage alcoholic cirrhosis. It is not recommended in patients who present with alcoholic hepatitis or have not achieved 6 months or more of sobriety.

Alcoholic Liver Disease and Hepatitis C Infection

The prevalence of hepatitis C infection is as high as 45 percent in patients with alcoholism, being greatest in those with evidence of liver disease. In one study of alcoholics in Spain, the prevalence of antibody to hepatitis C virus was 20 percent in patients with steatosis, 21 percent in patients with alcoholic hepatitis, and 43 percent in those with alcoholic cirrhosis.[75] The heavy ingestion of alcohol in patients with chronic hepatitis C accelerates the progression of liver fibrosis and the development of cirrhosis (see Chap. 33).[76,77] In one study ingestion of more than 50 g of ethanol per day for 5 years in patients with hepatitis C was associated with cirrhosis in 58 percent of individuals after 10 to 20 years compared with an incidence of cirrhosis of 12 percent in patients ingesting lesser amounts or no alcohol at all.[77] In addition, the quantity of alcohol ingested correlates directly with the levels of hepatitis C RNA in the blood.[78] Hence it is mandatory that all patients with chronic hepatitis C be abstinent from alcohol. The liver pathology in patients with chronic hepatitis C who ingest alcohol heavily is usually that of chronic viral hepatitis, rather than of alcoholic liver disease. The treatment of patients with alcoholic liver disease and hepatitis C requires sobriety before the initiation of interferon and ribavirin therapy and continued sobriety during the treatment (see Chap. 33).

NON-ALCOHOLIC STEATOHEPATITIS

Clinical Features

Non-alcoholic steatohepatitis (NASH) is a chronic form of liver disease of unknown etiology characterized histologically by fatty infiltration often accompanied by hepatocellular damage with inflammation resembling alcoholic hepatitis. A careful history of a lack of significant alcohol intake is essential to establish this diagnosis. NASH is one of the most common causes of elevated aminotransferases in patients referred for evaluation to hepatologists. The age of most patients ranges between 36 and 65 years with a mean age of 53 years[79]; 65 percent to 81 percent of the patients are female.[80] Obesity defined as greater than 30 percent over ideal weight was found in 70 percent of patients in one study.[78] In another study, however, obesity defined as weight greater than 10 percent over ideal weight was present in only 39 percent of the patients.[81] Non-insulin-dependent diabetes mellitus was found in 34 percent to 75 percent of patients.[80] Most of the patients are asymptomatic and liver disease is discovered by finding elevated serum aminotransferases. The principal symptoms, when present, are fatigue and right upper abdominal discomfort.[81,82] Hepatomegaly is found in 90 percent of cases, but splenomegaly is rare. The principal and often sole laboratory abnormality is an elevation of the serum aminotransferases. Characteristically the elevation of the serum aminotransferases is mild (usually less than 3 times above the normal values) and the serum ALT levels are usually higher than the AST level, which helps in differentiating non-alcoholic from alcoholic steatohepatitis.[83] The serum alkaline phosphatase is elevated in approximately 50 percent of patients, whereas serum bilirubin, albumin, and prothrombin time are usually normal. Hyperlipidemia (hypertriglyceridemia, hypercholesterolemia, or both) has been reported in 20 percent to 81 percent of patients with NASH.[80] Hyperglycemia is common because many of these patients are known to have diabetes at presentation. Serum ferritin and transferrin saturation were elevated in 55 percent and 6 percent of patients, respectively, in one series from the United States[81] and in 62 percent and 22 percent, respectively, in a study from Australia.[84] Of note is that in the Australian study 31 percent of the patients with NASH were either homozygous (8 percent) or heterozygous (23 percent) for the hereditary hemochromatosis (HFE) gene. All four patients homozygous for the HFE gene had elevated serum transferrin saturation but one of them did not have significant iron deposition in the liver. On the other hand 20 percent of the patients with increased stainable hepatic iron stores did not have the HFE mutation. The authors also noted an association between hepatic iron accumulation and the severity of hepatic fibrosis.

Diagnosis and Pathogens

Ultrasonography is the best method for detection of fatty infiltration of the liver as described previously in the section on alcoholic fatty liver. Liver biopsy is indicated in symptomatic patients with serum aminotransferase elevations of more than 6 months' duration. The histologic features of NASH, which are mostly indistinguishable from those of alcoholic hepatitis, include macrovesicular fatty infiltration, hepatocellular necrosis and ballooning degeneration, alcoholic hyalin, and an inflammatory reaction with many polymorphonuclear leukocytes (see Figures 30-1, 30-2, and 30-3). Fibrosis, when present, is initially detected around the central hepatic venules and in the perisinusoidal spaces. In more advanced cases septal fibrosis and cirrhosis may have developed.

The pathogenesis of NASH remains to be determined but appears to be multi-factorial.[82] Possible factors in the pathogenesis include carbohydrate and insulin excess leading to increased accumulation of fatty acids, endotoxemia with increase in TNFα-mediated injury, formation of oxygen radicals resulting in lipid peroxidation, and mitochondrial dysfunction.

Prognosis

The prognosis of patients with NASH is dependent on whether the patient has significant hepatic fibrosis or cirrhosis when first diagnosed. A review of nine series of patients with NASH revealed that 15 percent to 50 percent of patients have evidence of significant hepatic fibrosis or cirrhosis.[82] An analysis of 42 patients followed for a median of 4.5 years in which initially only 2 subjects had marked fibrosis and 1 had cirrhosis showed the progression of fibrosis to cirrhosis in only 1 case.[85] Although clinical course appears to be benign in patients with fatty infiltration and minimal or no fibrosis, patients with moderate to severe fibrosis were estimated to have at least a 5 percent risk of progressing to cirrhosis.[82] In one study liver-related deaths occurred in 11 percent of patients with evidence of hepatocellular damage in addition to fatty infiltration over a 10-year period.[86] NASH is a cause of some cases of cryptogenic cirrhosis. In a case-controlled study the prevalence of obesity and type II diabetes was 55 percent and 47 percent, respectively, in cryptogenic cirrhosis as compared with 24 percent and 22 percent in controls with cirrhosis of known causes.[87] Both obesity and type II diabetes were found in 23 percent of patients with cryptogenic cirrhosis as compared with 5 percent in those with cirrhosis of known causes. Thus a significant number of patients with cryptogenic cirrhosis may have NASH as the cause of their liver disease.

Treatment

Treatment in overweight patients consists of gradual moderate weight loss by placing the patient on a low-fat, low-carbohydrate, and high-protein diet. Weight loss often results in a fall in serum aminotransferases and in a decrease in fatty infiltration assessed by ultrasonography or by liver biopsy, but does not change the amount of fibrosis on liver biopsy.[88,89] Very rapid weight reduction, such as occurs after jejunoileal bypass, accelerates the progression of the disease.[90] Hyperglycemia and hyperlipidemia are controlled with medication. A few investigational drugs such as antibiotics, ursodeoxycholic acid, and vitamin E are under evaluation. Gemfibrozil, given as 600 mg/day for 4 weeks, was evaluated in a controlled trial in 46 patients.[91] ALT decreased in 74 percent of patients on gemfibrozil versus 30 percent of controls, whereas there were no significant differences in serum triglyceride levels. Vitamin E in doses of 400 to 1200 IU per day normalized elevated serum aminotransferases and alkaline phosphatase in 11 children with NASH aged 8.3 to 14.2 (mean 12.4) years.[92] However, despite the improvement in liver tests, fatty infiltration detected by ultrasonography remained unchanged. Ursodeoxycholic acid in a dose of 13 to 15 mg/kg/day for 1 year in a pilot study of 24 patients resulted in a decrease in hepatic steatosis on repeat liver biopsy in 12 of 19 patients, but there were no changes in mean ALT levels or in the histologic grade of inflammation or fibrosis.[93] By contrast, treatment with clofibrate, 2 g/day for 1 year, was without benefit.[93]

Liver transplantation is indicated for patients with NASH who have developed advanced cirrhosis. In one study of eight patients who underwent transplantation for NASH, six developed recurrent NASH. In three of these six patients, perivenular fibrosis recurred.[94] The recurrences appear to be related to post-transplant hyperlipidemia and increases in body weight.

Obesity and Liver Disease

Obesity, as noted previously, is a risk factor for alcoholic liver disease and a common factor in patients with NASH. Obesity in non-alcoholic patients with elevated serum aminotransferases was shown to be associated with a septal fibrosis in 30 percent and cirrhosis in 11 percent of patients.[95] A study from Italy shows that obesity is a greater risk factor for steatosis than alcohol ingestion because the prevalence of steatosis was 1.6-fold higher in obese nondrinking patients than in non-obese heavy drinkers.[96] Furthermore, the prevalence of steatosis increases markedly in obese heavy drinkers. Most likely the more severe alcoholic liver disease in obese alcoholic patients is related to the worse steatosis caused by the combination of obesity and heavy alcohol ingestion.

References

1. Mezey E: Alcoholic liver disease. Prog Liver Dis 7:555-572, 1982.
2. Pequignot G, Tuyns AJ: Compared toxicity of ethanol on various organs. In Stock C, Sarles H, eds: Alcohol and the Gastrointestinal Tract. Paris, INSERM, 1980:17-32.
3. Naveau S, Giraud V, Borotto E, et al: Excess weight risk factor for alcoholic liver disease. Hepatology 25:108-111, 1997.
4. Iturriaga H, Bunout D, Hirsh S, et al: Overweight as a risk factor or a predictive sign of histological liver damage in alcoholics. Am J Clin Nutr 47:235-238, 1988.
5. Zwiebel WJ: Sonographic diagnosis of diffuse liver disease. Semin Ultrasound CT MRI 16:8-15, 1995.
6. Foster KJ, Dewbury KC, Griffith AH, et al: The accuracy of ultrasound in the detection of fatty infiltration of the liver. Br J Radiol 53:440-442, 1980.
7. Mendenhall CL: Anabolic steroid therapy as an adjunct to diet in alcoholic hepatic steatosis. Am J Dig Dis 13:783-791, 1968.
8. Fenster LF: The nonefficacy of short-term anabolic steroid therapy in alcoholic liver disease. Ann Int Med 65:738-744, 1966.
9. Reeves HL, Burt AD, Wood S, et al: Hepatic stellate cell activation occurs in the absence of hepatitis in alcoholic liver disease and correlates with the severity of steatosis. J Hepatol 25:677-683, 1966.
10. Sorensen TIA, Orholm M, Bentsen KD, et al: Prospective evaluation of alcohol abuse and alcoholic liver injury in men as predictors of development of cirrhosis. Lancet 2:241-244, 1984.
11. Nakano M, Worner TM, Lieber CS: Perivenular fibrosis in alcoholic liver injury: ultrastructure and histologic progression. Gastroenterology 83:777-785, 1982.
12. Rotily M, Durbec JP, Berthezene P, et al: Diet and alcohol in liver cirrhosis: a case control study. Eur J Clin Nutr 44:595-603, 1990.
13. Nanji, AA, French SW: Dietary factors in alcoholic cirrhosis. Alcohol Clin Exp Res 10:271-273, 1986.
14. Galambos JT: Alcoholic hepatitis: its therapy and prognosis. Prog Liver Dis 4:567-588, 1972.
15. Goldberg SJ, Mendenhall CL, Connell AM, et al: "Nonalcoholic" chronic hepatitis in the alcoholic. Gastroenterology 72:598-604, 1977.
16. Levin DM, Baker AL, Riddel RH, et al: Nonalcoholic liver disease. Overlooked causes of liver injury in patients with heavy alcohol consumption. Am J Med 66:429-434, 1979.
17. Schiff ER: Hepatitis C and alcohol. Hepatology 26:39S-42S, 1999.
18. Jacobson JM, Worner TM, Sacks HS, et al: Human immunodeficiency virus and hepatitis B virus infection in a New York City alcoholic population. J Stud Alcohol 53:76-79, 1992.
19. Maddrey WC, Boitnott JK, Bedine MS, et al: Corticosteroid therapy of alcoholic hepatitis. Gastroenterology 75:193-199, 1978.

20. Carithers RL Jr, Herlong FH, Diehl AM, et al: Methylprednisone therapy in patients with severe alcoholic hepatitis. A randomized multicenter trial. Ann Intern Med 110:685-690, 1989.
21. Orrego H, Israel Y, Blake JE, et al: Assessment of prognostic factors in alcoholic liver disease: toward a global quantitative expression of severity. Hepatology 3:896-905, 1983.
22. Chistensen E, Schlichting P, Fauerholt L, et al: The Copenhagen study group for liver diseases. Prognostic value of Child-Turcotte criteria in medically treated cirrhosis. Hepatology 4:430-435, 1994.
23. Orrego H, Blake JE, Blendis LM, et al: Prognosis of alcoholic cirrhosis in the presence and absence of alcoholic hepatitis. Gastroenterology 92:208-214, 1987.
24. Shull HJ Jr, Wilkinson GR, Johnson R, et al: Normal disposition of oxazepam in acute viral hepatitis and cirrhosis. Ann Intern Med 84:420-425, 1976.
25. Mezey E: Interaction between alcohol and nutrition in the pathogenesis of alcoholic liver disease. Semin Liver Dis 11:340-348, 1991.
26. Mendenhall CL, Tosch T, Weesner RE, et al: VA cooperative study on alcoholic hepatitis. II. Prognostic significance of protein-calorie malnutrition. Am J Clin Nutr 213-218, 1986.
27. Calvey H, Davis M, Williams R: Controlled trial of nutritional supplementation with and without branched chain amino acid enrichment, in treatment of acute alcoholic hepatitis. J Hepatol 1:141-151, 1985.
28. Mendenhall C, Bongiovanni G, Goldberg S, et al: VA cooperative study on alcoholic hepatitis. III Changes in protein-calorie malnutrition associated with 30 days of hospitalization with and without enteral nutritional therapy. JPEN 9:590-596, 1985.
29. Cabre E, Gonzales-Huix A, Abad-Lacruz A, et al: Effect of total enteral nutrition on the short-term outcome of severely malnourished alcoholics. A randomized controlled trial. Gastroenterology 98:715-720, 1990.
30. Kearns PJ, Young H, Garcia G: Accelerated improvement of alcoholic liver disease with enteral nutrition. Gastroenterology 102:200-205, 1992.
31. Diehl AM, Boitnott JK, Herlong HF, et al: Effect of parenteral amino acid supplementation in alcoholic hepatitis. Hepatology 5:57-63, 1985.
32. Bonkovsky HL, Fiellin DA, Smith GS, et al: A randomized, controlled trial of treatment of alcoholic hepatitis with parenteral nutrition and oxandrolone. I. Short effects on liver function. Am J Gastroenterol 86:1200-1208, 1991.
33. Bonkovsky HL, Singh RH, Jafri IH, et al: A randomized, controlled trial of treatment of alcoholic hepatitis with parenteral nutrition and oxandrolone. II. Short effects on nitrogen metabolism, metabolic balance and nutrition. Am J Gastroenterol 86:1206-1218, 1991.
34. Naveau S, Pelletier G, Poynard T, et al: A randomized clinical trial of supplementary parenteral nutrition in jaundiced alcoholic cirrhotic patients. Hepatology 6:270-274, 1986.
35. Nasrallah SM, Galambos JT: Amino acid therapy of alcoholic hepatitis. Lancet 2:1276-1277, 1980.
36. Mezey E, Caballeria J, Mitchell MC, et al: Effect of parenteral amino acid supplementation on short-term and long-term outcomes in severe alcoholic hepatitis. A randomized controlled trial. Hepatology 14:1090-1096, 1991.
37. Leevy CM, Baker H, ten Hove W, et al: B-complex vitamins in liver disease of the alcoholic. Am J Clin Nutr 16:339-346, 1965.
38. Helman RA, Temko MH, Nye SW, et al: Alcoholic hepatitis. Natural history and evaluation of prednisolone therapy. Ann Intern Med 74:311-321, 1971.
39. Ramond MJ, Poynard T, Rueff B: A randomized trial of prednisolone in patients with severe alcoholic hepatitis. N Engl J Med 326:507-512, 1992.
40. Imperiale TF, McCullough AJ: Do corticosteroids reduce mortality from alcoholic hepatitis? A meta-analysis of the randomized trials. Ann Intern Med 113:299-307, 1990.
41. Daures JP, Peray P, Bories P, et al: Place de la corticotherapie dans le traitement des hepatites alcooliques aigues. Resultats d'une meta-analyse. Gastroenterol Clin Biol 15:223-228, 1991.
42. Lesesne HR, Bozymski EM, Fallon HJ: Treatment of alcoholic hepatitis with encephalopathy. Comparison of prednisolone with caloric supplements. Gastroenterology 73:169-173, 1978.
43. Cabre E, Rodriguez-Iglesias P, Caballeria J, et al: Short- and long-term outcome of severe alcohol-induced hepatitis treated with steroids or enteral nutrition: A multicenter randomized trial. Hepatology 32:36-42, 2000.
44. Strieter RM, Remick DG, Ward RV, et al: Cellular and molecular regulation of tumor necrosis factor-alpha production by pentoxifylline. Biochem Biophys Res Comm 155:1230-1236, 1988.
45. Felver ME, Mezey E, McGuire M, et al: Plasma tumor necrosis factor-α predicts long-term survival in severe alcoholic hepatitis. Alcohol Clin Exp Med 14:255-259, 1990.
46. Akriviadis E, Botla R, Briggs W, et al: Pentoxifylline improves short-term survival in severe acute alcoholic hepatitis: a double-blind, placebo controlled trial. Gastroenterology 119:1637-1648, 2000.
47. Israel Y, Kalant H, Orrego H, et al: Experimental alcohol-induced hepatic necrosis. Suppression by propylthiouracil. Proc Natl Acad Sci U S A 72:1137-1141, 1975.
48. Orrego H, Kalant H, Israel Y, et al: Effect of short-term therapy with propylthiouracil in patients with alcoholic liver disease. Gastroenterology 76:105-115, 1979.
49. Orrego H, Blake JE, Blendis LM, et al: Long-term treatment of alcoholic liver disease with propylthiouracil. N Engl J Med 317:1421-1427, 1987.
50. Halle P, Pare P, Kaptein E, et al: Double-blind controlled trial of propylthiouracil in patients with severe acute alcoholic hepatitis. Gastroenterology 82:925-931, 1982.
51. Mendenhall CL, Anderson S, Garcia-Pont P, et al: Short-term and long-term survival in patients with alcoholic hepatitis treated with oxandrolone and prednisolone. N Engl J Med 311:1464-1470, 1984.
52. Mendenhall C, Moritz T, Roselle G, et al: A study of oral nutritional support with oxandrolone in malnourished patients with alcoholic hepatitis: results of a Veterans Affairs cooperative study. Hepatology 17: 564-576, 1993.
53. Baker AL, Jaspan JB, Haines NW, et al: A randomized clinical trial of insulin and glucagon infusion for the treatment of alcoholic hepatitis: Progress report in 50 patients. Gastroenterology 80:1410-1414, 1981.
54. Bird G, Lau JYN, Koskinas J, et al: Insulin and glucagon infusion in acute alcoholic hepatitis: a prospective randomized controlled trial. Hepatology 14:1097-1101, 1991.
55. Trinchet JC, Balkau B, Poupon RE, et al: Treatment of severe alcoholic hepatitis by infusion of insulin and glucagon: a multicenter sequential trial. Hepatology 15:76-81, 1992.
56. Resnick RH, Boitnott J, Iber FL, et al: Preliminary observations of d-penicillamine therapy in acute alcoholic liver disease. Digestion 11:257-265, 1974.
57. Herlong HF, Boitnott JK, Maddrey WC: D-penicillamine in the treatment of alcoholic hepatitis. Gastroenterology 75:968, 1978.
58. Mezey E, Potter JJ, Iber FL, et al: Hepatic collagen proline hydroxylase in alcoholic hepatitis. Effect of D-penicillamine. J Lab Clin Med 93:92-100, 1970.
59. Morgan MY: Hepatoprotective agents in alcoholic liver disease. Acta Med Scand Suppl 703:225-233, 1985.
60. Keiding S, Badsberg JH, Becker U, et al: The prognosis of patients with alcoholic liver disease. An international randomized, placebo-controlled trial on the effect of malotilate on survival. J Hepatol 20:454-460, 1994.
61. Lieber CS, DeCarli LM, Mak KM, et al: Attenuation of alcohol-induced hepatic fibrosis by polyunsaturated lecithin. Hepatology 12:1390-1398, 1990.
62. Smith J, Horowitz J, Henderson JM, et al: Enteral hyperalimentation in undernourished patients with cirrhosis and ascites. Am J Clin Nutr 35:56-72, 1982.
63. Horst D, Grace ND, Conn HO, et al: Comparison of dietary protein with an oral, branched chain-enriched amino acid supplement in chronic portal systemic encephalopathy: a randomized controlled trial. Hepatology 4:279-287, 1984.
64. Christie ML, Sack DM, Pomposelli J, et al: Enriched branched-chain amino acids formula versus a casein-based supplement in the treatment of cirrhosis. JPEN 9:671-678, 1985.
65. Kershenobich D, Vargas F, Garcia-Tsao G, et al: Colchicine in the treatment of cirrhosis of the liver. N Engl J Med 218:1709-1713, 1988.
66. Abdi W, Millan JC, Mezey E: Sampling variability on percutaneous liver biopsy. Arch Intern Med 139:667-669, 1979.
67. Trinchet JC, Beaugrand M, Callard P, et al: Treatment of alcoholic hepatitis with colchicine. Results of a randomized double blind trial. Gastroenterol Clin Biol 13:551-555, 1989.

68. Akriviadis EA, Steidel H, Pinto PC, et al: Failure of colchicine to improve short-term survival in patients with alcoholic hepatitis. Gastroenterology 99:811-818, 1990.
69. Mato JM, Camara J, Fernadez de Paz J, et al: S-adenosylmethionine in alcoholic liver cirrhosis: A randomized, placebo controlled, double-blind, multicenter clinical trial. J Hepatol 30:1081-1089, 1999.
70. Kumar S, Stauber RE, Gavaler JS, et al: Orthotopic liver transplantation for alcoholic liver disease. Hepatology 11:159-164, 1990.
71. Lucey MR, Merion RM, Henley KS, et al: Selection for and outcome of liver transplantation in alcoholic liver disease. Gastroenterology 102:1736-1741, 1992.
72. Bonet H, Manez R, Kramer D, et al: Liver transplantation for alcoholic liver disease: survival of patients transplanted with alcoholic hepatitis plus cirrhosis as compared with those with cirrhosis alone. Alcoholism Clin Exp Res 17:1102-1106, 1993.
73. Lee RG: Recurrence of alcoholic liver disease after liver transplantation. Liver Transplant Surg 3:292-285, 1997.
74. Conjeevaram HS, Hart J, Lissoos TW, et al: Rapidly progressive liver injury and fatal alcoholic hepatitis occurring after liver transplantation in alcoholic patients. Transplantation 67:1562-1568, 1999.
75. Pares A, Barrera JM, Caballeria J, et al: Hepatitis virus antibodies in chronic alcoholic patients: association with severity of liver injury. Hepatology 12:1295-1299, 1990.
76. Poynard T, Bedossa P, Opolon P: Natural history of liver fibrosis progression in patients with chronic hepatitis C. Lancet 349:825-832, 1997.
77. Wiley TE, McCarthy M, Breidi L, et al: Impact of alcohol on the histological and clinical progression of hepatitis C infection. Hepatology 28:805-809, 1998.
78. Pessione F, Degos F, Marcellin P, et al: Effect of alcohol consumption on serum hepatitis C virus RNA and histological lesions in chronic hepatitis C. Hepatology 27:1717-1722, 1998.
79. Lee RG: Nonalcoholic steatohepatitis: a study of 49 patients. Hum Pathol 20:594-598, 1989.
80. Sheth SG, Gordon FD, Chopra S: Nonalcoholic steatohepatitis. Ann Intern Med 126:137-145, 1997.
81. Bacon BR, Farahvash MJ, Janney CG, et al: Nonalcoholic steatohepatitis: An expanded clinical entity. Gastroenterology 107:1103-1109, 1994.
82. James OFW, Day CP: Non-alcoholic steatohepatitis (NASH): a disease of emerging identity and importance. J Hepatol 29:495-501, 1998.
83. Sorbi D, Boynton J, Lindor KD: The ratio of aspartate aminotransferase to alanine aminotransferase: potential value in differentiating nonalcoholic steatohepatitis from alcoholic liver disease. Am J Gastroenterol 94:1018-1022, 1999.
84. George DK, Goldwurm S, MacDonald GA, et al: Increased hepatic iron concentration in nonalcoholic steatohepatitis is associated with increased fibrosis. Gastroenterology 114:311-318, 1998.
85. Powell EE, Cooksley GE, Hanson R, et al: The natural history of non-alcoholic steatohepatitis: A follow-up study of forty-two patients for up to 21 years. Hepatology 11:74-80, 1990.
86. Matteoni CA, Younossi ZM, Gramlich T, et al: Nonalcoholic fatty liver disease: A spectrum of clinical and pathologic severity. Gastroenterology 116:1413-1419, 1999.
87. Poonawala A, Nair SD, Thuluvath PJ: Prevalence of obesity and diabetes in patients with cryptogenic cirrhosis: A case controlled study. Hepatology 32:689-692, 2000.
88. Ericksson S, Ericksson K, Bondesson L: Nonalcoholic steatohepatitis. Acta Med Scand 220:83-88, 1986.
89. Rozental P, Biava C, Spencer H, et al: Liver morphology and function tests in obesity and during total starvation. Am J Dig Dis 12:198-208, 1967.
90. Moxley RT III, Posefsky T, Lockwood DH: Protein nutrition and liver disease after jejunoileal bypass for morbid obesity. N Engl J Med 290:921-925, 1974.
91. Basaranoglu M, Acbay O, Sonsuz A: A controlled trial of gemfibrozil in the treatment of nonalcoholic steatohepatitis. J Hepatol 31:384, 1999.
92. Lavine JE: Vitamin E treatment of nonalcoholic steatohepatitis in children: A pilot study. J Pediatr 136:734-738, 2000.
93. Laurin J, Lindor KD, Crippin JS, et al: Ursodeoxycholic acid or clofibrate in the treatment of non-alcoholic steatohepatitis: A pilot study. Hepatology 23:1464-1467, 1996.
94. Kim WR, Poterucha JJ, Porayko et al: Recurrence of nonalcoholic steatohepatitis following liver transplantation. Transplantation 96:1802-1805, 1996.
95. Ratziu V, Giral P, Charlotte F, et al: Liver fibrosis in overweight patients. Gastroenterology 118:1117-1123, 2000.
96. Bellentani S, Saccoccio G, Masutti, et al: Prevalence of and risk factors for hepatic steatosis in Northern Italy. Ann Intern Med 132:112-117, 2000.

SECTION

IV B

Diagnosis and Management of Liver Disease Due to Infectious Agents

CHAPTER

31

Hepatitis A and E

Raymond S. Koff, MD

INTRODUCTION

Outbreaks of jaundice resulting from enterically transmitted viral hepatitis have been recognized for centuries, although serologic identification of the responsible agents only became possible in the past 25 years. Hepatitis A and E, the two predominant forms of enterically transmitted hepatitis, are the most common forms of acute viral hepatitis in many parts of the world. In the United States hepatitis A has accounted for 55 percent to 60 percent of all reported cases of acute viral hepatitis. Whether a third form of enterically transmitted hepatitis resulting from a currently unidentified agent actually exists remains to be determined but seems likely. The responsible agents of hepatitis A and E are unrelated, but both are non-enveloped, ribonucleic acid (RNA)-containing viruses and both have been transmitted experimentally to non-human primates and propagated in tissue culture. Safe and effective vaccines for the prevention of hepatitis A are available. Vaccines against hepatitis E are under development. Specific drug treatment is unavailable for either hepatitis A or E infection. The annual costs of symptomatic hepatitis A virus (HAV) infection among adolescents and adults have been estimated to be just under $500 million in the United States when evaluated from a societal perspective.[1] Hepatitis A and E usually cause self-limited and asymptomatic infections in children; in adults they generally cause clinical disease, often with jaundice and other typical constitutional and hepatic symptoms. Fatal acute liver failure resulting from severe hepatitis A is not uncommon in middle-aged and older individuals[2] (Figure 31-1), and in patients with underlying chronic liver disease.[3] Although acute liver failure is a rare complication of hepatitis A during pregnancy, fatal acute liver failure is seen in a substantial proportion of pregnant women with hepatitis E. Acute liver failure in the non-pregnant patient with hepatitis E is uncommon. Neither hepatitis A nor hepatitis E has been identified as a cause of chronic liver disease, nor do they result in prolonged viremia or in an intestinal carrier state. Because most patients with hepatitis E are already immune to hepatitis A, hepatitis A seems to be more efficiently transmitted than hepatitis E. The greater thermal and chemical stability of HAV compared to hepatitis E virus (HEV) may be responsible. Human reservoirs of their infection are unknown. Thus it seems likely that both infections are maintained in nature by serial transmission from acutely infected to susceptible individuals. Transmission of hepatitis A to human beings from recently infected non-human primates has been described but an extrahuman reservoir of hepatitis A infection in nature has not been demonstrated. The host range of hepatitis A includes humans, chimpanzees, and marmosets (tamarins). The host range of hepatitis E appears to be wider; and, in contrast to hepatitis A, it is suggested, but not proved, that hepatitis E is a zoonotic disease.

HEPATITIS A

Virology

Viral Characteristics

HAV is the prototype member of the Hepatovirus genus within the family of picornaviruses (Picornaviridae), distinct from the enteroviruses.[4] One human HAV serotype and one simian serotype have been identified. Four human genotypes have been recognized and shown to breed true.[5] In fact, molecular sequencing has been used to define the genetic relatedness of HAV isolated from

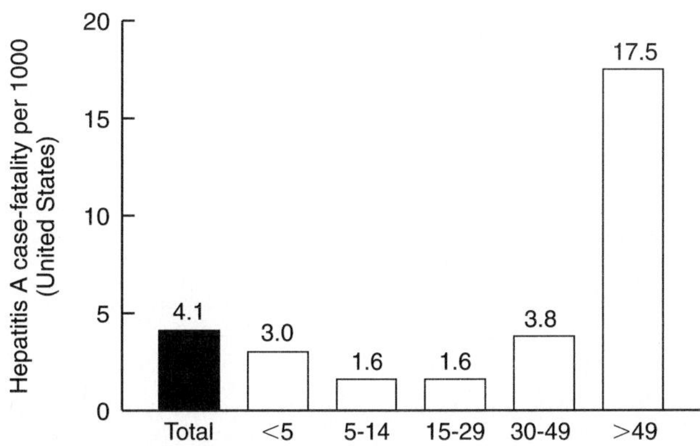

Figure 31-1 Reported case-fatality rates for acute hepatitis A in the United States as a function of age.

outbreak-related cases and their sources to thereby reliably elucidate the chain of HAV transmission.

HAV vaccine prepared from any of the human HAV genotypes provides protection against infection by all strains.

HAV is a small, non-enveloped spherical and icosahedral particle with a diameter of about 27 to 33 nm. Physical properties of this thermostable and acid-resistant RNA-containing virus are listed in Table 31-1. HAV can be inactivated by heating at 100° C for 20 minutes and by dry heat at 160° C for 60 minutes. HAV survives heating at 60° C for 60 minutes. As suggested by the variation in the size of the virion, HAV particles are heterogeneous and include intact mature virions, provirions that differ in virion polypeptide composition, and non-infectious procapsids (empty HAV particles similar to provirions but lacking HAV RNA). The provirions may have a lower specific infectivity and delayed uncoating kinetics as compared to mature virions.[6] Their precise role in the pathogenesis of infection remains to be determined. Dense HAV particles, detected in cell lysates after infection, may be an intermediate in the viral uncoating process.[7] Direct intrahepatic inoculation of HAV RNA transcribed from HAV complementary deoxyribonucleic acid (cDNA) clones induces acute hepatitis in non-human primates.[8] HAV replication appears to be limited to hepatocytes.

HAV RNA Genome. HAV RNA is a single-stranded, linear, positive-sense molecule with a length of about 7.5 kb. It serves as a messenger RNA for translation into a single polyprotein (Figure 31-2). At the 5′ end of the genome a long non-translated region of about 735 nucleotides is involved in internal initiation of protein synthesis—the internal ribosomal entry site. Although nucleotide substitutions in the 5′-non-translated region have been linked with virulence, substitutions elsewhere in the genome may be more closely associated with virulence and efficiency of HAV replication.[9] At the 3′ end, a short, 63-nucleotide, polyadenylated non-translated region is present. The large open-reading frame is translated into both structural and non-structural viral proteins. P1 is the region encoding structural proteins. P2 and P3 encode the non-structural proteins. The structural capsid proteins of the virus are thought to be the site of the immunodominant neutralization epitopes. The cleavages that produce the HAV proteins are mediated by the only proteinase known to be encoded by the virus: cysteine proteinase 3C; however, host cell proteases may participate in the generation of certain virion proteins, namely the maturation of the HAV VP1 capsid protein.[10,11] Whether cysteine proteinase 3C serves a replicative function, as has been suggested,[12] remains to be established. The development of inhibitors of HAV cysteine proteinase has been reported but clinical studies of therapeutic efficacy are not available.[13]

TABLE 31-1

Characteristics of Hepatitis A Virus

Family	Picornaviridae
Genus	Hepatovirus
Serotypes	One human
Genotypes	Four human
Nucleic acid	Linear, single-strand RNA
Genome size	7.5 kb
Open reading frame	Single, 6.7 kb
Size	27-33 nm in diameter
Morphology	Spherical particle
Symmetry	Icosahedral
Buoyant density in cesium chloride	1.33 g/cm^3
Buoyant density in sucrose	1.34 g/cm^3
Sedimentation coefficient	156S-160S
Physicochemical properties	Chemical/thermal resistance
Envelope	None
Replication	Hepatocyte cytoplasm
Capsomeric structural proteins	Four, VP1-4
Nonstructural proteins	Seven
Primate host range	Human beings, chimpanzees, marmosets

RNA, Ribonucleic acid.

HAV Propagation in Cell Culture. HAV can be propagated in vitro in cell lines of human and non-human primate origin but growth is usually slow and virus yields are low. Typically, a cytopathic effect is absent in permissive cell lines, and the virus is unable to inhibit host cell macromolecular synthesis. Nonetheless, cytopathic HAV strains have been identified; and for some of these, cell death appears to be induced by apoptosis rather than by cytopathology.[14] A membranous tubular-vesicular network has been identified in cell-culture infected with adapted and cytopathic strains cells.[14] These vesicles may be associated with replication of HAV RNA. HAV within vesicles may be present in the circulation and in stool, as well as in the cytoplasm of infected hepatocytes. Whether the vesicles protect virus from antibody remains uncertain.

Attenuated HAV strains adapted to cell culture have been used in vaccine development. The slow replication of HAV in cell culture, which results in relatively low virus yields in the MRC-5 cells used for vaccine production, appears to be a consequence of low translation efficiency. In these cells viral translation is rate-limiting for HAV replication.[15]

HAV Life Cycle. After peroral inoculation, HAV is believed to be transferred from the lumen of the intestine to intestinal epithelial cells and from there into the portal circulation. The vectorial process permitting intestinal entry into epithelial cells and release of HAV remains ill-defined.[16] Hepatocyte uptake of HAV may involve cell-surface receptors, but the nature and specificity of such have yet to be determined. One putative cellular receptor for HAV has been identified in a cell line.[17] Further work is necessary to determine its role in infection in vivo. In a mouse hepatocyte model, HAV-specific immunoglobulin A (IgA anti-HAV) appears to mediate HAV infection by serving as a carrier of HAV and by binding to the asialoglycoprotein receptor, which internalizes IgA.[18] HAV replication within the infected hepatocyte occurs exclusively in the cytoplasm. An RNA-dependent RNA polymerase is involved, but the precise steps in HAV replication are unknown. It seems likely that an uncoated intermediate may be formed early after infection.[7] The mechanisms responsible for the intracellular transport of HAV particles to the hepatocyte bile canaliculi for excretion also are not fully understood. The virus is resistant to inactivation by bile. After biliary excretion HAV re-enters the intestine. Resistance to inactivation by intestinal proteinases permits HAV to survive contact with the intestinal contents and to be shed in feces.

Epidemiology

Incubation Period

The incubation period of enterically transmitted hepatitis A is probably not related to the size of the inoculum. In contrast, the incubation period seems to correlate with inoculum size after intravenous inoculation of HAV. The usual incubation period of HAV transmitted by the fecal-oral route is between 15 and 50 days with a mean of about 28 to 30 days.

Fecal Shedding of HAV

As shown in Figure 31-3, concentrations of HAV in feces are considerably higher than those in other body fluids, including urine. HAV is shed in the feces as early as 2 weeks after exposure and for 1 to 2 weeks before the onset of illness. The peak period of viral shedding occurs at the onset of symptoms and then declines rapidly during the first week of illness (Figure 31-4). However, using highly sensitive techniques such as polymerase chain reaction (PCR), it is possible to detect HAV RNA in feces for several months after the peak of liver enzyme abnormalities.[19,20] In limited studies stool specimens positive for HAV RNA by PCR but negative by the less sensitive enzyme immunoassay for HAV antigen failed to induce infection in susceptible tamarins.[20] The latter observation and the bulk of epidemiologic data indicating that most secondary cases occur within one incubation period after exposure to the index case suggest that the risk of

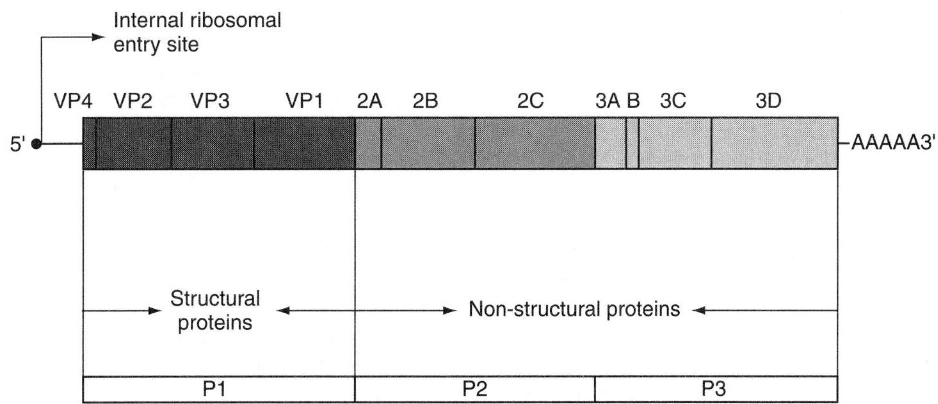

Figure 31-2 Genomic organization of HAV RNA. *HAV,* Hepatitis A virus; *RNA,* ribonucleic acid.

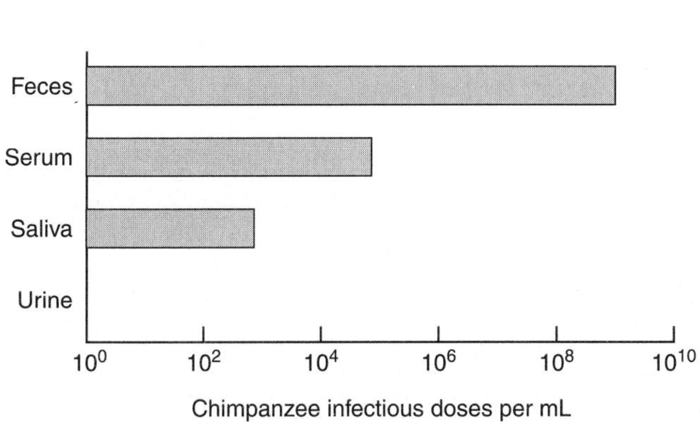

Figure 31-3 Concentrations of HAV in body fluids and excretions. *HAV,* Hepatitis A virus.

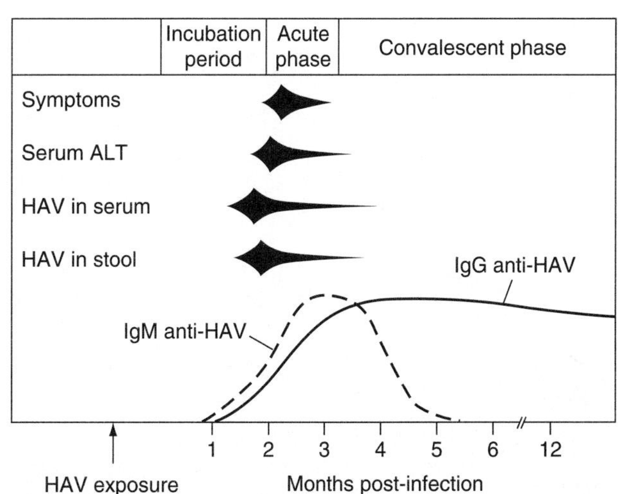

Figure 31-4 Sequence of clinical, biochemical, virologic, and serologic events in acute hepatitis A.

person-to-person transmission during the late convalescent phase must be exceedingly low. Hence prolonged fecal excretion of HAV in minute but detectable amounts appears to be of limited epidemiologic importance.

Period of Viremia

HAV has been detected in the blood of infected patients during the incubation period, acute phase of illness, and for several months during convalescence. Viremia in HAV infection has been demonstrated by PCR as early as 30 days before the onset of symptoms and, on average, 17 days before the peak serum alanine aminotransferase (ALT) level.[21] As shown in Figure 31-4, HAV RNA may be present before the appearance of IgM anti-HAV. Viremia in this study, persisted for about 80 days, on average, after the peak of serum ALT. The duration of viremia ranged from 36 to 391 days, with a mean of 95 days. In another study of viremia in hepatitis A, the mean duration of viremia was 30 days with a range of 5 to 59 days.[22] The persistence of viremia for more than a year in one of these studies is surprising but consistent with the occurrence, albeit rare, of bloodborne hepatitis A. The mechanisms responsible for persistent or intermittent viremia are poorly understood.

Incidence and Prevalence

Estimates of HAV infection rates in the United States often have been confounded by high rates of underreporting and failure to recognize anicteric infections, particularly among children. The current incidence of hepatitis A in the United States may be as high as 130,000 new infections and 70,000 cases annually (Table 31-2). Hepatitis A is now the most common cause of acute viral hepatitis in the United States but infection has declined dramatically from the 250,000 cases estimated to have occurred annually during the 1990s. Not unexpectedly, the prevalence of hepatitis A in the United States, as measured by the presence of circulating antibodies to HAV, also appears to be declining. The proportion of the population now susceptible to infection is increasing. Although the overall prevalence may currently be no higher than about 30 percent, age-specific prevalence rates of 20 percent are found in those between 20 and 29 years, 25 percent in those between age 30 and 39 years, 33 percent in the 40 to 49 year group, and 47 percent in those 50 years of age or older. As a consequence the average age at the time of acquisition of infection may be increasing, resulting in a higher frequency of icteric disease that is more severe.

The heterogeneity of socioeconomic conditions in the United States is such that in some communities, largely those in which substandard water and sewage sanitation systems continue to exist (see the following section), HAV infection rates have approached those found in the developing world.[23] States with high prevalence rates (mainly in the west and southwest) account for about 50 percent of reported cases of hepatitis A but only 20 percent of the United States population. National use of HAV vaccines should lower the national incidence of HAV even in high-risk communities because accumulating data show a reduced incidence of hepatitis A since the introduction of routine vaccination of children in some states with high attack rates.

In the economically developing countries of Africa, Asia, and Latin America, hepatitis A continues to be an exceedingly common infection in the early years of life (Figure 31-5). Most infections occur during the first 5 years of life, and seroprevalence rates are nearly 100 percent in adolescents and young adults. Seroprevalence rates in western and southern Europe have been declining in recent decades and in some populations no more than 10 percent of people have evidence of previous infection.

TABLE 31-2

Acute Hepatitis A in the United States (1999)

Infections	Cases	Deaths
130,000	70,000	200

Modes of Transmission

Fecal-oral spread of HAV by person-to-person contact within the household is the major mode of transmission. The secondary attack rate of clinically apparent infection among household contacts of acutely infected index cases may approach 20 percent to 50 percent. As mentioned, most secondary household infections occur just one incubation period apart from the index case. Household transmission to susceptibles often involves children, and infection rates are correlated with household size. In community-wide outbreaks, children with unrecognized infection appear to play an important role in transmission within and between households.[24]

As shown in Table 31-3, no risk factor can be identified in nearly half of cases of HAV. Many of these cases occur in the setting of community-wide outbreaks. School-age children, adolescents, and young adults are the predominantly recognized infected groups but younger children are likely to be the major transmitters of infection. Large household size, low socioeconomic status, low educational attainment, inadequate domestic water supplies, defective sewage systems, and the presence of young children in the household appear to be correlated with

TABLE 31-3

Risk Factors for Hepatitis A in the United States

Factor	Percent
Unknown	48
Personal contact	21
Day care associated	13
International travel	8
Homosexual/bisexual men	5
Injecting drug users	3
Common-source outbreaks	2

both community-wide outbreaks and sporadic cases. Day care centers for preschool, diapered children and infants have been linked repeatedly with hepatitis A transmission in the form of outbreaks and sporadic cases in endemic regions.[25] Recognition of day care centers as a source of HAV transmission may be difficult because clinically apparent cases may be absent in the children or the staff. The appearance of cases among relatives in contact with children attending the day care center may be the only clue to the source of infection[26] in such circumstances. Fecal contamination of the environment appears to be responsible for HAV transmission in this setting, in neonatal intensive care units, and in institutions for the developmentally disadvantaged.

For a number of years common-source outbreaks of variable size have been linked to contamination of domestic drinking water and even to swimming in contaminated waters.

Sewage-contaminated well water has been associated with multiple outbreaks of hepatitis A, and it has been possible to detect HAV in the contaminated water. Furthermore, the chain of transmission has been strengthened by the demonstration of the genetic relatedness of HAV isolates from infected patients and well water.[27] In some countries with high attack rates of hepatitis A the source of domestic water has been correlated with rates of exposure to HAV: rates are higher in households with external sources when compared to those with indoor plumbing.[28] Although data are conflicting, wastewater and sewage workers may have an increased risk of HAV infection. Absence of protection of face and skin from contact with sewage (at least once daily) appears to be associated with infection.[29]

Seafood harvested from contaminated waters and consumed uncooked or undercooked, such as raw or steamed clams, oysters, and mussels, has been implicated in outbreaks and sporadic cases, particularly in some Mediterranean countries.[30] Thermal resistance of HAV appears to be increased in bivalve mollusk tissues.[31] Depuration of bivalve mollusks in an attempt to reduce the risk of infection is unlikely to be successful. Hence only appropriate cooking before consumption can eliminate the risk.

Contamination during harvesting or processing of foods before distribution appears responsible for outbreaks linked to consumption of fruits and vegetables.[32] Similarly, the use of nightsoil for crop fertilization in some countries may contribute to transmission of HAV. Infected food handlers have been responsible for some outbreaks linked to consumption of food in restaurants. Studies of HAV transfer from fingers to food indicate that hand washing with water and topical agents can significantly reduce HAV levels on fingers.[33] Use of plastic disposable gloves may be even more effective in the interruption of HAV transfer from fingers to food.

International travel to areas with high attack rates of hepatitis A represents a risk for individuals from regions of low prevalence who travel to endemic regions. Most viral hepatitis imported into developed countries in the form of travelers returning from endemic regions is hepatitis A. Poor local sanitation and inadequate hygienic standards promote the risk of transmission to the susceptible traveler. Consumption of contaminated food or water is the likely source of infection for the traveler.

An increased risk of hepatitis A has been associated with a high number of sexual partners. Although a number of outbreaks of HAV infection have been reported in men who have sex with men, and oral-anal and digital-anal sexual practices have been linked with transmission,[34] in some studies the prevalence of infection has not exceeded that in heterosexual men.[35]

Individuals who share illicit drugs and associated equipment for injection are at increased risk of HAV. Among injecting drug users who acquire hepatitis A, the precise modes of transmission remain ill-defined. Evidence for person-to-person spread both by fecal-oral routes and percutaneous routes is available.[36] Poor personal hygiene and poor handling of the injection equipment may result in a high frequency of contamination. Contamination of the illicit drugs is also possible.

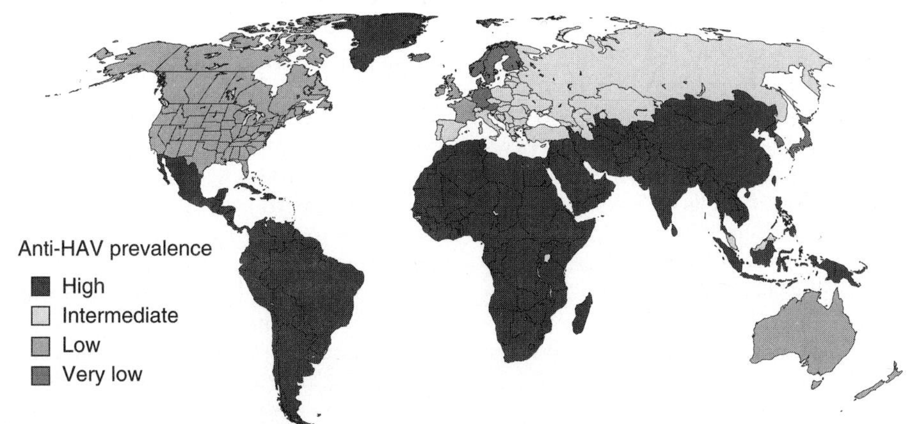

Figure 31-5 Global distribution of HAV infection. *HAV*, Hepatitis A virus. (Redrawn from CDC, National Center for Infectious Diseases Slideset. Slide 11—Geographic Distribution of HAV Infections, 2000. http://www.cdc.gov/ncidod/disease/hepatitis/slideset/hep_a/slide_11.htm.)

Maternal-neonatal transmission is possible, but its epidemiologic importance seems minimal. Blood transfusion-associated hepatitis A has been rare in the United States. Outbreaks of hepatitis A also have been associated with clotting factor concentrates,[37] but transmission by these products contributes little to the overall epidemiology of infection. Factor concentrates are now inactivated by pasteurization, vapor heating, or psoralen and ultraviolet A treatment. HAV nucleic acid testing of blood donor minipools has been used by some blood derivative manufacturers, but blood bank testing of individual donors for HAV RNA is unlikely to become a routine screening procedure.

Immunopathogenesis

Cell-mediated immune mechanisms, mediated via CD8+ and natural killer cells and possibly gamma-interferon, are believed to be responsible for the hepatocyte injury seen in hepatitis A. A direct cytopathic effect of HAV on hepatocytes has not been established and the presence of circulating immune complexes also appears to be unrelated to the necroinflammatory lesions found in the liver. Apoptosis also may contribute to hepatocyte death. In experimental infection of non-human primates, expression of inducible nitric oxide synthase was observed in hepatocytes, Kupffer cells, and splenic macrophages before the onset of necroinflammatory changes and reached maximal levels coincident with liver injury. These observations suggest a role of nitric oxide in the HAV-induced hepatic injury.[38] Cytokine-mediated inhibition of viral replication and the induction of serum neutralizing antibodies may contribute to resolution of infection.

In the case of relapsing hepatitis A, it has been postulated that secretory IgA directed against HAV and derived from gastrointestinal mucosa-associated lymphoid tissue may transport HAV from the intestine to the liver and permit hepatocyte reinfection.

Humoral Response to HAV Infection

A dominant IgM and IgG immune response against VP1, a major HAV capsid polypeptide, has been recognized during the acute phase of hepatitis A. The IgM anti-HAV is thought to have neutralizing activity. Subsequently, in the late convalescent phases, antibodies to VP3 and VP0 also are present in the circulation.[39] IgM anti-HAV may reduce the intrahepatic spread of HAV from infected hepatocytes to contiguous susceptible cells. It is also possible that this IgM anti-HAV can impede the development of secondary viremia. Antibody to HAV of the IgG class rises in titer during the acute phase of infection and remains present indefinitely. IgG anti-HAV is believed to be responsible for the lifelong immunity that follows recovery from hepatitis A.

Serologic Diagnosis

The detection of IgM anti-HAV during the acute phase of symptomatic or anicteric hepatitis and for 3 to 6 months thereafter is generally diagnostic of acute hepatitis A. An IgG anti-HAV also may be present early in the acute phase of infection, but the IgM anti-HAV antibody is always present in high titers at this time. The presence of IgG anti-HAV without IgM anti-HAV strongly suggests that another disorder is responsible for the hepatitis and that the individual had been exposed previously to HAV and is now immune to reinfection. Measurement of HAV RNA in blood or stool remains a research technique, too expensive and labor intensive for use in diagnosis.

Pathologic Features of Hepatitis A

Although liver biopsy is rarely undertaken today in the evaluation of patients with hepatitis A, earlier studies defined the histopathologic features of the acute infection and recovery. The major changes observed in the fully developed, active phase of infection are the presence of ballooning and acidophilic (apoptotic) degeneration of hepatocytes. Progressive acidophilic degeneration leads to the formation of the acidophilic body (Councilman-like body), readily identified by its oval or round shape and its hyaline, deep eosinophilic but waxy cast. These degenerative changes and evidence of necrosis are usually accompanied by lymphocytic inflammation within the lobule and portal and periportal areas. The portal infiltrate is often dense and comprises both lymphocytes and plasma cells. Lobular disarray is a characteristic feature. It results from loss of uniformity of the hepatocyte plates resulting from the ballooning of the cells, smudging of the cell membranes, increased cellularity from Kupffer cell and endothelial cell enlargement and hyperplasia, and the presence of focal collections of lymphocytes and macrophages. The reticulin framework is generally well preserved despite occasional focal disruption. In some patients pericentral cholestasis is the most prominent feature with minimal necroinflammatory changes. Unusual lesions in hepatitis A include fibrin-ring granulomas and microvesicular change in hepatocytes.

Hepatocyte regeneration may begin during the active phase of infection. It is recognized by thickening of the hepatocyte plates, the presence of mitotic figures, many binucleated cells, cytoplasmic basophilia, and hepatocyte rosette formation.

Clinical Features of Typical Hepatitis A

In most infected children and perhaps in as many as 10 percent of adults, hepatitis A may be asymptomatic or accompanied by only minor and non-specific constitutional or gastrointestinal symptoms that abate within a few days. In rare instances acute pancreatitis has been reported in children and adults with hepatitis A.[40] Jaundice is uncommon in children with hepatitis A but is characteristic of symptomatic disease in adults. In patients with symptomatic hepatitis A, the onset is often abrupt with a prodrome of fever, malaise, anorexia, nausea and vomiting, arthralgias, and myalgias before the onset of dark urine and jaundice. Upper respiratory and influenza-like symptoms, including coryza, pharyngitis, cough, headache, and photophobia may be present. The prodromal features generally resolve with the onset of jaundice but continuing weakness and anorexia may be prominent in some patients. Commonly reported symptoms of icteric hepatitis A are shown in Table 31-4.

Darkening of the urine usually is noted before jaundice is recognized. Pruritus may accompany the jaundice but is not invariably present. Extrahepatic manifestations of hepatitis A are distinctly uncommon and may cause confusion with other systemic diseases.

For example, the fever, rash, and arthritis seen in hepatitis A may resemble Still's disease.[41] Acute cholecystitis, with viral invasion of gallbladder epithelium, has also been reported.[42] Rarely, in the absence of acute liver failure, hepatitis A has been linked with transient renal failure that may require hemodialysis. The underlying mechanism is unknown. Another rare manifestation, seen before, during, or after the acute phase of illness, is a transient sensory neuropathy.[43] Its pathogenesis also remains obscure. Other rare manifestations include the development of cutaneous necrotizing vasculitis and mononeuritis multiplex. Putative associations of hepatitis A with the development of diabetes mellitus and coronary artery disease[44] are very speculative with little biologic plausibility.

Physical examination may reveal the presence of scleral or buccal icterus. The liver may be mildly enlarged and punch tenderness may be elicited. The spleen tip may be palpated in about 20 percent of patients, and shotty posterior cervical lymphadenopathy may be present.

Laboratory Features

Although there is considerable variability, elevations of the serum aminotransferase levels are usually the most prominent laboratory finding. Peak levels of between 400 and 5000 U/ml are commonly reported. In general the ALT is slightly higher than the aspartate aminotransferase. Serum bilirubin levels are variable. Levels of total serum bilirubin above 10 mg/dl with a predominance of conjugated bilirubin are uncommon and suggest more severe disease (e.g., acute liver failure resulting from hepatitis A or the development of cholestatic hepatitis A). Striking elevations of unconjugated bilirubin also may be seen as a consequence of hemolysis in hepatitis A patients with underlying glucose-6-phosphate dehydrogenase deficiency. In typical self-limited hepatitis A, serum albumin levels may be normal or slightly diminished and prothrombin times are either normal or slightly prolonged. Mild leukopenia is common; atypical lymphocytes may be present. Neither anemia nor thrombocytopenia is to be expected. Very rarely, aplastic anemia has been seen as a sequela to resolving hepatitis A.

TABLE 31-4

Symptoms Reported in More than 50 Percent of Patients with Icteric Hepatitis A

Symptom	Frequency (%)
Dark urine	94
Lassitude	91
Anorexia	90
Nausea	87
Weakness	77
Fever	76
Vomiting	71
Headache	70
Abdominal pain/discomfort	65
Myalgia	52

Adapted from Koff RS: Viral hepatitis. In Schiff L, Schiff ER, eds: Diseases of the Liver. Philadelphia, Lippincott, 1993.

Treatment of Typical Hepatitis A

Hospitalization is required infrequently and is usually reserved for patients with persistent vomiting or severe anorexia leading to dehydration or those who present with features of acute liver failure (see the following section). No specific dietary recommendations can be made other than to attempt to maintain adequate fluid and calorie intake. Alcohol intake should be prohibited during the acute phase of illness. Non-essential drugs are best avoided although oral contraceptives may be continued. Unusually, strenuous physical activity also should be avoided during the acute phase. The need for rest is best assessed by the patient based on the level of fatigue and malaise experienced. Strict bed rest has no particular value but the need for it is also best determined by the degree of weakness and fatigue as perceived by the patient. Clinical and laboratory recovery generally begin within 2 or 3 weeks after onset of symptoms and are anticipated to be complete within 3 to 6 months.

Clinical Features of Atypical Hepatitis A

Acute Liver Failure

Acute liver failure from hepatitis A is generally a consequence of infection in the middle-aged and the elderly,[45] and case fatality rates are highest in the oldest patients. Hospitalization rates for hepatitis A increase with increasing age because of increased severity of disease, as reflected by higher serum bilirubin levels, prolonged prothrombin times, and diagnostic uncertainty in older patients. Increased severity of disease is also likely in patients with co-morbid diseases, such as diabetes and chronic cardiac and pulmonary diseases. However, because hepatitis A knows no age boundaries and can be severe at any age, acute liver failure resulting from hepatitis A is not rare in young children.[46] Although somewhat controversial, acute liver failure appears to be more common when hepatitis A superinfection occurs in the setting of preexisting chronic liver disease (e.g., chronic hepatitis C).[47]

The clinical features of acute liver failure resulting from hepatitis A include progressive jaundice, changes in mental status, and coagulopathy, reflected in prolongation of the prothrombin time, usually occurring within 2 weeks of the onset of symptoms or jaundice. The serum aminotransferases may decline despite progression of disease. Cerebral edema, renal failure with hypotension, metabolic abnormalities, sepsis, and the development of multi-organ failure (respiratory and cardiac) are common. Cerebral edema may be responsible for about 50 percent of the mortality in acute hepatic failure. Typical metabolic changes include hypoglycemia, hypokalemia, respiratory alkalosis, and hyponatremia. Terminally, lactic acidosis may supervene. No specific treatment is available and survival rates have been as low as 5 percent to 30 percent with only supportive management. Early referral to a liver transplantation center may permit survival in as many as 65 percent.

Cholestatic Hepatitis A

The course of cholestatic hepatitis A is prolonged and marked by persistent and striking jaundice that may last from 2 to 8 months.[48] Despite the hyperbilirubinemia, which may exceed 20 mg/dl but rarely exceeds 30 mg/dl, the serum aminotransferases are generally similar to those seen in typical hepatitis A and may decline despite prolonged and deep jaundice. Pruritus is often a prominent feature and also may persist for several months before resolution. Anorexia and diarrhea accompany the jaundice in some patients. The serum alkaline phosphatase levels and serum cholesterol levels may be elevated, but striking elevations of the former are infrequent. Complete recovery is the rule of thumb with or without a short course of corticosteroid therapy or treatment with ursodeoxycholic acid. Although no controlled trial has been undertaken, corticosteroids appear to shorten the duration of symptoms and ursodeoxycholic acid may hasten resolution of laboratory abnormalities.

Relapsing Hepatitis

Relapsing hepatitis has been recognized in just under 3 percent to as many as 20 percent of patients with hepatitis A[49] and may be more common in children than in adults. Multiple episodes also may be more common in children; however, no specific predisposing factor has been identified. Typically, after symptoms and laboratory studies suggest apparent recovery of the initial episode of otherwise unremarkable hepatitis A, a recurrence is noted after a period of 1.5 to 18 weeks. HAV again may be shed in the feces during a relapse and viremia may be present. Symptoms may mirror those seen in the initial episode and maximal levels of serum bilirubin and aminotransferases may resemble those seen during the initial illness. In some patients laboratory abnormalities may be more severe, whereas in others they are less striking. The duration of the relapse is variable and laboratory abnormalities may persist for weeks even after clinical remission. A syndrome of transient, self-limited arthritis, vasculitis, and cryoglobulinemia has been seen in a small number of patients with relapsing hepatitis A.[50] Even without intervention, complete clinical, laboratory, and histologic recovery is anticipated in all affected patients.

Immunoprophylaxis

Prevention of HAV infection in the developed world requires maintenance of high hygienic standards and the appropriate use of immunoprophylaxis. In developing countries improvements in sanitary standards with emphasis on safe, potable water and food supplies are long-term goals. Immunoprophylaxis should be a concomitant control measure. For travelers to HAV-endemic regions, pretravel immunoprophylaxis and the avoidance of drinking water or ice of uncertain origin and uncooked bivalve mollusks, fruits, and vegetables seems reasonable.

Immunoprophylaxis of hepatitis A may be achieved by passive transfer of anti-HAV in the form of immunoglobulin or by the administration of hepatitis A vaccine to elicit endogenous formation of antibodies. Some of the differences between the two are shown in Table 31-5.

Immunoglobulin

Human immunoglobulin has been used for nearly five decades in the prevention of hepatitis A. Remarkably, its effectiveness was demonstrated well before IgG anti-HAV, the protective antibody, could be identified and be-

TABLE 31-5

Immunoprophylaxis of Hepatitis A: Comparisons of Immunoglobulin and Inactivated Hepatitis A Vaccine

	Immunoglobulin	Hepatitis A vaccine
Serum-derived biological	Yes	No
Tissue-culture propagation	No	Yes
Passive acquisition of anti-HAV	Yes	No
Induction of endogenous anti-HAV	No	Yes
Time to appearance of first antibodies	Immediate	1-2 weeks
Peak anti-HAV titer (GMT)	150 mIU/ml	4000 mIU/ml
Efficacy of protection preexposure	90%	>95%-100%
Duration of protection	4-6 months	>10 years
Efficacy of protection postexposure	Limited	Unknown
Adverse effects	Mild, transient pain at injection site	Mild, transient pain at injection site
Anaphylaxis	Rare	Rare
Cost	Low	High
Availability	Limited	Unlimited

HAV, Hepatitis A virus; *GMT,* geometric mean titer.

fore HAV was visualized, classified, and grown in tissue culture. Intramuscular injection of immunoglobulin results in the appearance within a day or so of relatively low levels of circulating IgG anti-HAV. These levels are sufficient to provide preexposure protection against clinical disease for a number of months in a substantial proportion of recipients. However, the subsequent decline and then disappearance of antibody is accompanied by a return of susceptibility. Immunoglobulin for intramuscular administration produced in the United States has an excellent safety record but in recent years has been in short supply. In the United States immunoglobulin usage for preexposure prophylaxis is currently limited largely to children younger than 2 years of age and to travelers leaving shortly for endemic regions. Vaccine-induced protection may require 2 weeks to reach optimal levels.

The major current use of immunoglobulin is for postexposure prophylaxis of household contacts of infected individuals. Although this may change in the future (see the following section), household or intimate contacts of patients with hepatitis A should receive immunoglobulin in a dose of 0.02 ml/kg body weight as soon as possible after recognition of infection in the index case. Efficacy declines or disappears if the injection is given more than 2 weeks after exposure.

There is no current role for immunoglobulin in the control of community-wide or common-source outbreaks. In fact, administration of immunoglobulin during the incubation period of HAV might adversely alter and extend the duration of HAV excretion. Limited data suggest, for example, that HAV RNA could not be detected in stools obtained a median of 8 days after peak elevations of liver enzymes in patients not receiving immunoglobulin. However, HAV RNA could be detected in this setting in patients who did receive immunoglobulin.[51]

Hepatitis A Vaccine

A live, attenuated HAV vaccine has been developed and used extensively in China.[52] Information about this vaccine remains scant. Other attenuated live virus vaccines are under study in the United States.[53] In part because of concern for potential reversion to wild-type virus, attenuated live virus vaccines are unlikely to be introduced into the United States in the near future. Currently, two highly immunogenic, purified, safe and effective, whole-particle HAV vaccines are U.S. Food and Drug Administration (FDA)-approved and in use in the United States.[54,55] These are Havrix (manufactured by SmithKline Beecham and first approved in the United States in 1995) and Vaqta (manufactured by Merck and approved in 1996). Both are produced by growth of attenuated HAV strains in tissue culture followed by inactivation with formaldehyde. Both have been well tolerated. Transient pain and tenderness at the intramuscular deltoid injection site have been the major side effects. Headache and fever occur in no more than 15 percent of vaccine recipients.

Inactivated HAV vaccine products available outside the United States include a formaldehyde-inactivated product, Avaxim (Pasteur Merieux Connaught, Lyon, France), which is licensed in more than 40 countries[56] and a formaldehyde-inactivated vaccine in which the HAV antigen is bound to immunopotentiating, reconstituted influenza virosome membranes.[57] Features of the four inactivated vaccines available globally are shown in Table 31-6. Other inactivated HAV vaccines are under evaluation.[58]

Immunogenicity. The inactivated HAV vaccines are stable; storage for 2 years at 4° C does not affect immunogenicity. The induction of neutralizing antibodies and specific-memory B cells is thought to be responsible for the protection provided by HAV vaccines. The concept of immunologic memory is based on observations that the inactivated vaccines induce an early proliferative T-cell response that persists for at least 5 months.[59] This HAV-specific, cell-mediated response suggests that after a viral challenge immune vaccinees should develop a rapid anamnestic response resulting in an early, rapid, and high level of neutralizing antibody. After a single intramuscular dose, nearly 100 percent of vaccine recipients develop protective levels of antibody within a month of immunization. Anti-HAV is detectable in serum as early as 15 days in 70 percent to 98 percent of vaccinees. After intramuscular inoculation of two doses, serum levels of anti-HAV may approach those seen after natural infection. In fact, vaccine-induced levels of anti-HAV may be about 15 times higher than those usually attained with doses of immunoglobulin known to confer protection. The inactivated HAV vaccines have been shown to be highly immunogenic in children, adolescents, and adults, including those who are middle-aged and overweight.[60]

TABLE 31-6
Commercially Available, Inactivated Hepatitis A Virus Vaccines (Global)

	Havrix	Vaqta	Epaxal Berna	Avaxim
Manufacturer	SmithKline Beecham	Merck	Berna	Pasteur Merieux
Formaldehyde inactivation	Yes	Yes	Yes	Yes
Strain	HM-175	CR326F	RG-SB	GBM
Cell line	MRC-5	MRC-5	MRC-5	MRC-5
Virosomal	No	No	Yes	No
Two-dose schedule	0,6-12 months	0,6 months	0,12 months	0,6 months
Licensed in United States	Yes	Yes	No	No

Subcutaneous administration of inactivated HAV vaccine appears to be safe in children with hemophilia, although geometric mean titers of antibody were lower than in their non-hemophilic siblings vaccinated intramuscularly.[61] In a study comparing a jet-injector with needle injection of HAV vaccine, those who received the vaccine by jet-injector had higher seroconversion rates but more local reactivity.[62] Intradermal injections also may elicit anti-HAV. These cannot be recommended because multiple injections are probably necessary and information about titer and duration of antibody persistence is limited.

The long-term persistence of anti-HAV after vaccination has been estimated by mathematical models based on geometric mean titers and on individual anti-HAV titers.[63] Based on these methods antibody levels above or equal to 20 mIU/ml on average will persist for at least 10 years in fully vaccinated subjects. Concurrent administration of HAV vaccine does not impair the response to other vaccines commonly given to travelers.[64] However, peak anti-HAV titers may be a little lower after simultaneous administration of HAV and immunoglobulin than after administration of vaccine alone during the first 24 weeks after immunization.[65] After the second vaccine dose at 24 weeks, geometric mean titers of anti-HAV were not significantly different whether or not immunoglobulin was administered with the first dose of vaccine. Although the concentrations of anti-HAV in those receiving vaccine and immunoglobulin simultaneously were reduced after the first administration of vaccine, levels were thought to be sufficiently high to provide immediate and short-term protection. They were higher, for example, than levels seen in recipients of immunoglobulin alone. Therefore the injection of both immunoglobulin and vaccine at separate deltoid sites is appropriate for travelers leaving within too short a period to be certain of vaccine-induced immunity. Long-term protection, extending for years, which is presumably dependent on immune memory rather than serum levels of anti-HAV, also is likely to be unimpaired in those who receive both vaccine and immunoglobulin. Data to support this conclusion are unavailable, however.

Field trial, head-to-head comparisons of the two United States–approved, inactivated vaccines are not currently available. However, both vaccines have been reported to have similar immunogenicity when identical immunoassays are used for their evaluation.[66] Seroconversion rates of 100 percent were observed 4 to 8 weeks after a single dose of either vaccine. It seems likely that the kinetics for appearance and decline of postvaccination neutralizing antibody, over time, are also similar.

Immunogenicity in Patients with Liver Disease. Not surprisingly, immunosuppressed patients and human immunodeficiency virus (HIV)–positive individuals may be somewhat less responsive to HAV vaccines as compared with healthy subjects, but the immune response is usually adequate in most of the former patients. Information about the immunogenicity of HAV vaccine in patients with liver disease is limited. The immune response to inactivated HAV vaccine among Chinese children who were carriers of hepatitis B virus (HBV) appeared to be reduced when compared to the response in non-carrier children. The differences were not statistically significant through 5 years of follow-up; however, all recipients had detectable anti-HAV at year 5.[67] In a study of young Italian children who were HBV carriers or in those with chronic hepatitis B, inactivated HAV vaccine was highly immunogenic.[68] In adult patients with mild to moderately severe chronic liver disease, particularly those with chronic hepatitis C, HAV vaccine appeared to be slightly less immunogenic than in healthy controls.[69] Nonetheless, the height of the anti-HAV immune response after the second vaccine dose appeared adequate to provide protection from infection, and nearly 95 percent of vaccinees were seropositive for anti-HAV at the completion of the vaccination course (Table 31-7).

In patients with decompensated liver disease, post-HAV vaccine seroconversion rates and anti-HAV titers are low.[70] Among 100 liver transplant recipients only 24 had detectable anti-HAV before transplantation and 30 percent of these became anti-HAV negative at 2 years after transplantation.[71] Collectively, these findings support the notion that immunization of HAV susceptible chronic liver disease patients should be provided early rather than late after diagnosis.

Immunogenicity in the First Year of Life. In early studies the response to HAV vaccine appeared to be diminished in infants in whom maternal antibodies to HAV were acquired passively by the newborn. Recent studies have failed to establish reduced immunogenicity. In one study in which the first vaccine dose was given at 5 months of age and the second at 11 months, a 100 percent sero-

TABLE 31-7

Immunogenicity of Hepatitis A Virus Vaccine in Healthy Adults and Patients with Chronic Liver Diseases

Vaccinated subjects	Seroconversion rate 1 month after second vaccine dose	Geometric mean anti-HAV titer
Healthy adults	98.2%	1315 mIU/ml
Chronic hepatitis B	97.7%	749 mIU/ml
Chronic hepatitis C	94.3%	467 mIU/ml
Other liver diseases	95.2%	562 mIU/ml

Adapted from Keeffe EB, Iwarson S, McMahon BJ, et al: Safety and immogenicity of hepatitis A vaccine in patients with chronic liver disease. Hepatology 27:881-886, 1998.
HAV, Hepatitis A virus.

conversion rate was reported after the second dose. Nonetheless, the geometric mean titer of anti-HAV was lower in infants with maternal antibodies as compared with those without.[72] A second study also suggested that, although vaccination beginning at 2 months of age produced a lower geometric mean titer in infants seropositive before vaccination, priming nonetheless occurred.[73] Until more information is available, HAV vaccine is not likely to be recommended in the United States for children before age 2 years. However, it seems probable that passively acquired maternal antibodies will have disappeared by the end of the first year of life and that vaccine immunogenicity would be satisfactory during the second year of life.

Efficacy of HAV Vaccine. In a large field trial undertaken in Thai children, the cumulative preexposure protective efficacy rates for Havrix were 95 percent for both symptomatic and asymptomatic HAV infection.[54] In an epidemic setting in upstate New York, preexposure administration of Vaqta conferred 100 percent protection 16 days after vaccination.[55] The effectiveness of HAV vaccine in postexposure immunoprophylaxis is uncertain. Its use is not currently recommended. Studies in chimpanzees experimentally infected with HAV and then vaccinated suggested efficacy for vaccination but the small number of animals tested and the interval between exposure and vaccine administration were quite short.[74] Possible efficacy for vaccination postexposure was also suggested in the trial of vaccine in upstate New York because no cases occurred in any vaccinated child more than 16 days after vaccination,[55] for an illness with a typical incubation period of 30 days.

Although data are sparse, abrupt reductions in clinical cases after the use of vaccine in the control of community-wide outbreaks also supports the concept that vaccine is effective in the postexposure setting. To date, no prospective, randomized, controlled clinical trials have compared HAV vaccine to immunoglobulin for postexposure immunoprophylaxis. In one trial from Italy, household contacts of hospitalized patients with HAV infection were randomized to receive HAV vaccine within 8 days of onset of symptoms in the index case or to remain unvaccinated.[75] An efficacy rate of 82 percent was reported from the vaccine, with 95 percent confidence intervals of 20 percent to 96 percent for individual contacts. Because postexposure immunoprophylaxis with immunoglobulin is currently the conventional choice, a head-to-head comparison of vaccine to immunoglobulin administration is needed.

Levels of anti-HAV sufficient to ensure protection for at least 1 year have been found in about 95 percent of vaccine recipients after a single priming dose of HAV vaccine.[76] One priming dose of HAV vaccine appeared to provide protection for children at risk who were exposed before the second dose.[77] Thus a single dose of vaccine might be sufficient to provide prolonged protection, especially if memory B cells capable of responding to HAV exposure by the rapid production of neutralizing antibodies to HAV were activated. Because it is not yet clear that a single dose of vaccine is always effective in inducing an anamnestic humoral response on reexposure, the two-dose regimen probably should be used until more data about the efficacy of a single dose become available.

Prevaccination Screening. Strategies of prevaccination testing to identify susceptibles have been assessed in cost-decision analyses. When immunity is less than 50 percent in a selected population, one such analysis suggested that universal vaccination appeared to be a less costly strategy than one involving prevaccination testing for immunity.[78] In low-prevalence, developed countries, screening for anti-HAV before vaccination is rational for older individuals and for those with a history of probable HAV infection or in immigrants from a high-prevalence area.

Indications

Vaccination of Young Children. As mentioned previously, the prevalence of clinically recognized HAV infection in children in the United States is low. Nevertheless, there are geographic areas in the United States with attack rates approaching those in developing countries. Vaccination of children has been recommended for those residing in states, counties, or regions in which HAV attack rates are increased by at least twice the national average of 10/100,000 population. Where rates are above the national average but do not meet the twofold threshold, the decision about vaccination of children has been left to local health authorities. Routine vaccination of young children over the age of 2 and catch-up vaccination of unvaccinated older children have been ongoing among native peoples of Alaska and the Americas for several years. Attack rates for HAV are decreasing in these communities.

Hepatitis A vaccination of adolescents residing in states with high incidence rates for hepatitis A has been reported to be cost-effective.[79] The current high susceptibility of children in the United States, the key role played by children in spreading infection in households, and the knowledge that clinically apparent HAV infection is more severe with increasing age together argue for early, universal immunization. Mass HAV vaccination of very young children also may be cost-effective in developed countries.[80] It seems likely, but has not been proved, that immunization of young children will provide prolonged protection, lasting through adolescence and young adulthood.

In developing countries, in which hepatitis A is endemic or hyperendemic, universal vaccination of very young children has rarely been attempted, in part because of the cost of vaccine and in part because of the lack of appropriate health care infrastructure for delivery of vaccine. Vaccination is undoubtedly essential, however, for controlling infection in these areas, especially where improvements in water supplies and sanitary standards cannot be readily initiated. When improvements in economic and hygienic conditions are made in the absence of childhood vaccination programs, HAV infection rates are likely to decrease. Unfortunately, this may result in an increase in the number of susceptibles present in the non-vaccinated population, and may be followed by an increase in the average age of infected individuals, increased morbidity, and the possibility of resurgence with major community-wide outbreaks.[81]

The development of a combined hepatitis A and B vaccine may resolve the issue for those developing countries in which hepatitis B vaccine already has been incorporated into immunization programs. Two such bivalent vaccines have been developed. The initial combination hepatitis A and B vaccine produced by Merck appeared to produce acceptable levels of anti-HAV but not acceptable levels of anti-HBs.[82] The SmithKlineBeecham bivalent vaccine (Twinrix) elicited good immunogenicity for both immunogens and was well tolerated.[83,84] When given to healthy adults in a three-dose schedule, 100 percent of the recipients were anti-HAV positive and more than 95 percent had seroprotective levels of anti-HBs 4 years after the first dose.[85] Twinrix has been approved for use in several European countries and Canada. It became available in the United States in 2002.

Travelers to Endemic Regions. Because HAV is the most important vaccine-preventable disease among international travelers, HAV vaccine should be targeted to this group. Travelers from low-prevalence, developed countries who visit high-endemicity regions (Mexico, the Caribbean, Southeast Asia, South and Central America, and Africa) should receive the first dose of HAV vaccine at least 2 weeks before travel. Regardless of duration of travel, candidates for HAV vaccine include tourists, business travelers, diplomats, foreign service personnel, military and peacekeeping forces, health care workers, missionaries, travel industry workers, and accompanying household and family members. Vaccination of frequent travelers and military personnel assigned to endemic regions appears to be more cost-effective than passive immunization. The cost-effectiveness of vaccination is dependent on the immune status and incidence of infection in the target population as well as the cost of the vaccine.[86]

Patients with Chronic Liver Disease. Patients with chronic liver diseases and those with end-stage liver disease or patients who have received liver transplants are candidates for HAV vaccine if they lack circulating anti-HAV. Early vaccination after the diagnosis of chronic liver disease is appropriate because patients with decompensated liver disease and awaiting liver transplantation and those who have received transplants and are on immunosuppressive regimens may respond less well than those with milder disease.[70] One analysis suggested that vaccination of patients with chronic hepatitis C[87] may not be cost-effective, but many of the assumptions underlying that conclusion have been criticized,[88] and vaccination has become standard practice in many hepatology centers.

Patients with Clotting Factor Disorders. Because recipients of solvent/detergent-treated clotting factor concentrates are at some risk, HAV vaccine should be given to individuals with clotting factor disorders for whom treatment with recombinant or heat-treated products is unlikely. For those patients who have received concentrates at risk, testing for susceptibility before vaccination makes sense. For all others, vaccination without testing would be appropriate unless a history of prior hepatitis A is obtained.

Community Outbreaks. Studies of the effectiveness of HAV vaccine in interrupting ongoing community-wide or common-source outbreaks are limited. Vaccination programs may be effective in interrupting community outbreaks if a sufficiently large proportion of the population at risk is immunized.[89] Vaccine coverage rates of 70 percent to 80 percent may be required to stem outbreaks. In some outbreaks the effectiveness of vaccination has been difficult to determine.[90] Controlled field trials are not yet available, and in many instances delays in implementation of vaccination programs may blunt their effectiveness. The role of HAV vaccine in the control of common-source outbreaks remains uncertain.

Other Candidates. Preexposure immunoprophylaxis with HAV vaccine has been recommended by the Advisory Committee on Immunization Practices (ACIP) of the United States Public Health Service for additional groups at risk for HAV exposure.[91] HAV vaccine is recommended for adolescent males and men who have sex with men, for users of illicit injection and non-injection drugs, and for individuals who work with or handle HAV directly or HAV-infected or newly imported nonhuman primates (e.g., virology laboratory technicians, zoo workers, veterinarians). Sewage and waste water treatment plant workers, health care workers in neonatal intensive care units, and employees and attendees of day care centers and institutions for the mentally disadvantaged also seem to be appropriate candidates for vaccination.

A case could be made for preemployment and preexposure HAV vaccination of food handlers. These people are not necessarily at increased risk, but an infected food handler can amplify the incidence of infection by contaminating foods served to hundreds of consumers. Obstacles to wide-scale vaccination of food handlers include high employment turnover and the frequent absence of health insurance for part-time workers in the food industry. ACIP recommends that vaccination of food handlers should be considered whenever local conditions suggest that it would be cost-effective to do so.

HEPATITIS E

Virology

Viral Characteristics and Heterogeneity

HEV is a RNA-containing, non-enveloped, 27 to 34 nm in diameter spherical virus-like particle with icosahedral symmetry and indentations and spikes on its surface. It is relatively stable to acidic and mildly alkaline conditions. Physicochemical and other characteristics of the virus are shown in Table 31-8. Although HEV had been classified tentatively as a member of the *Caliciviridae* species, its genomic organization appears to be distinct from the caliciviruses. A possible relationship to positive-strand RNA plant viruses and rubella virus seemed more likely. However, the virus has been placed into an "unassigned" classification status.[92]

TABLE 31-8
Characteristics of Hepatitis E Virus

Family	Unclassified
Genus	Unknown
Genotypes	Four or more
Nucleic acid	Single-stranded RNA
Genome size	7.5 kb
Morphology	Spherical particles
Symmetry	Icosahedral
Open reading frames	Three, overlapping
Surface structure	Indentations and spikes
Envelope	None
Size	27-34 nm in diameter
Buoyant density	1.290 g/cm^3
Sedimentation coefficient	183S
Antigenic sites	Two immunodominant epitopes
Physicochemical properties	Relatively stable to acid and mild alkaline states
Replication site	Hepatocyte cytoplasm
Primate host range	Human beings, chimpanzees, rhesus monkeys, cynomolgus macaques, owl monkeys, marmosets

RNA, Ribonucleic acid.

Only one HEV serotype is known, but four main human HEV genotypes have been identified. Others may exist. The recognized genotypes include an Asian cluster named genotype I, which may have an African subtype; a US genotype named genotype II; a Mexican genotype named genotype III; and a Chinese-Beijing genotype named genotype IV. Genotypes I and III may co-exist in Africa.[93] Separate subtypes within the major genotypes have been identified. In general, HEV isolates from the same country or region are closely related,[94] but diversity has been reported.[95]

The host range of HEV includes but may not limited to human and non-human primates. A number of mammalian species may be infected by a very similar, if not identical, virus. Most attention has been focused on HEV infection in swine. Swine herds in both HEV-endemic and non-endemic countries have been shown to be seropositive.[96] Sequencing studies indicate that swine and human HEV share between 84 percent and 95 percent of nucleotides.[97] A difference of 20 amino acids in the products of open reading frame (ORF)-2 may separate the swine and human HEV.

It is not yet understood whether human HEV can infect pigs and whether swine HEV is pathogenic for human beings. The role of swine as a reservoir for HEV infection remains ill-defined and cross-reactivity of commercially available reagents for anti-HEV may be responsible in part for the unexpected finding of anti-HEV in non-endemic, developed areas. Nonetheless, populations with occupational exposure to wastes from swine or domestic animals have higher prevalences of anti-HEV than healthy blood donors from the same geographic region.[98]

Anti-HEV also has been found in domestic rats, sheep, and chickens. The specificity of these positive antibody tests and the significance of these animals for spreading human infection remains to be determined.

HEV RNA Genome. The isolation of HEV was reported in 1990[99]; cloning and sequencing of the HEV genome were reported one year later.[100] HEV is a positive sense, single-stranded, polyadenylated RNA of about 7.5 kb. Three discontinuous, partially overlapping ORFs and a capped 5′ non-translated region of about 27 to 35 nucleotides and a 65 to 74 nucleotide 3′ poly (A) tail have been identified (Figure 31-6). ORF-1 is about 5 kb in length and encodes the non-structural polyprotein, which has been expressed as a 186-kDa protein.[101] The ORF-1 motifs are more rubivirus-like than calicivirus-like. The large polyprotein encoded by ORF-1 possesses motifs for a cysteine protease, methyltransferase, helicase, "Y" and "X" domains, a proline-rich "hinge" region, and an RNA-dependent RNA polymerase. It is cleaved into individual, non-structural proteins, presumably by viral proteases. ORF-2 is shorter, at about 2 kb, and encodes for the structural capsid protein. Antibodies elicited by a vaccine containing ORF-2 recognize native HEV,[102] suggesting that the major capsid protein contains an immunodominant epitope capable of stimulating protective antibody. The third and shortest open reading frame (ORF-3) overlaps ORF-1 and ORF-2 and is just about 370 nucleotides long. It encodes a phosphoprotein. Although its function remains unsettled, an association of the ORF-3 phosphoprotein with the cytoskeleton suggests that it may serve as a membrane anchor region and is involved in cell signaling.[103] A second potential immunodominant epitope at the carboxyl end of ORF-3 has been recognized.[104] In the absence of the first and third ORFs, the ORF-2 peptide self-assembles into virus-like particles, thereby suggesting that neither ORF-1 nor ORF-3 is essential for particle assembly.[105]

Although point mutations in HEV have been observed in different patients within discrete outbreaks,[106] the mutation rate for HEV has not been established. Most

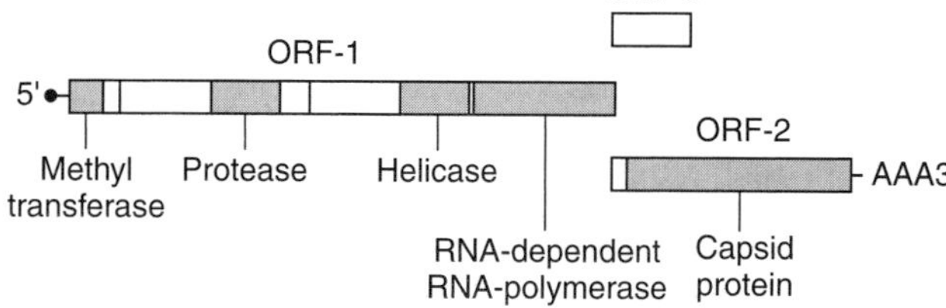

Figure 31-6 Genomic organization of HEV RNA. *HEV,* Hepatitis E virus; *RNA,* ribonucleic acid.

nucleotide substitutions occur in the third base of the codon and the amino acid sequence is unaffected. However, in HEV genotype IV, a single nucleotide insertion in ORF-3 changes the initiation of ORF-3 and possibly also ORF-2.[107]

HEV RNA is infectious. Transfection of cells with genomic RNA synthesized in vitro from a full-length HEV cDNA clone resulted in the production of viable HEV particles capable of inducing infection in a rhesus monkey.[108]

HEV Propagation in Tissue Culture. Cell culture of HEV has been reported in a variety of continuous cell lines derived from human lung or liver and in primary macaque hepatocytes. Cytopathic effects that could be neutralized by antibodies have been described in some lines but cytopathic effects are not present invariably and appear to be cell line–dependent.[109,110] Whether any of the systems for culture in vitro will prove reliable and yield sufficient virus for development of a vaccine or prove useful for studies of HEV replication remains to be determined.

HEV Life Cycle. The pathophysiologic changes induced during the course of HEV infection are not well characterized. The liver is probably the sole site of HEV replication, however. In most non-experimental settings, the virus is thought to enter the circulation through the intestine via contaminated water or, less commonly, contaminated food. The precise mechanisms and sequence of events permitting the transfer of ingested HEV from the intestinal lumen to the liver remain in debate and studies in human volunteers directed at this issue remain unlikely to be undertaken. In a single volunteer study, HEV was detected in serum after oral inoculation before clinical signs of infection were observed.[111] In experimentally infected non-human primates, HEV-associated antigen could be detected in hepatocyte cytoplasm as early as 10 days after intravenous inoculation.[112] HEV antigen persisted for about 3 weeks after its initial appearance. The transfer of HEV RNA from hepatocytes to bile has been studied in experimentally infected rhesus monkeys after intravenous inoculation.[113] HEV RNA positive and negative strands were found in hepatocytes early after infection (during the incubation period). Virus-like particles were found in bile before histologic evidence of hepatitis and during the acute and convalescence phases of hepatitis. HEV RNA appeared in the canalicular side of biliary epithelial cells and then diffusely in the cytoplasm of these cells. With recovery, HEV RNA disappeared from biliary epithelium.

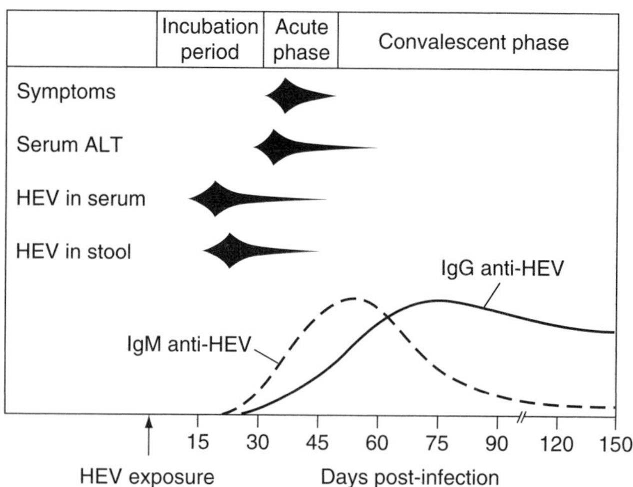

Figure 31-7 Sequence of clinical, biochemical, virologic, and serologic events in acute hepatitis E.

Epidemiology

Incubation Period and Fecal Shedding

The incubation period for hepatitis E ranges between 2 and 9 weeks with a mean of about 6.5 weeks. Biochemical evidence of hepatitis, namely elevation of serum aminotransferase levels, persists for 3 to 13 weeks. HEV excretion in stools may begin during the latter half of the incubation period or occur at the onset of illness or 2 to 3 weeks later. The precise duration of fecal shedding is not known (Figure 31-7). In one recent study the maximal duration of fecal excretion of HEV RNA, measured by PCR, was 30 days after onset of the first symptom.[114]

Period of Viremia

HEV appears in the blood of infected patients but the precise onset and duration of viremia are uncertain. HEV may appear in serum before its appearance in stool. In one recent study viremia was short-lived with a maximal duration of 45 days after the onset of the first symptom.[114] These observations suggest that viremia extending beyond the duration of the biochemical features of hepatitis E is probably very uncommon.

Incidence and Prevalence

The incidence of HEV infection in the United States is so low that accurate figures are impossible to estimate. Documented, clinically apparent cases also are exceedingly rare. Most reported cases have been in travelers returning from endemic regions. Nonetheless, sporadic cases not associated with international travel have been identified. Two HEV isolates have been identified and sequenced from patients with acute viral hepatitis in the United States, in whom no risk factors could be identified. These isolates were related and genetically distinct from other non–United States isolates.[115,116]

Clinically overt hepatitis E has a worldwide distribution with a predominance in Southeast and Central Asia, the Middle East, and North Africa (Figure 31-8). Frequent

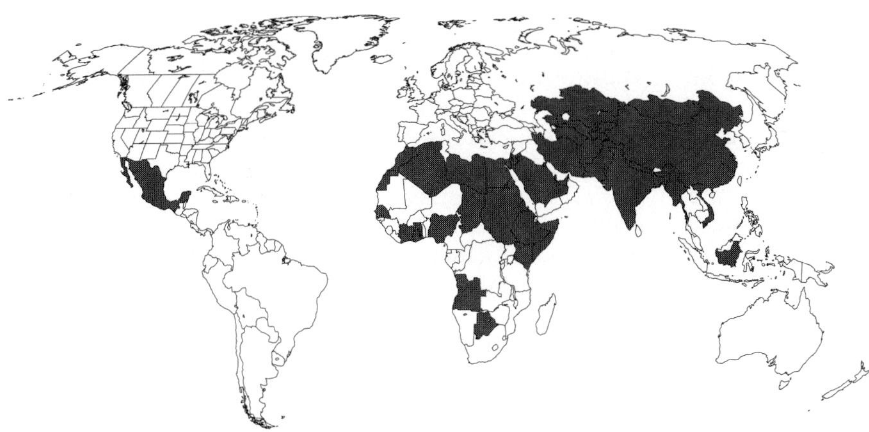

Figure 31-8 Countries with high endemicity for HEV or sites of reported outbreaks. *HEV,* Hepatitis E virus. (Data from Aggarwal R, Krawczynski K: Hepatitis E: An overview and recent advances in clinical and laboratory research. J Gastroenterol Hepatol 15:9-20, 2000.)

outbreaks and a high prevalence of infection have been reported from the Indian subcontinent, Nepal, Burma, and China. In Africa hepatitis E has been documented in Egypt, Algeria, Morocco, Tunisia, Chad, in the Sudan, Kenya, Ethiopia, Somalia, Djibouti, South Africa, and Namibia. In the western hemisphere, outbreaks have been reported in Mexico, and endemic HEV has been described in Mexico, Brazil, Venezuela, and Cuba.[117] The African isolates appear to be closely related and differ from those from Burma, Mexico, China, and probably the United States.[118]

Outbreaks are variable in length, occasionally lasting for many months. Peak attack rates as high as 30 percent have been described in adults, and the highest rates of clinically apparent disease generally occur in young and middle-aged adults. Anicteric or subclinical infections may be more common in younger individuals. Men are more often affected than women in most outbreaks. Clinically apparent attack rates are often less than 10 percent in children. In endemic regions acute hepatitis E may account for more than half of all sporadic viral hepatitis in adults and children. In non-endemic regions where outbreaks do not occur, HEV accounts for less than 1 percent of clinically apparent viral hepatitis. As in the United States, HEV infection is very uncommon in Western Europe and is most often related to travel to an endemic area. However, community-acquired HEV infection may occur sporadically without linkage to travel or contact with travelers in developed nations.[119]

The specificity of anti-HEV assays used in seroprevalence studies remains uncertain. In most Western, developed, non-endemic countries, seroprevalence studies indicate the presence of antibodies in 0.5 percent to 2.5 percent, whereas in endemic regions, average prevalence rates are between 10 percent and 25 percent. The range, however, is extraordinarily wide. Within the United States, the prevalence of anti-HEV generally has been less than 2 percent among healthy populations. Higher seroreactivity rates for anti-HEV have been reported in blood donors (21 percent), men who have sex with men (16 percent), and injection drug users (23 percent).[120] These findings may not represent valid infection with HEV because serologic cross-reaction with a related antigen is possible. Non-pathogenic HEV infection seems unlikely but cannot be totally excluded. The lack of concordance between serologic assays developed for HEV suggests that current assays have imperfect specificity.[121] Differences in the antigenic strains used in the assays may be responsible.

Within individual endemic regions, widely varying infection rates also have been reported and are biologically more plausible. Differences in living conditions related to sources of drinking water are probably responsible. For example, in Malaysia, only 2 percent of urban blood donors but 44 percent to 50 percent of individuals in aboriginal communities were anti-HEV positive.[122]

Modes of Transmission

Fecal-oral spread, mainly via contaminated drinking water, is the predominant mode of HEV transmission in endemic regions. Use of river water for drinking, cooking, personal washing, and disposal of human excreta in Southeast Asia appears to be highly associated with the prevalence of infection. In contrast, boiling of river water has been reported to be negatively associated with high seroprevalence of HEV.[123] Person-to-person transmission may occur, but intrafamilial spread of HEV appears to be unusual.[124] Secondary attack rates of clinically apparent hepatitis E among household contacts are often less than 5 percent.

Percutaneous, bloodborne modes of transmission also may contribute to the spread of HEV in endemic regions. The finding of HEV RNA in asymptomatic blood donors in endemic areas suggests that bloodborne transmission may occur,[125] and transfusion-associated hepatitis E infection has been reported. In one study of 56 transfused patients, two individuals seroconverted to IgM and IgG anti-HEV 4 and 5 weeks after transfusion and one developed elevated serum aminotransferase levels but neither reported symptoms of hepatitis.[126] The prevalence of HEV infection was higher in hemodialysis patients (6.3 percent) when compared with blood donors (2.8 percent) in Spain but no relation to number of blood transfusions was found.[127]

Transmission from a patient hospitalized with acute hepatitis E and liver failure to health care workers has been reported,[128] but the precise routes of spread and the frequency of nosocomial transmission remain uncertain. Similarly, vertical transmission has been described[129]; its epidemiologic importance also remains to be established.

Immunopathogenesis and Immunity

Although still poorly understood, a variety of patterns of infection have now been reported in experimentally infected chimpanzees.[130] Liver injury is evident in some animals after intravenous inoculation of HEV, whereas in others infection occurs without evidence of liver involvement. Viremia occurred in some chimpanzees, but anti-HEV could not be detected. In others, viremia, fecal shedding of virus, elevated aminotransferase levels, and seroconversion to anti-HEV positive were observed. The role of inoculum size, the presence of non-infectious defective particles, routes of infection, and host factors affecting immunocompetency (e.g., age, body weight, nutritional status) remain ill-defined for both chimpanzees and human patients. These observations, if fully generalizable to human infection, suggest that subclinical infection may be more common than previously believed and fit with observations of the presence of anti-HEV in residents of endemic and non-endemic regions in whom no history of clinical disease is recognized. In one recent study from Taiwan, a non-endemic area, 11 percent of healthy subjects were anti-HEV positive.[131]

Serologic Diagnosis

Serologic testing for evidence of acute HEV infection includes assays for both IgM and IgG anti-HEV (see Figure 31-7). IgM, IgA, and IgG antibodies to HEV appear after HEV infection and are detectable in most acute specimens. Limited studies of the sensitivities and specificities of the IgM and IgG enzyme immunoassays have been reported in acute hepatitis E. Relative to testing for HEV RNA, the IgM and IgG had sensitivities of 53 percent and 87 percent, respectively, whereas the specificities were 99 percent and 92 percent, respectively.[131] Levels of IgM anti-HEV decline rapidly during the convalescent phase. The IgG anti-HEV may persist in some patients although declining in titer. IgG anti-HEV is believed to be responsible for short-term humoral immunity to reinfection. Enzyme immunoassays for IgM and IgG anti-HEV are available in commercial laboratories but none of the assays have been FDA-approved. An immunofluorescent antibody blocking assay for antibody to HEV in serum and liver tissue has been available at the Centers for Disease Control and Prevention. PCR tests for the detection of HEV RNA in serum and stool samples are also research techniques but are not widely available, and not conventionally used in diagnosis.

Pathology

The histopathologic features of acute hepatitis E resemble those seen in acute hepatitis A, with lobular disarray, ballooning degeneration, acidophilic bodies, and spotty lobular necrosis. Cholestatic features may be prominent in some patients with canalicular bile plugs, rosette formation, portal and periportal inflammation, and preserved lobular architecture. Bridging necrosis, submassive necrosis, and massive necrosis may be seen in some severe cases. In other severe cases endothelial inflammation and cholestasis have been the most prominent features. In patients who recover, complete resolution is anticipated.

Clinical and Laboratory Features

Clinical signs and symptoms of hepatitis E are similar to those seen in acute hepatitis A and include malaise, anorexia, dark urine, jaundice, nausea, vomiting, fever, and abdominal discomfort. Arthralgias, diarrhea, rashes, and pruritus may be seen. Common clinical features and their frequencies are shown in Table 31-9. Although the course of acute hepatitis E may resemble that of hepatitis A in most patients and is usually self-limited, acute, fatal liver failure has been seen in as many as 10 percent to 20 percent of infected pregnant women, particularly if the infection is acquired in the third trimester. Additionally, a severe course has been identified, albeit rarely, in non-pregnant patients co-infected with HAV and HEV.[132]

Treatment of HEV Infection

No specific drug therapy is available. As in the case of hepatitis A, management is largely symptomatic and supportive. Early delivery of the pregnant woman with acute hepatitis E is probably reasonable but whether it will reduce fetal and maternal mortality remains to be determined.

Immunoprophylaxis

Prevention of HEV infection in developing countries in which the disease is currently endemic requires the availability of clean water supplies. Travelers from non-endemic to endemic regions should avoid water or ice of uncertain origin and uncooked bivalve mollusks, fruits, and vegetables.

Immunoglobulin

Immunoglobulin prepared in non-endemic regions is not effective in the prevention of HEV infection; immunoglobulin prepared in endemic regions is probably ineffective, although in one study immunoglobulin administration appeared to reduce the incidence of infections in pregnant women.[133] In experimentally infected non-human primates, passive transfer of anti-HEV reduced fecal shedding and ameliorated the disease.[134] Monoclonal antibodies to the HEV ORF-2–encoded capsid protein have been reported to neutralize HEV in vitro.[135] Whether immunoglobulin preparations of mon-

TABLE 31-9
Common Clinical Features of Icteric Hepatitis E

Symptom	Frequency
Malaise	95%-100%
Anorexia	66%-100%
Abdominal pain	37%-82%
Nausea, vomiting	29%-100%
Fever	23%-97%
Pruritus	14%-59%

Adapted from Aggarwal R, Krawczynksi K. Hepatitis E: An overview and recent advances in clinical and laboratory research. J Gastroenterol Hepatol 15:9-20, 2000.

oclonal antibodies could provide preexposure or post-exposure protection remains to be determined. Neither hyperimmunoglobulin nor monoclonal antibody preparations are available.

Hepatitis E Vaccine

Subunit or naked DNA HEV vaccines are currently under development; low virus yields in tissue culture have hampered development of an inactivated, whole virus particle vaccine. Similarly, a live, attenuated HEV vaccine is not likely in the immediate future. It is not yet certain that a vaccine prepared from one HEV isolate would provide protection against all isolates although the use of a highly conserved immunogen, such as the ORF-2 protein, might be cross-reactive among the different genotypes. After an inexpensive, effective HEV vaccine becomes available it would be used in endemic regions to reduce HEV-associated morbidity. Targeting of a HEV vaccine to susceptible pregnant women, whether resident within or travelers to endemic regions, would make good sense.

The protein expressed from ORF-2 of HEV appears to be the most promising immunogen described to date. In a study in mice, a purified recombinant plasmid vector containing ORF-2 elicited a long-term humoral immune response. The antibodies produced have been shown to recognize native HEV.[136] The antibody response to DNA immunization with a plasmid expressing the HEV ORF-2 structural protein was enhanced with the use of plasmids expressing IL-2 and granulocyte-macrophage colony-stimulating factor or with virus-like particles expressed through a baculovirus expression system.[137]

In rhesus monkeys a prototype recombinant ORF-2 protein vaccine given after exposure reduced the duration and extent of viremia and fecal shedding of HEV after challenge with live HEV but did not provide sterilizing immunity.[138] Preexposure vaccination similarly did not reduce the frequency of infection after intravenous challenge with homologous or heterologous strains but it did provide protection from hepatitis as defined by serum ALT levels and histopathology.[138] Circulating levels of HEV and fecal excretion of HEV were lower in vaccinated animals. In cynomolgus macaques, in contrast to intradermal inoculation, gene gun delivery of a plasmid construct expressing ORF-2 protected the monkeys from challenge with a heterologous HEV strain.[139]

Studies of a candidate, two-dose recombinant ORF-2 HEV vaccine have been initiated in healthy volunteers in the United States and a field trial of this vaccine given in a three-dose schedule is in progress in Nepal.

References

1. Berge JJ, Drennan DP, Jacobs J, et al: The cost of hepatitis A infection in American adolescents and adults in 1997. Hepatology 31:469-473, 2000.
2. Wilner IR, Uhl MD, Howard SC, et al: Serious hepatitis: an analysis of patients hospitalized during an urban epidemic in the United States. Ann Intern Med 128:111-114, 1998.
3. Vento S, Garofano T, Renzini C, et al: Fulminant hepatitis associated with hepatitis A virus superinfection in patients with chronic hepatitis C. N Engl J Med 338:286-290, 1998.
4. Francki RIB, Fauquet CM, Knudson DL, Brown F: Classification and nomenclature of viruses. Fifth report of the International Committee on Taxonomy of Viruses. Arch Virol Suppl 2:320-326, 1991.
5. Robertson BH, Jansen RW, Khanna B, et al: Genetic relatedness of hepatitis A virus strains recovered from different geographical regions. J Gen Virology 73:1365-1377, 1992.
6. Bishop NE, Anderson DA: Uncoating kinetics of hepatitis A virus virions and provirions. J Virology 74:3423-3426, 2000.
7. Bishop NE: Hepatitis A replication: an intermediate in the uncoating process. Intervirology 43:36-47, 2000.
8. Emerson SU, Lewis M, Govindarajan S, et al: In vivo transfection by hepatitis A virus synthetic RNA. Arch Virol 9(suppl):205-209, 1994.
9. Yokosuka O: Molecular biology of hepatitis A virus: significance of various substitutions in the hepatitis A virus genome. J Gastroenterol Hepatol 15(suppl):D91-D97, 2000.
10. Graff J, Richards OC, Swiderek KM, et al: Hepatitis A virus capsid protein VP1 has a heterogeneous C terminus. J Virology 73:6015-6023, 1999.
11. Martin A, Benichou D, Chao S-F, et al: Maturation of the hepatitis A virus capsid protein VP1 is not dependent on processing by the 3Cpro proteinase. J Virology 73:6220-6227, 1999.
12. Kusov YY, Gauss-Muller V: In vitro RNA binding of the hepatitis A virus proteinase 3C (HAV 3C pro) to secondary structure elements within the 5′ terminus of the HAV genome. RNA 3:291-302, 1997.
13. Hill RD, Vederas JC: Azodicarboxamides: a new class of cysteine proteinase inhibitor for hepatitis A virus and human rhinovirus 3C enzymes. J Org Chem 64:9538-9546, 1999.
14. Gosert R, Egger D, Bienz K: A cytopathic and a cell culture adapted hepatitis A virus strain differ in cell killing but not in intracellular membrane rearrangements. Virology 266:157-169, 2000.
15. Funkhouser AW, Schultz DE, Lemon SM, et al: Hepatitis A virus translation is rate-limiting for virus replication in MRC-5 cells. Virology 254:268-278, 1999.
16. Shavrina Asher LV, Binn LN, et al: Pathogenesis of hepatitis A in orally inoculated owl monkeys *(Aotus trivirgatus)*. J Med Virol 47:260-268, 1995.
17. Kaplan G, Totsuka A, Thompson P, et al: Identification of a surface glycoprotein on African green monkey kidney cells as a receptor for hepatitis A virus. EMBO J 15:4282-4296, 1996.
18. Bishop NE: Hepatitis A virus replication: an intermediate in the uncoating process. Intervirology 43:36-47, 2000.
19. Yotsuyanagi H, Koike K, Yasuda K, et al: Prolonged fecal excretion of hepatitis A virus in adult patients with hepatitis A as determined by polymerase chain reaction. Hepatology 24:10-13, 1996.
20. Polish LB, Robertson BH, Khanna B, et al: Excretion of hepatitis A virus (HAV) in adults: comparison of immunologic and molecular detection methods and relationship between HAV positivity and infectivity in tamarins. J Clin Microbiol 37:3615-3617, 1999.
21. Bower WA, Nainan OV, Han X, Margolis HS: Duration of viremia in hepatitis A virus infection. J Infect Dis 182:12-17, 2000.
22. Kwon OS, Byun KS, Yeon JE, et al: Detection of hepatitis A viral RNA in sera of patients with acute hepatitis A. J Gastroenterol Hepatol 15:1043-1047, 2000.
23. Leach CT, Koo FC, Hilsenbeck SG, Jenson HB: The epidemiology of viral hepatitis in children in South Texas: increased prevalence of hepatitis A along the Texas-Mexico border. J Infect Dis 180:509-513, 1999.
24. Staes CJ, Schlenker TL, Risk I, et al: Sources of infection among persons with acute hepatitis A and no identified risk factors during a sustained community-wide outbreak. Pediatrics 106:E54, 2000.
25. Redlinger T, O'Rourke K, VanDerslice J: Hepatitis A among schoolchildren in a US-Mexico border community. Am J Public Health 87:1715-1717, 1997.
26. Sadetzki S, Rostmi N, Modan B: Hepatitis A outbreak originating in a day care center: a community case report. Eur J Epidemiology 15:549-551, 1999.
27. De Serres G, Cromeans TL, Levesque B, et al: Molecular confirmation of hepatitis A virus from well water: epidemiology and public health implications. J Infect Dis 179:37-43, 1999.
28. Brown MG, Lindo JF, King SD: Investigations of the epidemiology of infections with hepatitis A virus in Jamaica. Ann Trop Med Parasitol 94:497-502, 2000.
29. Weldon M, VanEgdom MJ, Hendricks KA, et al: Prevalence of antibody to hepatitis A virus in drinking water workers and wastewater workers in Texas from 1996 to 1997. J Occup Environ Med 42:821-826, 2000.

30. Divizia M, Gabrieli R, Donia D, et al: Concomitant poliovirus infection during an outbreak of hepatitis A. J Infection 19:227-230, 1999.
31. Croci L, Ciccozzi M, De Medici D, et al: Inactivation of hepatitis A virus in heat-treated mussels. J Appl Microbiol 87:884-888, 1999.
32. Hutin YJF, Pool V, Cramer EH, et al: A multistate, foodborne outbreak of hepatitis A. N Engl J Med 340:595-602, 1999.
33. Bidawid S, Farber JM, Sattar SA: Contamination of foods by food handlers: experiments on hepatitis A virus transfer to food and its interruption. Appl Environm Microbiol 66:2759-2763, 2000.
34. Henning KJ, Bell E, Braun J, Barker ND: A community-wide outbreak of hepatitis A: risk factors for infection among homosexual and bisexual men. Am J Med 154:828-831, 1995.
35. Corona R, Stroffilini T, Giglio A, et al: Lack of evidence for increased risk of hepatitis A infection in homosexual men. Epidemiol Infect 123:89-93, 1999.
36. Hutin YJ, Sabin KM, Hutwagner LC, et al: Multiple modes of hepatitis A virus transmission among methamphetamine users. Am J Epidemiol 152:186-192, 2000.
37. Chudy M, Budek I, Keller-Stanislawksi B, et al: A new cluster of hepatitis A infection in hemophiliacs traced to a contaminated plasma pool. J Med Virol 57:91-99, 1999.
38. Pinto MA, Marchevsky RS, Pelajo-Machado M, et al: Inducible nitric oxide synthase (iNOS) expression in liver and splenic T lymphocyte rise are associated with liver histological damage during experimental hepatitis A virus (HAV) infection in *Callithrix jacchus*. Exp Toxicol Pathol 52:3-10, 2000.
39. Wang C-H, Tschen S-Y, Heinricy U, et al: Immune response to hepatitis A virus capsid proteins after infection. J Clin Microbiol 34:707-713, 1996.
40. Shrier LA, Karpen SJ, McEvoy C: Acute pancreatitis associated with acute hepatitis A in a young child. J Pediatrics 126:57-59, 1995.
41. Sridharan S, Mossad S, Hoffman G: Hepatitis A infection mimicking adult onset Still's disease. J Rheumatol 27:1792-1795, 2000.
42. Mourani S, Dobbs SM, Genta RM, et al: Hepatitis A virus-associated cholecystitis. Ann Intern Med 120:398-400, 1994.
43. Islam S, McDonald JA: Sensory neuropathy in the prodromal phase of hepatitis A and review of the literature. J Gastroenterol Hepatol 15:809-811, 2000.
44. Zhu J, Quyyumi AA, Normal JE, et al: The possible role of hepatitis A virus in the pathogenesis of atherosclerosis. J Infect Dis 182:1583-1587, 2000.
45. Forbes A, Williams R: Increasing age—an important adverse prognostic factor in hepatitis A virus infection. J Royal Coll Phys London 22:237-239, 1988.
46. Debray D, Cullufi P, Devictor D, et al: Liver failure in children with acute hepatitis A. Hepatology 26:1018-1022, 1997.
47. Lefilliatre P, Villenueve JP: Fulminant hepatitis A in patients with chronic liver disease. Can J Publ Health 91:168-170, 2000.
48. Gordon SC, Reddy KR, Schiff L, et al: Prolonged intrahepatic cholestasis secondary to acute hepatitis A. Ann Intern Med 101:635-637, 1984.
49. Glikson M, Galun E, Oren R, et al: Relapsing hepatitis A. Review of 14 cases and literature survey. Medicine 71:14-23, 1992.
50. Inman RD, Hodge M, Johnson ME, et al: Arthritis, vasculitis and cryoglobulinemia associate with relapsing hepatitis A virus infection. Ann Intern Med 105:700-703, 1986.
51. Polish LB, Robertson BH, Khanna B, et al: Excretion of hepatitis A virus (HAV) in adults: comparison of immunologic and molecular detection methods and relationship between HAV positivity and infectivity in tamarins. J Clin Microbiol 37:3615-3617, 1999.
52. Mao JS, Chai SA, Xie RY, et al: Further evaluation of the safety and protective efficacy of live attenuated hepatitis A vaccine (H2-strain) in humans. Vaccine 15:944-947, 1997.
53. Emerson SU, Tsarev SA, Govindarajan S, et al: A simian strain of hepatitis A virus, AGM-27, functions as an attenuated vaccine for chimpanzees. J Infect Dis 173:592-597, 1996.
54. Innis BL, Snitbhan R, Kyunasol P, et al: Protection against hepatitis A by an inactivated vaccine. JAMA 271:1328-1334, 1994.
55. Werzberger A, Mensch B, Kuter B, et al: A controlled trial of a formalin-inactivated hepatitis A vaccine in healthy children. N Engl J Med 327:453-457, 1992.
56. Castillo de Febres O, Chacon de Petrola M, Casanova de Escalona L, et al: Safety, immunogenicity and antibody persistence of an inactivated hepatitis A vaccine in 4 to 15 year old children. Vaccine 18:656-664, 2000.
57. Zurbriggen R, Novak-Hofer I, Seelig A, Gluck R: IRIV-adjuvanted hepatitis A vaccine: in vivo absorption and biophysical characterization. Prog Lipid Res 39:3-18, 2000.
58. Minutello M, Zotti C, Orecchia S, et al: Dose range evaluation of a new inactivated hepatitis A vaccine administered as a single dose followed by a booster. Vaccine 19:10-15, 2000.
59. Cederna JB, Klinzman D, Stapleton JT: Hepatitis A virus-specific humoral and cellular immune responses following immunization with a formalin-inactivated hepatitis A vaccine. Vaccine 18:893-898, 2000.
60. Bertino JS, Thoelen S, Van Damme P, et al: A dose response study of hepatitis A vaccine in healthy adults who are > 30 years old and weigh > 77 kg. J Infect Dis 178:1181-1184, 1998.
61. Ragni MV, Lusher JM, Koerper MA, et al: Safety and immunogenicity of subcutaneous hepatitis A vaccine in children with haemophilia. Haemophilia 6:98-103, 2000.
62. Williams J, Fox-Leyva L, Christensen C, et al: Hepatitis A vaccine administration: comparison between jet-injector and needle injection. Vaccine 18:1939-1943, 2000.
63. Van Herck K, Beutels P, Van Damme P, et al: Mathematical models for assessment of long-term persistence of antibodies after vaccination with two inactivated hepatitis A vaccines. J Med Virol 60: 1-7, 2000.
64. Bock HL, Kruppenbacher JP, Bienzle U, et al: Does the concurrent administration of an inactivated hepatitis A vaccine influence the immune response to other travelers vaccines. J Travel Med 7:74-78, 2000.
65. Walter EB, Hornick RB, Poland GA, et al: Concurrent administration of inactivated hepatitis A vaccine with immune globulin in healthy adults. Vaccine 17:1468, 1999.
66. Ashur Y, Adler R, Rowe M, et al: Comparison of immunogenicity of two hepatitis A vaccines—VAQTA and HAVRIX—in young adults. Vaccine 17:2290, 1999.
67. Chan C-Y, Lee S-D, Yu M-I, et al: Long-term followup of hepatitis A vaccination in children. Vaccine 17:369, 1999.
68. Nebbia G, Giacchino R, Soncini R, et al: Hepatitis A vaccination in chronic carriers of hepatitis B virus. J Pediatrics 134:784, 1999.
69. Keeffe EB, Iwarson S, McMahon BJ, et al: Safety and immunogenicity of hepatitis A vaccine in patients with chronic liver disease. Hepatology 27:881-886, 1998.
70. Dumot JA, Barnes DS, Younossi Z, et al: Immunogenicity of hepatitis A vaccine in decompensated liver disease. Am J Gastroenterol 94:1601, 1999.
71. Arslan M, Wiesner RH, Poterucha JJ, et al: Hepatitis A antibodies in liver transplant recipients: evidence for loss of immunity posttransplantation. Liver Transpl 6:191-195, 2000.
72. Piazza M, Safary A, Vegnente A, et al: Safety and immunogenicity of hepatitis A vaccine in infants: a candidate for inclusion in the childhood vaccination programme. Vaccine 17:585-588, 1999.
73. Dagan R, Amir J, Mijalovsky A, et al: Immunization against hepatitis A in the first year of life: priming despite the presence of maternal antibody. Pediatr Infect Dis J 19:1045-1052, 2000.
74. Robertson BH, D'Hondt EH, Spelbring J, et al: Effect of postexposure vaccination in a chimpanzee model of hepatitis A virus infection. J Med Virology 43:249, 1994.
75. Sagliocca L, Amoroso P, Stroffolini T, et al: Efficacy of hepatitis A vaccine in prevention of secondary hepatitis A infection: a randomised trial. Lancet 353:1136, 1999.
76. Clemens R, Safary A, Hepburn A: Clinical experience with an inactivated hepatitis A vaccine. J Infect Dis 171:44, 1995.
77. Werzberger A, Kuter B, Nalin D: Six years' follow-up after hepatitis A vaccination. N Engl J Med 338:1160, 1998.
78. Saab S, Martin P, Yee HF Jr: A simple cost-decision analysis model comparing two strategies for hepatitis A vaccination. Am J Med 109:241-244, 2000.
79. Jacobs RJ, Margolis HS, Coleman PJ: The cost-effectiveness of adolescent hepatitis A vaccination in states with the highest disease rates. Arch Pediatr Adolesc Med 154:763-770, 2000.
80. Das A: An economic analysis of different strategies of immunization against hepatitis A in developed countries. Hepatology 29:548-552, 1999.
81. Gay NJ: A model of long-term decline in the transmissibility of an infectious disease: implications for the incidence of hepatitis A. Int J Epidemiol 25:854-861, 1996.

82. Frey S, Dagan R, Ashur Y, et al: Interference of antibody production to hepatitis B surface antigen in a combination hepatitis A/B vaccine. J Infect Dis 180:2018-2022, 1999.
83. Knoll A, Hottentrager B, Kainz J, et al: Immunogenicity of a combined hepatitis A and B vaccine in healthy young adults. Vaccine 18:2029-2032, 2000.
84. Kallinowski B, Knoll A, Lindner E, et al: Can monovalent hepatitis A and B vaccines be replaced by a combined hepatitis A/B vaccine during the primary immunization course? Vaccine 19:16-22, 2000.
85. Thoelen S, Van Damme P, Leentvaar-Kuypers A, et al: The first combined vaccine against hepatitis A and B: an overview. Vaccine 17:1657, 1999.
86. Rajan E, Shattock AG, Fielding JF: Cost-effective analysis of hepatitis A prevention in Ireland. Am J Gastroenterol 95:223-226, 2000.
87. Myers RP, Gregor JC, Marotta PJ: The cost-effectiveness of hepatitis A vaccination in patients with chronic hepatitis C. Hepatology 31:834-839, 2000.
88. Jacobs RJ, Koff RS: Cost-effectiveness of hepatitis A vaccination in patients with chronic hepatitis C. Hepatology 32:873-874, 2000.
89. McMahon BJ, Beller M, Williams J, et al: A program to control an outbreak of hepatitis A in Alaska by using an inactivated hepatitis A vaccine. Arch Pediatr Adoles Med 150:733-739, 1996.
90. Craig AS, Sockwell DC, Schaffner W, et al: Use of hepatitis A vaccine in a community-wide outbreak of hepatitis A. Clin Infect Dis 27:531, 1998.
91. Centers for Disease Control and Prevention: Prevention of hepatitis A through active or passive immunization: recommendations of the Advisory Committee on Immunization Practices (ACIP). MMWR 45 (No. RR-15):1-30, 1996.
92. Green KY, Ando R, Balayan MS, et al: Taxonomy of the caliciviruses. J Infect Dis 181(suppl 2): S322-S330, 2000.
93. Buisson Y, Grandadam M, Nicand E, et al: Identification of a novel hepatitis E virus in Nigeria. J Gen Virology 81:903-909, 2000.
94. He J, Binn LN, Tsarev SA, et al: Molecular characterization of a hepatitis E virus isolate from Namibia. J Biomed Sci 7:334-338, 2000.
95. Wu JC, Sheen IJ, Chang TY, et al: The impact of traveling to endemic areas on the spread of hepatitis E virus infection. Hepatology 27:1415-1420, 1998.
96. Meng X-J, Dea S, Engle RE, et al: Prevalence of antibodies to the hepatitis E virus in pigs from countries where hepatitis E is common or is rare in the human population. J Med Virology 59:297-302, 1999.
97. Wu JC, Chen CM, Chiang TY, et al: Clinical and epidemiological implications of swine hepatitis E virus infection. J Med Virol 60:166-171, 2000.
98. Karetnyi YV, Gilchrist MJ, Naides SJ: Hepatitis E virus infection prevalence among selected populations in Iowa. J Clin Virol 14:51-55, 1999.
99. Reyes G, Purdy MA, Kim JP, et al: Isolation of a cDNA from the virus responsible for enterically transmitted non-A, non-B hepatitis. Science 247:1335-1339, 1990.
100. Tam AW, Smith MM, Guerra ME, et al: Hepatitis E virus (HEV): molecular cloning and sequencing of the full-length viral genome. Virology 185:120-131, 1991.
101. Ansari IH, Nanda SK, Durgapal H, et al: Cloning, sequencing, and expression of the hepatitis E virus (HEV) nonstructural open reading frame 1 (ORF 1). J Med Virol 60:275-283, 2000.
102. He J, Binn LN, Caudill JD, et al: Antiserum generated by a DNA vaccine binds to hepatitis E virus (HEV) as determined by PCR and immune electron microscopy (IEM): application for HEV detection by affinity-capture RT-PCR. Virus Research 62:59-65, 1999.
103. Zafrullah M, Ozdener MH, Panda SK, et al: The ORF 3 protein of hepatitis E virus is a phosphoprotein that associates with the cytoskeleton. J Virol 71:9043-9053, 1997.
104. Riddell MA, Li F, Anderson DA: Identification of immunodominant and conformational epitopes in the capsid protein of hepatitis E virus by using monoclonal antibodies. J Virol 74:8011-8017, 2000.
105. Xing L, Kato K, Tiancheng L, et al: Recombinant hepatitis E capsid protein self-assembles into a dual-domain T=1 particle presenting native virus epitopes. Virology 265:35-45, 1999.
106. Aggarwal R, McCaustland KA, Dilawari JB, et al: Genetic variability of hepatitis E virus within and between three epidemics in India. Virus Res 59:35-48, 1999.
107. Wang Y, Zhang H, Ling R, et al: The complete sequence of hepatitis E virus genotype 4 reveals an alternative strategy for translation of open reading frames 2 and 3. J Gen Virol 81:1675-1686, 2000.
108. Panda SK, Ansari IH, Durgapal H, et al: The in vitro-synthesized RNA from a cDNA clone of hepatitis E virus is infectious. J Virol 74:2430-2437, 2000.
109. Huang R, Li D, Wei S, et al: Cell culture of sporadic hepatitis E virus in China. Clin Diag Laboratory Immunol 6:729-733, 1999.
110. Divizia M, Gabrielli R, Degener AM, et al: Evidence of hepatitis E virus replication on cell cultures. Microbiologica 22:77-83, 1999.
111. Chauhan A, Jameel S, Dilawari JB, et al: Hepatitis E transmission to a volunteer. Lancet 341:149-150, 1993.
112. Krawczynski K, Bradley DW: Enterically transmitted non-A, non-B hepatitis: identification of virus-associated antigen in experimentally infected cynomologous macaques. J Infect Dis 159:1042-1049, 1989.
113. Kawai HF, Koji T, Iida F, et al: Shift of hepatitis E RNA from hepatocytes to biliary epithelial cells during acute infection of rhesus monkey. J Viral Hepat 6:287-297, 1999.
114. Aggarwal R, Suni D, Sofat S, et al: Duration of viraemia and faecal viral excretion in acute hepatitis E. Lancet 356:1081-1082, 2000.
115. Erker JC, Desai SM, Schlauder GG, et al: A hepatitis E virus variant from the United States: molecular characterization and transmission in cynomolgus macaques. J Gen Virol 80:681-690, 1999.
116. Kwo PY, Schlauder GG, Carpenter HA, et al: Acute hepatitis E by a new isolate acquired in the United States. Mayo Clin Proc 72:1133-1136, 1997.
117. Lemos G, Jameel S, Panda S, et al: Hepatitis E virus in Cuba. J Clin Virol 16:71-75, 2000.
118. He J, Binn LN, Tsarev SA, et al: Molecular characterization of a hepatitis E virus isolate from Namibia. J Biomed Sci 7:334-338, 2000.
119. McCrudden R, O'Connell S, Farrant T, et al: Sporadic acute hepatitis E in the United Kingdom: an underdiagnosed phenomenon? Gut 46:732-733, 2000.
120. Thomas DL, Yarbrough PO, Vlahov D, et al: Seroreactivity to hepatitis E virus in areas where the disease is not endemic. J Clin Microbiol 35:1244-1247, 1997.
121. Mast EE, Alter MJ, Holland PV, et al: Evaluation of assays for antibody to hepatitis E virus by a serum panel. Hepatitis E virus antibody serum panel evaluation group. Hepatology 27:857-861, 1998.
122. Seow H-F, Mahomed NMB, Mak J-W, et al: Seroprevalence of antibodies to hepatitis E virus in the normal blood donor population and two aboriginal communities in Malaysia. J Med Virology 59:164-168, 1999.
123. Corwin AL, Nguyen T, Tien K, et al: The unique riverine ecology of hepatitis E virus transmission in South-East Asia. Trans Roy Soc Trop Med Hyg 93:255-260, 1999.
124. Arankalle VA, Chadha MS, Mehendale SM, et al: Epidemic hepatitis E: serological evidence for lack of intrafamilial spread. Indian J Gastroenterol 19:24-28, 2000.
125. Arankalle VA, Chobe LP: Hepatitis E virus: can it be transmitted parenterally? J Viral Hepat 6:161-164, 1999.
126. Arankalle VA, Chobe LP: Retrospective analysis of blood transfusion recipients: evidence for post-transfusion hepatitis E. Vox Sang 79:72, 2000.
127. Mateos ML, Camarero C, Lasa E, et al: Hepatitis E virus: relevance in blood donors and risk groups. Vox Sang 76:78-80, 1999.
128. Robson SC, Adams S, Brink N, et al: Hospital outbreak of hepatitis E. Lancet 339:1424-1425, 1992.
129. Khuroo M, Kamili S, Jameel S: Vertical transmission of hepatitis E. Lancet 345:1025-1026, 1995.
130. McCaustland KA, Krawczynski K, Ebert JW, et al: Hepatitis E virus infection in chimpanzees: a retrospective analysis. Arch Virol 145:1909-1918, 2000.
131. Lin CC, Wu JC, Chang TT, et al: Diagnostic value of immunoglobulin G (IgG) and IgM anti-hepatitis E virus (HEV) tests based on HEV RNA in an area where hepatitis E is not endemic. J Clin Microbiol 38:3915-3918, 2000.
132. Zanetti AR, Schlauder GG, Romano L, et al: Identification of a novel variant of hepatitis E virus in Italy. J Med Virol 57:356-360, 1999.
133. Arankalle VA, Chadha MS, Dama BM, et al: Role of immune serum globulin in pregnant women during an epidemic of hepatitis E. J Viral Hepat 5:199-214, 1998.
134. Tsarev SA, Tsareva TS, Emerson SU, et al: Successful passive and active immunization of cynomolgus monkeys against hepatitis E. Proc Natl Acad Sci U S A 91:10198-10202, 1994.

135. Schofield DJ, Glamann J, Emerson SU, Purcell RH: Identification by phage display and characterization of two neutralizing chimpanzee monoclonal antibodies to the hepatitis E virus capsid protein. J Virology 74:5548-5555, 2000.
136. He J, Binn LN, Caudill JD, et al: Antiserum generated by a DNA vaccine binds to hepatitis E virus (HEV) as determined by PCR and immune electron microscopy (IEM): application for HEV detection by affinity-capture RT-PCR. Virus Research 62:59-65, 1999.
137. Tuteja R, Li TC, Takeda N, Jameel S: Augmentation of immune responses to hepatitis E virus ORF2 DNA vaccination by codelivery of cytokine genes. Viral Immunol 13:169-178, 2000.
138. Tsarev SA, Tsareva TS, Emerson SU, et al: Recombinant vaccine against hepatitis E: dose response and protection against heterologous challenge. Vaccine 15:1834, 1997.
139. Kamili S, Spelbring J, Krawczynski K: DNA vaccination protects non-human primates against hepatitis E virus. Hepatology 32:380a, 2000.

CHAPTER

32

Hepatitis B and D

Satheesh Nair, MD, and Robert P. Perrillo, MD

ABBREVIATIONS

AFP	alpha fetoprotein
ALT	alanine aminotransferase
anti-HBc	antibody to HBcAg
anti-HBe	antibody to HBeAg
anti-HBs	antibody to HBsAg
anti-HDV	antibody to hepatitis delta virus
AST	aspartate aminotransferase
BCP	basal core promoter
cccDNA	covalently closed circular deoxyribonucleic acid
CTLs	cytotoxic T lymphocytes
HAV	hepatitis A virus
HBcAg	hepatitis B core antigen
HBeAg	hepatitis B e antigen
HBIG	hepatitis B immunoglobulin
HBsAg	hepatitis B surface antigen
HBV	hepatitis B virus
HBV DNA	hepatitis B virus deoxyribonucleic acid
HBX	hepatitis B X antigen
HCV	hepatitis C virus
HDAg	hepatitis delta antigen
HDV	hepatitis delta virus
HIV	human immunodeficiency virus
HLA	histocompatibility locus antigen
IFN	interferon
M-CSF	macrophage colony-stimulating factor
MHC	major histocompatibility complex
PAN	polyarteritis nodosa
PCR	polymerase chain reaction
TNF	tumor necrosis factor
YMDD	tyrosine-methionine-aspartate-aspartate

IMPORTANCE AS A GLOBAL HEALTH PROBLEM

Five percent of the Earth's population have hepatitis B, making it one of the most common infectious diseases in the world today. There are an estimated 400 million carriers of hepatitis B virus (HBV) worldwide, 75 percent to 80 percent of whom reside in Asia and the Western Pacific. Effective vaccines have been available for nearly 20 years, but perinatal exposure continues to be a major source of exposure in high prevalence areas, and high-risk behavior, particularly in young adults, accounts for a significant number of new cases each year in the Western world. The medical importance of this disorder is best understood by considering the increased mortality associated with acute and chronic HBV infection. Fulminant HBV infection is an important cause of acute liver failure and is responsible for approximately 100 to 200 deaths per year in the United States alone. Chronic HBV infection accounts for 1 million deaths annually and is the chief cause of cirrhosis and hepatocellular carcinoma in the world today.

EPIDEMIOLOGY

Geographic Distribution and Sources of Exposure

The prevalence of hepatitis B infection varies greatly around the world (Figure 32-1). In highly endemic regions, such as Southeast Asia (excluding Japan), China, and much of Africa, the lifetime risk of infection is greater than 60 percent, and 8 percent or more of the population are chronic HBV carriers.[1,2] In these areas vertical transmission from an infected mother to neonate and horizontal spread among children are the major ways that the infection is spread. High endemicity areas account for a total of 45 percent of the global population and harbor more than half of the HBV carriers in the world.[3] Areas of intermediate endemicity include parts of Southern and Eastern Europe, the Middle East, Japan, the Indian subcontinent, much of the former Soviet Union, and Northern Africa. Taken together, these regions constitute approximately 40 percent of the Earth's population. Individuals of all age groups are infected in areas of intermediate endemicity, but chronic HBV infection is generally caused by transmission during infancy or early childhood. The lifetime risk of infection in these areas is 20 percent to 60 percent.[3] Regions of low prevalence include North America, Western Europe, certain parts of South America, and Australia. Here the lifetime risk of HBV infection is less than 20 percent and transmission is primarily horizontal (between individuals). Sexual transmission is the main mode of transmission in Europe and

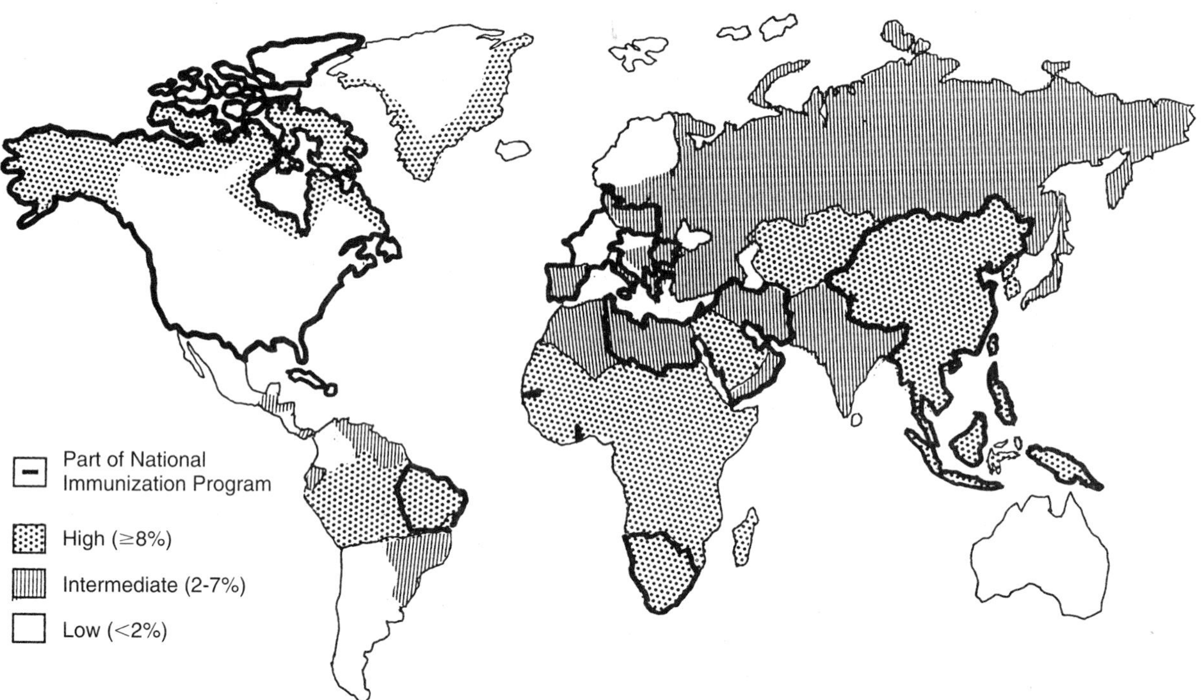

Figure 32-1 Geographic prevalence of hepatitis B throughout the world. The vast majority of chronic infections occur in Asia. Dark bordered areas represent those in which national immunization programs are available. Boxes refer to low-, intermediate-, and high-incidence areas according to the World Health Organization, 1997.

North America and occurs predominantly in individuals younger than age 50, although needle sharing among injecting drug users and occupational exposure to contaminated blood and blood products continue to be important modes of exposure.[4]

Transmission of infection from an HBV carrier mother to neonate accounts for the majority of new infections in the world today. From 60 percent to 90 percent of hepatitis B surface antigen (HBsAg)-positive mothers with active HBV infection (i.e., hepatitis B e [HBe] antigen-positive) will transmit the disease to their offspring, whereas HBsAg-positive asymptomatic carriers with antibody to HBeAg (anti-HBe) do so less frequently (15 percent to 20 percent).[5,6] Other, less frequent, sources of infection include household contact with an HBV carrier,[7] hemodialysis,[8] exposure to infected health care workers,[9] tattooing, body piercing,[10] artificial insemination,[11] and receipt of blood products or organs.[12,13] Transfusion-associated hepatitis B has become rare in the United States since routine screening of the blood supply has been in place. The persistence of a small number of cases may reflect the use of blood or blood products from patients in the incubation phase of infection. Several studies have also indicated a higher rate of infection in recipients of anti-hepatitis B core (anti-HBc)-positive blood that is due to a small amount of circulating virus in the donor.[14,15] These studies argue for continuation of the policy of routine anti-HBc screening to prevent post-transfusion hepatitis B.

HBV is very efficiently transmitted, primarily by percutaneous and mucous membrane exposure to infectious body fluids. The presence of HBeAg positivity indicates a higher risk of transmission from mother to child, after needlestick exposure, and in the setting of household contact.[5,7,16] HBV deoxyribonucleic acid (DNA) has been detected by sensitive techniques such as polymerase chain reaction (PCR) in saliva and most body fluids, with the notable exception of stool that has not been contaminated with blood. Although HBV replicates primarily in hepatocytes the presence of replicative intermediates and virally encoded proteins in other sites such as adrenal glands, testis, colon, nerve ganglia, and skin suggests that there is a vast extrahepatic reservoir for infectious virus.[17] Small amounts of HBV can be sequestered in peripheral mononuclear cells of HBsAg-negative donors and liver tissue for prolonged periods.[18,19] Taken together, these findings have potentially important implications for transmission of HBV infection by organ donation.

Rates of Infection in the United States

Infection rates in the United States have been closely monitored by the Centers for Disease Control and Prevention (CDC) (Figure 32-2). After a period of relative stability ended in 1987, the incidence of hepatitis B declined by more than 70 percent in the United States. This is probably the result of vaccination programs, changes in sexual lifestyle, refinements in blood screening procedures, and the availability of virus-inactivated blood components.[20] Nonetheless, an estimated 185,000 new HBV infections occurred in 1997, with the highest incidence

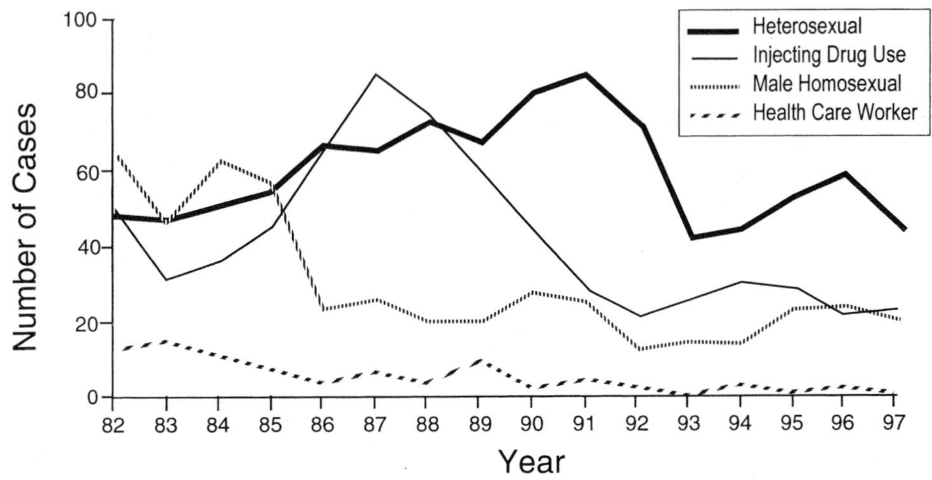

Figure 32-2 Trends in selected risk factors for hepatitis B, United States, 1982-1997. Data according to Centers for Disease Control. (Courtesy of Dr. Miriam Alter.)

of disease among young adults (20-29 years old), and higher rates among blacks and Hispanics compared with whites.[21] Currently, nearly 50 percent of the cases of acute hepatitis B reported to the CDC are attributable to intimate contact among heterosexuals and approximately 20 percent are due to injecting drug use. No identifiable source of exposure can be demonstrated in 10 percent to 15 percent of cases, and infection in these cases is presumed to be due to intimate contact or non-admitted injecting drug use.

According to the third National Health and Nutrition Examination Survey (1988-1994), one or more serologic markers of HBV infection were demonstrated in 4.9 percent of the US population, although the prevalence of chronic infection was 0.4 percent.[22] Traditional estimates based upon the results of blood donation screening in the late 1970s also indicated a prevalence rate for chronic infection of 0.2 percent to 0.4 percent in the US population.[23] In a screening program of nearly 14,000 individuals in 40 US medical centers the prevalence of HBV infection was 17.8 percent, with 2.1 percent of patients determined to be HBV carriers.[24] Even given the possibility of self-selection bias, it is clear from this survey that hepatitis B is not an uncommon medical disorder in the US population at large.

CLINICAL OUTCOME OF HBV INFECTION

Definition of the HBV Carrier State

Patients in whom HBsAg persists in serum for more than 6 months are referred to as "chronic HBsAg carriers." In common usage the term "carrier" often has been used to refer to persistently infected individuals with normal serum aminotransferase levels (sometimes also referred to as healthy HBV carriers).[25] The term "healthy carrier" seems to be a poor one in that these patients may have evidence for hepatic inflammation on biopsy, particularly when serologic markers of viral replication are evident.[26,27] Because of potentially confusing nomenclature, it has been proposed that the carrier state be categorized as inactive or active, with the former referring to patients who have evidence for HBV replication by PCR-based assay only and normal or only mildly abnormal serum aminotransferase levels. Long-term follow-up of inactive carriers suggests that the majority of patients do not have progressive liver disease and do not develop complications.[26,27] There are two major exceptions to this rule, however: some of these patients have periodic reactivations of their liver disease in association with an increase in viremia and immunologic responses; moreover, some patients with the inactive carrier state may develop hepatocellular carcinoma. Active carriers, in contrast, have evidence for HBV replication by standard hybridization assays, abnormal serum aminotransferase levels, and evidence for chronic hepatitis, with or without concomitant cirrhosis.

Clinical Sequelae of Acute HBV Infection

The age at which the individual becomes infected with HBV correlates with clinical outcome and the possible route of exposure.[1,28] Liver injury and extrahepatic disorders are caused by cell-mediated and humoral patterns of response to HBV infection (see Immunopathogenesis and Clinical Features of Chronic Hepatitis B). The severity of the liver injury reflects the activity of the immune response: the strongest response causes the greatest hepatocellular injury and higher likelihood of viral clearance. Thus HBV infection in adults with intact immune systems is likely to cause clinically apparent acute hepatitis B, with only 1 percent to 5 percent of cases becoming chronically infected.[4] By contrast, as much as 95 percent of infected neonates become chronic HBV carriers and generally develop subclinical infection because of their immature immune systems.[3,4]

In adults fulminant liver failure resulting from acute hepatitis B occurs in less than 1 percent of cases but this still accounts for 400 deaths in the United States each year.[29] The Acute Liver Failure study group found that acute hepatitis B accounted for 5 percent of all cases of acute liver failure in the United States.[30] Spontaneous survival in acute liver failure resulting from hepatitis B is between 20 and 30 percent.[31] Liver transplantation has resulted in a 50 percent to 60 percent survival rate, and recurrent disease in the allograft is infrequent in this situation.[32,33] Anti-viral therapy has little rationale for fulminant hepatitis B because most of the immunologically mediated liver damage and elimination of HBV has already occurred by the time of presentation. Patients in whom the diagnosis of acute fulminant hepatitis B is suspected are often HBeAg-negative and may be HBsAg-negative when first seen. Thus the accurate diagnosis of fulminant liver failure resulting from hepatitis B may require testing with immunoglobulin (Ig)M antibody to HBc antigen (HBcAg) (see Serologic Markers of HBV Infection).[34]

Clinical Sequelae of Chronic HBV Infection

Chronic hepatitis B is a serious consequence of HBV infection. Between one third and one quarter of people chronically infected with HBV are expected to develop progressive liver disease (including cirrhosis and primary liver cancer).[35] An estimated 15 percent to 25 percent of all age groups with chronic HBV infection will die prematurely from these conditions.

Patients with chronic HBV infection may be considered as active or inactive carriers of infection. The former consist of individuals with abnormal serum aminotransferase levels, active liver histology, and high viral replication (HBeAg is often measurable; HBV DNA is detectable by molecular hybridization assay). Inactive carriers, often inappropriately termed "healthy carriers," are asymptomatic individuals who have normal serum aminotransferase levels, normal or minimally abnormal liver histology, and very low viral replication (i.e., undetectable HBeAg and HBV DNA detected by PCR testing only).[25] HBsAg carriers who lack evidence for HBeAg and have normal serum aminotransferase levels rarely transmit the infection to others and usually do not have progressive liver disease even after prolonged follow-up.[27,36]

Several large cohort studies have demonstrated that the presence of active viral replication and long-standing necroinflammatory liver disease resulting from HBV strongly influence the rate of progression to cirrhosis (Table 32-1). The major determinant of survival for patients with chronic hepatitis B is the extent of the liver disease when patients first come to medical attention.[37-42] Cirrhosis is associated with decreased survival and higher frequency of complications, including hepatocellular carcinoma. In one study overall mortality in 302 patients with clinically stable chronic hepatitis B was shown to be increased fivefold over that of the general population, with a standardized mortality ratio of 6.2 for patients without cirrhosis and 18.6 for those with cirrhosis.[42] In another study 45 (12 percent) of 366 patients with compensated HBV-related cirrhosis died of liver failure during a 6-year observation period and 23 (6 percent) succumbed to hepatocellular carcinoma.[41] The investigators in that study reported a cumulative probability of survival of 84 percent and 68 percent, respectively, at 5 and 10 years. Five-year and twenty-year survival rates of 55 percent and 25 percent, respectively, have been reported in 131 HBV-infected cirrhotics in contrast to 97 percent and 63 percent at the same time-points for those with mild disease.[37,38] The most dramatic difference in survival seems to exist between patients with compensated versus decompensated cirrhosis. One group of investigators found an 84 percent 5-year survival in 77 patients with compensated HBV-related cirrhosis but a 14 percent survival in the subset who had ascites, jaundice, encephalopathy, or a history of variceal bleeding.[40] A second study indicated that after the first episode of hepatic decompensation the probability of survival was 35 percent at 5 years.[43] Multi-variate analyses in several of these large cohort studies have identified that age, ascites, hyperbilirubinemia, and other features of advanced liver disease independently correlate with survival in cirrhotics (Table 32-1). Longer survival without complications or need for transplantation has been reported after successful anti-viral therapy.[44] These studies affirm the need to treat patients with chronic hepatitis B early in the disease process. It is not clear, however, to what extent survival or the rate of hepatic complications is affected by reduction in viral replication once cirrhosis and features of hepatic decompensation are evident (see Anti-viral Therapy of Chronic HBV Infection).[40,45-48]

MOLECULAR ASPECTS OF HBV

Life Cycle of HBV

HBV belongs to a group of viruses termed *hepadna*. Other members of this virus family include the woodchuck hepatitis virus, the ground squirrel hepatitis virus, and the duck hepatitis virus. Hepadnaviruses have also been found in tree squirrels and in herons. All hepadnaviruses share common characteristics, and several have been useful as animal models to study HBV.[49]

HBV is a small (3.2 Kb) DNA virus with four open reading frames in which several genes overlap and use the same DNA to encode viral proteins.[50] The four viral genes are core, surface, X, and polymerase. The core gene encodes the core nucleocapsid protein and a large part of the non-structural (secreted) HBeAg. The surface gene encodes the pre-S1, pre-S2, and S protein (large [L], middle [M], and small [S] surface proteins, respectively). The X gene encodes the X protein, which has transactivating properties and may be important in hepatic carcinogenesis. Unlike the other genes, the biologic function of the X gene in the viral life cycle remains largely unknown. The polymerase gene has a large open reading frame (approximately 800 amino acids) and overlaps the entire length of the surface open reading frame. It encodes a large protein with functions critical for packaging and DNA replication (including priming, ribonucleic acid [RNA]- and DNA-dependent DNA polymerase, and RNAse H activities).

Although HBV is a DNA virus, replication is through an RNA intermediate requiring an active viral reverse transcriptase/polymerase enzyme. The reverse transcriptase is believed to lack a proofreading function, which results in a higher mutation rate than other DNA viruses (approximately 1 nucleotide per 10,000 bases/infection

TABLE 32-1
Extended Follow-Up Studies of Chronic HBV

Author, year (reference no.)	Type of patient	Number of patients	Duration of follow-up	Major findings
Weissberg et al, 1984-1999 (37, 38)	Compensated and decompensated chronic hepatitis B	378	Mean, 18.7 yr	Survival rate of 65% with no fibrosis, 58% with fibrosis, and 25% with cirrhosis at entry
Fattovich et al, 1991 (39)	Non-cirrhotic chronic hepatitis B: 66 HBeAg/HBV DNA-positive, 38 anti-HBe-positive, 26 HBV DNA-positive	105	Mean, 5.5 yr, range, 1-16 yr	Cirrhosis correlates with older age, bridging fibrosis, persistence of HBV DNA in serum
de Jongh et al, 1992 (40)	HBV-related cirrhosis, 77 compensated, 21 decompensated	98	Mean, 4.3 yr, range, 0.1-18 yr	84% 5-yr survival if clinically stable; 14% if decompensated. Survival correlates with increasing age, hyperbilirubinemia, and ascites at entry
Realdi et al, 1994 (41)	Compensated cirrhosis: 35% HBeAg-positive, 48% HBV DNA-positive, 20% anti-HDV-positive	366	Mean, 6 yr, range, 0.5-17 yr	84% survival at 5 yr, 68% at 10 yr. Survival correlates with age, albumin. splenomegaly, bilirubin, and HBeAg status at entry
Di Marco et al, 1999 (42)	Compensated chronic hepatitis B including 86 with cirrhosis—29% HBeAg-positive, 27% HBeAg-negative/HBV DNA-positive, 25% anti-HDV-positive	302	Median, 7.8 yr ± 3.1 yr	Decompensation in 15.2%, death in 11.4%. Survival predicted by young age, absence of cirrhosis, and sustained ALT normalization. Survival without decompensation predicted by above and interferon treatment
Fattovich et al, 1995 (43)	Compensated cirrhosis	349	Mean, 6 yr	Hepatocellular carcinoma develops in 9% and decompensation in 28%. Five-year survival 35% after decompensation
Niederau et al, 1996 (44)	Compensated chronic hepatitis B all treated with IFN	103	Mean, 4.1 yr, range, 1-7.5 yr	Overall survival and survival without complications significantly longer after HBeAg loss.

HBeAg, Hepatitis B e antigen; *HBV,* hepatitis B virus; *DNA,* deoxyribonucleic acid; *anti-HBe,* antibody to HBeAg; *anti-HDV,* antibody to hepatitis delta virus; *ALT,* alanine aminotransferase.

year).[51] In addition, replication fidelity by reverse transcriptase has been shown to vary with concentrations of intracellular deoxynucleotide triphosphate.[52] Use of complete HBV genomic sequencing has identified a large number of mutations within the HBV genome, many of which are silent or do not alter the amino acid sequence of encoded proteins. Because of genomic overlap, however, some of the silent mutations in one open reading frame may result in an amino acid substitution in an overlapping reading frame. For example, nucleotide substitutions in the polymerase gene that occur during nucleoside analog therapy can cause a stop codon in the surface open reading frame and thus affect production of HBsAg.[53]

The life cycle of HBV has been deduced from studies in animal models and tissue cultures (Figure 32-3). The initial phase of hepadnaviral infection involves the attachment of mature virions (Dane particles) onto hepatocyte membranes. Binding studies of hepatocyte membranes with duck hepatitis B virus have demonstrated specific interaction with the pre-S domain of the surface protein. Carboxypeptidase D has been found to facilitate viral entry in the duck model, but the human receptor for HBV remains unknown. Studies with HBV suggest that its pre-S domain also participates in binding to cells but the S protein may also be important.[54] Entry of the virus results from fusion of the viral and host membranes when the nucleocapsid is released into the cytoplasm.

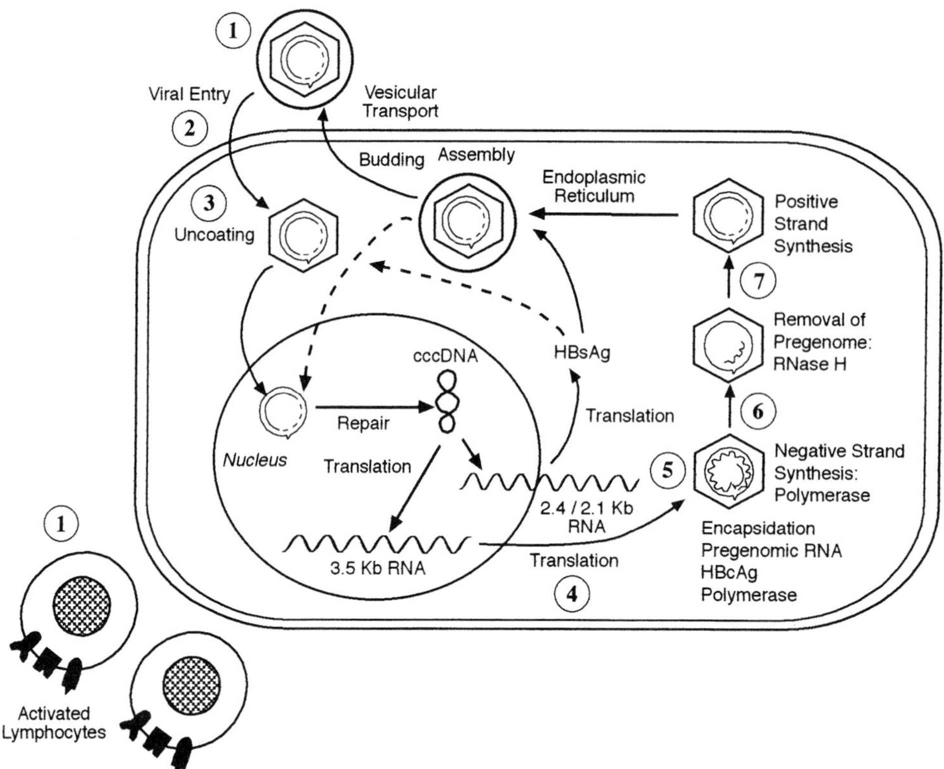

Figure 32-3 Life cycle of hepatitis B virus and sites for therapeutic intervention. Numbers indicate areas of potential drug effects. *1,* Neutralization of HBsAg-containing viral particles by hepatitis B immunoglobulin and hepatitis B vaccination.T-cell responses to virally infected liver cells stimulated by interferon. *2,* Viral entry into hepatocyte inhibited by interferon and possibly pre-S vaccine. *3,* Uncoating inhibited by interferon. *4,* Translation of mRNA is blocked by anti-sense oligonucleotides.This is the site of action of ribozymes, which degrade viral mRNA. Interferon activates ribonucleases, which degrade viral mRNA.Translation is blocked by antisense oligonucleotides. *5,* Packaging of RNA pregenome into core particles is inhibited by interferon. *6,* Priming of first-strand HBV DNA synthesis is inhibited by certain nucleoside analogs. Reverse transcriptase function of HBV DNA polymerase inhibited by lamivudine and other nucleosides resulting in impaired synthesis of first-strand HBV DNA from RNA pregenome. *7,* Lamivudine and other nucleoside analogs competitively inhibit HBV DNA polymerase, resulting in termination of second HBV DNA strand. *HBsAg,* Hepatitis B surface antigen; *mRNA,* messenger ribonucleic acid; *HBV,* hepatitis B virus; *DNA,* deoxyribonucleic acid.

Mechanisms of intracellular transport of viral genome into the nucleus are poorly understood but the first step in genomic replication involves conversion of the relaxed circular form of HBV DNA into a double-stranded covalently closed circular form of DNA (cccDNA).[55] These cccDNA molecules serve as the template for viral transcription and are the major form of viral DNA in the nucleus of the infected hepatocytes.[56] Subgenomic (0.7-2.4 Kb) and pregenomic (3.5 Kb) RNA molecules are transcribed from this template. The L protein is translated from the 2.4-Kb RNA, the M and S proteins from the 2.1-Kb message, and the hepatitis B X antigen (HBx) protein from the 0.7-Kb transcript. The pregenomic RNA serves as the template for reverse transcription and the messenger RNA (mRNA) for core and polymerase; the precore RNA codes for the precore gene product.

HBV replication begins with encapsidation of the pregenome RNA through complex interactions between host and viral proteins. The pregenomic RNA is the only genomic RNA species that is packaged. HBV DNA polymerase reverse transcribes this pregenomic RNA into a negative-strand HBV DNA, which in turn serves as the template for positive-strand synthesis to form a partially double-stranded genome. Concurrent with DNA synthesis, the nucleocapsid also undergoes maturation and, through a yet incompletely understood mechanism, interaction occurs with the S protein to initiate viral assembly in the endoplasmic reticulum. The signal for nucleocapsid-surface protein association appears to reside in the pre-S1 domain of the L protein.

S protein is synthesized in the endoplasmic reticulum, where monomer aggregates that exclude host membrane proteins subsequently bud into the lumen as subviral particles. Once formed, the HBsAg undergoes glycosylation in the endoplasmic reticulum and the Golgi apparatus. Of the three S gene products, the L protein is often absent in 20-nm particles and, when overexpressed, tends to build up within the endoplasmic reticulum. In the presence of

TABLE 32-2
Clinical Relevance of HBV Mutants

Type mutant	Relative frequency	Setting	Major associations
HBsAg	Rare	After HBIG and vaccination infection	Lack of neutralization by anti-HBs False negative HBsAg
Precore	Common	HBeAg-negative chronic HBV infection	High rate of relapse with conventional nucleoside analog and interferon regimens
Core promoter	Uncommon	HBeAg-positive or HBeAg-negative chronic hepatitis	Increase in viral replication, fulminant hepatitis (Japan)
Core	Common	HBeAg-positive or HBeAg-negative chronic hepatitis	May affect response to interferon and contribute to disease activity after HBeAg seroconversion
HBV DNA polymerase	Common	Treatment with nucleosides	Resistance to lamivudine, famciclovir, and other nucleosides
X gene	Unknown	Chronic HBV infection	Promotion of hepatocellular carcinoma

HBsAg, Hepatitis B surface antigen; *HBIG,* hepatitis B immunoglobulin; *anti-HBs,* antibody to HBsAg; *HBeAg,* hepatitis B e antigen; *HBV,* hepatitis B virus; *DNA,* deoxyribonucleic acid.

excess L protein, M and S proteins are not secreted. In the transgenic mouse model, retention of the L protein has been associated with hepatocyte injury and transition to hepatocellular carcinoma.[57,58]

Genomic Variation

In a chronically infected patient 10^{11} to 10^{13} HBV virions are produced each day. This high rate of virion production, together with a high frequency of misincorporation of nucleotides (10^{-4} per base per replication cycle), leads to substantial HBV genomic variation. The nomenclature in this area is evolving. HBV variants are viral strains with mutations in the genome that arise under natural circumstances. The term *HBV mutant,* on the other hand, is best reserved for viral variants that have emerged under a selection pressure often related to therapeutic intervention—for example, vaccine-induced surface antibody escape mutants or anti-viral drug-induced polymerase mutants (see the following section).

HBV Genotypes

The serologic heterogeneity of the HBsAg has been well established. HBV isolates have been classified into nine different subtypes according to the antigenic determinants of their HBsAg.[59] Alternatively, a genetic classification based on the comparison of complete genomes has defined seven genotypes of HBV—A through G.[60] Genotypically these differences are based on an intergroup divergence of 8 percent or more in the complete nucleotide sequence. Several studies have defined the geographic distribution of each genotype.[61] Genotype A is the predominant genotype in northern Europe and the United States. Genotypes B and C are confined to populations in eastern Asia and the Far East. Genotype D is found worldwide but prevails in the Mediterranean area, and the Near and Middle East. Genotype E is indigenous to western sub-Saharan areas; genotype F prevails in Central America. The geographic distribution for genotype G is yet to be determined. There appear to be clinical associations with the various genotypes. Recent studies in Taiwan have shown that genotype C is associated with more severe liver disease, and genotype B associated with the development of hepatocellular carcinoma.[62] In a Swiss study, genotype A was found to be associated with chronic hepatitis and genotype D with acute resolving hepatitis.[63] Genotyping may also have implications for the prevalence of precore and core mutations. In a recent case-control study from Japan patients with genotypes B and C commonly had precore mutation at nucleotide position 1896, but patients with genotype C were more likely to have a double mutation in the basic core promoter and this was associated with the age of the patient and more advanced liver disease (see Mutations in the Precore, Core Promoter, and Core Genes).[64]

Mutation of the HBV Genome

Various types of mutations in the viral genome, such as single nucleotide substitutions (point mutations), deletions, or insertions, have been described in patients with HBV infection. Point mutations occur more frequently and some of these are silent and do not alter the amino acid sequence in a particular open reading frame, whereas others result in amino acid changes. If the mutant strain becomes a dominant part of the viral population in a patient, this may impair the diagnosis of HBV infection or allow for viral escape from the neutralizing effect of host-derived or exogenous antibody to HBsAg (anti-HBs). Other mutations can affect the replication capacity of the virus or confer resistance to treatment with nucleoside analogs (Table 32-2). The more common mutants with clinical implications are discussed in the following section.

HBsAg Mutants

Mutations in the surface gene can result in amino acid changes in the antibody binding domain. Accordingly, both virus neutralization by polyclonal antibody to HBsAg and testing for HBsAg by methods that depend on antibody binding can be affected. The "a" determinant is a region of the surface protein of HBV located between amino acids 121 and 149 that is the major target of polyclonal antibody to HBsAg.[65] Large-scale vaccination programs in endemic regions have revealed a 2 percent to 3 percent incidence of vaccine escape mutants, resulting from alterations in the "a" determinant of the HBsAg protein. Typically, this results in the substitution of glycine for arginine at amino acid position 145, which prevents binding of neutralizing antibodies (i.e., anti-HBs). In patients infected with the HBV mutant HBsAg is not detectable by commonly used HBsAg assays. As a result, these mutations have public health significance because patients harboring them do not exhibit quantifiable HBsAg but remain infectious nonetheless. HBV infection remains detectable by HBV DNA or HBeAg testing in these patients.

Neonatal HBV vaccination provides a selection pressure for HBV surface gene mutants. In studies in which age-matched children not receiving HBV vaccine were compared to those who did, none of the non-vaccinated compared to 27 percent of the vaccinated had mutations in the "a" determinant. None of the mothers of the children harboring these mutants had similar sequences in the surface gene, indicating that the mutants were host rather than viral dependent and likely to have emerged or become selected under immune pressure.[66] An increasing number of "a" determinant mutants has been observed since the implementation of universal vaccination of infants in Taiwan, raising concerns that current vaccines may ultimately prove less effective.[67] The clinical significance of these mutants remains highly controversial at this time; further study is needed.

Another setting where "a" determinant mutants have been shown to have clinical relevance is after liver transplantation for hepatitis B. Recurrent HBV infection despite the use of HBIg can be due to these "escape" mutants in as many as 50 percent of cases, and the rate at which they can be detected appears to correlate with the duration of passive immunization.[65,68] As with neonatal vaccination, the pathogenicity of these surface gene mutants remains to be determined.

Other studies have demonstrated the presence of mutations in the preS2 region of the HBV genome, an area that affects immune recognition. Mutations of this type have been associated with increased virulence in a small series; additional data are awaited to confirm these observations.[69]

Mutations in the Precore, Core Promoter, and Core Genes

The synthesis of HBeAg is doubly controlled at transcription and translation levels. The precore mRNA encodes HBeAg. The core promoter resides in the overlapping X open reading frame region and controls transcription of the two core gene products: core and precore RNA. Thus mutations in either region can affect the production of HBeAg. It has been suggested that mutation in the core promoter may enhance viral replication.[70,71]

The best-defined precore mutation occurs at nucleotide 1896 and results in a stop codon that abolishes the synthesis of HBeAg.[72] Mutations in the core promoter at nucleotides 1762 and 1764 decrease HBeAg synthesis by approximately 70 percent while maintaining pregenomic RNA levels.[73] Both types of mutations have been associated with severe or fulminant hepatitis in some studies. This has been attributed to the fact that HBeAg appears to induce immunologic tolerance and is cross-reactive with HBcAg at the T-cell level.[74] It should be stressed, however, that precore stop mutations have also been detected in isolates from healthy HBV carriers and patients with severe disease.

Core gene mutations seem to occur more frequently in patients with precore mutant HBV. The core gene mutations are epidemiologically associated with disease activity and the precore mutation may have little clinical relevance in this situation.[70] Core gene mutations can block recognition of HBV by cytotoxic T cells.[75] Mutations in the core promoter, on the other hand, increase viral replication and appear capable of enhancing disease activity independent of other mutations.[73] Precore and core promoter mutations have also been described in the same patients.[76]

In patients with perinatally acquired chronic hepatitis B a prolonged immune tolerant phase with minimal to absent hepatic necroinflammatory activity is typically seen for the first 20 to 30 years of HBV infection. Sequencing studies have shown stable core gene sequences during this phase.[77] Precore mutations are also uncommon during this period. Core gene mutations become more common as patients pass from the immune tolerant phase, at which time an increasing number of mutations are observed in the region of the core gene that includes many B- and T-cell epitopes. Both precore stop codon mutants and core gene mutants have been associated with a poor response to interferon (IFN) therapy.[78-80] After HBeAg seroconversion to anti-HBe, individuals may develop either a precore mutant–dominant phase of infection or retain precore wild-type virus, and patients who remain precore-dominant have a consistently higher rate of mutations in the core gene and continuing liver injury.[81] Why these different genotypic events occur in some patients at the time of HBeAg seroconversion and the relative frequency with they occur are not well understood.

There are marked geographic differences in the prevalence of precore stop codon mutant viruses. For example, only 10 percent of HBV isolates from US patients with fulminant hepatitis and 12 percent to 27 percent of isolates from US and Western European patients with chronic hepatitis B exhibit these stop mutants, whereas this is found in 47 percent to 60 percent of isolates from patients in Asia, Africa, Southern Europe, and the Middle East.[82] The prevalence of the precore stop codon mutant has been associated with genotypes B through D and absent with genotype A.[83] It has been hypothesized that precore stop mutations at nucleotide 1896 are less frequent in genotype A. This is related to the base-pairing with the nucleotide at position 1858, which is situated opposite position 1896 in the precore stem loop structure.[83a] Further studies are needed to confirm these relationships. A clear-cut geographic dispersion for core gene mutants and core promoter mutants has not been described.

HBV DNA Polymerase Mutants

The polymerase gene product is needed for encapsidation of viral RNA into core particles and conversion of the pregenomic viral RNA into genomic viral DNA.[70] In general, the HBV reverse transcriptase activity is highly conserved because major mutations in this region would impair viral replication. The advent of nucleoside analog therapy has drawn a clear focus on the clinical importance of mutations in this gene. After prolonged exposure to lamivudine, a nucleoside analog that inhibits HBV DNA polymerase, nucleotide substitutions have been observed in domain B (the template binding site of the polymerase) and domain C (the catalytic site of the polymerase). There are two types of mutations at codon 552 of domain C that result in substitution of the amino acid methionine either for isoleucine or valine (designated M552I and M552V, respectively). The M552V tends to occur in conjunction with a mutation in domain B that results in substitution of leucine to methionine (L528M).[70] The M552I mutation or the combined M552V and L528V mutations result in marked resistance to the antiviral effect of lamivudine. Mutations occur in these sites in a time-dependent manner and are found in approximately 15 percent to 20 percent of patients after 1 year of treatment, 30 percent to 40 percent of those treated for 2 years, 50 percent after 3 years, and in greater than 65 percent in whom treatment has been continued for 4 years.[84,84a] These mutant viruses appear to be less replication competent, and although patients with these mutants have a lower chance of HBeAg seroconversion, patients may continue to exhibit clinical improvement.[85] HBV DNA polymerase mutations are not unique to lamivudine and have also been observed at codon 528 during famciclovir therapy.[86] These mutations also markedly decrease famciclovir efficacy. A revised classification system for these mutants has recently been proposed and further studies on their natural history are needed.[86a]

X Gene Mutation

Although the viral regulatory X protein is essential for infection, its mode of action remains obscure, and much of the work on its function has been done in cell culture. The X protein up-regulates gene expression, functions to sensitize cells to apoptotic killing, and deregulates cell growth arrest in certain cancer cell types. It is suspected that the X gene plays a role in hepatocarcinogenesis, but how it does this is uncertain. HBx binds the human tumor suppressor protein, p53, and this may affect the development of hepatic malignancy by inhibiting p53 effects on cellular DNA repair.[87] Mutations in the HBx gene have been shown to abolish growth arrest and apoptosis in vitro.[88] It is also possible that the X gene may be involved in hepatocarcinogenesis by potentiating oncogenes.[88a] How the multiple functions of the X gene are associated with the viral life cycle is not clear but mutations in the X gene have been shown to abolish productive hepadnavirus infection in woodchucks.[89]

IMMUNOPATHOGENESIS OF ACUTE AND CHRONIC HBV INFECTION

HBV is generally not a cytopathic virus. The existence of an HBV carrier state for many years without evidence of parenchymal liver damage and the presence of variable numbers of infiltrating mononuclear cells in chronic hepatitis B suggest that the pathogenesis of the latter disorder is mediated by immune mechanisms. The immunopathogenetic mechanisms that account for the development of acute and chronic hepatitis, cirrhosis, and hepatocellular carcinoma in patients with HBV infection are only partly defined because of the limited host range and lack of an in vivo culture system. Woodchucks and ducks do not appear to have similar immunologic responses to their respective hepadnaviruses as humans have to HBV; therefore, this imposes limitations in understanding the immunopathogenesis of hepatitis B.[90] Whereas both humoral and cellular immune responses are needed for effective viral clearance, the cellular immune response appears to be primarily involved in disease pathogenesis.

Immunologic response to HBV encompasses both a non-viral antigen-specific or innate response (e.g., natural killer cells, IFNs) and an adaptive immune response, including antibodies to viral antigens, class II restricted $CD4^+$ T cells, and class I restricted $CD8^+$ cytotoxic T lymphocytes (CTLs). Induction of the antigen-specific T-cell response is thought to occur in lymphoid organs where the host T cells encounter viral peptide antigens (or epitopes) that are presented by antigen-presenting cells such as dendritic cells, B cells, and macrophages. This process results in the maturation and expansion of T cells specific for these viral epitopes and is followed by their migration to the liver where they perform their effector function. Recent data indicate that a significant number of inflammatory cells in liver tissue are also non-antigen-specific (e.g., natural killer cells).[91]

To be recognized by the $CD8^+$ CTL, targeted hepatocytes must present viral epitopes as short peptides that have been endogenously processed and fit within the peptide-binding groove of the class I major histocompatibility complex (MHC) molecules.[92] The binding of the CTL T-cell receptor to the peptide-MHC complex on the hepatocyte surface can then result in the direct killing of the infected cell and the release of potent anti-viral cytokines by the activated CTL.[93] Recognition by class II restricted CD4 helper T cells requires the appropriate presentation of viral peptides in the context of class II MHC molecules. The CD4 cells produce anti-viral cytokines and provide help in neutralizing antibody production. Antibody neutralization limits spread during primary infection and serves an important role in preventing reinfection.

Acute HBV Infection

In acute, self-limited hepatitis, most HBV DNA molecules are cleared in the incubation phase (i.e., before the onset of liver damage and clinical symptoms of acute hepatitis B).[94] This rapid reduction in viral load has been attributed to inhibition of viral gene expression and replication by cytokines such as IFN-γ and tumor necrosis factor (TNF) alpha, which are detectable in the liver even before infiltration of large numbers of HBV-specific T cells.[94] HBV-specific CTLs that become detectable during the incubation phase are thought to be the primary source of these cytokines, but helper T cells, natural killer cells, and natural killer T cells are also potentially important.[95] Natural killer cells may play a particularly important role because they are readily detectable during the incubation period of viral hepatitis and rapidly decline after regression of serum HBV DNA levels.[96] The cytokines that are elaborated by these cells inhibit HBV gene expression by activating the hepatocytes to actively degrade the viral RNA and inhibit HBV replication by preventing the assembly or destabilizing the viral nucleocapsid particles within which replication occurs. Experiments in chimpanzees have demonstrated a decline in serum and liver HBV DNA levels by fiftyfold and 500-fold, respectively, that is coincident with the induction of IFN-γ and TNFα and occurs earlier than the influx of lymphocyte mRNA, suggesting that the cytokines are produced by non–T cells in the liver.[97]

Whereas early clearance of HBV viremia coincides with the non-cytolytic mechanisms defined previously, the necroinflammatory changes in liver tissue characteristic of acute viral hepatitis are considered to be a response to a vigorous, polyclonal, and multi-specific CD4 helper and CD8 CTL response. Virtually all patients with acute self-limited hepatitis B display a vigorous multi-specific CD4 cell response against several epitopes in the HBcAg and HBeAg, including strongly immunodominant epitopes that are recognized by patients with different histocompatibility locus antigen (HLA) backgrounds.[98] These patients also display a vigorous, polyclonal HLA class I–restricted CTL response against multiple epitopes in the HBV envelope, nucleocapsid, and polymerase epitopes. These viral antigen-specific responses ultimately lead to clearance of HBe and HBs antigens and development of neutralizing antibodies. It has recently been shown that the HBV-specific CTL response is maintained for decades after the loss of conventional viral markers (e.g., HBsAg, HBeAg) in the peripheral blood, and this is thought to be stimulated by trace amounts of HBV DNA in the peripheral blood and mononuclear cells.[99] The persistence of this cell-mediated immunity may be one reason why late reactivation of hepatitis occurs rarely, and that when it does, often requires an immunosuppressive event to trigger it (see Acute Flares in Chronic Hepatitis B).

Chronic HBV Infection

Chronic hepatitis B results from a partial deficiency in the immunologic response to HBV. It has been hypothesized that if the T-cell response directed against HBV is quantitatively weak or late or produces insufficient amounts of the viral inhibitory cytokines, cytotoxic T cell effector functions dominate, giving rise to persistent necroinflammatory change in the liver. This process can be viewed as a maladaptation to incomplete viral clearance by the first phase of the immunologic response. In contrast to the findings observed in acute self-limited acute hepatitis B, patients with chronic hepatitis B display a much less vigorous HBV-specific CD4 T-cell and CD8 T-cell response. HBV-specific CD4$^+$ T cells are present in very low frequencies in the peripheral blood and liver of patients with chronic hepatitis B.[100,101] One of the events that occurs during acute and chronic hepatitis B is the recruitment or local proliferation of non-specific T cells, which may result from stimulation of cross-reactive viral antigens or by cytokine-mediated bystander activation.[102] One group has shown that the number of CD8$^+$ HBc specific T cells in the liver was not different in patients with chronic HBV infection and normal serum aminotransferase levels when compared to those with abnormal aminotransferase levels.[103] However, the total number of CD8$^+$ T cells in the liver was much higher in those with liver damage, suggesting that the continued presence of an incompletely effective immune response led to recruitment of non-specific T cells. Thus it is likely that non-specific T cells also contribute in a significant way to the inflammatory changes characteristic of chronic hepatitis B.

The strength of the CD4 and CD8 T-cell responses is modifiable during chronic HBV infection under certain circumstances. For example, a nucleocapsid-specific CD4 T-cell response is accentuated during flares of chronic hepatitis in reaction to increased HBV replication; this response decreases as the disease subsides, suggesting that it may contribute to liver injury in this setting.[104] In a recent study HBV-specific proliferative CD4 T-cell responses were partially restored after 2 weeks of nucleoside analog therapy, which suggests that high viral burden may be a co-factor in the diminished T-cell response characteristic of chronically infected patients.[101] Patients with chronic HBV infection who clear the virus after IFNα therapy display a vigorous and multi-specific HBV-specific CTL response similar to that observed in self-limited acute hepatitis B.[105] Reconstitution of CD8-specific CTL responses has also been observed during lamivudine therapy.[106]

Apoptosis and Viral Hepatitis

Apoptosis is a morphologically and biochemically distinct form of cell death that is defined by cell shrinkage, cellular injury, and nuclear fragmentation.[107] It is the final common pathway of hepatocyte destruction in acute and chronic viral hepatitis, and activation of apoptotic pathways may be anticipated to interrupt viral replication and eliminate virally infected cells. The end result of apoptosis is recognizable on routine microscopy as Councilman or acidophilic bodies. There is accumulating evidence that this plays a significant role in the pathogenesis of viral hepatitis and is directly influenced by activated lymphocytes during acute and chronic viral hepatitis.[108] Apoptosis associated with hepatitis B is thought to be effected by CTL and is mediated through Fas ligand/Fas antigen and perforin/granzyme B pathways. Binding of Fas ligand to Fas receptors on the virus-infected hepatocytes triggers the release of intracellular proteases termed caspases; this ultimately leads to apoptosis. In addition, CTLs release perforin after engagement of the T-cell receptor. The result is damage to the cellular membrane that allows easy entry of cytotoxic granules containing granzyme B. The latter cleaves procaspases that also promote apoptosis. Cytokines released by inflammatory cells such as TNFα may also induce apoptosis after binding to specific receptors on hepatocytes.[108]

Evidence has accumulated that HBV may sensitize hepatocytes to apoptosis. For example, in a rat hepatocyte cell line TNFα-induced apoptosis only occurs in cells expressing a high level of HBV. The sensitization of liver cells to apoptotic stimuli during HBV infection has been linked to the X-gene product of HBV.[109] Although seemingly incompatible with the life cycle of HBV, stimulation of apoptotic pathways by the virus may allow completed viral particles to spread to neighboring cells that endocytose cellular fragments. In this way, the virus may escape immune recognition and neutralization by antibodies.

CLINICAL FEATURES OF ACUTE AND CHRONIC HBV INFECTION

Acute Hepatitis B

There is nothing specific about the clinical features of acute hepatitis B, and this may be totally indistinguishable from other forms of acute viral hepatitis. The incubation period varies from a few weeks to 6 months depending on the amount of replicating virus in the inoculum.[110] Approximately 70 percent of patients with acute hepatitis B have subclinical or anicteric hepatitis, whereas 30 percent develop icteric hepatitis. The disease may be more severe in patients co-infected with other hepatitis viruses or with underlying liver disease.[111] Acute infections are heralded by a serum sickness–like prodrome in 10 percent to 20 percent of patients with fever, arthralgias or arthritis, and skin rash, most frequently being of the maculopapular or urticarial variety. This prodrome results from circulating HBsAg/anti-HBs complexes that activate complement and deposit in the synovium and walls of cutaneous blood vessels.[112] These features generally abate early in the illness before the manifestations of liver disease and peak aminotransferase elevations. Less frequently, they may persist for more lengthy periods during the course of the acute illness.

Non-specific constitutional symptoms may develop and appear insidiously or abruptly. These symptoms include malaise, unusual fatigue, myalgia, anorexia, nausea, and, occasionally, vomiting. Clinical symptoms and jaundice generally disappear after 1 to 3 months, but some patients have prolonged fatigue even after normalization of alanine aminotransferase (ALT) levels.

In general, elevated ALT and serum HBsAg levels decline and disappear together. In approximately 80 percent of instances HBsAg disappears by 12 weeks after the onset of illness.[113] In 5 percent to 10 percent of cases, HBsAg is cleared early and is no longer detectable by the time the patient first presents to the physician. Persistence of HBsAg after 6 months implies the existence of a carrier state with only a small likelihood of recovery during the next 6 to 12 months.[114]

Elevation of ALT and aspartate aminotransferase (AST) are the hallmark of acute viral hepatitis. Values up to 1000 to 2000 IU/L are typically seen, with ALT being higher than AST. In patients with icteric hepatitis, increase in bilirubin levels often lags behind increase in ALT levels. The peak ALT level has no correlation with prognosis; prothrombin time is the best indicator of prognosis.

The frequency of progression from acute to chronic HBV infection is primarily determined by the age at infection, with approximately 90 percent for perinatally acquired infection,[115] 20 percent to 50 percent for infections between the age of 1 and 5 years,[116] and less than 5 percent for adult-acquired infection.[117]

After clinical recovery from acute hepatitis B, HBV DNA often remains detectable using PCR assays (see Serologic Diagnosis), despite the presence of anti-HBs and HBV-specific cytotoxic T cells.[118,119] These data suggest that viral eradication is seldom achieved in patients who have apparently recovered from acute hepatitis B, and that traces of HBV DNA are contained by humoral and cellular immune responses.[119]

Fulminant hepatitis occurs in less than 1 percent of cases. It generally occurs within 4 weeks of symptom onset and is associated with encephalopathy, multi-system organ failure, and a high mortality (greater than 80 percent) if not treated by liver transplantation (see Chap. 16). Patients older than age 40 appear to be more susceptible to "late-onset liver failure" in which encephalopathy, renal dysfunction, and other extrahepatic disorders associated with severe liver insufficiency become manifest over several months.[120] This may reflect impaired hepatic regeneration.[121] The pathogenic mechanisms for fulminant hepatitis are not clear but are believed to be caused by massive immune-mediated lysis of infected hepatocytes. This explains why many patients with fulminant hepatitis B have no evidence of viral replication at presentation.[122] Fulminant hepatitis has been reported in association with core promoter and precore HBV mutants but further studies are needed to determine the strength of this association.[123]

Chronic Hepatitis B

General Features

A history of acute or symptomatic hepatitis is obtained in only a small percentage of patients with chronic HBV infection. In low- or intermediate-prevalence areas, where HBV infection is predominantly acquired during adult or childhood years, approximately 30 percent to 50 percent of patients with chronic HBV infection have a history of acute hepatitis. Clinically evident hepatitis is also lacking in most patients in high-prevalence areas, where HBV infection is predominantly acquired perinatally.

Many patients with chronic HBV infection are asymptomatic unless they have severe chronic hepatitis or decompensated cirrhosis. When symptoms are present fatigue tends to predominate over other constitutional symptoms, such as poor appetite and malaise. Right upper quadrant pain may also be found. Patients may remain asymptomatic even during periods of reactivated hepatitis. In other instances, particularly when superimposed on cirrhosis, patients may demonstrate frank jaundice and signs of liver failure.

With chronic hepatitis B, physical examination may be normal or there may be hepatosplenomegaly. In decompensated cirrhosis, spider angiomata, jaundice, ascites, and peripheral edema are common. Biochemical tests are usually completely normal in patients with long-standing non-replicative infection, but most patients with replicative infection (except for patients in the immune tolerant phase who have acquired their infection perinatally) have mild to moderate elevation in serum AST and ALT. During exacerbations ALT levels may be as high as 1000 IU/L or more, and the patient may have a clinical and laboratory picture that is indistinguishable from acute hepatitis B, even including the presence of IgM anti-HBc.[124] In addition, alpha-fetoprotein levels in excess of 200 ng/ml may be seen.[125] Progression to cirrhosis should be suspected whenever there is evidence of hypersplenism, hypoalbuminemia in the absence of nephropathy, or prolongation of the prothrombin time. Hyperbilirubinemia also is a frequent feature in patients with decompensated cirrhosis, but other causes, such as Gilbert's syndrome and obstructive cholelithiasis, may on occasion obscure the significance of this finding. AST is frequently elevated out of proportion to ALT in patients with advanced cirrhosis.[126] Such patients also tend to have low serum HBV DNA levels.[46]

Extrahepatic Manifestations

Extrahepatic syndromes are seen in association with acute or chronic hepatitis B (Table 32-3) and are important to recognize because they may occur without clinically apparent liver disease and can be mistaken for independent disease processes. In the acute setting these non-hepatic disorders tend to be self-limited, whereas in chronic HBV infection these disorders often contribute significantly to the morbidity and mortality associated with infection. Thus their recognition is also important because anti-virals can be used to treat the more serious disorders. The pathogenesis of these extrahepatic disorders has not been fully elucidated, but it has been demonstrated that HBV replicative intermediates and viral proteins can be found in the bone marrow, kidney, skin, colon, stomach, testes, and periadrenal ganglia.[17] These extrahepatic reservoirs of infection may facilitate the expression of the extrahepatic disease syndromes. Many of the non-hepatic manifestations (e.g., arthritis, dermatitis, glomerulonephritis, polyarteritis nodosa, mixed cryoglobulinemia, papular acrodermatitis, polymyalgia rheumatica) are observed in association with circulating immune complexes. Other disorders (e.g., pleural effusion, pancreatitis, Guillain-Barré syndrome) may be manifestations of severe or fulminant hepatitis and are not believed to be due to immune complex disease.

Arthritis-Dermatitis. Approximately 10 percent to 20 percent of patients develop a serum sickness-like syndrome as a prodromal manifestation of acute hepatitis B. This disorder consists of fever, arthralgia, rash, angioneurotic edema, and, less commonly, hematuria and proteinuria.[127] Frank arthritis is uncommon. These symptoms usually begin in the late incubation period and often disappear 2 to 3 weeks before the onset of hepatitis-related symptoms. The joints that are most commonly afflicted are the proximal interphalangeal joints, knees, ankles, shoulders, and wrists.[127] During the period of acute joint

TABLE 32-3
Extrahepatic Manifestations of Acute and Chronic HBV

	Immune complex association	Clinical course
Acute Disorder		
Serum sickness-like illness	Yes	Prodromal manifestation, resolves
Polyarteritis nodosa	Yes	May resolve or persist
Glomerulonephritis	Yes	May resolve
Cryoglobulinemia	Yes	Seen with serum sickness prodrome
Papular acrodermatitis	Yes	Pediatric disease; may persist along with chronic HBV infection
Chronic Disorder		
Polyarteritis nodosa	Yes	Tends to be progressive; liver disease often mild
Glomerulonephritis Membranous Mesangial proliferative Membranoproliferative	Yes	Resolution usual in children; often progressive in adults
Essential mixed cryoglobulinemia*	Yes	Frequently asymptomatic or paucisymptomatic

HBV, Hepatitis B virus.
*Association is uncertain.

symptoms, HBsAg titers in the blood are high and complement levels are low. HBsAg has been detected in synovial membranes, and complement levels in synovial fluid are low.[128] There is evidence for activation of the complement system by surface antigen-antibody complexes, which have been isolated from cryoglobulins.[129] After the joint symptoms subside complement levels normalize and HBsAg titers in serum begin to decline. This syndrome may be mistaken for rheumatoid arthritis, but in acute hepatitis B there is little erythema or warmth over the affected joints, synovial thickening can not be appreciated, and deformity or destructive joint changes are absent. Arthritis and dermatitis may also appear in conjunction with a multi-system vasculitis in patients with chronic HBV infection. Various combinations of fever and renal, cardiac, gastrointestinal and neurologic disease are found, the symptoms are often prolonged, and fatalities have been reported.[130]

Polyarteritis Nodosa. One of the most serious extrahepatic syndromes associated with chronic HBV infection is systemic necrotizing vasculitis or polyarteritis nodosa. As much as 30 percent to 70 percent of patients with polyarteritis nodosa are infected with HBV,[131] but only less than 1 percent of patients with HBV develop this disorder.[132] This may occur after acute or recent hepatitis B, in which case HBsAg seroconversion and spontaneous recovery have been reported.[127,133] The manifestations of vasculitis may precede the development of acute hepatitis B but most often they follow it by weeks to months. Polyarteritis nodosa is more commonly seen in association with chronic HBV infection. Symptoms include arthralgias, mononeuritis, fever, abdominal pain, renal disease, hypertension, central nervous system (CNS) abnormalities, and rash. Medium to small arteries and arterioles are involved by fibrinoid necrosis and perivascular infiltration. The disease is thought to be due to circulating immune complexes that contain HBsAg; for this reason, plasmapheresis has been used as part of a combined therapeutic regimen.[134] In patients with HBV-associated polyarteritis nodosa the clinical complications are very similar to those observed in cases without a specific triggering event. Some investigators have found that malignant hypertension, renal infarction, and orchiepididymitis are more commonly associated with HBV infection.[135] There is no apparent relationship between the severity of the vasculitis and the severity of the hepatic disease, and often the hepatic disease is relatively quiescent.[131] The course of the disease is variable; however, 30 percent to 50 percent of patients may die as a result of the vasculitis, which is similar to the mortality rate observed in HBV-unassociated polyarteritis nodosa.[136] Prognosis is gravest for those with significant proteinuria (more than 1 g/day), renal insufficiency (serum creatinine levels higher than 1.6 mg percent), gastrointestinal involvement, cardiomyopathy, and CNS involvement.[137]

Glomerulonephritis. Prerenal azotemia and acute tubular necrosis are the most common causes of acute renal failure in patients with acute hepatitis B. Glomerulonephritis may rarely be manifested at the same time as acute hepatitis B, in which case spontaneous resolution of both disorders may occur.[138] Renal biopsies in patients with acute hepatitis B have found glomerular involvement, as shown by immune complex deposition and cytoplasmic inclusions in the glomerular basement membrane.[139] These complexes activate complement and cytokine production with a subsequent inflammatory response.[140] In a retrospective study of 59 patients who died of either acute fulminant hepatitis or subacute hepatitis (most of whom had hepatitis B), glomerular deposits were found in 15 percent of the renal tissue specimens examined,[141] irrespective of the clinical presence of renal disease. Several types of glomerular lesions have been described in chronic HBV infection, with membranous glomerulonephritis and membranoproliferative glomerulonephritis being the most common.[142-144]

HBV-associated glomerulonephritis occurs mainly in children, predominantly males, in areas of the world where HBV infection is endemic. Only occasionally, cases of HBV-associated glomerulonephritis have been reported in the United States, in both adults and children. The prevalence of this disorder is not known. Whereas some patients with chronic renal disease may circulate HBsAg, only a small percentage of these patients demonstrate glomerular deposits containing HBV antigens.

Nephrotic syndrome is the most frequent presentation of HBV-associated glomerulonephritis. During childhood, significant renal failure at presentation is infrequent, and a prior history of clinical liver disease is uncommon. Nevertheless, liver biopsies almost always demonstrate varying degrees of chronic viral hepatitis. The diagnosis of HBV-associated glomerulonephropathy is usually established by serologic evidence of HBV antigens or antibodies, by the presence of immune-complex glomerulonephritis on renal biopsy, and by the demonstration of glomerular deposits of one or more HBV antigens, such as HBsAg, HBcAg, or HBeAg, by immunohistochemistry.[145] Most patients have detectable HBeAg in serum and will demonstrate activation of the classic complement cascade, with low serum C3 and occasionally C4 levels. The renal disease often resolves in months to several years, especially in children who have membranous glomerulonephritis. Often this resolution occurs with seroconversion of HBeAg. Rarely, however, renal failure may ensue. The natural history of HBV-related glomerulonephritis in adults has not been well defined but several reports from Asia suggest that the course is not as benign as in children, and the glomerular disease is often slowly and relentlessly progressive.[146] The glomerulonephritis secondary to chronic HBV infection may appear histologically similar to that which is unassociated with infection. The presence of persistent HBV antigenemia, the evidence for chronic liver disease, and the localization of HBV antigens in glomerular deposits by immunocytochemical means confirm the diagnosis of HBV-associated disease.

Essential Mixed Cryoglobulinemia. Type II cryoglobulins consist of a polyclonal IgG and monoclonal IgM, whereas type III cryoglobulins contain polyclonal IgG and rheumatoid factor. Type II and type III cryoglobulinemia has been associated with hepatitis B, but more recent evidence suggests that the association was likely related to an unrecognized chronic C hepatitis.[147] Cryoglobulinemia may be associated with systemic vasculitis (purpura, arthralgia, peripheral neuropathy, and glomerulonephritis[148]) but is often not associated with any symptoms. Cryoglobulins do not contribute to the pathogenesis of liver disease. Recently, the association of chronic HBV infection and mixed cryoglobulinemia has been further clarified. In a large series of patients with various forms of chronic liver disease the overall prevalence of mixed cryoglobulinemia was high (42 percent) when all patients were assessed.[149] The frequency of cryoglobulinemia was significantly higher in chronic hepatitis C virus infection (54 percent) when compared to patients with chronic HBV infection (15 percent).

PATHOLOGY OF HBV INFECTION

Acute Hepatitis B

Acute hepatitis B (see Chap. 25) is characterized by degeneration of hepatocytes, acidophilic bodies, lobular necrosis, and inflammation of the portal triads and parenchyma. Kupffer cell hyperplasia is characteristically seen, and disruption of lobular architecture is evident. Cells undergoing ballooning degeneration are swollen, with obscure cell margins and rarefied cytoplasm. In contrast, cells undergoing acidophilic degeneration are shrunken, angulated, and eosinophilic. The inflammatory cells infiltrating the liver substance are predominantly lymphocytes. Occasionally eosinophils and neutrophils can be seen. Plasma cells are rare. The extent of necrosis varies according to clinical disease severity. In submassive necrosis there is hepatocyte dropout in the central and midzonal areas, with condensation of the reticulum framework and sinusoidal dilation. Adjacent necrotic areas may be linked to form bridging necrosis. The area of hepatocyte dropout is more extensive in fulminant hepatic failure, and massive necrosis is present involving all three zones. Cholangiolar proliferation may accompany massive necrosis. Ultrastructurally, there is enlargement of the endoplasmic reticulum, ribosomes, and mitochondria in cells undergoing ballooning degeneration. Loss of organelles is seen in cells undergoing acidophilic degeneration. Further changes of acidophilic degeneration result in the formation of Councilman or apoptotic bodies that are often demonstrable in the space of Disse.

Chronic Hepatitis B

Chronic hepatitis B infection is characterized by the presence of inflammatory cells, mainly lymphocytes, in the portal triad. Periportal inflammation may lead to the disruption of the limiting plate of hepatocytes (piecemeal necrosis or interface hepatitis) (Plate 32-1). Histologic features of chronic hepatitis B had been previously classified as chronic persistent and chronic active hepatitis depending on the degree of interface hepatitis and presence of fibrosis. These findings are two ends of a spectrum of pathologic changes in chronic hepatitis. Depending on the progression of the disease or treatment interventions, the pathologic findings may change from one pattern to the other. During reactivated hepatitis B there is more intense lobular inflammation reminiscent of the features of acute viral hepatitis (Plate 32-2).

The only histologic feature on routine light microscopy that is specific for chronic hepatitis B is the presence of ground-glass hepatocytes (Plate 32-3). These were first described in chronic carriers of hepatitis B in 1973.[150] The morphologic findings are due to HBsAg particles (20-30 nm in diameter) that accumulate in the dilated endoplasmic reticulum.[151] Because of high levels of cystine in HBsAg, ground-glass cells have a high affinity toward certain dyes such as orcein, Victoria blue, and aldehyde fuchsin. These stains can identify the HBsAg in paraffin-embedded specimens stored for extended periods.[152] Ground-glass hepatocytes are seen in chronic hepatitis B and may also be seen in HBsAg carriers, in whom they may be detected in up to 5 percent of cells. When present in abundance they are often indicative of a state of active viral replication.[152] Immunofluorescence and electron microscopic studies have shown HBcAg inside the hepatocyte nuclei of affected cells.[153] Hepatitis B surface and core antigens can be demonstrated in hepatocytes by immunohistochemical staining (Plate 32-4, *A-C*). Hepatitis B surface antigen is found in the cytoplasm and sometimes can be seen in a submembranous distribution (Plate 32-4, *A*). Core antigen can be detected in both the cytoplasm and hepatocyte nuclei. The presence of cytoplasmic core correlates with active viral proliferation, and when it is the predominant finding it correlates with active liver histology (Plate 32-4, *B*).[153a]

ACUTE FLARES IN CHRONIC HBV INFECTION

Acute flares in chronic hepatitis B occur in association with a number of circumstances and clinical situations (Figure 32-4). Most of these flares are due to a change in the balance between immunologic responses to HBV and the extent of viral proliferation. Key to understanding flares is the concept that the persistent hepatic inflammation that characterizes chronic hepatitis B is the result of a suboptimal or inadequate cellular immune response to nucleocapsid antigens.[154] The greater the extent of the cell-mediated immune deficiency to HBV, the more likely the host will be immunotolerant to the virus and lack significant histologic disease. The opposite situation also applies; that is, the more robust the immunologic response to virally encoded antigens, the greater the likelihood of substantial inflammatory changes and replacement of damaged hepatocytes with fibrous tissue. Acute flares in chronic hepatitis B that are not explainable by infection with other hepatotropic viruses often occur as a secondary response to increased levels of replicating wild-type or mutant virus or as a result of therapeutic intervention with immunologic modifiers such as IFN, corticosteroids, or cancer chemotherapy. In some instances the initiating events for the acute exacerbations in chronic hepatitis B may not be readily identifiable; these flares are considered to be spontaneous in nature.

Spontaneous Flares in the Natural History of Chronic HBV Infection

The natural history of chronic hepatitis B is punctuated by spontaneous flares of the disease in which substantial elevation of serum aminotransferase levels occurs.[155] The acute episodes are precipitated by reactivated infection,

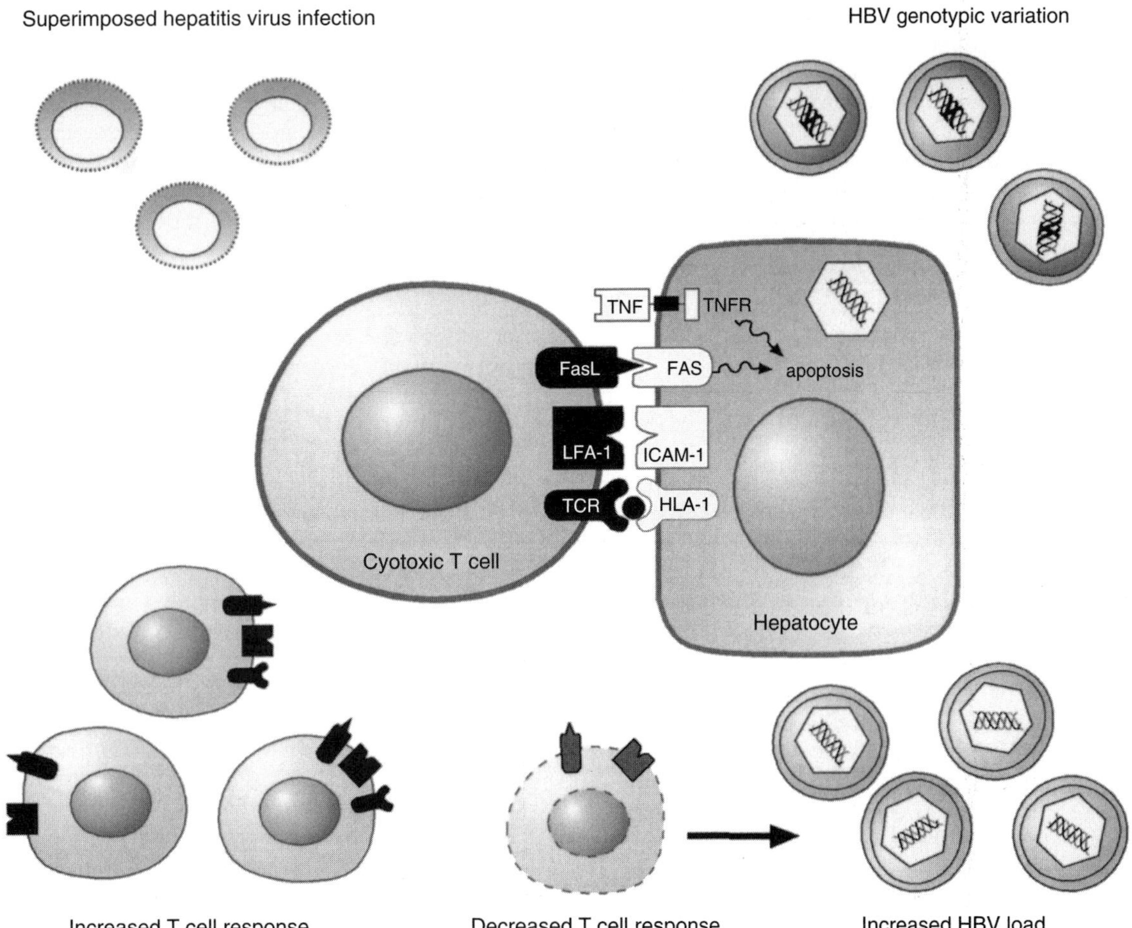

Figure 32-4 Immunopathogenesis of hepatocyte injury during chronic hepatitis B and the factors that contribute to acute flares. (From Perrillo RP: Gastroenterology 120:1009, 2001.) (See Acute Flares in Chronic Hepatitis B for details).

and it has been shown that low basal viremia increases markedly before an increase in serum aminotransferase level is observed.[156] Histologic evidence of acute lobular hepatitis superimposed on the changes of chronic viral hepatitis is frequently observed during these flares.[157] IgM antibody to HBcAg, a marker often diagnostic of acute viral hepatitis, also may appear at this time and is generally in lower titer than in acute infection.[156]

The reasons for reactivated infection are unknown but are likely explained by subtle changes in the immunologic control of viral replication. Reactivation seems to occur more commonly in male homosexuals, in individuals infected with human immunodeficiency virus (HIV), and concurrently with prolonged physical stress or serious infections.[157,158] The flares are important clinically because they can have severe or even fatal consequences.[117,159] In one study from Greece spontaneous reactivation was shown to account for 27 percent of cases of apparent acute hepatitis in HBsAg carriers; this was associated with a mortality rate of 18 percent.[117] An estimated 10 percent to 30 percent of hepatitis B carriers experience such episodes each year.[160] It is not uncommon to encounter episodes of abrupt elevation of AST and ALT to 2 to 5 times previous levels. Less intense elevations have been shown to occur even more frequently if patients are monitored closely.[157] In individuals who acquire their infection early in life, flares become more common during adulthood because of a breakdown of immunotolerance to HBV.[161] Patients may experience fatigue, nausea, and anorexia during an acute flare, but many individuals, particularly those who have mild or early disease, remain asymptomatic. Occasionally signs of frank liver failure will become obvious, particularly when it is superimposed on advanced chronic hepatitis B.[162]

Most clinically recognizable flares occur in patients who are in the non-replicative phase of infection (i.e., initially anti-HBe–positive and serum HBV DNA negative by molecular hybridization assay). During these episodes serum aminotransferase levels increase in response to the sudden re-emergence of viral replication. HBV DNA and HBeAg are often detectable when the patient is first seen, but if the flares have been ongoing for several weeks or months, the accompanying enhancement of the immune response may make it difficult to detect serum HBV DNA by relatively insensitive molecular hybridization assays. Frequently these hepatitis flares precede loss of serum HBV DNA and HBeAg.[157,159] Similar observations have been found in HBeAg-positive children.[163] Flares also can occur in patients who are in the replicative stage of infection (i.e., already positive for serum HBV DNA and HBeAg). In these instances HBV replication intensifies, serum HBV DNA levels increase, and biochemical deterioration occurs without subsequent loss of HBeAg. These episodes can be viewed as an abortive attempt at seroconversion. Some patients undergo multiple episodes in which flares precede HBeAg seroconversion only to have a second flare months later in which reactivated infection occurs.[157] Multiple episodes of reactivation and remission have been shown to accelerate the progression of chronic hepatitis B.[157,159]

The frequency of acute flares of hepatitis differs in Asian and Western patients. Studies in Asian patients with chronic hepatitis B have shown more serologic fluctuation than that occurring in patients in the United States and Western Europe. In a study of 224 HBeAg-positive Asian carriers flares of disease activity occurred in 40 percent of the study's population, but this seldom led to seroconversion or a sustained virologic response.[164] Instead, reactivated infection subsequently developed in more than 30 percent of patients who lost HBeAg. The rate of reactivation was lowest in patients who initially developed anti-HBe, but even in this group reactivation occurred relatively frequently (16 percent). These differences in the natural history of infection in Asian and Western patients become important when deciding on the need for anti-viral treatment.

Immunosuppressive Therapy and Viral Reactivation

Reactivation of HBV replication is a well-recognized complication in patients with chronic HBV infection who receive cytotoxic or immunosuppressive therapy.[165] Suppression of the normal immunologic responses to HBV leads to enhanced viral replication and is thought to result in widespread infection of hepatocytes.[166] Upon discontinuation of immunosuppressive medications such as cancer chemotherapy, anti-rejection drugs, or corticosteroids, immune competence is restored and infected hepatocytes are rapidly destroyed.[167] The more potent the immunosuppression, the greater the level of viral replication, and thus the greater the potential for serious clinical consequences of sudden withdrawal.

The first references to the deleterious effects of immunosuppressive therapy in chronic HBV infection were in patients with myeloproliferative disorders, lymphoproliferative diseases, and choriocarcinoma.[168,169] Several case series subsequently described exacerbations of hepatitis and reactivation of hepatitis B in patients who were given chemotherapy for other malignancies, including testicular cancer, small cell lung cancer, and neuroendocrine tumors.[170] The biochemical and clinical deterioration has been most intense after withdrawal of cancer chemotherapy.[166,167,169,171] Most reports have included some patients with evidence of serious or massive liver injury. Postmortem study of liver tissue in cases of severe liver injury has documented sparse staining of viral antigens suggesting that patients were in an active state of immune clearance.[167,171]

The majority of patients have been HBsAg-positive before treatment but some studies have emphasized the reappearance of this marker in patients who were initially positive for anti-HBs or anti-HBc, either alone or in combination.[172-174] The frequency with which hepatitis in HBsAg carriers undergoing cancer chemotherapy is due to reactivation of hepatitis B has varied widely (14 percent-72 percent).[170,172] Reactivated hepatitis tends to occur more frequently and is usually more severe in patients who are HBsAg-positive before treatment.[172,174] Chemotherapy given to cancer patients who are chronic hepatitis B carriers clearly leads to an increased risk of liver-related morbidity and mortality.[175]

Reactivated hepatitis B also occurs in patients who are given immunosuppressive medications for organ transplantation. The first cases were described in patients who underwent renal transplantation, but reactivation has also been described in HBsAg-positive or anti-HBs/anti-HBc- positive patients who undergo bone marrow, liver, renal, heart, or lung transplantation.[33,175-180] Reactivated hepatitis in HBsAg-negative patients with anti-HBc or anti-HBs is explainable by the possible latency of HBV in liver and mononuclear cells and the large extrahepatic reservoir of HBV.[17-19] The prevalence of reactivated hepatitis appears to be particularly common in patients undergoing bone marrow transplantation because of the extensive immunologic conditioning before transplantation and treatment regimens for graft-versus-host reactions.[181] The clinical spectrum in organ recipients with reactivated hepatitis B has varied from asymptomatic anicteric hepatitis to fulminant hepatitis and fibrosing cholestatic hepatitis, a rapidly progressive form of injury associated with inordinately high levels of HBsAg and HBcAg in liver tissue.[182,183]

Acute flares of hepatitis B resulting from cancer chemotherapy and other immunosuppressive drugs are often detected relatively late. The use of anti-viral treatment after major biochemical abnormalities have been detected should be anticipated to have relatively little effect on reducing liver injury because much of the immunologic response to HBV and viral elimination has already occurred. Thus the key to management of this situation lies in anticipating its occurrence and in early anti-viral treatment (see Anti-viral Therapy).

Anti-viral Therapy–induced Hepatic Flares

Anti-viral treatment of chronic hepatitis B can be associated with flares of hepatitis in three ways. Flares may occur during IFN therapy, in response to treatment with nucleoside analogs, and after withdrawal of corticosteroids.

Interferon

IFN-induced flares are explainable by the immunostimulatory properties of this drug. IFN increases T-cell cytolytic activity and natural killer cell function, and flares typically occur during the second to third month of treatment (Figure 32-5).[184-186] In a study involving 169 patients with chronic hepatitis B, a twofold or greater elevation in ALT activity relative to baseline occurred in 33 percent of patients given 5 million units of IFN-2b. Flares were associated with a higher likelihood of a virologic response, and a sustained loss of HBV DNA occurred in 54 percent of treated patients who demonstrated a flare as compared to 28 percent of those without a flare. Unfortunately, IFN-related flares tend to be particularly common in patients

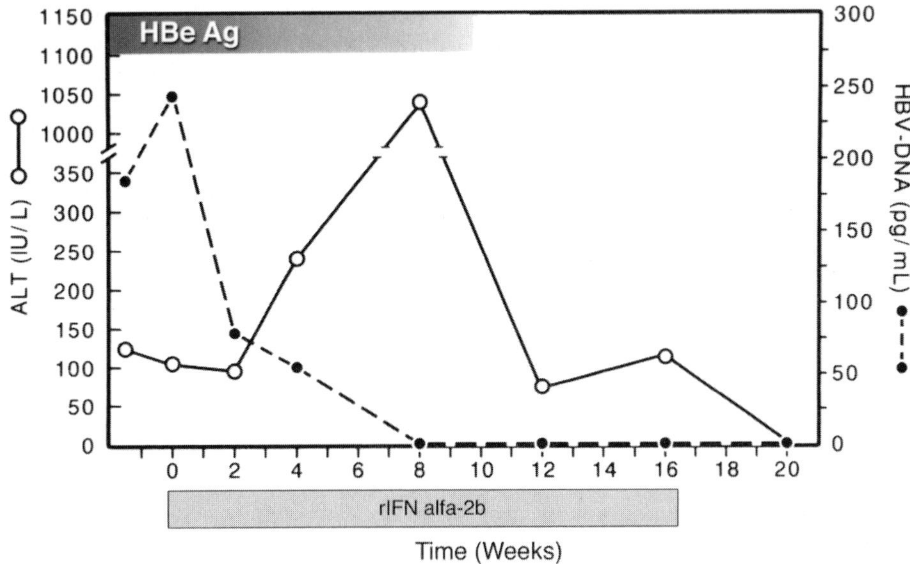

Figure 32-5 Interferon-induced biochemical flare. Such flares have been associated with a higher rate of virologic response and typically occur during the second or third month of treatment.

who have decompensated liver disease, having occurred in 50 percent of patients in one series.[187] This may be associated with clinical deterioration in these patients.[46,187]

Nucleoside Analogs

Acute flares in serum aminotransferase levels occur with nucleoside analog therapy. The treatment of chronic hepatitis B with lamivudine has been associated with an increase in serum aminotransferase levels to 3 to 10 times baseline values in 10 percent of patients.[188] Flares in ALT have also been observed with famciclovir.[189] Unlike the late ALT elevations that occur with IFN, flares during lamivudine treatment tend to occur within the first 4 to 6 weeks, often after a major decline in serum HBV DNA. They are generally not associated with symptoms and tend not to be sustained despite continued treatment. Review of the phase III lamivudine trials has indicated that these flares do not occur any more commonly with this drug than they do with placebo.[188,190] The mechanism behind these flares during the early part of treatment is not known but it has been postulated that they are due to a restoration of T-cell responsiveness that accompanies a decline in viral proliferation.[101,106,191]

Of greater importance are the uncommon flares in hepatitis that occur upon withdrawal of lamivudine. These have been attributed to resurgence of wild-type virus and have been associated with serious clinical exacerbations in Asians with advanced liver disease.[192,193] Phase III trial data revealed that post-treatment ALT elevations greater than 3 times baseline occurred in 41 (19 percent) of 215 lamivudine-treated patients as compared to 5 (8 percent) of 66 placebo-treated controls.[190] After discontinuation of treatment there was a slightly greater frequency of ALT levels that were 2 or more times baseline and in excess of 500 IU/L in treated patients (14 percent versus 9 percent) but no difference was observed in the number of patients having twofold or greater ALT elevations in conjunction with a twofold elevation in serum bilirubin (1 percent and 2 percent, respectively). It is unknown if these post-treatment flares should be managed with reinstitution of lamivudine therapy but this therapy has reportedly induced a prompt decline in elevated serum HBV DNA and aminotransferase levels.

Prednisone Withdrawal. A pronounced elevation of serum aminotransferase levels associated with an inverse decline in HBsAg titers and HBV DNA polymerase has been observed in chronic hepatitis B after withdrawal of corticosteroids.[194-196] These observations led to a series of clinical trials in which a short course of corticosteroids was used with adenine arabinoside, IFN, and, more recently, lamivudine.[186,197-201] The apparent immune rebound after withdrawal from a 4- to 8-week course of corticosteroids may be due to increased activation of lymphocytes that promote Th-1 cytokine responses at a time when there is increased viral antigen expression.[200,201] Peak ALT values typically occur 4 to 6 weeks after withdrawal, and the intensity of the flare may be modifiable by increasing the initial dose and shortening the duration of corticosteroid treatment.[202,203] In a US multi-center IFN alfa-2b trial 43 patients were treated with a 6-week course of prednisone followed in sequence by a 2-week non-treatment interval and 16 weeks of IFN alfa-2b.[186] ALT flares occurred in 53 percent of these patients and were associated with a virologic response in 50 percent. The mean level for the increase in ALT was 3.4-fold (range: twofold to 6.5-fold) when compared to pretreatment values. Flares occurred at a mean interval of 4.9 weeks after initiation of IFN in the combined therapy group versus 7.7 weeks in a group given the identical dose of IFN alone preceded by a placebo. These flares are generally well tolerated in patients with mild to moderate hepatitis but serious hepatic decompensation has been reported in patients with advanced disease.[203-205] One study reported that the relative risk of hepatic decompensation in Asian cirrhotic patients was 16 times that of non-cirrhotic patients after withdrawal from a 4- to 6-week course of corticosteroids.[203]

Flares Resulting from HBV Genotypic Variation

Acute flares in chronic hepatitis B may also occur in response to HBV genotypic variation. Chronic infection with precore mutant HBV (also called HBeAg-minus HBV) is often associated with multiple flares of liver cell necrosis interspersed with periods of asymptomatic HBV carriage.[206] Episodic flares in patients with chronic hepatitis B have been attributed to increases in the concentration of precore mutants and changes in the proportion of precore to wild-type HBV.[207,208] It has been suggested that disease exacerbations are uncommon during the earliest phase of chronic HBV at a time when wild-type HBV predominates and that flares become common with the gradual emergence of the precore variant.[207] These flares are thought to subside with time as genetic heterogeneity disappears and patients become exclusively infected with precore HBV.

Mutations at the basal core promoter (BCP) region of the HBV genome are associated with decreased HBeAg synthesis, active liver histology, and increased viral replication.[70,209] Multiple exacerbations of hepatitis resulting from reactivated HBV infection have been described in patients with BCP mutation, either alone or in association with precore mutation.[210] Sometimes these exacerbations have been fatal, presenting as fulminant liver failure.[211] HBeAg-negative patients who harbor both precore and core promoter mutants may be particularly predisposed to severe reactivation episodes after chemotherapy for malignancies.[212]

Mutations in domains B and C of the HBV DNA polymerase gene occur during lamivudine therapy in a time-dependent manner. These mutations occur in approximately 15 percent of patients after 1 year of treatment and in more than 50 percent after 3 to 4 years of continuous treatment.[70,213] Some of these mutants confer high-level resistance to lamivudine and should be suspected whenever serum HBV DNA reappears in a patient who was previously negative on treatment.[70,213] The HBV DNA polymerase mutants can be rapidly selected during repeat courses of treatment (Figure 32-6). A mild to moderate increase in ALT often precedes or accompanies the reappearance of HBV DNA but this is generally transient, and aminotransferase levels often remain below pretreatment levels.[70,214] The polymerase mutants have been found to be not as replication-competent as are wild-type HBV, which may explain the lower ALT and HBV DNA levels.[85] There are occasional notable exceptions to these general findings, however. In one study 13 of 32 Asian patients (41 percent) who were maintained on lamivudine after resistance was confirmed had one or more exacerbations of hepatitis (median: 24 weeks after first detection of polymerase mutants).[215] During these episodes ALT levels ranged from 247 to 2010 IU/L with the majority of peak values in excess of 10 times the upper limit of normal, and HBeAg seroconversion subsequently occurred in 75 percent of cases. Further study by the same group of investigators demonstrated the emergence of new polymerase mutants that replaced the original mutants in some cases—this event was also often associated with flares in ALT.[53]

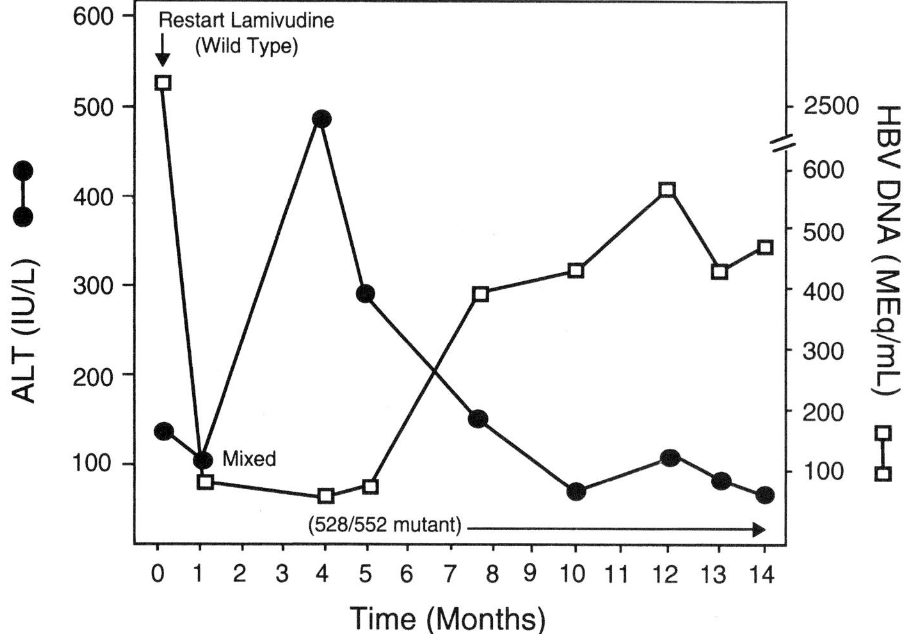

Figure 32-6 Hepatitis flare induced by lamivudine-resistant HBV DNA polymerase gene mutant. The patient had previously received a 6-month course of lamivudine and the mutant virus (here abbreviated as the 528/552 mutant) was rapidly selected during a second course of treatment. *HBV,* Hepatitis B virus; *DNA,* deoxyribonucleic acid. (From Perrillo RP: Gastroenterology 120:1009, 2001.)

Hepatitis Flares Resulting from Infection with Other Viruses

Patients with chronic HBV infection may exhibit pronounced flares in serum aminotransferases and even frank liver failure when superinfected with other hepatotropic viruses such as hepatitis A virus (HAV), hepatitis C virus (HCV), and hepatitis delta virus (HDV). Increased mortality has been reported when hepatitis A is superimposed on chronic hepatitis B, although this has not been a consistent finding in the available studies.[216-219] The discrepancy in findings may be based on differences in the severity of the underlying hepatitis B.[220] Fulminant liver failure frequently occurs when delta virus superinfection is superimposed on chronic hepatitis B and chronic HDV infection is associated with multiple fluctuations in serum aminotransferase levels (see Hepatitis Delta Virus).[221,222] Acute hepatitis C has also been shown to predispose patients with chronic hepatitis B to fulminant liver failure.[223] Similar to delta infection, infection with HCV frequently becomes chronic, and the subsequent course may be characterized by frequent fluctuations in ALT and AST values.[224]

The degree to which acute flares in chronic HBsAg carriers can be explained by superinfection with other viruses in contrast to flares resulting from HBV is contingent on a number of factors, including the background prevalence of these other viral infections, the frequency of spontaneous HBV reactivation in a given population, and the underlying HBeAg status of the individual. In one study acute flares in serum aminotransferase levels (at least 10 times the normal value) were detected in 76 asymptomatic Asian HBsAg carriers, and the etiology for these was determined by testing for HBeAg, anti-HBe, serum HBV DNA, IgM antibody to hepatitis A virus, and anti-delta.[225] Nearly 90 percent of patients who were initially HBeAg-positive either were initially or became HBV DNA–negative, suggesting immune clearance of HBV as the cause for the flare. In contrast, 55 percent of anti-HBe–positive patients were diagnosed as having delta superinfection, 21 percent were suspected of having non-A, non-B virus superinfection, and only 24 percent were considered to have reactivation of HBV.

Patients with chronic hepatitis B who become infected with other hepatotropic viruses may become HBeAg-negative and serum HBV DNA–negative by non-PCR–based assays because of a process of viral interference.[226] This has been described with superimposition of HAV, HCV, and HDV infections[227-229] and combined infections with HCV and HDV.[230] In some instances, these secondary infections result in HBeAg and HBsAg seroconversion.[227,231] Thus serologic assessment for other hepatitis viruses and markers for HBV replication may be necessary to correctly interpret or recognize the cause of acute exacerbations in patients with chronic hepatitis B.

The interrelationship between human HIV infection and HBV infection is complex. Abnormal levels of liver enzymes are common among people infected with HIV and may be caused by multiple factors, including medication toxicity and co-infection with HBV or HCV. Early reports emphasized that patients co-infected with HIV and HBV had high serum HBV DNA levels, but acute hepatitis flares, implying an active cell-mediated immune response to HBV, were seldom reported.[232,233] The development of more effective antiretroviral regimens has led to immune reconstitution in many HIV-infected patients, however, and the clinical spectrum of chronic hepatitis B, including flares of serum aminotransferase levels, observed in these patients has more recently been described to be similar to that which occurs in non–HIV-infected hosts.[234-236]

SERODIAGNOSIS OF ACUTE AND CHRONIC HBV INFECTION

The diagnosis of hepatitis B virus infection relies on the detection of viral antigens and antibodies, and viral replication status is indicated by measurement of serum HBV DNA and HBeAg. Liver disease tends to be active when viral replication markers are detectable and quiescent when they are absent.

Serologic Markers of HBV Infection

HBsAg is the serologic hallmark of HBV infection. HBsAg appears in serum 2 to 10 weeks after exposure to the virus and before the onset of symptoms or the elevation of serum aminotransferase levels. In patients who subsequently recover, HBsAg usually becomes undetectable after 4 to 6 months. Persistence of HBsAg for more than 6 months implies progression to chronic HBV infection.

The disappearance of HBsAg is followed by the appearance of anti-HBs. In most patients, anti-HBs persists for life, conferring long-term immunity. In some patients anti-HBs may not become detectable, but these patients do not appear to be susceptible to recurrent infection.[237] Anti-HBs may not be detectable during a window period of several weeks to months after the disappearance of HBsAg.[113,170] During this period diagnosis of HBV infection is made by the detection of IgM antibodies against HBcAg (IgM anti-HBc, see the following section).[238]

Co-existence of HBsAg and anti-HBs has been reported in approximately 25 percent of HBsAg-positive individuals.[239] In most instances the antibodies are low-level, non-neutralizing, and heterotypic (i.e., directed against a different subtype of HBsAg than that present in the infected patient).[173] The presence of these heterotypic antibodies is not associated with specific risk factors or change in clinical course and may occur in the setting of active liver disease and viral replication.[239,240]

Anti-HBc is detectable in acute and chronic HBV infection. During acute infection anti-HBc is predominantly of the IgM class. When the manufacturer's recommendations for serum preparation are used, this antibody is usually detectable for 4 to 6 months after an acute episode of hepatitis and may rarely persist for up to 2 years. IgM anti-HBc may become detectable during exacerbations of chronic hepatitis B.[241] Because of an association with active viral replication, IgM anti-HBc has also been used as a monitoring tool during anti-viral therapy.[242] IgG anti-HBc persists in those who recover from acute hepatitis B and in association with HBsAg in those who progress to chronic infection.

Isolated presence of anti-HBc in the absence of HBsAg and anti-HBs has been reported to occur in 0.6 percent of blood donors in low prevalence areas and in 3 percent to 12 percent of the population in endemic countries.[243-245] Isolated detection of anti-HBc can occur in four settings: during the window period of acute hepatitis B when it is predominantly of the IgM class; many years after recovery from acute hepatitis B when anti-HBs has fallen to undetectable levels; as a false positive serologic test; and after many years of chronic infection when the HBsAg titer has decreased below the level of detection.[12] False positive anti-HBc reactions are not an infrequent occurrence, even in endemic areas of the world, because as many as two thirds of individuals with isolated detection of anti-HBc react to vaccination as though they were having a primary rather than an anamnestic response.[244,245]

Serologic studies have shown that 0 percent to 30 percent of patients with isolated anti-HBc have HBV DNA in serum by PCR.[243,246,247] The frequency of HBV DNA positivity in patients with anti-HBc alone reflects the background frequency of infection in a particular population.[175,179] Using a commercially available quantitative PCR assay with a detection limit of 100 copies/ml, levels below 1000 copies/ml have been found in HBsAg-negative patients with anti-HBc compared with median serum levels of $10^{8.6}$ and $10^{4.3}$ copies/ml, respectively, in HBeAg-positive and HBeAg-negative HBsAg carriers.[248] The presence of viremia in these HBsAg-negative subjects has clinical implications with regard to potential infectivity. As an example, it has been shown that the serum of HBsAg-negative but HBV DNA–positive patients can transmit infection to chimpanzees,[249] and anti-HBc testing of blood donors prevents some cases of post-transfusion hepatitis B.[250] Also, the risk of transmission of HBV infection from an anti-HBc–positive liver donor has been observed to be as high as 50 percent to 70 percent in some series, and lower rates of infection also have been observed in other forms of solid organ transplantation.[251,252] Low-level viral replication also has implications with regard to the possibility of underlying liver disease. HBV DNA in serum and liver tissue has been confirmed by PCR in HBsAg-negative patients with cirrhosis and hepatocellular carcinoma,[253,254] and PCR has confirmed an association in some cases of fulminant non-A to non-C hepatitis.[255]

HBeAg is a soluble viral protein that is found in serum early during acute infection. HBeAg positivity 3 or more months after the onset of illness indicates a high likelihood of transition to chronic infection.[113,256,257] The finding of HBeAg in the serum of an HBsAg carrier indicates a high level of viral replication and greater infectivity.[5,7,16] Most HBeAg-positive patients also have active liver disease, the exception being HBeAg-positive children and young adults with perinatally acquired HBV infection, who usually have normal ALT levels and minimal inflammation in the liver.[258] In general, seroconversion from HBeAg to anti-HBe is associated with the disappearance of HBV DNA in serum and remission of liver disease.[45,259] Some patients, however, continue to have active liver disease and detectable HBV DNA in serum resulting from either low levels of wild-type virus or the presence of precore mutation that impairs e antigen secretion.[260-262]

HBV DNA can be measured in serum using qualitative or quantitative assays. The clinical evaluation of serum HBV DNA has been hampered by the absence of a licensed test in the United States and an accepted international reference standard. Three types of commercially available assays are available: a branched nucleotide assay or signal amplification method (Quantiplex HBV, Bayer Diagnostics), a hybridization format in which a labeled probe is allowed to hybridize to HBV DNA either on a solid phase (Hybrid Capture II, Digene) or in a gel solution medium (Genostics, Abbott Laboratories), and a target amplification or quantitative PCR assay (Amplicor HBV Monitor, Roche Diagnostics). The signal amplification method quantitates virus titers from 7×10^5 to 5×10^9 DNA equivalents per ml. Results of the solid-phase hybridization assay are quantitative in the range of 1.4×10^5 to 5.6×10^9 copies per ml (0.5-20,000 pg/ml). The lower detection limit of the solution hybridization assay is 1 to 2 pg/ml (approximately 6×10^5 copies/ml) and the upper limit of the dynamic range has not been defined. The commercially licensed PCR assay quantitates virus titers from 4×10^2 to 4×10^7 copies per ml. Although less sensitive than PCR, the results of the non–PCR-based assays tend to correlate with a clinical response to anti-viral therapy.[186] Unfortunately, the number of viral genomes measured by the non–PCR-based assays is not strictly comparable, which limits the clinical interpretation of changes in viral load by more than one assay.[263] In addition to these considerations, there may be considerable differences in sensitivity of the various assays across all genotypes.[264]

The sensitivity of the non-PCR–based assays varies according to whether the patient is HBeAg-positive. The signal amplification method detects HBV DNA in serum in 73 percent to 100 percent of HBeAg-positive specimens and in 25 percent to 31 percent of HBeAg-negative specimens.[265] The solution hybridization assay is slightly less sensitive, but for all intents and purposes can be used interchangeably in clinical practice. The detection limits of both assays, however, are 10,000-fold to 100,000-fold less than PCR.[266] In most clinical circumstances, the increased sensitivity of PCR-based assays offers no real advantage over the less-sensitive hybridization assays (Table 32-4). The quantitative PCR assay may provide better discrimination of the risk for recurrent HBV infection after liver transplantation.

The development of PCR methods of detecting HBV DNA has altered traditional concepts of clearance of HBV DNA in acute and chronic infection. For example, recovery from acute hepatitis B is marked by the disappearance of HBV DNA from serum as measured by hybridization assay. PCR, on the other hand, can detect HBV DNA in serum and peripheral mononuclear cells years after recovery from acute viral hepatitis.[118,119] Similarly, the disappearance of HBeAg in chronically infected patients is generally associated with the absence of HBV DNA in serum by hybridization but not PCR assays. Using PCR, the disappearance of HBsAg is followed by the loss of HBV DNA from serum in chronic hepatitis B.[19] Even then, HBV DNA persists in small amounts in liver tissue and peripheral mononuclear cells years after subsidence of infection.[19,267]

Quantitation of serum HBV DNA is clinically useful in several situations (see Table 32-4). Most of the clinical

TABLE 32-4
Clinical Utility of HBV DNA Serum Testing

	PREFERRED METHOD*			
Clinical situation	**Qualitative**	**Quantitative**	**Non-PCR**	**PCR**
Candidacy for anti-viral treatment		+	+	
Response to anti-viral treatment		+	+	
Determining the etiology of biochemical flares		+	+	
Detection of phenotypic resistance to lamivudine and other nucleosides		+	+	
Detection of genotypic resistance to lamivudine and other nucleosides				+†
Identification of precore mutant‡		+	+	
Detection of relative risk for recurrent infection post-transplantation		+	+	
Cryptic HBV infection	+			+
Determining infectivity of anti-HBc-positive donor§	+			+

HBV, Hepatitis B virus; *DNA,* deoxyribonucleic acid; *PCR,* polymerase chain reaction; *anti-HBc,* antibody to HBcAg.
*Based upon general usage patterns in published literature.
†Non-PCR detection followed in turn by PCR and molecular analysis of sequence.
‡Hepatitis B e antigen–negative chronic hepatitis B patient with positive HBV DNA may have core promoter mutant or precore mutant requiring PCR and molecular analysis for further clarification.
§As applicable to organ transplantation.

treatment trials have used non-PCR methods of detection, but this is apt to change in the future because of the commercial availability of PCR methods of detection. Measurement of the level of HBV DNA in serum is an important determinant of the likelihood of response to antiviral therapy in patients with chronic HBV infection. High pretreatment serum HBV DNA correlates with a low probability of response to IFN therapy[186,268] but seems to be less important in predicting response to nucleoside agents such as lamivudine.[269,270] In one study patients with a baseline serum HBV DNA level in excess of 200 pg/ml by the solution hybridization assay uniformly failed to respond to 16 weeks of IFN alfa-2b in comparison to a 33 percent response for those with levels between 100 and 200 pg/ml.[186] Reappearance of HBV DNA in serum by non-PCR assays during lamivudine treatment suggests that genotypic resistance to this drug has occurred[70]; multi-variate analysis has confirmed that high pretreatment serum HBV DNA levels are associated with a significantly greater likelihood that lamivudine resistance will develop.[70,84] High levels of serum HBV DNA (in excess of 10 million copies) by quantitative PCR have also been shown to correlate with a higher rate of recurrent infection in liver transplant recipients who are treated with lamivudine.[271] Furthermore, serial measurement of HBV DNA level can be helpful in determining whether spontaneous or treatment-induced flares will result in a virologic remission[157] or whether anti-viral treatment is indicated.

Qualitative testing for HBV DNA can be clinically useful in several situations also. Detection of HBV DNA in serum by hybridization assay before liver transplantation identifies patients with a higher rate of recurrence.[271] PCR detection of serum HBV DNA may allow identification of HBV as the cause of liver disease in HBsAg-negative patients.[272] This may be a particularly important consideration in patients with fulminant hepatitis B who frequently have cleared HBsAg by the time they obtain medical attention.[122]

Anti-viral Therapy of Chronic HBV Infection

The major goal of anti-viral therapy is to permanently limit viral replication and thereby obtain a remission of the liver disease and prevent the long-term complications of this disorder. Major advances in the treatment of chronic hepatitis B have been made in the last several years. Two licensed approaches are available—IFN alfa and lamivudine, a nucleoside analog. IFN alfa and lamivudine have comparable rates of virologic and clinical response, and the ease of administration and absence of adverse effects of the latter have stimulated the development of a number of newer analogs. Because IFN and nucleoside analogs have different mechanisms of action, the potential exists for additive or synergistic effects when used in combination. Studies employing a combination of IFN and nucleoside analog therapy and multiple nucleoside analogs used together are currently under way. Table 32-5 lists the suggested approaches to the management of chronic hepatitis B.

Interferon

IFN was licensed for hepatitis B in 1992 after it was proven to be effective in promoting HBeAg loss, seroconversion to anti-HBe, HBsAg seroconversion, and diminishing histologic activity. A virologic response, defined as the sustained disappearance of HBeAg and loss

TABLE 32-5
Suggested Treatment Regimens for Chronic Hepatitis B

Type patient	Treatment	Dose	Duration	Comments
HBeAg/HBV DNA-positive and clinically stable				
Normal ALT	None, observation	—	—	Treatment only in investigational protocol
ALT > 1 but < 2.5 × ULN	Interferon, consider pretreatment with corticosteroids*	5 MU daily or 10 MU TIW	4-6 months	Low response rate
ALT 2.5-10 × ULN	Interferon	5 MU daily or 10 MU TIW	4-6 months†	Virologic, biochemical, and histologic response: 30%-35% of cases
	Lamivudine	100 mg	52 weeks‡	20%-30% of cases
ALT > 10 × ULN	Observation for 1-2 months§, if persistently high, interferon or lamivudine	Same as above	Same as above	May undergo spontaneous seroconversion
HBeAg-positive or HBeAg-negative/ HBV DNA-positive, decompensated cirrhosis	Lamivudine	100 mg	52 weeks or longer‖	Consider liver transplantation
	Interferon¶	1-2 MU on alternate days	4-6 months or longer	
HBeAg-negative, DNA-positive, clinically stable	Interferon	6 MU/m² TIW	12-18 months	High rate of relapse
	Lamivudine	100 mg daily	12-18 months or longer	

HBeAg, Hepatitis B e antigen; *HBV,* hepatitis B virus; *DNA,* deoxyribonucleic acid; *ALT,* alanine aminotransferase; *ULN,* upper limit of normal; *MU,* million units; *TIW,* three times a week.
*Patients should lack evidence for cirrhosis on liver biopsy. Prednisone or prednisolone is usually given in tapered fashion over 4-6 weeks.
†Patients who are HBV DNA-negative by non-PCR-based assay may benefit from an additional 4-6 months of interferon.
‡Patients who remain HBeAg-positive but HBV DNA-negative by non-PCR-based assay may benefit from additional treatment based upon severity of liver disease.
§High rate of spontaneous seroconversion to anti-HBe is to be anticipated. Decision when to treat should also be based upon persistent laboratory or clinical abnormalities.
‖Lamivudine is safer than interferon but early use may encourage development of drug resistance before transplantation is possible.
¶Should only be given to patients with very mild decompensation (Child's A status). Inordinate risk of complications has been observed in more advanced disease.

of serum HBV DNA by non-PCR-based assays, occurs in 35 percent to 40 percent of treated patients, and a complete virologic response, defined as clearance of HBsAg, occurs in 8 percent to 10 percent.[186,273] Because persistence of HBV infection is dependent on virus-host interactions and IFN affects cell-mediated immunity to HBV, the immunomodulatory effects of this agent appear to be key in achieving a lasting response to therapy. Its major disadvantages continue to be the unpleasant adverse effects associated with its administration and its high cost.

Mechanisms of Action. IFNs are proteins produced by host nucleated cells in response to viral infection. Three different types of are identified. Alpha-IFN is produced by B-lymphocytes and monocytes, beta-IFN by fibroblasts, and gamma-IFN by helper T and natural killer cells.[274,275] IFN has both anti-viral and immunomodulatory effects. The anti-viral effect is due in part to viral mRNA degradation mediated through the release of proteins (such as 2′,5′-oligoadenylate synthetase), which can activate ribonucleases.[274] IFN also leads to the production of a protein kinase that activates eukaryotic initiation factor (E,F)-2 and inhibits peptide chain initiation.[276,277] It also inhibits viral entry, uncoating, and mRNA translation and assembly.[278]

The immunomodulatory effects of IFNs are mediated in part by an increase in the expression of HLA class I antigen on the surface of hepatocytes. These membrane-associated proteins are important in the appropriate presentation of virally encoded peptides to sensitized CTL.[279] Moreover, IFNs increase FC receptor expression, CD4/CD8 ratio, and non-specific (natural killer cell) pathways.[274,280,281] Unlike IFN-α and IFN-β, IFN-γ has a predominant immunomodulatory effect. Gamma IFN enhances HLA class II expression and cytocidal activity of macrophages and B and T cells.[282,283]

Currently, IFN-α is the only approved type used in treating chronic hepatitis B. Virtually all patients treated with IFN-α show an initial decrease in HBV replication, presumably as a result of a direct anti-viral effect. The immunomodulatory effect of exogenous IFN therapy appears to be maximal at the time of HBeAg seroconversion.[281]

Approximately 60 percent to 70 percent of IFN responders exhibit a sudden increase in serum aminotransferase levels during the second or third month of therapy, which is thought to reflect the immune-stimulating properties of this agent (see Figure 32-5). In addition to these effects IFN alfa-n1 (lymphoblastoid) therapy has been shown to have an anti-fibrogenic effect. Lymphoblastoid IFN results in a decrease in serum procollagen type III peptide and hepatic transforming growth factor–beta-1 mRNA expression.[284] The former is a marker for hepatic fibrosis and the latter is thought to play a critical role in the production of extracellular matrix proteins such as collagen.[285]

Patient Selection and Indications. Candidates for IFN therapy should have evidence of ongoing viral replication (presence of serum HBeAg or HBV DNA), persistently elevated serum aminotransferase activity, and evidence of chronic hepatitis B on liver biopsy. Before initiating IFN, it may be beneficial to monitor HBV DNA and serum aminotransferase levels in clinically stable patients for several months when clear-cut documentation of the duration of elevated liver chemistries is not known. This enables the identification of individuals who have frequent fluctuations in disease intensity or those who may be entering into a period of spontaneous seroconversion of HBeAg to anti-HBe. Spontaneous seroconversion occurs in about 5 percent to 10 percent of patients annually, and this may be precipitated by sudden flares in serum aminotransferase levels.[157,186,286,287]

IFN is generally contraindicated in patients with decompensated cirrhosis for several reasons. Patients with ascites, a history of variceal bleeding, encephalopathy, or marginal synthetic function are at increased risk of further decompensation or serious infections with therapy.[46,187] Furthermore, there is no evidence to suggest that IFN protects against the risk of hepatocellular carcinoma in hepatitis B–associated cirrhosis.[288,289] Instead, patients with advanced liver disease are often better treated by transplantation. IFN is also contraindicated in patients with severe neuropsychiatric illness, and caution must be taken in treating patients with autoimmune diseases that can be exacerbated by IFN therapy.[290] Appropriate patient selection is critical to maximizing the risk-benefit ratio of treatment.

Predictors of Response. The clinical variables that have been shown to be consistently associated with a favorable response to therapy include high pretherapy serum aminotransferases (more than 3 to 4 times the upper limit of normal), low HBV DNA (less than 200 pg/ml by solution hybridization), and active disease on liver biopsy.[186,291,292] Each of these features has been interpreted as reflecting a greater immunologic response to HBV. In a large US multi-center IFN trial, low baseline HBV DNA by solution hybridization was found to be the most reliable independent predictor of response.[186] Other variables that are less useful but are also associated with a higher rate of response include female sex, acquisition of infection in adulthood, heterosexuality, HIV antibody negativity, history of acute hepatitis, and short duration of infection.[283,291-295]

The relative predictive value of these features with regard to IFN therapy has been questioned. The inherent value of a variety of patient and viral features was analyzed in a meta-analysis of 10 controlled trials including more than 750 patients.[296] When HIV-positive status was excluded, the overall HBeAg disappearance rate was higher in patients with high transaminases and a history of acute hepatitis irrespective of whether or not patients had received IFN therapy.

It is still unclear why most patients do not respond to IFN therapy. In some instances resistance to IFN is probably the result of an inability to stimulate cellular immune responses to HBV appropriately, whereas in other instances it may be due to natural selection of viral mutants that confer resistance to IFN. It is known that the translational products of the HBV precore and core regions represent the major target for the host immune response, and several mutations in the precore region of HBV have been discovered. The most common precore mutant is characterized by anti-HBe positivity and evidence of active HBV replication (see Mutation of the HBV Genome). These precore mutants tend to have a low rate of sustained response to IFN. The relationship between specific precore sequences and response to IFN remains unclear, however, because it has been demonstrated that the A1896 precore mutation may be seen in patients with a high rather than a low rate of response.[297]

It has been hypothesized that variability in the core gene may also result in an unfavorable response to therapy. This is based upon the observation that substitutions in the amino acids 21 through 27 of the core protein, known to affect CTL function, occur in patients with more advanced chronic hepatitis B and seem to be detected more frequently in IFN non-responders.[79] Also, anti-HBe–positive patients with active disease have more variability in the core gene.[80] Despite these apparent associations, there are no specific recommendations on viral genomic heterogeneity and patient selection for IFN treatment.

Various virologic and immunologic parameters have been evaluated to determine the likelihood of response to IFN. Significantly lower HBeAg levels have been noted in IFN responders.[298] Also, elevated IgM anti-HBc levels have been associated with a sustained response to therapy.[281] Although a significant rise in CD4/CD8 ratio and a fall in peripheral CD8 count and natural killer cell activity have been observed in IFN responders, no correlation has been established between a response to IFN and pretreatment CD4/CD8 ratio, NK activity, or lymphocyte proliferative response.[281] Whereas therapy with IFN may induce neutralizing antibody to IFN, the presence of this antibody does not appear to preclude a response.[186] High rates of IFN antibody (39 percent) have been reported in Chinese adults who were treated with IFN alfa-2b; however, the role that the antibody plays in the low rates of response to IFN remains a matter of controversy.[299]

It is important to realize that the "predictive" variables for response have been established from a retrospective analysis of treated patients. Knowledge of these parameters enables the clinician to have a more realistic expectation of response to anti-viral therapy, but the presence of one or more features correlating with a lower likelihood of response should not deter consideration for treatment in an otherwise acceptable patient.

Anti-viral Efficacy. The major goal of therapy is the permanent suppression of viral replication or elimination of infection. Clinical trials of IFN have shown that biochemical, clinical, and histologic remission occurs whenever there is a sustained disappearance of markers of viral replication (HBV DNA and HBeAg).

In most studies a response to IFN has been defined as a sustained loss of HBeAg and HBV DNA with normalization or near normalization of ALT for at least 6 months after therapy. This has been observed in 25 percent to 40 percent of patients.[273] After therapy, aminotransferase normalization occurs in approximately 80 to 90 percent of patients who demonstrate a sustained loss of HBV DNA.[202] HBsAg seroconversion, implying a termination of the HBV carrier state, occurs in approximately one third of patients who lose HBeAg.[186] In a meta-analysis of 15 randomized controlled trials that included more than 800 patients, IFN increased the sustained loss of HBeAg by 20 percent when compared to untreated controls.[273] Also the rate of HBsAg loss was found to be 6 percent higher in the IFN-treated patients when compared to untreated controls. Another meta-analysis of 22 published randomized controlled trials encompassing more than 1200 patients demonstrated that IFN increased the rates of serum HBV DNA clearance and aminotransferase normalization by threefold at 1 year after therapy.[300]

Long-term Response. Virologic response has been generally maintained during post-treatment intervals of 3 to 11 years.[301-304] Responders to IFN demonstrate biochemical, histologic, and symptomatic improvement.[305] The disease can reactivate but the rate of reactivated hepatitis B after IFN treatment is similar to that occurring in patients who spontaneously seroconvert from HBeAg to anti-HBe.[301,302,306] Reactivation usually occurs within 1 year of completion of therapy but it may on rare occasion be delayed for several years after therapy.[304]

The loss of HBsAg after a sustained response to IFN occurs sooner and at a higher rate when compared to spontaneous seroconversion.[302] HBsAg loss occurs in 10 percent to 12 percent of patients during treatment or in the first 3 months after therapy.[186] After HBsAg loss 75 percent to 90 percent of cases have detectable anti-HBs, although frequently it is found in low titers.[307] With long-term follow-up, the delayed clearance of HBsAg has been reported in a high proportion (more than 70 percent) of IFN responders.[308] In approximately 80 percent of patients who become HBsAg-negative, serum HBV DNA is no longer detectable by PCR.[19,302,305] Low levels of HBV DNA, however, often remain detectable by PCR in the liver tissue for several years after spontaneous or treatment-induced HBsAg seroconversion.[19] There is evidence that in some cases, ongoing low-level viral replication may be detectable in serum despite the loss of HBsAg but the clinical significance of this is uncertain.[19] The clearance of HBsAg with IFN results in marked improvement (but not necessarily total disappearance) of necroinflammatory changes within the liver tissue even after intervals as long as 9 years after therapy.[267,309] This long-term histologic improvement is even greater than that observed in biopsy material taken within 1 year of completion of therapy.[267,309]

To examine the long-term clinical benefit of IFN treatment, several studies have compared cohorts of responders with untreated controls. After a mean follow-up of 50 months, it was noted that the frequency of death, liver transplantation, and severe clinical complications resulting from cirrhosis was lower in patients who lost HBeAg.[44] Also the overall length of survival without clinical complications was longer in this group of patients, and the clearance of HBeAg was found to be the strongest predictor of survival. However, this degree of benefit may not be evident in all responders. In one study a higher survival and lower risk for complications of liver disease were only observed in responders with compensated cirrhosis.[303] Some of the discrepancies reported in the literature may be due to differences in patient selection; long-term follow-up studies with appropriate controls will be necessary to demonstrate differences in survival in patients with mild or moderate disease.

Combined Therapy with Corticosteroids. Because a short course of corticosteroids tends to result in acute elevation of serum aminotransferase levels with a transient decline of viral replication markers, it has been used in combination with IFN to increase response rates.[196,292] The immunologic events after the withdrawal of corticosteroids have not been extensively studied; therefore, the mechanisms involved are poorly understood. It has been hypothesized that corticosteroids enhance the membrane expression of hepatitis B core peptides, which can serve as a target for cytotoxic T-cell responses.[305,310] In vitro studies have demonstrated a glucocorticoid-responsive element in the HBV genome, which enhances viral replication independent of immune response against the virus.[311] It has also been observed that the serum concentration of macrophage colony-stimulating factor (M-CSF) is significantly increased after prednisolone withdrawal; this increase is similar to that observed during an acute exacerbation of chronic hepatitis B.[312] This could be important because increased serum M-CSF is closely associated with increased serum IFN or proinflammatory cytokine production by peripheral blood cells, and a peak in M-CSF has been found to precede seroconversion to anti-HBe.[312] Taken together, the clinical and immunologic observations provide a rationale for the use of IFN in combination with corticosteroids.

In a large randomized, controlled multi-center US trial nearly identical rates of HBeAg loss and disappearance of HBsAg were observed when IFN was given alone in a dose of 5 million units daily for 16 weeks versus an identical regimen preceded by a 6-week course of prednisone.[186] However, patients with low pretherapy ALT (less than 100 IU/L) tended to respond more frequently to combination therapy (44 percent versus 17 percent). Similar results were observed in a European multi-center study that employed the same entry criteria and treatment groups.[313] A meta-analysis evaluated seven randomized trials involving more than 350 patients in which a combination of prednisone and IFN was compared to IFN alone.[314] The addition of prednisone did not increase the overall rate of loss of HBeAg, HBV DNA, or HBsAg. In the three trials that allowed comparison of the two treatments after stratification for ALT level, however, a significant benefit was seen when patients with low pretherapy ALT (defined as either less than 100 or 200 IU/L) were pretreated with prednisone.

Krogsgaard and colleagues subsequently compared a combination of a 4-week course of prednisolone or matching placebo followed by 12 weeks of lymphoblastoid IFN in a randomized multi-center, controlled study of 200 patients.[198] The results of the clinical trial revealed a significantly higher rate of HBeAg disappearance and anti-HBe seroconversion with the prednisolone and IFN combination. HBeAg disappearance rates at the end of treatment were 17 percent and 5 percent, respectively, for the combination therapy and IFN-alone groups and 42 percent and 26 percent, respectively, at 1-year post-treatment. In contrast to previous studies, a priming course of corticosteroid was effective in all patient groups irrespective of the level of serum aminotransferases at baseline.

It is important to recognize that corticosteroid withdrawal should not be used in patients with marginal synthetic liver function or overt hepatic decompensation. In such cases the lobular inflammatory response superimposed on the chronic liver disease may result in further decompensation.[315]

Adverse Effects. Treatment with IFN is frequently associated with adverse events. Dose reduction is required in at least 20 percent of patients who are treated with the recommended regimen of 5 million units daily or 10 million units three times weekly. Discontinuation of treatment, however, is necessary in less than 5 percent of clinically stable patients.[186,316-321] Most patients experience an influenza-like illness with fever, chills, myalgia, and headaches 6 to 8 hours after the first injection. These symptoms tend to improve or disappear with subsequent injections. Patients often benefit by premedication with acetaminophen or a low dose of non-steroidal anti-inflammatory medications. With prolonged therapy the most frequent adverse events are fatigue and myalgias. Psychiatric side effects, especially depression, occur in about 15 percent of patients and tend to occur more commonly in patients receiving the 10 million-unit dose.[317] Mild-to-moderate depression can be treated with anti-depressants and psychiatric counseling. Frank delirium and suicidal ideation have rarely been reported and are more likely to occur in patients with preexisting organic brain injury or dysfunction.[317]

At doses used to treat chronic hepatitis B, IFN results in a 30 percent to 50 percent decrease in platelet count, a 20 percent to 40 percent reduction in total white blood cell count, and a slight fall (3 percent-5 percent) in hematocrit levels.[186,283,318] These changes are usually clinically insignificant and often return to normal after discontinuation of treatment. Profound thrombocytopenia (less than 25,000 per mm^3) or granulocytopenia (less than 500 per mm^3), serious mood or behavior changes, frequent nausea and vomiting, diarrhea (more than eight stools per day), or debilitating fatigue should be cause for discontinuation of therapy.[283,305] If adverse events are less severe and tolerable, consideration should be given to adjusting the dose of IFN by 50 percent, with readjustment to previous levels when side effects subside.

IFN can induce an autoimmune diathesis and has been associated with clinically significant worsening or unmasking of autoimmune conditions.[319,320] More than 50 percent of patients treated for 4 months develop autoantibodies, such as anti-nuclear, anti-smooth muscle, anti-thyroid, and insulin antibodies.[305,321,322] Although hypothyroidism and, less commonly, hyperthyroidism, have been reported with IFN therapy, clinically evident thyroid dysfunction is relatively uncommon and autoimmune thyroiditis has occurred in 2 percent to 5 percent of cases.[316,322] In a few cases treatment has been reported to result in autoimmune hepatitis,[319,323] hemolytic anemia, autoimmune thrombocytopenia, systemic polyarthropathy,[290,320] lupus erythematosus-like syndromes,[320] and type I diabetes.[324] Moreover, there are reports of worsening psoriasis and rheumatoid arthritis during therapy. Thus caution should then be taken when treating patients with preexisting autoimmune conditions.

Treatment of Special Populations

HBeAg-negative Chronic Hepatitis B. Patients with a precore glycine (G) to arginine (A) mutation at position 1896 of the HBV genome have been treated with IFN. Serum HBV DNA levels are frequently below the level of detectability by molecular hybridization techniques and are only detected by PCR, yet these patients have been difficult to manage. Early treatment trials of HBeAg-negative patients with active disease indicated that loss of serum HBV DNA and normalization of ALT were observed in as many as 75 percent of patients treated with IFN-α compared to 10 percent of untreated controls.[325,326] A significant proportion of patients, however, relapsed after therapy, with an overall sustained response rate of 20 percent at 5 years of follow-up.[326,327] Sustained response rates as low as 9.4 percent have also been reported after 7 years of follow-up.[328] As with wild-type HBV, the majority of relapses have occurred during the first year after therapy. In one study there was no significant difference between varying doses of IFN-α, but prolonged therapy to 12 months was more effective in preventing relapse.[329] The overall HBsAg clearance rate in responders has been calculated to be 12 percent at 4 years.[326] However, higher rates of HBsAg clearance (16 percent at 1 year and 44 percent at 3 years of follow-up) have also been reported.[328,329] Significant improvement in hepatic inflammation has been reported in 40 percent to 50 percent of patients after IFN therapy.[330-332]

The response rate to IFN in HBeAg-negative patients has been shown to be independent of initial serum HBV DNA level and IFN dose.[333] It has been suggested, however, that a high proportion of precore mutant HBV (more than 20 percent of circulating virus) at baseline may result in a lower rate of response.[328] Recently, longer duration of IFN treatment and re-treatment was found to be more effective in inducing sustained biochemical responses in approximately 20 percent of patients.[333]

Decompensated Cirrhosis. Serum HBV DNA levels are frequently low in patients with decompensated cirrhosis. These patients with decompensated cirrhosis resulting from chronic HBV infection have been shown to benefit from IFN therapy both clinically and histologically.[46,187,334] Nonetheless, IFN is generally not recommended because of a higher risk for serious side effects such as spontaneous bacterial peritonitis and flares of hepatitis.[46,187,335] A study conducted at the National Institutes of Health reported beneficial responses including normalization of synthetic liver function followed by sustained disappearance of HBV DNA in 33 percent of subjects.[187] In this study patients with higher pretherapy transaminases, lower prothrombin times, Child's score A and B, and no encephalopathy tended to respond better. Fifty percent of patients, however, had one or more serious adverse effects, such as bacterial infections (peritonitis, pneumonia), an acute flare of hepatitis, or acute psychiatric syndromes that required discontinuation of therapy. Other investigators have analyzed the safety and potential efficacy of a 6-month course of low-dose, titrable IFN alfa-2b in 26 patients with decompensated cirrhosis. In that study therapy was commenced with a dose of 5×10^5 units on alternate days and upward adjustments were made every 2 weeks according to tolerability. The rate of hepatitis flares was substantially lower than that reported in other studies but serious bacterial infections still occurred in 12 percent of Child's class B and C patients.[46] A sustained loss of HBV DNA by direct hybridization was associated with improved survival. Taken together, these studies indicate that patients with Child's A cirrhosis can be treated with low doses of IFN. In Child's B and C patients, the risk-benefit ratio is such that other forms of treatment such as lamivudine should be considered to stabilize the patient clinically (see Nucleoside Analogs). Liver transplantation is often a more appropriate therapeutic option in these patients.

Co-infection with HIV. Patients with advanced HIV co-infection may have a poor response to IFN because they often have high levels of HBV DNA, relatively low serum alanine aminotransferase levels, and depressed immune function.[232,273] Also, in the past death was more likely to occur in these patients as a result of complications of acquired immunodeficiency syndrome rather than chronic hepatitis B. Accordingly, there has been a reluctance to treat patients who are co-infected with HBV and HIV. Improved survival in HIV-infected patients, however, has led to increased interest in treatment of the underlying hepatitis B. Additional support for treatment can be seen from reports of lethal liver failure from hepatitis B in HIV-co-infected patients before the appearance of any complication of HIV infection[336] and the theoretic possibility that chronic HBV infection may accelerate the course of HIV infection.[337] Responses to IFN have been described in early HIV infection.[292,338] A lack of correlation between the response to treatment and the pretreatment CD4 cell count and p24 antigenemia has been described.[338] There are very few data with regard to long-term follow-up of treated patients with HIV and HBV co-infection.[339] Many HIV-infected patients are currently treated with lamivudine (see Nucleoside Analogs); this has made IFN therapy less important as a therapeutic option.

Co-infection with Hepatitis C. The data with regard to IFN treatment of combined chronic hepatitis B and C infection are also limited. Co-infection with HBV and HCV has been associated with more severe histologic injury and a relatively low response to therapy.[340,341] In one study a loss of HBV DNA and HBeAg occurred in only 1 of 15 patients (6.7 percent) with dual HBV and HCV infection, whereas a similar type of response was observed in 46 (28 percent) of 164 HCV-negative patients.[340] The converse also seems to be true in that a lower response to IFN treatment of chronic hepatitis C has been documented when HCV infection occurs in association with inapparent HBV infection (HBV DNA–positive by PCR only).[342,343] Further studies are needed in patients with hepatitis B and C co-infection to validate these observations.

Non-responders to IFN. The majority (60 to 70 percent) of patients with chronic hepatitis B do not respond to a 4- to 6-month course of IFN. The largest group of non-responders has normal or low-level serum alanine aminotransferase levels (more than twofold the upper limit of normal). These patients may benefit from a preceding short course of corticosteroids provided that cirrhosis is absent.[186,292,313,314] Other approaches to immune augmentation, however, are needed in this large subgroup of patients. IFN is ineffective in patients with normal serum aminotransferases because these patients are immunologically tolerant.

Extension of IFN treatment beyond 16 weeks may be helpful in some patients who remain HBeAg-positive but HBV DNA–negative in serum by direct hybridization assay.[344] Studies are needed to evaluate the effects of higher doses and longer durations of therapy. A recent study did not reveal any additional therapeutic benefit for a combination anti-viral protocol in which a 16-week course of IFN-α was preceded by an 8-week course of lamivudine, a potent nucleoside analog that inhibits HBV replication.[345] It is theoretically possible, however, that nucleoside analog therapy may abrogate the immunologic activating properties of IFN when initiated at the same time or when given before IFN, as has been done in the available studies. If this is the case, initiating IFN a few months before nucleoside analog therapy may ultimately prove to be a more effective approach.[345a]

Polyarteritis Nodosa. Conventional treatment of polyarteritis nodosa with immunosuppressive agents and corticosteroids can have a deleterious effect on the underlying liver disease because it enhances HBV replication.[311] Also, liver disease may be exacerbated upon withdrawal of corticosteroids and other immunosuppressive medications.[169,315] Treatment of polyarteritis nodosa with plasma exchange in combination with IFN-α has met with variable success.[135] The development of nucleoside analogs that have potent effects on HBV replication may in the future relegate the use of IFN to being more of historic importance in the treatment of polyarteritis related to HBV infection.

Glomerulonephritis. Many adult patients with HBV-associated glomerulonephritis ultimately develop end-stage renal failure. Treatment with corticosteroids and immunosuppressants has been disappointing for this disorder because of only transient or incomplete remissions. One report suggests that therapy may actually worsen morbidity and mortality.[346] IFN-induced reduction in viral replication has been associated with improvement of renal and hepatic disease.[347-349] In one series 8 of 15 patients (53 percent) had a lasting (1-7 year) virologic response, with marked improvement in renal function and diminution of proteinuria in 7 of the 8 patients.[347] A study in Asian patients with membranous nephropathy had a disappointing response to IFN-α with only 1 of 5 HBeAg-positive patients securing a complete remission with seroconversion to anti-HBe.[146] The poor response to IFN therapy may reflect the recognized limited response to this therapy by adult Asians with chronic hepatitis B.[350] It is not clear whether eradication of the HBV virus is needed to induce a remission of HBV-associated membranous glomerulonephritis.[143] Response to IFN appears to be more efficacious in patients with membranous glomerulonephritis than in those with membranoproliferative glomerulonephritis.[347,351] There is no indication that treatment of patients who lack evidence for viral replication offers any benefit.

Essential Mixed Cryoglobulinemia. Data on the treatment of HBV-associated essential mixed cryoglobulinemia are very limited. Several case reports have documented a response to IFN.[352,353] In one patient vasculitis-induced purpura was successfully treated with IFN-α.[352] In a second report a decrease in circulating immune complexes and cryoglobulins with a complete remission of vasculitis was sustained at 3 to 4.5 years post-treatment.[353] Similar to polyarteritis nodosa, IFN seems preferable to immunosuppressive therapy. More experience is necessary, however, before the role of anti-viral therapy for the mixed cryoglobulinemic syndromes associated with chronic HBV infection can be accepted.

Arthritis. There are very limited data with respect to the management of joint manifestations of chronic HBV infection with IFN. A case has been described in which a patient with chronic hepatitis B had HBV DNA in serum and synovial fluid in association with migratory polyarthralgia and synovial effusion. The patient was treated with a 14-week course of lymphoblastoid IFN, which resulted in clearance of HBeAg and HBsAg and resolution of the arthritic complaints.[354] In a second case a rheumatoid factor–positive mono-arthritis appeared after the treatment of chronic hepatitis B with a 3-month course of IFN.[355]

Nucleoside Analogs

A number of nucleoside analog derivatives are either commercially available or under study to treat chronic hepatitis B (Table 32-6). Many of the nucleoside analogs were found to be inhibitory to HBV replication when used against HIV. After intracellular phosphorylation, these agents inhibit HBV DNA polymerase and act as obligatory chain terminators.[355a] The nucleoside analogs may directly inhibit either first- or second-strand HBV DNA synthesis, or both, and some (e.g., penciclovir) also inhibit the priming step for reverse transcription. The drugs have high bioavailability when given orally and 1 month of treatment results in a $\log_2$ to $\log_4$ reduction in serum HBV DNA.

The first generation nucleoside analogs were first tested more than two decades ago.[356,357] The use of adenine arabinoside and its aqueous soluble salt, adenine arabinoside monophosphate, resulted in a marked decline in serum HBV DNA but could not be used long enough to induce a clinically significant rate of HBeAg seroconversion because of neuromuscular toxicity. Moreover, they had to be administered parenterally. Fialuridine, a fluoro-iodo-arabinofuranosyl-uracil nucleoside, was subsequently shown to markedly suppress HBV DNA,[358,359] but this agent caused severe multi-organ failure resulting from inhibition of mitochondrial function in patients treated for more than 2 months.[360] This resulted in more intensive preclinical investigation of the second-generation nucleoside analogs famciclovir and lamivudine that have proven to be extremely safe in large clinical trials.

TABLE 32-6
Nucleoside Analogs to Treat Chronic Hepatitis B

Agent	Resistance demonstrated*	Activity against YMDD mutant
Lamivudine	Yes	None
Famciclovir	Yes	None
Adefovir dipivoxil†	No	Yes, in vivo and in vitro
Entecavir†	No	Yes in vivo and in vitro,
Emtricitabine (FTC)†‡	Likely	Not likely
DAPD†	Not known	Not known
Clevudine (FMAU)†	Not known	Not known
LdT†	Not known	Not known

YMDD, Tyrosine-methionine-aspartate-aspartate; *DAPD,* I-B-D-2,6-diaminopurine dioxolane; *LdT,* B-L-2′-deoxythymidine.
*When used as monotherapy.
†Currently investigational only.
‡Structurally similar to lamivudine.

Nucleoside analogs offer a number of advantages to IFN-α and some disadvantages as well (Table 32-7). In contrast to IFN, the nucleoside analogs have not been shown to have direct immunoregulatory activity, although a number of in vitro studies have suggested that lamivudine is capable of restoring both CD4 and CD8 cellular-mediated immune responses to HBV.[101,106] Although the rate of HBeAg loss and sustained disappearance of serum HBV DNA occur with comparable frequency to that observed with IFN, the rate of HBsAg seroconversion is lower with nucleoside analogs. This can be explained by the relative resistance of the covalently closed, circular, HBV DNA to the effects of nucleoside derivatives and the possibility that IFN-induced hepatocytolysis more effectively eliminates this genomic template.[361,361a]

Nucleoside analogs have activity against other viruses, such as herpes and varicella, which make them particularly suitable in co-infected immunosuppressed patients. Lamivudine and famciclovir are commercially available for the treatment of hepatitis B. Only lamivudine, however, has been specifically licensed for this purpose. A number of third-generation nucleoside analogs (e.g., entecavir, adefovir, emtricitabine, clevudine) are under development. Entecavir and adefovir appear to be active against lamivudine-resistant variants and wild-type HBV (see Lamivudine). Most experts believe that combinations of nucleoside analogs will provide greater efficacy and reduce the frequency of drug resistance that occurs when these agents are used alone. Early studies using combination nucleoside analog therapy are under way. Combination treatment with IFN and nucleoside analogs also deserves further study because these agents have different mechanisms of action and the potential exists for additive or synergistic effects.

Ganciclovir. Ganciclovir is a synthetic analog of 2′ deoxyguanosine that inhibits replication of herpesviruses and has activity against HBV. It must be given parenterally because its oral form has limited bioavailability. Ganciclovir was the first nucleoside derivative to be applied to the treatment of recurrent hepatitis B after liver transplantation and is currently only of historic importance as a treatment for hepatitis B. Dosage-related neutropenia is associated with its use. There is some evidence that it may be active against lamivudine-resistant HBV in the transplant setting,[362] but safer and more effective nucleoside analogs will most likely become available in the next few years.

Famciclovir. Famciclovir is a synthetic acyclic guanine derivative that is a prodrug of penciclovir. It is licensed worldwide as treatment for acute herpes zoster and recurrent genital herpes. Famciclovir has been shown to be less inhibitory to HBV replication than lamivudine (see the following section). Famciclovir has not been used as extensively in clinical trials as lamivudine, but a 16-week course of treatment at a dose of 500 mg three times daily has resulted in consistent inhibition of HBV DNA and appears to be well tolerated.[363] In a preliminary trial in patients with chronic hepatitis B, however, famciclovir resulted in HBeAg seroconversion in only a small minority of patients.[364] In addition, a recently reported 12-week comparison of lamivudine and famciclovir demonstrated that famciclovir resulted in a high frequency of non-responders, and most responses were only partial.[365] In vitro studies have shown that a combination of penciclovir and lamivudine results in synergistic inhibition of duck hepatitis B virus replication.[361] The use of famciclovir and lamivudine in combination has been shown to result in a more rapid decline in serum HBV DNA levels than either agent alone.[366] Further studies are needed to assess whether a more prolonged course of treatment can lead to a higher rate of sustained virologic response. Unfortunately, sequential use of famciclovir and lamivudine has been associated with a more rapid development of resistance to the latter drug because both drugs can lead to HBV DNA polymerase mutation in domain B of the polymerase gene.[367]

Lamivudine. Lamivudine (100 mg once daily) is more active against HBV than famciclovir or ganciclovir and results in higher HBeAg seroconversion rates. Lamivudine was licensed in the United States, Asia, and Europe after phase III clinical trials demonstrated similar rates of HBeAg loss, HBeAg seroconversion, biochemical response, and histologic improvement to that obtained with IFN. Lamivudine was given for 52 weeks in these

TABLE 32-7

Comparison Between Interferon and Nucleoside Analog Therapy

	Advantages	Disadvantages
Interferon	Well-characterized short- and long-term response Virologic response in 30%-40% of cases Need only be given for 4-6 months No drug-resistant viral mutants	Not effective in patients with high baseline HBV DNA Expensive Frequent adverse effects Many problem patients
Nucleoside analog	Virologic response frequency similar to interferon Well tolerated Inexpensive Can be used safely in decompensated cirrhosis	Not as likely to result in loss of HBsAg Acquisition of drug-resistant HBV mutants Long-term therapy (>1 yr) often required Occasional postwithdrawal flares of hepatitis

HBV, Hepatitis B virus; *DNA,* deoxyribonucleic acid; *HBsAg,* hepatitis B surface antigen.

clinical trials. When compared to placebo a higher rate of HBeAg seroconversion has been demonstrated for patients with mild histologic and biochemical markers of disease.[188,368] It is considerably more potent than IFN in reducing viral replication and is free of serious adverse effects, which make it particularly suitable for patients with decompensated cirrhosis. Patients who are successfully treated with lamivudine have less progression of fibrosis than do untreated controls.[369] Moreover, when patients are maintained on treatment for 2 or more years, there appears to be significant histologic improvement in preexisting cirrhosis.[370] A 4-year follow-up of patients who have continued on treatment has indicated that HBeAg seroconversion rates continue to improve. Higher responses are achieved in patients with elevated ALT levels at baseline, and the pretreatment ALT level has been shown to be the best independent predictor of response to treatment.[269,270] Although the development and licensing of this drug has been a significant advance in the medical treatment of hepatitis B, the frequent occurrence of drug- resistant HBV mutants has led to questions on how long to treat and in what clinical situations this should be considered first line therapy.

Lamivudine-resistant Mutants. The major downside of lamivudine has been the emergence of drug-resistant HBV variants when this agent is used as monotherapy. A high level of serum HBV DNA is the best independent predictor that drug resistance will occur.[84,271] Although a high level of HBV replication in immunosuppressed patients facilitates the emergence of lamivudine resistance, this has also been observed in immunocompetent people as well. For example, in a US multi-center study resistance was observed in nearly 40 percent of patients,[188] whereas in a large study conducted in Asia, resistance was observed in 14 percent of patients after 52 weeks of treatment.[368] The rate of resistance increases with the duration of treatment, being detected in approximately 50 percent of patients after 3 years and 65 percent to 75 percent after 4 years of continuous treatment.[84,371]

During lamivudine treatment, one or more mutations occur in the highly conserved portion of the HBV DNA polymerase gene designated as the Tyrosine-methionine-aspartate-aspartate (YMDD) motif.[70] This genomic region affects nucleotide binding, and it has been hypothesized that mutations that change the amino acid composition of this region enlarge the nucleotide binding pocket, reducing its affinity for lamivudine.[372] The specific nucleotide mutations that have been associated with resistance to lamivudine result in substitution of either valine or isoleucine for methionine at residue 552 (M552V and M552I) in domain C of the polymerase gene. A second mutation often occurs upstream in the polymerase gene (domain B) and results in the substitution of methionine for leucine. In vitro studies suggest that the M552V mutation confers only partial resistance to lamivudine and that it confers high-level resistance only in conjunction with the L528M mutation. Whereas the presence of these mutations can be conclusively demonstrated by molecular studies, lamivudine resistance is highly suggested by the reappearance of HBV DNA by non-PCR-based assays after several previously negative tests in a patient who has been on more than 12 months of treatment. There is in vitro evidence that the drug-resistant variants are less replication-competent and that they are frequently associated with lower ALT and HBV DNA levels than those observed before treatment.[85,188,214] In one study, however, the emergence of these mutants was associated with flares in hepatitis that were severe enough to induce HBeAg seroconversion.[215] Although the long-term natural history of hepatitis B resulting from the YMDD variants remains unclear, cases have been described in which significant histologic deterioration has occurred.[214,271,373] Most of these reports have involved patients who were transplanted for hepatitis B.

There are several possible options to diminish the frequency or clinical impact of drug resistance to lamivudine. The first way would be to use lamivudine in combination with one or more nucleoside analogs with activity against HBV (see Table 32-6 and Alternative Nucleoside Analogs), a tactic that has worked well in HIV infection. This strategy seems most promising at this time but will have to await the availability of other nucleosides that do not induce or select for similar mutations in the HBV DNA polymerase gene. A second strategy to minimize the emergence of lamivudine resistance would be to combine lamivudine with a therapy that has immunomodulatory properties such as IFN. This could permit a shorter exposure to lamivudine, thereby decreasing the likelihood of drug-induced viral mutation. When lamivudine use has preceded IFN, the clinical results have been inconclusive.[345,374] Studies in which IFN is either given simultaneously or before lamivudine are needed to properly evaluate this form of combined therapy. A short course of corticosteroids provides another potentially useful mechanism for manipulating the immune response to HBV. In one study involving 30 patients with HBeAg-positive chronic hepatitis B, a flare of ALT, presumed to reflect immunologic activation, occurred in 67 percent of patients who were treated with a 9-month course of lamivudine preceded by a 4-week course of prednisolone.[200] High rates of HBeAg seroconversion (60 percent) were observed in patients who demonstrated an immunologic rebound. These data need further confirmation in larger randomized, controlled trials. A third way of dealing with lamivudine resistance would be to use an alternate drug that is active against the YMDD mutant and wild-type HBV such as adefovir dipivoxil. This could either be used as primary treatment or as salvage therapy should lamivudine resistance occur.

Adefovir Dipivoxil. Adefovir dipivoxil is a monophosphorylated nucleotide derivative with activity against wild-type HBV and lamivudine-resistant mutants. Preliminary reports indicate that this drug can be effective in reducing HBV replication and improving biochemical parameters in patients with advanced hepatitis B who are infected with the YMDD mutants (Figure 32-7).[375,376] Four patients with recurrent hepatitis B and one patient with compensated cirrhosis demonstrated a sustained $\log_2$ to $\log_4$ reduction in HBV DNA level by quantitative PCR during a mean treatment interval in excess of 1 year.[375] This drug is currently under study as a means of rescuing patients who have acquired lamivudine resistance and as

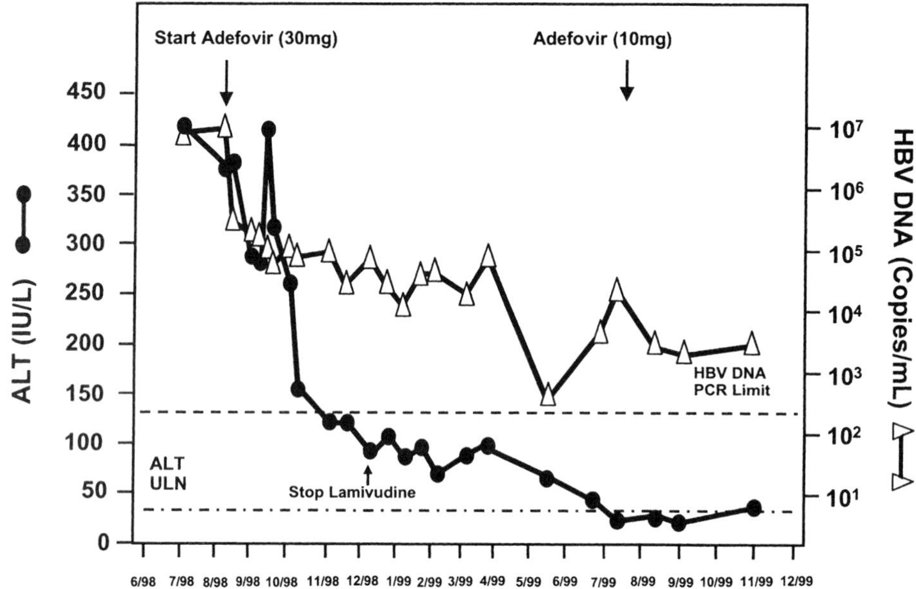

Figure 32-7 Treatment of lamivudine-resistant HBV mutant with adefovir dipivoxil. The patient was successfully treated with adefovir after emergence of lamivudine resistance. This patient had also been treated with interferon alfa before initiation of adefovir. *HBV,* Hepatitis B virus. (From Perrillo RP, Schiff E, Yoshida E, et al: Hepatology 32:129, 2000.)

primary therapy when given in low doses (10 mg daily). Studies are also under way in which lamivudine and adefovir are used in combination in previously untreated patients. Adefovir has been associated with renal toxicity at higher doses (30, 60, and 120 mg), however, and the long-term safety and efficacy of this approach require further study.

Alternative Nucleoside Analogs. Among the newer nucleoside derivatives, adefovir dipivoxil, entecavir, and emtricitabine appear to be at least as potent as lamivudine in suppressing HBV replication. Famciclovir appears less potent. In vitro studies show that YMDD mutations confer cross-resistance between lamivudine and emtricitabine. However, adefovir dipivoxil and entecavir suppress replication of YMDD mutant HBV, and wild-type HBV. Beta-D-2,6-diaminopurine dioxolane (DADD) and clevudine may also have some activity against the YMDD variant although the data appear less conclusive. It is likely that combinations of these agents will prove more effective than either alone.[377]

Treatment of Special Populations

HBeAg-negative Chronic Hepatitis B. Similar to the experience with IFN, patients with precore mutant HBV infection often have transient responses to nucleoside analog therapy. In one study 65 percent of patients who were treated with lamivudine for 52 weeks versus 6 percent given placebo had a complete virologic and biochemical response, but this was only maintained in 11 percent of the treated patients after lamivudine was discontinued.[378] More extended treatment may provide better results in this population but resistance will most likely become a limitation of this approach. Resistance to lamivudine appears to occur with equal frequency in precore mutant infection as it does with wild-type HBV.[378-380] YMDD mutants were observed in 27 percent of precore patients treated for 1 year and 37 percent who were treated for 2 years.[378,379] Histologic response has been documented during therapy,[378,379] but it is not clear how often this is maintained after resistance to lamivudine emerges. There are currently no reports of multi-drug therapy in this population and little published information on nucleoside analog treatment of decompensated cirrhosis resulting from precore mutant infection.[381] Using an in vitro means of determining sensitivity to a variety of anti-viral agents, it has been found that precore mutant HBV is more sensitive to lamivudine and penciclovir when compared to wild-type HBV.[382] Adefovir, by contrast, was less inhibitory.

Decompensated Cirrhosis. Nucleoside analogs are the preferred treatment for patients with advanced cirrhosis (see Table 32-5). The majority of clinical experience has been with lamivudine, but famciclovir has also been used successfully in patients with decompensated cirrhosis.[383] In one study 35 patients with advanced cirrhosis (10 Child's B, 25 Child's C) were treated with lamivudine monotherapy.[47] Twenty of the 23 patients (87 percent) treated for 6 or more months demonstrated progressive clinical and biochemical improvement, as defined by a decrease in the Child-Pugh score of at least 2 points. Improvement tended to be more noticeable after 9 months of treatment. In this study the majority of patients who died from complications of liver disease (5 of 7) did so within the first 6 months of treatment. Other studies also suggest that the first 6 months of treatment may be a critical interval for determining the likelihood of long-term survival during lamivudine treatment. In a recent analysis of 133 patients with advanced cirrhosis who were treated in 3 multi-center North American lamivudine

TABLE 32-8

Genetic and Immunologic Approaches to Treatment of Chronic HBV Infection

Gene therapy	Immune intervention
Ribozymes	Thymosin-α
Anti-sense oligonucleotides	DNA vaccine
Dominant negative core mutants	Pre-S vaccine
	Core-peptide vaccine
	Interleukin-12, interleukin-2, interferon-γ
	Allogeneic bone marrow transplantation

DNA, Deoxyribonucleic acid.

trials, 23 of the 30 deaths (77 percent) occurred within the first 6 months of treatment.[384] In this study survival was related to the degree of preexisting liver damage (as reflected by the level of serum bilirubin and albumin) rather than early differences in anti-viral response. These data raise the question of whether there is a point in the disease process where treatment may have little effectiveness and only transplantation can be looked upon as a viable option.

The point at which lamivudine should be initiated in patients with decompensated cirrhosis has become an important question. Too-early initiation can be associated with a high rate of drug resistance and an uncertain prognosis before and after transplantation. Too-late initiation may fail to stabilize the patient and prevent disease progression. Although several studies have demonstrated that treatment with lamivudine can forestall the need for liver transplantation, this has been observed in a minority of patients and it is not clear how this type of outcome can be predicted.

Extrahepatic Disorders. There are very limited data with respect to the management of the extrahepatic manifestations of hepatitis B with nucleoside analogs. Adenine arabinoside has been used with some success in conjunction with IFN and immunosuppression as therapy for polyarteritis nodosa.[135] With the development of safer nucleoside derivatives, this treatment can no longer be advocated. In individual case reports immunosuppressive treatment has been used in conjunction with lamivudine[385] or as a combined regimen with IFN and lamivudine.[386,387] In one report a patient had limited improvement in neuropathy associated with polyarteritis nodosa until the addition of lamivudine.[387] HBeAg and HBsAg seroconversion occurred and clinical improvement was sustained.

Molecular and Immunomodulatory Therapy

The development of new anti-viral strategies for the treatment of chronic hepatitis B remains a major goal because HBV cannot be successfully managed with IFN or nucleoside analog therapy in many instances. Two major types of alternative therapy have been proposed: gene therapy that is designed to block viral gene expression or function at different levels of the viral life cycle and therapeutic vaccines and cytokines that result in a change in immunologic response against HBV (Table 32-8).[388]

Gene Therapy. A number of gene-based therapies such as ribozymes, anti-sense oligonucleotides, and dominant negative core mutants are under exploration as treatment for chronic hepatitis B. To optimize the anti-viral effects of these agents, various novel expression systems such as adenoviral vectors have been developed to deliver the agents to infected cells. Ribozymes are ribonucleic acid enzymes that catalyze the sequence-specific cleavage of RNA and RNA-splicing reactions. In theory this is an attractive approach because one ribozyme can cleave many target RNAs. Several studies have shown that ribozymes can specifically cleave HBV RNA in vitro, but in vivo studies are still lacking.[389] Anti-sense oligonucleotides are designed to specifically bind to viral RNA, resulting in the formation of RNA-DNA or RNA-RNA hybrids (anti-sense RNA) with an arrest of RNA replication, reverse transcription, or mRNA translation. The anti-sense strategy has been successfully applied in vitro to HBV infection.[390,391] In addition, in vivo experimentation in hepadnavirus animal models has shown the applicability of this approach. Although no toxic effects have been observed, the contribution of non–anti-sense effects to the inhibition of viral replication or gene expression has not been systematically assessed in most studies. Another genetically based approach that has been used involves the intracellular synthesis of interfering peptides or whole proteins, including non-secreted antibodies aimed at the interference with the assembly or function of viral structural or non-structural proteins. This approach has proven effective for both mammalian and avian hepadnaviruses in cell culture, in which case the fusion of different polypeptides to the HBV core protein yields dominant negative core mutants.[392,393] These mutants are species-specific and suppress viral replication by at least 90 percent at an appropriate effector-to-target ratio. The potential advantage of dominant negative mutants over ribozymes or anti-sense oligonucleotides is their relative independence from viral sequence variations, minimizing the risk of selecting escape mutants.

Although these genetic approaches are conceptually attractive and may complement existing or future therapeutic strategies, further studies in experimental animal models are necessary before human trials can be approached. Several key issues remain, such as the specificity of gene therapy for the targeted gene and the stability and potential toxicity of the therapeutic nucleic acids or proteins and their delivery to and expression in infected hepatocytes and non-hepatocytes. Moreover, it is possible that viral or immune-mediated resistance to genetic anti-viral strategies could develop.

Immune-based Therapy. Because cytokines play a crucial role in the natural clearance of HBV, they have been used as possible therapeutic agents for chronic hepatitis B. Cytokine responses are characterized as $T_H{}^1$, which induce HBV-specific cytotoxic T lymphocytes and virucidal cytokines such as TNFα and IFN-γ, or $T_H{}^2$, which induce antibody responses to viral antigens. The cytokine profile shown to promote viral eradication is $T_H{}^1$, which is induced by interleukin (IL)-12. Consideration of therapies that may alter the $T_H{}^1/T_H{}^2$ balance has led to pilot studies of IL-2 and other cytokines, such as IL-12 and IFN-γ.[394,396] Of these, IL-12 has seemed to be the most promising.[396,397] IL-12 directly stimulates IL-2 and IFN-γ secretion by $CD4^+$ T cells and has been shown to have therapeutic effects in different tumor cell lines and infectious disease models, including the transgenic mouse model of HBV infection. IL-12 also has been shown to stimulate alpha IFN in humans. In phase I and II studies, weekly injections of IL-12 have resulted in decreases in serum HBV DNA levels in a dose-dependent manner.[397] Moreover, treatment resulted in measurable increases in serum levels of IFN-γ, IL-10 (an anti-inflammatory cytokine) and β_2 microglobulin (part of the HLA–class I antigen molecular complex expressed on the surface of hepatocytes). Although these observations indicate that IL-12 was capable of increasing $T_H{}^1$ activity in vivo, it did not result in a lasting virologic response. Further studies using IL-12 in combination with more traditional anti-viral therapies may offer greater promise.

Thymic peptides have immunomodulatory effects, and synthetic peptides such as thymosin alpha 1 have been used in an attempt to stimulate appropriate cell-mediated immune responses to HBV. Early studies in chimpanzees demonstrated that thymosin increased indices of cell-mediated immunity but had no effect on viral clearance.[398] Pilot studies in humans revealed a decline in HBV replication and improvement in serum aminotransferase levels.[399] In a larger, controlled trial, however, HBeAg seroconversion rates in those receiving thymosin were not significantly different from the rates in placebo recipients.[400] The experience with this drug in Asian trials has been more optimistic. In one study there was a trend for HBeAg seroconversion to increase or accumulate gradually after the end of treatment, and blinded histologic assessment showed a significant improvement in lobular inflammation in treated patients versus placebo recipients.[401] Studies in patients with anti-HBe, HBV DNA–positive chronic hepatitis B have not been able to confirm efficacy although prolonged effects on improvement of serum aminotransferase levels have been observed.[402,403] Thymosin does appear to have immunologic activity; further studies in combination with IFN and nucleoside analogs appear warranted.

Recently, a case has been reported in which an S gene mutant arose during treatment with thymosin, further attesting to its immunologic effects.[404]

Conventional vaccination against HBV has not proven effective in promoting viral clearance, but a number of innovative strategies using therapeutic vaccines have been tried. In one trial patients with chronic hepatitis B were given four doses of a vaccine that contained a cytotoxic T lymphocyte epitope and a T-helper cell epitope. Although this proved ineffective in inducing a virologic response, it did demonstrate a low-level cytotoxic T-cell response that was dose-dependent.[405] It is conceivable that a similar approach could be more effective when used in combination with drugs that inhibit viral replication or when multiple core epitopes are incorporated into the vaccine. Immunization of HLA transgenic mice with a DNA minigene encoding several CTL epitopes has been shown to result in the induction of a cytotoxic T-cell response to multiple epitopes that better simulates responses occurring during natural viral clearance.[406] An alternate approach to therapeutic vaccination involves the intramuscular injection of viral genes in which the antigen is synthesized in vivo after direct introduction of its encoding sequences incorporated into plasmid DNA expression vectors. By virtue of the sustained in vivo antigen synthesis, these vaccines offer strong and long-lasting humoral and cell-mediated immune responses to HBV. In animal models DNA vaccines give immunity superior to that of the current traditional antigen-based vaccines and can overcome tolerance to HBV antigens in a transgenic mouse model.[407,408] Additional studies are needed in preclinical testing before this approach can be used in humans.

Pre-S 1- and pre-S 2-containing vaccines have also been employed because they are more immunogenic in humans and may interrupt tolerance to HBsAg.[409] In the transgenic mouse model multiple doses of pre-S-containing vaccines have been shown to result in elimination of HBsAg and HBeAg from serum and reduction in HBV DNA titer.[410] Trials in humans are very limited but a preliminary study from France has indicated that pre-S/S vaccination results in a decline in viral replication, and when followed by IFN a sustained disappearance of HBV DNA has been observed.[411] It has been shown that the pre-S 2 vaccine results in the induction of viral antigen-specific $CD4^+$ T-cell responses and increased IFN-γ levels in conjunction with a measurable decline in serum HBV DNA. It is likely that the important role that helper T cells play in secreting anti-viral cytokines such as IFN-γ allows an optimal activation of protective cytotoxic T-cell responses. Administration of a unique adjuvanted pre-S 2-containing vaccine has shown promise in early clinical trials.[411a]

Serologic clearance of HBsAg has been described after receipt of marrow from anti-HBc/anti-HBs–positive and anti-HBs–positive donors.[412-415] In one study in which 21 HBsAg carriers underwent bone marrow transplantation, 2 of 5 individuals who received bone marrow allografts from anti-HBs–positive donors cleared HBsAg versus none of 16 receiving marrow from anti-HBs–negative donors. In some instances clearance of HBsAg is accompanied by flares of ALT, suggesting that the clearance is immunologically mediated. Vaccination of the anti-HBs–positive bone marrow donor has been proposed as a means of providing further assurances that the HBsAg-positive recipient will undergo serologic clearance of infection.

PREVENTION OF HBV INFECTION

Immune prophylaxis against hepatitis B can be achieved by passive immunization with Ig preparations that contain high titers of antibody to HBsAg, active immunization with HBsAg-containing vaccines, or a combination of the two (active-passive immunization). Hepatitis B immunoglobulin (HBIG) is used exclusively in postexposure prophylaxis whereas the vaccine is used in both preexposure and postexposure settings.

Immunoglobulins

HBIG is prepared from plasma that is known to contain high titers of anti-HBs and is derived from healthy adults who have recovered from hepatitis B infection. Plasmapheresis of healthy people who are immunized with highly immunogenic HBV vaccines containing pre-S antigens may be used in the future as a safer alternative.[416] The efficacy of immunoglobulins in preventing hepatitis B is well established.A number of preexposure and postexposure trials in the last two decades have clearly demonstrated the efficacy of immunoglobulin in preventing HBV infections in adults.[417-423] Similarly, four controlled trials have established the efficacy of HBIG in decreasing perinatal transmission of hepatitis B from infected mothers to their neonates.[423-426]

HBIG is currently marketed by several manufacturers. These preparations vary considerably in the concentration of anti-HBs and amount of protein.The anti-HBs concentration of intramuscular preparations of HBIG in the United States and Europe is usually between 200 and 300 U/ml. For example, the anti-HBs concentration in HyperHep Bayhep (Bayer Corporation,West Haven, Ct.) is 217 to 250 U/ml, and this has a protein concentration of 15 percent to 18 percent, whereas the concentration of anti-HBs in NABI-HB (NABI, Boca Raton, Fla.) is 312 U/ml with 4 percent to 6 percent protein. The concentration of anti-HBs in the intravenous preparations is usually in the order of 50 U/ml with somewhat lower protein concentrations than the intramuscular preparations. In the setting of liver transplantation—in which a large amount of anti-HBs is used—intramuscular preparations have been given intravenously after dilution with normal saline.

In general, HBIG preparations have proven to be very safe. Administration of Ig intramuscularly or intravenously may occasionally be associated with hypersensitivity reactions (or very rarely, anaphylaxis). In patients who are HBsAg-positive, administration of HBIG can potentially lead to immune complex formation.[427,428] Although there is no direct evidence to support clinically important immune complex formation, findings such as arthralgias, myalgias, skin rash, and CNS disorders after administration of HBIG provide indirect evidence of a role for immune complexes.These side effects may be related to the concentration of anti-HBs in the preparations and are more likely to occur when intramuscular preparations with high concentration of anti-HBs are given intravenously. A relatively high frequency of symptoms such as back pain (90 percent), headache (20 percent), and flushing (5 percent) has been reported in liver transplant recipients when intramuscular preparations of HBIG are given intravenously.[429] The risk of transmission of HIV and other viruses has been virtually eliminated because of mandatory serologic screening of donors and inactivating chemical procedures.[430,431] The current viral inactivation procedures with solvent and detergent treatment using tri-n-butyl phosphate and sodium cholate are effective in inactivating known enveloped viruses such as HBV, HIV, and HCV.[432]

HBV Vaccine

Types

Two types of hepatitis B vaccines are available in the United States, both of which are produced by recombinant DNA technology. In most countries plasma-derived vaccine has been replaced by recombinant vaccines.The former vaccines were derived from the plasma of chronically infected carriers; the source material was biophysically purified and inactivated by sequential treatment with pepsin digestion, 8 M urea, and formalin.[433,434] Manufacture of the recombinant vaccines depends upon the insertion of a plasmid containing the HBs or S gene into *Saccharomyces cerevisiae* (common baker's yeast).[435,436] The product of the inserted gene (HBsAg) is harvested from the yeast cell cultures, purified, and inactivated by treatment with formaldehyde. Aluminum hydroxide is added as an adjuvant, and thimerosal (1:20,000 concentration) is added as a preservative.The vaccine may contain up to 4 percent yeast protein but this has not been associated with harmful effects in vaccine recipients. Two companies have marketed the recombinant vaccines in the United States and elsewhere. Recombivax HB (Merck & Co., West Point, Penn.) was licensed in 1986 and Engerix-B (SmithKline Beecham, Pittsburgh, Penn.) was licensed in 1989.These vaccines are similar in efficacy, duration of immunity, and cost but differ in HBsAg concentration (Recombivax HB has 10 μg/ml; Engerix-B has 20 μg/ml). Recombivax HB has been licensed for only three doses; Engerix-B is approved for four doses.

Immunogenicity and Efficacy

The immunogenicity of the plasma-derived and recombinant DNA vaccines is excellent, with the latter achieving a slightly better antibody response rate.The prophylactic efficacy of these vaccines is dependent on neutralizing activity against the "a" epitope in the HBsAg gene (aa 124-148). Hepatitis B vaccine induces HBsAg-specific T-helper cells and T-cell–dependent B cells as early as 2 weeks after the first immunization.[437,438] Anti-HBs titers greater than 100 mIU/ml confer uniform protection against HBV infection. Because the vaccine contains only HBsAg, not the nucleocapsid antigen, anti-HBc is not detectable unless the individual has been previously infected.

Three clinical trials in the early 1980s established the efficacy of HBV vaccines in preventing HBV infection.[439-441] In a study involving 1083 homosexual men high titer of anti-HBs was seen in 77 percent of vaccinees within 2 months. This rate increased to 96 percent after the booster dose.[439] Only 1.4 percent to 3.4 percent of vaccinees developed a clinically apparent hepatitis B or subclinical infection during the follow-up period, in contrast to 18 percent to 27 percent of placebo recipients. In addition, none of the vaccinees with a detectable antibody response developed clinical hepatitis B or asymptomatic antigenemia. In another randomized control study among 1402 homosexual men two doses of vaccine induced antibody responses in 80 percent of vaccinees, and the third dose increased the response to 85 percent.[440] Excellent antibody responses also have been observed in neonates and infants after three doses of vaccine.[442-444]

The indicator of successful vaccination is the presence of an anti-HBs titer of greater than 10 mIU/ml. Long-term follow-up data on vaccinees have shown that the risk of HBV infection increases several-fold when the anti-HBs titer falls below 9.9 sample ratio units (SRU comparable to 10 mIU/ml).[445,446] In one study the risk of HBV infection with a low anti-HBs titer (less than 9.9 SRU) was 7 times higher than the risk with a higher antibody titer.[445] In the same study the estimated risk of HBV infection in people with an anti-HBs level during a given 6-month interval of less than 9.9 SRU was 6.9/100 patient-years exposed. These studies have also revealed that the risk of HBV infection was inversely related to the maximal antibody titer achieved with the initial vaccination series. During a 5-year follow-up evaluation of 635 vaccine recipients the rate of HBV infection was 8.9/100 patient-years of follow-up in people with a peak antibody response of 10 to 49 SRU as compared to 0.74/100 patient-years of follow-up in those with peak antibody levels greater than 100 SRU.[445] Most of the infections in vaccine recipients with low-titer anti-HBs were clinically silent, with anti-HBc positivity being the only evidence of infection. In the 5-year follow-up period 38 vaccinees developed HBV infection but only 2 had clinically apparent infection with detectable HBsAg and elevated transaminases.[445] Similar observations were made in a 10-year follow-up evaluation of 1630 vaccinees in which only 13 patients developed HBV infection.[446] None of the infected patients had clinical hepatitis.

The titer of anti-HBs in responders generally declines to non-protective levels with prolonged follow-up. Two studies in different patient populations demonstrated that anti-HBs titers decreased to non-protective levels in at least 25 percent to 50 percent of vaccine recipients over a period of 5 to 10 years.[445,446] The rate of decline in antibody titers is principally influenced by the maximal antibody levels achieved with the initial vaccination. People with higher peak anti-HBs levels are more likely to have protective titers for a longer duration. Five-year follow-up studies have demonstrated that anti-HBs disappears in 70 percent of individuals who have peak anti-HBs titers of less than 50 mIU/ml, and in almost all others the levels decrease to less than 10 mIU/ml during the same interval. In contrast, among people with a peak antibody titer greater than 100 mIU/ml, anti-HBs disappeared in only 7 percent at the end of 5 years.[445]

A number of factors influence the immunogenicity of the current vaccines. The response rate is low in smokers, obese individuals, and those with chronic liver diseases.[447-449] Older individuals have lower seroconversion rates and generally have lower peak anti-HBs titers.[449,450] The response rate of neonates is excellent compared to other vaccines but slightly lower than that observed in older children and adults. There seems to be no difference in response rate between male and females. Typically the response rate in hemodialysis and immunocompromised patients (e.g., organ transplant recipients, HIV-infected patients, those receiving chemotherapy) is 40 percent to 60 percent.[451-453] These patients may respond to higher doses or a second vaccine series. Injection of vaccine into the buttocks elicits a significantly lower antibody titer and seroconversion rate when compared to injection in the deltoid or anterolateral thigh (as for infants), probably because a larger volume of fat in the buttocks impedes vaccine absorption.[454]

Route of Administration

The hepatitis vaccine is administered intramuscularly in the deltoid area of adults and the anterolateral thigh in infants or neonates. Intradermal administration of vaccine is associated with a lower antibody response. Three doses of intradermal injection are associated with a lower rate of seroconversion (55 percent-80 percent) when compared to an identical regimen delivered by intramuscular injection (90 percent seroconversion).[455-458] Four doses delivered intradermally have, however, been shown to have an equivalent antibody response.[459] In animal studies and in a small clinical trial in humans intradermal injection was shown to produce a stronger humoral and cellular immunity than conventional intramuscular doses.[460-464] These studies have shown that intradermal injection, by recruiting "professional" dendritic cells, may be able to stimulate primary major HLA class I- and class II–restricted T-cell responses.[460-464] One of the studies also included nine "non-responders" to conventional vaccination, all of whom responded to two to five doses of intradermally delivered recombinant vaccine.[464] Despite these encouraging results, there are no recommendations for intradermal vaccination in either adults or infants—it should be considered for research purposes only.

Booster Doses

Considering the strong immunologic memory and evidence that clinical hepatitis is rare even in patients with a low or undetectable anti-HBs titer, there does not appear to be a role for booster doses in immunocompetent people. The only official recommendation from the US Public Health Service (USPHS) for booster doses is for patients undergoing hemodialysis. In these patients anti-HBs antibody titer should be tested annually and a booster dose given if the titer is less than 10 mIU/ml.[465]

Serologic Testing Before and After Vaccination

Serologic confirmation of susceptibility is not indicated for children or adolescents because of the low likelihood of HBV infection and the relatively low cost of vaccine for each pediatric versus adult dose.[465] In adults prevaccination testing should be based on the relative likelihood of exposure. Serologic testing may be offered to high-risk patients who are likely to have become infected in the past (homosexual men, injecting drug users, patients from areas of high endemicity). Even in these patients the cost of testing should be balanced against the cost of vaccine saved by not giving the vaccine. If routine testing is considered cost-effective, either anti-HBs or anti-HBc testing can be performed. In populations anticipated to have a low HBV carrier rate (less than 2 percent), neither test has any advantage. However, in groups with a higher carrier rate, anti-HBc testing may be useful in identifying previously undetected HBV carriers.

Non-responders

Non-responders are immunocompetent individuals who fail to demonstrate detectable anti-HBs after a full course of vaccine. This situation occurs in about 3 percent to 8 percent of vaccinees. Those people who develop detectable antibody responses with the maximal level below the protective range (less than 10 mIU/ml) are called hyporesponders. Certain histocompatibility haplotypes are more frequent among non-responders. These include HLA B8, HLA B44, HLA DR3, and HLA DQ2.[466-470] This is probably because of a lack of a dominant gene required for a humoral response to HBsAg.[470] Such non-responders may respond to a repeat dose of vaccination. Adequate antibody response is seen in 30 percent to 50 percent of non-responders after three additional doses.[445,465] Hyporesponders respond better than non-responders to a second vaccine series (79 percent versus 41 percent after three additional doses of vaccine).[445] The response may not be sustained, however, and for this reason periodic monitoring of the antibody titer and repetition of the vaccination series may be required.

Vaccination in Patients with Chronic Liver Disease

In general, hepatitis B vaccination is recommended for patients with chronic liver disease.[471] Vaccination of patients with hepatitis C is particularly advisable because hepatitis B can worsen the clinical status of the patient and increase the risk of cirrhosis and hepatocellular carcinoma.[472-474] Studies have shown that anti-HCV–positive patients may have a lower response to vaccination.[475,476] In a recent prospective study involving 117 patients (59 with chronic hepatitis C and 58 healthy controls) 31 percent of the HCV-infected patients were non-responders (defined in the study as those with an anti-HBs antibody titer of less than 10 mIU/ml) compared to 9 percent of controls.[477] This was not related to the level of HCV viremia or the severity of liver disease. Haplotypes HLA B8DR3 and HLA DR7DQ2 were, however, 3 times more common among non-responders and 4 to 5 times more frequent than in the general population. Patients with cirrhosis, particularly those with more advanced disease (e.g., those awaiting liver transplantation), may not achieve high anti-HBs titers after vaccination.[478]

Vaccination in the Setting of Hemodialysis

Only 50 percent to 60 percent of patients on hemodialysis achieve a satisfactory response to hepatitis B vaccination because of immune system depression.[479] In a study involving 80 patients with chronic renal failure the factors that predicted a poor response were old age, presence of DR3 and DR7DQ2, and absence of A2 alleles.[480] Hemodialysis regimen or nutritional status did not influence the response rate. It is probably advisable to vaccinate these patients early in the course of renal failure to improve the response rate.[481] Even though the overall response rate is low, patients who develop protective titers of anti-HBs after vaccination appear to be protected against HBV infection.[482] The USPHS recommends annual anti-HBs testing for hemodialysis patients and booster doses if the titer falls to less than 10 mIU/ml. Enhancing the antibody response using colony stimulating factor appeared promising in animal studies although a recent clinical trial failed to show any benefit.[483] Repeat doses with intradermal vaccination (5 μg every 2 weeks to provide a titer of more than 1000 IU/L) have been recently shown to achieve a response rate of 97.6 percent in chronic hemodialysis patients.[484] Further studies are needed before the efficacy of intradermal vaccination strategy can be established in this subset of patients.

Adverse Effects

Plasma-derived and recombinant vaccines are safe, and other viral infections have not been reported in vaccine recipients. The most commonly reported adverse event is pain at the injection site. This was the only side effect observed in a higher frequency among patients who received vaccine as compared to placebo in the phase III controlled trials.[439,440] Other minor side effects include low-grade fever, fatigue, headache, and myalgias. There have been reports of Guillain-Barré syndrome in some vaccinees after administration of plasma-derived vaccine. These occurrences were rare (0.5/100,000 vaccinees). In more than 850,000 US vaccinees who received plasma-derived vaccine between June 1982 and May 1985, Guillain-Barré syndrome was seen in 9 patients, which slightly exceeded the expected frequency.[485] Other neurologic adverse events reported included convulsions (5 cases), Bell's palsy (10 cases), optic neuritis (5 cases), transverse myelitis (4 cases), and lumbar or brachial neuropathy (8 cases).[485] Occurrence of these neurologic events did not exceed the expected frequency. Among the 2.5 million adults who received recombinant vaccination between 1986 and 1990, no increase in neurologic adverse events was noted.[465] From the available data it appears that Guillain-Barré syndrome and other reported neurologic disorders such as aseptic meningitis, transverse myelitis, and grand mal seizures are not associated with hepatitis B vaccine. A recent case-control study indicated a lack of association between hepatitis B vaccination and the development of multiple sclerosis.[486]

Preexposure Prophylaxis

Preexposure prophylaxis against hepatitis B is aimed at preventing the transmission of hepatitis B from an infected person or contaminated source to a susceptible individual. Preexposure prophylaxis can be targeted to a selected population that is at high risk of exposure to HBV or to be part of a universal vaccination strategy toward eradication of hepatitis B (see Figure 32-1). Preexposure prophylaxis is usually achieved by three doses of hepatitis B vaccine except in special circumstances. Table 32-9 provides the dose recommendations for vaccination in neonates and adults. The typical vaccination schedule is 0, 1, and 6 months. The first two priming doses have little effect on the final antibody titer. The third dose acts as a booster to achieve anti-HBs titers that are generally in excess of 100 mIU/ml in immunocompetent individuals. Because studies have shown that the risk of subsequent infection is inversely related to the maximal antibody titers, the third dose is essential to achieve the long-term goals of vaccination. Vaccination is considered successful if the vaccinee achieves an anti-HBs titer greater than 10 mIU/ml. In immunocompromised patients, including those on hemodialysis, four doses are recommended to provide greater certainty that a protective level is achieved. If the vaccination series is interrupted, the second dose should be administered as soon as possible.[465] If the third dose is interrupted, it should be given when convenient but within 12 months of the second dose. Ideally, the second and third doses should be separated at least by 2 months.[465] When vaccines from different manufacturers are combined to complete a vaccination schedule, the immune response achieved is comparable to that obtained when vaccine from a single manufacturer.[465] Accelerated vaccination with three doses given at 0, 1, and 2 months followed by a fourth dose at 6 to 12 months may be used in people traveling to endemic areas—provided the first three doses can be given before departure.[465]

Targeted High-risk Groups

Hepatitis B vaccination is recommended in certain individuals who are at high risk of exposure to hepatitis B. Table 32-10 delineates the high-risk adult groups in whom vaccination is strongly recommended. Targeted vaccination has not achieved its objective in certain

TABLE 32-9

Recommended Doses of the Currently Available Vaccines[465]*

	Recombivax HB 10 μg/ml	Engerix-B 20 μg/ml
Infants† and children < 11 yr	2.5 μg	10 μg
Children/adolescents 11-19 yr	5 μg	20 μg
Adults > 20 yr	10 μg	20 μg
Hemodialysis patients	40 μg (1.0 ml)‡	40 μg (2.0 ml)§
Immunocompromised patients	40 μg (1.0 ml)‡	40 μg (2.0 ml)§

*The standard schedule is 0, 1, and 6 months.
†Infants born to hepatitis B surface-negative mothers.
‡Special formulation.
§Two 1-ml doses administered at one site in four-dose schedule: 0, 1, 2, and 6 months.

TABLE 32-10

High-Risk Groups

1. Health care workers
2. Public safety workers with likelihood of exposure to blood
3. Staff and clients of institutions for developmentally disabled
4. Hemodialysis patients
5. Patients with hematologic disorders requiring frequent transfusions or blood products
6. Household contacts and sex partners of HBV carriers or patients with acute HBV
7. International travelers to endemic areas who may have intimate contact with local populations or may take part in medical activities in endemic areas
8. Injecting drug users
9. Sexually active bisexual and homosexual men
10. Sexually active heterosexual men and women if they have more than one partner
11. Inmates of correctional facilities
12. Patients awaiting liver transplantation*

HBV, Hepatitis B virus.
*Most transplant centers vaccinate all patients awaiting liver transplantation. This has become particularly relevant with the greater use of anti-HBc-positive donors in an attempt to expand the donor pool.

high-risk people, such as injecting drug users. In an epidemiologic survey of four sentinel counties from 1981 to 1988, the overall incidence of hepatitis B has remained relatively constant although there were some changes in the epidemiologic pattern of the disease. The proportion of hepatitis B among male homosexuals and health care workers decreased, whereas cases related to parenteral drug use increased.[487] Vaccination in health care professionals has resulted in substantial reductions in the rate of new infections. The impact of universal infant vaccination on new cases of infection has not been completely defined but has been shown to markedly decrease the incidence of hepatocellular cancer in Taiwanese children.[488]

Perinatal Exposure

The risk of perinatal transmission of HBV infection varies from 10 percent to 80 percent depending on the HBeAg and HBV DNA status of the mother. Infected infants have a 90 percent likelihood of developing chronic hepatitis B. A combination of immunoglobulin (HBIG) and vaccination (active-passive immunization) has proven to be more than 90 percent effective in preventing infection in exposed neonates. Because selected screening of pregnant women for HBsAg has failed to identify a high proportion of HBV-infected mothers, universal prenatal testing for all pregnant women is recommended.[489,490] The immunization strategy in preventing perinatal transmission is outlined in Table 32-11.[465] If prenatal HBsAg screening is not possible, all infants should be vaccinated within 12 hours of birth with the second dose given at 2 months of age and the third given at 6 months of age. If the mother is found to be HBsAg-positive, further evaluation for chronic liver disease and appropriate follow-up of sexual partners should be initiated.

Adolescent Vaccination Recommendations

All adolescents 11 to 12 years of age, if not previously vaccinated, should be vaccinated with the doses recommended in Table 32-9 at the time of routine physician visits. The impact of adolescent vaccination on the incidence of new cases should, in theory, be realized more quickly. Also, school-based immunization programs can be effective in ensuring adequate vaccination coverage.[491] Unvaccinated adolescents more than 12 years of age should be vaccinated if they are at risk of acquiring hepatitis B.[492] The typical schedule is three doses at 0, 1 to 2 months, and 6 months.

Postexposure Prophylaxis

Postexposure vaccination should be considered for any percutaneous, ocular, or mucous membrane exposure. The type of immunoprophylaxis is determined by the HBsAg status of the source and the vaccination response status of the exposed person. Table 32-12 outlines the recommended regimen for postexposure prophylaxis after a percutaneous or mucosal exposure.[493] All exposed

TABLE 32-11
HBV Prophylaxis to Prevent Perinatal Transmission

	VACCINE			
	Recombivax HB	Engerix-B	HBIG	Age of Infant
Infants Born to HBsAg-positive Mother				
First dose	5 μg (0.5 ml)	10 μg (0.5 ml)	0.5 ml IM*	Within 12 hr of birth
Second dose	5 μg (0.5 ml)	10 μg (0.5 ml)	—	1 month
Third dose	5 μg (0.5 ml)	10 μg (0.5 ml)	—	6 months
Mother Whose HBsAg Status is Unknown at the Time of Delivery but Later Found to be HBsAg-positive				
First dose	5 μg (0.5 ml)	10 μg (0.5 ml)	0.5 ml IM* not later than 7 days†	Within 12 hr of birth
Second dose	5 μg (0.5 ml)	10 μg (0.5 ml)	—	1-2 months
Third dose	5 μg (0.5 ml)	10 μg (0.5 ml)	—	6 months
	VACCINE			
	Recombivax HB	Engerix-B	Follow-up doses	
Mother Whose HBsAg Status is Negative by Prenatal Testing				
First dose	2.5 μg (0.5 ml)	10 μg (0.5 ml)	Birth or before hospital discharge	
Second dose	2.5 μg (0.5 ml)	10 μg (0.5 ml)	1-2 months	
Third dose	2.5 μg (0.5 ml)	10 μg (0.5 ml)	6 months	

HBIG, Hepatitis B immunoglobulin; *HBsAg,* hepatitis B surface antigen; *IM,* intramuscular.
*HBIG should be administered at a site different from that used for vaccine.
†Protective efficacy of HBIG given after 48 hours is not known.
‡Hepatitis B vaccine can be administered simultaneously with diphtheria-tetanus pertussis, *Haemophilus influenzae* type b conjugate, measles-mumps-rubella, and oral polio vaccine at the same visit.

TABLE 32-12

Postexposure Prophylaxis: Percutaneous or Mucous Membrane Exposure[493]

Vaccination status of exposed person	Immune prophylaxis
Source HBsAg-Positive	
Unvaccinated	HBIG (0.06 ml/kg) and initiate vaccination series
Previously vaccinated	
Known responder*	No treatment
Known non-responder	HBIG × 2 dose or HBIG × 1 dose and initiate revaccination
Antibody response unknown	Test antibody response—
	If adequate*: no treatment
	If inadequate†: HBIG × 1 dose and provide vaccine booster
Source HBsAg-Negative	
Unvaccinated	Initiate HBV vaccination series
Previously vaccinated	
Known responder	No treatment
Known non-responder	No treatment
Antibody response unknown	No treatment
Source HBsAg Status Unknown	
Unvaccinated	Initiate vaccination series
Previously vaccinated	
Known responder*	No treatment
Known non-responder	If source is high risk, treat as if source is HBsAg-positive
Antibody response unknown	Test antibody response—
	If adequate*: no treatment
	If inadequate†: initiate revaccination

HBsAg, Hepatitis B surface antigen; *HBIG,* hepatitis B immunoglobulin; *HBV,* hepatitis B virus.
*Antibody to hepatitis surface titer > 10 mIU/ml.
†Antibody to hepatitis surface titer < 10 mIU/ml.

people should have anti-HBs testing within 1 to 2 months of the vaccination series. Those who do not respond to primary vaccine should be tested for HBsAg and, if negative, complete a second three-dose vaccine series. Those who are non-responders should be counseled about the need for HBIG for subsequent exposure.

Sexual partners of HBsAg-positive people are at high risk of acquiring hepatitis B, and HBIG has been shown to be 75 percent effective in preventing such infections.[421] The exact period after sexual contact during which HBIG remains effective is not clear. It is generally considered effective when given within 14 days after contact. All those who are susceptible should be given HBIG (0.06 ml/kg) within 14 days of contact and be vaccinated with three doses of vaccine.[461] Unvaccinated household contacts of patients who are HBsAg-positive should be vaccinated. If they have blood exposure, they should be treated as with sexual exposure.[465] Infants whose primary care giver has developed hepatitis B must be treated with HBIG (0.5 ml) and a full vaccination series.[465]

Recent Developments

Immunization using HBV DNA genetic sequences encoding for HBsAg and nucleoprotein has been developed. These DNA-based vaccines elicit both humoral and cellular immunity and stimulate both $CD4^+$ and $CD8^+$ T-cell responses when given to antigen-processing tissues by the intradermal or intramuscular route.[494-496] In a recently reported study 12 healthy volunteers who received DNA vaccine developed anti-HBs titers of at least 10 mIU/ml and expressed antigen-specific $CD8^+$ T cells that bound HLA-A2/HBsAg tetramers.[497] A novel delivery of vaccine to immunize the fetus in utero was successfully performed in fetal lambs.[498] When introduced into the amniotic fluid, HBV DNA vaccine resulted in high serum antibody titers and strong cell-mediated immune responses.[498]

Triple antigen vaccines (S, pre-S 1, pre-S 2, Hepacare, Medeva Pharma, United Kingdom) have undergone clinical trials and may be more immunogenic than the presently available vaccines.[498a] In a recently reported study, health care workers who were known to be inadequate responders to prior immunization were vaccinated either with a single dose of a triple antigen vaccine or with a single dose of conventional vaccine. Triple antigen vaccine induced protective antibody titers in more vaccinees than the conventional vaccine.[498b] Recently, the Food and Drug Administration has approved a combination hepatitis vaccine (hepatitis A and B). The antibody responses and safety have been shown to be comparable to the corresponding monovalent vaccines.[498c]

Edible vaccine for hepatitis B is another area of interest. The DNA fragment encoding for HBsAg was used to obtain transgenic lupin and transgenic lettuce. Human volunteers fed with transgenic lettuce expressing HBsAg developed specific serum IgG responses to plant-derived protein.[499] Efforts to increase the immunogenicity of the vaccine using a different adjuvant such as monophosphoryl lipid A are under way. These vaccines could potentially elicit a higher degree of antibody response and may eliminate the need for multiple doses of vaccine.

DELTA VIRUS

Delta virus or HDV is a small RNA-containing virus that requires the concomitant presence of HBV in an obligate manner for its survival and pathogenicity. It was first described in 1977 in HBsAg-positive patients.[500] Within a few short years of its discovery it was linked to cases of progressive chronic hepatitis B and fulminant hepatitis B.[501-503]

Epidemiology of HDV

HDV is distributed worldwide with the highest endemicity in South America.[504] It is believed that at least 5 percent of hepatitis B carriers worldwide are infected with HDV, although considerable regional variation exists, with some countries reporting a much higher co-infection rate. This is particularly true for Mediterranean countries, northern Africa, and the Middle East. HDV is also endemic in countries of the Amazon basin. The prevalence of HDV in the Far East is probably lower than in these regions despite a high endemicity of HBV. In countries with a low prevalence of HBV, such as North America and northern Europe, the HDV co-infection rate is much lower. Based on blood donor screening, the seropositive rate among HBsAg-positive blood donors in the United States has been found to be 3.8 percent.[505] Infection with HDV is much more prevalent among intravenous drug users (20 percent-53 percent) and hemophiliacs (48 percent-80 percent).[506]

Three distinct genotypes of hepatitis D have been identified. Genotype I, the most prevalent type, is the most common genotype in the Mediterranean countries, Africa, Europe, and North America.[507-509] It is believed that different subtypes within this genotype may exist in certain parts of Africa. Genotype II is mostly reported in Japan and Taiwan.[510] Genotype II is associated with a milder disease compared to genotype I. Genotype III was isolated from epidemics in South America.[511] Genotypic variations in hepatitis D may also reflect variations in the prevalent HBV subtypes in a particular area. Several reports over the last decade have suggested that the incidence of hepatitis D is decreasing.[512-514] Many epidemiologists have observed that the HDV epidemic that began in the 1970s is declining.[515] In a recent report from Italy the prevalence of antibody to HDV (anti-HDV) was 8.3 percent among 834 patients with chronic hepatitis B[516] in contrast to a 25 percent and 14 percent prevalence reported in 1987 and 1992, respectively.[517,518] The decreasing prevalence of HDV is probably related to vaccination against HBV, use of disposable needles, and improvement in socioeconomic standards. Even though it is on the decline, HDV infection still remains a significant problem among intravenous drug abusers.[519,520] Moreover, areas with high HDV prevalence are being newly identified.

HDV infection is transmissible only if the recipient is a carrier of HBV. In cases of acute co-primary infection, HBV infection needs to be established in the host before HDV infection can occur. In this situation the infectivity of HDV depends on the titer of infecting HBV. Superinfection in a host with previously established HBV infection is much more common than co-infection. Co-primary and superinfections occur because the mode of transmission of HDV is similar to that of HBV. Parenteral transmission is the most efficient mode of spread in non-endemic areas of HBV infection. There is a definite risk of transmitting HDV through blood and blood products. Because of widespread usage of hepatitis B vaccination and screening donor blood for HBsAg, however, the risk of transfusion-associated HDV infection has markedly decreased.[521] Inadvertent parenteral transmission has been reported in households with overcrowding, as evidenced from the genomic homology among members of a household. This is probably a common mode of spread in underdeveloped countries. In the endemic countries of northern South America the most likely route of transmission to children is contact with infected individuals who have skin breaks. The risk of perinatal transmission is extremely low, and infection with HDV is also very uncommon in populations with high rates of childhood and infant HBV infection. In contrast to HBV, sexual transmission is uncommon in developed nations, although it is a significant mode of transmission in endemic areas.[522]

Virology

The HDV genome is a 1.7-Kb single-stranded RNA that is very similar to plant viroids.[523] The genome is folded on itself because of extensive intramolecular base pairing (70 percent) and appears rod-like in configuration. This base pairing is seen among many plant viroids. HDV also contains ribozymes, which are functionally similar to "hammerhead" ribozymes of plant viruses. Unlike these plant agents, however, HDV RNA encodes for a protein-hepatitis delta antigen (HDAg). The virion comprises the HDV genome complexed with several copies of HDAg (approximately 70 copies), surrounded by an envelope protein composed of lipids and HBsAg. The protein envelope protects the HDV RNA–HDAg complex but is not required for replication of HDV.

HDV RNA encodes for only one protein, HDAg, which is produced in two forms—a short form (HDAg-S) and a long form (HDAg-L). The HDAg is translated from an 800-nucleotide (nt) poly-adenylated mRNA. The short form promotes viral replication, whereas the long form inhibits it.[524,525] The exact mechanism by which HDAg-S promotes HDV RNA replication is not clear. HDAg-L is required for packaging the viral RNA in complete virions.[526,527] Even though both forms are encoded by the same region in the anti-genomic sense RNA, they differ in 19 or 20 amino acids at the C terminus. The extra amino acids for HDAg-L are the result of RNA editing that is a unique and essential event in the life cycle of the virus.[528,529] The RNA editing that takes place exclusively in anti-genomic RNA is carried out by double-stranded RNA adenosine deaminase (Figure 32-8) at nucleotide 1012 of the amber/W site.[530,531] This enzyme converts the nucleotide sequence uracil adenosine guanine (UAG) to uracil inosine guanine in the anti-genomic sense RNA that, after a round of initial viral replication, transcribes mRNA in which the HDAg-S stop codon has been converted to a tryptophan codon (UGG), thus allowing synthesis of HDAg-L (Figure 32-12). The extent of RNA editing determines the amount of HDAg-L formed, consequently influencing the rate of replication. In states of high replication no change occurs at nt position 1012 and only HDAg-S is synthesized. Ultimately the intracellular ratio of the S and L forms determines the rate of replication, assembly, and transport out of the infected hepatocyte. Hence RNA editing is a critical step in the replication of HDV genome. HDV RNA is one of the very few RNAs known to be a substrate for editing. Several functional domains of HDAg have been recently elucidated. These include (1) a nuclear localization signal (between 68 and 88 amino acids from the N terminus) involved in intracellular transport of the HDAg-HDV genome complex into the nucleoplasm; (2) an arginine-rich motif for HDV RNA binding (between 95 and 146 amino acids from N terminus); (3) an isoprenylation site, which allows HDAg-L to attach to HBsAg and initiate packaging; and (4) regions for assembly formation of dimers and oligomers.[524,532-537]

HDV enters the host along with its HBsAg envelope. The HDAg/HDV RNA complex migrates to the nucleoplasm aided by the nuclear localization signal. The initial replication takes place in the nucleus of the hepatocyte. HDV is not known to replicate outside hepatocytes. The circular genomic RNA, which is of negative polarity, is transcribed into a linear anti-genomic transcript and mRNA for HDAg. The replication then proceeds according to a double rolling model.[524,532,533] The mechanism of replication and transcription by HDV RNA is unclear but is most likely dependent on host DNA-dependent RNA polymerases because HDV itself does not encode a polymerase and there is no known RNA-dependent RNA polymerase in humans. It is not known how HDV RNA corrupts the host DNA-dependent RNA polymerase to read from an RNA template. The anti-genomic transcript undergoes autocatalytic cleavage by HDV ribozymes and ligation by host-encoded ligase to produce a circular genome of opposite polarity (anti-genomic RNA). This, in turn, replicates and generates negative genomic RNA, thus completing the cycle (see Figure 32-8). As the cycle proceeds further the RNA editing of the anti-genomic RNA changes the stop codon of HDAg-S (U<u>A</u>G) to a tryptophan codon (U<u>G</u>G), allowing continued translation and the synthesis of HDAg-L. The predominance of HDAg-L switches the mode of replication from synthesis to packaging. To accomplish this the C terminus of HDAg-L complexes with proteins in HBsAg and directs the packaging of HDV-genomic RNA and HDAg-S into complete virions.

Taxonomy

HDV is classified under a separate genus of the Deltaviridae family. No other virus has been identified in this genus. The consensus is that HDV is a satellite virus,[538,539]

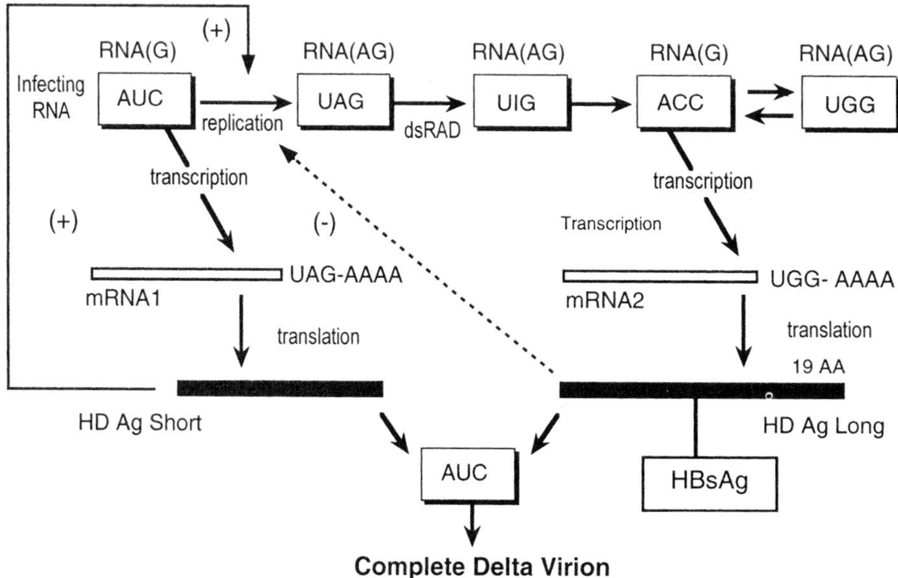

Figure 32-8 Schematic representation of HDV replication and synthesis of delta antigen. mRNA-1 is mRNA for HDsAg-S with a stop codon UAG; mRNA-2 is mRNA for HDAg-L in which stop codon above is changed to UGG, allowing continued translation for another 19 amino acids (see text for details). Boxes represent viral RNA with the nucleotide sequence for editing. *HDV,* Hepatitis delta virus; *mRNA,* messenger ribonucleic acid; *HDsAg-S,* hepatitis delta surface antigen; *G,* genomic RNA; *Ag,* antigenomic RNA; *A,* adenosine; *U,* uracil; *G,* guanosine; *C,* cytosine; *I,* inosine; *AAAA,* polyadenylated tail; *dsRAD,* double-stranded adenosine deaminase; +, positive effect; −, negative effect.

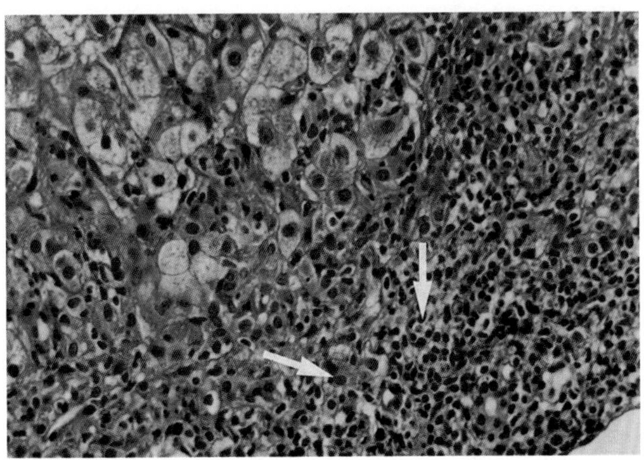

Plate 32-1 Interface hepatitis in a patient with chronic hepatitis B. Arrows indicate areas where Periportal cells are trapped in an inflammatory infiltrate and undergo degenerative changes. (Hematoxylin and eosin; ×400.) (Courtesy of Dr. G. Farr, Ochsner Medical Institutions.)

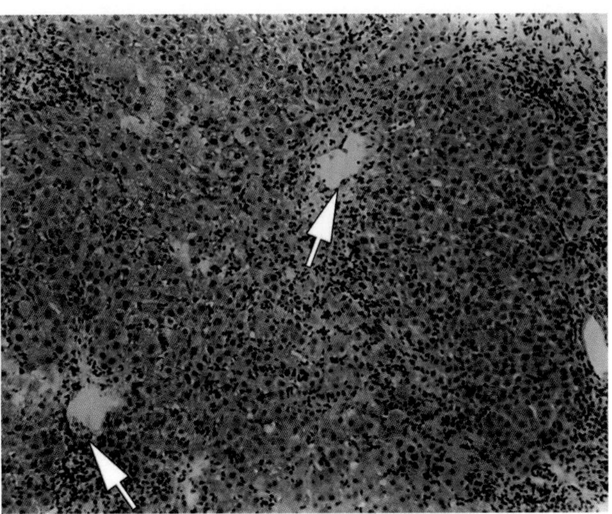

Plate 32-2 Reactivated hepatitis B. Note the diffuse infiltration of liver parenchyma with mononuclear cells and accentuation around central veins *(arrows)* that are reminiscent of changes seen in acute viral hepatitis. (From Perrillo RP: Gastroenterology 120:1009, 2001.)

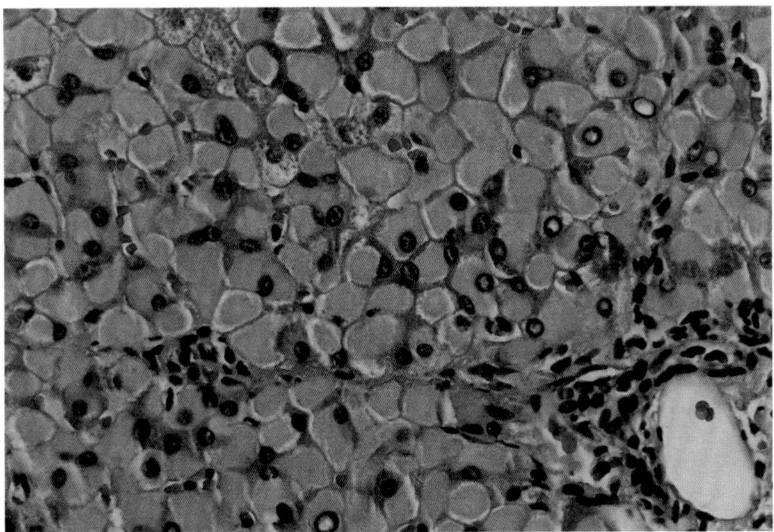

Plate 32-3 Ground-glass hepatocytes in a patient with chronic hepatitis B. (Hematoxylin and eosin; ×400.) (Courtesy of Dr. G. Farr, Ochsner Medical Institutions.)

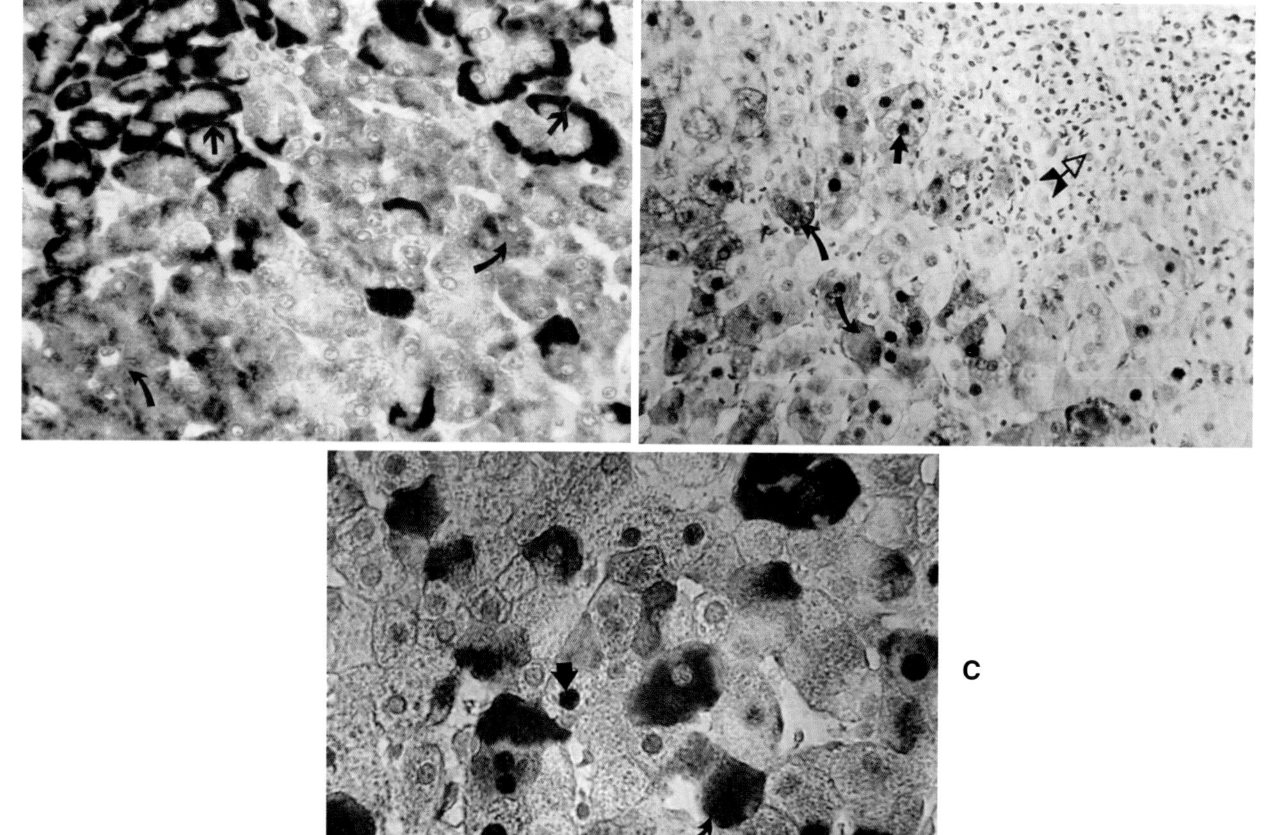

Plate 32-4 Immunohistochemical stains for core and surface antigens in chronic hepatitis B. **A,** Hepatitis B surface antigen is demonstrated in the cytoplasm of hepatocytes *(curved arrows)* with submembranous distribution in some cells *(straight arrows)* (immunoperoxidase stain; ×400.) **B,** Hepatitis B core antigen is found in the cytoplasm *(curved arrows)* and nuclei *(straight arrow)* of hepatocytes. Cytoplasmic core antigen is frequently observed in cases with active liver histology *(open-tip arrow)* (immunoperoxidase stain; ×400). **C,** Hepatitis B core antigen predominantly in nuclei *(straight arrow)* and hepatitis B surface antigen in cytoplasm *(curved arrow)* using rabbit polyclonal antibody to hepatitis B core antigen and murine monoclonal antibody to hepatitis B surface antigen. Note that most hepatocytes demonstrate one or the other antigen and a few stain for both (×400). (**A,** Courtesy of Dr. G. Farr, Ochsner Medical Institutions; **B** and **C,** courtesy of Dr. Nikolai Nauomov, University College, London, England.)

which is a subviral particle that carries a distinct nucleic acid, usually RNA, that requires a helper virus for transmission and multiplication. Satellite viruses should have a nucleic acid that is substantially distinct from the nucleic acid of the helper virus. No other animal virus has been identified as a satellite virus. HDV is not a viroid as previously believed because its RNA codes for the structural protein HDAg.[540]

HDV Genotypes

Three genotypes of HDV are identified: type I, type II, and type III (Table 32-13). As mentioned previously these genotypes have different geographic distribution. In addition, they differ in the disease severity, possibly because of differences in replication ability.[541] Type III produces the most severe disease. Type II is associated with a less severe disease than type I.[542]

A 30 percent to 40 percent sequence variation is observed between different genotypes; a 10 percent to 15 percent variation is observed within genotypes. The genotype specific variations occur at the N terminus of HDAg-S, C terminus of HDAg-L, and around the amber/W RNA editing site.[543] In contrast to this variability, some regions such as the autocleavage sites and sequence-encoding RNA binding sites are highly conserved among all isolates. It is believed that different genotypes may interact variably with different HBV genotypes. The interaction between HDAg-L and HBsAg is mediated by the C-terminal 19 amino acids of HDAg-L. These amino acids are very highly conserved in a genotype but vary considerably between genotypes. The genomic variability may explain specific interactions of certain HDV genotypes with particular HBV genotypes. For example, in northern South America HDV genotype III interacts with HBV genotype F in a consistent pattern.[511] Although infection with HDV genotype III and HBV genotype F has been associated with a clinically severe form of hepatitis, it is not clear if the interaction with HBV genotype F specifically increases the virulence of HDV genotype III.

Pathogenesis of HDV Infection

The pathogenic mechanism of HDV infection remains poorly understood. Because HBV is not known to be directly cytotoxic to hepatocytes, the severity of a combined infection of HBV and HDV may be attributed to either a direct cytotoxic effect of HDV or an enhanced immune response against two viruses. Theoretically, because of similarities between HDV RNA and human RNA, the viral RNA could disrupt the translation process and hence have a direct cytotoxic effect. Reports of small-droplet steatosis in patients with HDV infection,[544] cytoplasmic eosinophilia in chronic carriers,[545] and an apoptotic promoting effect of HDAg in vitro in HeLa and Hep G2 continuous cell lines[546] gave credence to a possible cytotoxic effect of HDV. Recent studies in transgenic mice expressing either long or short forms of the HDAg showed no evidence of hepatocyte injury.[547] In addition, there is no evidence of hepatocyte injury in liver transplant recipients expressing HDAg in the allograft without concurrent HBV expression, raising doubts about the direct cytotoxic potential of the virus.[548,549] The presence of lobular infiltration with lymphocytes in chronic hepatitis D and the finding of liver-kidney microsomal antibodies suggest a role for the host immune system in causing liver injury in HDV infection.[550,551] Other autoantibodies that have been elucidated in HDV infection include antibodies against thymocytes and nuclear lamin C.[552,553] The clinical relevance of the autoantibodies is not clear, and there is no correlation between the antibody titers and severity of infection. Liver-specific autoimmune reactivity was not found to be a mechanism for hepatocyte injury in HDV infection.[554] Epidemiologic data showing severe HDV infection by genotype III, particularly in association with HBV F genotype, underscore the potential importance of HBV in modifying the pathogenicity of HDV. This is further illustrated by the sequence of events occurring after liver transplantation in which HDV infection becomes pathogenic only when recurrent HBV infection develops.[544,545]

Diagnosis of HDV Infection

The most useful markers of HDV infection include HDV antigen, anti-HDV antibody, HDV RNA, and immunohistochemistry in the liver (Table 32-14, Figure 32-9). Detection of HDV RNA by reverse transcriptase PCR amplification (RT-PCR) is the most reliable technique, with nearly 100 percent sensitivity.[555-558] It is also a reliable marker for monitoring the efficacy of treatment and documenting viral eradication. The detection limit of RT-PCR is 50 to 100 copies/ml of virus. Viral RNA can also be detected in the serum and liver by hybridization techniques, which are generally less sensitive than RT-PCR.[558-560] Molecular techniques for partial-sequence homology with the viral genome are available. These are less reliable because of heterogeneity of the viral genome. Among these the most

TABLE 32-13
Genotypes of HDV

Genotype	Efficiency of virion formation*	Disease severity	Distribution
I	2%	Moderate	Worldwide except South America
II	—	Mild	Japan, Taiwan
III	20%	Severe	South America

*As determined by experiments using transfected human hepatoma cell lines.

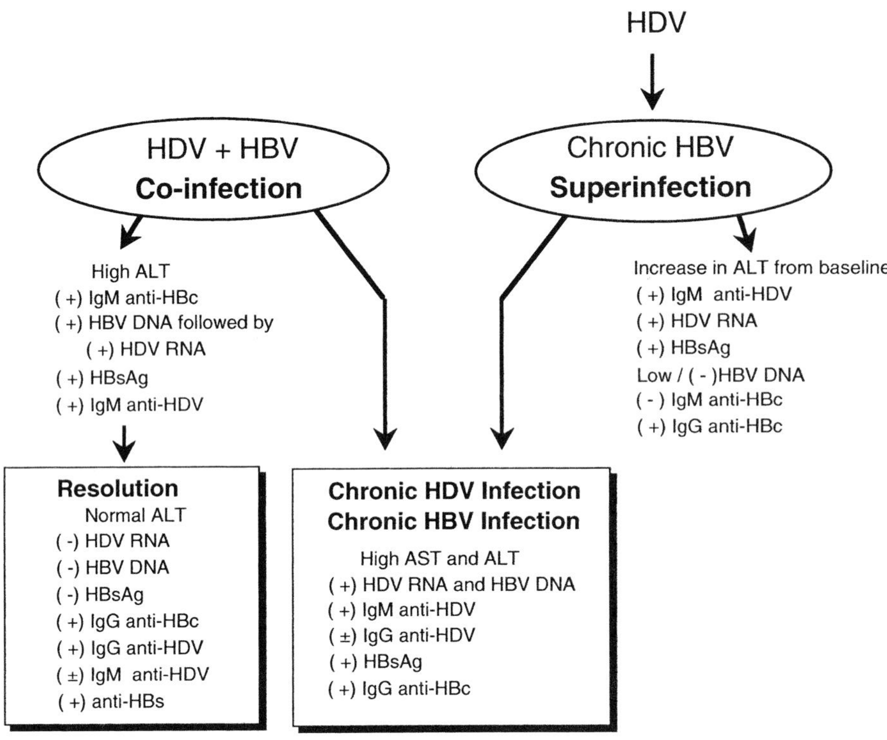

Figure 32-9 Serologic markers in HDV infection (see text for details).

TABLE 32-14

Serologic Tests in HDV Infection

Test	Clinical Utility	Advantages/disadvantages
RT-PCR	Diagnosis Evaluating response to treatment and viral eradication	Sensitive (50-100 copies) but problems with specificity
HDsAg	None	Cumbersome, high rate of false negatives
IgM HDV	Diagnose acute infection	Good sensitivity High titer indicates more severe disease but may be detected in convalescent phase
IgG HDV	Chronic infection	May be detected for prolonged period after resolved infection
IgM anti-HBc	To differentiate co-infection and superinfection	Reliable, readily available but sometimes seen with severe chronic hepatitis B

HDV, Hepatitis D virus; *RT-PCR,* reverse transcriptase PCR amplification; *HDsAg,* hepatitis delta surface antigen; *IgM,* immunoglobulin M; *HDV,* hepatitis D virus; *anti-HBc,* antibody to hepatitis B core.

reliable are the assays using amplification of C-terminal segments of the HDAg coding region of the genome.[561,562]

The HDV genome product, HDAg, is another marker of HDV infection. HDAg can be demonstrated in the hepatocytes by immunohistochemistry, the predictive value of which decreases with chronicity of the disease. Many hepatocytes fail to produce adequate amounts of HDAg as the chronic HDV infection progresses; hence immunohistochemistry may yield negative results. Determination of serum HDAg is also problematic because of the presence of high titers of binding antibodies that interfere with its detection. Immunoblot assays have been shown to be considerably more sensitive when compared to enzyme-linked immunosorbent assays.[563]

The most readily available marker for HDV infection is anti-HDV. Anti-HDV can be detected either as IgM anti-HDV[564] or as total HDV antibody that comprises both IgM and IgG antibodies. IgM anti-HDV appears at the time of acute infection; IgG anti-HDV develops later.[565,566] IgM antibody persists as the infection becomes chronic, which is when it is often detectable in high titers. IgM anti-HDV has been regarded as a marker for serious liver damage.[567] It has been shown that as the infection evolves from an acute form to chronicity, the type of IgM anti-

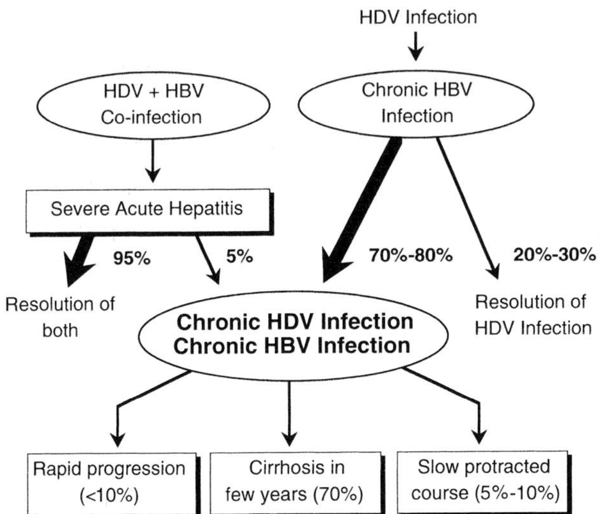

Figure 32-10 Natural history of HDV infection. Note that the vast majority of acute co-primary infections resolve, whereas the majority of superinfections evolve to chronic HDV infection. *HDV,* Hepatitis delta virus.

body also changes from a monomeric (7S) form to a multi-meric form (19S).[568] IgG antibody persists for years in immunocompetent patients and may represent a chronic infection or previous infection. HDV antibodies do not confer any protection against the virus. In a study of 79 patients with detectable HDV RNA in serum by RT-PCR a total anti-HDV titer of 1:100 or greater was found to be an excellent cut off to differentiate acute HDV infection from chronic superinfection.[569] IgM and IgG antibodies can persist even after the infection has resolved and are seen in the absence of detectable HDV RNA. In 43 patients who were positive for total HDV antibody only 21 (49 percent) were found to be positive for HDV RNA by PCR.[570] Similarly, among 199 patients with total HDV antibody only 79 had HDV RNA in the serum.[571] Hence detection of anti-HDV alone may lead to overestimation of the frequency of an active infection.

Natural History of HDV Infection

HDV requires HBV for host infection to occur. As a result, two types of HDV infection are possible. One is a co-primary infection in which there is a simultaneous infection of HBV and HDV. The other represents a superinfection in which HDV is superimposed on an already-established chronic HBV infection (Figure 32-10). Because of its obligate relationship to HBV infection, the natural history of HDV infection is dependent on the clinical course of HBV infection.

Early epidemiologic data suggested that HDV infection increases the severity of hepatitis B and that patients with combined infection had a rapidly progressive course compared to patients with isolated HBV infection.[501-503,572,573] In many parts of the world the prevalence of HDV infection among HBV carriers with severe disease was initially shown to be high. Subsequent studies, however, demonstrated that some patients with hepatitis B and high titer of anti-HDV had normal or near-normal serum aminotransferase levels and normal or minimally disordered hepatic architecture.[571] In a Japanese study of 375 HBsAg-positive patients 13 were HDV RNA–positive (3.5 percent) and all had normal or near-normal liver tests.[574] In a large European multi-center study on prognostic features in patients with chronic hepatitis B and compensated cirrhosis, HDV infection was shown not to influence the prognosis.[41] Also, in a recently published long-term follow-up study of 302 patients with chronic hepatitis B (76 with HDV infection) HDV infection was not found to be an independent predictor of mortality.[42] From these reports it is evident that HDV infection has a variable influence on the course of hepatitis B. The clinical severity of dual infection probably depends on a number of factors, including the endemicity of HDV in a specific area, the degree of HBV viremia, and the genotypes of HBV and of HDV.

In patients developing acute co-infection the natural history of HDV depends on the evolution of HBV infection. Co-infection is most often seen in intravenous drug abusers and less commonly in patients receiving multiple transfusions. Because hepatitis B infection resolves in a majority of patients, HDV also disappears in most patients. Acute HDV infection tends to aggravate the course of acute HBV infection and is more likely to lead to acute fulminant failure. In a European study involving 28 patients with acute fulminant hepatitis B, 14 (50 percent) had evidence of HDV infection, in contrast to 13 of 71 patients (18 percent) with non-fulminant acute hepatitis B.[575] In another report from Greece HDV infection was seen in 52 percent of patients with acute fulminant hepatitis B.[576] Fulminant non-fatal hepatitis was reported in less than 5 percent of 42 patients with HBV and HDV co-infection but because underlying HBV infection was self-limited in the vast majority of cases, almost all patients made a full recovery.[577]

Superinfection of chronic HBV infection with HDV often leads to a very high degree of HDV viremia because HBV infection is already established. Because of high-intensity replication, HDV superinfection leads to a more severe acute hepatitis; on occasion this may lead to fulminant hepatic failure. Appearance of anti-HDV coincides with the peak level of viremia, and HDV replication exerts an inhibitory effect on HBV replication that results in a marked decline in HBV DNA levels in the serum.[578] The rate of HBeAg loss has been reported to be higher in HBV carriers who become superinfected with HDV. For example, in a study in which 28 HBV carriers were superinfected with HDV, 18 (64.3 percent) cleared HBeAg compared to 70 of 214 (32.7 percent) carriers who remained uninfected.[579] Very rarely HDV superinfection may lead to the disappearance of HBsAg.[579]

Chronic HDV infection occurs in 70 percent of superinfected patients; this is characterized by persistent HDV viremia and detectable HDV RNA in the serum. In chronic HDV infection the clinical course can be varied. The most common pattern is persistent replication of HDV and HBV leading to progressive hepatitis that culminates in cirrhosis within a few years. Rarely, particularly among illicit drug users, rapidly progressive liver disease may occur, leading to end-stage liver disease within 2 years.[580,581] In a minority of patients liver disease is slowly progressive. Based on PCR studies in 185 patients it has been proposed that HDV superinfection can be divided into the following three stages: (1) acute phase, characterized by active HDV replication and suppression of HBV with high ALT; (2) chronic phase, with decreasing HDV and reactivating HBV with moderate ALT levels; and (3) late phase, in which patients either develop cirrhosis and hepatocellular carcinoma or enter into a remission resulting from a marked reduction of both viruses.[578]

The role of genotype in determining the course of HDV infections has been recently studied. In northern South America genotype III has been observed to be associated with a particularly severe form of liver disease.[543] Similarly, the chronic healthy HDV carrier state has been reported in Greek patients who are infected with a mutant HDV in which there has been a change from serine to asparagine at amino acid position 170.[582] The clinical course of a triple infection with HBV, HDV, and HCV is usually dominated by HCV. Such triple infection presents with a more severe acute hepatitis in the context of HDV or HCV superinfection, but the chronic stage is slowly progressive and does not substantially differ from chronic HCV infection alone.[583]

In liver transplant recipients a latent type of HDV infection has been reported in which HDV is expressed in hepatocytes in the absence of HBV.[548,584] Such cases are due to very low expression of HBV in the allograft rather than a true autonomous infection.[584] The latent infection is usually silent but develops into clinical hepatitis after HBV infection becomes established in the allograft.[548]

Clinical Features

Clinical features of HDV infection vary depending on whether it is a co-infection or a superinfection. In addition, the replication status of HBV also influences HDV infection and expression of HDV markers.

Acute co-primary infection typically presents with a self-limited acute hepatitis, which is clinically indistinguishable from other types of viral hepatitis. Some patients may show a double peaking in serum aminotransferase levels resulting from a delay in HDV replication after HBV replication. Acute hepatitis usually resolves in a few weeks with gradual normalization of liver tests. Serologic markers that are detectable at this time include anti-IgM HBc antibody, IgM anti-HDV, HDV RNA, HBV DNA, and HBsAg. As the infection resolves, the HDV RNA and HBV DNA titers steadily decrease and anti-HBs appears. IgM anti-HDV may persist for a longer time, even after the appearance of anti-HBs and normalization of aminotransaminases. On certain occasions, the replication markers of HBV may not be evident because of a profound inhibitory effect of HDV on HBV replication.[549] In such cases the only clue in diagnosing recent HBV infection may be the presence of IgM anti-HBc. In less than 5 percent of patients the illness evolves into a chronic hepatitis characterized by persistently abnormal transaminase levels, persistence of HBsAg, rising titer of antibodies to HDV, and persistent detection of HDV RNA in serum (see Figure 32-9).

Superinfection is characterized clinically as an acute hepatitis in an otherwise stable chronic HBV carrier. The hepatitis may be very severe because of high-intensity HDV replication in a host with already-established HBV infection. Hepatitis may at times progress into fulminant failure.[585] An acute flare in serum aminotransferase levels may also be due to reactivated HBV infection and needs to be distinguished on serologic grounds. The serologic features for superinfection include HDV RNA, IgM anti-HDV, and HBsAg and IgG anti-HBc. HBV DNA is usually suppressed and may be seen only in low levels. In both acute co-infection and superinfection, IgM anti-HDV is detected; hence the distinguishing serologic feature for co-infection is the presence of IgM anti-HBc.[586]

Chronic HDV infection is almost always the result of a superinfection because co-infection seldom leads to chronic infection. Histologically, chronic delta hepatitis is characterized by periportal inflammation, interface hepatitis, lobular inflammation, and varying degree of fibrosis. Cirrhosis is not an uncommon finding. Significant liver disease may be seen in asymptomatic patients.[587,588]

Treatment

Because HDV requires an established and active HBV infection, therapies for chronic HDV have centered on an effective treatment for hepatitis B. Because anti-viral therapy often fails to eradicate HBsAg, the only protein of HBV on which HDV depends, it may compromise the ability of these treatments to be effective against HDV.

Several clinical trials have examined the efficacy of IFN and lamivudine in the treatment of chronic HDV infection (Table 32-15).[589-597] Farci and colleagues randomized 42 patients with chronic HDV hepatitis into three arms: 14 patients received 9 million units of IFN alfa-2a three times weekly for 48 weeks; a second group of patients received IFN alfa-2a 3 million units three times a week for 48 weeks; and the third group did not receive treatment.[589] At the end of treatment 71 percent of patients who received 9 million units normalized serum ALT levels and 50 percent had a complete response (normalization of ALT and disappearance of HDV RNA). These patients also had marked improvement in periportal necrosis and lobular inflammation. Most patients, however, had a virologic relapse, although some (5 of 14) had a sustained biochemical response during 4 years of follow-up. In another study 61 patients were randomized to either IFN alfa-2b (5 million units/m^2 three times weekly for 4 months followed by 3 million units/m^2 three times weekly for 8 months) or no treatment.[590] Most of the treated patients failed to show any improvement in HDV RNA levels or intrahepatic HDAg despite biochemical and histologic improvement. Other smaller studies also have yielded similar results, with biochemical improvement in 50 percent to 70 percent of patients without any sustained virologic remission.[592-594] In many trials, especially those using higher dosages of IFN, psychiatric alterations were the major adverse event reported.

IFN treatment of chronic HDV infection in children has been disappointing.[598,599] The biochemical response and virologic response were similar to those of the adult patients with a significant relapse after cessation of treatment. Long-term treatment (24 months) did not show a greater therapeutic benefit. Treatment response

TABLE 32-15

Summary of Clinical Trials in Chronic HDV Infection

Investigator, year (patient no.) (reference no.)	Treatment	Dosage	Results
Rosina et al, 1991 (n = 61)* (590)	IFN alfa-2b	5 MU/m^2 TIW for 4 months Followed by 3 MU/m^2 TIW for 8 months	Decrease in hepatic inflammation (ALT) No effect on HDV RNA or HDAg in liver cells
Madejon et al, 1994 (n = 32)* (593)	IFN alfa-2a	18 MU TIW × 6 months followed by 9 MU TIW, 6 MU TIW (each × month) then 3 MU TIW × 4 months versus 3 MU daily for 3 months followed by 1.5 MU daily for 9 months	Normalization of ALT (31% in high dose, 12% in low dose) but no change in HDV RNA
Di Bisceglie et al, 1990 (n = 12) (594)	IFN alfa-2b	5 MU/day for at least 4 months	Decrease in ALT and HDV RNA Relapse within 6 months
Farci et al, 1994 (n = 42)* (589)	IFN alfa-2a	9 MU TIW for 48 weeks versus 3 MU TIW for 48 weeks	Normalization in ALT and HDV RNA in 50% of patients Improvement in histology Relapse common
Gaudin et al, 1995 (n = 22)* (592)	IFN alfa-2b	5 MU TIW for 4 months followed by 3 MU TIW for 8 months	Significant decrease in ALT and RNA High rate of relapse
Lau et al, 1999 (n = 5) (596)	Lamivudine	100 mg/day for 12 months	Decrease in HBV DNA but no effect on RNA or histology
Wolters et al, 2000 (n = 8) (595)	Lamivudine IFN + lamivudine	100 mg/day for 24 weeks followed by high-dose IFN and 9 MU TIW maintenance	Transient decrease in HDV RNA without meaningful change in histology

HDV, Hepatitis D virus; *IFN,* interferon; *TIW,* three times a week; *ALT,* alanine aminotransferase; *RNA,* ribonucleic acid; *HDAg,* hepatitis delta antigen: *DNA,* deoxyribonucleic acid.
*Randomized controlled trials.

in patients with HDV and HIV is very poor. Biochemical response is only seen in 10 percent to 15 percent of patients. In an open-labeled study using high-dose IFN (10 million units three times weekly for 6 months and 6 million units three times weekly for the next 6 months) 16 patients with HIV and HDV infection and 21 with HDV infection alone were treated. A sustained response was noted in one patient in the HIV-infected group.[600] Patients who are co-infected with HCV also appear to have low response rates.[341]

The currently preferred treatment strategy for chronic HDV infection is 5 to 9 million units of IFN three times a week for 12 months. It may be prudent to prolong treatment for a longer time (18-24 months) to prevent the relapse. There is no consensus, however, on the dosage and duration of IFN treatment necessary to achieve an optimal sustained virologic response.

The clinical experience with IFN has not led to identification of variables that are predictive of a biochemical or virologic response. Unlike the situation with HBV infection, there is no relationship of response to the pretreatment ALT or viral load. Therapy should be continued for a year before considering the patient a treatment failure. In several studies IFN treatment of patients who are HDV infected has resulted in suppression of HBV replication as evidenced by disappearance of HBV DNA and HBeAg. This treatment, however, has had limited effects on inducing a sustained clearance of HDV RNA. Because HDV depends on HBsAg, only therapies that can result in the disappearance of the HBV envelope protein are likely to achieve sustained HDV clearance.[341,597]

Two small studies have evaluated the efficacy of lamivudine either alone or in combination with IFN.[596,597] Both of these studies have failed to show any benefit in eradicating HDV despite effective suppression of HBV DNA. Considering the limited ability of lamivudine to result in HBsAg clearance, it is unlikely to be an effective treatment for chronic HDV. Other anti-virals such as acyclovir and ribavirin have been tried without any success. Suramin prevents entry of HDV into the hepatocyte but is too toxic to be used as a viable treatment option.[601] Advances in molecular biology may help to identify specific inhibitors of viral replication.[602] Prenylation of HDAg-L is a critical determinant of HDV particle assembly, and in vitro studies have shown that inhibition of prenylation can effectively abolish particle production in a dose-dependent manner.[603]

Prevention

Successful vaccination with hepatitis B vaccine effectively prevents HDV transmission. The recently described decline in HDV prevalence in Southern Europe is attributed mainly to widespread vaccination. No vaccine is currently available for HDV infection although experiments in woodchucks using recombinant HDAg and vaccinia virus expressing either large or small HDAg have shown some promise.[604,605]

References

1. Maynard JE: Hepatitis B: global importance and need for control. Vaccine 8(suppl):S18, 1990.
2. Gust ID: Epidemiology of hepatitis B infection in the Western Pacific and South East Asia. Gut 38(suppl 2):S18, 1996.
3. Alter M: Epidemiology and disease burden of hepatitis B and C. Antiviral Ther 1(suppl 3):9, 1996.
4. Lee WM: Hepatitis B virus infection. N Engl J Med 337:1733, 1997.
5. Okada K, Kamiyama I, Inomata M, et al: E antigen and anti-E in the serum of asymptomatic carrier mothers as indicators of positive and negative transmission of hepatitis B virus to their infants. N Engl J Med 294:746, 1976.
6. Hwang LY, Roggendorf M, Beasley RP, et al: Perinatal transmission of hepatitis B virus: role of maternal HBeAg and anti-HBc IgM. J Med Virol 15:265, 1985.
7. Perrillo RP, Gelb L, Campbell C, et al: Hepatitis B e antigen, DNA polymerase activity, and infection of household contacts with hepatitis B virus. Gastroenterology 76:1319, 1979.
8. Alter MJ, Ahtone J, Maynard JE: Hepatitis B virus transmission associated with a multiple-dose vial in a hemodialysis unit. Ann Intern Med 99:330, 1983.
9. Harpaz R, Von Seidlein L, Averhoff FM, et al: Transmission of hepatitis B virus to multiple patients from a surgeon without evidence of inadequate infection control. N Engl J Med 334:549, 1996.
10. Limentani AE, Elliott LM, Noah ND, et al: An outbreak of hepatitis B from tattooing. Lancet 2:86, 1979.
11. Berry WR, Gottesfeld RL, Alter HJ, et al: Transmission of hepatitis B virus by artificial insemination. JAMA 257:1079, 1987.
12. Hoofnagle JH: Posttransfusion hepatitis B. Transfusion 30:384, 1990.
13. Dickson RC, Everhart JE, Lake JR, et al: Transmission of hepatitis B by transplantation of livers from donors positive for antibody to hepatitis B core antigen. The National Institute of Diabetes and Digestive and Kidney Diseases Liver Transplantation Database. Gastroenterology 113:1668, 1997.
14. Katchaki JN, Siem TH, Brouwer R, et al: Detection and signficance of anti-HBc in the blood bank; preliminary results of a controlled prospective study. J Virol Methods 2:119, 1980.
15. Cossart YE, Kirsch S, Ismay SL: Post-transfusion hepatitis in Australia. Report of the Australian Red Cross Study. Lancet 1:208, 1982.
16. Alter HJ, Seeff LB, Kaplan PM, et al: Type B hepatitis: the infectivity of blood positive for e antigen and DNA polymerase after accidental needlestick exposure. N Engl J Med 295:909, 1976.
17. Mason A, Wick M, White H, et al: Hepatitis B virus replication in diverse cell types during chronic hepatitis B virus infection. Hepatology 18:781, 1993.
18. Mason A, Yoffe B, Noonan C, et al: Hepatitis B virus DNA in peripheral-blood mononuclear cells in chronic hepatitis B after HBsAg clearance. Hepatology 16(1):36, 1992.
19. Kuhns M, McNamara A, Mason A, et al: Serum and liver hepatitis B virus DNA in chronic hepatitis B after sustained loss of surface antigen. Gastroenterology 103:1649, 1992.
20. Hollinger FB: Comprehensive control (or elimination) of hepatitis B virus transmission in the United States. Gut 38(suppl 2):S24, 1996.
21. Alter M: Presented at 51st Annual Meeting of the American Association for the Study of Liver Disease, Dallas, Tex., 2000.
22. McQuillan GM, Coleman PJ, Kruszon-Moran D, et al: Prevalence of hepatitis B virus infection in the United States: the National Health and Nutrition Examination Surveys, 1976 through 1994. Am J Public Health 89:14, 1999.
23. Szmuness W, Harley EJ, Ikram H, et al: Sociodemographic aspects of the epidemiology of hepatitis B. In Vyas GN, Cohen SN, Schmid R, eds: Viral Hepatitis. Philadelphia, Franklin Institute Press, 1978:297.
24. Kaur S, Rybicki L, Bacon BR, et al: Performance characteristics and results of a large-scale screening program for viral hepatitis and risk factors associated with exposure to viral hepatitis B and C: results of the National Hepatitis Screening Survey. National Hepatitis Surveillance Group. Hepatology 24:979, 1996.
25. Hoofnagle JH, Shafritz DA, Popper H: Chronic type B hepatitis and the "healthy" HBsAg carrier state. Hepatology 7:758, 1987.
26. Feinman SV, Cooter N, Sinclair JC, et al: Clinical and epidemiological significance of the HBSAg (Australia antigen): carrier state. Gastroenterology 68:113, 1975.
27. De Franchis R, D'Arminio A, Vecchi M, et al: Chronic asymptomatic HBsAg carriers: histologic abnormalities and diagnostic and prognostic value of serologic markers of the HBV. Gastroenterology 79:521, 1980.
28. Chang M-H: Hepatitis B: long-term outcome and benefits from mass vaccination in children. Acta Gastroenterol Belg 61:210-213, 1998.
29. Lee WM: Acute liver failure. N Engl J Med 329:1862-1872, 1993.
30. Lee WM: Acute viral hepatitis in the United States. Presented at the AASLD Postgraduate Course Oct 27, 2000, Dallas, Tex.
31. Schiodt FV, Atillasoy E, Shakil AO, et al: Etiology and outcome for 295 patients with acute liver failure in the United States. Liver Transpl Surg 5:29, 1999.
32. Samuel D, Muller R, Alexander G, et al: Liver transplantation in European patients with the hepatitis B surface antigen. N Engl J Med 329:1842, 1993.
33. Todo S, Demetris AJ, Van Thiel D, et al: Orthotopic liver transplantation for patients with hepatitis B virus-related liver disease. Hepatology 13:619, 1991.
34. Chau KH, Hargie MP, Decker RH, et al: Serodiagnosis of recent hepatitis B infection by IgM class anti-HBc. Hepatology 3:142, 1983.
35. Zuckerman AJ: Progress towards the comprehensive control of hepatitis B. Gut 38(suppl 2):S1, 1996.
36. Villeneuve JP, Desrochers M, Infante-Rivard C, et al: A long-term follow-up study of asymptomatic hepatitis B surface antigen-positive carriers in Montreal. Gastroenterology 106:1000, 1994.
37. Weissberg JI, Andres LL, Smith CI, et al: Survival in chronic hepatitis B. An analysis of 379 patients. Ann Intern Med 101:613, 1984.
38. Cardenas CL, Soetikno R, Robinson WS, et al: Long-term follow-up of patients with chronic hepatitis B: a 25 year prospective study. Hepatology 30:300A, 1999 (abstract).
39. Fattovich G, Brollo L, Giustina G, et al: Natural history and prognostic factors for chronic hepatitis type B. Gut 32:294, 1991.
40. de Jongh FE, Janssen HLA, de Man RA, et al: Survival and prognostic indicators in hepatitis B surface antigen-positive cirrhosis of the liver. Gastroenterology 103:1630, 1992.
41. Realdi G, Fattovich G, Hadziyannis S, et al: Survival and prognostic factors in 366 patients with compensated cirrhosis type B: a multicenter study. The Investigators of the European Concerted Action on Viral Hepatitis (EUROHEP). J Hepatol 21:656, 1994.
42. Di Marco V, Lo Iacono O, Camma C, et al: The long-term course of chronic hepatitis B. Hepatology 30:257, 1999.
43. Fattovich G, Giustina G, Schalm SW, et al: Occurrence of hepatocellular carcinoma and decompensation in Western European patients with cirrhosis type B. The EUROHEP Study Group on Hepatitis B Virus and Cirrhosis. Hepatology 21:77, 1995.
44. Niederau C, Heintgen T, Lange S, et al: Long-term follow-up of HBeAg-positive patients treated with interferon alfa for chronic hepatitis B. N Engl J Med 334:1422, 1996.
45. Realdi G, Alberti A, Rugge M, et al: Seroconversion from hepatitis B e antigen to anti-HBe in chronic hepatitis B virus infection. Gastroenterology 79:195, 1980.
46. Perrillo RP, Tamburro C, Regenstein F, et al: Low-dose, titratable interferon alfa-2b in decompensated liver disease caused by chronic infection with hepatitis B virus. Gastroenterology 109:908, 1995.
47. Villeneuve JP, Condreay LD, Willems B, et al: Lamivudine treatment for decompensated cirrhosis resulting from chronic hepatitis B. Hepatology 31:207, 2000.
48. Perrillo RP, Wright T, Rakela J, et al: A multicenter US-Canadian trial to assess lamivudine monotherapy before and after liver transplantation for chronic hepatitis B. Hepatology 33:424, 2001.
49. Robinson WS: Hepadnaviridae and their replication. In Fields BN, Knipe DM, eds: Fields Virology, vol 2. New York, Raven Press, 1990:2137.
50. Tiollais P, Pourcel C, Dejean A: The hepatitis B virus. Nature 317:489, 1985.
51. Nowak MA, Bonhoeffer S, Hill AM, et al: Viral dynamics in hepatitis B virus infection. Proc Natl Acad Sci U SA 93:4398, 1996.

52. Gunther S, Sommer G, Plikat U, et al: Naturally occurring hepatitis B virus genomes bearing the hallmarks of retroviral G to A hypermutation. Virology 235:104, 1997.
53. Yeh CT, Chien RN, Chu CM, et al: Clearance of the original hepatitis B virus YMDD-motif mutants with emergence of distinct lamivudine-resistant mutants during prolonged lamivudine therapy. Hepatology 31:1318, 2000.
54. De Meyer S, Gong ZJ, Suwandhi W, et al: Organ and species specificity of hepatitis B virus (HBV) infection: a review of the literature with a special reference to preferential attachment of HBV to human hepatocytes. J Viral Hepatol 4:145, 1997.
55. Tuttleman JS, Pourcel C, Summers JW: Formation of the pool of covalently closed circular viral DNA in hepadnavirus-infected cells. Cell 47:451, 1986.
56. Mason WS, Aldrich C, Summers J, et al: Asymmetric replication of duck hepatitis B virus DNA in liver cells: free minus strand DNA. Proc Natl Acad Sci U S A 79:3997, 1982.
57. Chisari FV, Filippi P, Buras J, et al: Structural and pathological effects of synthesis of hepatitis B virus large envelope polypeptide in transgenic mice. Proc Natl Acad Sci U S A 84:6909, 1987.
58. Nakamoto Y, Guidotti LG, Kuhlen C, et al: Immune pathogenesis of hepatocellular carcinoma. J Exp Med 188:341, 1998.
59. Nishioka K, Levin AG, Simmons MJ: Hepatitis B antigen, antigen subtypes, and hepatitis B antibody in normal subjects and patients with liver disease. Bull World Health Organ 52:293, 1975.
60. Norder H, Courouce AM, Magnius LO: Complete genomes, phylogenetic relatedness, and structural proteins of six strains of the hepatitis B virus, four of which represent two new genotypes. Virology 198:489, 1994.
61. Lindh M, Andersson AS, Gusdal A: Genotypes, nt 1858 variants, and geographic origin of hepatitis B virus—large-scale analysis using a new genotyping method. J Infect Dis 175:1285, 1997.
62. Kao J-H, Chen P-J, Lai M-Y, Chen D-S: Hepatitis B genotypes correlate with clinical outcomes in patients with chronic hepatitis B. Gastroenterology 118:554, 2000.
63. Mayerat C, Mantegani, Frei PC: Does hepatitis B virus (HBV) genotype influence the clinical outcome of HBV infection? J Viral Hepat 6:299, 1999.
64. Orito E, Mizokami M, Sakugawa H, et al: A case-control study for clinical and molecular biological differences between hepatitis B viruses of genotypes B and C. Hepatology 33:218, 2001.
65. Carman WF, Trautwein C, Van Deursen FJ, et al: Hepatitis B virus envelope variation after transplantation with and without hepatitis B immune globulin prophylaxis. Hepatology 24:489, 1996.
66. Hsu H-Y, Chang M-H, Ni Y-H, et al: Surface gene mutants of hepatitis B virus in infants who develop acute or chronic infections despite immunoprophylaxis. Hepatology 26:786, 1997.
67. Hsu H-Y, Chang M-H, Liaw S-H, et al: Changes of hepatitis B surface antigen variants in carrier children before and after universal vaccination in Taiwan. Hepatology 30:1312, 1999.
68. Ghany MG, Ayola B, Villamil FG, et al: Hepatitis B virus S mutants in liver transplant recipients who were reinfected despite hepatitis B immune globulin prophylaxis. Hepatology 27:213, 1998.
69. Pollicino T, Zanetti AR, Cacciola I, et al: Pre-S2 defective hepatitis B virus infection in patients with fulminant hepatitis. Hepatology 26:495, 1997.
70. Hunt CM, McGill JM, Allen MI, et al: Clinical relevance of hepatitis B viral mutations. Hepatology 31:1037, 2000.
71. Buckwold VE, Xu Z, Chen M, et al: Effects of a naturally occurring mutation in the hepatitis B virus basal core promoter on precore gene expression and viral replication. J Virol 70:5845, 1996.
72. Brunetto MR, Stemler M, Schodel F, et al: Identification of HBV variants which cannot produce precore derived HBeAg and may be responsible for severe hepatitis. Ital J Gastroenterol Hepatol 21:151, 1989.
73. Li J, Buckwold VE, Hon MW, Ou JH: Mechanism of suppression of hepatitis B virus precore RNA transcription by a frequent double mutation. J Virol 73:1239, 1999.
74. Milich DR, Jones JE, Hughes JL, et al: Is a function of the secreted hepatitis B e antigen to induce immunologic tolerance in utero? Proc Natl Acad Sci U S A 87:6599, 1990.
75. Bertoletti A, Sette A, Chisari FV, et al: Natural variants of cytotoxic epitopes are T-cell receptor antagonists for antiviral cytotoxic T cells. Nature 369:407, 1994.
76. Hou J, Lau GK, Cheng J, et al: T1762/A1764 variants of the basal core promoter of hepatitis B virus; serological and clincal correlations in Chinese patients. Liver 19:411, 1999.
77. Bozkaya H, Akarca US, Ayola B, et al: High degree of conservation in the hepatitis B virus core gene during the immune tolerant phase in perinatally acquired chronic hepatitis B infection. J Hepatol 26:508, 1997.
78. Brunetto MR, Giarin M, Saracco G, et al: Hepatitis B virus unable to secrete e antigen and response to interferon in chronic hepatitis B. Gastroenterology 105:845, 1993.
79. Naoumov NV, Thomas MG, Mason AL, et al: Genomic variations in the hepatitis B core gene: a possible factor influencing response to interferon alfa treatment. Gastroenterology 108:505, 1995.
80. Fattovich G, McIntyre G, Thursz M, et al: Hepatitis B virus precore/core variation and interferon therapy. Hepatology 22:1355, 1995.
81. Maruyama T, Mitsui H, Maekawa H, et al: Emergence of the precore mutant late in chronic hepatitis B infection correlates with the severity of liver injury and mutations in the core region. Am J Gastroenterol 95:2894, 2000.
82. Lindh M, Horal P, Dhillon AP, et al: Hepatitis B virus carriers without precore mutations in hepatitis B e antigen-negative stage show more severe liver damage. Hepatology 24:494, 1996.
83. Grandjacques C, Pradat P, Stuyver L, et al: Rapid detection of genotypes and mutations in the pre-core promoter and the pre-core region of hepatitis B virus genome: correlation with viral persistence and disease severity. J Hepatol 33:430, 2000.
83a. Lok AS, Akarca U, Greene S: Mutations in the pre-core region of hepatitis B virus serve to enhance the stability of the secondary structure of the pre-genome encapsidation signal. Proc Natl Acad Sci U S A 91:4077, 1994.
84. Atkins M, Hunt CM, Brown N, et al: Clinical significance of YMDD mutant hepatitis B virus (HBV) in a large cohort of lamivudine-treated hepatitis B patients. Hepatology 28:398A, 1998.
84a. Chang TT, Liaw YF, Guan R, et al: Incremental increases in HBeAg seroconversion and continued ALT normalization in Asian chronic HBV patients treated with lamivudine for four years (abstract). Antivir Ther 5(suppl 1):44, 2000.
85. Melegari M, Scaglioni PP, Wands JR: Hepatitis B virus mutants associated with 3TC and famciclovir administration are replication defective. Hepatology 27:628, 1998.
86. Aye TT, Bartholomeusz AI, Shaw T, et al: Hepatitis B virus polymerase mutations during antiviral therapy in a patient following liver transplantation. J Hepatol 26 (5):1148, 1997.
86a. Stuyver LJ, Locarnini SA, Lok A, et al: Nomenclature for antiviral-resistant human hepatitis virus mutations in the polymerase region. Hepatology 33:751, 2001.
87. Prost S, Ford JM, Taylor C, et al: Hepatitis B x protein inhibits p53-dependent DNA repair in primary mouse hepatocytes. J Biol Chem 273:33327, 1998.
88. Sirma H, Giannini C, Poussin K, et al: Hepatitis B virus X mutants, present in hepatocellular carcinoma tissue abrogate both the antiproliferative and transactivation effects of HBx. Oncogene 18:4848, 1999.
88a. Wei Y, Tiollais P: Molecular biology of hepatitis B virus. Clin Liver Dis 3:189, 1999.
89. Sitterlin D, Bergametti F, Tiollais P, et al: Correct binding of viral X protein to UVDDB-p127 cellular protein is critical for efficient infection by hepatitis B viruses. Oncogene 19:4427, 2000.
90. Menne S, Tennant B: Unraveling hepatitis B infection of mice and men (and woodchucks and ducks). Nat Med 5:1125, 1999.
91. Curry MP, Koziel M: The dynamics of the immune response in acute hepatitis B: new lessons using new techniques. Hepatology 32:117, 2000.
92. Bertoletti A, Ferrari C, Fiaccadori F, et al: HLA claa I-restricted human cytotoxic T cells recognize endogenously synthesized hepatitis B virus nucleocapsid antigen. Proc Natl Acad Sci U S A 88:10445, 1991.
93. Koziel M: The immunopathogenesis of HBV infection. Antivir Ther 3(suppl 3):13-24, 1998.
94. Guidotti LG, Rochford R, Chung J, et al: Viral clearance without destruction of infected cells during acute HBV infection. Science 284:825, 1999.
95. Koziel MJ: Cytokines in viral hepatitis. Semin Liv Disease 19:157, 1999.

96. Webster GJM, Reignat S, Maini MK, et al: Incubation phase of acute hepatitis B in man: dynamic of cellular immune mechanisms. Hepatology 32:1117, 2000.
97. Chisari FV: Immunopathogenesis of hepatitis B. Presented at AASLD Postgraduate Course, Oct 28, 2000, Dallas, Tex.
98. Ferrari C, Bertoletti A, Penna A, et al: Identification of immunodominant T cell epitopes of the hepatitis B virus nucleocapsid antigen. J Clin Invest 88:214, 1991.
99. Penna A, Artini M, Cavalli A, et al: Long-lasting memory T cell responses following self-limited acute hepatitis B. J Clin Invest 98:1185, 1996.
100. Ferrari C, Mondelli MU, Penna A, et al: Functional characterization of cloned intrahepatic, hepatitis B virus nucleoprotein-specific helper T cell lines. J Immunol 139:539, 1987.
101. Boni C, Bertoletti A, Penna A, et al: Lamivudine treatment can restore T cell responsiveness in chronic hepatitis B. J Clin Invest 102:968, 1998.
102. Tough DF, Borrow P, Sprent J: Induction of bystander T cell proliferation by viruses and type I interferons in vivo. Science 272:1947, 1996.
103. Maini MK, Boni C, Lee CK, et al: The role of virus-specific CD8+ cells in liver damage and viral control during persistent hepatitis B infection. J Exp Med 191:1269, 2000.
104. Marinos G, Torre F, Chokshi S, et al: Induction of T-helper cell reponse to hepatitis B core antigen in chronic hepatitis B: a major factor in activation of the host immune response to the hepatitis B virus. Hepatology 22:1040, 1995.
105. Rehermann B, Lau D, Hoofnagle JH, et al: Cytotoxic T lymphocyte responsiveness after resolution of chronic hepatitis B virus infection. J Clin Invest 97:1655, 1996.
106. Boni C, Penna A, Ogg GS, et al: Lamivudine treatment can overcome cytotoxic T cell hyporesponsiveness in chronic hepatitis B: new perspectives for immune therapy. Hepatology 33:963, 2001.
107. Patel T, Gores GJ: Apoptosis and hepatobiliary disorders. Hepatology 21:1725, 1995.
108. Lau JYN, Xie X, Lai MMC, et al: Apoptosis and viral hepatitis. Semin Liver Dis 18:169, 1998.
109. Kim H, Lee H, Yun Y: X-gene product of hepatitis B virus induced apoptosis in liver cells. J Biol Chem 273:381, 1998.
110. Tabor E, Purcell RH, London WT, et al: Use of and interpretation of results using inocula of hepatitis B virus with known infectivity titers. J Infect Dis 147:531, 1983.
111. Liaw YF, Yeh CT, Tsai SL: Impact of acute hepatitis B superinfection on chronic hepatitis C virus infection. Am J Gastroenterol 95:2978, 2000.
112. Gocke DJ: Extrahepatic manifestations of viral hepatitis. Am J Med Sci 270:49, 1975.
113. Krugman S, Overby LR, Mushahwar IK, et al: Viral hepatitis type B. Studies on natural history and prevention-re-examined. N Engl J Med 300:101, 1979.
114. Lindsay KL, Redeker AG, Ashcavai M: Delayed HBsAg clearance in chronic hepatitis B viral infection. Hepatology 1:586, 1981.
115. Stevens CE, Beasley RP, Tsui J, et al: Vertical transmission of hepatitis B antigen in Taiwan. N Engl J Med 292:771, 1975.
116. Beasley RP, Hwang LY, Lin CC, et al: Incidence of hepatitis B virus infections in preschool children in Taiwan. J Infect Dis 146:198, 1982.
117. Tassopoulos NC, Papaevangelou GJ, Sjogren MH, et al: Natural history of acute hepatitis B surface antigen-positive hepatitis in Greek adults. Gastroenterology 92:1844, 1987.
118. Rehermann B, Folwler P, Sidney J, et al: The cytotoxic T lymphocyte response to multiple hepatitis B virus polymerase epitopes during and after acute viral hepatitis. J Exp Med 181:1047, 1995.
119. Rehermann B, Ferrari C, Pasquinelli C, et al: The hepatitis B virus persists for decades after patients' recovery from acute viral hepatitis despite active maintenance of a cytotoxic T-lymphocyte response. Nat Med 2:1104, 1996.
120. Gimson AE, O'Grady J, Ede RJ, et al: Late onset hepatic failure: clinical, serologic and histologic features. Hepatology 6:288, 1986.
121. Peters RL: Viral hepatitis: a pathologic spectrum. Am J Med Sci 270:17, 1975.
122. Wright TL, Mamish D, Combs C, et al: Hepatitis B virus and apparent fulminant non-A, non-B hepatitis. Lancet 339:952, 1992.
123. Omata M, Ehata T, Yokosuka O, et al: Mutations in the precore region of hepatitis B virus DNA in patients with fulminant and severe hepatitis. N Engl J Med 324:1699, 1991.
124. Tassopoulos NC, Sjogren MH, Purcell RH: 19S and 7-8S forms of IgM antibody to hepatitis B core antigen in acute icteric hepatitis superimposed on hepatitis B surface antigen carriage. Infection 18(6):376, 1990.
125. Lok ASF, Lai CL: alpha-Fetoprotein monitoring in Chinese patients with chronic hepatitis B virus infection: role in the early detection of hepatocellular carcinoma. Hepatology 9:110, 1989.
126. Williams AL, Hoofnagle JH: Ratio of serum aspartate to alanine aminotransferase in chronic hepatitis. Relationship to cirrhosis. Gastroenterology 95:734, 1988.
127. Seeff LB: Diagnosis, therapy, and prognosis of viral hepatitis. In Zakim, D, Boyer TD, eds: Hepatology. A Textbook of Liver Disease, ed 3. Philadelphia, WB Saunders Company, 1996:1067-1145.
128. Onion DK, Crumpacker CS, Gilliland BC: Arthritis of hepatitis associated with Australia antigen. Ann Intern Med 75:29, 1971.
129. Wands JR, Mann E, Alpert E, et al: The pathogenesis of arthritis associated with acute-hepatitis-B surface antigen-positive hepatitis. Complement activation and characterization of circulating immune complexes. J Clin Invest 55:930, 1975.
130. Duffy J, Lidsky MD, Sharp JT, et al: Polyarthritis, polyarteritis and hepatitis B. Medicine (Baltimore) 55:19, 1976.
131. Willson RA: Extrahepatic manifestations of chronic viral hepatitis. Am J Gastroenterol 92:3, 1997.
132. Guillevin L, Lhote F, Jarrousse B, et al: Polyarteritis nodosa related to hepatitis B virus. A prospective study of 66 patients. Ann Med Interne (Paris) 143:63, 1992.
133. McMahon BJ, Heyward WL, Templin DW, et al: Hepatitis B-associated polyarteritis nodosa in Alaskan Eskimos: clinical and epidemiologic features and long-term follow-up. Hepatology 9:97, 1989.
134. Michalak T: Immune complexes of hepatitis B surface antigen in the pathogenesis of periarteritis nodosa. A study of seven necropsy cases. Am J Pathol 90:619, 1978.
135. Guillevin L, Lhote F, Cohen P, et al: Polyarteritis nodosa related to hepatitis B virus. A prospective study with long-term observation of 41 patients. Medicine (Baltimore) 74:238, 1995.
136. Scott DGI, Bacon PA, Elliott PJ, et al: Systemic vasculitis in a district general hospital 1972-1980: clinical and laboratory features, clarification and prognosis in 80 cases. Q J Med 51(203):292, 1982.
137. Guillevin L, Lhote F, Gayraud M, et al: Prognostic factors in polyarteritis nodosa and Churg-Strauss syndrome. Medicine 75:17, 1996.
138. Safadi R, Almog Y, Dranitzki-Elhalel M, et al: Glomerulonephritis associated with acute hepatitis B. Am J Gastroenterol 91:138, 1996.
139. Eknoyan G, Gyorkey F, Dichoso C, et al: Renal morphological and immunological changes associated with acute viral hepatitis. Kidney Int 1:413, 1972.
140. Glassock RJ: Immune complex induced glomerular injury in viral diseases: an overview. Kidney Int 40(suppl 35):5, 1991.
141. Morzycka M, Slusarczyk J: Kidney glomerular pathology in various forms of acute and chronic hepatitis. Arch Pathol Lab Med 103:38, 1979.
142. Takehoshi Y, Tanaka M, Shida N, et al: Strong association between membranous nephropathy and hepatitis-B surface antigenemia in Japanese children. Lancet 2:1065, 1987.
143. Johnson RJ, Couser WG: Hepatitis B infection and renal disease: clinical, immunopathogenetic and therapeutic considerations. Kidney Int 37:663, 1990.
144. Venkataseshan VS, Liberman K, Kim DU, et al: Hepatitis-B-associated glomerulonephritis: pathology, pathogenesis, and clinical course. Medicine 69:200, 1990.
145. Dienstag JL: Hepatitis B as an immune complex disease. Semin Liver Dis 1:45, 1981.
146. Lai KN, Li PK, Lui SF, et al: Membranous nephropathy related to hepatitis B virus in adults. N Engl J Med 324:1457, 1991.
147. Popp JW, Dienstag JL, Wands JR, et al: Essential mixed cryoglobulinemia without evidence for hepatitis B virus infection. Ann Intern Med 92:379, 1980.
148. Monti G, Galli M, Invernizzi F, et al: Cryoglobulinaemias: a multicenter study of the early clinical and laboratory manifestations of primary and secondary disease. GISC. Italian Group for the Study of Cryoglobulinaemias. Q J Med 88:115, 1995.
149. Lunel F, Musset L, Cacoub P, et al: Cryoglobulinemia in chronic liver diseases: role of hepatitis C virus and liver damage. Gastroenterology 106:1291, 1994.

150. Hadziyannis S, Gerber MA, Vissoulis C, et al: Cytoplasmic hepatitis B antigen in "ground-glass" hepatocytes of carriers. Arch Pathol 96:327-30, 1973.
151. Gerber MA, Hadziyannis S, Vissoulis C, et al: Electron microscopy and immunoelectronmicroscopy of cytoplasmic hepatitis B antigen in hepatocytes. Am J Pathol 75:489-502, 1974.
152. Shikata T, Uzawa T, Yoshiwara N, et al: Staining methods of Australia antigen in paraffin section—detection of cytoplasmic inclusion bodies. Jpn J Exp Med 44:25-36, 1974.
153. Gerber MA, Hadziyannis S, Vernace S, et al: Incidence and nature of cytoplasmic hepatitis B antigen in hepatocytes Lab Invest 32:251, 1975.
153a. Chu C-M, Liaw Y-F: Intrahepatic distribution of hepatitis B surface and core antigens in chronic hepatitis B virus infection. Gastroenterology 92:220, 1987.
154. Rehermann B: Immunopathogenesis of viral hepatitis. Baillieres Clin Gastroenterol 10:483, 1996.
155. Davis GL, Hoofnagle JH: Reactivation of chronic type B hepatitis presenting as acute viral hepatitis. Ann Intern Med 102:762, 1985.
156. Mels GC, Bellati G, Leandro G, et al: Fluctuations in viremia, aminotransferases and IgM antibody to hepatitis B core antigen in chronic hepatitis B patients with disease exacerbations. Liver 14:175, 1994.
157. Perrillo RP, Campbell CR, Sanders GE, et al: Spontaneous clearance and reactivation of chronic hepatitis B virus infection among male homosexuals with chronic type B hepatitis. Ann Intern Med 100:43, 1984.
158. Davis GL, Hoofnagle JH: Reactivation of chronic hepatitis B virus infection. Gastroenterology 92:2028, 1987.
159. Hoofnagle JH, Seeff LB: Natural history of chronic type B hepatitis. Prog Liver Dis 7:469, 1982.
160. Seeff LB, Koff RS: Evolving concepts of the clinical and serologic consequences of hepatitis B virus infection. Semin Liver Dis 6:11, 1986.
161. Liaw YF, Tsai SL: Pathogenesis and clinical significance of spontaneous exacerbations and remissions in chronic hepatitis B virus infection. Viral Hepatitis 3:143, 1997.
162. Gupta S, Govindarajan S, Fong TL, Redeker AG: Spontaneous reactivation in chronic hepatitis B: patterns and natural history. J Clin Gastroenterol 12:562, 1990.
163. Bortolotti F, Cadrobbi P, Crivellaro C, et al: Long-term outcome of chronic type B hepatitis in patients who acquire hepatitis B virus infection in childhood. Gastroenterology 99:805, 1990.
164. Lok ASF, Lai CL, Wu PC, et al: Spontaneous hepatitis B e antigen to antibody seroconversion and reversion in Chinese patients with chronic hepatitis B virus infection. Gastroenterology 92:1839, 1987.
165. Liaw YF: Hepatitis viruses under immunosuppressive agents. J Gastroenterol Hepatol 13:14, 1998.
166. Hoofnagle JH, Dusheiko GM, Schafer DF, et al: Reactivation of chronic hepatitis B virus infection by cancer chemotherapy. Ann Intern Med 96:447, 1982.
167. Thung SN, Gerber MA, Klion F, et al: Massive hepatic necrosis after chemotherapy withdrawal in a hepatitis B virus carrier. Arch Intern Med 145:1313, 1985.
168. Wands JR, Chura CM, Roll FJ, et al: Serial studies of hepatitis-associated antigen and antibody in patients receiving antitumor chemotherapy for myeloproliferative and lymphoproliferative disorders. Gastroenterology 68:105, 1975.
169. Galbraith RM, Eddleston AL, Williams R, et al: Fulminant hepatic failure in leukaemia and choriocarcinoma related to withdrawal of cytotoxic drug therapy. Lancet 2:528, 1975.
170. Alexopoulos CG, Vaslamatzis M, Hatzidimitriou G: Prevalence of hepatitis B virus marker positivity and evolution of hepatitis B virus profile, during chemotherapy, in patients with solid tumors. Br J Cancer 81:69, 1999.
171. Lau JYN, Lai CL, Lin HJ, et al: Fatal reactivation of chronic hepatitis B virus infection following withdrawal of chemotherapy in lymphoma patients. Q J Med 73:911, 1989.
172. Lok ASF, Liang RHS, Chiu EKW, et al: Reactivation of hepatitis B virus replication in patients receiving cytotoxic therapy. Report of a prospective study. Gastroenterology 100:182, 1991.
173. Perrillo RP: Acute flares in chronic hepatitis B: the natural and unnatural history of an immunologically mediated liver disease. Gastroenterology 120:1009, 2001.
174. Liang RHS, Lok ASF, Lai CL, et al: Hepatitis B infection in patients with lymphomas. Hematol Oncol 8:261, 1990.
175. Liang R, Lau GKK, Kwong YL: Chemotherapy and bone marrow transplantation for cancer patients who are also chronic hepatitis B carriers: a review of the problem. J Clin Oncol 17:394, 1999.
176. Nagington J: Reactivation of hepatitis B after transplantation operations. Lancet 1:558, 1977.
177. Pariente EA, Goudeau A, Dubois F, et al: Fulminant hepatitis due to reactivation of chronic hepatitis B virus infection after allogeneic bone marrow transplantation. Dig Dis Sci 33:1185, 1988.
178. Marcellin P, Giostra E, Martinot-Peignoux M, et al: Redevelopment of hepatitis B surface antigen after renal transplantation. Gastroenterology 100:1432, 1991.
179. Blanpain C, Knoop C, Delforge ML, et al: Reactivation of hepatitis B after transplantation in patients with pre-existing anti-hepatitis B surface antigen antibodies: report on three cases and review of the literature. Transplantation 66:883, 1998.
180. Stamenkovic SA, Alphonso N, Rice P, et al: Recurrence of hepatitis B after single lung transplantation. J Heart Lung Transplant 18:1246, 1999.
181. Lau GKK, Liang R, Chiu EKW, et al: Hepatic events after bone marrow transplantation in patients with hepatitis B infection: a case controlled study. Bone Marrow Transplant 19:795, 1997.
182. Davies SE, Portmann BC, O'Grady JG, et al: Hepatic histological findings after transplantation for chronic hepatitis B virus infection, including a unique pattern of fibrosing cholestatic hepatitis. Hepatology 13:150, 1991.
183. Mason AL, Wick M, White HM, et al: Increased hepatocyte expression of hepatitis B virus transcription in patients with features of fibrosing cholestatic hepatitis. Gastroenterology 105:237, 1993.
184. Peters M, Davis GL, Dooley JS, et al: The interferon system in acute and chronic viral hepatitis. Prog Liver Dis 8:453, 1986.
185. Alexander GJM, Brahm J, Fagan EA, et al: Loss of HBsAg with interferon therapy in chronic hepatitis B virus infection. Lancet 2:66, 1987.
186. Perrillo RP, Schiff ER, Davis GL, et al: A randomized, controlled trial of interferon alfa-2b alone and after prednisone withdrawal for the treatment of chronic hepatitis B. The Hepatitis Interventional Therapy Group. N Engl J Med 323:295, 1990.
187. Hoofnagle JH, Di Bisceglie AM, Waggoner JG, et al: Interferon alfa for patients with clinically apparent cirrhosis due to chronic hepatitis B. Gastroenterology 104:1116, 1993.
188. Dienstag JL, Schiff ER, Wright TL, et al: Lamivudine as initial treatment for chronic hepatitis B in the United States. N Engl J Med 341:1256, 1999.
189. Seigneres B, Pichoud C, Ahmed SS, et al: Evolution of hepatitis B virus polymerase gene sequence during famciclovir therapy for chronic hepatitis B. J Infect Dis 181:1221, 2000.
190. Glaxo Wellcome, data on file.
191. Hultgren C, Weiland O, Milich DR, et al: Cell-mediated immune responses and loss of hepatitis B e-antigen (HBeAg) during successful lamivudine and famciclovir combination therapy for chronic replicating hepatitis B virus infection. Clin Infect Dis 29:1575, 1999.
192. Honkoop P, de Man RA, Heijtink RA, et al: Hepatitis B reactivation after lamivudine (letter). Lancet 346:1156, 1995.
193. Chayama K, Suzuki Y, Kobayashi M, et al: Emergence and takeover of YMDD motif mutant hepatitis B virus during long-term lamivudine therapy and re-takeover by wild type after cessation of therapy. Hepatology 27:1711, 1998.
194. Scullard GH, Smith CI, Merigan TC, et al: Effects of immunosuppressive therapy on viral markers in chronic active hepatitis B. Gastroenterology 81:987, 1981.
195. Nair PV, Tong MJ, Stevenson D, et al: Effects of short-term, high-dose prednisone treatment of patients with HBsAg-positive chronic active hepatitis. Liver 5:8, 1985.
196. Rakela J, Redeker AG, Weliky B: Effect of short-term prednisone therapy on aminotransferase levels and hepatitis B virus markers in chronic type B hepatitis. Gastroenterology 84:956, 1983.
197. Perrillo RP, Regenstein FG, Bodicky CJ, et al: Comparative efficacy of adenine arabinoside 5′ monophosphate and prednisone withdrawal followed by adenine arabinoside 5′ monophosphate in the treatment of chronic active hepatitis type B. Gastroenterology 88:780, 1985.
198. Krogsgaard K, Marcellin P, Trepo C, et al: Prednisolone withdrawal therapy enhances the effect of human lymphoblastoid interferon

in chronic hepatitis B. INTREPED Trial Group. J Hepatol 25:803, 1996.
199. Liaw YF, Chien RN: Case report: dramatic response to lamivudine therapy following corticosteroid priming in chronic hepatitis B. J Gastroenterol Hepatol 14:804, 1999.
200. Liaw YF, Tsai SL, Chien RN, et al: Prednisolone priming enhances Th1 response and efficacy of subsequent lamivudine therapy in patients with chronic hepatitis B. Hepatology 32:604, 2000.
201. Hanson RG, Peters MG, Hoofnagle JH: Effects of immunosuppressive therapy with prednisolone on B and T lymphocyte function in patients with chronic type B hepatitis. Hepatology 6:173, 1986.
202. Perrillo RP: Antiviral therapy of chronic hepatitis B: past, present, and future. J Hepatol 17(suppl 3):S56, 1993.
203. Sheen IS, Liaw YF, Lin SM, et al: Severe clinical rebound upon withdrawal of corticosteroid before interferon therapy: incidence and risk factors. J Gastroenterol Hepatol 11:143, 1996.
204. Buti M, Esteban R, Esteban JI, et al: Severe hepatic failure after ARA-A prednisolone for chronic type B hepatitis (letter). Gastroenterology 92:274, 1987.
205. Laskus T, Slusarczyk J, Cianciara J, et al: Exacerbation of chronic active hepatitis type B after short-term corticosteroid therapy resulting in fatal liver failure. Am J Gastroenterol 85:1414, 1990.
206. Brunetto MR, Giarin MM, Oliveri F, et al: Wild-type and e antigen-minus hepatitis B viruses and course of chronic hepatitis. Proc Natl Acad Sci U S A.88:4186, 1991
207. Brunetto MR, Gorin JM, Civitico G, et al: Pre-core/core gene mutants of hepatitis B virus: pathogenetic implications. In Rizzetto M, Purcell RH, Gerin JL, Verme G, eds: Viral Hepatitis and Liver Disease: Proceedings of IX Triennial International Symposium on Viral Hepatitis and Liver Disease. Turin, Italy, Edizioni Minerva Medica, 1997:127.
208. Oketani M, Oketani K, Xiaohong C, et al: Low level wild-type and pre-core mutant hepatitis B viruses and HBeAg negative reactivation of chronic hepatitis B. J Med Virol 58:332, 1999.
209. Lindh M, Gustavson C, Mardberg K, et al: Mutation of nucleoside 1,762 in the core promoter region during hepatitis B e seroconversion and its relation to liver damage in hepatitis B e antigen carriers. J Med Virol 55:185, 1998.
210. Gerner P, Lausch E, Friedt M, et al: Hepatitis B virus core promoter mutations in children with multiple anti-HBe/HBeAg reactivations result in enhanced promoter activity. J Med Virol 59:415, 1999.
211. Inoue K, Yoshiba M, Sekiyama K, et al: Clinical and molecular virological differences between fulminant hepatic failures following acute and chronic infection with hepatitis B virus. J Med Virol 55:35, 1998.
212. Steinberg JL, Yeo W, Zhong S, et al: Hepatitis B virus reactivation in patients undergoing cytotoxic chemotherapy for solid tumours: precore/core mutations may play an important role. J Med Virol 60:249, 2000.
213. Allen MI, Gauthier J, DesLauriers M, et al: Two sensitive PCR-based methods for detection of hepatitis B virus variants associated with reduced susceptibility to lamivudine. J Clin Microbiol 37:3338, 1999.
214. Perrillo R, Rakela J, Dienstag J, et al: Multicenter study of lamivudine therapy for hepatitis B after liver transplantation. Lamivudine Transplant Group. Hepatology 29:1581, 1999.
215. Liaw YF, Chien RN, Yeh CT, et al: Acute exacerbation and hepatitis B virus clearance after emergence of YMDD motif mutation during lamivudine therapy. Hepatology 30:567, 1999.
216. Fukumoto Y, Okita K, Konishi T, et al: Hepatitis A infection in chronic carriers of hepatitis B virus. In Sung JL, Chen DS, eds: Viral Hepatitis and Hepatocellular Carcinoma. Amsterdam: Excerpta Medica, 1990:46.
217. Vento S, Garofano T, Renzini C, et al: Fulminant hepatitis associated with hepatitis A virus superinfection in patients with chronic hepatitis C. N Engl J Med 338:286, 1998.
218. Zachoval R, Roggendorf M, Deinhardt F: Hepatitis A infection in chronic carriers of hepatitis B virus. Hepatology 3:528, 1983.
219. Tassopoulos N, Papaevangelou G, Roumeliotou-Karayannis A, et al: Double infections with hepatitis A and B viruses. Liver 5:348, 1985.
220. Yao G: Clinical spectrum and natural history of viral hepatitis A in a 1988 Shanghai epidemic. In Hollinger FB, Lemon SM, Margolis H, eds: Viral Hepatitis and Liver Disease: Proceedings of the 1990 International Symposium on Viral Hepatitis and Liver Disease: Contemporary Issues and Future Prospects. Baltimore, Williams & Wilkins, 1991:76.
221. Medile A, Farci P, Verme G, et al: Influence of delta infection on severity of hepatitis B. Lancet 2:945, 1982.
222. Hadziyannis SJ: Hepatitis delta: an overview. In Rizzetto M, Purcell RH, Gerin JL, Verme G, eds: Viral Hepatitis and Liver Disease: Proceedings of IX Triennial International Symposium on Viral Hepatitis and Liver Disease. Turin, Italy, Edizioni Minerva Medica, 1997:283.
223. Chu CM, Yeh CT, Liaw YF: Fulminant hepatic failure in acute hepatitis C: increased risk in chronic carriers of hepatitis B virus. Gut 45:613, 1999.
224. Liaw YF, Tsai SL, Chang JJ, et al: Displacement of hepatitis B virus by hepatitis C virus as the cause of continuing chronic hepatitis. Gastroenterology 106:1048, 1994.
225. Chu CM, Liaw YF, Pao CC, et al: The etiology of acute hepatitis superimposed upon previously unrecognized asymptomatic HBsAg carriers. Hepatology 9:452, 1989.
226. Dulbecco R, Ginsberg HS: Interference with viral multiplication. In Davis BD, Dulbecco R, Eisen HN, et al, eds: Microbiology. New York: Harper and Row, 1973:1172.
227. Keeffe EB: Is hepatitis A more severe in patients with chronic hepatitis B and other chronic liver diseases? Am J Gastroenterol 90:201, 1995.
228. Fong TL, Di Bisceglie AM, Waggoner JG, et al: The significance of antibody to hepatitis C virus in patients with chronic hepatitis B. Hepatology 14:64, 1991.
229. Krogsgaard K, Kryger P, Aldershvile J, et al: Delta-infection and suppression of hepatitis B virus replication in chronic HBsAg carriers. Hepatology 7:42, 1987.
230. Liaw YF, Chien RN, Chen TJ, et al: Concurrent hepatitis C virus and hepatitis delta virus superinfection in patients with chronic hepatitis B virus infection. J Med Virol 37:294, 1992.
231. Sheen IS, Liaw YF, Chu CM, et al: Role of hepatitis C virus infection in spontaneous hepatitis B surface antigen clearance during chronic hepatitis B virus infection. J Infect Dis 165:831, 1992.
232. Perrillo RP, Regenstein FG, Roodman ST: Chronic hepatitis B in asymptomatic homosexual men with antibody to the human immunodeficiency virus. Ann Intern Med 105:382, 1986.
233. Krogsgaard K, Lindhardt BO, Nielson JO, et al: The influence of HTLV-III infection on the natural history of hepatitis B virus infection in male homosexual HBsAg carriers. Hepatology 7:37, 1987.
234. Caredda F, Antinori S, Coppin P, et al: The influence of human immunodeficiency virus infection on acute and chronic HBsAg-positive hepatitis. Prog Clin Biol Res 364:365, 1991.
235. Carr A, Cooper DA: Restoration of immunity to chronic hepatitis B infection in an HIV-infected patient on protease inhibitor (letter). Lancet 349:995, 1997.
236. Proia LA, Ngui SW, Kaur S, et al: Reactivation of hepatitis B in patients with human immunodeficiency virus infection treated with combination antiretroviral therapy. Am J Med 108:249, 2000.
237. Hoofnagle JH, Schafer DF: Serologic markers of hepatitis B virus infection. Semin Liver Dis 6:1, 1986.
238. Perrillo RP, Chau KH, Overby LR, et al: Anti-hepatitis B core immunoglobulin M in the serologic evaluation of hepatitis B virus infection and simultaneous infection with type B, delta agent, and non-A, non-B viruses. Gastroenterology 85:163, 1983.
239. Tsang TK, Blei AT, O'Reilly DJ, et al: Clinical significance of concurrent hepatitis B surface antigen and antibody positivity. Dig Dis Sci 31:620, 1986.
240. Shiels MT, Taswell HF, Czaja AJ, et al: Frequency and significance of concurrent hepatitis B surface antigen and antibody in acute and chronic hepatitis. Gastroenterology 93:675, 1987.
241. Bonino F, Colloredo Mels G, Bellati G, et al: Problems in diagnosing viral hepatitis. Gut 34(suppl 2):S36, 1993.
242. Brunetto MR, Cerenzia MT, Oliveri F, et al: Monitoring the natural course and response to therapy of chronic hepatitis B with an automated semi-quantitative assay for IgM anti-HBc. J Hepatol 19:431, 1993.
243. Douglas DD, Taswell HF, Rakela J, et al: Absence of hepatitis B virus DNA detected by polymerase chain reaction in blood donors who are hepatitis B surface antigen negative and antibody to hepatitis B core antigen positive from a United States population with a low prevalence of hepatitis B serologic markers. Transfusion 33:212, 1993.

244. McMahon BJ, Parkinson AJ, Helminiak C, et al: Response to hepatitis B vaccine of persons positive for antibody to hepatitis B core antigen. Gastroenterology 103:590, 1992.
245. Lok AS, Lai CL, Wu PC: Prevalence of isolated antibody to hepatitis B core antigen in an area endemic for hepatitis B virus infection: implications in hepatitis B vaccination programs. Hepatology 8: 766, 1988.
246. Wang J-T, Wang T-H, Sheu J-C, et al: Detection of hepatitis B virus DNA by polymerase chain reaction in plasma of volunteer blood donors negative for hepatitis B surface antigen. J Infect Dis 163:397, 1991.
247. Jilg W, Sieger E, Zachoval R, et al: Individuals with antibodies against hepatitis B core antigen as the only serological marker for hepatitis B infection: high percentage of carriers of hepatitis B and C virus. J Hepatol 23:14, 1995.
248. Noborg U, Gusdal A, Horal P, et al: Levels of viraemia in subjects with serological markers of past or chronic hepatitis B virus infection. Scand J Infect Dis 32:249, 2000.
249. Thiers V, Nakajima E, Kremsdorf D, et al: Transmission of hepatitis B from hepatitis-B-seronegative subjects. Lancet ii:1273, 1988.
250. Mosley JW, Stevens CE, Aach RD, et al: Donor screening for antibody to hepatitis B core antigen and hepatitis B virus infection in transfusion recipients. Transfusion 35:5, 1995.
251. Wachs ME, Amend WJ, Ascher NL, et al: The risk of transmission of hepatitis B from HBsAg(-), HBcAb(+), HBIgM(-) organ donors. Transplantation 59:230, 1995.
252. Dodson SF, Issa S, Araya V, et al: Infectivity of hepatic allografts with antibodies to hepatitis B virus. Transplantation 64:1582, 1997.
253. Paterlini P, Gerken G, Nakajima E, et al: Polymerase chain reaction to detect hepatitis B virus DNA and RNA sequences in primary liver cancers from patients negative for hepatitis B surface antigen. N Engl J Med 323:80, 1990.
254. Brechot C, Jaffredo F, Lagorce D, et al: Impact of HBV, HCV, and GBV-C/HGV on hepatocellular carcinomas in Europe: results of a European concerted action. J Hepatol 29:173, 1998.
255. Fukai K, Yokosuka O, Fujiwara K, et al: Etiologic considerations of fulminant non-A, non-B viral hepatitis in Japan: analyses by nucleic acid amplification method. J Infect Dis 178(2):325, 1998.
256. Nielsen JO, Juhl E, Dietrichson O: Incidence and meaning of the "e" determinant among hepatitis-B-antigen positive patients with acute and chronic liver diseases. Lancet ii: 913, 1974.
257. Aikawa T, Furuta S, Shikata T, et al: Seroconversion from hepatitis B e antigen to anti-HBe in acute hepatitis B virus infection. N Engl J Med 298:439, 1978.
258. Lok ASF, Lai CL: A longitudinal follow-up of asymptomatic hepatitis B surface antigen-positive Chinese children. Hepatology 8:1130, 1988.
259. Hoofnagle JH, Dusheiko GM, Seeff LB, et al: Seroconversion from hepatitis B e antigen to antibody in chronic type B hepatitis. Ann Intern Med 94:744, 1981.
260. Bonino F, Rosina F, Rizzetto M, et al: Chronic hepatitis in HBsAg carriers with serum HBV-DNA and anti-HBe. Gastroenterology 90:1268, 1986.
261. Carman WF, Hadziyannis S, McGarvey MJ, et al: Mutation preventing formation of hepatitis B e antigen in patients with chronic hepatitis B infection. Lancet 2:588, 1989.
262. Lok ASF, Hadziyannis SJ, Weller IV, et al: Contribution of low level HBV replication to continuing inflammatory activity in patients with anti-HBe positive chronic hepatitis B virus infection. Gut 25:1283, 1984.
263. Kapke G, Watson G, Sheffler S, et al: Comparison of the Chiron Quantiplex branched DNA (bDNA) assay and the Abbott Genostics solution hybridization assay for quantification of hepatitis B viral DNA. J Viral Hepat 4:67, 1997.
264. Krajden M, Waldron J, Comanor L, et al: Effect of HBV genotype on viral load quantification. J Hepatol 30(suppl 1): 125, 1999 (abstract).
265. Hendricks DA, Stowe BJ, Hoo BS, et al: Quantitation of HBV DNA in human serum using a branched DNA (bDNA) signal amplification assay. Am J Clin Pathol 104:537, 1995.
266. Zaaijer HL, ter Borg F, Cuypers HT, et al: Comparison of methods for detection of hepatitis B virus DNA. J Clin Microbiol 32(9):2088, 1994.
267. Fong TL, Di Bisceglie AM, Gerber MA, et al: Persistence of hepatitis B virus DNA in the liver after loss of HBsAg in chronic hepatitis B. Hepatology 18:1313, 1993.
268. Hope RL, Weltman M, Dingley J, et al: Interferon alfa for chronic active hepatitis B. Long term follow-up of 62 patients: outcomes and predictors of response. Med J Aust 162(1):8, 1995.
269. Perrillo RP, Schalm SW, Schiff ER, et al: Predictors of HBeAg seroconversion in chronic hepatitis B patients treated with lamivudine. Hepatology 30:317A, 1999 (abstract).
270. Chien R-N, Liaw Y-F, Atkins M: Pretherapy alanine aminotransferase level as a determinant for hepatitis B e antigen seroconversion during lamivudine therapy in patients with chronic hepatitis B. Asian Hepatitis Lamivudine Trial Group. Hepatology 30:770, 1999.
271. Mutimer D, Pillay D, Dragon E, et al: High pre-treatment serum hepatitis B virus titre predicts failure of lamivudine prophylaxis and graft re-infection after liver transplantation. J Hepatol 30:715, 1999.
272. Brechot C, Degos F, Lugassy C, et al: Hepatitis B virus DNA in patients with chronic liver disease and negative tests for hepatitis B surface antigen. N Engl J Med 312:270, 1985.
273. Wong DK, Cheung AM, O'Rourke K, et al: Effect of alpha-interferon treatment in patients with hepatitis B e antigen-positive chronic hepatitis B. A meta-analysis. Ann Intern Med 119:312, 1993.
274. Davis GL, Hoofnagle JH: Interferon in viral hepatitis: role in pathogenesis and treatment. Hepatology 6:1038, 1986.
275. Peters M, Vierling J, Gershwin ME, et al: Immunology and the liver. Hepatology 13:977, 1991.
276. Baglioni C: 2′5′-oligo (A) pathway of interferon action. In Baron S, Stanton GJ, Freischmann WR, eds: The Interferon System: A Current Review to 1987. Austin, Tex., University of Texas Press, 1987.
277. Peters M: Mechanisms of action of interferons. Semin Liver Dis 9:235, 1989.
278. Peters M: Immunological aspects of antiviral therapy. Springer Semin Immunopathol 12:47, 1990.
279. Pignatelli M, Waters J, Brown D, et al: HLA class I antigens of the hepatocyte membrane during recovery from acute hepatitis B infection and during interferon therapy in chronic hepatitis B virus infection. Hepatology 6:349, 1986.
280. Kirchner H: Interferons, a group of multiple lymphokines. Springer Semin Immunopathol 7:347, 1984.
281. Scully LJ, Brown D, Lloyd C, et al: Immunological studies before and during interferon therapy in chronic HBV infection: identification of factors predicting response. Hepatology 12:1111, 1990.
282. Ijzermans JN, Marquet RL: Interferon-gamma: a review. Immunobiology 179:456, 1989.
283. Perrillo RP: Interferon in the management of chronic hepatitis B. Dig Dis Sci 38:577, 1993.
284. Castilla A, Prieto J, Fausto N: Transforming growth factors beta 1 and alpha in chronic liver disease. Effects of interferon alfa therapy. N Engl J Med 324:933, 1991.
285. Rothstein KD, Munoz SJ: Interferon and other therapies for hepatitis B and C infections. Clin Lab Med 16:465, 1996.
286. Wong DKH, Heathcote J: The role of interferon in the treatment of viral hepatitis. Pharmacol Ther 63:177, 1994.
287. Wright TL, Lau JYN: Clinical aspects of hepatitis B virus infection. Lancet 342:1340, 1993.
288. Oliveri F, Colombatto P, Bonino F, et al: Impact of interferon-alpha therapy on the development of hepatocellular carcinoma in patients with liver cirrhosis: results of an international survey. J Viral Hepat 4(suppl 2):79, 1997.
289. Mazzella G, Accogli E, Sottili S, et al: Alpha interferon treatment may prevent hepatocellular carcinoma in HCV-related cirrhosis. J Hepatol 24:141, 1996.
290. Conlon KC, Urba WJ, Smith JW, et al: Exacerbation of symptoms of autoimmune disease in patients recieving alpha-interferon therapy. Cancer 65:2237, 1990.
291. Brook MG, Karayiannis P, Thomas HC: Which patients with chronic hepatitis B virus infection will respond to alpha-interferon therapy? A statistical analysis of predictive factors. Hepatology 10:761, 1989.
292. Perrillo RP, Regenstein FG, Peters MG, et al: Prednisone withdrawal followed by recombinant alpha interferon in the treatment of chronic type B hepatitis: a randomized controlled trial. Ann Intern Med 109:95, 1988.
293. Lok ASF, Lai CL, Wu PC, et al: Alpha-interferon treatment in Chinese patients with chronic hepatitis B. J Hepatol 11:S121, 1990.
294. McDonald JA, Caruso L, Karayiannis P, et al: Diminished responsiveness of male homosexual chronic hepatitis B virus carriers

with HTLV-III antibodies to recombinant alpha-interferon. Hepatology 7:719, 1987.

295. Novick DM, Lok ASF, Thomas HC: Diminished responsiveness of homosexual men to antiviral therapy for HBsAg-positive chronic liver disease. J Hepatol 1:29, 1985.
296. Krogsgaard K, Bindslev N, Christensen E, et al: The treatment effect of alpha interferon in chronic hepatitis B is independent of pre-treatment variables. Results based on individual patient data from 10 clinical controlled trials. European Concerted Action on Viral Hepatitis (Eurohep). J Hepatol 21:646, 1994.
297. Lok ASF, Akarca US, Greene S: Predictive value of precore hepatitis B virus mutations in spontaneous and interferon-induced hepatitis B e antigen clearance. Hepatology 21:19, 1995.
298. Hayashi PH, Beames MP, Kuhns MC, et al: Use of quantitative assays for hepatitis B e antigen and IgM antibody to hepatitis B core antigen to monitor therapy in chronic hepatitis B. Am J Gastroenterol 91:2323, 1996.
299. Lok ASF, Lai C-L, Leung EK: Interferon antibodies may negate the antiviral effects of recombinant alpha-interferon treatment in patients with chronic hepatitis B virus infection. Hepatology 12:1266, 1990.
300. Tine F, Liberati A, Craxi A, et al: Interferon treatment in patients with chronic hepatitis B: a meta-analysis of the published literature. J Hepatol 18:154, 1993.
301. Carreno V, Bartolome J, Castillo I: Long-term effect of interferon therapy in chronic hepatitis B. J Hepatol 20:431, 1994.
302. Korenman J, Baker B, Waggoner J, et al: Long-term remission of chronic hepatitis B after alpha-interferon therapy. Ann Intern Med 114:629, 1991.
303. Lau DTY, Everhart J, Kleiner DE, et al: Long-term follow-up of patients with chronic hepatitis B treated with interferon alfa. Gastroenterology 113:1660, 1997.
304. Teuber G, Dienes HP, Meyer Zum Buschenfelde KH, et al: Long-term follow-up of patients with chronic hepatitis B after interferon treatment. Z Gastroenterol 34:230, 1996.
305. Perrillo RP, Mason AL: Therapy for hepatitis B virus infection. Gastroenterol Clin North Am 23:581, 1994.
306. Levy P, Marcellin P, Martinot-Peignoux M, et al: Clinical course of spontaneous reactivation of hepatitis B infection in patients with chronic hepatitis B. Hepatology 12:570, 1990.
307. Karayiannis P, Kanatakis S, Thomas HC: Anti-HBs response in seroconverting chronic HBV carriers following alpha-interferon treatment. J Hepatol 10:350, 1990.
308. Di Bisceglie AM: Long-term outcome of interferon-alpha therapy for chronic hepatitis B. J Hepatol 22(suppl 1):65, 1995.
309. Perrillo RP, Brunt EM: Hepatic histologic and immunohistochemical changes in chronic hepatitis B after prolonged clearance of hepatitis B e antigen and hepatitis B surface antigen. Ann Intern Med 115:113, 1991.
310. Sagnelli E, Manzillo G, Maio G, et al: Serum levels of hepatitis B surface and core antigens during immunosuppressive treatment of HBsAg-positive chronic active hepatitis. Lancet 2:395, 1980.
311. Tur-Kaspa R, Burk RD, Shaul Y, et al: Hepatitis B virus DNA contains a glucocorticoid-responsive element. Proc Natl Acad Sci U S A 83:1627, 1986.
312. Itoh Y, Okanoue T, Sakamoto S, et al: The effects of prednisolone and interferons on serum macrophage colony stimulating factor concentrations in chronic hepatitis B. J Hepatol 26:244, 1997.
313. Fevery J, Elewaut A, Michielsen P, et al: Efficacy of interferon alfa-2b with or without prednisone withdrawal in the treatment of chronic viral hepatitis B. A prospective double-blind Belgian-Dutch study. J Hepatol 11(suppl 1):S108, 1990.
314. Cohard M, Poynard T, Mathurin P, et al: Prednisone-interferon combination in the treatment of chronic hepatitis B: direct and indirect metanalysis. Hepatology 20:1390, 1994.
315. Hess G, Manns M, Hutteroth TH, et al: Discontinuation of immunosuppressive therapy in hepatitis B surface antigen-positive chronic hepatitis: effect on viral replication and on liver cell damage. Digestion 36:47, 1987.
316. Fentiman IS, Thomas BS, Balkwill FR, et al: Primary hypothyroidism associated with interferon therapy of breast cancer. Lancet 1:1166, 1985.
317. Renault PF, Hoofnagle JH, Park Y, et al: Psychiatric complications of long-term interferon alfa therapy. Arch Intern Med 147:1577, 1987.
318. Hoofnagle JH: Thrombocytopenia during interferon alfa therapy. JAMA 266:849, 1991.
319. Cianciara J, Laskus T: Development of transient autoimmune hepatitis during interferon treatment of chronic hepatitis B. Dig Dis Sci 40:1842, 1995.
320. Ronnblom LE, Alm GV, Oberg KE: Autoimmunity after alpha-interferon therapy for malignant carcinoid tumors. Ann Intern Med 115:178, 1991.
321. di Cesare E, Previti M, Russo F, et al: Interferon-alpha therapy may induce insulin autoantibody development in patients with chronic viral hepatitis. Dig Dis Sci 41:1672, 1996.
322. Fried MW: Therapy of chronic viral hepatitis. Med Clin North Am 80:957, 1996.
323. Shindo M, Di Bisceglie AM, Hoofnagle JH: Acute exacerbation of liver disease during interferon alfa therapy for chronic hepatitis C. Gastroenterology 102:1406, 1992.
324. Waguri M, Hanafusa T, Itoh N, et al: Occurrence of IDDM during interferon therapy for chronic viral hepatitis. Diab Res Clin Prac 23:33, 1994.
325. Brunetto MR, Oliveri F, Rocca G, et al: Natural course and response to interferon of chronic hepatitis B accompanied by antibody to hepatitis B e antigen. Hepatology 10:198, 1989.
326. Hadziyannis SJ: Natural course and therapy of anti-HBe-positive chronic hepatitis B. In Arroyo V, Jaume B, Miquel B, Rodes J, eds: Therapy In Liver Diseases: The Pathophysiological Basis of Therapy. Barcelona, Masson, SA, 1997:301.
327. Rizzetto M, Borghesio E: Interferon therapy for chronic hepatitis B and D: an overview. In Arroyo V, Jaume B, Miquel B, Rodes J, eds: Therapy In Liver Diseases: The Pathophysiological Basis of Therapy. Barcelona, Masson, SA, 1997:295.
328. Brunetto MR, Oliveri F, Colombatto P, et al: Treatment of chronic anti-HBe-positive hepatitis B with interferon-alpha. J Hepatol 22(1 suppl):42, 1995.
329. Lopez-Alcorocho JM, Bartolome J, Cotonat T, et al: Efficacy of prolonged interferon-alpha treatment in chronic hepatitis B patients with HBeAb: comparison between 6 and 12 months of therapy. J Viral Hepat 4(suppl 1):27, 1997.
330. Alberti A, Fattovich G: Interferon therapy for anti-HBe positive form of chronic hepatitis B. Antiviral Res 24:145, 1994.
331. Fattovich G, Farci P, Rugge M, et al: A randomized controlled trial of lymphoblastoid interferon-alpha in patients with chronic hepatitis B lacking HBeAg. Hepatology 15:584, 1992.
332. Pastore G, Santantonio T, Milella M, et al: Anti-HBe-positive chronic hepatitis B with HBV-DNA in the serum response to a 6-month course of lymphoblastoid interferon. J Hepatol 14:221, 1992.
333. Manesis EK, Hadziyannis SJ: Interferon a treatment and retreatment of hepatitis B e antigen-negative chronic hepatitis B. Gastroenterology 121:101, 2001.
334. Marcellin P, Giuily N, Loriot MA, et al: Prolonged interferon-alpha therapy of hepatitis B virus-related decompensated cirrhosis. J Viral Hepat 4(suppl 1):21, 1997.
335. Perrillo RP: Chronic hepatitis B: problem patients (including patients with decompensated disease). J Hepatol 22(1 suppl):45, 1995.
336. Housset C, Pol S, Carnot F, et al: Interactions between human immunodeficiency virus-1, hepatitis delta virus and hepatitis B virus infection in 260 chronic carriers of hepatitis B virus. Hepatology 15:578, 1992.
337. Scharschmidt BF, Held MJ, Hollander HH, et al: Hepatitis B in patients with HIV infection: relationship to AIDS and patient survival. Ann Intern Med 117:837, 1992.
338. Zylberberg H, Jiang J, Pialoux G, et al: Alpha-interferon for chronic active hepatitis B in human immunodeficiency virus-infected patients. Gastroenterol Clin Biol 20:968, 1996.
339. di Martino V, Lunel F, Cadranel JF, et al: Long-term effects of interferon-alpha in five HIV-positive patients with chronic hepatitis B. J Viral Hepat 3:253, 1996.
340. Liaw YF, Chien RN, Lin SM, et al: Response of patients with dual hepatitis B virus and C virus infection to interferon therapy. J Interferon Cytokine Res 17:449, 1997.
341. Weltman MD, Brotodihardjo A, Crewe EB, et al: Coinfection with hepatitis B and C or B, C and delta viruses results in severe chronic liver disease and responds poorly to interferon-alpha treatment. J Viral Hepat 2:39, 1995.
342. Zignego AL, Fontana R, Puliti S, et al: Relevance of inapparent coinfection by hepatitis B virus in alpha interferon-treated patients with hepatitis C virus chronic hepatitis. J Med Virol 51:313, 1997.

343. Zignego AL, Fontana R, Puliti S, et al: Impaired response of alpha interferon in patients with an inapparent hepatitis B and hepatitis C virus coinfection. Arch Virol 142:535, 1997.
344. Janssen HLA, Berk L, Schalm SW, et al: Antiviral effect of prolonged intermittent lymphoblastoid alpha interferon treatment in chronic hepatitis B. Gut 33:1094, 1992.
345. Schiff E, Karayalcin S, Grimm I, et al: A placebo controlled study of lamivudine and interferon alpha-2b in patients with chronic hepatitis B who previously failed interferon therapy. Hepatology 28:388A, 1998 (abstract).
345a. Perrillo R: How will we use the new anti-viral agents for hepatitis B. Current Gastroenterology Reports. 4:63, 2002.
346. Lai KN, Tam JS, Lin HJ, et al: The therapeutic dilemma of the usage of corticosteroid in patients with membranous nephropathy and persistent hepatitis B surface antigenaemia. Nephron 54:12, 1990.
347. Conjeevaram HS, Hoofnagle JH, Austin HA, et al: Long-term outcome of hepatitis B virus–related glomerulonephritis after therapy with interferon alfa. Gastroenterology 109:540, 1995.
348. de Man RA, Schalm SW, van der Heijden AJ, et al: Improvement of hepatitis B-associated glomerulonephritis after antiviral combination therapy. J Hepatol 8:367, 1989.
349. Lisker-Melman M, Webb D, Di Bisceglie AM, et al: Glomerulonephritis caused by chronic hepatitis B virus infection: treatment with recombinant human alpha-interferon. Ann Intern Med 111:479, 1989.
350. Lok ASF: Antiviral therapy of the Asian patient with chronic hepatitis B. Semin Liver Dis 13:360, 1993.
351. Chung DR, Yang WS, Kim SB, et al: Treatment of hepatitis B virus associated glomerulonephritis with recombinant human alpha interferon. Am J Nephrol 17:112, 1997.
352. Lohr H, Goergen B, Weber W, et al: Mixed cryoglobulinemia type II in chronic hepatitis B associated with HBe-minus HBV mutant: cellular immune reactions and response to interferon treatment. J Med Virol 44:330, 1994.
353. Nityanand S, Holm G, Lefvert AK: Immune complex mediated vasculitis in hepatitis B and C infections and the effect of antiviral therapy. Clin Immunol Immunopathol 82:250, 1997.
354. Scully LJ, Karayiannis P, Thomas HC: Interferon therapy is effective in treatment of hepatitis B-induced polyarthritis. Dig Dis Sci 37:1757, 1992.
355. Chan GC, Lee SS, Yeoh EK: Mono-arthritis in a chronic hepatitis B patient after alpha-interferon treatment. J Gastroenterol Hepatol 7:432, 1992.
355a. Torresi J, Locarnini S: Antiviral chemotherapy for the treatment of hepatitis B virus infections. Gastroenterology 118:S83, 2000.
356. Hess G, Arnold W, Meyer zum Buschenfelde KH: Inhibition of hepatitis B virus deoxyribonucleic acid polymerase by the 5'-triphosphates of 9-beta-D-arabinofuranosyladenine and 1-beta-D-arabinofuranosylcytosine. Antimicrob Agents Chemother 19:44, 1981.
357. Hoofnagle JH, Minuk GY, Dusheiko GM, et al: Adenine arabinoside 5'-monophosphate treatment of chronic type B hepatitis. Hepatology 6:784, 1982.
358. Paar DP, Hooton TM, Smiles KA, et al: The effect of FIAU on chronic hepatitis B virus (HBV) infection in HIV-infected subjects (ACTG 122b) (abstract). In Programs and Abstracts of the 32nd Interscience Conference on Antimicrobial Agents and Chemotherapy, Anaheim, Calif., 10-14 October 1992. Washington, DC, American Society for Microbiology, 1992:264.
359. Fried MW, Di Bisceglie AM, Straus SE, et al: FIAU, a new oral antiviral agent, profoundly inhibits HBV DNA in patients with chronic hepatitis B. Hepatology 16:127A, 1992 (abstract).
360. McKenzie R, Fried MW, Sallie R, et al: Hepatic failure and lactic acidosis due to fialuridine (FIAU), an investigational nucleoside analogue for chronic hepatitis B. N Engl J Med 333:1099, 1995.
361. Colledge D, Locarnini S, Shaw T: Synergistic inhibition of hepadnaviral replication by lamivudine in combination with penciclovir in vitro. Hepatology 26:216, 1997.
361a. Dandri M, Burda MR, Will H, et al: Increased hepatocyte turnover and inhibition of woodchuck hepatitis B virus replication by adefovir in vitro do not lead to reduction of the closed circular DNA. Hepatology 32:139, 2000.
362. Mutimer D, Pillay D, Shields P, et al: Outcome of lamivudine resistant hepatitis B virus infection in the liver transplant recipient. Gut 46:107, 2000.
363. Trepo C, Jezek P, Atkinson GF, et al: Efficacy of famciclovir in chronic hepatitis B: results of a dose finding study. Hepatology 24:188A, 1997.
364. Main J, Brown JL, Howells C, et al: A double-blind, placebo-controlled study to assess the effect of famciclovir on virus replication in patients with chronic hepatitis B virus infection. J Viral Hepat 3:211, 1996.
365. Jaeckel E, Tillmann HL, Krueger M, et al: Resistance against nucleoside analogues in patients after liver transplantation for hepatitis B cirrhosis. Hepatology 28:235, 1998 (abstract).
366. Lau GK, Tsiang M, Hou J, et al: Combination therapy with lamivudine and famciclovir for chronic hepatitis B-infected Chinese patients: a viral dynamics study. Hepatology 32:394, 2000.
367. Tillmann HL, Trautwein C, Bock T, et al: Mutational pattern of hepatitis B virus on sequential therapy with famciclovir and lamivudine in patients with hepatitis B virus reinfection occurring under HBIg immunoglobulin after liver transplantation. Hepatology 30:244, 1999.
368. Lai CL, Chien RN, Leung NW, et al: A one-year trial of lamivudine for chronic hepatitis B. Asia Hepatitis Lamivudine Study Group. N Engl J Med 339:61, 1998.
369. Kweon Y-O, Goodman ZD, Dienstag JL, et al: Lamivudine decreases fibrogenesis in chronic hepatitis B: an immunohistochemical study of paired liver biopsies. Hepatology 32:377A, 2000 (abstract).
370. Schiff ER, Heathcote J, Dienstag JL, et al: Improvements in liver histology and cirrhosis with extended lamivudine therapy. Hepatology 32:296A, 2000 (abstract).
371. Lau DT, Khokhar MF, Doo E, et al: Long-term therapy of chronic hepatitis B with lamivudine. Hepatology 32:828, 2000.
372. Allen MI, Deslauriers M, Andrews CW, et al: Identification and characterization of mutations in hepatitis B virus resistant to lamivudine. Lamivudine Clinical Investigation Group. Hepatology 27:1670, 1998.
373. Ben-Ari Z, Pappo O, Zemel R, et al: Association of lamivudine resistance in recurrent hepatitis B after liver transplantation with advanced hepatic fibrosis. Transplantation 68:232, 1999.
374. Schalm SW, Heathcote J, Cianciara J, et al: Lamivudine and alpha interferon combination treatment of patients with chronic hepatitis B infection: a randomised trial. Gut 46:562, 2000.
375. Perrillo R, Schiff E, Yoshida E, et al: Adefovir dipivoxil for the treatment of lamivudine-resistant hepatitis B mutants. Hepatology 32:129, 2000.
376. Peters M, Angus P, Dickson R, et al: Adefovir dipivoxil treatment of hepatitis B virus disease in patients failing lamivudine therapy (abstract 079). Presented at 10th International Symposium on Viral Hepatitis and Liver Disease Atlanta, Ga, April, 2000:45.
377. Farrell GC: Clinical potential of emerging new agents in hepatitis B. Drugs 60:701, 2000.
378. Tassopoulos NC, Volpes R, Pastore G, et al: Efficacy of lamivudine in patients with hepatitis B e antigen-negative/hepatitis B virus DNA-positive (precore mutant) chronic hepatitis B. Lamivudine Precore Mutant Study Group. Hepatology 29:889, 1999.
379. Tassopoulos NC, Anagnostopoulos GD, Delladetsima JK, et al: Extended lamivudine treatment in patients with HBeAg negative/HBV DNA positive chronic hepatitis B (CHB). Hepatology 32:456, 2000 (abstract).
380. Santantonio T, Mazzola M, Sinisi E, et al: Long term lamivudine treatment in anti-HBe positive chronic hepatitis B: an interim analysis. Hepatology 32:458A, 2000.
381. Ben-Ari Z, Zemel R, Kazetsker A, et al: Efficacy of lamivudine in patients with hepatitis B virus precore mutant infection before and after liver transplantation. Am J Gastroenterol 94:663, 1999.
382. Chen RY, Desmond PV, Delaney WE, et al: Antiviral sensitivity of pre-core mutant HBV to nucleoside analogues in vitro using a novel recombinant HBV-baculovirus system. Hepatology 32:456A, 2000 (abstract).
383. Benner KG, Rosen HR, Flora KD: Famciclovir treatment of decompensated HBV cirrhosis. Hepatology 24:282A, 1996 (abstract).
384. Fontana RJ, Perrillo R, Hann HWL, et al: Determinants of survival in 133 patients with decompensated chronic hepatitis B treated with lamivudine. Hepatology 32:221A, 2000 (abstract).
385. Maclachlan D, Battegay M, Jacob AL, et al: Successful treatment of hepatitis-B associated polyarteritis nodosa with a combination of lamivudine and conventional immunosuppressive therapy: a case report. Rheumatology (Oxford) 39(1):106, 2000 (letter).

386. Wicki J, Olivieri J, Pizzolato G, et al: Successful treatment of polyarteritis nodosa related to hepatitis B virus with a combination of lamivudine and interferon alpha. Rheumatology (Oxford) 38:183, 1999 (letter).
387. Erhardt A, Sagir A, Guillevin L, et al: Successful treatment of hepatitis B virus associated polyarteritis nodosa with a combination of prednisolone, alpha-interferon and lamivudine. J Hepatol 33(4):677, 2000.
388. von Weizsacker F, Wieland S, Kock J, et al: Gene therapy for chronic viral hepatitis: ribozymes, antisense oligonucleotides, and dominant negative mutants. Hepatology 26:251, 1997.
389. von Weizsacker F, Blum HE, Wands JR: Cleavage of hepatitis B viral RNA by three ribozymes transcribed from a single DNA template. Biochem Biophys Res Commun 189:743, 1992.
390. Wu GY, Wu CH: Specific inhibition of hepatitis B viral gene expression in vitro by targeted antisense oligonucleotides. J Biol Chem 267:12436, 1992.
391. Nakazono K, Ito Y, Wu CH, et al: Inhibition of hepatitis B virus replication by targeted pretreatment of complexed antisense DNA *in vitro*. Hepatology 23:1297, 1996.
392. Delaney MA, Goyal S, Seeger C: Design of modified core genes that inhibit replication of woodchuck hepatitis virus. In Hollinger FB, Lemon SM, Margolis H, eds: Viral Hepatitis and Liver Disease. Baltimore, Williams & Wilkins, 1991:667.
393. Scaglioni P, Melegari M, Takahashi M, et al: Use of dominant negative mutants of the hepadnaviral core protein as antiviral agents. Hepatology 24:1010, 1996.
394. Artillo S, Pastore G, Alberti A, et al: Double-blind, randomized trial of interleukin-2 treatment of chronic hepatitis B. J Med Virol 54:167, 1998.
395. Di Bisceglie AM, Rustgi VK, Kassianides C, et al: Therapy of chronic hepatitis B with recombinant human alpha and gamma interferon. Hepatology 11:266, 1990.
396. Naoumov NV, Rossol S: Studies of interleukin-12 in chronic hepatitis B virus infection. J Viral Hepat 4(suppl 2):87, 1997.
397. Carreno V, Zeuzem S, Hopf U, et al: A phase I/II study of recombinant human interleukin-12 in patients with chronic hepatitis B. J Hepatol 32:317, 2000.
398. Eichberg JW, Seeff LB, Lawlor DL, et al: Effect of thymosin immunostimulation with and without corticosteroid immunosuppression on chimpanzee hepatitis B carriers. J Med Virol 21:25, 1987.
399. Mutchnick MG, Appelman HD, Chung HT, et al: Thymosin treatment of chronic hepatitis B: a placebo-controlled pilot trial. Hepatology 14:409, 1991.
400. Mutchnick MG, Lindsay KL, Schiff ER, et al: Thymosin alpha 1 treatment of chronic hepatitis B: results of a phase III multicentre, randomized, double-blind and placebo-controlled study. J Viral Hepatol 6:397, 1999.
401. Chien RN, Liaw YF, Chen TC, et al: Efficacy of thymosin alpha 1 in patients with chronic hepatitis B: a randomized, controlled trial. Hepatology 27:1383, 1998.
402. Andreone P, Cursaro C, Gramenzi A, et al: A randomized controlled trial of thymosin-alpha-1 versus interferon alfa treatment in patients with hepatitis B e antigen antibody- and hepatitis B virus DNA-positive chronic hepatitis B. Hepatology 24:774, 1996.
403. Zavaglia C, Severini R, Tinelli C, et al: A randomized, controlled study of thymosin-alpha 1 therapy in patients with anti-HBe, HBV-DNA-positive chronic hepatitis B. Dig Dis Sci 45:690, 2000.
404. Tang JH, Yeh CT, Chen TC, et al: Emergence of an S gene mutant during thymosin alpha1 therapy in a patient with chronic hepatitis B. J Infect Dis 178:866, 1998.
405. Heathcote J, McHutchison J, Lee S, et al: A pilot study of the CY-1899 T-cell vaccine in subjects chronically infected with hepatitis B virus. The CY1899 T Cell Vaccine Study Group. Hepatology 30:531, 1999.
406. Ishioka GY, Fikes J, Hermanson G, et al: Utilization of MHC class I transgenic mice for development of minigene DNA vaccines encoding multiple HLA-restricted CTL epitopes. J Immunol 162:3915, 1999.
407. Mancini M, Hadchouel M, Davis HL, et al: DNA-mediated immunization in a transgenic mouse model of the hepatitis B surface antigen chronic carrier state. Proc Natl Acad Sci U S A 93:12496, 1996.
408. Koziel MJ, Liang JT: DNA vaccines and viral hepatitis: are we going around in circles? Gastroenterology 112:1410, 1997.
409. Zuckerman JN: Hepatitis B third-generation vaccines: improved response and conventional vaccine non-response—third generation pre-S/S vaccines overcome non-response. J Viral Hepat 5(suppl 2):13, 1998.
410. Akbar SM, Kajino K, Tanimoto K, et al: Placebo-controlled trial of vaccination with hepatitis B virus surface antigen in hepatitis B virus transgenic mice. J Hepatol 26:131, 1997.
411. Couillin I, Pol S, Mancini M, et al: Specific vaccine therapy in chronic hepatitis B: induction of T cell proliferative responses specific for envelope antigens. J Infect Dis 180:15, 1999.
411a. Wright TL, Tong MJ, Hsu HH: Phase I study of a potent adjuvanted hepatitis B vaccine (HBV/M59) for therapy of chronic hepatitis B. Hepatology 30:421A, 1999 (abstract).
412. Reed EC, Myerson D, Corey L, et al: Allogeneic marrow transplantation in patients positive for hepatitis B surface antigen. Blood 77:195, 1991.
413. Ilan Y, Nagler A, Adler R, et al: Ablation of persistent hepatitis B by bone marrow transplantation from a hepatitis B-immune donor. Gastroenterology 104:1818, 1993.
414. Shouval D, Ilan Y: Immunization against hepatitis B through adoptive transfer of immunity. Intervirology 38:41, 1995.
415. Lau GK, Lok AS, Liang RH, et al: Clearance of hepatitis B surface antigen after bone marrow transplantation: role of adoptive immunity transfer. Hepatology 25:1497, 1997.
416. Branger M, Elias A, Vitrano L, et al: Collection of anti-HBs hyperimmune plasma: stimulation by Genhevac B in weakly immunized donors. Rev Fr Transfus Hemobiol 35:325, 1992.
417. Desmyter J, Bradburne AF, Vermylen C, et al: Hepatitis-B immunoglobulin in prevention of HBs antigenaemia in haemodialysis patients. Lancet 2:376, 1975.
418. Iwarson S, Ahlmen J, Ericksson E, et al: Hepatitis B immune globulin in prevention of hepatitis B among hospital staff members. J Infect Dis 135:473, 1977.
419. Kleinknecht D, Courouce AM, Delons S, et al: Prevention of hepatitis B in hemodialysis patients using hepatitis B immunoglobulin. A controlled study. Clin Nephrol 8:373, 1977.
420. Prince AM, Szmuness W, Mann MK, et al: Hepatitis B immune globulin: final report of a controlled, multicenter trial of efficacy in prevention of dialysis-associated hepatitis. J Infect Dis 137:131, 1978.
421. Redeker AG, Mosley JW, Gocke DJ, et al: Hepatitis B immune globulin as a prophylactic measure for spouses exposed to acute type B hepatitis. N Engl J Med 293:1055, 1975.
422. A combined Medical Research Council and Public Health Laboratory Service Report, The incidence of hepatitis B infection after accidental exposure and anti-HBs immunoglobulin prophylaxis. Lancet 1:1:6, 1980.
423. Kohler PF, Dubois RS, Merrill DA, et al: Prevention of chronic neonatal hepatitis B virus infection with antibody to the hepatitis B surface antigen. N Engl J Med 291:1378, 1974.
424. Dosik H, Jhaveri R: Prevention of neonatal hepatitis B infection by high-dose hepatitis B immune globulin. N Engl J Med 298:602, 1978.
425. Iwarson S, Norkrans G, Hermodsson S, et al: Passive-active immunization in a neonate treated with repeated doses of high-titred hepatitis B immune globulin. Scand J Infect Dis 11:167, 1979.
426. Reesink HW, Reerink-Brongers EE, Lafeber-Schut BJT, et al: Prevention of chronic HBsAg carrier state in infants of HBsAg-positive mothers by hepatitis B immunoglobulin. Lancet 2:436, 1979.
427. Reed WD, Eddleston AL, Cullens H, et al: Infusion of hepatitis B antibody in antigen-positive active chronic hepatitis. Lancet 2:1347, 1973.
428. Gateau P, Opolon P, Nusinovici V, et al: Passive immunotherapy in HBs Ag fulminant hepatitis. Results on antigenaemia and survival. Digestion 14:304, 1976.
429. al-Hemsi B, McGory RW, Shepard B, et al: Liver transplantation for hepatitis B cirrhosis: clinical sequela of passive immunization. Clin Transplant 10(6 Pt 2):668, 1996.
430. Wells MA, Wittek AE, Epstein JS, et al: Inactivation and partition of human T-cell lymphotropic virus, type III, during ethanol fractionation of plasma. Transfusion 26:210, 1986.
431. Dodd RY: Infectious risk of plasma donations: relationship to safety of intravenous immune globulins. Clin Exp Immunol 104(suppl 1):31, 1996.
432. Horowitz B: Investigations into the application of tri(n-butyl)phosphate/detergent mixtures to blood derivatives. Curr Stud Hematol Blood Transfus 56:83, 1989.

433. Buynak EB, Roehm RR, Tytell AA, et al: Vaccine against human hepatitis B. JAMA 235:2832, 1976.
434. Buynak EB, Roehm RR, Tytell AA, et al: Development and chimpanzee testing of a vaccine against human hepatitis B. Proc Soc Exp Biol Med 151:694, 1976.
435. Valenzuela P, Medina A, Rutter WJ, et al: Synthesis and assembly of hepatitis B virus surface antigen particles in yeast. Nature 298:347, 1982.
436. Emini EA, Ellis RW, Miller WJ, et al: Production and immunological analysis of recombinant hepatitis B vaccine. J Infect 13(suppl A):3, 1986.
437. Bocher WO, Herzog-Hauff S, Herr W, et al: Regulation of the neutralizing anti-hepatitis B surface (HBs) antibody response in vitro in HBs vaccine recipients and patients with acute or chronic hepatitis B virus (HBV) infection. Clin Exp Immunol 105:52, 1996.
438. Bocher WO, Herzog-Hauff S, Schlaak J, et al: Kinetics of hepatitis B surface antigen-specific immune responses in acute and chronic hepatitis B or after HBs vaccination: stimulation of the in vitro antibody response by interferon gamma. Hepatology 29:238, 1999.
439. Szmuness W, Stevens CE, Harley EJ, et al: Hepatitis B vaccine: demonstration of efficacy in a controlled clinical trial in a high-risk population in the United States. N Engl J Med 303:833, 1980.
440. Francis DP, Hadler SC, Thompson SE, et al: The prevention of hepatitis B with vaccine. Report of the centers for disease control multi-center efficacy trial among homosexual men. Ann Intern Med 97:362, 1982.
441. Szmuness W, Stevens CE, Harley EJ, et al: Hepatitis B vaccine in medical staff of hemodialysis units: efficacy and subtype cross-protection. N Engl J Med 307:1481, 1982.
442. Maupas P, Chiron JP, Barin F, et al: Efficacy of hepatitis B vaccine in prevention of early HBsAg carrier state in children: Controlled trial in an endemic area (Senegal). Lancet 1:289, 1981.
443. McLean AA, Hilleman MR, McAleer WJ, et al: Summary of worldwide clinical experience with H-B-Vax (B, MSD). J Infect 7(suppl 1):95, 1983.
444. Prozesky OW, Stevens CE, Szmuness W, et al: Immune response to hepatitis B vaccine in newborns. J Infect 7(suppl 1):53, 1983.
445. Hadler SC, Francis DP, Maynard JE, et al: Long-term immunogenicity and efficacy of hepatitis B vaccine in homosexual men. N Engl J Med 315:209, 1986.
446. Wainwright RB, Bulkow LR, Parkinson AJ, et al: Protection provided by hepatitis B vaccine in a Yupik Eskimo population—results of 10-year study. J Infect Dis 175:674, 1997.
447. Weber DJ, Rutala WA, Samsa GP, et al: Obesity as a predictor of poor antibody response to hepatitis B plasma vaccine. JAMA 254:3187, 1985.
448. Shaw FE, Guess HA, Roets JM, et al: Effect of anatomic injection site, age and smoking on the immune response to hepatitis B vaccination. Vaccine 7:425, 1989.
449. Wood RC, MacDonald KL, White KE, et al: Risk factors for lack of detectable antibody following hepatitis B vaccination of Minnesota health care workers. JAMA 270:2935, 1993.
450. Clements ML, Miskovsky E, Davidson M, et al: Effect of age on the immunogenicity of yeast recombinant hepatitis B vaccines containing surface antigen (S) or PreS2 + S antigens. J Infect Dis 170:510, 1994.
451. Stevens CE, Szmuness W, Goodman AI, et al: Hepatitis B vaccine: immune responses in haemodialysis patients. Lancet 2:1211, 1980.
452. Xu ZY, Liu CB, Francis DP, et al: Prevention of perinatal acquisition of hepatitis B virus carriage using vaccine: preliminary report of a randomized, double-blind placebo-controlled and comparative trial. Pediatrics 76:713, 1985.
453. Weitberg AB, Weitzman SA, Watkins E, et al: Immunogenicity of hepatitis B vaccine in oncology patients receiving chemotherapy. J Clin Oncol 3:718, 1985.
454. Suboptimal response to hepatitis B vaccine given by injection into the buttock. MMWR Morb Mortal Wkly Rep 34:105, 1985.
455. Redfield RR, Innis BL, Scott RM, et al: Clinical evaluation of low-dose intradermally administered hepatitis B vaccine. A cost reduction strategy. JAMA 254:3203, 1985.
456. Coleman PJ, Shaw FE, Serovich J, et al: Intradermal hepatitis B vaccination in a large hospital employee population. Vaccine 9:723, 1991.
457. Gonzalez ML, Usandizaga M, Alomar P, et al: Intradermal and intramuscular route for vaccination against hepatitis B. Vaccine 8:402, 1990.
458. Lancaster D, Elam S, Kaiser AB: Immunogenicity of the intradermal route of hepatitis B vaccination with the use of recombinant hepatitis B vaccine. Am J Infect Control 17:126, 1989.
459. King JW, Taylor EM, Crow SD, et al: Comparison of the immunogenicity of hepatitis B vaccine administered intradermally and intramuscularly. Rev Infect Dis 12:1035, 1990.
460. Bohm W, Schirmbeck R, Elbe A, et al: Exogenous hepatitis B surface antigen particles processed by dendritic cells or macrophages prime murine MHC class I-restricted cytotoxic T lymphocytes in vivo. J Immunol 155:3313, 1995.
461. Schirmbeck R, Melber K, Mertens T, et al: Antibody and cytotoxic T-cell responses to soluble hepatitis B virus (HBV) S antigen in mice: implication for the pathogenesis of HBV-induced hepatitis. J Virol 68:1418, 1994.
462. Wilson CC, Olson WC, Tuting T, et al: HIV-1 specific CTL responses primed in vitro by blood-derived dendritic cells and Th1-biasing cytokines. J Immunol 162:3070, 1999.
463. Bachmann MF, Lutz MB, Layton GT, et al: Dendritic cells process exogenous viral proteins and virus-like particles for class I presentation to CD8+ cytotoxic T lymphocytes. Eur J Immunol 26:2595, 1996.
464. Rahman F, Dahmen A, Herzog-Hauff S, et al: Cellular and humoral immune responses induced by intradermal or intramuscular vaccination with the major hepatitis B surface antigen. Hepatology 31:521, 2000.
465. Hepatitis B virus: a comprehensive strategy for eliminating transmission in the United States through Universal Childhood Vaccination. Recommendations of the Immunization Practices Advisory Committee (ACIP). MMWR Morb Mortal Wkly Rep 40(RR-13):1, 1991.
466. McDermott AB, Zuckerman JN, Sabin CA, et al: Contribution of human leukocyte antigens to the antibody response to hepatitis B vaccination. Tissue Antigens 50:8, 1997.
467. Desombere I, Willems A, Leroux-Roels G: Response to hepatitis B vaccine: multiple HLA genes are involved. Tissue Antigens 51:593, 1998.
468. Hohler T, Meyer CU, Notghi A, et al: The influence of major histocompatibility class II genes and T-cell Vbeta repertoire on response to immunization with HBsAg. Hum Immunol 59:212, 1998.
469. Lango-Warensjo A, Cardell K, Lindblom B: Haplotypes comprising subtypes of the DQB1*06 allele direct the antibody response after immunisation with hepatitis B surface antigen. Tissue Antigens 52:374, 1998.
470. Kruskall MS, Alper CA, Awdeh Z, et al: The immune response to hepatitis B vaccine in humans: inheritance pattern in families. J Exp Med 175:495, 1992.
471. Lemon SM, Thomas DL: Vaccine to prevent viral hepatitis. N Engl J Med 336:196, 1997.
472. Zarski JP, Bohn B, Bastie A, et al: Characteristics of patients with dual infection by hepatitis B and C viruses. J Hepatol 28:27, 1998.
473. Kaklamani E, Trichopoulos D, Tzonou A, et al: Hepatitis B and C viruses and their interaction in the origin of hepatocellular carcinoma. JAMA 265:1974, 1991.
474. Simonetti RG, Camma C, Fiorello F, Cottone M, et al: Hepatitis C virus infection as a risk factor for hepatocellular carcinoma in patients with cirrhosis. A case-control study. Ann Intern Med 116:97, 1992.
475. Keeffe EB, Iwarson S, McMahon BJ, et al: Safety and immunogenicity of hepatitis A vaccine in patients with chronic liver disease. Hepatology 27:881, 1998.
476. Keeffe EB, Krause DS: Hepatitis B vaccination of patients with chronic liver disease. Liver Transpl Surg 4:437, 1998.
477. Wiedmann M, Liebert UG, Oesen U, et al: Decreased immunogenicity of recombinant hepatitis B vaccine in chronic hepatitis C. Hepatology 31:230, 2000.
478. Villenuve E, Vincelette J, Villeneuve JP: Ineffectiveness of hepatitis B vaccination in cirrhotic patients waiting for liver transplantation. Can J Gastroenterol 14(suppl B):59B, 2000.
479. Stevens CE, Alter HJ, Taylor PE, et al: Hepatitis B vaccine in patients receiving hemodialysis. Immunogenicity and efficacy. N Engl J Med 311:496, 1984.
480. Peces R, de la Torre M, Alcazar R, et al: Prospective analysis of the factors influencing the antibody response to hepatitis B vaccine in hemodialysis patients. Am J Kidney Dis 29:239, 1997.
481. Seaworth B, Drucker J, Starling J, et al: Hepatitis B vaccines in patients with chronic renal failure before dialysis. J Infect Dis 157:332, 1988.

482. Moyer LA, Alter MJ, Favero MS: Hemodialysis-associated hepatitis B: revised recommendations for serologic screening. Semin Dialyis 3:201, 1990.
483. Evans TG, Schiff M, Graves B, et al: The safety and efficacy of GM-CSF as an adjuvant in hepatitis B vaccination of chronic hemodialysis patients who have failed primary vaccination. Clin Nephrol 54:138, 2000.
484. Charest AF, McDougall J, Goldstein MB: A randomized comparison of intradermal and intramuscular vaccination against hepatitis B virus in incident chronic hemodialysis patients. Am J Kidney Dis 36:976, 2000.
485. Shaw FE, Graham DJ, Guess HA, et al: Postmarketing surveillance for neurologic adverse events reported after hepatitis B vaccination. Experience of the first three years. Am J Epidemiol 127:337, 1988.
486. Ascherio A, Zhang SM, Hernan MA, et al: Hepatitis B vaccination and the risk of multiple sclerosis. N Engl J Med 344:327, 2001.
487. Alter MJ, Hadler SC, Margolis HS, et al: The changing epidemiology of hepatitis B in the United States. Need for alternative vaccination strategies. JAMA 263:1218, 1990.
488. Chang MH, Chen CJ, Lai MS: Universal hepatitis B vaccination in Taiwan and incidence of hepatocellular carcinoma in children. Taiwan Childhood Hepatoma Study Group. N Engl J Med 336:1855, 1997.
489. Jonas MM, Schiff ER, O'Sullivan MJ, et al: Failure of Centers for Disease Control criteria to identify hepatitis B infection in a large municipal obstetrical population. Ann Intern Med 107:335, 1987.
490. Centers for Disease Control and Prevention: Protection against viral hepatitis: recommendations of the Immunization Practice Advisory Committee MMWR 39:5-22, 1990.
491. Kollar LM, Rosenthal SL, Biro FM: Hepatitis B vaccine series compliance in adolescents. Pediatr Infect Dis J 13:1006, 1994.
492. Immunizations for adolescents: Centers for Disease Control and Prevention: MMWR, 4-5, 1996.
493. Immunization of health care workers: Centers for Disease Control and Prevention: MMWR, 23, 1997.
494. Davis HL, Michel ML, Mancini M, et al: Direct gene transfer in skeletal muscle: plasmid DNA-based immunization against the hepatitis B virus surface antigen. Vaccine 12:1503, 1994.
495. Geissler M, Tokushige K, Chante CC, et al: Cellular and humoral immune response to hepatitis B virus structural proteins in mice after DNA based immunization. Gastroenterology 112:1307, 1997.
496. Loirat D, Lemonnier FA, Michel ML : Multiepitopic HLA-A*0201-restricted immune response against hepatitis B surface antigen after DNA-based immunization. J Immunol 165:4748, 2000.
497. Roy MJ, Wu MS, Barr LJ, et al: Induction of antigen-specific CD8+ T cells, T helper cells, and protective levels of antibody in humans by particle-mediated administration of a hepatitis B virus DNA vaccine. Vaccine 19:764, 2000.
498. Gerdts V, Babiuk LA, van Drunen Littel-van den Hurk, et al: Fetal immunization by a DNA vaccine delivered into the oral cavity. Nat Med 6:929, 2000.
498a. Young MD, Schneider DL, Zuckerman AJ, et al: The US Hepacare Study Group. Adult hepatitis B vaccination using a novel triple antigen recombinant vaccine. Hepatology 34:372, 2001.
498b. Zuckerman JN, Zuckerman AJ, Symington I, et al: UK Hepacare Study Group. Evaluation of a new hepatitis B triple-antigen vaccine in inadequate responders to current vaccines. Hepatology 34:798, 2001.
498c. Joines RW, Blatter M, Abraham B, et al: A prospective, randomized, comparative US trial of a combination hepatitis A and B vaccine (Twinrix) with corresponding monovalent vaccines (Havrix and Engerix-B) in adults. Vaccine 19:4710, 2001.
499. Kapusta J, Modelska A, Figlerowicz M, et al: A plant-derived edible vaccine against hepatitis B virus. FASEB J 13:1796, 1999.
500. Rizzetto M, Canese MG, Arico S, et al: Imunofluorescence detection of new antigen-antibody system (delta/anti-delta) associated to hepatitis B virus in liver and in serum of HBsAg carriers. Gut 18:997, 1977.
501. Rizzetto M, Shih JW, Gocke DJ, et al: Incidence and significance of antibodies to delta antigen in hepatitis B virus infection. Lancet 2:986, 1979.
502. Hadler SC, Monzon M, Ponzetto A, et al: Delta virus infection and severe hepatitis. An epidemic in the Yucpa Indians of Venezuela. Ann Intern Med 100:339, 1984.
503. Govindarajan S, Chin KP, Redeker AG, et al: Fulminant B viral hepatitis: role of delta agent. Gastroenterology 86:1417, 1984.
504. Torres JR: Hepatitis B and hepatitis delta virus infection in South America. Gut 38(suppl 2):S48, 1996.
505. Nath N, Mushawar IK, Fang CT, et al: Antibodies to delta antigen in asymptomatic hepatitis B surface antigen-reactive blood donors in the United States and their association with other markers of hepatitis B virus. Am J Epidemiol 122:218, 1985.
506. Rizzetto M, Purcell RH, Gerin JL: Epidemiology of HBV-associated delta agent: geographical distribution of anti-delta and prevalence of polytransfused HBsAg carriers. Lancet 1:1215, 1980.
507. Shakil AO, Hadziyannis S, Hoofnagle JH, et al: Geographic distribution and genetic variability of hepatitis delta virus genotype I. Virology 234:160, 1997.
508. Zhang YY, Hansson BG: Introduction of a new hepatitis agent in retrospect: genetic studies of Swedish hepatitis D virus strains. J Clin Microbiol 34:2713, 1996.
509. Zhang YY, Tsega E, Hansson BG: Phylogenetic analysis of hepatitis D viruses indicating a new genotype I subgroup among African isolates. J Clin Microbiol 34:3023, 1996.
510. Lee CM, Changchien CS, Chung JC, et al: Characterization of a new genotype II hepatitis delta virus from Taiwan. J Med Virol 49:145, 1996.
511. Casey JL, Niro GA, Engle RE, et al: Hepatitis B virus (HBV)/hepatitis D virus (HDV) coinfection in outbreaks of acute hepatitis in the Peruvian Amazon Basin: the roles of HDV genotype III and HBV genotype F. J Infect Dis 174:920, 1996.
512. Sakugawa H, Nakasone H, Shokita H, et al: Seroepidemiological study on hepatitis delta virus infection in the Irabu Islands, Okinawa, Japan. J Gastroenterol Hepatol 12:299, 1997.
513. Hadziyannis SJ: Decreasing prevalence of hepatitis D virus infection. J Gastroenterol Hepatol 12:745, 1997.
514. Hadziyannis SJ, Dourakis SP, Papaionnou C, et al: Changing epidemiology and spreading modalities of hepatitis delta virus infection in Greece. Prog Clin Biol Res 382:259, 1993.
515. Giusti G, Sagnelli E, Gallo C, et al: The etiology of chronic hepatitis in Italy: a multicenter study. Hepatogastroenterology 41:397, 1994.
516. Gaeta GB, Stroffolini T, Chiaramonte M, et al: Chronic hepatitis D: a vanishing disease? An Italian multicenter study. Hepatology 32:824, 2000.
517. Sagnelli E, Stroffolini T, Ascione A, et al: Decrease in HDV endemicity in Italy. J Hepatol 26:20, 1997.
518. Navascues CA, Rodriguez M, Sotorrio NG, et al: Epidemiology of hepatitis D virus infection: changes in the last 14 years. Am J Gastroenterol 90:1981, 1995.
519. Coppola RC, Manconi PE, Piro R, et al: HCV, HIV, HBV and HDV infections in intravenous drug addicts. Eur J Epidemiol 10:279, 1994.
520. Tennant F, Moll D: Seroprevalence of hepatitis A, B, C and D markers and liver function abnormalities in intravenous heroin addicts. J Addict Dis 14:35, 1995.
521. Rosina F, Saracco G, Rizzetto M: Risk of post-transfusion infection with the hepatitis delta virus. A multicenter study. N Engl J Med 312:1488, 1985.
522. Liaw YF, Chiu KW, Chu CM, et al: Heterosexual transmission of hepatitis delta virus in the general population of an area endemic for hepatitis B virus infection: a prospective study. J Infect Dis 162:1170, 1990.
523. Wang KS, Choo QL, Weiner AJ, et al: Structure, sequence and expression of hepatitis delta viral genome. Nature 323:508, 1986.
524. Kuo MY, Chao M, Taylor J: Initiation of replication of the human hepatitis delta virus genome from cloned DNA: role of delta antigen. J Virol 63:1945, 1989.
525. Chao M, Hsieh SY, Taylor J: Role of two forms of hepatitis delta virus antigen: evidence for a mechanism of self-limiting genome replication. J Virol 64:5066, 1990.
526. Wu JC, Chen PJ, Kuo MY, et al: Production of hepatitis delta virus and suppression of helper hepatitis B virus in a human hepatoma cell line. J Virol 65:1099, 1991.
527. Ryu WS, Bayer M, Taylor J: Assembly of hepatitis delta virus particles. J Virol 66:2310, 1992.
528. Luo GX, Chao M, Hsieh SY, et al: A specific base transition occurs on replicating hepatitis delta virus RNA. J Virol 64:1021, 1990.
529. Casey JL, Bergmann KF, Brown TL, et al: Structural requirements for RNA editing in hepatitis delta virus: evidence for a uridine-to-

cytidine editing mechanism. Proc Natl Acad Sci U S A 89:7149, 1992.
530. Polson AG, Bass BL, Casey JL: RNA editing of hepatitis delta virus antigenome by dsRNA-adenosine deaminase. Nature 380:454, 1996.
531. Casey JL, Gerin JL: Hepatitis D virus RNA editing: specific modification of adenosine in the antigenomic RNA. J Virol 69:7593, 1995.
532. Chen PJ, Kalpana G, Goldberg J, et al: Structure and replication of the genome of hepatitis delta virus. Proc Natl Acad Sci U S A 83:8774, 1986.
533. Taylor IM: Hepatitis delta virus: cis and trans functions needed for replication. Cell 61:508, 1990.
534. Chang MF, Sun CY, Chen CJ, et al: Functional motifs of delta antigen essential for RNA binding and replication of hepatitis delta virus. J Virol 67:2529, 1993.
535. Lazinski DW, Taylor JM: Relating structure to function in the hepatitis delta virus antigen. J Virol 67:2672, 1993.
536. Cullen JM, David C, Wang JG, et al: Subcellular distribution of large and small hepatitis delta antigen in hepatocytes of hepatitis delta virus superinfected woodchucks. Hepatology 22:1090, 1995.
537. Glenn JS, Watson JA, Havel CM, et al: Identification of a prenylation site in delta virus large antigen. Science 256:1331, 1992.
538. Smedile A, Rizzetto M, Gerin JL: Advances in hepatitis D virus biology and disease. Progress Liver 12:157, 1994.
539. Diener TO: Hepatitis delta virus-like agents: an overview. Prog Clin Biol Res 382:109, 1993.
540. Mayo MA: Current ideas about the taxonomy of sub-viral virus-like agents. Prog Clin Biol Res 382:117, 1993.
541. Wu JC, Choo KB, Chen CM, et al: Genotyping of hepatitis D virus by restriction-fragment length polymorphism and relation to outcome of hepatitis D. Lancet 346:939, 1995.
542. Wu JC, Chen CM, Sheen IJ, et al: Evidence of transmission of hepatitis D virus to spouses from sequence analysis of the viral genome. Hepatology 22:1656, 1995.
543. Casey JL, Brown TL, Colan EJ, et al: A genotype of hepatitis D virus that occurs in northern South America. Proc Natl Acad Sci U S A 90:9016, 1993.
544. Popper H, Thung SN, Gerber MA, et al: Histologic studies of severe delta agent infection in Venezuelan Indians. Hepatology 3:906, 1983.
545. Verme G, Amoroso P, Lettieri G, et al: A histological study of hepatitis delta virus liver disease. Hepatology 6:1303, 1986.
546. Cole SM, Gowans EJ, Macnaughton TB, et al: Direct evidence for cytotoxicity associated with expression of hepatitis delta virus antigen. Hepatology 13:845, 1991.
547. Guilhot S, Huang SN, Xia YP, et al: Expression of the hepatitis delta virus large and small antigens in transgenic mice. J Virol 68:1052, 1994.
548. Ottobrelli A, Marzano A, Smedile A, et al: Patterns of hepatitis delta virus reinfection and disease in liver transplantation. Gastroenterology 101:1649, 1991.
549. Samuel D, Zignego AL, Reynes M, et al: Long-term clinical and virological outcome after liver transplantation for cirrhosis caused by chronic delta hepatitis. Hepatology 21:333, 1995.
550. Crivelli O, Lavarini C, Chiaberge E, et al: Microsomal autoantibodies in chronic infection with the HBsAg associated delta agent. Clin Exp Immunol 54:232, 1983.
551. Philipp T, Durazzo M, Trautwein C, et al: Recognition of uridine disphosphate glucuronosyl transferases by LKM-3 antibodies in chronic hepatitis D. Lancet 344:578, 1994.
552. Amengual MJ, Catalfamo M, Pujol A, et al: Autoantibodies in chronic delta virus infection recognize a common protein of 46 kD in rat forestomach basal cell layer and stellate thymic epithelial cells. Clin Exp Immunol 78:80, 1989.
553. Wesierska-Gadek J, Penner E, Hitchman E, et al: Antibodies to nuclear lamin C in chronic hepatitis delta virus infection. Hepatology 12:1129, 1990.
554. McFarlane BM, Bridger CB, Smith HM, et al: Autoimmune mechanisms in chronic hepatitis B and delta virus infections. Eur J Gastroenterol Hepatol 7:615, 1995.
555. Zignego AL, Deny P, Feray C, et al: Amplification of hepatitis delta virus RNA sequences by polymerase chain reaction: a tool for viral detection and cloning. Mol Cell Probes 4:43, 1990.
556. Madejon A, Castillo I, Bartolome J, et al: Detection of HDV-RNA by PCR in serum of patients with chronic HDV infection. J Hepatol 11:381, 1990.
557. Tang JR, Cova L, Lamelin JP, et al: Clinical relevance of the detection of hepatitis delta virus RNA in serum by RNA hybridization and polymerase chain reaction. J Hepatol 21:953, 1994.
558. Jardi R, Buti M, Cotrina M, et al: Determination of hepatitis delta virus RNA by polymerase chain reaction in acute and chronic delta infection. Hepatology 21:25, 1995.
559. Smedile A, Rizzetto M, Denniston K, et al: Type D hepatitis: the clinical significance of hepatitis D virus RNA in serum as detected by a hybridization-based assay. Hepatology 6:1297, 1986.
560. Smedile A, Bergmann KF, Baroudy BM, et al: Riboprobe assay for HDV RNA: A sensitive method for the detection of the HDV genome in clinical serum samples. J Med Virol 30:20, 1990.
561. Negro F, Rizzetto M: Diagnosis of hepatitis delta virus infection. J Hepatol 22(1 suppl):136, 1995.
562. Cariani E, Ravaggi A, Puoti M, et al: Evaluation of hepatitis delta virus RNA levels during interferon therapy by analysis of polymerase chain reaction products with a nonradioisotopic hybridization assay. Hepatology 15:685, 1992.
563. Buti M, Esteban R, Jardi R: Chronic delta hepatitis: detection of hepatitis delta virus antigen in serum by immunoblot and correlation with other markers of delta viral replication. Hepatology 10:907, 1989.
564. Smedile A, Lavarini C, Crivelli O, et al: Radioimmunoassay detection of 1gM antibodies to the HBV-associated delta antigen; clinical significance in delta infection. J Med Virol 9:131, 1982.
565. Aragona M, Macagno S, Caredda F, et al: Serological response to the hepatitis delta virus in hepatitis D. Lancet 1:478, 1987.
566. Farci P, Gerin JL, Aragona M, et al: Diagnostic and prognostic significance of the 1gM antibody to the hepatitis delta virus. JAMA 225:1443, 1986.
567. Borghesio E, Rosina F, Smedile A, et al: Serum immunoglobulin M antibody to hepatitis D as a surrogate marker of hepatitis D in interferon-treated patients and in patients who underwent liver transplantation. Hepatology 27:873, 1998.
568. Macagno S, Smedile A, Caredda F, et al: Monomeric (7S) immunoglobulin M antibodies to hepatitis delta virus in hepatitis type D. Gastroenterology 98:1582, 1990.
569. Huang YH, Wu JC, Sheng WY, et al: Diagnostic value of anti-hepatitis D virus (HDV) antibodies revisited: a study of total and IgM anti-HDV compared with detection of HDV-RNA by polymerase chain reaction. J Gastroenterol Hepatol 13:57, 1998.
570. Rosina F, Pintus C, Meschievitz C, et al: A randomized controlled trial of a 12-month course of recombinant human interferon-alpha in chronic delta (type D) hepatitis: a multicenter Italian study. Hepatology 13:1052, 1991.
571. Hadziyannis SJ, Hatzakis A, Papaioannou C, et al: Endemic hepatitis delta virus infection in a Greek community. Prog Clin Biol Res 234:181, 1987.
572. Fattovich G, Boscaro S, Noventa F, et al: Influence of hepatitis delta virus infection on progression to cirrhosis in chronic hepatitis type B. J Infect Dis 155:931, 1987.
573. Saracco G, Rosina F, Brunetto MR, et al: Rapidly progressive HBsAg-positive hepatitis in Italy. The role of hepatitis delta virus infection. J Hepatol 5:274, 1987.
574. Arakawa Y, Moriyama M, Taira M, et al: Molecular analysis of hepatitis D virus infection in Miyako island, a small Japanese island. J Viral Hepat 7:375, 2000.
575. Krosgaard K, Mathiesen LR, Aldershvile J, et al: Delta infection and hepatitis B virus replication in Danish patients with fulminant hepatitis B. Scand J Infect Dis 20:127, 1988.
576. Tassopoulos NC, Koutelou MG, Macagno S, et al: Diagnostic significance of IgM antibody to hepatitis delta virus in fulminant hepatitis B. J Med Virol 30:174, 1990.
577. Buti M, Esteban R, Jardi R, et al: Clinical and serological outcome of acute delta infection. J Hepatol 5:59, 1987.
578. Wu JC, Chen TZ, Huang YS, et al: Natural history of hepatitis D viral superinfection: significance of viremia detected by polymerase chain reaction. Gastroenterology 108:796, 1995.
579. Ichimura H, Tamura I, Tsubakio T, et al: Influence of hepatitis delta virus superinfection on the clearance of hepatitis B virus (HBV) markers in HBV carriers in Japan. J Med Virol 26:49, 1988.

580. Shakil AO, Casey IL, Hoofnagle J, et al: Fifth International Symposium on Hepatitis Delta Virus and Liver Disease (abstract). Gold Coast, Australia 1995:D9.
581. Tan WI, Zhan MY: Molecular cloning and sequencing of HDAg-coding fragments of six Chinese hepatitis delta virus isolates. Fifth International Symposium on Hepatitis Delta Virus and Liver Disease (abstract). Gold Coast, Australia 1995:D10.
582. Yang A, Papaioannou C, Hadziyannis S, et al: Base changes at positions 1014 and 578 of Delta virus RNA in Greek isolates maintain base pair in rod conformation with efficient RNA editing. J Med Virol 47:113, 1995.
583. Liaw YF, Tsai SL, Sheen IS, et al: Clinical and virological course of chronic hepatitis B virus infection with hepatitis C and D virus markers. Am J Gastroenterol 93:354, 1998.
584. Smedile A, Rizzetto M, Gerin JL: Advances in hepatitis D virus biology and disease. In Boyer IL, Ockner RK, eds: Progress Liver Disease. New York, WB Saunders, 1994:157.
585. Caredda F, Antinori S, Pastecchia C, et al: Incidence of hepatitis delta virus infection in acute HBsAg-negative hepatitis. J Infect Dis 159:977, 1989.
586. Saracco G, Macagno S, Rosina F, et al: Serologic markers with fulminant hepatitis in persons positive for hepatitis B surface antigen. A worldwide epidemiologic and clinical survey. Ann Intern Med 108:380, 1988.
587. Farci P, Smedile A, Lavarini C, et al: Delta hepatitis in inapparent carriers of hepatitis B surface antigen. A disease simulating acute hepatitis B progressive to chronicity. Gastroenterology 85:669, 1983.
588. Arico S, Aragona M, Rizzetto M, et al: Clinical significance of antibody to the hepatitis delta virus in symptomless HBsAg carriers. Lancet 2:356, 1985.
589. Farci P, Mandas A, Coiana A, et al: Treatment of chronic hepatitis D with interferon alfa-2a. N Engl J Med 330:88, 1994.
590. Rosina F, Pintus C, Meschievitz C, et al: A randomized controlled trial of a 12-month course of recombinant human interferon-alpha in chronic delta (type D) hepatitis: a multicenter Italian study. Hepatology 13:1052, 1991.
591. Lau JY, King R, Tibbs CJ, et al: Loss of HBsAg with interferon-alpha therapy in chronic hepatitis D virus infection. J Med Virol 39:292, 1993.
592. Gaudin JL, Faure P, Godinot H, et al: The French experience of treatment of chronic type D hepatitis with a 12-month course of interferon alpha-2B. Results of a randomized controlled trial. Liver 15:45, 1995.
593. Madejon A, Cotonat T, Bartolome J, et al: Treatment of chronic hepatitis D virus infection with low and high doses of interferon-alpha 2a: utility of polymerase chain reaction in monitoring antiviral response. Hepatology 19:1331, 1994.
594. Di Bisceglie AM, Martin P, Lisker-Melman M, et al: Therapy of chronic delta hepatitis with interferon alfa-2b. J Hepatol 11(suppl 1):S151, 1990.
595. Wolters LM, van Nunen AB, Honkoop P, et al: Lamivudine-high dose interferon combination therapy for chronic hepatitis B patients coinfected with hepatitis D virus. J Viral Hepat 7:428, 2000.
596. Lau DT, Doo E, Park Y, et al: Lamivudine for chronic delta hepatitis. Hepatology 30:546, 1999.
597. Battegay M, Simpson LH, Hoofnagle JH, et al: Elimination of hepatitis delta virus infection after loss of hepatitis B surface antigen in patients with chronic delta hepatitis. J Med Virol 44:389, 1994.
598. Di Marco V, Giacchino R, Timitilli A, et al: Long-term interferon-alpha treatment of children with chronic hepatitis delta: a multicentre study. J Viral Hepat 3:123, 1996.
599. Dalekos GN, Galanakis E, Zervou E, et al: Interferon-alpha treatment of children with chronic hepatitis D virus infection: the Greek experience. Hepatogastroenterology 47:1072, 2000.
600. Puoti M, Rossi S, Forleo MA, et al: Treatment of chronic hepatitis D with interferon alpha-2b in patients with human immunodeficiency virus infection. J Hepatol 29:45, 1998.
601. Petcu DJ, Aldrich CE, Coates L, et al: Suramin inhibits in vitro infection by duck hepatitis B virus, Rous sarcoma virus, and hepatitis delta virus. Virology 167:385, 1988.
602. Madejon A, Bartlome J, Carreno V: In vitro inhibition of the hepatitis delta virus replication mediated by interferon and trans-ribozyme or antisense probes. J Hepatol 29:385, 1998.
603. Glenn JS, Marsters JC, Greenberg HB: Use of a prenylation inhibitor as a novel antiviral agent. J Virol 72:9303, 1998.
604. Eckart MR, Dong C, Houghton M, et al: The effects of using recombinant vaccinia viruses expressing either large or small HDAg to protect woodchuck hepadnavirus carriers from HDV superinfection. Prog Clin Biol Res 382:201, 1993.
605. Ponzetto A, Eckart M, D'urso N, et al: Towards a vaccine for the prevention of hepatitis delta virus superinfection in HBV carriers. Prog Clin Biol Res 382:207, 1993.

CHAPTER

33

Hepatitis C

Jay H. Hoofnagle, MD, and Theo Heller, MB, BCh

Hepatitis C is the result of infection with the hepatitis C virus (HCV) and is a common cause of both acute and chronic liver disease.[1,2] Chronic HCV infection is estimated to affect 170 million people worldwide, including 2 to 3 million Americans.[3] Although frequently a silent disease with few clinical manifestations, chronic hepatitis C is, nonetheless, a common cause of cirrhosis, end-stage liver disease, and hepatocellular carcinoma.[4,5] In the United States chronic hepatitis C is the single major reason for liver transplantation in adults.[6] Indeed, hepatitis C is now the most commonly made chronic liver disease diagnosis, accounting for more than half of cases.[7]

HCV

History and Background

The existence of a third form of viral hepatitis was first shown in 1974 when epidemiologic findings combined with newly developed tests for hepatitis A virus showed that most cases of post-transfusion hepatitis that were not the result of hepatitis B were also not the result of hepatitis A.[8,9] The disease was given the name non-A, non-B hepatitis and subsequently shown to be due to a transmissible agent that could cause both acute and chronic hepatitis.[10-13] Studies in chimpanzees demonstrated that the agent of non-A, non-B hepatitis was a virus that was approximately 60 nm.[14,15] Ultrastructural changes were seen in hepatocytes in infected livers from chimpanzees,[16,17] but the virus itself remained elusive.

The landmark breakthrough in hepatitis C occurred in 1989 when Houghton and colleagues at the Chiron Corporation isolated a viral complementary deoxyribonucleic acid (cDNA) clone from the serum of a chimpanzee experimentally infected with non-A, non-B hepatitis.[18] This cDNA encoded a small protein fragment that reacted with antibodies from patients with this disease. This discovery provided the first identification of the genome of the HCV and the means of developing serologic assays for anti-HCV.[19] Hepatitis C was soon shown to be the major cause of post-transfusion hepatitis and an important cause of chronic liver disease, cirrhosis, and hepatocellular carcinoma. Enzyme immunoassays (EIAs) for anti-HCV were developed providing for a simple and reliable means of diagnosis and of screening blood donations for hepatitis C. The HCV was identified to be a single-stranded, positive sense ribonucleic acid (RNA) virus with a single, large open reading frame (ORF) that encoded a polyprotein of approximately 3000 amino acids.[20] HCV was classified in the family *Flaviviridae* and given its own genus: hepacivirus.

Since the first description of HCV there have been major advances in the understanding the molecular virology of this virus. Six major genotypes have been identified and the nature of HCV quasispecies and their relationship to progressive and chronic liver disease has been studied.[21,22] The polyprotein processing has been elucidated, many of the protein functions are known, and infectious cDNA clones have been constructed.[23-26] Most recently a replicon system for analysis of replication has been developed,[27, 28] although robust growth of full-length HCV in tissue culture remains elusive. Few discoveries in medicine have had such an immediate and profound effect on the understanding and control of an important liver disease.

Virus Structure

HCV circulates in serum at relatively low levels, which has made direct visualization of hepatitis C difficult. The structure of the virus has been deduced largely from molecular analyses. Filtration studies suggest that the virus is 30 to 60 nm in diameter.[15] Infectivity is abolished by chloroform, suggesting that the virus has a lipid envelope.[14] Analyses of particle density have produced variable results, possibly because of the heterogeneity of the virus and the association of some particles with lipoproteins (decreasing density) and others with antibody (increasing density). HCV particles 50 nm in size have been seen by electron microscopy in Daudi cells infected with HCV.[29] From 55 to 65 nm double-shelled particles with spike-like projections and a structure similar to flaviviruses have been visualized by electron microscopy of serum of patients with hepatitis C and high levels of HCV RNA.[30] Virus-like particles have also been produced in a baculovirus expression system using HCV structural proteins.[31] These studies suggest that HCV is a double-shelled RNA virus, approximately 50 to 60 nm. The virus may circulate complexed with antibody and with lipoprotein-rich particles.

Genome Structure

The genomic organization of HCV has similarities to flaviviruses and pestiviruses. The genome is a molecule of single-stranded RNA that averages 9.6 Kb in length (Figure 33-1). The RNA genome is of positive polarity and contains a single ORF that encodes a polyprotein of approximately 3000 amino acids. The structural proteins are encoded at the 5′ end and the non-structural proteins at the 3′ end of the ORF. The single ORF is flanked at the 5′ and 3′ ends by untranslated regions (UTR) that are necessary for the translation of viral proteins and replication of viral genome and are highly conserved in nucleotide sequence and secondary structure.

The 5′ UTR

The 5′ UTR is 341 nucleotides in length and binds ribosomes via an internal ribosomal entry site (IRES), a cap-independent mechanism of translation initiation (which is typical of pestiviruses but not flaviviruses). The 5′ UTR has four major domains,[32] all of which are probably important in translation of viral proteins. The third domain is made up of six individual stem loops, secondary structures that appear to be important for the function of the IRES. The fourth domain contains the initiating codon. These structures are highly conserved and the minor sequence differences have been used for development of genotype specific assays. Several proteins bind to and alter the activity of the HCV IRES,[33-36] although the in vivo importance of these reactions is not known. The HCV 5′ UTR also has several short ORFs, but it is uncertain whether these regions encode any polypeptides.

The 3′ UTR

The 3′ UTR of HCV is variable in length and consists of three distinct regions.[37,38] The first region is immediately downstream of 3′ end of the polyprotein and is variable in length (28 to 40 nucleotides) and sequence. The second region is a polypyrimidine stretch, also of variable length. The third region is highly conserved and consists of three stem loop structures 98 nucleotides in length. This third region is essential for replication[39] but also affects IRES-initiated translation.[40-42] The 3′ UTR also initiates synthesis of the HCV minus strand.[43] These results and others show that the 3′ UTR plays a critical role both in translation and replication of HCV.

Translation and Polyprotein Processing

As the HCV polyprotein is translated by ribosomes in the cytoplasm, it is cleaved into smaller viral proteins. The initial cleavages are in the structural proteins (core, E1, and E2) and are mediated by host signal peptidases in the endoplasmic reticulum.[44,45] This is followed by cleavage of the non-structural proteins by virally encoded proteases, including NS2 that cleaves the NS2/NS3 junction in *cis* and NS3 that cleaves the NS3/NS4 junction, also in *cis*. NS3 then cleaves the remaining polyprotein in *trans* to release NS4A, NS4B, NS5A, and NS5B. Both of the NS5 proteins undergo phosphorylation.

The Structural Proteins

The structural proteins include a single core protein and two envelope proteins (E1 and E2). The core protein has a molecular weight of 21 Kd and is the putative nucleocapsid of the virus. The nucleotide sequence of the core region is highly conserved.[46,47] The core protein localizes

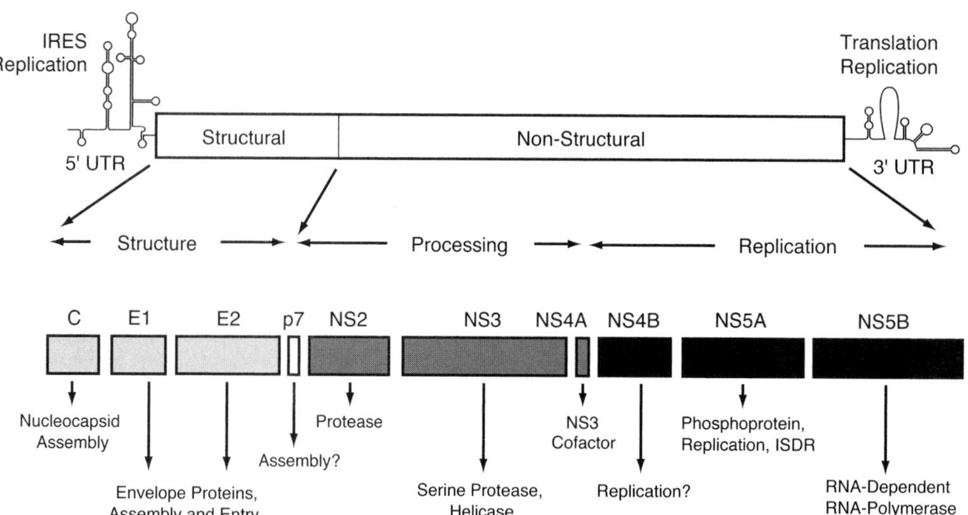

Figure 33-1 The genomic structure of HCV RNA. The genome is a single-stranded molecule of RNA with 5′ and 3′ UTRs and a single, large ORF. The 5′ end of the ORF encodes three structural proteins: C (nucleocapsid), E1, and E2 (two glycosylated envelope proteins). The 3′ end of the ORF encodes multiple NS proteins that are important for protein processing and replication. The postulated function of each protein is shown. *HCV,* Hepatitis C virus; *RNA,* ribonucleic acid; *UTRs,* untranslated regions; *ORF,* open reading frame; *NS,* non-structural.

to the cytoplasm and its N terminal portion binds non-specifically to RNA.[48,49] In addition to providing the protective nucleocapsid structure for HCV, core protein may also have other functions that allow the virus to escape immune surveillance or immune attack and promote viral replication. Thus core protein has been shown to bind the cytoplasmic domain of the lymphotoxin-B receptor, to activate cellular apoptosis,[50] potentiate nuclear factor-kappa B activation,[51] sensitize to fas-mediated apoptosis,[52] and inhibit c-myc induced apoptosis.[53] These other functions of core protein are controversial and of uncertain biologic significance.

The putative viral envelope glycoproteins, E1 (31 Kd) and E2 (70 Kd), provide the coat protein of the virus and therefore are likely to contain the neutralizing epitopes and the attachment sites for viral uptake into hepatocytes. E1 and E2 are separated co-translationally and are targeted to the endoplasmic reticulum where they undergo N-linked glycosylation.[54-57] The E1 and E2 form a stable heterodimer by non-covalent association, a process that requires cellular chaperones.[58,59] E1 and E2 are retained in the endoplasmic reticulum until viral assembly occurs.

The E2 protein has two highly variable regions (HVR1 and HVR2) that are candidates for the major neutralizing epitopes of the virus.[60,61] HVR1 consists of the first 27 amino acids of E2. Antibodies specific to HVR1 have been reported to be protective against re-infection,[62,63] and spontaneous mutations in this region are believed to play a role in immune escape.[64-67] E2 also contains a conserved region known as the PePHD, which may interact with intracellular protein kinase R, an interferon-induced enzyme. These findings suggest that the PePHD region may confer interferon resistance.[68] The receptor binding sites on the envelope proteins, the cellular receptor, and entry into hepatocytes remain unclear for HCV.

The Non-structural Proteins

The various non-structural proteins of HCV provide the enzymatic activity necessary for viral replication. These proteins include NS2, NS3, NS4A, NS4B, NS5A, and NS5B. HCV does not have an NS1 region, a domain found in the flaviviruses upon which the nomenclature is based. The function and structure of most, but not all, of the HCV non-structural proteins have been defined.

The NS2 polypeptide is a short 23-Kd transmembrane protein that acts as a metalloprotease requiring zinc for function.[69] NS2 is active in cleavage of the NS3 protein and may also play a role in the phosphorylation of NS5A.[70]

The NS3 region encodes a 67-Kd protein with two distinct and important enzymatic activities, a 181-amino acid protease at the N-terminus and a 465-amino acid helicase and nucleotide triphosphatase (NTPase) domain at the C-terminus.[71] Both the protease and the helicase domains are of considerable interest as potential targets for anti-viral activity. Both viral enzymes have been resolved by x-ray crystallography.[72-74] In addition, functional assays have been developed for the protease[75,76] and NTPase[77] activities.

The NS3 protease domain has the typical serine protease amino acid triad—serine, histidine, and aspartic acid—at its active center, a zinc binding site required for correct folding, and a chymotrypsin-like fold. Amino acid side chains in the substrate binding site determine the substrate specificity. The NS3 protease cleaves the remainder of the HCV polyprotein, including NS4A that subsequently binds to NS3 and serves as a co-factor for protease activity.[78]

The NS3 helicase domain forms a Y-shaped molecule that unwinds double-stranded viral RNA, the NTPase providing energy for the reaction. Although there is no known DNA stage in the HCV life cycle, the viral NS3 helicase can also unwind double-stranded DNA and RNA-DNA duplexes.[77] The exact role of the helicase in HCV replication is not yet clearly defined but this molecule is also an attractive target for development of anti-viral agents.

NS4 protein is cleaved into two products, NS4A and NS4B, which are 6 and 27 Kd in mass. NS4A is a co-factor for NS3 protease activity[72,79] and may also bind to NS4B and NS5A.[80] The function of NS4B is unknown, although it was recently shown to be a co-factor for the phosphorylation of NS5A.[81]

The NS5 protein is also cleaved into two products known as NS5A and NS5B. The function of NS5A is unknown, although mutations in this region appear to enhance replication.[28,82] NS5A exists in phosphorylated and hyperphosphorylated forms, the degree of which varies among genotypes.[83,84] NS5A contains a putative interferon sensitivity-determining region[85] that in vitro interacts with the interferon-induced protein kinase R.[86] Lack of variability in the interferon sensitivity-determining region has been reported to correlate with lack of response to alpha interferon therapy. Thus NS5A is probably a requisite part of the replication complex of HCV.

NS5B is a 68-Kd, RNA-dependent RNA polymerase responsible for replication of the virus.[87] NS5B shares structural similarities with other viral polymerases and contains the characteristic GDD motif.[88] The NS5B polypeptide has been expressed in both insect cells[87] and *Escherichia coli*[89]; the resultant recombinant proteins have been shown to synthesize RNA in a primer-dependent[87] and primer-independent manner.[90] The NS5B is also a potential target of anti-viral compounds.

Replication

Replication of HCV at the molecular level remains poorly understood and what is known derives largely from study of other flaviviruses. HCV appears to replicate largely in the liver. The basis for hepatocyte tropism is unknown. The first step in replication is the binding of HCV to a cell-surface receptor followed by entry into the hepatocyte and uncoating of the viral genome (Figure 33-2). The receptor for HCV has yet to be definitely identified, but two candidates are CD81 and the low-density lipoprotein (LDL) receptor. CD81 is a ubiquitous cell surface marker that binds specifically to C-terminally truncated E2. However, it is not clear whether CD81 binds to intact virions, and by itself CD81 does not appear to be

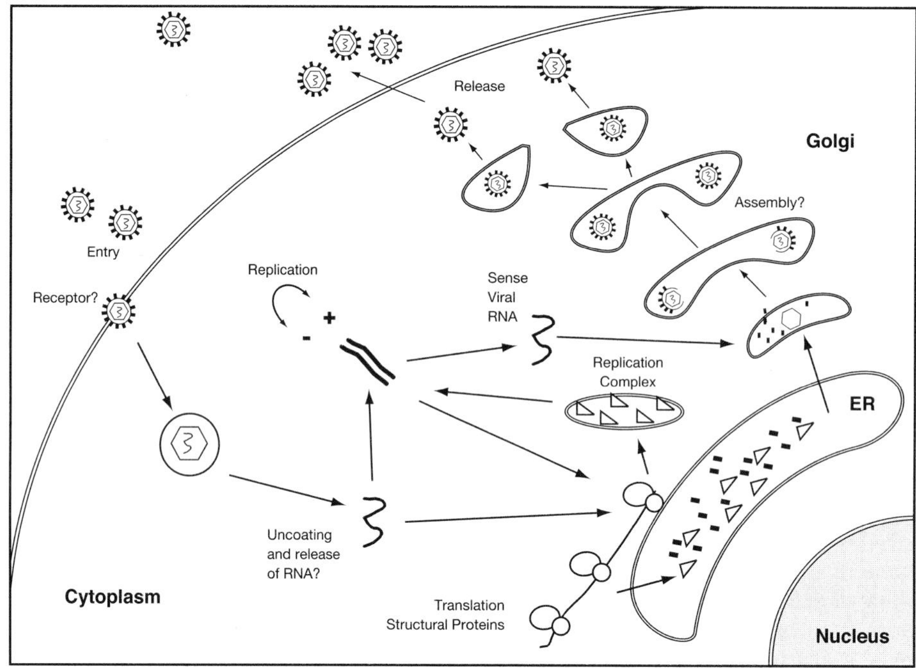

Figure 33-2 Current concept of the replicative cycle of HCV. HCV virions attach to and enter the hepatocyte via an unknown receptor. Possibly in vesicles the envelope and core proteins are disrupted and HCV RNA released. RNA serves as the template for translation of both structural and non-structural proteins. The non-structural proteins assemble into a replication complex that binds to HCV RNA molecules and initiates replication of the RNA into anti-sense (negative strands) and sense (positive stands) HCV RNA molecules. Positive stranded HCV RNA is taken up into assembling HCV core particles that are then encapsidated by addition of E1 and E2 proteins. These progeny virions are then released from the hepatocyte, possibly by exocytosis. *HCV,* Hepatitis C virus; *RNA,* ribonucleic acid.

sufficient for viral entry into cells.[91,92] The LDL receptor binds HCV particles in vitro and could account for liver tropism, but it has yet to be shown to be necessary for viral entry into cells.[92]

Uncoating of HCV probably occurs in acidic endosomes, in which pH changes cause the shedding of the viral envelope and nucleocapsid followed by release of RNA. The viral RNA associates with ribosomes and other cellular proteins leading to IRES-mediated translation of viral proteins. After the replicative complex of viral enzymes is synthesized and assembled, HCV RNA molecules bind to the viral polymerase and negative-strand RNA molecules are produced. The negative-strand daughter RNA molecules are then used as templates for positive-strand RNA synthesis in the same replicative complex. Assembly of the virion requires formation of a nucleocapsid consisting of the core protein that binds to the positive-strand viral RNA. The envelope proteins retained in the endoplasmic reticulum membrane then associate with the nucleocapsid. After the virion is assembled it is probably released from the cell via host cellular exocytosis pathways.

Cell Culture of HCV

Tissue culture growth of HCV remains elusive. HCV has been reported to propagate in a number of mammalian cells, but the level of replication in these systems has been too low to allow for reliable analysis of the replicative cycle or its control. A recent important advance has been the description of HCV replicons—incomplete HCV genomes that are, nevertheless, capable of autonomous replication in mammalian cells.[27] These replicons lack the structural regions of HCV, but have fully functional non-structural regions and both the 5′ and 3′ UTR. Inclusion of a neomycin resistance gene allows for selection of cells containing the replicon, and a more potent IRES allows for a higher level of replication. The replicon system can be used to study HCV replication and to screen anti-viral agents for activity against HCV. Reintroduction of the structural genes into replicons has led to diminished replication in these systems. Adaptive mutations that confer a replicative advantage in tissue culture and the anti-viral effects of interferon in this system have been described.[28,82] Further modification of this system may eventually lead to a fully representative tissue system for HCV.

Animal Models of HCV

The traditional animal model for HCV has been the chimpanzee (*Pan troglodyte*). The chimpanzee has the advantages of an immune system that is similar to humans, thus allowing study of acute and chronic infection. This model has the disadvantages of being based upon a rare, precious endangered species that is difficult and expensive to maintain. In addition, chronic HCV infection in the chimpanzee is rarely associated with liver disease, so that cirrhosis and hepatocellular carcinoma (HCC) occur at a far lower frequency than in humans. However, the chimpanzee model has been invaluable, providing the first evidence that HCV was a viral infection that could cause acute and chronic hepatitis[11-13] and providing the resources for the eventual identification of HCV.[18] More recently, the chimpanzee has allowed for the development of infectious cDNA clones.[23,24] The chimpanzee model will ultimately be crucial for development of HCV vaccines.

Other animal models of HCV replication include the tree shrew *(Tupaia belangeri chinensis),* which develops a transient viremia when inoculated with HCV,[93] and various mouse models including transgenic mice that express one or more HCV proteins.[94,95] In most of these animal models, however, there is little evidence of liver injury or hepatitis.[96,97] Immunodeficient mice have been used to assess HCV replication by transplantation of either hematopoietic cells[98] or fragments of human liver.[99] Recently, a severe combined immunodeficiency mouse transgenic for plasminogen activator has been developed that allows transplantation and growth of human hepatocytes that are susceptible to HCV infection.[100] This system may allow study of HCV infectivity and replication and permit rapid screening of anti-viral compounds.

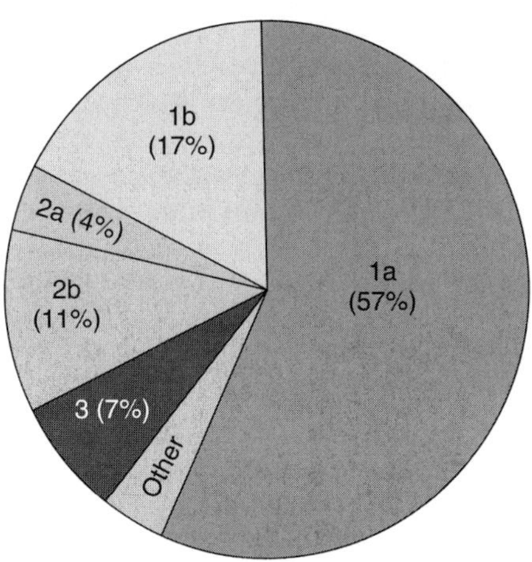

Figure 33-3 Genotypes of HCV in the United States. Proportions identified in testing of samples from the NHANES survey.[3] *HCV,* Hepatitis C virus; *NHANES,* National Health and Nutrition Evaluation Surveys.

TABLE 33-1
Heterogeneity of HCV

Classification	Average degree of diversity*
Quasispecies	<1% to 5%
Isolate	2%-15%
Subtype a, b, c	10%-30%
Genotype 1, 2, 3, 4, 5, 6	>30%

*Variability in nucleotide sequence in representative regions of the viral ribonucleic acid.

Genotypes, Quasispecies, and Viral Heterogeneity

A distinctive feature of HCV is its sequence diversity or heterogeneity. HCV, as with many RNA viruses, circulates not as a single species of virions with identical RNA sequences, but rather as a collection of distinct but closely related RNA sequences.[101] This variability is called quasispecies diversity. The sequence variability can occur in any region of the viral genome, although some regions are more highly conserved (the 5′ and 3′ UTRs and core regions) and some more variable (particularly the HVR1 and HVR2 regions of E2) than others. Replicative fitness and immune pressure probably dictate which variations in sequence are more likely to persist.

HCV can be classified into genotypes, subtypes, and isolates based on sequence diversity of the genome (Table 33-1). Greater than 30 percent sequence divergence indicates different genotypes, designated 1 to 6.[21,22] Variation between 10 percent and 30 percent is characteristic of different subtypes of HCV, which are designated by lower case letters after the genotype, such as 1a or 3b. More than 50 subtypes of HCV have been described. Sequence variation of 2 percent to 15 percent is found among different isolates from patients with the same subtype. Variability of 1 percent to 5 percent is typical of the quasispecies diversity found in a single infected patient.

The classification system of HCV into genotypes and subtypes is based on phylogenetic analyses.[21] Genotypes are stable in a particular patient, although infection with multiple genotypes or subtypes can occur. There are distinct geographic variations in frequencies of different genotypes. Genotypes 1 and 2 are found worldwide; genotype 3 is common in the Indian subcontinent and Southeast Asia; 4 is the major genotype of Africa and the Middle East; genotype 5 has been found largely in South Africa; and 6 in Hong Kong and Viet Nam. In the United States 1a is the most common genotype and genotypes 1a and 1b account for at least 70 percent of infections (Figure 33-3). Genotype 2 is found in 10 percent to 15 percent and genotype 3 in 5 percent to 10 percent of patients in the United States. As population shifts occur and modes of transmission change, changes in HCV genotype distributions occur. Genotypes 1a and 3a were probably rather recently introduced in the United States and European populations, perhaps as a result of the spread of injection drug use in the 1960s and 1970s. Testing for genotypes can be important in epidemiologic studies. The clinical importance of genotypes relates to response to anti-viral therapy. Patients with genotypes 1 and 4 are more likely to be resistant to interferon-based therapy than are patients with genotypes 2 or 3.[102,103,132-134]

Viral diversity and sequence variation may play a major role in determining the course and outcome of HCV infection, but the precise role of these factors remains unclear. The basis for sequence variability appears to be the inaccuracy and lack of proofreading ability of the viral RNA polymerase. As a result, mutant progeny viral

RNA are produced that may replace or replicate along with the parental strains. Evolution of quasispecies diversity may account in part for persistence of HCV infection,[104] but this may be the result rather than the cause of chronicity. Selection pressure for specific variants may be caused by host immune responses to different HCV epitopes,[105] which may account for why some regions of the virion have greater sequence variability. However, purely viral factors may determine shifts in viral variants because some quasispecies may have replicative advantage.[106-108] There is conflicting information about the correlation between quasispecies diversity and severity or outcome of chronic infection, such as in development of cirrhosis or HCC.

Although it is clear that understanding of HCV at a molecular level has progressed remarkably, there is much that is not known about the replication of HCV and the natural history of infection and virus-host interactions. Development of better cell culture and animal models of HCV is needed for a more complete elucidation of the nature of this virus and the disease it causes. Most importantly, these advances are needed for the ultimate development of an effective HCV vaccine.

EPIDEMIOLOGY AND SPREAD

Acute Hepatitis C

Acute hepatitis C currently accounts for 12 percent to 16 percent of cases of acute viral hepatitis in the United States, considerably below the proportion attributable to hepatitis A (40 percent to 55 percent) or hepatitis B (30 percent to 35 percent).[109] Similar proportions have been reported from Europe. Importantly, the proportion of acute cases attributable to HCV and the overall incidence of acute hepatitis C have been falling markedly in the last decade (Figure 33-4). Estimated numbers of cases of acute HCV infection (or non-A, non-B hepatitis as it was known then) rose steadily beginning in the mid-1960s and peaking in the mid-1980s, when there were an average of 240,000 cases per year in the United States. After 1989 and concurrent with the discovery of HCV the estimated incidence of new cases fell markedly and currently is less than 40,000 cases per year, an overall decrease of 80 percent.

The fluctuations in incidence of hepatitis C are attributable to changes in major risk behaviors for acquiring this disease. Thus the rise in incidence of hepatitis C from the 1960s to the 1980s followed the rise in injection drug use in the United States. Furthermore, the decrease in hepatitis C during the 1990s was largely the result of fewer new cases among injection drug users. The introduction of routine screening of blood donations for anti-HCV in 1991-1992 has led to the disappearance of post-transfusion hepatitis C,[110] which has also contributed to the decrease in cases of acute hepatitis C. Finally, with the identification of HCV and the introduction of universal blood precautions in the 1990s,[111] nosocomial and accidental exposures may have also decreased and contributed to the overall decrease in acute hepatitis C. The relative contribution of these changes has been difficult to demonstrate.

Chronic Hepatitis C

The epidemiology of chronic hepatitis C has been more difficult to characterize than that of acute disease. The major reason for this is that chronic hepatitis C is frequently subclinical and a high proportion of patients are not aware that they have chronic infection. With the introduction of tests for hepatitis C, the diagnosis has become easier to make and cases readily identified. Population-based surveys of newly diagnosed cases of chronic liver disease indicate that between 50 percent and 60 percent are attributable to HCV and that the incidence averages 72 per 100,000 population.[7] Many newly diagnosed patients, however, have had chronic infection for years or decades and represent newly discovered rather than newly acquired cases. Because of the increased attention paid to hepatitis C in the lay and

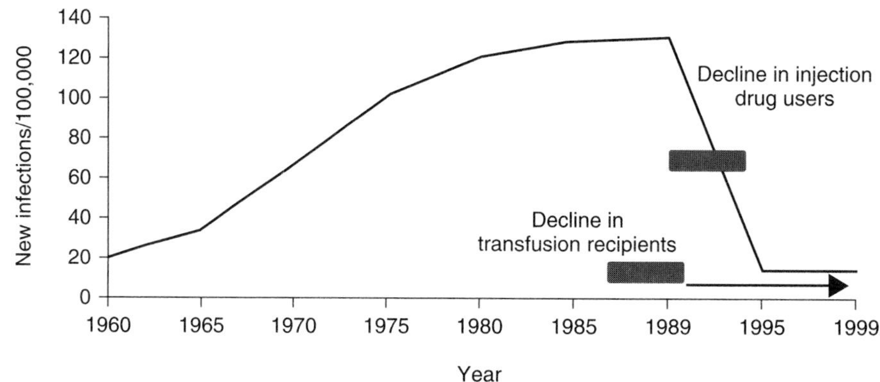

Figure 33-4 Annual rate of new cases of HCV infection in the United States between 1960 and 1999 based upon estimates from both active and passive reporting systems. There was a gradual sixfold rise in incidence between 1960 and the late 1980s, followed by an 80 percent decrease between 1989 to 1999 resulting mostly to a decline in cases of hepatitis C among injection drug users and to a lesser extent to a decline in post-transfusion hepatitis.[109] *HCV,* Hepatitis C virus.

scientific press, the high rate of newly discovered cases is likely to persist for another decade.

The prevalence of chronic hepatitis C can be estimated from population-based serologic surveys. Testing of blood donors demonstrates that 0.1 percent to 0.6 percent are positive for anti-HCV and approximately 70 percent of these also harbor HCV RNA and thus have chronic infection.[112] Volunteer blood donors, however, are not representative of the general population, but rather a highly selected group typically screened for the major risk factors for acquiring hepatitis. The best estimates of the prevalence of hepatitis C in the general US population come from testing of stored serum samples from the National Health and Nutrition Evaluation Surveys (NHANES), conducted at approximately 10-year intervals.[3] In these surveys a carefully constructed, random cohort of non-institutionalized, non-military US citizens are selected for interview, examination, and serum collection. In the NHANES-III population who were surveyed between 1991 and 1994 anti-HCV testing was done on more than 4000 specimens. The frequency of anti-HCV overall was 1.8 percent. Extrapolation to the US population based upon age, sex, and racial or ethnic distribution suggests that this represents 3.9 million Americans. The rate of anti-HCV varied considerably by age, race, and gender. Thus anti-HCV was uncommonly found in pediatric age groups (fewer than 0.1 percent) and rose with age, peaking between age 30 and 50 years. The prevalence of anti-HCV was two times higher in men than women (Figure 33-5, *A*) and approximately twice as high among African-Americans as in whites (Figure 33-5, *B*). The highest rates of anti-HCV positivity were found in African-American men between the ages of 30 and 49 in whom the overall rate was 9 percent.

Not all people with anti-HCV have active HCV infection; some have antibody without detectable viremia. In the NHANES population 74 percent of anti-HCV–positive samples were HCV RNA–positive by polymerase chain reaction (PCR).[3] This proportion suggests that 1.5 percent of the population has chronic HCV infection, or approximately 2.7 million Americans. The proportion of antibody-positive samples that were HCV RNA–reactive also varied with age, gender, and race or ethnic background. Chronic infection was more frequent among men than women and in African-Americans than in non-Hispanic whites. Thus 86 percent of anti-HCV–positive African-Americans, but only 68 percent of non-Hispanic whites, were HCV RNA–positive. Indeed, among African-American men, 98 percent of anti-HCV positive subjects were also HCV RNA–positive, compared with only 70 percent of women.[113] The proportion of HCV RNA–reactive to anti-HCV–reactive samples estimates the chronicity rate of hepatitis C, which is usually estimated as 75 percent to 85 percent. Clearly, however, the chronicity rate as estimated by such cross-sectional testing varies with age, sex, and race, being higher in older than younger subjects, in men than women, and in blacks than whites.

The actual prevalence of hepatitis C in the United States may be higher than was estimated from the NHANES cohort. Hepatitis C is more common in institutionalized and imprisoned populations than in the non-institutionalized populations surveyed in the NHANES study. Studies in United States prisons, for instance, show that 30 percent to 40 percent of inmates are infected with HCV.[114] Because there are 2 million Americans in prison, jails may harbor 600,000 to 800,000 infected individuals. Thus the overall number of Americans with chronic HCV infection may be as high as 4 million.

Only a small proportion of infected individuals are aware of having hepatitis C, although with the growing awareness and availability of testing, this proportion may be increasing. This issue was not addressed in the NHANES study, but in studies tracing people who received blood from donors who later tested positive for anti-HCV, only one third of HCV-infected individuals that were identified were aware of their infection.[115] Thus chronic hepatitis C affects between 1 percent and 2 percent of Americans and probably only one third are aware of the presence of liver disease.

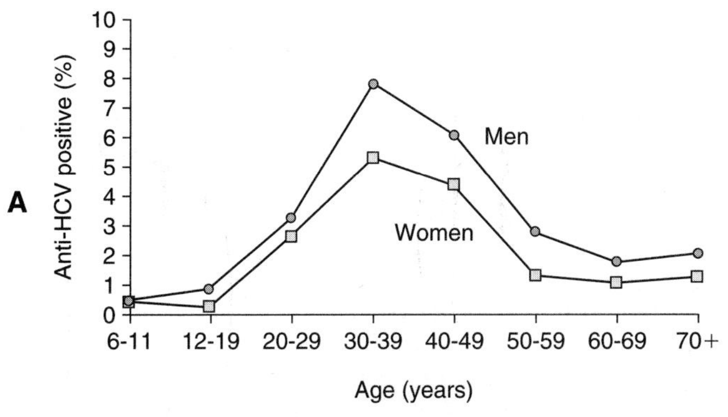

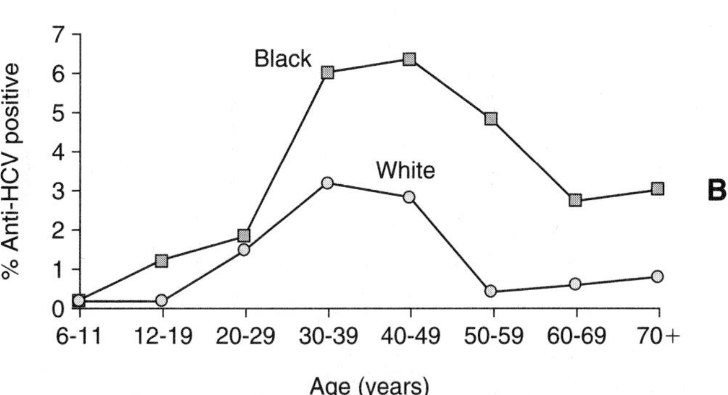

Figure 33-5 A, Prevalence of anti-HCV in the United States by sex and age based upon testing of serum samples from the NHANES survey. Anti-HCV is uncommon among children, and peak rates (between 4 percent and 8 percent) are found in people between the ages of 30 and 49 years. Rates are higher among men than women in all age groups.[3] **B,** Prevalence of anti-HCV in the United States by race and age based upon testing of serum samples from the NHANES survey. Rates are higher and the rise of anti-HCV prevalence with age occurs earlier among African-Americans than Caucasians.[3] *HCV,* Hepatitis C virus; *NHANES,* National Health and Nutrition Evaluation Surveys.

Risk Factors for Acquiring Hepatitis C

At present, the single major risk factor for acquiring acute hepatitis C is injection drug use, which accounts for between 50 percent and 60 percent of cases.[109] Another 20 percent to 30 percent of cases of acute hepatitis C are probably sexually acquired,[110] but history of sexual exposure may be difficult to elicit, particularly in patients with chronic hepatitis C in whom the exposure occurred years before clinical presentation. Other risk factors include accidental needlestick exposure, medical procedures, hemodialysis, and household and perinatal spread, which collectively account for 10 percent of cases of acute hepatitis C (Table 33-2). Acute hepatitis C is also associated with low socioeconomic status, but the mode of transmission in most cases is probably parenteral or sexual exposure.

The relative contribution of different risk factors for acquiring HCV infection is somewhat different for chronic than acute hepatitis C. Thus in most series describing large numbers of cases of chronic hepatitis C, 20 percent of cases are attributable to blood transfusion, 50 percent to injection drug use, and relatively few to sexual exposure.[102,103,116-119] A large proportion (averaging 30 percent) of patients do not report a history of parenteral or other exposure to hepatitis C. A significant proportion of these cases of unknown source may represent sexually transmitted infection.

Transmission by Blood and Blood Products

Transmission of hepatitis C by blood and blood products is the best characterized mode of transmission of this disease. Indeed, the study of post-transfusion hepatitis and use of the chimpanzee model of transmission was the basis not only for the first descriptions of non-A, non-B hepatitis,[8,9] but also the isolation and identification of the virus.[18] Institution of screening of all blood donations for anti-HCV in 1990 led to a marked decrease in the incidence of post-transfusion hepatitis.[110] The improvement of EIA assays in 1992 led to a virtual disappearance of post-transfusion hepatitis C. Nevertheless, estimates made on the basis of testing for HCV RNA in blood donor populations suggested that cases might still occur because of donors with viremia but without antibody. In 1998 nucleic acid testing for both human immunodeficiency virus (HIV) and HCV RNA was introduced by many blood testing laboratories with which the probability of transmission of hepatitis C is estimated to be less than 1 per 100,000 units.[120] However, testing of donor blood for anti-HCV is not performed in all countries of the world; in developing nations, post-transfusion hepatitis C still occurs.

Pooled blood and plasma products are also capable of transmitting hepatitis C; chronic infection with HCV is common among recipients of these products, such as people with hemophilia A and B.[121] Hepatitis C can be inactivated by heat, and heat-inactivation methods were introduced into production of anti-hemophilic factors in 1986. With that modification and particularly with the introduction of routine anti-HCV screening of blood, transmission of hepatitis C by these products has been rare. Accordingly, people with hemophilia who were almost universally infected by HCV are now at low risk for this infection. Nevertheless, there is a large cohort of patients with hemophilia born before 1991 who have chronic hepatitis C, and in whom chronic liver disease and cirrhosis and major causes of morbidity and mortality.

Exposure to blood and blood products also probably explains the high rate of hepatitis C among patients with thalassemia and oncology patients who were treated before the availability of blood donor screening for hepatitis.[122-124] Exposure to blood and blood products is also responsible for the high rate of hepatitis C among renal dialysis and transplant patients.[125] Although the role of blood transfusions is probably no longer important, nosocomial spread by medical injections and contamination of reusable equipment used in dialysis and infusion therapy may play a continuing role in spread of this disease.[126,127]

Immunoglobulin is a plasma product usually prepared from pools of plasma from thousands of donors. Standard immunoglobulin is given by intramuscular injection and has had a long history of being free from hepatitis even when prepared from infectious pools. Shortly after introduction of routine screening of plasma for anti-HCV and elimination of antibody-positive units, an outbreak of hepatitis C occurred in the United States that was attributed to intravenous immunoglobulin from a single US manufacturer.[128] This product differed from other commercially available products in not being heat-inactivated. The outbreak was attributed to the inclusion of HCV RNA–positive units without the neutralizing effects of other anti-HCV–positive units and the absence of chemical or heat inactivation. With the subsequent requirement that immunoglobulins undergo either chemical or heat viral-inactivation, cases of hepatitis C from intravenous immunoglobulin have not been reported.

TABLE 33-2
Modes of Transmission of Hepatitis C

Blood transfusion*
Administration of blood products* (anti-hemophilic factor, factor IX, intravenous immunoglobulin)
Injection drug use
Cocaine snorting
Accidental occupational exposure (i.e., needlestick)
Exposure to contaminated medical equipment (reusable syringes, inadequately unsterilized medical instruments, contamination of intravenous fluids or injectable medications)
Tattooing or body piercing*
Sexual spread
Maternal-infant spread

*Currently uncommon

Injection Drug Use

Injection drug use is the most common mode of spread of hepatitis C in Western countries.[109,129] In most studies between 40 percent and 60 percent of cases of acute or chronic hepatitis C have a history of injection drug use.

In cross-sectional surveys of injection drug users, 75 percent to 95 percent are found to have anti-HCV, rates that are far higher than those for hepatitis B or HIV infection.[130,131] These studies indicate that the majority of injection drug users acquire HCV infection within the first few years of illicit drug use. Prospective studies of new injection drug users have shown that a history of needle sharing, frequent drug use, and attending a "shooting gallery" are the major correlates of acquiring HCV infection. In some instances of chronic hepatitis C, patients relate a single episode of injection drug use decades before the diagnosis. Clearly, hepatitis C is unlikely to be eradicated or come under control until means are available to prevent spread by injection drug use. The efficacy of needle exchange programs in decreasing spread of hepatitis C is still unproven. HCV vaccines would be most appropriate for this population at risk.

Snorting cocaine in the absence of injection drug use has been linked to spread of hepatitis C in at least one retrospective study,[132] but as a risk factor it is difficult to separate it reliably from unacknowledged use of injection drugs or multiple sexual partners.

Sexual Spread

Transmission of acute hepatitis C has been attributed to sexual exposure in several cross-sectional studies and in surveillance studies and case reports.[129,132-138] Nevertheless, sexual spread appears to be uncommon and is certainly less common than in hepatitis B or HIV infection. Cross-sectional serologic surveys show that only 2 percent to 10 percent of spouses or long-term sexual partners of patients with chronic hepatitis C have anti-HCV, and in many cases the seropositive partner has other risk factors for hepatitis C, such as drug use or nosocomial exposures.[134,137] Prospective study of sexual partners of patients with chronic hepatitis C demonstrates minimal transmission, with new onset infections occurring in less than 1 percent of exposed partners yearly.[132] Thus transmission of hepatitis C appears to be uncommon among monogamous partners of patients with chronic hepatitis C.

Despite the rarity with which hepatitis C is spread between sexual partners, studies in acute hepatitis C indicate that up to 30 percent of cases have a history of having multiple sexual partners or recent sexual exposure to a person with hepatitis C.[109] The actual mode of spread has not been well characterized in these studies, and it remains unclear what form of sexual activity predisposes to transmission. It is also unclear why transmission of hepatitis C is more frequently associated with a history of multiple sexual partners rather than with a long-term monogamous relationship with an HCV-infected person. One explanation of this discrepancy is that other sexually transmitted infections promote the spread of hepatitis C, perhaps by causing breaks in the surface of mucosal membranes.

Recommendations to HCV-infected people regarding sexual practices are difficult. Patients with multiple sexual partners should be instructed in safe sexual practices and use of condoms. Patients with a stable sexual partner should be told of the low (but not absent) risk of transmission of hepatitis C. In the situation of a long-term stable sexual relationship, it is best to encourage the couple not to change their sexual practices.

Household and Workplace Spread

Household and workplace spread of hepatitis C is rare and has not been documented in most prospective studies.[132] There is no evidence that hepatitis C is spread by food preparation or sharing of eating utensils or bathing items such as towels or soap. Spread of hepatitis C in the workplace and in schools has not been documented and no restriction should be placed on the person with hepatitis C in either situation.

Occupational Spread

Medical care workers are at increased risk of acquiring hepatitis B as a result of exposure to blood and bodily secretions. However, in cross-sectional surveys of physicians, nurses, and dentists, rates of anti-HCV are low (0.5 percent to 2.0 percent) and similar to those of the general population.[109,139,140] Similarly, rates of anti-HCV among police, firefighters, and emergency medical technicians are similar to those of age- and sex-matched populations.[141,142] Nevertheless, accidental needlestick exposure is a well-documented mode of transmission. Prospective studies of people with well-documented accidental percutaneous exposure to anti-HCV–positive blood show that approximately 5 percent of exposures are followed by HCV infection.[126] The rate of transmission of hepatitis C after needlestick accident is well below that of hepatitis B, but is higher than that for HIV.

Medical care workers with hepatitis C have rarely been implicated in spread of this disease to patients. A single instance of spread of hepatitis C from a cardiovascular surgeon to several patients was reported from Spain,[143] but this mode of transmission is far less common than that occurring with hepatitis B. There are no recommendations at present to restrict the activities of medical care workers who are infected with hepatitis C. These individuals should follow strict aseptic techniques and barrier practices as is recommended for all medical care workers.

Nosocomial Spread of Hepatitis C

Much more common causes of spread of hepatitis C in medical situations are errors in aseptic techniques and sterilization of medical equipment.[144-147] Thus the use of multi-dose vials of medications has been implicated in several outbreaks of hepatitis C, probably as a result of contamination of the vial by reinsertion of a needle or syringe after administration of some of the drug or solution to a patient. Nosocomial spread has been a common cause of hepatitis C in Egypt because of injections of anti-schistosomal medications and in Italy because of reusable glass syringes. With the introduction of non-reusable medical equipment, this mode of transmission should decrease, but lack of adherence to strict universal precautions remains an important cause of spread of this disease.

Another source of nosocomial spread occurs as a result of criminal behavior when an HCV-positive medical care worker illicitly takes narcotic or controlled substances meant for the patient, self-injects the drug, and then purposefully or inadvertently contaminates the intravenous line or drug-administration intravenous solution with his or her own plasma. Outbreaks of hepatitis C resulting from contamination of medical solutions or injection drugs as a result of illicit drug use have been reported and may account for episodes of what appears to be spread of hepatitis C from a medical care worker to a patient.

Maternal-Infant Spread

Hepatitis C can be spread from HCV-positive mother to newborn, but such spread is uncommon. Furthermore, chronic hepatitis C does not appear to worsen the outcome of pregnancy or predispose to fetal abnormalities. Indeed, serum aminotransferase levels tend to decrease during pregnancy, whereas levels of HCV RNA remain stable.[148,149] Thus hepatitis C is not a reason to avoid childbearing.

In large prospective studies 5 percent to 10 percent of infants born to anti-HCV–positive mothers acquire hepatitis C during the first 1 to 2 years of life.[148,150-156] The transmission appears to occur in the postnatal period, although instances of HCV infection detected at the time of birth have been reported. Proof of transmission and actual diagnosis of HCV infection during the first year of life are difficult. All infants born to anti-HCV–positive mothers have anti-HCV in serum as a result of passive transfer of immunoglobulin in utero. The passively transferred anti-HCV can persist for 12 months and possibly longer, which makes anti-HCV testing unreliable for documenting transmission. Most studies have relied upon HCV RNA testing to detect transmission, but HCV RNA positivity may be transient and detectable only by frequent monitoring. Also complicating the issue is the occurrence of false-positive HCV RNA results from PCR, particularly when testing cord blood at the time of delivery. Thus proof of transmission of hepatitis C usually requires the presence of detectable HCV RNA on two separate occasions or persistence of anti-HCV after 12 months of age. Using these criteria the rate of transmission ranges from 5 percent to 10 percent and up to 50 percent of infected newborns clear HCV RNA spontaneously, so that chronic infection eventuates in only 2 percent to 5 percent of children.

Most infants who acquire infection are HCV RNA–negative at birth and become reactive within the first 1 to 3 months of life. Serum alanine aminotransferase (ALT) levels are usually minimally elevated, although high levels can occur, particularly in children who have self-limited infection. Only rarely is neonatal infection associated with symptoms or jaundice. Chronicity develops in at least half of cases. The importance of maternal-infant transmission is shown by studies of hepatitis C in children that demonstrate that vertical transmission now accounts for the majority of cases of chronic hepatitis C in children.[157]

Maternal-infant transmission of hepatitis C occurs only if the mother has HCV RNA in addition to anti-HCV in serum. Other factors that are reported to correlate with a higher likelihood of transmission of hepatitis C are high maternal titers of HCV RNA, co-infection with HIV, a prolonged or difficult delivery, and the use of internal fetal monitoring during delivery.[148,150-158] These factors indicate that amniocentesis and invasive fetal monitoring should be avoided in HCV-positive mothers. Caesarean delivery has not been associated with a lower (or higher) rate of HCV transmission, but may be indicated in the mother with early rupture of membranes and a prolonged or difficult delivery.

Transmission of HCV has not been associated with breast-feeding, but the numbers of cases studied have been few. If breast-feeding is elected, careful breast hygiene and avoidance of feeding if there are cracks in the nipples are appropriate. There is no evidence to suggest that use of anti-viral therapy during the last trimester will decrease transmission of HCV, and the safety of interferon in this situation is unproven and of considerable concern.

Other Modes of Spread

Other possible parenteral modes of spread of hepatitis C include tattooing, body piercing, religious scarification, and bodily injuries with blood exposure. Some of these practices are common and clearly might be a source of spread, but they are rarely identified as important in large cross-sectional studies.[109,129] Tattooing is often cited as a risk factor for developing hepatitis C, but is rarely associated with spread of this disease and is probably a risk only when done unprofessionally using poor sterile technique.[159,160]

CLINICAL COURSE OF HEPATITIS C

Acute Hepatitis C

The course and outcome of acute hepatitis C are variable and largely unpredictable. In adults only 30 percent to 35 percent of cases are symptomatic or icteric and fewer than 1 percent are fatal.[161] The clinical, biochemical, and serologic course of a "typical" case of acute hepatitis C is shown in Figure 33-6. The course of acute hepatitis C can be separated into four phases: incubation, preicteric, icteric, and convalescence.

The incubation period of acute hepatitis C lasts for 15 to 75 days, averaging 50 days. During this period and within a week or two of exposure, HCV RNA becomes detectable in serum and levels of virus gradually rise, peaking at levels of 10^5 to 10^7 genomes/ml within the next 4 to 10 weeks.[162] Patients are without symptoms, and anti-HCV is usually not detectable. The preicteric phase of illness usually begins with the rise of serum aminotransferase levels, occurring within 2 to 4 weeks of appearance of HCV RNA. Symptoms appear somewhat after aminotransferase elevations and are generally nonspecific, consisting of malaise, weakness, poor appetite, nausea, low-grade fever, muscle aches, and right-upper-quadrant pain or tenderness. Extrahepatic manifestations are uncommon in acute hepatitis C, but can include skin rash, hives, and arthralgias. The icteric phase of illness

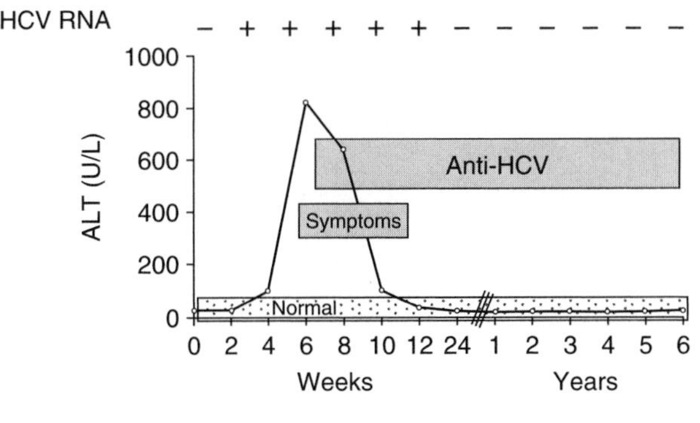

Figure 33-6 Typical course of acute hepatitis C. HCV RNA is detectable by polymerase chain reaction within 2 weeks of exposure. ALT levels rise thereafter, and symptoms appear 6 to 8 weeks after viremia. Anti-HCV generally arises late, after onset of ALT elevations and symptoms. In self-limited disease HCV RNA is cleared and ALT returns to normal levels with resolution of the clinical disease.[161] *HCV,* Hepatitis C virus; *RNA,* ribonucleic acid; *ALT,* serum alanine aminotransferase.

starts with the appearance of dark urine followed by jaundice. Symptoms typically worsen, and it is at this point that the patient is likely to seek medical care. Most patients are HCV RNA–positive at the time of onset of symptoms and jaundice, but only 50 percent to 70 percent have anti-HCV.[163-166] This feature makes testing for anti-HCV relatively unreliable in establishing the diagnosis of acute hepatitis C. The icteric phase of acute hepatitis C is variable in duration and severity, the illness usually lasts 4 to 6 weeks, but the disease can be prolonged and relapsing in course. Some patients develop marked cholestasis and itching that may last several months. Clinical recovery, however, is the usual outcome. Fulminant and subfulminant hepatitis resulting from hepatitis C is rare. The convalescent phase of acute hepatitis C begins with resolution of symptoms and return of appetite and stamina. Serum aminotransferases usually fall to normal within a few weeks of HCV RNA, becoming undetectable. Titers of anti-HCV rise, but rarely to high levels.

The duration of viremia in acute hepatitis C is quite variable. A high proportion of patients with acute infection do not recover and develop chronic hepatitis C.[164,167] However, resolution in acute, self-limited infection can be slow. Most patients with acute resolving hepatitis C remain HCV RNA–positive for 2 to 4 months, so that the finding of HCV RNA 3 months after onset of symptoms suggests but does not prove that chronic infection has become established. Instances of late resolution of viremia after 8, 12, and even 24 months of HCV RNA positivity have been reported.[168] The opposite also occurs, with patients becoming HCV RNA–negative during early convalescence and subsequently redeveloping detectable viral RNA and ultimately developing chronic hepatitis C. These features of the variable course of hepatitis C make it important to assess patients at least 12 months after onset to demonstrate resolution of infection.

Clinical convalescence and disappearance of symptoms and signs of hepatitis do not always indicate resolution of the infection or disease. In hepatitis C between 50 percent and 90 percent of patients develop chronic HCV infection, averaging 75 percent among adults and 55 percent in children.[3,169-172] Titers of anti-HCV tend to be low during the acute phase of hepatitis C and gradually rising thereafter, particularly in patients who develop chronic infection. There have been few studies addressing the issue of whether anti-HCV titers or profiles during the acute illness can distinguish patients who ultimately recover from those who develop chronic infection. A proportion of patients with self-limited hepatitis C either do not produce anti-HCV or produce anti-HCV for a short time only.[166] In long-term follow-up studies at least 10 percent of patients ultimately lose anti-HCV reactivity and are left without serologic evidence of previous hepatitis C.[170] In these patients without anti-HCV, T-cell responses to HCV can be detected.[173]

Patients who have acute self-limited hepatitis C appear in follow-up to have truly recovered from the infection: serum aminotransferase levels are normal and there are no symptoms of liver disease and no long-term consequences.[166] Interestingly, patients with anti-HCV without HCV RNA may have minor abnormalities on liver biopsy, spotty inflammation, and occasional areas of focal necrosis.[174] The reason for these abnormalities is not clear, whether they represent residual viral replication, presence of low levels of viral antigens, an autoimmune phenomenon induced by the previous hepatitis, or an incidental and non-specific finding unrelated to hepatitis C. The persistence of low levels of virus or integrated genomic material that occurs in many viral infections including hepatitis B does not appear to occur with hepatitis C.

Diagnosis of Acute Hepatitis C

The diagnosis of acute hepatitis C is suggested by the presence of clinical or biochemical evidence of acute hepatitis accompanied by anti-HCV or HCV RNA in serum. None of the clinical symptoms or signs or biochemical laboratory features is reliably characteristic to allow for separation of hepatitis C versus other forms of hepatitis or acute liver injury. Thus diagnosis requires serologic (anti-HCV) or virologic testing (HCV RNA by PCR). In most instances the diagnosis can be made based upon anti-HCV testing alone. However, exclusion of hepatitis C may require repeat testing 4 to 6 weeks later or direct assays for HCV RNA. In this situation the most sensitive test—the qualitative PCR—should be used.

The presence of anti-HCV or HCV RNA in a patient with biochemical evidence of acute hepatitis is suggestive but not completely diagnostic of acute hepatitis C. Neither anti-HCV nor HCV RNA testing can reliably distinguish between acute and chronic hepatitis C with a superimposed form of acute liver injury or acute exacerbation. Assays for immunoglobulin (Ig)M anti-HCV are not widely available, nor have they been found to be reliable in separating acute from chronic infection (unlike in hepatitis A and B).[175] Definitive proof of the diagnosis of acute hepatitis C requires the de novo development of anti-HCV or HCV RNA; however, such documentation is rarely possible and is usually not needed in clinical practice. Because anti-HCV frequently appears late during the course of the acute disease, proof of acute hepatitis C can be based upon finding HCV RNA in serum during the acute illness, with later development of anti-HCV. In addition, spontaneous resolution of infection with loss of HCV RNA is also indicative of acute hepatitis C. In some instances the pattern of development of anti-HCV reactivity can suggest acute hepatitis C. Thus the initial antibody reactivities during acute infection are present in low levels and are directed to the core and NS3 regions of the viral genome (anti-22c and anti-c33c). Antibodies to NS4 and the envelope regions (anti-E1 and anti-E2) arise somewhat later. These reactivities can be separated using current anti-HCV recombinant immunoblot assay, which is used for confirmatory testing, but is expensive and only semiquantitative in assessing levels of antibody reactivity.

A more common issue in managing patients with acute hepatitis is the need to rule out hepatitis C as a cause of acute liver injury in a patient who lacks other serologic markers for hepatitis A (IgM anti-HAV) and B (hepatitis B surface antigen [HBsAg] and IgM anti-HBc). In this situation testing for HCV RNA during the acute illness or testing for anti-HCV both during the acute illness and during convalescence effectively rules out acute hepatitis C.

Clinical Course of Chronic Hepatitis C

The course of a patient developing chronic hepatitis C is shown in Figure 33-7. The initial clinical, biochemical, and virologic features are similar to what occurs with acute, self-limited disease. Approximately one third of patients who develop chronic hepatitis C have clinical symptoms or signs that are compatible with the diagnosis of acute hepatitis C at the time of onset of infection.[164-167,170] During this phase, there are no clinical or biochemical features that distinguish whether the patient is developing chronic infection. In general, titers of HCV RNA reach higher and more sustained levels during the acute phase of infection in patients who develop chronic viremia, but the amount of variability in the quantitative assays for HCV RNA and the spontaneous fluctuations in levels of viremia make this clinically unhelpful.[162,176] Indeed, may patients become transiently HCV RNA–negative, despite having chronic viremia during follow-up. This typically occurs during the later phases of acute infection. After the infection is chronic, levels of HCV RNA tend to be stable and spontaneous clearance of virus is uncommon.

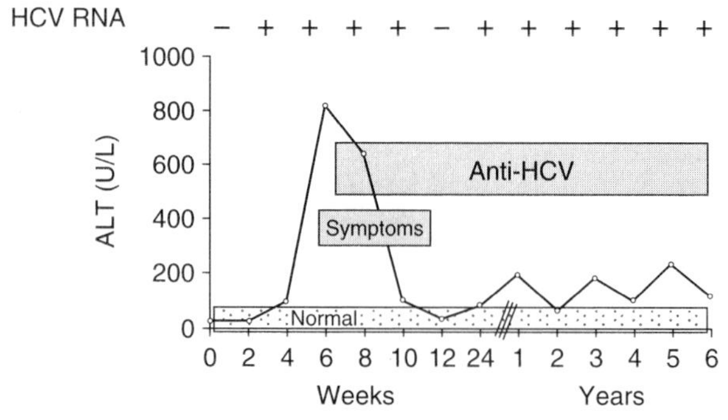

Figure 33-7 Typical course of chronic hepatitis C. HCV RNA is detectable by polymerase chain reaction within 2 weeks of exposure. ALT levels rise thereafter and symptoms appear 6 to 8 weeks after viremia. Anti-HCV generally arises late, after onset of ALT elevations and symptoms. With development of chronic disease, serum ALT and HCV RNA levels fluctuate, being intermittently normal or undetectable. Chronic infection is shown by persistence of HCV RNA positivity with or without ALT elevations.[161] *HCV,* Hepatitis C virus; *RNA,* ribonucleic acid; *ALT,* serum alanine aminotransferase.

Not all patients who develop chronic hepatitis C persist in having elevations in serum aminotransferase levels. In prospective and retrospective-prospective studies, between 25 percent and 50 percent of patients who develop chronic HCV infection have persistently normal ALT values.[166,168,177] These patients are sometimes referred to as "healthy HCV carriers," but the term is inappropriate because almost all patients have chronic hepatitis with at least some degree of active inflammatory component on liver biopsy.[174,178-180] In most patients with moderate or severe hepatitis by liver biopsy despite normal ALT levels, there are other features that indicate significant disease, such as elevations in aspartate aminotransferase (AST) or gamma glutamyl transpeptidase (GGTP) levels or abnormalities of serum albumin, bilirubin, prothrombin time, or platelet counts.

Diagnosis of Chronic Hepatitis C

The diagnosis of chronic hepatitis C is generally made on the basis of persistence of ALT elevations or HCV RNA in serum for 6 months or longer. Follow-up of humans at high risk of developing HCV infection and experimental animals inoculated with infectious material demonstrates that self-limited infection may be associated with delayed clearance of HCV RNA. However, loss of HCV RNA more than 12 months after onset of hepatitis C is relatively uncommon and may be best described as early spontaneous recovery from chronic hepatitis C rather than late recovery from acute (self-limited) disease.

SEROLOGIC AND VIROLOGIC MARKERS OF HEPATITIS C

Anti-HCV Assays

The most widely used tests for anti-HCV are EIAs. Several third-generation EIAs are commercially available and approved for use in screening blood. The assays consist of multiple recombinant HCV antigens immobilized on a solid phase.[166,181] Anti-HCV from the serum sample binds to the viral antigens and is detected using enzyme, labeled anti-human IgG. Substrate is then added to the reaction and the enzyme catalyzes the development of a colored product that is measured by spectrophotometry. Comparison of the sample optical density to that of negative controls yields a ratio that correlates with the amount of anti-HCV. EIAs typically are only semiquantitative and results are read as positive or negative (or "gray-zone"). Current assays have a high degree of sensitivity and specificity. At least 70 percent of patients with acute hepatitis will be anti-HCV-positive when they present with symptoms. The remaining patients become positive within the next 1 to 2 months. More than 98 percent of patients with chronic hepatitis C test positive for anti-HCV by EIA. The remaining patients usually have some form of immunodeficiency, such as hypo- or agammaglobulinemia, HIV infection, renal failure, or treatment with immunosuppressive agents. Research EIAs for specific HCV antibody reactivities (e.g., anti-E1, anti-E2, anti-core, anti-NS3) have been developed, but defining the pattern of antibodies is generally not helpful either in diagnosis or in assessment of severity of disease. Similarly, assays for IgM anti-HCV are not helpful in distinguishing acute from chronic infection.[175]

Immunoblot Assays

Immunoblot assays for anti-HCV are available for confirmation of EIA test results.[182,183] These assays employ recombinant HCV antigens immobilized on nitrocellulose strips. Binding of anti-HCV can then be demonstrated by enzyme-labeled anti-IgG, the pattern of binding indicating the specific anti-HCV reactivity such as anti-core (anti-c22), anti-NS3 (anti-c33c), anti-NS4 (anti–c100-3), or anti-NS5. Reactivity with one specific band is considered an "indeterminate" reaction and reactivity with two or more a confirmed positive. Immunoblot assays are helpful in confirming anti-HCV reactivity found by EIA. In patients with biochemical evidence of liver disease, testing for HCV RNA is a more appropriate approach to confirming anti-HCV reactivity.[184,185] In assessing blood donors found to be anti-HCV positive, however, positive reactions may require confirmation because of the presence of anti-HCV without HCV RNA. This pattern can represent resolved hepatitis C, but also may indicate a false-positive reaction that would be demonstrated by a negative immunoblot assay.

HCV RNA Tests (Qualitative)

Testing for HCV RNA is the most direct method of demonstrating active HCV infection.[184,185] The levels of HCV RNA found in serum are generally too low to be detected using direct hybridization techniques, but can be readily detected after amplification by PCR.[186] Commercially available assays include the Amplicor assay (Roche Molecular Diagnostics), which has a lower limit of detection of approximately 100 copies per milliliter.[187,188] The assay has a built-in step to decrease false-positive reactions caused by contamination with PCR products from previous tests, a frequent problem with laboratory-based assays. Most patients with acute or chronic hepatitis will test positive for HCV RNA. Two exceptions need to be mentioned: patients during recovery from acute hepatitis C (when HCV RNA levels can fluctuate in and out of the detectable range) and patients with end-stage liver disease (in whom HCV RNA levels may fall below detectability despite persistence in the liver). False-positive reactions can occur with any PCR for HCV RNA, but probably at a rate of less than 1 in 100 samples.[189,190] These may be due to contamination of the specimen or technical error.

HCV RNA Levels (Quantitative Assays)

Testing for the level of HCV RNA can be helpful in assessing the likelihood of a response before or during therapy. Two major commercial assays are widely available, one being based upon competitive qualitative PCR (qPCR) and one using signal amplification of branched DNA (bDNA). PCR-based assays include the Monitor assay (Roche Molecular Diagnostics), which has a lower limit of sensitivity of 1000 IU/ml and an upper dynamic, linear range of 850,000 IU/ml, samples above that level requiring a 1/100 dilution for quantitation.[188] A bDNA assay relying upon amplification of the probe rather than the sample RNA (Quantiplex, Bayer Corporation, Emeryville, CA) has a lower limit of detection of 160,000 copies per milliliter and an upper range of linear detection to above 50 million copies per milliliter. All of these assays yield reproducible results; however, they usually yield different results. Thus levels determined by the qPCR assay typically average 0.8 logs lower than levels determined by the bDNA test. Use of international units to define HCV RNA levels may help to circumvent the different results, but most publications on hepatitis C use copies per milliliter and do not carefully define comparable results. Thus 2 million copies per milliliter as measured by the bDNA test (the number that is usually used to separate high from low levels) is equivalent to approximately 800,000 IU/ml as measured by qPCR.[188]

Other quantitative assays for HCV RNA include a commercial competitive PCR assay (SuperQuant, National Genetics Institute, Los Angeles, CA),[191] which has a lower limit of detection of 50 copies/ml and a transcription-mediated amplification assay with a dynamic range from approximately 8 to 10 million copies/ml.

HCV levels can also be quantified using assays for HCV core in serum.[192] These assays rely upon removal of serum proteins and anti-HCV and the viral envelope by detergents and then measurement of the amount of HCV core by EIA. The sensitivity of these assays appears to be similar to those of competitive PCR for HCV RNA levels. These tests have not been extensively evaluated and are not generally available.

Genotyping Assays

Testing for HCV genotype is important in epidemiologic studies and in evaluating patients for therapy. Genotyping can be done by sequence analysis of various regions of the virus, by restriction fragment length polymorphism analysis, by probe-specific hybridization, or by line probe assay (LiPA).[193,194] A widely used commercial assay is the LiPA assay, in which PCR products are incubated on a nitrocellulose strip with genotype-specific hybridization probes.[195,196] The pattern of reactive lines on the strip defines the HCV genotype. The use of sequence analysis is the gold standard and the method required in the case of defining new genotypes, but all methods of genotyping are reasonably reliable, and discrepant results are uncommon. Approximately 5 percent of patients appear to have more than one genotype. A higher proportion of patients have multiple serotype antibody, suggesting infection with several genotypes, some of which are cleared.

PATHOLOGY OF HEPATITIS C

Liver histology of chronic hepatitis C is characterized by hepatocellular injury, necrosis, and unrest, accompanied by both portal and parenchymal inflammation and variable degrees of fibrosis.[197,198] The hepatocyte injury is typically spotty and focal with accompanying chronic inflammatory cells and macrophages. Periportal injury (interface hepatitis or piecemeal necrosis) is often prominent and is characterized by irregularity of the limiting plate, drop-out of hepatocytes, ballooning or eosinophilic degeneration, and prominent lymphocytic infiltrates. The portal inflammation in chronic hepatitis C usually consists predominantly of $CD4^+$ lymphocytes, histocytes, and macrophages. The parenchymal infiltrate consists largely of $CD8^+$ lymphocytes and macrophages.

Prominent portal lymphoid aggregates are more common in chronic hepatitis C than in other forms of chronic hepatitis. The lymphoid aggregates can form into germinal centers and often occur in association with apparent bile duct injury ("Poulsen lesion").[199,200] Actual bile duct loss is uncommon. Also typical of chronic hepatitis C is steatosis, which is more likely to be present and to be moderate to severe in degree in HCV-related as opposed to HBV-related or other forms of chronic hepatitis. The reasons for these typical findings are not clear.

A consequence of chronic hepatitis is hepatic fibrosis that typically starts in the periportal areas with expansion of the portal tracts. Thereafter, septae develop between portal areas and between portal areas and central veins. These septae include bridging hepatic fibrosis, which is usually the preceding lesion to the development of cirrhosis, characterized by distortion of the hepatic architecture by fibrosis and regenerative nodules. The rate of progression of hepatic fibrosis is the major determinant of the prognosis of chronic hepatitis C and the likelihood of ultimately developing cirrhosis and end-stage liver disease.[201] However, initially, hepatic fibrosis is irregularly distributed and needle biopsy may not be reliable in assessing fibrosis because of sampling error.

There are no diagnostic histologic features of hepatitis C. Liver biopsy, indeed, is not so helpful in diagnosis as much as in grading and staging of the chronic hepatitis. "Grading" refers to the assessment of the activity of the liver disease and the amount of hepatocellular injury and inflammation. "Staging" refers to assessment of the degree of fibrosis or permanent architectural damage.[202] Scoring systems have been developed for the grading and staging of chronic hepatitis C (which are also applicable to chronic hepatitis B and autoimmune hepatitis). The most commonly used scoring systems are the histology activity index (HAI or Knodell Score)[203] and the Metavir system (Table 33-3).[204] Modifications of the HAI scoring system have been published and referred to as the Ishak scoring system (Table 33-4).[205] Four general elements are scored in these systems: periportal necrosis and inflammation (piecemeal necrosis), lobular inflammation and necrosis, portal inflammation, and fibrosis. These scoring systems are only semiquantitative and the significance of changes in scores of disease activity or fibrosis remain unclear. In general the degree of piecemeal necrosis and lobular inflammation best reflect serum aminotransferase elevations and the likelihood of disease progression.[180,201,206] All three features are improved by suc-

TABLE 33-3

Metavir Histologic Grading and Staging System[204]

Feature	Score	Description
Periportal necrosis	0	Absent
	1	Mild: focal piecemeal necrosis in some portal areas
	2	Moderate: diffuse in some portal areas or focal in all
	3	Severe: diffuse in all portal areas
Bridging necrosis	0	Absent
	1	Present
Lobular necrosis	0	None or mild: <1 necroinflammatory focus per lobule
	1	Moderate: at least 1 focus per lobule
	2	Severe: several foci per lobule or bridging necrosis
Portal inflammation	0	Absent
	1	Mild: mononuclear aggregates in some portal areas
	2	Moderate: aggregates in all portal areas
	3	Marked: large & dense aggregates in all portal areas
Fibrosis	0	Absent
	1	Stellate enlargement of portal tracts without septae
	2	Enlargement of portal tracts with rare septae
	3	Numerous septae without cirrhosis
	4	Cirrhosis

cessful therapy with alpha interferon. Fibrosis, although generally considered irreversible, does seem to improve gradually in patients who have resolution of the chronic viral infection.[207-209] Although the improvement in fibrosis is sometimes attributed to the anti-fibrotic effects of alpha interferon, it more likely is due to natural reparative processes that occur once the chronic necroinflammatory disease is resolved.

IMMUNOPATHOGENESIS OF HEPATITIS C

The course and outcome of HCV infection are defined by both viral and host factors. Indeed, HCV replication appears to have little direct cytotoxicity on hepatocytes. The severity and complications of both acute and chronic hepatitis C are independent of serum levels, genotype, or strain of virus. Many patients with hepatitis C have mild or minimal disease and escape chronic sequelae of the disease despite persistence of high levels of virus in serum and liver. For these reasons, the immune response to HCV infection is believed to be a major determinant of severity, course, and outcome of acute and chronic hepatitis C.

The immune response to most infection comprises an early innate response and a later adaptive arm. The innate arm consists of non-specific immunologic factors including cytokines, neutrophils, macrophages, natural killer (NK), and natural killer T (NKT) cells. The adaptive arm is made up of the virus-specific responses, including B- and T-cell responses, production of anti-viral antibody, and antigen-specific cellular cytotoxicity (Figure 33-8).

Early immunologic events during acute hepatitis C have been analyzed in chimpanzees experimentally infected with HCV. Within a week of inoculation most chimpanzees have HCV RNA detectable in serum. At the same time, changes can be detected in expression of genes in the liver, reflecting activation of the innate immune system.[210] These early changes include increases in the interferon response genes such as 2′5′ oligoadenylate synthetase and RNA-dependent protein kinase R (PKR), indicating the induction of type 1 interferons that act to stimulate NK and $CD8^+$ cells and up-regulate the expression of major histocompatibility complex (MHC) molecules.[211,212] At the same time, NK and NKT cells are increased in the liver and cytokines such as IL-6, tumor necrosis factor alpha, and interferon-γ are detectable. The role of the innate immune response has not been fully defined in hepatitis C, particularly its relative contribution to the course of the disease. The adaptive arm of the immune system in hepatitis C includes specific

TABLE 33-4
Ishak Histologic Grading and Staging System [205]

Feature	Score	Description
Periportal necrosis	0	Absent
	1	Mild: focal piecemeal necrosis in a few portal areas
	2	Mild/moderate: focal, most portal areas
	3	Moderate: <50% portal areas
	4	Severe: >50% portal areas
Confluent necrosis	0	Absent
	1	Focal
	2	Zone 3 necrosis, some areas
	3	Zone 3 necrosis, most areas
	4	Zone 3 necrosis, some portal-central bridges
	5	Zone 3 necrosis, multiple portal-central bridges
	6	Panacinar or multi-acinar necrosis
Lobular necrosis	0	Absent
	1	Mild: 1 focus or less per 10× objective
	2	Mild/moderate: 2-4 foci per 10× objective
	3	Moderate: 5-10 foci per 10× objective
	4	Severe: >10 foci per 10× objective
Portal inflammation	0	None
	1	Mild: mononuclear cells in some or all portal areas
	2	Moderate: cells in some or all portal areas
	3	Moderate/marked: aggregates cells in all portal areas
	4	Marked: dense aggregates in all portal areas
Fibrosis	0	Absent
	1	Portal fibrosis, some portal areas
	2	Portal fibrosis, most portal areas
	3	Occasional portal-portal bridging
	4	Marked portal-portal bridging
	5	Marked bridging and occasional nodules (incomplete cirrhosis)
	6	Cirrhosis, probable or definite

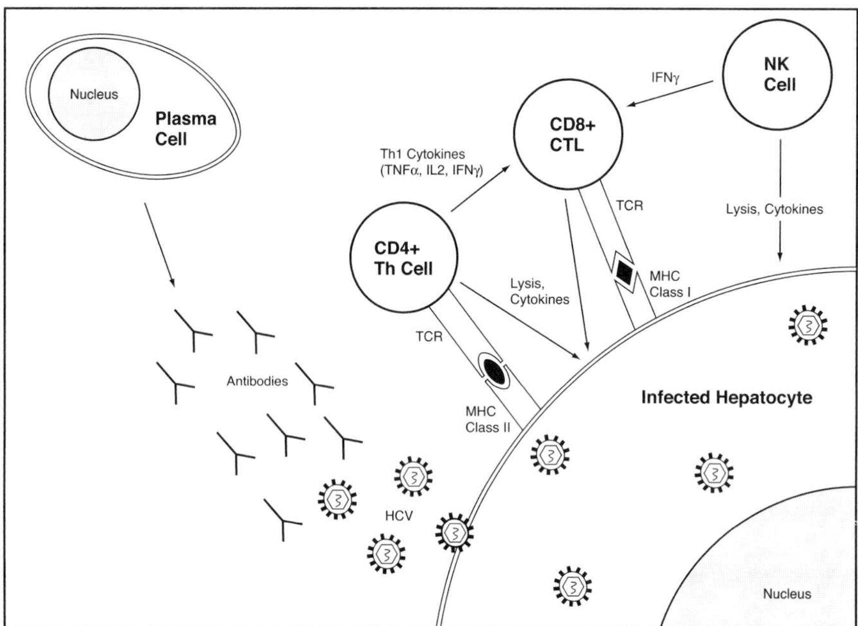

Figure 33-8 The effector phase of the immune response to hepatitis C. In the adaptive immune response plasma cells make anti-HCV directed against different HCV epitopes. In addition, infected hepatocytes present viral peptides in association with MHC molecules that are recognized by the TCR on activated CD4 or CD8 T cells, which result in cytokine secretion (TNF-α, IL-2, and IFN-γ) and, in some instances, cell lysis by CTL. In the innate immune response NK cells secrete cytokines and can cause lysis of infected cells but without the requirement of antigen presentation by MHC molecules or priming. *HCV,* Hepatitis C virus; *MHC,* major histocompatibility complex; *TCR,* T-cell receptor; *TNF-α*, tumor necrosis factor alpha; *IL-2,* interleukin 2; *IFN-γ,* gamma interferon; *CTL,* cytotoxic T cells; *NK,* natural killer.

B- and T-cell responses, development of antibody to HCV, and antigen-specific CD4 and CD8 T-cell reactivity.

Humoral Immunity to Hepatitis C

The role of antibody in determining the outcome of hepatitis C is complex. More than 90 percent of patients develop anti-HCV at some time during the course of acute hepatitis C, although antibody often appears late. Anti-HCV is not necessary for recovery because patients with agammaglobulinemia with acute, resolving hepatitis C have been described.[213] Furthermore, some patients have a mild, self-limited course of infection and never develop antibody. Titers of anti-HCV rise late during acute hepatitis C and achieve higher and more sustained levels in patients who develop chronic infection than in those with acute resolving hepatitis C. Indeed, long-term follow-up on patients with resolved hepatitis C indicate that levels of anti-HCV gradually decline and can become undetectable years or decades after infection.[173] In contrast, anti-HCV levels remain high in most patients with chronic hepatitis C, although the titer and pattern of antibody reactivities do not appear to correlate with severity of disease.

Anti-HCV also does not appear to be completely protective against hepatitis C. Re-infection despite presence of anti-HCV has been reported both in experimentally inoculated chimpanzees[214] and in humans after multiple exposures.[215] The second episode of infection is not necessarily attenuated and can lead to chronic hepatitis. These findings suggest that anti-HCV does not prevent HCV infection and is not required for clearance of virus. Nevertheless, antibody may be partially protective, as shown in studies of immunoglobulin in chimpanzees,[216] as well as partial attenuation of disease in chimpanzees vaccinated with recombinant E1 and E2 proteins[217] or during reinfection[218] and partial protection against reinfection with convalescent serum.[219] In addition, the course of hepatitis C appears to be more severe and rapidly progressive in patients with agammaglobulinemia and other immune deficient states.[220-222] Thus antibody to hepatitis C may be partially protective and antibody responses may attenuate disease progression.

Cellular Immunity in Hepatitis C

Cellular immunity and T cells may play a greater role than humoral immunity and B cells in the course and outcome of hepatitis C. Thus in acute hepatitis C in both chimpanzees and humans, resolution of the infection is associated with a vigorous and broadly based CD8 cytotoxic T-lymphocyte (CTL) response.[153,223] T-cell responses are detectable against multiple HCV structural and nonstructural epitopes at the time of viral clearance,[224,225] which may be the result of both cytolytic and noncytolytic (cytokine-mediated) mechanisms.[226] CD4 T-cell responses are also important. Thus in a study of acute hepatitis C in humans, patients who recovered had a vigorous T-cell proliferative response to NS3 epitopes accompanied by a Th1 cytokine profile.[227] In contrast, patients who developed chronic infection had weak or no detectable CD4 or Th1 responses. An interesting third group of patients initially displayed a strong CD4 response with loss of virus but then relapsed and became HCV RNA–positive when they lost the specific T-cell response.

Both CD4 and CD8 T-cell responses persist for decades after acute infection, even when anti-HCV titers fall to undetectable levels.[173] In contrast, patients with chronic hepatitis C usually have persistence of a weak and narrowly focused T-cell response to HCV.[228-230] The low but persistent T-cell response may underlie the continued hepatocellular injury in chronic hepatitis C. The reasons for the poor T-cell responses to HCV antigens (despite strong B-cell responses) during chronic hepatitis C are not known. When a vigorous T-cell response appears to an HCV epitope, the predominant HCV quasispecies may mutate, escaping the immune surveillance. Alternatively, some HCV variants may down-regulate the CTL response.[231] Presentation of an agonist and antagonist epitope may result in prevention of T-cell activation.[232] In hepatitis C antagonistic HCV variants have been demonstrated for both CD4 and CD8 T-cell responses.[105,231,233-236] Finally, there is the possibility that HCV may actively block the immune response directed against itself by interference with the function of antigen-presenting dendritic cells,[237] by viral proteins interacting with effector pathways (such as complement C1q receptor),[238] or by hiding immunogenic viral epitopes by association with serum lipoproteins.[239]

Thus there are multiple mechanisms by which HCV can circumvent the immune response. Of greatest importance in recovery and clearance of HCV infection is a strong, broadly directed, and durable cellular immune response. Persistence of viremia appears to be accompanied by a T-cell immune response that is weaker and directed against fewer epitopes. The persistence of a low-level, ineffective immune response to HCV is likely to be responsible for chronic hepatic injury rather than a direct cytopathic effect of HCV. Antibody to HCV with or without a cellular immune response may also provide a protective immunity. Better characterization of the immune response during acute and chronic hepatitis is needed for the ultimate development of a successful HCV vaccine.

NATURAL HISTORY OF CHRONIC HEPATITIS C

After chronic HCV infection is established, spontaneous resolution is uncommon.[161,240] Disease activity in chronic hepatitis C may improve or worsen spontaneously, but loss of viremia is rare. This was shown in the early studies of alpha interferon therapy of chronic hepatitis C in which untreated control groups were used; normalization of aminotransferases occurred in approximately 5 percent of untreated controls and liver histology improved in up to half, but loss of HCV RNA was rare.[241] In natural history studies of patients with chronic hepatitis C, persistence of detectable HCV RNA has been the rule except with evolution to end-stage liver disease and hepatic failure.[240] Indeed, among patients undergoing liver transplantation for end-stage liver disease, absence of HCV RNA is found in a proportion of patients with cirrhosis and anti-HCV in serum; after transplantation, these same patients usually develop re-infection in the graft.[242] These results suggest that tests for HCV RNA in patients with hepatic failure may be unreliable and that viral levels decrease with hepatic failure and can fall below the level of detection by current assays.

Thus spontaneous resolution of HCV infection, after it has become chronic, is uncommon. On the other hand, chronic infection is not always associated with progressive liver disease or the complications of cirrhosis, end-stage liver disease, or HCC.[243] The proportion of patients who ultimately develop each of these complications is not well defined, largely because of the lack of large, unselected cohorts of patients with chronic hepatitis C who have been followed carefully on no therapy for prolonged periods. With the steady improvement of treatments for chronic hepatitis C, there are unlikely ever to be such well-characterized cohorts. Most of the quantitative information on complication rate of chronic hepatitis C has come from retrospective studies done on patients infected during an outbreak of hepatitis C or patients who were followed after blood transfusion or known exposure. These studies were not truly prospective and patients were not followed at regular intervals, yet they have provided a fairly consistent picture of the overall natural history of HCV infection from onset to development of clinically important complications.

Natural History Studies of Hepatitis C

Studies of post-transfusion hepatitis have shown that 70 percent to 75 percent of patients infected with HCV develop chronic infection, but only two thirds of these developed chronic serum aminotransferase elevations.[170,243] Liver biopsies taken during the course of the ensuing chronic hepatitis C revealed that 5 percent to 10 percent of those with chronic HCV infection develop cirrhosis within 10 years and up to 20 percent by 20 years of onset.[169] Death from liver disease or HCC was rare during the first two decades of infection. In the largest long-term study of patients developing post-transfusion hepatitis, mortality rates during the first 20 years were the same among patients who developed hepatitis C and those who underwent transfusion but who did not develop hepatitis.[170] These studies, however, did not separate patients with hepatitis C from those with other forms of non-A, non-B hepatitis and included patients with acute, self-limited hepatitis in the long-term analyses of outcome.

Several studies have documented the rates of chronicity and development of significant liver disease after epidemics of hepatitis C caused by use of contaminated plasma products. Large outbreaks of hepatitis C occurred in Ireland[172] and Germany[173,244] as a result of HCV-contaminated immunoglobulins in the late 1970s. In 10- to 20-year follow-up of these outbreaks 55 percent to 60 percent of anti-HCV positive women still had HCV RNA in their serum, indicating a lower rate of chronicity in these young women than has been reported in studies of post-transfusion hepatitis, in which most patients were older and many were men. In addition, rates of cirrhosis were low in both studies, being less than 5 percent after 15 to 20 years of follow-up. In neither study were there instances of end-stage liver disease or hepatocellular carcinoma. These results indicate that the course of chronic hepatitis C may be milder in younger individuals and in women and that severe complications are rare during the first two decades of infection.

Supportive of the relatively benign natural history of chronic hepatitis C in young individuals are studies of children infected with hepatitis C as a result of maternal-infant exposure or blood transfusion.[245] In a large study from Germany 10- to 20-year follow-up was available on a cohort of children who underwent open heart surgery in the 1980s.[171] Sixty-seven children with anti-HCV were identified, but only 37 had HCV RNA, a chronicity rate of 55 percent. None of the 37 children with chronic HCV infection had clinically apparent liver disease and the majority had normal serum aminotransferase levels. Liver biopsies in 17 children showed cirrhosis in 1 and portal fibrosis in 2, a rate of cirrhosis of less than 5 percent in the first two decades of infection. Similar results have been found in young adults who survived childhood leukemia but received multiple transfusions before the availability of anti-HCV testing.[124] It must be stressed, however, that a small proportion of children do develop significant degrees of fibrosis and cirrhosis.

In summary, studies of cohorts of patients from the onset of HCV infection have suggested that only a small proportion of patients develop severe complications of chronic hepatitis C during the first one to two decades of infection. Even though a proportion of patients develop cirrhosis, few develop disability from chronic liver disease, HCC, or death. At issue is whether the slow rate of development of cirrhosis and mortality from liver disease during the first two decades of infection continues thereafter.

Natural History of Established Chronic Hepatitis C

Natural history studies of patients with established chronic hepatitis C provide a less benign picture of the natural course of this disease. In a study of 131 patients with chronic hepatitis C presenting to a referral hospital in Los Angeles 51 percent had cirrhosis on liver biopsy when first evaluated.[246] During follow-up over the next 4 years, 5 percent developed HCC and 15 percent died of end-stage liver disease. Cirrhosis on biopsy was the most significant poor prognostic finding. In a more representative study from Germany 838 patients with chronic hepatitis C (only 17 percent of whom had cirrhosis) were followed for an average of 4 years.[247] During this time 21 (5 percent) died from either end-stage liver disease or HCC. Compared to an age- and sex-matched control group, however, excess deaths occurred only in patients with cirrhosis. Thus short-term poor prognosis in chronic hepatitis C appears to be largely confined to patients with cirrhosis.

Multi-center studies from Europe have more clearly defined the natural history of chronic hepatitis C after cirrhosis is present. Among 384 patients with compensated cirrhosis resulting from hepatitis C, 5-year survival was 92 percent and 10-year survival 81 percent.[248] Hepatic decompensation occurred in 2 percent to 4 percent of patients per year (average = 3.2 per 100 person-years) and HCC in 1 percent to 2 percent of patients per year (average = 1.6 per 100 person-years). After hepatic decompensation arose, prognosis was extremely poor, with the 5-year survival being less than 50 percent. Factors that correlated with likelihood of decompensation were age, signs and symptoms of cirrhosis, high serum bilirubin, and low platelet counts. Factors correlating with likelihood of HCC were similar, but also included male sex.

Clearly, natural history studies suggest that the short-term prognosis of chronic hepatitis C is good unless cirrhosis is present. Cirrhosis generally develops only after several decades of infection and occurs insidiously, frequently with minimal or no symptoms and with few clinical signs or serum biochemical test abnormalities indicative of the severity of the hepatic fibrosis. For this reason, liver biopsy and methods of staging the degree of hepatic fibrosis are of central importance in defining the natural history of hepatitis C, providing information on prognosis, and possibly intervening to prevent the long-term consequences of the disease.

Fibrosis Progression

Cross-sectional studies of large numbers of liver biopsies from patients referred for evaluation for anti-viral therapy have identified factors that predict the presence of advanced fibrosis or cirrhosis on liver biopsy and have attempted to define the risk factors for subsequent development of cirrhosis. The major factors found to correlate with the presence of fibrosis on liver biopsy are patient age, age at onset of infection, male sex, and history of heavy alcohol intake.[249] The height of the serum aminotransferase levels, duration of known infection, history of acute hepatitis, source of infection, and body weight or obesity have generally not correlated with the stage of fibrosis. Age has most consistently been found to correlate with amount of fibrosis, but strangely, known duration of disease as predicted by a history of blood transfusion or initiation of injection drug use has not generally correlated with fibrosis. The lack of correlation with duration of infection is difficult to explain because fibrosis is viewed as a progressive condition and as worsening with duration of infection. The lack of correlation with duration of infection is probably the result of inaccuracy of estimation of duration and the limited duration of infection in most studies (the majority of patients being infected for 10 to 25 years).

A more accurate reflection of the natural progression of fibrosis is derived from prospective studies in which patients undergo repeat liver biopsies after 1 to 10 years.[180,206,250-252] These studies have identified different factors that correlate with progression in fibrosis: mainly age, serum aminotransferase elevations, and degree of piecemeal necrosis on the initial liver biopsy. The effect of age is quite striking and progression of fibrosis being minimal or nil before the age of 40, and escalating considerably after the age of 60 years. Serum ALT and AST values at the time of initial liver biopsy as well as degree of piecemeal necrosis probably reflect the activity of the liver disease. Interestingly, patients with normal serum aminotransferases and those with minimal elevations, generally demonstrate little or no progression of fibrosis over a period of 3 to 5 years.[180] These studies also demonstrate that prediction of the rate of progression of fibrosis from an initial liver biopsy is a poor predictor of subsequent progression.

The correlation of fibrosis progression with disease activity (ALT elevations and periportal inflammation and necrosis on liver biopsy) and with patient age provides insights into some of the variability in the natural history of chronic hepatitis C. Thus the lack of evidence of progression in the majority of children and young women with chronic HCV infection from studies in Germany and Ireland is also reflected by the lack of severe disease activity on liver biopsies from these patients and the frequency with which ALT levels are minimally elevated or normal. Indeed, in the study of Irish women exposed to Rh immunoglobulins, more than 50 percent had normal serum ALT levels and less than 10 percent had values greater than 5 times the upper limit of the normal range.[172] Similarly, among the children exposed to blood products during open heart surgery, all except two had normal ALT levels when identified and evaluated 10 to 25 years later.[171]

Both cross-sectional and prospective studies of liver biopsy histology have failed to identify reliable markers for the presence of significant fibrosis. In the progression from portal fibrosis to bridging hepatic fibrosis to cirrhosis the earliest changes from laboratory tests are decreases in platelet count. Values fall from mid to high normal to low normal or slight decreases as patients develop bridging hepatic fibrosis. Often the decrease in platelet count occurs rapidly, over the course of 6 to 12 months. Thus monitoring of platelet count can be helpful in defining when significant hepatic fibrosis is occurring. The heights of serum aminotransferase values are poor indicators of the degree of hepatic fibrosis, although, as discussed previously, they may be helpful in predicting future worsening of fibrosis. Serum bilirubin and albumin levels and prothrombin time usually remain normal until cirrhosis is present and the finding of elevations in direct bilirubin, decreases in serum albumin and prolongation of the prothrombin time are reliable markers for the presence of cirrhosis. Other indications of the presence of cirrhosis are a reversal of the ALT/AST ratio that often occurs as platelet counts decrease and mild increases in GGTP and alkaline phosphatase levels, serum enzymes that are typically normal during the precirrhotic course of hepatitis C.[253] Finally, intermittent elevations in serum alpha fetoprotein levels are common in patients with cirrhosis, typically occurring during transient exacerbations of disease.[254]

Alcohol Use and Chronic Hepatitis C

A major factor that correlates with degree of fibrosis found on liver biopsy is history of heavy alcohol use. Studies of the US general population indicate that patients with hepatitis C are more likely to drink alcohol (65 percent versus 46 percent) and to be heavy drinkers (21 percent versus 5.8 percent) than patients without HCV infection.[255] In addition, patients with hepatitis C who are found to have cirrhosis on liver biopsy are more likely to have a history of heavy alcohol intake than patients without cirrhosis.[256,257] Among patients with chronic hepatitis C, development of HCC is also associated with alcohol use independent of the role of cirrhosis.[258] In small studies patients who were actively drinking alcohol had higher HCV RNA and serum aminotransferase levels than those who were not drinking.[259] Yet in population-based surveys, there is little correlation between ALT elevations and drinking history in patients with HCV infection, and the level of alcohol intake associated with worsening of hepatitis C has not been defined.[255] In most studies the worsening of liver disease is seen largely among patients who are heavy drinkers, defined as consuming more than 50 to 60 grams (five drinks) per day. Less clear is whether moderate alcohol consumption is harmful. The difficulty in accurately measuring alcohol intake particularly over a prolonged period and the uncertain relationship with hepatitis C make these analyses difficult. In most prospective studies patients are advised not to drink, particularly when embarking upon a course of therapy.

EXTRAHEPATIC MANIFESTATIONS OF HEPATITIS C

Chronic hepatitis C is associated with several extrahepatic manifestations, the most common of which is mixed cryoglobulinemia. Other HCV-related syndromes include low-grade B-cell lymphoma, glomerulonephritis, keratoconjunctivitis sicca, seronegative arthritis, lichen planus, and porphyria cutanea tarda.

Cryoglobulinemia

The association of "essential" mixed cryoglobulinemia with hepatitis C was made shortly after the identification of the virus and development of serologic tests for HCV infection.[260] Retrospective testing of serum samples showed that 80 percent to 98 percent of patients with the previous diagnosis of essential mixed cryoglobulinemia had anti-HCV and HCV RNA in serum.[261-263] Furthermore, complexes of anti-HCV, HCV RNA, and rheumatoid factor were found in cryoprecipitates. On the basis of these associations this condition is probably best described as HCV-related cryoglobulinemia.

Clinical symptoms and signs include vasculitic skin rash, arthralgias, renal disease and glomerulonephritis, neuropathies, Raynaud's phenomenon, and sicca syndrome. The most common and distinctive symptom is palpable purpura, typically occurring on the lower extremities, with intermittent appearance of an erythematous raised pruritic rash that on biopsy shows a leukoclastic vasculitis. Also common are non-specific arthralgias, fatigue and weakness that is out of proportion to the severity of the accompanying liver disease. Indeed, the chronic hepatitis C that accompanies cryoglobulinemia is typically mild and subclinical. More severe cases of cryoglobulinemia will have sialadenitis, glomerulonephritis, nephrotic syndrome, progressive renal failure, or neuropathy.[264] Severe systemic vasculitis similar to polyarteritis nodosa can also occur in association with chronic hepatitis C.[265]

Laboratory findings confirm the diagnosis. Most patients will have high levels of cryoglobulins and rheumatoid factor in serum. Serum complement levels may also be low. The detection of cryoglobulins in serum is not difficult but requires proper collection and processing of samples. Blood should be drawn in prewarmed syringes, and allowed to clot and centrifuged at 37° C. Serum is then stored at 4° C for at least 72 hours and amount of cryoprecipitate is quantified (the "cryocrit"). The typical patient will have a cryocrit of 3 percent to 12 percent. Cryoglobulinemia is often classified as either type I having a single monoclonal immunoglobulin, type II having polyclonal IgG and monoclonal IgM rheumatoid factor, and type III having polyclonal IgG and polyclonal IgM rheumatoid factor. HCV-related cryoglobulinemia is typically associated with type II or type III cryoglobulins.[261]

Testing of cohorts of patients reveals that 30 percent to 50 percent of adults with chronic hepatitis C harbor low levels of cryoglobulins (generally less than 3 percent).[263,266,267] A high proportion of these patients also have rheumatoid factor although most have no signs of extrahepatic disease. Such patients should not be labeled as having cryoglobulinemia unless clinical signs and symptoms of vasculitis are present. The clinical significance of low levels of cryoglobulins in hepatitis C is not known.

The natural history of mixed cryoglobulinemia is not well defined. The disease rarely resolves spontaneously, but can respond to anti-viral therapy. A proportion of patients with cryoglobulinemia eventually develops proliferation of B cells in the bone marrow and liver and appear to have a low-grade B-cell lymphoma.[268] Although this condition is not truly a malignancy, the expansion of B cells can replace bone marrow elements and lead to progressive anemia and decrease in white cells and platelets. Descriptions of correlations of hepatitis C with B-cell lymphomas may actually represent the end-stage of cryoglobulinemia rather than a malignant B-cell lymphoma.[269,270]

Glomerulonephritis

A proportion of patients with chronic hepatitis C develop either membranous or membrano-proliferative glomerulonephritis.[271] The majority of these patients have cryoglobulinemia as the underlying etiology. This condition can lead to progressive renal failure and need for dialysis or renal transplantation. Patients with glomerulonephritis, at least in the early stages, may respond to anti-viral therapy of the hepatitis C with improvements in proteinuria and renal function.

Sjögren's Syndrome

Keratoconjunctivitis sicca has been associated with chronic hepatitis C, particularly among middle-aged women with long-standing disease.[272] The pathogenesis of the progressive loss of salivary and lacrimal glands is not known. This syndrome is a secondary form of Sjögren's syndrome and is often related to cryoglobulinemia. Patients with typical primary Sjögren's syndrome rarely have HCV infection.[273] Salivary gland biopsies in unselected patients with chronic hepatitis C often show lymphocytic sialadenitis.

Seronegative Arthritis

Also common among patients with chronic hepatitis C is seronegative, non-specific arthritis. The frequency of rheumatoid factor in patients with chronic hepatitis C may lead to the erroneous diagnosis of rheumatoid arthritis. HCV-related forms of arthritis rarely cause cartilage or joint destruction.

Porphyria Cutanea Tarda

A small proportion of patients with chronic hepatitis C develop porphyria cutanea tarda (PCT). This syndrome is associated with many forms of liver disease and is usually accompanied by excess hepatic iron, although not necessarily in the range found in primary hemochromatosis. The most common symptoms are blistering and erosions of the skin in response to minor trauma, usually in sun-exposed areas. The diagnosis is made by the finding of increased excretion of uroporphyrin in urine. In the United States approximately half of patients with PCT have chronic hepatitis C.[274] Phlebotomy to remove excess iron leads to resolution of symptoms even in patients with chronic hepatitis C. Phlebotomy is best done before anti-viral therapy is initiated.

THERAPY OF HEPATITIS C

Anti-viral Therapy of Hepatitis C

Alpha interferon was first shown to improve serum aminotransferase levels and liver histology in chronic hepatitis C in 1986, well before the discovery of HCV and at a time that the disease was known as non-A, non-B hepatitis.[275] Identification of HCV[18] and development of assays for viral RNA[186] showed that the improvements in disease during therapy were associated with decrease or loss of HCV RNA from serum and that sustained remissions were accompanied by sustained loss of viral RNA.[276] These studies also showed that the rate of response to a 24-week course of alpha interferon was poor—in the range of only 5 percent to 12 percent.[241,277,278] Nevertheless, alpha interferon was approved for use in chronic hepatitis C in 1990 with a recommended duration of therapy of 24 weeks. Subsequent studies showed that extending therapy to 48 weeks increased the sustained response rate to the range of 12 percent to 20 percent.[241] A major improvement in therapy came with the discovery that the addition of ribavirin to alpha interferon increased the rate of sustained responses by twofold to threefold (to 35 percent to 45 percent).[116,117,279] Most recently, the development of pegylated forms of alpha interferon appears to have improved response rates further.[118,119,280-282] Two large multicenter trials showed that a 48-week course of peginterferon and ribavirin yielded an overall sustained response rate of 54 percent to 56 percent.[102,103] Thus in the 10 years after the initial approval of alpha interferon therapy for chronic hepatitis C there has been remarkable improvement in response rates (Figure 33-9).[2] Nevertheless, considerable controversy remains regarding the appropriate indications for therapy, the optimal doses of pegylated interferon and ribavirin, and optimal duration of therapy for different subsets of patients.

Patterns of Response to Therapy in Chronic Hepatitis C

Responses to therapy can be categorized on the basis of normalization in serum aminotransferase levels (biochemical response), disappearance of HCV RNA (virologic response), and improvement in histology (histologic response).[283] These three patterns often occur together, but not always. Some patients have a full biochemical response but remain viremic. Others clear HCV RNA but continue to have mild elevations in serum aminotransferases. Responses can also be classified on the basis of timing as either initial (occurring within 6 months), maintained (being present as long as therapy is continued), end-of-treatment (being present when therapy is stopped), and sustained (remaining present for at least 6 or 12 months after stopping therapy). The primary end-point for most trials of anti-viral therapy has been the 6-month post-treatment sustained virologic response rate, representing the proportion of patients who remain HCV RNA-negative 6 months after stopping therapy. However, each type of response has meaning and can be used to guide management of patients and evaluation of new therapies.

Sustained Virologic Response

Patients with a sustained virologic response most typically have a rapid and immediate decrease in aminotransferase levels accompanied by disappearance of detectable serum HCV RNA within 1 to 3 months of starting treatment (Figure 33-10, *A*). Patients with higher initial levels of HCV RNA and particularly those with genotype 1 may take longer to become HCV RNA-negative. Some patients, and particularly those with advanced fibrosis or cirrhosis, may continue to have abnormal serum ALT levels during therapy that fall into the normal range only when treatment is stopped (Figure 33-10, *B*). The critical element in a sustained response is that once undetectable, HCV RNA remains negative for the duration of treatment and follow-up. A 6-month, post-treatment, sustained virologic response is a surrogate marker for the success of therapy but has proven to be reliable. In most studies more than 90 percent of patients who have a sustained virologic response also have normal serum aminotransferase levels and 80 percent to 90 percent have improved histology.[116,117] Long-term follow-up studies on patients who remain HCV RNA-negative 6 months after stopping therapy have shown that the response is durable, that serum aminotransferase levels usually remain normal, and that HCV RNA rarely returns.[207-209]. Liver biopsies have shown resolution of all but small amounts of inflammation and actual reversal of fibrosis, at least in patients with portal and early bridging hepatic fibrosis initially. Furthermore, testing of liver biopsy tissue using sensitive PCR techniques demonstrates the absence of detectable HCV RNA, suggesting that virus has been eradicated and patients are cured. Although progression of liver disease does not occur, HCC may arise in patients who have had a sustained virologic response to alpha interferon therapy, but usually only in patients with preexisting cirrhosis or advanced fibrosis at the time of therapy. The rate of development of HCC in patients with a sustained virologic response has been far less than in similar cohorts of non-responder patients.[284-288]

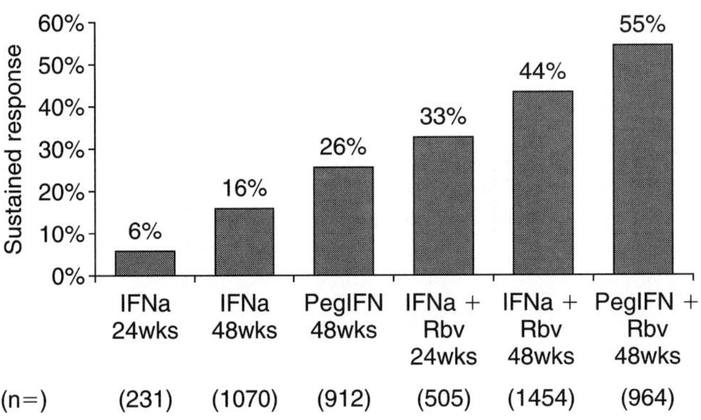

Figure 33-9 Sustained virologic response rates in patients with chronic hepatitis C (all genotypes) treated with 24- or 48-week courses of alpha interferon or pegylated interferon with or without ribavirin. Combined data are from five large randomized controlled trials.[102,103,116-118]

Transient Response and Relapse

A response to therapy but subsequent relapse occurs in a proportion of patients treated with alpha interferon, occurring most commonly with interferon monotherapy and with short courses of treatment. These patients may have a rapid loss of HCV RNA and improvement in serum ALT levels (Figure 33-11, *A*), but more typically have a delayed loss of viremia (Figure 33-11, *B*). The return of HCV RNA after stopping therapy is usually rapid; at least 90 percent of patients who relapse will be found to have HCV RNA detectable 4 weeks after stopping interferon.[289] In some instances, however, relapse occurs later, either at 16 or 24 weeks. Relapse more than 6 months after discontinuation of therapy is uncommon, which is the basis for using the 6-month post-treatment HCV RNA result as a definition for a sustained response. Nevertheless, occasional late relapses occur.[208] Late relapses may sometimes represent re-exposure and reinfection.[290] With relapse, the disease usually returns to the pretreatment level of activity, but some patients have a transient worsening when the HCV RNA returns, such that serum aminotransferases rise twofold to threefold above pretreatment levels. These biochemical relapses are rarely severe or symptomatic.

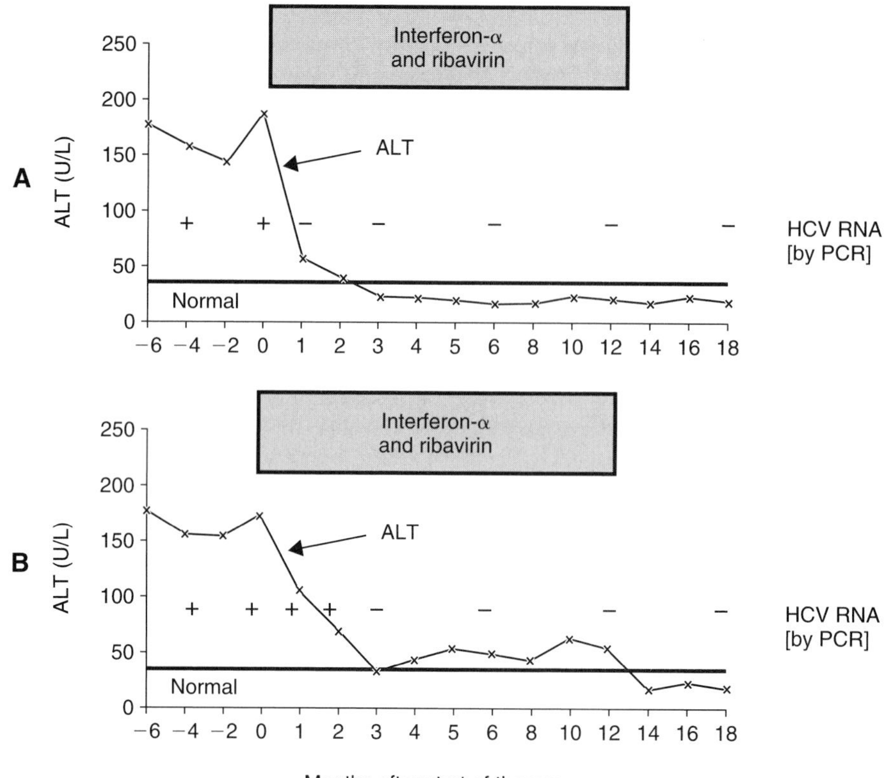

Figure 33-10 **A,** Typical course of a sustained response to antiviral therapy in chronic hepatitis C. With initiation of therapy, serum HCV RNA becomes undetectable by PCR and serum ALT levels fall into the normal range. A sustained virologic response is defined by the lack of HCV RNA at least 6 months after stopping therapy. Most patients also continue to have normal serum ALT levels. **B,** Somewhat atypical course of a sustained response to antiviral therapy in chronic hepatitis C as shown by late normalization of serum aminotransferase levels. With initiation of therapy, serum HCV RNA levels fall and become undetectable by PCR. Serum ALT levels decrease, but remain slightly above the normal range for the duration of treatment. A sustained virologic response is defined by the lack of HCV RNA at least 6 months after stopping therapy. With discontinuation of treatment, ALT levels fall to normal. *HCV,* Hepatitis C virus; *RNA,* ribonucleic acid; *PCR,* polymerase chain reaction; *ALT,* alanine aminotransferase.

Non-response

As many as half of patients treated with alpha interferon and ribavirin are virologic non-responders and never become HCV RNA–negative during treatment (Figure 33-12, *A, B*) or become negative only transiently and have a breakthrough during therapy (Figure 33-12, *C*). There is great variability in the degree of decline in HCV RNA levels and ALT levels in non-responders. Some have little or no change in HCV RNA levels and are truly resistant to alpha interferon.[113] Others have substantial decreases in HCV RNA levels, but never into the undetectable range. In a similar manner serum aminotransferase levels decrease to normal or near normal in some non-responders and remain unchanged in others. There is some degree of correlation between changes in ALT and changes in HCV RNA levels in non-responder patients. A biochemical without a virologic response occurs in at least half of non-responders (see Figure 33-12, *B*). It has been proposed that these patients might benefit from long-term, continuous interferon therapy aimed at suppressing disease activity and perhaps slowing progression of disease.[291] Long-term use of alpha interferon in non-responder patients is currently being evaluated in large scale randomized, controlled trials and at present must be considered experimental.

Optimal Anti-viral Regimen

Currently, the optimal regimen of therapy of chronic hepatitis C is a 24- or 48-week course of the combination of alpha interferon and ribavirin.[1,2] The usual dose of ribavirin is 1200 mg daily (given orally in two divided doses) for patients who weigh more than 75 kilograms (165 pounds) and 1000 mg daily for those who weigh less than 75 kilograms. Lower doses of ribavirin have been used in some trials,[292] but may be suboptimal, particularly in patients with genotype 1 and higher body weights.[102] Further modification of dose of ribavirin by weight (to as high as 1400 mg) has been suggested by recent studies, but has not been systematically evaluated. Hemolytic anemia usually limits the dose of ribavirin that can be used even in large patients.

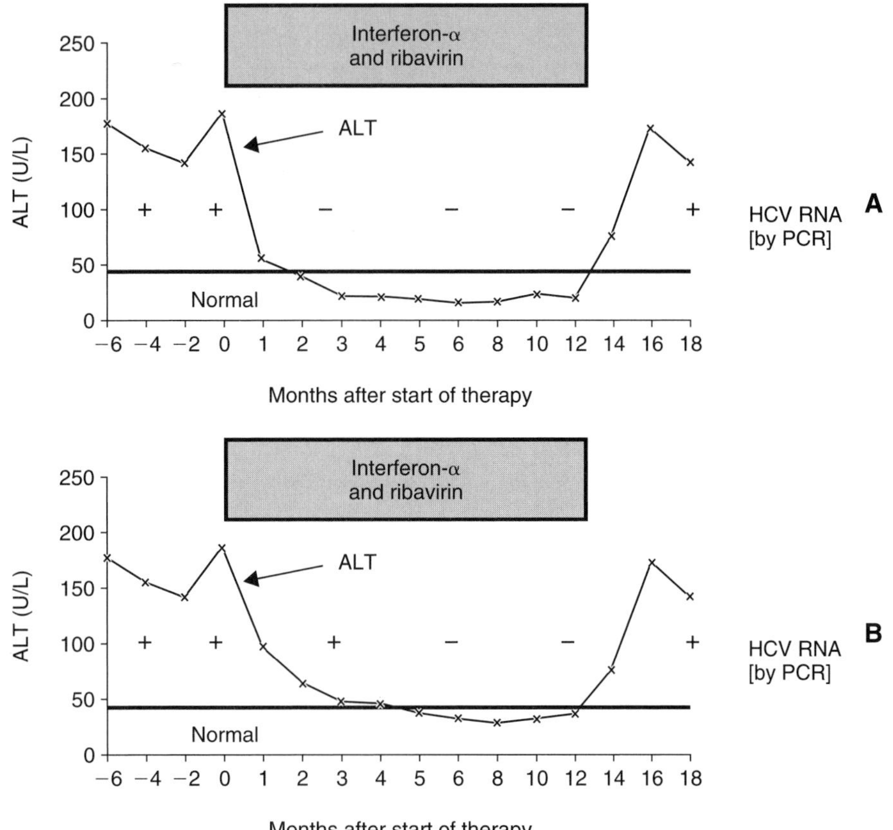

Figure 33-11 **A,** Course of a patient with chronic hepatitis C who has a virologic response to antiviral therapy but subsequent relapse. With initiation of therapy, serum HCV RNA becomes undetectable by PCR, and serum ALT levels fall into the normal range. After treatment is stopped, however, serum HCV RNA becomes detectable again and serum ALT levels rise. **B,** Course of a patient with chronic hepatitis C who has a delayed virologic response to antiviral therapy but subsequent relapse. With initiation of therapy, serum HCV RNA decreases slowly and eventually becomes undetectable by PCR. Serum ALT levels also decrease. After treatment is stopped, however, serum HCV RNA becomes detectable again and serum ALT levels rise. *HCV,* Hepatitis C virus; *RNA,* ribonucleic acid; *PCR,* polymerase chain reaction; *ALT,* alanine aminotransferase.

The usual dose of interferon depends upon the formulation and product. Typically, standard alpha interferon (alfa-2a, alfa-2b, and alfa-n1) is given in doses of 3 million units three times weekly by subcutaneous (SC) injection.[116,117,293,294] Consensus interferon, in contrast, is administered in a dose of 9 μg SC three times weekly.[294] The pegylated forms of alpha interferon are given once weekly and in doses of either 180 μg per injection (peginterferon alfa-2a: Pegasys)[119,281,282] or 1.0 to 1.5 μg per kilogram (peginterferon alfa-2b: PegIntron).[102,118] Pegylated interferons have usually yielded a higher rate of response than standard formulations, but are approximately twice as expensive and may have more side effects.

The optimal duration of therapy is still controversial and not well defined for all regimens. In two large scale studies of 24 and 48 weeks of combination therapy using standard interferon and ribavirin, a 24-week course of therapy was found to be similar in efficacy to a 48-week course in patients with genotypes 2 or 3 regardless of initial viral level (sustained response rates being 62 percent with either regimen) (Figure 33-13, *B*). In addition, among patients with genotype 1 and low levels of HCV RNA (below 2 million copies/ml) the response rate to a 24-week course (32 percent) was similar to that with a 48-week course (33 percent) (Figure 33-13, *A*).[116,117] Indeed, only in patients with genotype 1 and high levels of HCV RNA was a 48-week course of therapy clearly better than a 24-week course (yielding response rates of 27 percent versus 10 percent). On the bases of these studies a 24-week course of combination therapy was recommended for all patients with chronic hepatitis C except those with genotype 1 and high levels of HCV RNA.[2,295] Because virtually all long-term responders to therapy become HCV RNA–negative before 24 weeks, it was also recommended that patients who remained viremic at 24 weeks discontinue therapy at that point. This overall approach appeared to be the most effective and efficient. The ability to discontinue therapy after 24 weeks in patients unlikely to respond spares expense and the side effects of prolonging therapy.

At present, the major difficulty with recommending 24 weeks of therapy for subgroups of patients with hepatitis C is that studies of the newer pegylated forms of

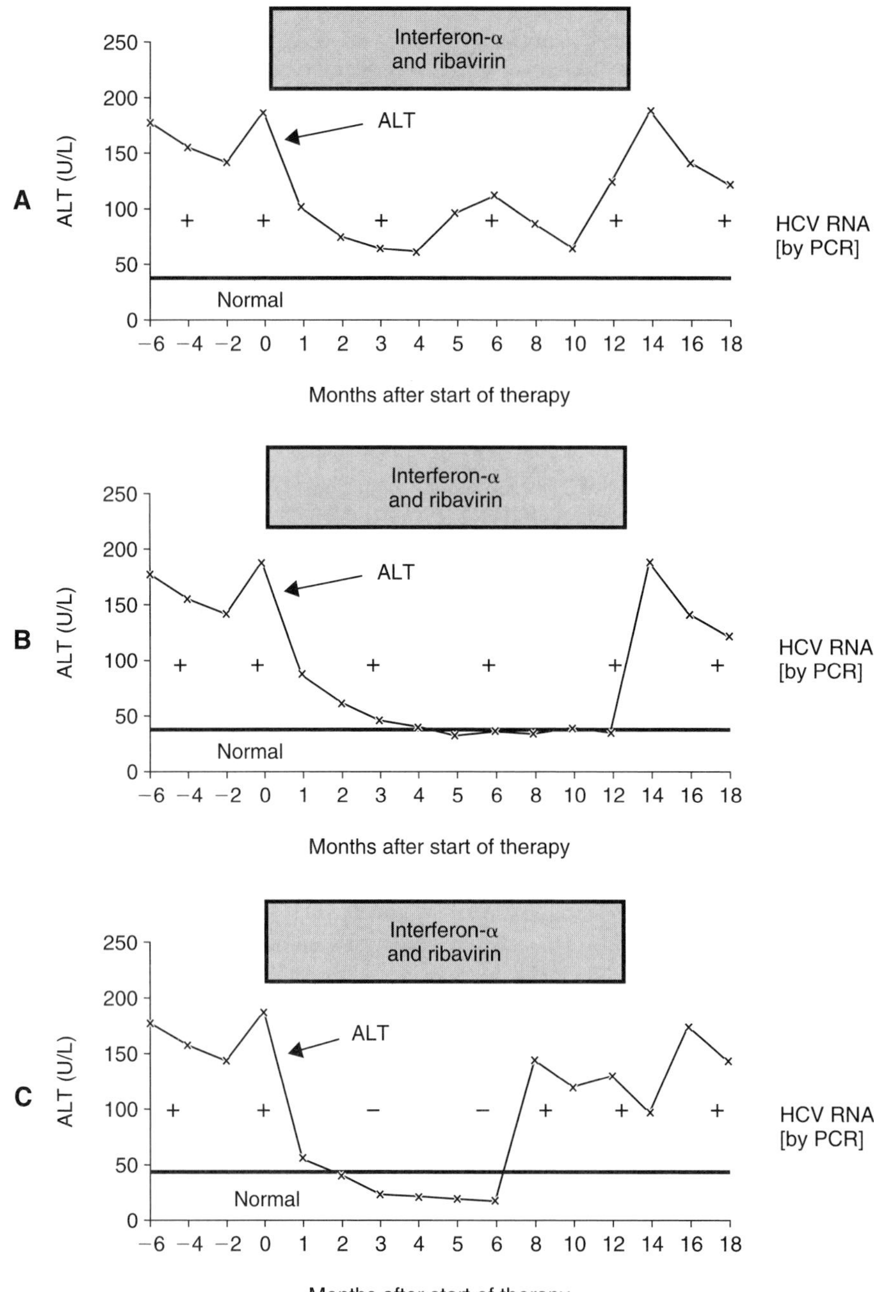

Figure 33-12 **A,** Typical course of a patient with chronic hepatitis C who has neither a virologic nor a biochemical response to antiviral therapy. HCV RNA levels decrease minimally and remain detectable for the duration of treatment. Serum ALT levels also decrease but do not fall into the normal range. HCV RNA remains present and ALT elevations persist when therapy is stopped. **B,** Typical course of a patient with chronic hepatitis C who has a biochemical but not virologic response to antiviral therapy. HCV RNA levels decrease minimally and remain detectable for the duration of treatment and follow up. Serum ALT levels decrease into the normal range and remain normal for the duration of treatment, but rise to pretreatment values after therapy is stopped. **C,** Typical course of a patient with chronic hepatitis C who has a transient virologic response to antiviral therapy but subsequent breakthrough during treatment. With initiation of therapy, serum HCV RNA becomes undetectable by PCR. Serum ALT levels also decrease. During the later phase of therapy, however, HCV RNA again becomes detected and ALT levels rise, remaining abnormal after therapy is stopped. *HCV,* Hepatitis C virus; *RNA,* ribonucleic acid; *ALT,* alanine aminotransferase; *PCR,* polymerase chain reaction.

Low < 2 million/ml

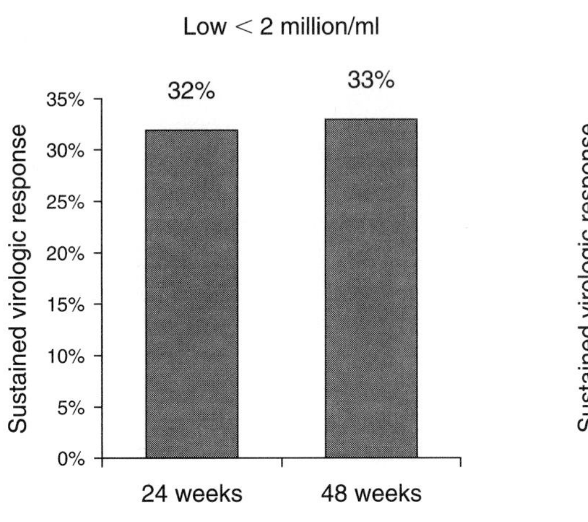

High > 2 million/ml

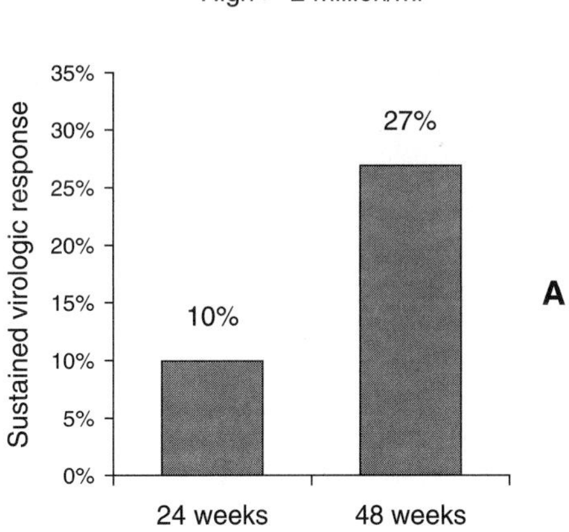

A

U.S. and international trials: n = 1195

Low < 2 million/ml

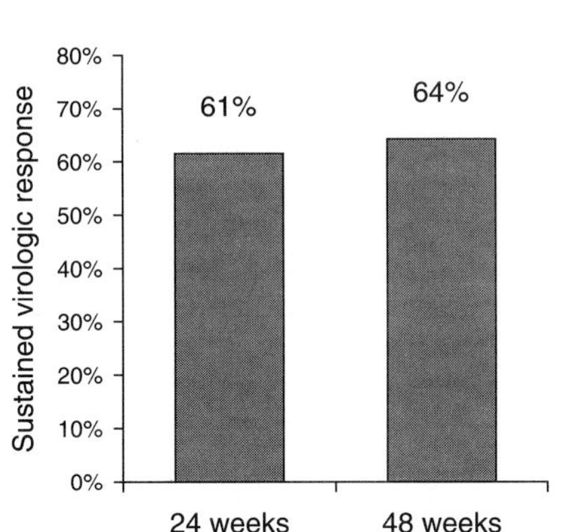

High > 2 million/ml

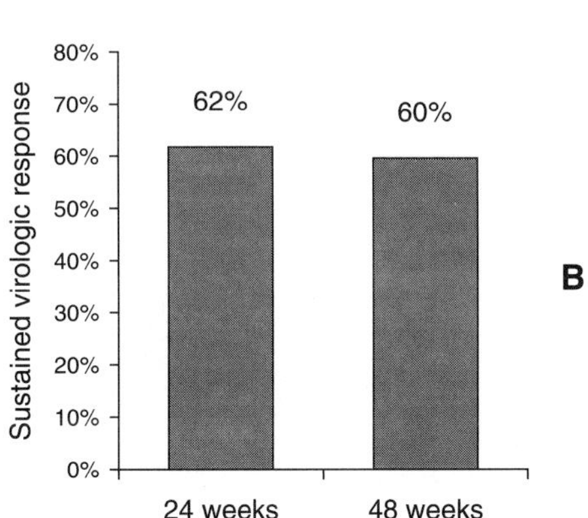

B

U.S. and international trials: n = 548

Figure 33-13 **A,** Sustained virologic response rate to either a 24- or 48-week course of combination therapy with alpha interferon and ribavirin in patients with chronic hepatitis C, genotype 1 with either low (left panel) or high (right panel) levels of HCV RNA on testing before therapy. The 48-week course of therapy was clearly more beneficial only in patients with high initial levels of HCV RNA. Summary of results from two large randomized controlled trials.[116 117] **B,** Sustained virologic response rate to either a 24- or 48-week course of combination therapy with alpha interferon and ribavirin in patients with chronic hepatitis C, genotypes 2 and 3 with either low (left panel) or high (right panel) levels of HCV RNA on testing before therapy. The 48-week course of therapy was no more effective than the 24-week course in patients with either high or low initial levels of HCV RNA. This figure is the summary of results from two large randomized controlled trials.[116,117] *HCV,* Hepatitis C virus; *RNA,* ribonucleic acid.

interferon used 48-week courses only.[102,103] Recently reported preliminary results from studies that have directly compared 24 and 48 week courses of combination therapy using peginterferon (alfa-2a) and ribavirin indicate that 24 weeks of therapy is adequate for patients with genotypes 2 and 3, yielding a sustained virological response rate of 78 percent. In contrast, a full 48 weeks of therapy is optimal for patients with genotype 1, regardless of initial viral level, yielding a sustained response rate of 51 percent. In addition, use of a slightly lower dose of ribavirin (800 mg daily) was adequate for patients with genotypes 2 and 3, but the full, standard dose of ribavirin (1000 to 1200 mg daily) was needed to achieve optimal response rates in patients with genotype 1.

A second difficulty in recommending a shorter course of therapy in subgroups of patients with hepatitis C is that the definition of "high" and "low" levels of HCV RNA has been somewhat arbitrary and variable. Furthermore, different assays can yield differing results for HCV RNA levels and few studies have standardized the reporting of viral titers using international units.[188,296-298] In studies of interferon alfa-2b high levels were defined as above 2 million copies/ml using a competitive PCR assay (SuperQuant, National Genetics Institute, Los Angeles, CA). Similar levels are obtained using the branched DNA signal amplification assay (Quantiplex HCV RNA, Bayer Diagnostics, Emeryville, CA).[297] These levels are roughly equivalent to 0.8 million IU/ml as measured in the non-competitive PCR-based Amplicor Monitor assay (Roche Molecular Systems, Pleasanton, CA).[188] Because of the lack of standardization among assays and the week-to-week and test-to-test sample variation in results, limitation of a course of therapy to 24 weeks on the basis of initial viral level should be done with caution and only in patients with HCV RNA levels clearly below the values cited above.

The combined sustained virologic response rates to 24- and 48-week courses of standard and pegylated interferon given alone or in combination with ribavirin as described in five large multi-center trials[102,103,116-118,281] are shown in Figure 33-14, *A* for patients with genotype 1 and in Figure 33-14, *B* for those with genotypes 2 and 3 (or non-1).

Thus whereas further confirmation is needed, at present the optimal duration of therapy for chronic hepatitis C appears to be for 48 weeks in patients with genotype 1 and for 24 weeks in patients with genotypes 2 and 3. Shortening the duration of therapy in patients with genotype 1 on the basis of viral level should be done with caution. The optimal duration of therapy for patients with genotypes 4, 5, and 6 has yet to be established. The response rates in patients with these less common genotypes appear to be more similar to those with genotype 1 than with genotypes 2 and 3. The optimal dose of ri-bavirin in combination therapy depends upon genotype and body weight; being 800 mg daily for all patients with genotypes 2 or 3; 1000 mg daily for patients with genotype 1 who weigh less than 75 kg; and 1200 mg daily for patients with genotype 1 who weigh 75 kg or more. Ribavirin is given orally in two divided doses daily and dose adjustments may be needed because of hemolysis and anemia. The optimal dose of peginterferon has not been well defined in all situations and varies by the product used: the recommended regimen for peginterferon alfa-2a is a fixed dose of 180 μg once weekly while that for peginterferon alfa-2b is a weight-adjusted dose of 1.5 μg/kg once weekly. These doses of peginterferon are high and may need to be decreased based on side effects and tolerance.

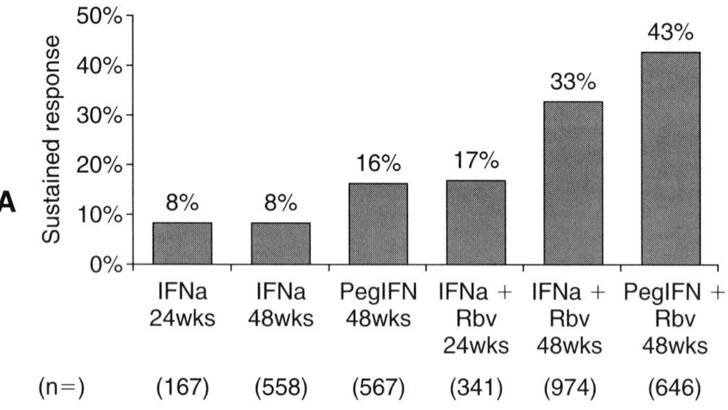

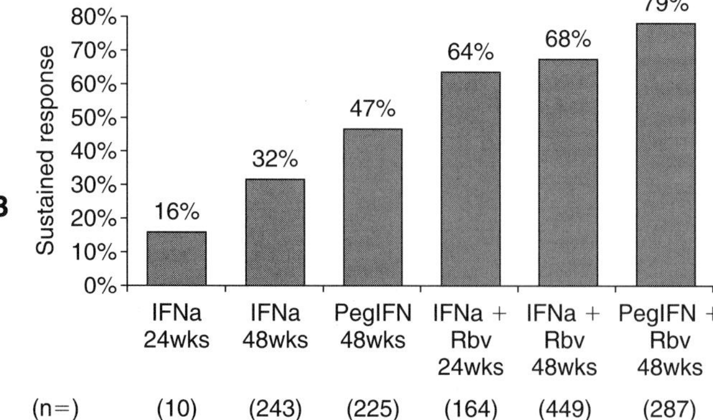

Figure 33-14 **A,** Sustained virologic response rates to either 24- or 48-week courses of standard IFN-α or PegIFN, with or without Rbv in patients with chronic hepatitis C, genotype 1. Numbers of patients treated with each regimen are shown in parentheses. Combined data are from five large randomized controlled trials.[102,103,116-118] **B,** Sustained virologic response rates to either 24- or 48-week course of standard IFN-α or PegIFN with or without Rbv in patients with chronic hepatitis C, genotypes 2 and 3. Combined data are from five large randomized controlled trials.[102,103,116-118] *IFN-α*, Alpha interferon; *PegIFN*, pegylated interferon; *Rbv*, ribavirin.

Viral Kinetics of HCV RNA During Anti-viral Therapy of Hepatitis C

Detailed analysis of HCV RNA levels and mathematical modeling of viral kinetics during therapy with alpha interferon and ribavirin have provided important insights into the mechanisms of action of these anti-viral agents.[299,301] These analyses may also provide clinically useful guidelines regarding the duration of treatment and early termination in patients who have no or minimal likelihood of having a response.

Mathematical modeling of HCV RNA levels after initiation of therapy identifies two distinct phases of decline in viral levels: an initial rapid decline that occurs within the first 24 to 48 hours and a second, slower decline that occurs thereafter.[299,301] The degree and slopes of the first and second phase decline in HCV RNA depend upon dose and anti-viral agent or agents used, whether they are standard or pegylated interferon, whether they are given daily or every other day or weekly, and whether combined with ribavirin.

Four general patterns of anti-viral kinetic response are shown in Figure 33-15. For most patients, the first phase decline starts approximately 8 to 12 hours after the first injection of interferon, after which levels fall by 0.5 to 1.5 logs within 24 to 48 hours. This first phase decline has been interpreted as representing the anti-viral efficacy of interferon and to be directly related to dose.[299] The pattern of the first phase decline may be slightly delayed with pegylated interferon, but differences in dose and absorption as well as the great individual variation in response may also account for differences. In general, the first-phase response can be assessed by testing for HCV RNA levels just before the first injection and again 24 to 48 hours later. The decline in $\log_{10}$ IU can be used as the first phase decline, efficacy or ϵ. The second phase decline is usually measured after 24 or 48 hours and several points over the ensuing weeks define its slope, usually expressed as $\log_{10}$ IU decline per day. There is great individual variation in the slope of the second phase decline of HCV RNA, which can be categorized as either rapid, slow, or flat (Figure 33-15, first three patterns). If there is no phase one or phase two decline, the pattern can be referred to as a nil response. In initial reports the phase two decline was interpreted as representing the death of infected hepatocytes, but the data to support this are scant and the decline is probably better characterized as the clearance of infected hepatocytes (whether by cell death or eradication of virus and establishment of viral resistance inside of the cell).

The slope of the phase 2 decline correlates well with the likelihood of a sustained virologic response; indeed, it is not an independent marker of this response, but rather the early phase of the response. Patients with a rapid response have the highest sustained response rate (75 percent-90 percent) and those with a slow response a lower rate (25 percent-50 percent). Patients with a flat or null response obviously rarely have either an end-of-treatment or sustained virologic response. Indeed, detection of this pattern of response early during therapy may be highly predictive of a non-response allowing for early termination of therapy. These findings suggest that viral kinetic studies may eventually be helpful in guiding therapy and in identifying patients who require higher doses of anti-virals or alternative treatments.

Predicting Non-response During Therapy

Predicting non-response is important in limiting the duration of therapy in the face of a poor likelihood of ultimate response. The best characterized factor that allows for early discontinuation is the continued presence of HCV RNA after 24 weeks of treatment. In all large clinical trials of combination therapy using either standard or pegylated interferon 98 percent to 99 percent of patients who ultimately had a sustained virologic response became HCV RNA-negative by 24 weeks of treatment.[102,302] For these reasons a 24-week "stop rule" is appropriate. For interferon monotherapy an early stop rule of 12 weeks is often used, although the data in support of this are less than the data for stopping at 24 weeks during combination therapy.[116,118,302]

In two recent studies of pegylated interferon and ribavirin, quantitative assays for HCV RNA were used to try to better refine an early stop rule and the likelihood of relapse.[102,103] In both trials the continued presence of HCV RNA at 12 weeks with less than a 2 log decrease in level was highly associated with a lack of sustained virologic response. To use these criteria to stop therapy early, however, requires that HCV RNA levels be tested immediately before therapy and at 12 weeks using a single, reliable, and standardized assay. Furthermore, this algorithm misclassified some sustained responders and would have allowed for early discontinuation of therapy in less than 15 percent of patients. Criteria using viral levels for early determination of a non-response should be used with caution, weighing other factors such as tolerance and severity of the underlying hepatitis.

Use of Virologic Testing to Determine the Duration of Therapy

Testing for HCV RNA during therapy can also be used to estimate the likelihood of relapse and the appropriate duration of therapy. The difference in response rates between 24 and 48 weeks of therapy is not the proportion of patients who become HCV RNA-negative on treatment, but rather the proportion who subsequently relapse.[116,117] Prolongation of therapy increases the sustained response rate largely by decreasing the relapse rate. Although usually not reported in clinical trials of therapy, the relapse rate is actually the major challenge that the clinician faces after the patient becomes HCV RNA-negative on therapy. The purpose of continuing therapy after HCV RNA has become undetectable is to increase the likelihood it will remain negative when therapy is stopped. Although therapy is currently recommended for fixed periods (24 or 48 weeks), it would be preferable to be able to continue therapy until virus is eradicated and when relapse will not occur.

There are no specific tests that can reliably demonstrate that virus is no longer present. Current assays for HCV RNA have a lower limit of detection of 50 to 200 viral copies per milliliter. However, virus eradication must depend upon viral levels being completely absent and less than one in any cell or any amount of body fluid. Mathematically, this level is probably in the range of 10^{-4}

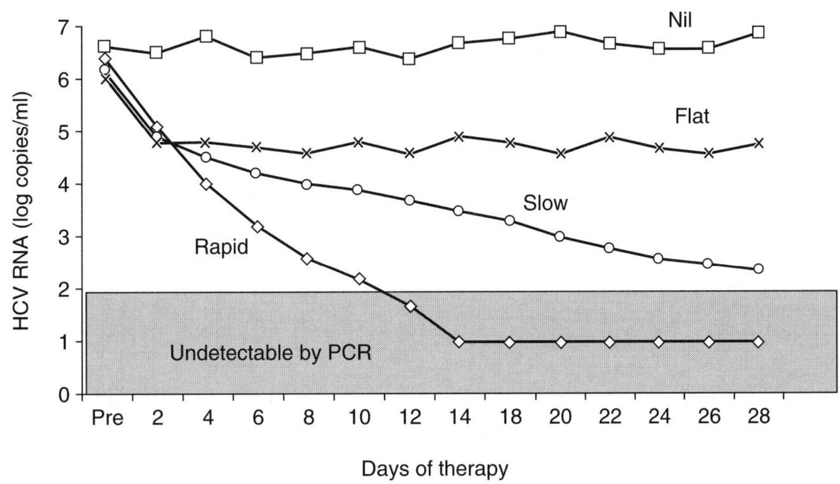

Figure 33-15 Four patterns of change in HCV RNA levels during alpha interferon therapy of chronic hepatitis C, showing either rapid, slow, flat, or nil response to treatment.[299] *HCV,* Hepatitis C virus; *RNA,* ribonucleic acid.

to 10^{-6} viral copies per milliliter. Obviously there are no assays with this degree of sensitivity. On the other hand, these levels might be estimated based upon serial testing of HCV RNA during therapy and calculating the slope of decrease in HCV RNA and the time that would be required for levels to fall below 10^{-6} given a continued linear decrease. Indeed, studies of time to HCV RNA-negativity demonstrate that the likelihood of relapse correlates with the duration of therapy required for HCV RNA to fall to undetectable levels. Thus sustained virologic responses were highest in patients who became HCV RNA-negative by week 4 (77 percent to 86 percent), lower in those who only became HCV RNA-negative by week 12 (32 percent to 52 percent), and lowest in those who first became negative at week 24 (13 to 20 percent).[118] The time of HCV RNA negativity correlated both with initial virus level and genotype—the two major determinants of a sustained virologic response. This provides the theoretic basis for use of time to HCV RNA negativity as a determinant of duration of therapy. Most patients with genotypes 2 or 3 become HCV RNA-negative within 1 to 2 months of starting therapy, whereas patients with genotype 1 and particularly those with high initial levels of HCV RNA often require longer. This approach to therapy has not been evaluated in a prospective manner, but might be best applied to patients who relapse after an initial course of treatment.

Current Indications

Current recommendations for therapy of hepatitis C are based largely upon the 1997 National Institutes of Health (NIH) Consensus Development Conference entitled "Management of Hepatitis C."[303] The Consensus Panel recommended that therapy be offered for all adult patients between 18 and 60 years of age who have HCV RNA in serum, raised serum aminotransferase levels, a liver biopsy showing fibrosis or moderate-to-severe necroinflammatory activity, and no contraindications to treatment (Table 33-5). The Panel also concluded that children, older patients, and patients with mild underlying hepatitis C can be safety treated, but the long-term benefit of therapy in these groups has not been demonstrated, and the decision to treat should be based upon careful review of the risks and benefits with the individual patient. The Consensus Panel recommended caution in treating patients with decompensated liver disease, an organ transplant, renal failure, active alcohol or substance abuse, severe neuropsychiatric disease, and any specific contraindication to therapy such as inability to practice birth control. These indications are still widely accepted, but are likely to be revised by the upcoming Consensus Development Conference Update on management of chronic hepatitis C scheduled for June 2002.

Contraindications

The relative contraindications to interferon therapy of hepatitis C include decompensated liver disease, coronary or cerebrovascular disease, renal insufficiency, solid organ transplantation, severe neuropsychiatric disease, anemia or bone marrow insufficiency, active substance abuse, and active autoimmune disease (Table 33-6). In each of these situations interferon with or without ribavirin is usually poorly tolerated and can be harmful; efficacy has not been clearly demonstrated. Unfortunately, these contraindications eliminate a large number of patients with this disease. Furthermore, there are instances of excellent responses to therapy in patients with some of the relative contraindications, such as decompensated liver disease, renal insufficiency, neuropsychiatric disease, and active substance abuse. It is important to stress that these are all *relative* contraindications and should not be used to exclude patients who otherwise are good candidates for therapy. The *absolute* contraindications include pregnancy, breast-feeding, and inability to practice birth control.

Therapy of Children

The treatment of children with hepatitis C is still controversial. Neither interferon nor ribavirin has been adequately evaluated for pediatric use and neither is ap-

TABLE 33-5

Usual Indications for Therapy of Chronic Hepatitis C

Age greater than 18 years*
Raised serum aminotransferase levels†
HCV RNA detectable in serum
Chronic hepatitis on liver biopsy with moderate or severe inflammatory activity or any fibrosis‡
No contraindications

HCV, Hepatitis C virus; *RNA,* ribonucleic acid.
*Neither interferon nor ribavirin has been approved for use in children, but published studies have demonstrated rates of response that are equivalent if not better than in adults.
†In some situations patients with normal serum aminotransferase levels warrant therapy.
‡Liver biopsy is helpful in making a decision to treat patients, but is not an absolute requisite for therapy if there are contraindications or obstacles to obtaining a liver biopsy.

TABLE 33-6

Contraindications to Combination Therapy

Both Interferon and Ribavirin
Pregnancy
Breast-feeding, inability to practice birth control

Ribavirin
Anemia (hemoglobin less than 11 g/dl)
Coronary or cerebrovascular disease
Renal failure
Allergic or hypersensitivity reaction to ribavirin

Interferon
Continued and unstable neuropsychiatric disease
Continued and unstable drug or alcohol abuse
History of allergy, hypersensitivity, or severe adverse reaction to interferon

proved for this indication in the United States. Chronic hepatitis C tends to be mild and non-progressive in children and the need for treatment can be questioned.[171] Nevertheless, preliminary uncontrolled studies suggest that children have a better rate of response to interferon therapy than adults and that they tend to have fewer side effects.[304-306] Chronic hepatitis C rarely resolves spontaneously; children with this disease are likely to have the infection for life. For these reasons, early treatment may be appropriate and is often requested. Because of the lack of information on dose and safety of ribavirin in children, monotherapy with interferon might be considered most appropriate at present, but neither the dose nor the duration of therapy has been defined in children, particularly with the newer pegylated interferons.

Therapy of the Elderly

On the other side of the age spectrum, therapy of the elderly with chronic hepatitis C is often problematic because of a higher rate of side effects and a lower rate of response with increasing age. Nevertheless, hepatitis C tends to be more rapidly progressive in older patients[250,201] and successful therapy has been accomplished in people in their late 70s and early 80s. For these reasons, therapy of hepatitis C in people above age 60 is probably appropriate if the chronic liver disease appears progressive and there are no other significant co-morbidities or contraindications to therapy. Increased attention should be given to the possibility of side effects in this age group, particularly neuropsychiatric adverse events.

Therapy of Patients with Mild Disease

Because therapy is associated with side effects and is effective in only a proportion of patients, the 1997 NIH Consensus Panel recommended that therapy be limited to patients with moderate or severe disease.[303] Criteria used to define severity were serum aminotransferase levels and liver biopsy. Therapy was not recommended for patients with normal serum aminotransferase levels or with no fibrosis and only mild activity on liver biopsy. These criteria were developed when overall response rates were less than 20 percent and are now overly restrictive. For instance, liver biopsy studies have shown that some patients with normal serum aminotransferase levels have severe and potentially progressive histologic disease.[307-309] Furthermore, some patients are symptomatic despite having no fibrosis or only mild degrees of inflammation and necrosis on liver biopsy. In addition, response rates to therapy are similar if not better in patients with normal aminotransferase levels and mild disease. For these reasons therapy might be offered to all patients with chronic hepatitis C with the caveat that patients with mild disease can safely defer treatment until therapeutics improve and the optimal regimen for their disease, genotype, and viral level is more clearly defined. Monitoring patients on no specific therapy while awaiting advances in this rapidly evolving field is an entirely appropriate approach for many patients without symptoms and without clinical or histologic features of rapidly progressive disease.

Therapy of Patients with Advanced Disease

Patients with compensated cirrhosis resulting from hepatitis C can be safely treated. Indeed, most of the controlled trials of various forms of interferon and combination therapy have included patients with cirrhosis.[102,116-119] Retrospective analyses have shown that patients with advanced fibrosis and cirrhosis have a lower rate of sustained response than those with milder forms of hepatic fibrosis. However, this predictive factor is not always shown to be independent of other more important factors such as genotype, viral level, and age. In the most recent studies of combination therapy with pegylated interferon and ribavirin, response rates in patients with cirrhosis or advanced fibrosis were 41 percent to 44 percent.[102,103] In a study of pegylated interferon monotherapy among patients with cirrhosis or advanced fibrosis the overall response rate among patients with cirrhosis receiving the highest dose of pegylated interferon was 32 percent.[119]

Thus between 30 and 40 percent of patients with compensated cirrhosis resulting from hepatitis C can be successfully and safely treated with combination therapy. For patients with HCV-related cirrhosis who do not respond or who relapse after an initial response, options are limited. In patients with significant underlying liver disease long-term therapy with either ribavirin or alpha interferon or both may be effective in suppressing disease activity and preventing further progression of fibrosis and worsening liver function.[291,310] Currently, there are several prospective controlled trials of continuous pegylated interferon or ribavirin focusing upon their long-term tolerance and safety and whether long-term treatment is effective in preventing hepatic decompensation and death from end-stage liver disease. At present, however, prolongation of therapy with interferon with or without ribavirin beyond 24 weeks in a patient who remains HCV RNA–positive must be considered experimental.

Patients with decompensated cirrhosis resulting from hepatitis C are a greater challenge for management and treatment. End-stage liver disease resulting from hepatitis C is currently the single major indication for liver transplantation in adults.[6] Modeling of rates of HCV in the US population suggests that deaths from chronic hepatitis C and HCC are likely to increase substantially in the next 10 to 20 years.[311] At present, however, the only effective therapy of patients with decompensated cirrhosis resulting from hepatitis C is liver transplantation. Small pilot studies have shown that interferon is poorly tolerated in this population.[312,313] Patients with decompensated cirrhosis have a high rate of serious adverse events during interferon therapy, including sudden worsening of liver disease, neuropsychiatric syndromes, bleeding complications, and severe infections. Thrombocytopenia, anemia, and neutropenia frequently accompany end-stage liver disease and often limit the dose and duration of interferon and ribavirin therapy. Fatalities resulting from complications of interferon treatment have been reported in patients with end-stage liver disease. For these reasons, patients with decompensated cirrhosis resulting from hepatitis C should be referred to liver transplant centers and only treated with interferon with or without ribavirin in the context of prospective controlled trials.

Therapy of hepatitis C in the liver transplant patient, either before or after transplantation, is discussed in Chap. 56.

Therapy of Patients with Renal Disease

Hepatitis C is common in patients with renal disease, before and while on dialysis and after renal transplantation.[125,127,314-316] The reasons for the co-occurrence of HCV infection and renal disease are many. Chronic HCV infection can cause glomerulonephritis, nephrotic syndrome, and progressive renal failure, either as a complication of cryoglobulinemia or independently.[271] In addition, chronic hepatitis C can be a complication of the management of renal disease as a result of blood transfusions or nosocomial transmission of HCV during dialysis or medical procedures.[126,127] Strict universal precautions and avoidance of multi-use vials and reusable medical devices have helped to decrease the incidence of hepatitis C in dialysis and transplant patients. Nevertheless, chronic hepatitis C remains a common complication of end-stage renal disease and is an increasing cause of morbidity and mortality in renal transplant patients.[317]

The presence of renal disease complicates diagnosis, management, and therapy of hepatitis C. Studies in US peritoneal and hemodialysis centers show that approximately 9 percent of dialysis patients have anti-HCV, but the rate is as high as 40 percent in some centers. The majority of patients with anti-HCV are also reactive for HCV RNA. Importantly, both false-positive and false-negative results of anti-HCV testing are more common in patients with renal disease than in those without. False-positive anti-HCV reactions can be excluded by confirmatory testing using recombinant immunoblot testing or assays for HCV RNA. Patients with renal disease may also have false-negative results of anti-HCV testing as a result of lack of antibody development during chronic HCV infection. Thus a proportion of patients with end-stage renal disease and hepatitis C may escape detection in routine screening using commercially available anti-HCV EIA assays.[318] In addition, renal dialysis may alter serum ALT levels, making aminotransferase elevations less reliable as markers for the presence of hepatitis. Most dialysis centers screen patients on a regular basis for ALT elevations and anti-HCV and then confirm the presence of chronic infection by HCV RNA testing. Patients with HCV RNA are not isolated routinely. Strict adherence to proper infection control practice is usually adequate to prevent spread of hepatitis C in dialysis centers. Awareness of the issue and attention to details are important in maintaining prevention.

Treatment of hepatitis C in the patient with renal disease is difficult. Both alpha interferon and ribavirin are cleared by the kidneys, and renal disease can be expected to alter the pharmacokinetics of both agents. Ribavirin is the most affected and accumulates rapidly in patients with renal compromise. The hemolysis induced by ribavirin can be severe in renal disease patients, particularly because they usually have preexisting anemia and bone marrow compromise. For these reasons, ribavirin should not be used in patients with creatinine clearance below 50 ml/min and should be used with caution and frequent determinations of hemoglobin in patients with milder degrees of renal insufficiency. Small-scale pilot studies using minimal doses of ribavirin (200 to 400 mg daily or every other day) in combination with alpha interferon in patients with renal disease have been undertaken[319] but this approach should be considered experimental because there is no evidence that these low doses of ribavirin increase the efficacy of interferon alone in eradicating HCV.

Thus patients with renal disease and hepatitis C are candidates for anti-viral therapy. Although there have been no randomized controlled trials of alpha interferon of adequate size to demonstrate efficacy in patients with end-stage renal disease, small pilot studies have shown that sustained responses can be achieved. The overall rate of response to interferon monotherapy in patients with renal disease is low, reported rates ranging from 0 percent to 25 percent and averaging 12 percent.[315]

Nevertheless, this rate is not greatly lower than the rate of response to interferon monotherapy in patients without renal disease. Trials of pegylated interferon in patients with renal disease have not been reported. Because pegylation increases the half-life of interferon largely by reducing its renal clearance, pegylated interferon may not provide additional benefit over standard interferon in this population.

Treatment of hepatitis C after renal transplantation has been reported in small case series, usually with use of alpha interferon alone. Initial studies indicated that interferon therapy exacerbated or induced acute cellular rejection, which led to be abandonment of studies of therapy of hepatitis C in renal transplant patients and placed additional focus on treatment of patients before transplantation.[320,321] At present therapy of chronic hepatitis C in patients with a renal transplant must be considered experimental and potentially harmful.

Treatment of Patients with HCV-related Cryoglobulinemia

Randomized controlled trials of alpha interferon in patients with HCV-related cryoglobulinemia showed that therapy reduced cryoglobulin levels and induced clinical remissions in more than half of patients.[322-324] Unfortunately, relapse was common when interferon was stopped, particularly in trials of interferon monotherapy given for 24 weeks only. Small studies of combination therapy have shown similar rates of response in patients with cryoglobulinemia as in those without.[325,326] Several reports of long-term therapy with alpha interferon resulting in maintained remission of cryoglobulinemia have been published,[327] and chronic therapy with ribavirin monotherapy has been reported to sustain remissions in patients who failed to clear HCV RNA with interferon therapy.[328] Thus patients with cryoglobulinemia deserve a trial of combination therapy in a regimen suitable for the infecting genotype. Patients who relapse when therapy is stopped may benefit from long-term continuous therapy with interferon to ameliorate symptoms and complications.

Therapy of Patients with Active or Recent Alcohol or Drug Abuse

Virtually all of the large randomized controlled trials of combination therapy of hepatitis C excluded patients with recent or ongoing alcohol or drug abuse. This practice, which was appropriate for the initial large efficacy trials, unfortunately has been translated into dictums regarding treatment in patients with alcohol and drug abuse problems.[295,303,329] One reason for avoiding interferon therapy in patients who have recently stopped using drugs or alcohol is that relapse of substance abuse is a common side effect of treatment, probably as a result of the side effects of irritability and depression. In addition, patients with ongoing alcohol and drug abuse may be less likely to complete therapy or comply with a suitable regimen. Finally, patients with ongoing drug abuse may suffer relapse after successful therapy because of re-exposure and re-infection. Nevertheless, there are examples of patients who have ongoing problems with drugs or alcohol who have successfully completed therapy and responded to treatment.[330,331]

Furthermore, re-infection after successful therapy has not been reported in prospective studies. Serious side effects such as seizures, psychosis, depression, and suicide may be more common among people with ongoing or recent drug and alcohol abuse, which argues in favor of more active monitoring for side effects in these patients.[331,332] Therapy of patients with a history of alcohol or drug abuse is best carried out in collaboration with an alcohol or drug abuse counselor or with support from a group such as Alcoholics Anonymous; indeed, the structure and rigor of methadone clinic attendance may provide an excellent framework for applying combination therapy.

Treatment of Patients with Hemophilia and Coagulation Disorders

Hepatitis C is common among patients with hemophilia and other coagulation disorders as a consequence of the receipt of pooled plasma products made before the introduction of methods of viral inactivation. Recipients of anti-hemophilic factors made before 1986 were at high risk of acquiring hepatitis C, hepatitis B, and HIV; subsequent routine testing showed that 70 percent to 90 percent of patients with hemophilia A or B who were diagnosed and treated before 1986 have anti-HCV and 20 percent to 30 percent have anti-HIV.[121,333] Although management of HIV infection has been the major focus of medical treatment in this cohort, hepatitis C is becoming a major cause of morbidity and mortality in this group.

Treatment of hepatitis C in patients with hemophilia has been reported from case series and randomized controlled trials.[305,334-337] These studies demonstrate that response rates in patients with hemophilia are no different from those in patients without coagulation disorders. Liver biopsy, which is considered routine in evaluating patients with hepatitis C for therapy, can be done in patients with hemophilia given adequate coagulation factor support. However, liver biopsy should not be considered a requisite for therapy.

Treatment of Patients Co-infected with HIV

Hepatitis C shares some of the modes of transmission with HIV, and co-infection with HIV and HCV is common. Co-infection occurs most frequently among HIV-infected injection drug users and patients with hemophilia, but can also be found in patients with transfusion-acquired and sexually transmitted HIV infection. Prospectively followed cohorts of patients with HCV and HIV infection have shown that hepatitis C is more rapidly progressive in patients with HIV co-infection, and the disease tends to worsen as immune deficiency worsens[333,338-340] In the period before the availability of highly active antiretroviral therapies (HAART) hepatitis C was not considered a major problem for HIV-infected patients. With the dramatic decrease in mortality that accompanied the introduction of HAART, the role of hepatitis C in morbidity and mortality has become more evident. Several recent studies have shown that 25 percent to 50 percent of deaths in patients with HIV infection now result from liver disease.[341,342] Both hepatitis B and D and drug hepatotoxicity play a role in causing liver-related deaths in HIV-infected people, but the single major cause of significant liver disease in HIV-positive people is hepatitis C. Indeed, liver transplantation for end-stage liver disease resulting from hepatitis C has become a significant issue in HIV-infected patients. Unfortunately, in preliminary studies HCV infection has been reported to be associated with poor long-term survival in HIV-positive patients undergoing liver transplantation.[343]

Obviously, therapy of hepatitis C should be considered in the long-term management of patients with HIV-HCV co-infection. Furthermore, the usual concerns of avoiding the expense and side effects of therapy in patients with early or mild disease should not weigh as greatly in the decision to treat patients who have HCV-HIV co-infection. Case series of patients with HIV who have been treated for hepatitis C with alpha interferon alone or with combination therapy have shown that response rates in HIV-infected patients with normal or near-normal CD4 counts (at least 400 cells/mm^3) are similar to those in patients without HIV, whereas the response rate is decidedly poor in patients with more advanced immune deficiency and in more advanced chronic liver disease.[344-347] For these reasons, patients with HIV infection and HCV co-infection should be treated early regardless of the severity of the underlying hepatitis C: with worsening of immune deficiency from HIV infection, hepatitis C is likely to become more rapidly progressive and more difficult to eradicate.

There have been few reports on the use of combination therapy of hepatitis C in HIV co-infected individuals. Small case series show a sustained virologic response rate that averages 29 percent to 40 percent.[348,349] Combination therapy may not be well tolerated in patients with HIV infection who are also receiving multiple other antiviral agents. Recently, cases of lactic acidosis with microvesicular fatty liver have been reported in patients receiving ribavirin-interferon combination therapy while on HAART.[350] Ribavirin can interact with other anti-viral nucleosides and should be used with caution in patients receiving agents that have been linked to cases of lactic acidosis, pancreatitis, and microvesicular steatosis such as zalcitabine, didanosine, stavudine, or zidovudine. Regular testing for lactate, amylase, and lipase is prudent in patients receiving both ribavirin-interferon combination therapy and HAART. The dose of ribavirin may need to be modified in patients receiving other nucleosides.

A final issue in treating patients with HIV-HCV co-infection is the possible effect of interferon therapy on the GBV-C virus (also known as the hepatitis G virus), a newly recognized human flavivirus similar to the HCV but that by itself appears to cause little or no hepatic injury.[351] Several studies on the natural history of HIV infection have shown that co-infection with the GBV-C virus is associated with a slower progression of HIV infection to AIDS and lower mortality rates.[352,353] Alpha interferon therapy suppresses GBV-C RNA levels, and prolonged treatment can result in sustained viral clearance.[354] Thus therapy of HCV may also result in clearance of GBV-C, which may negatively affect the natural history of HIV infection. These are theoretical concerns but point to the critical need for careful prospective studies and long-term follow up of therapy of patients with HIV-HCV co-infection.

Treatment of Patients with Serious Co-morbidities

A high proportion of patients with chronic hepatitis C have other serious co-morbidities such as diabetes, hypertension, obesity, cardiovascular or cerebrovascular disease, pulmonary conditions, immune deficiencies, or autoimmune disorders. These other medical conditions can complicate therapy, affecting both tolerance and efficacy.

Psychiatric co-morbidities of hepatitis C are particularly difficult because of the many psychologic side effects of alpha interferon therapy, which constitute the major reason for dose modification and early termination of therapy. Unfortunately, hepatitis C is more common among people with severe mental illness, particularly institutionalized individuals.[355] Concerns about exacerbation of psychiatric illness in these patients are valid, but in prospective studies the psychiatric side effects of interferon were found to be largely unpredictable and not occurring necessarily in patients with preexisting depression or psychosis.[356] Indeed, with adequate management of the preexisting psychiatric condition, alpha interferon therapy can be successfully completed.[357] Patients with a history of acute psychosis, manic-depressive disorder, severe depression, or suicide should be treated with caution and psychiatric symptoms frequently monitored.

The presence of severe and active autoimmune disease is generally considered a contraindication to alpha interferon therapy. There have been many instances of worsening of ulcerative colitis, Crohn's disease, psoriasis, rheumatoid arthritis, and autoimmune hepatitis during therapy with alpha interferon.[327,358] On the other hand, if the condition can be adequately managed, combination therapy of hepatitis C is sometimes possible and can be successful.

Acute Hepatitis C

Most cases of acute hepatitis C are mild and self-limited, but evolution to chronic infection is common. The chronicity rate of acute hepatitis C averages 75 percent, but varies considerably in different cohorts, being lower in younger patients and women and higher in older people, men, and African-American patients. The rationale for therapy of acute hepatitis C is not to shorten the course of disease and ameliorate symptoms as much as to prevent chronicity. There have been no prospective randomized controlled trials of alpha interferon for acute hepatitis C, largely because of the sporadic and uncommon nature of the disease. Recently several case series have shown that a high proportion of patients who are treated during the acute phase of hepatitis C resolve the viral infection.

In a recent multi-center study from Germany 44 patients presenting with acute hepatitis C were treated with a 6-month course of alpha interferon (given in a dose of 5 million units daily for 2 weeks and then thrice weekly for another 22 weeks).[359] Overall 98 percent of patients had a sustained virologic response and had normal serum aminotransferase levels and no detectable HCV RNA during long-term follow-up. The one patient who did not respond was later successfully re-treated with combination therapy. Therapy did not result in transient worsening of the disease; indeed, within 2 to 4 weeks of starting therapy serum aminotransferases were improving and HCV RNA had become undetectable in most patients. These findings suggest that patients with acute hepatitis C should be treated with interferon monotherapy. Use of pegylated interferon is a reasonable alternative to the higher doses of standard interferon used in this initial clinical report. The high rate of response would indicate that ribavirin is not needed and that a 24-week course is adequate.

An important issue in treatment of acute hepatitis C is when to start therapy. Some patients are identified with acute infection before the onset of symptoms, for instance, as a result of monitoring after accidental needlestick exposure. HCV RNA is detectable in serum within 1 to 2 weeks of exposure and well before onset of symptoms or ALT elevations. It is important to stress that the reported high rates of response to anti-viral therapy in acute hepatitis C were achieved in patients who were already symptomatic and jaundiced for several weeks when treatment was started. Thus there is no reason to start treatment before onset of symptoms. Indeed, delay of therapy may be preferable; thus in several recent studies of acute hepatitis C, therapy was delayed for several months during which time a high proportion of patients resolved the infection spontaneously and would have been treated unnecessarily if therapy was started early.[360] Furthermore, small case series have reported nonresponses occurring in patients identified during the incubation period and started on therapy before onset of clinical disease.[176] Thus there is no need to initiate this expensive and prolonged therapy before the patient develops clinically apparent disease and has been shown to have persistence of HCV RNA. Because recovery from hepatitis C is due in part to a vigorous immune response to the viral infection, it also may be appropriate to wait for several weeks after the onset of clinical disease, the time that vigorous T-cell responses to HCV antigens typically appear.

Re-treatment

Because response rates are higher with combination therapy using pegylated interferon and ribavirin than with other regimens, it is reasonable to assume that some patients who relapsed or failed to respond after a course of monotherapy or combination therapy with standard interferon might benefit from re-treatment using pegylated interferon and ribavirin.[309,361-366] Re-treatment is more likely to be successful if the patient had a virologic response and relapsed after the previous course, particularly if the previous course employed interferon monotherapy and was for 24 weeks only. However, in all situations the need for therapy should be reassessed and consideration given to whether the patient might better wait for further improvement in therapeutics over the next 5 to 10 years. Re-treatment of patients with the identical regimen is rarely effective and should be avoided. Patients who relapsed after a previous course may benefit from a longer course of treatment. Patients who failed to respond and remained HCV RNA-positive during the previous course of treatment are least likely to respond to re-treatment and should only be re-treated if the regimen is clearly different. Re-treatment with a different form of standard interferon or with a different pegylated interferon should not be undertaken. Furthermore, use of higher doses of interferon is rarely successful in improving response rates in non-responder patients and is associated with significantly higher rates of adverse events.

Management of the Non-Responder Patient

For the patient who has failed to respond to an optimal regimen of combination therapy of hepatitis C, the options are few. Monitoring on no therapy is appropriate for such patients who have early or mild disease. Attention should be focused upon avoidance of further injury including avoidance of alcohol use and minimizing exposure to other medications. For patients with more advanced disease, with early cirrhosis or bridging hepatic fibrosis on liver biopsy, other options include long-term maintenance treatment with interferon or with ribavirin. These are currently experimental approaches that are being subjected to randomized controlled trials.

Patients with viral resistance to interferon represent the major single challenge to anti-viral therapy of hepatitis C. Analyses of genomic sequences from patients who have failed to respond to interferon have suggested that there are interferon sensitivity-determining regions (ISDRs) in the viral sequence that correlate with a response or lack of response to therapy. The best described ISDR is a 29-amino acid sequence found in the NS5A region of HCV genotype 1b.[85,367] Investigators from Japan reported that the presence of conserved wild-type sequences in this region correlated with a lack of sustained response to interferon therapy; in contrast, the presence of multiple mutations in the ISDR correlated with a high likelihood of a sustained virologic response.[368] These results have not been reproduced in all studies, particularly those from the United States and Europe.[369] In support of the NS5A region playing a role in susceptibility and resistance to interferon effects has been the in vitro finding that the NS5A polypeptide binds to and inactivates interferon-induced enzymatic activity in cells (the protein kinase PKR).[370,371] This inhibitory activity, however, does not correlate well with clinical responses to interferon in patients.[372] More recent reports have focused upon the structural E2 region of the HCV genome that encodes a polypeptide that also binds to the interferon-induced PKR.[373,374] At issue is whether these in vitro findings have relevance to HCV infection in humans. Preliminary analyses of HCV replication using subgenomic replicons and chimeric viruses have yet to demonstrate a role of these regions in determining response to interferon or ribavirin.[28] The molecular basis of viral resistance remains poorly defined, and other immunologic, racial, genetic, and environmental factors are under investigation.[113]

SIDE EFFECTS OF COMBINATION THERAPY

Both alpha interferon and ribavirin have significant side effects (Table 33-7). Patients should be fully informed of the range of side effects that can occur and be provided with some indication of their frequency. Patient-friendly descriptions of the risks of therapy are available with the medication and package insert for alpha interferon and combination therapy.

Initial Constitutional Symptoms

Most patients experience an influenza-like syndrome after the initial injection of alpha interferon. The most common symptoms include fever (to as high as 104° F), chills, malaise, muscle aches, headaches, nausea (more rarely vomiting), diarrhea, and poor appetite. These symptoms usually arise 6 to 8 hours after the first injection and persist for 8 to 16 hours. The symptoms may be delayed and more prolonged with pegylated interferon. Symptoms are helped by acetaminophen or non-steroidal anti-inflammatory agents that can be administered expectantly at the time of the first injection. With subsequent injections this syndrome is much abated, but it may arise again if there is temporary interruption of therapy. Because of the potential severity of this reaction, patients should be advised to stay at home for the 24 hours after the initial injection of interferon.

Fatigue and Malaise

The most common side effect with continued interferon or combination therapy is fatigue or malaise. These symptoms are often accompanied by muscle aches and, in some patients, nausea, diarrhea, or headaches. These constitutional side effects of alpha interferon are usually mild and tolerable but can be unpredictable in severity

TABLE 33-7
Side Effects of Alpha Interferon and Ribavirin Combination Therapy

Constitutional Symptoms*
Fatigue, malaise, lethargy
Increased need for sleep
Muscle aches
Headaches
Fever and chills
Nausea
Vomiting
Diarrhea

Psychologic Side Effects
Anxiety
Irritability
Depression
Emotionality
Personality change

Bone Marrow Suppression
Anemia†
Neutropenia‡
Thrombocytopenia

Skin Problems
Itching†
Skin rash†
Photosensitivity†
Local erythema‡
Local abscess formation

Neurologic
Tinnitus
Hearing loss
Retinal hemorrhages§
Decrease in visual acuity§
Visual field loss§
Seizures
Difficulty concentrating
Insomnia
Memory Loss
Confusion
Coma

Autoimmunity
Induction of autoantibodies
Induction of autoimmune condition§ (e.g., hyperthyroidism or hypothyroidism, diabetes, autoimmune hemolytic anemia, thrombocytopenic purpura, celiac disease, myasthenia gravis, lupus-like syndrome, psoriasis)

Miscellaneous Severe Adverse Events
Relapse in alcohol or drug abuse§
Acute renal failure
Acute congestive heart failure
Severe bacterial infection§

Side Effects that Can Be Triggered by Hemolysis and Anemia†
Shortness of breath
Palpitations
Headache
Arrhythmia§
Angina pectoris§
Myocardial infarction§
Transient ischemic attack§
Stroke§

Hepatic
Exacerbation of hepatitis

*Most prominently occurring 6 to 12 hours after the initial injection of interferon; these symptoms can later reappear during continuation of therapy.
†Caused or particularly exacerbated by ribavirin.
‡More prominent with pegylated interferons.
§Occur particularly in patients with predisposition to these complications—such as genetic predisposition to autoimmune disease or preexisting atherosclerosis for angina pectoris, myocardial infarction, or stroke.

and intermittent in timing in relationship to injections. In up to 10 percent of patients these side effects are sufficiently severe and problematic to require early discontinuation of therapy. The fatigue and muscle aches of interferon can be partially alleviated by acetaminophen or non-steroidal anti-inflammatory drugs. Regular physical activity, careful sleep hygiene, and attention to diet and hydration are recommended to help with these constitutional symptoms.

Psychologic Side Effects

More challenging with interferon therapy are the psychologic side effects of this cytokine. Between 20 percent and 35 percent of patients receiving a 24- or 48-week course of combination therapy develop some degree of depression, irritability, anxiety, or moodiness.[102,103,116] The most common psychologic problem is depression or sadness.[356] The depression is often accompanied by fatigue, lethargy, and lack of interest in usual activities. This side effect is idiosyncratic and can occur in patients who have no history of depression and who describe themselves as cheerful and optimistic. Depression usually appears after 1 to 2 months of therapy. Selective serotonin-reuptake inhibitors can be helpful,[357] but in some instances therapy must be discontinued. Severe depression and attempted and even successful suicide have occurred during interferon therapy.

Other psychologic side effects of interferon therapy are irritability, emotionality, anxiety, sleeplessness, encephalopathy, confusion, and frank coma or acute psychosis. Patients may become short-tempered and easily upset, side effects that can cause marital or workplace problems that are not typically reported by the patient. Patients' families are best advised to consider a change in behavior to be related to interferon therapy and report it to the health care providers. A separate syndrome of emotionality and tearfulness occurs in some patients receiving interferon. This side effect can be very distressing and require dose modification or early discontinuation of therapy. Finally, acute psychosis or mania can occur on interferon therapy, particularly with higher doses. This severe neuropsychiatric syndrome occurs most frequently in patients with previous brain injury or a preexisting neurologic condition.[356]

Bone Marrow Suppression

Alpha interferon is myelosuppressive and the doses used to treat chronic hepatitis C regularly result in decreases in red cell, white cell, and platelet counts. Ribavirin causes a dose-dependent red cell hemolysis apparently resulting from a concentration of ribavirin triphosphate inside of red cells. Ribavirin also causes mild lymphopenia.[375] Combination therapy using either standard or pegylated interferon and ribavirin regularly results in a 30 percent to 50 percent decrease in white blood cell and platelet counts and a 10 percent to 20 percent decrease in hematocrit or hemoglobin. The decrease in white blood cells includes both neutrophils and lymphocytes and generally begins within 1 week and reaches an equilibrium within 2 to 4 weeks. Dose modification is occasionally needed, particularly in using pegylated interferon if absolute neutrophil counts fall below 500 cells/mm^3. However, bacterial infections caused by neutropenia during interferon therapy are rare even with absolute neutrophil counts of 300 to 400 cells/mm^3.

The platelet count can also decrease by as much as half during combination therapy, although thrombocytopenia tends to be more severe with monotherapy (ribavirin induces thrombocytosis as a result of the hemolytic anemia). Dose modification is rarely needed because of thrombocytopenia. Sudden, marked drops in platelet counts (by more than 50 percent of baseline) should, however, suggest the induction of thrombocytopenic purpura and prompt immediate discontinuation of therapy.

Anemia is a more difficult problem with combination therapy, with the decrease in red cell counts occurring between weeks 2 and 8 and leveling off thereafter. Anemia during combination therapy is due both to hemolysis induced by ribavirin and myelosuppression caused by interferon. The decrease in hemoglobin averages 2 to 3 g/dl or an overall decrease of 10 percent to 20 percent from baseline. Patients may become symptomatic and complain of shortness of breath, palpitations, and headaches. The presence of symptoms or hemoglobin levels falling below 8.5 g/dl should lead to withholding ribavirin or lowering of the dosage by 200 to 400 mg daily. Ribavirin has a long half-life and therapy can be withheld for several days before restarting drug at a lower dose. Ribavirin therapy is contraindicated in patients with preexisting anemia, hemolysis, renal failure, or any condition that would be seriously affected by anemia. Patients with coronary or cerebral artery disease can suffer from an acute myocardial infarction or stroke as a consequence of the sudden onset of anemia and should only be treated either with interferon monotherapy or combination therapy with lower doses of ribavirin (600 mg daily).

Autoimmunity

Alpha interferon can induce autoantibodies, and 1 percent to 2 percent of patients treated for 24 to 48 weeks develop an autoimmune disorder while on therapy.[356,376,377] The most common autoimmune condition is thyroiditis, accompanied by either hyperthyroidism (Graves' disease with antibodies to the thyroid-stimulating hormone [TSH] receptor) or hypothyroidism (Hashimoto's thyroiditis with antimicrosomal or antithyroperoxidase antibodies). Surveillance with regular measurement of serum TSH levels at 24 and 48 weeks is warranted when treating patients with hepatitis C. Sudden onset of hyperthyroidism can be severe and even life-threatening.

Other autoimmune conditions that can be induced by interferon therapy include type I diabetes, celiac disease, myasthenia gravis, autoimmune hepatitis, hemolytic anemia, and thrombocytopenic purpura. The induction of these autoimmune conditions probably occurs in patients with an underlying autoimmune diathesis. Known preexisting autoimmune conditions can be worsened by interferon therapy, including rheumatoid arthritis, psoriasis, and ulcerative colitis. Finally, a fairly high proportion of patients (between 10 percent and 50 percent, depending upon the assays used) will develop new onset of autoantibodies during interferon therapy, but only a small proportion of these are associated with development of disease.[376]

Dermatologic Side Effects

Chronic ribavirin therapy can cause pruritus and skin rash.[310] This may represent photosensitivity. Itching can be severe enough to require dose modification or discontinuation. Ribavirin also can cause nasal and throat congestion with chronic rhinitis, sinusitis, throat irritation, and ear ache; the mechanism of this side effect is unknown, but it appears to be a histamine-like reaction.

Other Rare Severe Adverse Events

Severe adverse events on combination therapy are not common but can be life-threatening and sudden. These complications include local abscesses, systemic bacterial infections, idiopathic pneumonitis, congestive heart failure, seizures, encephalopathy, coma, hearing loss, visual loss, and renal failure. Vision and hearing can be affected. Retinal hemorrhages and cotton wool spots occur commonly on therapy but are not commonly associated with visual loss and usually resolve spontaneously despite continuation of treatment.[378] Similar small vessel hemorrhages may also account for occasional sudden hearing loss, vertigo, and seizures.[379,380] These small vascular side effects are more common in patients with an underlying predisposition, such as to hypertension or diabetes. Bacterial infections are common in patients who are treated with alpha interferon who have an underlying predisposition to infections, such as advanced cirrhosis (bacterial peritonitis), bronchitis (pneumonia or lung abscess), or recurrent urinary tract infections.

Exacerbation of Hepatitis

Finally, an uncommon but distinctive and important side effect of interferon therapy is a paradoxical worsening of the underlying hepatitis. This side effect occurs in fewer than 1 percent of treated patients and is most common in patients with preexisting autoantibodies, such as antinuclear antibodies (ANA) or anti-liver-kidney microsomal antibodies. An increase in serum aminotransferases more than two to three times baseline should lead to prompt discontinuation of therapy and evaluation for autoimmune liver disease. The worsening of liver disease tends to be transient, but instances of evolution to chronic autoimmune hepatitis have been reported.[381,382]

Dose Modification

Side effects of therapy may necessitate dose modification. In large clinical trials 10 percent to 14 percent of patients receiving pegylated interferon and ribavirin required dose discontinuation, and 40 percent to 42 percent required dose reduction of either interferon or ribavirin.[102,103] In modifying dosages the first decision to be made is whether interferon or ribavirin is causing the side effect.

Anemia is the most common reason for modification of the dose of ribavirin.[375] A decrease in hemoglobin of 2 to 3 g/dl is common during combination therapy. If the drop in hemoglobin is to 8.5 g/dl or lower or particularly sudden in onset, symptoms may arise and the dose should be reduced. Depending upon the circumstances, it may be advisable to withhold ribavirin until the symptoms or anemia resolve and then restart at a lower dose (200 or 400 mg or less per day). Skin rash and severe and recurrent nasal and throat congestion are other side effects that may lead to dose modification or early discontinuation of ribavirin. In many of these circumstances interferon can be continued at the previous dose.

The major side effects of interferon that lead to dose modification are fatigue, depression, psychiatric side effects, and severe thrombocytopenia or neutropenia. The amount of dose reduction depends upon the interferon product used, but it is generally a reduction of one third to one half the starting dose. For standard interferon, the usual reduction is from 3 to 2 million units thrice weekly: this reduced dose, however, is probably suboptimal for most patients. For pegylated alpha 2a, the usual dose reduction is from 180 to 135 μg per week and, if need be, to 90 mcg per week. For pegylated alpha 2b a practical approach is to lower the dose from 1.5 to 1.0 to 0.5 mcg/wk per week. Although response rates may be slightly lower, these pegylated interferons are clearly effective even at these lower doses.[102,118,282]

OTHER RECOMMENDATIONS

Non-specific Recommendations to Prevent Transmission

Recommendations on prevention and interruption of spread of hepatitis C are based largely on the US Public Health Service (USPHS) recommendations published and updated regularly in *Morbidity and Mortality Weekly Reports* and on summaries and guidelines published by the Centers for Disease Control and Prevention.[111] Spread of hepatitis C is largely through exposure to blood and contaminated needles, syringes or medical equipment, and less commonly through person-to-person contact.

People with hepatitis C should refrain from donating blood, tissue, and semen and should inform people possibly exposed to their blood and secretions of their potential infectivity (medical care deliverers, nurses, physicians, dentists, phlebotomists). There is no need to restrict other activities or access to medical procedures. Universal precautions are recommended for handling all blood and potentially infectious secretions and the procedures taken should be the same whether or not the patient is known or not known to harbor hepatitis C.

Patients should be educated regarding transmission of hepatitis C and the importance of not sharing personal items that might be contaminated with blood or secretions such as toothbrushes and razors. Patients who have multiple sexual partners should be advised on safe sexual practices. Patients with a stable sexual relationship should be informed of the current understanding regarding sexual transmission: the possibility of sexual transmission exists, but the rate is low, the incidence being less than 1 percent per year. Testing of the sexual partner for anti-HCV can be helpful in defining the risk and answering questions about risk. Prevention of sexual transmission to partners is often a reason given for wanting to receive therapy for hepatitis C.

Accidental Percutaneous Exposure

People who have an occupational accidental percutaneous exposure to hepatitis C should be managed according to USPHS guidelines.[126] HCV is not transmitted efficiently through accidental needlestick exposure, with the risk of infection after a known exposure being less than 3 percent.[383-385] If an exposure occurs the wound should be washed thoroughly with soap and water or Betadine solution and the mucous membranes flushed with water. The type of fluid and exposure should be noted and the risk of transmission assessed by clinical information and by testing for HBsAg, anti-HCV, and anti-HIV. People with an exposure to anti-HCV–positive blood or secretions should be monitored with retesting for HCV RNA and ALT levels at baseline and after 4 weeks with follow-up testing for anti-HCV and ALT levels at 4 to 6 months. Most people who develop HCV infection after a defined parenteral exposure become HCV RNA–positive within 1 to 2 weeks. There are no known means of postexposure prevention of spread of hepatitis C. Immunoglobulin is not effective (and most current preparations lack anti-HCV). Prophylactic therapy with antiviral agents to prevent hepatitis C has not been evaluated prospectively. Because the rate of infection is so low (reported rates are 0 percent to 7 percent),[126] use of anti-viral agents in this situation is not practical. Furthermore, several studies have shown a high rate of response to a course of alpha interferon initiated at the time of acute disease.[359]

Non-specific Recommendations

There are no specific diets or dietary restrictions that are appropriate for patients with chronic hepatitis C unless advanced cirrhosis is present. Use of alcohol should be discouraged, particularly if there is a history of alcohol dependence or abuse. Regular physical activity and healthy diet should be advised. Vaccination against hepatitis A and B is appropriate, and prescreening for immunity (anti-HAV and anti-HBs or anti-HBc) is reasonable before vaccination in patients with a history of high-risk behaviors.

Finally, patients with hepatitis C should be encouraged to have regular follow-ups of their liver disease. Monitoring at 6-month intervals for serum aminotransferase levels is appropriate. Patients with cirrhosis are at risk of developing HCC. At present, the effectiveness of routine surveillance for HCC is not well defined. Alpha-fetoprotein testing and regular ultrasound examination have been evaluated in several studies of patients with cirrhosis from hepatitis C without evidence that this approach improves survival.[386,387] Nevertheless, ultrasound screening and alpha-fetoprotein testing at 6-month intervals is usually recommended for patients with hepatitis C and cirrhosis. For patients with lesser degrees of fibrosis, routine screening is generally not recommended.

FUTURE APPROACHES TO THERAPY AND PREVENTION

The importance of hepatitis C as a liver disease and the limited efficacy of even optimal therapies have led to search for more effective and better tolerated therapies. These approaches have included non-specific therapies and recommendations, immune modulatory agents and cytokines, molecular approaches, and specific anti-viral drugs.

Non-specific Therapies

Non-specific approaches to therapy include use of complementary and alternative therapies, antioxidants, milk thistle, and hepatic iron reduction through phlebotomy. None of these approaches have been proven beneficial in prospective controlled clinical trials, but neither have they been found to be harmful.[388] Milk thistle is a botanical widely used for liver disease, largely based on natural food stores, the Internet, and advice from friends. The major active ingredient in milk thistle preparations is silymarin, a naturally occurring flavonoid and antioxidant. Milk thistle is widely used among patients with liver disease, but prospective studies have shown that milk thistle preparations have no effect on HCV RNA levels and little if any effect on serum aminotransferase levels in hepatitis C.[389]

Phlebotomy to reduce hepatic iron often leads to decreases in serum ALT levels in patients with hepatitis C, but the improvements are usually transient and have not been shown to be accompanied by improvements in hepatic histology or changes in HCV RNA levels or increased rates of response to subsequent anti-viral therapy.[390,391] Iron reduction should be recommended in any patient with hepatitis C and iron overload even in the absence of genetic hemochromatosis. An appropriate criterion for phlebotomy is 3+ iron staining on liver biopsy. Generally, iron depletion is achieved in patients without hemochromatosis by withdrawal of 3 to 10 units of blood.

Anti-viral Agents

Several broad spectrum anti-viral drugs have been evaluated in small numbers of patients with chronic hepatitis C. Amantadine was reported to lower serum ALT levels and increase the rate of response to alpha interferon in patients with hepatitis C.[392] Subsequent experience and randomized controlled trials, however, have failed to show an effect of amantadine in hepatitis C, either by itself or in combination with alpha interferon.[393-396]

Ribavirin is a broad spectrum anti-viral agent with activity against several flaviviruses. Ribavirin by itself was shown to lower serum aminotransferase levels in approximately 50 percent of patients[375,397] but to have little or no effect on serum HCV RNA levels and did not result in sustained improvements or remissions in disease.[310,398] Continuous, long-term ribavirin therapy may ameliorate the underlying liver disease in patients whose serum ALT levels become normal, but the degree of improvement is less than occurs with successful therapy with interferon.[310] The mechanism of action of ribavirin against HCV is unknown, although in vitro studies suggest that it has activity against the HCV polymerase,[399] and analysis of viral kinetics suggests that it has mild anti-viral activity against HCV in humans.

Cytokines

The effectiveness of alpha interferon in hepatitis C led naturally to a search for other cytokines or immunomodulatory agents that might be beneficial in this disease. Pilot studies of gamma interferon,[400] thymosin,[401] and interleukin (IL)-12[402] showed minimal, if any, effects on HCV RNA levels or disease activity in hepatitis C. A pilot study of recombinant IL-10 suggested that it had beneficial effects on serum aminotransferase elevations and hepatic fibrosis without effects on levels of HCV RNA.[403] A subsequent, larger randomized controlled trial failed to show any benefit from IL-10 therapy.

Newer Anti-viral Approaches to Therapy

Understanding of the genomic structure and replicative cycle of HCV has identified potential targets for anti-viral therapy. The most promising targets are the enzymic activities of HCV, such as the NS3 helicase or protease or the NS-5B polymerase activities.[72-74,404] To date, no small molecule with virus-specific protease, helicase, or polymerase inhibitory activity has been developed.

Other promising approaches to treat hepatitis C are the inactivation of the internal ribosomal initiation site of HCV and molecular interruption of viral replication or translation. In vitro studies have already demonstrated the activity of specific antisense oligonucleotides[405] and synthetic ribozymes[406] directed against HCV, and pilot phase trials of each have been initiated. These molecular approaches either alone or in combination with other anti-virals may provide important further advances in the therapy of this disease.

Hepatitis C Vaccines

Despite efforts from investigators throughout the world, there has been little progress made in developing a safe and effective vaccine against hepatitis C. Impediments to development of a HCV vaccine are many and include the lack of a vigorous tissue culture system for propagating the virus, the absence of methods for detection of neutralizing antibody, the lack of a simple animal model of infection, and the lack of detailed understanding of the immunology of hepatitis C. A central problem appears to be the lack of absolute immunity to reinfection with this virus and the frequency with which the virus can mutate and escape immune clearance. Candidate vaccines using recombinant E1 and E2 proteins have provided only partial protection against infection in the chimpanzee model of hepatitis C.[217] Approaches being pursued include immunization against multiple epitopes, application of special adjuvants, use of virus-like particles as immunogens, induction of T-cell immunity, application of DNA vaccines, and use of chimeric viruses.[2]

Thus current therapies of chronic hepatitis C are effective in approximately half of patients but are limited by poor tolerability and lack of applicability for special populations of patients that are deserving of treatment. The rapid advances in knowledge of HCV and availability of new tools to evaluate virus replication and inhibition promise to provide new, more effective, and better tolerated approaches to the treatment and prevention of this important liver disease.

References

1. Hepatitis C virus infection. N Engl J Med 345:41-52, 2001.
2. Liang TJ, Rehermann B, Seeff LB, Hoofnagle JH: Pathogenesis, natural history, treatment, and prevention of hepatitis C. Ann Intern Med 132:296-305, 2000.
3. Alter MJ, Kruszon-Moran D, Nainan OV, et al: The prevalence of hepatitis C virus infection in the United States, 1988 through 1994. N Engl J Med 341:556-562, 1999.
4. Armstrong GL, Alter MJ, McQuillan GM, Margolis HS: The past incidence of hepatitis C virus infection: implications for the future burden of chronic liver disease in the United States. Hepatology 31:777-782, 2000.
5. Di Bisceglie AM, Carithers RL Jr, Gores GJ: Hepatocellular carcinoma. Hepatology 28:1161-1165, 1998.
6. Seaberg EC, Belle SH, Beringer KC, et al: Liver transplantation in the United States from 1987-1998: updated results from the Pitt-UNOS Liver Transplant Registry. Clin Transplant 17-37, 1998.
7. Bell BP, Navarro VJ, Manos MM, et al: The epidemiology of newly-diagnosed chronic liver disease in the United States: findings of population-based sentinel surveillance. Hepatology 34:468A, 2001.
8. Prince AM, Brotman B, Grady GF, et al: Long-incubation post-transfusion hepatitis without serological evidence of exposure to hepatitis-B virus. Lancet 2:241-246, 1974.
9. Feinstone SM, Kapikian AZ, Purcell RH, et al: Transfusion-associated hepatitis not due to viral hepatitis type A or B. N Engl J Med 292:767-770, 1975.
10. Hoofnagle JH, Gerety RJ, Tabor E, et al: Transmission of non-A, non-B hepatitis. Ann Intern Med 87:14-20, 1977.
11. Tabor E, Gerety RJ, Drucker JA, et al: Transmission of non-A, non-B hepatitis from man to chimpanzee. Lancet 1:463-466, 1978.
12. Alter HJ, Purcell RH, Holland PV, Popper H: Transmissible agent in non-A, non-B hepatitis. Lancet 1:459-463, 1978.
13. Hollinger FB, Gitnick GL, Aach RD, et al: Non-A, non-B hepatitis transmission in chimpanzees: a project of the transfusion-transmitted viruses study group. Intervirology 10:60-68, 1978.
14. Bradley DW, McCaustland KA, Cook EH, et al: Posttransfusion non-A, non-B hepatitis in chimpanzees. Physicochemical evidence that the tubule-forming agent is a small, enveloped virus. Gastroenterology 88:773-779, 1985.
15. He LF, Alling D, Popkin T, et al: Determining the size of non-A, non-B hepatitis virus by filtration. J Infect Dis 156:636-640, 1987.
16. Shimizu YK, Feinstone SM, Purcell RH, et al: Non-A, non-B hepatitis: ultrastructural evidence for two agents in experimentally infected chimpanzees. Science 205:197-200, 1979.
17. Pfeifer U, Thomssen R, Legler K, et al: Experimental non-A, non-B hepatitis: four types of cytoplasmic alteration in hepatocytes of infected chimpanzees. Virchows Arch B Cell Pathol Incl Mol Pathol 33:233, 1980.
18. Choo QL, Kuo G, Weiner AJ, et al: Isolation of a cDNA clone derived from a blood-borne non-A, non-B viral hepatitis genome. Science 244:359-362, 1989.
19. Kuo G, Choo QL, Alter HJ, et al: An assay for circulating antibodies to a major etiologic virus of human non-A, non-B hepatitis. Science 244:362, 1989.
20. Major ME, Feinstone SM: The molecular virology of hepatitis C. Hepatology 25:1527-1538, 1997.
21. Bukh J, Miller RH, Purcell RH: Genetic heterogeneity of hepatitis C virus: quasispecies and genotypes. Semin Liver Dis 15:41-63, 1995.
22. Simmonds P: Variability of hepatitis C virus. Hepatology 21:570-583, 1995.
23. Kolykhalov AA, Agapov EV, Blight KJ, et al: Transmission of hepatitis C by intrahepatic inoculation with transcribed RNA. Science 277:570, 1997.
24. Yanagi M, Purcell RH, Emerson SU, Bukh J: Transcripts from a single full-length cDNA clone of hepatitis C virus are infectious when directly transfected into the liver of a chimpanzee. Proc Natl Acad Sci U S A 94:8738-8743, 1997.
25. Beard MR, Abell G, Honda M, et al: An infectious molecular clone of a Japanese genotype 1b hepatitis C virus. Hepatology 30:316-324, 1999.
26. Hong Z, Beaudet-Miller M, Lanford RE, et al: Generation of transmissible hepatitis C virions from a molecular clone in chimpanzees. Virology 256:36-44, 1999.
27. Lohmann V, Korner F, Koch J, et al: Replication of subgenomic hepatitis C virus RNAs in a hepatoma cell line. Science 285:110, 1999.
28. Blight KJ, Kolykhalov AA, Rice CM: Efficient initiation of HCV RNA replication in cell culture. Science 290:1972, 2000.
29. Shimizu YK, Feinstone SM, Kohara M, et al: Hepatitis C virus: detection of intracellular virus particles by electron microscopy. Hepatology 23:205-209, 1996.
30. Kaito M, Watanabe S, Tsukiyama-Kohara K, et al: Hepatitis C virus particle detected by immunoelectron microscopic study. J Gen Virol 75:1755-1760, 1994.
31. Baumert TF, Ito S, Wong DT, Liang TJ: Hepatitis C virus structural proteins assemble into viruslike particles in insect cells. J Virol 72:3827-3836, 1998.
32. Honda M, Beard MR, Ping LH, Lemon SM: A phylogenetically conserved stem-loop structure at the 5′ border of the internal ribosome entry site of hepatitis C virus is required for cap-independent viral translation. J Virol 73:1165-1174, 1999.
33. Pestova TV, Kolupaeva VG, Lomakin IB, et al: Molecular mechanisms of translation initiation in eukaryotes. Proc Natl Acad Sci U S A 98:7029-7036, 2001.
34. Fukushi S, Okada M, Kageyama T, et al: Specific interaction of a 25-kilodalton cellular protein, a 40S ribosomal subunit protein, with

the internal ribosome entry site of hepatitis C virus genome. Virus Genes 19:153-161, 1999.
35. Ali N, Pruijn GJ, Kenan DJ, et al: Human La antigen is required for the hepatitis C virus internal ribosome entry site-mediated translation. J Biol Chem 275:27531, 2000.
36. Hahm B, Kim YK, Kim JH, et al: Heterogeneous nuclear ribonucleoprotein L interacts with the 3' border of the internal ribosomal entry site of hepatitis C virus. J Virol 72:8782, 1998.
37. Kolykhalov AA, Feinstone SM, Rice CM: Identification of a highly conserved sequence element at the 3' terminus of hepatitis C virus genome RNA. J Virol 70:3363-3371, 1996.
38. Tanaka T, Kato N, Cho MJ, et al: Structure of the 3' terminus of the hepatitis C virus genome. J Virol 70:3307-3312, 1996.
39. Yanagi M, St Claire M, Emerson SU, et al: In vivo analysis of the 3′ untranslated region of the hepatitis C virus after in vitro mutagenesis of an infectious cDNA clone. Proc Natl Acad Sci U S A 96:2291-2295, 1999.
40. Wood J, Frederickson RM, Fields S, Patel AH: Hepatitis C virus 3′X region interacts with human ribosomal proteins. J Virol 75:1348-1358, 2001.
41. Ito T, Tahara SM, Lai MM: The 3'-untranslated region of hepatitis C virus RNA enhances translation from an internal ribosomal entry site. J Virol 72:8789-8796, 1998.
42. Tsuchihara K, Tanaka T, Hijikata M, et al: Specific interaction of polypyrimidine tract-binding protein with the extreme 3'-terminal structure of the hepatitis C virus genome, the 3'X. J Virol 71:6720, 1997.
43. Hong Z, Cameron CE, Walker MP, et al: A novel mechanism to ensure terminal initiation by hepatitis C virus NS5B polymerase. Virology 285:6-11, 2001.
44. Martire G, Viola A, Iodice L, et al: Hepatitis C virus structural proteins reside in the endoplasmic reticulum as well as in the intermediate compartment/cis-Golgi complex region of stably transfected cells. Virology 280:176-182, 2001.
45. Wu JZ: Internally located signal peptides direct hepatitis C virus polyprotein processing in the ER membrane. IUBMB Life 51:19-23, 2001.
46. Hijikata M, Kato N, Ootsuyama Y, et al: Gene mapping of the putative structural region of the hepatitis C virus genome by in vitro processing analysis. Proc Natl Acad Sci U S A 88:5547-5551, 1991.
47. Bukh J, Purcell RH, Miller RH: Sequence analysis of the core gene of 14 hepatitis C virus genotypes. Proc Natl Acad Sci U S A 91:8239-8243, 1994.
48. Santolini E, Migliaccio G, La Monica N: Biosynthesis and biochemical properties of the hepatitis C virus core protein. J Virol 68:3631-3641, 1994.
49. Shimoike T, Mimori S, Tani H, et al: Interaction of hepatitis C virus core protein with viral sense RNA and suppression of its translation. J Virol 73:9718-9725, 1999.
50. Matsumoto M, Hsieh TY, Zhu N, et al: Hepatitis C virus core protein interacts with the cytoplasmic tail of lymphotoxin-beta receptor. J Virol 71:1301, 1997.
51. You LR, Chen CM, Lee YH: Hepatitis C virus core protein enhances NF-kappaB signal pathway triggering by lymphotoxin-beta receptor ligand and tumor necrosis factor alpha. J Virol 73:1672-1681, 1999.
52. Ruggieri A, Harada T, Matsuura Y, Miyamura T: Sensitization to Fas-mediated apoptosis by hepatitis C virus core protein. Virology 229:68-76, 1997.
53. Ray RB, Meyer K, Ray R: Suppression of apoptotic cell death by hepatitis C virus core protein. Virology 226:176-182, 1996.
54. Matsuura Y, Harada S, Suzuki R, et al: Expression of processed envelope protein of hepatitis C virus in mammalian and insect cells. J Virol 66:1425-1431, 1992.
55. Grakoui A, Wychowski C, Lin C, et al: Expression and identification of hepatitis C virus polyprotein cleavage products. J Virol 67:1385-1395, 1993.
56. Ralston R, Thudium K, Berger K, et al: Characterization of hepatitis C virus envelope glycoprotein complexes expressed by recombinant vaccinia viruses. J Virol 67:6753-6761, 1993.
57. Cocquerel L, Wychowski C, Minner F, et al: Charged residues in the transmembrane domains of hepatitis C virus glycoproteins play a major role in the processing, subcellular localization, and assembly of these envelope proteins. J Virol 74:3623-3633, 2000.
58. Dubuisson J, Hsu HH, Cheung RC, et al: Formation and intracellular localization of hepatitis C virus envelope glycoprotein complexes expressed by recombinant vaccinia and Sindbis viruses. J Virol 68:6147-6160, 1994.
59. Choukhi A, Ung S, Wychowski C, Dubuisson J: Involvement of endoplasmic reticulum chaperones in the folding of hepatitis C virus glycoproteins. J Virol 72:3851, 1998.
60. Weiner AJ, Brauer MJ, Rosenblatt J, et al: Variable and hypervariable domains are found in the regions of HCV corresponding to the flavivirus envelope and NS1 proteins and the pestivirus envelope glycoproteins. Virology 180:842, 1991.
61. Kato N, Ootsuyama Y, Ohkoshi S, et al: Characterization of hypervariable regions in the putative envelope protein of hepatitis C virus. Biochem Biophys Res Commun 189:119-127, 1992.
62. Habersetzer F, Fournillier A, Dubuisson J, et al: Characterization of human monoclonal antibodies specific to the hepatitis C virus glycoprotein E2 with in vitro binding neutralization properties. Virology 249:32-41, 1998.
63. Farci P, Shimoda A, Wong D, et al: Prevention of hepatitis C virus infection in chimpanzees by hyperimmune serum against the hypervariable region 1 of the envelope 2 protein. Proc Natl Acad Sci U S A 93:15394, 1996.
64. Kato N, Sekiya H, Ootsuyama Y, et al: Humoral immune response to hypervariable region 1 of the putative envelope glycoprotein (gp70) of hepatitis C virus. J Virol 67:3923, 1993.
65. Manzin A, Solforosi L, Petrelli E, et al: Evolution of hypervariable region 1 of hepatitis C virus in primary infection. J Virol 72:6271, 1998.
66. McAllister J, Casino C, Davidson F, et al: Long-term evolution of the hypervariable region of hepatitis C virus in a common-source-infected cohort. J Virol 72:4893-4905, 1998.
67. Farci P, Shimoda A, Coiana A, et al: The outcome of acute hepatitis C predicted by the evolution of the viral quasispecies. Science 288:339-344, 2000.
68. Taylor DR, Shi ST, Romano PR, et al: Inhibition of the interferon-inducible protein kinase PKR by HCV E2 protein. Science 285:107-110, 1999.
69. Santolini E, Pacini L, Fipaldini C, et al: The NS2 protein of hepatitis C virus is a transmembrane polypeptide. J Virol 69:7461-7471, 1995.
70. Tanji Y, Kaneko T, Satoh S, Shimotohno K: Phosphorylation of hepatitis C virus-encoded nonstructural protein NS5A. J Virol 69:3980-3986, 1995.
71. Gallinari P, Brennan D, Nardi C, et al: Multiple enzymatic activities associated with recombinant NS3 protein of hepatitis C virus. J Virol 72:6758-6769, 1998.
72. Kim JL, Morgenstern KA, Lin C, et al: Crystal structure of the hepatitis C virus NS3 protease domain complexed with a synthetic NS4A cofactor peptide. Cell 87:343-355, 1996.
73. Kim JL, Morgenstern KA, Griffith JP, et al: Hepatitis C virus NS3 RNA helicase domain with a bound oligonucleotide: the crystal structure provides insights into the mode of unwinding. Structure 6:89-100, 1998.
74. Love RA, Parge HE, Wickersham JA, et al: The crystal structure of hepatitis C virus NS3 proteinase reveals a trypsin-like fold and a structural zinc binding site. Cell 87:331-342, 1996.
75. Lin C, Rice CM: The hepatitis C virus NS3 serine proteinase and NS4A cofactor: establishment of a cell-free trans-processing assay. Proc Natl Acad Sci U S A 92:7622, 1995.
76. Bouffard P, Bartenschlager R, Ahlborn-Laake L, et al: An in vitro assay for hepatitis C virus NS3 serine proteinase. Virology 209:52-59, 1995.
77. Tai CL, Chi WK, Chen DS, Hwang LH: The helicase activity associated with hepatitis C virus nonstructural protein 3 (NS3). J Virol 70:8477-8484, 1996.
78. Failla CM, Pizzi E, Francesco RD, Tramontano A: Redesigning the substrate specificity of the hepatitis C virus NS3 protease. Fold Des 1:35-42, 1995.
79. Failla C, Tomei L, De Francesco R: Both NS3 and NS4A are required for proteolytic processing of hepatitis C virus nonstructural proteins. J Virol 68:3753, 1994.
80. Lin C, Wu JW, Hsiao K, Su MS: The hepatitis C virus NS4A protein: interactions with the NS4B and NS5A proteins. J Virol 71:6465-6471, 1997.
81. Neddermann P, Clementi A, De Francesco R: Hyperphosphorylation of the hepatitis C virus NS5A protein requires an active NS3 protease, NS4A, NS4B, and NS5A encoded on the same polyprotein. J Virol 73:9984-9991, 1999.

82. Krieger N, Lohmann V, Bartenschlager R: Enhancement of hepatitis C virus RNA replication by cell culture-adaptive mutations. J Virol 75:4614-4624, 2001.
83. Koch JO, Bartenschlager R: Modulation of hepatitis C virus NS5A hyperphosphorylation by nonstructural proteins NS3, NS4A, and NS4B. J Virol 73:7138, 1999.
84. Hirota M, Satoh S, Asabe S, et al: Phosphorylation of nonstructural 5A protein of hepatitis C virus: HCV group-specific hyperphosphorylation. Virology 257:130-137, 1999.
85. Enomoto N, Sakuma I, Asahina Y, et al: Mutations in the nonstructural protein 5A gene and response to interferon in patients with chronic hepatitis C virus 1b infection. N Engl J Med 334:77-81, 1996.
86. Gale M Jr, Kwieciszewski B, Dossett M, et al: Antiapoptotic and oncogenic potentials of hepatitis C virus are linked to interferon resistance by viral repression of the PKR protein kinase. J Virol 73:6506, 1999.
87. Lohmann V, Korner F, Herian U, Bartenschlager R: Biochemical properties of hepatitis C virus NS5B RNA-dependent RNA polymerase and identification of amino acid sequence motifs essential for enzymatic activity. J Virol 71:8416, 1997.
88. Poch O, Sauvaget I, Delarue M, Tordo N: Identification of four conserved motifs among the RNA-dependent polymerase encoding elements. EMBO J 8:3867, 1989.
89. Ferrari E, Wright-Minogue J, Fang JW, et al: Characterization of soluble hepatitis C virus RNA-dependent RNA polymerase expressed in Escherichia coli. J Virol 73:1649, 1999.
90. Oh JW, Ito T, Lai MM: A recombinant hepatitis C virus RNA-dependent RNA polymerase capable of copying the full-length viral RNA. J Virol 73:7694-7702, 1999.
91. Pileri P, Uematsu Y, Campagnoli S, et al: Binding of hepatitis C virus to CD81. Science 282:938-941, 1998.
92. Wunschmann S, Medh JD, Klinzmann D, et al: Characterization of hepatitis C virus (HCV) and HCV E2 interactions with CD81 and the low-density lipoprotein receptor. J Virol 74:10055-10062, 2000.
93. Xie ZC, Riezu-Boj JI, Lasarte JJ, et al: Transmission of hepatitis C virus infection to tree shrews. Virology 244:513-520, 1998.
94. Kawamura T, Furusaka A, Koziel MJ, et al: Transgenic expression of hepatitis C virus structural proteins in the mouse. Hepatology 25:1014, 1997.
95. Pasquinelli C, Shoenberger JM, Chung J, et al: Hepatitis C virus core and E2 protein expression in transgenic mice. Hepatology 25:719-727, 1997.
96. Moriya K, Fujie H, Shintani Y, et al: The core protein of hepatitis C virus induces hepatocellular carcinoma in transgenic mice. Nat Med 4:1065, 1998.
97. Wakita T, Taya C, Katsume A, et al: Efficient conditional transgene expression in hepatitis C virus cDNA transgenic mice mediated by the Cre/loxP system. J Biol Chem 273:9001, 1998.
98. Bronowicki JP, Loriot MA, Thiers V, et al: Hepatitis C virus persistence in human hematopoietic cells injected into SCID mice. Hepatology 28:211, 1998.
99. Galun E, Burakova T, Ketzinel M, et al: Hepatitis C virus viremia in SCID→BNX mouse chimera. J Infect Dis 172:25-30, 1995.
100. Mercer DF, Schiller DE, Elliott JF, et al: Hepatitis C virus replication in mice with chimeric human livers. Nat Med 7:927-933, 2001.
101. Holland J, Spindler K, Horodyski F, et al: Rapid evolution of RNA genomes. Science 215:1577-1585, 1982.
102. Manns MP, McHutchison JG, Gordon SC, et al: Peginterferon alfa-2b plus ribavirin compared with interferon alfa-2b plus ribavirin for initial treatment of chronic hepatitis C: a randomised trial. Lancet 358:958-965, 2001.
103. Fried MW, Shiffman M, Reddy RK, et al: Pegylated (40kDa) interferon alfa-2a (PegasysTM) in combination with ribavirin: efficacy and safety results from a phase III, randomized, actively-controlled, multicenter study. Gastroenterology 120:289A, 2001.
104. Ray SC, Wang YM, Laeyendecker O, et al: Acute hepatitis C virus structural gene sequences as predictors of persistent viremia: hypervariable region 1 as a decoy. J Virol 73:2938-2946, 1999.
105. Erickson AL, Kimura Y, Igarashi S, et al: The outcome of hepatitis C virus infection is predicted by escape mutations in epitopes targeted by cytotoxic T lymphocytes. Immunity 15:883, 2001.
106. Forns X, Thimme R, Govindarajan S, et al: Hepatitis C virus lacking the hypervariable region 1 of the second envelope protein is infectious and causes acute resolving or persistent infection in chimpanzees. Proc Natl Acad Sci U S A 97:13318, 2000.
107. Major ME, Mihalik K, Fernandez J, et al: Long-term follow-up of chimpanzees inoculated with the first infectious clone for hepatitis C virus. J Virol 73:3317, 1999.
108. Thomson M, Nascimbeni M, Gonzales S, et al: Emergence of a distinct pattern of viral mutations in chimpanzees infected with a homogeneous inoculum of hepatitis C virus. Gastroenterology 121:1226, 2001.
109. Alter MJ: Hepatitis C virus infection in the United States. J Hepatol 31:88-91, 1999.
110. Alter MJ, Hadler SC, Judson FN, et al: Risk factors for acute non-A, non-B hepatitis in the United States and association with hepatitis C virus infection. JAMA 264:2231, 1990.
111. Recommendations for prevention and control of hepatitis C virus (HCV) infection and HCV-related chronic disease. Centers for Disease Control and Prevention. MMWR Recomm Rep 1998. 47:1-39.
112. Glynn SA, Kleinman SH, Schreiber GB, et al: Trends in incidence and prevalence of major transfusion-transmissible viral infections in US blood donors, 1991 to 1996. Retrovirus Epidemiology Donor Study (REDS). JAMA 284:229, 2000.
113. Howell C, Jeffers L, Hoofnagle JH: Hepatitis C in African Americans: summary of a workshop. Gastroenterology 119:1385-1396, 2000.
114. Ruiz JD, Molitor F, Sun RK, et al: Prevalence and correlates of hepatitis C virus infection among inmates entering the California correctional system. West J Med 170:156-160, 1999.
115. Culver DH, Alter MJ, Mullan RJ, Margolis HS: Evaluation of the effectiveness of targeted lookback for HCV infection in the United States—interim results. Transfusion 40:1176, 2000.
116. McHutchison JG, Gordon SC, Schiff ER, et al: Interferon alfa-2b alone or in combination with ribavirin as initial treatment for chronic hepatitis C. Hepatitis Interventional Therapy Group. N Engl J Med 339:1485, 1998.
117. Poynard T, Marcellin P, Lee SS, et al: Randomised trial of interferon alpha2b plus ribavirin for 48 weeks or for 24 weeks versus interferon alpha2b plus placebo for 48 weeks for treatment of chronic infection with hepatitis C virus. International Hepatitis Interventional Therapy Group (IHIT). Lancet 352:1426-1432, 1998.
118. Lindsay KL, Trepo C, Heintges T, et al: A randomized, double-blind trial comparing pegylated interferon alfa-2b to interferon alfa-2b as initial treatment for chronic hepatitis C. Hepatology 34:395-403, 2001.
119. Heathcote EJ, Shiffman ML, Cooksley WG, et al: Peginterferon alfa-2a in patients with chronic hepatitis C and cirrhosis. N Engl J Med 343:1673-1680, 2000.
120. Kleinman SH, Busch MP: The risks of transfusion-transmitted infection: direct estimation and mathematical modelling. Baillieres Best Pract Res Clin Haematol 13:631-649, 2000.
121. Soucie JM, Richardson LC, Evatt BL, et al: Risk factors for infection with HBV and HCV in a large cohort of hemophiliac males. Transfusion 41:338-343, 2001.
122. Prati D, Zanella A, Farma E, et al: A multicenter prospective study on the risk of acquiring liver disease in anti-hepatitis C virus negative patients affected from homozygous beta-thalassemia. Blood 92:3460, 1998.
123. Wonke B, Hoffbrand AV, Brown D, Dusheiko G: Antibody to hepatitis C virus in multiply transfused patients with thalassanemia major. J Clin Pathol 43:638-640, 1990.
124. Strickland DK, Riely CA, Patrick CC, et al: Hepatitis C infection among survivors of childhood cancer. Blood 95:3065, 2000.
125. Tokars JI, Alter MJ, Favero MS, et al: National surveillance of dialysis associated diseases in the United States, 1992. ASAIO J 40:1020, 1994.
126. Updated US Public Health Service Guidelines for the Management of Occupational Exposures to HBV, HCV, and HIV and Recommendations for Postexposure Prophylaxis. MMWR Recomm Rep 50:1-52, 2001.
127. Forns X, Fernandez-Llama P, Pons M, et al: Incidence and risk factors of hepatitis C virus infection in a haemodialysis unit. Nephrol Dial Transplant 12:736, 1997.
128. Bresee JS, Mast EE, Coleman PJ, et al: Hepatitis C virus infection associated with administration of intravenous immune globulin. A cohort study. JAMA 276:1563, 1996.

129. Murphy EL, Bryzman SM, Glynn SA, et al: Risk factors for hepatitis C virus infection in United States blood donors. NHLBI Retrovirus Epidemiology Donor Study (REDS). Hepatology 31:756-762, 2000.
130. Galeazzi B, Tufano A, Barbierato E, Bortolotti F: Hepatitis C virus infection in Italian intravenous drug users: epidemiological and clinical aspects. Liver 15:209-212, 1995.
131. Villano SA, Vlahov D, Nelson KE, et al: Incidence and risk factors for hepatitis C among injection drug users in Baltimore, Maryland. J Clin Microbiol 35:3274, 1997.
132. Conry-Cantilena C, VanRaden M, Gibble J, et al: Routes of infection, viremia, and liver disease in blood donors found to have hepatitis C virus infection. N Engl J Med 334:1691, 1996.
133. Alter MJ, Coleman PJ, Alexander WJ, et al: Importance of heterosexual activity in the transmission of hepatitis B and non-A, non-B hepatitis. JAMA 262:1201, 1989.
134. Thomas DL, Villano SA, Riester KA, et al: Perinatal transmission of hepatitis C virus from human immunodeficiency virus type 1-infected mothers. Women and Infants Transmission Study. J Infect Dis 177:1480, 1998.
135. Eyster ME, Alter HJ, Aledort LM, et al: Heterosexual co-transmission of hepatitis C virus (HCV) and human immunodeficiency virus (HIV). Ann Intern Med 115:764, 1991.
136. Akahane Y, Kojima M, Sugai Y, et al: Hepatitis C virus infection in spouses of patients with type C chronic liver disease. Ann Intern Med 120:748, 1994.
137. Stroffolini T, Lorenzoni U, Menniti-Ippolito F, et al: Hepatitis C virus infection in spouses: sexual transmission or common exposure to the same risk factors? Am J Gastroenterol 96:3138, 2001.
138. Sciacca C, Pellicano R, Berrutti M, et al: Sexual transmission of hepatitis C virus: the Turin study. Panminerva Med 43:229-231, 2001.
139. Thomas DL, Factor SH, Kelen GD, et al: Viral hepatitis in health care personnel at The Johns Hopkins Hospital. The seroprevalence of and risk factors for hepatitis B virus and hepatitis C virus infection. Arch Intern Med 153:1705, 1993.
140. Thomas DL, Gruninger SE, Siew C, et al: Occupational risk of hepatitis C infections among general dentists and oral surgeons in North America. Am J Med 100:41, 1996.
141. Werman HA, Gwinn R: Seroprevalence of hepatitis B and hepatitis C among rural emergency medical care personnel. Am J Emerg Med 15:248-251, 1997.
142. Roome AJ, Hadler JL, Thomas AL, et al: Hepatitis C virus infection among firefighters, emergency medical technicians, and paramedics—selected locations, United States, 1991-2000. MMWR Morb Mortal Wkly Rep 49:660, 2000.
143. Esteban JI, Gomez J, Martell M, et al: Transmission of hepatitis C virus by a cardiac surgeon. N Engl J Med 334:555-560, 1996.
144. Knoll A, Helmig M, Peters O, Jilg W: Hepatitis C virus transmission in a pediatric oncology ward: analysis of an outbreak and review of the literature. Lab Invest81:251-262. 2001.
145. Mele A, Spada E, Sagliocca L, et al: Risk of parenterally transmitted hepatitis following exposure to surgery or other invasive procedures: results from the hepatitis surveillance system in Italy. J Hepatol 35:284, 2001.
146. Maio G, d'Argenio P, Stroffolini T, et al: Hepatitis C virus infection and alanine transaminase levels in the general population: a survey in a southern Italian town. J Hepatol 33:116-120, 2000.
147. Frank C, Mohamed MK, Strickland GT, et al: The role of parenteral antischistosomal therapy in the spread of hepatitis C virus in Egypt. Lancet 355:887, 2000.
148. Conte D, Fraquelli M, Prati D, et al: Prevalence and clinical course of chronic hepatitis C virus (HCV) infection and rate of HCV vertical transmission in a cohort of 15,250 pregnant women. Hepatology 31:751, 2000.
149. Hunt CM, Carson KL, Sharara AI: Hepatitis C in pregnancy. Obstet Gynecol 89:883-890, 1997.
150. Ceci O, Margiotta M, Marello F, et al: Vertical transmission of hepatitis c virus in a cohort of 2,447 HIV-seronegative pregnant women: a 24-month prospective study. J Pediatr Gastroenterol Nutr 33:570, 2001.
151. Tajiri H, Miyoshi Y, Funada S, et al: Prospective study of mother-to-infant transmission of hepatitis C virus. Pediatr Infect Dis J 20:10-14, 2001.
152. Ruiz-Extremera A, Salmeron J, Torres C, et al: Follow-up of transmission of hepatitis C to babies of human immunodeficiency virus-negative women: the role of breast-feeding in transmission. Pediatr Infect Dis J 19:511, 2000.
153. Zanetti AR, Tanzi E, Romano L, et al: A prospective study on mother-to-infant transmission of hepatitis C virus. Intervirology 41:208-212, 1998.
154. Spencer JD, Latt N, Beeby PJ, et al: Transmission of hepatitis C virus to infants of human immunodeficiency virus-negative intravenous drug-using mothers: rate of infection and assessment of risk factors for transmission. J Viral Hepat 4:395-409, 1997.
155. Hershow RC, Riester KA, Lew J, et al: Increased vertical transmission of human immunodeficiency virus from hepatitis C virus-coinfected mothers. Women and Infants Transmission Study. J Infect Dis 176:414-420, 1997.
156. Tovo PA, Palomba E, Ferraris G, et al: Increased risk of maternal-infant hepatitis C virus transmission for women coinfected with human immunodeficiency virus type 1. Italian Study Group for HCV Infection in Children. Clin Infect Dis 25:1121, 1997.
157. Bortolotti F, Iorio R, Resti M, et al: An epidemiological survey of hepatitis C virus infection in Italian children in the decade 1990-1999. J Pediatr Gastroenterol Nutr 32:562, 2001.
158. Ohto H, Terazawa S, Sasaki N, et al: Transmission of hepatitis C virus from mothers to infants. The Vertical Transmission of Hepatitis C Virus Collaborative Study Group. N Engl J Med 330:744-750, 1994.
159. Haley RW, Fischer RP: Commercial tattooing as a potentially important source of hepatitis C infection. Clinical epidemiology of 626 consecutive patients unaware of their hepatitis C serologic status. Medicine (Baltimore) 80:134-151, 2001.
160. Balasekaran R, Bulterys M, Jamal MM, et al: A case-control study of risk factors for sporadic hepatitis C virus infection in the southwestern United States. Am J Gastroenterol 94:1341, 1999.
161. Hoofnagle JH: Hepatitis C: the clinical spectrum of disease. Hepatology 26:15S-20S, 1997.
162. Alter HJ, Sanchez-Pescador R, Urdea MS, et al: Evaluation of branched DNA signal amplification for the detection of hepatitis C virus RNA. J Viral Hepat 2:121-132, 1995.
163. Alter MJ, Margolis HS, Krawczynski K, et al: The natural history of community-acquired hepatitis C in the United States. The Sentinel Counties Chronic non-A, non-B Hepatitis Study Team. N Engl J Med 327:1899-1905, 1992.
164. Farci P, Alter HJ, Wong D, et al: A long-term study of hepatitis C virus replication in non-A, non-B hepatitis. N Engl J Med 325:98-104, 1991.
165. Aach RD, Stevens CE, Hollinger FB, et al: Hepatitis C virus infection in post-transfusion hepatitis. An analysis with first- and second-generation assays. N Engl J Med 325:1325, 1991.
166. Alter HJ, Purcell RH, Shih JW, et al: Detection of antibody to hepatitis C virus in prospectively followed transfusion recipients with acute and chronic non-A, non-B hepatitis. N Engl J Med 321:1494-1500, 1989.
167. Hino K, Sainokami S, Shimoda K, et al: Clinical course of acute hepatitis C and changes in HCV markers. Dig Dis Sci 39:19-27, 1994.
168. Villano SA, Vlahov D, Nelson KE, et al: Persistence of viremia and the importance of long-term follow-up after acute hepatitis C infection. Hepatology 29:908, 1999.
169. Di Bisceglie AM, Goodman ZD, Ishak KG, et al: Long-term clinical and histopathological follow-up of chronic posttransfusion hepatitis. Hepatology 14:969-974, 1991.
170. Seeff LB, Hollinger FB, Alter HJ, et al: Long-term mortality and morbidity of transfusion-associated non-A, non-B, and type C hepatitis: a National Heart, Lung, and Blood Institute collaborative study. Hepatology 33:455, 2001.
171. Vogt M, Lang T, Frosner G, et al: Prevalence and clinical outcome of hepatitis C infection in children who underwent cardiac surgery before the implementation of blood-donor screening. N Engl J Med 341:866, 1999.
172. Kenny-Walsh E: Clinical outcomes after hepatitis C infection from contaminated anti-D immune globulin. Irish Hepatology Research Group. N Engl J Med 340:1228, 1999.
173. Takaki A, Wiese M, Maertens G, et al: Cellular immune responses persist and humoral responses decrease two decades after recovery from a single-source outbreak of hepatitis C. Nat Med 6:578-582, 2000.
174. Shakil AO, Conry-Cantilena C, Alter HJ, et al: Volunteer blood donors with antibody to hepatitis C virus: clinical, biochemical,

virologic, and histologic features. The Hepatitis C Study Group. Ann Intern Med 123:330, 1995.
175. Chau KH, Dawson GJ, Mushahwar IK, et al: IgM-antibody response to hepatitis C virus antigens in acute and chronic post-transfusion non-A, non-B hepatitis. J Virol Methods 35:343, 1991.
176. Thimme R, Oldach D, Chang KM, et al: Determinants of viral clearance and persistence during acute hepatitis C virus infection. J Exp Med 194:1395-1406, 2001.
177. Barrera JM, Bruguera M, Ercilla MG, et al: Persistent hepatitis C viremia after acute self-limiting posttransfusion hepatitis C. Hepatology 21:639-644, 1995.
178. Alberti A, Morsica G, Chemello L, et al: Hepatitis C viraemia and liver disease in symptom-free individuals with anti-HCV. Lancet 340:697, 1992.
179. Puoti C, Magrini A, Stati T, et al: Clinical, histological, and virological features of hepatitis C virus carriers with persistently normal or abnormal alanine transaminase levels. Hepatology 26:1393, 1997.
180. Martinot-Peignoux M, Boyer N, Cazals-Hatem D, et al: Prospective study on anti-hepatitis C virus-positive patients with persistently normal serum alanine transaminase with or without detectable serum hepatitis C virus RNA. Hepatology 34:1000, 2001.
181. Chien DY, Choo QL, Tabrizi A, et al: Diagnosis of hepatitis C virus (HCV) infection using an immunodominant chimeric polyprotein to capture circulating antibodies: reevaluation of the role of HCV in liver disease. Proc Natl Acad Sci U S A 89:10011, 1992.
182. Marcellin P, Martinot-Peignoux M, Boyer N, et al: Second generation (RIBA) test in diagnosis of chronic hepatitis C. Lancet 337:551-552, 1991.
183. Alter HJ, Tegtmeier GE, Jett BW, et al: The use of a recombinant immunoblot assay in the interpretation of anti-hepatitis C virus reactivity among prospectively followed patients, implicated donors, and random donors. Transfusion 31:771, 1991.
184. Gretch DR: Diagnostic tests for hepatitis C. Hepatology 26:43S-47S, 1997.
185. Lok AS, Gunaratnam NT: Diagnosis of hepatitis C. Hepatology 26:48S-56S, 1997.
186. Weiner AJ, Truett MA, Rosenblatt J, et al: HCV testing in low-risk population. Lancet 336:695, 1990.
187. Albadalejo J, Alonso R, Antinozzi R, et al: Multicenter evaluation of the COBAS AMPLICOR HCV assay, an integrated PCR system for rapid detection of hepatitis C virus RNA in the diagnostic laboratory. J Clin Microbiol 36:862, 1998.
188. Pawlotsky JM, Bouvier-Alias M, Hezode C, et al: Standardization of hepatitis C virus RNA quantification. Hepatology 32:654, 2000.
189. Zaaijer HL, Cuypers HT, Reesink HW, et al: Reliability of polymerase chain reaction for detection of hepatitis C virus. Lancet 341:722, 1993.
190. Damen M, Cuypers HT, Zaaijer HL, et al: International collaborative study on the second EUROHEP HCV-RNA reference panel. J Virol Methods 58:175-185, 1996.
191. Tong MJ, Blatt LM, Conrad A, et al: The changes in quantitative HCV RNA titers during interferon alpha 2B therapy in patients with chronic hepatitis C infection. Am J Gastroenterol 93:601, 1998.
192. Shiratori Y, Kato N, Yokosuka O, et al: Quantitative assays for hepatitis C virus in serum as predictors of the long-term response to interferon. J Hepatol 27:437-444, 1997.
193. Mahaney K, Tedeschi V, Maertens G, et al: Genotypic analysis of hepatitis C virus in American patients. Hepatology 20:1405, 1994.
194. Pawlotsky JM, Prescott L, Simmonds P, et al: Serological determination of hepatitis C virus genotype: comparison with a standardized genotyping assay. J Clin Microbiol 35:1734, 1997.
195. Stuyver L, Rossau R, Wyseur A, et al: Typing of hepatitis C virus isolates and characterization of new subtypes using a line probe assay. J Gen Virol 74:1093-1102, 1993.
196. van Doorn LJ, Kleter B, Stuyver L, et al: Analysis of hepatitis C virus genotypes by a line probe assay and correlation with antibody profiles. J Hepatol 21:122, 1994.
197. Goodman ZD, Ishak KG: Histopathology of hepatitis C virus infection. Semin Liver Dis 15:70-81, 1995.
198. Scheuer PJ, Ashrafzadeh P, Sherlock S, et al: The pathology of hepatitis C. Hepatology 15:567-571, 1992.
199. Vyberg M: The hepatitis-associated bile duct lesion. Liver 13:289-301, 1993.
200. Lefkowitch JH, Schiff ER, Davis GL, et al: Pathological diagnosis of chronic hepatitis C: a multicenter comparative study with chronic hepatitis B. The Hepatitis Interventional Therapy Group. Gastroenterology 104:595-603, 1993.
201. Yano M, Kumada H, Kage M, et al: The long-term pathological evolution of chronic hepatitis C. Hepatology 23:1334, 1996.
202. Desmet VJ, Gerber M, Hoofnagle JH, et al: Classification of chronic hepatitis: diagnosis, grading and staging. Hepatology 19:1513, 1994.
203. Knodell RG, Ishak KG, Black WC, et al: Formulation and application of a numerical scoring system for assessing histological activity in asymptomatic chronic active hepatitis. Hepatology 1:431, 1981.
204. Bedossa P, Poynard T: An algorithm for the grading of activity in chronic hepatitis C. The METAVIR Cooperative Study Group. Hepatology 24:289-293, 1996.
205. Ishak K, Baptista A, Bianchi L, et al: Histological grading and staging of chronic hepatitis. J Hepatol 22:696, 1995.
206. Fontaine H, Nalpas B, Poulet B, et al: Hepatitis activity index is a key factor in determining the natural history of chronic hepatitis C. Hum Pathol 32:904, 2001.
207. Lau DT, Kleiner DE, Ghany MG, et al: 10-year follow-up after interferon-alpha therapy for chronic hepatitis C. Hepatology 28:1121, 1998.
208. Marcellin P, Boyer N, Gervais A, et al: Long-term histologic improvement and loss of detectable intrahepatic HCV RNA in patients with chronic hepatitis C and sustained response to interferon-alpha therapy. Ann Intern Med 127:875-881, 1997.
209. Shiratori Y, Imazeki F, Moriyama M, et al: Histologic improvement of fibrosis in patients with hepatitis C who have sustained response to interferon therapy. Ann Intern Med 132:517-524, 2000.
210. Bigger CB, Brasky KM, Lanford RE: DNA microarray analysis of chimpanzee liver during acute resolving hepatitis C virus infection. J Virol 75:7059, 2001.
211. Cella M, Jarrossay D, Facchetti F, et al: Plasmacytoid monocytes migrate to inflamed lymph nodes and produce large amounts of type I interferon. Nat Med 5:919-923, 1999.
212. Kadowaki N, Antonenko S, Lau JY, Liu YJ: Natural interferon alpha/beta-producing cells link innate and adaptive immunity. J Exp Med 192:219, 2000.
213. Adams G, Kuntz S, Rabalais G, et al: Natural recovery from acute hepatitis C virus infection by agammaglobulinemic twin children. Pediatr Infect Dis J 16:533, 1997.
214. Farci P, Alter HJ, Govindarajan S, et al: Lack of protective immunity against reinfection with hepatitis C virus. Science 258:135-140, 1992.
215. Lai ME, Mazzoleni AP, Argiolu F, et al: Hepatitis C virus in multiple episodes of acute hepatitis in polytransfused thalassaemic children. Lancet 343:388-390, 1994.
216. Krawczynski K, Alter MJ, Tankersley DL, et al: Effect of immune globulin on the prevention of experimental hepatitis C virus infection. J Infect Dis 173:822, 1996.
217. Abrignani S, Houghton M, Hsu HH: Perspectives for a vaccine against hepatitis C virus. J Hepatol 31:259-263, 1999.
218. Bassett SE, Guerra B, Brasky K, et al: Protective immune response to hepatitis C virus in chimpanzees rechallenged following clearance of primary infection. Hepatology 33:1479, 2001.
219. Farci P, Alter HJ, Wong DC, et al: Prevention of hepatitis C virus infection in chimpanzees after antibody-mediated in vitro neutralization. Proc Natl Acad Sci U S A 91:7792-7796, 1994.
220. Bjoro K, Froland SS, Yun Z, et al: Hepatitis C infection in patients with primary hypogammaglobulinemia after treatment with contaminated immune globulin. N Engl J Med 331:1607, 1994.
221. Rossi G, Tucci A, Cariani E, et al: Outbreak of hepatitis C virus infection in patients with hematologic disorders treated with intravenous immunoglobulins: different prognosis according to the immune status. Blood 90:1309, 1997.
222. Bjoro K, Skaug K, Haaland T, Froland SS: Long-term outcome of chronic hepatitis C virus infection in primary hypogammaglobulinaemia. QJM 92:433-441, 1999.
223. Cooper S, Erickson AL, Adams EJ, et al: Analysis of a successful immune response against hepatitis C virus. Immunity 10:439-449, 1999.
224. Lechner F, Wong DK, Dunbar PR, et al: Analysis of successful immune responses in persons infected with hepatitis C virus. J Exp Med 191:1499-1512, 2000.
225. Gruener NH, Gerlach TJ, Jung MC, et al: Association of hepatitis C virus-specific CD8+ T cells with viral clearance in acute hepatitis C. J Infect Dis 181:1528, 2000.

226. Guidotti LG, Chisari FV: Noncytolytic control of viral infections by the innate and adaptive immune response. Annu Rev Immunol 19:65-91, 2001.
227. Gerlach JT, Diepolder HM, Jung MC, et al: Recurrence of hepatitis C virus after loss of virus-specific CD4(+) T-cell response in acute hepatitis C. Gastroenterology 117:933-941, 1999.
228. Rehermann B, Chang KM, McHutchinson J, et al: Differential cytotoxic T-lymphocyte responsiveness to the hepatitis B and C viruses in chronically infected patients. J Virol 70:7092-7102, 1996.
229. Hiroishi K, Kita H, Kojima M, et al: Cytotoxic T lymphocyte response and viral load in hepatitis C virus infection. Hepatology 25:705-712, 1997.
230. Nelson DR, Marousis CG, Davis GL, et al: The role of hepatitis C virus-specific cytotoxic T lymphocytes in chronic hepatitis C. J Immunol 158:1473, 1997.
231. Chang KM, Rehermann B, McHutchison JG, et al: Immunological significance of cytotoxic T lymphocyte epitope variants in patients chronically infected by the hepatitis C virus. J Clin Invest 100:2376, 1997.
232. Lanzavecchia A: Understanding the mechanisms of sustained signaling and T cell activation. J Exp Med 185:1717, 1997.
233. Weiner A, Erickson AL, Kansopon J, et al: Persistent hepatitis C virus infection in a chimpanzee is associated with emergence of a cytotoxic T lymphocyte escape variant. Proc Natl Acad Sci U S A 92:2755, 1995.
234. Tsai SL, Chen YM, Chen MH, et al: Hepatitis C virus variants circumventing cytotoxic T lymphocyte activity as a mechanism of chronicity. Gastroenterology 115:954-965, 1998.
235. Frasca L, Del Porto P, Tuosto L, et al: Hypervariable region 1 variants act as TCR antagonists for hepatitis C virus-specific CD4+ T cells. J Immunol 163:650, 1999.
236. Wang H, Eckels DD: Mutations in immunodominant T cell epitopes derived from the nonstructural 3 protein of hepatitis C virus have the potential for generating escape variants that may have important consequences for T cell recognition. J Immunol 162:4177, 1999.
237. Bain C, Fatmi A, Zoulim F, et al: Impaired allostimulatory function of dendritic cells in chronic hepatitis C infection. Gastroenterology 120:512-524, 2001.
238. Kittlesen DJ, Chianese-Bullock KA, Yao ZQ, et al: Interaction between complement receptor gC1qR and hepatitis C virus core protein inhibits T-lymphocyte proliferation. J Clin Invest 106:1239, 2000.
239. Thomssen R, Bonk S, Propfe C, et al: Association of hepatitis C virus in human sera with beta-lipoprotein. Med Microbiol Immunol 181:293-300, 1992.
240. Yokosuka O, Kojima H, Imazeki F, et al: Spontaneous negativation of serum hepatitis C virus RNA is a rare event in type C chronic liver diseases: analysis of HCV RNA in 320 patients who were followed for more than 3 years. J Hepatol 31:394, 1999.
241. Carithers RL Jr, Emerson SS: Therapy of hepatitis C: meta-analysis of interferon alfa-2b trials. Hepatology 26:83S-88S, 1997.
242. Everhart JE, Wei Y, Eng H, et al: Recurrent and new hepatitis C virus infection after liver transplantation. Hepatology 29:1220, 1999.
243. Alter HJ, Seeff LB: Recovery, persistence, and sequelae in hepatitis C virus infection: a perspective on long-term outcome. Semin Liver Dis 20:17-35, 2000.
244. Muller R: The natural history of hepatitis C: clinical experiences. J Hepatol 24:52, 1996.
245. Bortolotti F, Resti M, Giacchino R, et al: Hepatitis C virus infection and related liver disease in children of mothers with antibodies to the virus. J Pediatr 130:990, 1997.
246. Tong MJ, el-Farra NS, Reikes AR, Co RL: Clinical outcomes after transfusion-associated hepatitis C. N Engl J Med 332:1463, 1995.
247. Niederau C, Lange S, Heintges T, et al: Prognosis of chronic hepatitis C: results of a large, prospective cohort study. Hepatology 28:1687, 1998.
248. Fattovich G, Giustina G, Degos F, et al: Morbidity and mortality in compensated cirrhosis type C: a retrospective follow-up study of 384 patients. Gastroenterology 112:463-472, 1997.
249. Poynard T, Ratziu V, Charlotte F, et al: Rates and risk factors of liver fibrosis progression in patients with chronic hepatitis C. J Hepatol 34:730, 2001.
250. Poynard T, Bedossa P, Opolon P: Natural history of liver fibrosis progression in patients with chronic hepatitis C. The OBSVIRC, METAVIR, CLINIVIR, and DOSVIRC groups. Lancet 349:825-832, 1997.
251. Morris K, Bharucha C: Completed hepatitis C lookback in Northern Ireland. Transfus Med 7:269, 1997.
252. Poynard T, McHutchison J, Davis GL, et al: Impact of interferon alfa-2b and ribavirin on progression of liver fibrosis in patients with chronic hepatitis C. Hepatology 32:1131, 2000.
253. Williams AL, Hoofnagle JH: Ratio of serum aspartate to alanine aminotransferase in chronic hepatitis. Relationship to cirrhosis. Gastroenterology 95:734, 1988.
254. Di Bisceglie AM, Hoofnagle JH: Elevations in serum alpha-fetoprotein levels in patients with chronic hepatitis B. Cancer 64:2117-2120, 1989.
255. Everhart JE, Herion D: Hepatitis C virus infection and alcohol. In Liang TJ, Hoofnagle JH, eds: Hepatitis C, vol 1. San Diego, Academic Press, 2000:363-388.
256. Serfaty L, Chazouilleres O, Poujol-Robert A, et al: Risk factors for cirrhosis in patients with chronic hepatitis C virus infection: results of a case-control study. Hepatology 26:776, 1997.
257. Ostapowicz G, Watson KJ, Locarnini SA, Desmond PV: Role of alcohol in the progression of liver disease caused by hepatitis C virus infection. Hepatology 27:1730, 1998.
258. Donato F, Tagger A, Chiesa R, et al: Hepatitis B and C virus infection, alcohol drinking, and hepatocellular carcinoma: a case-control study in Italy. Brescia HCC Study. Hepatology 26:579-584, 1997.
259. Pessione F, Degos F, Marcellin P, et al: Effect of alcohol consumption on serum hepatitis C virus RNA and histological lesions in chronic hepatitis C. Hepatology 27:1717-1722, 1998.
260. Pascual M, Perrin L, Giostra E, Schifferli JA: Hepatitis C virus in patients with cryoglobulinemia type II. J Infect Dis 162:569, 1990.
261. Agnello V, Chung RT, Kaplan LM: A role for hepatitis C virus infection in type II cryoglobulinemia. N Engl J Med 327:1490, 1992.
262. Misiani R, Bellavita P, Fenili D, et al: Hepatitis C virus infection in patients with essential mixed cryoglobulinemia. Ann Intern Med 117:573, 1992.
263. Pawlotsky JM, Ben Yahia M, Andre C, et al: Immunological disorders in C virus chronic active hepatitis: a prospective case-control study. Hepatology 19:841, 1994.
264. Heckmann JG, Kayser C, Heuss D, et al: Neurological manifestations of chronic hepatitis C. J Neurol 246:486-491, 1999.
265. Cacoub P, Maisonobe T, Thibault V, et al: Systemic vasculitis in patients with hepatitis C. J Rheumatol 28:109-118, 2001.
266. Cicardi M, Cesana B, Del Ninno E, et al: Prevalence and risk factors for the presence of serum cryoglobulins in patients with chronic hepatitis C. J Viral Hepat 7:138-143, 2000.
267. Cacoub P, Renou C, Rosenthal E, et al: Extrahepatic manifestations associated with hepatitis C virus infection. A prospective multicenter study of 321 patients. The GERMIVIC. Groupe d'Etude et de Recherche en Medecine Interne et Maladies Infectieuses sur le Virus de l'Hepatite C. Medicine (Baltimore) 79:47-56, 2000.
268. Zuckerman E, Zuckerman T, Levine AM, et al: Hepatitis C virus infection in patients with B-cell non-Hodgkin lymphoma. Ann Intern Med 127:423, 1997.
269. Monteverde A, Rivano MT, Allegra GC, et al: Essential mixed cryoglobulinemia, type II: a manifestation of a low-grade malignant lymphoma? Clinical-morphological study of 12 cases with special reference to immunohistochemical findings in liver frozen sections. Acta Haematol 79:20, 1988.
270. Hausfater P, Cacoub P, Sterkers Y, et al: Hepatitis C virus infection and lymphoproliferative diseases: prospective study on 1,576 patients in France. Am J Hematol 67:168-171, 2001.
271. Johnson RJ, Gretch DR, Yamabe H, et al: Membranoproliferative glomerulonephritis associated with hepatitis C virus infection. N Engl J Med 328:465-470, 1993.
272. Pawlotsky JM, Roudot-Thoraval F, Simmonds P, et al: Extrahepatic immunologic manifestations in chronic hepatitis C and hepatitis C virus serotypes. Ann Intern Med 122:169-173, 1995.
273. King PD, McMurray RW, Becherer PR: Sjogren's syndrome without mixed cryoglobulinemia is not associated with hepatitis C virus infection. Am J Gastroenterol 89:1047, 1994.
274. Bonkovsky HL, Poh-Fitzpatrick M, Pimstone N, et al: Porphyria cutanea tarda, hepatitis C, and HFE gene mutations in North America. Hepatology 27:1661, 1998.
275. Hoofnagle JH, Mullen KD, Jones DB, et al: Treatment of chronic non-A, non-B hepatitis with recombinant human alpha interferon. A preliminary report. N Engl J Med 315:1575, 1986.

276. Shindo M, Di Bisceglie AM, Cheung L, et al: Decrease in serum hepatitis C viral RNA during alpha-interferon therapy for chronic hepatitis C. Ann Intern Med 115:700, 1991.
277. Di Bisceglie AM, Martin P, Kassianides C, et al: Recombinant interferon alfa therapy for chronic hepatitis C. A randomized, double-blind, placebo-controlled trial. N Engl J Med 321:1506-1510, 1989.
278. Davis GL, Balart LA, Schiff ER, et al: Treatment of chronic hepatitis C with recombinant interferon alfa. A multicenter randomized, controlled trial. Hepatitis Interventional Therapy Group. N Engl J Med 321:1501, 1989.
279. Reichard O, Norkrans G, Fryden A, et al: Randomised, double-blind, placebo-controlled trial of interferon alpha-2b with and without ribavirin for chronic hepatitis C. The Swedish Study Group. Lancet 351:83-87, 1998.
280. Glue P, Rouzier-Panis R, Raffanel C, et al: A dose-ranging study of pegylated interferon alfa-2b and ribavirin in chronic hepatitis C. The Hepatitis C Intervention Therapy Group. Hepatology 32:647-653, 2000.
281. Zeuzem S, Feinman SV, Rasenack J, et al: Peginterferon alfa-2a in patients with chronic hepatitis C. N Engl J Med 343:1666, 2000.
282. Reddy KR, Wright TL, Pockros PJ, et al: Efficacy and safety of pegylated (40-kd) interferon alpha-2a compared with interferon alpha-2a in noncirrhotic patients with chronic hepatitis C. Hepatology 33:433, 2001.
283. Lindsay KL: Therapy of hepatitis C: overview. Hepatology 26:71S-77S, 1997.
284. Yoshida H, Shiratori Y, Moriyama M, et al: Interferon therapy reduces the risk for hepatocellular carcinoma: national surveillance program of cirrhotic and noncirrhotic patients with chronic hepatitis C in Japan. IHIT Study Group. Inhibition of Hepatocarcinogenesis by Interferon Therapy. Ann Intern Med 131:174-181, 1999.
285. Bruno S, Battezzati PM, Bellati G, et al: Long-term beneficial effects in sustained responders to interferon-alfa therapy for chronic hepatitis C. J Hepatol 34:748-755, 2001.
286. Camma C, Giunta M, Andreone P, Craxi A: Interferon and prevention of hepatocellular carcinoma in viral cirrhosis: an evidence-based approach. J Hepatol 34:593-602, 2001.
287. Toyoda H, Kumada T, Tokuda A, et al: Long-term follow-up of sustained responders to interferon therapy, in patients with chronic hepatitis C. J Viral Hepat 7:414, 2000.
288. Shindo M, Hamada K, Oda Y, Okuno T: Long-term follow-up study of sustained biochemical responders with interferon therapy. Hepatology 33:1299-1302, 2001.
289. Shiratori Y, Yokosuka O, Nakata R, et al: Prospective study of interferon therapy for compensated cirrhotic patients with chronic hepatitis C by monitoring serum hepatitis C RNA. Hepatology 29:1573, 1999.
290. Kao JH, Lai MY, Chen PJ, Chen DS: Probable reinfection with hepatitis C virus in a chronic hepatitis C patient with a sustained response to combination therapy. J Formos Med Assoc 100:824, 2001.
291. Shiffman ML, Hofmann CM, Contos MJ, et al: A randomized, controlled trial of maintenance interferon therapy for patients with chronic hepatitis C virus and persistent viremia. Gastroenterology 117:1164, 1999.
292. Bonkovsky HL, Stefancyk D, McNeal K, et al: Comparative effects of different doses of ribavirin plus interferon- alpha2b for therapy of chronic hepatitis C: results of a controlled, randomized trial. Dig Dis Sci 46:2051, 2001.
293. Lee WM: Therapy of hepatitis C: interferon alfa-2a trials. Hepatology 26:89S-95S, 1997.
294. Farrell GC: Therapy of hepatitis C: interferon alfa-n1 trials. Hepatology 26:96S-100S, 1997.
295. EASL International Consensus Conference on hepatitis C: Paris, 26-27 February 1999. Consensus statement. J Hepatol 31:3-8, 1999.
296. Martinot-Peignoux M, Le Breton V, Fritsch S, et al: Assessment of viral loads in patients with chronic hepatitis C with AMPLICOR HCV MONITOR version 1.0, COBAS HCV MONITOR version 2.0, and QUANTIPLEX HCV RNA version 2.0 assays. J Clin Microbiol 38:2722, 2000.
297. Fang JW, Albrecht JK, Jacobs S, Lau JY: Quantification of serum hepatitis C virus RNA. Hepatology 29:997, 1999.
298. Saldanha J, Lelie N, Heath A: Establishment of the first international standard for nucleic acid amplification technology (NAT) assays for HCV RNA. WHO Collaborative Study Group. Vox Sang 76:149-158, 1999.
299. Neumann AU, Lam NP, Dahari H, et al: Hepatitis C viral dynamics in vivo and the antiviral efficacy of interferon-alpha therapy. Science 282:103, 1998.
300. Zeuzem S, Lee JH, Franke A, et al: Quantification of the initial decline of serum hepatitis C virus RNA and response to interferon alfa. Hepatology 27:1149, 1998.
301. Zeuzem S, Herrmann E, Lee JH, et al: Viral kinetics in patients with chronic hepatitis C treated with standard or peginterferon alpha2a. Gastroenterology 120:1438, 2001.
302. McHutchison JG, Shad JA, Gordon SC, et al: Predicting response to initial therapy with interferon plus ribavirin in chronic hepatitis C using serum HCV RNA results during therapy. J Viral Hepat 8:414-420, 2001.
303. National Institutes of Health Consensus Development Conference Panel statement: management of hepatitis C. Hepatology 26:2S-10S, 1997.
304. Jacobson KR, Murray K, Zellos A, Schwarz KB: An analysis of published trials of interferon monotherapy in children with chronic hepatitis C. J Pediatr Gastroenterol Nutr 34:52-58, 2002.
305. Ko JS, Choe YH, Kim EJ, et al: Interferon-alpha treatment of chronic hepatitis C in children with hemophilia. J Pediatr Gastroenterol Nutr 32:41-44, 2001.
306. Jonas MM, Ott MJ, Nelson SP, et al: Interferon-alpha treatment of chronic hepatitis C virus infection in children. Pediatr Infect Dis J 17:24, 1998.
307. Haber MM, West AB, Haber AD, Reuben A: Relationship of aminotransferases to liver histological status in chronic hepatitis C. Am J Gastroenterol 90:1250, 1995.
308. Lee SS, Sherman M: Pilot study of interferon-alpha and ribavirin treatment in patients with chronic hepatitis C and normal transaminase values. J Viral Hepat 8:202, 2001.
309. Di Bisceglie AM, Thompson J, Smith-Wilkaitis N, et al: Combination of interferon and ribavirin in chronic hepatitis C: re- treatment of nonresponders to interferon. Hepatology 33:704, 2001.
310. Hoofnagle JH, Lau D, Conjeevaram H, et al: Prolonged therapy of chronic hepatitis C with ribavirin. J Viral Hepat 3:247-252, 1996.
311. Wong JB, McQuillan GM, McHutchison JG, Poynard T: Estimating future hepatitis C morbidity, mortality, and costs in the United States. Am J Public Health 90:1562, 2000.
312. Crippin JS, Sheiner P, Terrault NA, et al: A pilot study of the tolerability and efficacy of antiviral therapy in patients awaiting liver transplantation for hepatitis C. Hepatology 32:308A, 2000.
313. Berenguer M, Lopez-Labrador FX, Wright TL: Hepatitis C and liver transplantation. J Hepatol 35:666-678, 2001.
314. Chan TM, Lok AS, Cheng IK, Chan RT: Prevalence of hepatitis C virus infection in hemodialysis patients: a longitudinal study comparing the results of RNA and antibody assays. Hepatology 17:5-8, 1993.
315. Zacks S, Fried MW: Hepatitis C and renal disease. In Liang TJ, Hoofnagle JH, eds: Hepatitis C, vol 1. San Diego, Academic Press, 2000:329-349.
316. Recommendations for preventing transmission of infections among chronic hemodialysis patients. MMWR Recomm Rep 50:1-43, 2001.
317. Mathurin P, Mouquet C, Poynard T, et al: Impact of hepatitis B and C virus on kidney transplantation outcome. Hepatology 29:257-263, 1999.
318. Bukh J, Wantzin P, Krogsgaard K, et al: High prevalence of hepatitis C virus (HCV) RNA in dialysis patients: failure of commercially available antibody tests to identify a significant number of patients with HCV infection. Copenhagen Dialysis HCV Study Group. J Infect Dis 168:1343, 1993.
319. Bruchfeld A, Stahle L, Andersson J, Schvarcz R: Ribavirin treatment in dialysis patients with chronic hepatitis C virus infection—a pilot study. J Viral Hepat 8:287-292, 2001.
320. Therret E, Pol S, Legendre C, Gagnadoux MF, et al: Low-dose recombinant leukocyte interferon-alpha treatment of hepatitis C viral infection in renal transplant recipients. A pilot study. Transplantation 58:625, 1994.
321. Rostaing L, Izopet J, Baron E, et al: Treatment of chronic hepatitis C with recombinant interferon alpha in kidney transplant recipients. Transplantation 59:1426, 1995.

322. Ferri C, Marzo E, Longombardo G, et al: Interferon-alpha in mixed cryoglobulinemia patients: a randomized, crossover-controlled trial. Blood 81:1132, 1993.
323. Misiani R, Bellavita P, Fenili D, et al: Interferon alfa-2a therapy in cryoglobulinemia associated with hepatitis C virus. N Engl J Med 330:751, 1994.
324. Dammacco F, Sansonno D, Han JH, et al: Natural interferon-alpha versus its combination with 6-methyl-prednisolone in the therapy of type II mixed cryoglobulinemia: a long-term, randomized, controlled study. Blood 84:3336, 1994.
325. Zuckerman E, Keren D, Slobodin G, et al: Treatment of refractory, symptomatic, hepatitis C virus related mixed cryoglobulinemia with ribavirin and interferon-alpha. J Rheumatol 27:2172, 2000.
326. Calleja JL, Albillos A, Moreno-Otero R, et al: Sustained response to interferon-alpha or to interferon-alpha plus ribavirin in hepatitis C virus-associated symptomatic mixed cryoglobulinaemia. Aliment Pharmacol Ther 13:1179, 1999.
327. Lunel F, Cacoub P: Treatment of autoimmune and extrahepatic manifestations of hepatitis C virus infection. J Hepatol 31:210, 1999.
328. Durand JM, Cacoub P, Lunel-Fabiani F, et al: Ribavirin in hepatitis C related cryoglobulinemia. J Rheumatol 25:1115, 1998.
329. Edlin BR, Seal KH, Lorvick J, et al: Is it justifiable to withhold treatment for hepatitis C from illicit-drug users? N Engl J Med 345:211, 2001.
330. Backmund M, Meyer K, Von Zielonka M, Eichenlaub D: Treatment of hepatitis C infection in injection drug users. Hepatology 34:188-193, 2001.
331. Jowett SL, Agarwal K, Smith BC, et al: Managing chronic hepatitis C acquired through intravenous drug use. QJM 94:153, 2001.
332. Schafer M, Boetsch T, Laakmann G: Psychosis in a methadone-substituted patient during interferon-alpha treatment of hepatitis C. Addiction 95:1101, 2000.
333. Eyster ME, Diamondstone LS, Lien JM, et al: Natural history of hepatitis C virus infection in multitransfused hemophiliacs: effect of coinfection with human immunodeficiency virus. The Multicenter Hemophilia Cohort Study. J Acquir Immune Defic Syndr 6:602-610, 1993.
334. Rumi MG, Santagostino E, Morfini M, et al: A multicenter controlled, randomized, open trial of interferon alpha2b treatment of anti-human immunodeficiency virus-negative hemophilic patients with chronic hepatitis C. Hepatitis Study Group of the Association of Italian Hemophilia Centers. Blood 89:3529, 1997.
335. Makris M, Preston FE, Triger DR, et al: A randomized controlled trial of recombinant interferon-alpha in chronic hepatitis C in hemophiliacs. Blood 78:1672, 1991.
336. Hanley JP, Jarvis LM, Andrew J, et al: Interferon treatment for chronic hepatitis C infection in hemophiliacs—influence of virus load, genotype, and liver pathology on response. Blood 87:1704, 1996.
337. Beurton I, Bertrand MA, Bresson-Hadni S, et al: Interferon alpha therapy in haemophilic patients with chronic hepatitis C: a French multicentre pilot study of 58 patients. Eur J Gastroenterol Hepatol 13:859, 2001.
338. Di Martino V, Rufat P, Boyer N, et al: The influence of human immunodeficiency virus coinfection on chronic hepatitis C in injection drug users: a long-term retrospective cohort study. Hepatology 34:1193, 2001.
339. Yee TT, Griffioen A, Sabin CA, et al: The natural history of HCV in a cohort of haemophilic patients infected between 1961 and 1985. Gut 47:845-851, 2000.
340. Ragni MV, Belle SH: Impact of human immunodeficiency virus infection on progression to end-stage liver disease in individuals with hemophilia and hepatitis C virus infection. J Infect Dis 183:1112, 2001.
341. Monga HK, Rodriguez-Barradas MC, Breaux K, et al: Hepatitis C virus infection-related morbidity and mortality among patients with human immunodeficiency virus infection. Clin Infect Dis 33:240, 2001.
342. Bica I, McGovern B, Dhar R, et al: Increasing mortality due to end-stage liver disease in patients with human immunodeficiency virus infection. Clin Infect Dis 32:492, 2001.
343. Prachalias AA, Pozniak A, Taylor C, et al: Liver transplantation in adults coinfected with HIV. Transplantation 72:1684, 2001.
344. Boyer N, Marcellin P, Degott C, et al: Recombinant interferon-alpha for chronic hepatitis C in patients positive for antibody to human immunodeficiency virus. Comite des Anti-Viraux. J Infect Dis 165:723, 1992.
345. Marriott E, Navas S, del Romero J, et al: Treatment with recombinant alpha-interferon of chronic hepatitis C in anti-HIV-positive patients. J Med Virol 40:107, 1993.
346. Soriano V, Garcia-Samaniego J, Bravo R, et al: Efficacy and safety of alpha-interferon treatment for chronic hepatitis C in HIV-infected patients. HIV-Hepatitis Spanish Study Group. J Infect 31:9-13, 1995.
347. Mauss S, Klinker H, Ulmer A, et al: Response to treatment of chronic hepatitis C with interferon alpha in patients infected with HIV-1 is associated with higher CD4+ cell count. Infection 26:16-19, 1998.
348. Landau A, Batisse D, Piketty C, et al: Long-term efficacy of combination therapy with interferon-alpha 2b and ribavirin for severe chronic hepatitis C in HIV-infected patients. AIDS 15:2149, 2001.
349. Sauleda S, Juarez A, Esteban JI, et al: Interferon and ribavirin combination therapy for chronic hepatitis C in human immunodeficiency virus-infected patients with congenital coagulation disorders. Hepatology 34:1035, 2001.
350. Lafeuillade A, Hittinger G, Chadapaud S: Increased mitochondrial toxicity with ribavirin in HIV/HCV coinfection. Lancet 357:280, 2001.
351. Kleinman S: Hepatitis G virus biology, epidemiology, and clinical manifestations: implications for blood safety. Transfus Med Rev 15:201-212, 2001.
352. Tillmann HL, Heiken H, Knapik-Botor A, et al: Infection with GB virus C and reduced mortality among HIV-infected patients. N Engl J Med 345:715-724, 2001.
353. Xiang J, Wunschmann S, Diekema DJ, et al: Effect of coinfection with GB virus C on survival among patients with HIV infection. N Engl J Med 345:707-714, 2001.
354. Lau DT, Miller KD, Detmer J, et al: Hepatitis G virus and human immunodeficiency virus coinfection: response to interferon-alpha therapy. J Infect Dis 180:1334, 1999.
355. Rosenberg SD, Goodman LA, Osher FC, et al: Prevalence of HIV, hepatitis B, and hepatitis C in people with severe mental illness. Am J Public Health 91:31-37, 2001.
356. Renault PF, Hoofnagle JH, Park Y, et al: Psychiatric complications of long-term interferon alfa therapy. Arch Intern Med 147:1577, 1987.
357. Musselman DL, Lawson DH, Gumnick JF, et al: Paroxetine for the prevention of depression induced by high-dose interferon alfa. N Engl J Med 344:961, 2001.
358. Dusheiko G: Side effects of alpha interferon in chronic hepatitis C. Hepatology 26:112S-121S, 1997.
359. Jaeckel E, Cornberg M, Wedemeyer H, et al: Treatment of acute hepatitis C with interferon alfa-2b. N Engl J Med 345:1452, 2001.
360. Gerlach JT, Zachoval R, Gruener NH, et al: Acute hepatitis C: natural course and response to antiviral treatment. Hepatology 34:341A, 2001.
361. Davis GL, Esteban-Mur R, Rustgi V, et al: Interferon alfa-2b alone or in combination with ribavirin for the treatment of relapse of chronic hepatitis C. International Hepatitis Interventional Therapy Group. N Engl J Med 339:1493, 1998.
362. Chapman BA, Stace NH, Edgar CL, et al: Interferon-alpha2a/ribaviran versus interferon-alpha2a alone for the retreatment of hepatitis C patients who relapse after a standard course of interferon. N Z Med J 114:103, 2001.
363. Cheng SJ, Bonis PA, Lau J, et al: Interferon and ribavirin for patients with chronic hepatitis C who did not respond to previous interferon therapy: a meta-analysis of controlled and uncontrolled trials. Hepatology 33:231-240, 2001.
364. Enriquez J, Gallego A, Torras X, et al: Retreatment for 24 vs 48 weeks with interferon-alpha2b plus ribavirin of chronic hepatitis C patients who relapsed or did not respond to interferon alone. J Viral Hepat 7:403, 2000.
365. Marco VD, Almasio P, Vaccaro A, et al: Combined treatment of relapse of chronic hepatitis C with high-dose alpha2b interferon plus ribavirin for 6 or 12 months. J Hepatol 33:456-462, 2000.
366. Teuber G, Berg T, Hoffmann RM, et al: Retreatment with interferon-alpha and ribavirin in primary interferon-alpha non-responders with chronic hepatitis C. Digestion 61:90, 2000.
367. Enomoto N, Sakuma I, Asahina Y, et al: Comparison of full-length sequences of interferon-sensitive and resistant hepatitis C virus

1b. Sensitivity to interferon is conferred by amino acid substitutions in the NS5A region. J Clin Invest 96:224-230, 1995.
368. Chayama K, Tsubota A, Kobayashi M, et al: Pretreatment virus load and multiple amino acid substitutions in the interferon sensitivity-determining region predict the outcome of interferon treatment in patients with chronic genotype 1b hepatitis C virus infection. Hepatology 25:745, 1997.
369. Zeuzem S, Lee JH, Roth WK: Mutations in the nonstructural 5A gene of European hepatitis C virus isolates and response to interferon alfa. Hepatology 25:740, 1997.
370. Gale MJ Jr, Korth MJ, Tang NM, et al: Evidence that hepatitis C virus resistance to interferon is mediated through repression of the PKR protein kinase by the nonstructural 5A protein. Virology 230:217, 1997.
371. Gale M Jr, Blakely CM, Kwieciszewski B, et al: Control of PKR protein kinase by hepatitis C virus nonstructural 5A protein: molecular mechanisms of kinase regulation. Mol Cell Biol 18:5208, 1998.
372. Mihm S, Monazahian M, Grethe S, et al: Lack of clinical evidence for involvement of hepatitis C virus interferon-alpha sensitivity-determining region variability in RNA-dependent protein kinase-mediated cellular antiviral responses. J Med Virol 61:29-36, 2000.
373. Taylor DR, Shi ST, Lai MM: Hepatitis C virus and interferon resistance. Microbes Infect 2:1743, 2000.
374. Chayama K, Suzuki F, Tsubota A, et al: Association of amino acid sequence in the PKR-eIF2 phosphorylation homology domain and response to interferon therapy. Hepatology 32:1138, 2000.
375. Di Bisceglie AM, Conjeevaram HS, Fried MW, et al: Ribavirin as therapy for chronic hepatitis C. A randomized, double- blind, placebo-controlled trial. Ann Intern Med 123:897-903, 1995.
376. Mayet WJ, Hess G, Gerken G, et al: Treatment of chronic type B hepatitis with recombinant alpha-interferon induces autoantibodies not specific for autoimmune chronic hepatitis. Hepatology 10:24, 1989.
377. Lisker-Melman M, Di Bisceglie AM, Usala SJ, et al: Development of thyroid disease during therapy of chronic viral hepatitis with interferon alfa. Gastroenterology 102:2155-2160, 1992.
378. Guyer DR, Tiedeman J, Yannuzzi LA, et al: Interferon-associated retinopathy. Arch Ophthalmol 111:350, 1993.
379. Kanda Y, Shigeno K, Kinoshita N, et al: Sudden hearing loss associated with interferon. Lancet 343:1134, 1994.
380. Shakil AO, Di Bisceglie AM, Hoofnagle JH: Seizures during alpha interferon therapy. J Hepatol 24:48-51.1996.
381. Garcia-Buey L, Garcia-Monzon C, Rodriguez S, et al: Latent autoimmune hepatitis triggered during interferon therapy in patients with chronic hepatitis C. Gastroenterology 108:1770, 1995.
382. Shindo M, Di Bisceglie AM, Hoofnagle JH: Acute exacerbation of liver disease during interferon alfa therapy for chronic hepatitis C. Gastroenterology 102:140, 1992.
383. Lanphear BP, Linnemann CC Jr, Cannon CG, et al: Hepatitis C virus infection in healthcare workers: risk of exposure and infection. Infect Control Hosp Epidemiol 15:745-750, 1994.
384. Puro V, Petrosillo N, Ippolito G: Risk of hepatitis C seroconversion after occupational exposures in health care workers. Italian Study Group on Occupational Risk of HIV and Other Bloodborne Infections. Am J Infect Control 23:273, 1995.
385. Mitsui T, Iwano K, Masuko K, et al: Hepatitis C virus infection in medical personnel after needlestick accident. Hepatology 16:1109, 1992.
386. Colombo M: Screening for cancer in viral hepatitis. Clin Liver Dis 5:109-122, 2001.
387. Sherman M: Surveillance for hepatocellular carcinoma. Semin Oncol 28:450, 2001.
388. Seeff LB, Lindsay KL, Bacon BR, et al: Complementary and alternative medicine in chronic liver disease. Hepatology 34:595-603, 2001.
389. Liu JP, Manheimer E, Tsutani K, Gluud C: Medicinal herbs for hepatitis C virus infection (Cochrane Review). Cochrane Database Syst Rev 4, 2001.
390. Di Bisceglie AM, Bonkovsky HL, Chopra S, et al: Iron reduction as an adjuvant to interferon therapy in patients with chronic hepatitis C who have previously not responded to interferon: a multicenter, prospective, randomized, controlled trial. Hepatology 32:135, 2000.
391. Fong TL, Han SH, Tsai NC, et al: A pilot randomized, controlled trial of the effect of iron depletion on long-term response to alpha-interferon in patients with chronic hepatitis C. J Hepatol 28:369, 1998.
392. Smith JP: Treatment of chronic hepatitis C with amantadine. Dig Dis Sci 42:1681, 1997.
393. Andant C, Lamoril J, Deybach JC, et al: Amantadine for chronic hepatitis C: pilot study in 14 patients. Eur J Gastroenterol Hepatol 12:1319, 2000.
394. Tabon M, Laudi C, Delmastro B, et al: Interferon and amantadine in combination as initial treatment for chronic hepatitis C patients. J Hepatol 35:517-521, 2001.
395. Caronia S, Bassendine MF, Barry R, et al: Interferon plus amantadine versus interferon alone in the treatment of naive patients with chronic hepatitis C: a UK multicentre study. J Hepatol 35:512, 2001.
396. Teuber G, Berg T, Naumann U, et al: Randomized, placebo-controlled, double-blind trial with interferon-alpha with and without amantadine sulphate in primary interferon-alpha nonresponders with chronic hepatitis C. J Viral Hepat 8:276-283, 2001.
397. Dusheiko G, Main J, Thomas H, et al: Ribavirin treatment for patients with chronic hepatitis C: results of a placebo-controlled study. J Hepatol 25:591, 1996.
398. Zeuzem S, Schmidt JM, Lee JH, et al: Hepatitis C virus dynamics in vivo: effect of ribavirin and interferon alfa on viral turnover. Hepatology 28:245-252, 1998.
399. Maag D, Castro C, Hong Z, Cameron CE: Hepatitis C virus RNA-dependent RNA polymerase (NS5B) as a mediator of the antiviral activity of ribavirin. J Biol Chem 276:46094, 2001.
400. Saez-Royuela F, Porres JC, Moreno A, et al: High doses of recombinant alpha-interferon or gamma-interferon for chronic hepatitis C: a randomized, controlled trial. Hepatology 13:327-331, 1991.
401. Andreone P, Cursaro C, Gramenzi A, et al: A double-blind, placebo-controlled, pilot trial of thymosin alpha 1 for the treatment of chronic hepatitis C. Liver 16:207-210, 1996.
402. Zeuzem S, Hopf U, Carreno V, et al: A phase I/II study of recombinant human interleukin-12 in patients with chronic hepatitis C. Hepatology 29:1280, 1999.
403. Nelson DR, Lauwers GY, Lau JY, Davis GL: Interleukin 10 treatment reduces fibrosis in patients with chronic hepatitis C: a pilot trial of interferon nonresponders. Gastroenterology 118:655-660, 2000.
404. Yao N, Hesson T, Cable M, et al: Structure of the hepatitis C virus RNA helicase domain. Nat Struct Biol 4:463, 1997.
405. Alt M, Eisenhardt S, Serwe M, et al: Comparative inhibitory potential of differently modified antisense oligodeoxynucleotides on hepatitis C virus translation. Eur J Clin Invest 29:868, 1999.
406. Macejak DG, Jensen KL, Jamison SF, et al: Inhibition of hepatitis C virus (HCV)-RNA-dependent translation and replication of a chimeric HCV poliovirus using synthetic stabilized ribozymes. Hepatology 31:769-776, 2000.

CHAPTER

34

Other Hepatitis Viruses

Mahmoud M. Yousfi, MD, David D. Douglas, MD, and Jorge Rakela, MD

Apart from hepatotrophic viruses, there are viral agents that may involve the liver as part of systemic involvement. This hepatic involvement may be indistinguishable from that caused by hepatitis viruses, although the systemic involvement and other organ involvement could be better defined. These agents usually cause only transient, mild hepatitis but may lead to fulminant hepatic failure and usually do not cause chronic hepatitis or liver disease.

These agents that may cause a hepatitis-like picture include herpes simplex virus (HSV); varicella-zoster virus (VZV); Epstein-Barr virus (EBV); cytomegalovirus (CMV); human herpesvirus (HHV)6, 7, and 8; human parvovirus (HPV)B19; and adenoviruses.

HERPES SIMPLEX VIRUS

Herpes simplex virus (HSV-1 and HSV-2) is a common infection in humans and produces a variety of illnesses, including mucocutaneous infection, infections of the central nervous system, and an occasional infection of the visceral organs; many of these may be life-threatening. The clinical manifestations and course of HSV infections depend mainly on the site involved and the host's age and immune status. Primary herpes infections, in which the host lacks HSV antibodies, occur in children and young adults and manifest as mucocutaneous vesicular and ulcerated lesions. These are usually accompanied by regional lymphadenopathy and systemic signs and symptoms, such as fever and malaise. HSV-1 is frequently associated with oral-labial infections (mainly pharyngitis and gingivostomatitis), whereas HSV-2 is associated with genital infections. Reactivation of infection occurs periodically, especially genital herpes, and causes mucocutaneous vesicular lesions without systemic features.[1,2]

Occasionally, HSV viremia results in visceral involvement, affecting mainly three organs: the esophagus, lungs, and liver. Liver involvement occurs in the following settings: neonatal infections, pregnancy, immunocompromised hosts, and, rarely, immunocompetent adults.

In neonates, hepatitis occurs with multi-organ involvement and usually carries a high mortality rate. Fulminant hepatitis caused by HSV was first described by Hass in 1935 in a neonate with liver and adrenal necrosis associated with distinctive intranuclear inclusions.[3] Several subsequent reports have shown that acute fulminant hepatitis and adrenal insufficiency remain the most common causes of death in neonates with disseminated HSV infection.[4] In most reports infection results from contact with infected genital secretions at the time of delivery but sometimes no pre-existing risk factors were established. The delay in instituting anti-viral therapy against HSV, while awaiting confirmation of diagnosis, results in a catastrophic outcome.[5] In children beyond the neonatal period, HSV hepatitis has been reported with underlying kwashiorkor or severe malnutrition, Wiskott-Aldrich syndrome, acquired immunodeficiency syndrome (AIDS), and inflammatory bowel disease (treated with corticosteroids).[6]

HSV hepatitis in pregnant females was first reported in 1969 and was seen in the context of disseminated primary infection, usually late in gestation, 65 percent of cases in one study occurred in third trimester and usually manifests as acute fulminant hepatitis.[7-9] Differential diagnosis includes conditions associated with hepatic dysfunction in the third trimester of pregnancy, such as severe preeclampsia, acute fatty liver of pregnancy, HELLP (hemolysis, elevated liver enzymes, and low platelets) syndrome, and cholestasis of pregnancy. Mucocutaneous lesions are present in only half of cases; therefore, the clinical suspicion for diagnosis of this condition must be high. Twenty-five percent of cases were not diagnosed until autopsy. Maternal and perinatal mortality approaching 39 percent for both mother and fetus was reported in some studies. Early recognition with initiation of anti-viral therapy may reverse an otherwise fatal process.[10-14]

HSV is an uncommon cause of hepatitis in immunocompetent patients. A mild asymptomatic elevation of transaminase levels can be detected in 14 percent of healthy adults with acute genital herpes infection.[15] Fulminant hepatitis with more than 100-fold rise in transaminases was reported and associated with a favorable outcome after anti-viral therapy.[16-18] In immunocompromised hosts, HSV hepatitis has occurred during primary and rarely during recurrent infection, with a triad of fever, leukopenia, and markedly elevated aminotransferases suggestive of the diagnosis. An abrupt rise in bilirubin and disseminated intravascular coagulation may develop without concurrent mucocutaneous lesions.[2,16,19-33]

Computed tomography scan abnormalities are nonspecific and may reveal multiple low-density areas that do not enhance, implying non-perfused liver parenchyma resulting from hemorrhagic hepatic necrosis. HSV serologic studies are not helpful in establishing the diagnosis.

Liver biopsy is essential to establish the diagnosis of HSV hepatitis, especially in pregnancy. It usually shows focal, sometimes extensive, hemorrhagic or coagulative necrosis of the hepatocytes with limited inflammatory response (usually mononuclear and scattered lymphocytes) (Figure 34-1). Typical intranuclear inclusions (Cowdry A type) are often identified at the margins of the foci of necrosis (Figure 34-2). Some periportal hepatocytes with multi-nucleated forms may show a "ground-glass" appearance of the nuclei, suggesting the presence of viral inclusions. Electron microscopy and immunohistochemical studies in the liver with specific HSV antibodies may also identify typical HSV viral particles. The diagnosis is confirmed by the detection of HSV deoxyribonucleic acid (DNA) sequences by polymerase chain reaction (PCR) techniques, which are more sensitive than tissue culture methods.[1,10,16,34]

HSV hepatitis is one of the infectious disease emergencies associated with a rapid and lethal course and requires early recognition and institution of anti-viral therapy to improve outcome while awaiting confirmation of diagnosis. At the Mayo Clinic the incidence of HSV hepatitis was reported to be 6 percent among all fulminant hepatitis patients reviewed from 1974 to 1982.[35] High-dose acyclovir is the anti-viral drug of choice (at least 10 mg/kg/day every 8 hours) and has been successfully used in pregnancy.[10,23,36,37] Shanley reported a case of a healthy female who developed disseminated HSV-2 infection and fulminant hepatitis during the third trimester of pregnancy requiring high-dose anti-viral therapy, which resulted in eradication of HSV mucocutaneous lesions. However, the patient's condition continued to deteriorate, and she survived only after orthotopic liver transplantation without evidence of recurrence, suggesting that disseminated HSV infection should not be an absolute contraindication to transplantation in certain clinical settings.[38]

VARICELLA-ZOSTER VIRUS

VZV causes two distinct clinical diseases. Varicella (commonly called chickenpox) is the primary infection and is characterized as a benign generalized exanthematous rash. Recurrence of infection results in a more localized phenomenon known as herpes zoster (often called shingles).[39] Rare non-cutaneous manifestation, such as encephalitis, pneumonitis, myocarditis, and hepatitis, may accompany the skin rash, especially in immunocompromised patients, and may be life-threatening.[40]

Mild and transient liver enzyme abnormalities are not uncommon in varicella infection in children and can occur in up to 25 percent of cases.[41,43] During the convalescent phase of infection and especially with the administration of aspirin, microvesicular fatty infiltration of the liver may occur, associated with hyperammonemia, coagulopathy, and cerebral edema. This uncommon phenomenon, known as Reye's syndrome, is fatal about 30 percent of the time.[44,45]

Primary infection in immunocompetent adults may cause severe acute hepatitis with a more than tenfold increase in transaminases[8] and, sometimes, fulminant hepatic failure with evidence of varicella in the liver and other organs only revealed on autopsy.[46]

In contrast to the rather benign course of zoster (reactivation of infection) in the setting of organ transplantation, primary varicella infection can be quite virulent.[47] Visceral involvement, including the liver, may occur in the immediate postoperative period or may be delayed several months after transplantation. Usually it is associated with rapid onset and fatal fulminant hepatitis.[48,52] Other immunocompromised patients tend to have a similar life-threatening course.[53,54] Therefore any exposure to VZV in these patients or development of vesicular skin rash should prompt early diagnostic testing and institu-

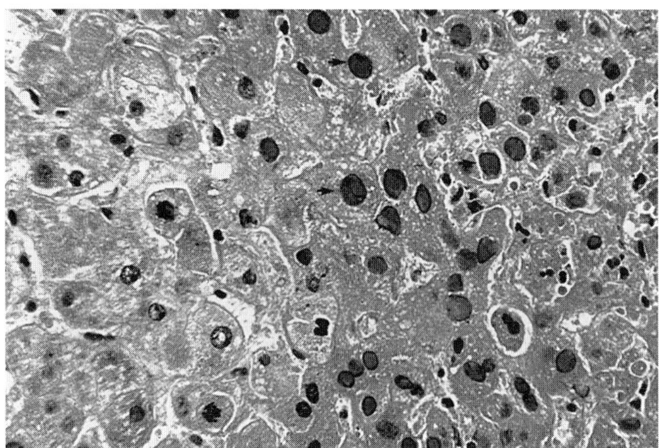

Figure 34-1 HSV hepatitis liver biopsy. HSV hepatitis with focal neurosis and coagulative neurosis with limited inflammatory response.

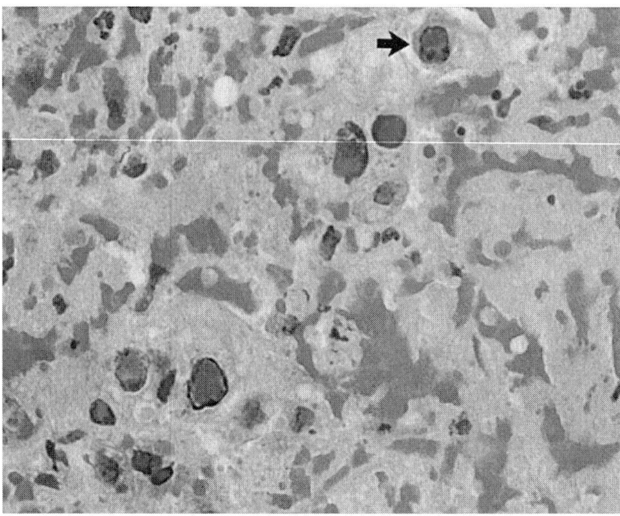

Figure 34-2 HSV hepatitis. Typical intranuclear inclusions (Cowdry A type).

tion of anti-viral therapy while awaiting confirmation of diagnosis.[55,56]

Serologic testing is of little use, especially in immunocompromised patients. Confirmation of diagnosis is possible through the isolation of VZV from the skin lesions or other affected organ. Liver biopsy often shows foci of coagulative necrosis and intranuclear inclusions with an inflammatory response. PCR and immunoperoxidase techniques may be needed to distinguish VZV from HSV hepatitis.

Centers for Disease Control and Prevention (CDC) guidelines for the prevention and control of nosocomial infections must be instituted for infection control in hospital personnel.[57] Early administration of anti-viral therapy is critical in the setting of VZV hepatitis, especially in immunocompromised patients. The drug of choice is intravenous acyclovir 30 mg/kg/day in three divided doses for 7 to 10 days.[58,59] Other agents such as vidarabine or interferon have been used but acyclovir was more effective with fewer side effects.[60,61]

EPSTEIN-BARR VIRUS

EBV shares the characteristic morphologic features of the *Herpesviridae* family of viruses. It was first identified by an electron microscopy of cells cultured from Burkitt's lymphoma tissue by Epstein, Achong, and Barr in 1964.[62] A few years later EBV was established as the causative agent of heterophile-positive infectious mononucleosis.[63] The EBV genome consists of a linear DNA molecule that encodes nearly 100 viral proteins, which are important for regulating the expression of viral genes. During viral DNA replication, these proteins form structural components of the virion and modulate the host immune response. In vitro cultivation of the virus has been primarily described in nasopharyngeal epithelial cells and B lymphocytes. Infection of epithelial cells by EBV in vitro results in active replication, with production of virus and lysis of the cell. In contrast, infection of B cells by EBV in vitro results in a latent infection, with immortalization of the cells. After infecting B-lymphocytes the linear EBV genome becomes circular and forms an episome, which usually remains latent in these B cells. Viral replication is spontaneously activated in only a small percentage of latently infected B cells.[64]

Transmission of EBV infection usually occurs by contact with oral secretions (saliva droplets or possibly cells in saliva). The postulated association with kissing is well known. Transmission by blood transfusion has been reported but is very unusual.[65] The virus replicates in the nasopharyngeal epithelial cells, and nearly all seropositive people actively shed virus in the saliva. B cells in the oropharynx may be the primary site of infection.[66] Shedding of EBV from the oropharynx is abolished in patients treated with acyclovir, whereas the number of EBV-infected B cells in the circulation remains the same as before treatment. Resting memory B cells are thought to be the site of persistence of EBV within the body. The diseases associated with latent EBV infection depend on the type of gene expression of EBV-encoded proteins. Researchers were able to identify three general patterns of expression resulting in various clinical conditions associated with EBV, such as infectious mononucleosis, Burkitt's lymphoma, nasopharyngeal carcinoma, Hodgkin's disease, peripheral T-cell lymphoma, and lymphoproliferative disease.[67]

EBV infection is very common, infecting more than 90 percent of humans worldwide and persisting for the lifetime of the person. Whereas most EBV infections of infants and children are asymptomatic or have non-specific symptoms, infections of adolescents and adults frequently result in infectious mononucleosis. More than 50 percent of patients with infectious mononucleosis manifest the triad of fever, lymphadenopathy, and pharyngitis. Prodromal non-specific symptoms may occur 2 to 5 days before specific symptoms. Hepatosplenomegaly and palatal petechiae may be present in more than 10 percent of patients. Most patients with infectious mononucleosis recover uneventfully. Less common complications may occur, including autoimmune hemolytic anemia, thrombocytopenia, aplastic anemia, myocarditis, hepatitis, genital ulcers, splenic rupture, rash, and neurologic complications such as Guillain-Barré syndrome, encephalitis, and meningitis.[67-69]

Liver involvement is well recognized in EBV infections. Manifestations of liver involvement range from the most commonly encountered mild, self-limiting acute hepatitis to occasional reports of fatal, acute, fulminant hepatitis.

Long before the discovery of EBV as the causative agent in heterophile antibody-positive infectious mononucleosis, liver tests and liver histology were observed to be abnormal in nearly all cases of infectious mononucleosis. Mild elevation of transaminases 2 to 3 times the upper limit of normal and elevated lactate dehydrogenase levels are seen in up to 90 percent of the cases of infectious mononucleosis. Typically, transaminases rise gradually to a peak, lower than commonly encountered in active viral hepatitis, over a 1- to 2-week period and decline gradually over a 3- to 4-week period.[70-75] Patients older than 30 years generally have more severe disease than children. Mild elevation of alkaline phosphatase levels is also seen in 60 percent and mild hyperbilirubinemia in about 45 percent of cases.[70]

Severe cholestatic jaundice and right upper quadrant abdominal pain may occur in elderly patients. Jaundice may occasionally be the initial clinical presentation, in combination with fever and abdominal pain, and can be mistaken for extrahepatic biliary obstruction. Jaundice predominantly occurs when EBV infection is complicated with autoimmune hemolytic anemia, and occasionally as a direct result of virus-induced cholestasis.[76-80]

Other occasional clinical settings for EBV liver involvement include post-transfusion hepatitis, granulomatous hepatitis, chronic hepatitis, and fatal fulminant hepatitis. An outbreak of post-transfusion hepatitis secondary to EBV infection was reported in a hemodialysis unit in 1973 after exposure to a single venous-pressure monitor; 11 of 40 patients in that hemodialysis unit had clinical or biochemical evidence of hepatitis during a 5-week period. The clinical disease was mild and was limited solely to dialysis patients.[81] Chronic active EBV infection is a very rare disorder in which illness of more than 6 months' duration that begins as a primary EBV infection is associated with histologic evidence of organ disease (e.g., pneumonitis, hepatitis) and demonstration of EBV antigens or EBV DNA in tissue.[82] In some cases of granulomatous hepatitis, serologic evidence of chronic EBV infection was found.[83,84] A detailed clinicopathologic analysis of 30 patients with sporadic fatal infectious mononucleosis was described by Markin and colleagues. Hepatic dysfunction was uniformly present and caused death in 13 of these patients, with a median survival of 8 weeks.[84] Cases of fatal fulminant hepatitis with massive hepatic necrosis and disseminated intravascular coagulation were reported in both immunocompromised and immunocompetent hosts.[85-88] Gallbladder wall thickening on ultrasound maybe an early indicator of the severity of hepatitis.[89]

The diagnosis of infectious mononucleosis is established on the basis of the clinical features and laboratory and serologic findings indicative of a recent EBV infection. The most common hematologic findings include leukocytosis in 70 percent of cases, with predominantly lymphocytosis and monocytosis, and mild thrombocytopenia in up to 50 percent of cases. The "monospot" test detects heterophile antibodies, although it is sensitive but not very specific. EBV-specific immunoglobulin (Ig)G and IgM antibodies, directed against the viral capsid antigens, early antigens (EBV anti-D and anti-R), nuclear antigen, and soluble complement-fixing antigens (anti-S), improve sensitivity and specificity in detecting the infection.[68,90,91] With liver involvement, abdominal ultrasound may show a fatty liver appearance or gallbladder wall thickening.[89-92] In the vast majority of cases there is no indication for liver biopsy. The presence of a pleomorphic inflammatory infiltrate without disruption of the liver architecture is the main feature. There may be portal and sinusoidal mononuclear cell infiltration with focal hepatic necrosis or fatty infiltration. Multi-nucleated giant cells are not seen.[65] Of particular utility is in situ hybridization, Southern blot analysis, and PCR as diagnostic methods to identify specific ribonucleic acid (RNA) or DNA sequences in organs involved.[93-94] However, cultivation of EBV is not routinely available in most diagnostic virology laboratories.

The differential diagnosis of EBV hepatitis includes viral hepatitis forms A through E, CMV hepatitis, and drug-induced hepatitis. Cervical lymphadenopathy is less common, and peripheral monocytosis is encountered with CMV hepatitis.[95]

There is no specific drug or treatment of EBV infection. Acyclovir inhibits EBV in vitro replication and reduces viral shedding in the oropharynx but has no effect on the symptoms of infectious mononucleosis (which are primarily the result of immune response to the virus) and therefore is not recommended.[96] In EBV hepatitis no anti-viral agent has proven to be effective. Corticosteroids are indicated for patients with upper airway obstruction; they may be helpful in patients with neurologic, hematologic, or cardiac complications.[69] Corticosteroid role in hepatitis has not been studied. A single report of fulminant hepatic failure in an immunocompetent young girl caused by primary EBV infection was treated by orthotopic liver transplantation.[97] Concerns are rising about increased EBV replication after transplantation and the development of post-transplant lymphoproliferative disorders, especially in pediatric patients.[98] A vaccine against EBV is being developed, but the clinical utility of vaccination for immunocompromised hosts is still under investigation.

CYTOMEGALOVIRUS

Human CMV is the largest member of the β Herpesviridae family of viruses and is in fact the largest virus to infect human beings. Cytomegaly (giant cell) and prominent intranuclear inclusion bodies characterize the cellular response to CMV infection. It was first isolated in 1954 from a human salivary gland and was first called salivary gland virus or cytomegalic inclusion disease virus. A syndrome of CMV mononucleosis was later reported after transfusion with blood products.[99,100] CMV infections are common in all human populations, reaching 60 percent to 70 percent in urban US cities. CMV infection plays a significant role as a common opportunistic pathogen in immunocompromised hosts. Early recognition of infection, institution of therapy, and prevention of infection are critical in altering the outcome in these patients.[101,102]

Several factors determine the manifestations and severity of CMV infection, including the route of transmission, age, and immune status of the host. Infection is acquired either in the perinatal period and infancy or in adulthood through sexual contact, blood transfusions, or organ transplantation. Most primary CMV infections in immunocompetent adults are either asymptomatic or associated with a mild mononucleosis-like syndrome. As with other herpesviruses, all primary infections resolve and enter a state of lifelong latency in which live virus is sequestered in a non-replicative state. People with latent infection and an intact immune system have no symptoms but exhibit antibodies to CMV. Circulating lymphocytes, monocytes, and polymorphonuclear leukocytes may serve as the predominant sites of viral latency. The risk for intermittent reactivation is increased with diminished host immune status. CMV disease in immunocompromised patients can be the result of either a primary infection in a previously uninfected (seronegative) host, reinfection with a new virus, or more commonly reactivation of latent infection. Although adequate anti-CMV antibodies are detected during episodes of reactivation of infection, cell-mediated immunity (characterized by decreased numbers of cytotoxic T lymphocytes and natural killer cells) is defective. The incidence and severity of CMV disease closely parallel the degree of cellular immune dysfunction.[103,104]

CMV disease syndromes range from asymptomatic infection, life-threatening congenital CMV syndrome in neonates, infectious mononucleosis syndrome in young adults, to severe pulmonary, retinal, neurologic, gastrointestinal, and hepatic diseases in immunocompromised hosts, in whom CMV is a very common opportunistic pathogen.[105]

Congenital CMV infection occurs as a result of intrauterine transmission in the pregnant non-immune mother, with primary CMV infection causing a fulminant cytomegalic inclusion disease with multi-organ involvement. This form of congenital infection is associated with substantial morbidity and mortality and manifested, shortly after birth, by jaundice, hepatosplenomegaly, thrombocytopenic purpura, and severe neurologic symptoms. Multi-focal hepatic necrosis with cytomegalic cells, intranuclear inclusion, inflammatory response, and marked bile stasis may be detected on liver biopsy. If the child survives, the jaundice and hepatosplenomegaly may subside but the neurologic sequelae and mental retardation persist.[106-108]

A different form of neonatal CMV infection occurs as a result of perinatal (from the mother's cervix during delivery) or postnatal (from breast-feeding) transmission of the virus, resulting in a clinical picture resembling mild infectious mononucleosis syndrome without neurologic involvement. Mild, self-limiting hepatitis or ascites may occur but usually resolves during the first year of life.[109,110] Chang and colleagues studied 50 infants with neonatal hepatitis and detected the CMV genome by PCR in 46 percent of the liver tissues of these patients, whereas none of 30 infants without neonatal hepatitis had a positive PCR, suggesting that CMV may play a major role in the pathogenesis of neonatal hepatitis.[111]

In immunocompetent children and adults, CMV infection is usually subclinical but sometimes can cause a disease that resembles EBV infectious mononucleosis syndrome. Constitutional symptoms (fever, malaise, and nausea), lymphadenopathy, and relative lymphocytosis constitute the predominant clinical presentation. Unlike EBV mononucleosis, pharyngitis and cervical lymphadenopathy are absent and the heterophile response is negative (negative monospot).[95] It is estimated that EBV is responsible for about 80 percent of infectious mononucleosis cases and the remaining 20 percent are caused by acute CMV infection.[112] The mode of transmission for these patients is through intimate sexual contact, kissing, intrafamilial transmission (sharing objects with contaminated saliva among family members), and blood transfusion. However, sometimes no clear source can be identified.[104-113] In surgical patients requiring massive blood transfusions CMV infection should be considered as a source of postoperative fever (sometimes called postperfusion syndrome).[114]

Liver dysfunction is commonly associated with CMV mononucleosis. It is usually mild and rarely symptomatic in the immunocompetent patient. Hepatosplenomegaly and laboratory evidence of mild to moderate hepatic dysfunction are the predominant features, with increased transaminases and alkaline phosphatase values in 88 percent and 64 percent of cases, respectively, but still lower than commonly encountered in active viral hepatitis.[75,115] Rare manifestations of CMV hepatitis include tender hepatomegaly, granulomatous hepatitis (with scattered microscopic granulomas found on liver biopsy), anicteric or icteric cholestatic form of hepatitis, and acute hepatitis with massive hepatic necrosis.[116,118,119,123]

In patients with impaired cell-mediated immunity, disseminated CMV infection results in life-threatening diseases. CMV is the most common opportunistic viral infection in AIDS patients, causing retinitis, central nervous system infections, esophagitis, and colitis. CMV may also invade the hepatobiliary tract in AIDS patients, causing hepatitis, pancreatitis, and acute acalculous gangrenous cholecystitis.[124-126] The presence of CMV retinitis, gastrointestinal disease, or viremia in AIDS patients increases the risk for the development of a cholestatic syndrome caused by papillary stenosis and sclerosing cholangitis, which does not usually respond to anti-viral therapy.[127] Other immunocompromised patients at risk are organ transplant recipients. This topic is discussed in detail in Chapter 55.

The diagnosis of CMV hepatitis always requires confirmatory laboratory tests because clinical presentation alone is not sufficient. Serologic studies of CMV-IgM antibodies may be helpful in primary infections.[128] Viral culture technique could be greatly speeded up with the use of "shell vial" assays, in which monoclonal antibodies are used to detect CMV early antigens.[129-130] Shell vial assay is the most rapid and sensitive method of determining CMV infection, especially in immunocompromised patients in whom viremia preceeds organ involvement.[131] Using PCR techniques to detect CMV early antigen or the CMV DNA polymerase increases the sensitivity of detecting CMV infection in the blood or tissue.[132,133]

Liver biopsy with characteristic histopathologic findings is important in establishing the diagnosis in CMV hepatitis, especially in the immunocompromised host. Giant multi-nucleated cell reaction with an inflammatory response, multi-focal necrosis, and biliary stasis can be seen in liver biopsy. Giant cells can be seen in the parenchyma and bile duct epithelium. Large nuclear inclusion-bearing cells, which are called sometimes owl's eye inclusions, can be found in some hepatocytes or bile duct epithelium.[134,135]

Treatment of CMV with anti-viral agents is not always indicated, especially in self-limited disease in immunocompetent adults. For severe and worrisome cases, particularly in those patients with impaired cell-mediated immunity, therapy can be life-saving. Acyclovir is ineffective.[136] Ganciclovir is a nucleoside analogue of guanosine and a homolog of acyclovir that has a long intracellular half-life. It is considered the anti-viral agent of choice against CMV; however, significant bone marrow toxicity may occur, especially granulocytopenia, which requires dose reduction, discontinuation of other marrow-suppressing drugs, or even concomitant administration of granulocyte growth factors. The severity of CMV viremia determines the extent of tissue damage; therefore, the duration of therapy should be guided by repeated measurement of CMV in blood samples. Emerging strains resistant to ganciclovir are cumbersome; foscarnet or cidofovir may become alternative anti-viral agents but significant nephrotoxicity is a major problem with these drugs.[137]

There should be a high index of clinical suspicion of CMV, particularly in solid-organ transplant recipients who have risk factors for the development of CMV disease, including donor CMV seropositivity, the use of anti-lymphocyte preparations, and retransplantation. The availability of effective anti-viral therapy to treat CMV disease has emphasized the importance of an aggressive approach to the prophylactic protocols, early diagnosis, and treatment of this viral infection.[138]

HUMAN HERPESVIRUS 6, 7, AND 8

HHV-6 infects nearly all humans by the age of 2 years and usually causes exanthem subitum (roseola infantum; sixth disease), infantile fever without rash, febrile seizures, and occasionally encephalitis.[139,140] Liver involvement with HHV-6 infection has been previously investigated, but attempts to prove an etiologic association of HHV-6 with liver injury have been inconclusive because of the high prevalence of primary infection at a young age. Elevated transaminase levels were not appreciated as a common feature of roseola in a large case series.[141] HHV-6 was isolated from the peripheral blood mononuclear cells in sporadic case reports of patients with acute hepatitis and fulminant hepatic failure.[142-144] PCR techniques and in situ hybridization led to isolation of HHV-6 from the liver tissue of infants with chronic hepatitis, suggesting HHV-6 as a causative agent.[145,146] Reactivation of infection may occur after solid-organ transplantation with questionable clinical significance.[147] Foscarnet has a better in vitro virus sensitivity than acyclovir and ganciclovir against HHV-6.[148]

HHV-7 also infects all humans by the age of 5 years, causing febrile syndromes. Hepatitis in association with HHV-7 was infrequently reported in the literature with questionable clinical relevance.[149]

HHV-8 (also called Kaposi's sarcoma–associated HHV-8) has been detected consistently in Kaposi's sarcoma, body cavity lymphoma, and multi-centric Castleman's disease, mainly in human immunodeficiency virus (HIV)–positive patients but occasionally in HIV-negative patients. Liver involvement may occur in the visceral type of Kaposi's sarcoma. Life-threatening extensive disease is usually treated with chemotherapy alone or in combination with surgery and radiation therapy. Antiviral drugs have no established role in treating HHV-8–associated malignancies, but recombinant interferon-α may be used for treating cutaneous non–life-threatening disease.[139,150]

HUMAN PARVOVIRUS B19

HPV-B19 is a small DNA virus (*parvum* is the Latin ward for "small") and is the only parvovirus known to be a human pathogen. It was discovered incidentally in 1974 when parvovirus-like particles were noted in serum specimens from asymptomatic blood donors being tested for hepatitis B surface antigen. Sample number 19 in panel B (hence B19) gave an anomalous, "false positive" result that was recognized later as a member of the parvoviridae.[151,152]

HPV-B19 infection produces a spectrum of clinical manifestations including: (1) erythema infectiosum, "fifth disease," in children; (2) hydrops fetalis and fetal death; (3) an arthritis syndrome associated with acute infections in adults; (4) hematologic disorders such as leukopenia, thrombocytopenia, transient aplastic crisis in patients with chronic hemolytic anemia, and chronic anemia in immunocompromised patients including those with AIDS; and (5) rarely, other organ involvement including neurologic, cardiac, liver, and vasculitis.[152]

Hepatic manifestations range from a transient elevation of serum transaminases[153,154] sometimes seen during the course of erythema infectiosum[155,156] to fulminant hepatic failure (FHF).[157] HPV-B19 DNA has been found in liver samples from 67 percent of patients with non–A-C FHF and aplastic anemia and in 50 percent of patients with cryptogenic FHF without aplastic anemia, compared to 15 percent of control subjects with chronic liver failure. This led some investigators to suggest that HPV-B19 is a possible causative agent of fulminant liver failure.[158] Sokal reported that children with fulminant hepatitis caused by acute HPV-B19 infection had particularly low bilirubin concentrations and rapid recovery of liver function without transplantation and therefore a favorable outcome compared to fulminant hepatitis caused by other etiologies.[159] The pathogenesis is not very well understood.

Definitive diagnosis of acute HPV-B19 infection relies on the detection of HPV-B19 IgM or viral DNA. Assays for serum HPV-B19 IgM and IgG, as detected by radioimmunoassay or enzyme-linked immunosorbent assay, are now available.[152] PCR is much more sensitive for detecting viral DNA in the serum, other body fluid, and fresh- and paraffin-embedded tissue. Electron microscopy can also identify HPV-B19 virus in serum or tissue.[160]

The prevalence of antibody to HPV-B19 (anti-B19 IgG) in England and Wales was measured in more than 2000 serum specimens. It was found that the presence of anti–HPV-B19 IgG increased with age. The antibody was found in 5 percent to 15 percent of children 1 to 5 years old; 50 percent to 60 percent of older children, young adults, and women of child-bearing age; and more than 85 percent of those older than 70 years.[161] In another study the prevalence of anti–HPV-B19 IgG was 61 percent in hepatitis C–infected patients compared to 4 percent in the control group.[162] Anti–HPV-B19 IgG was also found in the serum of patients with vasculitis and mixed cryoglobulinemia, but studies suggested that it was neither an etiologic factor nor a co-factor in the pathogenesis.[163] However, HPV-B19 DNA was only detected in 6 of 1000 serum samples from blood donors (incidence, 0.6 percent).[164]

In most cases HPV-B19 infection is benign and self-limited and results in life-long immunity and requires no treatment other than symptomatic relief.[152] At the Mayo Clinic we reported two cases of a less severe form of hepatitis-associated aplastic anemia. One patient also had autoimmune hepatitis and responded well to steroid therapy; the other improved spontaneously with supportive care.[165]

ADENOVIRUSES

Adenoviruses were first isolated from surgically removed adenoidal tissues in the middle of the last century. Currently, there are close to 50 serotypes causing mainly acute infections of the respiratory system, conjunctivae, and gastrointestinal tract, and occasionally hemorrhagic cystitis, infantile diarrhea, intussusception, and central nervous system infections.[166] Emerging concerns in immunocompromised patients are rising, particularly after organ transplantation, in which infections tend to occur in the organ transplanted (e.g., hepatitis after liver transplantation and hemorrhagic cystitis after renal transplantation).[167-171] Disseminated disease with multi-organ involvement has also been reported in immunocompromised patients and is associated with an increased mortality rate.[172]

The role of adenovirus as an etiologic agent of hepatic damage has been controversial. Adenoviral hepatitis was reported in severe combined immunodeficiency disease, DiGeorge's syndrome, and HIV infection and after chemotherapy for acute lymphoblastic leukemia.[173,174] Fatal cases of adenoviral infection with fulminant hepatitis were reported in these immunosuppressed adult patients. The postmortem liver pathology revealed widespread hepatic necrosis with intranuclear inclusions within viable hepatocytes. Electron microscopy may show crystalline arrays of virions within hepatocytes.[175,176] Viral tissue cultures help confirm the diagnosis. No specific therapy for adenoviral hepatitis is currently available.

ADDITIONAL HEPATITIS AGENTS

Additional hepatitis agents have been suggested from transfusion-associated hepatitis studies, CDC Sentinel Counties studies, and in the majority of patients with fulminant hepatitis in whom no agent has been identified. In all these conditions, a viral agent is suspected to exist but no specific virus has been identified.

The GB agent and the hepatitis G virus (HGV) are RNA viruses that belong to the Flaviviridae family.[45] Extensive investigations have failed to show that these agents play any etiologic role in acute or chronic liver disease.[177,178]

The TT virus (TTV) has been shown to be a small, nonenveloped, single-stranded, circular DNA virus in the family of Circoviridae.[179,180] It is now clear that TTV is a heterogeneous agent that can be transmitted to humans by both parenteral and non-parenteral routes. The agent is of particularly high prevalence in Japan where TTV has been detected in healthy people. Although initially implicated in fulminant hepatitis and cryptogenic chronic liver disease, these associations have not been confirmed and presently there are no proven hepatic diseases associated with the agent.[181,182]

The newly described viruses in this family have been designated SANBAN and YONBAN.[183-186] These agents have similar properties to TTV but also have sufficient nucleotide differences to make them distinct members of the Circoviridae family.

SEN virus (SEN-V), named after the initials of the patient in whom it was discovered, was discovered independently using amplification strategies with highly degenerate TTV primers.[183] Two SEN-V variants (SEN-D and SEN-C/H) have been studied and been found as acute infections in 11 of 12 (93 percent) of transfusion-transmitted non-A to E hepatitis cases. There is no current evidence that SEN-V is truly a hepatitis virus; further work is needed.

Novel genetic sequences and new viral agents will continue to be discovered. The challenge will be to establish causality between these new agents and the presence of liver disease in a patient. Fredricks and Relman[187] have suggested that the sequences of a putative pathogen should be present in most cases of the disease; the sequences should be found preferentially in the target organ; fewer or no copies should be found in hosts or tissues without disease; sequences should be found in areas of pathology; with resolution of disease, the copy number of sequences should decrease and become undetectable; and temporality should be demonstrated between sequence detection and disease and disease severity.

These criteria are particularly pertinent in the field of transfusion medicine and transfusion-transmitted viruses[188] in which these novel sequences and potential new agents have mostly been described.

References

1. Corey L: Herpes simplex virus. In Mandell G, Bennett J, Dolin R: Principles and Practice of Infectious Diseases, vol 2. Philadelphia, Churchill Livingstone, 2000:1564-1580.
2. Corey L, Spear PG: Infections with herpes simplex viruses (2). N Engl J Med 314(12):749-757, 1986.
3. Hass G: Hepato-adrenal necrosis with intranuclear inclusion bodies. Am J Pathol 11:127-142, 1935.
4. Hanshaw J: Herpesvirus hominis infections in the fetus and the newborn. Am J Dis Child 126(4):456-555, 1973.
5. Benador N, et al: Three cases of neonatal herpes simplex virus infection presenting as fulminant hepatitis. Eur J Pediatr 149:555-559, 1990.
6. Barton LL, et al: Herpes simplex virus hepatitis in a child: case report and review. Pediatr Infects Dis J 18(11):1026, 1999.
7. Flewett T, Parker R, Phillip W: Acute hepatitis due to herpes simplex virus in an adult. J Clin Pathol 22:60-66, 1969.
8. Mudido P, et al: Disseminated herpes simplex virus infection during pregnancy. A case report. J Reprod Med 38(12):964, 1993.
9. Fink CG, et al: Acute herpes hepatitis in pregnancy [see comments]. J Clin Path 46(10):968-971, 1993.
10. Klein NA, et al: Herpes simplex virus hepatitis in pregnancy. Two patients successfully treated with acyclovir. Gastroenterology 100(1):239-244, 1991.
11. Wertheim RA, et al: Fatal herpetic hepatitis in pregnancy. Obstet Gynecol 62:3(suppl):38s-42s, 1983.
12. Fairley I, Wilson J: Herpes hepatitis in pregnancy [letter; comment] [published erratum appears in J Clin Pathol 47(10):964, 1994]. J Clin Pathol 47(5):478, 1994.
13. Kang AH, Graves CR: Herpes simplex hepatitis in pregnancy: a case report and review of the literature. Obstet Gynecol Surv 54(7):463-468, 1999.
14. Yaziji H, et al: Gestational herpes simplex virus hepatitis. South Med J 90(3):347-351, 1997.
15. Minuk G, Nicolle L: Genital herpes and hepatitis in healthy young adults. J Med Virol 19:269-275, 1986.
16. Chase RA, et al: Herpes simplex viral hepatitis in adults: two case reports and review of the literature. Rev Infect Dis 9(2):329-333, 1987.
17. Velasco M, et al: Fulminant herpes hepatitis in a healthy adult: a treatable disorder? J Clin Gastroenterol 28(4):386-389, 1999.
18. Farr RW, Short S, Weissman D: Fulminant hepatitis during herpes simplex virus infection in apparently immunocompetent adults: report of two cases and review of the literature. Clin Infect Dis 24(6):1191, 1997.
19. Aboguddah A, et al: Herpes simplex hepatitis in a patient with psoriatic arthritis taking prednisone and methotrexate. Report and review of the literature. J Rheumatol 18(9):1406-1412, 1991.
20. Anuras S, Summers R: Fulminant herpes simplex hepatitis in an adult: report of a case in renal transplant recipient. Gastroenterology 70(3):425-428, 1976.
21. Berglin E, et al: A case of lethal herpes simplex hepatitis in a diabetic renal transplant recipient. Transplant Proc 14(4):765-769, 1982.
22. Elliott WC, et al: Herpes simplex type 1 hepatitis in renal transplantation. Arch Intern Med 140(12):1656-1660, 1980.
23. Gabel H, Flamholc L, Ahlfors K: Herpes simplex virus hepatitis in a renal transplant recipient: successful treatment with acyclovir. Scand J Infect Dis 20(4):435-438, 1988.
24. Hayashi M, et al: Severe herpes simplex virus hepatitis following autologous bone marrow transplantation: successful treatment

with high dose intravenous acyclovir. Jpn J Clin Oncol 21(5):372-376, 1991.
25. Isobe H, et al: An association of acute herpes simplex hepatitis and erythema multiforme. Am J Gastroenterol 89(10):1905, 1994.
26. Johnson JR, et al: Hepatitis due to herpes simplex virus in marrow-transplant recipients. Clin Infect Dis 14(1):38-45, 1992.
27. Kusne S, et al: Herpes simplex virus hepatitis after solid organ transplantation in adults. J Infect Dis 163(5):1001, 1991.
28. Luchtrath H, Totovic V, de Leon F: A case of fulminant herpes simplex hepatitis in an adult. Pathol Res Pract 179(2):235-241, 1984.
29. Markin RS, et al: Opportunistic viral hepatitis in liver transplant recipients. Transplant Proc 23:1 (Pt 2):1520, 1991.
30. Seksik P, et al: Fatal herpetic hepatitis in adult following short corticotherapy: a case report. Intern Care Med 25(4):415-417, 1999.
31. Shlien RD, et al: Fulminant herpes simplex hepatitis in a patient with ulcerative colitis. Gut 29(2):257-261, 1988.
32. Takebe N, et al: Fatal herpes simplex hepatitis type 2 in a post-thymectomized adult. Gastroenterol Japon 28(2):304-311, 1993.
33. Taylor RJ, et al: Primary disseminated herpes simplex infection with fulminant hepatitis following renal transplantation. Arch Intern Med 141(11):1519, 1981.
34. Pellise M, Miquel R: Liver failure due to herpes simplex virus. J Hepatol 32(1):170, 2000.
35. Rakela J, et al: Fulminant hepatitis: Mayo Clinic experience with 34 cases. Mayo Clin Proc 60(5):289-292, 1985.
36. Glorioso DV, et al: Successful empiric treatment of HSV hepatitis in pregnancy. Case report and review of the literature. Dig Dis Sci 41(6):1273, 1996.
37. Kaufman B, et al: Herpes simplex virus hepatitis: case report and review [see comments]. Clin Infect Dis 24(3):334-338, 1997.
38. Shanley CJ, et al: Fulminant hepatic failure secondary to herpes simplex virus hepatitis. Successful outcome after orthotopic liver transplantation. Transplantation 59(1):145-149, 1995.
39. Whitley R: Varicella-zoster virus. In Mandell G, Bennett J, Dolin R, eds: Principles and Practice of Infectious Diseases, vol 2. Philadelphia, Churchill Livingstone, 2000:1685-1693.
40. Phuah HK, et al: Complicated varicella zoster infection in 8 paediatric patients and review of literature. Sing Med J 39(3):115-120, 1998.
41. Plotkin SA: Clinical and pathogenetic aspects of varicella-zoster. Postgrad Med J 61(suppl 4):7-14, 1985.
42. Ey J, Smith S, Fulginiti V: Varicella hepatitis without neurologic symptoms or findings. Pediatrics 67(2):285-287, 1981.
43. Pitel P, et al: Subclinical hepatic changes in varicella infection. Pediatrics 65:631-633, 1980.
44. Reye R: Encephalopathy and fatty degeneration of the viscera: a disease entity in childhood. Lancet 2:749, 1963.
45. Linnemann CJ, et al: Reye's syndrome: epidemiologic and viral studies, 1963-1974. Am J Epidemiol 101(6):517-526, 1975.
46. Anderson D, et al: Varicella hepatitis: a fatal case in a previously healthy, immunocompetent adult. Report of a case, autopsy, and review of the literature. Arch Intern Med 154(18):2101-2106, 1993.
47. Rubin R, Tolkoff-Rubin N: Viral infection in the renal transplant patient. Proc Eur Dialysis Transplant Assoc 19:513-526, 1983.
48. Schiller GJ, et al: Abdominal presentation of varicella-zoster infection in recipients of allogeneic bone marrow transplantation [see comments]. Bone Marrow Transplant 7(6):489-491, 1991.
49. Alonso EM, et al: Postnecrotic cirrhosis following varicella hepatitis in a liver transplant patient. Transplantation 49(3):650-653, 1990.
50. Bensousan TA, et al: Fulminant hepatitis revealing primary varicella in a renal graft recipient. Transplant Proc 27(4):2512, 1995.
51. Morishita K, et al: Fulminant varicella hepatitis following bone marrow transplantation [letter]. JAMA 253(4):511, 1985.
52. Patti ME, Selvaggi KJ, Kroboth FJ: Varicella hepatitis in the immunocompromised adult: a case report and review of the literature [see comments]. Am J Med 88(1):77-80, 1990.
53. Soriano V, Bru F, Gonzalez-Lahoz J: Fatal varicella hepatitis in a patient with AIDS [letter]. J Infect 25(1):107, 1992.
54. Ross JS, et al: Fatal massive hepatic necrosis from varicella-zoster hepatitis. Am J Gastroenterol 74(5):423-427, 1980.
55. Kusne S, et al: Varicella-zoster virus hepatitis and a suggested management plan for prevention of VZV infection in adult liver transplant recipients. Transplantation 60(6):619-621, 1995.
56. Morales JM: Successful acyclovir therapy of severe varicella hepatitis in an adult renal transplant recipient [letter; comment]. Am J Med 90(3):401, 1991.
57. Williams WW: CDC guidelines for the prevention and control of nosocomial infections. Guideline for infection control in hospital personnel. Am J Infect Control 12(1):34-63, 1984.
58. Alford CA: Acyclovir treatment of herpes simplex virus infections in immunocompromised humans. An overview. Am J Med 73(1A):225-228, 1982.
59. Shulman ST: Acyclovir treatment of disseminated varicella in childhood malignant neoplasms. Am J Dis Child 139(2):137-140, 1985.
60. Ho M: Interferon for the treatment of infections. Ann Rev Med 38:51-59, 1987.
61. Whitley RJ, et al: Disseminated herpes zoster in the immunocompromised host: a comparative trial of acyclovir and vidarabine. The NIAID Collaborative Antiviral Study Group. J Infect Dis 165(3):450, 1992.
62. Epstein M, Achong B, Barr Y: Virus particles in cultured lymphoblasts from Burkitt's lymphoma. Lancet 1:702-703, 1964.
63. Henle G, Henle W, Diehl V: Relation of Burkitt's tumor-associated herpes-type virus to infectious mononucleosis. Proc Nat Acad Sci U S A 59(1):94-101, 1968.
64. Sixbey J, et al: Replication of Epstein-Barr virus in human epithelial cells infected in vitro. Nature 306:480-483, 1983.
65. White NJ, Juel-Jensen BE: Infectious mononucleosis hepatitis. Semin Liver Dis 4(4):301-306. 1984.
66. Yao Q, Rickinson A, Epstein M: A re-examination of the Epstein-Barr virus carrier state in healthy seropositive individuals. Intl J Cancer 35:35-42, 1985.
67. Cohen J: Epstein-Barr virus Infections. N Engl J Med 343(7):481-492, 2000.
68. Schooly A: Epstein-Barr virus. In Mandell G, Bennett J, Dolin R, eds: Principles and Practice of Infectious Diseases, vol 2. Philadelphia, Churchill Livingstone, 2000:1599-1613.
69. Chetham MM, Roberts KB: Infectious mononucleosis in adolescents. Pediatr Ann 20(4):206-213, 1991.
70. Hoagland R: The clinical manifestations of infectious mononucleosis. A report of two hundred cases. Am J Med Sci 240:55-63, 1960.
71. Baron D, Bell J, Demmett W: Biochemical studies on hepatic involvement in infectious mononucleosis. J Clin Pathol 1965(18):209-211, 1960.
72. Rosalki S, Jones T, Verney A: Transaminases and liver function studies in infectious mononucleosis. BMJ 1:929-932, 1960.
73. Reichman S, Burke A, Davis WJ: Hepatic involvement of infectious mononucleosis. Am J Dig Dis 2:430-436, 1957.
74. Nelson R, Darragh J: Infectious mononucleosis hepatitis. A clinicopathologic study. Am J Med 21:26-33, 1956.
75. Horwitz C, et al: Hepatic function in mononucleosis induced by Epstein-Barr virus and cytomegalovirus. Clin Chem. 26(2):243-246, 1980.
76. Madigan N, Newcomer A, Taswell H: Intense jaundice in infectious mononucleosis. Mayo Clin Proc 48:857-862, 1973.
77. Edoute Y, et al: Severe cholestatic jaundice induced by Epstein-Barr virus infection in the elderly. J Gastroenterol Hepatol 13(8):821-824, 1998.
78. Fuhrman S, et al: Marked hyperbilirubinemia in infectious mononucleosis. Analysis of laboratory data in seven patients. Arch Intern Med 147(5):850-853, 1987.
79. Horwitz C, et al: Infectious mononucleosis in patients aged 40 to 72 years: report of 27 cases, including 3 without heterophil-antibody responses. Medicine 62(4):256-262, 1983.
80. Jacobson IM, Gang DL, Schapiro RH: Epstein-Barr viral hepatitis: an unusual case and review of the literature. Am J Gastroenterol 79(8):628-632, 1984.
81. Corey L, et al: HBs-Ag-negative hepatitis in a hemodialysis unit: relation to Epstein-Barr virus. N Engl J Med 293(25):1273-1278, 1975.
82. Straus S: The chronic mononucleosis syndrome. J Infect Dis 157:405-412, 1988.
83. Biest S, Schubert TT: Chronic Epstein-Barr virus infection: a cause of granulomatous hepatitis? J Clin Gastroenterol 11(3):343-346, 1989.
84. Harrington P, et al: Granulomatous hepatitis. Rev Infect Dis 4(3):638-655, 1982.

85. Donhuijsen-Ant R, et al: Aggressive hepatitis in a patient with acute myeloid leukaemia during complete remission and detection of Epstein-Barr virus DNA in a liver biopsy. Br J Haematol 76(4):557, 1990.
86. Papatheodoridis GV, et al: Fulminant hepatitis due to Epstein-Barr virus infection. J Hepatol 23(3):348, 1995.
87. Davies M, et al: A fatal case of Epstein-Barr virus infection with jaundice and renal failure. Postgrad Med J 56:794-795, 1980.
88. Pelletier L, et al: Disseminated intravascular coagulation and hepatic necrosis. Complications of infectious mononucleosis. JAMA 235(11):1144-1146, 1976.
89. Sainsbury R, et al: Gallbladder wall thickening with infectious mononucleosis hepatitis in an immunosuppressed adolescent. J Pediatr Gastroenterol Nutr 19(1):123, 1994.
90. Edwards JM, et al: Laboratory diagnosis of EB virus infection in some cases presenting as hepatitis. J Clin Pathol 31(2):179-182, 1978.
91. Lloyd-Still JD, Scott JP, Crussi F: The spectrum of Epstein-Barr virus hepatitis in children. Pediatr Pathol 5(3-4):337-351, 1986.
92. Kilpatrick Z: Structural and functional abnormalities of liver in infectious mononucleosis. Arch Intern Med 117(1):47-53, 1966.
93. Markin R: Manifestations of Epstein-Barr virus-associated disorders in liver. 14(1):1-13, 1994.
94. Gan YJ, Sullivan JL, Sixbey JW: Detection of cell-free Epstein-Barr virus DNA in serum during acute infectious mononucleosis. J Infect Dis 170(2):436, 1994.
95. Watanabe S, et al: Comparison between sporadic cytomegalovirus hepatitis and Epstein-Barr virus hepatitis in previously healthy adults. Liver 17(2):63-69, 1997.
96. van der Horst C, et al: Lack of effect of peroral acyclovir for the treatment of acute infectious mononucleosis. J Infect Dis 164(4):788-792, 1991.
97. Feranchak AP, et al: Fulminant Epstein-Barr viral hepatitis: orthotopic liver transplantation and review of the literature. Liver Transplant Surg 4(6):469-476, 1998.
98. Sokal E, et al: Early signs and risk factors for the increased incidence of Epstein-Barr virus-related posttransplant lymphoproliferative diseases in pediatric liver transplant recipients treated with tacrolimus. Transplantation 64(10):1438, 1997.
99. Smith M: Propagation of salivary gland virus of the mouse in tissue cultures. Proc Soc Exp Biol Med 86:435-440, 1954.
100. Kaariainen L, Klemola E, Paloheimo J: Rise of cytomegalovirus antibodies in an infectious-mononucleosis-like syndrome after transfusion. BMJ 5498:1270-1272, 1966.
101. Kim W, et al: The economic impact of cytomegalovirus infection after liver transplantation. Transplantation 69(3):357-361, 2000.
102. Paya C, et al: Incidence, distribution, and outcome of episodes of infection in 100 orthotopic liver transplantations. Mayo Clin Proc 64(5):555-564, 1989.
103. Goodgame R: Gastrointestinal cytomegalovirus disease. Ann Intern Med 119(9):924-935, 1993.
104. Crumpacker C: Cytomegalovirus. In Mandell G, Bennett J, Dolin R, eds: Principles and Practice of Infectious Diseases, vol 2. Philadelphia, Churchill Livingstone, 2000:1586-1599.
105. Carey WD, Patel G: Viral hepatitis in the 1990s, part III: hepatitis C, hepatitis E, and other viruses. Cleve Clin J Med 59(6):595-601, 1992.
106. Stagno S, et al: Congenital cytomegalovirus infection: The relative importance of primary and recurrent maternal infection. N Engl J Med 306(16):945-949, 1982.
107. Fowler K, et al: The outcome of congenital cytomegalovirus infection in relation to maternal antibody status. N Engl J Med 326(10):663-667, 1992.
108. Stagno S, Whitley R: Herpesvirus infections of pregnancy. Part I: cytomegalovirus and Epstein-Barr virus infections. N Engl J Med 313(20):1270-1274, 1985.
109. Griffiths P: Cytomegalovirus and the liver. Semin Liver Dis 4(4):307-313, 1984.
110. Levy I, et al: Recurrent ascites in an infant with perinatally acquired cytomegalovirus infection [see comments]. Eur J Pediatr 148(6):531-532, 1989.
111. Chang MH, et al: Polymerase chain reaction to detect human cytomegalovirus in livers of infants with neonatal hepatitis [see comments]. Gastroenterology 103(3):1022, 1992.
112. Klemola E, et al: Infectious-mononucleosis-like disease with negative heterophil agglutination test. Clinical features in relation to Epstein-Barr virus and cytomegalovirus antibodies. J Infect Dis 121(6):608-614, 1970.
113. Pass R, et al: Increased rate of cytomegalovirus infection among parents of children attending day-care centers. N Engl J Med 314(22):1414-1418, 1986.
114. Lang D, Scolnick E, Willerson J: Association of cytomegalovirus infection with the postperfusion syndrome. N Engl J Med 278(21):1147-1149, 1968.
115. Kunno A, et al: Clinical and histological features of cytomegalovirus hepatitis in previously healthy adults. Liver 17(3):129-132, 1997.
116. Carter A: Cytomegalovirus disease presenting as hepatitis. BMJ 3:986, 1968.
117. Henson D: Cytomegalovirus hepatitis in an adult. An autopsy report. Arch Pathol Lab Med 88(2):199-203, 1969.
118. Bonkowsky H, Lee R, Klatskin G: Acute granulomatous hepatitis. Occurrence in cytomegalovirus mononucleosis. JAMA 233(12):1284-1288, 1975.
119. Reller LB: Granulomatous hepatitis associated with acute cytomegalovirus infection. Lancet 1(7793):20-22, 1973.
120. Toghill PJ, et al: Cytomegalovirus hepatitis in the adult. Lancet 1(7504):1351, 1967.
121. Mosley JW, et al: Multiple hepatitis viruses in multiple attacks of acute viral hepatitis. N Engl J Med 296(2):75-78, 1977.
122. Stern H: Cytomegalovirus and EB virus infections of the liver. Br Med Bull 28(2):180-185, 1972.
123. Shusterman N, Frauenhoffer C, Kinsey M: Fatal massive hepatic necrosis in cytomegalovirus mononucleosis. Ann Intern Med 88(6):810-812, 1978.
124. Teixidor H, et al: Cytomegalovirus infection of the alimentary canal: radiologic findings with pathologic correlation. Radiology 163(2):317-323, 1987.
125. Roulot D, et al: Cholangitis in the acquired immunodeficiency syndrome: report of two cases and review of the literature. Gut 28(12):1653-1660, 1987.
126. Blumberg R, et al: Cytomegalovirus- and Cryptosporidium-associated acalculous gangrenous cholecystitis. Am J Med 76(6):1118-1123, 1984.
127. Jacobson M, Cello J, Sande M: Cholestasis and disseminated cytomegalovirus disease in patients with the acquired immunodeficiency syndrome. Am J Med 84(2):218-224, 1988.
128. Eeckhout E, et al: The importance of a specific IgM antibody assay in the early detection of cytomegalovirus hepatitis [letter]. Am J Gastroenterol 84(1):79-80, 1989.
129. Shuster E, et al: Monoclonal antibody for rapid laboratory detection of cytomegalovirus infections: characterization and diagnostic application. Mayo Clin Proc 60(9):577-585, 1985.
130. Martin WI, Smith T: Rapid detection of cytomegalovirus in bronchoalveolar lavage specimens by a monoclonal antibody method. J Clin Microbiol 23(6):1006-1008, 1986.
131. Paya C, et al: Rapid shell vial culture and tissue histology compared with serology for the rapid diagnosis of cytomegalovirus infection in liver transplantation. Mayo Clin Proc 64(6):670-675, 1989.
132. Mendez J, et al: Evaluation of PCR primers for early diagnosis of cytomegalovirus infection following liver transplantation. J Clin Microbiol 36(2):526-530, 1999.
133. Persing DH, Rakela J: Polymerase chain reaction for the detection of hepatitis viruses: panacea or purgatory? [editorial; comment]. Gastroenterology 103(3):1098, 1992.
134. Espy M, et al: Diagnosis of cytomegalovirus hepatitis by histopathology and in situ hybridization in liver transplantation. Diagn Microbiol Infect Dis 14(4):293-296, 1991.
135. Snover DC, Horwitz CA: Liver disease in cytomegalovirus mononucleosis: a light microscopical and immunoperoxidase study of six cases. Hepatology 4(3):408-412, 1984.
136. Plotkin S, Starr S, Bryan C: In vitro and in vivo responses of cytomegalovirus to acyclovir. Am J Med 73(1A):257-261, 1982.
137. Balfour HJ: Antiviral drugs. N Engl J Med 340(16):1255-1268, 1999.
138. Wiesner R, et al: Advances in the diagnosis, treatment, and prevention of cytomegalovirus infections after liver transplantation. Gastroenterol Clin North Am 22(2):351-366, 1993.
139. Straus S: Human herpesvirus types 6, 7, and 8. In Mandell G, Bennett J, Dolin R, eds: Principles and Practice of Infectious Diseases, vol 2. Philadelphia, Churchill Livingstone, 2000:1613-1621.

140. Pruksananonda P, et al: Primary human herpesvirus 6 infection in young children. N Engl J Med 326(22):1445-1450, 1992.
141. Hall C, et al: Human herpesvirus-6 infection in children. A prospective study of complications and reactivation. N Engl J Med 33(7):432-438, 1994.
142. Sobue R, et al: Fulminant hepatitis in primary human herpesvirus-6 infection [letter]. N Engl J Med 324(18):1290, 1991.
143. Asano Y, et al: Fatal fulminant hepatitis in an infant with human herpesvirus-6 infection [letter]. Lancet 335(8693):862, 1990.
144. Dubedat S, Kappagoda N: Hepatitis due to human herpesvirus-6 [letter]. Lancet 2(8677):1463, 1989.
145. Tajiri H, et al: Chronic hepatitis in an infant, in association with human herpesvirus-6 infection. J Pediatr 131(3):473, 1997.
146. Schmitt K, et al: Autoimmune hepatitis and adrenal insufficiency in an infant with human herpesvirus-6 infection. Lancet 348(9032):966, 1996.
147. Lunel F, et al: Hepatitis virus infections in heart transplant recipients. Biomed Pharmacother 49(3):125, 1995.
148. Reymen D, et al: Antiviral activity of selected acyclic nucleoside analogues against human herpesvirus 6. Antiviral Res 28(4):343-357, 1995.
149. Hashida T, et al: Hepatitis in association with human herpesvirus-7 infection. Pediatrics 96(4 Pt 1):783, 1995.
150. Antman K, Chang Y: Medical progress: Kaposi's sarcoma. N Engl J Med 342(14):1027-1038, 2000.
151. Cossart Y, et al: Parvovirus-like particles in human sera. Lancet 1(Jan 11):72-73, 1975.
152. Brown K, Parvoviruses. In Mandell G, Bennett J, Dolin R, eds: Principles and Practice of Infectious Diseases, vol 2. Philadelphia, Churchill Livingstone, 2000:1685-1693.
153. Tsuda, H., Liver dysfunction caused by parvovirus B19 [letter]. American Journal of Gastroenterology, 1993. 88(9)(1993 Sep):1463.
154. Yoto Y, et al: Transient disturbance of consciousness and hepatic dysfunction associated with human parvovirus B19 infection. Lancet 344(27 August):624-625, 1994.
155. Yoto Y, et al: Human parvovirus B19 infection associated with acute hepatitis. Lancet 347(30 March):868-869, 1996.
156. Drago F, et al: Parvovirus B19 infection associated with acute hepatitis and a purpuric exanthem. Br J Dermatol 141:160-161, 1999.
157. Karetnyi Y, et al: Human parvovirus B19 infection in acute fulminant liver failure. Arch Virol 144(9):1713-1724, 1999.
158. Langnas A, et al: Parvovirus B19 as a possible causative agent of fulminant liver failure and associated aplastic anemia. Hepatology 22:1661-1665, 1995.
159. Sokal E, et al: Acute parvovirus B19 infection associated with fulminant hepatitis of favourable prognosis in young children. Lancet 35:1739-1741, 1998.
160. Clewley J: Polymerase chain reaction assay of parvovirus B19 DNA in clinical specimens. J Clin Microbiol 27:2647-2651, 1989.
161. Cohen B, Buckley M: The prevalence of antibody to human parvovirus B19 in England and Wales. J Med Microbiol 25:151-153, 1988.
162. Lavorino C, et al: Antibodies anti-parvovirus B19 in chronic hepatitis C virus infection [letter]. Am J Gastroenterol 90(April):676-677, 1995.
163. Cacoub P, et al: Parvovirus B19 infection, hepatitis C virus infection, and mixed cryoglobulinaemia. Ann Rheum Dis 57(7):422-424, 1998.
164. Yoto Y, et al: Incidence of human parvovirus B19 DNA detection in blood donors. Br J Haematol 9:1017-1018, 1995.
165. Pardi D, et al: Hepatitis-associated aplastic anemia and acute parvovirus B19 infection: a report of two cases and a review of the literature. Am J Gastroenterol 93:468-470, 1998.
166. Baum S: Adenovirus. In Mandell G, Bennett J, Dolin R, eds: Principles and Practice of Infectious Diseases, vol 2. Philadelphia, Churchill Livingstone, 2000:1624-1630.
167. Carrigan D: Adenovirus infections in immunocompromised patients. Am J Med 102(3A):71-74, 1997.
168. Michaels M, et al: Adenovirus infection in pediatric liver transplant recipients. J Infect Dis 165(1):170-174, 1992.
169. Yagisawa T, et al: Acute hemorrhagic cystitis caused by adenovirus after kidney transplantation. Urol Intl 54:142, 1995.
170. Koneru B, et al: Serological studies of adenoviral hepatitis following pediatric liver transplantation. Transplant Proc 22(4):1547-1548, 1990.
171. Saad R, et al: Adenovirus hepatitis in the adult allograft liver. Transplantation 64(10):1483-1485, 1997.
172. Zahradnik J, Spencer M, Porter D: Adenovirus infection in the immunocompromised patient. Am J Med 68(5):725-732, 1980.
173. Krilov R, et al: Disseminated adenovirus infection with hepatic necrosis in patients with HIV infection and other immunodeficiency states. Rev Infect Dis 12:303, 1990.
174. Washington K, Gossage D, Gottfried M: Pathology of liver in severe combined immunodeficiency and DiGeorge syndrome. Pediatr Pathol 13(4):485, 1993.
175. Carmichael GJ, et al: Adenovirus hepatitis in an immunosuppressed adult patient. Am J Clin Pathol 71(3):352-355, 1979.
176. Wigger H, Blanc W: Fatal hepatic and bronchial necrosis in adenovirus infection with thymic alymphoplasia. N Engl J Med 275(16):870-874, 1966.
177. Laskus T, et al: Hepatitis G virus infection in American patients with cryptogenic cirrhosis: no evidence for liver replication. J Infect Dis 176(6):1491, 1997.
178. Laskus T, et al: Lack of evidence for hepatitis G virus replication in the livers of patients coinfected with hepatitis C and G viruses. J Virol 71(10):7804, 1997.
179. Nishizawa T, et al: A novel DNA virus (TTV) associated with elevated transaminase levels in posttransfusion hepatitis of unknown etiology. Biochem Biophys Res Commun 241(1):92, 1997.
180. Mushahwar IK, et al: Molecular and biophysical characterization of TT virus: evidence for a new virus family infecting humans. Proc Natl Acad Sci U S A 96(6):3177, 1999.
181. Naoumov NV, et al: Presence of a newly described human DNA virus (TTV) in patients with liver disease. Lancet 352(9123):195-197, 1998.
182. Matsumoto A, et al: Transfusion-associated TT virus infection and its relationship to liver disease. Hepatology 30(1):283, 1999.
183. Tanaka Y, et al: Genomic and molecular evolutionary analysis of a newly identified infectious agent (SEN virus) and its relationship to the TT virus family. J Infect Dis 183(3):359-367, 2001.
184. Takahashi K, Hijikata M, Samokhvaler EI, et al: Full or near full length nucleotide sequences of TT virus variants (Types SANBAN and YONBAN) and the TT virus-like mini virus. Intervirology 43(2):119-123, 2000.
185. Biagini P, et al: Complete sequences of two highly divergent European isolates of TT virus. Biochem Biophys Res Commun 271(3):837-841, 2000.
186. Hijikata M, Takahashi K, Mishiro S: Complete circular DNA genome of a TT virus variant (isolate name SANBAN) and 44 partial ORF2 sequences implicating a great degree of diversity beyond genotypes. Virology 260(1):17-22, 1999.
187. Fredericks DN, Relman DA: Sequence-based identification of microbial pathogens: a reconsideration of Koch's postulates. Clin Microbiol Rev 9(1):18-33, 1996.
188. Mosley JW, Rakela J: Foundling viruses and transfusion medicine [editorial]. Transfusion 39(10):1041, 1999.

CHAPTER

35

Parasitic Diseases of the Liver

Carlos A. DiazGranados, MD, Wayne A. Duffus, MD, PhD, and Helmut Albrecht, MD

Multiple parasites affect the liver. Some cause significant liver disease, whereas others use the hepatocyte as part of their life cycle but cause little damage to the organ itself. Because the liver is a major organ of the reticulo-endothelial system, it is also involved in the immune response against many microorganisms, including parasites. Reactive hyperplasia or granulomatous reactions are therefore observed in many of these infections.

Protozoa are simple parasites, most of them unicellular, microscopic, and free-living. Several protozoan infections are characterized by significant liver involvement. Liver disease is most severe in amebiasis, malaria (*Plasmodium* species), toxoplasmosis, trypanosomiasis, and leishmaniasis.

Additionally, various helminthic infections also affect the liver. Helminths are large, multi-cellular parasitic organisms, commonly referred to as worms. They are grouped in different categories (Annelids, nematodes, and platyhelminths). Nematodes are commonly known as roundworms, and among them, *Ascaris lumbricoides, Toxocara canis/cati, Strongyloides stercoralis,* and *Capillaria hepatica* can affect the liver. Platyhelminths are subclassified in trematodes and cestodes. Trematodes (commonly known as flukes) of importance in hepatology include *Schistosoma* species, *Fasciola* species, *Clonorchis* species, and *Opisthorchis.* Relevant cestodes (tapeworms) in hepatology are *Echinococcus granulosus* and *Echinococcus multilocularis,* the etiologic agents of cystic and alveolar hydatid disease.

Multiple clinical syndromes are associated with these microorganisms. Parasitic infections therefore have to be included in the differential diagnosis of the major liver syndromes in the appropriate epidemiologic and clinical settings (Table 35-1).

In this chapter the important parasitic diseases involving the liver are discussed. Parasitic diseases of the liver in human immunodeficiency virus (HIV)-infected and immunocompromised hosts are discussed elsewhere (see Chap. 51).

INFECTIONS CAUSED BY PROTOZOAN AMEBIASIS

Background and Epidemiology

Entamoeba histolytica is the etiologic agent for the widespread parasitic infection amebiasis. The organism is a pseudopod-forming non-flagellated protozoan parasite with an estimated genome size of approximately 20 megabases.[1] *E. histolytica* has two life forms: trophozoite and cyst. The infective cyst form contains four nuclei. It can withstand the acidic pH of the stomach and can survive in a moist or dry environment for several weeks. Cysts are 10 to 16 μm diameter and contain four nuclei when mature.

The trophozoite form is capable of mucosal invasion and subsequent spread.[2,3] The size of the trophozoite ranges from 10 to 60 μm. Its cytoplasm has a clear outer ectoplasm with a central granular endoplasm containing food vacuoles (Plate 35-1). The single spherical nucleus is approximately one sixth the diameter of the entire ameba. An unstained halo surrounds a small, distinct central karyosome. The nuclear membrane is lined by small aggregations of chromatin.[4] The genome of the organism has a low guanosine/cytosine content (22.4 percent) and consists of both linear chromosomes along with many circular plasmid-like molecules. It is on these circular deoxyribonucleic acids (DNAs) that the ribosomal ribonucleic acid (rRNA) genes are found.[5,6]

Of all the amebae normally inhabiting the human colon, only *E. histolytica* is capable of invading tissue. Non-pathogenic amebae frequently isolated from the gastrointestinal tract include *Entamoeba dispar, Entamoeba moshkovskii, Entamoeba coli, Entamoeba hartmanni,* and *Endolimax nana.* Species occasionally associated with diarrhea include *Dientamoeba fragilis* and *Entamoeba polecki. Entamoeba gingivalis* has been linked to periodontal disease in HIV type 1-infected patients.[7]

Colonization with *E. dispar* and the differentiation between "pathogenic" and "non-pathogenic" strains of *Entamoeba* organisms have been the source of much confusion. Older literature has been misleading in

TABLE 35-1
Major Parasitic Liver Syndromes

	Elevated AST/ALT (hepatitis)	Cholestasis	Jaundice	Hepatomegaly	Cirrhosis	Portal hypertension	Acute liver failure	Mass occupying lesions
Amebiasis	++	−	+	+	−	−	−	++
Malaria	+	−	++	+	−	−	+	−
Toxoplasmosis	++	−	++	+	−	−	+	+/−
American trypanosomiasis	+	−	+/−	+	+/− (Cardiac)	−	−	−
African trypanosomiasis	+	−	+	+/−	−	−	−	−
Leishmaniasis	+	−	+	+	−	−	−	−
Ascariasis*	+/−	+	++	+	−	−	−	+
Strongyloidiasis*	+	+	+	+	+/− (Thiab)	−	−	−
Toxocariasis*	+	−	+/−	+	−	−	−	+
Capillariasis*	+	−	+/−	+	−	−	−	+
Schistosomiasis*	+/−	−	+/−	+	−	++	−	−
Liver flukes*	+	+	+	+	+/−	−	−	+/−
Echinococcosis*	+/−	+/−	+/−	+	−	+/− (*E. multil.*)	−	++

AST, Aspartate aminotransferase; *ALT,* alanine aminotransferase; ++, very common, +, common; +/−, uncommon; −, absent.
*May present with significant eosinophilia.

documenting the prevalence of amebiasis because it did not distinguish between the morphologically identical but genetically distinct *E. histolytica* and the non-pathogenic *E. dispar.*[8-12] Earlier reports even conveyed that they could convert in culture. This has been shown to be artifactual because of inadvertent contamination of the cultures. *E. histolytica* and *E. dispar* can now be reliably differentiated by isoenzyme analysis,[13] restriction fragment length polymorphism, and monoclonal antibodies typed to surface antigens. With the availability of specific tests, *E. dispar* has been shown to be 3 times more prevalent in developing countries and at least 10 times more common in developed regions of the world.[14,15]

Worldwide, *E. histolytica* ranks second only to malaria in mortality resulting from protozoan infections that cause an estimated 100,000 deaths yearly.[16] Areas with the highest endemic activity include India, Mexico, East and South Africa, and regions of Central and South America.

The majority of infected people never becomes symptomatic and clears the infection spontaneously. In most cases *E. histolytica* lives as a harmless commensal in the lumen of the gut, a state referred to as *asymptomatic amebiasis.*[17-19] In this state the parasite feeds on the debris and bacteria and not on the host tissues without causing colitis or extraintestinal manifestation.

The consequences of immigration and the ease of international travel have contributed to an increased incidence and awareness of the complications of amebiasis in developed countries. Accordingly, immigrants from and tourists to developing countries are those most likely to become diagnosed with amebiasis in the United States. The Centers for Disease Control and Prevention documented 2970 cases of *E. histolytica* infection in 1993 alone. Of these, 33 percent of the patients were Hispanic immigrants and 17 percent were immigrants from Asia or the Pacific Islands.[20] Incidence rates peak between the third and fifth decades of life.[21,22] Travelers to warm climates are at a low but definite risk for developing amebic infection.[23,24] One study of 2700 German citizens returning from tropical regions showed a 0.3 percent incidence of *E. histolytica* infection.[23] Mentally retarded, institutionalized patients are also at increased risk of acquiring amebic colitis and liver abscess.[25,26] In addition, experimental studies suggest that the pathogenesis of amebic liver abscesses can be enhanced by impaired immunity.[27-29] Thymectomy or splenectomy in animal models results in an increased incidence of amebic liver abscess and larger size of the lesions.[27,28] Conversely, stimulation of the immune system with bacillus Calmette-Guérin decreased the risk of developing amebic liver abscess.[29] Immunocompromised patients, including HIV-infected patients, patients on systemic corticosteroid therapy, and pregnant women, are at increased risk of developing serious complications of amebiasis (see Pathogenesis and Pathology). Heavy alcohol consumption is a common finding in patients with amebic liver abscess and has been reported in up to 40 percent of patients.[30] It is hypothesized that alcohol makes the liver more susceptible to infection by directly impairing Kupffer cell function in the liver. Alternatively, long-standing alcohol use could also impair the cellular and humoral immunologic response to *E. histolytica* infection.

Life Cycle and Transmission

Humans are the principal host for *E. histolytica,* and infection occurs via the ingestion of the cyst form of the parasite. Fecal-oral transmission via contaminated food products is the most common route of infection.[31] Food-borne outbreaks are not uncommon and are usually caused by unsanitary handling of food or its preparation by infected individuals. This is especially prevalent where human feces are used for fertilizer. A large epidemic has been linked to a waterborne outbreak in Tblisi, Republic of Georgia.[32] On ingestion the quadrinucleated cyst excysts, liberating the trophozoite form of the parasite in the neutral or alkaline environment of the small intestine. The cyst wall is digested in the lumen of the gut by digestive enzymes and the amebae rapidly divide to yield eight metacystic trophozoites. These are carried with the intestinal juices into the cecum where they mature into trophozoites.

In 90 percent of individuals no disease or only colonization occurs. Colonization is facilitated by enteric bacteria, which provide a low oxygen potential and satisfy other metabolic needs. While traveling down the colon the trophozoites assume a precystic spherical shape as the fecal stream becomes progressively dehydrated. A thin but tough cyst wall is secreted, forming an immature cyst. Within this structure four nuclei are generated from two mitotic divisions. This now represents the infective cyst form, which is liberated into the environment with passage of the feces.

Pathogenesis and Pathology

Only 5 percent to 10 percent of individuals develop invasive disease. In these patients trophozoites manage to adhere to the colonic mucin glycoproteins via a galactose and N-acetyl-galactosamine (Gal/GalNAc) specific lectin.[19,33] This initiates a superficial lytic necrosis of the mucosal wall. The organisms then spread superficially along the basement membrane of the mucosa. They also penetrate the interstitial tissue between the glandular cells.[34] Invasion into the muscularis may result in colonic perforation. Trophozoites reaching mesenteric venules travel to the liver via the portal vein and may later reach the systemic circulation.

Amebic liver abscess is the most common extraintestinal manifestation of *E. histolytica* infection. When retained by thrombi the organisms cause lytic necrosis of the vessel walls, allowing translocation into hepatic sinusoids. The amebic cytolytic and proteolytic activity destroys the hepatocytes and is accompanied by a striking polymorphonuclear (PMN) leukocytic infiltration within the first 24 hours. This is followed by progressive lysis of PMNs on contact with the living parasites.[35,36] The pathophysiology involves three distinct consecutive stages: acute inflammation, granuloma formation, and progressively advancing necrosis with periportal fibrosis or necrotic abscess formation.[2,36] Imaging studies, histology, and clinical findings indicate that this process is reversible upon institution of appropriate treatment.[36,37]

Microscopically the amebic liver abscess contains an outer zone consisting of normal hepatic tissue being invaded by the organism; the center is filled with an acellular, proteinaceous debris.[2,3,38] The resulting abscess size is highly variable.

E. histolytica uses many as-yet undefined cellular and biochemical mechanisms to enhance its pathogenesis. Among them are secretion of toxic substances and the ability to phagocytose liver or previously killed target cells. Important virulence factors of *E. histolytica* include cysteine proteinases,[39,40] surface lectins, calmodulin, cytolytic ion channel-forming proteins or amoebapores, and phospholipases.[41] The relative contribution of each of the components to the overall virulence of the ameba parasite is an area of ongoing research. It is clear, however, that the interaction between *E. histolytica* and the host cell can be divided into two main stages. The first is the precise recognition and binding between surface adhesions of *E. histolytica* and receptors on the target cell. This is followed by the release of several intracellular components into the immediate environment with destructive effects on the host cell.[42]

The exact mechanism by which *E. histolytica* causes liver cell death (i.e., necrosis versus programmed cell death or both) has been matter of an ongoing debate.[11,43-45] Because apoptotic mechanisms are associated with minimal inflammatory response their use could potentially enhance survival of *E. histolytica* within the host.

A commonly used modality of distinguishing between apoptosis and necrosis is morphology. Characteristic changes of apoptosis include cell shrinkage, surface blebbing, and chromatin condensation.[45] In addition DNA of apoptotic cells usually displays a so-called ladder pattern on gel electrophoresis. In comparison, necrotic cells are characterized by cell swelling, rupture of plasma membrane, and the release of cell contents detectable by microscopy. In one study *E. histolytica* trophozoites were incubated with a murine myeloid cell line expressing Bcl-2, a protein, which confers resistance to apoptotic cell death. The results demonstrated a DNA ladder fragmentation pattern in the target cells suggesting killing via Bcl-2–independent apoptotic mechanisms.[43] By contrast, studies by Berninghausen and Leippe[45] only identified microscopic and morphologic characteristics associated with necrosis when HL-60 and Jurkat target cell lines were incubated with viable trophozoites or isolated amoebapores. Seydel and Stanley[44] have demonstrated that *E. histolytica* does in fact induce apoptosis in both inflammatory cells and hepatocytes in a SCID mouse model of amebic liver abscess. In this system cell death did not use the Fas/Fas ligand pathway of apoptosis or the tumor necrosis factor alpha–dependent pathway of programmed cell death.[44]

The reason for the capability of *E. histolytica* but not other amebae to invade tissue is not entirely clear. Studies have, however, demonstrated a unique cysteine proteinase gene (ACP1) that is present only in pathogenic strains of *E. histolytica* that has amino acid sequence homology with the cysteine proteinases released by invasive cancer cells and activated macrophages.[39] Anti-sense expression of cystein proteinases does not affect cytopathic or hemolytic activity but inhibits phagocytosis.[46] Neutral cysteinase has also been shown to degrade immunoglobulin (Ig)G and prevent its binding.[47] This virulence factor also facilitates escape from the host immune system via cleavage of secretory immunoglobulin A and lack of activation of complement.[40] When human intestinal xenografts in SCID mice are infected with a trophozoite carrying an anti-sense message to the cysteine proteinase gene, infection results in less intestinal inflammation and destruction of the mucosal barrier.[48] It appears that the cysteine proteinase possesses interleukin (IL)-1B–converting enzyme activity that contributes to inflammation by activating human IL-1B, released by damaged intestinal epithelium.[48] Invasion of the gastrointestinal tract requires adhesion to the colonic epithelium by the trophozoite after the lysis of the cell. This adhesion is facilitated by a 260 Kd Gal/GalNAc lectin consisting of 170 Kd and 35 Kd subunits.[49] The 170 Kd galactose- and N-acetylgalactosamine– inhibitable lectin has both protective and exacerbating epitopes that make attractive vaccine candidates.[50] Host-cell destruction is prevented by incubation of the parasite lectin with Gal/GalNAc, and cells that lack surface Gal/GalNAc are resistant to adherence and cytolysis.[51,52]

The 170 Kd subunit has striking immunologic similarity to the so-called beta 2 integrins, which are human cell surface glycoproteins expressed exclusively on leucocytes. Beta 2 integrins are important for various adhesive and signaling functions. The immunologic similarity between the 170 Kd subunit and the beta 2 integrins may offer an explanation for the trophozoites' ability to bind to and invade colonic epithelium,[53] as demonstrated in experiments using dominant negative mutants. The inducible expression of the lectin cytoplasmic tail interfered with the internal regulation of lectin activity and consequently decreased abscess size by 90 percent in experimental models.[54] The 170 Kd heavy subunit carbohydrate recognition domain sequence is also identical to the receptor-binding domain of hepatocyte growth factor. It competes with hepatic growth factor for binding to the c-Met hepatic growth factor receptor.[55] The parasites that have invaded human tissue can also evade destruction by the complement arm of the host immune system by lectin-mediated inhibition of assembly of the membrane attack complex.[56]

The small acidic calcium-binding protein, calmodulin, has been demonstrated to be important in the pathogenesis of several protozoa such as *Plasmodium falciparum, Trypanosoma* organisms, and *Giardia lamblia.* The 19 Kd calmodulin facilitates the secretion of collagenases contained in the electron-dense granule components, which are important in the cytotoxicity and erythrophagocytosis of *E. histolytica* trophozoites. Calmodulin inhibitors such as trifluoperazine and N-(6-aminohexyl)-5-chloro-1-naphthalene-sulfonamide inhibit cytotoxicity and growth of *E. histolytica* in a time- and concentration-dependent manner.[57]

Amoebapores are 77-residue peptides that reside inside cytoplasmic granules of the amebic trophozoite. They are structural and functional analogs of natural killer (NK)-lysin and granulysin of porcine and human cytotoxic T lymphocytes and NK cells. Amoebapores have the ability to oligomerize and form ion channels or pores in lipid membranes and thus lyse target cells when released into the contact zone.[45] The pAP-R2 transfectant of pathogenic *E. histolytica* strain HM-1:IMSS, which carries an anti-sense plasmid that specifically inhibits amoebapore synthesis, demonstrated significantly reduced virulence both in vivo and in vitro.[58]

Little is known about the host response to an acute infection except that the majority of individuals remain asymptomatic and spontaneously clear the infection.[59] Human saliva secretory IgA extracted from a pool of antiprotease-positive samples exhibited a strong in vitro inhibitory effect on *E. histolytica* proteolytic activity.[60] This suggests that the human secretory immune response may influence the outcome of intestinal amebiasis by disrupting some of the factors involved in pathogenesis, such as cysteine proteinases and lectins. The acute amebic lesions in animal models are characterized by infiltration with inflammatory cells, particularly neutrophils.[2,61,62] In vitro studies using co-culture of human epithelial and stromal cells and cell lines with trophozoites have demonstrated an increased expression and secretion of many proinflammatory cytokines and chemoattractants. These cytokines are known to govern PMN localization and function. These include IL-8, growth-related oncogene (GRO), alpha, granulocyte-macrophage colony-stimulating factor (CSF), IL-1 alpha, and IL-6 whose high level secretion is controlled by the paracrine action of cytolytically released IL-1 alpha.[63]

With immunosuppression, invasive amebiasis can be particularly severe, suggesting a role for cell-mediated immunity in limiting disease. Pregnant women in Nigeria have one of the highest incidences of colonic amebiasis,[64] and the disease is particularly fulminant in the setting of inappropriate corticosteroid use.[65,66] Infants tend to succumb rapidly to amebiasis.[65-68] Cases of symptomatic amebiasis, including hepatic abscesses, have been associated with malnutrition, a recognized immunodeficiency state.[68,69]

Patients who are receiving corticosteroids appear to also be at risk for the development of extraintestinal amebiasis or worsened amebic liver abscess lesions.[70] Other co-morbid medical conditions associated with the development of amebic liver abscess include pregnancy, hepatitis, peptic ulcer disease, and malaria. Even though T-cell–mediated immunity is an important defense mechanism against amebiasis, organ transplant recipients with pronounced T-cell depression do not appear to be at increased risk for acquisition of invasive *Entamoeba* organism infection. It may also be that such patients tend to be more careful in avoiding contaminated food and water. Nevertheless, the first report of a liver transplant patient with invasive amebiasis was treated successfully with metronidazole without modification of immunosuppressive regimen.[71]

Of importance is whether HIV infection with its attendant CD4 T-cell deficiency is a risk factor for development of extraintestinal amebiasis and hence worsened disease course.[33] During the 1970s the incidence of amebiasis increased exponentially in men who have sex with men in San Francisco over a 10-year period.[72] Other studies at that time showed that up to 40 percent of patients in a New York hospital with amebiasis were homosexual.[73-76] It appears that the homosexual lifestyle may enhance transmission but it is still unresolved if this increases the risk of amebic liver abscess formation.

Studies to date have failed to demonstrate a significant difference in other gastrointestinal symptoms between diarrheal HIV-infected patients with or without *E. histolytica* infection. This finding was reported in a series that examined the clinical course of 19 acquired autoimmune deficiency syndrome (AIDS) patients with positive *Entamoeba* isolates matched to AIDS patients whose stool culture was negative for *E. histolytica.*[77] In most patients other potential pathogens were identified. Another study of 100 homosexual patients, seronegative or seropositive for HIV, failed to detect symptomatic, microscopic, or serologic evidence of invasive amebiasis.[78,79] This benign clinical course is perhaps explained by infection with the non-pathogenic *E. dispar.* The Adult and Adolescent Spectrum of HIV Disease Project has reported that, among HIV-infected patients in the United States, the incidence of diagnosed *E. histolytica* disease was low (13.5 cases per 10,000 person-years [95 percent confidence interval, 7.7-22.2]). This diagnosis was more common in men who have sex with men, however.[80]

Clinical Manifestations

Invasive amebiasis can produce a variety of intestinal and extraintestinal manifestations. For intestinal colitis a review of 295 cases showed that 52.9 percent of patients sought medical attention within 1 week of symptom onset and 72.9 percent within 2 weeks. Nine patients in this series, however, had symptoms for longer than a year before obtaining medical intervention, with the longest duration being 12 years.[65] The clinical spectrum of intestinal disease is quite variable: *Amebic rectocolitis* is usually a milder, non-bloody diarrheal illness. Patients often complain of abdominal discomfort, colicky pain, and tenesmus but usually do not have fever or other systemic manifestations.[65,67,73,81-83] On pathology small ulcers are detected most commonly in the cecum, sigmoid colon, and rectum.[83]

Acute necrotizing colitis is a more fulminant disease.[84] Patients usually have marked constitutional and abdominal symptoms, including pain, rebound tenderness, distention, fever, anorexia, and weakness. Of these patients 0.5 percent will progress to toxic megacolon with perforation and hypovolemic hypotension, which carries a significant mortality and usually requires surgical intervention. The indications for surgical intervention include failure of resolution while on medical therapy and perforation.[85,86] Primary anastomosis is contraindicated because the bowel wall is usually highly friable. Partial or total colectomy with temporary exteriorization is the preferred approach.[85,86] On pathology there is thrombosis of the colonic wall venules with ischemia of the intestine, infarction, and tissue necrosis and a purulent peritonitis.[87]

Amebomas are rare colonic pseudotumors characterized by necrosis, granulomatous inflammation, and edema of the mucosa and submucosa of the colon. Macroscopically they are not easily distinguished from malignant colon neoplasms. Histologically neovascularity, inflammatory cells, granulation tissue, and live organisms are seen. Patients may present with multiple amebomas measuring 5 to 30 cm in diameter,[88] which on occasion may cause intussusception. Amebic appendicitis is often indistinguishable from conventional acute appendicitis but is usually preceded by a history of bloody diarrhea.

Amebic liver abscess remains the most common extraintestinal manifestation of *E. histolytica* infection.[30,89] Hepatic abscesses result from the travel of the amebae via the mesenteric-splanchnic circulation into the portal venous system. Initially, the trophozoites cause minimal sinusoidal dilation with significant infiltration by PMNs into the liver tissue (Plate 35-2). Eventually, the leukocytes undergo lysis with progressive necrosis of the surrounding parenchyma. As time progresses, extensive necrosis with minimal inflammatory reaction is noted.[36] Abscess size is variable but on average is between 5 and 15 cm in diameter. Most amebic abscesses are located in the right lobe of the liver and more often tend to be single lesions.[30,90,91] Autopsy specimens show that the lesion is well demarcated, with the liver parenchyma replaced by necrotic material that is yellowish in color with a creamy texture. In some cases the center can also be solid, bland, or semiliquid with mucus. This abscess is surrounded by congested liver tissue. Rupture is the most feared complication of a hepatic abscess. This may occur into the peritoneal cavity causing acute peritonitis, into abdominal visceral organs (stomach, duodenum, colon, biliary ducts, portal vessels), toward the retroperitoneum, and even into the thoracic cavity.[83]

Only a minority of patients with liver abscesses present with active intestinal disease. In 59 percent of cases, there is no prior history of diarrhea[92] or the diarrhea has already resolved.

A review of 400 admissions with amebic liver abscess has shown that 95 percent of patients may experience symptoms for up to 12 weeks before presentation.[82] The average duration of symptoms before presentation ranges from a few days to several weeks but typically is less than 2 to 4 weeks.[70,90,91,93] Generally, most patients will present with fever and pain in the right upper quandrant.[30] In some patients pain is referred or radiates to the right chest, epigastrium, or right shoulder. Pain is often exacerbated by cough, right lateral decubitus position, and deep inspiration. In left-sided disease the pain may radiate to the retrosternal area and to the precordium. Patients may experience weight loss, myalgias, nausea, vomiting, abdominal distention and cramping, diarrhea, or constipation. In rare cases obstructive jaundice can result from compression of the biliary system from a large liver lesion. Typically, there is tender hepatomegaly with point tenderness to palpation or intercostal tenderness with dullness to percussion at the right lung base. Some patients present with a localized swelling over the liver.[82]

Cases of hepatic liver abscesses have been classified into acute and chronic disease, benign or aggressive forms.[90] Elevation of the aspartate aminotransferase (AST) correlates with parenchymal necrosis and is the best indicator of aggressive disease. The acute form presents abruptly or over less than 10 days with fever and significant leukocytosis. In acute benign disease AST is normal, alkaline phosphatase is normal or minimally elevated, and hepatic tenderness is present but mild. In acute aggressive disease AST, serum bilirubin, and alkaline phosphatase levels are elevated, and signs of peritoneal irritation and hepatomegaly are commonly observed.[90] A more chronic presentation occurs over 2 to 12 weeks with low-grade intermittent fever, weight loss, and abdominal pain. In chronic benign disease marked leukocytosis is uncommon. Alkaline phosphatase level is often elevated, whereas AST is usually within the normal range. A chronic illness that suddenly worsened characterizes the aggressive form, with high fevers and leukocytosis and diffuse peritoneal signs. Additional laboratory values include abnormal AST and elevated alkaline phosphatase with more severe anemia.

A review of the medical history of 56 patients in San Francisco identified distinct clinical features in patients who developed amebic liver abscess after travel to an endemic area compared to controls who have lived in an endemic region. Patients with travel-related amebic complications were older, more likely to be male, and tended to have an insidious onset of illness, larger abscesses, more marked hepatomegaly, and a greater proportion of multiple, often bilateral, lesions.[30] Other rare manifestations of invasive amebiasis include peritonitis,[65,67,82,90] thoracic amebiasis, genital amebiasis,[94] cutaneous amebiasis,[67] pericarditis,[82] and brain abscesses resulting from hematogenous spread of the trophozoites.[95-97]

Differential Diagnosis

A thorough history, including travel and attention to clinical signs and symptoms, is crucial in establishing the diagnosis of invasive amebiasis. Amebic colitis needs to be distinguished from other causes of colitis, including ulcerative colitis, Crohn's disease, ischemic or pseudomembranous colitis, and tuberculosis.[98-101]

Amebic liver abscesses need to be differentiated from pyogenic abscess in many instances (Table 35-2). The most common location for a pyogenic abscess is also the right lobe of the liver and the patients are likely to be older with underlying medical conditions. A pyogenic abscess frequently presents with a palpable mass, jaundice, pruritus, sepsis, or shock. Amebic liver abscess may be confused with viral hepatitis, echinococcal infection, ascending cholangitis, *Mycobacterium tuberculosis*, cholecystitis, or appendicitis.[102-104] It is also important to exclude malignancy as a cause of the patient's complaint, in particular, hepatoma, lymphoma, primary hepatic carcinoma, or metastatic disease to the liver.[82,102,105]

Diagnostic Tests

Radiologic Imaging

Abdominal plain radiographs are of little value in the diagnosis of ulcerative amebic colitis except in the presence of a perforation.[98,106-108] Hepatomegaly on plain film may be a clue to the presence of a hepatic abscess.[109] Approximately 50 percent of patients will have an abnormal chest radiograph manifested as focal elevation of the right hemidiaphragm, pleural effusion, pneumonitis, or atelectasis of the lower lung lobes with diminished excursion of the right hemidiaphragm.[109-111] The differential

TABLE 35-2
Differentiating Characteristics of Pyogenic and Amebic Liver Abscesses

	Pyogenic abscess	Amebic abscess
Location	Right lobe predominance	Right lobe predominance
Age	More common in elderly	Peak age 20-40 yr
Gender	Equal distribution	Male predominance
Number of lesions	>50% with multiple lesions	Chronic disease: >80% with single lesion; 50% solitary abscess
Positive blood culture	Yes	No
Positive amebic serology	No	Yes
History of travel	No	Yes
Jaundice	Common	Unusual
Alcohol use	Common	Common
Diabetes mellitus	Increased incidence	No increased risk
Pruritus	Common	Unusual
Bilirubin elevation	Common	Unusual
AST elevation	Common	Unusual
Alkaline phosphatase elevation	Common	Common

AST, Aspartate aminotransferase.

diagnosis includes phrenic nerve paralysis, hepatic neoplasm, acute cholecystitis, or subphrenic abscess.

Technetium-99 sulfur colloid and dimethyl iminodiacetic acid imaging can confirm the presence of a hepatic abscess and often be helpful in excluding other hepatobiliary pathology.[112,113] The typical finding that corresponds well with computed tomography (CT) or magnetic resonance imaging (MRI) is a halo of radioactivity surrounding a photopenic or "cold defect" because amebic abscesses do not contain leukocytes.[113] In contrast, the presence of leukocytes in pyogenic abscesses creates a typically "hot" lesion on radionuclide scanning. This represents increased isotope uptake resulting from concentration within leukocytes.[114] In an analysis of 2500 cases of amebiasis by liver scanning, 4286 abscesses were detected in 3379 imaging sessions.[112] Sensitivity was somewhat dependent on the projection used but was generally comparable to ultrasound.[90] Limitations of radionuclide imaging include false-positive results caused by a prominent portal area, when the gallbladder overlies the liver, or when there is a subjective defect caused by a thin liver edge.[112]

Ultrasound is sensitive at detecting a hepatic abscess but is often not capable of differentiating amebic from pyogenic abscesses. Because sonograms are inexpensive, usually readily available, non-invasive, and useful for the diagnosis of other causes of right upper quadrant pain they are the modality of choice for initial screening.[109,112] Characteristics that are highly suggestive of amebic abscess include a peripheral location adjacent to the liver capsule, homogenous appearance, hypoechoic compared with normal liver parenchyma, rounded or oval shape, and transmission deep to the lesion.[93,95,115,116]

On CT scans amebic abscesses characteristically appear as hypodense lesions that are most often round or oval. The walls commonly enhance and the abscess may demonstrate nodular borders and internal septations.[116,117] CT scans are also helpful in distinguishing other lesions, such as hepatic cysts, solid tumors, or hemangiomas, from an abscess.[109] Major limitations include cost and potential complications of dye application to hypersensitive patients.

MRI is even more sensitive than ultrasonography or CT scan at detecting small lesions. It is incapable, however, of differentiating a pyogenic abscess from an amebic abscess. It has the disadvantage of relatively high cost, need for trained personnel, and limited availability. An MRI scan should demonstrate a homogenous hypointense signal with well-defined margins on T1-weighted imaging.[81] Depending on the internal composition of the necrotic exudates, a hyperintense signal that can appear heterogenous is seen on T2-weighted imaging.[81]

The optimal timing for follow-up imaging has not been determined. Some studies have suggested that within 6 months only one third to two thirds of amebic abscesses have resolved, depending on the initial size of the lesion.[83]

Laboratory Tests

The standard chemistry panel may reflect several abnormalities in patients with amebiasis. These include derangements in albumin, alkaline phosphatase, prothrombin time, AST, or bilirubin levels. However, these liver tests are not helpful in establishing the diagnosis or eliminating other diseases. In a study of 67 consecutive cases in San Diego alkaline phosphatase and AST levels correlated with the duration of the disease. In chronic illness the alkaline phosphatase was frequently abnormal and the AST normal, whereas the reverse was observed in acute cases. In addition, the AST level appeared predictive of severity of disease in either category of patients.[90] Another typical finding is an anemia of chronic infection whose severity is dependent on the duration of symptoms. In one series of 400 consecutive admissions of patients with amebic liver abscess 77 percent had a leukocytosis greater than 10,000/mm^3 and 63 percent had anemia lower than 12 g/100 ml hemoglobin.[82] The presence of eosinophilia is unusual in this illness.[102] The differential white count will show a predominance of PMN leukocytes with toxic granulation and band forms.[90]

Aspiration was previously the preferred modality to establish the diagnosis of amebiasis. Although it has largely been replaced by less invasive serologic testing, aspiration still has a therapeutic role if medical treatment is ineffective.[89,118,119] This is especially true if the abscess is very large (defined as a cavity size greater than 5 cm) and at risk of rupture. Because large lesions in the left lobe of the liver can potentially erode into the pericardium with devastating consequences, these abscesses are often considered for therapeutic aspiration.[115] The fluid obtained has no specific appearance and may be dirty brown, pink, reddish, or opaque. Only in a minority of cases are amebae detected in the pus.

Serologic tests have become the diagnostic procedure of choice. Circulating *E. histolytica*-specific antibodies appear approximately 7 days after the initiation of symptoms of invasive amebiasis.[120] Consequently, the failure to detect serum antibodies 7 or more days after the onset of presumptive symptoms of amebiasis virtually eliminates this infectious etiology. Several laboratory diagnostic tests are available to enable diagnosis of this parasitic disease and include indirect immunofluorescence, indirect hemagglutination (IHA), latex agglutination, enzyme-linked immunosorbent assay (ELISA), counterimmunoelectrophoresis, and agar gel diffusion,[117,121-131] which are generally positive in over 90 percent of cases.

Currently, the ELISA for the detection of the galactose-inhibitable adherence protein of *E. histolytica* is considered the most sensitive test. It is rapid, easy to perform, and fairly inexpensive. The drawback with all serologic testing has been that they do not differentiate current from past infection. They may also remain positive for many months or years after treatment and are thus of limited diagnostic value in highly endemic areas. However, Hung and colleagues have shown that in patients living in an endemic area who are also HIV-infected, IHA has a sensitivity of 72.7 percent and a specificity of 99.1 percent. In this patient population the positive predictive value for invasive amebiasis was 92.9 percent and the negative predictive value was 95.5 percent.[132]

Recombinant DNA technology has made use of the serine-rich *E. histolytica* surface protein (SREHP) to make the diagnosis of active invasive amebiasis with a sensitivity of 79 percent and a specificity of 87 percent.[133-135] Immunofluorescence using samples of fresh stool with specific monoclonal antibodies allows the differentiation between the invasive and non-invasive abilities of the parasite with a reported 100 percent correlation.[124] Immunoblot methods have been used successfully to establish the diagnosis of invasive amebiasis.[125] Also available is a home latex agglutination test for patients that have invasive intestinal amebiasis; the test is reported to have excellent concordance with serologic tests.[126] However, stool examination and stool antigen detection tests in patients with amebic liver abscess are usually negative because most will not have detectable parasites in their stools.[81]

Evangelopoulos and colleagues have developed a nested, multiplex polymerase chain reaction (PCR) assay that can be used to differentiate between *E. histolytica* and *E. dispar*.[136] The detection limit is 1000 trophozoites of *E. histolytica* or 200 trophozoites of *E. dispar* per gram of stool sample. The advantage of this methodology is that mixed infections can be demonstrated even in the presence of 20,000 trophozoites of the other species per gram of stool sample.[136]

Colonoscopy is preferred over sigmoidoscopy because disease may be localized to the cecum or ascending colon. Endoscopic examinations should be reserved for patients in whom antigen detection tests are negative or in whom a second pathology is suspected. The differential includes inflammatory bowel disease because granular, friable, pseudomembranes or ulceration may be seen and are not pathognomonic for amebiasis. Biopsy specimens are best taken from the edge of the ulcers; the organisms are detected by a magenta color with periodic acid-Schiff (PAS) staining.[137] Diagnostic confusion has resulted from *E. histolytica* trophozoites invading carcinomas.[138]

Therapy

Treatment for complicated or uncomplicated *E. histolytica* infection is well established and highly effective (Table 35-3).[139] Importantly, *E. dispar* infection does not require treatment. The asymptomatic colonization of the intestine should be treated with a luminal agent alone. Choices include iodoquinol 650 mg three times per day for 20 days or paromomycin 25-35 mg/kg per day in three doses for 7 days. Alternatively, diloxanide furoate 500 mg three times per day for 10 days is effective but is available only from the Centers for Disease Control and Prevention. It should be considered if clinical failure to iodoquinol or paromomycin is observed. Common gastrointestinal side effects of iodoquinol include nausea, vomiting, diarrhea, and abdominal cramps. It rarely causes optic neuritis and atrophy with prolonged use. It is contraindicated in patients with abnormal hepatic function or documented allergies to iodine or 8-hydroxyquinolones. Paromomycin may also cause gastrointestinal side effects. Diloxanide furoate has also been associated with nausea, vomiting, flatulence, and, rarely, diplopia.

Invasive amebiasis, whether colitis or liver abscess, should be treated with metronidazole (1-(2-hydroxyethyl)-2-methyl-5-nitroimidazole). The drug enters the cell through passive diffusion in an anaerobic or microaerophilic environment. Here it encounters ferredoxin and flavodoxin, which function as electron acceptors of pyruvate-ferredoxin oxidoreductase, hydrogenase, and other enzymes. The nitro group of metronidazole is reduced to reactive cytotoxic nitro radicals by reduced ferredoxin or flavodoxin. In vitro resistance to metronidazole is associated with decreased expression of ferredoxin and flavin reductase and increased expression of iron-containing superoxide dismutase and peroxiredoxin.[140] The recommended dosage is 750 mg three

TABLE 35-3
Treatment of Amebiasis

Syndrome	Pathogen	Therapy	Additional measures/alternatives
Asymptomatic colonization	*Entamoeba histolytica*	Paromomycin 25-35 mg/kg/day in 3 doses × 7 days Iodoquinol 650 mg tid × 10 days Diloxanide furoate 500 mg tid × 10 days	
	E. dispar	No treatment required	
Amebic colitis	*E. histolytica*	Metronidazole 750 mg tid × 10 days *or* Tinidazole 600 mg bid (or 800 mg tid) × 5 days *or* Secnidazole 500 mg tid × 5 days Followed by luminal agent	Chloroquine 600 mg q day × 2 days then 300 mg q day × 14-21 days if no response; may be substituted or added
Amebic liver abscess	*E. histolytica*	Metronidazole 750 mg tid × 10 days *or* Tinidazole 600 mg bid (or 800 mg tid) × 5 days *or* Secnidazole 500 mg tid × 5 days Followed by luminal agent	Poor response: aspirate or add chloroquine

tid, Three times per day; *q,* every; *bid,* two times per day.

times per day for 10 days. Treatment should be followed by a course of a luminal agent in the dosage used to treat asymptomatic disease. Failure to institute this luminal course has been estimated to result in relapse in approximately 10 percent of patients.[141] Metronidazole has some rare, unpleasant side effects, including nausea, vomiting, diarrhea, anorexia, abdominal discomfort, or a metallic taste. It occasionally produces a disulfiram-like reaction to alcohol. Infrequently, neurologic complications, including neuropathy, seizures, confusion, vertigo, or irritability, are observed.

Response to metronidazole is expected within 72 hours of institution of therapy; more than 90 percent of patients are expected to be cured.[102,110,142] Of all factors evaluated to predict metronidazole treatment failures, only timing of clinical response correlated with successful therapy.[102,142] For the rare patient who does not respond, alternative medical therapy or surgical options including percutaneous drainage[143] or open aspiration should be considered. Other nitroimidazoles such as tinidazole or secnidazole appear to be at least as effective as metronidazole but are better tolerated. The dosing of tinidazole is 600 mg by mouth twice per day (or 800 mg by mouth three times per day) for 5 days and secnidazole, is 500 mg by mouth three times per day for 5 days. These drugs, however, are not currently marketed in the United States. Alternatively, chloroquine base 600 mg by mouth each day for 2 days, then 300 mg by mouth each day for 14 to 21 days, can be substituted for or added to metronidazole therapy. Chloroquine alone is somewhat less effective than the nitroimidazoles.[110] Surgery is not recommended for uncomplicated hepatic amebic abscesses. Indications for surgery are rupture, impending rupture, or failure to respond after 72 hours of medical therapy.[105,144]

Prevention

Only humans and some higher non-human primates are susceptible to infection by *E. histolytica.* This suggests that an anti-amebic vaccine should theoretically be able to eradicate the organism. The feasibility of such a vaccine is corroborated by uncontrolled epidemiologic investigations demonstrating acquired immunity to amebic infection. Between 1963 and 1968 in Mexico City the hospital charts of 1021 patients cured of amebic liver abscess were reviewed. During this time only three patients were readmitted to the study hospital for recurrent abscess formation. This rate was significantly lower than the expected rate in the total population,[145] especially because these patients were considered at high risk to reacquire the disease.[146] Limitations of this study, however, include the failure to investigate admissions to other hospitals or the patients' current whereabouts.[147] Patients in hyperendemic areas with serum anti-amebic antibodies implying previous infection were also less likely to become colonized than seronegative individuals.[18,148] The level of the serum antibodies was not correlated with resistance to reinfection.

Barriers to vaccine development include insufficient understanding of the mechanisms of immunity development and the lack of a suitable animal model for the asymptomatic carrier state or amebic colitis. Vaccine development needs to target antigens that are not only conserved and highly immunogenic, but that also are inexpensive to produce.[147,149,50] Potential candidates include the Gal/GalNac lectin, the cysteine proteinases, the amoebapores, SREHP, and the 29-kDa cysteine-rich *E. histolytica* antigen. The latter two were isolated using complementary DNA libraries.[151,152] The cysteine proteinases and amoebapores have yet to be evaluated as potential vaccine components.

Until an effective human vaccine becomes available, prevention of amebiasis needs to rely on interrupting the fecal-oral spread of the cyst stage of the parasite. Contaminated water and fresh vegetables are the two major sources for acquisition of infection. Uncooked vegetables or unpeeled fruits should be washed with a detergent and then soaked in vinegar or acetic acid for 15 minutes before they are eaten.[31] Boiling water is the most definite means of neutralizing the infectivity of the cyst; low doses of chlorine or iodine are ineffective.[31,81] Improvements in waste disposal and proper water purification methods in developing countries are necessary to reduce continued spreading of infection.[153] Screening of household contacts of index cases of intestinal *E. histolytica* infection has also been recommended.

MALARIA

Background and Epidemiology

Malaria is a major public health problem in the world, accounting for 200 to 300 million cases and 3 million deaths per year.[154,155] The areas of the world affected by malaria are commonly also overwhelmed with poverty and underdevelopment. Malaria is caused by protozoan parasites of the genera *Plasmodium.*[156] The two main species that affect humans are *Plasmodium falciparum* and *Plasmodium vivax,* with *Plasmodium ovale* and *Plasmodium malariae* having regional importance. Malaria is a vectorborne disease transmitted by an arthropod. Only female mosquitos from several *Anopheles* species are capable of transmitting the disease. Certain environmental characteristics are required for the natural transmission of the disease, with tropical areas near sea level meeting all the requirements. Malaria is infrequent at altitudes higher than 1600 meters (5250 feet) because of poor adaptation of the vector. Humidity requirements are in excess of 60 percent. These factors are in part responsible for the geographic distribution of the disease.[156]

Life Cycle and Transmission

The life cycle of all human pathogenic *Plasmodium* parasites consists of two separate phases: the sporogonic phase takes place inside the vector, whereas the schizogonic phase occurs in the human host. The sporogonic cycle starts with the infection of the female anopheline mosquito after the ingestion of human blood from a patient with the disease. The life forms infectious to the mosquito are sexually differentiated and are called macrogametocytes and microgametocytes. Inside the mosquito's gut they evolve into male and female gametes that mate to form the ookinete. The ookinete invades the gut where it develops into the oocyst. Meiotic divisions create sporozoites, which travel to the salivary gland of the vector. The schizogonic cycle starts when the female mosquito bites humans, inoculating sporozoites into the blood stream via the capillary vessels of the skin. Sporozoites circulate in the blood stream for approximately 30 minutes before they penetrate hepatocytes where they form the tissue schizont (exoerythrocytic schizogony). After 6 to 12 days the deformed hepatocyte ruptures and liberates thousands of tissue merozoites, which invade erythrocytes initiating the erythrocytic schizogony. In infection caused by *P. vivax* and *P. ovale* some of the tissue forms develop very slowly and may remain silent for months (hypnozoites), which may cause late relapses of the disease. Inside the red blood cells the merozoites evolve into ring forms and then trophozoites, which multiply to form a second schizont. Schizonts lyse the erythrocytes, releasing multiple merozoites that are able to invade uninfected red blood cells and start a new erythrocytic schizogony. Some intraerythrocytic parasites, however, may alternatively differentiate into microgametocytes and macrogametocytes, which are the infectious forms for the anopheline vector.[155,156] Malaria has also been observed as the result of congenital transmission, blood transfusion, or needle sharing with blood containing merozoites. In these cases there is no exoerythrocytic schizogony and therefore hypnozoites are not formed. This condition is commonly referred to as induced malaria.

Pathogenesis and Pathology

Many of the injuries and the subsequent clinical manifestations in *P. falciparum* infection are derived from the effect of the parasite on the microvasculature. Infected erythrocytes with mature *P. falciparum* parasites have knobs that facilitate adherence to endothelial cells. Receptors in the parasite surface and the endothelial cells that are responsible for cytoadherence have been reviewed elsewhere.[155,157] Obstruction of microvasculature leads to end-organ damage. Additionally, hyperparasitemia may result in hypoglycemia (from depletion of glycogen storage secondary to fasting and consumption of glucose by the parasite), lactic acidosis, possible lipid peroxidation with generation of free radicals, and systemic inflammation secondary to the release of tumor necrosis factor (TNF) and other cytokines. These mechanisms act in concert to produce the renal, cerebral, pulmonary, hepatic, and gastrointestinal injuries seen in severe *P. falciparum* malaria.[155,157]

Anemia in malaria is a result of direct hemolysis as a consequence of the erythrocytic schizogony and of myelosuppressive effects of TNF.[155,158] Erythrocyte sequestration may also play an important role in the pathogenesis of anemia in *P. falciparum* infection.[158] Tissue section in *P. falciparum* infection may show parasitized red blood cells adherent to the microvessels, scattered ring hemorrhages, and perivascular inflammation. For further details on the interactions between malaria and the liver see the following section.

Clinical Manifestations

The main clinical manifestation of malaria is cyclic fever, which is evoked by synchronized release of merozoites into the blood stream. If synchronization is achieved patients experience fever bouts every 48 hours (tertian fever) for *P. ovale, P. vivax,* and *P. falciparum* infections, and every 72 hours (quartan fever) for *P. malariae* infection. *P. falciparum* may present also with intermittent fevers. The febrile episode (fever paroxysm) is usually preceded by shaking chills and followed by severe diaphoresis and fatigue. Other non-specific signs and symptoms include nausea, vomiting, cough, tachycardia, headache, backache, hepatosplenomegaly, and abdominal pain. Patients with flu-like illness returning from endemic areas should be investigated for malaria. Malaise, fatigue, and anorexia may be the result of anemia. In general, clinical manifestations of tourists and expatriates are much more severe than those seen in residents of malarious areas.[155,156,158] Severe *P. falciparum* malaria can present with a variety of clinical manifestations. These include, but are not limited to, central nervous system (CNS) complications, respiratory distress, renal failure, and occasionally liver failure (see the following section). Malaria has also been linked with chronic clinical syndromes such as the hyperactive malarial splenomegaly (HMS) syndrome, previously referred to as tropical splenomegaly syndrome, nephrotic syndrome, and Burkitt's lymphoma.[158]

Diagnostic Tests

Findings of hemolytic anemia (e.g., increased low-density lipoprotein [LDH], low haptoglobin, reticulocyte response) are commonly detected. Laboratory abnormalities resulting from end-organ damage can also be present in patients with falciparum malaria (e.g., increased blood urea nitrogen and creatinine, hypoglycemia, lactic acidosis, thrombocytopenia, hypoxemia, increased liver enzymes).

The classic method used for the diagnosis of malaria is to test thin and thick smears of peripheral blood. The thick smear is more sensitive but requires more expertise. Because of significant differences in prognosis and therapy, it is important to exactly determine the species of *Plasmodium* responsible for infection. Clues to identify *P. falciparum* include presence of small ring forms, presence of banana-shaped gametocytes, high-level parasitemias, presence of multiple-infected red blood cells, absence of schizonts, and infection of normal-size erythrocytes.[158] Determining the level of parasitemia has prognostic and therapeutic implications. New rapid or more sensitive tests for the diagnosis of malaria have been developed but are still quite expensive or not widely available. These techniques include ELISAs for histidine-rich protein 2 or parasite lactate dehydrogenase, DNA hybridization, and DNA and RNA amplification.[155,159,160]

Treatment and Prevention

P. vivax, P. ovale, P. malariae, and chloroquine-susceptible *P. falciparum* are treated with chloroquine 600 mg base initially, followed by 300 mg doses 6 hours later and on days 2 and 3. The therapy of choice for chloroquine-resistant *P. falciparum* is quinine 650 mg by mouth every 8 hours for 3 to 7 days, plus doxycycline 100 mg by mouth twice per day for 7 days. Other medications active against chloroquine-resistant *P. falciparum* include sulfadoxine-pyrimethamine, clindamycin, mefloquine, halofantrine, atovaquone, and artesunate.[139] Areas suspicious for chloroquine-resistant *P. falciparum* include all endemic areas except Central America west of the Panama Canal, and the Caribbean. For patients with severe disease and those unable to tolerate oral medications, parenteral therapy with intravenous quinine or quinidine is indicated. If available, arthemether is a viable alternative. After patients have completed therapy for *P. vivax* and *P. ovale,* a course of primaquine must be administered to prevent relapses resulting from activation of hypnozoites, except in cases of "induced malaria."

Despite ongoing research, an effective malaria vaccine is not yet available. Therefore prevention relies on basic measures such as vector control, use of insecticide-impregnated mosquito nets, appropriate clothing, insect repellents, elimination of collections of standing water, and chemoprophylaxis. Chloroquine is recommended for prophylaxis of people traveling to areas endemic for chloroquine-sensitive *P. falciparum.* For those traveling to areas with chloroquine-resistant *P. falciparum* mefloquine is recommended. Chemoprophylaxis with chloroquine or mefloquine should commence 1 week before and continue for 4 weeks after traveling to an endemic area. Doxycycline or chloroquine plus proguanil are other alternatives.[139] Recently the combination of atovaquone and proguanil (Malarone) was approved in the United States for the treatment and prevention of *P. falciparum* malaria. It is a safe and effective drug combination but it is also more expensive than other regimens.[161]

Malaria and the Liver

It is important to recognize that the liver is the primary target organ in the life cycle of the parasite after a mosquito bite.[162,163] In 1948 Shortt and Garham[164] elucidated the hepatocyte stage of the life cycle, and in 1980 Krotoski and colleagues were the first to demonstrate the hypnozoite stage of the *P. vivax* infection.[165] The mechanisms by which malaria sporozoites invade the liver after injection into the blood stream by the female anopheline mosquito are only partially elucidated.[162,163,166,167] In vitro culture of exo-erythrocytic stages in human embryonic cells (WI38) and hepatoma cells (HepG2-A16) has been possible since the early 1980s.[163] This has allowed for intensive research into the interactions between hepatocyte and sporozoite. Some evidence suggests that sporozoites are initially trapped by Kupffer cells and then transported to hepatocytes. Others have provided evidence supporting the hypothesis that sporozoites home to hepatocytes directly. The major surface protein of malaria sporozoites, the circumsporozoite (CS) protein, has been shown to bind to heparan sulfate proteoglycans on the surface of hepatocytes.[166,167] Thrombospondin-related adhesive protein and sporozoite surface protein 2 are other sporozoite proteins likely to be involved in hepatocyte invasion, binding to hepatocytes in a fashion similar to that of the CS protein.[167] Although the hepatocyte is a crucial component in the early plasmodial life cycle, this is not associated with significant morphologic or functional changes.[162] Overt clinical disease is therefore not observed during this phase. Later, however, the liver can become acutely and chronically affected in patients with malaria (Plate 35-3). This is not the result of the exoerythrocytic schizogony mentioned previously, but mainly is secondary to the activation of the reticuloendothelial system by plasmodial organisms and significant reductions in hepatic blood flow in severe, complicated *P. falciparum* infection.[162,168] When the hepatic and splenic reticulo-endothelial system is activated parasites, parasitized erythrocytes, and malaria pigment (hemozoin; Plate 35-4) are phagocytized.[158,162,163] Reduction of hepatic blood flow is a multi-factorial process, including sympathetic overactivity and endothelial sequestration of infected erythrocytes causing mechanical obstruction.[158,162] In severe cases this may result in significant centrolobular necrosis. Hepatomegaly is observed in about 60 percent of patients with falciparum or vivax malaria[169] and is often associated with splenomegaly. The hyperreactive malarial splenomegaly seen in some individuals living in endemic areas is also frequently accompanied by significant hepatomegaly.[170] Although jaundice is common it is usually the consequence of hemolysis.[162,171] In chronic or severe cases falciparum malaria can mimic liver failure with jaundice (with a significant component of conjugated hyperbilirubinemia in chronic stages), marked elevation of transaminases and alkaline phosphatase, prolonged prothrombin time, hypoalbuminemia, hypoglycemia, lactic acidosis, encephalopathy, and renal failure.[156,162,172,173] Hepatitis with mild elevations of transaminases, alkaline phosphatase, and γ-glutamyl transpeptidase is observed frequently in patients infected with other plasmodium species.[174]

Despite initial concerns regarding a proposed link between malaria and chronic hepatitis, cirrhosis, or hepatoma, aside from the hepatosplenomegaly observed in HMS, there is no conclusive evidence of long-term sequelae after malaria infection.[162,175] Liver impairment can also be the consequence of anti-malaria medications. Amodiaquine, sulfadoxine-pyrimethamine, quinine, and mefloquine have been responsible for overt liver toxicity or hepatic laboratory abnormalities. Chloroquine and primaquine may interfere with hepatic drug metabolism.[162,163,176]

Finally, the hepatic phase of the malaria parasite life cycle appears to be essential for the induction of protection against the exo-erythrocytic stage of infection; therefore, much current effort is focused on developing malaria vaccines targeting exo-erythrocytic parasites.[177-179] It appears that non-parenchymal liver cells are crucial for the development of cellular immune response.[179] A specific protein called liver-stage antigen 1 is known to be expressed during the liver phase and may contribute to protective immunity; it therefore has been considered as a vaccine candidate.[177]

TOXOPLASMOSIS

Background and Epidemiology

Toxoplasma gondii is a protozoan parasite with three main life stages[180]:

1. Oocyst (containing sporozoites)
2. Tissue cyst (containing bradyzoites)
3. Tachyzoite

The oocysts are formed in the small intestine of felines and are excreted in the feces of these animals. Tissue cysts are the result of intracellular replication and encystation that occurs in different tissues. The tachyzoite, which has a crescentic form, multiplies rapidly inside the host's cells, causing cell disruption and cell death; their presence is the hallmark of active infection. Conversion from one stage to another has been observed. Tachyzoites can evolve into cyst-forming bradyzoites and vice versa, according to the immune status of the host.

A large proportion of the world's population is infected with *T. gondii.* In many areas of the world, seropositivity reaches 60 percent to 70 percent and may be as high as 90 percent in selected areas.[180-183] Seroprevalence studies have generally shown that seropositivity rates correlate with age. Even though *T. gondii* is not a common cause of disease in immunocompetent individuals, it is a significant cause of morbidity and mortality when it affects immunodeficient patients or pregnant women. The definite hosts are cats and other felines, in which the full life cycle of *T. gondii* can be completed. Many other animals can serve as intermediate hosts, including herbivorous, omnivorous, and carnivorous animals. Soil can serve as an environmental reservoir because of the ability of the oocysts to remain viable for many months. Coprophagous invertebrates (e.g., flies, cockroaches) can act as transport hosts for the oocyst.[180]

Life Cycle and Transmission

The definitive host can ingest oocysts from the soil, tachyzoites from tissues of animals with active infection, or cysts from tissues of animals with latent infection.[181] Once inside the gut of the feline, all of the parasite stages evolve into an enteroepithelial phase, during which sexual reproduction takes place, with the production of different life forms, including tachyzoites and oocysts. Tachyzoites migrate outside the gut and produce remote tissue involvement. Oocysts are shed in feces. Oocysts sporulate in the environment and are ingested by intermediate or definitive hosts. Intermediate hosts can also become infected when ingesting cysts contained in tissues of affected animals. After oocysts or tissue cysts are ingested by intermediate hosts, they become tachyzoites, which have the ability to invade any cell type, and travel with lymph, blood, or inside blood or immune cells to various organs. In the target tissues the tachyzoites can cause further damage or can become bradyzoites contained inside cysts.

Humans become infected mainly by the ingestion of oocysts or tissue cysts. Oocyst-mediated infection is more common in young children as a result of ingestion of contaminated food or soil. Tissue-cyst mediated infection seems to be more common in countries in which the ingestion of raw meat is a common practice (e.g., France). Infected pork may be one of the major sources of infection in humans, much more than ingestion of lamb, beef, or poultry. Infection can be transmitted congenitally when tachyzoites invade the placenta. Less common mechanisms of transmission include transplantation of an infected organ,[184,185] transfusion of contaminated blood, inoculation as a result of a needle stick injury, or exposure of open wounds or mucosal surfaces to the parasite.[180,181,186]

Pathogenesis and Pathology

T. gondii multiplies intracellularly in the gastrointestinal tract. Tachyzoites travel to different organs with blood, lymph, or blood cells, where they trigger inflammatory responses and tissue injury responsible for the clinical manifestations of acute infection. Because a competent host's immune response is capable of controlling parasite proliferation the parasite's phenotype is switched to bradyzoite with formation of tissue cysts in various organs. It is believed that interferon γ and nitric oxide are important triggers for the conversion of tachyzoites to bradyzoites.[180,187,188] In the absence of an adequate immune response tachyzoites continue to proliferate and invade, causing significant tissue damage, largely via direct cell destruction but, in part, secondary to vascular involvement with subsequent coagulation necrosis. Autopsies of adults with active infection have shown lymphadenitis, chorioretinitis, pneumonitis, focal hepatitis, myocarditis, myositis, and encephalitis associated with tachyzoites and few cysts. Lymph node biopsies show reactive germinal centers, histiocyte infiltration of the germinal center, and sinus distention by monocytoid B cells.[180] Liver biopsies show acute, generalized hepatitis with necrosis of hepatocytes and infiltration by lymphocytes, histiocytes, and granulocytes. Staining with specific antibodies may demonstrate the parasite. Granuloma formation has been observed but is rare.[189,190] Recrudescent lesions show a significant number of tachyzoites in target-like focal lesions.[181] Congenital toxoplasmosis produces multi-organ involvement, but in autopsy either central nervous lesions or generalized lesions predominate.[181] Mononuclear inflammatory reaction and tachyzoites at the periphery of the lesions can be detected in the liver, lungs, and heart. Liver histology may show giant cell hepatitis and extramedullary hematopoiesis.

Clinical Manifestations

The clinical spectrum of toxoplasmosis is quite variable and dependent on the host's immunocompetence. Toxoplasmosis can be categorized as follows: (1) infection in the immunocompetent patient, (2) infection in the immunodeficient patient, (3) infection in pregnancy, and (4) congenital infection.

Most immunocompetent patients with toxoplasmosis are asymptomatic. The most common presentation is asymptomatic cervical lymphadenopathy. Other clinical syndromes seen in immunocompetent individuals include a mononucleosis-like syndrome, *Toxoplasma* chorioretinitis, and rarely, severe disseminated disease with myocarditis, pneumonitis, hepatitis, and encephalitis (with clinical manifestations predominating in one or more organs). Hepatosplenomegaly is present in the mononucleosis-like syndrome, and hepatomegaly can be found in patients with toxoplasmosis hepatitis as the predominant target organ in cases of disseminated disease.[180,186,189,190] In a study in Atlanta 11 percent of a group of 37 patrons of a riding stable with acute acquired toxoplasmosis had hepatitis.[191] Jaundice may be noted by the patient or in the physical exam.[189]

In contrast with immunocompetent patients, immunodeficient individuals often have severe, life-threatening disease. Patients with organ transplants or underlying malignancies can present with serious CNS disease, myocarditis, and pneumonitis as a result of newly acquired or reactivated *T. gondii* infection.[180] Disseminated toxoplasmosis and chorioretinitis have been described after liver transplantation.[184,185] In patients with AIDS the most common clinical syndromes produced by *T. gondii* are encephalitis, pneumonitis, and chorioretinitis.[183,192] Acute hepatic failure, although very uncommon, has been reported.[192,193] *T. gondii* infection in pregnancy has been implicated in spontaneous abortion, stillbirth, and premature births.[180]

Congenital toxoplasmosis can result from acute infection or reactivated infection of a pregnant woman. The infection is transmitted more frequently when the mother is infected in the third trimester. The disease in the newborn, however, tends to be more severe if the infection is acquired in the first or second trimester. Infection transmitted in early pregnancy usually produces disseminated involvement, with retinitis, brain involvement, intracranial calcifications, lymphadenopathy, and hepatosplenomegaly.[180,181,186] Infection late in pregnancy usually produces more protracted clinical manifestations, mainly chorioretinitis that can manifest years after infection.

Diagnostic Tests

Routine laboratory tests may show a low white blood cell count, lymphocytosis, and monocytosis. Anemia may be present in patients with prolonged illness. In cases with hepatic involvement elevated transaminases are detected, sometimes exceeding 2000 IU/ml,[189,190,193] and hyperbilirubinemia. Patients with muscle involvement will have elevated creatine phosphokinase levels. LDH is usually markedly elevated in AIDS patients with disseminated disease.[183,192] Radiologic studies are particularly useful in patients with encephalitis, in whom a presumptive diagnosis can be made by the combination of the clinical presentation and the radiologic findings.[180] Delayed-type hypersensitivity responses reflected by positive skin test to toxoplasma antigen have been useful in epidemiologic studies but have largely been replaced by sensitive serologic tests.[181,186] Serologic tests are the primary diagnostic test. The Sabin-Feldman dye test is specific and sensitive and is considered the gold standard. It primarily detects IgG antibodies quantified by dilution. The test is no longer readily available in many laboratories because of the requirement for live organisms. ELISA tests are used to detect IgM or IgG antibodies with good sensitivity and specificity. The modified agglutination test incorporating mercaptoethanol is simple, accurate, and inexpensive. Indirect fluorescent antibody (IFA) tests are also widely used, with acceptable sensitivity and specificity compared to the dye test and with the ability to detect IgM antibodies in acute infections. IgM enzyme-linked immunosorbent agglutination assay is more sensitive for acute infection than are IgM ELISA and IgM-IFA.[180,186]

Recent developments have allowed the application of the PCR technique for the diagnosis of toxoplasmosis. PCR can be done in different body fluids and tissues, including cerebrospinal fluid, amniotic fluid, fluid from broncho-alveolar lavage, intraocular samples, and even blood. In particular, PCR has revolutionized the diagnosis of intrauterine toxoplasmosis.[180,194] Definitive demonstration of the parasite can be performed by histologic examination of tissue samples or body fluids or by isolation of the parasite by mouse inoculation or tissue cell cultures.[180,186,192,193]

Treatment and Prevention

Immunocompetent patients should receive therapy when visceral disease is present and when symptoms are severe or persistent. Disease acquired by transfusion of blood products or as a result of laboratory accidents should also be treated given the more severe course that usually follows these types of transmissions. Pregnant women and babies with congenital infection should be treated as well. Immunocompromised individuals always require therapy. The decision whether to treat ocular toxoplasmosis depends on the size and number of the lesions, the degree of associated vitreous inflammation, the duration of active disease, and the acuity of the infection.[180]

The therapy of choice for toxoplasmosis is the combination of pyrimethamine and sulfadiazine. The usual regimens for adults are pyrimethamine 75 mg for 3 days followed by 25 to 50 mg/day for 2 to 4 weeks, combined with sulfadiazine 500 mg four times daily. Folinic acid is given to prevent or treat the bone marrow toxicity resulting from pyrimethamine. Other antimicrobials active against *T. gondii* include trimethoprim-sulfamethoxazole, clindamycin, clarithromycin, spiramycin, azithromycin, atovaquone, and dapsone. Treatment of infection in immunocompromised patients requires prolonged therapy, lasting usually more than 6 months. In AIDS patients with *Toxoplasma* encephalitis the doses required are higher and initial duration is 3 to 6 weeks at full dose, followed by maintenance therapy with lower doses or alternative regimens. Pregnant women have been traditionally treated with spiramycin. Because spiramycin does not cross the placenta, pyrimethamine and sulfadiazine should be used if fetal infection is documented. Fetal infection diagnosed at a gestational age of less than 12 to 14 weeks is treated with sulfadiazine alone. Congenital infections are treated for a minimum of 12 months.[180,181,186]

Prevention is very important for pregnant women and immunodeficient patients. It is based on education of the patients and their families about mechanisms of transmission. Feeding habit modification, vector control, and pet and personal hygiene are recommended. Primary prophylaxis of HIV patients is effective and can be achieved with trimethoprim-sulfamethoxazole. Serologic screening may be important in pregnant women and before transfusion of blood products to toxoseronegative immunodeficient patients.[180]

Summary of Toxoplasmosis and the Liver

Liver transplantation has uncommonly resulted in the transmission of toxoplasmosis. *Toxoplasma* infection produces focal hepatitis associated with tachyzoites and few cysts (Plate 35-5), and tissue sections may reveal acute, generalized hepatitis with hepatocyte necrosis and infiltration by lymphocytes, histiocytes, and granulocytes. Granulomas can be seen infrequently. Recrudescent lesions show multiple tachyzoites in a target-like focal pattern. Liver tissue in congenital toxoplasmosis shows mononuclear cell inflammation with tachyzoites at the periphery of the lesions and extramedullary hematopoiesis. In the immunocompetent host toxoplasmosis can present as hepatitis, with hepatomegaly, jaundice, and non-specific symptoms. Hepatosplenomegaly can be seen in patients with the mononucleosis-like syndrome and in disseminated toxoplasmosis affecting multiple organs. Disseminated toxoplasmosis and chorioretinitis have been described after liver transplant. Acute hepatic failure uncommonly can be seen in patients with AIDS and toxoplasmosis.

AMERICAN TRYPANOSOMIASIS

Background and Epidemiology

American trypanosomiasis, or Chagas' disease, is caused by the protozoan parasite *Trypanosoma cruzi*. American trypanosomiasis is endemic in all countries of the Americas from the southwestern United States to Argentina and Chile. The majority of cases are reported from central and southern Brazil, but the highest seroprevalence is found in Bolivia. About one quarter of the population in Latin America is considered at risk.[195] It is estimated that 16 to 18 million people are currently infected with *T. cruzi*. Up to 45,000 people die of Chagas' disease each year.[196]

Life Cycle and Transmission

The invertebrate host and vector is a reduviid bug of the triatome species (*Rhodnius prolixus* and *Triatoma infestans*), better known as kissing the bug.[197] The vertebrate hosts are humans and multiple wild and domestic mammals.[195,197] The parasite passes through different morphologic stages known as epimastigote, amastigote, and trypomastigote during its cycle in vertebrate and invertebrate hosts.[197]

The insects become infected by sucking blood from the vertebrate hosts carrying trypomastigotes. Once inside the gut of the bug the parasites multiply and change morphology, becoming epimastigotes and then metacyclic trypomastigotes that are discharged with defecation when the insect takes a blood meal from another vertebrate host. Humans (and other mammals) become infected when the metacyclic trypomastigotes present in the feces of the insect penetrate a break in the skin or intact mucous membranes to infect local tissue histiocytes. Inside the cell, the parasite evolves into an amastigote, which multiplies several times until the cell ruptures and releases many trypomastigotes into the lymphatic and systemic circulation that can reach and invade other tissue cells or can be ingested by a reduviid bug to initiate a new cycle.[195,197]

Aside from vector-borne transmission, *T. cruzi* can be transmitted through blood transfusions,[195,198] with organ transplants, congenitally,[199] or after laboratory accidents.[200] Outbreaks of disease after ingestion of food contaminated with insect feces have been described in Brazil.[195]

Pathogenesis and Pathology

After intracellular reproduction and release of parasites at the port of entry, local inflammation associated with a mixed cellular, predominantly lymphoplasmocytotic infiltrate. This may give rise to the formation of an inoculation granuloma, also known as "chagoma." When the inflammation extends to the regional lymphatics, obstruction with significant interstitial edema may ensue. Via lymph and blood, the parasites reach other tissue cells (e.g., reticulo-endothelial cells, myocytes) and cause cell destruction by rupture after reproduction and by elicitation of inflammatory responses that damage infected and non-infected cells. The organs showing the most marked pathology are the heart, brain, and liver. Marked inflammation and focal hemorrhage can be observed in affected hearts. Brain and meninges may show congestion and petechiae and, occasionally, small inflammatory foci containing parasites. The liver is usually enlarged. Fatty degeneration is common and parasites can be detected inside Kupffer cells.[195,201] It seems possible that some strains have preferential tropism for certain tissues and therefore produce different clinical and pathologic pictures.[202-204]

After the acute phase patients enter an indeterminate phase in which immune responses are able to limit parasitemia and patients remain asymptomatic. The immune response to *T. cruzi* is complex. Initially the parasite is resistant to the alternate complement pathway, but after antibodies develop the parasite becomes sensitive to the classic complement pathway. Cellular responses are also important and interferon γ is instrumental in activating macrophages capable of killing intracellular amastigotes. Immune-suppressive cytokines such as IL-10 and transforming growth factor beta are believed to play a role in disease progression.[195]

During the chronic phase chronic inflammation and fibrosis predominate. The organs most severely affected are the heart and the gastrointestinal tract. Although the parasite load is significantly lower than during the acute phase, parasites and parasite DNA have repeatedly been detected in chronically affected organs. The heart suffers dilation, thinning of the walls, and formation of apical aneurysms. The conduction system is also affected. As a result, heart failure and arrhythmias develop. The liver is affected during this stage by passive congestion, as in other forms of heart failure. Secondary inflammation of the intestinal walls with consecutive denervation megasyndromes may develop in the gastrointestinal system.[195,197,201]

Clinical Manifestations

Most acute infections are asymptomatic. The acute syndromes can follow any mode of transmission after an incubation period of 7 to 14 days. This includes inoculation granulomas or chagomas, as mentioned previously (observed in approximately 50 percent of patients after vector-transmitted disease), or the Romaña sign (characterized by unilateral bipalpebral edema secondary to interstitial edema after conjunctival inoculation of the parasite). One fifth of the infected patients experience a nonspecific syndrome that is variable in severity and characterized by fever, malaise, adenopathy, and hepatosplenomegaly. Approximately 5 percent of infected patients develop early severe disease characterized by acute myocarditis or meningoencephalitis.[195,197,201]

The indeterminate phase is usually asymptomatic and on average lasts 10 years.[201] The chronic phase is characterized by evolving cardiomyopathy with heart failure, conduction system disturbances, or the megasyndromes—most commonly mega-esophagus or megacolon. It is worth mentioning that patients in the indeterminate or chronic phase may relapse into a more acute disease if they suffer immunosuppression (e.g., post-transplant, cytotoxic therapy, AIDS).

Diagnostic Tests

Routine tests during the acute phase can show mild anemia, initial leukocytosis followed by leukopenia with a relative increase of mononuclear cells. Modest elevations of liver and muscle enzymes are common. Non-specific electrocardiogram changes can be observed, as can varying degrees of cardiomegaly on chest x-ray.[195,201] The diagnosis of Chagas' disease can be established by microbiologic test or immunodiagnostic assays, or with the use of molecular techniques. Microbiologic tests are the mainstay of the diagnosis of acute disease. They include wet preparations of anti-coagulated blood or buffy coat, Giemsa stains of thin and thick smears, xenodiagnostic tests (in which uninfected laboratory bugs feed on the affected patient), culture of blood or other clinical specimens using special media, or animal inoculation. Only the first two tests are clinically used because the others require much more time before yielding results. Overall the sensitivities of these tests are low (50 percent or less). Therefore new molecular techniques are becoming increasingly useful to establish the diagnosis.

Immunodiagnostic assays are useful for the diagnosis of indeterminate and chronic Chagas' disease. IgG antibodies can be detected using different methods (i.e., IFA, complement fixation, ELISA). A drawback of these tests is the relative low specificity.

Molecular techniques have been developed in response to the need for better tests for the confirmation of both acute and chronic Chagas' disease.[195] Studies using PCR-based techniques report increased sensitivity and specificity in acute and chronic infection.[205] This complex technology, however, may not be available in the developing countries in which Chagas' disease is endemic.[197,205]

Treatment and Prevention

Two drugs are considered effective for the specific therapy of Chagas' disease. Nifurtimox, at a dose of 10 mg/kg/day in four divided doses for 3 to 4 months, is somewhat effective in the majority of cases but side effects are common (mainly gastrointestinal and neurologic). Benznidazol at a dose of 5 mg/kg/day for 2 months is also effective, with adverse events that include neuropathy, rash, and granulocytopenia.[197,206,207] An international panel of experts recently recommended that all *T. cruzi*-infected patients be treated with either of these medications regardless of their clinical status or the time elapsed since infection. Some of the new azoles may be effective in the therapy of Chagas' disease but they are not yet available. Interferon γ has been a used as adjuvant therapy and may be particularly helpful in patients with immunosuppression.[197]

Non-specific treatment modalities include supportive therapy for heart failure, arrhythmias, and gastrointestinal disease. Prevention involves avoiding dilapidated dwellings, use of insect repellent, and mosquito nets in endemic areas and safety measures for laboratory personnel and blood banks.

Summary of American Trypanosomiasis and the Liver

Hepatosplenomegaly is not uncommon in the acute phase of Chagas' disease and is mainly the result of interstitial edema, fatty degeneration, inflammatory cell, parasitic infiltration of the parenchyma, and activation of the reticulo-endothelial system. During the acute phase elevated liver enzymes are common. During the chronic phase of Chagas' disease, the liver is involved through chronic passive congestion secondary to heart failure. Reactivation of acute Chagas' disease after immunosuppression has been documented in patients with HIV infection or after solid organ transplantation. Nevertheless, *T. cruzi* infection is not considered a contraindication to organ transplantation. Periodic monitoring for signs and symptoms of the disease, however, is mandatory in such cases.[197,208]

AFRICAN TRYPANOSOMIASIS

Background and Epidemiology

African trypanosomiasis, or sleeping sickness, is caused by two subspecies of a protozoan parasite: *Trypanosoma brucei rhodesiense* and *Trypanosoma brucei gambiense*. They are endemic in sub-Saharan areas of southeast and west central Africa, respectively. Approximately 50 million individuals are at risk for acquiring the disease and thousands of new cases occur each year.[209,210] This distribution is determined by the interaction of humans with the invertebrate hosts and the vectors of the disease, flies of the genus *Glossina*—better known as tsetse flies. The gambiense subspecies only uses humans as their vertebrate host whereas, other hosts such as antelope and cattle may act as reservoirs for the rhodesiense subspecies.

Life Cycle and Transmission

The tsetse fly becomes infected when taking a blood meal from a vertebrate host with circulating trypomastigotes. Inside the gut of the insect trypomastigotes transform into procyclic trypomastigotes that multiply and migrate to the salivary glands. Here they differentiate into epimastigotes that transform into metacyclic trypomastigotes.

Humans become infected when the metacyclic trypomastigotes are released into salivary secretions and injected during an insect bite. The trypomastigotes go on to multiply in the blood and other tissues.[209,210] Very rarely the parasite is transmitted via blood transfusions, congenitally, or as a result of a laboratory accident.

Pathogenesis and Pathology

After inoculation the parasites multiply in the interstitium and produce an acute inflammatory lesion characterized by edema, tissue destruction, and intense mononuclear reaction. This may give rise to a clinically apparent inoculation chancre. Subsequently the parasites travel to regional lymph nodes, where they proliferate and cause further inflammation. Through the lymphatics they reach the blood stream, where multiplication continues, and eventually enter interstitial spaces in other tissues. When the CNS is invaded the ensuing inflammation causes meningoencephalitis or meningomyelitis. Heart, spleen, and systemic lymph nodes are also frequently affected. Serositis and liver involvement have also been documented. Histology characteristically shows mononuclear infiltration (including lymphocytes and plasma cells including characteristically vacuolated plasma cells, the so-called morular cells), nests of organisms, and varying degrees of fibrosis.[209,210]

Immune response to African trypanosomes includes cellular and humoral responses, but the parasite has developed sophisticated strategies to evade attacks by the immune system. During multiplication trypanosomes undergo antigenic variations in their surface glycoproteins,[210] allowing for ongoing proliferation for prolonged periods.

High levels of circulating antigen-antibody complexes are uniformly present. These may play a major role in some of the clinical and laboratory abnormalities observed, including anemia, tissue damage, and increased intravascular permeability.[209]

Clinical Manifestations

The clinical picture of *Trypanosoma brucei gambiense* is characterized by an early and a late stage, which may last months to years, whereas *T. brucei rhodesiense* is a much more acute disease, lasting 1 to 3 months. Lymphadenopathy is more prominent in gambiense trypanosomiasis, whereas visceral complications are more pronounced in rhodesiense trypanosomiasis.

Initially, an inoculation chancre may develop 1 to 2 weeks after the insect bite. Chancres are more frequently observed in rhodesiense trypanosomiasis. This is followed by the hemolymphatic stage in which patients experience intermittent fevers, lymphadenopathy, headaches, malaise, and fatigue. Most patients develop cervical lymphadenopathy (including the characteristic Winterbottom's sign when the posterior cervical lymph nodes are involved). Some patients develop splenomegaly but hepatomegaly is rare. Pruritus, edema, and rashes are other manifestations during this stage of the illness.

The meningoencephalitic stage is characterized by personality and mental status changes and progressive daytime somnolence. Extrapyramidal signs and ataxia are frequent. CNS involvement often progresses to coma and death. In rhodesiense trypanosomiasis hemolymphatic and meningoencephalitic stages are usually more severe and often occur simultaneously.

Diagnostic Tests

Routine laboratory tests usually show a normocellular anemia with reticulocytosis, thrombocytopenia, leukocytosis, an elevated erythrocyte sedimentation rate, and occasionally disseminated intravascular coagulation.[209] Hyperbilirubinemia and elevated transaminases and alkaline phosphatase levels are seen in both types of African trypanosomiasis, but are usually more severe in Rhodesian trypanosomiasis. Hepatic involvement can be significant and may present remarkably similarly to viral hepatitides.[211-213] Other laboratory abnormalities include hypergammaglobulinemia; presence of heterophile, antinuclear, and anti-DNA antibodies; and positive rheumatoid factors. Anti-liver antibodies have been found in a significant proportion of vertebrate hosts infected with African trypanosomiasis.[214] CSF analysis during the meningoencephalitic phase is characterized by increased protein, a predominantly mononuclear pleocytosis, vacuolated plasmocytes ("morular" cells), and eosinophils.[209] A definite diagnosis can be established using microbiologic or immunodiagnostic tests. Microbiologic tests are based on the identification of the parasite in clinical specimens (e.g., fluid from chancre, lymph nodes, CSF, ascitic fluid, blood, buffy coat smears, bone marrow aspiration) using Giemsa stain. At least in Rhodesian trypanosomiasis, laboratory animals (i.e., mice, rats) can be inoculated, resulting in parasitemia 1 to 2 weeks later.[209] Serologic tests are available but they have varying degrees of sensitivity and specificity and are mainly used for epidemiologic purposes. Agglutination methods are also available. The role of PCR is currently undergoing evaluation.[209]

Treatment and Prevention

Suramine and eflornithine are effective for the hemolymphatic stage of sleeping sickness. Because of its widespread availability pentamidine has emerged as an attractive alternative. Eflornithine is also effective for the treatment of patients with the meningoencephalitic stage of gambiense trypanosomiasis. Alternatively these patients may be treated with a combination of the organic arsenical tryparsamide and suramine. The only available treatment for the meningoencephalitic stage of Rhodesian trypanosomiasis is the highly toxic organic arsenic melarsoprol. Prevention has focused on the control of the vector and therapy of affected humans. Humans can reduce the risk of becoming infected by avoiding areas known to harbor vectors, using appropriate clothing and insect repellent. Chemoprophylaxis is not an option because of the toxicity of the available agents. A vaccine is not currently available.[209]

Summary of African Trypanosomiasis and the Liver

During the hemolymphatic stage of African trypanosomiasis, hepatomegaly is observed occasionally. The clinical and laboratory picture can be confused with viral hepatitis. Liver involvement with mononuclear infiltration, nests of organisms, and varying degrees of fibrosis can be demonstrated in histologic specimens. Hypergammaglobulinemia is a constant feature of the disease, and anti-liver antibodies are not uncommonly detected. The detection of the primary biliary cirrhosis (PBC) antigen has led to speculations regarding the role of parasitic organisms in the etiology of PBC.[215]

VISCERAL LEISHMANIASIS (KALA-AZAR)

Background and Epidemiology

Visceral leishmaniasis is a chronic disease caused by protozoa of the genus *Leishmania.* It is also known by the Hindi expression *kala-azar,* meaning "black sickness."[216] The three most common species causative of human visceral disease are *Leishmania donovani* (India), *Leishmania infantum* (Mediterranean coast, China, Middle East, and Africa), and *Leishmania chagasi* (South America). The organism has an oval amastigote stage in the reticulo-endothelial cells of the vertebrate host and an elongated flagellated promastigote stage in the gut of the invertebrate host. The global annual incidence of visceral leishmaniasis has been estimated at more than 100,000 cases per year.[216] In the past two decades the disease has received increased attention because of several large epidemics and its emergence as an opportunistic disease in immunocompromised patients (e.g., HIV, post-transplant).[217-221] The epidemiology depends on the interaction of sandflies, reservoir hosts, and susceptible humans. The vectors of the disease are phlebotomine sandflies of the genera *Phlebotomus* in the Old World and *Lutzomyia* in the New World. In some areas of the world other vertebrate hosts including dogs, foxes, jackals, and rodents serve as reservoirs.[216]

Life Cycle and Transmission

Promastigotes in the gut of the female sandfly are introduced into the skin of the vertebrate host during a blood meal. The parasites invade cells of the reticulo-endothelial system and transform into amastigotes. Amastigotes multiply and invade other reticulo-endothelial cells. Amastigotes in the infected vertebrate host are transmitted to the sandfly during a blood meal where they evolve into promastigotes and continue to multiply.[216,217,220] Aside from vector-borne transmission, leishmania can be transmitted by blood transfusions, sexual contact, congenitally, and occupational exposure.[216]

Pathogenesis and Pathology

After inoculation the promastigotes invade cells of the reticulo-endothelial cells. This initial encounter often results in an inoculation granuloma characterized by accumulation of epithelioid, giant cell, and amastigote-filled histiocytes. From the inoculation site parasites spread to local lymphatics and then hematogenously to liver, spleen, and bone marrow where they stimulate a cell-mediated immune response with granuloma formation. Depending on the quality of the immune response this process can result in cure, subclinical disease, or ongoing multiplication with clinical disease. In the spleen the parasites cause hyperplasia of reticulo-endothelial cells and occasionally splenic infarcts. In the lymphatics they can lead to granuloma formation and overt lymphadenopathy. The bone marrow contains many parasite-laden macrophages. The liver is usually enlarged with multiple amastigote-laden Kupffer cells (Plate 35-6). Cellular reaction is often minimal or even absent. In subclinical cases non-caseating granulomas can be found.[216]

Clinical Manifestations

The site of inoculation is usually not apparent but occasionally a small papule may be noticed. The incubation period varies but is often in the range of 3 to 8 months.[217] The clinical presentation can be acute or of gradual onset. It is characterized by fever, chills, weakness, loss of appetite, pallor, hepatosplenomegaly, and weight loss. With time, liver and spleen may become massively enlarged. As the disease progresses patients may develop a grayish skin discoloration. Secondary bacterial infections are common. Hepatic cirrhosis is an uncommon complication of kala-azar, but when present can lead to persistent splenomegaly despite appropriate therapy of the underlying infection.[216]

Laboratory Tests and Diagnosis

Routine laboratory tests show pancytopenia. Elevated liver enzymes and bilirubin are occasionally observed. Hypergammaglobulinemia is common.[216,217,220,221] In non-immunocompromised hosts serologic methods generally show a good sensitivity (more than 90 percent) but poor specificity, especially in endemic areas.[216,217,222,223] Serologic methods are considered unreliable in immunocompromised patients.[221] Sensitive PCR techniques have been developed but are not widely available.[224] Direct visualization of the parasite in clinical specimens is the most commonly used diagnostic test. Splenic puncture is the most sensitive method (approaching 98 percent) but in few cases has caused life-threatening organ rupture.[216,217,225] Bone marrow aspiration has a sensitivity of 54 percent to 86 percent and is safer.[217] Liver biopsy is less sensitive than splenic puncture or bone marrow aspiration and also carries a minor risk of bleeding. In patients with clinical adenopathy lymph nodes may also be aspirated. Material obtained by puncture, aspiration, or biopsy can be stained with Giemsa or Wright stains (see Plate 35-6), inoculated into uninfected phlebotomine vectors, or cultured using special media. The leishmanin skin test (Montenegro reaction) is positive in patients who have been treated successfully and in patients with spontaneous resolution. It is useful for epidemiologic studies but not for clinical purposes.[217]

Treatment and Prevention

Pentavalent antimony remains the initial treatment of choice for visceral leishmaniasis in many areas. Either stibogluconate sodium or meglumine antimonate can be used. Liposomal amphotericin is at least as effective as pentavalent antimony and less toxic but much more expensive; it is the only approved therapy for visceral leishmaniasis in the United States. Alternatives include amphotericin B liposomal and pentamidine isethionate.[217] Prevention is based on the control of sandfly vectors, extermination of animal reservoirs, and treatment of infected humans. Use of insect repellent and fine mesh netting at night provides partial protection. An effective vaccine is not available.

Summary of Visceral Leishmaniasis and the Liver

Leishmania parasites can produce a granulomatous reaction in the liver. Hepatomegaly is frequent, usually accompanied by significant splenomegaly. Elevated liver enzymes and bilirubin levels are occasionally present. Liver biopsy may be useful in the diagnosis, but it is considered somewhat less sensitive than splenic biopsy or bone marrow aspirate.

INFECTIONS CAUSED BY NEMATODES—ASCARIASIS

Background and Epidemiology

Ascaris is an intestinal roundworm affecting more than 1 billion people worldwide, making ascariasis the most common helminthic infection.[226] Despite a global distribution, prevalence is much higher in developing countries, with most cases reported from Africa, Latin America, India, and the Far East.[227] Infection commonly affects preschool and young school-age children.[228] The adult worm has a life span of 10 to 24 months, is white or reddish-yellow, measures 15 to 35 cm in length, and lives in the small intestine, mainly the jejunum and ileum. The adult female worm produces up to 200,000 ova daily. *Ascaris* eggs can survive in the environment for years.[228] It is unclear if pigs can serve as a reservoir for the infection.[229]

Life Cycle and Transmission

Adult worms inhabit the lumen of the human small intestine. Eggs produced by female worms are shed with feces. Under favorable environmental conditions infective embryos (second-stage larva) develop inside the eggs. After ingestion the larvae hatch in the intestine, penetrate the intestinal wall, and migrate with the venous blood, eventually reaching the lungs. Inside the lungs they penetrate alveoli and advance to the bronchi, the trachea, and eventually the larynx via active movement and cough. After aspiration they again reach the small bowel where they mature into adult worms. Adult worms copulate, resulting in production of large numbers of ova in the female, reinitiating the cycle.[228,230] Transmission is caused by ingestion of embryonated eggs, usually via fecal-oral transmission.

Pathogenesis and Pathology

The pulmonary phase may produce hypersensitivity reactions and inflammation, resulting in bronchoconstriction. Histology shows eosinophilic infiltration and granuloma formation in the lungs, and in severe instances, vasculitis with perivascular granulomatous reactions. Larvae can sometimes be recovered in the sputum.

While in the intestine, worms affect health in several ways. They can interfere with absorption of nutrients, adversely affecting growth, physical fitness, and cognitive development in children. Heavy worm burdens can cause bowel obstruction and intestinal volvulus. Adult worms also have the tendency to migrate. Proposed stimuli for migration include fever, anesthesia, certain medications, and diets. Migration into the biliary tree, pancreatic ducts, and appendix has been documented in many patients.[230] Intrahepatic and extrahepatic adult worms have caused cholangitides and pyogenic liver abscesses.[228,230-232] A rare case of granulomatous hepatitis caused by ova of *Ascaris lumbricoides* presenting as a liver mass has been reported.[233] A relationship between high worm burden and certain hemoglobin types and blood group A carriers has been described.[234] Antibodies to adult and larval antigens are not protective.[230]

Clinical Manifestations

Most patients infected with *Ascaris* parasites are asymptomatic. Sensitized patients can present with asthma-like symptoms during the pulmonary phase of the infection, occasionally accompanied by hemoptysis, chest pain, and cyanosis.[230] This stage of the illness can resemble Löffler's syndrome with transient respiratory symptoms, pulmonary infiltrates, and eosinophilia.[228] Occasionally urticaria and other allergic reactions are seen.

The intestinal phase usually does not produce overt symptoms but can result in cognitive and nutritional impairment in children. Asymptomatic shedding of adult worms can occur. Heavy worm burden can result in intestinal obstruction. In some cases this has resulted in worm emesis. Migration of the worm can result in clinical syndromes of recurrent abdominal pain, biliary colic, acute cholecystitis, cholangitis, obstructive jaundice, pancreatitis, appendicitis, and pyogenic liver abscesses (Plate 35-7). Most patients (98 percent) with pancreatic-biliary ascariasis present with abdominal pain, one fourth have a history of worm emesis, and another 25 percent have previously undergone cholecystectomy or endoscopic sphincterotomy.[233] Hepatomegaly may be found in 50 percent of patients with uncomplicated biliary ascariasis, and the liver may be exquisitely tender to palpation. Rupture of bile ducts may give rise to chemical peritonitis. Rupture of liver abscesses containing worms through the diaphragm can result in the development of an empyema. Invasion of hepatic veins can produce inflammation and further migration of the worms, resulting in symptoms mimicking massive pulmonary embolism.[236] In non-endemic areas the clinical presentation may be confused with pancreatic or biliary neoplasms.[237]

An unusual case of hemobilia secondary to an intrahepatic pseudoaneurysm after treatment of biliary ascariasis in a 5-year-old girl has been described.[238]

Diagnostic Tests and Diagnosis

Routine laboratory tests may show leukocytosis with eosinophilia. Hyperbilirubinemia may be seen in 10 percent to 20 percent of patients with biliary ascariasis. The diagnosis of intestinal ascariasis is based on the detection of characteristic eggs in fecal specimens. Shed adult worms can be identified by the examination of the characteristic anterior worm segment.[239]

Radiologic tests are helpful, but are usually only required for the diagnosis of complications. Contrast studies can demonstrate luminal helminths, which may be useful in rare cases in which infection is limited to male worms.[230,239] Complicated ascariasis can be diagnosed with ultrasonography, CT scan, or MRI. Ultras onography is particularly useful for the diagnosis of biliary-pancreatic ascariasis. Ultrasound has a good sensitivity when performed by experienced individuals.[233,240] Detection of helminthic movement within the biliary tree is diagnostic of biliary ascariasis. Other sonographic clues for the detection of ascariasis include "spaghetti-like appearance," "inner-tube sign," "double-tube sign," "bull's-eye sign," and "impacted worms sign."[241] A "bull's eye" or "inner-tube" appearance of biliary ascariasis has also been observed on CT scans or MRI.[242] Magnetic resonance cholangiopancreatography (MRCP) can provide tridimensional images equivalent to endoscopic retrograde cholangiopancreatography(ERCP).[241,243] ERCP is useful for the diagnosis of inconclusive cases and therapeutically. Worms can be seen protruding from the papillary orifice or can be detected during the contrast cholangiographic phase.[233]

Treatment and Prevention

Several drugs are effective for the treatment of ascariasis. The treatment of choice is mebendazole 100 mg twice per day for 3 days, or 500 mg as a single dose. Pyrantel pamoate 10 mg/kg as a single dose has also been used successfully. Albendazole in a single dose of 400 mg is effective in most cases. In cases of suspected intestinal or biliary obstruction piperazine citrate has been recommended.[139,228,230]

Obstruction of the biliary tree or pancreatic duct usually requires endoscopic extraction via ERCP using forceps or Dormia baskets.[230,232,244] Although ERCP is associated with a very low incidence of procedure-related complications, endoscopic extraction is not always successful. In these cases surgery is indicated. Surgery also remains important in the management of infections complicated by biliary or pancreatic strictures or stones and worms in the gallbladder.[245,246] Adjunctive antibiotics are helpful in the management of patients with cholangitis, liver abscess, appendicitis, and peritonitis. Mass chemotherapy or chemotherapy targeted at school-age children is considered feasible and effective for worm control.[230,247]

Summary of Ascariasis and the Liver

Most hepatobiliary complications are caused by the ability of the parasite to migrate from the small intestine into the biliary tree, resulting in tender hepatomegaly, recurrent abdominal pain, classic biliary colic, obstructive jaundice, cholangitis, cholecystitis, pancreatitis, and liver abscesses. Liver abscesses containing dead or living worms have been described (see Plate 35-7). *Ascaris* ova can also cause hepatic granuloma formation. In nonendemic areas in which the diagnosis is not suspected and physicians are not familiar with typical radiologic findings, hepatobiliary ascariasis has been confused for hepatic, biliary, and pancreatic neoplasms. A cholecystectomy or sphincterotomy may predispose the patient to the development of biliary-pancreatic ascariasis.

STRONGYLOIDIASIS

Background and Epidemiology

Strongyloides stercoralis is widely distributed in tropical and subtropical areas, including the southeast United States and southern and eastern Europe. It has been estimated that 50 to 100 million people are infected worldwide. Higher incidence rates are found in human T-cell lymphotropic virus (HTLV-1)–infected patients in regions in which this virus is endemic.[248] The worms can survive and reproduce as parasites in humans or as free-living forms in the soil.[249] The female is 2.2 mm long; the male 0.7 mm long. Although *S. stercoralis* and other species may be found in dogs, cats, or monkeys, humans are the main reservoir. Because infection can be maintained for 40 years or more, affected individuals may remain at risk of episodic symptoms of chronic infection or severe hyperinfection as a consequence of immunosuppression.[248]

Life Cycle and Transmission

Adult worms in the human intestine deposit ova, which usually hatch in the mucosa, releasing the rhabditiform larvae that are shed in the feces. Under favorable conditions rhabditiform larvae transform into infectious filariform larvae in the soil or in the perianal region after defecation. Autoinfection may occur as a result of accelerated transformation of rhabditiform larvae to filariform larvae inside the gut lumen or by penetration of the perianal skin. Pending favorable soil conditions rhabditiform larvae can also directly transform into free-living adult worms in the soil. Filariform larvae are able to penetrate intact skin or mucous membranes. After penetration these larvae invade venous blood vessels and travel to the lungs. In the pulmonary capillary bed they penetrate the alveolar membrane and start ascending the airways. After aspiration they reach the small intestine, where they mature into adult worms. Females burrow through the mucosa and start producing new ova.[228,248]

Pathogenesis and Pathology

The initial penetration and migration of the larvae causes an immediate hypersensitivity reaction responsible for the clinical syndromes of urticarial rash and pulmonary infiltrates with wheezing and eosinophilia. Mechanical damage of alveoli during the pulmonary migration phase can result in minor hemorrhages, exudation, and inflammation, causing affected patients to experience cough and hemoptysis.[239,248] In the intestine, adult worms cause mechanical trauma and microscopic ulceration affecting mucosa and superficial submucosa, usually associated with minimal inflammation. Heavy infection can result in a significant increase in epithelial cell turnover, causing protein-losing enteropathy and malnutrition. Progressive infection can result in mucosal atrophy with subsequent malabsorption, confluent ulceration with enteritis, and risk of secondary bacterial superinfection. In rare cases granulomas may form. Histology may show adult worms, ova, and larvae. Usually the duodenum and jejunum are affected, but in severe cases, particularly in the hyperinfection syndrome, pathology is more widespread and may become confluent, resulting in mucosal necrosis involving both small and large bowel.[239,248]

Occasionally larvae are detected in biliary or pancreatic ducts, liver, urine, or various inflammatory exudates. In patients with the hyperinfection syndrome larva-induced damage and bacterial superinfection may affect any organ.[248] Histology typically shows inflammation with plasmocytes, macrophages, giant cells, and eosinophils that occasionally forms granulomas. These changes may also affect the liver, with prominent cellular infiltrates in the portal tracts and hepatic lobules. A diffuse, moderate hepatic steatosis has been described in severe cases. Intrahepatic cholestasis is common.[250,251]

Cellular immunity is important in order to contain the parasite. It is well-recognized that illnesses resulting in loss of cellular immunity, including corticosteroid therapy, may lead to uncontrolled parasite multiplication and migration, resulting in the hyperinfection syndrome.[248] Extraintestinal strongyloidiasis, however, has not been reported as a common complication of patients with AIDS in areas of Africa highly endemic for *S. stercoralis*.[248,252] Recent studies suggest that IgA and IgE are important in regulating larval output and autoinfection, whereas IgG4 is able to block IgE-mediated responses to the parasite.[253]

Clinical Manifestations

The clinical manifestations of strongyloidiasis can be classified in acute, chronic, and hyperinfection syndromes. Approximately one third of patients remain asymptomatic. Acute manifestations of strongyloidiasis mainly affect skin, lungs, or the intestinal tract. The cutaneous migration of filariform larvae causes the syndrome termed *larva currens.* Caused by external autoinfection it is mainly seen in the perianal area and buttocks. A pruritic maculo-papular rash or migrating linear urticaria is observed in affected patients. The pulmonary syndrome is characterized by eosinophilia, pulmonary infiltrates, and various respiratory symptoms, including cough, wheezing, chest pain, and occasional hemoptysis. Intestinal infection manifests as burning or colicky epigastric or abdominal pain and diarrhea. In patients with severe infections malabsorption and small bowel obstruction can be seen.[228,239,248] The chronic syndrome is characterized by recurrent urticaria, abdominal pain, and diarrhea. Some patients manifest respiratory symptoms, and cough is the most commonly reported symptom in some series.[248,254] The hyperinfection syndrome affects patients with iatrogenic or otherwise compromised cellular immune systems. In these patients rapid transformation of rhabditiform larvae to filariform larvae occurs, followed by hematogenous dissemination of the filariform larvae to virtually all organ systems. More recently hyperinfection syndrome has been described in association with the administration of ribavirin to patients with hepatitis C virus infection.[255] The hyperinfection syndrome is characterized by severe generalized abdominal pain, profound diarrhea, vomiting, malabsorption, electrolyte disturbances, pulmonary infiltrates (sometimes with cavitation) with varying degrees of respiratory failure, and sepsis syndrome secondary to bacterial superinfection. Meningitis caused by gram-negative or intestinal gram-positive organisms is not uncommon. Bacteremia, endocarditis, and peritonitis are other well-described complications. Patients may become mildly jaundiced. Isolated hepatomegaly without splenomegaly may also be present.[228,239,248-250]

Diagnostic Tests

Routine laboratory tests frequently show eosinophilia and hypoalbuminemia. Importantly, eosinophilia may be absent in patients taking steroids or suffering from a hyperinfection syndrome. Its absence is an adverse prognostic sign.[248] In patients with hyperinfection syndrome larval infiltration of the liver may result in elevation of liver enzymes. Blood cultures may be positive for enteric gram-negative or gram-positive organisms. The diagnosis is based on the identification of larvae or adult worms. Ova are rarely present, unless diarrhea is massive. Rhabditiform larvae, filariform larvae, and adult worms may be found in feces or duodenal samples. The Entero-Test uses a gelatin capsule that is attached to a nylon line and swallowed by the patient to be retrieved 4 hours later. The detection of the parasite forms in stool may prove difficult. Repeated and occasionally alternative tests are often required to establish the diagnosis. The formalin-ether concentration method may increase the sensitivity of stool examination. The Baermann funnel gauze method has proven to be more efficient than most conventional techniques, including the Entero-Test.[248] In vitro culture presents another diagnostic option. Some experts consider the modified agar plate technique as the test of choice in the diagnosis of strongyloidiasis, in which larvae are identified through detection of characteristic burrows. Reported sensitivities of this test range from 70 percent to 96 percent.[248,256,257] Rarely, larvae are detected in other clinical samples, including biopsies or sputum samples. Despite recent advances parasitologic diagnosis of strongyloidiasis remains difficult. Some authors advocate the use of combining stool studies with serologic test to improve the diagnostic yield.[258,259] Immunofluorescence and ELISA tests have been developed, which may prove useful, especially in patients with chronic syndromes or immunodeficiencies. False-positive tests have been observed in patients with filarial infections.[248]

Treatment and Prevention

For a long time thiabendazole 25 mg/kg by mouth twice per day for 2 to 3 days remained the treatment of choice for patients with asymptomatic infection and acute and chronic syndromes. Some authorities recommend retreatment after 1 week. Patients with hyperinfection syndrome require therapy for 5 to 14 days. Side effects include nausea, vomiting, dizziness, and malodorous urine.[248] One patient developed severe cholestasis and subsequent biliary cirrhosis after thiabendazole therapy.[260] Alternatives include ivermectin 200 μg/kg/day, with excellent cure rates and few side effects, and albendazole 400 mg/day for 3 days, which is less toxic than thiabendazole but also less efficacious.[248,261] Prevention is based on improvement of sanitary conditions and personal hygiene.[239,248] In some areas endemic for intestinal helminths, periodic albendazole therapy has been used for worm control.[247] The prevention of hyperinfection syndrome relies on empiric administration of anthelmintic medications or the screening for asymptomatic infection followed by therapy of affected patients scheduled to receive immunosuppressive therapy.

Summary of Strongyloidiasis and the Liver

Liver involvement in strongyloidiasis most commonly is a component of the hyperinfection syndrome. In these cases the patients may manifest hepatomegaly and usually mild elevations of transaminases, alkaline phosphatase, and bilirubin. Microscopic examination of liver tissue of affected patients reveals inflammation with plasmocytes, macrophages, giant cells, and eosinophils with or without granuloma formation. Cellular infiltration of portal tracts and hepatic lobules may be present. A diffuse but usually mild to moderate steatosis has been described in severe cases. Intrahepatic cholestasis is common. The hyperinfection syndrome has anecdotally been linked to ribavirin administration in patients with hepatitis C virus infection. Severe cholestasis and subsequent development of liver cirrhosis have been described after the administration of thiabendazole, even though a causal relationship has not definitely been established.

TOXOCARIASIS

Background and Epidemiology

The animal roundworms *Toxocara canis* and *Toxocara catis* cause human toxocariasis. Toxocariasis has a worldwide distribution and is more prevalent in areas of the world where dogs and cats are found and *Toxocara* eggs find favorable conditions for prolonged survival.[262-264] Toxocariasis is one of the most common helminthic infections in developed countries.[265,266] Infective *Toxocara* eggs have been found in the soil of urban and suburban parks and public playgrounds.[262] Because of undeveloped sanitary habits, their propensity to geophagia (pica), and their close association with domestic pets, children are most frequently affected.[267] In animals infection is more common in puppies, with a progressive reduction of infectivity after 6 months of age.[262]

Life Cycle and Transmission

Adult worms live in the intestine of dogs or cats and produce eggs that are shed in the feces. After 2 to 3 weeks in moist soil temperatures, eggs embryonate and become infective. Humans ingest embryonated eggs directly from the soil or from contaminated hands, toys, or food. After ingestion larvae are released in the proximal intestine, penetrate the mucosa, and travel to the liver via the portal circulation. Some larvae are retained in the liver. Others continue migration to the lungs or other organs until they reach a vessel too small for passage. Here they penetrate the vessel and migrate into the surrounding tissue.[262-264] Infrequently transmission to humans has been reported after ingestion of larvae present in liver, meats, or other tissues of the definitive hosts (i.e., dogs or cats). In humans the life cycle cannot be completed. In the definitive hosts larvae reach the airway, ascend to the pharynx, and enter the gastrointestinal tract where they mature to adult worms. After mating, large numbers of eggs are liberated via animal feces.

Pathogenesis and Pathology

When larvae are liberated from ingested eggs and reach the capillary bed of a target organ, penetration of the vessel and invasion of surrounding tissues cause hemorrhage, necrosis, and inflammation. Frequently an eosinophilic infiltrate can be seen in portal triads.[268] Although larvae are usually surrounded by eosinophilic granulomas[262] the degree of inflammation seems to be independent of IL-5 and eosinophilic responses. Based on a murine model of toxocariasis, trapping of larvae is also not dependent on the presence of eosinophils.[269] In later stages fibrosis and calcification may ensue.[262]

Larvae have been detected in multiple organs, including liver (Plate 35-8, *A* and *B*), lungs, heart, eyes, and brain. Most larvae die whereas others become latent and may reactivate years later. Despite eliciting a vigorous immunologic response larvae may survive for prolonged periods. This is apparently mediated through production of protective factors and the shedding of antigenic components from the larval surface.

Clinical Manifestations

Most infections are asymptomatic or go unrecognized. The two main clinical syndromes are visceral and ocular larva migrans. Visceral larva migrans is usually seen in young children and is characterized by persistent fever, hepatomegaly, eosinophilia, and cough. Hepatomegaly is present in more than 70 percent of reported cases.[270] This syndrome must be distinguished from other diseases causing eosinophilia, hepatomegaly, and fever, including ascariasis, schistosomiasis, clonorchiasis, opisthorchiasis, echinococcosis, and capillariasis.[263] Some patients with hepatic toxocariasis were initially misdiagnosed as other granulomatous hepatitides[271] or non-infectious conditions such as juvenile rheumatoid arthritis[272] and neoplastic liver lesions.[273] It has been hypothesized that liver involvement in toxocariasis may predispose to formation of pyogenic liver abscesses in children, presumably via down-regulation of the TH1 response or because the granulomatous reaction around the larvae could facilitate trapping of bacteria in the liver.[270] Other organs are also commonly affected.[268,274] Ocular larva migrans is most commonly seen in older children and is characterized by endophthalmitis with granuloma formation.[262]

Diagnostic Tests

Routine laboratory tests show leukocytosis with eosinophilia, anemia, and abnormal liver tests.[262-264,270,271,275] Hypergammaglobulinemia is frequently observed. Visceral larva migrans should be considered in any person with persistent eosinophilia. Parasitologic diagnosis requires the demonstration of typical larvae in histologic specimens (see Plate 35-8, *A* and *B*). In many cases diagnosis is established by a combination of typical laboratory (eosinophilia) and radiologic findings with serologic tests. Abdominal ultrasonography reveals hypoechoic lesions in the liver.[270] MRI usually shows an ill-defined necrotic area with concentric thick walls accompanied by perifocal edema in the surrounding liver parenchyma.[276] Specific *Toxocara* organism ELISAs are considered the most accurate serologic test.[262-264,270] PCR-based techniques have been useful in the evaluation of liver biopsy specimens.[277]

Treatment and Prevention

Asymptomatic toxocariasis does not require anthelmintic therapy. Effective medications include diethylcarbamazine, thiabendazole, albendazole, and mebendazole. Severe pulmonary, myocardial, or CNS involvement may warrant corticosteroid therapy.[262] Local and systemic steroids are also considered the treatment of choice of patients with ocular larva migrans. Laser photocoagulation may provide additional benefit. Improvement of personal hygiene, elimination of pet parasitism, and child education are the mainstays of prevention. Restriction of certain children activities in playgrounds and periodic anthelmintic therapy for pets are considered beneficial.[262]

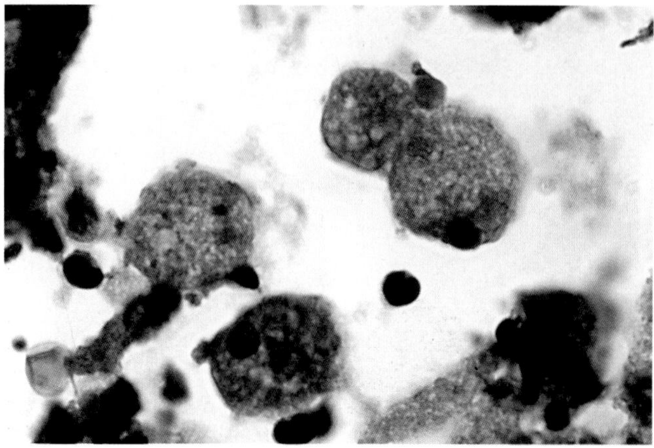

Plate 35-1 *Entamoeba histolytica* trophozoites displaying erythrophagocytosis. (Courtesy of David A. Schwartz, MD, Atlanta, Ga.)

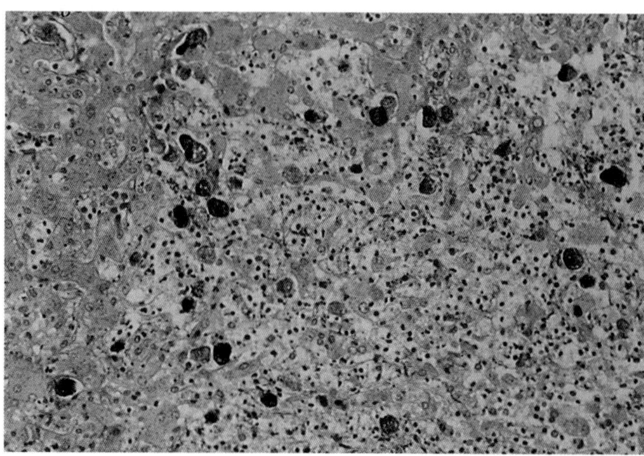

Plate 35-2 PAS stain of biopsy specimen of patient with amebic liver abscess showing multiple *Entamoeba histolytica* trophozoites. *PAS,* Periodic acid-Schiff. (Courtesy of David A. Schwartz, MD, Atlanta, Ga.)

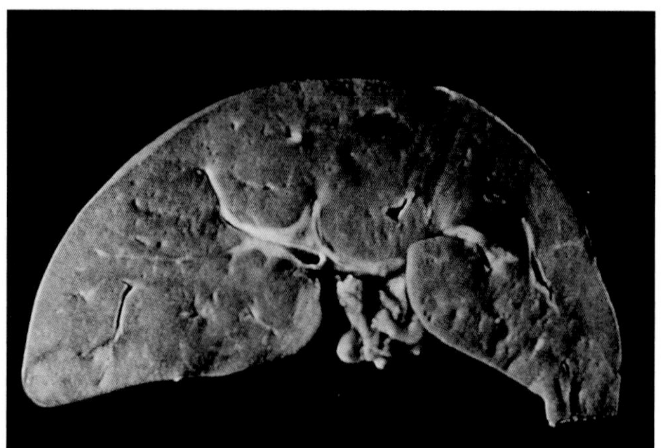

Plate 35-3 Hepatomegaly and hepatic hyperpigmentation in severe malaria. (Courtesy of David A. Schwartz, MD, Atlanta, Ga.)

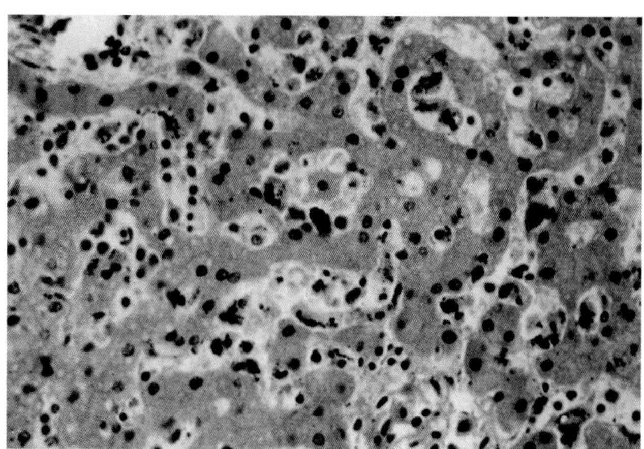

Plate 35-4 Chronic hepatic deposition of hemozoin in patient with recurrent malaria. (Courtesy of David A. Schwartz, MD, Atlanta, Ga.)

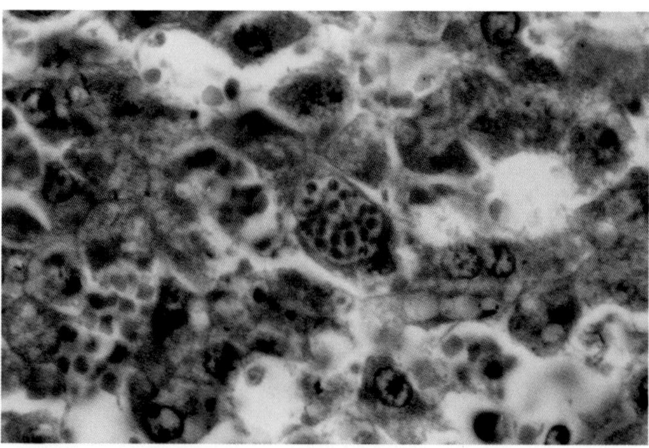

Plate 35-5 *Toxoplasma gondii* cyst in liver tissue. (Courtesy of David A. Schwartz, MD, Atlanta, Ga.)

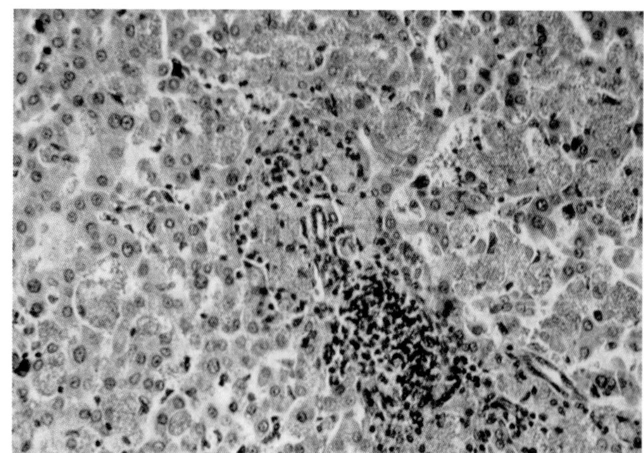

Plate 35-6 Multiple amastigote-laden Kupffer cells in visceral leishmaniasis. (Courtesy of David A. Schwartz, MD, Atlanta, Ga.)

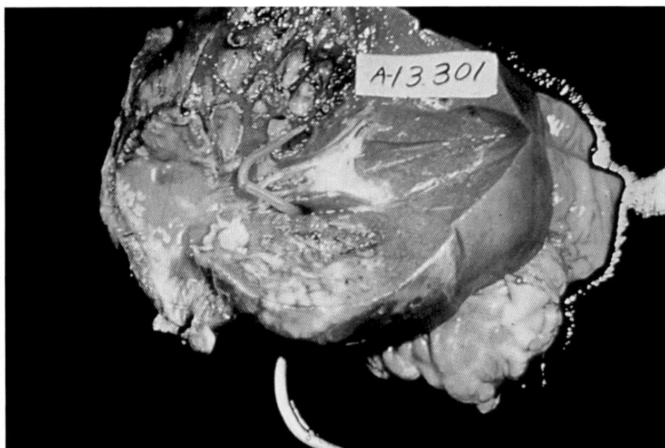

Plate 35-7 Pyogenic liver abscess secondary to ascariasis with *Ascaris lumbricoides* in situ. (Courtesy of David A. Schwartz, MD, Atlanta, Ga.)

A

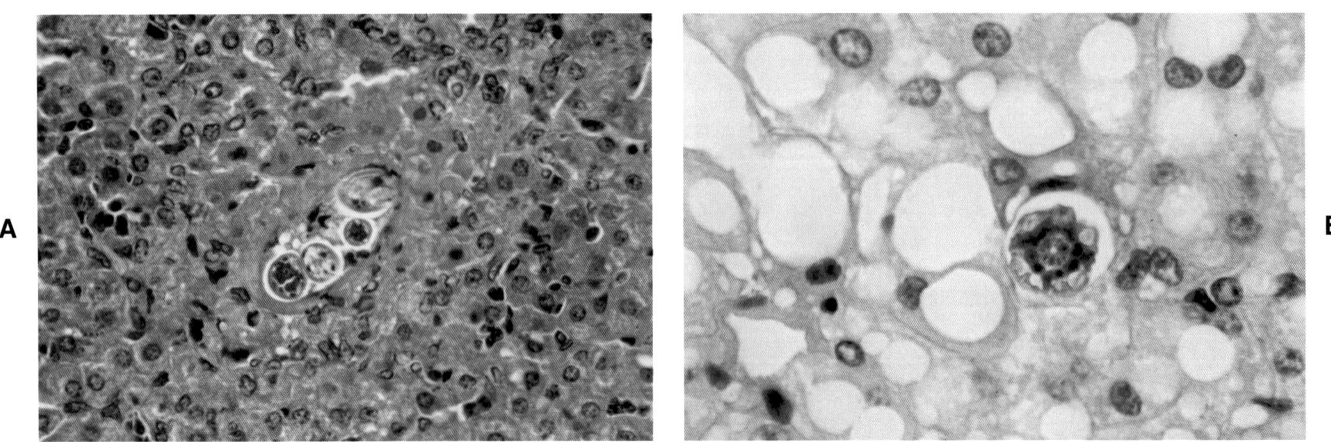

B

Plate 35-8 Hepatic visceral larva migrans with cross section of **A,** *Toxocara canis* or **B,** *Toxocara cati.* (Courtesy of David A. Schwartz, MD, Atlanta, Ga.)

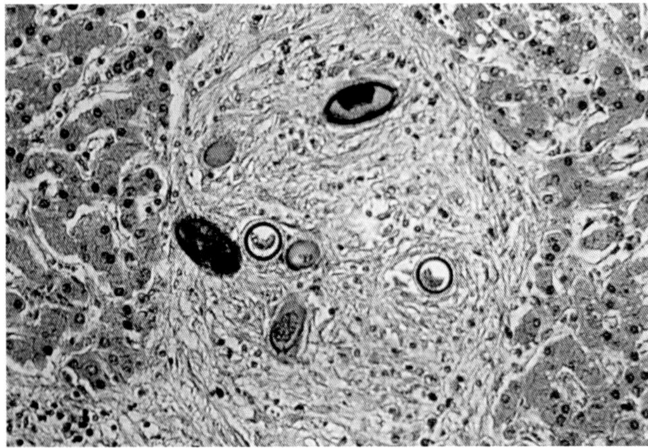

Plate 35-9 Capillaria hepatica in liver tissue. (Courtesy of David A. Schwartz, MD, Atlanta, Ga.)

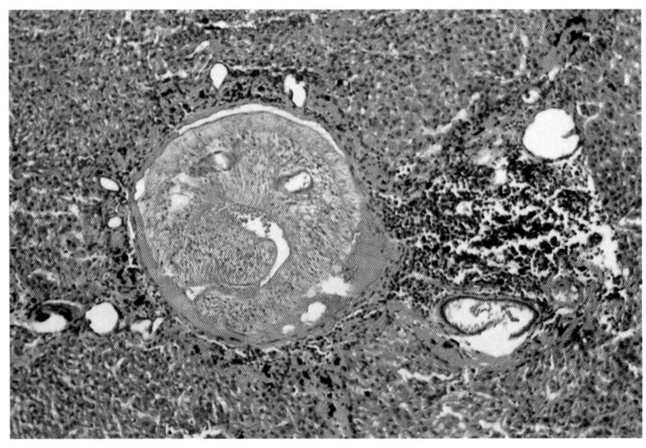

Plate 35-10 Mature schistosome lodged in portal vein. (Courtesy of David A. Schwartz, MD, Atlanta, Ga.)

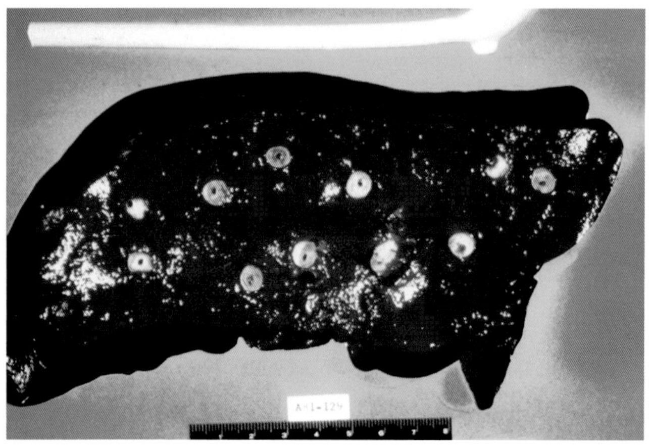

Plate 35-11 Pipe stem fibrosis in schistosomiasis. (Courtesy of David A. Schwartz, MD, Atlanta, Ga.)

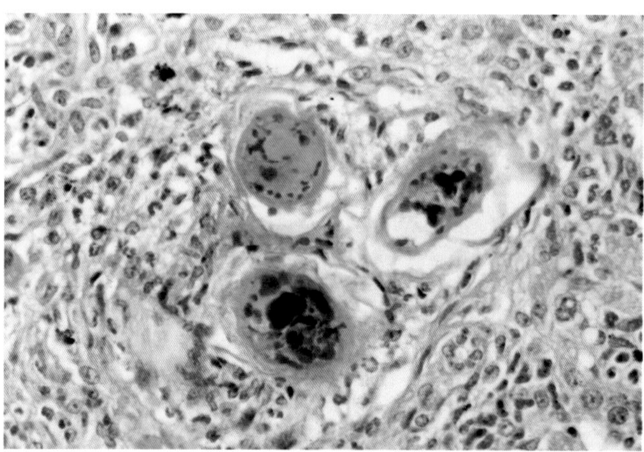

Plate 35-12 "Egg granulomas" in schistosomiasis. (Courtesy of David A. Schwartz, MD, Atlanta, Ga.)

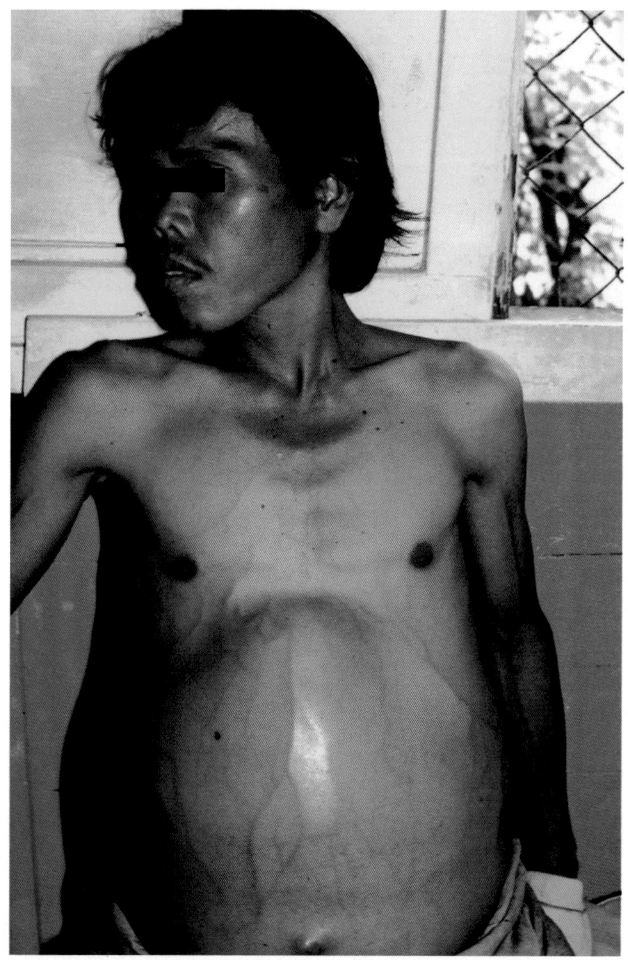

Plate 35-13 Patient with decompensated portal hypertension secondary to schistosomiasis. (Courtesy of David A. Schwartz, MD, Atlanta, Ga.)

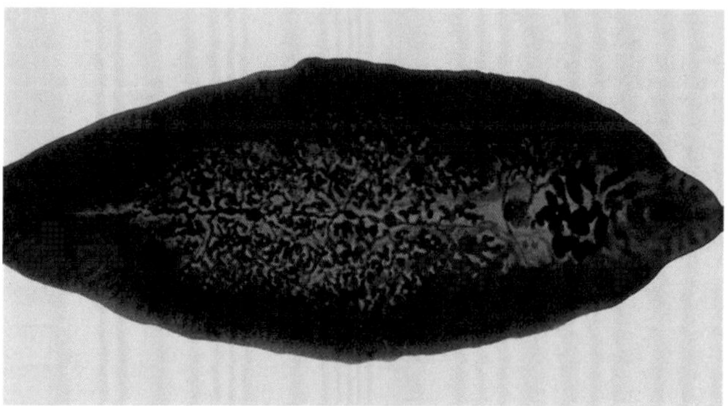

Plate 35-14 *Fasciola hepatica.* (Courtesy of David A. Schwartz, MD, Atlanta, Ga.)

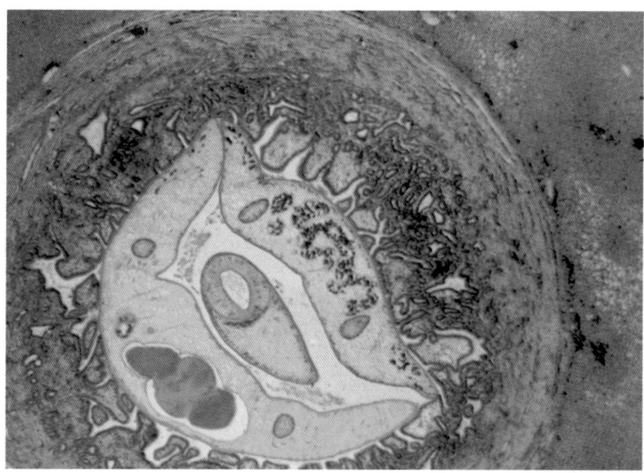

Plate 35-15 *Clonorchis sinensis* in bile duct. (Courtesy of David A. Schwartz, MD, Atlanta, Ga.)

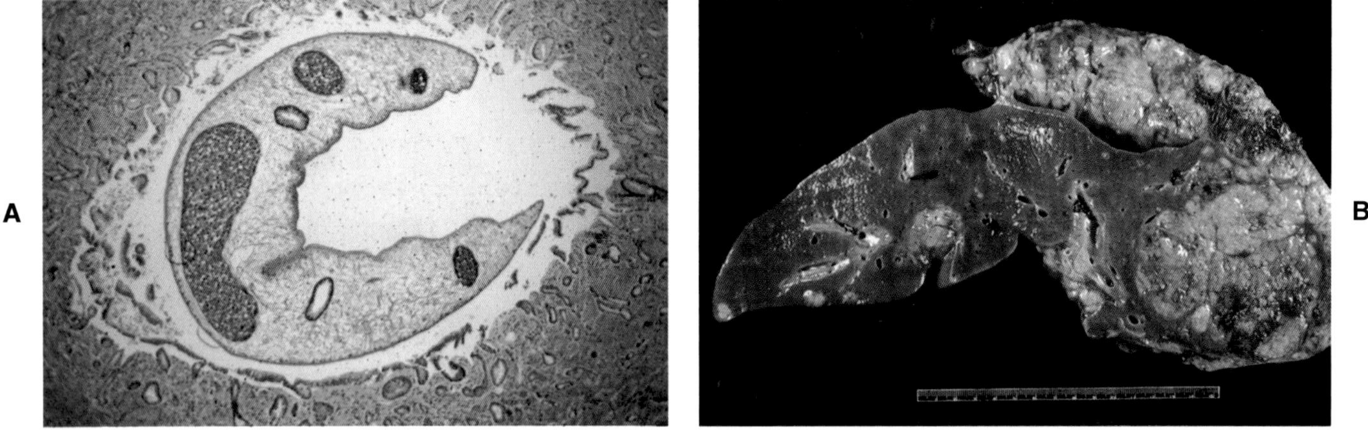

Plate 35-16 Autopsy **(A)** and histologic specimens **(B)** of patients with *Clonorchis sinensis* infection and associated cholangiocarcinoma. (Courtesy of David A. Schwartz, MD, Atlanta, Ga.)

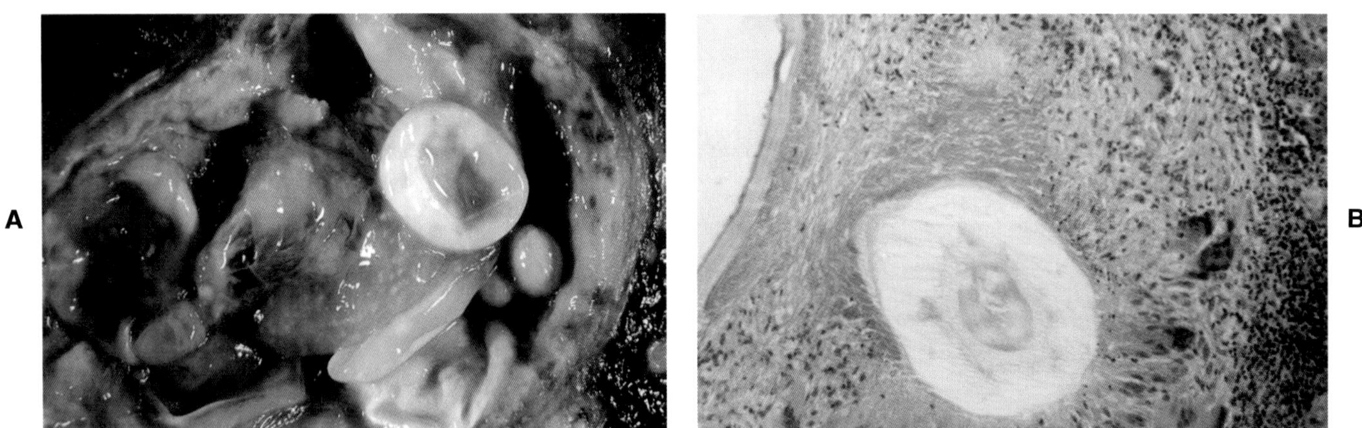

Plate 35-17 **A** and **B,** Hepatic echinococcal cysts. (Courtesy of David A. Schwartz, MD, Atlanta, Ga.)

Summary of Toxocariasis and the Liver

Toxocariasis is a well-described cause of liver granulomas. Granuloma formation is usually accompanied by a local and systemic eosinophilic response. Abnormal liver tests and sonographic evidence of hypoechoic lesions are common. Toxocariasis has to be distinguished from other causes of hepatomegaly, fever, and eosinophilia.

Even though a parasitologic diagnosis is not required in most cases, liver biopsy may reveal typical larvae (see Plate 35-8, *A* and *B*). Toxocariasis may be an important predisposing factor for the development of pyogenic liver abscesses in children.

HEPATIC CAPILLARIASIS

Background and Epidemiology

Capillaria hepatica is a nematode of the *Trichuroidea* family. Despite its name it is a rare cause of hepatic disease in humans, with less than 50 cases reported in the literature. More than half of these cases were diagnosed in children.[278] Cases have been reported from the Far and Middle East, Europe, Africa, and the Americas.[278-285] *Capillaria hepatica* is a parasite mainly affecting rodents but has also been found in other vertebrates, including cats and dogs. Humans acquire the infection by ingesting embryonated eggs in food contaminated with feces or soil. In the intestine released larvae penetrate the mucosa and travel to the liver via the portal circulation. Many larvae are retained in the liver, whereas others continue migration to lungs, kidneys, and other organs. The life cycle is only completed in non-human hosts.

Pathogenesis and Pathology

Tissue sections of affected liver tissue show granulomatous inflammation, including giant cells predominantly in the portal spaces, confluent eosinophilic microabscesses, and degenerated *Capillaria hepatica* parasites (Plate 35-9).[278,279]

Clinical Manifestations

The triad of persistent fever, eosinophilia, and hepatomegaly is virtually always present.[279] Splenomegaly is found in 50 percent to 60 percent of the cases. Because the main differential diagnosis is toxocariasis, a negative *Toxocara* serology may be helpful for establishing the diagnosis.[280] Massive destruction of the liver with hepatic failure has been described.[278] Other non-specific symptoms include anorexia, nausea, vomiting, night sweats, and change in bowel habits.

Diagnostic Tests

Laboratory tests frequently show anemia, eosinophilia, moderate elevation of liver enzymes, increased erythrocyte sedimentation rate, and hypergammaglobulinemia.[278,281,284] Hepatic ultrasonography shows non-specific hyperechogenicities in the portal spaces.[278] Until recently serology was used mainly to rule out alternative diseases. Recently, a specific indirect immunofluorescence assay has been developed, but availability is limited.[286] Currently the detection of the parasite in liver biopsy specimens is the only way to establish a definitive diagnosis. Because hepatic involvement in most cases is diffuse and massive, percutaneous liver biopsy is usually sufficient.[278,281]

Treatment and Prevention

Recommendations for antihelmintic therapy are solely based on anecdotal case reports. Several medications have been used, including thiabendazole, mebendazole, albendazole, and ivermectin.[278,283,285] Based on treatment failures of alternative drugs, thiabendazole for at least 3 weeks is considered the therapy of choice by some experts.[278] Steroids are occasionally used to reduce hepatic inflammation.[278,283,285] Prevention is based on the restriction of geophagia, the improvement of sanitary conditions, and the eradication of rats.[278]

Summary of Capillariasis and the Liver

Capillaria hepatica produces a granulomatous inflammation of the liver. Eosinophilic infiltration and formation of microabscesses are commonly detected. More than 90 percent of the infected patients will have hepatomegaly. The clinical syndrome may simulate other forms of hepatitis with fever, hepatomegaly, and elevated transaminases. Liver enzymes are usually mildly or moderately elevated. Liver failure is rare but has been described. In most cases a definitive diagnosis requires a liver biopsy (see Plate 35-9).

INFECTIONS CAUSED BY TREMATODES—SCHISTOSOMIASIS

Background and Epidemiology

Schistosomiasis causes approximately 200 million human infections and 200,000 deaths yearly.[287-290] It is endemic in tropical and subtropical areas of Africa, Asia, South America, and the Caribbean. Schistosomiasis has been reported from 77 countries, all situated between 36° north and south of the equator. Requirements include optimal freshwater temperatures (25°-30° C) for the survival of different snail populations, which serve as intermediate hosts for the parasite.[287,288]

The prevalence of schistosomiasis continues to increase as more patients are exposed to contaminated water secondary to increased use of irrigation for agricultural development, urbanization, and inadequate control measures.[288] In endemic areas infection often occurs early in childhood with prevalence peaking between 8 and 10 years of age in heavily affected communities.[288] Even though schistosomiasis is not transmitted in Europe and North America because of the absence of the intermediate host, immigration and travel have resulted in the diagnosis of several thousand cases in the developed world.[287-289]

Humans are the main vertebrate host for schistosomes but other animal species, including non-human primates, rodents, dogs, cats, pigs, horses, sheep, goats, and water buffaloes, can serve as reservoirs.[287] Adult worms are 1 to 2 cm in length, have oral and ventral suckers, and prominent reproductive organs.[289] Important species that cause human disease are *Schistosoma mansoni, Schistosoma japonicum, Schistosoma intercalatum, Schistosoma mekongi,* and *Schistosoma haematobium. S. haematobium* is predominantly associated with urinary tract pathology and will therefore not be discussed here. All others cause significant disease in intestine, the portal vein and its tributaries, and the liver. *S. mekongi* and *S. intercalatum* are of regional importance, whereas *S. mansoni* and *S. japonicum* are widely distributed.[287,288]

Life Cycle and Transmission

Adult worms inhabit the venous plexus of the intestines (*S. mansoni, S. japonicum, S. intercalatum, S. mekongi*) or the bladder (*S. haematobium*) of their vertebrate host (Plate 35-10). Motile schistosomal eggs are able to penetrate the walls of bladder and intestine and are excreted in the urine or the stool. If they reach static or slow-moving fresh water, eggs release ciliated miracidia, which swim until they reach a susceptible snail or die. After penetrating the snail the miracidium evolves into a sporocyst, which replicates and forms secondary sporocysts. These replicate for several weeks and mature into hundreds of cercaria that exhibit a forked tail. Cercaria exit the snail and actively swim in search of the vertebrate host. They are capable of penetrating intact skin and migrate through the dermis where they evolve to schistosomula. These reach the venous circulation, the systemic circulation, and finally the mesenteric capillaries and venules where they mature into adult worms. Adult worms copulate in the portal vein, and the female worm migrates against the portal flow to deposit the eggs in the mesenteric circulation. These eggs can be carried by the portal circulation into the liver or they can remain in the mesenteric plexus. After inciting an inflammatory response, eggs penetrate the wall of the intestine and reach the intestinal lumen to be excreted with the stool.[287,288,291]

Pathogenesis and Pathology

Most pathology of schistosomiasis is the result of the host reaction to the schistosome. This reaction varies according to the life cycle stage of the parasite, which correlates with distinct clinical syndromes. When cercaria penetrate the skin they use proteases and elastases, which may produce mild edema and localized eosinophilic and mononuclear infiltration.[288] Unless exposed to a heavy cercarial load, most patients remain asymptomatic until eggs are released by the adult parasite. Egg release can result in an acute serum sickness–type reaction secondary to the formation of large immune-complexes resulting in activation of the reticulo-endothelial system. This acute reaction is usually self-limiting. Long-term sequelae, however, are frequent, because eggs that remain in mesenteric venules may cause granulomatous enteritis or intestinal erosions. Eggs migrating into the liver via the portal flow may cause pyelophlebitis, peripylephlebitis, and periportal fibrosis. Pathologically, egg granulomas are formed. Despite progressive periportal fibrosis the lobular architecture and the arterial and ductal structures are usually well preserved.[287,288] This pattern of scarring is often referred to as "Symmers' pipestem fibrosis" (Plate 35-11).[287,288,292] Ultimately presinusoidal portal hypertension evolves. Other affected areas, including the lungs, the pulmonary vasculature, the CNS, the bowel, and the kidneys, may be involved when ectopic eggs reach the systemic circulation.

Schistosomal egg granulomas are well-circumscribed aggregates of inflammatory cells, including eosinophils, macrophages, lymphocytes, and neutrophils (Plate 35-12). In early stages of the infection a cellular TH1 type immune response with increased IL-2 and interferon γ levels are observed.[287,293] In later stages immune activation is switched toward a predominantly humoral response, with activation of TH2 type lymphocytes and secretion of IL-4, IL-5, IL-10, and IL-13, causing B-cell activation and eosinophil recruitment.[287,294] Granulomas formed when humoral responses are dominant seem to be beneficial and capable of limiting the spread of the eggs, whereas granulomas formed during TH1 predominance are inefficient and associated with undesirable hepatic microvesicular changes, inflammation, and necrosis.[287] The humoral response to schistosomes plays a role in susceptibility and resistance to reinfection. IgM, IgG2, and IgG4 seem to block eosinophil-dependent killing of the schistosomula,[295,296] whereas IgE and IgA are considered protective.[287,297,298] Because IgM and IgG responses wane and IgE and IgA responses tend to increase with age, susceptibility to reinfection is lower in older individuals.

Clinical Manifestations

Schistosomiasis manifests clinically in distinct acute and chronic syndromes. Acute manifestations include cercarial dermatitis, larval pneumonitis, and Katayama fever. Cercarial dermatitis correlates with cercarial migration through the skin, is seen mainly in people already sensitized to cercarial antigens, and is characterized by a pruritic papular rash.[288] Larval pneumonitis is a self-limiting process that correlates with the migration of schistosomula through the pulmonary vasculature. Pulmonary infiltrates and eosinophilia are characteristics of this stage. Katayama fever is a self-limiting serum sickness–like phenomenon, which correlates with early ovideposition. Characteristic symptoms include fever, chills, arthralgia, myalgia, dry cough, wheezing, diarrhea, abdominal pain, hepatomegaly, splenomegaly, lymphadenopathy, and eosinophilia.[287-289,291]

Chronic manifestations can involve multiple organ systems. The CNS can be affected when egg granulomas form in brain or spine, resulting in seizures or other focal neurologic events, including transverse myelitis.[288] Uncommonly eggs in the pulmonary vasculature can cause pulmonary hypertension and cor pulmonale.[288,291] The most common manifestations of chronic schistosomiasis are the intestinal and the hepatosplenic forms of the disease.[287] Both syndromes, which may occur simultaneously in the same host, correlate with a vigorous granulomatous immune response to egg deposition. Although the entire intestine can be affected, lesions are predominantly found in the large bowel. Symptoms include mucoid or bloody diarrhea, tenesmus, and abdominal pain with symptoms and complications similar to those seen in patients with inflammatory bowel disease. Hepatosplenic schistosomiasis is clinically characterized by hepatomegaly (mainly of the left lobe of the liver) and portal hypertension and its complications (Plate 35-13). Signs of advanced liver dysfunction such as jaundice, spider angiomata, palmar erythema, testicular atrophy, or gynecomastia are usually absent.[287-289,291] Despite the wide spectrum of schistosomal disease, most infections are asymptomatic. Common reasons for seeking medical care include anemia and complications of portal hypertension.[287]

Laboratory Tests and Diagnosis

Routine laboratory tests usually reveal normal transaminases and coagulation profiles, but may be noteworthy for mild elevations of alkaline phosphatase, cytopenias, and heme-positive stools. Radiologic tests, including abdominal ultrasonography, CT, and MRI, are useful for staging purposes. Accurate measurements of liver and spleen size, grading of portal fibrosis, and degree of portal hypertension are prognostically important.[299,300] The diagnosis can be confirmed through demonstration of eggs in stool samples, biopsies, or with immunodiagnostic assays. Stool examination using the Kato-Katz thick smear preparation has a sensitivity of 90 percent if three specimens obtained on different days are examined.[287,288,291,301] Rectal biopsies may be helpful and examination of six biopsy specimens using a crush technique has proven more sensitive than two Kato-Katz smears.[287,302] Immunodiagnostic assays include the use of specific antisera to *S. mansoni* and ELISAs for circulating schistosomal antigens. Antibody assays are useful for the diagnosis in patients who have recently visited endemic areas, but are of limited utility for the evaluation of patients from these areas.[287,303] Urine and serum ELISA tests have been developed that are capable of detecting various circulating antigens (e.g., circulating cationic antigen, circulating anionic antigen, circulating soluble egg antigens). These tests are considered very specific. Furthermore, quantitative assays correlate with intensity of infection and can be used to monitor response to therapy.[287,304,305]

Treatment and Prevention

Chemotherapy of schistosomiasis decreases morbidity, reduces disease transmission in the community, and may even result in some improvement of periportal fibrosis.[287] Pharmacologic options include praziquantel (active against all species) and oxamniquine (active against *S. mansoni*). Praziquantel causes spastic paralysis of the parasite. Side effects include abdominal discomfort, fever, dizziness, and headache. Depending on the infecting species 20 mg/kg are taken twice or three times per day for 1 to 3 days. Oxamniquine kills adult worms by causing lethal tegumental alterations. A single dose of 15 to 20 mg/kg is sufficient for patients returning from Latin America, whereas 60 mg/kg is used for African cases. Side effects are rare and transient and may include dizziness, headache, vomiting, diarrhea, and seizures.[287-289,291] Adjunctive surgical and endoscopic procedures may benefit patients presenting with complications of portal hypertension.[287] Preventive measures are directed toward the control of snail populations using molluscicides, improved sanitation, health education, and mass or targeted chemotherapy campaigns.[287]

Summary of Schistosomiasis and the Liver

Four of the five most common species of schistosomes affecting humans are characterized by significant liver involvement. Even during early stages such as Katayama fever, patients may present with hepatomegaly. Hepatosplenic schistosomiasis is one of the most common chronic syndromes associated with long-standing infection. Affected patients present with hepatomegaly (mainly of the left lobe) and portal hypertension caused by periportal fibrosis, whereas synthetic liver functions are usually preserved (see Plate 35-13). Histologic examination of the liver reveals egg granulomas (see Plate 35-12). Some authors have reported a higher incidence of concurrent hepatitis B and C infection in patients with schistosomiasis.[287,306,307] Although this is still considered controversial, in a few series co-infection was associated with a more severe and rapid course toward fibrosis, cirrhosis, and cancer.[307]

LIVER FLUKES (FASCIOLIASIS, CLONORCHIASIS, OPISTORCHIASIS)

Background and Epidemiology

Fascioliasis is caused by either *Fasciola hepatica* or *Fasciola gigantica*. *F. hepatica* (Plate 35-14) is a flat, leaflike trematode, 20 to 30 mm long and 10 mm wide, with large, ovoid eggs. *F. gigantica* may reach 7.5 cm in length and has even larger operculated eggs.[291,308] *F. hepatica* is mainly found in temperate climates. It has a cosmopolitan distribution, being prevalent in most sheep-raising areas, with reported cases from South America, Europe, Africa, China, and Australia.[289] More than 2 million people are estimated to be infected worldwide. Numerous species of amphibious snails of the genus *Lymnaea* serve as the first intermediate hosts. The second intermediate hosts are various kinds of aquatic vegetation. The most important definitive hosts are sheep but other herbivores are commonly infected. *F. gigantica* infection is found in Africa, southern Europe, the southern United States and Hawaii, the former Soviet Union, the Middle East, and South East Asia.[308] A wide range of mammals such as cattle, goats, and water buffaloes act as definitive hosts. As in *F. hepatica* snails constitute the intermediate host.

Clonorchiasis is caused by the Chinese liver fluke (*Clonorchis sinensis*), which measures 10 to 25 mm by 3 to 5 mm and produces small operculated eggs. It is endemic in Japan, Korea, China, Taiwan, and Vietnam, where the intermediate hosts are found and people eat raw fish.

It is believed that more than 7 million people are infected. Snails and fish are intermediate hosts for this parasite. The definitive hosts are mammals, including dogs, cats, pigs, mink, rats, and other fish-eating animals.[308] Opisthorchiasis is caused by *Opisthorchis viverrini* and *Opisthorchis felineus.* Both are approximately 10 mm long and produce small operculated eggs. *O. viverrini* is endemic in northern and northeastern Thailand and Laos. *O. felineus* is found in Poland, Germany, Siberia, and the former Soviet Union. Approximately 1.6 million people are affected. The two intermediate hosts are different snail species and fish. Domestic cats, dogs, and fish-eating mammals are definitive hosts.[308]

Life Cycle and Transmission

Eggs shed in feces of the definitive host reach fresh water where they transform into miracidia, which penetrate various snail species and evolve to sporocysts, rediae, and cercariae. Mature cercariae emerge from the snail and reach the second intermediate host. In the case of fascioliasis aquatic vegetation serves as the second intermediate host, whereas in clonorchiasis and opisthorchiasis different fish species are implicated.

Definitive hosts, including humans and other mammals, become infected when they ingest the second intermediate host. In fascioliasis, metacercaria excyst in the duodenum and migrate through the intestinal wall into the peritoneal cavity, then penetrate the liver capsule and parenchyma to enter the bile ducts, where they mature into adult flukes. In clonorchiasis and opisthorchiasis, metacercaria excyst in the duodenum or jejunum and migrate through the ampulla of Vater and the common bile duct and finally reach intrahepatic bile ducts where they mature and begin to produce eggs (Plate 35-15).

Pathogenesis and Pathology

In fascioliasis, migrating metacercariae cause parenchymal necrosis, hemorrhage, and abscesses. Adult flukes result in hyperplasia, desquamation, thickening, dilation, and fibrotic changes of bile ducts. It is speculated that parasite-derived proline is responsible for some of these changes. The degree of tissue destruction correlates with the worm load.[308] In clonorchiasis and opisthorchiasis excessive mucin production, desquamation, and adenomatous hyperplasia of the duct epithelium are observed. A multi-factorial etiology including mechanical irritation, production of toxic substances, immunologic responses of the host, and bacterial superinfection has been postulated. More severe disease may result in biliary obstruction caused by periductal infiltration with inflammatory cells as well as necrosis and atrophy of surrounding hepatocytes. Dilation of intrahepatic bile ducts is common. The gallbladder is frequently enlarged and dysfunctional. Opisthorchiasis has been associated with cirrhosis, cholangitis, pancreatitis, and cholangiocarcinoma (Plate 35-16, *A* and *B*).[308,309]

Clinical Manifestations

The metacercarial migratory phase in fascioliasis correlates with an acute illness characterized by dyspepsia, anorexia, nausea, vomiting, fevers, abdominal pain, hepatomegaly, and urticaria. Rarely, prostration and jaundice are seen. These symptoms can persist for months. In some areas asymptomatic infection is common. In chronic disease, after the lodging of the adult worms in the biliary tract, most patients are asymptomatic but others present with right upper quadrant pain, diarrhea, nausea, vomiting, hepatomegaly, and jaundice.[289,308] Most people with clonorchiasis and opisthorchiasis are asymptomatic.[289,310] Although infections are often acquired in childhood, symptomatic disease is rarely observed before the third decade of life. Only a few patients present with acute symptoms resembling serum sickness, facial edema, or allergic hepatitis. The onset of symptoms of chronic disease is usually insidious. Symptomatic disease may be heralded by dull discomfort in the right upper quadrant, followed by anorexia, flatulence, occasional diarrhea, low-grade fever, and hepatomegaly. Urticaria, jaundice, and ascites are rare. Weight loss has been reported in patients with high parasite loads. Other complications include cholangitis, pancreatitis, and cholangiocarcinoma (see Plate 35-16, *A* and *B*).

Diagnostic Tests

In fascioliasis, laboratory tests may show anemia, leukocytosis, eosinophilia, hypergammaglobulinemia, and elevated liver enzymes. Imaging studies may be helpful; ultrasonography is often normal but may detect flukes in the biliary tree.[311] CT scans frequently show small, often peripheral hypodense, nodules, which decrease in size after successful therapy.[311,312] Cholangiography can demonstrate flukes in bile ducts or gallbladder.[308] Serologic tests including ELISA, hemagglutination, complement fixation, and counterimmunoelectrophoresis are available. Serology is useful in patients with ectopic fascioliasis or with acute disease before eggs appear in the feces.[308,311] Definitive diagnosis usually relies on the detection of eggs in the fecal samples or duodenal aspirates. Rarely, adult flukes are detected at surgery or autopsy.[308]

In clonorchiasis and opisthorchiasis, results of routine laboratory tests show findings similar to what is seen in fascioliasis. Serologic tests (ELISA) and antigen-detection tests may assist in the diagnosis, but the definitive diagnosis is made by detecting eggs in fresh samples of stool or bile.[308]

Treatment and Prevention

Therapeutic options for fascioliasis include bithionol, triclabendazole, praziquantel, chloroquine, and emetine. Emetine has been used extensively in the past but has only limited efficacy.[291,308] Similarly, chloroquine has been found to be of little value in controlled trials.[308] Praziquantel is effective in some cases, but has demonstrated poor efficacy in a trial in Egypt.[308] Bithionol[139,289,313] or triclabendazole[308,314] is therefore considered the treatment of choice. Praziquantel is very effective for the treatment of clonorchiasis and opisthorchiasis, even when used in single-day or single-dose regimens. Mebendazole for 3 to 4 weeks and albendazole for 7 days are alternatives. Prevention relies on education regarding eating habits associated with an increased risk of infection. Avoiding watercress salad for fascioliasis and cooking freshwater fish for other liver flukes is recommended. The use of molluscicides and other measures to eliminate snails is theoretically attractive but may prove difficult and expensive.

Summary of Liver Flukes and the Liver

Liver flukes can produce right upper quadrant symptoms. Hepatomegaly is a common finding on physical examination of affected patients. Liver enzymes are frequently elevated. Biliary obstruction, associated jaundice, and complications including cholangitis, pancreatitis, and cholangiocarcinoma (see Plate 35-16, *A* and *B*) have been reported. Patients presenting with right upper quadrant symptoms, fever, elevated liver enzymes, and jaundice are commonly tested for viral hepatitides. In such cases the presence of eosinophilia and a good knowledge of the epidemiologic background are helpful clues in the diagnosis.

INFECTIONS CAUSED BY CESTODES ECHINOCOCCOSIS (HYDATID CYST AND ALVEOLAR CYST)

Background and Epidemiology

Echinococcosis is a zoonotic disease caused by the larval stage of the tapeworms *Echinococcus granulosus, Echinococcus vogeli,* and *Echinococcus multilocularis.* The adult tapeworm of this parasite infects a variety of carnivores, including dogs, foxes, and wolves, which are considered the definitive hosts. The intermediate hosts for *E. granulosus* and *E. vogeli* are farm animals such as sheep, cattle, swine, and horses that acquire the parasite via ingestion of eggs deposited in the pasture. In the case of *E. multilocularis* intermediate hosts comprise voles, lemmings, shrews, and mice. Humans are accidental hosts.[315-317] *E. granulosus* and *E. vogeli* infections are prevalent in regions of the world where dogs are used to herd large flocks of sheep. They are widely distributed in South America, the Mediterranean basin, central Russia, Asia, Australia, and Africa.[315] *E. multilocularis* has adapted to cold climates and is able to thrive even in arctic and alpine climates.[317] Cases have been reported from the United States, Switzerland, France, Germany, Austria, the former Soviet Union, Siberia, northern Japan, and China.

Life Cycle and Transmission

Adult tapeworms live in the intestine of their carnivorous definitive hosts. Eggs are shed into the environment with feces and are ingested by intermediate hosts. In the intestinal lumen oncospheres hatch, penetrate the mucosa, and enter the portal circulation. When they reach a target organ, oncospheres transform into mature larval cysts. The definitive host, acquires the parasite by ingestion of infected viscera containing larval forms. In the intestines of the definite hosts, larvae mature into adult tapeworms.[316,318]

Human disease is caused by larval forms. Humans acquire the parasite via ingestion of eggs in food contaminated with feces or soil.

Pathogenesis and Pathology

Oncospheres penetrate the intestinal mucosa and reach the mesenteric and portal circulation. From there they reach the liver and various other organs, forming larval cysts (Plate 35-17, *A*). This is accompanied by an initial inflammatory reaction characterized by infiltration with mononuclear and eosinophilic cells. Larval cysts of *E. granulosus* and *E. vogeli* are most commonly found in the liver (50 percent-70 percent of patients) or the lungs (20 percent-30 percent) and only rarely affect other organs such as brain, heart, or bones.[315,316] Liver cysts more frequently affect the right lobe. Cysts usually remain asymptomatic until complications arise secondary to mass effect, rupture, invasion of adjacent structures, or bacterial superinfection. Growing cysts have eroded into the biliary tree, suprahepatic veins, vena cava, or bronchi. Microscopic sections of the cyst wall reveal an outer layer of neutrophils, lymphocytes, and eosinophils; an external laminated membrane; a central fibroblastic zone; and an inner germinal membrane containing scoleces (Plate 35-17, *B*). Atrophy of surrounding hepatocytes may be observed. The fluid of the cyst is a potent antigen, and small leaks can result in sensitization and later cause allergic reactions of varying severity.

E. multilocularis produces multi-loculated tumor-like cystic lesions with a firm, solid, and yellow to grayish appearance in a variety of different organs.[316,317] Cysts are primarily found in the liver, but the parasite has a tendency to metastasize to distant body sites via lymphatic and hematogenous spread. Lesions are often multiple and affect all parts of the liver. Larval proliferation is most active at the periphery of the cysts, whereas central areas can degenerate, resulting in necrosis, calcification, and frank abscess formation. Microscopically the masses show multiple vesicles of varying sizes lined by the external laminated membrane of the parasite. The multitude of vesicles is the consequence of asexual reproduction by lateral budding. Usually a dense layer of scar tissue and inflammatory cells surrounds the vesicles.

Clinical Manifestations

Disease produced by *E. granulosus* and *E. vogeli* (cystic hydatid disease) is often asymptomatic, and clinical syndromes arise as a consequence of mass effect, rupture, or superinfection. Many asymptomatic cysts are detected incidentally in patients undergoing radiologic studies. Mass effect can result in a palpable mass, obstructive jaundice, chest pain, cough, fever, and hemoptysis. Bacteria may secondarily superinfect cysts and result in formation of pyogenic abscesses within the cyst. Bacterial superinfection can also complicate bronchial and biliary erosion. Cyst rupture can result in formation of peritoneal cysts and occasionally causes peritonitis. Leakage or rupture can also trigger allergic reactions in previously sensitized patients, ranging from a mild erythematous rash to a life-threatening anaphylactic reaction.[315,316]

E. multilocularis infection (alveolar hydatid disease) behaves like a malignant tumor and is often manifested by abdominal pain, a palpable mass, hepatomegaly, jaundice, shortness of breath, and CNS symptoms when brain disease is present. Complications include portal and suprahepatic vein compression, biliary obstruction with jaundice and cholangitis, and portal system involvement with portal hypertension and its consequences. Bacterial superinfection has been associated with septic illness or formation of pyogenic liver abscesses.[316,317]

Diagnostic Tests

Routine laboratory tests may show an elevated alkaline phosphatase, slight leukocytosis, and eosinophilia.[315] Elevations of transaminase levels are rare, as is cholestatic hyperbilirubinemia. Imaging studies are a mainstay of the diagnostic work-up. Even plain abdominal x-rays may be able to detect the presence of a liver cyst or mass, especially if the cyst wall shows calcifications. Chest radiography is the method of choice for the diagnosis of lung cysts. Ultrasonography, nuclear imaging, CT scanning, and MRI are useful to confirm the diagnosis and rule out alternative diagnoses. Cysts may appear as solitary lesions containing echogenic structures or as multi-loculated cysts. Some authors consider MRI more sensitive than CT.[319] In the case of *E. multilocularis* results of imaging studies may mimic polycystic disease[320] or malignancy.[316,317]

Suspected hydatid disease can be confirmed using serologic or parasitologic tests. Serologic tests include indirect hemagglutination test, ELISA, immune-electrophoresis, Western blot, and enzyme- linked immunoelectrotransfer blot test, which have high specificity (88 percent-96 percent) but in some series were noted to have suboptimal sensitivity (80 percent-100 percent) in patients with documented liver cysts.[321,322] A negative serologic test is therefore not considered sufficient to rule out hydatid disease in patients with characteristic lesions on imaging studies.[316,323] The sensitivity of serologic tests is even lower for patients with disease involving other organs. Hemagglutination tests often suffer from cross reactivity to *E. multilocularis* infection, with sensitivities around 90 percent. ELISA and Western blot analysis are more specific and can differentiate between *E. granulosus* and *E. multilocularis,* and some may be useful in distinguishing active and inactive disease.[324-326] Antigen detection tests using recombinant echinococcal antigens may increase specificity and may be able to distinguish between *E. granulosus* and *E. vogeli* infections.[316,318] Parasitologic tests are based on the examination of expectorated, aspirated, or surgical specimens, which may reveal protoscolices, hooklets, or hydatid membranes.[315] Aspiration of *E. granulosus* and *E. vogeli* cysts carries a risk of anaphylactic reactions and inadvertent seeding of infection.[318] Because of the tumor-like appearance of *E. multilocularis* disease, many lesions are biopsied. The characteristic multi-laminar cyst membrane shows up well using a PAS stain.[317]

Treatment and Prevention

Asymptomatic cystic hydatid disease can be observed for prolonged periods.[316] Completely calcified cysts do not require any therapy.[315] Symptomatic or complicated cysts should be treated. Chemotherapy with albendazole (10-15 mg/kg, or 400 mg twice per day, in 3 to 12 cycles of 28 days with 14-day periods of rest) is indicated for the treatment of inoperable disease and for pre- and post-surgical treatment (including before and after percutaneous drainage) to prevent or reduce the risk of recurrence after cyst spillage during operation.[315] Some authorities favor combination therapy with ivermectin. Percutaneous aspiration of hepatic cysts under ultrasonographic guidance in conjunction with albendazole has been used with good results and is considered more cost-effective than surgery.[327,328] Cyst contents are aspirated and the cavity is filled with hypertonic saline (20 percent-30 percent), which is left in place for 20 minutes before reaspiration. It is considered the method of choice in centers with expertise.[315] Adequate monitoring is critical to detect and treat potential life-threatening anaphylactic reactions. Some centers consider surgical removal of the cyst the treatment of choice for symptomatic cysts.[316] The recommended approach is visualization of the cyst, removal of some of the fluid, instillation of a cysticidal agent followed by re-aspiration, opening of the cyst, removal of the membranes, and filling of the cavity with omentum.[315,316] Perioperative use of steroids is recommended to prevent serious allergic reactions. Superinfected cysts usually require drainage. For alveolar hydatid disease, surgical resection including hepatic lobectomy or liver transplantation is recommended.[329,330] Adjuvant therapy with albendazole was beneficial in case series.[316] For inoperable cases long-term chemotherapy with albendazole or mebendazole is associated with a 10-year survival rate approaching 90 percent.[317] Regression of cysts can be expected in almost 50 percent of conservatively treated patients and stabilization or halting of progression is observed in an additional 30 percent of these patients. However, 15 percent will likely experience progressive disease despite chemotherapy.[331] Severe late complications of chemotherapy include cholestatic jaundice and esophageal variceal bleeding secondary to hilar fibrosis.[317] Prevention includes periodic treatment of dogs with praziquantel, avoiding feeding raw viscera to dogs, and behavior-modifying education. In some areas control was achieved after extermination of non-domestic canines.[315,317]

Summary of Echinococcosis and the Liver

E. granulosus and *E. vogeli* cause cystic hydatid disease characterized by liver cysts (see Plate 35-17, *A* and *B*). Many of these cases are detected incidentally when patients undergo imaging studies for unrelated symptoms. Complications include cholestasis, superinfection, and rupture. Laboratory tests may reveal increases of alkaline phosphatase, AST, alanine aminotransferase (ALT), and hyperbilirubinemia. *E. multilocularis* causes alveolar hydatid disease characterized by tumor-like lesions primarily involving the liver that commonly metastasize to other organs. Clinical appearance and progression may mimic malignant tumors. Complications include cholangitis, obstruction of hepatic veins, portal hypertension with its sequelae, and bacterial superinfection with a sepsis-like syndrome. Long-term chemotherapy with albendazole has been associated with cholestasis and variceal bleeding resulting from treatment-induced hilar fibrosis.

References

1. Willhoeft U, Tannich E: The electrophoretic karyotype of *Entamoeba histolytica.* Mol Biochem Parasitol 99:41-53, 1999.
2. Brandt H, Perez Tamayo R: Pathology of human amebiasis. Hum Pathol 1:351-385, 1970.
3. Prathap K, Gilman R: The histopathology of acute intestinal amebiasis. Am J Pathol 60:229-239, 1970.
4. Beaver PC, Jung RC, Cupp EW: Amebae inhibiting the alimentary canal. In Goldman IS, Brandborg LL, eds: Clinical Parasitology. Philadelphia, Lea & Febiger, 1984:101.
5. Bhattacharya A, Satish S, Bagchi A, et al: The genome of *Entamoeba histolytica.* Int J Parasitol 30(4):401-410, 2000.
6. Bagchi A, Bhattacharya A, Bhattacharya S: Lack of a chromosomal copy of the circular rDNA plasmid of *Entamoeba histolytica.* Int J Parasitol 29(11):1775-1783, 1999.
7. Lucht E, Evengard B, Skott J, et al: *Entamoeba gingivalis* in human immunodeficiency virus type 1-infected patients with periodontal disease. Clin Infect Dis 27:471-473, 1998.
8. Ravdin JI: Diagnosis of invasive amoebiasis—time to end the morphology era. Gut 35:1018-1021, 1994.
9. Clark CG, Diamond LS: *Entamoeba histolytic*—an explanation for the reported conversion of nonpathogenic ameba to the pathogenic form. Exp Parasitol 77:456-460, 1993.
10. Clark CG, Diamond LS: Ribosomal RNA genes of "pathogenic" and "nonpathogenic" *Entamoeba histolytica* are distinct. Mol Biochem Parasitol 49:297-302, 1991.
11. Huston CD, Hahn CS, Petri WA Jr: Role of host cell caspase 3 in apoptotic killing by *Entamoeba histolytica* (abstract 203). In Program and Abstracts of the Annual Meeting of the American Society of Tropical Medicine and Hygiene, Nov 29-Dec 2, 1999, Washington, DC.
12. Tannich E, Horstmann RD, Knobloch J, et al: Genomic DNA differences between pathogenic and non-pathogenic *Entamoeba histolytica.* Proc Natl Acad Sci U S A 86:5118-5122, 1989.
13. Sargeaunt PG, Williams JE, Grene JD: The differentiation of invasive and non-invasive *Entamoeba histolytica* by isoenzyme electrophoresis. Trans R Soc Trop Med Hyg 72(5):519-521, 1978.
14. Haque R, Ali IM, Petri WA Jr: Prevalence and immune response to *Entamoeba histolytica* infection in preschool children in Bangladesh. Am J Trop Med Hyg 60:1031-1034, 1999.
15. Martinez-Garcia MC, Munoz O, Garduno G, et al: Pathogenic and non-pathogenic zymodemes of *Entamoeba histolytica* in a rural area of Mexico: concordance with serology. Arch Invest Med Mex 21(suppl 1):147-152, 1990.
16. WHO: Amoebiasis. WHO Weekly Epidemiol Rec 72(14):97-99, 1997.
17. Nanda R, Anand BS, Baveja U: *Entamoeba histolytica* cyst passers: clinical features and outcome in untreated subjects. Lancet 2:301-303, 1984.
18. Gaithiram V, Jackson TFGH: A longitudinal study of asymptomatic carriers of pathogenic zymodemes of *Entamoeba histolytica.* S Afr Med J 72:669-672, 1987.
19. Petri WA: Recent advances in amebiasis. Crit Rev Clin Lab Sci 33(1):1-37, 1996.
20. Anonymous: Summary of notifiable diseases, United States. MMWR 43(53):1-80, 1994.
21. Thompson JE Jr, Glasser AJ: Amebic abscess of the liver: diagnostic features. J Clin Gastroenterol 8:550-554, 1986.
22. Thorsen S, Ronne-Rasmussen J, Petersen E, et al: Extra-intestinal amebiasis. Clinical presentation in a non-endemic setting. Scand J Infect Dis 25:747-750, 1993.
23. Weinke T, Friedrich-Janicke B, Hopp P, et al: Prevalence and clinical importance of *Entamoeba histolytica* in two high-risk groups: travelers returning from the tropics and male homosexuals. J Infect Dis 161:1029-1031, 1989.
24. de Lalla F, Rinaldi E, Santoro D, et al: Outbreak of *Entamoeba histolytica* and *Giardia lamblia* infections in travelers returning from the tropics. Infection 20:78-82, 1992.
25. Gatti S, Lopes R, Cevini C, et al: Intestinal parasitic infections in an institution for the mentally retarded. Ann Trop Med Parasitol 94(5):453-460, 2000.
26. Nagakura K, Tachibana H, Tanaka T, et al: An outbreak of amebiasis in an institution for the mentally retarded in Japan. Jpn J Med Sci Biol 42:63-76, 1989.
27. Ghadirian E, Meerovitch E: Effect of immunosuppression on the size and metastasis of amoebic liver abscesses in hamsters. Parasite Immunol 3:329-338, 1981.
28. Ghadirian E, Meerovitch E: Effect of splenectomy on the size of the amoebic liver abscesses and metastatic foci in hamsters. Infect Immunol 31:571-573, 1981.
29. Ghadirian E, Meerovitch E: Macrophage requirement for host defense against experimental hepatic amebiasis in the hamster. Parasite Immunol 4:219-225, 1982.
30. Seeto RK, Rockey DC: Amebic liver abscess: epidemiology, clinical features, and outcome. West J Med 170:104-109, 1999.
31. Walsh JA: Transmission of *Entamoeba histolytica* infection. In Ravdin JL, ed: Amebiasis: Human Infection by *Entamoeba histolytica.* New York, John Wiley & Sons, 1988:126.
32. Barwick RS, Uzicanin A, Lareau S, et al: Outbreak of amebiasis in Tbilisi, Republic of Georgia, 1998. In Program and Abstracts of the Annual Meeting of the American Society of Tropical Medicine and Hygiene, Nov-2 Dec 29, 1999, Washington, DC.
33. Gottle MU, Keller K, Belley A, et al: Functional heterogeneity of colonic adenocarcinoma mucins for inhibition of *Entamoeba histolytica* adherence to target cells. J Eukaryot Microbiol 45:17S-23S, 1998.
34. Leroy A, Lauwaet T, De Bruyne G, et al: *Entamoeba histolytica* disturbs the tight junction complex in human enteric T84 cell layers. FASEB J 14(9):1139-1146, 2000.
35. Salata RA, Ravdin JL: The interaction of human neutrophils and *Entamoeba histolytica* increase cytopathogenicity for liver cell monolayers. J Infect Dis 154:19-26, 1986.
36. Tsutsumi V, Mena-Lopez R, Anaya-Velazquez F, et al: Cellular basis experimental amebic liver abscess formation. Am J Pathol 117:81-91, 1984.
37. Sharma MP, Sushma S, Verma N: Long term follow-up of amebic liver abscess. Clinical and ultrasound patterns of resolution. Trop Gastroenterol 16:24-28, 1995.
38. Joyce MP, Ravdin JI: Pathology of human amebiasis. In Ravdin JI, ed: Amebiasis: Human infection by *Entamoeba histolytica.* New York, John Wiley & Sons, 1988:132.
39. Reed S, Bouvier J, Pollack AS, et al: Cloning of a virulence factor of *Entamoeba histolytica:* pathogenic strains possess a unique cysteine proteinase gene. J Clin Invest 91(4):1532-1540, 1993.
40. Que X, Reed SL: Cysteine proteinases and the pathogenesis of amebiasis. Clin Microbiol Rev 13(2):196-206, 2000.
41. Long-Krug SA, Fischer KJ, Hysmith RM, et al: Phospholipase A enzymes of *Entamoeba histolytica:* description and subcellular localization. J Infect Dis 152:536-541, 1985.
42. Espinosa-Cantellano M, Martinez-Palomo A: Pathogenesis of intestinal amebiasis: from molecules to disease. Clin Microbiol Rev 13(2):318-331, 2000.
43. Ragland BD, Ashley LS, Vaux DL, et al: *Entamoeba histolytica* target cells killed by trophozoites undergo apoptosis which is not blocked by bcl-2. Exp Parasitol 79:460-467, 1994.
44. Seydel KB, Stanley SL Jr: *Entamoeba histolytica* induces host cell death in amebic liver abscess by a non-fas-dependent, non-tumor necrosis factor alpha-dependent pathway of apoptosis. Infect Immunol 66:2980-2983, 1998.
45. Berninghausen O, Leippe M: Necrosis versus apoptosis as the mechanism of target cell death induced by *Entamoeba histolytica.* Infect Immunol 65:3615-3621, 1997.
46. Ankri S, Stolarsky T, Mirelman D: Antisense inhibition of expression of cysteine proteinases does not affect *Entamoeba histolytica* cytopathic or haemolytica activity but inhibits phagocytosis. Mol Microbiol 28:777-785, 1998.
47. Tran VQ, Herdman DS, Torian BE, et al: The neutral cysteine proteinase of *Entamoeba histolytica* degrades IgG and prevents its binding. J Infect Dis 177:508-511, 1998.
48. Zhang Z, Yan L, Wang L, et al: *Entamoeba histolytica* cysteine proteinases with interleukin-1 beta converting enzyme (ICE) activity cause intestinal inflammation and tissue damage in amoebiasis. Mol Microbiol 37(3):542-548, 2000.
49. Petri WA Jr, Chapman MD, Snodgrass T, et al: Subunit structure of the galactose and N-acetyl-D-galactosamine-inhibitable adherence lectin of *Entamoeba histolytica.* J Biol Chem 264:3007-3012, 1989.
50. Lotter H, Zhang T, Seydel KB, et al: Identification of an epitope on the *Entamoeba histolytica* 170-kD lectin conferring antibody-

mediated protection against invasive amebiasis. J Exp Med 185(10):1793-1801, 1997.
51. Ravdin JL, Guerrant RL: Role of adherence in cytopathogenic mechanisms of *Entamoeba histolytica.* Study with mammalian tissue culture cells and human erythrocytes. J Clin Invest 68:1305-1313, 1981.
52. Li E, Becker A, Stanley SL: Use of Chinese hamster ovary cells with altered glycosylation patterns to define carbohydrate specificity of *Entamoeba histolytica* adhesions. J Exp Med 167:1725-1730, 1988.
53. Adams SA, Robson SC, Gathiram V, et al: Immunological similarity between the 170 kD amoebic adherence glycoprotein and human *Beta 2* integrins. Lancet 341(8836):17-19, 1993.
54. Vines RR, Ramakrishnan G, Rogers JB, et al: Regulation of adherence and virulence by the *Entamoeba histolytica* lectin cytoplasmic domain, which contains a *B*2 integrin motif. Mol Biol Cell 9:2069-2079, 1998.
55. Dodson JM, Leukowski PW Jr, Eubanks AC, et al: Infection and immunity mediated by the carbohydrate recognition domain of the *Entamoeba histolytica* Gal/GalNac lectin. J Infect Dis 179:460-466, 1999.
56. Jacobs T, Bruchhaus I, Dandekar T, et al: Isolation and molecular characterization of a surface-bound proteinase of *Entamoeba histolytica.* Mol Microbiol 27:269-276, 1998.
57. Arias-Negrete S, De Lourdes-Munoz M, Murillo-Jasso F: Expression of *in vitro* virulence by *Entamoeba histolytica:* effect of calmodulin inhibitors. APMIS 107(9):875-881, 1999.
58. Bracha R, Nuchamowitz Y, Leippe M, et al: Antisense inhibition of amoebapore expression in *Entamoeba histolytica* causes a decrease in amoebic virulence. Mol Microbiol 34(3):463-472, 1999.
59. Salata RA, Ravdin JI: Review of the human immune mechanisms directed against *Entamoeba histolytica.* Rev Infect Dis 8(2):261-272, 1986.
60. Guerrero-Manriquez GG, Sanchez-Ibarra F, Avila EE: Inhibition of *Entamoeba histolytica* proteolytic activity by human salivary IgA antibodies. APMIS 106(11):1088-1094, 1998.
61. Martinez-Palomo A, Tsutsumi F, Anaya-Velazquez F, et al: Ultrastructure of experimental intestinal invasive amebiasis. Am J Trop Med Hyg 41:273-279, 1989.
62. Tsutsumi V, Martinez-Palomo A: Inflammatory reaction in experimental hepatic amebiasis: an ultrastructural study. Am J Pathol 130:112-119, 1988.
63. Eckmann L, Reed S, Smith JR, et al: *Entamoeba histolytica* trophozoites induce an inflammatory cytokine response by cultured human cells through the paracrine action of cytolytically released interleukin-1 alpha. J Clin Invest 96(3):1269-1279, 1995.
64. Abioye AA: Fatal amoebic colitis in pregnancy and puerperium: a new clinico-pathological entity. J Trop Med Hyg 76:97-100, 1973.
65. Lewis EA, Antia AU: Amoebic colitis: review of 295 cases. Trans R Soc Trop Med Hyg 63(5):633-638, 1969.
66. Eisert J, Hannibal JE Jr, Sanders SL: Fatal amebiasis complicating corticosteroid management of pemphigus vulgaris. N Engl J Med 261:843-845, 1959.
67. Adams EB, Macleod IN: Invasive amebiasis. I. Amebic dysentery and its complications. Medicine 56:315-323, 1977.
68. Rode H, Davies MRQ, Cywes S: Amoebic liver abscesses in infancy and childhood. S Afr J Surg 16:131-138, 1978.
69. Chandra RK: Cell-mediated immunity in nutritional imbalance. Fed Proc 39:3088-3092, 1980.
70. Ahmed M, McAdam KPWJ, Sturm AW, et al: Systematic manifestations of invasive amebiasis. Clin Infect Dis 15:974-982, 1991.
71. Palau LA, Kemmerly SA: First report of invasive amebiasis in an organ transplant recipient. Transplantation 64(6):936-937, 1997.
72. Pearce RB: Intestinal protozoal infections in AIDS. Lancet 2:51, 1983.
73. Pomerantz BM, Marr JS, Goldman WD: Amebiasis in New York City, 1958-1978: identification of the male homosexual high risk population. Bull N Y Acad Med 56:232-244, 1980.
74. William DC, Shookfoff HB, Feldman YM, et al: High rates of enteric protozoal infections in selected homosexual males attending a venereal disease clinic. Sex Transm Dis 5:155-157, 1978.
75. Phillips SC, Mildvan D, Willliam DC, et al: Sexual transmission of enteric protozoa and helminthes in a venereal disease clinic population. N Engl J Med 305:603-606, 1981.
76. Schmerin MJ, Gelston A, Jones TC: Amebiasis. An increasing problem among homosexuals in New York City. JAMA 238;1386-1387, 1977.
77. Reed SL, Wessel DW, Davis CE: *Entamoeba histolytica* infection and AIDS. Am J Med 90:269-271, 1991.
78. Allason-Jones E, Mindel A, Sargeaunt PG, et al: *Entamoeba histolytica* as a commensal intestinal parasite in homosexual men. N Engl J Med 315:353-356, 1986.
79. Allason-Jones E, Mindel A, Sargeaunt PG, et al: Outcome of untreated infection with *Entamoeba histolytica* in homosexual men with and without HIV antibody. BMJ 297:654-657, 1988.
80. Lowther SA, Sworkin MS, Hanson DL: *Entamoeba histolytica/ Entamoeba dispar* infections in human immunodeficiency virus-infected patients in the United States. Clin Infect Dis 30(6):959-959, 2000.
81. Petri WA, Singh U: Diagnosis and management of amebiasis. Clin Infect Dis 29:1117-1125, 1999.
82. Adams EB, Macleod IN: Invasive amebiasis. II. Amebic liver abscess and its complications. Medicine 56:325-334, 1977.
83. Kimura K, Stoopen M, Reeder MM, et al: Amebiasis: modern diagnostic imaging with pathological and clinical correlation. Semin Roentgenol 32(4):250-275, 1997.
84. Ellyson JH, Bezmalinovic Z, Parks SN, et al: Necrotizing amebic colitis: a frequently fatal complication. Am J Surg 152:21-26, 1986.
85. Turner GR, Millikan M, Carter R: Surgical significance of fulminating amebic colitis. Am Surg 31(11):759-763, 1965.
86. Aristizabal H, Acevedo J, Botero M: Fulminant amebic colitis. World J Surg 15:216-221, 1991.
87. Luvuno FM, Mtshali Z, Baker LW: Toxic dilatation complicating fulminant amebic colitis. Br J Surg 69:56-57, 1982.
88. Levine SM, Stover JF, Warren JG, et al: Amoeboma forgotten granuloma. JAMA 215:1461-1464, 1971.
89. Chuah SK, Chang-Chien CS, Sheen IS, et al: The prognostic factors of severe amebic liver abscess: a retrospective study of 125 cases. Am J Trop Med Hyg 46(4):398-402, 1992.
90. Katzenstein D, Rickerson V, Braude A: New concepts of amebic liver abscess derived from hepatic imaging, serodiagnosis, and hepatic enzymes in 67 consecutive cases in San Diego. Medicine 61(4):237-246, 1982.
91. Greenstein AJ, Barth J, Dicker A, et al: Amebic liver abscess: a study of 11 cases compared with a series of 38 patients with pyogenic abscess. Am J Gastroenterol 80:472-478, 1985.
92. Gonzalez MF, Lee Ramos AF, Aguirre GJ: Influencia del sexo y la edad en la amibiasis invasora del higado. Arch Invest Med Mex 5(suppl 1):395-400, 1971.
93. Barnes PF, De Cock KM, Reynolds TN, et al: A comparison of amebic and pyogenic abscess of the liver. Medicine 66:472-483, 1987.
94. Citronberg RJ, Semel JD: Severe vaginal infection with *Entamoeba histolytica* in a woman who recently returned from Mexico: case report and review. Clin Infect Dis 20:700-702, 1995.
95. Ralls PW: Focal inflammatory disease of the liver. Radiol Clin North Am 36:377-389, 1998.
96. Reddy DR, Rao JJ, Krishna RV: Amoebic brain abscess. J Indian Med Assoc 63(2):61-62, 1974.
97. De Villers JP, Durra G: Amoebic abscess of the brain. Clin Radiol 53:307-309, 1998.
98. Krogstad DJ, Spencer HC, Healy GR, et al: Amebiasis: epidemiologic studies in the United States, 1971-1974. Ann Intern Med 88:89-97, 1978.
99. Fishman EK, Kavuru M, Jones B, et al: Pseudomembraneous colitis: CT evaluation of 26 cases. Radiology 180:57-60, 1991.
100. Caroline DF, Evers K: Colitis: radiographic features and differentiation of idiopathic inflammatory bowel disease. Radiol Clin North Am 25:47-66, 1987.
101. Leder RA, Low VH: Tuberculosis of the abdomen. Radiol Clin North Am 33:691-705, 1995.
102. Thompson JE Jr, Forlenza S, Verma R: Amebic liver abscess: a therapeutic approach. Rev Infect Dis 7:171-179, 1985.
103. Yeoh KG, Yap I, Wong ST, et al: Tropical liver abscess. Postgrad Med J 73:89-92, 1996.
104. Kammerer WS, Schantz PM: Echinococcal disease. Infect Dis Clin North Am 7:605-618, 1993.
105. Nordestgaard AG, Stapleford L, Worthen N, et al: Contemporary management of amebic liver abscess. Am Surg 58:315-320, 1992.
106. Cardoso JM, Kimura K, Stoopen M, et al: Radiology of invasive amebiasis of the colon. Am J Roentgenol 128:935-941, 1977.

107. Hardy R, Scullen DR: Thumbprinting in a case of amebiasis. Radiology 98:147-148, 1971.
108. Faengerbur D, Chiat H, Mandel P, et al: Toxic megacolon in amebic colitis: report of a case. Am J Roentgenol 99:74-76, 1967.
109. Kimura K, Stoopen M, Reeder MM, et al: Amebiasis: modern diagnostic imaging with clinical and pathological correlation. Semin Roentgenol 32:250-275, 1997.
110. Maltz G, Knauer CM: Amebic liver abscess. A 15-year experience. Am J Gastroenterol 86:704-710, 1991.
111. Sharma OP, Maheshwari A: Lung diseases in the tropics, part 2. Common tropical lung diseases: diagnosis and management. Tuber Lung Dis 74:359-370, 1993.
112. Cuaron A, Gordon F: Liver scanning, analysis of 2500 cases of amebic hepatic abscesses. J Nucl Med 11:435-439, 1970.
113. Remedios PA, Colletti PM, Ralls PW: Hepatic amebic abscess: cholescintigraphic rim enhancement. Radiology 160:395-398, 1986.
114. Ralls PW, Colletti PM, Halls JM: Imaging in hepatic amebic abscess. In Ravdin JL, ed: Amebiasis: Human infection by *Entamoeba histolytica.* New York, John Wiley & Sons, 1988:675.
115. Sharma MP, Dasarathy S: Amoebic liver abscess. Trop Gastroenterol 14:3-9, 1993.
116. Barreda R, Ros PR: Diagnostic imaging of liver abscess. Crit Rev Diag Imag 33:29-58, 1992.
117. Reitano M, Masci JR, Bottone EJ: Amebiasis: clinical and laboratory perspectives. Crit Rev Clin Lab Sci 28:357-385, 1991.
118. Rajak CL, Gupta S, Jain S, et al: Percutaneous treatment of liver abscesses: needle aspiration versus catheter drainage. AJR Am J Roentgenol 170:1035-1039, 1998.
119. Baek SY, Lee MG, Cho KS, et al: Therapeutic percutaneous aspiration of hepatic abscesses: effectiveness in 25 patients. AJR Am J Roentgenol 160:799-802, 1993.
120. Morris CN, Berbari EF, Steckelberg JM: 69-year-old man with fever, diarrhea, and abdominal pain. Mayo Clin Proc 73(12):1201-1204, 1998.
121. Gonzalez-Ruiz A, Bendall RP: Diagnosis of invasive amoebiasis: renaissance of the morphology era. Gut 36(5):800, 1995.
122. Ravdin JL: Reply: diagnosis of invasive amoebiasis: renaissance of the morphology era. Gut 36(5):800-801, 1995.
123. Haque R, Ali IKM, Akther S, et al: Comparison of PCR, isoenzyme analysis, and antigen detection for diagnosis of *Entamoeba histolytica* infection. J Clin Microbiol 36(2):449-452, 1998.
124. Gonzalez-Ruiz A, Haque R, Rehman T, et al: Further diagnostic use of an invasive-specific monoclonal antibody against *Entamoeba histolytica.* Arch Med Res 23:281-283, 1992.
125. Ganayi GA, Attia RA, Naggar HM: Some immunological studies on amebiasis. J Egypt Soc Parasitol 24:357-362, 1994.
126. Cummins AJ, Moody AH, Lalloo K, et al: Rapid latex agglutination test for extraluminal amebiasis. J Clin Pathol 47:647-664, 1994.
127. Ghandi BM, Irshad M, Chawla TC, et al: Enzyme-linked protein A: an ELISA for detection of amoebic antibody. Trans R Soc Trop Med 81:183-185, 1985.
128. Jalan KN, Maitra TK: Amebiasis in the developing world. In Ravdin JL, ed: Amebiasis: Human Infection by *Entamoeba histolytica.* New York, John Wiley & Sons, 1988:545.
129. Proctor EM: Laboratory diagnosis of amebiasis. Clin Lab Med 11:829-859, 1991.
130. Despommier DD: The laboratory diagnosis on *Entamoeba histolytica.* Bull N Y Acad Med 57(3):212-216, 1981.
131. Shamsuzzaman SM, Haque R, Hasin SK, et al: Evaluation of indirect fluorescent antibody test and enzyme-linked immunosorbent assay for diagnosis of hepatic amebiasis in Bangladesh. J Parasitol 86(3):611-615, 2000.
132. Hung CC, Chen PJ, Hsieh SM, et al: Invasive amoebiasis: an emerging parasitic disease in patients infected with HIV in an area endemic for amoebic infection. AIDS 13(17):2421-2428, 1999.
133. Myung K, Burch P, Jackson T, et al: Serodiagnosis of invasive amebiasis using a recombinant *Entamoeba histolytica* antigen-based ELISA. Arch Med Res 23:285-288, 1992.
134. Ravdin JL, Jackson TFGH, Petri WA Jr, et al: Association of serum antibodies to adherence lectin with invasive amebiasis and asymptomatic infection with pathogenic *Entamoeba histolytica.* J Infect Dis 162:768-772, 1990.
135. Stanley SL, Jackson TFGH, Foster L, et al: Longitudinal study of the antibody response to recombinant *Entamoeba histolytica* antigens in patients with amebic liver abscess. Am J Trop Med Hyg 58:414-416, 1998.
136. Evangelopoulos A, Spanakos G, Patsoula E, et al: A nested, multiplex, PCR assay for the simultaneous detection and differentiation of *Entamoeba histolytica* and *Entamoeba dispar* in faeces. Ann Trop Med Parasitol 94(3):233-240, 2000.
137. Gilman R, Islam M, Paschi S, et al: Comparison of conventional and immunofluorescent techniques for the detection of *Entamoeba histolytica* in rectal biopsies. Gastroenterology 78:435-439, 1980.
138. Mhlanga BR, Lanoie LO, Norris HJ, et al: Amebiasis complicating carcinomas: a diagnostic dilemma. Am J Trop Med Hyg 46:759-764, 1992.
139. Anonymous: Drugs for parasitic infections. Med Lett Drugs Ther 40 (1017):1-12, 1998.
140. Wassman C, Hellberg A, Tannich E, et al: Metronidazole resistance in the protozoan parasite *Entamoeba histolytica* is associated with increased expression of iron-containing superoxide dismutase and peroxiredoxin and decreased expression of ferredoxin 1 and flavin reductase. J Biol Chem 274(37):26051-26056, 1999.
141. Irusen EM, Jackson TFHG, Simjee AE: Asymptomatic intestinal colonization by pathogenic *Entamoeba histolytica* in amebic liver abscess: prevalence, response to therapy, and pathogenic potential. Clin Infect Dis 14:889-893, 1992.
142. Sharma MP, Ahuja V: Management of amebic liver abscess. Arch Med Res 31(4 suppl):S4-S5, 2000.
143. Hanna RM, Dahniya MH, Badr SS, et al: Percutaneous catheter drainage in drug-resistant amoebic liver abscess. Trop Med Int Health 5(8):578-581, 2000.
144. Eggleston FC, Verghese M, Handa AK, et al: The results of surgery in amebic liver abscess: experiences in eighty-three patients. Surgery 83:536-539, 1978.
145. Kagan IG: Pathogenicity of *E. histolytica.* Arch Invest Med Mex 5(suppl 2):457-464, 1974.
146. De Leon A: Pronostico tardio en el abscesco hepatico amibiano. Arch Invest Med Mex 1(suppl):205-206, 1970.
147. Huston CD, Petri WA Jr: Host-pathogen interaction in amebiasis and progress in vaccine development. Eur J Clin Microbiol Infect Dis 17:601-614, 1998.
148. Choudhuri G, Prakash V, Kumar A, et al: Protective immunity to *Entamoeba histolytica* infection in subjects with antiamoebic antibodies residing in hyperendemic zone. Scand J Infect Dis 23:771-776, 1991.
149. Ginny Soong CJ, Kain KC, Abd-Alla M, et al: A recombinant cysteine-rich section of the *Entamoeba histolytica* galactose-inhibitable lectin is efficacious as a subunit vaccine in the gerbil model of amebic liver abscess. J Infect Dis 171:645-651, 1995.
150. Stanley SL Jr: Progress towards development of a vaccine for amebiasis. Clin Microbiol Rev 10(4):637-649, 1997.
151. Stanley SL, Becker A, Kunz-Jenkins C, et al: Cloning and expression of a membrane antigen of *Entamoeba histolytica* possessing multiple tandem repeats. Proc Natl Acad Sci U S A 87:4976-4980, 1990.
152. Torian BE, Flores BM, Stroeher VL, et al: cDNA sequence analysis of a 29-kDa cysteine-rich surface antigen of pathogenic *Entamoeba histolytica.* Proc Natl Acad Sci U S A 87:6358-6362, 1990.
153. Reed SL, Davis CE, Jinich H: Amebiasis from the "Miraculous Water of Tlacote." N Engl J Med 332(10):687-688, 1995.
154. World malaria situation in 1994, Parts I-III. Wkly Epidemiol Rec 72:269-274, 277-283, 285-291, 1997.
155. Krogstad DJ: Plasmodium species (malaria). In Mandell GL, Bennett JE, Dolin R, eds: Principles and Practice of Infectious Diseases, ed 5, vol II. Philadelphia, Churchill Livingstone, 2000:2817-2831.
156. Botero D, Restrepo M: Malaria. In Botero D, Restrepo M, eds: Parasitosis Humanas, ed 3. Medellin (Colombia), CIB, 1998:158-202.
157. Miller LH, Good MF, Milton G: Malaria pathogenesis. Science 264:1878-1883, 1994.
158. Taylor TE, Strickland GT: Malaria. In Strickland DT, ed: Hunter's Tropical Medicine and Emerging Infectious Diseases, ed 8. Philadelphia, WB Saunders Co., 2000:614-642.
159. Parra ME, Evans CB, Taylor DW: Identification of *Plasmodium falciparum* histidine-rich protein 2 in the plasma of humans with malaria. J Clin Microbiol 29:1629-1634, 1991.
160. Palmer CJ, Lindo JF, Klaskala WI, et al: Evaluation of the OptiMAL test for rapid diagnosis of *Plasmodium vivax* and *Plasmodium falciparum* malaria. J Clin Microbiol 36: 203, 1998.

161. Nosten F: Prophylactic effect of Malarone against malaria: all good news? Lancet 356:1864, 2000.
162. Cook GC: Malaria in the liver. Postgrad Med J 70:780, 1994.
163. Hollingdale MR: Malaria and the liver. Hepatology 5(2):327-335, 1985.
164. Shortt HE, Garnham PCC, Covell G, Shute PG: The pre-erythrocytic stage of human malaria, *Plasmodium vivax*. BMJ 1:547, 1948.
165. Krotoski WA, Collins WE, Bray RS, et al: Demonstration of a hypnozoites in sporozoite-transmitted *Plasmodium vivax* infection. Am J Trop Med Hyg 31:1291, 1982.
166. Frevert U: Malaria sporozoite-hepatocyte interactions. Exp Parasitol 79:206-210, 1994.
167. Sinnis P: The malaria sporozoite journey into the liver. Infect Agents Dis 5:182-189, 1996.
168. Molyneux ME, Looareesuwan S, Menzies IS, et al: Reduced hepatic blood flow and intestinal malabsorption in severe falciparum malaria. Am J Trop Med Hyg 40:470-476, 1989.
169. Ramachandras S, Perera MV: Jaundice and hepatomegaly in primary malaria. J Trop Med Hyg 79:207, 1976.
170. Crane GG: Hyperreactive malarious splenomegaly (tropical splenomegaly syndrome). Parasitol Today 2:4-9, 1986.
171. Chawla LS, Sidhu G, Sabharwal BD, Bhatia KL, et al: Jaundice in *Plasmodium falciparum*. J Assoc Physicians India 37:390-391, 1989.
172. Joshi YK, Tandon BN, Acharya SK, et al: Acute hepatic failure due to *Plasmodium falciparum* liver injury. Liver 6:357-360, 1986.
173. Warrell DA, Francis N: Malaria. In McIntyre N, Benhamou J, Bircher J, et al, eds: Oxford Textbook of Clinical Hepatology. Oxford, Oxford University Press, 1991:701-706.
174. Anand AC, Ramji C, Narula AS, et al: Malarial hepatitis: a heterogeneous syndrome? Natl Med J India 5:59-62, 1992.
175. Welsh JD, Brown JD, Mathews HM, et al: Hepatitis BS antigen, malaria titers, and primary liver cancer in South Vietnam. Gastroenterology 70(3):392-396, 1976.
176. Back DH, Purba HS, Staiger C, et al: Inhibition of drug metabolism by the antimalarial drugs chloroquine and primaquine in the rat. Biochem Pharmacol 32:257-263, 1983.
177. Hollingdale MR, McCormick CJ, Heal KG, et al: Biology of malarial liver stages: implications for vaccine design. Ann Trop Med Parasitol 92(4):411-417, 1998.
178. Kamboj KK: Current trends in research on tissue stage of malaria. Indian J Med Res 106:120, 1997.
179. Mazier D, Renia L, Nussler A, et al: Hepatic phase of malaria is the target of cellular mechanisms induced by the previous and the subsequent stages. A crucial role for liver nonparenchymal cells. Immunol Lett 25:65-70, 1990.
180. Montoya JG, Remington JS: *Toxoplasma gondii*. In Mandell GL, Bennett JE, Dolin R, eds: Principles and Practice of Infectious Diseases, ed 5, vol II. Philadelphia, Churchill Livingstone, 2000:2558-2588.
181. Frenkel JK, Fishback JL: Toxoplasmosis. In Strickland DT, ed: Hunter's Tropical Medicine and Emerging Infectious Diseases, ed 8. Philadelphia, WB Saunders Co., 2000:691-701.
182. Stellbrink HJ, Führer-Burow R, Raedler A, et al: Risk factors for severe disease due to *Toxoplasma gondii* in HIV-positive patients. Eur J Epidemiol 9:633, 1993.
183. Albrecht H, Skörde J, Arasteh K, et al: Disseminated toxoplasmosis in AIDS-patients—report of 16 cases. Scand J Infect Dis 27:71-74, 1995.
184. Chiquet C, Fleury J, Blanc-Jouvan M, et al: Acquired ocular toxoplasmosis (panuveitis) after liver transplantation. J Fr Ophtalmol 23: 375, 2000.
185. Patel R: Disseminated toxoplasmosis after liver transplantation. Clin Infect Dis 29(5):705-706, 1999.
186. Botero D, Restrepo M: Toxoplasmosis. In Botero D, Restrepo M, eds: Parasitosis Humanas, ed 3. Medellin (Colombia), CIB, 1998:252-270.
187. Bohne W, Roos DS: Stage-specific expression of a selectable marker in *Toxoplasma gondii* permits selective inhibition of either tachyzoites or bradyzoites. Mol Biochem Parasitol 88:115-126, 1997.
188. Khan IA, Matsuura T, Kasper LH: Inducible nitric oxide synthase is not required for long-term vaccine-based immunity against *Toxoplasma gondii*. J Immunol 161(6):2994-3000, 1998.
189. Visher TL, Bernheim C, Engelbrecht E: Two cases of hepatitis due to *Toxoplasma gondii*. Lancet 2: 919, 1967.
190. Weitberg AB, Alper JC, Diamond I, et al: Acute granulomatous hepatitis in the course of acquired toxoplasmosis. N Engl J Med 300:1093-1096, 1979.
191. Teutsch SM, Juranek DD, Sulzer A, et al: Epidemic toxoplasmosis associated with infected cats. N Engl J Med 300:695-699, 1979.
192. Brion JP, Pelloux H, Le Marc'hadour F, et al: Acute toxoplasmic hepatitis in a patient with AIDS. Clin Infect Dis 15:183, 1992.
193. Albrecht H, Sobottka I, Stellbrink HJ, et al: Diagnosis of disseminated toxoplasmosis using a peripheral blood smear. AIDS 10:799-800, 1996.
194. Pujol-Rique M, Derouin F, Garcia-Quintanilla A, et al: Design of a one-tube hemi-nested PCR for detection of *Toxoplasma gondii* and comparison of the DNA purification methods. J Med Microbiol 48: 857-862, 1999.
195. Magill AJ, Reed S: American trypanosomiasis. In Strickland DT, ed: Hunter's Tropical Medicine and Emerging Infectious Diseases, ed 8. Philadelphia, WB Saunders Co., 2000:653-664.
196. Anonymous: Chagas' disease—interruption of transmission, Brazil. Wkly Epidemiol Rec 72:1-4, 1997.
197. Kirchhoff LV: Trypanosoma species (American Trypanosomiasis, Chagas' disease): biology of trypanosomes. In Mandell GL, Bennett JE, Dolin R, eds: Principles and Practice of Infectious Diseases, ed 5, vol II. Philadelphia, Churchill Livingstone, 2000:2845-2853.
198. Schmunis GA: *Trypanosoma cruzi*, the etiologic agent of Chagas' disease: status in the blood supply in endemic and non-endemic countries. Transfusion 31:547-557, 1991.
199. Freilij H, Altcheh J: Congenital Chagas' disease: diagnostic and clinical aspects. Clin Infect Dis 21:551, 1995.
200. Hofflin JM, Sadler RH, Araujo FG: Laboratory-acquired Chagas' disease. Trans R Soc Trop Med Hyg 81:437-440, 1987.
201. Botero D, Restrepo M: Trypanosomosis. In Botero D, Restrepo M, eds: Parasitosis Humanas, ed 3. Medellin (Colombia), CIB, 1998:203-227.
202. Melo RC, Brener Z: Tissue tropism of different *Trypanosoma cruzi* strains. J Parasitol 64(3):475-482, 1978.
203. Cano RC, Hilba E, Rubiolo ER: Creatine kinase and lactate dehydrogenase levels as potential indicators of *Trypanosoma cruzi* infectivity and histotropism in experimental Chagas' disease. Parasitol Res 86(3):244-252, 2000.
204. Metze K, Lorand-Metze I: Relationships between histopathological findings and phylogenetic divergence in *Trypanosoma cruzi*. Trop Med Int Health 4(3):238, 1999.
205. Russomando G, Figueredo A, Almiron M, et al: Polymerase chain reaction-based detection of *Trypanosoma cruzi* DNA in serum. J Clin Microbiol 30:2864, 1992.
206. Levi GC, Lobo IM, Kallas EG, et al: Etiological drug treatment of human infection by *Trypanosoma cruzi*. Rev Inst Med Trop Sao Paulo 38:35, 1996.
207. Coura JR: Current prospects of specific treatment of Chagas' disease. Bol Chil Parasitol 51:69-75, 1996.
208. Lopez-Blanco OA, Cavalli NH, Jasovich A, et al: Chagas' disease and kidney transplantation—follow-up of nine patients for 11 years. Transplant Proc 24:3089-3090, 1992.
209. Kirchhoff LV: Agents of African trypanosomiasis (sleeping sickness). In Mandell GL, Bennett JE, Dolin R, eds: Principles and Practice of Infectious Diseases, ed 5, vol II. Philadelphia, Churchill Livingstone, 2000:2853-2858.
210. Pepin J: African trypanosomiasis. In Strickland DT, ed: Hunter's Tropical Medicine and Emerging Infectious Diseases, ed 8. Philadelphia, WB Saunders Co., 2000:643-653.
211. Francis TI: Visceral complications of Gambian trypanosomiasis in a Nigerian. Trans R Soc Trop Med Hyg 66:140, 1972.
212. Robertson DHH, Jenkins AR: Hepatic dysfunction in human trypanosomiasis. 1. Abnormalities of excretory function, seroflocculation phenomena and other tests of hepatic function with observations on the alterations of these tests during treatment and convalescence. Trans R Soc Trop Med Hyg 53:511, 1959.
213. Gelfand M, Friedlander J: Jaundice in Rhodesian sleeping sickness. Report on two European cases. Trans R Soc Trop Med Hyg 57:290, 1963.
214. Mackenzie AR, Boreham PFL, Facer CA: Autoantibodies in African trypanosomiasis. Trans R Soc Trop Med Hyg 67(2):268, 1973.
215. Uzoegwu PN, Baum H, Williamson J: The occurrence and localization in trypanosomes and other endo-parasites of an antigen cross-reacting with mitochondrial antibodies of primary biliary cirrhosis. Comp Biochem Physiol B Biochem Mol Biol 88:1181, 1987.

216. Magill AJ: Leishmaniasis. In Strickland DT, ed: Hunter's Tropical Medicine and Emerging Infectious Diseases, ed 8.Philadelphia, WB Saunders Co., 2000:665-687.
217. Pearson RD, de Queiroz Sousa A, Jeronimo SMB: Leishmania species: visceral (Kala-Azar), cutaneous, and mucosal leishmaniasis. In Mandell GL, Bennett JE, Dolin R, eds: Principles and Practice of Infectious Diseases, ed 5, vol II. Philadelphia, Churchill Livingstone, 2000:2831-2844.
218. Alvar J, Canavate C, Gutierrez-Solar B, et al: Leishmania and human immunodeficiency virus coinfection: the first 10 years. Clin Microbiol Rev 10:298-319, 1997.
219. Moulin B, Ollier J, Bouchouareb D, et al: Leishmaniasis: a rare cause of unexplained fever in a renal graft recipient. Nephron 60:360, 1992.
220. Botero D, Restrepo M: Leishmaniosis. In Botero D, Restrepo M, eds: Parasitosis Humanas, ed 3. Medellin (Colombia), CIB, 1998:228-251.
221. Albrecht H, Sobottka I, Emminger C, et al: Visceral leishmaniasis emerging as an important opportunistic infection in HIV-infected persons living in areas nonendemic for *Leishmania donovani*. Arch Pathol Lab Med 120:189-198, 1996.
222. Badaro R, Reed SG, Carvalho EM: Immunofluorescent antibody test in American visceral leishmaniasis: sensitivity and specificity of different morphological forms of two Leishmania species. Am J Trop Med Hyg 32:480-484, 1983.
223. Kar K: Serodiagnosis of leishmaniasis. Crit Rev Microbiol 21:123-152, 1995.
224. Katakura K, Kawazu S, Naya T, et al: Diagnosis of Kala-azar by nested PCR based on amplification of the Leishmania mini-exon gene. J Clin Microbiol 36(8):2173, 1998.
225. Chulay JD, Bryceson ADM: Quantitation of amastigotes of *Leishmania donovani* in smears of splenic aspirates from patients with visceral leishmaniasis. Am J Trop Med Hyg 32:475, 1983.
226. DeSilva NR, Chan MS, Bundy DA: Morbidity and mortality due to ascariasis: reestimation and sensitivity analysis of global numbers at risk. Trop Med Int Health 2:519-528, 1997.
227. Bratton RL, Nesse RE: Ascariasis. An infection to watch for in immigrants. Postgrad Med 93:171-178, 1993.
228. Mahmoud A: Intestinal nematodes (roundworms). In Mandell GL, Bennett JE, Dolin R, eds: Principles and Practice of Infectious Diseases, ed 5, vol II. Philadelphia, Churchill Livingstone, 2000:2938-2943.
229. Anderson TJ: Ascaris infections in humans from North America: molecular evidence for cross-infection. Parasitology 110:215-219, 1995.
230. Bundy DAP, DeSilva N: Intestinal nematodes that migrate through lungs (ascariasis). In Strickland DT, ed: Hunter's Tropical Medicine and Emerging Infectious Diseases, ed 8. Philadelphia, WB Saunders Co., 2000:726-730.
231. Ferreyra NP, Cerri GG: Ascariasis of the alimentary tract, liver, pancreas and biliary system: its diagnosis by ultrasonography. Hepatogastroenterology 45(22):932, 1998.
232. Botembe N, Cabrera-Alvarez G, Le Moine O, et al: A rare cause of biliary pain in Belgium. Acta Gastroenterol Belg 62(4):443, 1999.
233. Fogaca HS, Oliveira CS, Barbosa HT, et al: Liver pseudotumor: a rare manifestation of hepatic granulomata caused by *Ascaris lumbricoides* ova. Am J Gastroenterol 95(8):2099-2101, 2000.
234. Morales G, Loaiza L, Pino LA: Risk markers in subjects with loads of *Ascaris lumbricoides* in a rural community of the Cojedes state, Venezuela. Bol Chil Parasitol 54:88-96, 1999.
235. Sandouk F, Haffar S, Zada MM, et al: Pancreatic-biliary ascariasis: experience of 300 cases. Am J Gastroenterol 92:2264, 1997.
236. Arean VM, Crandall CA: Ascariasis. In Marcial-Rojas RA, ed: Pathology of protozoal and helminthic diseases with clinical correlation. Baltimore, Williams & Wilkins, 1971:769.
237. Amog G, Lichtenstein J, Sieber S, et al: A case report of ascariasis of the common bile duct in a patient who had undergone cholecystectomy. Arch Pathol Lab Med 124(8):1231, 2000.
238. Corr P, Smit J, Hadley GL: An unusual cause of haemobilia: biliary ascariasis. Pediatr Radiol 27:348, 1997.
239. Botero D, Restrepo M: Parasitosis intestinales por nematodos. In Botero D, Restrepo M, eds: Parasitosis Humanas, ed 3. Medellin (Colombia), CIB, 1998:89-135.
240. Shulman A: Ultrasound appearances of intra- and extrahepatic ascariasis. Abdom Imaging 23:60, 1998.
241. Ng KK, Wong HF, Kong MS, et al: Biliary ascariasis: CT, MR cholangiopancreatography, and navigator endoscopic appearance—report of a case of acute biliary obstruction. Abdom Imaging 24:470, 1999.
242. Rocha MS, Costa NS, Costa JC, et al: CT identification of ascaris in the biliary tract. Abdom Imaging 20:317, 1995.
243. Fitoz S, Atasoy C: MR cholangiography in massive hepatobiliary ascariasis. A case report. Acta Radiol 41:273, 2000.
244. Misra SP, Dwivedi M: Clinical features and management of biliary ascariasis in a non-endemic area. Postgrad Med J 76:29-32, 2000.
245. Beckingham IJ, Cullis SN, Krige JE, et al: Management of hepatobiliary and pancreatic Ascaris infestation in adults after failed medical treatment. Br J Surg 85:907-910, 1998.
246. Osman M, Lausten SB, El-Sefi T, et al: Biliary parasites. Dig Surg 15(4):287-296, 1998.
247. Mascie-Taylor CG. Alam M, Montanari RM, et al: A study of cost effectiveness of selective health interventions for the control of intestinal parasites in rural Bangladesh. J Parasitol 85(1):6-11, 1999.
248. Gilman RH: Intestinal nematodes that migrate through skin and lung. In Strickland DT, ed: Hunter's Tropical Medicine and Emerging Infectious Diseases, ed 8. Philadelphia, WB Saunders Co., 2000:730-740.
249. Grove DI: Human strongyloidiasis. Adv Parasitol 38:251-309, 1996.
250. Poltera AA, Katsimbura N: Granulomatous hepatitis due to Strongyloides stercoralis. J Pathol 113:241, 1974.
251. DePaola D, Braga-Diaz L, Rodrigues da Silva J: Enteritis due to Strongyloides stercoralis. A report of 5 fatal cases. Am J Dig Dis 7:1086, 1962.
252. Petithory JC, Derouin F: AIDS and strongyloidiasis in Africa. Lancet 1:921, 1987.
253. Atkins NS, Conway DJ, Lindo JF, et al: L3 antigen-specific antibody isotype responses in human strongyloidiasis: correlations with larval output. Parasite Immunol 21(10):517-526, 1999.
254. Rodriguez Calabuig D, Oltra Alcaraz C, Igual Adell R, et al: 30 cases of strongyloidiasis at a primary care center: characteristics and possible complications. Aten Primaria 21(5):271-274, 1998.
255. Parana R, Portugal M, Vitvitski L, et al: Severe strongyloidiasis during interferon plus ribavirin therapy for chronic HCV infection. Eur J Gastroenterol Hepatol 12(2):245, 2000.
256. Moustafa MA: An evaluation of the modified agar plate method for diagnosis of *Strongyloides stercoralis*. J Egyp Soc Parasitol 27(2):571, 1997.
257. Jongwutiwes S, Charoenkorn M, Sitthichareonchai P, et al: Increased sensitivity of routine laboratory detection of *Strongyloides stercoralis* and hookworm by agar-plate culture. Trans R Soc Trop Med Hyg 93(4):398-400, 1999.
258. van der Feltz M, Slee PH, van Hees PA, et al: Strongyloides stercoralis infection: how to diagnose best? Neth J Med 55(3):128-131, 1999.
259. de Paula FM, de Castro E, Goncalves-Pires MD, et al: Parasitological and immunological diagnosis of strongyloidiasis in immunocompromised and non-immunocompromised children at Uberlandia, State of Minas Gerais, Brazil. Rev Inst Med Trop Sao Paulo 42:51-55, 2000.
260. Skandrani K, Richardet JP, Duvoux C, et al: Hepatic transplantation for severe ductopenia related to ingestion of thiabendazole. Gastroenterol Clin Biol 21:623-625, 1997.
261. Adenusi AA: Cure by ivermectin of a chronic, persistent, intestinal strongyloidosis. Acta Trop 66(3):163-166, 1997.
262. Schantz PM: Toxocariasis. In Strickland DT, ed: Hunter's Tropical Medicine and Emerging Infectious Diseases, ed 8. Philadelphia, WB Saunders Co., 2000: 787-790.
263. Nash TE: Visceral larva migrans and other unusual helminth infections. In Mandell GL, Bennett JE, Dolin R, eds: Principles and Practice of Infectious Diseases, ed 5, vol II. Philadelphia, Churchill Livingstone, 2000:2965-2969.
264. Botero D, Restrepo M: Parasitosis tisulares por larvas de helmintos. In Botero D, Restrepo M, eds: Parasitosis Humanas, ed 3. Medellin (Colombia), CIB, 1998:335-372.
265. Barriga OO: A critical look at the importance, prevalence and control of toxocariasis and the possibilities of immunological control. Vet Parasitol 29:195-234, 1988.
266. Schantz PM: Toxocara larva migrans now. Am J Trop Med Hyg 41:21-34, 1989.
267. Worley G, Green JA, Frothingham TE, et al: Toxocara canis infection: clinical and epidemiological associations with seropositivity in kindergarten children. J Infect Dis 149:591-597, 1984.

268. Pereira FE, Musso C, Castelo JS: Pathology of pyogenic liver abscess in children. Pediatr Dev Pathol 2:537-543, 1999.
269. Parsons JC, Coffman RL, Grieve RB: Antibody to interleukin 5 prevents blood and tissue eosinophilia but not liver trapping in murine larval toxocariasis. Parasite Immunol 15:501-508, 1993.
270. Baldisserotto M, Conchin CF, Soares MD, et al: Ultrasound findings in children with toxocariasis: report on 18 cases. Pediatr Radiol 29:316-319, 1999.
271. Kaushik SP, Hurwitz M, McDonald C, et al: Toxocara canis infection and granulomatous hepatitis. Am J Gastroenterol 92(7):1223, 1997.
272. de Corral VR, Lozano-Garcia J, Ramos-Corona LE: An unusual case of systemic toxocariasis. Bol Med Hosp Infant Mex 47(12):841, 1990.
273. Almeida MT, Ribeiro RC, Kauffman WM, et al: Toxocariasis simulating hepatic recurrence in a patient with Wilm's tumor. Med Pediatr Oncol 22(3):211, 1994.
274. Moreira-Silva SF, Pereira FE: Intestinal nematodes, Toxocara infection, and pyogenic liver abscess in children: a possible association. J Trop Pediatr 46(3):167-172, 2000.
275. Gonzalez MT, Ibanez O, Balcarce N, et al: Toxocariasis with liver involvement. Acta Gastroenterol Latinoam 30(3):187-190, 2000.
276. Jain R, Sawhney S, Bhargava DK, et al: Hepatic granulomas due to visceral larva migrans in adults: appearance on US and MRI. Abdom Imaging 19(3):253, 1994.
277. Rai SK, Uga S, Wu Z, et al: Use of polymerase chain reaction in the diagnosis of toxocariasis: an experimental study. Southeast Asian J Trop Med Public Health 28(3):541-544, 1997.
278. Terrier P, Hack I, Hatz C, et al: Hepatic capillariasis in a 2-year-old boy. J Pediatr Gastroenterol Nutr 28(3):338-340, 1999.
279. Govil H, Desai M: Capillaria hepatica parasitism. Indian J Pediatr 63(5):698-700, 1996.
280. Kumar V, Brandt J, Mortelmans J: Hepatic capillariasis may simulate the syndrome of visceral larva migrans, an analysis. Ann Soc Belg Med Trop 65:101, 1985.
281. Choe G, Lee HS, Seo JK, et al: Hepatic capillariasis: first case report in the Republic of Korea. Am J Trop Med Hyg 48:610-625, 1993.
282. Cislaghi F, Radice C: Infection by *Capillaria hepatica.* First report in Italy. Helv Pediatr Acta 25:647-654, 1970.
283. Berger T, Degremónt A, Gebbers JO, et al: Hepatic capillariasis in a 1-year old child. Eur J Pediatr 149:333, 1990.
284. Silverman NH, Katz JS, Levin SE: Capillaria hepatica infestation in a child. S Afr Med J 47:219-221, 1973.
285. Sawamura R, Fernandes MI, Peres LC, et al: Hepatic capillariasis in children: report of 3 cases in Brazil. Am J Trop Med Hyg 61(4):642, 1999.
286. Juncker-Voss M, Prosl H, Lussy H, et al: Serologic detection of Capillaria hepatica by indirect immunofluorescence assay. J Clin Microbiol 38(1):431, 2000.
287. Bica I, Hamer DH, Stadecker MJ: Hepatic schistosomiasis. Infect Dis Clin North Am 14(3):583-604, 2000.
288. Strickland GT, Ramirez BL: Schistosomiasis. In Strickland DT, ed: Hunter's Tropical Medicine and Emerging Infectious Diseases, ed 8. Philadelphia, WB Saunders Co., 2000:804-832.
289. Mahmoud AAF: Trematodes (schistosomiasis) and other flukes. In Mandell GL, Bennett JE, Dolin R, eds: Principles and Practice of Infectious Diseases, ed 5, vol II. Philadelphia, Churchill Livingstone, 2000:2950-2955.
290. The control of schistosomiasis. Report of a WHO expert committee. World Health Org Tech Rep Ser 728:1-113, 1985.
291. Botero D, Restrepo M: Parasitosis tisulares por trematodos. In Botero D, Restrepo M, eds: Parasitosis Humanas, ed 3. Medellin (Colombia), CIB, 1998:319-334.
292. Symmers WC: Note on a new form of liver cirrhosis due to the presence of the eggs of *Bilharzia haematobia.* J Pathol Bacteriol 9:237, 1904.
293. Stadecker MJ: The development of granulomas in schistosomiasis: genetic backgrounds, regulatory pathways, and specific egg antigen responses that influence the magnitude of disease. Microbes Infec 1:505-510, 1999.
294. Pearce EJ, Caspar P, Grzych JM, et al: Down regulation of Th-1 cytokine production accompanies induction of Th-2 responses by a parasite helminth Schistosoma mansoni. J Exp Med 173:159-166, 1991.
295. Demeure CE, Rihet P, Abel L, et al: Resistance to *Schistosoma mansoni* in humans: influence of the IgE/IgG4 balance and IgG2 in immunity to reinfection after chemotherapy. J Infect Dis 168:1000, 1993.
296. Naus CWA, Kimani G, Ouma JH, et al: Development of antibody isotype responses to *Schistosoma mansoni* in an immunologically naïve immigrant population: influence of infection duration, infection intensity and host age. Infect Immunol 67:3444, 1999.
297. Grzych JM, Grezel D, Xu CB, et al: IgA antibodies to a protective antigen in human *Schistosomiasis mansoni.* J Immunol 150:527-535, 1993.
298. Butterworth AE, Dunne DW, Fulford AJ, et al: Immunity and morbidity in human Schistosomiasis mansoni infection: quantitative aspects. Am J Trop Med Hyg 55:109-115, 1996.
299. The use of diagnostic ultrasound in schistosomiasis—attempt at standardization of methodology. Cairo Working Group. Acta Trop 51:45-63, 1992.
300. Palmer PE: Schistosomiasis. Semin Roentgenol 33:6-25, 1998.
301. Engels D, Sinzinkayo E, Gryseels B: Day-to-day egg count fluctuation in *Schistosoma mansoni* infection and its operational implications. Am J Trop Med Hyg 54:319-324, 1996.
302. Abdel-Hafez MA, Bolbol AH: Fibre-optic sigmoidoscopy compared to Kato technique in diagnosis and evaluation of the intensity of Schistosoma mansoni infection. Trans R Soc Trop Med Hyg 86:641, 1992.
303. Bergquist NR: Present aspects of immunodiagnosis of schistosomiasis. Mem Inst Oswaldo Cruz 87(suppl 4):29-38, 1992.
304. Nibbeling HA, Van Lieshout L, Deelder AM: Levels of circulating soluble egg antigen in urine of individuals infected with *Schistosoma mansoni* before and after treatment with Praziquantel. Trans R Soc Trop Med Hyg 92:675, 1998.
305. Van Lieshout L, De Jonge N, el Masry NA, et al: Improved diagnostic performance of the circulating antigen assay in human schistosomiasis by parallel testing for circulating anodic and cathodic antigens in serum and urine. Am J Trop Med Hyg 47:463-469, 1992.
306. Helal TE, Danial MF, Ahmed HF: The relationship between hepatitis C virus and schistosomiasis: histopathologic evaluation of liver biopsy specimens. Hum Pathol 29:743, 1998.
307. Madwar MA, El Tahawy ME, Strickland GT: The relationship between uncomplicated schistosomiasis and hepatitis B infection. Trans R Soc Trop Med Hyg 83:233-236, 1989.
308. Bunnag D, Cross JH, Bunnag T: Liver fluke infections. In Strickland DT, ed: Hunter's Tropical Medicine and Emerging Infectious Diseases, ed 8. Philadelphia, WB Saunders Co, 2000:840-846.
309. Moller H, Heseltine E, Vainio H: Working group report on schistosomes, liver flukes and *Helicobacter pylori.* Int J Cancer 60:587, 1995.
310. Liu LX, Harinasuta KT: Liver and intestinal flukes. Gastroenterol Clin North Am 5:627-636, 1996.
311. Price TA, Tuazon CU, Simon GL: Fascioliasis: case reports and review. Clin Infect Dis 17:426-430, 1993.
312. Pulpiero JR, Armesto V, Vrela J, et al: Fascioliasis: findings in 15 patients. Br J Radiol 64:798-801, 1991.
313. Bacq Y, Besnier JM, Doung TH, et al: Successful treatment of acute fascioliasis with bithionol. Hepatology 14:1066, 1991.
314. Apt W, Aguilera X, Vega F, et al: Treatment of human chronic fascioliasis with triclabendazole: drug efficacy and serologic response. Am J Trop Med Hyg 52:532-535, 1995.
315. Moro PL, Gonzalez AE, Gilman RH: Cystic hydatid disease. In Strickland DT, ed: Hunter's Tropical Medicine and Emerging Infectious Diseases, ed 8. Philadelphia, WB Saunders Co., 2000:866-871.
316. King CH: Cestodes (tapeworms). In Mandell GL, Bennett JE, Dolin R, eds: Principles and Practice of Infectious Diseases, ed 5, vol II. Philadelphia, Churchill Livingstone, 2000:2956-2964.
317. Gilman RH, Lee BH: Alveolar hydatid cyst disease. In Strickland DT, ed: Hunter's Tropical Medicine and Emerging Infectious Diseases, ed 8. Philadelphia, WB Saunders Co., 2000:872-875.
318. Botero D, Restrepo M. Hidatidosis et al: Parasitosis tisulares por trematodos. In Botero D, Restrepo M, eds: Parasitosis Humanas, ed 3. Medellin (Colombia), CIB, 1998:358-366.
319. Taourel P, Marty-Ane B, Charasset S, et al: Hydatid cyst of the liver: comparison of CT and MRI. J Comput Assist Tomogr 17:80-85, 1993.

320. Beggs I:The radiologic appearances of hydatic disease of the liver. Clin Radiol 34:555-563, 1983.
321. Force L, Torres JM, Carrillo A, et al: Evaluation of eight serologic tests in the diagnosis of human echinococcosis and follow-up. Clin Infect Dis 15:473-480, 1992.
322. Verastegui M, Moro P, Guevara A, et al: Enzyme-linked immunoelectrotransfer blot test for the diagnosis of human hydatid disease. J Clin Microbiol 30:1557-1561, 1992.
323. MacPherson CN, Roming T, Zeyhle E, et al: Portable ultrasound scanner versus serology screening for hydatid cyst in a nomadic population. Lancet 2:259-261, 1987.
324. Gottstein B, Tschudi K, Eckert J, et al: Em2-ELISA for the follow-up of alveolar *Echinococcus* after complete surgical resection of liver lesions. Trans R Soc Trop Med Hyg 83:389-393, 1989.
325. Ito A, Wang XG, Liu YH: Differential serodiagnosis of alveolar and cystic hydatid disease in the People's Republic of China. Am J Trop Med Hyg 49:208-213, 1993.
326. Rausch RL, Wilson JF, Schantz PM, et al: Spontaneous death of *Echinococcus multilocularis* cases diagnosed serologically (by Em2 ELISA) and clinical significance. Am J Trop Med Hyg 36:576-585, 1987.
327. Salama H, Farid Abdel-Wahab MF, Strickland GT: Diagnosis and treatment of hepatic hydatid cysts with the aid of echo-guided percutaneous cyst puncture. Clin Infect Dis 21:1372, 1995.
328. Khuroo MS, Wani NA, Javid G, et al: Percutaneous drainage compared with surgery for hepatic hydatid cysts. N Engl J Med 337:881, 1997.
329. Guidelines for treatment of cystic and alveolar echinococcosis in humans. WHO Informal Working Group on Echinococcosis. Bull World Health Organ 74:231-242, 1996.
330. Mboti B, Van de Stadt J, Carlier Y, et al: Long-term disease-free survival after liver transplantation for alveolar echinococcosis. Acta Chir Belg 96:229-232, 1996.
331. Ammann RW, Ilisch N, Marincek B, et al: Effect of chemotherapy on the larval mass and the long-term course of alveolar echinococcosis. Swiss Echinococcosis Study Group. Hepatology 19:735-742, 1994.

CHAPTER

36

Bacterial and Miscellaneous Infections of the Liver

Helmut Albrecht, MD

PYOGENIC ABSCESS OF THE LIVER

Liver abscesses were already known to Hippocrates, who reported an association between prognosis and the type of fluid contained within the lesion:

> When abscess of the liver is treated by cautery or incision, if the pus which is discharged be pure and white the patients recover (for in this case it is situated in the coats of the liver) but if it resembles the lees of oil as it flows they die.[1]

Incidence and Mortality

Despite an apparent recent increase in incidence, pyogenic liver abscesses remain a relatively uncommon clinical entity responsible for between 7 and 20 per 100,000 hospital admissions.[2-14] The prevalence in autopsy series ranges from 0.29 percent to 1.47 percent.[6] In contrast to amebic liver abscess there are no significant gender differences reported in patients with pyogenic liver abscess. Almost 50 percent of patients will present with more than one abscess. Solitary abscesses involve the right lobe in 75 percent, the left in 20 percent, and the caudate in approximately 5 percent. Multiple abscesses follow a similar pattern of distribution. Although this is likely the result of the relative mass of each lobe it remains unclear if other factors such as hepatic blood flow contribute to this distribution.

Over the last 20 to 30 years significant changes in etiology, microbiology, diagnostics, therapies, and outcome have occurred.[2-14] The perceived increase in incidence in recent years is likely secondary to improved quality and availability of imaging methods. Additionally, prolonged survival of patients with increased susceptibility to liver abscess, such as iron overload states, sickle cell disease, diabetes mellitus, advanced cardiovascular disease, or metastatic cancer also contributes to the growing patient load. The increasing number of immunocompromised patients has added another new dimension to this problem. Hepatic abscesses have been reported in patients with a multitude of immunodeficiency states, including primary immunodeficiencies, especially patients with neutrophil deficiencies (e.g., Job's syndrome or chronic granulomatous disease), acquired immunodeficiencies (e.g., human immunodeficiency virus [HIV] infection), and iatrogenic immunodeficiencies (e.g., patients undergoing chemotherapy). Patients undergoing orthotopic liver transplantation are also at risk for the formation of hepatic abscesses posttransplant. In these patients liver abscesses commonly develop secondary to hepatic arterial thrombosis.[15]

Although the incidence seems to be on the increase, mortality has decreased dramatically from close to 100 percent to 5 percent to currently 31 percent. This improvement has been observed despite larger numbers of patients with underlying diseases in recent studies.[9-14,16] Underlying malignancies (especially cholangiocarcinoma), severe hepatic dysfunction, and multiple versus singular abscesses are associated with an increased mortality.[11,14,16,17] Compared with earlier cases, however, a large study from John Hopkins recently reported that the reduction in mortality was most apparent for patients with multiple abscesses when compared with earlier cases (44 percent versus 88 percent, respectively; $P < .05$) and for patients with a biliary etiology (38 percent versus 90 percent, respectively; $P < .05$).[10] Mortality of patients with cryptogenic liver abscesses is low (5 percent).[9]

Etiology

Bacterial pathogens can reach the liver by five different routes: portal vein, hepatic artery, biliary, penetrating trauma, and direct extension from a contiguous, usually intra-abdominal, but rarely pleural focus. Infection via any of these routes can potentially lead to formation of liver abscesses but the associated scope of pathogens may be quite different. Since the classic report of Ochsner in 1938[2] the etiology of hepatic abscesses has changed significantly. In the pre-antibiotic era, liver abscesses were typically encountered in patients with appendicitis and associated pyelophlebitis. Incidence was highest in the third to fourth decades of life. Mortality, especially in patients who did not undergo prompt surgical drainage, approached 100 percent.[2] The peak incidence of pyogenic abscesses has shifted into the older age group with most recent case series reporting an average patient's age of more than 60 years. Pyelophlebitis has become rare but is still observed. Diverticulitis has surpassed appendicitis as the most common cause of pyelophlebitis. Cryptogenic and biliary tract-associated liver abscesses are most common in more recent case series.[9-14]

Suppurative ascending cholangitis has become the most frequent identifiable cause of pyogenic liver abscesses. Although cholelithiasis is by far the most common cause of biliary tract-derived pyogenic abscesses, patients with Caroli's disease and sclerosing cholangitis are also at increased risk. In developing countries biliary ascariasis is a not infrequent cause of liver abscesses. Patients with biliary disease as the cause of liver abscesses often present with multiple abscesses.

Cryptogenic abscesses now account for up to 60 percent of cases in recent series.[9,11] The reason for this observation is not entirely clear. Improved diagnostic modalities resulting in earlier intervention including the use of empiric antibiotic therapy may allow eradication of focal infectious foci before they become clinically apparent. On the other hand improved management of biliary tract disease including endoscopic retrograde cholangiopancreatography (ERCP) and stent placement may have reduced the incidence of biliary-derived abscesses resulting in proportionally more cryptogenic cases. Host factors predisposing patients to pyogenic abscess development may increase the likelihood of "cryptogenic" abscesses. In patients with iron overload states, sickle cell disease, diabetes mellitus, cirrhosis, advanced cardiovascular disease, metastatic cancer, or immunodeficiency states, trivial bacterial insults may manifest as hepatic abscesses.

Any bacteremic episode, including line-associated septicemia or endocarditis, may seed the liver via the hepatic artery. Extensive formation of microabscesses is not an infrequent finding at autopsy, especially in patients succumbing to overwhelming sepsis. These patients, however, have traditionally been excluded from most case series of patients with pyogenic liver abscesses unless they also had evidence of macroscopic abscesses. In one series only 22 percent of patients with microabscesses were diagnosed before death.[5]

Spread from a contiguous focus has included subphrenic, paracolic, or perinephric abscesses; empyema; cholecystitis; and necrotizing pancreatitis. Pyogenic abscess formation associated with penetrating trauma often involves skin flora but may be associated with intestinal flora if the gastrointestinal tract was lacerated at the same time. The initial insult may be as trivial as the incidental ingestion of toothpicks or fish bones.[18-20] Children and patients with psychiatric disorders such as pica or suicidal ideation are at highest risk because they are more likely to swallow sharp items.[19,21,22] Liver abscesses in rare cases have even been observed after blunt trauma to the abdomen, presumably as a result of secondary superinfection of liver hematomas.

Other new etiologic entities include modern therapeutic interventions such as transhepatic chemoembolization.[23] Hepatic abscesses are also observed as a late complication of endoscopic sphincterotomy for biliary duct stones. Case series have shown rates of up to 2 percent of patients undergoing sphincterotomy.[24] Most cases were associated with recurrent stones; the mortality was surprisingly high at 40 percent.[24] Biliary-intestinal anastomosis has also been described as a risk factor for the subsequent development of pyogenic liver abscesses.[25] Patients who underwent anastomosis using subsegmental bile ducts or who had vascular reconstruction were at highest risk. In all affected patients surgery was performed to resect a malignant lesion. Abscess formation was uniformly detected 3 to 6 weeks after surgery. In the largest case series mortality approached 50 percent.[25]

Microbiology

The organisms recovered from patients with pyogenic liver abscesses vary greatly (Table 36-1). This is not surprising given the diverse etiologies discussed previously. Results of single studies should not be generalized because they are highly dependent on the culture methods used and the patient population studied. Despite these difficulties recent studies have improved our understanding of the microbiology of pyogenic liver abscesses. Early studies reported a high rate of "sterile" abscesses, often exceeding 50 percent. Despite the increased use of empiric and more effective antibiotic therapy recent studies commonly report positive abscess cultures in 80 percent to 100 percent of patients presenting with pyogenic liver abscesses.[10,12,26] Gram stains are mandatory and may provide the only clue to a mixed infection in patient pretreated with antibiotics. Thirty-five percent to 70 percent of patients will also have positive blood cultures. Because blood cultures are often the only cultures obtained before antibiotic administration, in 5 percent to 10 percent of patients they provide the only positive culture data.

Using strict anaerobic techniques, recent studies have found that 45 percent to 75 percent of hepatic abscesses are caused by anaerobic or mixed aerobic/anaerobic infections.[26-28] Even these high detection rates may represent underestimates secondary to the fastidious nature of some anaerobes. Anaerobes are especially common in polymicrobial abscesses. It is generally believed that many abscesses are polymicrobial but estimates range from 10 percent to 75 percent. Solitary abscesses are more likely to be polymicrobial than are multiple abscesses.

Escherichia coli and *Klebsiella pneumoniae* are the most common specific pathogens isolated. Whereas *E. coli* dominated virtually all early series, *K. pneumoniae* has recently emerged as a major cause of pyogenic liver abscesses. In a large series 160 patients with abscesses resulting solely from *K. pneumoniae* were compared with patients with polymicrobial abscesses.[29] In the group of patients with *K. pneumoniae* liver abscesses there was a striking increase in the prevalence of diabetes or glucose intolerance (75 percent versus 4.5 percent), a lower rate of co-existing intra-abdominal infection (0.6 percent versus 95.5 percent), a lower death rate (11.3 percent versus 41 percent), and a lower relapse rate (4.4 percent versus 41 percent). A number of patients with *K. pneumoniae* abscesses had other foci of infection, including pneumonia, skin lesions, meningitis, or endophthalmitis.[29] Alkaline phosphatase and bilirubin levels were higher in patients with polymicrobial abscesses, but on other grounds (i.e., signs and symptoms)

TABLE 36-1
Microbial Pathogens Isolated from Pyogenic Liver Abscesses

Gram-negative Aerobic Bacteria
*Escherichia coli**
*Klebsiella pneumoniae**
Pseudomonas aeruginosa
Proteus species
Enterobacter species
Citrobacter freundii
Morganella species
Serratia species
Haemophilus species
Legionella pneumophila
Yersinia species
Gram-positive Aerobic Bacteria
*Staphylococcus aureus**
Enterococcus species*
Viridans streptococci*
Beta-hemolytic streptococci
Streptococcus pneumoniae
Listeria monocytogenes
Anaerobes
Anaerobic streptococci*
Bacteroides species*
Fusobacterium species
Peptostreptococcus species
Actinomyces (Plate 36-2)
Eubacterium
Propionibacterium acnes
Clostridium species
Lactobacillus species
Peptococcus species
Eubacterium species
Capnocytophaga species (facultatively anaerobic)
Microaerophilic Organisms
Streptococcus milleri group
Miscellaneous
Mycobacterium species*
Chlamydia species
Candida species

*Commonly isolated pathogens (more than 5% of cases).

the groups were indistinguishable. In addition, *K. pneumoniae* abscesses are frequently gas-forming.[30] Although the intrinsic characteristics of the *Klebsiella* abscesses including size, loculation, or complexity were often not well documented, it appears that liver abscesses caused by *K. pneumoniae* represent a clinical unique entity characterized by a relatively benign course.[29] Several questions remain unanswered, including the pathogenesis of this disorder, its relationship with diabetes mellitus, and whether the strains found in liver abscesses are unique or similar to other *K. pneumoniae* strains.

Of the gram-positive pathogens, staphylococci are more commonly found in monomicrobial abscesses whereas streptococci and especially enterococci are most often associated with polymicrobial abscesses. In one large series isolation of *Staphylococcus aureus* and beta-hemolytic streptococci was associated with trauma; *Streptococcus* group D, *K. pneumoniae,* and *Clostridium* species with biliary disease; and *Bacteroides* species and *Clostridium* species with colonic disease.[26] Disturbingly, highly resistant nosocomial pathogens such as multi-drug-resistant *Pseudomonas* isolates,[10] vancomycin-resistant enterococci, and even vancomycin-intermediate *S. aureus* are now being isolated from hepatic abscesses.[31] Other disturbing trends include the increased frequency of fungal or mixed bacterial and fungal abscesses probably reflecting recent shifts in the etiology of nosocomial infections.[10,32] In one large series mortality was significantly increased (50 percent) in patients with mixed bacterial and fungal abscesses ($p < .02$).[10]

Clinical Features

Only 10 percent of patients present with the "characteristic" symptom triad of fever, jaundice, and right upper quadrant (RUQ) tenderness. The most common presentation is a mildly symptomatic patient with fever and other non-specific constitutional symptoms, including malaise, anorexia, and weight loss (Table 36-2). Localizing symptoms such as nausea and vomiting, diarrhea, and abdominal pain may be present are also not specific. Some patients present only with respiratory symptoms, including pleuritic pain and cough. Pain may be felt in the left upper quadrant by patients with abscesses of the left lobe or may be diffuse in patients with secondary peritonitis. Patients with subphrenic abscesses may present with right shoulder pain. A high index of suspicion is therefore required to make a timely diagnosis. Furthermore, patients with necrotic hepatocellular carcinomas may present with classic symptoms and signs of pyogenic liver abscess, namely fever, chills, abdominal pain, leukocytosis, and hepatomegaly.[16,17] The pathogenesis is presumed to involve spontaneous tumor necrosis or biliary obstruction caused by tumor thrombi with or without bacterial superinfection. Major clues to the possibility of underlying hepatocellular carcinoma are the presence of hepatitis B surface antigen or hepatitis C viral RNA and evidence of cirrhosis (i.e., ascites, low albumin, prolonged protein).[17] Because significant underlying liver disease is uncommon in patients with uncomplicated pyogenic (or amebic) liver abscesses, evidence of cirrhosis should result in a work-up to rule out hepatocellular carcinoma.

Hepatomegaly is the most common finding on physical exam (Table 36-3). Other clues may include a palpable liver mass and RUQ tenderness. Abnormal physical findings on chest exam are common and may include an upwardly displaced and fixed lower pulmonary border on the right, evidence of consolidation or pleural effusions, friction rubs, or rales. Jaundice is noted in 10 percent to 50 percent of patients and is associated with a

TABLE 36-2
Symptoms Associated with Pyogenic Liver Abscess[2-14]

Symptom	Range
Fever and chills	45%-100%
Anorexia and weight loss	28%-100%
Malaise and weakness	11%-97%
Abdominal pain	27%-91%
Nausea and vomiting	9%-53%
Diarrhea	8%-48%
Cough	4%-28%
Chest pain	2%-24%

TABLE 36-3
Physical Signs Associated with Pyogenic Liver Abscess[2-14]

Sign	Range
Hepatomegaly	7%-91%
Right upper quadrant tenderness	14%-71%
Jaundice	4%-54%
Chest findings	11%-52%
Splenomegaly	1%-21%
Sepsis	3%-18%
Ascites	2%-6%

TABLE 36-4
Laboratory Findings Associated with Pyogenic Liver Abscess[2-14]

Finding	Range
Elevation of alkaline phosphatase	66%-100%
Leukocytosis	65%-99%
Anemia	45%-91%
Prolonged prothrombin time	44%-87%
Albumin < 3.0 g/dl	20%-87%
Bilirubin elevation	21%-74%
Hypergammaglobulinemia	33%-66%
Transaminase elevation	15%-60%

biliary etiology or advanced disease. Splenomegaly has become uncommon in recent series.

Leukocytosis is detected in most patients and the increase can be dramatic (720,000/mm^3). Anemia also is common. Although aminotransferase bilirubin and albumin levels and prothrombin time are often abnormal, they are seldom marked. Normal results do not exclude the diagnosis of pyogenic liver abscess. Alkaline phosphatase levels are commonly elevated and tend to be increased more than other liver tests. In summary, laboratory studies may suggest liver disease but are neither sensitive nor specific for the diagnosis of pyogenic liver abscess (Table 36-4).

Chest x-ray findings may be abnormal in up to 80 percent of patients with pyogenic liver abscess. Findings include pneumonitis, consolidation, pleural effusions, and elevation or immobility of the right diaphragm. Air fluid levels may be visible on plain films of the abdomen.

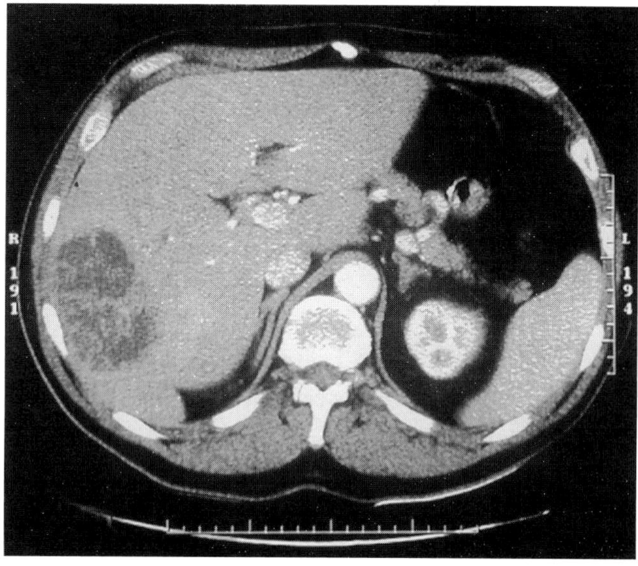

Figure 36-1 Computed tomography image of an early pyogenic abscess.

Diagnosis

Patients with hepatic abscesses commonly present with non-specific symptoms, are often elderly, or have underlying illnesses that may mask their symptoms. Empiric antibiotic therapy may prevent timely recovery of the etiologic pathogen. Diagnosis is therefore often delayed. In many series patients had been symptomatic for at least 2 weeks before the diagnosis was established. The availability of modern imaging, however, has enabled physicians to streamline the diagnostic work-up of affected patients. A study comparing the period from 1981 to 1989 with 1990 to 1998 found a clear reduction in time to diagnosis (13 versus 3 days) that was explained by the earlier and more frequent use of modern imaging modalities.[12]

Radionuclide scanning with technetium-99^m sulfur colloid was commonly used in early studies. Sensitivity for lesions larger than 2 cm was 50 percent to 90 percent but specificity was low. Ultrasonography and computed tomography (CT) have replaced radionuclide scanning as the diagnostic procedures of choice for liver imaging. Both modalities offer excellent sensitivity and may be used for guidance of percutaneous drainage procedures. Hepatic abscesses are usually less echogenic than the surrounding liver tissue on ultrasound. Sensitivity of ultrasonography ranges from 65 percent to 95 percent, with higher detection rates in patients with larger lesions. Microabscesses and singular lesions high in the dome of the liver are missed or misdiagnosed more easily. Hepatic abscesses generally appear less dense on CT images than does surrounding liver tissue (Figures 36-1 to 36-3). Administration of contrast medium often enhances these attenuation differences. Contrast-enhanced CT scanning offers improved sensitivity over ultrasonography (range, 75 percent to 100 percent) and is superior to ultrasound for performance of complex drainage procedures.

Available technologies for imaging of the liver are rapidly evolving. The introduction of new contrasting

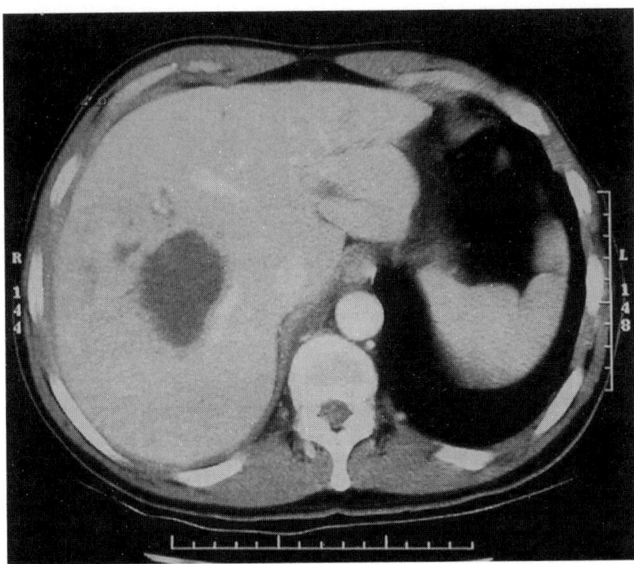

Figure 36-2 Computed tomography image of a mature abscess resulting from *Klebsiella pneumoniae* infection.

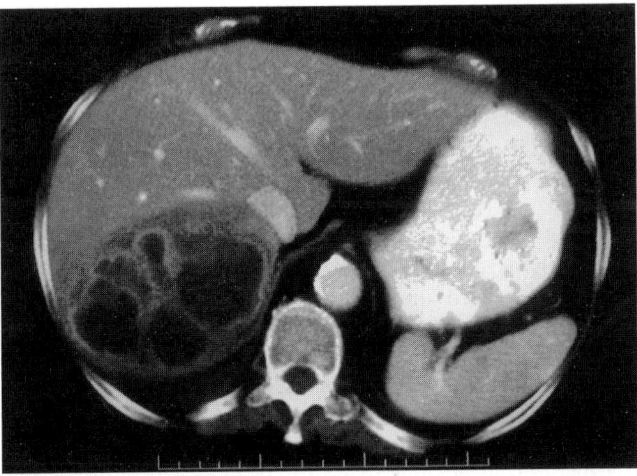

Figure 36-3 Computed tomography image of a multi-loculated abscess resulting from *Staphylococcus aureus infection.*

agents, spiral CT scanning, and fast magnetic resonance imaging (MRI) are among the promising technologies that continue to improve the diagnostic evaluation of patients with suspected hepatic abscesses.[33,34] Infectious liver diseases such as pyogenic liver abscess, but also echinococcal disease and fungal infections, are often characterized by low attenuation on CT and high signal intensity on T2-weighted MRI.[33]As further experience with these newer techniques is gained, further improvements in diagnostic capabilities are anticipated.

Whether and to what extent patients should be evaluated in an attempt to identify the source of the abscess is a controversial area. In one series 53 percent of patients without an obvious source of infection underwent colonoscopy. Endoscopy failed to detect lesions in any of these patients. Likewise in patients without jaundice, elevated bilirubin, or dilated biliary ducts, ERCP revealed cholelithiasis in only 3 of 10 patients. No other abnormality was detected in any of the 10 patients examined.[9] Appropriate and, if necessary, invasive evaluations should therefore be restricted to patients with localizing clinical or laboratory findings.

Therapy

Untreated hepatic abscesses carry a mortality approaching 100 percent. Before modern imaging techniques became available treatment consisted of open surgical drainage and antibiotics. Initial management has notably shifted from a primarily surgical approach[1] to antibiotic management with or without the use of percutaneous drainage or aspiration.[10]

A retrospective meta-analysis concluded in 1986 that percutaneous drainage is safe and associated with a success rate of 90 percent and is comparable to open surgical drainage.[35] Nowadays surgical intervention is usually reserved for patients failing percutaneous drainage. Relative contraindications to percutaneous drainage include large amounts of ascites and severe coagulopathy. Drainage catheters are left in place until drainage has subsided, which usually requires 5 to 10 days. Potential complications include hemorrhage, sepsis, catheter dislodgement, leakage, and perforation of other organs. In one series analyzing patients diagnosed between 1973 and 1993, mortality was lower (14 percent versus 26 percent) with open surgical as opposed to percutaneous abscess drainage, but the numbers were too small to reach statistical significance ($P = .19$).[10] Laparoscopic drainage of complicated abscesses has been used successfully.[36,37] More experience will be required before this modality can replace laparotomy as the intervention of choice. Already, however, laparoscopy offers a viable alternative for some patients who are poor surgical candidates.[37]

Although continuous drainage has become the mainstay of therapy, over the past 15 years more and more centers have switched to percutaneous aspiration without drainage. In combination with antibiotic therapy success rates ranging from 58 percent to 96 percent have been reported, similar to what has been reported for percutaneous drainage.[9-11,13,14,38,39] In a large series the number of patients treated with a primary surgical approach dropped from 92 percent from 1972 and 1973 to 0 percent from 1990 to 1994. During the latter period all patients had percutaneous aspiration with or without drainage. In this series the success rate of this approach was excellent, with complete resolution in 90 percent of cases and a mortality rate of 5 percent.[9] Although a randomized trial comparing drainage versus aspiration has not been performed, a number of case series confirms high success rates using aspiration alone. Giorgio reported success in 113 of 115 consecutive patients with 147 abscesses.[39] Two patients with large viscous abscesses required open drainage. Repeat aspiration was required in a majority of patients but no complications or deaths were reported. In another series 59 of 63 patients were treated successfully with aspiration and antibiotics. Two patients died from septic complications, two required surgical drainage, and one suffered a liver laceration requiring laparotomy. In large abscesses aspiration alone is less likely to succeed, but overall success rates in experienced hands may approach 100 percent.[14] Multiloculated abscesses also pose more problems for both drainage and aspiration.

A controversial area of treatment has been the use of antibiotics without aspiration or drainage of the abscess. Although this approach may not be sufficient in many cases it has proven highly effective in selected patients, with reported success rates ranging from 75 percent to 85 percent.[9,13,14] A major problem of empiric antibiotic therapy without aspiration is the lack of microbiologic data, which allows for a more targeted selection of antimicrobial agents. Although conservative medical therapy may be a reasonable option for certain patients, most patients will benefit from a combined approach. Until indications for exclusive antibiotic therapy are better defined, this approach should be reserved for patients with small abscesses not amenable to drainage or those in whom drainage is associated with an unacceptable risk.

Initial antibiotics should provide coverage against aerobic gram-negative bacilli, microaerophilic streptococci, and anaerobes, including *Bacteroides fragilis.* Metronidazole offers the advantage of good coverage of anaerobes and *Entamoeba histolytica.* The suspected origin of infection should be considered when choosing empiric antibiotic therapy because this will help predict the most likely pathogens. Blood cultures, and if at all possible, a diagnostic aspiration should be performed before or shortly after initiating therapy. Antibiotic coverage should be readjusted after culture results become available. Optimal duration of therapy depends on size of the abscesses, extent of prior drainage, virulence of the organism, response to therapy, and immune status of the affected patient. In general parenteral antibiotics should be given for at least 7 to 14 days, followed by a prolonged course of oral therapy. Follow-up ultrasound or CT scans are often helpful in determining required length of treatment.

PYELOPHLEBITIS

Pyelophlebitis or septic thrombophlebitis of the portal vein used to be common in the pre-antibiotic era and was frequently associated with appendicitis. In early series pyelophlebitis was the most common cause of hepatic abscesses. In recent years it has become a very uncommon entity with approximately 20 cases reported between 1979 and 2000.[39-41] Now a precipitating focus of infection, most commonly diverticulitis, can be identified in approximately two thirds of affected patients. Bacteremia (often polymicrobial) was present in 88 percent of patients in recent series. The most common blood isolate was *B. fragilis.* Overall mortality was 32 percent, but most of the patients who died had severe refractory sepsis before initiation of antibiotic therapy. Heparin was used in one fourth of the patients, all of whom survived, but no clear benefit of this agent could be detected because of the small number of evaluable patients.

PARAINFECTIOUS HEPATITIS

Jaundice and liver function abnormalities are well-described complications of severe bacterial infections ("bilirubin of bacterial badness") (see Chap. 28). This is especially common in neonates and infants, but has also been documented in adults with severe bacterial infections. The exact incidence of this phenomenon remains unknown but Franson and colleagues reported bilirubin elevations in 54 percent of 82 consecutive bacteremic patients.[43] Another study of 84 bacteremic patients found bilirubin levels elevated in only 6 percent, but serum aspartate aminotransferase elevations in 53 percent.[44]

Numerous organisms have been implicated in parainfectious hepatitis, including *E. coli, K. pneumoniae, Bacteroides* species, *Pseudomonas aeruginosa, Streptococcus pneumoniae, Haemophilus influenzae, Proteus* species, aerobic and anaerobic streptococci, *Clostridium* species, *Salmonella* species, *Shigella* species, *S. aureus,* and many others. Implicated primary infection sites are quite diverse and include endocarditis, pneumonia, appendicitis, diverticulitis, pyelonephritis, distant abscesses, septic abortion, and a myriad of other infections. Jaundice associated with lobar pneumonia (known as *pneumonia biliosa*) was reported as early as 1836.[45]

Jaundice secondary to generalized sepsis syndrome must be differentiated from primary infections of the liver. Clinical manifestations and laboratory findings are sufficiently characteristic to distinguish the underlying disease from jaundice due to other causes. In sepsis-associated jaundice, hepatomegaly may be present, but pruritus and abdominal pain are rare. Fever, leukocytosis or leukopenia, and a left shift of the white blood cell differential are common. Bilirubin commonly is elevated to a level of less than 10 mg/dl but may be much higher in neonates, reflecting their immature biliary excretory mechanisms. Most of the bilirubin is conjugated. Alkaline phosphatase and aminotransferase levels may also be increased. Elevations exceeding four times the upper limit of normal are rare unless prolonged hypotension occurred. Histologically, there is intrahepatic cholestasis but little or no necrosis of hepatocytes is seen. Kupffer cell hyperplasia, mild to moderate non-specific inflammatory cell infiltrates predominantly in portal areas, and mild fatty changes have been described. Electron microscopy shows dilation of bile canaliculi, flattening and diminution of microvilli, prominent bile-containing Golgi complexes, and peculiarly enlarged mitochondria.[46]

In prospective studies comparing patients suffering from severe extrahepatic infection with or without jaundice the presence of jaundice does not seem to correlate with survival.[44,47] Duration of jaundice is dependent on control of the underlying infection. The principal underlying metabolic abnormality is a decreased organic anion transport, whereas synthetic, cytosolic, and microsomal functions remained preserved.[47]

There is evidence to suggest that endotoxinemia or, rather, endotoxin-induced cytokine secretion may be the cause of parainfectious liver function abnormalities.[43,48-50] Accordingly, jaundice often manifests before bacteremia is detected.[43] In the rat model administration of endotoxin results in impaired hepatic uptake and secretion of bile acids, presumably because of inhibition of sodium-dependent bile acid uptake or both membrane-potential-dependent and ATP-dependent transport of bile acids.[48,49]

Endotoxins and other bacterial components also affect hepatic microvasculature. Activation of sinusoidal endothelial cells and Kupffer cells results in production of proinflammatory mediators, including tumor necrosis factor alpha, interleukin (IL)-1, IL-6, reactive oxygen metabolites, and eicosanoids. Although these mediators are critical for microbial killing, they are also associated with structural and functional liver damage. Hepatocyte function and hepatic circulation are affected by a very complex interaction of these mediators and multiple modifying factors, including IL-18, granulocyte elastase, α_1-antitrypsin, eglin C, aprotinin, capsase 3-like proteases, hormones, adhesion molecules, including p-selectin and intracellular adhesion molecule (ICAM-1), and hormones, among others.[51-55]

Secretions of chemoattractants eventually result in binding of leukocytes and platelets to sinusoidal endothelial cells, which are in a procoagulant state of inflammatory activation. This leads to a decrease of blood flow through the sinusoids, which is further aggravated by endothelin-1-induced constriction of hepatic stellate cells in the sinusoids. During the early hyperdynamic phase of sepsis, characterized by an increased cardiac output and moderate peripheral vasodilation, adequate sinusoidal perfusion is maintained via the hepatoprotective action of two natural antagonists of endothelin-1, nitric oxide (NO) and carbon monoxide (CO). NO and CO cause relaxation of sinusoidal vessels. However, during the late, hypodynamic phase of sepsis, massive overproduction of NO by the inducible NO synthase results in circulatory collapse, which inevitably includes breakdown of the liver circulation as part of an often-fatal multi-organ failure.[56]

In a porcine model of postburn septicemia, infusion of endotoxin resulted in a significant reduction of portal blood flow (51 percent of baseline). The hepatic arterial blood supply was also significantly reduced to 12 percent to 67 percent of baseline, indicating loss of the hepatic arterial response. Postburn endotoxinemia resulted in a significant decrease in hepatic oxygen delivery (88 percent) and hepatic oxygen consumption (79 percent). Although the burn injury did not affect the portal venous pressure, postburn endotoxinemia caused significant portal hypertension (225 percent of baseline).[57] Additionally, accumulating evidence indicates that circulating endotoxin from intestinal gram-negative bacteria may be involved in alcohol-induced liver injury, including fatty liver. A histochemical study revealed that continuous treatment with alcohol and unsaturated fatty acids caused fatty liver in controls, but not in rats immunized against bacterial endotoxin.[58]

Bacterial infections may not only affect liver function; patients with severe liver dysfunction manifest a significantly increased susceptibility to bacterial infections, presumably as a result of impaired phagocytic function, reduced immunoglobulin and complement levels, and the need for invasive procedures. Bacteriologically proven infections are recorded in up to 80 percent of patients with advanced liver disease or frank liver failure. Clinical signs such as high temperature and elevated white blood cell counts are absent in 30 percent of the cases. Pneumonia accounts for 50 percent of infective episodes, and bacteremia and urinary tract infection for a further 20 percent to 25 percent, respectively. Selective parenteral and enteral antimicrobial regimens have been evaluated in prospective controlled studies of patients with acute liver failure, and early systemic antibiotics alone were as effective as combined treatment modalities. With early use of antibiotics, the incidence of infective episodes was reduced to 20 percent and the overall mortality to 44 percent. Additional benefits included a reduction in progression to encephalopathy and an increased opportunity for transplantation (see Chap. 22).[59,60]

Small-bowel bacterial overgrowth (SBO) has been speculated to cause liver damage in rodents, possibly because of increased small intestinal permeability to proinflammatory bacterial polymers. A recent human study revealed, however, that SBO per se is not a major risk factor for liver damage in humans, even when the overgrowth flora includes obligate anaerobes.[61]

BACTERIAL HEPATITIS

Several bacterial infections affect the liver directly.[62] A case report of meningococcal hepatitis with clinical features suggestive of viral hepatitis[63] underscores the need to perform blood cultures in the jaundiced, febrile patient.

Staphylococcal and Streptococcal Toxic Shock Syndromes

Scarlatiniform rash, hypotension, fever or hypothermia, vomiting, and rapid progression to multi-organ failure are hallmarks of the toxic shock syndrome. Etiologic agents possess superantigens capable of eliciting an unusually broad and potentially fatal immune response. Hepatic involvement is almost universally present and may be extensive with high transaminase levels and deep jaundice. In one study deposition teichoic acid on hepatocyte membranes was demonstrated using indirect immunofluorescent staining.[64] The authors speculated that teichoic acid, a common component of the bacterial cell wall, might exert an endotoxin-like effect on hepatocytes.

Listeriosis

Listeria monocytogenes is a zoonotic gram-positive bacterium, which may cause meningoencephalitis, endocarditis, gastrointestinal disease, and pneumonitis in humans. The propensity of *L. monocytogenes* to affect the liver is well documented in animals and human neonates. Interestingly, one of the initial names proposed for the organism was *Listerella hepatolytica* in recognition of the characteristic focal hepatic necrosis it causes in some animals.[65] Hepatic involvement in adults is rare, but may be severe with transaminase levels in excess of 5000 IU/ml.[66] Most patients with clinically significant liver involvement have underlying liver disease. Histology shows microabscesses and granulomas.[66-68]

Clostridial Infections

Jaundice is detected in 20 percent of patients with *Clostridium perfringens* infections that is the result mostly of intravascular hemolysis secondary to toxin release. Liver involvement with abscess formation and gas in the portal vein or biliary tract has been described.

Meliodosis

Burkholderia pseudomallei is a water- and soil-borne gram-negative bacterium predominantly found in Southeast Asia, Madagascar, and regions of Central America. It is the causative agent of meliodosis.[69-71] The clinical spectrum of meliodosis may range from asymptomatic infection to fulminant overwhelming multi-organ disease involving the liver.[72] A chronic indolent disease has also been described. Inflammatory infiltrates, microabscesses, and focal necrosis may be seen on histology. Intracellular organisms can often be demonstrated. In chronic disease granulomas may form. Cultures are the standard diagnostic test, and immunohistochemistry and serologic testing may aid in localized or chronic disease.

Salmonellosis

Hepatocellular injury resembling viral hepatitis has been described in patients with acute salmonellosis, especially with *Salmonella typhi.* "Typhoid hepatitis" was first described by William Osler as early as 1899.[73] Patients usually present with a chief complaint of fever. A history of recent travel or the finding of relative bradycardia may provide diagnostic clues. The clinical symptoms may be indistinguishable from acute viral hepatitis. Differentiating features are listed in Table 36-5.[74] Hepatomegaly and tender splenomegaly are not uncommon. Abnormal liver tests are frequent in patients with typhoid fever. Bilirubin levels are elevated in one fifth of affected patients, but frank jaundice is present in less than 10 percent of patients with typhoid fever. Transaminase levels are usually not as high as in viral hepatitis, but in rare cases may exceed 1000 U/L, with aspartate aminotransferase (AST) levels exceeding alanine aminotransferase (ALT) levels in 66 percent of affected patients. Periportal thickening may be detectable on ultrasound.[75]

Liver histology shows hepatocyte swelling, non-specific inflammatory changes, and occasionally steatosis. The term *Mallory* or *typhoid nodules* refers to a rare but characteristic focal area of hepatocyte necrosis with aggregation of hyperplastic Kupffer cells with eosinophilic cytoplasm. *S. typhi* antigens and intact *Salmonella* organisms have been demonstrated in liver tissue.[76] *Salmonella* organisms are relatively resistant to phagocytosis and reticuloendothelial killing. Prolonged exposure to endotoxins is the likely pathogenesis for the observed hepatic injury.

Unrecognized typhoid hepatitis carries a mortality rate of 20 percent. Mortality is low, however, with appropriate antibiotic therapy, including quinolones, ampicillin, or third-generation cephalosporins.[74,77] Defervescence may require 3 to 5 days.

Shigellosis

Cholestatic hepatitis is not uncommon in severe shigellosis. Histologic finding include portal and periportal infiltrates (usually with polymorphonuclear leukocytes), cholestasis, and hepatocyte necrosis.[78-80]

Yersiniosis

Diabetes and conditions associated with iron overload predispose to *Yersinia enterocolitica* extra-intestinal infections. Abscess formation is not uncommon in these patients. *Yersiniosis* organisms are also an underappreciated cause of granulomatous hepatitis.[81-85]

Brucellosis

Several species of *Brucella,* small gram-negative coccobacilli, cause brucellosis. Brucellosis is a universal

TABLE 36-5

Differential Diagnosis of Typhoid versus Viral Hepatitis[74]

	Typhoid hepatitis (n = 27)	Viral hepatitis (n = 27)	*P*
Jaundice	33%	89%	<0.0001
Fever >104° F	44%	4%	<0.0001
Relative bradycardia	42%	4%	<0.002
Rigors	44%	33%	NS
Hepatomegaly	44%	66%	NS
Splenomegaly	7%	11%	NS
Peak ALT	296 U/L	3234 U/L	<0.0001 peak AST
	535 U/L	2844 U/L	<0.0003
AP	500 U/dl	228 U/dl	<0.004
Admission ALT/LDH ratio (expressed as multiples of upper limit of normal value)	100% <4	100% >5	<0.0001
Left shift	83%	37%	<0.004
Hospitalization in days	14.8	6.5	<0.0001

ALT, Alanine aminotransferase; *AST,* aspartate aminotransferase; *AP,* alhaline phosphatase; *LDH,* lactic dehydrogenase.

zoonosis and typically presents as prolonged or recurrent fevers. Headaches, malaise, arthralgia, backache, and night sweats are common. Hepatic abnormalities are frequently encountered. The presence of jaundice correlates with severity of the illness. Hepatosplenomegaly is detected in more than half of affected patients.[86] Imaging studies may show typical lesions characterized by central calcification surrounded by a necrotic rim.[87,88] Infection, especially with *Brucella abortus,* is associated with formation of non-caseating or necrotizing hepatic granulomas (Plate 36-1). Focal mononuclear infiltrate may be detected in portal tracts or lobules.[86-90] Positive blood or tissue cultures are diagnostic. Serum agglutination tests are helpful in chronic disease. Prolonged treatment with rifampin and doxycycline provides cure in most cases.

Legionellosis

About half of the patients with documented *Legionella pneumophila* infection will have elevated transaminase and alkaline phosphatase levels, and a few will have frank jaundice.[91-96] Liver histology shows microvesicular steatosis and focal necrosis. Organisms can occasionally be detected.[91-94]

Q Fever

Coxiella burnetti causes the zoonosis Q fever, which is characterized by myalgia, headache, relapsing fevers, pneumonitis, and occasionally culture-negative endocarditis. The liver commonly is affected.[62,97] Frank hepatitis is seen in 3 percent to 4 percent of affected patients, jaundice in 30 percent, and hepatosplenomegaly in more than 70 percent. Alkaline phosphatase is elevated out of proportion to the usually mild increase of transaminases and bilirubin. Histologically, the characteristic "fibrin-ring granulomas" may be seen.[97-100] A ring of fibrinoid necrosis encircled by histiocytes and lymphocytes surrounds a central fat vacuole. This lesion, often referred to as *doughnut or lipogranuloma lesion,* is suggestive, but not pathognomonic, of Q fever. The same lesion may be seen in malignant lymphoma, visceral leishmaniasis, allopurinol hypersensitivity, and several other clinical entities.[99] Widening of the portal tracts by lymphoplasmacellular infiltrate has been observed.[100] Hepatic steatosis is not uncommon.

Rocky Mountain Spotted Fever

The classic triad of fever, headache, and characteristic rash occurring 1 to 2 weeks after a tick bite or a potential exposure in an endemic area should raise suspicions for Rocky Mountain spotted fever (RMSF).[101] RMSF is caused by *Rickettsia rickettsii.* Effects of this organism on endothelial cells include increased vascular permeability, edema, hypovolemia, hypotension, prerenal azotemia, and, in life-threatening cases, pulmonary edema, shock, acute tubular necrosis, and meningoencephalitis. Jaundice is common and occasionally accompanied by various degrees of transaminase and alkaline phosphatase increases.[102,103] The diagnosis is based on clinical suspicion, and treatment is empiric. Laboratory findings are usually not helpful because antibodies are often detected only in convalescence, and immunohistologic methods for detection of rickettsiae are unavailable in most clinics. The hepatic lesion in RMSF is portal triaditis, in which large mononuclear cells and neutrophils predominate. Sinusoidal erythrophagocytosis and portal vasculitis can be demonstrated in severe cases, but hepatocellular necrosis is uncommon. In two series of fatal cases rickettsiae were identified in the portal tracts of 8 of 9 adults, and 7 of 16 pediatric patients.[104,105] Doxycycline is the treatment of choice. Pregnant and tetracycline-allergic patients are treated with chloramphenicol.[101] Other rickettsiae, including *Rickettsia typhi, Rickettsia conorii,* and *Rickettsia tsutsugamushi,* may also affect the liver.[97,106-108]

Ehrlichiosis

Human ehrlichiosis is a tick-borne, zoonotic infection caused by members of the genus *Ehrlichia,* which can affect multiple organs, including the gastrointestinal tract and liver.[109-111] *Ehrlichia* organisms are rickettsia-like, obligate intracellular, gram-negative bacteria. Signs and symptoms include abdominal pain, nausea, vomiting, diarrhea, jaundice (40 percent), hepatosplenomegaly, leukopenia, thrombocytopenia, and, rarely, a faint macular rash. Patients usually present with rapidly increasing levels of AST and ALT. Even with successful therapy transaminase levels normalize slowly. Bilirubin elevations may exceed 10 mg/dl. Immunocompromised and asplenic patients are at risk for more severe and protracted disease.

Human monocytic ehrlichiosis is caused by *Ehrlichia chaffeensis,* whereas human granulocytic ehrlichiosis is caused by *Ehrlichia granulocytophilia.* Both diseases can produce intracytoplasmic morulae in either monocytes or neutrophils, which are occasionally visualized on Wright-stained peripheral smears. The diagnosis is confirmed by demonstrating seroconversion, a positive polymerase chain reaction (PCR), or growth of the organism in tissue culture. If not diagnosed and treated in a timely fashion, ehrlichiosis can progress to multi-organ failure, which is associated with significant mortality. Doxycycline provides rapid and effective treatment. Therapy should not be delayed pending confirmation of the diagnosis. Rifampin or chloramphenicol may be tried in patients in whom use of tetracyclines is contraindicated.

Actinomycosis

Actinomycosis caused by *Actinomyces israelii* and rarely by other Actinomycetales may involve the liver.[112-114] Although some patients have oral disease or intra-abdominal infections, the majority of cases are cryptogenic. Most patients with hepatic disease will develop frank pyogenic abscesses but some have chronic indolent infection. In these patients the organism infiltrates the liver without causing frank necrosis mimicking malignant liver disease.

The typical patient is male and between 30 and 50 years of age. Common presenting symptoms include fever, abdominal pain, and anorexia with weight loss.

Findings on physical examination include fever, RUQ pain, and hepatomegaly. Leukocytosis with a left shift, anemia, an elevated serum erythrocyte sedimentation rate, and an elevated level of alkaline phosphatase are almost universally present. Many patients undergo exploratory laparotomy to rule out malignancy, but most recent cases have been diagnosed with percutaneous biopsy. Histologically characteristic sulfur granules and the characteristic gram-positive branching rods may be demonstrated (Plate 36-2). Anaerobic cultures usually result in growth of the organism. Treatment consists of prolonged administration of penicillin or tetracycline and is associated with complete recovery in the majority of cases.

Leptospirosis

Leptospirosis is presumed to be the most widespread zoonosis in the world and has a wide range of domestic and wild animal reservoirs. Leptospires are tightly coiled spirochetes. Humans usually acquire the spirochete from water contaminated with urine from an infectious animal. The incidence is higher in warmer and humid climates, presumably because of prolonged survival of the organisms in the environment.[115]. A majority of infections are subclinical or mild enough not to result in medical attention. Anicteric leptospirosis accounts for 90 percent of all recognized cases. Affected patients characteristically suffer a biphasic illness. The first phase (leptospiremic or acute stage) is characterized by the abrupt onset of an influenza-like illness with fever, myalgia, headache, and malaise. Conjunctival suffusion, if present, may provide an early diagnostic clue. After a brief period of improvement, the second phase (leptospiruric or immune stage), characterized by myalgia, potentially severe headache, abdominal pain, nausea, vomiting, and, occasionally, aseptic meningitis commences. During this phase elevations of transaminase and bilirubin levels are rare, but hepatomegaly is not uncommon. A maculo-papular rash and iridocyclitis may be present. Mortality is extremely rare in anicteric leptospirosis.

From 5 percent to 10 percent of infected patients develop the more severe icteric form, which is often referred to as Morbus Weil or Weil's syndrome. The first phase, which may last for weeks, is characterized by jaundice. During the second phase, which commonly follows without interceding improvement, high fevers ensue. Hepatic and renal dysfunction predominate this phase. Jaundice may be marked, with bilirubin levels in excess of 80 mg/dl. Aminotransferase levels are usually only mildly or moderately elevated. Acute tubular necrosis is common and may result in acute renal failure. Hemorrhagic complications are frequent and probably immune-complex mediated.

Hepatic histology is generally non-specific. Intrahepatic cholestasis, hypertrophy, and hyperplasia of Kupffer cells are found frequently. Erythrophagocytosis has been documented in severe or fatal cases.[115] Electron microscopy shows mitochondrial alterations and disruption of the hepatocyte membrane. Frank hepatocyte necrosis, however, is uncommon.

Diagnosis can be made by positive blood (first phase) or urine (second phase) cultures. More commonly, serologic or molecular tests are used to confirm the diagnosis of leptospirosis. Doxycycline is effective if administered early and has also been shown to be effective for prophylaxis before or after exposure in high-risk environments or laboratory accidents. Long-term sequelae in survivors are extremely rare.

Borreliosis

This arthropod-transmitted infection is caused by several spirochetal organisms of the genus *Borrelia.* Diseases include relapsing fever and Lyme disease. Incubation time of relapsing fever is 3 to 15 days. Onset of symptoms is usually abrupt with high fevers, headache, and myalgia. Epistaxis, profound prostration, bronchial symptoms, and a rash or conjunctival injection may be present. In severe attacks jaundice and tender hepatosplenomegaly may develop. Defervescence may be dramatic, with fatal collapses reported in the literature.

Borrelia organisms multiply in organs of the reticulo-endothelial system. They invade liver cells, causing focal necrosis. Before crisis, *Borrelia* organisms coil tightly and are ingested by cells of the reticulo-endothelial system, where they may survive and cause relapsing infection. Several relapses may occur in weekly intervals. Spirochetes may be visualized in thick blood films,[116] cutaneous biopsies, or lymph node aspirates, but diagnosis is often established using agglutination or complement fixation-based serologic tests. Treatment with doxycycline is curative.

Hepatic involvement has also been described in Lyme disease caused by infection with the tick-transmitted spirochete *Borrelia burgdorferi.* Liver test abnormalities are common in patients with erythema migrans, but are usually mild in asymptomatic patients, and improved or resolved by 3 weeks after the onset of antibiotic therapy in most patients. In a prospective study of patients with early Lyme disease 40 percent of patients had at least one liver test abnormality compared with 19 percent of controls. Gamma-glutamyl transpeptidase (28 percent) and ALT (27 percent) were the most frequently elevated liver tests. Patients with early disseminated Lyme disease were more likely to have elevated liver studies (66 percent) compared with patients with localized disease (34 percent). Gastrointestinal symptoms, including anorexia, nausea, or vomiting, were reported by 30 percent of patients, but were not associated with elevated liver tests.[117] In later stages of the illness, presumably after invasion of the reticulo-endothelial system, hepatitis-type illnesses have been described.[118] These are rare and usually overshadowed by other manifestations of the disease but may become diagnostic pitfalls.

Syphilis

Jaundice complicating early syphilis was first described by Paracelsus in 1585.[119] Liver disease has been reported accompanying congenital, primary, secondary, and tertiary syphilis, treatment of syphilis (Jarisch-Herxheimer reaction),[120] and lues maligna. Some early reports, however, must be viewed with caution as testing for concurrent hepatitis C virus (HCV) infection was not available.

Congenital syphilis is associated with the formation of small epithelioid granulomas and variable, but occasionally significant, portal and interstitial fibrosis.[121,122] Coiled treponemes are usually easily detected in vascular structures, fibrous tissue, and liver parenchyma using a silver stain, such as Warthin-Starry. Extensive granulomatous disease can cause hepatomegaly (hepar lobatum), portal hypertension, and ascites. Hepatic calcifications may be extensive.

Patients with secondary syphilis often present with a maculo-papular rash involving their palms and soles and non-specific symptoms including malaise, weight-loss, fever, and anorexia. Jaundice, RUQ tenderness, or hepatomegaly is uncommon. Laboratory testing usually shows an isolated or disproportionate elevation of alkaline phosphatase levels. Lymphocytic infiltration in and around portal tracts is common; in some patients there is evidence of focal intralobular necrosis (Plate 36-3). Kupffer cell hyperplasia may be seen. Spirochetes have been demonstrated on silver staining in up to 50 percent of affected patients.[120,123-125]

Tertiary syphilis with the exception of central nervous system disease is now rare. Patients may be asymptomatic or present with non-specific symptoms, including malaise, anorexia, weight loss, abdominal pain, or fever. Hepatic lesions are common.[126] Tender nodular hepatomegaly has been reported, resulting in work-up for suspected malignancy. The characteristic lesion is the gumma, a centrally necrotic granuloma of rubbery consistency. Histologically, extensive scarring surrounding granulation tissue consisting of a lymphoplasmacytic infiltrate can be seen. Endarteritis is common.

In most cases syphilis is diagnosed serologically. There is some evidence for cross-reactivity between serologic tests for HCV infection and syphilis.[127] Penicillin is effective for all stages. Desensitization, tetracyclines, and cephalosporins may be used in penicillin-allergic patients.

Gonorrhea

The liver is commonly involved in gonococcal bacteremia, with up to 50 percent of patients manifesting abnormal liver tests. Frank jaundice is rare (less than 10 percent) but increased levels of aminotransferases (33 percent) and alkaline phosphatase (50 percent to 100 percent) are relatively common. Liver biopsy often shows a dense inflammatory infiltrate most pronounced in portal areas and focal necrosis of hepatocytes. Perihepatitis (Fitz-Hugh-Curtis syndrome) is the most common hepatic complication of disseminated gonococcal infection.[128] This syndrome has a striking gender predilection for women. Abrupt onset of sharp RUQ pain is the typical presenting symptom. Most patients are febrile. The liver tends to be tender and a friction rub may be present. Most patients have a history of pelvic inflammatory disease. Laparoscopic detection of violin string-like adhesions between liver capsule and peritoneal wall are highly suggestive of the diagnosis. Although gonococcal infection tends to respond dramatically to antimicrobial therapy, abnormal liver tests may initially worsen during therapy. Within a month, however, all laboratory tests tend to normalize. A similar perihepatitis can also accompany chlamydial infections.[129,130]

Mycobacteria

Mycobacterium tuberculosis

Liver involvement in tuberculosis is well documented and may present in several different ways. Liver involvement in miliary tuberculosis is common and present in up to 50 percent of patients dying from pulmonary tuberculosis.[131] Localized lesions, such as tuberculomas or tuberculous abscesses, are much less common and frequently misdiagnosed initially. Tuberculosis of the liver without disseminated disease is uncommon. In a review of 341 patients with tuberculous liver disease only 39 patients had hepatic involvement without widespread miliary tuberculosis.

Symptoms are often non-specific (Table 36-6). RUQ pain is not uncommon, and generalized abdominal pain usually indicates concurrent peritoneal involvement. Ascites may be present in patients with peritoneal involvement. In these latter patients a "doughy" feel is described on abdominal examination.

Elevation of alkaline phosphatase and aminotransferases are common with liver involvement. Hyperbilirubinemia is present in less than 25 percent of patients. Jaundice is usually caused by adenopathy in the porta hepatis obstructing the common bile duct or by postinflammatory strictures.[132,133] Hypoalbuminemia and hyponatremia are noted in 88 percent and 65 percent of patients, respectively. The ascitic fluid white blood cell in patients with peritoneal involvement is elevated and more than 80 percent of the cells are mononuclear. The serum to ascites albumin gradient is <1.1 (see Chap. 22).

The presence of hepatic calcification and evidence of concurrent pulmonary disease are helpful in distinguishing hepatic tuberculosis from other liver diseases. Radiologic evidence of pulmonary disease, however, may be absent in as many as one third of affected patients.[134,135] Hepatic lesions are usually hypoechoic on ultrasound, but may occasionally be hyperechoic.[136] Because signs and symptoms of hepatic tuberculosis are nonspecific, diagnosis requires histologic or bacteriologic confirmation. Percutaneous, laparoscopic, or open biopsies have all been used successfully.[137] In rare cases bile fluid obtained via endoscopic retrograde cholangiography (ERC) is diagnostic.

TABLE 36-6
Clinical Features in Hepatic Tuberculosis[131,133-135]

Hepatomegaly	91%
Fever	75%
Weight loss	64%
Abdominal pain	52%
Splenomegaly	39%
Digestive symptoms	33%
Night sweats	25%
Jaundice	12%

The finding of hepatic granulomas with central necrosis on biopsy is characteristic and should be considered diagnostic of tuberculosis until proven otherwise. Acid-fast bacilli can only be detected in about two thirds of affected patients. Culture and PCR tests are more sensitive.

FUNGAL HEPATITIS

Many fungal infections affect the liver. Some, such as *Histoplasma capsulatum,* are taken up by the reticuloendothelial system. In fungemic patients organisms reach the liver via the hepatic artery. Disruption of the gastrointestinal lining also may result in invasion of the portal venous system by *Candida* species that are part of the normal human intestinal flora. Most fungal infections of the liver occur in immunocompromised patients. HIV-infected patients suffer from opportunistic mycoses, including histoplasmosis, blastomycosis, cryptococcosis, penicilliosis, coccidioidomycosis, and paracoccidioidomycosis. Patients with prolonged neutropenia after transplantation or chemotherapy are at risk for candidiasis, aspergillosis, mucormycosis, trichosporonosis, and other rare fungal infections. Fungal infections of the liver in patients infected with HIV or after liver transplantation are reviewed in separate chapters (see Chaps. 51 and 55). The following reviews fungal infections in immunocompromised patients.

Candidiasis

Candida species are currently the fourth most common cause of nosocomial bloodstream infections. Patients with indwelling lines, abdominal surgery, or neutropenia are at highest risk. Seeding of the liver is common in candidemic patients but is usually not clinically apparent in immunocompetent patients. Autopsies of fatal cases often reveal microabscesses in virtually all organs, including the liver. As *Candida* species are part of the normal intestinal flora, disruption of the intestinal wall may also result in heptic candidiasis.

Coccidioidomycosis

Coccidioides immitis is endemic in southwest United States and the San Joaquin Valley of California. Males, especially African-Americans and immigrants, and immunocompromised patients appear more susceptible to infection. In the disseminated form hepatic involvement is common, occurring in 40 percent to 60 percent of cases. In many patients liver disease is asymptomatic but some manifest a hepatitis-like picture, which is characterized by a disproportionate elevation of alkaline phosphatase. Hepatic granulomas may be found.[138]

Cryptococcosis

Infections with the yeast *Cryptococcus neoformans* usually present as a self-limited pneumonia, fever of unknown origin, or, most commonly, as meningitis. Hepatic cryptococcosis is rare with the exception of patients suffering from acquired immunodeficiency syndrome. In non–HIV-infected patients liver infiltration may result in focal granulomatous hepatitis, which may clinically mimic viral hepatitis. Very rarely, the liver is extensively involved, resulting in hepatic failure.[139] Another rare presentation is obstructive jaundice secondary to sclerosing cholangitis with recovery of yeast from the common bile duct.[140]

Microscopic examination of affected tissues or body fluids may suggest the correct diagnosis. Staining with India ink or nigrosin-based stains emphasizes the capsule. Confirmation requires a positive culture or the detection of fungal antigen using latex agglutination. Amphotericin B in doses of 0.3 to 0.6 mg/kg daily is usually sufficient therapy unless the patient is infected with HIV. Fluconazole is a promising alternative and has been used successfully in mild illnesses. Experience with the use of azoles outside this setting, however, is still scarce.

Histoplasmosis

Histoplasma capsulatum is a dimorphic fungus that can be found in soil contaminated with bird or bat excreta. Histoplasmosis is endemic in the eastern and central United States, Central and South America, Africa, India, and Asia. Infection occurs via inhalation but subsides without clinical disease in most patients. Occasionally the infection may disseminate from the lungs to involve organs of the reticuloendothelial system, including the liver. In non-immunocompromised hosts, infection is commonly self-limiting. Many patients from endemic areas who are without a history of primary infection are found to have hepatic calcifications, some of which may contain *H. capsulatum* organisms. Progressive dissemination is not uncommon in immunocompromised patients, but rarely occurs in normal hosts.[141] Approximately two thirds of affected patients will present with tender hepatomegaly.[91] Several reports have documented histoplasmosis as a common cause of infection-associated hemophagocytic syndrome.[142] Affected patients present with hepatosplenomegaly, high fever, and abnormal liver tests. Histoplasmosis may also present as an isolated liver lesion.[143]

The most common histologic finding is a portal lympho-histiocytic infiltrate. Discrete hepatic granulomas were seen in less than 20 percent of involved livers.[144] Diagnosis is based on demonstration of the organism in histologic specimens, growth in fungal culture media, or detection of fungal antigen in serum or urine. Serologic tests are only helpful in non-endemic settings. Treatment of patients with severe disease consists of amphotericin B in doses of 0.8 to 1 mg/kg daily followed by prolonged treatment with itraconazole.

Paracoccidioidomycosis

Paracoccidioidomycosis is a systemic infection caused by the dimorphic fungus *Paracoccidioides brasiliensis.* The infection is only seen in parts of South and Central America, including Mexico, and most commonly affects adult men. Infection is common in endemic areas, but clinical disease is extremely rare.

Evidence of hepatic involvement in immunocompetent patients is largely based on autopsy series, in which up to 50 percent of patients who die of paracoccidioidomycosis are found to have liver involvement.[145,146]

Hepatomegaly is reported in 40 percent of patients with clinical disease but jaundice is found in fewer than 6 percent of affected individuals. One case of obstructive jaundice secondary to infection of hilar lymph nodes has been reported.[147] Aminotransferase levels are commonly elevated, whereas bilirubin and alkaline phosphatase levels are only elevated in patients with severe disease. Biopsy specimens show lesions ranging from small granulomas to diffuse infiltration of yeast forms and fibrosis. The bile ducts are commonly involved. Positive fungal cultures are diagnostic. Itraconazole is the treatment of choice.

PELIOSIS HEPATIS

Peliosis hepatis is characterized by cystic, blood-filled spaces in the liver and is seen in patients with chronic infections or advanced cancer and as a consequence of therapy with certain medications, including anabolic steroids. In patients with HIV infection, and rarely in other immunocompromised patients, peliosis hepatis is a sequela of infection by certain *Bartonella* species.[148,149] In immunocompetent patients bartonellosis manifests as cat-scratch disease, trench fever, bacteremia, or endocarditis. In immunocompromised patients bartonellosis presents as bacillary angiomatosis, peliosis, bacteremia, and endocarditis. *Bartonella henselae* has been cultured from peliotic liver lesions.

Affected patients present with prolonged fever and hepatomegaly, which in 75 percent of cases is accompanied by splenomegaly. Other symptoms or findings may include the presence of bony lesions, lymphadenopathy, and abdominal or RUQ pain. Cutaneous lesions of bacillary angiomatosis are seen in 40 percent of the cases. Anemia is common, but thrombocytopenia or pancytopenia have also been reported. Aminotransferase levels are rarely increased, but elevations of alkaline phosphatase, by an average of fivefold above the normal limit, are regularly detected. Subcutaneous and lytic bone lesions are more common in infections with *Bartonella quintana,* whereas peliosis hepatis is exclusively associated with *B. henselae*. *B. henselae* infection is epidemiologically linked to cat and flea exposure, whereas infection with *B. quintana* occurs in clusters and is associated with low-income status, homelessness, and exposure to lice.[150]

On CT, peliotic lesions appear as scattered hypodense lesions. Histopathologically, the characteristic lesions contain dilated capillaries and larger, occasionally macroscopically visualized cystic, blood-filled spaces. They are scattered throughout the hepatic parenchyma. The lining of these cystic spaces is often thin. Peliosis hepatis associated with *Bartonella* organism infection, but not in unrelated cases, is additionally characterized by a myxoid stroma and clumps of a granular purple material, which on Warthin-Starry staining and electron microscopy can be identified as bacilli. Because culture remains difficult, serologic tests have become the mainstay of diagnosis. PCR-based tests are being evaluated. *Bartonella*-associated peliosis hepatis rarely has been reported in patients with cancer or after transplants.[151,152]

Peliosis hepatis responds to treatment with macrolides and doxycycline. Other drugs with in vitro activity against *Bartonella* species but no established clinical efficacy include rifampin, third-generation cephalosporins, trimethoprim-sulfamethoxazole, and quinolones. Results of in vitro susceptibility tests do not necessarily correlate with clinical efficacy because treatment failures with penicillins and first-generation cephalosporins are common despite several reports documenting in vitro susceptibility.[153] Patients with hepatic bartonellosis should be treated for at least 4 months. Relapsing patients should receive life-long treatment. Jarisch-Herxheimer–like reactions have been reported after the first dose of antibiotics in patients with peliosis hepatis.[153]

References

1. Adams F: The Genuine Works of Hippocrates, vol 1, 2. New York, William Wood & Co., 1886:57-58, 266-267.
2. Ochsner A, DeBaley M, Murray S: Pyogenic abscess of the liver. Am J Surg 40:292-319, 1938.
3. Reyes AI, Reyes DA: Hepatic abscess. An analysis of 86 cases. Int Surg 52(2):173-178, 1969.
4. Lazarchick J, De Souza e Silva NA, Nichols DR, Washington JA 2nd: Pyogenic liver abscess. Mayo Clin Proc 48(5):349-355, 1973.
5. Rubin RH, Swartz MN, Malt R: Hepatic abscess: changes in clinical, bacteriologic and therapeutic aspects. Am J Med 57(4):601-610, 1974.
6. Greenstein AJ, Lowenthal D, Hammer GS, et al: Continuing changing patterns of disease in pyogenic liver abscess: a study of 38 patients. Am J Gastroenterol 79(3):217-226, 1984.
7. McDonald MI, Corey GR, Gallis HA, Durack DT: Single and multiple pyogenic liver abscesses. Natural history, diagnosis and treatment, with emphasis on percutaneous drainage. Medicine 63(5):291-302, 1984.
8. Barnes PF, De Cock KM, Reynolds TN, Ralls PW: A comparison of amebic and pyogenic abscess of the liver. Medicine 66(6):472-483, 1987.
9. Seeto RK, Rockey DC: Pyogenic liver abscess. Changes in etiology, management, and outcome. Medicine 75(2):99-113, 1996.
10. Huang CJ, Pitt HA, Lipsett PA, et al: Pyogenic hepatic abscess. Changing trends over 42 years. Ann Surg 223(5):600-607, 1996.
11. Chu KM, Fan ST, Lai EC, et al: Pyogenic liver abscess. An audit of experience over the past decade. Arch Surg 131(2):148-152, 1996.
12. Corredoira Sanchez JC, Casariego Vales E, et al: (Pyogenic liver abscess: changes in etiology, diagnosis and treatment over 18 years). Rev Clin Esp 199(11):705-710, 1999.
13. Barakate MS, Stephen MS, Waugh RC, et al: Pyogenic liver abscess: a review of 10 years' experience in management. Aust N Z J Surg 69(3):205, 1999.
14. Chou FF, Sheen-Chen SM, Chen YS, Chen MC: Single and multiple pyogenic liver abscesses: clinical course, etiology, and results of treatment. World J Surg 21(4): 384-388, 1997.
15. Rabkin JM, Orloff SL, Corless CL, et al: Hepatic allograft abscess with hepatic arterial thrombosis. Am J Surg 175(5):354, 1998.
16. Jan YY, Yeh TS, Chen MF: Cholangiocarcinoma presenting as pyogenic liver abscess: is its outcome influenced by concomitant hepatolithiasis? Am J Gastroenterol 93(2):253-255, 1998.
17. Yeh TS, Jan YY, Jeng LB, et al: Hepatocellular carcinoma presenting as pyogenic liver abscess: characteristics, diagnosis, and management. Clin Infect Dis 26(5):1224, 1998.
18. Tsai JL, Than MM, Wu CJ, et al: Liver abscess secondary to fish bone penetration of the gastric wall: a case report. Chung Hua I Hsueh Tsa Chih 62(1):51-54, 1999.
19. Tsui BC, Mossey J: Occult liver abscess following clinically unsuspected ingestion of foreign bodies. Can J Gastroenterol 11(5):445, 1997.
20. Drnovsek V, Fontanez-Garcia D, Wakabayashi MN, Plavsic BM: Gastrointestinal case of the day. Pyogenic liver abscess caused by perforation by a swallowed wooden toothpick. Radiographics 19(3):820-822, 1999.
21. Lowry P, Rollins NK: Pyogenic liver abscess complicating ingestion of sharp objects. Pediatr Infect Dis J 12(4):348-350, 1993.
22. Perkins M, Lovell J, Gruenewald S: Life-threatening pica: liver abscess from perforating foreign body. Australas Radiol 43(3):349-352, 1999.

23. de Baere T, Roche A, Amenabar JM, et al: Liver abscess formation after local treatment of liver tumors. Hepatology 23(6):1436-1440, 1996.
24. Tanaka M, Takahata S, Konomi H,, et al: Long-term consequence of endoscopic sphincterotomy for bile duct stones. Gastrointest Endosc 48(5):465-469, 1998.
25. Kubo S, Kinoshita H, Hirohashi K, et al: Risk factors for and clinical findings of liver abscess after biliary-intestinal anastomosis. Hepatogastroenterology 46(25):116-120, 1999.
26. Brook I, Frazier EH: Microbiology of liver and spleen abscesses. J Med Microbiol 47(12):1075-1080, 1998.
27. Lee JF, Block GE: The changing clinical pattern of hepatic abscesses. Arch Surg 104(4):465-470, 1972.
28. Sabbaj J, Sutter VL, Finegold SM: Anaerobic pyogenic liver abscess. Ann Intern Med 77(4):627-638, 1972.
29. Wang JH, Liu YC, Lee SS, et al: Primary liver abscess due to *Klebsiella pneumoniae* in Taiwan. Clin Infect Dis 26(6):1434, 1998.
30. Chou FF, Sheen-Chen SM, Chen YS, Lee TY: The comparison of clinical course and results of treatment between gas-forming and non-gas-forming pyogenic liver abscess. Arch Surg 130(4):401, 1995.
31. Hageman J, Pegues D, Jepson C, et al: Vancomycin-intermediate *Staphylococcus aureus* hepatic abscess arising in a home healthcare patient, Nevada. Abstract L-3, presented at the 40th Interscience Conference for Antimicrobial Agents and Chemotherapy, 2000.
32. Lipsett PA, Huang CJ, Lillemoe KD, et al: Fungal hepatic abscesses: characterization and management. J Gastrointest Surg 1(1):78-84, 1997.
33. Kawamoto S, Soyer PA, Fishman EK, Bluemke DA: Nonneoplastic liver disease: evaluation with CT and MR imaging. Radiographics 18:827-848, 1998.
34. Runge VM, Wells JW, Williams NM: Hepatic abscesses. Magnetic resonance imaging findings using gadolinium-BOPTA. Invest Radiol 31(12):781, 1996.
35. Bertel CK, van Heerden JA, Sheedy PF 2nd: Treatment of pyogenic hepatic abscesses. Surgical vs percutaneous drainage. Arch Surg 121(5):554-558, 1986.
36. Marks J, Mouiel J, Katkhouda N, et al: Laparoscopic liver surgery. A report on 28 patients. Surg Endosc 12(4):331-334, 1998.
37. Siu WT, Chan WC, Hou SM, Li MK: Laparoscopic management of ruptured pyogenic liver abscess. Surg Laparosc Endosc 7(5):426, 1997.
38. Ch Yu S, Hg Lo R, Kan PS, Metreweli C: Pyogenic liver abscess: treatment with needle aspiration. Clin Radiol 52(12):912-916, 1997.
39. Giorgio A, Tarantino L, Mariniello N, et al: Pyogenic liver abscesses: 13 years of experience in percutaneous needle aspiration with US guidance. Radiology 195(1):122-124, 1995.
40. Plemmons RM, Dooley DP, Longfield RN: Septic thrombophlebitis of the portal vein (pylephlebitis): diagnosis and management in the modern era. Clin Infect Dis 21(5):1114-1120, 1995.
41. Baddley JW, Singh D, Correa P, Persich NJ: Crohn's disease presenting as septic thrombophlebitis of the portal vein (pylephlebitis): case report and review of the literature. Am J Gastroenterol 94(3):847-849, 1999.
42. Saxena R, Adolph M, Ziegler JR, et al: Pylephlebitis: a case report and review of outcome in the antibiotic era. Am J Gastroenterol 91(6):1251-1253, 1996.
43. Franson TR, Hierholzer WJ Jr, LaBrecque DR: Frequency and characteristics of hyperbilirubinemia associated with bacteremia. Rev Infect Dis 7:1-9, 1985.
44. Sikuler E, Guetta V, Keynan A, et al: Abnormalities in bilirubin and liver enzyme levels in adult patients with bacteremia. A prospective study. Arch Intern Med 149:2246-2248, 1989.
45. Garvin IP: Remarks on pneumonia biliosa. South Med Surg 1:536-544, 1836.
46. Fahrlander H, Huber F, Gloor F: Intrahepatic retention of bile in severe bacterial infections. Gastroenterology 47:590-594, 1964.
47. Pirovino M, Meister F, Rubli E, Karlaganis G: Preserved cytosolic and synthetic liver function in jaundice of severe extrahepatic infection. Gastroenterology 96:1589-1595, 1989.
48. Bolder U, Ton-Nu HT, Schteingart CD, et al: Hepatocyte transport of bile acids and organic anions in endotoxemic rats: impaired uptake and secretion. Gastroenterology 112:214-225, 1997.
49. Moseley RH, Wang W, Takeda H, et al: Effect of endotoxin on bile acid transport in rat liver: a potential model for sepsis-associated cholestasis. Am J Physiol 271:G137-G146, 1996.
50. Nolan JP: Intestinal endotoxins as mediators of hepatic injury—an idea whose time has come again. Hepatology 10:887-891, 1989.
51. Sauer A, Hartung T, Aigner J, Wendel A: Endotoxin-inducible granulocyte-mediated hepatocytotoxicity requires adhesion and serine protease release. J Leukoc Biol 60:633-643, 1996.
52. Essani NA, Fisher MA, Simmons CA, et al: Increased P-selectin gene expression in the liver vasculature and its role in the pathophysiology of neutrophil-induced liver injury in murine endotoxin shock. J Leukoc Biol 63:288-296, 1998.
53. Jaeschke H, Fisher MA, Lawson JA, et al: Activation of caspase 3 (CPP32)-like proteases is essential for TNF-alpha-induced hepatic parenchymal cell apoptosis and neutrophil-mediated necrosis in a murine endotoxin shock model. J Immunol 160:3480-3486, 1998.
54. Ikejima K, Enomoto N, Iimuro Y, et al: Estrogen increases sensitivity of hepatic Kupffer cells to endotoxin. Am J Physiol 274:G669, 1998.
55. Weigand MA, Schmidt H, Pourmahmoud M, et al: Circulating intercellular adhesion molecule-1 as an early predictor of hepatic failure in patients with septic shock. Crit Care Med 27:2656, 1999.
56. Ring A, Stremmel W: The hepatic microvascular responses to sepsis. Semin Thromb Hemost 26:589-594, 2000.
57. Tadros T, Traber DL, Herndon DN: Hepatic blood flow and oxygen consumption after burn and sepsis. J Trauma 49:101-108, 2000.
58. Nishimura G, Nakahara K, Misawa N, et al: Immunization against intestinal bacterial endotoxin prevents alcoholic fatty liver in rats. J Vet Med Sci 63(3):275-280, 2001.
59. Rolando N, Philpott-Howard J, Williams R: Bacterial and fungal infection in acute liver failure. Semin Liver Dis 16(4):389-402, 1996.
60. Navasa M, Rimola A, Rodes J: Bacterial infections in liver disease. Semin Liver Dis 17(4):323-333, 1997.
61. Riordan SM, McIver CJ, Williams R: Liver damage in human small intestinal bacterial overgrowth. Am J Gastroenterol 93(2):234, 1998.
62. Cunha BA: Systemic infections affecting the liver. Some cause jaundice, some do not. Postgrad Med 84:148-158, 1988.
63. Cowan GO: Meningococcal hepatitis: a case report. J Trop Med Hyg 90:95-96, 1987.
64. Rose HD, Lentino JR, Mavrelis PG, Rytel MW: Jaundice associated with nonhepatic *Staphylococcus aureus* infection. Does teichoic acid have a role in pathogenesis? Dig Dis Sci 27:1046-1050, 1982.
65. Pirie JHH: Listeria. Change of a name for a genus of bacteria. Nature 145:264-265, 1940.
66. Yu VL, Miller WP, Wing EJ, et al: Disseminated listeriosis presenting as acute hepatitis. Case reports and review of hepatic involvement in listeriosis. Am J Med 73:773-777, 1982.
67. Desprez D, Blanc P, Larrey D, et al: Acute hepatitis caused by *Listeria monocytogenes* infection. Gastroenterol Clin Biol 18:516-519, 1994.
68. Hardie R, Roberts W: Adult listeriosis presenting as acute hepatitis. J Infect 8:256-258, 1984.
69. Dance DA: Melioidosis as an emerging global problem. Acta Trop 74:115-119, 2000.
70. Brett PJ, Woods DE: Pathogenesis of and immunity to melioidosis. Acta Trop 74:201-210, 2000.
71. Zysk G, Splettstosser WD, Neubauer H: A review on melioidosis with special respect on molecular and immunological diagnostic techniques. Clin Lab 46:119-113, 2000.
72. Vatcharapreechasakul T, Suputtamongkol Y, Dance DA, et al: *Pseudomonas pseudomallei* liver abscesses: a clinical, laboratory, and ultrasonographic study. Clin Infect Dis 14:412-417, 1992.
73. Osler W: Hepatic complications of typhoid fever. Johns Hopkins Hosp Rev 8:373-387, 1899.
74. El-Newihi HM, Alamy ME, Reynolds TB: Salmonella hepatitis: analysis of 27 cases and comparison with acute viral hepatitis. Hepatology Sept;24(3):516, 1996
75. Medhat A, Nafeh M, Swifee Y, et al: Ultrasound-detected hepatic periportal thickening in patients with prolonged pyrexia. Am J Trop Med Hyg 59:45-48, 1998.
76. Calva JJ, Ruiz-Palacios GM: Salmonella hepatitis: detection of salmonella antigens in the liver of patients with typhoid fever. J Infect Dis 154:373-374, 1986.
77. Khosla SN: Typhoid hepatitis. Postgrad Med J 66:923-925, 1990.

78. Horney JT, Schwarzmann SW, Galambos JT: Shigella hepatitis. Am J Gastroenterol 66:146-149, 1976.
79. Stern MS, Gitnick GL: Shigella hepatitis. JAMA 235:2628, 1976.
80. Squires RH, Keating JP, Rosenblum JL, et al: Splenic abscess and hepatic dysfunction caused by Shigella flexneri. J Pediatr 98:429-430, 1981.
81. Saebo A: Liver affection associated with *Yersinia enterocolitica* infection. Acta Chir Scand 143:445-450, 1977.
82. Stjernberg U, Silseth C, Ritland S: Granulomatous hepatitis in *Yersinia enterocolitica* infection. Hepatogastroenterology 34:56-57, 1987.
83. Saebo A, Lassen J: Acute and chronic liver disease associated with *Yersinia enterocolitica* infection: a Norwegian 10-year follow-up study of 458 hospitalized patients. J Intern Med 231:531, 1992.
84. Strungs I, Farrell DJ, Matar LD, et al: Multiple hepatic abscesses due to *Yersinia enterocolitica.* Pathology 27:374-377, 1995.
85. Albrecht H, Stellbrink HJ, Nägele HH, et al: Leber Abszesse durch *Yersinia enterocolitica.* Deutsch Med Wochenschr 116:331-334, 1991.
86. Cervantes F, Bruguera M, Carbonell J, et al: Liver disease in brucellosis. A clinical and pathological study of 40 cases. Postgrad Med J 58:346-350, 1982.
87. Cosme A, Barrio J, Ojeda, 2001.
88. Halimi C, Bringard N, Boyer N, et al: Hepatic brucelloma: 2 cases and a review of the literature. Gastroenterol Clin Biol 23:513, 1999.
89. Janbon F: The liver and brucellosis. Gastroenterol Clin Biol 23:431, 1999.
90. Williams RK, Crossley K: Acute and chronic hepatic involvement of brucellosis. Gastroenterology 83:455, 1982.
91. Kirby BD, Snyder KM, Meyer RD, et al: Legionnaires' disease: clinical features of 24 cases. Ann Intern Med 89:278-283, 1978.
92. Cunha BA: Clinical features of Legionnaires' disease. Semin Respir Infect 13:116-127, 1998.
93. Cunha A, Jensen L, Calubrian O, et al: Cytomegalovirus and legionella species as the cause of liver enzyme elevations in haemodialysis patients. J Hosp Infect 14:95-98, 1989.
94. Verneau A, Beaugrand M, Dournon E, et al: Severe jaundice in Legionnaires' disease: a case with early hepatic biopsy. Gastroenterol Clin Biol 11:254-257, 1987.
95. Schurmann D, Grosse G, Horbach I, et al: Pulmonary and extrapulmonary manifestations of *L. pneumophila.* Zentralbl Bakteriol Mikrobiol Hyg (A) 255:120-126, 1983.
96. Garcia Diaz JJ, Pena Somovilla JL, Salcedo Aguilar FJ, et al: Jaundice as a presentation of pneumonia caused by Legionella. Ann Med Interna 8:152-153, 1991.
97. Abril Lopez de Medrano V, Ortega Gonzalez E, Ruiz Cavanilles C, et al: Liver involvement in Q fever and Mediterranean boutonneuse fever. A comparative study. Rev Esp Enferm Dig 86:891-893, 1994.
98. Arrebola Garcia JD, Magro Ledesma D, Montero Leal C,, et al: Hepatic granulomatosis caused by Q fever: a cause of erroneous tuberculosis diagnosis. Ann Med Interna 10:595-8, 1993.
99. Marazuela M, Moreno A, Yebra M, et al: Hepatic fibrin-ring granulomas: a clinicopathologic study of 23 patients. Hum Pathol 22:607-613, 1991.
100. Westlake P, Price LM, Russell M, Kelly JK: The pathology of Q fever hepatitis. A case diagnosed by liver biopsy. J Clin Gastroenterol 9:357-363, 1987.
101. Thorner AR, Walker DH, Petri WA Jr: Rocky Mountain spotted fever. Clin Infect Dis 27:1353-1359, 1998.
102. Verne GN, Myers BM: Jaundice in Rocky Mountain spotted fever. Am J Gastroenterol 89:446-448, 1994.
103. Ramphal R, Kluge R, Cohen V, Feldman R: Rocky Mountain spotted fever and jaundice. Two consecutive cases acquired in Florida and a review of the literature on this complication. Arch Intern Med 138:260-263, 1978.
104. Adams JS, Walker DH: The liver in Rocky Mountain spotted fever. Am J Clin Pathol 75:156-161, 1981.
105. Jackson MD, Kirkman C, Bradford WD, et al: Rocky mountain spotted fever: hepatic lesions in childhood cases. Pediatr Pathol 5:379-388, 1986.
106. Silpapojakul K, Mitarnun W, Ovartlarnporn B, et al: Liver involvement in murine typhus. QJM 89:623-629, 1996.
107. Kanno A, Yamada M, Murakami K, Torinuki W: Liver involvement in Tsutsugamushi disease. Tohoku J Exp Med 179:213-217, 1996.
108. Walker DH, Staiti A, Mansueto S, Tringali G: Frequent occurrence of hepatic lesions in boutonneuse fever. Acta Trop 43:175-181, 1986.
109. McQuiston JH, Paddock CD, Holman RC, Childs JE: The human ehrlichioses in the United States. Emerg Infect Dis 5:635-642, 1999.
110. Bakken JS, Dumler JS: Human granulocytic ehrlichiosis. Clin Infect Dis 31:554-560, 2000.
111. Nutt AK, Raufman J: Gastrointestinal and hepatic manifestations of human ehrlichiosis: 8 cases and a review of the literature. Dig Dis 17:37-43, 1999.
112. Miyamoto MI, Fang FC: Pyogenic liver abscess involving Actinomyces: case report and review. Clin Infect Dis 16:303-309, 1993.
113. Vargas C, Gonzalez C, Pagani W, et al: Hepatic actinomycosis presenting as liver mass: case report and review of the literature. P R Health Sci J 11:19-21, 1992.
114. Kacem C, Puisieux F, Kammoun A, et al: Abdominal actinomycosis. Report of three cases and review of the literature. Ann Med Interne (Paris) 151:243-247, 2000.
115. Levett PN: Leptospirosis. Clin Microbiol Rev 14:296-326, 2001.
116. Newton JA, Pepper PV: Images in clinical medicine. Relapsing fever. N Engl J Med 335:1197, 1996.
117. Horowitz HW, Dworkin B, Forseter G, et al: Liver function in early Lyme disease. Hepatology 23:1412, 1996.
118. Dadamessi I, Brazier F, Smail A, et al: Hepatic disorders related to Lyme disease. Study of two cases and a review of the literature. Gastroenterol Clin Biol 25:193-196, 2001.
119. While UJ, Karshner RG: Icterus gravis syphiliticus. JAMA 68:1311-1314, 1917.
120. Taniguchi Y, Nakae Y, Ikoma K, et al: Subclinical syphilitic hepatitis, which was markedly worsened by a Jarisch-Herxheimer reaction. Am J Gastroenterol 94:1694-1696, 1999.
121. Shah MC, Barton LL: Congenital syphilitic hepatitis. Pediatr Infect Dis J 8:891-892, 1989.
122. Herman TE: Extensive hepatic calcification secondary to fulminant neonatal syphilitic hepatitis. Pediatr Radiol 25:120-122, 1995.
123. Relvas S, Carreira F, Castro B: Liver involvement in secondary syphilis. Am J Gastroenterol 87:1528, 1992.
124. Young MF, Sanowski RA, Manne RA: Syphilitic hepatitis. J Clin Gastroenterol 15:174-176, 1992.
125. Relvas S, Carreira F, Castro B: Liver involvement in secondary syphilis. Am J Gastroenterol 87:1528, 1992.
126. Maincent G, Labadie H, Fabre M, et al: Tertiary hepatic syphilis. A treatable cause of multinodular liver. Dig Dis Sci 42:447-450, 1997.
127. Sonmez E, Ozerol IH, Senol M, et al: False-positive reaction between syphilis and hepatitis C infection. Isr J Med Sci Nov; 33(11):724-727, 1997.
128. Litt IF, Cohen MI: Perihepatitis associated with salpingitis in adolescents. JAMA 240(12):1253, 1978.
129. Haight JB, Ockner SA: Chlamydia trachomatis perihepatitis with ascites. Am J Gastroenterol 83(3):323, 1988.
130. Wolner-Hanssen P, Westrom L, Mardh PA: Perihepatitis and chlamydial salpingitis. Lancet 26(8174):901-903, 1980.
131. Morris E: Tuberculosis of the liver. Am Rev Tuberc 22:585-592, 1930.
132. Hickey N, McNulty JG, Osborne H, Finucane J: Acute hepatobiliary tuberculosis: a report of two cases and a review of the literature. Eur Radiol 9:886-889, 1999.
133. Bearer EA, Savides TJ, McCutchan JA: Endoscopic diagnosis and management of hepatobiliary tuberculosis. Am J Gastroenterol 91:2602, 1996.
134. Alvarez SZ: Hepatobiliary tuberculosis. J Gastroenterol Hepatol 13:833-839, 1998.
135. Kok KY, Yapp SK: Isolated hepatic tuberculosis: report of five cases and review of the literature. J Hepatobiliary Pancreat Surg 6:195-198, 1999.
136. Tan TC, Cheung AY, Wan WY, Chen TC: Tuberculoma of the liver presenting as a hyperechoic mass on ultrasound. Br J Radiol 70:1293, 1997.
137. Martin-Vivaldi Martinez R, Espinosa Aguilar MD, Nogueras Lopez F, et al: Pseudotumorous hepatic tuberculosis: laparoscopic appearance. Gastroenterol Hepatol 19:456-458, 1996.
138. Zangerl B, Edel G, von Manitius J, Schmidt-Wilcke HA: Coccidioidomycosis as the cause of granulomatous hepatitis. Med Klin 93:170, 1998.

139. Sabesin SM, Fallon HJ, Andriole VT: Hepatic failure as a manifestation of cryptococcosis. Arch Intern Med 111:661-669, 1963.
140. Bucuvalas JC, Bove KE, Kaufman RA, et al: Cholangitis associated with *Cryptococcus neoformans*. Gastroenterology 88:1055-1059, 1985.
141. Reddy P, Gorelick DF, Brasher CA, Larsh H: Progressive disseminated histoplasmosis as seen in adults. Am J Med 48:629-636, 1970.
142. Kumar N, Jain S, Singh ZN: Disseminated histoplasmosis with reactive hemophagocytosis: aspiration cytology findings in two cases. Diagn Cytopathol 23:422-424, 2000.
143. Martin RC 2nd, Edwards MJ, McMasters KM: Histoplasmosis as an isolated liver lesion: review and surgical therapy. Am Surg 67:430-431, 2001.
144. Lamps LW, Molina CP, West AB, et al: The pathologic spectrum of gastrointestinal and hepatic histoplasmosis. Am J Clin Pathol 113:64-72, 2000.
145. Teixeira F, Gayotto LC, De Brito T: Morphological patterns of the liver in South American blastomycosis. Histopathology 2:231-237, 1978.
146. Raphael A, Campana AO, Waiman J: Hepatic coma in South American blastomycosis. Amb Rev Assoc Med Bras 10:151-154, 1964.
147. Chaib E, de Oliveira CM, Prado PS, et al: Obstructive jaundice caused by blastomycosis of the lymph nodes around the common bile duct. Arq Gastroenterol 25:198-202, 1988.
148. Perkocha LA, Geaghan SM, Yen TS, et al: Clinical and pathological features of bacillary peliosis hepatis in association with human immunodeficiency virus infection. N Engl J Med 323:1581, 1990.
149. Mohle-Boetani JC, Koehler JE, et al: Bacillary angiomatosis and bacillary peliosis in patients infected with human immunodeficiency virus: clinical characteristics in a case-control study. Clin Infect Dis 22:794-800, 1996.
150. Koehler JE, Sanchez MA, Garrido CS, et al: Molecular epidemiology of Bartonella infections in patients with bacillary angiomatosis-peliosis. N Engl J Med 337:1876-1883, 1997.
151. Liston TE, Koehler JE: Granulomatous hepatitis and necrotizing splenitis due to *Bartonella henselae* in a patient with cancer: case report and review of hepatosplenic manifestations of Bartonella infection. Clin Infect Dis 22:951-957, 1996.
152. Ahsan N, Holman MJ, Riley TR, et al: Peliosis hepatis due to *Bartonella henselae* in transplantation: a hemato-hepato-renal syndrome. Transplantation 65:1000-1003, 1998.
153. Spach DH, Koehler JE: Bartonella-associated infections. Infect Dis Clin North Am 12:137-155, 1998.

SECTION IV C

Diagnosis and Management of Chronic Forms of Liver Disease

CHAPTER

37

Immune Mechanisms in the Production of Liver Diseases

Karl Hermann Meyer zum Büschenfelde, MD, PhD, DrHC, FRCP and G. Gerken, MD

INTRODUCTION

During recent years, cell biology, biochemistry, molecular biology, immunology, immunogenetics, and gene technology have formed a more complete picture of the physiologic functions of the different cellular components of the liver. The importance of the structural-functional relationships between liver cells and matrix components also has been realized. The interactions between cells and the matrix components have an important role in determining the phenotypic and functional expression of cells (see Chaps. 12 and 13). In particular, cytokines, chemokines, adhesion molecules, hormone-like factors, and metabolites produced by cells within the liver are responsible for maintaining specific liver functions. A balance between regulatory factors produced by the hepatocytes and non-parenchymal liver cells as well and cells in other organs is of great importance in maintaining liver homeostasis. Disturbances of this balance may change the phenotype and numbers of different liver cells, leading to abnormalities in liver structure and function.

Among the different physiologic functions of the liver, maintenance of immunologic homeostasis is of central importance. Evidence for this comes from experimental studies and clinical observations.

The liver is an immune-privileged organ that favors the induction of peripheral tolerance rather than induction of immunity. Understanding the mechanisms of local regulation of immune responses in the liver requires a basic knowledge of the metabolic function of the liver and its functional microanatomy.

The liver has important functions in the metabolism of amino acids, carbohydrates and fatty acids, lipoproteins, plasma proteins, and vitamins (see Chaps. 3-7). To serve these many functions, the hepatocyte must efficiently extract nutrients, waste, or toxic products from the blood that circulates through the sinusoids. Blood from the gastrointestinal tract entering via the portal vein and blood from the systemic circulation entering the liver via the hepatic artery drain into the sinusoids. Thus liver cells are exposed to a mixture of portal venous and arterial blood.

Because the liver is involved in clearance of foreign antigens from the gastrointestinal tract and of toxic products, it is mandatory to avoid unnecessary activation of the immune system to prevent damage to hepatocytes. Delivery of antigen into the liver is not ignored by the immune system, but is followed by the induction of peripheral tolerance towards this antigen. Portal-venous application of an antigen[1-3] as well as drainage of an allogeneic organ transplant into the portal vein leads to antigen-specific tolerance that prevents a delayed-type hypersensitivity response upon challenge or rejection of the allotransplant.[4-6] Furthermore, allogeneic liver transplants across fully incompatible human leukocyte antigen (HLA) barriers sometimes survive without the need for immunosuppression.[7] This clearly shows that active regulation of the immune response occurs locally in the liver, which favors development of peripheral tolerance.

On the other hand, infection of the liver by pathogenic microorganisms must lead to induction of an effective immune response that clears infection from the liver and prevents development of chronic infection. How the immune response is regulated locally in the liver and which cell types and molecular mechanisms are involved in shaping the hepatic immune response are the subjects of this chapter.

IMMUNE RESPONSE AND HOST DEFENSE

The Role of Liver Cells

Besides the parenchymal hepatocytes, the liver contains other cell populations: sinusoidal endothelial cells (SEC), Kupffer cells, perisinusoidal (stellate) cells, biliary epithelial cells, dendritic cells, and liver-associated lymphocytes. Figure 37-1 shows that the liver SEC constitute the wall of the liver sinusoids.[8] Kupffer cells and liver-associated lymphocytes are found in the sinusoidal lumen adhering to the SEC. Kupffer cells are located mainly in the periportal area. This is a strategic position for Kupffer cells to phagocytose and eliminate particulate antigens or pathogens entering the liver in portal-venous blood.

Hepatocytes

Parenchymal cells represent about 80 percent of the total volume of the liver. Hepatocytes not only serve as

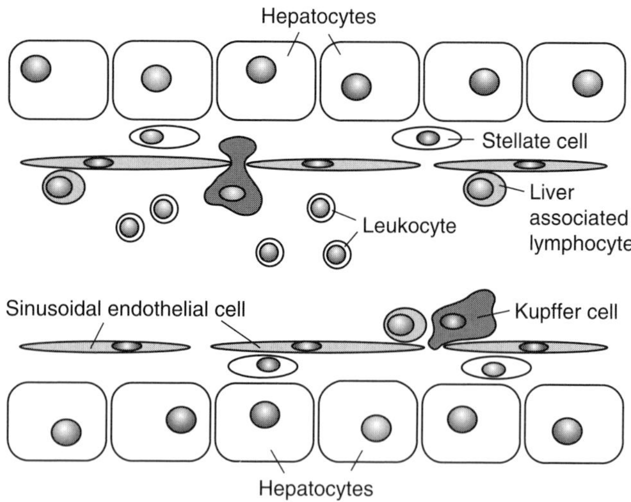

Figure 37-1 Microanatomy of the liver sinusoid. Schematic drawing of the microarchitecture of the liver showing the relative positions of hepatocytes, Kupffer cells, SEC, stellate cells, and liver-associated lymphocytes. *SEC,* Sinusoidal endothelial cells.

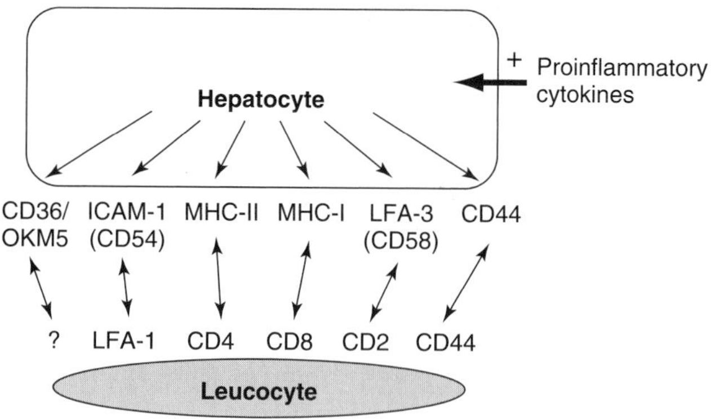

Figure 37-2 Accessory molecules on hepatocytes.

passive target cells for immunologic attacks by effector T cells, but may also participate in initiation and perpetuation of the immune response itself. Enhanced expression of major histocompatibility complex (MHC) class I antigens and the de novo expression of MHC class II antigens in acute and chronic hepatitis indicate that hepatocytes may undergo phenotypic changes during an immune response.[9] The induction of MHC class II antigens appears to be a fundamental step in interactions between antigen-presenting cells (APC) and target cells at inflammatory sites.[10] In addition to MHC antigens, hepatocytes in acute and chronic inflammatory states express a number of accessory molecules, which may serve to replace or bypass antigen-presenting cells (Figure 37-2).[11] These molecules were originally believed to have adhesive functions only and to strengthen the interactions between T cells and antigen-bearing cells. However, the binding of ligands to accessory molecules augments biochemical signals provided by the antigen-specific T-cell receptor (TCR) and appears to be necessary for effective antigen recognition and T-cell triggering.[12] In acute and chronic inflammatory liver disorders resulting from various causes, hepatocytes express several of these accessory molecules such as intercellular adhesion molecule-1 (ICAM-1), lymphocyte function-associated antigen-3 (LFA-3), and CD36 OKM5 antigen. The accessory molecules and HLA class II molecules act in concert to generate a local immune response.[13,14] Hepatocyte surface expression of these molecules correlates positively with the presence of liver-infiltrating T cells. These cells support the role of locally released T-cell–derived immune mediators in the modulation of the hepatocyte phenotype. In acute hepatitis, these activators and hepatocellular adhesion molecules are distributed diffusely throughout the inflamed liver parenchyma. Their expression is restricted to periportal and intralobular areas of inflammation in chronic hepatitis.[15] The immune adhesion and activation antigens are induced by various cytokines, which may be released by activated T cells or other cells of the liver-associated immune system. To exert their regulatory role, these cytokines have to interact with specific receptors displayed on the surface of target cells. The human interferon-γ receptor is lacking on normal hepatocytes, but variable hepatocellular expression of these receptors is observed in inflammatory liver diseases.[16] The receptors for tumor necrosis factor-α (TNF) also are up-regulated on hepatocytes in a diffuse manner in both acute and chronic hepatitis.[17] Thus hepatocytes can be target cells for the biologic effects of TNF-α, suggesting that release of these cytokines by monocyte/macrophages is involved in the early immune and acute phase response (APR). The later phase of the immune response seems to be under the control of interferon (IFN)-γ release by activated T lymphocytes. Hepatocytes also express another potential cytokine receptor, the CD40 antigen.[18] This is a glycoprotein found on many lymphoid and non-lymphoid cell types. Its expression is enhanced by cytokines, including IFN-γ and interleukin-4 (IL-4). CD40 is a member of a cytokine receptor family that may render hepatocytes more efficient antigen-presenting cells during the immune response.

Participation of hepatocytes in the generation of the immune response seems to be regulated by a series of events. Cytokines or antigenic material itself may be the initial stimulus for induction of an activated hepatic phenotype, followed by antigen-independent interactions between hepatocytes and T lymphocytes that further enable and modulate antigen-specific TCR-mediated recognition. The expression of accessory molecules is central to the accessory function of hepatocytes.

Sinusoidal Endothelial Cells

SEC represent only 2.8 percent of the parenchymal volume of the liver. They are involved in the clearance of components from the sinusoidal blood. Furthermore, they participate in biosynthesis of extracellular matrix (see Chap. 12).[19]

The SEC that line liver sinusoids display unique morphologic characteristics. They possess fenestrations with a mean diameter of approximately 100 nm.[8,20] The total area of the fenestrae accounts for approximately 10 percent of the entire surface of the SEC.[20] Numerous studies investigating receptor-mediated uptake of macromolecules in the liver show clearly that even protein-coated gold particles as small as 15 nm do not pass freely through the fenestrae of SEC to reach hepatocytes.[21-23] Thus SEC function as a barrier between hepatocytes and macromolecules or leukocytes in the sinusoidal lumen.[24] Direct contact between passenger leukocytes and hepatocytes is prevented by SEC.

Receptor-mediated uptake of macromolecules in SEC occurs quickly and efficiently via various pattern recognition receptors such as the scavenger receptor and the mannose receptor.[25-28] The expression of these receptors (23,000 binding sites per cell for mannose-terminated glycoproteins[27]) enables SEC to remove non-enzymatically glycosylated proteins called advanced glycation end products and other potentially harmful substances from the circulation.[29] After receptor-mediated endocytosis, efficient transport across the SEC to hepatocytes has been demonstrated for macromolecules such as transferrin and ceruloplasmin.[30-32] Although a vectorial transport across SEC as a physiologic mechanism to increase delivery of macromolecules from the sinusoidal lumen to hepatocytes has not been formally proven, this seems a possible scenario. One must assume that molecules endocytosed by SEC are delivered to the hepatocyte for metabolism and/or clearance.

SEC are efficient antigen-presenting cells and induce proliferation and cytokine expression in $CD4^+$ cells in vitro.[33,34] Similar to dendritic cells,[35] SEC express the mannose receptor[27] and use this receptor for efficient uptake of antigen.[34] Antigen presentation by endothelial cells is not a new phenomenon and has been demonstrated in macrovascular and microvascular endothelial cells from different organs.[36-39] But effective antigen presentation by these endothelial cells is present only after prestimulation with exogenous cytokines. Microvascular SEC, however, are unique because no prestimulation with proinflammatory stimuli, such as IFN-γ or TNF-α, is required to induce efficient antigen presentation to $CD4^+$ T cells.[33,34] SEC do not need to mature to acquire antigen-presenting function but can simultaneously and efficiently endocytose, process, and present antigen to T cells.[34] In this aspect SEC are similar to intermediate dendritic cells.

The SEC phenotype has further characteristics consistent with an antigen-presenting cell. SEC constitutively express MHC class II together with CD80, CD86, and CD40 (Table 37-1).[33,34] In humans SEC express CD58.[40] The ligand for CD2 triggers the alternative pathway of T-cell activation.[41] Moreover, SEC bear resemblance to dendritic cells in that they express CD4,[42] the mannose receptor,[27] and low levels of CD11c.[43] This phenotype suggests a myeloid origin of SEC, which has not been proved. Therefore it may be that repopulation of SEC occurs from within the liver from either resident SEC or hepatic stem cells.

TABLE 37-1
Phenotype of Resting Sinusoidal Endothelial Cells

Molecule	Expression
CD54 (ICAM-1)	+++
CD106 (VCAM-1)	+
CD80 (B7-1)	+
CD86 (B7-2)	+
CD40	++
MHC class II	+
CD62E	–
CD11c	(+)
CD4	+

ICAM, Intercellular adhesion molecule; *VCAM,* vascular cell adhesion molecule; *MHC,* major histocompatibility complex.

Kupffer Cells

Kupffer cells are hepatic macrophages that reside in the lumen of hepatic sinusoids. They are the first cells of the mononuclear phagocyte system exposed to immunoreactive material absorbed from the gastrointestinal tract. This position gives Kupffer cells a key function in host defense. The main properties of Kupffer cells are endocytosis, destruction of ingested material, antigen presentation, and secretion of biologically active products. They serve many functions, including clearance and destruction of bacteria, yeasts, parasites, endotoxins, tumor cells, and particulate cell debris; defense against viruses; modulation of immune and inflammatory responses; tissue and matrix remodeling; control of hepatocyte functions; metabolism of iron and bilirubin; and regulation of hematopoiesis and clotting.[44] Kupffer cells have a high phagocytic capacity but show low-level synthesis of superoxide.[45,46] Activated Kupffer cells can release cytokines such as TNF-α, interferons, interleukins, and transforming growth factors (TGF) alpha and beta. Thus Kupffer cells can activate hepatic natural killer cells. Clearance and modification of endotoxins are specialized functions of Kupffer cells, which pass endotoxins to hepatocytes for further modification and excretion into the bile.[47] Endotoxin activates phagocytosis by Kupffer cells and synthesis of biochemically active products, including prostaglandins, thromboxanes, leukotrienes, fibronectin, IL-1, IFNs, TNF-α, erythropoietin, procoagulants, collagenase, lysozymes, and plasminogen activator.[48] These responses support host defense but also are implicated in endotoxin-induced liver injury. Kupffer cells modulate immune and inflammatory responses via secretion of eicosanoids and cytokines in addition to a role in antigen presentation.[44] Furthermore, they may be important for remodeling connective tissue and fibrosis. Increased numbers of Kupffer cells are seen at the onset of liver fibrosis. It was demonstrated that antigens introduced into the portal venous system failed to produce an immune response, but injection into the vena cava did. Porta-caval anastomosis or blockade of Kupffer cell phagocytosis prevented immune tolerance.[49,50]

This suggests that Kupffer cells are effective scavengers of immunogenic antigens before they reach the peripheral lymphoid tissue. Kupffer cells express MHC class II antigens and present antigens. There is evidence for an increased number of HLA-DR–presenting Kupffer cells, perhaps indicative of a role in producing autoimmune phenomena in special forms of chronic liver disease.[51] Kupffer cells also are involved in the pathogenesis of experimental autoimmune hepatitis (AIH) in mice.[52]

Kupffer cells express IL-10 in response to physiologic concentrations of lipopolysaccharide (LPS).[53] Expression of IL-10 in Kupffer cells occurs within 2 hours.[54] IL-10 expression in monocytes is mainly observed 24 hours after challenge with LPS.[55] These data are consistent with experiments demonstrating the early appearance of IL-10 in whole liver extracts from LPS-challenged mice.[56] IL-10 expression in Kupffer cells is regulated by a negative, autoregulatory, feedback loop.[54] Because Kupffer cells are mainly located in the periportal area and release IL-10 into the sinusoidal lumen, blood flow distributes IL-10 along the sinusoids away from Kupffer cells. Prolonged release of IL-10 in response to a single exposure to LPS may ensue in vivo until a sufficient local concentration of IL-10 is reached for negative autoregulation of Kupffer cells.

IL-10 has potent effects on Kupffer cells and SEC. IL-10 down-regulated $CD4^+$ T cell activation by antigen-presenting Kupffer cells and SEC.[34] The immunoregulatory effect of IL-10 is achieved by down-regulation of receptor-mediated antigen uptake and down-regulation of MHC class II and the co-stimulatory molecules CD80 and CD86.[34] To achieve its potent effect, IL-10 must be present during antigen uptake and interaction with T cells.[34] The immunoregulatory potential of IL-10 in the liver is restricted to the time it is present in the sinusoids. Once washed away, IL-10 likely has no further influence on the development and quality of immune responses in the liver.

Kupffer cells constitutively express prostanoids[57] and show up-regulated prostanoid production after contact with LPS.[58] T-cell activation by antigen-presenting SEC is down-regulated dose-dependently by exogenous prostaglandin E2, demonstrating another paracrine control mechanism for antigen presentation in SEC.[34] Kupffer cell–derived mediators are important autocrine, but also paracrine, negative regulators of T-cell activation by antigen-presenting SEC. Regulation of antigen presentation by SEC is different from that for other antigen-presenting cell populations.

Liver-associated Lymphocytes

Liver-associated lymphocytes are considered to be a population of intrasinusoidal immune cells. The uninfected average liver of 1.2 to 1.5 kg contains approximately 10^9 to 10^{10} lymphocytes. A high percentage of these is considered to represent truly resident lymphocytes. Because liver and gut are derived from the endoderm, both organs can support tissue-specific lymphocyte differentiation as evidenced by expression of genes such as recombinase activation genes 1 and 2 that are otherwise expressed only by immature thymocytes undergoing gene rearrangement.[59-62] Similarly, expression of CD45, CD34, and CD7 indicates the presence in liver of hematopoietic stem cells and early lymphoid progenitors.[63] Indeed, hematopoiesis takes place in the fetal liver and liver grafts.[64]

The lymphocyte population of the liver, however, differs considerably from that found in the blood. Specifically, the CD4:CD8 ratio is reversed, and the $CD8^+$ T-cell population is extremely heterogeneous and contains a large percentage of unconventional lymphocytes that are not found frequently in the peripheral blood.[63] These include $CD4^-$ $CD8^-$ double-negative T cells,[65-67] $CD4^+$ $CD8^+$ double-positive T cells,[63] T cells that display the $\gamma\delta$ T-cell receptor instead of the $\alpha\beta$ T-cell receptor characteristic of peripheral blood T cells,[68] and cells that express both the natural killer (NK) cell marker CD56 and the T-cell marker CD3.[69] The latter have been termed NK T cells and have distinct functional characteristics, such as the ability to recognize non-peptide antigens presented by non-classic MHC molecules.[70]

According to a definition by Trinchieri,[71] NK cells (1) are large lymphoid cells with azurophilic granules (LGL), without surface immunoglobulin (Ig), $TCR/CD3^-$ $CD56^-$ (N-CAM), and $CD16^-$; (2) secrete a lymphokine repertoire consisting of IFN-γ, TNF-α, granulocyte-macrophage–colony-stimulating factor (GM-CSF), and IL-3; (3) probably originate from the bone marrow, but not thymus; (4) have a half-life of a few days up to a few weeks; (5) respond to IL-2 with proliferation; (6) kill virus-infected cells; (7) are important for hematopoiesis and in T-cell responses; (8) have cytotoxicity against sensitive tumor cells dependent on cell-to-cell contact, but independent of antibodies or MHC, probably involving LFA-1 and embryonic antigen.

LGL morphology is not restricted to NK cells, as some T cells, mostly cytotoxic T cells (CTL), are also LGL cells but certainly not NK cells.[72] T cells have a different function relative to NK cells, as described by Yokoyama: T cells search for the presence of foreign, whereas NK cells survey tissues for the absence of self.[73]

Stellate Cells (Fat-storing Cells)

Stellate cells (Ito cells, fat-storing cells, peri- or parasinusoidal cells, lipocytes)[74] are located in the space of Disse under the endothelial cell lining and are in close contact with hepatocytes (see Chap. 13). They contain characteristic fat droplets, whose number and diameter seem to vary between species and under different physiologic conditions. Lipocytes play an important part in intrahepatic processing and storage of retinol and retinyl esters.[75] These cells contribute to the production of connective tissue and have morphologic characteristics in common with fibroblasts. In a chronically injured liver, fat-storing cells acquire a new fibroblast-like phenotype and participate in fibrogenesis.[76-78] With respect to the topics presented in this chapter, the role of stellate cells in liver injury shall be mentioned briefly. In liver injury stellate cells undergo an activation that represents a cascade of cellular events secondary to all forms of liver damage. The initiation of activation results from paracrine mediators from SEC, Kupffer cells, and hepatocytes. Perpetuation of activation leads to several activation-dependent functional changes,[79] which are shown in Table 37-2.

TABLE 37-2

Transcriptional, Signaling Molecule, and Gene Activation of Stellate Cells and Consequences

Mediators, receptors, growth factors	Actions	Changes
Prostanoids: PGF2α, PGD2, PGI-2, PGE2, LTC4, LTB4	Proliferation	→ Cell increase
	Regeneration	→ Cell renewing
Leukocyte mediators: M-CSF, MCP-1, PAF	Chemotaxis	→ Cell recruitment and inflammation
Mitogens: HGF, EGF, PDGF, SCF, IgF I and II, FGF	Fibrogenesis	→ ECM increase
Extracellular matrix molecules: collagens, proteoglycans, glycoproteins, proteases	Matrix degeneration	→ ECM destruction
Vasoactive mediators: ET-1, nitric oxide	Contractility	→ Sinusoidal contraction, vasoregulation
Cytokines and cytokine receptors: TGFβ I, II, III, PDGF, ET-1, MCP-1, IL-6, ET-R, EGF-R	Acute phase response	→ Inflammation
Paracrine mediators of S from K, SEC, H	Retinoid metabolism	→ Loss of retinoid droplets

PGD, E, F, Prostaglandin D, E, F; *PGI-2,* prostacyclin; *LT C, B,* leukotriene C, B; *HGF,* hepatocyte growth factor; *EGF,* epidermal growth factor; *PDGF,* platelet derived growth factor; *SCF,* stem cell factor; *IGF,* insulin-like growth factor; *FGF,* fibroblast growth factor; *ET-1,* endothelin-1; *TGFβ,* transforming growth factor; *MCP-1,* monocyte chemotactic peptide-1; *IL-6,* interleukin-6; *ET-R,* endothelin receptor; *EGF-R,* epidermal growth factor receptor.

TABLE 37-3

Hepatic Cytokines that Modulate Liver Inflammation, Fibrogenesis, and Cell Growth

Cytokines	Cell source	Inflammation	Fibrogenesis	Growth/proliferation
TGF-α	H, K, S			+
TGF-β	SEC, K, S	+	+	−
HGF	SEC, K, S			+
IGF I	S			+
IGF II	H, SEC, K, S			+
HBGF I	H, SEC, K, S			+
HBGF II	SEC			+
PDGF	S	+	+	+
TNF-α/TNF-β	K/S	+	−	+
IL-1	K	+	+	−/+ (T- and B-cells)
IL-4	K	−	+	
IL-10	K	−	−	
IFN-γ	K	+	−	
ET-1	SEC, S		+	
MCP-1	K, S	+	+	
Chemokines	H, K, SEC, S	+	+	

HPGF, Heparin-binding growth factor; *H,* hepatocyte; *K,* Kupffer cell; *S,* stellate cell; *SEC,* sinusoidal endothelial cell; +, stimulation; −, down-regulation.

Cytokines Released by Liver Cells

The unique microenvironment within the sinusoid is the basis for cell-specific interactions between hepatocytes, sinusoidal endothelial cells, Kupffer cells, liver-associated lymphocytes, and stellate cells. Cytokines released by these cells are important mediators with physiologic and pathologic implications.[80] They are crucial for immunologic homeostasis, induction of tolerance, local immune cell development and activation, recruitment of immune cells to the liver, and induction of immunity. Furthermore, they are regulators of hepatic cell growth and regeneration (see Chap. 2), hepatic fibrogenesis (see Chaps. 12 and 13), and APR. The most important cytokines produced by hepatic cells plus their role in inflammation, fibrogenesis, and cell growth/proliferation are listed in Table 37-3. Responses to and production of cytokines by immune cells are shown in Figure 37-3.

Hepatic Acute Phase Response

The APR is a defense reaction of the organism to attacks against its integrity, which has the aim to restrict organ damage, to eliminate the causative agent, to maintain the vital functions of the liver, and to control the defense mechanisms themselves. The loss of tissue integrity caused by toxic agents induces a local inflammation. On

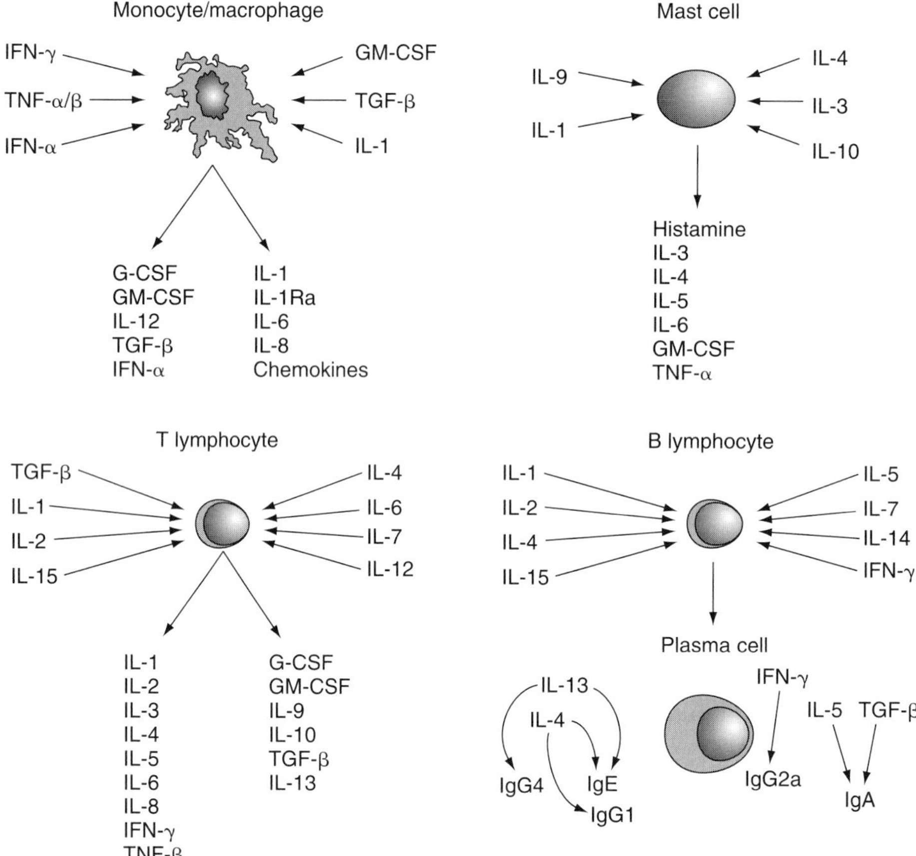

Figure 37-3 Response and production of cytokines by macrophages/monocytes, mast cells, and T- and B-lymphocytes.

the one hand inflammatory cells have the task of eliminating the injurious agents and the destroyed tissue, but on the other hand they produce mediators or induce the production of factors, particularly cytokines that are responsible for systemic reactions and for the induction of clinical symptoms of the APR. The quantity and quality of individual reactions depend on the toxic agent, the organ, and the extent of organ damage. Prominent features are increased plasma levels of α1-, α2-, β-globulins, and so-called "positive acute phase proteins" (i.e., C-reactive protein [CRP] and serum amyloid A [SAA]).[81]

The regulation of acute phase protein (APP) genes and cytokines mediating regulation has been characterized, receptors and receptor antagonists identified, and their mode of function analyzed.[82] The main mediators of APR are proinflammatory cytokines (i.e., IL-1β, TNF-α, IL-6). Figure 37-4 shows one way by which cells can interact in the initiation and progression of APR by production of cytokines. IL-6 induces the broadest pattern of APR in human and animal hepatocytes. IL-6 is produced not only by cells of the inflamed tissue like macrophages, endothelial cells, and fibroblasts, but also by a large number of cells of different origin. In human acute phase conditions, the serum concentration of IL-6 and TNF-α are increased, whereas IL-1β may be released later, probably during or after cell death.[81]

Many potent stimulators of the APR in liver cells have been identified: IL-6–type cytokines (IL-6, IL.11, leukemia inhibitory factor [LIF]), IL-1-type cytokines (IL-1α, IL-1β, TNF-α, TNF-β), glucocorticoids, and growth factors (insulin, hepatocyte growth factor [HGF], fibroblast growth factor, TGF-β). The sources of these cytokines are not completely known, but non-parenchymal liver cells certainly have a major role because they are situated adjacent to hepatocytes. Even the production of small amounts of cytokines may exert an important local effect.

IL-6, IL-1β, and TNF-α are inducers of APP gene expression in the liver. Members of the IL-6–type cytokine family such as LIF, oncostatin M (OSM), ciliary neurotropic factor (CNTF), cardiotropin-1 (CT-1), and IL-11 modulate the expression of APP in liver cells and regulate a spectrum of biologic functions in extrahepatic organs.[83-85] Whenever the qualitative and quantitative effects of cytokines involved in the regulation and modulation of APR in the liver are divergent, they exhibit overlapping biologic activities and functional redundancies. This ensures the species-specific rearrangement of the expression of the complete set of hepatic APP genes.[86-90] Stimulation of the expression of positive APP is due to activation of cytokine-stimulated transcription factors.[91-94]

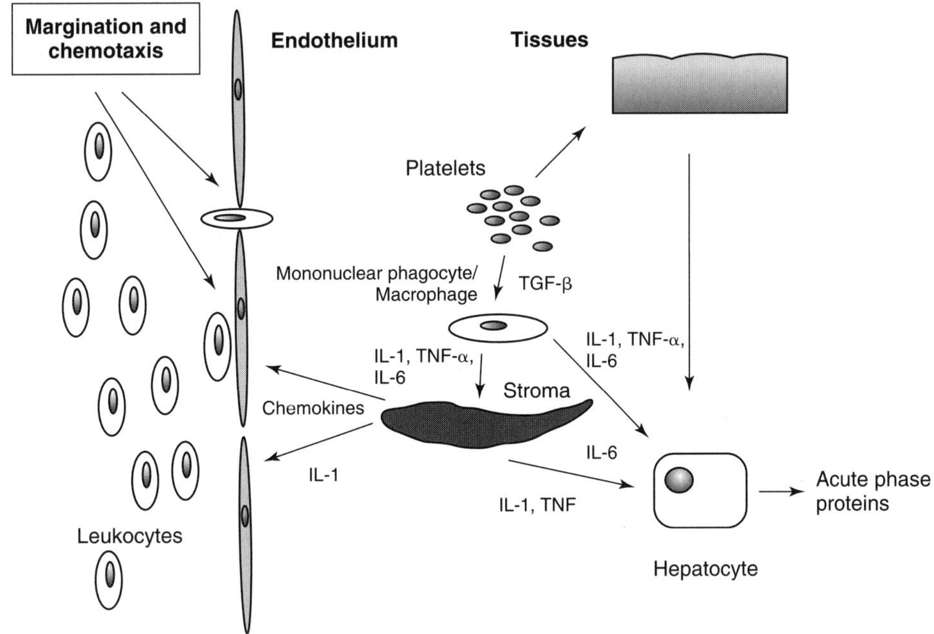

Figure 37-4 Cell and cytokine interactions in the acute phase response. (Modified from Baumann H, Gauldi F: The acute phase response. Immunol Today 15:74, 1994.)

The pattern of induction of APP can be divided into two groups. Type 1 APP genes, comprising the genes encoding CRP, SAA, α1 acid glycoprotein, and complement component TNF-α, are stimulated by cytokines of the IL-1 type such as IL-1β or TNF-α. The second group comprises cytokines of the IL-6 type such as IL-6, OSM, LIF, and CNTF, and stimulates the expression of the type 2 APP genes (i.e., the various fibrinogen chains, α2 macroglobulin, haptoglobin, hemopexin) and others depending on the species investigated. Type 2 APP genes contain response elements in their promoter deoxyribonucleic acid (DNA) that are stimulated by the transcription factors of the C/EBP family or the STAT family (Figure 37-5).[95] In most instance, IL-1- and TNF-mediated stimulation of type 1 APP genes is synergistically enhanced by IL-6-type cytokines. IL-1-type cytokines do not stimulate any of the type 2 APP genes, nor do they enhance the effect of IL-6-type cytokines. If there is any influence, it is inhibitory.[95]

Recently two new APP were identified, lipopolysaccharide binding protein[95] and P100.[97] P100 is a 100-kD serine protease that is structurally related to the C1r and C1s subcomponents of complement factor I. This protease activates complement by binding to bacterial polysaccharides.[98] Studies in vivo and in vitro show that P-100 gene expression is up-regulated in the liver of rats treated intramuscularly with turpentine and in isolated rat hepatocytes treated with IL-6.[98]

It has been suggested that the messenger ribonucleic acid (mRNA) of the APP might also be increased by posttranscriptional stabilization[99] during the APR, in addition to transcription stimulation of the expression of APP genes. The expression of the negative APP genes, which comprise prealbumin, albumin, transferrin, α1-inhibitor 3, and α1-lipoprotein,[100] but also components of the blood-clotting cascade, such as factor XII,[101] is reduced during the APR. Although it is clear that the inhibition of negative APP gene expression occurs mainly at the transcriptional level, nothing is known of the molecular events. There is also limited evidence for posttranscriptional regulation.[102]

Glucocorticoids directly stimulate the expression of some APPs. However, the principal action of glucocorticoids is to enhance the effect of IL-1- and IL-6-type cytokines on many APPs.[103] The mediators TGF-β, insulin-like growth factor, HGF, and insulin have the potential to modulate hepatic response to IL-1- and IL-6-type cytokines. Insulin attenuates IL-1- and IL-6-type cytokine stimulation of most APP genes in human and rat hepatoma cells.[104] In contrast, while suppressing IL-1 stimulation, TGF-β enhances the effects of IL-6 on type 2 APP genes, possibly by increasing the number of IL-6 receptors.[105]

Kupffer cells represent the bulk of tissue macrophages and an important source of acute phase mediators. Endotoxinemia is known to induce an increase in the plasma level of acute phase mediators, acute phase mediator receptors, and acute phase mediator receptor antagonists. Because intravenously administered endotoxin mainly accumulates in Kupffer cells and because endotoxin stimulates production of cytokines such as IL-1β and TNF-α in isolated Kupffer cells, it has been supposed that tissue macrophages enhance synthesis and secretion of acute phase mediators during the APR.[44]

Another important aspect of the APR is its termination and resolution.[81] Anti-inflammatory cytokines may down-regulate APP synthesis by hepatocytes. Inhibitory antibodies or antagonists of IL-1 and TNF-α limit the APR, as do naturally occurring antagonists, such as IL-1 receptor antagonists. In addition several inhibitory functions for other cytokines, including IL-4 and IL-10, have been newly

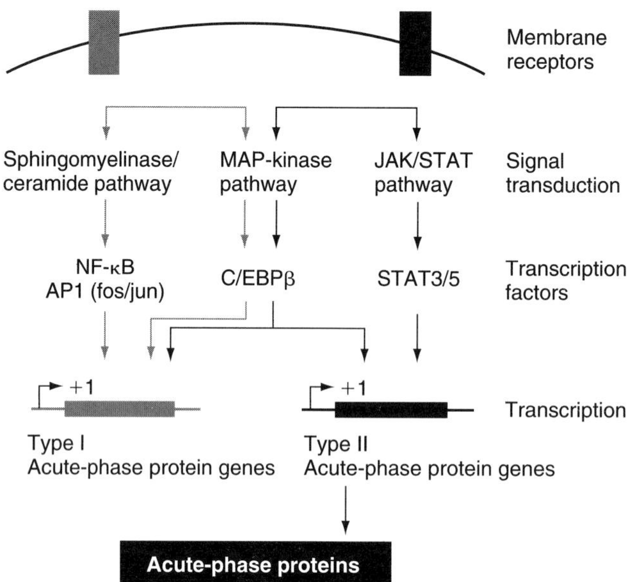

Figure 37-5 Induction of type 1 and type 2 acute phase protein gene expression by IL-1-like cytokines and IL-6-like cytokines resp. IL-1-type cytokines activate transcription factors NF-κB and AP1 via the ceramide pathway then stimulate transcription of type 1 acute phase protein genes. IL-6-like cytokines activate transcription factors of the STAT family via the JAK/STAT pathway then stimulate the transcription of type 2 acute-phase protein genes. IL-1-like and IL-6-like cytokines stimulate transcription factors of the C/EBP family via the MAP kinase pathway to activate type 1 acute phase protein genes and type 1 and type 2 acute phase protein genes, respectively. *IL,* Interleukin; *NF,* nuclear factor; *MAP,* mitogen activated protein. (From Ramadori G, Christ B: Cytokines and the hepatic acute-phase response. Semin Liver Dis 19(2):141, 1999.)

described. The IL-4 cytokines, primarily released by Th2 lymphocytes and originally described as a hematopoietic factor, appear to have a significant role in limiting acute inflammation. In an isolated monocyte/macrophage system, IL-4 caused down-regulation of proinflammatory cytokines such as TNF-α, IL-1, and IL-8, and decreased the release of prostaglandin and superoxide anion. IL-10 is produced by Th2 lymphocytes, monocytes, macrophages, and B cells, and is an inhibitor of cytokine synthesis. IL-10 inhibits monocyte/macrophage synthesis of IL-1, TNF-α, IL-6, IL-8, and the CSF and up-regulates IL-1 receptor antagonist expression. Recent data show that IL-10 regulates cytokine secretion and the surface expression of molecules involved in the generation of antigen-specific immune response (IL-12 and B7).[106] The activity of IL-4 and IL-10 cytokines released from cells in the vicinity of the inflammation and the activity of corticosteroids produced through stimulation of the adrenal-pituitary axis may be sufficient to terminate the APR (Figure 37-6).[81]

The APR is normally terminated after 24 to 48 hours. Sinusoidal cells are able to secrete IL-10 in response to lipopolysaccharides (LPS), with a maximum effect after 24 hours. However, the normal pathway can be prolonged, perhaps by persistence of stimulation or disruption of normal control mechanisms leading to a runaway or chronic phase of inflammation. It is not known which control step is crucial to this evolution, but elucidation of how acute inflammation becomes chronic will lead to new therapeutic approaches. Recent studies on the role of IL-1-receptor antagonists in blocking inflammation mediated by the APR cytokine IL-1 provide a basis for new therapeutic interventions in a variety of inflammatory diseases due to microbes and autoimmune mechanisms.[107]

Leukocyte-endothelial Interaction and Antigen Presentation in the Liver

The volume of blood passing through the human liver is substantial: 1500 ml/min. This means that the entire blood volume of the organism passes through the liver 360 times per day. Once in the liver, leukocytes have to pass through the sinusoids, which have a mean diameter of approximately 5 to 7 μm. The narrow diameter of the sinusoids and low velocity blood flow in the sinusoids (25-250 μm/min) promotes contact between leukocytes and the SEC that line the sinusoids. Furthermore, Kupffer cells patrol the sinusoids at low speed (2 μm/min) and can temporarily arrest the blood flow in an individual sinusoid by partially blocking the lumen.[108,109] In contrast to other organs, leukocyte adhesion to liver sinusoidal endothelium does not require the expression of selectins to induce leukocyte rolling but depends upon the endothelial expression of vascular adhesion protein-1[110] and interaction between the receptor-ligand pairs CD54-CD11a and CD106-CD49d. Because both CD54 and CD106 are expressed constitutively on SEC, adhesion of leukocytes to SEC can occur in the liver under physiologic situations. The number of leukocytes adhering to SEC under physiologic conditions is constant, irrespective of the total number of circulating leukocytes.[111] Thus control over

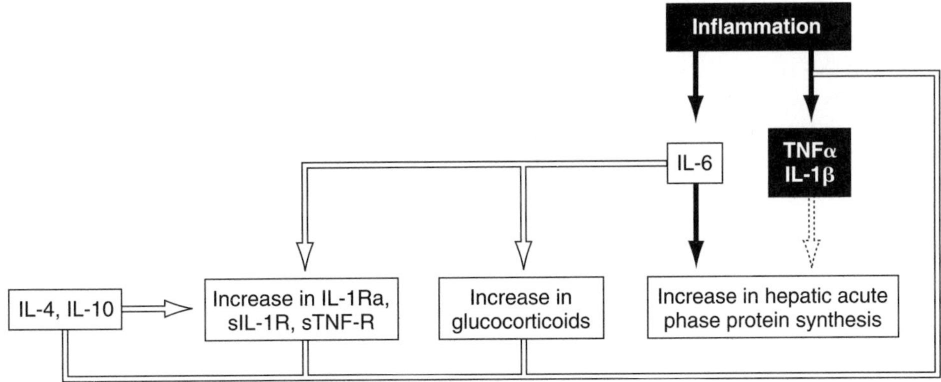

Figure 37-6 Counterregulatory mechanisms for the termination of the acute phase reaction. Inflammatory processes cause an increase in proinflammatory cytokines, which in the liver trigger the increase in the synthesis of the acute-phase proteins. During the late inflammatory response, IL-6 and the anti-inflammatory cytokines IL-4 and IL-10 stimulate the synthesis of IL-1 receptor antagonist and increase the proteolytic cleavage of the extracellular domain of the IL-1 receptor and the TNF receptors to yield their soluble forms. These decrease the biologically active forms of IL-1 and TNF in the circulation. In turn, they attenuate the acute phase reaction in the liver. IL-4, IL-10, and glucocorticoids inhibit the synthesis of IL-1 and TNF by decreasing the transcription of the genes encoding IL-1 and TNF. *IL,* Interleukin; *TNF,* tumor necrosis factor.(From Ramadori G, Christ B: Cytokines and the hepatic acute-phase response. Semin Liver Dis 19(2):141, 1999.)

leukocyte-endothelial interaction in the liver must be achieved at the level of the SEC and is necessary to avoid organ damage from non-specific immune-effector mechanisms. Many proinflammatory, adhesion-promoting substances are present physiologically in portal venous blood (e.g., bacterial antigens, LPS) and are cleared by Kupffer cells and SEC.[112] It is known that paracrine and autocrine control mechanisms operate in SEC to regulate leukocyte adhesion; leukocyte adhesion to SEC may also be influenced by local factors. The balance within the local microenvironment may be switched toward increased adhesion in case of strong inflammatory stimuli. The interaction between leukocytes and SEC seems to be a central mechanism of peripheral immune surveillance in the liver.[113]

On entering the liver, antigens and leukocytes contact sinusoidal cells first, particularly SEC and Kupffer cells. Both cell populations are efficiently involved in the uptake of antigens by receptor-mediated endocytosis and phagocytosis.[27,44,114] SEC seem to play a key role in the clearance of macromolecules. Both SEC and Kupffer cells eliminate antigens more efficiently if they are present in the form of immune complexes.

As the delivery of antigens into the liver induces immune responses, the sinusoidal cells involved in antigen clearance may simultaneously mediate the activation of the immune system. The dual function of SEC and Kupffer cells may be operative only under the control of local mediators. Endogenous prostanoids (PGE_2) produced by SEC are effective immunomodulators that control antigen-presenting activity of SEC.[115] Furthermore LPS that are physiologic constituents of the portovenous blood[116] seem to be important control factors of antigen presentation by SEC.[117] It has been shown that LPS can down-regulate antigen presentation by SEC to $CD4^+$ T cells in a dose-dependent fashion. Physiologic concentrations of LPS (100 pg/ml) already decrease IFN-γ release from activated T cells by more than 50 percent.[118] This effect is in contrast to bone marrow cells, which show increased antigen-presenting function when exposed to equivalent amounts of LPS. The negative effect of LPS on SEC is not mediated by increased prostanoid expression and the lack of co-stimulatory and modulatory cytokines. The down-regulated antigen presentation caused by LPS in liver does not influence the receptor-mediated antigen uptake by SEC. As Kupffer cells behave in the same manner in response to physiologic doses of LPS, the absence of antigen-specific activation of immune cells by LPS in the liver may be explained by a special reaction pattern of SEC or Kupffer cells towards LPS in the unique microenvironment of the sinusoid.[113,118]

The control of accessory functions of SEC and Kupffer cells is of vital importance for liver integrity and survival of the organism. One important control factor is TGF-β, which is expressed by SEC and Kupffer cells under physiologic conditions.[119] A breakdown of the barrier formed by SEC within the sinusoid leads to unrestricted access of activated immune cells to hepatocytes as shown in experimental models of fulminant hepatitis induced by concanavalin A.[52,120-122] These data demonstrate clearly that SEC are involved in an early step of the immune-mediated liver damage induced by pathogens. These studies also underline the importance of local regulatory mechanisms for limiting accessory function and antigen presentation by SEC and Kupffer cells.

The Role of the Liver in Tolerance Induction

Oral Tolerance

Specific induction of tolerance is necessary and is part of the physiologic function of the immune system. With respect to oral tolerance, the gastrointestinal immune system is involved primarily. The liver may function as a second security line to ensure tolerance towards dietary antigens coming from the gastrointestinal tract via the portal vein.[123] This notion is supported by portal-systemic shunting, which leads to a loss of tolerance towards dietary antigens.[124,125] Furthermore the spillover of dietary antigens into the systemic circulation may occur physiologically as shown by the detection of spleen cells, which present dietary antigens to T cells 6 hours after feeding.[126]

The hepatic mechanisms operative in oral tolerance are not fully understood. Experimental studies in vitro and in vivo support the idea that SEC, as natural barriers between hepatocytes and sinusoidal blood and physiologic levels of LPS, are the most important factors of the local "tolerogenic" microenvironment in gut and liver. Antigens derived from the gut are usually accompanied by LPS. It is known that physiologic levels of LPS down-regulate the antigen-presenting capacity of SEC for both memory $CD4^+$ T cells and naive $CD4^+$ T cells. Thus dietary antigen presentation by SEC may function in a dose-dependent manner regulated by LPS. The central role of LPS is shown in mice unresponsive to LPS, which fail to develop tolerance to dietary antigens. The physiologic intestinal and sinusoidal microenvironment of the organism seems to be crucial for the immune system to react in a well-balanced manner between tolerance and immunity.[43,113]

Induction of Peripheral Tolerance

The concept of peripheral induction of tolerance in the liver is based on the transfer of tolerance-mediating cells from a "tolerized" animal to a naive animal.[127] Additional evidence that the liver has central importance for induction of peripheral tolerance comes from apoptosis research, transplantation immunology, and functional studies of SEC.

Apoptosis. The role of apoptosis in induction of peripheral tolerance in the liver is not yet well elucidated. There are no convincing data to show that apoptosis occurs in the liver or that detection of apoptotic cells in the liver is not simply a reflection of dying lymphocytes.[113] Antigen specificity of apoptosis induction in the liver is a prerequisite for its involvement in induction of tolerance. Although some studies have shown apoptosis in T cells mediated by SEC, Kupffer cells, and hepatocytes,[128-132] the basic questions are not yet answered. Only one experimental model gives evidence that antigen specificity may be operative in apoptosis-mediated induction of peripheral tolerance. In MHC class I-restricted TCR transgenic mice, T cells bearing the transgenic TCR accumulate in the liver and become apoptotic after injection of specific peptides.[133] Thus apoptosis may be involved in the immune regulation in liver.[134,135]

Transplantation Immunology. Induction of donor-specific tolerance is a central aim in transplantation immunology. Several important observations support this concept:

- Prolongation of allograft survival by concomitant liver transplantation from the same donor[136]
- Prolongation of allograft survival as a consequence of venous drainage of the allograft into the portal vein[4-6]
- Induction of tolerance after portal-venous injection of donor-specific leukocytes[2,3]

Injection of donor-specific leukocytes via the portal vein but not via the lateral tail vein results in donor-specific acceptance of skin grafts.[137] Tolerance of skin grafts appears to be mediated by T cells that preferentially express IL-4 and IL-10 but not IL-2 upon contact with specific antigen in vitro.[138] Tolerance can be transferred from one animal to another by adoptive transfer of hepatic $\gamma\delta$ T cells, which suggests that tolerance is not mediated by clonal deletion but by immune deviation.[139] The functional phenotype of these cells is critically linked to the persistence of antigen. Prolonged absence of antigen results in loss of IL-4 and IL-10 expression and the ability to induce tolerance after adoptive transfer.

Recently a molecule termed OX-2 has been identified as involved in the non-MHC–restricted induction of tolerance.[140] It appears that OX-2–expressing cells inhibit stimulation of T cells by allogeneic dendritic cells. T cells activated in this way preferentially express IL-4 and IL-10 but not IL-2 or IFN-γ and are functionally capable of inhibiting allograft rejection in a model system of experimental kidney transplantation.[140] Thus a special subset of OX-2–expressing dendritic cells may be involved in induction of portal-venous tolerance in the liver.

Induction of tolerance to allogeneic cells may be different from induction of tolerance to soluble antigens. Different liver cells are involved in uptake and clearance of entire cells or subcellular components (Kupffer cells) versus soluble antigens (SEC). Kupffer cells are the only cell population in the liver that phagocytose particles larger than 0.2 μm.[28,141,142] Kupffer cells have been implicated in induction of tolerance toward portal-venous–injected allogeneic cells. Elimination of Kupffer cells by chemical compounds results in the loss of portal-venous tolerance.[143-146] It is possible that Kupffer cells contribute to induction of tolerance by releasing cytokines (e.g., IL-10, TGF-β), which promote induction of tolerance.[140,146]

The Role of Sinusoidal Endothelial Cells and Peripheral Tolerance

SEC may have a regulatory influence on peripheral induction of tolerance in the liver. SEC stimulate naive $CD4^+$ T cells to become T-helper (Th)-0 cells and to secrete cytokines IL-4 and IL-10 but not IFN-γ. The stimulated cells fail to differentiate to the Th1 phenotype. $CD4^+$ T cells primed by bone marrow–derived, antigen-presenting cells do not show expression of IL-4 or IL-10 upon restimulation.[43] SEC hence generate regulatory T cells that are involved in antigen-specific down-regulation of immune-reactive T cells. Although the molecular mechanisms of these findings are to be defined, some additional features of regulatory T-cell induction by SEC have been identified. Neutralization of IL-4 during the priming phase of naive $CD4^+$ T cells by SEC leads to a decrease of IL-4 and IL-10 expression by these cells upon restimulation. Thus IL-4 seems to be essential during the early priming phase of regulatory T cells. Cytokines promoting Th1-differentiation such as IL-12, IL-2, or IFN-γ show no effect on regulatory T cell differentiation by

SEC.[43] Very recently it was reported that SEC are organ-resident, non-myeloid APC capable of cross-presenting soluble exogenous antigen to $CD8^+$ T cells. Although SEC and dendritic cells use similar molecular mechanisms for cross-presentation, presentation of soluble antigen by SEC results in antigen-specific $CD8^+$-T-cell tolerance rather than immunity. It is likely that SEC may be key to hepatic induction of immune tolerance, particularly towards soluble antigens such as food and self-proteins.[147]

In conclusion the clearance of antigens, the elimination of pathogens, and the avoidance and control of systemic immune responses against harmful antigens require a microenvironment within the sinusoid that preferentially tries either to induce peripheral tolerance against antigens or to confine pathogen-host interactions locally. There is increasing evidence that SEC, Kupffer cells, liver dendritic cells, and liver-associated lymphocytes are involved in these complicated processes to keep the balance between induction of tolerance and immunity.

Innate Immune Responses

The innate immune system constitutes the early phase of immune defense and interacts with and controls adaptive immune responses.[148] The effector mechanisms of innate immunity, which include antimicrobial peptides, phagocytosis, and the alternative complement pathway, are activated immediately after infection and rapidly control the replication of the infected agent.[149,150] Thus innate immunity plays a crucial role in the early host defense. The main differences between the innate and the adaptive immune system are the mechanisms and repertoire used for immune recognition. During evolution the innate immune system appeared before the adaptive immune system[156] and seems to exist in all multi-cellular organs. In contrast to the adaptive immune response, innate immune recognition is mediated by germ-line encoded receptors and is thereby genetically predetermined. These receptors evolved by natural selection and have a defined specificity for infectious agents. Because the total number of receptors involved in innate immunity is limited (probably hundreds) as compared to somatically generated receptors of the adaptive immune response, strategies of both forms of immunity must be different. The innate immune response is directed to few highly conserved structures named pathogen-associated molecular patterns (PAMP), which have common features and are present in large groups of agents.[151] The three most important features of PAMP are that they are:

1. Produced by the pathogen and not by the host
2. Essential for survival and pathogenicity of the pathogens
3. Usually invariant structures shared by entire classes of pathogens

The receptors of the innate immune system are named pattern recognition receptors.[148,151] They differ substantially from other antigen receptors, are expressed on many effector cells of the innate immune system (macrophages, dendritic cells, and B cells), and belong to several families of proteins (leucin-rich repeated domains, calcium-dependent lectin domains, scavenger receptor protein domains). Functionally, they are divided into three classes: secreted, endocytic, and signaling. Secreted pattern recognition receptors function as opsonins. Endocytic receptors occur on the surface of phagocytes; signaling receptors recognize PAMP and activate signaling pathways (Figure 37-7). The recently identified receptors of the Toll family seem to have major significance for induction of immune and inflammatory responses.[152-157]

As mentioned before, receptors of the adaptive immune response recognize a broad spectrum of antigenic structures regardless of their origin—bacterial, environmental, or self. In contrast, receptors of the innate immunity are specific for structures expressed in pathogens and thereby can quickly signal the presence of infection. Control of the adaptive immune response by the innate immune system occurs via recognition signals through the innate immune system. The adaptive immune system is able to respond to pathogens only after recognition by the innate immune system. Particularly, the expression of the important accessory molecules CD80 and CD86 on the surface of antigen-presenting cells is controlled by the innate immune system. Toll-like receptors induce CD80 and CD86 molecules only in the presence of infection, which leads to induction of co-stimulatory molecules but also of cytokines and chemokines and thereby to activation of the innate immune response. Self-antigens are not recognized by receptors of the innate immune system. Dysfunctions of the components of the innate immune system (i.e., genetic alterations) may lead to immune abnormalities and diseases. Thus the innate immune system and immune recognition seem to control all major functions of the adaptive immune response.[158]

The role of the innate immune system in liver diseases is not well elucidated so far. The unique immunologic environment of the liver is enriched in cells of the innate immune response (i.e., NK cells, NK T cells, $\gamma\delta$-receptor-positive T cells, macrophages).[63] Therefore one can assume that the interaction of viral antigens with cells of the innate immune system may activate innate immunity locally, which may lead directly to inhibition of viral replication, gene expression, and protein synthesis. Furthermore, cytokines produced by macrophages, NK cells, and leukocytes (i.e., IL-12, TNF-α, IL-1α, IL-1β, IL-6, IL-10, TGF-β, IL-15, IL-18) function as part of the innate immune response and help to control infections locally.[159] Some of the cytokines modify the distribution and migration of immune cells and activate cells of innate immunity.[160,161] Recently it has been shown in the mouse system that IL-15 may be one of the most important stimulators of innate immunity.[162] IL-15 preferentially supports the development, activation, and homeostasis of innate immune cells. Figure 37-8 shows the pleiotropic effect of IL-15 in viral infections. After infection by a pathogen, conserved motifs result in a release of type 1 interferons (IFN-α and IFN-β) from infected host cells that lead to the induction of IL-15 by macrophages and to up-regulation of stimulatory molecules. IL-15 selectively activates NK cells, NK T cells, $\gamma\delta$-receptor-positive cells, and $CD8^+$ cells.[162] Stimulation of NK cells results in lysis of target cells by NK cells via

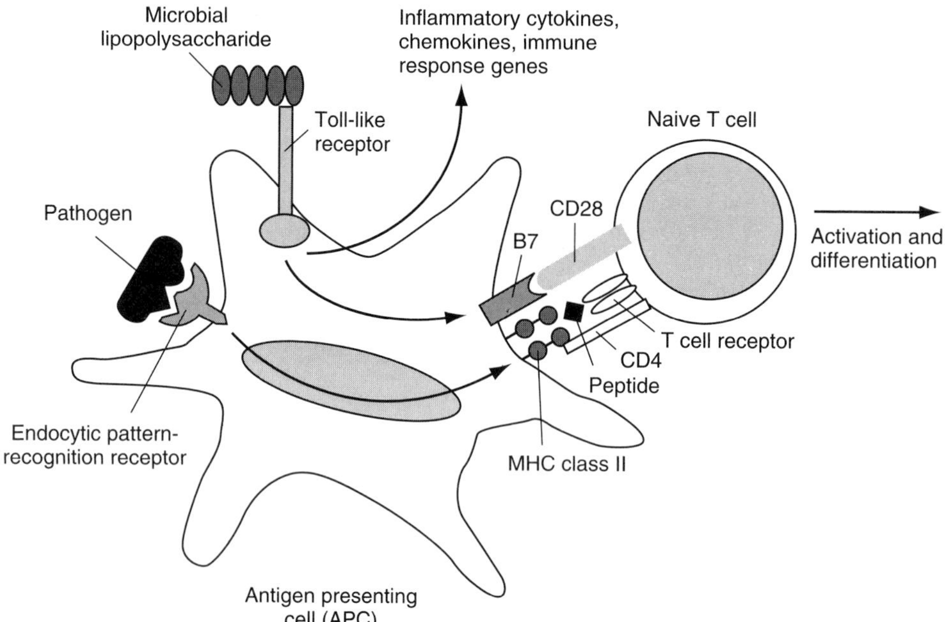

Figure 37-7 Innate receptors: Endocytic receptors bind to surface components of pathogens and mediate phagocytosis by APC. APC generate peptides that form a complex with MHC class II-molecules, which are recognized by T-cell receptors. Recognition of PAMP by signaling receptors (Toll-like receptors) leads to the induction of cytokines, chemokines, and co-stimulatory molecules and immune response genes. *APC,* Antigen-presenting cells; *PAMP,* pathogen-associated molecular patterns. (Modified from Medzhitov R, Janeway CA: Innate immunity. N Engl J Med 343:338, 2000.)

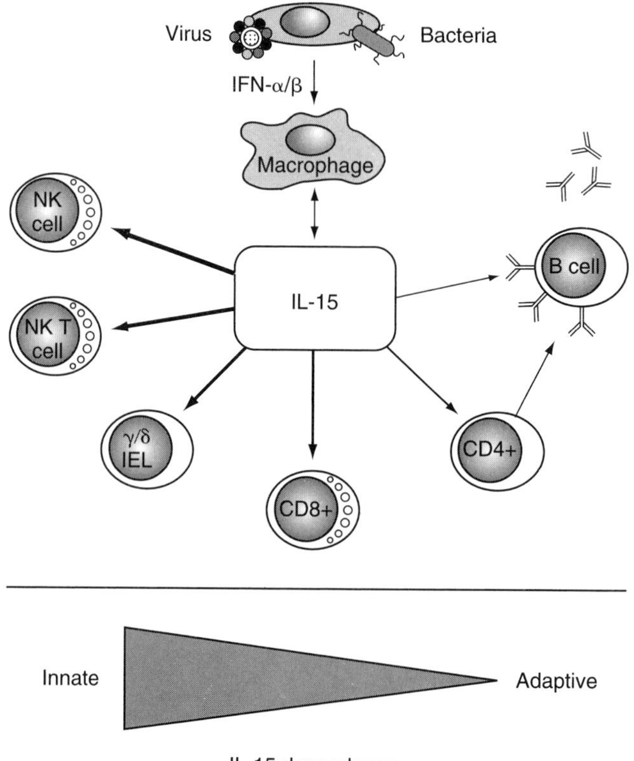

Figure 37-8 Role of IL-15 on cell development, activation and homeostasis of the innate immune response. Infection of host cells leads to release of type I interferons and induction of IL-15 secretion and up-regulation of accessory molecules. IL-15 selectively stimulates NK cells, NK T cells, intestinal γ/δT cells, and CD8$^+$ T cells. *IL,* Interleukin; *NK,* natural killer. (Modified from Ma A: Pleiotropic functions of IL 15 in innate and adoptive immunity. Mod Asp Immunobiol 1(3):102, 2000.)

perforin (Figure 37-9), mediates antibody-mediated cellular cytotoxicity (ADCC), and leads to production of cytokines (IFN-γ, TNF-α, and GM-CSF), chemokines (macrophage inflammatory proteins [MIP]-1α and MIP-1β), and RANTES (regulated upon activation normal cell expressed and secreted). The chemoattractant capacity of MIP-1α and TNF-α leads to accumulation of NK cells within the liver.[163-166]

Adaptive Immune Response

T- and B-Cell Responses

The adaptive immune response depends on two classes of specialized immune cells, T cells and B cells. In contrast to the cells of innate immunity, each lymphocyte of the adaptive immune system displays structurally unique receptors that are generated somatically during T- and B-cell development. Receptors thereby express binding sites that react not only with infectious but also with harmless environmental antigens and autoantigens. The number of antigen receptors in the whole lymphocyte population is very large and diverse, approximately 10^{14} and 10^{18} different somatically generated Ig and T-cell receptors, respectively. Antigen receptor interactions of individual lymphocytes lead to clonal selection and expansion. This is one of the most common and basic properties of the adaptive immune system. The adaptive immune response takes several days for induction of an adequate number of clones and for their differentiation into effector cells. This interval is too long to avoid organ or host damage. Furthermore, the adaptive immune response has the capacity to react against self or environmental antigens, which may lead to autoimmune and allergic disorders. Therefore interaction and control of the adaptive immune response by the innate immune system are of crucial importance in determining the origin of antigens (foreign or self) for the maintenance of host integrity and host defense.[63,158]

In liver diseases the adaptive immune response plays an important role in host defense against non-cytopathic agents and in organ damage.[150] Cells of adaptive immunity recognize agents in infected cells throughout the body because of the ubiquitous distribution of MHC class I molecule expression. Furthermore, the adaptive immune response has the capacity to induce and maintain immunologic memory. These functions are realized by antigen-specific $CD4^+$ Th cells and $CD8^+$ cytotoxic T cells (CTL). $CD4^+$ T helper cells recognize peptides of pathogens presented by various types of cells in association with MHC class II molecules. $CD8^+$ T cells respond to MHC class I peptide complexes. Peptides presented by MHC class II molecules are derived from internalized pathogens by antigen-presenting cells. Peptides presented on MHC class I molecules result from endogenously synthesized proteins in infected cells, as shown in Figure 37-10.

T helper cells that display Th1 or Th0 cytokine profiles support differentiation and proliferation of pathogen-specific $CD8^+$ cells and stimulate B cells for specific antibody production against a toxic agent. T helper cells and CTL secrete proinflammatory cytokines (i.e., IFN-γ and TNF-α) that inhibit replication and gene expression of the agent and may induce apoptosis and lysis of infected cells. Activated T cells are recruited to the liver continuously from the peripheral blood (Figure 37-11).

The Role of Cytokines

Cytokines are important proteins involved in many physiologic and pathologic processes in the liver. They are secreted by activated cells of the immune system. In Figure 37-12[167-170] regulatory checkpoints of naive T helper cells and the influence of the cytokine microenvironment on the pattern of T helper cell differentiation are shown.

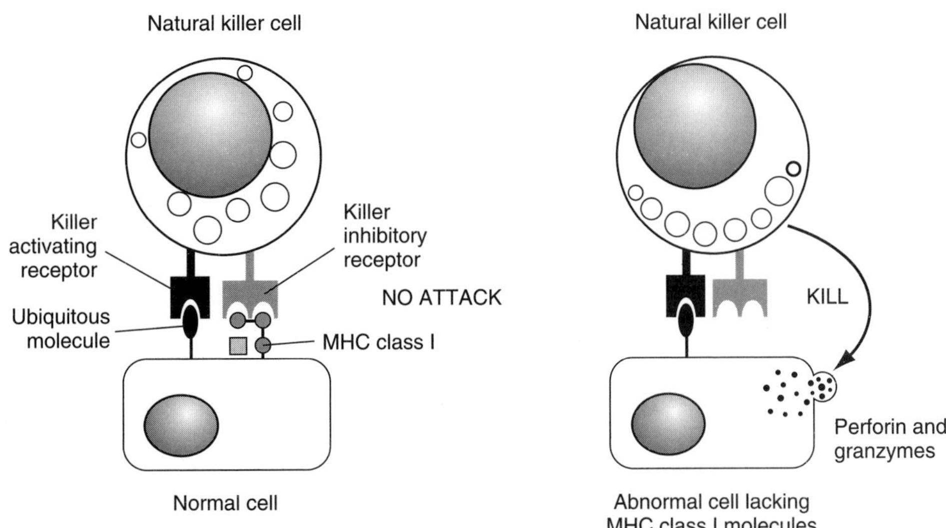

Figure 37-9 Interaction of NK cells with normal and abnormal cells. Abnormal cells lacking MHC class I molecules are killed by perforin and granzymes released from cytotoxic granules of NK cells. In the case of normal cells, the inhibitory receptor killing NK cells binds to MHC class I molecules and thus avoids an immune attack. *NK,* Natural killer; *MHC,* major histocompatibility complex.

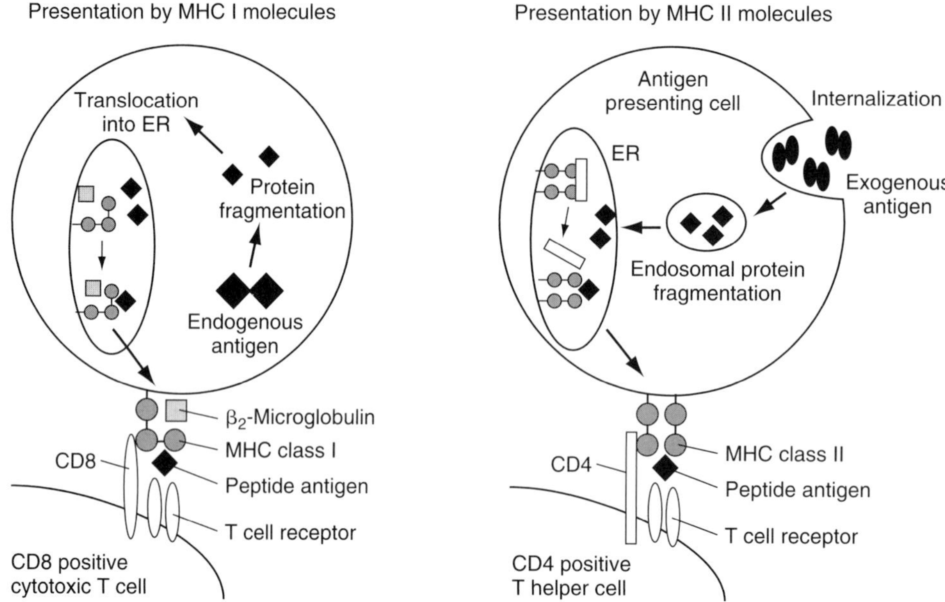

Figure 37-10 Pathways of antigen presentation by MHC class I and II molecules. *MHC,* Major histocompatibility complex.

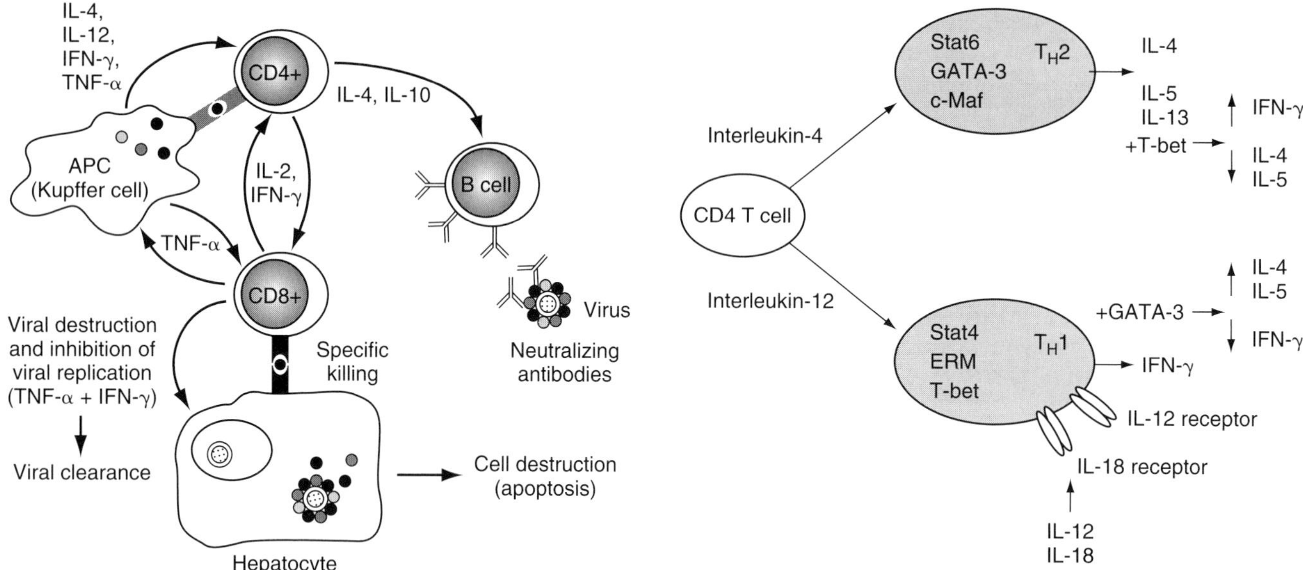

Figure 37-11 Host defenses against viruses: antigen presentation to CD4$^+$ T cell leads to differentiation and proliferation of CTL, proinflammatory cytokine secretion, and B-cell stimulation, resulting in killing of infected host cells, inhibition of viral replication and gene expression, and antiviral antibody production. *CTL,* Cytotoxic T cells.

Figure 37-12 Naive Th-cell differentiation to Th1 and Th2 cells, cytokine transcription and amplification, and the role of transcription factors T-bet, GATA3, and C-MAF on determining the fate of developing T cells. (Modified from O'Garra A: Commit ye helpers. Nature 404:719, 2000.)

The interaction between the TCR and the peptide MHC class II molecular complex leads to transcription of either IL-12 or IL-4 and induction of properties of a Th1 or Th2 cell (48 hours). Amplification of signaling by IL-12 or IL-4 and the action of co-stimulatory molecules (i.e., CD28, B7, CD4) and the activation of the STAT4 or STAT6 signaling proteins follow in 3 to 6 days. The transcription factors T-bet on the one side and the proteins $GATA_3$ and C-MAF on the other side are decisive for the final function and action of developing T cells. T-bet induces a Th1 cytokine profile and suppresses Th2 cytokines and is even able to convert Th2 cells to produce Th1 cytokines. In contrast $GATA_3$ supports Th2 cell differentiation, suppresses Th1 cytokines, and converts Th1-primed cells to Th2 cells. In addition, the transcription factor C-MAF simulates production of IL-4. The balance between T-bet and $GATA_3$ and the effects of C-MAF ultimately determine the fate of developing T cells. The molecular mechanisms that direct lineage commitment in the immune system are still unknown.[170] The most common factors that may influence the T-cell differentiation program are the TCR-peptide MHC complex,[171,172] immune response genes, and the structure of the MHC class II molecules on the various antigen-presenting cells. Furthermore, the characteristics and the load of the pathogen and the affinity of the ligands for the TCR may be decisive for the propagation of a Th1 or Th2 cytokine program in the various types of pathogens.[173] In general intracellular pathogens (i.e., viruses, bacteria, autoantigens) preferentially induce Th1 cell differentiation and cytokine secretion. Extracellular agents (i.e., parasites, worms, and allergens) usually support a Th2 cell program. Of particular influence may be the affinity of the ligand for TCR. Low affinity of the ligand supports differentiation to the Th2 phenotype; high affinity supports differentiation to Th1. Altered peptide ligands may have a crucial role in phenotypic differentiation.[174] After exchange of one amino acid, wild-type peptides change their affinity from high to low. Variants and mutants in viral liver diseases thus may convert from a proinflammatory cytokine secretion to an anti-inflammatory action profile and promote viral persistence.

Recruitment of Immune Cells to the Liver

Chemotactic cytokines or chemokines are important mediators of the immune system.[175] Based on their structure and target cell specificity, chemokines are divided into two major groups: CXC chemokines and CC chemokines.[176,177] (C denotes cysteine. CXC chemokines are named for the CXC motif close to the N-terminus of molecules.) They preferentially function as chemoattractants and activators of leukocytes. In the human, CXC chemokines are IL-8, PF-4, and IFN-γ inducible protein 10 (IP-10). C-C chemokines with two adjoined cysteines near the N-terminus of molecules are mainly chemoattractants of macrophages, monocytes, and T cells. The most important ligands are eotaxin, MIP-1α and MIP-1β, monocyte chemotactic protein 1 (MCP-1), and RANTES. The chemokines are produced by monocytes, macrophages, Kupffer cells, liver sinusoidal and vascular endothelial cells, various epithelial cells, and fibroblasts. Important inducers of chemokines are IL-1, TNF-α, bacterial endotoxin, and oxidant stress.[176] Table 37-4 summarizes the

TABLE 37-4

Some Important Chemokine Receptors and Their Ligands

Function	Receptor	Ligand
Migration of naive T cells within lymphoid tissue	CXCR4	SDF-1α
Migration of memory T cells to lymphoid tissues	CCR7	SLC, ELC
Migration of memory T cells to sites of inflammation	CCR2	MCP-1, MCP-3, MCP-4
	CCR5	RANTES, MIP-1α and MIP-1β
Migration of effector T cells (Th1)	CCR2	MCP-1, MCP-3, MCP-4
	CCR5	RANTES, MIP-1α and MIP-1β
	CXCR3	IP-10, MIG, 1-TAC
Migration of effector T cells (Th2)	CCR3	Eotaxin-1, Eotaxin-2, Eotaxin-3; RANTES; MCP-2, MCP-3, MCP-4; HCC-2
	CCR4	TARC, MDC-1
	CCR8	I-309
Migration of B cells	CCR7	SLC, ELC
	CXCR4	SDF-1α
	CXCR5	BLC
Migration of dendritic cells to lymphoid tissues	CCR7	SLC, ELC
Migration of dendritic cells to sites of inflammation	CCR1	RANTES, MIP-1α, MCP-3; HCC-1, HCC-2, HCC-4; MPIF-1
	CCR2	MCP-1, MCP-3, MCP-4
	CCR5	RANTES, MIP-1α; MCP-3, HCC-1, HCC-2, HCC-4; MPIF-1
	CXCR1	Interleukin-8, GCP-2
Recruitment of monocytes	CCR1	RANTES, MIP-1α; MCP-3; HCC-1, HCC-2, and HCC-4; MPIF-1
	CCR2	MCP-1, MCP-3, and MCP-4
	CCR5	RANTES, MIP-1α and MIP-1β
	CCR8	I-309
	CXCR1	Interleukin-8, GCP-2
	CX_3CR1	Fraktalkine
Recruitment of neutrophils	CXCR1	Interleukin-8, GCP-2
	CXCR2	Interleukin-8, Groa-α, Groa-β, Groa-γ; Nap-2
Recruitment of eosinophils	CCR3	Eotaxin-1, Eotaxin-2, Eotaxin-3; RANTES; MCP-2, MCP-3, MCP-4; HCC-2
Migration of hematopoietic progenitor cells and B-cell development	CXCR4	SDF-1α

CCR, Receptor for CC chemokines; *CCXR,* receptor for CXC chemokines; *SDF-α_1,* stroma-derived factor α_1; *SLC,* secondary lymphoid tissue chemokine; *MCP,* monocyte chemotactic protein; *RANTES,* regulated on activation normal T cell expressed and secreted; *MIP,* macrophage inflammatory protein; *IP10,* inducible protein of 10 kD; *MIG,* monokine induced by interferon-γ; *I-TAC,* interferon inducible T-cell alpha chemoattractant; *HCC-2,* human CC chemokine; *TARC,* thymus- and activation-regulated chemokine; *MDC-1,* macrophage-derived chemokine; *BLC,* B-cell chemoattractant; *ELC,* Epstein-Barr virus–induced gene I ligand chemokine; *GCP-2,* granulocyte chemotactic protein-2; *MPIF-1,* myeloid progenitor inhibitor factor 1; *Groa,* growth-related activity; *Nap,* neutrophil-activating protein; *ENA,* epithelial cell–derived neutrophil attractant.

functions of the most important chemokine receptors and their ligands.

Chemokine receptor expression and tissue-specific migration are related to the type and activation status of T cells.[178] Liver-associated lymphocytes express higher amounts of CXC receptor 3 and the CC-receptor 5 than lymphocytes in the peripheral blood. T-cell subsets are characterized by different chemokine receptors (i.e., the CXC receptor 4 is expressed on naive T helper cells). The CXC receptor 3 is found preferentially on memory and activated T cells, Th0, and Th1 cells but at low levels on Th2 cells. T helper 2 cells are characterized by the CC receptors 3, 4, and 8.[179,180]

The ligands of the CXC receptor 3 and the CC receptor 5 are IP10 and the monokine induced by IFN-γ (MIG). Eotaxin is the ligand of the CC receptor 3 and 4. Of special importance for the induction of inflammation in the portal area of the liver may be the ligands of the CC receptor 5 (i.e., the chemokines MIP-1α, MIP-1β, and RANTES). They are expressed on vascular endothelial cells within the portal tract in normal and viral infected livers.[181-183] Chemokines are also released by cytotoxic CD8$^+$ T cells.[183] Thus CD8$^+$ T cells not only mediate cytotoxicity. They have chemoattractant functions for T helper cells and CD8$^+$ T cells.

IMMUNE-MEDIATED LIVER DISEASES

Immunogenetics and Liver Diseases

Immunogenetics have focused primarily on genes that encode members of the Ig super gene family, the MHC, and the TCR, and on genes controlling Ig production (Figure 37-13). HLA typing has permitted recognition of three highly polymorphic class I gene loci, which encode the heavy chain of the classic HLA class IA, B, and C glycoproteins. Molecular analysis of the region has revealed 6 functional genes (A, B, C, E, F, and G) and 12 pseudogenes or gene fragments.[184] The classic HLA class I antigens are glycoproteins, mainly found on the surface of almost all nucleated cells, and are required for T-cell cytotoxicity. HLA class II antigens are composed of two peptide chains, an alpha chain of approximately 32 kD, and an alpha/beta chain of approximately 28 kD. HLA class II molecules are expressed at the cell surface as heterodimers of either α or $\gamma\delta$ chains each encoded, as is Ig, by the rearrangement of V(D)J-gene segments and the C-region. Three hypervariable regions for the β chains of TCR are reported: the complementary determining region CDR/1, CDR/2, and CDR/3. CDR/1 and CDR/2 regions encoded within V genes are classified in 20 subfamilies. Both CDR1 and CDR2 regions bind to α helices of MHC molecules. The CDR3 region formed by the conjunction of V-, D-, and J-gene segment recognizes the antigenic peptide present in the groove of the MHC molecules.[185] Both the alpha and beta polypeptides are encoded on the short arm of chromosome 6 and are expressed by a restricted number of cell types, including cells involved in antigen presentation and by endothelial and epithelial cells. There are more than 30 HLA class II genes. The production of these genes has amino acid sequence homology with both Ig and class I molecules; unlike HLA class I molecules, both the α chain and the β chain of class II molecules may be polymorphic.[187] Polymorphism of the class IIA and B genes is located within distinct regions.[187]

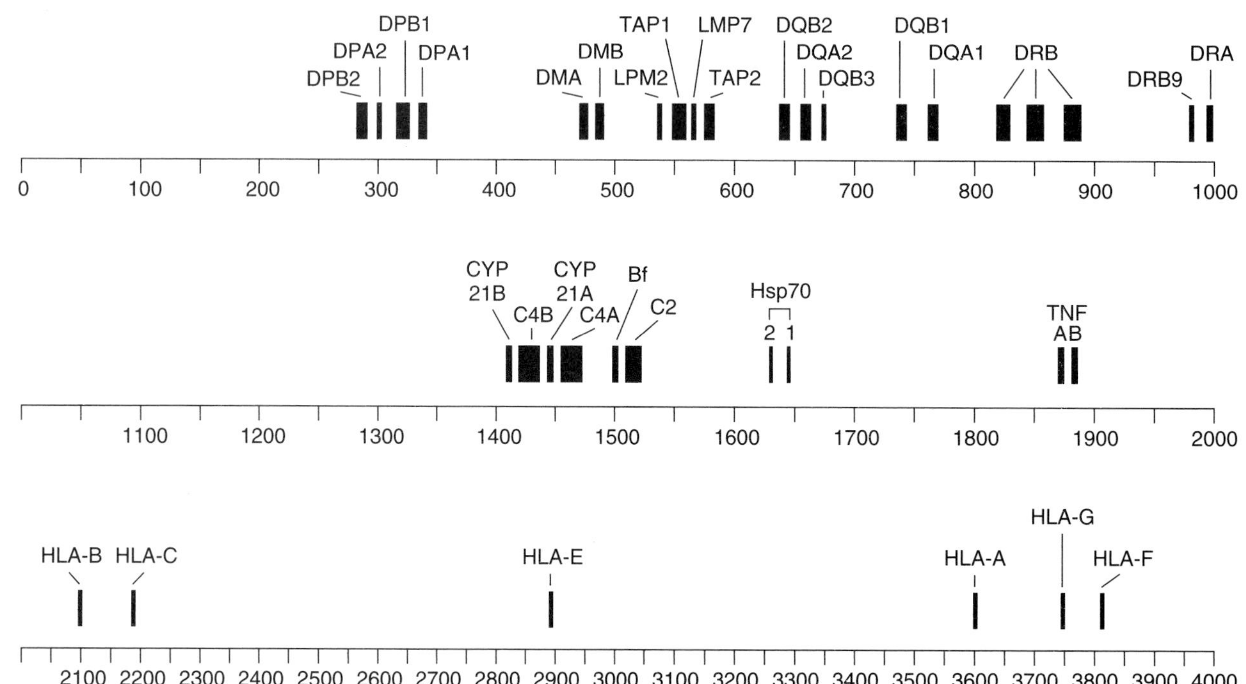

Figure 37-13 An abridged version of the gene map for the 6p21.3 band of the short arm of chromosome 6. The linear scale represents genetic distance in kilobases. (Adapted from Campbell RD, Trowsdale J: Map of the human MHC. Immunol Today 14:349, 1993.)

A third series of MHC genes, the so-called class III genes, describes a collection of non-HLA genes encoding a series of immune active polypeptides. The MHC class III region is located between the class II DR and the class IB loci. The region encodes several complement genes including C2, C4A, and C4B of the classic complement pathway and factor B of the alternative pathway.[188] Other immunoregulatory genes within this subregion include genes for TNF-α and TNF-β and three proteins of the heat shock protein 70 family.[189] Heat shock proteins may help to unfold tertiary structures of antigens before antigen presentation and therefore have been associated with autoimmunity.[190]

The MHC class I and II molecules have a fundamental role in the immune system by restricting the repertoire of activated T cells in an individual, which in turn orchestrates the humoral and cellular immune response.[191] T cells recognize antigens only through the interaction of the antigen receptor on the cell surface (TCR) and MHC peptide complex. MHC class I molecules present antigens derived from intracellular proteins to CD8-positive T cells, which are primarily involved in killing virus-infected cells. MHC class II molecules present antigens derived from endocytosed extracellular proteins to CD4-positive T cells, which may stimulate B lymphocytes in the cellular immune response and the autocrine IL-2 receptor pathway important in delayed-type hypersensitivity reactions. The specificity of a given T cell for a particular antigen is exclusively defined by the TCR.[192] The extreme diversity is generated by combinations of gene segments from large pools of genes and somatic recombinations that occur during interactive maturation.[193] The MHC molecules have the important function of selecting the T cells required for the generation of immune responses against foreign antigens. This process of clonal deletion is largely responsible for ensuring tolerance to self-antigens.[194] Self-tolerance in the periphery to antigens not present in the thymus may be maintained through clonal anergy. In most T-cell immune responses, interaction of the TCR of the effector cell with the peptide MHC complex is insufficient to cause a response. A second or co-signal is required. In the absence of the second signal, the TCR-MHC-peptide complex may induce clonal anergy.[195] The central role of the MHC peptide interaction in this process may underline the important relationship between HLA and disease susceptibility.

Autoimmune Hepatitis

Early studies found an increased frequency of the MHC haplotypes A1 and B8 in AIH.[196] These findings from Australia were later confirmed in Germany, the United Kingdom, and the United States. Recent studies confirmed the association with A1, B8, and DR3 haplotype and suggested that the susceptibility for AIH maps more closely to DR than either HLA-A or HLA-B. When the DR3-positive patients were excluded, the remaining patients were DR4 positive. Further analysis suggested that the age of onset of the disease was significantly lower in patients with DR3 than in patients with DR4. DR3-positive patients also were more likely to suffer a relapse while on immunosuppressive treatment.[197,198] In Japan, most patients with AIH have DR4, and the average age of onset is older than in European patients.[199] In recent studies it was reported that deleted C4A alleles are present in 50 percent of patients with AIH, mainly as a result of linkage dysequilibrium between DR3 and C4aQ0.[200] The associations found so far suggest that susceptibility to AIH lies closer to the DR locus than to either DQA or DQB and that DRB1$^+$401 and DRB3$^+$0101 are the most likely susceptibility alleles.

Most autoimmune disorders show a multiple allelic association, coding for antigens belonging to more than one class of HLA molecules. The specificity of antigen recognition by T cells and the variability in response to self-antigens and foreign antigens depend on the polymorphism at some amino acid positions of HLA antigens. The role of genetically polymorphic T cell–receptor molecules, but also of critical autoantigens as the third member of the effector-target cell binding complex, requires more attention that may help to extend our understanding of susceptibility and resistance to autoimmunity. In this context the findings of Doherty and colleagues[201] are particularly promising. The amino acid sequence Leu-Leu-Glu-Gln-Lys-Arg at position 67-72 on the DR polypeptide was found in 94 percent of DR3- or DR4-positive patients.[202] Further analysis suggests that the lysine (K) residue at position 71 is a key element in this motif. The site DRβ71 may be important in antigen binding and may have a critical role in the presentation of autoantigenic peptides. In Japan the DRB locus is the primary susceptibility locus for AIH. An association with broad serologic specificity for DR4 was stronger than the individual DR4 alleles. All DR4-negative patients had DR2. Because all DR4 alleles and DR2 encode a basic amino acid residue at position 13 of the DRβ polypeptide (Arg on DR2 and His on DR4), it was suggested that this residue is the basis for susceptibility to AIH in Japanese people.[203]

Keeping in mind the AIH-promoting factors in human and animal AIH, there seems no doubt that different environmental factors, such as viruses, toxins, drugs, and cytokines, are able to induce transient autoimmune phenomena. But it appears that autoimmune disease does not occur unless there is genetically determined background. Further advances in immunogenetic studies may have a key role in extending our knowledge on the immune pathogenesis of autoimmune liver disease.

Primary Sclerosing Cholangitis

Studies on HLA and primary sclerosing cholangitis (PSC) in the early 1980s showed increased frequencies of HLA-B8 (60-70 percent) and DR3 (approximately 70 percent) in PSC. These data were confirmed by several investigators. In addition, strong negative associations with HLA-B44-DR4 haplotype and a secondary positive association with DR2 in DR3-negative PSC patients from the United Kingdom were observed. Furthermore, an increased frequency of HLA B8 and DR3 was found in patients with hepatobiliary diseases (mostly PSC) and inflammatory bowel diseases, but not in ulcerative colitis patients without PSC.[205] Because the haplotype HLA-A1-B8 and DR3, present in about half of PSC patients, is also associated with susceptibility to a variety of organ-specific autoimmune disorders, there is increasing evidence that PSC may have an autoimmune basis.

A recent study, including patients from five European countries,[206] confirmed associations of PSC with three HLA class II haplotypes: DR3/DQ2, DR2/DQ6, and DR6. There are conflicting data published with respect to disease outcome and DR4. The findings that patients with DR3 may have a poorer prognosis and those with DR2 a more favorable outcome are in agreement with findings in AIH.[207]

Studies on HLA class I and class III molecules associated with PSC describe an association of a poor outcome with the inheritance of CW0701-B8-DRB1+ 03101 haplotype.[208] Furthermore, PSC was found to be associated with the TNFα-308A2 gene (HLA class II region), which is stronger than that for DR3 and B8.[207-209]

Taken together the present data show that four particular HLA haplotypes are associated strongly with PSC:

1. HLA1, B8, CW7, TNF+2, DRB3+0101, DRB1+0301, DRA1+0501, DQB1+0201. With the exception of HLA1, the same haplotype is associated with autoimmune hepatitis.[207]
2. DRB3+0101, DRB1+1301, DQA1+0102, DQB1+0603. This haplotype dominates in Swedish patients with PSC.[210,219]
3. B1*1501, DQB1+0602 is weakly associated with PSC in UK patients.[206]
4. DRB1+0401, DQA1+03, DQB1+0302 is thought to have a protective effect.[210]

Thus susceptibility to PSC seems to be mediated by more than one gene on the short arm of chromosome 6. Nevertheless, the role of HLA associations in the pathogenesis of PSC remains unclear and needs further investigation because there are conflicting results regarding HLA-DRW52A and HLA-DR4,[204] demographics, and whether PSC with or without inflammatory bowel diseases has the same pathogenesis and underlying genetic susceptibilities.

Primary Biliary Cirrhosis

Primary biliary cirrhosis (PBC), as with AIH and PSC, is thought to be an autoimmune disorder. Although many clinical and immunologic features support this notion, the response to immunosuppressive drugs is poor, and the only confirmed HLA association to DR8 is not strong. Other genetic associations between PBC and chromosome 6p21.3 are most likely the result of linkage with DR8.[213-216] The primary susceptibility allele is DRB1+0803 in Japan and Northern Europe.[213,217-220] But there are wide variations in associations of DR8 and PBC. Because stage 3 and 4 PBC show much stronger associations with DR8 than stage 1 and 2 PBC patients, it has been suggested that this genetic association is more likely to reflect progression than susceptibility. This also may be true for the linkage to TNF genes. The increased frequency of −308 TNF1/TNF1 genotype was seen only in patients with relatively advanced disease.[221]

Viral Liver Diseases

Hepatitis B Virus Infection. An association of the HLA class II allele DRB1+1302 with a self-limited course of acute hepatitis B (HBV) was reported in a large study in Gambia.[222] This was confirmed in Caucasian populations.[223-225] It was shown too that the HLA class II allele DRB1+1301-02 is associated with protection from chronic hepatitis.[225] Both 1301 and 1302 were decreased in frequency in patients with chronic hepatitis B. The allele DRB1+1302 also may influence response to interferon in chronic HBV. DR6, the serologic "super type" of DRB1+1302 and DR3 alleles, was associated with viral clearance in response to interferon.[224] The beneficial effect of the HLA-DR13 alleles on the outcome of hepatitis B infection is probably the result of a more vigorous HBV core-specific T-helper cell response.[226] This may be based either on better antigen presentation by HLA-DR13 molecules or on polymorphism of an adjacent immune regulatory gene. Furthermore, some studies have demonstrated that heterozygosity at MHC loci may be superior in viral clearance compared with full homozygosity.[227]

Viral clearance in HBV infection depends on factors that influence the production of IFN-γ and TNF-α. The TNF-α system is activated and TNF-α receptors are upregulated in the liver of patients with chronic HBV infections.[228] The gene for TNF-α is located within the class III region of MHC between HLA-B and HLA-DR. Two E versus A transitions in the promoter region at positions −308 and −238 have been shown to influence TNF-α expression. At position −308 TNF-α308.2 (A at −308) is associated with higher constitutive and inducible levels of TNF-α, whereas for the TNF-α238.2 allele (A at −238) the functional consequences are not yet clear. The TNF-α308.2 allele and TNF-α238.2 allele have been linked with susceptibility to some parasitic infections as well as tuberculosis. Recently it was shown that TNF-α promoter polymorphism at position −238 may be associated with chronic HBV infection, which appears to be linked to defective viral clearance. In addition, differential interaction of transactivation/inhibition factors of HBV with the TNF-α238.2 allele may cause decreased transcription of the TNF gene, TNF-α secretion, and thereby support viral resistance.[227-230]

No consistent result on MHC class I alleles in HBV-related liver diseases are reported. This is also true for complement and TAP/LMP genes.[224]

Recently associations between mutations of mannose-binding protein (MBP) and unusual or severe infections have been described.[231] MBP is an opsonizing protein that binds to mannose-terminated carbohydrate chains on agents. Because HBV bears this structure on the middle envelope protein (pre-S2-region), MBP may be a potential target for MBP binding and may enhance HBV clearance from the blood. The frequency of MBP mutations in patients with acute and chronic HBV infections differs significantly. The MBP codon 52-mutant was found more frequently in patients with HBV persistence.[232,233] German and Gambian HBV carriers are not associated with MBP polymorphisms.[234,235]

In conclusion, associations between host genetic factors and HBV infection so far only involve HLA class II alleles. The role of HLA class I alleles needs further clarification. Preliminary data in this field have to be confirmed in multi-cohort studies.

Hepatitis C Virus Infections. The outcome of hepatitis C virus (HCV)-related liver diseases varies substantially among individuals. Genetic factors, particularly polymorphisms of the MHC molecules and immune responses against HCV infections, are believed to influence this variability. Several studies have been performed to identify MHC class II alleles associated with different outcomes of HCV infections. Earlier results gave inconsistent results.[236-244] Recently the results of a large European study reported[245] that self-limited infection was associated with HLA-DRB1$^+$1101 and HLA-DQB1$^+$0301. The HLA DRB1 allele seemed to be dominant in determining the outcome of infection. Persistent HCV infection was associated with HLA-DRB1$^+$0701 and DRB4$^+$0101. This is a novel observation, which was confirmed in the second-stage study. No significant associations were found between MHC class II alleles and severe histologic injury or response to interferon therapy.[245] Two recent studies from Ireland[245,247] investigated the relationship between MHC class II alleles and HCV clearance in homogeneous cohorts of women, who received anti-D Ig contaminated with HCV type 1b. Both studies confirmed that HLA-DRB1$^+$0101 is associated with viral clearance. DRB1$^+$0301 and DQB1$^+$0201 occurred more frequently in chronically infected individuals than in those who cleared the virus. One study confirmed the role of DRB1$^+$0701 allele in persistence of HCV infection.[246]

These findings suggest a strong influence of host immunogenetic factors in determining the outcome of HCV infection. Furthermore, these studies demonstrated the value of defined and homogenous groups of patients stratified for clinical course, for identifying relevant pathogenetic factors.

IMMUNE RESPONSE IN AUTOIMMUNE LIVER DISEASES

Acute and chronic liver diseases resulting from autoimmunity are distinct entities in which immune-mediated reactions against self seem to be the major pathogenetic mechanism. This is believed to be true in AIH, PSC, and PBC. The availability of sensitive and specific techniques for the detection of the hepatitis viruses A, B, C, D, and E has led to a more definite characterization and understanding of autoimmune liver diseases (AILD).

Several studies have failed to show any significant associations between infection with hepatitis A, B, C, and D viruses and AILD.[248,250] The coexistence of viral hepatitis and AILD is a rare event and appears to be due to chance. Hepatitis viruses A, B, C, and D, however, are able to induce autoantibodies in a significant number of patients, most commonly antinuclear antibodies (ANA) or smooth muscle antibodies (SMA) but also anti-liver-specific membrane lipoprotein (LSP) and anti-asialoglycoprotein receptor (ASGPR) and to a lesser extent liver-kidney microsomal (LKM) autoantibodies in HCV, and more frequently in hepatitis D.[249] These autoantibodies usually tend to be low in titer in viral infections and mainly have one autoantibody subtype. Soluble liver antigen (SLA) autoantibodies are not found in viral liver diseases. They seem to be specific for AIH.[250] IFN-α therapy can induce a transient appearance of autoantibodies in viral liver diseases.[251] A special autoantibody observed in about 50 percent of patients with chronic HCV, named anti-Gor,[252] is a rare finding in AIH or other liver diseases. In HCV anti-Gor correlates with disease activity.[253]

In this context it is of special interest that anti-ASGPR autoantibodies are induced at high titers of between 1:600 and 1:1600 in patients with acute virus hepatitis A (68 percent) and in lower titers in HBV (60 percent), HCV (53 percent), and non-A-non-B-non-C-non-D (NA-NB-NC-ND) (48 percent),[254] but so far only three cases with AIH after acute hepatitis A[255] and one after acute HBV[256] have been reported.[254] This suggests a pathogen-non-specific or pathogen-unrelated induction of anti-ASGPR. Similar data were described for anti-LSP in the 1970s.[257,258] The viral trigger mechanism is of special interest pathophysiologically. Up-regulation of autoimmune reactions against membrane antigens of hepatocytes can be induced by all hepatitis viruses, but does not usually lead to self-perpetuating AILD. The same may be true for some non-hepatotropic viruses, such as Epstein-Barr and measles viruses (see ref. 257).

Autoimmune Hepatitis

Diagnostic Autoantigen/Autoantibody Systems

Autoantibodies targeted against nuclear, cytoplasmic, and membranous proteins are a hallmark of AIH (see refs. 258, 259). Several techniques have been developed to identify autoantigen/antibody systems in AILD. They include complement fixation tests, immunofluorescence (Figure 37-14), immunodiffusion, counterimmunoelectrophoresis, radioimmunoassays, enzyme immunoassays, immunoblotting, and, lately, recombinant DNA technologies.[259] If and how autoantibodies are involved in the pathogenesis of inflammatory liver disease remains unclear. However, the diagnostic importance of autoantibodies is essential for the differential diagnosis of chronic inflammatory diseases of the liver.

There are two main serologic subgroups of AIH (Table 37-5). The classic autoimmune-type (lupoid) hepatitis (type I AIH) is associated with ANA, SMA, and liver membrane autoantibodies (LMA). A second subgroup (type II AIH) is characterized by autoantibodies against microsomal antigens of liver and kidney, LKM, which are directed against cytochrome P450 enzymes.[259] Various subtypes of anti-P450 (LKM) autoantibodies are associated with autoimmune, viral, and drug-induced liver diseases[259] (Table 37-5). A third subgroup characterized by autoantibodies against SLA has been identified[260] that is identical clinically with type I AIH. Recently the target antigen of SLA has been identified as a liver/pancreas antigen named LP.[261] Furthermore, the target antigen (SLA/LP) has been cloned and a standardized enzyme immunoassay was developed using a recombinant antigen. The reliability of the assay was proven in a demographic study that showed that the autoantibodies against SLA/LP occur with similar frequencies in different geographic regions, races, and age groups, and count for about 15 to 20 percent of type I AIH (submitted article). Another subgroup, particularly of young patients (see Chap. 38), with disease clinically identical to AIH type I, expresses antibodies against F-actin, a constituent of the cytoskeleton of the liver cells with a close association to the plasma membrane.

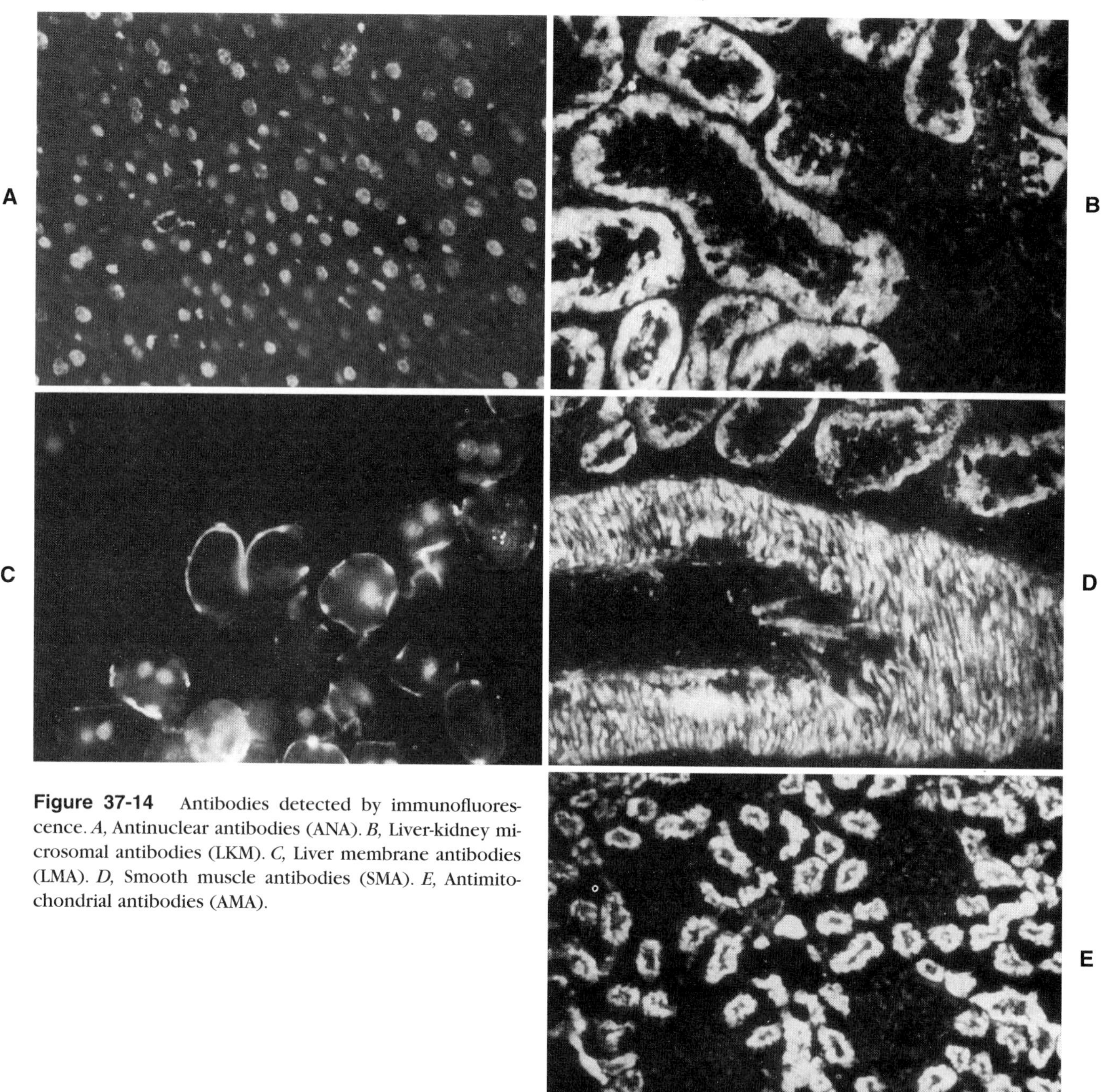

Figure 37-14 Antibodies detected by immunofluorescence. *A,* Antinuclear antibodies (ANA). *B,* Liver-kidney microsomal antibodies (LKM). *C,* Liver membrane antibodies (LMA). *D,* Smooth muscle antibodies (SMA). *E,* Antimitochondrial antibodies (AMA).

Liver Membrane Autoantigen-Autoantibody System

The lack of membrane expression of target antigens of marker autoantibodies has stimulated investigations to identify those autoantigens expressed on the plasma membrane of hepatocytes since the 1960s.[261] At that time a crude plasma membrane preparation with organ-specific components, later named LSP,[263] received clinical and experimental attention. It was possible to induce an autoimmune liver disease in experimental models, first in rabbits[264,265] and later in mice and rats.[266,267] Furthermore, T-cell reactivity to LSP and its components has been described in AIH but also, to a lesser extent, in other inflammatory liver diseases, in particular PBC (see ref. 258). In addition, several groups detected autoantibodies against LSP, more frequently in sera of patients with AIH. In follow-up studies, anti-LSP antibodies could predict the clinical outcome of AIH in men and received clinical relevance.[268] A further search for the relevant target antigens in LSP preparation has been started and led to the detection of liver membrane (LM)Ag[269] and ASGPR as part of LSP and its identification as autoantigens.[270] Meanwhile, several studies have demonstrated the clinical relevance of anti-ASGPR autoantibodies for both diagnosis and prognosis in AIH.[271] In addition to the ASGPR, several other liver-membrane autoantigens have been identified by autoantibodies,

TABLE 37-5
Classification of AIH According to Serum Autoantibody Profiles

Type	Subtypes	Auto-antibodies	Autoantigen	Other features
1	a	ANA/SMA	Nuclear/cytoskelet	LKM negative, LMA positive
	b	Anti-SLA/LP	Unidentified enzyme	LKM negative, LMA positive
	c	SMA/Antiactin	Cytoskelet	ANA negative or rarely positive, LMA?
	d	Anti-ASGPR	ASGPR	ANA/SMA/SLA negative, LMA positive
2	a	LKM_1	Cytochrome P450 IID6	Autoimmune hepatitis type 2 (hepatitis C)
	b	LKM_2	Cytochrome P450 IIC9	Ticrynafen-induced hepatitis
	c	LKM_3	Family 1 UGTs	Chronic hepatitis D
			Family 2 UGTs	Autoimmune hepatitis type 2
	d	LM	Cytochrome P450 IA2	Dihydralazine-induced hepatitis, autoimmune hepatitis, APS1
			Disulfide isomerase	Halothane hepatitis
			Carboxylesterase	Halothane hepatitis

ANA, Antinuclear autoantibodies; *SMA,* smooth muscle autoantibodies; *SLA,* soluble liver antigen; *LP,* liver/pancreas antigen; *LMA,* liver membrane autoantibodies; *LKM_1, LKM_2, LKM_3,* liver-kidney microsomal antibodies types 1, 2, and 3; *LMA,* liver microsomal antibodies; *UGTs,* uridinediphosphate-glucuronosyltransferases; *APS1,* autoimmune syndrome type 1.

but their clinical relevance remains questionable. Of special interest for further studies are a plasma membrane glycosphingolipid,[272] a 43-kD protein[273] located on the basolateral membrane of hepatocytes, a 26-kD LMA,[274] and a partially liver-specific 60-kD membrane antigen.[275] Further studies are needed to characterize the epitopes and their role as pathogens for AIH. The binding of liver-membrane autoantibodies to hepatocellular membrane antigens in vivo suggests that autoantibodies against epitopes expressed on the hepatocellular plasma membrane may be involved in the pathogenesis of AIH.[276,277]

Mechanism of Autoimmune-mediated Hepatocellular Injury

Theoretically both of the cellular and humoral autoimmune mechanisms described previously can cause hepatocellular damage. The direct cytotoxicity of T cells reacting with organ-specific antigens expressed on the liver plasma membrane is probably the most important mechanism in the initial phase of liver injury. Evidence for this comes from the murine model of AIH.[266,287] The essential role of T-cell recognition of liver antigens has been shown using a passive transfer of the disease by CD4-positive T cells in syngeneic mice. In this model autoantibodies appear at the time of spontaneous recovery from the disease.[278]

Acute onset with spontaneous recovery have rarely been observed in human disease. Immunologic studies need to be done in such patients. The most usual clinical picture is an acute or chronic progressive inflammatory course with cell-mediated autoreactivity, autoantibodies, hypergammaglobulinemia, and histopathologic features, which seem to have disease-specific characteristics.[279,280] Keeping in mind the monophasic course of experimental AIH, it is clear that there must be additional factors causing the chronic fluctuating self-perpetuating disease in humans.

Autoantibody-mediated Liver Injury

There is increasing evidence that liver-membrane autoantibodies are involved in the chronic phase of the disease. The first hint of this was the binding of IgG in vivo in a linear pattern to the surface of isolated hepatocytes taken from liver biopsies in AIH.[276,277] The essential role of the humoral autoimmune response in AIH received further support from an experimental rabbit model. A monoclonal antibody against the 43-kD liver-surface antigen induced acute liver injury and lysis of hepatocytes in vivo and in vitro in the absence of serum or T-cell components of the immune system.[273,281] It is likely that, in vivo, the monoclonal antibodies cooperate with NK cells via ADCC. Liver-perfusion studies using anti-ASGPR antibodies showed that anti-ASGPR binds or is consumed predominantly in the periportal zone of the hepatic lobule.[282] Because periportal inflammatory infiltrates dominate and are characteristic of AIH, ADCC may be responsible, in part, for the destruction of periportal hepatocytes. This notion is further supported by in vitro studies showing that non-T lymphocytes (NK cells) from the peripheral blood have cytotoxic activity to autologous hepatocytes isolated from biopsies in AIH.[283] Close correlations between anti-LSP and anti-ASGPR autoantibodies to disease activity and the disappearance of these autoantibodies under immunosuppression[268,284-286] further support their pathogenic role in vivo. In contrast, antinuclear and anticytosolic autoantibodies are detectable in AIH after many years in remission.

T-Cell–mediated Liver Injury

There is general agreement that autoimmune-mediated liver damage involves $CD4^+$ T cells that recognize liver-specific self-antigen peptides and epitopes.[288] Circulating T-lymphocytes that were sensitized against LSP and ASGPR in patients with AIH were described.[258,289] All patients showing T-cell reactivity against human ASGPR had signs of active disease at the time of study. T-cell clones from liver biopsies taken from patients with AIH responded specifically to human ASGPR. The response was restricted to autologous antigen-presenting cells and HLA class II recognition.[289] The majority of the T-cell clones exhibited the $CD4^+$, $CD8^-$ phenotype. The T cells were able to stimulate B cells in an antigen-specific manner to produce autoantibodies against the ASGPR.[290] Furthermore, it was shown that liver-infiltrating T cells from patients with AIH and non-AIH belong to different functional T-cell subsets.[291] The predominance of $CD4^+$ T cells among the T-cell clones from liver biopsies is in accordance with findings obtained from peripheral blood and in situ phenotyping of liver-infiltrating lymphocytes on tissue sections.[290,291] Furthermore, LKM-specific liver-infiltrating T cells were identified in LKM antibody-positive AIH.[292] Little is known about the physiologic expression of cytosolic autoantigens on the surface of hepatocytes. The LKM_1 antigen membrane expression may exist, but remains questionable yet.[259]

Cytokines

Cytokines secreted by activated immune cells and chemokines are important mediators that may function as stimulators and modifiers of the immunologic microenvironment of the liver (see Table 37-4, Figures 37-3 and 37-12). Circulating cytokine and cytokine receptor levels are high in AIH.[293,294] Cytokines may affect synthesis, function, and membrane expression of hepatocellular membrane glycoproteins such as the ASGPR.[295] ASGPR dysfunction has been reported in chronic active hepatitis and cirrhosis of the liver.[296] This can be explained by a loss of ASGPR as a consequence of reduced liver parenchyma, but should perhaps be interpreted more properly as an alteration of ASGPR during inflammation. Weiss and Ashwell speculated that a neuraminidase-producing pathogen may lead to an accumulation of desialysated lymphocytes.[297] The immunogenicity of liver-membrane lipoproteins may also be increased by dysfunction or alteration of the ASGPR, by excess ligands, by desialyzation by neuraminidases, by producing hyperasialoglycoproteinemia,[298] or by defects of resialyzation by liver-specific enzyme.[297,299] The effect of cytokine on hepatic injury could also be demonstrated in T-cell–mediated liver damage in mice induced by concanavalin A.[123,300,301]

TCR Vβ Repertoire

Three independent studies reported limited usage of TCR Vβ repertoire in liver-infiltrating T cells in AIH.[302-304] In one Japanese study,[303] Vβ3 was found in all clones of HLA-DR4–positive AIH patients. Moreover, they reported that Vβ3-positive/Jβ1.2-positive T cells bearing an Asp-Arg-Pro motif were associated with HLA-DR4. This suggests that shared CDR3 sequences rearranged to only one Jβ in HLA-DR4–positive AIH. The German study[304] confirmed these data in untreated active disease with both HLA-DR3 and HLA-DR4 AIH. The TCR Vβ3 T cells were enriched in liver tissue compared to autologous peripheral blood lymphocytes taken at the time of liver biopsy. In addition to Vβ3, overexpression increased TCR Vβ7, and Vβ13.1 T cells were observed. In a second study from Japan,[302] T-cell receptors Vβ2, Vβ3, and Vβ7 were enriched in DR4-positive AIH. Thus irrespective of the HLA-type TCR Vβ3, T cells seem to be involved in the development of autoimmune mediated liver injury. Preliminary data show that expression of the Vβ repertoire may vary during the natural course of AIH and under immunosuppressive medication.[307] Because only one study investigated a homogeneous, untreated, and clinically active group of patients,[304] it is difficult to compare the three reports. However there are more similarities than differences. It has been reported that the autoimmune TCR repertoire may evolve and change during the course of autoimmune disorders.[305] The so-called spreading of T-cell autoimmunity to cryptic determinants on autoantigens can regulate the response to the initial dominant epitopes.[306] If this is true for AIH, it could explain some of the differences discussed previously. Thus on the basis of the data available, the analysis of specific autoepitopes recognized by single TCR Vβ molecules should be possible, as recently shown in PBC.[369,379]

Considering the clinical, experimental, and immunologic findings, there is increasing evidence that autoimmune diseases are regulated by the patient's immune system.[287] This is also true for AIH.[278] In most cases AIH runs a subacute or chronic course with intermittent phases of acute disease and recovery. This clinical pattern can be explained only by an active interplay between disease-promoting factors (genetic predisposition and/or environmental factors) and counterregulatory elements of the immune system. Experimental data discussed previously give accumulating evidence that T-cell-mediated cytotoxicity may be the primary event of liver injury in AIH. The quality of down-regulation of T-cell responses involving antigen-specific and, to a lesser extent, non-specific suppression, may be a course-determining factor. In most cases of human AIH, the natural control and down-regulation of liver-specific T-cell responses may not be strong enough to control the autoimmune process. This may lead to the various courses seen in many autoimmune mediated disorders. In the chronic self-perpetuating phase of AIH, both cellular and humoral autoimmune reactions and cytokines, may shape the inflammatory picture, probably dominated by autoantibody-mediated cytotoxicity.

Primary Sclerosing Cholangitis

PSC is a chronic cholestatic liver disease of unknown etiology characterized by fibro-obliterative inflammation of the intrahepatic and extrahepatic bile ducts.[308] The usually progressive course leads to biliary cirrhosis and to cholangio-carcinoma in about 20 percent of the cases. Special features are male predominance (2:1) and association with inflammatory bowel diseases, in particular with ulcerative colitis (UC), that shows geographic variations between 20 percent and 90 percent. Recent studies have implicated genetic and immunologic factors as important pathogenetic mechanisms.[309]

Humoral Immune Abnormalities

Hypergammaglobulinemia with increased IgM levels occurs in about half the patients, but raised IgG levels are also a common feature. ANA and SMA in usually lower titers as compared to AIH are observed in 30 percent to

70 percent of patients. Autoantibodies do not correlate with clinical features and are not specifically related to the disease. They are immune markers without pathogenetic relevance.[309,310]

An early observation was the detection of increased levels of circulating immune complexes in serum and bile as a result of an impaired clearance function of the reticuloendothelial system.[311-316] But there is no evidence for an immune complex–mediated immune disorder as based on immune morphologic studies.

Antineutrophilic cytoplasmic antibodies (ANCA) are identified as immune markers of PSC. The disease specificity is not very high because ANCA are also associated with AIH and some other immune-mediated diseases.[317-325] About 70 percent to 80 percent of PSC patients are positive for ANCA irrespective of whether PSC is associated with UC.[317,318] Geographic variations of ANCA in PSC may be due to the techniques used to detect ANCA or may reflect ethnic differences. In one study ANCA were present in PSC (82 percent) and UC (70 percent) and in 25 percent and 30 percent of first-degree relatives, respectively.[326]

The target antigen of ANCA in PSC and AIH is neither the proteinase 3 nor myeloperoxidase that are associated with Wegener's granulomatosis and microscopic polyangiitis but several other target antigens (i.e., actin, catalase, enolase, cathepsin G, and lactoferrin).[327-329] The fluorescence pattern of autoantibodies against these target antigens is similar to the P-ANCA pattern induced by antimyeloperoxidase. The role of ANCA as a pathogenetic factor is not yet evident. Particularly, the lack of correlations with disease activity and its unchanged persistence after liver transplantation or colectomy suggest that ANCA in PSC and UC are epiphenomena.[330]

Recently the induction of ANCA was observed in a rat model of liver injury induced by intraportal administration of trinitrobenzinesulphonic acid (TNBS).[331] The target antigen of ANCA was mainly catalase, an autoantigen that has been identified in a high number of sera from patients with PSC and AIH. A similar ANCA pattern could be induced in a rat model of chronic fibrosing cholangitis induced by TNBS administered into dilated bile ducts in rats.[332] In this model ANCA showed specificity for myeloperoxidase, catalase, and actin. This model of a chronic fibrosing cholangitis shows some similarities to human PSC and may be useful in studying the mechanisms of inflammatory and fibrosing diseases of the bile ducts.

Autoantibodies reacting with target structures of the extrahepatic biliary tract and cells of the colon mucosa were found in 80 percent of patients with PSC and UC.[333] Furthermore, immune responses against cross-reacting peptides that share antigenic homologies between bile ducts and intestinal cells suggest that disease and organ-related immune mechanisms may be involved in the pathogenesis of PSC.[334] The identification of a cross-reacting monoclonal antibody with bile duct and colon cells supports the hypothesis of a common factor in the pathogenesis of PSC and associated UC.[335]

T-Cell Immunity

Periportal lymphocytic and mononuclear cell infiltrates are common findings in PSC, but the immunohistologic analysis of these infiltrates showed no consistent patterns in the distribution of T-cell subtypes that could be due to disease-specific, cell-mediated pathogenetic mechanisms. The histologic analysis rarely showed $CD4^+$ T cells adjacent to biliary epithelial cells. Furthermore, peribiliary $CD8^+$ T cells were uncommon in early stages of PSC. In addition, conflicting data about T-cell functions in PSC do not contribute to the understanding of the underlying immunopathogenesis.[336-339] The expression of aberrant MHC class II antigens (MHC DR) on biliary epithelial cells in PSC, but also in PBC, is an important finding, suggesting that these cells function as antigen-presenting cells of self or foreign antigens to $CD4^+$ T cells. So far it has not been shown whether or not co-stimulatory molecules such as B7-1 and B7-2 are expressed.[340] On the other hand, the expression of ICAM-1 on bile duct epithelial cells and high serum levels of circulating ICAM-1 in PSC are consistent with the notion that these cells are involved in immunoregulatory mechanisms in PSC.[341] In a recent histologic study, bile duct epithelia were identified as target cells in PSC and PBC. It is known that both diseases share common characteristics, including T-cell infiltration and progressive fibrosis.[342] The analysis of infiltrating lymphocytes may judge that hepatic T cells in PSC have oligoclonal restriction of the T-cell receptor repertoire preferentially to $V\beta3$, which was not observed in peripheral T cells of PSC patients.[343] This finding was confirmed by investigators, who demonstrated that T-cell lines from periportal infiltrates proliferate when exposed to enterocytes and become toxic to biliary epithelial cells.[344] With respect to the previously mentioned cross-reactive antigens between biliary cells and colon cells, this may be a first hint that T-cell–mediated mechanisms are involved in the pathogenesis of PSC.

In this context an interesting rat model of experimental cholangitis induced by oral administration of the biliary toxin α-naphthylisothiocyanate shows hepatic inflammation, bile duct damage and proliferation, and progressive fibrosis. The expression of MHC class II molecules, infiltration of $CD4^+$ and $CD8^+$ T cells, and a Th1 cytokine profile was associated with progressive morphologic bile duct injury.[345]

In summary there is increasing evidence that PSC is mediated by organ-specific autoimmune mechanisms. Susceptibility to PSC is strongly linked to MHC class II molecules, particularly HLA-B8 DR3 haplotypes, which are associated with other autoimmune disorder believed mediated by T-cell specificity. T-cell reactivity against bile duct epithelia and several humoral autoimmune epiphenomena support this notion. Finally, an overlap of PSC with autoimmune hepatitis[346,347] and inflammatory bowel diseases[318] fits with the presence of an immune-mediated, pathogenetic mechanism. But the question of whether PSC is an autoimmune disorder cannot yet be answered. The main problem is the lack of organ- and disease-specific autoantigens as targets of B- and T-cell immune responses.

Primary Biliary Cirrhosis

PBC is a chronic cholastatic liver disease characterized by progressive destruction of biliary epithelial cells lining the small intrahepatic bile ducts. PBC has all features of a classic autoimmune disorder, particularly a female predominance, disease-specific immune abnormalities, overlap with AIH, autoimmune cholangitis, and other autoimmune disorders, immunogenetic associations, and no link to viral liver diseases.[348]

Humoral Immune Abnormalities

The most important diagnostic markers of PBC are antimitochondrial antibodies (AMA). They are related to PBC in more than 90 percent of PBC patients. AMA were originally described by complement fixation test and later by indirect immunofluorescence (see Figure 37-14).[349] AMA detected by immunofluorescence are also present in non-hepatic autoimmune diseases. PBC-specific subtypes of AMA have been described.[350] Immunoblotting has characterized the target antigens of PBC-specific AMA. The molecular weights of the main mitochondrial antigens vary according to the organ or species used for antigen preparation and the method applied. For the main 70-kD antigen, molecular weights between 62 and 74 kD have been reported, and for the 50-kD antigen, between 48 and 52 kD. Radiolabeled IgGs that are purified from sera of patients with PBC and that react monospecifically with either the 70 (62 to 74)-kD or the 48-(48 to 52) kD antigen have been prepared, and it was shown that anti-70-kD and anti-48-kD antibodies do not block each other.[350] Thus these two major PBC-specific mitochondrial autoantigens are immunologically distinct.

Screening a rat liver complementary DNA (cDNA) expression library with AMA-positive PBC serum led to isolation of a cDNA clone by Gershwin and co-workers that specifically encodes for a protein reactive with anti-70-kD sera.[351] Yeaman and colleagues found that this cDNA encodes for the E2 subunit of the pyruvate dehydrogenase complex (PDC), a major mitochondrial enzyme.[352] From a series of recent reports, it has become evident that PBC sera react with epitopes of three mitochondrial enzymes (Table 37-6). These are the E2 subunits of the PDC (PDC-E2), the E2 subunit of the branched-chain oxoacid-dehydrogenase (BCOADC-E2), and the 2-oxoglutarate-dehydrogenase complex (OGDC-E2). Interestingly, some sera reacting with the 70-kD PDC-E2 also react with a 50-kD protein (component X of the PDC enzyme). As mentioned earlier, antibodies against the 48- to 52-kD BCOADC-E2 antigen are immunologically distinct from the PDH-E2 antigen.[353,354]

ANA of several different specificities (see ref. 355) are observed in patients with PBC, but only two of these seem to be highly specific for the disease: (1) ANA against integral proteins of the nuclear envelope membrane in particular nuclear pore membrane glycoprotein Gp210,[356,357] and (2) nuclear antigens recognized by antinuclear autoantibodies from individuals with PBC, most common being sp100.[358] The prevalence of Gp210 autoantibodies in PBC has ranged from 9.5 percent to 41 percent. In control subjects without PBC, Gp210 autoantibodies are observed in only up to 0.45 percent. Thus Gp210 autoantibodies are highly specific for PBC and may be of diagnostic value for the small number of patients with clinical and morphologic characteristics of PBC but without AMA. Gp210 autoantibodies persist after autotopic liver transplantation even though PBC is not apparent in the allograft. There are no reliable data on the prognostic value of Gp210 autoantibodies in PBC. Further autoantibodies against nuclear envelope epitopes are antibodies to antilamin B receptor. These are rare but PBC-specific. Anti-nuclear laminin antibodies have been detected in many different autoimmune disorders. The prevalence of these and several other autoantibodies directed against nuclear target structures is very low.

TABLE 37-6

Subunits of the 2-Oxoacid Dehydrogenase Complex, the Mitochondrial (M2) Autoantigens of Primary Biliary Cirrhosis—Frequency (percent) of AMA in PBC Sera Reacting with the Respective Components

OGDC	PDC	BCOADC
E2 73%	E2 95% X 95% E1-alpha 41% E2-beta 7%	E2 63%

OGDC, Oxoglutarate-dehydrogenase complex; *PDC,* pyruvate dehydrogenase complex; *BCOADC,* branched-chain oxoacid-dehydrogenase.

The nuclear envelope antigen sp100 recognized by autoantibodies in sera of patients with PBC shows multiple nuclear dot immunofluorescence patterns, which are different from those induced by antibodies against centromere. The sp100 first described by Scostecki and colleagues in 1987[358] has a nuclear mass of approximately 100 kD, sequence similarity to MHC class I domains, and several transacting regulatory proteins. There are three non-overlapping major autoantigenic domains of sp100 that are recognized by the majority of PBC sera. But sp100 appears to contain several different epitopes that are recognized by PBC sera. The prevalence of sp100 autoantibodies in PBC ranges from 18 to 44 percent. In other autoimmune disorders in healthy individuals this antibody is extremely rare; sp100 autoantibodies are rather specific for PBC. This is less true for antibodies against two other nuclear structures named sp140 and PCM (promyelocytic protein). So far, although some of them show high disease specificity, nuclear antibodies in sera of patients with PBC seem to be epiphenomena.[355]

T-Cell Immunity

The high specificity of bile duct damage, the presence of lymphoid infiltrates rich in activated $CD4^+$ and $CD8^+$ T cells, increased expression of MHC class I antigen and aberrant expression of MHC class II antigens, and the expression of adhesion molecules on the biliary epithelial cells suggest that autoantigens related to the small bile duct epithelium are the targets of autoimmune responses in PBC (see ref. 359). As mentioned previously, AMA are very closely associated with PBC. The main reactivity of AMA is to the E2 component of PDC. Purified PDC from different sources and recombinant components of PDC-E2 and PDC induce a proliferative response from T cells in patients with PBC.[360-365]

T cells recognize their antigen via T-cell receptors (TCR). MHC/peptide binding specificity is ensured by the complementary determining region 3 (CDR3) of TCR, which is encoded by the V-J or V-D-J junctions. Analysis of cells infiltrating the liver in PBC showed restricted usage of TCR Vβ chain (TCRVβ) elements,[366,367] conserved amino acid motifs in the CDR3 region,[367-369] and an accumulation of multiple clonotypic cells.[370] These data suggest that T cells infiltrating the liver are selected locally by autoantigens. Further studies analyzed PDC-specific T-cell clones and described heterogeneity in TCRVβ usage[372] and the presence of an immunodominant epitope within the PDC-E2 component that comprises amino acids 163 to 176 in patients expressing the HLA-DRB4^{+}0101 haplotype.[371,372] In this respect, it is of interest that a common T-cell autoantigen motif (ExETDK) in PBC patients expressing the DRB4^{+}0101 haplotype is included in the PDC peptides 163 through 176 and contains several negative charges. Even in PBC patient cohorts not matched for this MHC haplotype, a proliferative response to the PDC-E2 inner lipoyl domain, containing the epitope 163-176 or the peptide itself, was seen in about 35 percent of individuals responding to the whole PDC complex. This may be explained by additional binding motifs of the epitope peptide for other MHC class II alleles (i.e., DR1, DR3, DR7, and DR8).[373] Recently an accumulation of common clonal T cells specific for PBC in peripheral blood mononuclear cells (PBMC) and in the liver of PBC patients was shown. Single-strand conformation polymorphism (SSCP) analysis of the Vβ repertoire showed clonal expansions frequent for Vβ6, Vβ7, and Vβ13.2.[374] This underlines earlier findings that clonally expanded, disease-specific T cells of patients frequently include Vβ6, Vβ7, Vβ12, and Vβ13 bearing T cells with PBC specificity.

Analysis of the TCR α-chain repertoire revealed preferential usage of TCR AV2 in about one third of PBC-specific clones.[375] Furthermore, as expected,[376] rearrangement of two functional T-cell–receptor alpha V (TCRAV) genes has been observed.[375] Expression of two different TCRs by the same cell might be one of the causes of escape from self-tolerance and for the induction of autoimmunity.[377]

In addition to earlier findings by Shimada and colleagues,[378] a recent study provides evidence for molecular mimicry and cross-recognition among mitochondrial autoantigens by PDC-E2 163-176 reactive T cells in PBC.[379] The analysis of T-cell clones from three healthy subjects and five patients with PBC that recognize a single TCR ligand (PDC-E2 163-176/HLA-DR53) showed two major groups of cloned T-cell lines based on the recognition motifs of TCR ligands,[170] ExDK[173] and[168]EIExD,[172] in which x represents a variable amino acid. The reactivity of various mimicry peptides and the motif of the amino acid sequence in CDR3 of TCR Vβ differ between these two groups of T-cell lines. It is of interest that T cells of these groups were found in the peripheral blood of patients with PBC and healthy individuals and that reactivities to various mimicry peptides and to the motif of the amino acid sequence in the CDR3 of TCR Vβ were similar in both groups.

The identification of humoral autoepitopes present in nearly all patients with PBC and the characterization of an immunodominant autoreactive T-cell epitope (PDC-E2 163-176 peptide) give strong evidence that PBC is a T-cell–mediated autoimmune disorder closely related to a break of tolerance to epitopes of an autoantigen, which seems to be highly expressed on the apical surface of biliary epithelial cells in PBC as identified by monoclonal antibodies used to stain bile ducts in diseased patients and healthy individuals.[380,381] Although the nature and identity of the tissue-specific autoantigen that cross-reacts with PDC-E2 remain to be defined, the published data strongly suggest that cross-recognition and molecular mimicry among mitochondrial autoantigens may be the cause for the induction of a disease-specific autoimmunity. The etiology and the disease-promoting factors or agents of the disease-specific autoimmune response are not yet identified. But the fact that PDC-E2 is highly conserved among various species and is displayed on the cell surface of bacteria supports the notion that cross-reactivity or molecular mimicry at the T-cell level may be a decisive step for the break of tolerance to biliary autoantigens. This disease-promoting factor may mainly be effective in females with a special immunogenetic background. With respect to the defined autoepitope it is more likely that microbial infection may be crucial in the etiology of PBC rather than viral infections, which are shown to be unrelated to PBC, AIH, and PSC.[250] Recent observations in patients with scleroderma that shares characteristics of PBC encouraged investigation of microchimerisms as a disease-promoting factor in PBC. The available data could not support the hypothesis that microchimerism operates in PBC.[382]

IMMUNE RESPONSES IN VIRAL LIVER DISEASES

The liver is the primary site of viral replication of probably all clinically relevant hepatitis viruses. The early interaction between hepatitis viruses and the host determines the fate of viral infections. Although the relevance of the antigen non-specific (innate) immune response of the host is not well documented, it is likely that an early and strong innate immune reaction regulates the virus-specific adaptive cellular and humoral immune mechanisms and is a prerequisite for viral control and clearance. Because infected hepatocytes usually display no or little damage, the antiviral immune response is possibly not only responsible for viral clearance but also the most important factor in the pathogenesis of viral liver diseases (see ref. 383).

As mentioned previously, the normal liver eliminates activated immune cells after pathogen-induced expansion to restore homeostasis of the resident immune cells. In case of hepatic viral infection, intrahepatic induction of specifically primed Th0 cells and release of proinflammatory cytokines and chemokines by resident cells may be the primary, early response to control infection locally.[384,385] With respect to the incubation time, the local host-viral interaction may last about 3 months or more in HBV and about 2 months in HCV infections. The recruitment of specific Th1 cells, CTLs, and monocytes/macrophages from the peripheral blood may, in case of an insufficient local control of viral infection, lead to intrahepatic inflammation, tissue damage, and clinical disease.[386-388]

What is known about the dynamic of immune mechanisms during the usually long incubation time after infection with non-cytopathic viruses such as HBV and HCV in contrast to other viral diseases?[383] Study of a chimpanzee model of HBV infection shows that a marked reduction of viral load occurs before clinical disease.[389] A transgenic mouse model of HBV infection[390] shows that the CTL-mediated target cell lysis is associated with tissue injury and not viral clearance during the incubation time. Thus viral clearance or reduction of viral load may not be due to virus specific CTL but rather to other antiviral host defense mechanisms (i.e., cytokines). This notion is supported by a prospective analysis of cellular immune mechanisms during the incubation time of a single-source outbreak of HBV.[391] Reduction of viral replication was not related to tissue damage in acute hepatitis but occurred 4 weeks or more before clinical symptoms.[392] It is likely that antiviral cytokines released via resident and attracted immune cells may explain the long and individually different incubation times of HBV and HCV. The clinical disease that develops in only one third of individuals infected with HBV may result from an insufficient host defense at the sites of viral replication and activation of the adaptive immune mechanisms. Because of the wide distribution of MHC class I molecule expression, the adaptive cellular immune response has the ability to recognize viral antigens in infected cells throughout the body. At the site of viral replication, HLA class II restricted T helper cell responses are of particular importance for the outcome of infections. It has been shown by several investigators that in acute hepatic viral infections, T helper cells that display Th1 or Th0 cytokine profiles support differentiation and proliferation of virus-specific $CD8^+$ T cells. In addition, T helper cells stimulate B cells for specific neutralizing antiviral antibody production. Th cells and CTLs secrete proinflammatory cytokines, in particular IFN-γ and TNF-α, which inhibit replication and gene expression of viruses and induce apoptosis and lysis of infected cells (see Figure 37-11).[393]

Which factors influence viral persistence in HBV and HCV infections, and what makes the difference between HBV and HCV infections?

Immune Responses in HBV Infections

Host-defense mechanisms are effective in the majority of individuals after HBV inoculation. About 70 percent of HBV-infected subjects clear the virus without clinical disease. The remaining 30 percent develop acute hepatitis, but only 5 to 10 percent of them become chronic HBV carriers. The majority of individuals with long or life-long persistence of HBV result from vertical HBV transmission or from HBV infection during early childhood (i.e., in individuals with a poorly developed immune system). These HBV carriers seem to have a status of immune tolerance to HBV, as documented by the high rate (90 percent) of persistent infections, lack of disease activity in the presence of high viral load, and the very low rate of spontaneous or interferon-induced seroconversion from HBe antigen to anti-HBe. However, clinical and immunologic studies clearly show that HBV-specific T cells are present in so-called tolerant HBV carriers, as evidenced by the small number of carriers that develop HBV-specific T cell proliferation and seroconversion.[395] The trigger mechanisms that allow the immune system to overcome tolerance to HBV in patients with perinatally acquired HBV infections are unknown. Persistent HBV infections in adults are mainly related to male sex and various forms of T-cell immune deficiencies and immunosuppression. The majority of persistent HBV infections are associated with poor host defense mechanisms, which allow the virus to develop immune escape mechanisms. The latter include (1) the use of structural and non-structural proteins to alter the immune response; (2) the establishment of a pool of stable, extrachromosomal transcription templates that allow the virus to react sensitively to changes in its immune environment by up-and down-regulation of gene expression; (3) interference with cytokine response; (4) selective suppression of virus-specific immunity in immune-competent hosts; (5) development of antigenic variations and mutants[396]; and (6) HBV infections of intrahepatic and extrahepatic sites.

Patients with acute self-limited HBV infection display a vigorous polyclonal HLA class I-restricted CTL response against multiple epitopes of envelope, nucleocapsid, and polymerase genes of HBV.[397] Even after recovery and loss of HBV markers, T-cell memory and response are still present in the liver or peripheral immune cells for several decades.[398,399] Thus a complete elimination of HBV is a rare event and life-long low viral replication the rule. In patients with chronic HBV infections the HBV-specific $CD4^+$ Th and CTL response to viral antigens is rather weak and often limited to one or very few epitopes.[397,400,401] IL-12 seems to be a course-determining cytokine in chronic HBV, which may explain fluctuations of individual courses between mild, moderate, and severe clinical activity. Patients with chronic HBV who clear the virus or seroconvert from HBeAg to anti-HBe often have a high IL-12 level, a cytokine which activates Th1 cell differentiation and antigen-specific proliferation of CTL.[386,402]

Immune Mechanisms in HCV Infections

One of the most important features of HCV infections is the high rate of chronicity (70-90 percent). Chronic HCV infections resulting from vertical transmission are rare. In contrast to HBV viral, host factors seem to be of central importance for persistence of HCV and the outcome of the disease.[403] The genetic variability of HCV is very complex. Genotypes, subgenotypes, isolates, and quasispecies are the basis for the development of a large reservoir of biologically different variants.[403] Another important factor is the early extrahepatic expression and viral replication in cells of the immune system, including the immune-privileged sites of the liver. This feature of infection may alter and suppress innate and adaptive immune responses, especially during early phases of infection.[404] Extrahepatic manifestations of HCV infections, such as autoimmunity, immune abnormalities, and B cell lymphoproliferative disorders, are common.[405]

HCV appears to be non-cytopathic, and, as in HBV infection, the antiviral immune response is critical for viral clearance and the pathogenesis of the various courses of HCV-related liver diseases.[404] Self-limited HCV infections are associated with a strong, long-lasting HCV-specific $CD4^+$ T-cell response.[406-409] The HCV-specific $CD4^+$ T cells belong to the Th1/Th0 phenotype and seem to recognize only a limited number of highly conserved HCV epitopes. The central role of an early vigorous and particularly long-lasting $CD4^+$ T-cell response was also documented in patients with reappearance of HCV RNA and development of chronic hepatitis C. These patients show an early loss of $CD4^+$ HCV-specific T cells and a weak $CD8^+$ cytotoxic T-cell response, based on new immunologic techniques such as HLA class I tetramer and Elispot.[408,409]

Studies from the early 1990s suggested that HCV can persist despite the presence of an effective $CD4^+$ T cell proliferative response with reactivity to few viral epitopes.[410,411] These findings were not confirmed more recently. There is a weak HCV-specific $CD4^+$ T-cell response in chronic HCV associated with progressive liver injury.[409] The presence of HCV-specific CTLs in chronic HCV infections has been described by several investigators.[412-415] There is increasing evidence that HCV-specific CTLs are functionally deficient in the presence of poor HCV-specific $CD4^+$ T cell help.[412,416,417] In this context, association of HLA class II with outcome of HCV infection may be of interest. Particularly, the functional relationship between HLA alleles and the $CD4^+$ T cell reactivity has to be analyzed.

Because the HCV-specific T-cell response seems to be generally poor, non-specific immune reactions may account for mononuclear cell infiltrates in chronic HCV. Cytokine production at the sites of inflammation also may be a disease-determining factor. Unfortunately, the role of cytokines in persistent HCV infections is not completely understood. Correlations between proinflammatory Th1-associated cytokine production in chronic HCV infections and progressive liver injury are reported.[418,419] But with respect for the genetic variability of viral antigens, changes in the affinity of viral ligands to the T cell receptors, development of altered peptide ligands, and changes of viral load, it is more likely that an interplay between Th1 and Th2 cytokines explains the individual morphologic changes and courses of chronic HCV.[420] This notion received support by studies reporting elevated levels of IL-2, IL-4, IL-10, TNF-α, IFN-γ, and intrahepatic cytokine mRNA expression in chronic HCV.[418-423] Reduced levels of IL-10 seem to be associated with enhanced expression of IFN-γ and IL-2 mRNA and with portal inflammation.[419] Endogenous IL-10 is known to have anti-inflammatory and immunosuppressive properties and to down-regulate the immune response.[424-426] Thus the observed increase in expression of IL-10 may be an important pathogenetic factor and contribute to viral persistence.

Another cytokine that may be of pathogenetic importance is TGF-β1 produced by activated resident liver cells. TGF-β mRNA is high in chronic HCV and correlates with inflammatory activity and lobular necrosis.[419,427,428] TGF-β1 stimulates hepatic stellate cells and induces the initial step of fibrosis,[429] and may down-regulate the cytotoxic action of CTLs.[430] Finally, viral factors have to be considered, particularly in HCV infections with the known heterogeneity of viral genes. The viral mechanisms of immune evasion are multiple, including development of viral resistance to cytokines.[396]

In summary, the pathogenesis of the different courses of chronic HCV and hepatocellular injury is not yet fully understood, but there is increasing evidence that a loss of HCV-specific $CD4^+$ and $CD8^+$ T-cell responses is one of the central factors of HCV persistence and disease chronicity. With respect to the impaired HCV-specific T-cell function, disease progression and hepatocellular damage seem to be related to non-specific immune reactivity and proinflammatory cytokine production. But not only Th1 cytokines may be course-determining; changes in the secretion patterns of cytokine by Th1 to Th2/Th0 and vice versa—probably different compared with HBV[431]—are more likely to explain the different clinical pictures and development of fibrosis and cirrhosis in chronic HCV.[432]

References

1. Cantor H, Dumont A: Hepatic suppression of sensitization to antigen absorbed into the portal system. Nature 213:744, 1967.
2. May AG, Bauer S, Leddy JP, et al: Survival of allografts after hepatic portal venous administration of specific transplantation antigen. Ann Surg 170:824, 1969.
3. Gorczynski RM: Immunosuppression induced by hepatic portal venous immunization spares reactivity in IL-4 producing T lymphocytes. Immunol Lett 33:67, 1992.
4. Barker CF, Corrier JN Jr: Canine renal homotransplantation with venous drainage via the portal vein. Ann Surg 165:279, 1967.
5. Boeckx W, Sobis H, Lacqzet A, et al: Prolongation of allogeneic heart graft survival by pretransplant transfusion and/or by varying the route of allograft venous drainage. Transplantation 19:145, 1975.
6. Gorczynski RM, Chan Z, Chung S, et al: Prolongation of rat small bowel or renal allograft survival by pretransplant transfusion and/or by varying the route of allograft venous drainage. Transplantation 58:816, 1994.
7. Calne RY: Induction of immunological tolerance by porcine liver allografts. Nature 223:472, 1969.
8. Wisse E, De Zanger RB, Charels K, et al: The liver sieve: considerations concerning the structure and function of endothelial fenestrae, the sinusoidal wall and the space Disse. Hepatology 5:683, 1985.
9. Van den Oord JJ, De Vos R, Desmet VM: HLA expression in liver diseases. In Popper H, Schaffner F, eds: Progress in Liver Diseases, vol IX. Philadelphia, WB Saunders Co, 1990:73.
10. Geppert TD, Lipsky PE: Antigen presentation at the inflammatory site. Crit Rev Immunol 9:313, 1989.
11. Geppert TD, Davis LS, Gur H, et al: Accessory cell signals involved in T-cell activation. Immunol Rev 117:5, 1990.
12. Springer TA: Adhesion receptors of the immune system. Nature 346:425, 1990.
13. Volpes R, van den Oord JJ, Desmet VJ: Immunochemical study of adhesion molecules in liver inflammation. Hepatology 12:59, 1990.
14. Steinhoff G, Behrend M, Wonigkeit K: Expression of adhesion molecules on lymphocytes/monocytes and hepatocytes in human liver grafts. Hum Immunol 28:123, 1990.
15. Volpes R, van den Oord JJ, Desmet VJ: Hepatic expression of intercellular adhesion molecule 1 (ICAM-1) in viral hepatitis B. Hepatology 12:148, 1990.
16. Volpes R, van den Oord JJ, De Vos R, et al: Expression of interferon gamma receptor in normal and pathological human liver tissue. J. Hepatol 12:195, 1991.

17. Volpes R, van den Oord JJ, De Vos R, Desmet VJ: Hepatic expression of type A and type B receptors for tumor necrosis factor. J Hepatol 14:61, 1992.
18. Volpes R, van den Oord JJ, Desmet VJ: Expression of B-cell growth factor receptor (CDw40) on hepatocytes in areas of inflammation. J Hepatol 9(suppl):243, 1989.
19. Smedsrød B: Pathobiology of sinusoidal endothelial cells. In Gresner A, Ramadori G, eds: Molecular and Cell Biology of Liver Fibrogenesis. Dordrecht, Kluwer Academic Press, 1992:454.
20. Wisse E: An electron microscopic study of the fenestrated endothelial lining of rat liver sinusoids. J Ultrastruct Res 31:125, 1970.
21. Kolb-Bachofen V, Schlepper-Schafer J, Roos P, et al: GalNAc/Gal-specific rat liver lectins: their role in cellular recognition. Biol Cell 51:219, 1984.
22. Schlepper-Schafer J, Hulsmann D, Djovkar A, et al: Endocytosis via galactose receptors in vivo. Ligand size directs uptake by hepatocytes and/or liver macrophages. Exp Cell Res 165:494, 1986.
23. Kempka G, Kolb-Bachofen V: Binding, uptake and transcytosis of ligands for mannose-specific receptors in rat liver: an electron microscopic study. Exp Cell Res 176:38, 1988.
24. Fraser R, Dobbs BR, Rogers GW: Lipoproteins and the liver sieve: the role of the fenestrated sinusoidal endothelium in lipoprotein metabolism, atherosclerosis and cirrhosis. Hepatology 21:863, 1995.
25. Blomhoff R, Eskild W, Berg T: Endocytosis of formaldehyde treated serum albumin via scavenger pathway in liver endothelial cells. Biochem J 218:81, 1984.
26. Laurent TC: Scavenger functions of the liver endothelial cell. Biochem J 266:313, 1990.
27. Magnusson S, Berg T: Extremely rapid endocytosis mediated by the mannose receptor of sinusoidal endothelial rat liver cells. Biochem J 257:651, 1989.
28. Melkko J, Hellevik T, Risteli L, et al: Clearance of NH2-terminal propeptides of types I and III procollagen is a physiological function of the scavenger receptor in liver endothelial cells. J Exp Med 1879:405, 1994.
29. Horiuchi S: Advanced glycation end products are eliminated by scavenger-receptor-mediated endocytosis in hepatic sinusoidal Kupffer and endothelial cells. Biochem J 322:567, 1997.
30. Tavassoli M, Kishimoto T, Soda R, et al: Liver endothelium mediates the uptake of iron-transferrin complex by hepatocytes. Exp Cell Res 165:369, 1986.
31. Tavassoli M, Kishimoto T, Kataoka M: Liver endothelium mediates the hepatocyte's uptake of ceruloplasmin. J Cell Biol 102:1298, 1986.
32. Irie S, Kishimoto T, Tavassoli M: Desialation of transferrin by rat liver endothelium. J Clin Invest 82:508, 1988.
33. Lohse AW, Knolle PA, Bilo K, et al: Antigen-presenting function and B7 expression of murine sinusoidal endothelial cells and Kupffer cells. Gastroenterology 110:1175, 1996.
34. Knolle PA, Uhrig A, Hegenbarth S, et al: IL-10 down-regulates T cell activation by antigen-presenting liver sinusoidal endothelial cells through decreased antigen uptake via the mannose receptor and lowered surface expression of accessory molecules. Clin Exp Immunol 114:427, 1998.
35. Sallusto F, Cella M, Danieli C, Lanzavecchia A: Dendritic cells use macropinocytosis and the mannose receptor to concentrate macromolecules in the major histocompatibility complex class II compartment: downregulation by cytokines and bacterial products. J Exp Med 182:389, 1995.
36. Briscoe DM, Henauld LE, Geehan C, et al: Human endothelial cell costimulation of T cell IFN-γ production. J Immunol 159:3247, 1997.
37. Johnson DR, Hauser IA, Voll RE, Emmrich F: Arterial and venular endothelial cell costimulation of cytokine secretion by human T cell clones. J Leukoc Biol 63:613, 1998.
38. Ma W, Pober JS: Human endothelial cells effectively costimulate cytokine production by, but not differentiation of, naive $CD4^+$ T cells. J Immunol 161:2158, 1998.
39. Ferez VL, Henauld L, Lichtman AH: Endothelial antigen presentation: stimulation of previously activated but not naive TCR-transgenic mouse T cells. Cell Immunol 189:31, 1998.
40. Autschbach F, Meuer S, Moebius U, et al: Hepatocellular expression of lymphocyte function-associated antigen 3 in chronic hepatitis. Hepatology 14:223, 1991.
41. Meuer SC, Hussey RE, Fabbi M, et al: An alternative pathway of T-cell activation: a functional role for the 50 kd TI 1 sheep erythrocyte receptor protein. Cell 36:897, 1984.
42. Scoazec JY, Feldmann G: Both macrophages and endothelial cells of the human hepatic sinusoid express the CD4 molecule, a receptor for the human immunodeficiency virus. Hepatology 12:505, 1990.
43. Knolle P, Schmitt E, Jin S, et al: Induction of cytokine production in naive $CD4^+$ T cells by antigen-presenting murine liver sinusoidal endothelial cells but failure to induce differentiation toward Th1 cells. Gastroenterology 116:1428, 1999.
44. Winwood PJ, Arthur MJP: Kupffer cells: their activation and role in animal models of liver injury and human liver disease. Semin Liver Dis 13:50, 1993.
45. Laskin DL, Sirak AA, Pilaro AM: Functional and biochemical properties of rat Kupffer cells and peritoneal macrophages. J Leukoc Biol 44:71, 1988.
46. Lepay DA, Nathan CF, Steinmann RM: Murine Kupffer cells: mononuclear phagocytes deficient in the generation of reactive oxygen intermediates. J Exp Med 161:1079, 1985.
47. Van Vossuyt H, Zahger RB, Wisse E: Cellular and subcellular distribution of injected lipopolysaccharide in rat liver and its inactivation by bile salt. J Hepatol 7:325, 1988.
48. McCuskey RS, McCuskey PA, Urbaschek R, Urbaschek B: Kupffer cell function in host defense. Rev Infect Dis 9:616, 1987.
49. Rogoff TM, Lipsky PE: Role of the Kupffer cells in local and systemic immune response. Gastroenterology 80:854, 1981.
50. Callery MP, Kamei T, Flye MW: Kupffer cell blockade inhibits induction of tolerance by the portal venous route. Transplantation 47:1092, 1989.
51. Ballardini G, Faccani A, Fallani M, et al: Class II MHC antigen expression of sinusoidal lining cells in human chronic liver disease. In Kirn A, Knook DL, Wisse E, eds: Cells of the Hepatic Sinusoid, vol. 1. Leiden, Netherlands, Kupffer Cell Foundation 1986:41.
52. Tiegs G, Hentschel J, Wendel A: A T-cell dependent experimental liver injury in mice inducible by concanavalin A. J Clin Invest 90:196, 1992.
53. Knolle P, Schlaak J, Uhrig A, et al: Human Kupffer cells secrete IL-10 in response to lipopolysaccharide (LPS) challenge. J Hepatol 22:226, 1995.
54. Knolle PA, Uhrig A, Protzer U, et al: Interleukin-10 expression is autoregulated at the transcriptional level in human and murine Kupffer cells. Hepatology 27:93, 1998.
55. Figdor CG, de Vries JE: Interleukin 10 (IL-10) inhibits cytokine synthesis by human monocytes: an autoregulatory role of IL-10 produced by monocytes. J Exp Med 174:1209, 1991.
56. Wendel A: Lipopolysaccharide-induced interleukin-10 in mice: role of endogenous tumor necrosis factor-α. Eur J Immunol 25:2888, 1995.
57. Dieter P, Schulze-Specking A, Karck U, Decker K: Prostaglandin release but not superoxide production by rat Kupffer cells stimulated in vitro depends on Na^+/H^+ exchange. Eur J Biochem 170:201, 1987.
58. Grewe M, Duyster J, Dieter P, et al: Prostaglandin D2 and E2 syntheses in rat Kupffer cells are antagonistically regulated by lipopolysaccharide and phorbol ester. Biol Chem Hoppe Seyler 373:655, 1992.
59. Collins C, Norris S, McEntee G, et al: RAG1, RAG2 and pre-T cell receptor alpha chain expression by adult human hepatic T cells; evidence for extrathymic T cell maturation. Eur J Immunol 26:3114, 1996.
60. Lynch S, Kelleher D, McManus R, O'Farrelly C: RAG1 and RAG2 expression in human intestinal epithelium: evidence of extrathymic T cell differentiation. Eur J Immunol 25:1143, 1995.
61. Guy-Grand D, Vanden Broecke C, Briottet C, et al: Different expression of the recombination activity gene RAG-1 in various populations of thymocytes, peripheral T cells and gut thymus-independent intraepithelial lymphocytes suggests two pathways of T cell receptor rearrangement. Eur J Immunol 22:505, 1992.
62. Lundqvist C, Varanov V, Hammarstrom S, et al: Intra-epithelial lymphocytes. Evidence for regional specialization and extrathymic T cell maturation in the human gut epithelium. Int Immunol 7:1473, 1995.
63. O'Farrelly C, Crispe IN: Prometheus through the looking glass: reflections on the hepatic immune system. Immunol Today 20:394, 1999.

64. Schlitt HJ, Schafers S, Deiwick A, et al: Extramedullary erythropoiesis in human liver grafts. Hepatology 21:689, 1995.
65. Huang L, Sye K, Crispe IN: Proliferation and apoptosis of B220+CD4-CD8-TCR alpha beta intermediate T cells in the liver of normal adult mice: Implication for 1pr pathogenesis. Int Immunol 6:533, 1994.
66. Huang L, Solvevila G, Leeker M, et al: The liver eliminates T cells undergoing antigen-triggered apoptosis in vivo. Immunity 1:741, 1994.
67. Masuda T, Ohteki T, Abo T, et al: Expansion of the population of double negative CD4-CD8-T-alpha beta-cells in the liver is a common feature of autoimmune mice. J Immunol 147:2907, 1991.
68. Bandeira A, Itohara S, Bonneville M, et al: Extrathymic origin of intestinal intraepithelial lymphocytes bearing T-cell antigen receptor gamma delta. Proc Natl Acad Sci U S A 88:43, 1991.
69. MacDonald HR: NK1.1+ T cell receptor-alpha/beta+ cells: new clues to their origin, specificity, and function. J Exp Med 182:633, 1995.
70. Bendelac A, Lantz O, Quimby ME, et al: CD1 recognition by mouse NK1+ T lymphocytes. Science 268:863, 1995.
71. Trinchieri G: Definition and biology of natural killer cells. In Solan R, Pena J, eds: MHC Antigens and NK Cells. Austin, Tex, R.G. Landes Co, 1994:1.
72. Lotzova E, Ades EW: Natural killer cells: definition, heterogeneity, lytic mechanism, functions and clinical application. Mat Immunol Cell Growth Regul 8:1, 1989.
73. Yokoyama WM: Right-side-up and upside-down NK-cell receptors. Curr Biol 5:982, 1995.
74. Wake K: "Sternzellen" in the liver: perisinusoidal cells with special reference to storage of vitamin A. Am J Anat 132:429, 1971.
75. Hendriks HFJ, Verfoofstad WA, Brouwer A, et al: Perisinusoidal fat-storing cells are the main vitamin A storage sites in rat liver. Exp Cell Res 160:138, 1985.
76. Ramadori G: Kupffer cells and fibrogenesis. In Clement A, Guillozo EDS, eds: Cellular and Molecular Aspects of Cirrhosis. Paris, John Libbey Eurotext, 1992:215:169.
77. Knittel T, Kobold D, Salle B, et al: Rat liver myofibroblasts and hepatic stellate cells: different cell populations of the fibroblast lineage with fibrogenic potential. Gastroenterology 117:1205, 1999.
78. Friedman SL: The virtuosity of hepatic stellata cells. Gastroenterology 117:1244, 1999.
79. Friedman SL: Hepatic stellata cells. Prog Liver Dis 14:101, 1996.
80. Maher JJ: Cytokines: overview. Semin Liver Disease 19(2):109. 1999.
81. Ramadori G, Christ B: Cytokines and the hepatic acute-phase response. Semin Liver Disease 19(2):141, 1999.
82. Baumann H, Gauldi F: The acute phase response. Immunol Today 15:74, 1984.
83. Baumann H, Ziegler SF, Mosley B, et al: Reconstitution of the response to leukemia inhibitory factor, oncostatin M, and ciliary neurotrophic factor in hepatoma cells. J Biol Chem 268:8414, 1993.
84. Kishimoto T, Akira S, Narazaki M, Taga T: Interleukin-6 family of cytokines and gp130. Blood 86:1243, 1995.
85. Hibi M, Nakajima K, Hirano T: IL-6 cytokine family and signal transduction: a model of the cytokine system. J Mol Med 74:1, 1996.
86. Campos SP, Wang Y, Koj A, Baumann H: Divergent transforming growth factor-beta effects on IL-6 regulation of acute phase plasma proteins in rat hepatoma cells. J Immunol 151:7128, 1993.
87. Kordula T, Guttgemann I, Rose-John S, et al: Synthesis of tissue inhibitor of metalloproteinase-1 (TIMP-1) in human hepatoma cells (HepG2). Upregulation by interleukin-6 and transforming growth factor beta 1. FEBS Lett 313:143, 1992.
88. Guillen MI, Gomez-Lechon MJ, Nakamura T, Castell JV: The hepatocyte growth factor regulates the synthesis of acute-phase proteins in human hepatocytes: divergent effect on interleukin-6-stimulated genes. Hepatology 23:1345, 1996.
89. Schaper F, Siewert E, Gomez-Lechon MJ, et al: Hepatocyte growth factor/scatter factor (HGF/SF) signals via the STAT3/APRF transcription factor in human hepatoma cells and hepatocytes. FEBS Lett 405:99. 1997.
90. Wang Y, Kuropatwinski KK, White DW, et al: Leptin receptor action in hepatic cells. J Biol Chem 272:16216, 1997.
91. Birch HE, Schreiber G: Transcriptional regulation of genes encoding the acute-phase protein synthesis during inflammation. J Biol Chem 261:8077, 1986.
92. Goldberger G, Bing DH, Sipe JD, et al: Transcriptional regulation of genes encoding the acute-phase proteins CRP, SAA, and C3. J Immunol 138:3967, 1986.
93. Andus T, Geiger T, Hirano T, et al: Action of recombinant human interleukin 6, interleukin 1 beta and tumor necrosis factor alpha on the mRNA induction of acute-phase proteins. Eur J Immunol 18:739, 1988.
94. Morrone G, Ciliberto G, Oliviero S, et al: Recombinant interleukin 6 regulates the transcriptional activation of a set of human acute phase genes. J Biol Chem 263:12554, 1988.
95. Moshage H: Cytokines and the hepatic acute phase response. J Pathol 181:257, 1997.
96. Ramadori G, Meyer zum Büschenfelde KH, Tobias PS, et al: Biosynthesis of lipopolysaccharide-binding protein in rabbit hepatocytes. Pathobiology 58:89, 1990.
97. Ihara S, Takahashi A, Hatsue H, et al: Major component of RA-reactive factor, a complement activating bactericidal protein in mouse serum. J Immunol 146:1874, 1991.
98. Knittel TH, Fellmer P, Neubauer K, et al: The complement-activating protease P100 is expressed by hepatocytes and is induced by IL-6 in vitro and during the acute phase reaction in vivo. Lab Invest 77:221, 1997.
99. Sevaljevic L, Ivanovic MS, Petrovic M, et al: Regulation of plasma acute phase protein and albumin levels in the liver of scalded rats. Biochem J 258:663, 1989.
100. Milland J, Tsykin A, Thomas T, et al: Gene expression in regenerating and acute-phase rat liver. Am J Physiol 259:G340, 1990.
101. Citarella F, Felici A, Brouwer M, et al: Interleukin-6 downregulates factor XII production by human hepatoma cell lines (HepG2). Blood 80:1501, 1997.
102. Morrone G, Cortese R, Sorrentino V: Post-transcriptional control of negative acute phase genes by transforming growth factor beta. EMBO J 8:3767, 1989.
103. Fey GH, Gauldie J: The acute phase response of the liver in inflammation. Prog Liver Dis 9:89, 1990.
104. Campos SP, Baumann H: Insulin is a prominent modulator of the cytokine-stimulated expression of acute-phase plasma protein genes. Mol Cell Biol 12:1789, 1992.
105. Dimitris A, Papanicolau, Wilder RL, et al: The pathophysiologic roles of interleukin-6 in human diseases. Ann Intern Med 128:127, 1998.
106. Kubin M, Kamoun M, Trinchieri G: Interleukin 12 synergizes with B7/CD28 interaction in inducing efficient proliferation and cytokine production of human T-cells. J Exp Med 180:211, 1994.
107. Dinarello LHA: The role of the interleukin-1-receptor antagonist is blocking inflammation mediated by interleukin-1. N Engl J Med 343(10):732, 2000.
108. MacPhee PJ, Schmidt EE, Groom AC: Intermittence of blood flow in liver sinusoids, studied by high-resolution in vivo microscopy. Am J Physiol 269:G692, 1995.
109. MacPhee PJ, Schmidt EE, Groom AC: Evidence for Kupffer cell migration along liver sinusoids, from high resolution in vivo microscopy. Am J Physiol 263:G17, 1992.
110. McNab G, Reeves JL, Salmi M, et al: Vascular adhesion protein 1 mediates binding of T cells to human hepatic endothelium. Gastroenterology 110:522, 1996.
111. Wong J, Johnston B, Lee SS, et al: A minimal role for selectins in the recruitment of leukocytes into the inflamed liver microvasculature. J Clin Invest 99:2782, 1997.
112. Shnyra A, Lindberg AA: Scavenger receptor pathway for lipopolysaccharide binding to Kupffer and endothelial liver cells in vitro. Infect Immun 63:865, 1995.
113. Knolle PA, Gerken G: Local control of the immune response in the liver. Immunol Rev 174:21, 2000.
114. Steffan AM, Gendrault JL, McCuskey RS, et al: Phagocytosis, an unrecognized property of murine endothelial liver cells. Hepatology 6:830, 1986.
115. Rieder H, Ramadori G, Allmann KH, Meyer zum Büschenfelde KH: Prostanoid release of cultured liver sinusoidal endothelial cells in response to endotoxin and tumor necrosis factor. Comparison with umbilical vein endothelial cells. J Hepatol 11:359, 1990.
116. Jacob AI, Goldberg PK, Bloom N, et al: Endotoxin and bacteria in portal blood. Gastroenterology 72:1268, 1977.

117. Freudenberg MA, Freudenberg N, Galanos C: Time course of cellular distribution of endotoxin in liver, lungs and kidneys of rats. Br J Exp Pathol 63:56, 1982.
118. Knolle PA, Germann T, Treichel U, et al: Endotoxin downregulates T cell activation by antigen-presenting liver sinusoidal endothelial cells. J Immunol 162:1401, 1999.
119. Bissell DM, Wang SS, Jarnagin WR, Roll FJ: Cell-specific expression of transforming growth factor-β in rat liver: Evidence for autocrine regulation of hepatocyte proliferation. J Clin Invest 96:447, 1995.
120. Tiegs G, Küsters S, Künstle G: T cell-mediated experimental liver injury. In Berg P, Lohse AW, Tiegs G, Wendel A, eds: Autoimmune Liver Disease. Lancaster, Penn, Kluwer Academic Publishers, 1997:32.
121. Gantner F, Leist M, Lohse AW, et al: Concanavalin A-induced T cell-mediated hepatic injury in mice: the role of tumor necrosis factor. Hepatology 21:190, 1995.
122. Knolle PA, Gerken G, Löser E, et al: Role of sinusoidal endothelial cells of the liver in concanavalin A-induced hepatic injury in mice. Hepatology 24:824, 1996.
123. Weiner HL, Mayer LF: Oral tolerance: mechanisms and application. Ann NY Acad Sci 778:XIII-XVIII, 1996.
124. Yang R, Liu Q, Grosfeld JL, Pescovitz MD: Intestinal venous drainage through the liver is a prerequisite for oral tolerance induction. J Pediatr Surg 29:1145, 1994.
125. Callery MP, Kamei T, Flye MW: The effect of portacaval shunt on delayed-hypersensitivity responses following antigen feeding J Surg Res 46:391, 1989.
126. Gutgeman I, Fahrer AM, Altman JD, et al: Introduction of rapid T cell activation and tolerance by systemic presentation of an orally administered antigen. Immunity 8:667, 1998.
127. Gorczynski RM: Adoptive transfer of unresponsiveness to allogeneic skin grafts with hepatic $\gamma\delta$ T cells. Immunology 81:27, 1994.
128. Dini I, Caral EC: Hepatic sinusoidal endothelium heterogeneity with respect to the recognition of apoptotic cells. Exp Cell Res 240:388, 1998.
129. Müschen M, Warskulat U, Douillard P, et al: Regulation of CD95 (APO-1/Fas) receptor and ligand expression by lipopolysaccharide and dexamethasone in parenchymal and nonparenchymal rat liver cells. Hepatology 27:200, 1998.
130. Müschen M, Warskulat U, Peters-Regehr T, et al: Involvement of CD95 (APO-1/Fas) ligand expressed by rat Kupffer cells in hepatic immunoregulation. Gastroenterology 116:666, 1999.
131. Bertolino P, Trescol-Biemont MC, Rabourdin-Combe C: Hepatocytes induce functional activation of naive $CD8^+$ T lymphocytes but fail to promote survival. Eur J Immunol 28:221, 1998.
132. Galle PR, Hofmann WJ, Walczak M, et al: Involvement of the CD95 (APO-1/Fas) receptor and ligand in liver damage. J Exp Med 182:1223, 1995.
133. Huang L, Soldevila G, Leeker M, et al: The liver eliminates T cells undergoing antigen-triggered apoptosis in vivo. Immunity 1:741, 1994.
134. Cooper S, Erickson AL, Adams EJ, et al: Analysis of a successful immune response against hepatitis C virus. Immunity 10:439, 1999.
135. Crispe IN, Mehal WZ: Strange brew: T cells in the liver. Immunol Today 17:522, 1996.
136. Kamada N, Wight DG: Antigen-specific immunosuppression induced by liver transplantation in the rat. Transplantation 38:217, 1984.
137. Rossi-Bergman B: A subset of $\gamma\delta$ T-cell receptor-positive cells produce T-helper type-2 cytokines and regulate mouse skin graft rejection following portal venous pretransplant preimmunization. Immunology 87:381, 1996.
138. Gorczynski RM, Hozumi N, Wolf S, Chen Z: Interleukin 12 in combination with anti-interleukin 10 reverses graft prolongation after portal venous immunization. Transplantation 60:1337, 1995.
139. Gorczynski RM: Regulation of IFN-γ and IL-10 synthesis in vivo as well as continuous antigen exposure is associated with tolerance to murine skin allografts. Cell Immunol 160:224, 1995.
140. Gorczynski L, Chen Z, Hu J, et al: Evidence that an OX-2-positive cell can inhibit the stimulation of type 1 cytokine production by bone marrow-derived B7-1 and B7-2-positive dendritic cells. J Immunol 162:774, 1999.
141. Cosse L: Electron microscopy of Kupffer cells in the orthotopic porcine liver homograft during the late stage after transplantation (phagocytosis of host cells by Kupffer cells). Exp Pathol (Jena) 11:168, 1975.
142. Falsca L, Bergamini A, Serafino A, et al: Human Kupffer cell recognition and phagocytosis of apoptotic peripheral blood lymphocytes. Exp Cell Res 224:152, 1996.
143. Caliery MP, Kamei T, Flye MW: Kupffer cell blockade inhibits induction of tolerance by the portal venous route. Transplantation 47:1091, 1989.
144. Kamei T, Callery MP, Flye MW: Kupffer cell blockade prevents induction of portal venous tolerance in rat cardiac allograft transplantation. J Surg Res 48:393, 1990.
145. Roland CR, Mangino MJ, Duffy BF, Flye MW: Lymphocyte suppression by Kupffer cells prevents portal venous tolerance induction: a study of macrophage function after intravenous gadolinium. Transplantation 55:1151, 1993.
146. Steinbrink K, Wolf M, Jonuleit H, et al: Induction of tolerance by IL 10-treated dendritic cells. J Immunol 159:4772, 1997.
147. Limmer A, Ohl J, Kurts CH, et al: Efficient presentation of exogenous antigen by liver endothelial cells to $CD8^+$ T cells results in antigen-specific T-cell tolerance. Nature Medicine 6(12):1348, 1999.
148. Fearon DT, Locksley RM: The instructive role of innate immunity in the acquired immune response. Science 272:50, 1996.
149. Epstein J, Eichbaum Q, Sheriff S, Ezekowitz RA: The collectins in innate immunity. Curr Opin Immunol 8:29, 1996.
150. Biron CA: Role of early cytokines, including alpha and beta interferons (IFN-alpha/beta), in innate and adaptive immune responses to viral infections. Semin Immunol 10:383, 1998.
151. Medzhitov R, Janeway CA Jr: Innate immunity: impact on the adaptive immune response. Curr Opin Immunol 9:4, 1997.
152. Fraser IP, Koziel H, Ezekowitz RA: The serum mannose-binding protein and the macrophage mannose receptor are pattern recognition molecules that link innate and adaptive immunity. Semin Immunol 10:363, 1998.
153. Suzuki H, Kurihara Y, Takeya M, et al: A role for macrophage scavenger receptors in atherosclerosis and susceptibility to infection. Nature 386:292, 1997.
154. Thomas CA, Li Y, Kodama T, et al: Protection from lethal gram-positive infection by macrophage scavenger receptor-dependent phagocytosis. J Exp Med 191:147, 2000.
155. Hashimoto C, Hudson KL, Anderson KV: The Toll gene of Drosophila, required for dorsal-ventral embryonic polarity, appears to encode a transmembrane protein. Cell 52:269, 1988.
156. Hoffmann JA, Kafatos FC, Janeway CA, Ezekowitz RA: Phylogenetic perspectives in innate immunity. Science 284:1313, 1999.
157. Takeuchi O, Kaufmann A, Grote K, et al: Cutting edge: preferentially the R stereoisomer of the mycoplasmal lipopeptide macrophage-activating lipopeptide-2 activates immune cells through a Toll-like receptor 2- and MyD88-dependent signaling pathway. J Immunol 164:554, 2000.
158. Medzhitov R, Janeway CA: Innate immunity. N Engl J Med 343(5): 338, 2000.
159. Vilcek JSG: Interferons and other cytokines. In Fields BN, Howley PM, eds: Fundamental Virology, vol. 11. Philadelphia, Lippincott-Raven, 1996:341.
160. Ishikawa R, Biron CA: IFN induction and associated changes in splenic leukocyte distribution. J Immunol 150:3713, 1993.
161. Salazar-Mather TP, Ishikawa R, Biron CA: NK cell trafficking and cytokine expression in splenic compartments after IFN induction and viral infection. J Immunol 157:3054, 1996.
162. Ma A: Pleiotropic functions of IL 15 in innate and adoptive immunity. Mod Asp Immunobiol 1(3):102, 2000.
163. Salazar-Mather TP, Orange JS, Biron CA: Early murine cytomegalovirus (MCMV) infection induces liver natural killer (NK) cell inflammation and protection through macrophage inflammatory protein 1alpha (MIP-1alpha)-dependent pathways. J Exp Med 187:1, 1998.
164. Pilaro AM, Taub DD, McCormick KL, et al: TNF-alpha is a principal cytokine involved in the recruitment of NK cells to liver parenchyma. J Immunol 153:333, 1994.
165. Orange JS, Salazar-Mather TP, Opal SM, Biron CA: Mechanisms for virus-induced liver disease: Tumor necrosis factor-mediated pathology independent for natural killer and T cells during murine cytomegalovirus infection. J Virol 71:9248, 1997.
166. Lanier LL. NK receptors. Annu Rev Immunol 16:359, 1998.
167. Ihle JN: Cytokine receptor signaling. Nature 377:591, 1995.
168. Scabo SJ, Kim ST, Costa GL, et al: A novel transcription factor, T-bet, directs Th1 lineage commitment. Cell 100:655, 2000.

169. Ouyang W, Löhming M, Gao Z, et al: Stat6-independent Gata-3 autoactivation directs IL4-independent Th2 development and commitment. Immunity 12:27, 2000.
170. O'Garra A: Commit ye helpers. Nature 404:719, 2000.
171. Leitenberg D, Boutin Y, Lu DD, Bottomly K: Biochemical association of CD45 with the T cell receptor complex: regulation by CD45 isoform and during T cell activation. Immunity 10(6):701, 1999.
172. Tao X, Constant S, Jorritsma P, Bottomly K: Strength of TCR signal determines the costimulatory requirements for Th1 and Th2 $CD4^+$ T cell differentiation. J Immunol 159:5956, 1997.
173. Hsieh CS, Macatonia SE, O'Garra A, Murphy KM: Pathogen-induced Th1 phenotype development in $CD4^+$ $\alpha\beta$-TCR transgenic T cells is macrophage dependent. Int Immunol 5:371, 1993.
174. Boutin Y, Leitenberg D, Bottomly K: Distinct biochemical signals characterize agonist- and altered peptide ligand-induced differentiation of naive CD4+ T cells onto Th1 and Th2 subsets. J Immunol 159:5802, 1997.
175. Springer TA: Traffic signals for lymphocyte recirculation and leukocyte emigration: the multiple paradigma. Cell 76:304, 1994.
176. Shields PL, Morland CM, Salmon M, et al: Chemokine and chemokine receptor interactions provide a mechanism for selective T cell recruitment to specific liver compartments within hepatitis C-infected liver. J Immunol 163:6236, 1999.
177. Zlotnik A, Yoshic O: Chemokines: a new classification system and their role in immunity. Immunity 12:121, 2000.
178. Jung S, Littman DR: Chemokine receptors in lymphoid organ homeostasis. Curr Opin Immunol 11:319, 1999.
179. Sallusto F, Lenig D, Mackay CR, Lanzavecchia A: Flexible programs of chemokine receptor expression on human polarized T helper 1 and 2 lymphocytes. J Exp Med 187:875, 1998.
180. Bonechhi R, Bianchi G, Bordignon PP, et al: Differential expression of chemokine receptors and chemotactic responsiveness of type 1 T helper cells (Th1s) and Th2s. J Exp Med 187:129, 1998.
181. Murai M, Yoneyama H, Harada A, et al: Active participation of CCR5(+) T lymphocytes in the pathogenesis of liver injury in graft-versus-host disease. J Clin Invest 104:49, 1999.
182. Mehal WZ, Juedes AE, Crispe IN: Selective retention of activated CD8+ T cells by the normal liver. J Immunol 163:3202, 1999.
183. Cocchi F, DeVico AL, Garzino-Demo A, et al: Identification of RANTES, MIP-1 alpha, and MIP-1 beta as the major HIV-suppressive factors produced by $CD8^+$ T cells. Science 270:1811, 1995.
184. Geraghty DE: Structure of the class I region and expression of its resident genes. Curr Opin Immunol 5:3, 1993.
185. Hardy DA, Bell JI, Land EO, et al: Mapping of the class II region of the major histocompatibility complex. Nature 323:453, 1986.
186. Trowsdale J, Young JHI, Kelly AP, et al: Structure, sequence and polymorphism in the HLA-D region. Immunol Rev 85:5, 1985.
187. Trowsdale J, Campbell FD: Minireview. Complexity in the major histocompatibility complex. Eur J Immunol 19:45, 1992.
188. Carroll MC, Campbell DR, Bentley DR, Porter RR: A molecular map of the human major histocompatibility complex class III region linking complement genes C4, C2 and factor B. Nature 307:237, 1984.
189. Carroll MC, Katzman P, Alicot EM, et al: Linkage map of the human major histocompatibility complex including the tumor necrosis factor genes Proc Natl Acad Sci U S A 84:8535, 1987.
190. Kaufmann SHE: Heat shock proteins and the immune response. Immunol Today 11:129, 1990.
191. Zinkernagel RM, Doherty PC: Restriction of in vitro T-cell mediated cytotoxicity in lymphocytic choriomeningitis within a syngeneic or semi-allogeneic system. Nature 248:701, 1974.
192. Dembic Z, Hass W, Weiss S, et al: Transfer of specificity by murine alpha and beta T-cell receptor genes. Nature 320:232, 1986.
193. Kronenberg M, Siu G, Hood LE, Shasatri N: The molecular genetics of the T-cell antigen receptor and T-cell antigen recognition. Annu Rev Immunol 4:529, 1986.
194. Kappler JW, Roehm N, Marrack P: T-cell tolerance by clonal elimination in the thymus. Cell 49:273, 1987.
195. Morahan G, Allison J, Miller SF: Tolerance of class I histocompatibility antigens expressed extrathymically. Nature 339:622, 1989.
196. Mackay IR: Genetic aspects of immunologically mediated liver disease. Semin Liver Dis 4:13, 1984.
197. Krawitt EL, Albertini RJ: Immunogenetics of autoimmune chronic active hepatitis. In Meyer zum Büschenfelde KH, Hoofnagle JH, Manns M, eds: Immunology and the Liver. Boston, Kluwer Academic Press, 1993:240.
198. Donaldson P, Doherty D, Underhill J, Williams R: The molecular genetics of autoimmune liver disease. Hepatology 20:225, 1994.
199. Seki T, Kiyosawa K, Inoko H, Ota M: Association of autoimmune hepatitis with HLA-Bw54 and DR4 in Japanese patients. Hepatology 12:130, 1990.
200. Scully LJ, Toze C, Sengar DP, Goldstein R: Early onset autoimmune hepatitis is associated with a C4A gene deletion. Gastroenterology 104:1478, 1993.
201. Doherty DG, Donaldson PT, Underhill GA, et al: Allelic sequence variation in the class II genes and proteins in patients with autoimmune hepatitis. Hepatology 19:609, 1994.
202. Donaldson PD: Genetics of autoimmune liver disease. In Manns M, Paumgartner G, Leuschner U, eds: Immunology of the Liver. Lancaster, Penn, Kluwer Publishers, 2000:115.
203. Ota M, Seki T, Kiyosawa, et al: A possible association between basic amino acids at position 13 of DRB1 chains and autoimmune hepatitis. Immunogenetics 36:49, 2000.
204. Campbell RD, Trowsdale J: Map of the human MHC. Immunol Today 14:349, 1993.
205. Donaldson PT, Farrant JM, Wilkinson ML, et al: Dual association of HLA DR2 and DR3 with primary sclerosing cholangitis. Hepatology 14:129, 1991.
206. Spurkland A, Saarinen S, Bopberg KM, et al: HLA class II haplotypes in primary sclerosing cholangitis patients from five European populations. Tissue Antigens 53(5):459, 1999.
207. Chapman RW: Primary sclerosing cholangitis as an autoimmune disease: pros and cons. In Manns MP, Paumgartner G, Leuschner U, eds: Immunology of the Liver. Lancaster, Penn, Kluwer Academic Publishers, 2000:279.
208. Bernal W, Maloney M, Underhill J, Donaldson PT: Association of tumor necrosis factor polymorphism with primary sclerosing cholangitis. J Hepatol 30:237, 1999.
209. Wilson GA, Symons JA, McDowell TL, et al: Effects of a polymorphism in the human tumor necrosis factor α promoter on transcriptional activation. Immunology 94:3195, 1997.
210. Farrant JM, Doherty DG, Donaldson PT, et al: Amino acid substitutions at position 38 of the DR beta polypeptide confer susceptibility to and protection from primary sclerosing cholangitis. Hepatology 16:390, 1992.
211. Olerup O, Olsson R, Hultcrantz R, et al: HLA-DR and HLA-DQ are not markers for rapid disease progression in primary sclerosing cholangitis. Gastroenterology 108:870, 1995.
212. Mehal W, Lo Y, Wordsworth B, et al: HLA DR4 is a marker for rapid disease progression in primary sclerosing cholangitis. Gastroenterology 106:160, 1994.
213. Begovich A, Klitz W, Moonsamy PV, et al: Genes within the HLA class II region confer both predisposition and resistance to primary biliary cirrhosis. Tissue Antigens 43:71, 1994.
214. Briggs DC, Donaldson PT, Hayes P, et al: A major histocompatibility complex class III allotype C4B2 associated with primary biliary cirrhosis. Tissue Antigens 29:141, 1987.
215. Manns MP, Bremm A, Schneider PM, et al: HLA DRw8 and complement C4 deficiency as risk factors in primary biliary cirrhosis. Gastroenterology 101:1367, 1991.
216. Mella J, Roschmann E, Maier K, Volk B: Association of primary biliary cirrhosis with the allele HLA DPB1*0301 in a German population. Hepatology 21:398, 1995.
217. Maeda T, Onoshi S, Saibara T, et al: HLA DR8 and primary biliary cirrhosis. Gastroenterology 103:1118, 1992.
218. Seki T, Kiyosawa K, Ota M, et al: Association of primary biliary cirrhosis with human leukocyte antigen DPB1*0501 in Japanese patients. Hepatology 18:73, 1993.
219. Mukai T, Kimura A, Ishibashi H, et al: Association of HLA DRB1*0803 and *1602 with susceptibility to primary biliary cirrhosis. Int Hepat Commun 3:207, 1995.
220. Underhill JA, Donaldson PT, Bray G, et al: Susceptibility to primary biliary cirrhosis is associated with the HLA DR8-DQB1*0402 haplotype. Hepatology 16:1404, 1992.
221. Jones DEJ, Watt FE, Gove H, et al: Tumour necrosis factor—a promoter polymorphism in primary biliary cirrhosis. J Hepatol 30:232, 1999.
222. Thursz MR, Kwiatowski D, Allsopp CEM, et al: Association between an MHC class II allele and clearance of hepatic B virus in the Gambia. N Engl J Med 332:1065, 1995.

223. Thio CL, Carrington M, O'Brien SJ, et al:The association of HLA alleles and clearance of hepatitis B among African Americans. H Infect Dis 179(4):1004, 1999.
224. Almarri, A, Batchelor JR: HLA and hepatitis B infection. Lancet 344:1194, 1994.
225. Höhler T, Gerken G, Notghi A, et al: HLA-DRB1*1301 and *1302 protect against chronic hepatitis B. J Hepatol 26:503, 1997.
226. Diepholder HM, Jung MC, Keller E, et al: A vigorous virus-specific CD4+ T-cell response may contribute to the association of HLA-DR13 with viral clearance in hepatitis B. Clin Exp Immunol 113:244, 1998.
227. Thursz M, Thomas HC, Greenwood BM, Hill AVS: Heterozygote advantage for HLA class-II type in hepatitis B virus infection. Nature Genetics 17:111, 1997.
228. Höhler T, Kruger A, Gerken G, et al: A tumor necrosis factor-alpha (TNF-alpha) promoter polymorphism is associated with chronic hepatitis B infection. Clin Exp Immunol 111(3):579, 1998.
229. Sheron N, Lau J, Daniels H, et al: Increased production of tumour necrosis factor alpha in chronic hepatitis B virus infection. J Hepatol 12(2):241, 1991.
230. Marinos G, Naoumov NV, Rossol S, et al: Tumor necrosis factor receptors in patients with chronic hepatitis B virus infection. Gastroenterology 108(5):1453, 1995.
231. Summerfield JA, Ryder S, Sumiya M, et al: Mannose binding protein gene mutations associated with unusual and severe infections in adults. Lancet 345:886, 1995.
232. Thomas HC, Foster GR, Sumiya M, et al: Mutation of gene of mannose-binding protein associated with chronic hepatitis B viral infection. Lancet 348:1417, 1996.
233. Yuen MF, Lau CS, Lau YL, et al: Mannose binding lectin gene mutations are associated with progression of liver disease in chronic hepatitis B infection. Hepatology 29(4):1248, 1999.
234. Höhler T, Wunschel M, Gerken, G, et al: No association between mannose-binding lectin alleles and susceptibility to chronic hepatitis B virus infection in German patients. Exp Clin Immunogenet 15(3):130, 1998.
235. Bellamy R, Ruwende C, McAdam KP, et al: Mannose binding protein deficiency is not associated with malaria, hepatitis B carriage nor tuberculosis in Africans. Q J Med 91(1):13, 1998.
236. Cramp ME, Carucci P, Underhill J, et al: Association between HLA class II genotype and spontaneous clearance of hepatitis C viraemia. J Hepatol 29(2):207, 1998.
237. Alric L, For M, Izopet J, et al: Genes of the major histocompatibility complex class II influence the outcome of hepatitis C virus infection. Gastroenterology 113(5):1675, 1997.
238. Minton EJ, Smilie D, Neal KR, et al: Association between MHC class II alleles and clearance of circulating hepatitis C virus. J Infect Dis 178(1):39, 1998.
239. Kuzushita N, Hayashi N, Katayama K, et al: Increased frequency of HLA DR13 in hepatitis C virus carriers with persistently normal ALT levels. J Med Virol 48(1):1, 1996.
240. Peano G, Menardi G, Ponzetto A, Fenglio LM: HLA-DR5 antigen: a genetic factor influencing the outcome of hepatitis C virus infection. Arch Int Med 154:273, 1994.
241. Yasunami R, Miyamoto T, Kanda T: HLA-DRB1 is related to pathological changes of the liver in chronic hepatitis C. Hepatol Res 7:3, 1997.
242. Tibbs C, Donaldson P, Underhill JA, et al: Evidence that the HLA DQA1*03 allele confers protection from chronic HCV-infection in Northern European Caucasoids. Hepatology 24:1342, 1996.
243. Higashi Y, Kamikawaji N, Suko H, Ando M: Analysis of HLA alleles in Japanese patients with cirrhosis due to chronic hepatitis C. J Gastro Hepatol 11(3):241, 1996.
244. Höhler T, Gerken G, Notghi A, et al: MHC class II genes influence the susceptibility to chronic active hepatitis C. J Hepatol 27:259, 1997.
245. Thursz M, Yallop R, Goldin R, et al: Influence of MHC class II genotypes on the outcome of infection with hepatitis C virus. Lancet 354:2119, 1999.
246. Fanning LJ, Levis J, Kenny-Walsh E, et al: Viral clearance in hepatitis C (1b) infection: relationship with human leukocyte antigen class II in a homologous population. Hepatology 31(6):1334, 2000.
247. McKiernan SM, Hagan R, Curry M, et al: The MHC is a major determinant of viral status, but not fibrotic stage, in individuals infected with hepatitis C. Gastroenterology 118:1124, 2000.
248. Mitchel LS, Jeffers LJ, Reddy KR, et al: Detection of hepatitis C virus antibody by first and second generation assays and polymerase chain reaction in patients with autoimmune chronic active hepatitis types I, II, and III. Am J Gastroenterol 88:1027, 1993.
249. Philipp J, Durrazo M, Trautwein CH, et al: Recognition of uridine diphosphate glucuronosyl transferase by LKM_3 antibodies in chronic hepatitis D. Lancet 344:578, 1994.
250. Lohse AW, Gerken G, Mohr H, et al: Relation between autoimmune liver diseases and viral hepatitis: clinical and serological characteristics in 859 patients. Ger J Gastroenterol 33:527, 1995.
251. Mayet WH, Hess G, Gerken G, et al: Treatment of chronic type B hepatitis with recombinant alpha interferon induces autoantibodies not specific for autoimmune chronic hepatitis. Hepatology 10:24, 1989.
252. Michel G, Ritter A, Gerken G, et al: Anti-GOR and hepatitis C virus in autoimmune liver diseases. Lancet 339:267, 1992.
253. Löhr HF, Gerken G, Michel G, et al: In vitro secretion of anti-GOR protein and anti-hepatitis C virus antibodies in patients with chronic hepatitis C. Gastroenterology 107:1443, 1994.
254. Treichel U, Schreiter T, Tassopoulous N, et al: Zur Bedeutung des Nachweises zirkulierender Autoantikörper bei 257 Patienten mit akuter Hepatitis. Ger J Gastroenterol 1:96, 1996.
255. Huppertz HI, Treichel U, Gassel AM, et al: Autoimmune hepatitis following hepatitis A virus infection. J Hepatol 23:204, 1995.
256. Laskus T, Slusarczyk J: Autoimmune chronic active hepatitis developing after acute type B hepatitis. Dig Dis Sci 34:1294, 1989.
257. McFarlane IG: Autoimmunity and hepatotropic viruses. Semin Liver Dis 11:221, 1991.
258. Meyer zum Büschenfelde KH, Lohse AW, Manns M, Poralla T: Autoimmunity and liver disease. Hepatology 12:354, 1998.
259. Manns MP: Cytoplasmic autoantigens in autoimmune hepatitis: molecular analysis and clinical relevance. Semin Liver Dis 11:205, 1991.
260. Manns M, Gerken G, Kyriatsoulis A, et al: Characterization of a new subgroup of autoimmune chronic active hepatitis by autoantibodies against a soluble liver antigen. Lancet 1:292, 1987.
261. Wies I, Brunner S, Henninger J, et al: Identification of target antigen for SLA/LP autoantibodies in autoimmune hepatitis. Lancet 355:1510, 2000.
262. Meyer zum Büschenfelde KH, Schrank CH: Untersuchungen zur Frage organspezifischer Antigene der Leber. Klinische Wochenschr 44:654, 1966.
263. Meyer zum Büschenfelde KH, Miescher PA: Liver-specific antigens, purification and characterization. Clin Exp Immunol 10:89, 1972.
264. Meyer zum Büschenfelde KH, Kössling FK, Miescher PA: Experimental chronic active hepatitis in rabbits following immunization with human liver proteins. Clin Exp Immunol 10:99, 1972.
265. Hopf U, Meyer zum Büschenfelde KH: Studies on the pathogenesis of experimental chronic hepatitis in rabbits. II. Demonstration of immunoglobulin on isolated hepatocytes. Br J Exp Pathol 55:509, 1974.
266. Lohse AW, Manns M, Dienes HP, et al: Experimental autoimmune hepatitis: disease induction, time course and T-cell reactivity. Hepatology 11:24, 1990.
267. Takahashi H, Zeniya M. The Japanese animal models of autoimmune hepatitis. In: McFarlane IG, Williams R, ed: Molecular Basis of Autoimmune Hepatitis. London, Chapman and Hall, 1996:165.
268. McFarlane IG, Hegarty JE, McSorley CG, et al: Antibodies to liver-specific protein predict outcome of treatment withdrawal in autoimmune chronic active hepatitis. Lancet ii:954, 1984.
269. Meyer zum Büschenfelde KH, Manns M, Hütteroth T, et al: LM-Ag and LSP—two different target antigens involved in the immunopathogenesis of chronic active hepatitis? Clin Exp Immunol 37:205, 1979.
270. McFarlane BM, McSorley CG, Vergani D, et al: Serum autoantibodies reacting with the hepatic asialglycoprotein receptor protein (hepatic lectin) in acute and chronic liver disorders. J Hepatol 3:196, 1986.
271. Treichel U, McFarlane BM, Seki T, et al: Demographics of anti-asialoglycoprotein receptor autoantibodies in autoimmune hepatitis. Gastroenterology 107:799, 1994.
272. Toda G, Ikeda Y, Kashiwagi M, et al: Hepatocyte plasma membrane glycosphingolipid reactive with sera from patients with autoimmune chronic active hepatitis: its identification as sulfatide. Hepatology 12:664, 1990.

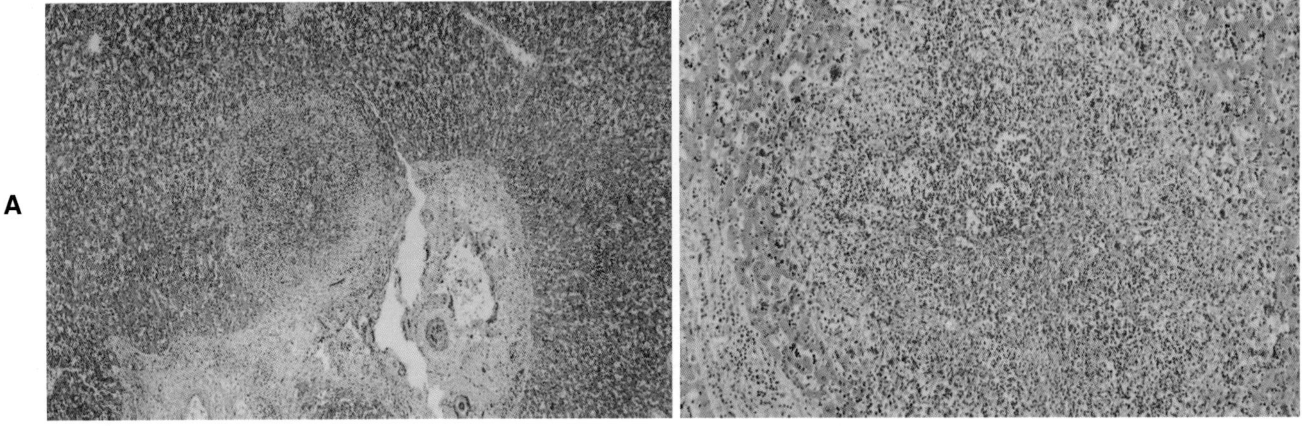

Plate 36-1 **A** and **B,** Granulomatous hepatitis resulting from *Brucella abortus* infection. (Courtesy David A. Schwartz, MD, Atlanta, Georgia.)

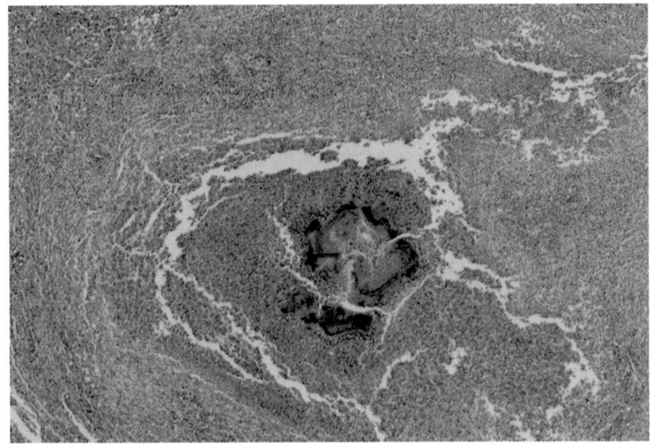

Plate 36-2 Hepatic necrosis and sulfur granules in actinomycosis. (Courtesy David A. Schwartz, MD, Atlanta, Georgia.)

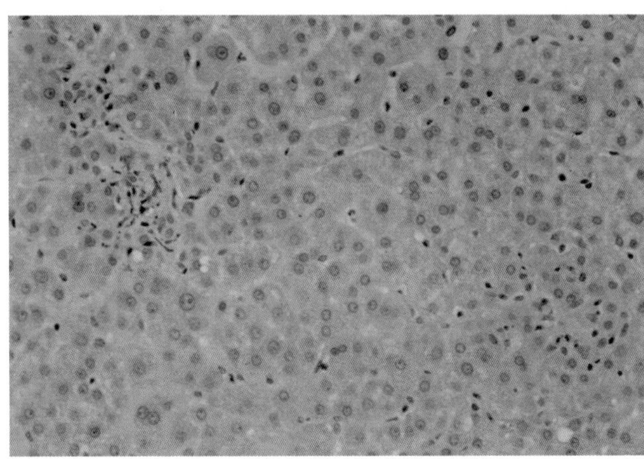

Plate 36-3 Portal triaditis in secondary syphilis. (Courtesy David A. Schwartz, MD, Atlanta, Georgia.)

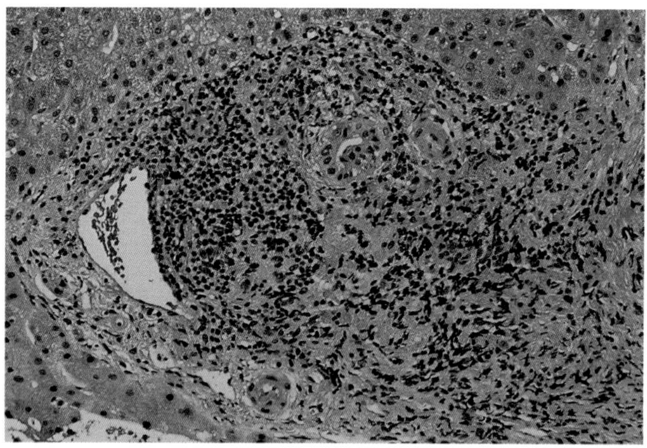

Plate 39-1 Florid duct lesion in stage I primary biliary cirrhosis. (Courtesy of Lawrence Burgart, MD. Mayo Foundation, Rochester, Minn.)

273. Poralla T, Ramadori G, Dienes HP, et al: Liver cell damage caused by monoclonal antibody against an organ-specific membrane antigen in vivo and in vitro. J Hepatol 4:373, 1987.
274. Hopf U, Jahn HU, Möller B, et al: Liver membrane antibodies (LMA) recognize a 26-kD protein on the hepatocellular surface. Clin Exp Immunol 79;54, 1990.
275. Swanson NR, Reed WD, Yarred LJ, et al: Autoantibodies to isolated plasma membranes in chronic active hepatitis. II. Specificity of antibodies. Hepatology 11:613, 1990.
276. Hopf U, Meyer zum Büschenfelde KH, Arnold W: Detection of a liver membrane autoantibody in HbsAg-negative chronic hepatitis. N Engl J Med 294:587, 1976.
277. Hopf U, Arnold W, Meyer zum Büschenfelde KH, et al: Studies on the pathogenesis of chronic inflammatory liver diseases. I. Membrane-fixed IgG on isolated hepatocytes from patients. Clin Exp Immunol 22:1, 1975.
278. Lohse AW, Kögel M, Meyer zum Büschenfelde KH: Evidence for spontaneous immunosuppression in autoimmune hepatitis. Hepatology 22:381, 1995.
279. Dienes HP, Popper H, Manns M, et al: Histologic features in autoimmune hepatitis. Z Gastroenterol 27:325, 1989.
280. Dienes HP, Autschbach F, Gerber MA: Ultrastructural lesion in autoimmune hepatitis and steps of the immune response in liver tissue. Semin Liver Dis 11:197, 1991.
281. Poralla T, Treichel U, Löhr H, Fleischer B: The asialoglycoprotein receptor as target structure in autoimmune liver diseases. Semin Liver Dis 11:215, 1991.
282. McFarlane BM, Sipos J, Gove CD, et al: Antibodies against the hepatic asialoglycoprotein receptor perfused in situ preferentially attach to periportal liver cells in the rat. Hepatology 11:408, 1990.
283. Mieli-Vergani G, Vergani D, Jenkins PJ, et al: Lymphocyte cytotoxicity to autologous hepatocytes in HBsAg-negative chronic active hepatitis. Clin Exp Immunol 38:16, 1979.
284. Jensen DM, McFarlane IG, Portmann BS, et al: Detection of antibodies directed against liver-specific membrane lipoprotein in patients with acute and chronic active hepatitis. N Engl Med 299:1, 1978.
285. Kakumu S, Arakawa Y, Goyi H, et al: Occurrence and significance of antibody to liver-specific membrane lipoprotein by double-antibody immunoprecipitation method in sera of patients with acute and chronic liver diseases. Gastroenterology 76:665, 1979.
286. Treichel U, Gerken G, Rossol S, et al: Autoantibodies against the human asialoglycoprotein receptor: effects of therapy in autoimmune and virus-induced chronic active hepatitis. J Hepatol 19:55, 1993.
287. Cohen IR, Miller A: Autoimmune disease models. New York, Academic Press, 1994.
288. Wen L, Peakman M, Lobo-Yeo A, et al: T-cell-directed hepatocyte damage in autoimmune chronic active hepatitis. Lancet 336:1527, 1990.
289. Löhr H, Treichel U, Poralla T, et al: The human hepatic asialoglycoprotein receptor is a target antigen for liver-infiltrating T cells in autoimmune chronic active hepatitis and primary biliary cirrhosis. Hepatology 12:1314, 1990.
290. Löhr H, Treichel U, Poralla T, et al: Liver-infiltrating T helper cells in autoimmune chronic active hepatitis stimulate the production of autoantibodies against the human asialoglycoprotein receptor in vitro. Clin Exp Immunol 88:45, 1992.
291. Löhr H, Schlaak JF, Gerken G, et al: Phenotypical analysis and cytokine release of liver-infiltrating and peripheral blood T lymphocytes from patients with chronic hepatitis of different etiology. Liver 14:161, 1994.
292. Löhr H, Manns M, Kyriatsoulis A, et al: Clonal analysis of liver-infiltrating T cells in patients with LKM-1 antibody-positive autoimmune chronic active hepatitis. Clin Exp Immunol 84:297, 1991.
293. Hussain MJ, Mowat AP, Miele-Vergani G, Vergani D: Circulating levels of interleukin-1α, tumor necrosis factor, interferon-γ and soluble interleukin-2 receptor are high in children with autoimmune chronic liver disease. Hepatology 12:937, 1990.
294. Schlaak JF, Löhr H, Gallati H, et al: Analysis of the in vitro cytokine production by liver-infiltrating T cells of patients with autoimmune hepatitis. Clin Exp Immunol 94:168, 1993.
295. Treichel U, Paietta E, Poralla T, et al: Effects of cytokines on synthesis and function of the hepatic asialoglycoprotein receptor. J Cell Physiol 158:527, 1994.
296. Kudo M, Todo A, Ikekubo K, et al: Evaluation of asialoglycoprotein receptor-binding, synthetic radiolabeled glycoprotein in estimating hepatic functional reserve. Acta Hepatol Jap 28:1277, 1987.
297. Weiss P, Ashwell G: Ligand-induced modulation of the hepatic receptor for asialoglycoproteins. Evidence for the role of cell surface hyposialylation. J Biol Chem 264:11572, 1989.
298. Sawamura T, Nakada H, Hazama H, et al: Hyperasialoglycoproteinemia in patients with chronic liver diseases and liver cell carcinoma. Gastroenterology 87:1217, 1984.
299. Paulson JC, Weinstein J, Schauer A: Tissue-specific expression of sialyltransferase. J Biol Chem 264:10931, 1989.
300. Leist M, Gantner F, Bohlinger I, et al: Tumor necrosis factor-induced hepatocyte apoptosis precedes liver failure in experimental murine shock models. Am J Pathol 146:5, 1995.
301. Leist M, Gantner F, Jilg S, Wendel A: Activation of the 55 kDa TNF receptor is necessary and sufficient for TNF-induced liver failure, hepatocyte apoptosis, and nitrite release. J Immunol 154:1307, 1995.
302. Zeniya M, Kuramoto A, et al: Immunologic mechanism of autoimmune hepatitis: a review on the molecular analysis of T-cell receptor. In Yamanaka M, Toda G, Tanaka T, eds: Progress in Hepatology, vol 5, Liver and Immunology, Excerpta Medica, 1999:95.
303. Hoshino YX, Enomoto N, Izumi N, et al: Limited usage of T cell receptor β chains and sequences of the complementarity determining region three of lymphocytes infiltrating in the liver of autoimmune hepatitis. Hepatology 22:142, 1995.
304. Arenz M, Meyer zum Büschenfelde KH, Löhr HF: Limited T cell receptor Vβ-chain repertoire of liver-infiltrating T cells in autoimmune hepatitis. J Hepatol 28:70, 1998.
305. Lehmann PV, Forsthuber T, Alexander M, et al: Determinant spreading and the dynamics of an autoantigen. Nature 358:155, 1992.
306. Lehmann PV, Sercarz EE, Forsthuber T, et al: Determinant spreading and the dynamics of the autoimmune T cell repertoire. Immunol Today 14:203, 1993.
307. Kuramoto A: Gene expression of liver infiltrating T cell receptor β chain variable region (TCR Vβ) in autoimmune hepatitis. Tokyo Jikeikai Med J 111:927, 1996.
308. Thorpe ME, Scheuer PJ, Sherlock S: Primary sclerosing cholangitis, the biliary tree and ulcerative colitis. Gut 8:435, 1967.
309. Chapman RW, Marborgh BA, Rhodes JM, et al: Primary sclerosing cholangitis: a review of its clinical features, cholangiography, and hepatic histology. Gut 21:870, 1980.
310. Zauli D, Schrumpf E, Crespi C, et al: An autoantibody profile in primary sclerosing cholangitis. J Hepatol 5:14, 1987.
311. Bodenheimer HC, LaRusso NF, Thayer WP Jr, et al: Elevated circulating immune complexes in primary sclerosing cholangitis. Hepatology 3:150, 1983.
312. Alberti-Flor JJ, de Medina M, Jeffeers L, et al: Elevated immunoglobulins and immune complexes in the bile of patients with primary sclerosing cholangitis. Hepatology 3:844, 1983.
313. Minuk GY, Angus M, Brickman CM, et al: Abnormal clearance of immune complexes from the circulation of patients with primary sclerosing cholangitis. Gastroenterology 88:166, 1985.
314. Lawley TJ, Hall RP, Fauci AS: Defective Fc-receptor functions associated with the HLA B8/DRW3 haplotype. N Engl J Med 304:185, 1981.
315. Brinch L, Teisberg P, Schrumpf E, et al: The in vivo metabolism of C3 in hepatobiliary disease associated with ulcerative colitis. Scand J Gastroenterol 17:523, 1982.
316. Senaldi G, Donaldson PT, Magrin S, et al: Activation of the complement system in primary sclerosing cholangitis. Gastroenterology 97:1430, 1989.
317. Snook JA, Chapman RW, Fleming K, et al: Anti-neutrophil nuclear antibody in ulcerative colitis, Crohn's disease, and primary sclerosing cholangitis. Clin Exp Immunol 76:30, 1989.
318. Duerr RH, Targan SR, Landers CJ, et al: Neutrophilic cytoplasmic antibodies: a link between primary sclerosing cholangitis and ulcerative colitis. Gastroenterology 100:1385, 1991.
319. Klein R, Eisenburg J, Weber P, et al: Significance and specificity of antibodies to neutrophils detected by Western blotting for the serological diagnosis of primary sclerosing cholangitis. Hepatology 14:1147, 1991.
320. Terjung B, Herzog V, Worman HJ, et al: Atypical antineutrophil antibodies with perinuclear fluorescence in chronic inflammatory bowel disease and the hepatobiliary disorders colocalize with nuclear envelope lamina proteins. Hepatology 28:332, 1998.

321. Mulder AHL, Horst G, Haagsma EB, et al: Prevalence and characterization of neutrophil cytoplasmic autoantibodies in autoimmune liver disease. Hepatology 17:411, 1993.
322. Ellerbroek PM, Oudkerk Pool M, Ridwan BU, et al: Neutrophil cytoplasmic antibodies (p-ANCA) in ulcerative colitis. J Clin Pathol 47:257, 1994.
323. Mulder AHL, Broskroelofs J, Horst G, et al: Anti-neutrophil cytoplasmic antibodies (ANCA) in inflammatory bowel disease: characterization and clinical correlates. Clin Exp Immunol 95:490, 1994.
324. Targan SR, Landers C, Vidrich A, Czaja AI: High-titer antineutrophil cytoplasmic antibodies in type-1 autoimmune hepatitis. Gastroentrology 108:1159, 1995.
325. Orth T, Gerken G, Kellner R, et al: Actin is a target antigen of antineutrophil cytoplasmic antibodies (ANCA) in autoimmune hepatitis type-1. J Hepatol 26:37, 1997.
326. Seibold F, Siametschka D, Gregor M, et al: Neutrophil autoantibodies. A genetic marker in primary sclerosing cholangitis and ulcerative colitis. Gastroentrology 107:532, 1994.
327. Orth T, Kellner R, Diekmann O, et al: Identification and characterization of autoantibodies against catalase and alpha-enolase in patients with primary sclerosing cholangitis. Clin Exp Immunol 112:507, 1998.
328. Roozendaal C, Zhao MH, Horst G, et al: Catalase and α-enolase: two novel granulocyte autoantigens in inflammatory bowel disease (IBD). Clin Exp Immunol 112:10, 1998.
329. Peen E, Almer S, Bodemar G, et al: Anti-lactoferrin antibodies and other types of ANCA in ulcerative colitis, primary sclerosing cholangitis, and Crohn's disease. Gut 34:56, 1993.
330. Lo SK, Fleming KA, Chapman RW: A 2-year follow-up study of antineutrophil antibody in primary sclerosing cholangitis: relationship to clinical activity, liver biochemistry and ursodeoxycholic acid treatment. J Hepatol 21(6):974, 1994.
331. Orth T, Neurath M, Schirmacher P, et al: Anti-neutrophil cytoplasmic antibodies in a rat model of trinitrobenzenesulphonic acid-induced liver injury. Eur J Clin Invest 29:929, 1999.
332. Ort T, Neurath M, Schirmacher P, et al: A novel rat model of chronic fibrosing cholangitis induced by local administration of a hapten reagent into the dilated bile duct is associated with increased TNF-α production and autoantibodies. J Hepatol 33:862, 2000.
333. Chapman RW, Cottone M, Selby WS, et al: Serum autoantibodies, ulcerative colitis, and primary sclerosing cholangitis. Gut 27:86, 1986.
334. Mandal A, Dasgupta A, Jeffers L, et al: Autoantibodies in sclerosing cholangitis against a shared peptide in biliary and colon epithelium. Gastroenterology 106:185, 1994.
335. Das KM, Vecchi M, Sakamaki S: A shared and unique epitope(s) on human colon, skin, and biliary epithelium detected by a monoclonal antibody. Gastroentrology 98:464, 1990.
336. Whiteside TL, Lasky S, Lusheng S, et al: Immunologic analysis of mononuclear cells in liver tissues and blood of patients with primary sclerosing cholangitis. Hepatology 5:468, 1985.
337. Lindor KD, Wiesner RH, Katzman JA, et al: Lymphocyte subsets in primary sclerosing cholangitis. Dig Dis Sci 32:720, 1987.
338. Snook JA, Chapman RW, Sachdev GK, et al: Peripheral blood and portal tract lymphocyte populations in primary sclerosing cholangitis. J Hepatol 9:36, 1989.
339. Lindor KD, Wiesner RH, LaRusso NF, et al: Enhanced autoreactivity in T-lymphocytes in primary sclerosing cholangitis. Hepatology 7:884, 1987.
340. Chapman RW, Kelly PM, Heryet A, et al: Expression of HLA-DR antigens on bile duct epithelium in primary sclerosing cholangitis. Gut 29(4):422, 1988.
341. Bloom S, Fleming K, Chapman R: Adhesion molecule expression in primary sclerosing cholangitis and primary biliary cirrhosis. Gut 36(4):604, 1995.
342. Dienes HP, Lohse AW, Gerken G, et al: Bile duct epithelia as target cells in primary biliary cirrhosis and primary sclerosing cholangitis. Virchows Arch 431:119, 1997.
343. Broomé U, Grunwald J, Scheynius A, et al: Preferential V beta3 usage by hepatic T lymphocytes in patients with primary sclerosing cholangitis. J Hepatol 26:527, 1997.
344. Probert CS, Christ AD, Saubermann LJ, et al: Analysis of human common bile duct-associated T cells: evidence of oligoclonality, T cell clonal persistence, and epithelial cell recognition. J Immunol 158:1941, 1997.
345. Tjandra K, Sharkey K, Swain MG: Progressive development of a Th-1-type hepatic cytokine profile in rats with experimental cholangitis. Hepatology 31:280, 2000.
346. Gohlke F, Lohse AW, Dienes HP, et al: Evidence for an overlap of autoimmune hepatitis and primary sclerosing cholangitis. J Hepatol 24:699, 1996.
347. Van Bauren HR, von Hoogstraten HJF, Terkivatan T, et al: High prevalence of autoimmune hepatitis among patients with primary sclerosing cholangitis. J Hepatol 33:543, 2000.
348. Mackay JR, Gershwin ME:. The nature of autoimmune disease. Semin Liver Dis 17:3, 1997.
349. Berg PA, Klein R, Lindenbom-Fontinos J: Antimitochondrial antibodies in primary biliary cirrhosis. J Hepatol 123:2, 1986.
350. Manns M, Gerken G, Kyriatsoulis A, et al: Two different subtypes of antimitochondrial antibodies are associated with primary biliary cirrhosis: identification and characterization by radioimmunoassay and immunoblotting. Hepatology 7:893, 1987.
351. Gershwin ME, Mackay JR, Sturgens A, Coppel RL: Identification and specificity of a cDNA encoding the 70 kD mitochondrial antigens recognized in primary biliary cirrhosis. J Immunol 138:3525, 1987.
352. Yeaman SJ, Fussey SPM, Mutimer DJ, et al: M2 autoantigens in primary biliary cirrhosis. Lancet 1:103, 1989.
353. Surh CD, Danner DJ, Ahmed A, et al: Reactivity of primary biliary cirrhosis sera with a human dehydrogenase dihydroliposamide acyltransferase, the 52 kD mitochondrial autoantigen. Hepatology 9:63, 1989.
354. Leung PSC, Coppel RL, Ansari A, et al: Antimitochondrial antibodies in primary biliary cirrhosis. Semin Liver Dis 17:61, 1997.
355. Worman HJ, Terjung B, Courvalin JC: Nuclear protein antigens in primary biliary cirrhosis. In Manns M, Paumgartner G, Leuschner U, eds: Immunology of the Liver. Dordrecht/Boston/London, Kluwer Academic Publishers, 2000:257.
356. Gerace L, Ottaviano Y, Kondor-Koch C: Identification of a major polypeptide of the nuclear pore complex. J Cell Biol 95:826, 1982.
357. Courvalin JC, Lassoned K, Bartnik E, et al: The 210 kD nuclear envelope polypeptide recognized by human autoantibodies in primary biliary cirrhosis is the major glycoprotein of the nuclear pore. J Clin Invest 86:279, 1990.
358. Szostecki C, Krippner H, Penner E, Boutz FA: Autoimmune sera recognize a 100 kD nuclear protein antigen (sp-100). Clin Exp Immunol 68:108, 1987.
359. Van de Water J, Shimoda S, Niko Y, et al: The role of T cells in primary biliary cirrhosis. Semin Liver Dis 17:105, 1997.
360. Van de Water J, Ansari A, Surh CD, et al: Evidence for the targeting by 2-oxo-dehydrogenase enzymes in the T cell response of primary biliary cirrhosis. J Immunol 146:89, 1991.
361. Löhr H, Fleischer B, Gerken G, et al: Autoreactive liver-infiltrating T cells in primary biliary cirrhosis recognize inner mitochondrial epitopes and the pyruvate dehydrogenase complex. J Hepatol 18:322, 1993.
362. Van de Water J, Ansari A, Prindiville T, et al: Heterogeneity of autoreactive T cell clones specific for the E2 component of the pyruvate dehydrogenase complex in primary biliary cirrhosis. J Exp Med 181:723, 1995.
363. Jones DEJ, Palmer JM, James OFW, et al: T cell responses to the components of pyruvate dehydrogenase complex in primary biliary cirrhosis. Hepatology 21:995, 1995.
364. Jones DEJ, Palmer JM, Yeaman SJ, et al: T cell responses to natural human proteins in primary biliary cirrhosis. Clin Exp Immunol 107:562, 1997.
365. Bassendine MF, Jones DEJ, Yeaman SJ: Biochemistry and autoimmune response to the 2-oxoacid dehydrogenase complexes in primary biliary cirrhosis. Semin Liver Dis 17:49, 1997.
366. Moebius U, Manns M, Hess G, et al: T cell receptor gene rearrangements of T lymphocytes infiltrating the liver in chronic active hepatitis B and primary biliary cirrhosis (PBC): oligoclonality of PBC-derived T cell clones. Eur J Immunol 20:889, 1990.
367. Mayo MJ, Combes B, Jenkins RN: T-cell receptor V beta gene utilization in primary biliary cirrhosis. Hepatology 24:1148, 1996.
368. Diu A, Moebius U, Ferradini L, et al: Limited T cell receptor diversity in liver-infiltrating lymphocytes from patients with primary biliary cirrhosis. J Autoimmunity 6:611, 1993.
369. Tsai SL, Lai MY, Chen DS: Analysis of rearranged T cell receptor (TCR) Vβ usage suggests antigen-driven selection. Clin Exp Immunol 103:99, 1996.

370. Ohmoto M, Yamamoto K, Nagano T, et al: Accumulation of multiple T cell clonotypes in the liver of primary biliary cirrhosis. Hepatology 25:33, 1997.
371. Shimoda S, Nakamura M, Ishibashi H, et al: HLA DRB4 0101-restricted immuno-dominant T cell autoepitope of pyruvate dehydrogenase complex in primary biliary cirrhosis: evidence of molecular mimicry in human autoimmune diseases. J Exp Med 181:1835, 1995.
372. Ichiki Y, Shimoda S, Hara H, et al: Analysis of T cell receptor β of the T cell clones reactive to the human PDC-E2 163-176 peptide in the context of HLA-DR53 in patients with primary biliary cirrhosis. Hepatology 26:728, 1997.
373. Palmer JM, Diamond AG, Yeaman SJ, et al: T cell responses to the putative dominant autoepitope in primary biliary cirrhosis (PBC). Clin Exp Immunol 116:133, 1999.
374. Ochiai H, Sekine H, Ohira H, et al: Analysis of peripheral blood mononuclear cells stimulated with pyruvate dehydrogenase complex, T cell receptors from patients with primary biliary cirrhosis. J Gastroenterol 33:694, 1998.
375. Pingel S, Arens M, Weyer S, et al: Pyruvate dehydrogenase specific T cells in primary biliary cirrhosis show restricted antigen recognition sites. Liver 2002, (in press).
376. Borgulyia P, Kishi H, Uematsu Y, von Boehmer H: Exclusion and inclusion of α and β T cell receptor alleles. Cell 69:529, 1992.
377. Sarukhan A, Garcia C, Lanoue A, von Boehmer H: Allelic inclusion of T cell receptor α genes poses an autoimmune hazard due to low-level expression of autospecific receptors. Immunity 8:563, 1998.
378. Shimoda S, Van de Water J, Ansari A, et al: Identification and precursor frequency analysis of a common T cell epitope motif in mitochondrial autoantigens in primary biliary cirrhosis. J Clin Invest 102:1831, 1998.
379. Shimoda S, Nakamura M, Shigematsu H, et al: Mimicry peptides of human PDC-E2 163-176 peptides, the immunodominant T-cell epitope of primary biliary cirrhosis. Hepatology 31:1212, 2000.
380. Tsuneyama K, Van de Water J, Leung PSC, et al: Abnormal expression of the E2 component of the pyruvate dehydrogenase complex on the luminal surface of biliary epithelium occurs before major histocompatibility complex class II and BB1/B7 expression. Hepatology 21:1031, 1995.
381. Joplin R, Gershwin ME: Ductular expression of autoantigens in primary biliary cirrhosis. Semin Liver Dis 17:97, 1997.
382. Tanaka A, Leung PSC, Van de Water J, et al: Clues to the etiology of primary biliary cirrhosis. In Manns M, Paumgartner G, Leuschner U, eds: Immunology of the Liver. Dordrecht/Boston/London, Kluwer Academic Publishers, 2000:244.
383. Zuckermann AJ, Zuckermann JN: Hepatitis viruses. In Weatherall DJ, Ledingham JGG, Warrell DA, eds: Oxford Textbook of Medicine, ed 2. Oxford: Oxford University Press, 1996:452
384. Biron CA, Nguyen KB, Pien GC, et al: Natural killer cells in antiviral defense: function and regulation by innate cytokines. Annu Rev Immunol 17:189, 1999.
385. Welsh RM, Brubaker JO, Vargas-Cortes M, O'Donnell CL: Natural killer (NK) cell response to virus infections in mice with severe combined immunodeficiency. The stimulation of NK cells and the NK cell-dependent control of virus infections occur dependently of T and B cell function. J Exp Med 173:1053, 1991.
386. Guidotti LG, Chisari FV: To kill or cure: options in host defense against viral infection. Curr Opin Immunol 8:478, 1996.
387. Maini MK, Boni C, Ogg GS, et al: Direct ex vivo analysis of hepatitis B virus-specific CD8(+) T cells associated with the control of infection. Gastroenterology 117:1386, 1999.
388. Maini MK, Boni C, Lee CK, et al: The role of virus-specific $CD8^+$ cells in liver damage and viral control during persistent hepatitis B virus (HBV) infection. J Exp Med 191:1269, 2000.
389. Guidotti LG, Rochford R, Chung J, et al: Viral clearance without destruction of infected cells during acute HBV infection. Science 284:825, 1999.
390. Guidotti LG, Ishikawa T, Hobbs MV, et al: Intracellular inactivation of the hepatitis B virus by cytotoxic T lymphocytes. Immunity 4:25, 1996.
391. Webster GJM, Hallett R, Whalley SA, et al: Molecular epidemiology of a large outbreak of hepatitis B linked to "autohaemotherapy." Lancet 356:379, 2000.
392. Webster GJM, Reignat S, Maini MK, et al: Incubation phase of acute hepatitis B in man: dynamics of cellular immune mechanisms. Hepatology 32:117, 2000.
393. Koziel MJ: Cytokines in viral hepatitis. Semin Liver Dis 19:157, 1999.
394. Lok AS: Natural history and control of perinatally acquired hepatitis B infection. Dig Dis 10:46, 1992.
395. Hsu HY, Chang MH, Lee CY, et al: Spontaneous loss of HBsAg in children with chronic hepatitis B virus infection. Hepatology 15:382, 1992.
396. Alcami A, Koszinowski UM: Viral mechanisms of immune evasion. Immunol Today 21(9):447, 2000.
397. Nayersina R, Fowler P, Guilhot S, et al: HLA A2 restricted cytotoxic T lymphocyte responses to multiple B surface antigen epitopes during hepatitis B virus infection. J Immunol 150:4659, 1993.
398. Oenna A, Artini M, Cavalli A, et al: Long-lasting memory T cell responses following self-limited acute hepatitis B. J Clin Invest 98:1185, 1996.
399. Rehermann B, Lau D, Hoofnagle JH, Chisari FV: Cytotoxic T lymphocyte responsiveness after resolution of chronic hepatitis B virus infection. J Clin Invest 97:1655, 1996.
400. Chisari FV: Cytotoxic T cells and viral hepatitis. J Clin Invest 99:1472, 1996.
401. Löhr HF, Gerken G, Schicht HJ, et al: Low frequency of cytotoxic liver-infiltrating T-lymphocytes specific for endogenous processed surface and core proteins in chronic hepatitis B. J Infect Dis 168:1133, 1993.
402. Rossol S, Marinos G, Carrucci P, et al: Interleukin-12 induction of Th1-cytokines is important for viral clearance in chronic hepatitis B. J Clin Invest 99:3025, 1997.
403. Farci P, Purcall RH: Clinical significance of hepatitis C virus. Genotypes and quasispecies. Semin Liver Dis 20:103, 2000.
404. Rehermann B: Interaction between the hepatitis C virus and the immune system. Semin Liver Dis 20:127, 2000.
405. Rammacco F, Sansonno D, Piccoli C, et al: The lymphoid system in hepatitis C infection: Autoimmunity, mixcoyoglobulinemia, and overt B cell malignancy. Semin Liver Dis 20:143, 2000.
406. Diepolder H, Zachoval R, Hoffmann R, et al: Possible mechanism involving T-lymphocyte response to non-structural protein 3 in viral clearance in acute hepatitis C virus infection. Lancet 346:1006, 1995.
407. Missale G, Bertoni R, Lamonaca V, et al: Different clinical behaviors of acute hepatitis C infection are associated with different vigor of the anti-viral cell-mediated immune response. J Clin Invest 98:706, 1996.
408. Cramp ME, Carucci P, Rossol S, et al: Hepatitis C virus (HCV) specific immune responses in anti-HCV positive patients with hepatitis C viraemia. Gut 44:424, 1999.
409. Gerlach JT, Diepolder HM, Jung MC, et al: Recurrence of hepatitis C virus after loss of virus-specific $CD4^+$ T-cell response in acute hepatitis C. Gastroenterology 117:933, 1999.
410. Botarelli P, Brunetto MR, Minutello MA, et al: T-lymphocyte response to hepatitis C virus in different clinical courses of infection. Gastroentrology 104:580, 1993.
411. Schupper H, Hayashi P, Scheffel J, et al: Peripheral-blood mononuclear cell responses to recombinant hepatitis C virus antigens in patients with chronic hepatitis C. Hepatology 18:1055, 1993.
412. Koziel JM, Dudley D, Afdhal N, et al: Hepatitis C virus (HCV)-specific cytotoxic T lymphocytes recognize epitopes in the core and envelope proteins of HCV. J Virol 67:7522, 1993.
413. He XS, Rehermann B, Lopez-Labrador FX, et al: Quantitative analysis of hepatitis C virus-specific $CD8^+$ T cells in peripheral blood and liver using peptide-MHC tetramers. Proc Natl Acad Sci U S A 96:5692, 1999.
414. Nelson DR, Marousis CG, Davis GL, et al: The role of hepatitis C virus-specific cytotoxic T lymphocytes in chronic hepatitis. J Immunol 158:1473, 1997.
415. Wong DK, Dudley DD, Afdhal NH, et al: Liver-derived CTL in hepatitis C virus infection: breadth and specificity of responses in a cohort of persons with chronic infection. J Immunol 160:1479, 1998.
416. Zajac AJ, Blattman JN, Murali-Krishna K, et al: Viral immune evasion due to persistence of activated T cells without effort function. J Exp Med 188:2205, 1998.
417. Kalams SA, Walker BD: The critical need for CD4 help in maintaining effective cytotoxic T lymphocyte responses. J Exp Med 188:2199, 1998.
418. Fukuda R, Ishimura N, Ishihara S, et al: Intrahepatic expression of pro-inflammatory cytokine mRNAs and interferon efficacy in chronic hepatitis C. Liver 16:390, 1996.

419. Napoli J, Bishop A, McGuinness PH, et al: Progressive liver injury in chronic hepatitis C infection correlates with increased intrahepatic expression of Th1-associated cytokines. Hepatology 24:759, 1996.
420. Nelson DR, Lau JYN: Pathogenesis of hepatocellular damage in chronic hepatitis C virus infection. Clin Liver Dis 1:515, 1997.
421. Tilg H, Wilmer A, Vogel W, et al: Serum levels of cytokines in chronic liver diseases. Gastroentrology 103:264, 1992.
422. Nelson DR, Lim HL, Marousis CG, et al: Activation of tumor necrosis factor α system in chronic hepatitis C virus infection. Dig Dis Sci 42:2487, 1997.
423. Dumoulin FL, Bach A, Leifeld L, et al: Semiquantitative analysis of intrahepatic cytokine mRNAs in chronic hepatitis C. J Infect Dis 175:681, 1997.
424. Kurilla MG, Swaminathan S, Welsch RM, et al: Effects of virally expressed interleukin-10 on vaccinia virus infection in mice. J Virol 67:7623, 1993.
425. Arai T, Hiromatsu H, Kobayashi N, et al: IL-10 is involved in the protective effect of dibutyryl cyclic adenosine monophosphate on endotoxin-induced inflammatory liver disease. J Immunol 155:5743, 1995.
426. Louis H, Le Moine O, Peny MO, et al: Production and role of interleukin-10 in concanavalin A-induced hepatitis in mice. Hepatology 25:1382, 1997.
427. Roulot D, Durand H, Coste T, et al: Quantitative analysis of transforming growth factor beta 1 messenger RNA in the liver of patients with chronic hepatitis C: absence of correlation between high levels and severity of disease. Hepatology 21:298, 1995.
428. Paradis V, Mathurin P, Laurent A, et al: Histological features predictive of liver fibrosis in chronic hepatitis C infection J Clin Pathol 49:998, 1996.
429. Gressner AM: Cytokine and cellular crosstalk involved in the activation of fat-storing cells. J Hepatol 22:28, 1995.
430. Kanto T, Takehara T, Katayama K, et al: Neutralization of transforming growth factor beta 1 augments hepatitis C virus-specific cytotoxic T lymphocyte induction in vitro. J Immunol 17:462, 1997.
431. Bertoletti A, D'Elios MM, Boni C, et al: Different cytokine profiles of intrahepatic T cells in chronic hepatitis B and hepatitis C virus infections. Gastroentrology 112:193, 1997.
432. Poynard T, Ratzin V, Bermanov Y, et al: Fibrosis in patients with chronic hepatitis C: detection and significance. Semin Liver Dis 20:47, 2000.

C H A P T E R

38

Autoimmune Liver Disease

Albert J. Czaja, MD

Autoimmune hepatitis is an unresolving inflammation of the liver characterized by interface hepatitis on histologic examination, hypergammaglobulinemia, and autoantibodies in serum.[1-3] There are no conventional immunoserologic markers pathognomonic of the disease,[2-4] and the clinical and histologic features at presentation may resemble those of other chronic hepatic diseases.[4,5] Indeed, the various immunoserologic markers typically found in autoimmune hepatitis can occur in acute and chronic liver diseases of a viral, drug, toxic, or immunologic nature,[2,5] and the histologic findings of interface hepatitis similarly lack disease specificity.[2,5] Consequently, the diagnosis of autoimmune hepatitis is one of exclusion, and it implies the absence of viral infection, hepatotoxic drugs, and hereditary disorders, such as Wilson disease, genetic hemochromatosis, and α_1-antitrypsin deficiency.[1,4-7]

The criteria for the diagnosis of autoimmune hepatitis have been codified by an international panel, and these criteria must now be applied to all patients (Table 38-1).[8,9] The propensity for an abrupt, rarely fulminant presentation has been recognized, and the temporal requirement for 6 months of disease activity to establish chronicity has been waived. The *definite* diagnosis requires manifestations of substantial immune reactivity reflected in high-titer autoantibodies and high concentrations of immunoglobulin G. The liver tissue must show features of lymphocytic, often lymphoplasmacytic, inflammatory infiltrates extending from portal tracts into acinar tissue in association with hepatocyte injury.[10] Panacinar (lobular) hepatitis may occur in acute onset disease or in autoimmune hepatitis that has relapsed after corticosteroid withdrawal, and panacinar hepatitis with bridging necrosis or multi-acinar necrosis is indicative of severe inflammatory activity.[10-12] Acinar zone 3 perivenular necrosis with and without sparing of the portal tracts is an unusual finding that is not yet included among the international criteria for diagnosis.[13,14] The

TABLE 38-1

Codified Diagnostic Criteria for Autoimmune Hepatitis

Probable autoimmune hepatitis	Definite autoimmune hepatitis
Partial α_1-antitrypsin deficiency	Normal α_1-antitrypsin phenotype
Abnormal serum copper or ceruloplasmin level if Wilson's disease excluded	Normal ceruloplasmin level
Non-specific serum iron or ferritin abnormalities	Normal serum iron and ferritin levels
No markers of active infection with hepatitis A, B, and C viruses	No markers of active infection with hepatitis A, B, and C viruses
Daily alcohol < 50 g/day and no recent use of hepatotoxic drugs	Daily alcohol < 25 g/day and no recent use of hepatotoxic drugs
Predominant serum aminotransferase abnormality	Predominant serum aminotransferase abnormality
ANA, SMA, or anti-LKM1 ≥1:40 in adults; other autoantibodies (anti-ASGPR, anti-SLA/LP, pANCA, anti-actin, anti-LC1)	ANA, SMA, or anti-LKM1 ≥ 1:80 in adults and ≥ 1:20 in children; no AMA
Interface hepatitis, moderate to severe	Interface hepatitis, moderate to severe
No biliary lesions, granulomas, or prominent changes suggestive of another disease	No biliary lesions, granulomas, or prominent changes suggestive of another disease

IgG, Immunoglobulin G; *ANA,* anti-nuclear antibodies; *SMA,* smooth muscle antibodies; *anti-LKM1,* antibodies to liver/kidney microsome type 1; *anti-ASGPR,* antibodies to asialoglycoprotein receptor; *anti-SLA/LP,* antibodies to soluble liver antigen/liver pancreas; *pANCA,* perinuclear anti-neutrophil cytoplasmic antibodies; *anti-LC1,* antibodies to liver cytosol type 1; *AMA,* anti-mitochondrial antibodies.

probable diagnosis of autoimmune hepatitis requires the same histologic findings as for definite disease but there may be less immunoreactivity and some exposure to potentially hepatotoxic drugs or alcohol (Table 38-1).[8,9] Furthermore, the probable diagnosis can be supported by the demonstration of antibodies to asialoglycoprotein receptor (anti-ASGPR), liver-specific cytosol antigen type 1 (anti-LC1), soluble liver antigen/liver pancreas (SLA/LP), or perinuclear anti-neutrophil cytoplasm (pANCA).[9]

Bile duct injury precludes the diagnosis if it is a destructive inflammatory reaction.[8,9] Concurrent, nondestructive biliary changes consisting of periductal lymphoid aggregates or pleomorphic or mixed inflammatory infiltrates are acceptable findings if interface hepatitis and other clinical features support the diagnosis.[15] A cholestatic form of autoimmune hepatitis is not recognized. The occurrence of destructive cholangitis or ductopenia generates alternative diagnoses, such as autoimmune cholangitis[16,17] or an autoimmune variant syndrome characterized by overlapping features of autoimmune hepatitis and primary biliary cirrhosis (PBC) or primary sclerosing cholangitis (PSC).[18-20]

A scoring system has been developed to facilitate the diagnosis in patients with mixed manifestations that provides a mechanism by which to assess the strength of the diagnosis in different populations (Table 38-2).[9] By weighing each component of the syndrome, discrepant features can be accommodated and biases associated with isolated inconsistencies avoided. The original scoring system has been validated[21] and has been recently revised to exclude cholestatic syndromes with more confidence.[9] An unintended but useful application of the scoring system has been to assess the resemblance of various chronic liver diseases to classic autoimmune hepatitis in a quantitative and objective fashion.[19,22]

TABLE 38-2

Scoring Criteria for the Diagnosis of Autoimmune Hepatitis

Category	Factor	Score
Gender	Female	+2
ALP:AST (or ALT) ratio	<1.5	+2
	1.5-3.0	0
	>3.0	−2
γ-Globulin or IgG levels above normal	>2.0	+3
	1.5-2.0	+2
	1.0-1.5	+1
	<1.0	0
ANA, SMA, or anti-LKM1 titers	>1:80	+3
	1:80	+2
	1:40	+1
	<1.40	0
AMA	Positive	−4
Viral markers	Positive	−3
	Negative	+3
Drugs	Yes	−4
	No	+1
Alcohol	<25 g/day	+2
	>60 g/day	−2
HLA	DR3 or DR4	+1
Immune disease	Thyroiditis, colitis, synovitis, others	+2
Other liver-defined autoantibody	Anti-SLA/LP, anti-actin, anti-LC1, pANCA	+2
Histologic features	Interface hepatitis	+3
	Plasma cells	+1
	Rosettes	+1
	None of above	−5
	Biliary changes	−3
	Other features	−3
Treatment response	Complete	+2
	Relapse	+3
Pretreatment Score		
Definite diagnosis		>15
Probable diagnosis		10-15
Posttreatment Score		
Definite diagnosis		>17
Probable diagnosis		12-17

ALP, Serum alkaline phosphatase level; *AST,* serum aspartate aminotransferase level; *ALT,* serum alanine aminotransferase level; *ANA,* anti-nuclear antibodies; *SMA,* smooth muscle antibodies; *anti-LKM1,* antibodies to liver/kidney microsome type 1; *AMA,* antimitochondrial antibodies; *anti-SLA/LP,* antibodies to soluble liver antigen/liver pancreas; *anti-LC1,* antibodies to liver cytosol type 1; *pANCA,* perinuclear anti-neutrophil cytoplasmic antibodies.

HISTORICAL PERSPECTIVE

Descriptions of hyperproteinemia and idiopathic, often recurrent, jaundice in association with severe chronic hepatocellular injury first appeared in the late 1930s and early 1940s.[23,24] The components of a syndrome, however, were not recognized until the 1950s when cirrhosis with plasma cell infiltration of the liver was described in young women who had hypergammaglobulinemia, fever of obscure origin, acne, cushingoid features, arthralgias, and amenorrhea.[25-28] The term "active chronic hepatitis" was applied in 1953[29] but was changed to "lupoid hepatitis" in 1956[30] when the association of the disease with the lupus erythematosus (LE) cell phenomenon was established.[31] The original deduction of Joske and King that the LE cell phenomenon was a by-product of excess gamma globulin production[31] yielded to arguments favoring an autoimmune disorder; in 1956, the LE cell phenomenon acquired a pathogenic connotation.[30]

Mackay and associates postulated that "lupoid hepatitis" was linked to systemic lupus erythematosus (SLE) by a common factor of disturbed immunologic response.[30] This proposal was especially exciting because it was an application of the theories of Burnet and Fenner that, in 1949, had focused attention on immunologic mechanisms of self-recognition. Indeed, the LE cell phenomenon was regarded as evidence of a failure of the antibody-producing mechanisms of the patient to recognize self-constituents; this failure of self-recognition was attributed to either a primary disorder of antibody production or a modification of cellular "self-markers" as a result of an infectious agent or noxious condition.[30,31] According to this hypothesis, components of the hepatocytes were rendered antigenic or were exposed to antibodies abnormally produced by B cells as a consequence of viral infection or nutritional damage. The pattern of liver cell injury was then perpetuated by an antibody-mediated cytotoxicity. Terms such as "autoclasia" were applied to the disease to connote a "self-breaking down" process,[32] and the "intrinsic" theory of pathogenesis was enlarged to include the possibility of spontaneous mutation and the creation of a B cell population ("forbidden clone") that was able to produce antibodies against normal host hepatocytic protein.[33]

The designation *lupoid hepatitis* connoted an autoimmune basis for the liver disease and emphasized an immunoserologic (and possibly pathogenic) similarity to SLE, which at that time was the prototypic immunologic disorder.[30,34] By the late 1950s these similarities were so closely drawn that the validity of lupoid hepatitis as a separate entity was threatened. Arthralgias, rash, hemolytic anemia, and nephropathy were recognized in both conditions, and the age and sex distributions were similar in both disorders. Although lupoid hepatitis infrequently co-existed with SLE, most series of patients with the liver disease or SLE showed some overlap (1 percent-10 percent concurrence)[35] and there was speculation that the liver disease might be an early prodrome of the systemic illness that would require years to finally evolve.[34]

Separation of lupoid hepatitis from SLE was ultimately established after multiple experiences emphasized the infrequency of concurrent diseases, the lack of an evolutionary pattern from lupoid hepatitis to SLE, and the absence of SLE features in the patients with the liver disease.[36] The absence of immunoglobulin G antibodies to double-stranded deoxyribonucleic acid (DNA) in patients with lupoid hepatitis was felt to be another important distinguishing feature,[37] although the specificity of this finding was subsequently challenged.[38]

In 1961 the concept of lupoid hepatitis was enlarged after studies indicated that the disease could afflict men (33 percent) and occur early in life (age 9 months).[39] Importantly, the disease seemed to behave differently in men, developing at an earlier age and progressing to cirrhosis and esophageal varices more slowly.[39] By 1963 experiences indicated that males had a poorer prognosis than females, and gender was defined as an important prognostic factor.[40] It was not yet possible, however, to link the poorer response to corticosteroid therapy in men to etiologic differences. Indeed, it was not until hepatitis B virus (HBV) testing became generally available and applied to these patient populations that the real reason for the prognostic differences became apparent.[41,42]

By 1964 the factors associated with responsiveness to corticosteroid therapy were clarified.[43] Acute onset of disease, concurrent extrahepatic immunologic diseases, extreme hypergammaglobulinemia, and the presence of the LE cell phenomenon separated the responders from the non-responders (and also the patients with autoimmune disease from the others).[44,45] Anecdotal experiences with corticosteroid regimens suggested that corticosteroid therapy could reduce early mortality if not prevent histologic progression.[43-45] The aggressiveness of untreated disease was recognized, and a 5-year survival of 65 percent was estimated in such patients.[46] Spontaneous resolution of inflammatory activity, however, was also described, and this outcome occurred in 41 percent of survivors (albeit usually with cirrhosis).[46] The possibility of spontaneous resolution confounded anecdotal attempts to assess the efficacy of corticosteroid therapy, and it was an important justification for the performance of controlled treatment trials that were launched in the late 1960s.[47-50]

In the mid 1960s the LE cell phenomenon was no longer required for the diagnosis of lupoid hepatitis because other autoantibodies, such as smooth muscle antibodies (SMA) and anti-nuclear antibodies (ANA), were described and linked to the disease.[51,52] Gamma globulin deposits (presumably newly synthesized as part of an immunologic reaction to hepatocytic components) were found in hepatic mesenchymal cells in the periphery of the liver lobule and in association with lymphocytes, plasma cells, histiocytes, and proliferated bile ductules.[53,54] The histologic picture of an immunologically mediated cytodestructive process was developed, and this pattern of "piecemeal necrosis" soon became the *sine qua non* for the diagnosis of autoimmune hepatitis. Indeed, the histologic findings were at least as important as the clinical and laboratory findings in making the diagnosis.

Autoimmune hepatitis became a histologic entity, nearly losing its clinical identity. Histologic patterns established the diagnosis, implied the prognosis, and determined treatment strategies.[55-60] Terms such as *chronic persistent hepatitis* and *chronic active hepatitis* connoted prognosis and need for treatment[55-60] and the clinical manifestations of these different histologic patterns were frequently secondary considerations.

Histologic patterns of bridging necrosis and multilobular necrosis were associated with an increased propensity for progression to cirrhosis,[11,55,56,58-61] and portal tract to central vein bridging in contrast to portal tract to portal tract bridging was recognized as a particularly aggressive lesion.[61] Spontaneous or treatment-induced transitions between periportal hepatitis, multi-lobular necrosis, bridging necrosis, portal hepatitis, and normal hepatic architecture were recognized,[11,49] and liver biopsy assessments became essential not only for diagnosis but also for assessing prognosis and response to treatment.[49,57,59-64] This was the era when inter- and intraobserver variation in the interpretation of histologic features was a key concern—as was the likelihood of sampling error in obtaining representative biopsy specimens.[65,66] Adjunctive diagnostic studies, including peritoneoscopy,[67] portal pressure determinations,[68] assessment of serum bile acid concentrations,[69] and measurements of aminopyrine metabolism,[70] were evaluated in the hope of identifying the aggressive histologic lesion more assuredly than did the pathologist.

During this same period, the autoimmune nature of autoimmune hepatitis was seriously questioned. Page and co-workers observed improvement in the disease during therapy with 6-mercaptopurine in the absence of immunosuppression.[44] They speculated that an unidentified virus had been affected by treatment and that clinical improvement had resulted from elimination of this agent. Mistilis and Blackburn supported this hypothesis by emphasizing the clinical heterogeneity of the disease, its frequent acute occurrence, its multi-systemic involvement, its occasional spontaneous resolution, and its infrequent occurrence after contact with acute viral hepatitis.[71] The stage, however, was not set to explore more fully the viral nature of autoimmune hepatitis until the discovery of "Australia antigen" by Blumberg and associates circa 1965.[72] The subsequent association of this antigen with HBV infection opened a new era of research and understanding.

The autoimmune nature of autoimmune hepatitis was thoroughly challenged in the early 1970s when hepatitis B surface antigen (HBsAg) testing disclosed that at least 25 percent of patients with chronic active hepatitis had evidence of HBV infection.[41,73,74] Soloway and colleagues demonstrated that the LE cell phenomenon could be detected in 10 percent of HBsAg-positive patients and that there was no difference in the laboratory features or frequency of concurrent immunologic diseases in patients with and without the LE cell phenomenon.[75] Furthermore, various drugs, including oxyphenisatin, alphamethyldopa, nitrofurantoin, and propylthiouracil, were implicated in the production of autoimmune hepatitis,[76-78] and it was estimated that 28 percent to 67 percent of patients in Scandinavia and Australia had drug-related, not idiopathic or autoimmune, disease.[76]

The rubric chronic active liver disease (CALD) was introduced during this period in an effort to encompass all patients of similar nature and disease severity and to emphasize their common features regardless of etiology.[79,80] This designation, however, was short-lived because experiences continued to indicate significant heterogeneity in various subpopulations of patients with CALD. Indeed, Bulkey and co-workers emphasized the importance of subclassification as a means of identifying patients with different presentations, prognosis, and pathogenic mechanisms,[81] and Schalm and colleagues recognized that patients with HBsAg responded less well to corticosteroids than did their HBsAg-negative counterparts.[41] The era of "splintering" CALD into small homogeneous subpopulations had begun.

By the late 1970s improved diagnostic techniques had diminished but not eliminated the population of patients with autoimmune hepatitis. The validity of the entity, however, was strengthened by the development of an animal model. New Zealand white rabbits that had been immunized with antigens prepared from normal human liver tissue developed histologic lesions similar to those of human disease and prolonged immunization was associated with progression to cirrhosis.[82,83] There also was evidence that the disease could perpetuate itself for up to 5 months after the last immunization.

Subsequent studies suggested that experimental autoimmune hepatitis was a lymphocyte-mediated cytotoxic reaction against hepatocytic proteins and that immunoglobulin G on the hepatocyte membrane surface could represent an antigen-antibody complex and a target for cytotoxic lymphocytes.[84] B-lymphocyte fractions were shown to be essential for cytotoxicity; aggregated immunoglobulin preparations blocked this cytotoxicity presumably by binding cytotoxic T-cell receptor sites; preincubation of liver-specific lipoprotein (LSP) with serum eliminated the cytotoxicity of the serum presumably by binding pathogenic autoantibodies; lymphocytes from patients showed an increased sensitization to LSP indicating increased immunoreactivity against normal hepatic membrane protein; and non–antigen-specific suppressor T-cell function was decreased in patients with the disease.[85,86] All of these findings justified the hypothesis that autoimmune hepatitis was an antibody-dependent, cell-mediated cytotoxic reaction that was self-perpetuated by inadequate immunoregulation and untempered antibody production against self-constituents.

Recognition that patients with autoimmune hepatitis were commonly human leukocyte antigen (HLA) B8 positive suggested that a genetic predisposition in some patients could heighten their immunoreactivity to auto- or extrinsic antigens and result in more active disease at an earlier age.[87-89] Furthermore, the findings that first degree relatives had an increased frequency of autoantibodies in serum, hypergammaglobulinemia, and non–antigen-specific suppressor cell dysfunction underscored the likelihood that autoimmune hepatitis had a familial predisposition and an inheritable genetic basis.[90] The relationship between the genetic predisposition of the host and the clinical behavior of the disease was also explored at this time, and HLA DR3 was found to be associated with treatment failure.

During the 1980s the number of organ-specific and non–organ-specific autoantibodies associated with the disease proliferated. Efforts were focused on the identification and isolation of a target antigen. Liver-specific protein was recognized as a complex liver membrane extract and it was the first of the contenders.[91] Unfortunately, it could not be characterized because a target autoantigen and antibodies to LSP were not disease specific. Reactivity was demonstrated in various human liver diseases, and cell-mediated immunity to the preparation could not be consistently shown in autoimmune hepatitis.[92,93] Furthermore, the animal model for autoimmune hepatitis that had been based on immunization with LSP could not be easily reproduced because antibodies induced by immunization were commonly unassociated with disease, immunogenicity of LSP depended on unphysiologic augmentation with adjuvants; protracted periods of immunization (almost 3 years) were required for disease manifestations, similar lesions were produced after injection of human skeletal muscle extract, the animals used in the model were highly selected (inbred genetic strains) or unnaturally perturbed (irradiated), and the consistent production of a lesion indistinguishable from the human disease could not be demonstrated.[94,95]

Liver membrane antigen (LMA) was less complex than LSP, but antibodies to LMA were found in normal individuals and various liver diseases other than autoimmune hepatitis.[96] Although levels of reactivity to LMA could distinguish autoimmune hepatitis and enhance the specificity of the assay, the broad overlap of values among different liver diseases and the arbitrary definition of significant seropositivity compromised the sensitivity and reliability of the determination.[96]

Asialoglycoprotein receptor (hepatic lectin) was the last of the hepatocytic membrane constituents to be advanced as a target autoantigen during this period of investigation, but antibodies to this protein also lacked disease specificity.[97] Indeed, none of the autoantibodies described during this period were shown to be pathogenic, and their production could not be linked to a disease-specific immunogenic stimulus. Investigators became increasingly concerned that the autoantibodies were the by-products of hepatocytic destruction rather than its cause and that the membrane antigens being isolated as targets of an immunologic reaction were simply membrane constituents released during cell death.

The modern era of research in autoimmune hepatitis began in the late 1980s when advances in molecular biology permitted the identification of the hepatitis C virus (HCV) and the cloning of hepatic autoantigens.[98,99] These developments now promise to enhance diagnostic precision and facilitate identification of pertinent liver autoantigens.

PREVALENCE

Autoimmune hepatitis is the principal form of chronic hepatitis in those geographic regions where the HLA B8 and DR3 phenotypes are common and the carriage frequency of chronic viral infection is low.[100] HLAs B8 and DR3 are found most frequently in the populations of Northern Europe, and the prevalence decreases with latitude toward the equator.[101] The frequency of autoimmune hepatitis seems to coincide with these regional changes in HLA prevalence[100] and the disease frequency is similar in the populations of North America that are largely derived from Northern Europe.

The prevalence of chronic viral infection also influences the frequency of autoimmune hepatitis.[100] In contrast to Hong Kong where only 1 percent of patients with chronic hepatitis have autoimmune disease and 86 percent have chronic hepatitis B,[102] the frequency of autoimmune hepatitis among patients with chronic hepatitis is 34 percent in Germany (versus 36 percent with chronic hepatitis B)[103] and 62 percent in Australia (versus 10 percent with chronic hepatitis B).[100] The rough inverse relationship between chronic viral infection and autoimmune hepatitis reflects the low prevalence of HLA B8 and DR3 phenotypes in Asia and the high frequency of chronic viral hepatitis in this base population.

The incidence of autoimmune hepatitis in North America is uncertain but it is probably similar to that in Northern Europe.[104] Among Caucasian Northern Europeans, the mean annual incidence of the disease is 1.9 per 100,000, and its point prevalence is 16.9 per 100,000.[105] This occurrence is greater than that for PBC and PSC in the same population. In the United States autoimmune hepatitis affects 100,000 to 200,000 individuals and accounts for 5.9 percent of liver transplants.[106] In the European Liver Transplant Registry, autoimmune hepatitis accounts for 2.6 percent of transplants.[107]

Despite its relative rarity, autoimmune hepatitis exemplifies a pathologic process that has an enormous impact on health and health care costs. In the United States 5 percent of the population have autoimmune disease, and the total annual health care expenditure for these diseases exceeds $83 billion. Autoimmunity in aggregate must be recognized as a major category of human disease that is chronic and incurable, and autoimmune hepatitis acquires a heavier mantle of importance if it can serve as a paradigm by which to understand mechanisms of autoimmunity and develop novel site-specific therapies.[108]

Estimates of prevalence mainly reflect disease that is sufficiently severe to justify medical evaluation or result in death and postmortem examination. Recent studies have indicated that asymptomatic patients with mild to moderate inflammatory activity may have autoimmune hepatitis of insufficient severity to be included in estimates of prevalence.[109] Of 47 such patients in whom liver biopsy examination was justified only by investigational protocol, 34 had histologic features of interface hepatitis (72 percent), including 16 who had features of cirrhosis.[109] Eighteen of those with interface hepatitis were ANA or SMA positive and they were classifiable as having asymptomatic autoimmune hepatitis. The actual size of this component of the "universe" is unknown but it is not represented in any estimates of disease prevalence.

SUBCLASSIFICATIONS

Three subclassifications of autoimmune hepatitis have been proposed based on distinctive immunoserologic markers[110,111] (Table 38-3). The clinical validity and utility of these subclassifications are unestablished but the designations have become part of the clinical jargon.[112,113]

Type 1 Autoimmune Hepatitis

Type 1 autoimmune hepatitis is the most common form of hepatitis in the United States, constituting at least 80 percent of cases in adults (Figure 38-1).[114] Type 1 disease is characterized by the presence of SMA or ANA; hypergammaglobulinemia; concurrent immunologic disorders; HLA DR3, HLA DR4, or the A1-B8-DR3 phenotype; and responsiveness to corticosteroid therapy (see Table 38-3).[1-3,114] The specificity of SMA for the diagnosis can be enhanced if anti-actin antibodies are sought,[115,116] and type 1 disease has been referred to as *anti-actin hepatitis*.[117]

Typically, type 1 autoimmune hepatitis afflicts women (71 percent) of age 40 years or less (48 percent).[114] An acute onset of illness occurs in 40 percent of patients[1-3]; these individuals may be misdiagnosed as having acute viral or toxic hepatitis.[118-121] The presence of hypoalbuminemia, hypergammaglobulinemia, or features of portal hypertension—such as thrombocytopenia, ascites, or esophageal varices—should raise the suspicion of autoimmune hepatitis in these patients.[119,121] Liver biopsy assessment may disclose fibrosis or cirrhosis and suggest exacerbation of a chronic indolent disorder.[122] Alternatively, the histologic findings may show a panacinar hepatitis that is indistinguishable from an acute infectious or toxic injury.[123] In all such instances, corticosteroid therapy can be lifesaving and therapy should not be deferred to satisfy arbitrary temporal criteria for chronicity.[119,121,123]

Thirty-two percent of patients with type 1 autoimmune hepatitis have concomitant immunologic diseases; of these, the majority have thyroiditis or Graves' disease (57 percent), ulcerative colitis (24 percent), or rheumatoid arthritis (12 percent).[114,124-127] The presence of ulcer-

TABLE 38-3
Subclassifications of Autoimmune Hepatitis

Features	Type 1	Type 2	Type 3
Signature autoantibodies	SMA, ANA	Anti-LKM1	Anti-SLA/LP
Associated autoantibodies	Anti-actin pANCA Anti-dsDNA Anti-ASGPR	Anti-LC1	Anti-actin SMA ANA
Onset	Adult	Pediatric	Adult
Women (%)	71	89	91
Immune diseases (%)	38	40	38
Common associated conditions	Autoimmune thyroiditis Graves' disease Ulcerative colitis Synovitis	Insulin-dependent diabetes Autoimmune thyroiditis Vitiligo	Autoimmune thyroiditis Graves disease Ulcerative colitis Synovitis
Genetic risk factors	*DRB1*0301* *DRB1*0401* *TNF*2A* *CTLA-4 GG*	*DRB1*0701* HLA B14 HLA DR3 *C4A-QO*	*DRB1*0301*
Target autoantigen	Unknown	P450 IID6 (CYP2D6)	50-kDA protein (tRNP$^{(Ser)Sec}$)
Low IgA level	No	Yes	No
Steroid responsive	Yes	Yes	Yes
Progression to cirrhosis (%)	40	80	Uncertain

SMA, Smooth muscle antibodies; *ANA,* anti-nuclear antibodies; *anti-LKM1,* antibodies to liver/kidney microsome type 1; *anti-SLA/LP,* antibodies to soluble liver antigen/liver pancreas; *pANCA,* perinuclear anti-neutrophil cytoplasmic antibodies; *anti-dsDNA,* antibodies to double-stranded DNA; *anti-ASGPR,* antibodies to asialoglycoprotein receptor; *tRNP$^{(Ser)Sec}$,* transfer ribonucleoprotein complex involved in the incorporation of selenocysteine in polypeptide chains.

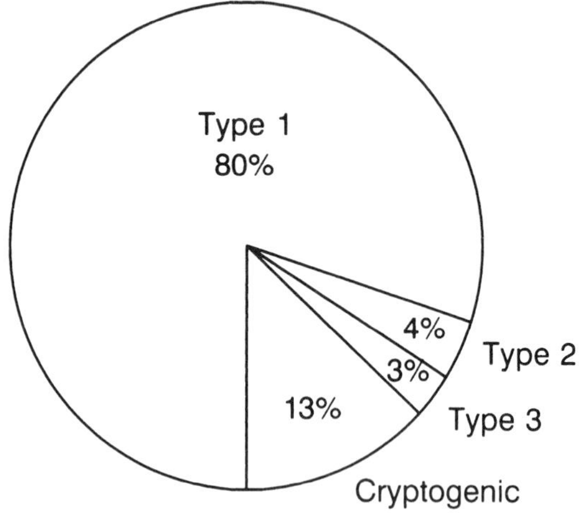

Figure 38-1 Frequencies of the different subclassifications of non-viral chronic hepatitis in Caucasian North American adults. Types 1, 2, and 3 connote subgroups of autoimmune hepatitis that are characterized by the presence of anti-nuclear or smooth muscle antibodies (type 1), antibodies to liver/kidney microsome type 1 (type 2), or antibodies to soluble liver antigen/liver pancreas, respectively. Cryptogenic connotes chronic hepatitis without viral or immunoserologic markers.

ative colitis does not compel the diagnosis of PSC nor does the presence of inflammatory bowel disease in these patients preclude a satisfactory response to corticosteroid therapy.[128] Cholangiography, however, is required in all such patients because PSC may resemble autoimmune hepatitis or coexist with it.[128-131]

Forty-one percent of patients with type 1 autoimmune hepatitis and ulcerative colitis have cholangiograms that suggest PSC; these patients commonly fail to respond to corticosteroid therapy.[128] Conversely, 59 percent of these patients have normal cholangiograms and respond to treatment in a fashion similar to individuals without ulcerative colitis. These findings indicate that cholangiography is essential to discount PSC in adult patients with ulcerative colitis; most adult patients with type 1 autoimmune hepatitis and inflammatory bowel disease do not have PSC, and ulcerative colitis is not an independent determinant of treatment outcome.[128]

Genetic predispositions strongly influence disease expression and behavior in type 1 autoimmune hepatitis. Caucasian Northern European and North American patients with HLA B8 are younger than counterparts with other HLA and they have greater degrees of inflammatory activity at presentation (Figure 38-2).[132] Furthermore, patients with HLA A1 and B8 commonly relapse after corticosteroid therapy.[132] Individuals with HLA DR3 fail corticosteroid treatment more frequently than patients with other HLA and they more commonly require liver transplantation (Figure 38-2).[125,133-135] In contrast, patients with HLA DR4 are older, more often female, and more commonly responsive to corticosteroid therapy.[125,127] They also have concomitant non-hepatic immunologic diseases and high-titer seropositivity for ANA more frequently than patients with other HLA (Figure 38-2).[124,125,127]

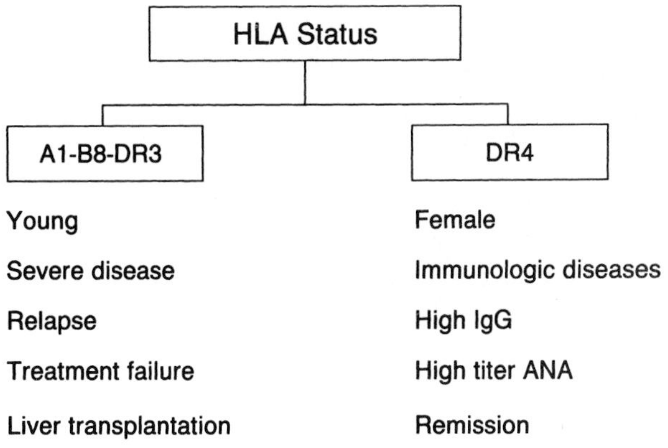

HLA Status

A1-B8-DR3	DR4
Young	Female
Severe disease	Immunologic diseases
Relapse	High IgG
Treatment failure	High titer ANA
Liver transplantation	Remission

Figure 38-2 Clinical and prognostic features associated with the human leukocyte antigen (HLA) DR3 and DR4 phenotypes. Immunoglobulin (Ig)G connotes serum IgG, and antinuclear antibodies (ANAs) connote serum ANAs.

High-resolution DNA-based technology has indicated that type 1 autoimmune hepatitis is a polygenic disorder involving the *DRB1* gene of chromosome 6.[136,137] Among Caucasian Northern European and North American patients, *DRB1*0301* and *DRB1*0401* are the alleles that affect susceptibility, clinical expression, and treatment outcome, whereas *DRB1*1501* confers resistance to the disease. Other alleles have been implicated in other ethnic groups. *DRB1*0404* is the susceptibility allele in Mestizo Mexicans[138] and *DRB1*0405* is the susceptibility allele in Japanese patients and Argentine adults.[139-142] Among Argentine children and Brazilian patients *DRB1*1301* predisposes to the disease.[141-143]

The target antigen for type 1 autoimmune hepatitis is unknown, but asialoglycoprotein receptor is a leading candidate because it resides on the hepatocyte surface, captures and transports foreign and self proteins, and is commonly associated with a disease-specific autoantibody.[97,144-147] Recently, a 50-kDa protein has been described in association with antibodies to anti-SLA/LP, which may also be a target autoantigen.[148] This antigen may be a transfer ribonucleic acid–protein complex (tRNP) involved in the incorporation of selenocysteine into polypeptide chains.[149]

The close association of type 1 autoimmune hepatitis with class II HLA suggests that a genetic predisposition may heighten immune reactivity to extrinsic and intrinsic antigens and foster an antibody-dependent, cell-mediated form of cytotoxicity.[3,85,86,150-155] Under such circumstances, it is easy to speculate that a viral infection or environmental factor could be a triggering agent in a genetically susceptible host.[153-157] Multiple etiologic triggers have been proposed for type 1 autoimmune hepatitis, including viruses, such as measles virus,[158-160] hepatitis A virus,[161,162] HBV,[163] HCV,[164,165] and drugs such as nitrofurantoin[77,78] and minocycline.[166-168] The multiplicity of triggers suggests that the antigenic epitope is short and easily mimicked. The long lag time between exposure to the trigger and recognition of the disease also means that understanding the nature of the disease is easier than understanding its cause.

Initial surveys from Spain using first-generation immunoassays for anti-HCV indicated that as many as 44 percent of patients with type 1 autoimmune hepatitis were HCV infected.[169] Subsequently, the first-generation assay was shown to be confounded by the high serum concentration of immunoglobulin G that characterizes patients with type 1 autoimmune hepatitis. Indeed, many of the patients in these early reports were undoubtedly falsely positive for anti-HCV.[170-174] In the United States only 5 percent to 7 percent of patients were seropositive for anti-HCV by first-generation immunoassay and of these, 40 percent were falsely positive.[172,173,175] A similar low prevalence of seropositivity for anti-HCV was reported in England[176] and Australia.[177] The frequency of anti-HCV seropositivity in type 1 autoimmune hepatitis decreased further (to 4 percent) with the availability of second-generation testing[126]; the application of polymerase chain reaction assays for the detection of HCV RNA in serum reconfirmed this estimate of low frequency.[164] Clearly, there are some patients with type 1 autoimmune hepatitis and true HCV infection[164-180] but the low frequency of this association suggests that HCV infection is either coincidental or an unimportant etiologic factor. Most patients with true HCV infection and autoimmune features have low-titer, background autoantibodies that should not alter the diagnosis of "chronic hepatitis C with autoimmune features" or dissuade antiviral therapy.[181-183]

Type 2 Autoimmune Hepatitis

Type 2 autoimmune hepatitis is characterized by the presence of antibodies to liver/kidney microsome type 1 (anti-LKM1) (see Table 38-3).[117] Sera react on Western blots with a 50-kDa microsomal protein, and the major antigen of anti-LKM1 is the cytochrome mono-oxygenase, P450 IID6 (CYP2D6), a drug-metabolizing enzyme system.[184-188] Clear understanding of the different immunofluorescent patterns associated with anti-LKM1 and anti-mitochondrial antibodies (AMA) is essential because 27 percent of patients with autoimmune hepatitis and seropositivity for AMA are actually anti-LKM1 rather than AMA positive.[189]

The diagnosis of anti-LKM1 seropositivity requires not only reactivity of serum by indirect immunofluorescence on the proximal tubule of the murine kidney but also reactivity by indirect immunofluorescence in the cytoplasm of murine hepatocytes (Figure 38-3).[189,190] Seropositivity for AMA requires reactivity of serum by indirect immunofluorescence on the distal tubules of the murine kidney and reactivity in the parietal cells of the murine stomach (Figure 38-3). An exuberant immunofluorescent reaction can obliterate distinctions between proximal and distal renal tubules and result in an indeterminate pattern of reactivity. The availability of enzyme immunoassays that detect the PBC-specific M2 antigens of the pyruvate dehydrogenase complex eliminates this possible confusion.

Patients with type 2 autoimmune hepatitis are mainly children (ages 2 to 14 years) (see Table 38-3).[117] In the United States the diagnosis is extremely unusual among adults, occurring in only 4 percent of patients with

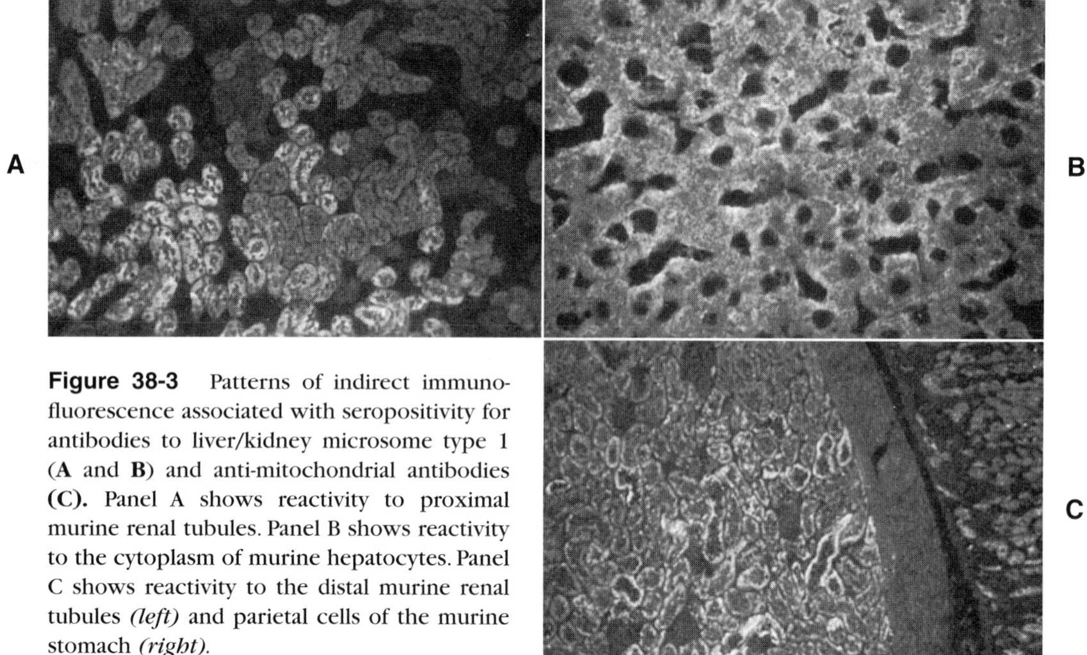

Figure 38-3 Patterns of indirect immunofluorescence associated with seropositivity for antibodies to liver/kidney microsome type 1 (**A** and **B**) and anti-mitochondrial antibodies (**C**). Panel A shows reactivity to proximal murine renal tubules. Panel B shows reactivity to the cytoplasm of murine hepatocytes. Panel C shows reactivity to the distal murine renal tubules *(left)* and parietal cells of the murine stomach *(right)*.

autoimmune hepatitis (see Figure 38-1).[191] In Europe, especially in Germany and France, 20 percent of patients with type 2 autoimmune hepatitis are adults.[117] In South America the disease is also more common than in the United States and affects mainly children.[143] Detection of antibodies to P450 IID6 (CYP2D6) supports the diagnosis but the recombinant assay is not generally available.[191] The current diagnostic requisite is the demonstration of anti-LKM1 in serum by indirect immunofluorescence. Genetic polymorphisms do occur, and 10 percent of normal adults lack P450 IID6 (CYP2D6).[99] This deficiency may explain in part the wide variation in disease occurrence in different geographic regions and ethnic groups.

Several subtypes of LKM antibodies have been described, and these must be distinguished because they define different clinical conditions.[99] Antibodies to LKM2 are associated with drug-induced (ticrynafen) hepatitis, and antibodies to LKM3 are associated with chronic hepatitis D (delta).[99] Furthermore, antibodies to LKM1 undoubtedly consist of subspecies that recognize different epitopes of the same antigen or similar epitopes in different antigens. Homologies exist between recombinant P450 IID6 (CYP2D6) and the genomes of HCV and herpes simplex virus. Rarely, this molecular mimicry can result in cross-reacting antibodies.[188]

In patients with HCV infection the antibodies to LKM1 recognize P450 IID6 (CYP2D6) less frequently than those from uninfected counterparts[192,193] or they recognize an epitope on P450 IID6 (CYP2D6) that is different from the core motif recognized by sera from uninfected patients.[194] These differences in reactivity to P450 IID6 (CYP2D6) suggest that anti-LKM1-positive patients with and without HCV infection have different diseases with different pathogenic mechanisms. The core motif within the P450 IID6 (CYP2D6) molecule recognized by anti-LKM1 associated with type 2 autoimmune hepatitis is the amino acid sequence 254-271. In contrast, the amino acid sequence recognized by anti-LKM1 associated with chronic hepatitis C is highly variable, with multiple epitopes within the region 208-273 of the P450 IID6 (CYP2D6) molecule.[194]

Associated immunologic disorders—including vitiligo, thyroiditis, insulin-dependent diabetes, autoimmune hemolytic anemia, idiopathic thrombocytopenic purpura, pernicious anemia, rheumatoid arthritis, and ulcerative colitis (Table 38-4)—are common (40 percent) in type 2 autoimmune hepatitis.[117] Hypergammaglobulinemia is less pronounced than in type 1 disease, and serum immunoglobulin A levels may be low. Non-organ-specific autoantibodies are rare, whereas organ-specific antibodies—including anti-thyroid microsome, anti-thyroglobulin, anti-islets of Langerhans, and anti-parietal cell antibodies—are common (30 percent).[117] Early experiences suggested that type 2 autoimmune hepatitis had a higher frequency of concurrent immune diseases than type 1 disease and that it progressed more rapidly to cirrhosis (82 versus 43 percent within 3 years).[117] These perceptions have not been corroborated, and both types respond well to corticosteroids. Successful cessation of treatment, however, is unlikely in patients with type 2 autoimmune hepatitis.[195]

Unlike type 1 autoimmune hepatitis, the target autoantigen of type 2 disease has been identified. P450 IID6 (CYP2D6) has a 33 amino acid linear sequence that is recognized by anti-LKM1.[186,188,194,196] Its activity is inhibited in vitro (but not in vivo) by anti-LKM1[187] and it is expressed on hepatocyte membrane surfaces.[197-199] Furthermore, liver-infiltrating immunocytes sensitized specifically against P450 IID6 (CYP2D6) have been recovered from the liver tissue of patients.[200] Susceptibility appears to relate to *DRB1*0701*,[143,201] but HLA B14, DR3, and *C4A-QO* have also been incriminated.[202]

A distinct form of LKM-positive autoimmune hepatitis occurs in association with the autoimmune polyen-

TABLE 38-4
Associated Immunologic Diseases

Common	Uncommon
Autoimmune thyroiditis	Celiac sprue
Graves' disease	Dermatitis herpetiformis
Synovitis	Erythema nodosum
Rheumatoid arthritis	Fibrosing alveolitis
Ulcerative colitis	Focal myositis
	Gingivitis
	Glomerulonephritis
	Hemolytic anemia
	Idiopathic thrombocytopenic purpura
	Insulin-dependent diabetes mellitus
	Leukocytoclastic vasculitis
	Myasthenia gravis
	Neutropenia
	Pericarditis
	Peripheral neuropathy
	Pernicious anemia
	Pleuritis
	Pyoderma gangrenosum
	Sjögren's syndrome
	Systemic lupus erythematosus
	Systemic sclerosis
	Urticaria
	Vitiligo

docrinopathy syndrome (APS).[203-205] This disorder is marked by the presence of numerous organ- and non-organ-specific autoantibodies and multiple concurrent autoimmune diseases. APS type 1 (APS1) is caused by a single gene mutation located on chromosome 21q22.3. The APS1 gene encodes for a transcription factor called the autoimmune regulator that is expressed in epithelial and dendritic cells within the thymus where it may regulate clonal deletion of autoreactive T cells and affect self-tolerance. Ectodermal dystrophy, mucocutaneous candidiasis, multiple endocrine gland failure (parathyroids, adrenals, ovaries), autoantibody production, and autoimmune hepatitis in various syndromatic combinations are features of the disease. Unlike other autoimmune diseases, APS1 has a Mendelian pattern of inheritance, complete penetrance of the gene, no HLA DR associations, and no female predominance. The target autoantigens of APS1 are P450 IA2, which occurs commonly in patients who have hepatitis as part of the syndrome, and P450 IIA6.[204,205] Reactivity to P450 IID6 (CYP2D6) has also been described in the hepatitis of APS1; this finding suggests that type 2 autoimmune hepatitis and the hepatitis of APS 1 may be similar.

HCV infection has been associated with the production of anti-LKM1, and this association has generated speculation that HCV is the etiologic agent of type 2 autoimmune hepatitis.[206-211] In Italy as many as 86 percent of patients with anti-LKM1 were seropositive for antibodies to HCV (anti-HCV),[206-208] and many of these individuals had true HCV infection as assessed by second-generation immunoassays and polymerase chain reaction.[207,208] In contrast, patients with chronic hepatitis C who were screened for anti-LKM1 were usually seronegative.[189,191,212] The association with HCV was manifested mainly in those patients with anti-LKM1 who were screened for HCV.[188,206-211] This finding suggested that a certain genotype or variant form of HCV might stimulate the production of anti-LKM1 or antibodies that cross-react with LKM1.[188]

Early studies supported this hypothesis. Genotype 3 of HCV was found more commonly in patients with anti-LKM1 than in counterparts without anti-LKM1 (22 percent versus 2 percent, $P \leq 0.05$), and deletions in the envelope region of HCV were present only in the virus strains infecting patients with anti-LKM1.[213] Subsequent analyses, however, demonstrated that ethnic heterogeneity was the principal factor contributing to differences in the virus genotype, and current understanding is that anti-LKM1 expression in chronic hepatitis C is a reflection of the host rather than the virus.[213,214] In Northern Europe and North America, this expression is exceedingly rare.[189,212]

Type 2 autoimmune hepatitis is not a viral syndrome. The presence of anti-LKM1 in chronic hepatitis C is rare in North American patients and it does not diminish the viral nature of the disease or alter treatment strategies. Patients with true HCV infection and anti-LKM1 have chronic viral hepatitis with autoimmune features and should be classified and treated as a viral illness.[215]

Type 3 Autoimmune Hepatitis

Type 3 autoimmune hepatitis is the least established of the subclassifications (see Table 38-3)[111] and is characterized by the presence of antibodies to soluble liver antigen/liver pancreas (anti-SLA/LP).[216] Antibodies to soluble liver antigen (anti-SLA) and antibodies to liver pancreas (anti-LP) were originally described in different laboratories but the reactivities were subsequently found to be identical and they are now designated anti-SLA/LP.[216,217] Glutathione S-transferases were originally proposed as the target autoantigens[218] but a 50-kDa cytosolic protein has been described that is the more likely target.[148] This antigen may be a transfer RNA-protein complex involved in the incorporation of selenocysteine in polypeptide chains ($tRNP^{(Ser)Sec}$ complex).[149] The identification of the target antigen has facilitated the development of an enzyme immunoassay based on recombinant protein, and a commercial assay for anti-SLA/LP has been developed.[219]

Patients with type 3 disease are mostly women (91 percent) with a mean age of 37 years (range, 17 years to 67 years) (see Table 38-3).[191,216] They lack antibodies to nuclear antigens, LKM1, thyroglobulin, and thyroid microsome, but only 26 percent are seronegative for all autoantibodies except anti-SLA/LP.[216] Indeed, SMA (35 percent), antibodies to liver membrane antigen (26 percent), and AMA (22 percent) may be present.[216] Recent studies have been unable to distinguish patients with and without anti-SLA/LP by clinical or laboratory features.[191,219] Consequently, it is uncertain if anti-SLA/LP are hallmarks of a unique disease with a variety of non-specific immunoserologic manifestations or unusual but non-specific markers of type 1 autoimmune hepatitis.[191,216,220] Preliminary studies from a large multi-center collaboration have suggested that anti-SLA/LP may be useful in identifying patients with type 1 autoimmune hepatitis who relapse after corticosteroid withdrawal.[221]

Importantly, anti-SLA/LP are expressed in patients from different geographic regions and ethnic backgrounds, and the frequency of detection worldwide by the recombinant enzyme immunoassay ranges from 7 percent in Japan to 19 percent in Germany.[221] At the Mayo Clinic type 3 autoimmune hepatitis constitutes 3 percent of the adult population with autoimmune hepatitis by the earlier inhibition assay (see Figure 38-1).[191]

Type 3 autoimmune hepatitis is a diagnostic consideration in those patients who are classified as having cryptogenic chronic hepatitis by conventional immunoserologic screening (see Figure 38-1).[191,219] Indeed, in 18 percent of patients with severe cryptogenic chronic hepatitis, seropositivity for anti-SLA/LP can be demonstrated, and these patients have been women, HLA B8 positive, and corticosteroid responsive.[191] By testing for anti-SLA/LP, patients with cryptogenic chronic hepatitis may be reclassifiable as autoimmune hepatitis. Assessments for novel immunoserologic markers in patients with cryptogenic chronic hepatitis, however, have not eliminated the diagnosis, and at the Mayo Clinic, cryptogenic chronic hepatitis still constitutes 13 percent of the patients with non-viral forms of chronic hepatitis. Indeed, cryptogenic chronic hepatitis remains the second most common diagnosis in adults with presumed non-viral disease (see Figure 38-1).[222,223]

Subclassification of patients into homogeneous populations is important because it facilitates communication between clinicians and investigators, emphasizes the diversity of the disease, and preserves the opportunity for meaningful insights into disease behavior and pathogenesis. Other subclassifications may evolve based on etiologic distinctions, HLA profiles, clinical expressions, and disease behavior. Etiologic differences have been the classic bases for subclassification of disease; further definition of pathogenic pathways in autoimmune hepatitis is necessary before this template can be applied.

VARIANT FORMS

Codification of the diagnostic criteria of autoimmune hepatitis has excluded many forms of the disease that had previously been accommodated within the diagnosis.[8,9] Patients with mixed features that resemble other liver diseases ("overlap syndromes") or that are insufficient for a definite diagnosis ("outlier syndromes") constitute the variant forms (Table 38-5).[16,18] The most common variant disorders are those with hybrid features of autoimmune hepatitis and cholestatic liver disease. The variant forms of autoimmune hepatitis lack an es-

TABLE 38-5
Variant Syndromes

Variant syndrome	Predominant features	Empiric treatment
Overlap Syndromes	Concurrent features of two established disorders	Appropriate for predominant disorder or each component
Autoimmune hepatitis and primary biliary cirrhosis	AMAs Cholestatic clinical features Histologic cholangitis	Prednisone, 20 mg daily, if serum alkaline phosphatase level ≤ twice normal Prednisone, 20 mg daily, and ursodeoxycholic acid, 13-15 mg/kg daily, if alkaline phosphatase > twice normal or florid duct lesion
Autoimmune hepatitis and primary sclerosing cholangitis	Inflammatory bowel disease Cholestatic clinical features Abnormal cholangiogram	Prednisone, 20 mg daily, and ursodeoxycholic acid, 13-15 mg/kg daily
Autoimmune hepatitis and viral hepatitis	True viral infection Autoantibodies	Antiviral therapy if minor immune features and histologic changes compatible with viral infection Prednisone and azathioprine if major immune features and histologic changes of autoimmune hepatitis
Outlier Syndromes	Autoimmune features insufficient for diagnosis	Appropriate for predominant manifestations
Autoimmune cholangitis	AMA-negative No bowel disease Cholestatic clinical features Bile duct injury or loss Normal cholangiogram	Ursodeoxycholic acid, 13-15 mg/kg daily Prednisone, 20 mg daily, added if marked hepatocellular component
Cryptogenic chronic hepatitis	No autoantibodies or virus Otherwise indistinguishable from autoimmune hepatitis	Standard prednisone and azathioprine therapy

AMAs, Anti-mitochondrial antibodies.

tablished diagnostic algorithm or confident management strategy. Treatment is empiric and typically directed at the predominant manifestations of the disease. Patients with equally mixed hepatitic and cholestatic features are commonly treated with combination regimens of corticosteroids and ursodeoxycholic acid.

Retrospective analyses of patients with classic diagnoses of autoimmune liver disease—including autoimmune hepatitis, PBC, and PSC—have indicated that the variant syndromes are common.[19] Five percent of patients with autoimmune hepatitis have features of PBC, 19 percent of patients with PBC have features of autoimmune hepatitis, and 54 percent of patients with PSC have features of autoimmune hepatitis. The frequency of variant syndromes in patients with autoimmune liver disease is 18 percent. This occurrence may distort perceptions of clinical expression, natural history, and treatment responsiveness of the classic disorders.

The diagnostic scoring system promulgated by the International Autoimmune Hepatitis Group allows objective assessment of the strength of the diagnosis of autoimmune hepatitis in each variant form.[9] The degree of similarity of the variant form to the classic disease can be determined in this fashion. Patients with autoimmune hepatitis and PBC most closely resemble definite autoimmune hepatitis, whereas patients with autoimmune cholangitis are the furthest from the classic disorder. Patients that most closely resemble autoimmune hepatitis are the most likely to respond to corticosteroid therapy. Typically, these patients have serum alkaline phosphatase levels less than twofold normal. The variant syndromes should be classified separately from the classic disorders because they may have different pathogenic mechanisms, therapies, and outcomes.

Autoimmune Hepatitis and Primary Biliary Cirrhosis

Autoimmune hepatitis and PBC is an overlap syndrome in which there are mixed features of hepatocellular inflammation, immune reactivity, and cholestasis. A requisite for the diagnosis is the presence of AMA (see Table 38-5).[191,124,225] A diagnostic algorithm that has been proposed for this variant requires the presence of at least two of three accepted criteria for each disease in the same patient.[226] This diagnostic formula is arbitrary and its sensitivity for the syndrome has not been established. Nevertheless, it does provide a diagnostic template that can be consistently applied. An alternative approach is to designate only those individuals who have scores sufficient for the probable diagnosis of autoimmune hepatitis (aggregate scores $\geq$ 10), seropositivity for AMA, and cholangitis on histologic examination as overlap variants. This strategy is compromised by revisions of the scoring system for autoimmune hepatitis that promise to eliminate incompatible diagnoses. More stringent diagnostic criteria for autoimmune hepatitis will enlarge the pool of individuals with non-diagnostic findings and increase the heterogeneity of patients with variant syndromes.

Features of cholestasis may be present in 50 percent of patients with autoimmune hepatitis,[227] AMA can be demonstrated in 20 percent of individuals with typical features of autoimmune hepatitis,[225] and bile duct lesions that suggest PBC can be identified in 12 percent.[15,19,228-230] The frequency of these disparate findings in individuals with classic autoimmune hepatitis mandates a diagnostic algorithm that can accommodate isolated inconsistent findings or recognize the non-specificity of mild atypical laboratory or histologic features. Serum titers of AMA in patients with autoimmune hepatitis are usually low, and only 12 percent of individuals have titers that exceed 1:160.[225] Histologic changes of cholangitis are typically non-destructive in nature; ductopenia is absent; and features of destructive cholangitis, when present, are commonly isolated background changes that do not affect clinical expression or treatment response.[15,228-230] Thresholds that distinguish subtle diagnostic inconsistencies from disease-significant changes must be refined to differentiate variant syndromes from an acceptable spectrum of classic disease expression.

Disease behavior and treatment response depend mainly on the disease component of the overlap syndrome that predominates. Patients with mostly autoimmune hepatitis have high serum aspartate aminotransferase levels, serum alkaline phosphatase concentrations less than twofold normal, moderate to severe interface hepatitis on histologic examination, and high diagnostic scores for autoimmune hepatitis (aggregate scores $\geq$ 10). These individuals commonly respond to corticosteroid therapy.[225,230,231] In contrast, patients with mainly features of PBC have pronounced cholestatic features manifested by serum alkaline phosphatase levels greater than twofold normal, serum γ-glutamyl transpeptidase concentrations at least fivefold normal, and florid bile duct lesions on histologic examination. These individuals commonly achieve a complete biochemical response on a combination of corticosteroids and ursodeoxycholic acid.[226] Cyclosporin A has also been used successfully in one patient who was recalcitrant to both corticosteroids and ursodeoxycholic acid.[232]

Treatment response may relate to the stage of PBC present at accession and the genetic factors that affect outcome in autoimmune hepatitis. Early-stage PBC may lack the classic histologic changes and resemble autoimmune hepatitis.[233] These patients may yet evolve to classic PBC but at the time of diagnosis they may be responsive to therapy with corticosteroids. Similarly, the genetic risk factors that affect the susceptibility and outcome of autoimmune hepatitis may influence the clinical expression and corticosteroid responsiveness of patients with hybrid features. Individuals with a "hepatitic" form of PBC frequently are positive for HLA B8, DR3, or DR4, and these genetic markers can be shared in all forms of autoimmune liver disease with a variable impact on disease behavior.[231]

The antibodies with high specificity for PBC are directed against the 70-kDa pyruvate dehydrogenase-E2 subunit or the 50-kDa branched-chain keto-dehydrogenase-E2 subunit.[234-242] These antigens are the dihydrolipoamide acetyltransferases (E2 components) of the pyruvate dehydrogenase enzyme complex and the branched chain alpha-ketoacid dehydrogenase complex within mitochondria.[235,240] Studies have indicated that 80 percent to 95 percent of serum samples from patients with PBC react with the 70-kDa protein, 30 percent to 50 percent of sera react with the 50-kDa protein, and less than 10 percent of sera either do not react or react with a 39-kDa peptide that has not as yet been fully characterized.[235]

Using an enzyme immunoassay with recombinant polypeptides coding for both the 70-kDa and 50-kDa mitochondrial antigens, 96 percent of patients with PBC are reactive to one or both antigens, whereas none of control sera from healthy individuals or patients with PSC is reactive.[235] Several studies have now confirmed the specificity of these immunoserologic markers for PBC,[236-242] and there have been only a few instances in which seropositivity by enzyme immunoassay has been described in patients with autoimmune hepatitis.[191,236,241,242] In the Mayo Clinic experience only 6 percent of patients with autoimmune hepatitis were seropositive for these PBC-specific antibodies, suggesting that they were either rare instances of diagnostic non-specificity or were patients with the overlap syndrome of autoimmune hepatitis and PBC.[191]

Autoimmune Hepatitis and Primary Sclerosing Cirrhosis

Clinical, biochemical, and histologic features of autoimmune hepatitis may be present in 6 percent of patients with ulcerative colitis and cholangiograms diagnostic of PSC (see Table 38-5).[128] Similarly, histologic features of lymphoid, fibrous, and pleomorphic cholangitis suggestive of PSC may be present in 20 percent of patients with autoimmune hepatitis.[15,17,225,230] Cholangiography to exclude PSC is justified in all patients with autoimmune hepatitis who have histologic changes of cholangitis, concurrent inflammatory bowel disease, or failure to respond to corticosteroids. As many as 41 percent of these individuals will have cholangiographic changes of PSC and they will be classifiable as an overlap syndrome of autoimmune hepatitis and PSC.[128] Similarly, 54 percent of patients with PSC have aggregate scores for autoimmune hepatitis that indicate the probability of coexistent diseases. PSC shares genetic risk factors with autoimmune hepatitis (HLA B8, DR3, and DRw52); this host-related propensity may result in similar clinical expressions or in transitions between the diseases.[243-247] Conversely, HLA DR4, which predisposes to autoimmune hepatitis, protects against PSC, and its presence dissuades a strong PSC component of the variant syndrome.[17,247]

In children with autoimmune hepatitis cholangiography is indicated even in the absence of inflammatory bowel disease because "autoimmune sclerosing cholangitis" cannot be reliably excluded by clinical and histologic findings.[248,249] Autoimmune sclerosing cholangitis is a disorder described in children who have the clinical phenotype of autoimmune hepatitis but also have abnormal cholangiograms. Because these children have features of autoimmune hepatitis and PSC, they satisfy criteria for an overlap syndrome. Cholestatic clinical, laboratory, and histologic features and inflammatory bowel disease are typically absent, and these children respond as well to corticosteroid therapy as counterparts with classic type 1 autoimmune hepatitis.[250] Consequently, they are distinct from the overlap syndrome reported in adults and are best categorized separately.

Adults with autoimmune hepatitis, cholestatic features, seronegativity for AMA, and normal cholangiograms may have small duct PSC or autoimmune cholangitis (AIC).[17] Liver biopsy assessment is important to evaluate ductopenia, destructive cholangitis, or fibrous obliterative cholangitis. High serum alkaline phosphatase activity or a ratio of serum alkaline phosphatase level to aspartate aminotransferase level that exceeds 1.5 suggests the existence of an overlap between autoimmune hepatitis and PSC, especially if biliary changes are evident on liver biopsy examination and inflammatory bowel disease is present. Currently, the only distinguishing clinical feature between small duct PSC and AIC is the presence or absence of inflammatory bowel disease.

The overlapping features of autoimmune hepatitis and PSC in some patients may reflect similarities in the immunopathogenesis of the disorders. Effector lymphocytes in both conditions react with antibody-coated target cells through their Fc receptors,[251] both conditions have similar frequencies of antibodies to liver membrane protein complex in serum,[251] and both disorders have similar HLA phenotypes.[243-247] These factors may account at times for similar clinical expressions, concurrence of the disorders, or the apparent evolution of PSC from autoimmune hepatitis.

There is no established treatment for the overlap variant of autoimmune hepatitis and PSC. Corticosteroid therapy has been associated with normalization of serum aminotransferase levels and improvement in the histologic features of inflammation in some patients.[252,253] In others, corticosteroid therapy has been ineffective.[19,128] As with the other variant syndromes, treatment is empiric and must be tailored to the predominant manifestations. The potential for a corticosteroid response is reserved for those individuals with serum alkaline phosphatase levels below twofold normal.[19] Ursodeoxycholic acid can be considered in individuals with dominant cholestatic features but it has generally not been useful in PSC.[254] The combination of corticosteroids and ursodeoxycholic acid manages all aspects of the disease and intuitively is the most appealing treatment. Its value, however, is uncertain.

Autoimmune Hepatitis and Viral Infection

The autoantibodies that characterize autoimmune hepatitis may occur in conjunction with antibodies to hepatitis A, B, or C viruses.[255-257] The concurrence of these markers can confound the diagnosis and complicate the management strategy. Anecdotal reports have indicated that the administration of interferon to patients with autoimmune hepatitis may exacerbate the disease,[258-261] whereas the administration of corticosteroids to patients with true viral infection is ineffective and increases the viral load.[262] Deterioration of patients with autoimmune features during interferon therapy is rare, but its occurrence in some patients has justified a wariness of antiviral treatment.[181,182] These concerns have underscored the importance of distinguishing autoimmune hepatitis with viral markers from chronic viral hepatitis with autoimmune features.

Autoimmune hepatitis is by definition a non-viral disease but there is an association between viral infection and the autoimmune response. Anti-nuclear antibodies or SMA occur in 20 percent to 40 percent of patients with chronic hepatitis B or C[256,263]; anti-LKM1 are detectable in up to 6 percent of patients with chronic hepatitis C[206,207]; antibodies to LKM3 are found in 13 percent of patients with chronic hepatitis D[264,265]; immune diseases that are viral-antigen driven (cryoglobulinemia) or autoantigen driven (autoimmune thyroiditis, Sjögren's syndrome) frequently co-exist[266-268]; and corticosteroids may be effective in some patients.[164,269-272] In most individuals the viral components predominate; these patients are best designated "chronic viral hepatitis with autoimmune features" and treated with anti-viral agents. Rarely, the autoimmune features predominate and the concurrent true viral infection is co-incidental or etiologic but non-essential for perpetuation of the disorder. These latter patients constitute the overlap syndrome of autoimmune hepatitis and true viral infection (see Table 38-5). Their diagnosis requires all the clinical, laboratory, and histologic features of classic autoimmune hepatitis and none of viral infection.[164]

Candidates for designation as an overlap of autoimmune hepatitis and viral hepatitis are patients with high titer SMA or ANA (titers ≥ 1:320) and hypergammaglobulinemia.[155,273] These patients commonly are HLA DR3 positive, and examination of the liver tissue typically discloses moderate to severe interface hepatitis with or without panacinar hepatitis. Viral features, such as steatosis and portal lymphoid aggregates, are typically absent. Retrospective analyses have indicated that these rare patients respond as well to corticosteroid treatment as to their uninfected counterparts.[164] Importantly, instances of deterioration during interferon treatment have been rare, and the routine precautionary use of corticosteroids in individuals without definite autoimmune hepatitis is unjustified. Similarly, the presence of anti-LKM1 in patients with true chronic hepatitis C infection has not contraindicated institution of anti-viral therapy.[274,275] The overlap syndrome of autoimmune hepatitis and true viral hepatitis is unusual and probably a serendipitous event rather than an important disease entity.

Cryptogenic Chronic Hepatitis

Second- and third-generation enzyme immunoassays for HCV have reduced the number of patients who qualify for the diagnosis of cryptogenic chronic hepatitis.[276,277] Twenty percent of patients with chronic hepatitis, however, still lack a formal designation.[16,278,279] These patients may have HCV infection that cannot be detected by current methods, another yet-undefined virus infection, or an autoimmune disease that has escaped detection by conventional immunoserologic testing.[280]

Patients with cryptogenic chronic hepatitis who are candidates for an autoimmune designation and corticosteroid therapy are commonly women (67 percent) and typically have hypergammaglobulinemia (75 percent) and elevated serum levels of immunoglobulin G (75 percent) (see Table 38-5).[222,223] Concurrent immunologic disorders may be present in 25 percent, and HLA B8 can be demonstrated in 75 percent.[223] The majority of patients (71 percent) will have HLA DR3, and 57 percent will have the HLA A1-B8-DR3 phenotype (see Table 38-5). Liver biopsy assessment typically discloses interface hepatitis with lymphocytic, occasionally lymphoplasmacytic, inflammatory infiltrates extending from portal tracts into acinar tissue, and 82 percent will enter remission during corticosteroid therapy.[223,281] Autoantibodies are fluctuating continuous variables, and serial assessments for these markers may ultimately demonstrate their presence in some patients. Other patients may remain seronegative for the conventional autoantibodies and await discovery by a novel marker, such as anti-SLA/LP. Patients with cryptogenic chronic hepatitis who resemble autoimmune hepatitis except for the conventional autoantibodies may well have "autoantibody-negative autoimmune hepatitis."

Patients with cryptogenic chronic hepatitis and autoimmune features should not be confused with patients who have cryptogenic cirrhosis.[276,277,280] This latter designation connotes an end-stage, inactive cirrhosis that has lost its identifying features. Such patients are not candidates for corticosteroid therapy.

Autoimmune Cholangitis

Autoimmune cholangitis is an outlier syndrome and probably a heterogeneous disorder that includes patients with small duct PSC, idiopathic adulthood ductopenia, and AMA-negative PBC (see Table 38-5).[17] Its major distinguishing feature from PBC is the absence of AMA, including antibodies against the E2 subunits of the pyruvate dehydrogenase complex. Typically, the biochemical profile is cholestatic with elevations of serum alkaline phosphatase and γ-glutamyl transpeptidase.[17] Hepatocellular inflammation, as reflected in serum aminotransferase elevations, can be pronounced, and elevations of serum immunoglobulin G are common in a fashion characteristic of autoimmune hepatitis.[17]

Retrospective analyses using PBC as a reference have emphasized its resemblance to PBC. In these studies patients with autoimmune cholangitis have been indistinguishable from those with PBC by histologic examination,[282] display of pyruvate dehydrogenase complexes on biliary epithelia,[283] presence of PBC-specific antibodies to 2-oxo-acid dehydrogenase complex in blood,[284-286] seropositivity for antibodies to carbonic anhydrase,[287,288] clinical and laboratory features,[289] and responsiveness to ursodeoxycholic acid.[290] Conversely, retrospective analyses using patients with autoimmune hepatitis as a reference for the diagnosis have emphasized its resemblance to autoimmune hepatitis. In these studies patients with autoimmune cholangitis have had ANA or SMA, interface hepatitis and portal plasma cell infiltration, high mean diagnostic scores for autoimmune hepatitis, and occasional improvement after corticosteroid therapy.[291-293] Prospective studies applying uniform criteria for diagnosis have indicated that autoimmune cholangitis is a heterogeneous disorder and not easily classifiable as simply AMA-negative PBC.[17]

ANA and SMA are usually present and histologic findings may include lymphocytic or lymphoplasmacytic portal infiltration, interface hepatitis, destructive cholangitis, lymphoid aggregates, or ductopenia in various combinations.[17,291,292] Patients with similar clinical profiles may have histologic changes that are indistinguishable from PBC or PSC. Other patients may have marked changes of interface hepatitis indistinguishable from autoimmune hepatitis in conjunction with destructive cholangitis. The variability of the histologic findings attests to the heterogeneity of autoimmune cholangitis or suggests that the disorder is a transition state within classic syndromes.[17] Autoimmune cholangitis does not have a reliable serologic marker. Early investigations suggesting that antibodies to carbonic anhydrase would be a useful marker of the disease have not been corroborated.[294]

Responsiveness to corticosteroids or ursodeoxycholic acid is variable and generally poor.[17] Most studies indicate an inability to induce histologic improvement with either drug.[291,292] Treatment is empiric and consists of corticosteroids, ursodeoxycholic acid, or a combination of both. It should be reserved for those individuals who are symptomatic with jaundice, pruritus, or malaise.[17]

NATURAL HISTORY

Early descriptions of the natural history of autoimmune hepatitis focused only on the most severe forms of the disease.[39,40,47-50] Retrospective studies failed to apply uniform criteria for diagnosis, assess drug histories, document epidemiologic risk factors, exclude viral disease, perform systematic evaluations, avoid haphazard use of medication, and maintain long-term follow-up. Cirrhosis was emphasized as a presenting feature or likely consequence of the disease,[39,40,46] and the 3-year survival was projected as 50 percent.[295] Only 10 percent of patients with autoimmune hepatitis lived for 10 years.[295]

Prospective clinical trials included control groups from which natural history could be assessed, but these studies were designed to evaluate life and death end points in the sickest patients.[48-50,296] In the Mayo Clinic experience 40 percent of untreated patients died within 6 months, whereas the remainder were switched to corticosteroids.[49] Individuals in untreated control groups had cirrhosis at presentation, died too rapidly after accession to progress to cirrhosis, or were reassigned to corticosteroid regimens soon after an effective treatment had been established. Under such circumstances, the prevention of cirrhosis by corticosteroid therapy could not be proven, nor could the natural history of less than severe disease be described.

The natural history of autoimmune hepatitis is defined by extrapolations from a diverse experience.[297] Patients with sustained elevation of the serum aspartate aminotransferase level to at least tenfold normal or fivefold normal in conjunction with a serum γ-globulin concentration of at least twice normal have a 3-year mortality of 50 percent (Figure 38-4).[295] Cirrhosis develops in 82 percent of patients with bridging necrosis or multi-acinar necrosis within 5 years; mortality during this period is 45 percent.[60] Bridging necrosis between portal tract and central vein progresses to cirrhosis more frequently than bridging necrosis between portal tract and portal tract (29 percent versus 10 percent), and interface hepatitis infrequently progresses to cirrhosis.[61] Cirrhosis is found at presentation in 25 percent of patients, who have a 5-year mortality of 58 percent.[60] Esophageal varices develop in 54 percent of individuals with cirrhosis within 2 years, and death from hemorrhage occurs in 20 percent of those with varices.[50] Hepatocellular carcinoma is possible in those patients with cirrhosis but is rare unless survival with cirrhosis is prolonged[298-301] or there is a concurrent viral infection.[302] Spontaneous resolution occurs in 13 percent to 20 percent of patients, and it is an unpredictable outcome.[49,297] Of patients who survive the early, most active stage of their disease, 41 percent attain inactive disease, albeit in the presence of cirrhosis.[46] Death from liver failure usually occurs within 2 years after presentation, and individuals who survive this critical period have an opportunity for prolonged survival.[46,303]

Wide fluctuations in inflammatory activity can occur, and recrudescence of the disease after years of remission has been described.[296] Exacerbations of inactive disease, however, are rare, and in such instances, a superimposed drug toxicity or viral infection must be sought. The stability of the inactive state that occurs spontaneously is different from that induced with medication. In the former instance the pathogenic mechanisms that perpetuate the inflammation have resolved, whereas in the latter instance, only their clinical manifestations have been suppressed.[297]

Transitions between the various histologic patterns of inflammatory activity may also occur spontaneously.[60] Interface hepatitis may progress to multi-acinar necrosis or bridging necrosis or improve to portal hepatitis in an unpredictable fashion. The inflammatory activity of autoimmune hepatitis can be variable in different regions of the liver, and histologic transitions may represent sampling variation. Sampling error for estimating inflammatory activity, however, is low, and fluctuations in histologic findings most commonly reflect the natural history of the disease.[65,66]

Patients with less severe inflammatory activity have better prognoses (see Figure 38-4).[297,303] In one experience with 71 patients who were followed for 7.5 years the frequencies of progression to cirrhosis (64 percent

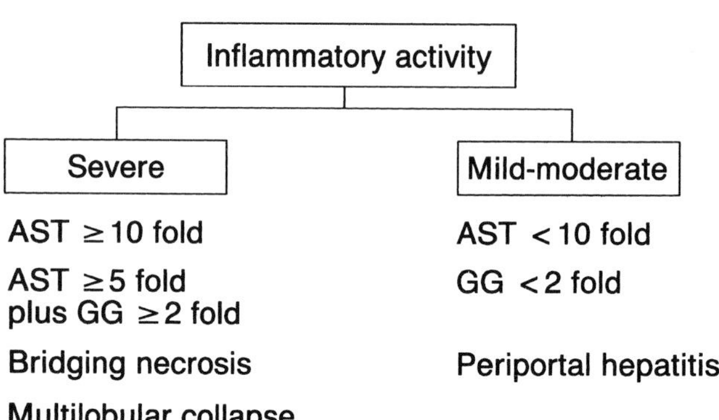

Figure 38-4 Biochemical and histologic features that reflect severity of inflammatory activity and prognosis in autoimmune hepatitis. Periportal hepatitis indicates the presence of interface hepatitis. *AST,* Aspartate aminotransferase activity; *GG,* serum γ-globulin concentration.

versus 83 percent) and death (23 percent versus 46 percent) were less in patients with mild-to-moderate as compared to severe disease.[303] In another experience cirrhosis developed in only 49 percent of patients with mild disease within 15 years and the 10-year mortality was only 10 percent.[304] Spontaneous improvement to features of portal hepatitis occurred in 50 percent of similar patients.[305] Asymptomatic patients who have been followed for an average of 6.3 years have a low frequency of progression to cirrhosis (19 percent) and death from liver failure (9 percent). The 5- and 10-year survivals are as high as 91 percent and 81 percent, respectively, in these patients.[306] In asymptomatic patients with mild to moderate disease activity the benefit-risk ratio of any therapy may be so low that treatment is unjustified.

CLINICAL FEATURES

Autoimmune hepatitis is typically an insidious disease of young women.[1] Women constitute at least 70 percent of cases and 50 percent are younger than age 40.[114] Onset is usually between the third and fifth decades, but patients may range in age from 9 months to 77 years.[1] Fifteen percent of patients have a history of contact with acute hepatitis or ancient blood transfusion; 40 percent have an abrupt onset of symptoms.[1,114] Importantly, a fulminant presentation is possible, especially in the young.[307] In such instances features of chronic liver disease, including hypergammaglobulinemia and histologic cirrhosis, must be sought[119-123] and all conventional immunoserologic markers must be assessed, especially antibodies to LKM1.[307]

Familial occurrences are rare but the disease has been reported in siblings, parents, and grandparents of afflicted individuals.[308-310] First-degree relatives may have abnormal serum immunoglobulin levels (47 percent), autoantibodies (42 percent), and hypergammaglobulinemia (34 percent).[308] In one series 3 of 55 families (5 percent) had more than one family member with chronic liver disease.[308]

Symptoms at Presentation

Easy fatigability is the most common symptom at presentation (85 percent) (Table 38-6).[1,303] The severity of the symptom does not correlate closely with the degree of inflammatory activity or histologic stage of the disease, and many patients never feel that they fully return to normal even after induction of remission. Recrudescence of the symptom is the earliest indication of relapse after drug withdrawal, whereas worsening of fatigue during therapy may be a sign that treatment has failed to suppress inflammatory activity.[311]

Features of jaundice during the prodrome of the disease (scleral icterus, dark urine, or light-colored stools) are described by as many as 77 percent of patients at presentation, but frank jaundice at accession can be documented in only 46 percent (see Table 38-6).[1,303]

Right upper quadrant pain is experienced by 48 percent of patients (see Table 38-6).[1,303] Typically, the discomfort is mild and manifested as a constant dull right upper quadrant ache or transient sharp pain with an unpredictable recurrence. Rarely, the pain may be the principal complaint and of sufficient severity to warrant analgesics. In these patients thorough assessments to exclude hepatic malignancy and biliary disease are warranted. Usually the pain subsides as disease activity declines, although improvement may lag behind the laboratory changes.

Polymyalgias (30 percent); anorexia (30 percent); diarrhea (28 percent); cosmetic changes including facial rounding, hirsutism, and acne (19 percent); and obscure fever (rarely as high as 40° C) are frequent complaints (see Table 38-6).[1,114,303] Delayed menarche and amenorrhea are common symptoms (89 percent) in women with severe inflammatory activity or advanced disease.[303] In adolescents delayed menarche may be the initial manifestation of the disease, whereas in adults the onset of amenorrhea may indicate the beginning of the disease or an exacerbation of inflammatory activity.

Pruritus may be present in 36 percent of patients but is typically an afterthought.[1,303] Intense pruritus is extremely unusual and suggests another diagnosis or complicating concurrent condition.[227] Weight loss is also unusual and is a disturbing sign that may reflect advanced-stage disease or occult malignancy. Many patients with autoimmune hepatitis actually gain weight because their diminished stamina and exercise tolerance may counterbalance the effects of their decreased appetite.[1,303]

Physical Findings at Presentation

Physical findings are reflective of the duration and severity of the disease, and therefore there are no features common to all presentations. Analyses have been restricted mainly to patients with severe disease, and the physical manifestations in these patients are undoubtedly more florid and more frequent than in individuals who are less ill.

Hepatomegaly is the most common physical finding at presentation (78 percent), and mild hepatic tenderness by palpation or punch may be present (see Table 38-6).[312]

TABLE 38-6
Major Clinical Features at Presentation

Features at presentation	Frequency (%)
Symptoms	85
Dark urine or light-colored stools	77
Right upper quadrant discomfort or pain	48
Generalized myalgias	30
Anorexia	30
Diarrhea	28
Physical Findings	
Hepatomegaly	78
Spider nevi	58
Palpable spleen	32-56
Scleral icterus	46
Ascites	20
Encephalopathy	14

Splenomegaly commonly accompanies cirrhosis (56 percent) but it may be present in the absence of this histologic finding (32 percent). Spider nevi are frequent findings (58 percent) but do not establish the presence of cirrhosis (see Table 38-6).[312]

Ascites (20 percent) and various degrees of hepatic encephalopathy (14 percent) are found infrequently and connote advanced liver disease and cirrhosis (see Table 38-6).[312] Hyperpigmentation and xanthelasmas are rare. Hirsutism, facial rounding, acne, and truncal obesity were originally described in young women with autoimmune hepatitis and cirrhosis.[26-28] The constellation of findings make up the syndrome of lupoid hepatitis and it still has specificity for the diagnosis although its sensitivity is low. Autoimmune hepatitis no longer has stereotypical physical findings as the diagnosis now spans all age groups and each gender.

Patients with active cirrhosis invariably have at least one physical finding that indicates the presence of chronic liver disease. Twenty-six percent of individuals without cirrhosis, however, may have entirely normal physical examinations despite severe inflammatory activity.[312]

Concurrent Immune Diseases

As many as 48 percent of patients with autoimmune hepatitis have concurrent immunologic diseases (see Table 38-4).[126,127,313,314] Patients with type 2 autoimmune hepatitis may have a higher frequency of co-existent disorders than those with type 1 disease (40 percent versus 10 percent), and the nature of these associated immunologic disorders may differ between the types.[117] Vitiligo and insulin-dependent diabetes mellitus are more common in type 2 autoimmune hepatitis, whereas autoimmune thyroiditis, chronic ulcerative colitis, and synovitis typify type 1 autoimmune hepatitis. Importantly, frequencies of concurrent disease determined at presentation underestimate true prevalence because many immunologic disorders evolve later in the course of the disease.

Autoimmune thyroiditis, ulcerative colitis, and synovitis are the most common extrahepatic features of autoimmune hepatitis (see Table 38-4).[126,127] Multiple non-hepatic immunologic diseases are present in 6 percent of patients. Of individuals with extrahepatic disorders 57 percent have autoimmune thyroid disease, including thyroiditis (43 percent) and Graves' disease (13 percent). Celiac sprue may be asymptomatic and present in 3 percent of patients. Its recognition is important because gluten restriction can improve the bowel disease and theoretically reduce liver inflammation.[315]

Individuals with HLA DR4 have concurrent immunologic diseases more commonly than those without these findings (65 percent versus 31 percent, $P = 0.0002$) (see Figure 38-2).[123,124] Autoimmune thyroid disease (65 percent versus 37 percent, $P = 0.02$) and the presence of microsomal thyroid antibodies (57 percent versus 35 percent, $P = 0.02$) are also found more commonly in patients with HLA DR4. In contrast, patients with ulcerative colitis and cholangiograms that exclude PSC are frequently heterozygous for HLA DR3 and DR4 (50 percent versus 10 percent, $P = 0.02$).[123,124] Importantly, the majority of the concurrent immunologic diseases associated with autoimmune hepatitis (68 percent) have known HLA-associations outside the context of autoimmune hepatitis; these may involve the same DR locus, as in the examples of autoimmune thyroiditis (HLA DR4), rheumatoid arthritis (HLA DR4), and secondary Sjögren's syndrome (HLA DR4).[123,124] Clustering of HLA-associated diseases may occur if each disease is caused by a common allele—one allele of a given haplotype is required for either disease or two linked loci each separately encode susceptibility to each disease.[316] The exact mechanisms that influence the expression of concurrent immunologic diseases in autoimmune hepatitis are unknown but it is apparent that a DR4 allele is involved.

Fifty-nine percent of patients with autoimmune hepatitis and ulcerative colitis have normal cholangiograms and enter remission during corticosteroid therapy as commonly as counterparts without ulcerative colitis (86 percent versus 94 percent).[128] Unfortunately, the reassurances acquired at presentation may not endure because large duct or small duct PSC may evolve during follow-up as a coexistent disease or one in transition from autoimmune hepatitis.[130,131] The emergence of a cholestatic biochemical profile or recalcitrance to corticosteroid therapy justifies repeat cholangiography.

Laboratory Findings at Presentation

The laboratory hallmarks of autoimmune hepatitis are abnormalities in serum aminotransferase activity and γ-globulin levels (Table 38-7).[1,8,9,317] These findings not only suggest the diagnosis but also are important indices of prognosis. In most cases the serum aminotransferase level at presentation does not exceed 500 U/L.[119] Sixteen percent of patients, however, have values of 1000 U/L or more. These patients may be confused with those who present with acute hepatocellular necrosis of viral, toxic, or ischemic origin. Fortunately, 92 percent of patients with autoimmune hepatitis who present in this fashion

TABLE 38-7

Major Laboratory and Histologic Findings at Presentation

Features at presentation	Frequency (%)
Laboratory Findings	
Hypergammaglobulinemia	80
Immunoglobulin G elevation	80
Bilirubin ≥ 3 mg/dl	46
Alkaline phosphatase ≥ twice normal limit	33
Aspartate aminotransferase ≥ 1000 U/L	16
Histologic Findings	
Interface hepatitis (severe)	23
Panacinar (lobular) hepatitis (moderate-severe)	47
Portal plasma cell infiltration	66
Cirrhosis	25

have other clinical and laboratory features that reflect their true nature.[119]

Hypergammaglobulinemia is present in more than 80 percent of cases and has been proposed as a requisite for the diagnosis.[1,8,9,21,317] A polyclonal increase in serum immunoglobulin concentrations is typical, and the immunoglobulin G fraction predominates.[1,21,317] In patients with type 2 autoimmune hepatitis, the serum immunoglobulin A level may be low, which may distinguish the condition from type 1 disease.[117]

Multiple paraproteins with antibody reactivity have been described in association with hypergammaglobulinemia, and the γ-globulin level is probably a barometer of immunoreactivity.[318] Antibodies to bacterial (*Escherichia coli*, *Bacteroides*, and *Salmonella*) and viral (measles, rubella, and cytomegalovirus) agents can frequently be demonstrated[319,320] and may reflect the inability of a damaged liver to clear exogenous antigens, a genetically determined non-specific increase in immune responsiveness, or an abnormal immunologic defense against bacterial and viral infection.[319] Rarely, extremely high levels of immunoglobulin may cause coagulation abnormalities, renal insufficiency, and mental disturbances consistent with the hyperviscosity syndrome.[321]

Hyperbilirubinemia is present in 83 percent of patients with severe inflammatory activity but the serum bilirubin level exceeds 3 mg/dl in only 46 percent of cases (see Table 38-7).[1,225,317] Similarly, abnormal elevation of the serum alkaline phosphatase level can be demonstrated in 81 percent of patients but it is greater than twofold normal in only 33 percent and more than fourfold normal in only 10 percent (see Table 38-7).[1,225,317] Urinary copper excretion may exceed normal values in nearly 50 percent of patients but is infrequently of a magnitude (greater than 100 μg/day) to suggest Wilson's disease.[322] Hepatic copper concentrations may also be increased but are rarely higher than 100 μg/g dry tissue weight.[322] Cholestatic indices are commonly present in autoimmune hepatitis but do not dominate the laboratory profile. Indeed, the diagnosis of autoimmune hepatitis is suspect if they do.[8,9]

AUTOANTIBODIES

A plethora of organ- and non–organ-specific autoantibodies has been described in autoimmune hepatitis; these immunoserologic markers are hallmarks of the disease (Tables 38-8 and 38-9).[8,9] Most autoantibodies are neither liver- or disease-specific, and none has been shown to be pathogenic.[190,323] The levels of autoantibody reactivity can change with the degree of hepatocellular inflammation and there are no objectively defined lower limits of significant seropositivity.[2,323] Furthermore, autoantibodies rarely "breed true" during the course of

TABLE 38-8

Standard Repertoire of Autoantibodies

Autoantibodies	Properties
Anti-nuclear	Traditional marker of type 1 autoimmune hepatitis
	Multiple nuclear targets, including centromere, ribonucleoproteins, and ribonucleoprotein complexes
	Not disease specific
	New enzyme immunoassay based on recombinant antigens
Double-stranded DNA	Common in ANA-positive patients
	Does not discriminate systemic lupus erythematosus
	Enzyme-linked immunosorbent assay defines ANA subgroup with high frequency of treatment failure
Smooth muscle	Marker of type 1 autoimmune hepatitis
	Co-exists or alternates with ANA expression
	Multiple reactivities, including actin, tubulin, vimentin, desmin, and skeletin
	Low disease specificity
Mitochondrial	Low titers by indirect immunofluorescence in type 1 disease
	Immunofluorescence pattern may be confused with anti-LKM1
	Antibodies to E2 subunits of pyruvate dehydrogenase complex in 8% with type 1 autoimmune hepatitis
Liver/kidney microsome type 1	Marker of type 2 autoimmune hepatitis
	Directed against P450 IID6 (CYP2D6)
	Infrequently associated with chronic hepatitis C
	Can occur in autoimmune polyglandular syndrome type 1
Perinuclear anti-neutrophil cytoplasm	Common in high titer in type 1 autoimmune hepatitis
	Rare in type 2 autoimmune hepatitis
	Immunoglobulin G_1 isotype
	Unknown target antigen
	Useful in evaluating cryptogenic chronic hepatitis

DNA, Deoxyribonucleic acid; *ANA*, anti-nuclear antibodies; *anti-LKM1*, antibodies to liver/kidney microsome type 1.

TABLE 38-9
Emerging Repertoire of Autoantibodies

Autoantibodies	Properties
Histones	Nuclear proteins complexed with DNA (nucleosome)
	Anti-H3 in young patients with active inflammation
Actin	High specificity for type 1 autoimmune hepatitis, especially F-actin
	Associated with early onset disease, poor response to corticosteroids, HLA DR3
	Lacks established assay
Liver cytosol type 1	Associated with early age onset, concurrent immunologic diseases, severe inflammation
	Fluctuates with disease activity
	Can co-exist with anti-LKM1
	Forminotransferase cyclodeaminase and argininosuccinate lyas are possible target antigens
Soluble liver antigen/liver pancreas	Associated with subgroup of type 1 autoimmune hepatitis
	Directed against 50-kDa cytosolic protein, possibly selenocysteine transfer ribonucleoprotein
	Associated with *DRB1*0301* and relapse propensity
	Useful in evaluating cryptogenic chronic hepatitis
Asialoglycoprotein receptor	Common in all types of autoimmune hepatitis
	Associated with disease activity and interface hepatitis
	Disappears during effective corticosteroid treatment
	Heralds relapse after corticosteroid withdrawal

DNA, Deoxyribonucleic acid; *HLA,* human leukocyte antigen; *anti-LKM1,* antibodies to liver/kidney microsome type 1.

autoimmune hepatitis, and one type may disappear and another appear or multiple types may be expressed simultaneously.[324] The cause-and-effect relationship between the autoantibodies and liver disease remains uncertain, and the specificity of the immunoserologic markers for the diagnosis depends on cut-off values that can be adjusted arbitrarily.[2,324] Autoantibodies continue to be characterized because they may be biologic probes by which the pathogenic mechanisms and target autoantigens can be discovered. Autoantibodies are also important diagnostic tools and some may be barometers of disease activity or indices of prognosis.[190,324]

Antinuclear Antibodies

The demonstration of ANA in serum is the traditional basis for the diagnosis of autoimmune hepatitis (see Table 38-8).[1] These antibodies can be found in 74 percent of patients with type 1 autoimmune hepatitis.[114,324] Typically, they coexist with SMA, occurring as the sole immunoserologic marker in only 9 percent to 14 percent of instances. Reactivity can appear and disappear during the disease and ANA can be replaced by SMA.[324]

The development of an enzyme immunoassay based on recombinant nuclear antigens has displaced previous assays based on indirect immunofluorescence.[190,325] Results from the enzyme immunoassay provide a quantification of positivity rather than a titer, and these findings cannot be converted into a titer. Results from the new assay system must be correlated with clinical features and disease outcome, and new correlations established. Clinical implications based on titer or on particular patterns of nuclear immunofluorescence (homogeneous versus speckled) must be reassessed in the context of the new technology.

The expression of ANA may be influenced by genetic factors linked to the major histocompatibility complex.[124] Patients with HLA DR4 have a higher frequency of strong ANA reactivity than counterparts with less reactivity (see Figure 38-2).[124] These findings suggest that marked ANA reactivity may be reflective of a genetic predisposition for immune reactivity associated with autoimmune hepatitis. The manifestation may be host-dependent rather than disease-specific, and ANA may be surrogate markers of an autoimmune phenotype.[127]

Recent studies assessing reactivities against recombinant nuclear proteins have indicated a high frequency of antibodies to recombinant centromere (Cenp-B) (42 percent) and 52-kDa ribonucleoprotein complexes (SSA/Ro) (23 percent) in patients with type 1 autoimmune hepatitis.[326,327] Forty-six percent of patients, however, had multiple reactivities and no antibodies to recombinant nuclear antigens that were associated with distinctive clinical or prognostic features. Consequently, it is unlikely that further subclassification of ANA by nuclear reactivity will have clinical value.

Antibodies to Histones

Histones are small basic nuclear proteins that are complexed with DNA in all eukaryotic cells and are subunits of the nucleosome (see Table 38-9).[328,329] Histones are probably important in the binding of DNA to the cell nucleus; theoretically, antibodies against histones could destabilize the nucleus and impair its function. The predominant antibody against histones in autoimmune hepatitis is the immunoglobulin G antibody to the H3 histone; preliminary studies have suggested that this antibody occurs mainly in younger patients with higher serum aspartate aminotransferase levels and greater frequency of HLA DR4 than seronegative patients.[328,329] There is still uncertainty that these determinations, including those for class specific antibodies, offer a diagnostic or prognostic advantage.

Antibodies to Double-stranded DNA

Antibodies to double-stranded DNA were initially considered to have high specificity for SLE and be a useful test to distinguish a systemic disease with hepatic manifestations from a primary liver disease (see Table 38-8).[37] These antibodies are now recognized to be common in ANA-positive patients with type 1 autoimmune hepatitis and may have prognostic value.[38,330] ANA-positive patients with antibodies to double-stranded DNA by enzyme immunosorbent assay exhibit HLA DR4 more commonly and fail corticosteroid treatment more often than seronegative patients with ANA. Antibodies to double-stranded DNA may define a subgroup of patients with ANA who respond less well to treatment. These associations, however, are assay-dependent, and the results of an enzyme immunosorbent assay have not correlated with those of an indirect immunofluorescence assay using *Crithidia luciliae* as substrate.[330]

Smooth Muscle Antibodies

SMAs typify type 1 autoimmune hepatitis (see Table 38-8).[51] They commonly co-exist with ANA but may be the only immunoserologic markers of type 1 autoimmune hepatitis in 26 percent of cases.[114] Concurrence of SMA and ANA is uncommon in chronic viral hepatitis, and the simultaneous expression of both autoantibodies provides reassurance about the non-viral nature of the disease.[180]

SMAs are detected by indirect immunofluorescence of murine stomach and kidney.[51,190,331] They are directed against actin and non-actin components, including tubulin, vimentin, desmin, and skeletin, and three types have been described using cultured fibroblasts treated with vinblastine.[332-333] Antibodies to actin, tubulin, and intermediate filaments constitute the principal types of SMA; antibodies to actin have specificity for autoimmune hepatitis.[333,334] The median titer of SMA at presentation is 1:160 (range, 1:40 to 1:5120), and 20 percent of patients have titers of only 1:40.[323] In 81 percent of patients with low titers, concurrent seropositivity for ANA reinforces the diagnosis. Patients with SMA more frequently have HLA DR4 than seronegative patients but this association is lost at high titers, suggesting that the relationship may be non-specific.[124]

The principal reactivity of SMA in type 1 autoimmune hepatitis is against actin cables, which span the long axis of cultured fibroblasts.[332-334] This reactivity is to polymerized F-actin, and it has a high specificity for autoimmune hepatitis. F-actin is closely associated with the hepatocyte membrane, and antibodies to F-actin may facilitate binding of immunoglobulin to the hepatocyte surface. Such binding may in turn promote an antibody-dependent, cell-mediated form of cytotoxicity. In other conditions, the patterns of staining on fibroblast monolayers may indicate reactivity to non-actin cytofilaments, and these reactions probably account for weak SMA reactions in acute and chronic viral hepatitis.[332-334]

Antibodies to Actin

Antibodies to actin, especially the polymerized F-actin, have greater specificity for type 1 autoimmune hepatitis than SMA but the method of detection has not been standardized (see Table 38-9).[335,337] A thermolabile F-actin depolymerizing factor has been described in serum; its effect on assay performance remains unclear.[337] Consequently, determinations of anti-actin have not been incorporated into conventional diagnostic algorithms. Preliminary studies using multiple assays for anti-actin have indicated their occurrence in patients who more commonly have HLA DR3, early-age onset disease, and a poorer response to corticosteroid therapy than patients without anti-actin.[339] The autoantibodies are less sensitive for type 1 autoimmune hepatitis than SMA, and testing for anti-actin is unlikely to replace testing for SMA as a screening tool.[339]

Anti-mitochondrial Antibodies

AMAs are found in 20 percent of patients with autoimmune hepatitis.[225] Serum titers, however, are low (less than 1:160 in 88 percent of instances); the histologic findings are indistinguishable from counterparts without AMA; tissue copper stains by rhodanine are negative or mildly positive; and patients respond satisfactorily to corticosteroid therapy (see Table 38-8).[225] Patients with high titers of AMA may actually have PBC or unrecognized anti-LKM1 seropositivity. Enzyme immunoassays for the more PBC-specific antibodies to the E2 subunits of the pyruvate dehydrogenase complex have improved diagnostic precision.[234-241] Those antibodies reacting against the dihydrolipoamide acyltransferase E2 subunits of the pyruvate dehydrogenase enzyme complex (anti–PDH-E2) have the highest specificity for PBC.[234-241]

Antibodies to Liver/Kidney Microsome Type 1

Antibodies to LKM1 are part of a family of immunoreactive molecules directed against microsomal autoantigens (see Table 38-8).[184-188] Antibodies to LKM1 have been associated with type 2 autoimmune hepatitis and are reactive against a 50-kDa antigen in the liver and kidney that has been identified as the cytochrome mono-oxygenase, P450 IID6 (CYP2D6).[188] Sera that are positive for anti-LKM1 can also recognize 55-kDa and 64-kDa antigens when tested against solubilized human liver microsomes, but these antigens have not yet been characterized.[99] Rarely, anti-LKM1 positive sera are monospecific for the 55-kDa or 64-kDa antigen. The diagnostic significance of these reactivities remains uncertain.

A minority of anti-LKM1 positive sera (10 percent) react with 50-kDa microsomal proteins that are different from P450 IID6 (CYP2D6).[99] One of these proteins has now been identified as P450 IA2, which is a liver-specific antigen responsible for the metabolism of phenacetin.[99] Antibodies to P450 IA2 inhibit enzyme function in vitro and are markers of the hepatitis associated with APS1.

P450 IA2 is the autoantigen common in patients with APS1 and hepatitis.[204]

Antibodies to Liver Cytosol Type 1

Antibodies to liver cytosol type 1 (anti-LC1) produce a homogeneous staining pattern of rat hepatocytes by indirect immunofluorescence (see Table 38-9).[340,341] They are present mainly in patients who are uninfected with HCV and have been used to discriminate anti–LKM1-positive patients with and without HCV infection (see Table 38-4). Anti-LC1 occur in young patients, typically less than 20 years old, and were initially thought to characterize individuals with an aggressive type of liver disease.[340,341] Anti-LC1 were associated with frequent concurrent immunologic diseases, marked hepatocellular inflammation, and rapid progression to cirrhosis. These early observations have not been fully corroborated, and anti-LC1 have been absent in children with fulminant autoimmune hepatitis, co-existent with SMA and ANA in type 1 autoimmune hepatitis and PSC, and present in chronic hepatitis C.[342] Serum levels do fluctuate with disease activity in contrast to anti-LKM1, and anti-LC1 may prove useful as markers of residual hepatocellular inflammation in type 2 autoimmune hepatitis or as probes of an autoantigen associated with disease severity.[343] Anti-LC1 are present in 32 percent of anti–LKM1-positive patients who are uninfected with HCV; in 14 percent of patients, they are the sole markers of autoimmune hepatitis. Formiminotransferase cyclodeaminase[344] and argininosuccinate lyase[345] have been proposed as the antigenic targets.

Antibodies to Soluble Liver Antigen/ Liver Pancreas

Antibodies to SLA/LP have high specificity for autoimmune hepatitis and have been proposed as the markers of type 3 autoimmune hepatitis (see Table 38-9).[216,217] They do not, however, define a clinically distinct subgroup of patients, and their greatest clinical value may be as diagnostic and prognostic aids. Antibodies to SLA/LP may be useful in re-classifying patients with cryptogenic chronic hepatitis as having autoimmune hepatitis and may identify patients who relapse after corticosteroid withdrawal.[219-221] A 50-kDa cytosolic protein is the prime candidate as target autoantigen,[148] and it may be a 48.8-kDa selenocysteine-specific protecting factor ($tRNP^{(Ser)Sec}$) that has 99 percent homology with the liver-pancreas antigen.[149] Previous studies have indicated than antibodies to the $tRNP^{(Ser)Sec}$ complex identify patients who relapse more commonly after corticosteroid treatment than seronegative counterparts.[346]

Antibodies to Asialoglycoprotein Receptor

Asialoglycoprotein receptor is a constituent of a liver-specific membrane lipoprotein complex (see Table 38-9); antibodies against this receptor (anti-ASGPR) have been demonstrated in autoimmune hepatitis characterized by SMA, ANA, and anti-LKM1.[144-146] Anti-human, anti-ASGPR occur in 88 percent of patients with autoimmune hepatitis compared to 7 percent of patients with chronic hepatitis B, 8 percent of patients with alcoholic liver disease, and 14 percent of patients with PBC. Their presence correlates with inflammatory activity, their disappearance connotes effective corticosteroid treatment, and their persistence after corticosteroid withdrawal heralds relapse.[347,348] Antibodies to ASGPR may be generic markers of autoimmune hepatitis, biologic probes of an important autoantigen, or important indices of treatment response. Their greatest clinical value may be to monitor patient responsiveness to corticosteroid therapy and to define an optimal end point of treatment. T lymphocytes harvested from patients with autoimmune hepatitis are sensitized to asialoglycoprotein receptor, and they have a genetically determined, antigen-specific T cell response to this protein.[145] The role of asialoglycoprotein receptor in the pathogenesis of autoimmune hepatitis is unclear but the protein remains a candidate as the target autoantigen of type 1 autoimmune hepatitis.

Perinuclear Anti-neutrophil Cytoplasmic Antibodies

pANCA are common in type 1 and rare in type 2 autoimmune hepatitis (see Table 38-8).[349,350] They are present in high titer in classic disease and may be useful in reclassifying patients with cryptogenic chronic hepatitis as having autoimmune hepatitis.[351] Despite uncertainties about their diagnostic specificity, pANCA have been incorporated into the repertoire of autoantibodies used to assess autoimmune liver disease. Their target antigen is unknown but myeloperoxidase, proteinase 3, and elastase have been eliminated as candidates.[349] Furthermore, the nomination of actin as target autoantigen has been challenged.[352] The reactivity of atypical pANCA in inflammatory bowel disease and hepatobiliary disorders is against granulocyte-specific antigens in the nuclear lamina; the search for target antigens for pANCA is probably best directed at this site.[353]

Patients with type 1 autoimmune hepatitis and those with ulcerative colitis commonly express the immunoglobulin G_1 isotype of pANCA, whereas most patients with PSC express the immunoglobulin G_1 and immunoglobulin G_3 isotypes.[349] Furthermore, the pANCA in type 1 autoimmune hepatitis react with neutrophils and monocytes, whereas the pANCA in PSC react only with neutrophils.[349] These observations suggest that the target autoantigens of pANCA are disease specific. Other studies have not found similar distinctions, and additional investigations in well-defined patient populations are necessary to resolve these issues.[354]

HUMAN LEUKOCYTE ANTIGEN ASSOCIATIONS

The HLAs A1, B8, and DR3 occur in from 34 percent to 82 percent of Caucasian Northern European and North American patients with autoimmune hepatitis.[134] HLA DR4 has also been recognized as a secondary but independent risk factor for autoimmune hepatitis, occurring in 43 percent of patients.[134] High-resolution DNA-based technology has indicated that *DRB1*0301* is the principal susceptibility allele and *DRB1*0401* is a secondary but independent risk factor.[136,137] Analyses of amino acid sequence variations encoded by these class II alleles of the major histocompatibility complex (MHC) indicate that *DRB1*0301* and *DRB1*0401* each encode a common (shared) six amino acid motif, LLEQKR, at positions 67-72 in the DRβ polypeptide chain of the HLA DR molecule. The presence of lysine (K) at DRβ position 71 appears to be critical.[136,137] *DRB1*1501* is protective against type 1 autoimmune hepatitis in this ethnic group and it encodes the sequence ILEQAR at DRβ positions 67 through 72.[355] The "disease resistance motif" differs from the "susceptibility motif" at two positions. Isoleucine (I) is encoded at DRβ67 and alanine (A) is encoded at DRβ71. The substitution of isoleucine for leucine (L) at DRβ67 is a neutral replacement because each amino acid is similarly charged. The substitution would have little or no effect on peptide binding and orientation. Alanine, however, is a neutral non-polar amino acid; its substitution for the highly charged polar amino acids lysine or arginine at DRβ71 would have a major impact on antigen binding and immunocyte recognition. This substitution could in turn affect antigen presentation and activation of CD4 T helper cells.[355]

The more alleles encoding lysine at DRβ71, the more intense the autoantigen display and the more robust the immunocyte reaction.[137,356] Because multiple class II MHC alleles can encode lysine at DRβ71, there is probably a "dosing effect" on disease susceptibility and behavior. *DRB1*0301* is in tight linkage dysequilibrium with *DRB3*0101*, which also encodes lysine-71. In contrast, *DRB1*0401* is in tight linkage dysequilibrium with *DRB4*0103*, which encodes an arginine (R) at DRβ71. Consequently, whereas *DRB1*0301* and *DRB1*0401* both share the same critical motif associated with increased disease susceptibility, they each may have different effects on clinical expression and disease severity. The *DRB1*0301-DRB3*0101* haplotype may be a greater risk factor for type 1 autoimmune hepatitis than the *DRB1*0401-DRB4*0103* haplotype because it provides a "double dose" of optimal binding sites for peptide and T cell antigen receptors (TCR). The *DRB1*0301-DRB3*0101* haplotype may contribute to a more robust activation of CD4 T helper cells than the *DRB1*0401-DRB4*0103* haplotype. These dosing effects may explain in part the observed differences between these haplotypes and disease onset and severity.

Not all patients with type 1 autoimmune hepatitis have *DRB1*0301 or DRB1*0401* nor do all patients with these alleles behave in the same fashion. These observations suggest that there are diverse susceptibility alleles or various autoimmune promoters that can affect susceptibility and severity in different and distinctive ways. Within the Caucasian Northern European population, 15 percent of individuals with type 1 autoimmune hepatitis lack *DRB1*0301* and *DRB1*0401*.[137,356] Among patients from other ethnic groups, the susceptibility alleles for type 1 autoimmune hepatitis are *DRB1*0405* in Japan, *DRB1*0405* in Argentine adults, *DRB1*1301* in Argentine children, *DRB1*13* and *DRB1*03* in Brazil, and *DRB1*0404* in Mestizo Mexicans.[355] This multiplicity of race-dependent allelic risk factors for type 1 autoimmune hepatitis suggests that different alleles encode one or more common determinants that are critical for disease expression. Alternatively, there may be other genetic promoters of type 1 autoimmune hepatitis that are or are not associated with the principal susceptibility alleles. These promoters may be selected by region-specific etiologic triggers and include both MHC-linked and MHC-independent loci.

The "shared motif hypothesis" predicts that diverse alleles associated with susceptibility to type 1 autoimmune hepatitis in different ethnic groups each encode the same or similar amino acid motifs at the critical site of antigen presentation and immunocyte activation. Multiple class II MHC alleles other than *DRB1*0301* and *DRB1*0401* encode lysine at position DRβ71, including *DRB1*0302*, **0303*, **0409*, **0413*, **0416*, and **1303* and *DRB3*0101*, **0201*, **0202*, and **0301*. Other alleles that encode slightly different motifs at DRβ67-72 may also confer susceptibility by encoding amino acid sequences that are insufficiently different to greatly alter antigen binding and TCR recognition. The class II MHC alleles, *DRB1*0404* and *DRB1*0405*, are associated with susceptibility to type 1 autoimmune hepatitis in Japan and Mexico and they each encode the motif LLEQRR at DRβ positions 67 through 72. In this sequence, arginine (R) occupies the critical position in place of lysine (K). Lysine and arginine, however, are very similar amino acids and possess a strong positive charge. Substitution of each for the other may have a minimal influence on which antigenic peptide is preferentially bound and how the peptides are presented to TCR.

The "shared motif hypothesis" of pathogenesis has recently been challenged by studies from South America that have identified *DRB1*1301* as the primary susceptibility allele in children with type 1 autoimmune hepatitis.[355] In these young patients from Argentina and Brazil, *DRB1*1301* encodes ILEDER at DRβ positions 67 through 72, with glutamic acid (E), aspartic acid (D), and glutamic acid (E) at DRβ positions 69, 70, and 71, respectively. Each of these amino acids is negatively charged and they greatly alter the antigen-binding characteristics of the MHC molecule. This failure of the "shared motif hypothesis" to fit all available data has stimulated the search for other autoimmune promoter genes both within the MHC and elsewhere in the human genome.

Determinations of HLA phenotype can be of value in assessing the candidacy of patients with cryptogenic chronic hepatitis for corticosteroid therapy, in strengthening the case for autoimmune hepatitis in patients with equivocal findings, or in estimating prognosis in patients with a suboptimal response to corticosteroid treatment. HLA typing, however, is not diagnostic of autoimmune hepatitis and should not be used as a conventional test.

Preliminary studies have suggested that patients with type 2 autoimmune hepatitis have different susceptibility alleles than do patients with type 1 autoimmune hepatitis.[143,201] These patients have increased frequencies of HLA DR3 (58 percent versus 19 percent), HLA DR7 (58 percent versus 23 percent), and C4AQO alleles (70 percent versus 35 percent) compared to controls.[202] Other studies in German and Brazilian populations suggest that *DRB1*0701* is an important susceptibility allele.[143,201]

HISTOLOGIC FINDINGS

Initial reports that emphasized the presence of periportal γ-globulin deposits in hepatic mesenchymal cells in association with lymphocytes, plasma cells, and histiocytes described the features of an immunologically mediated cytodestructive process but they lacked the diagnostic assays to exclude viral infection.[53,54] Consequently, the pattern of interface hepatitis lost diagnostic specificity because it was recognized in viral and cryptogenic forms of chronic hepatitis. Similarly, the plasma cell infiltrates in the portal tracts that had characterized patients with autoimmune hepatitis and so-called "plasma cell hepatitis"[44] did not retain their diagnostic value as monoclonal antibodies suggested that these infiltrates were rare.[2,357,358] Studies that depended on epidemiologic risk factors to identify viral disease lacked the sensitivity to appreciate subtle morphologic differences, and the descriptions of conspicuous changes, such as collapse and hydropic swelling, did not provide confident diagnostic criteria.[359] Second- and third-generation enzyme-linked immunosorbent immunoassays for the detection of antibodies to HCV now complement the sensitive and specific immunoassays for the detection of HBV infection. These tests facilitate the confident categorization of patients into viral and autoimmune categories and allow a more confident assessment of histologic differences.

Interface hepatitis (Figure 38-5) is seen as frequently in autoimmune hepatitis as in chronic hepatitis C (84 percent versus 76 percent, $P = 0.7$), but severe changes are found only in autoimmune hepatitis.[273,281,360] Similarly, moderate to severe panacinar inflammation (Figure 38-6) occurs mainly in autoimmune hepatitis (47 percent versus 16 percent, $P = 0.04$).[273,281] Plasma cells in the portal tracts are common to all diagnostic categories as part of a mixed inflammatory infiltrate, but moderate to severe plasma cell infiltration distinguishes patients with autoimmune hepatitis from those with chronic hepatitis C (66 percent versus 21 percent, $P = 0.005$) (Figure 38-7).[273,281]

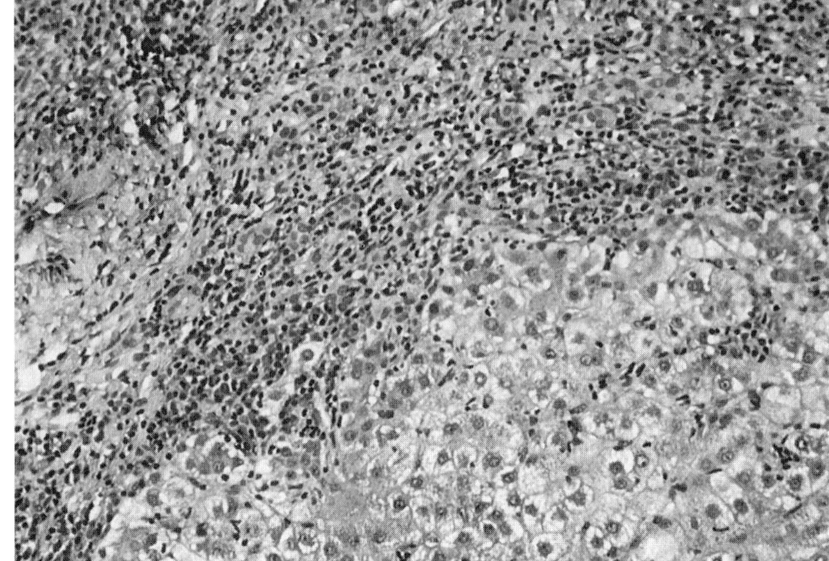

Figure 38-5 Interface hepatitis in autoimmune hepatitis (hematoxylin and eosin; ×200). The limiting plate of the portal tract is disrupted by mononuclear cells.

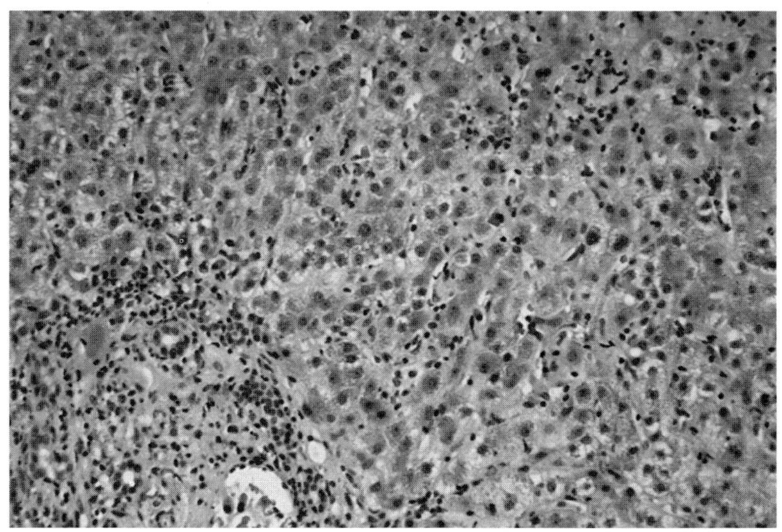

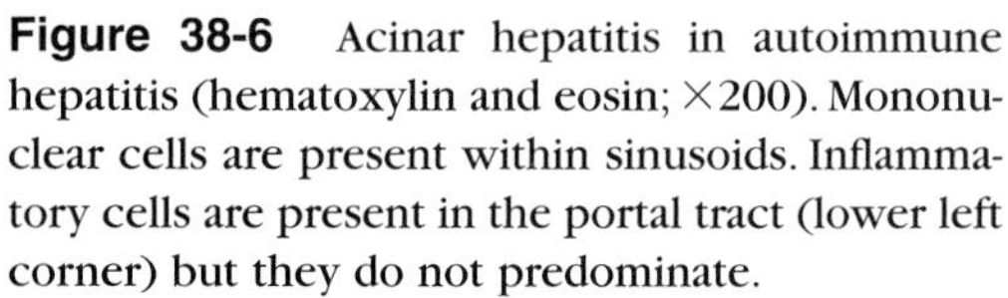

Figure 38-6 Acinar hepatitis in autoimmune hepatitis (hematoxylin and eosin; ×200). Mononuclear cells are present within sinusoids. Inflammatory cells are present in the portal tract (lower left corner) but they do not predominate.

Composite histologic patterns based on these individual distinctive, but not diagnostic, features have high specificity and predictability for autoimmune hepatitis.[273,281] The composite histologic pattern of moderate to severe interface hepatitis or panacinar hepatitis in the absence of portal lymphoid aggregates and steatosis has a specificity of 81 percent and positive predictability of 68 percent. The low negative predictability of 57 percent indicates that the absence of histologic features does not exclude the clinical diagnosis of autoimmune hepatitis in 43 percent of patients. Diagnostic sensitivity is also low in autoimmune hepatitis, and the histologic diagnosis of autoimmune hepatitis can be made in only 40 percent of individuals with the clinical diagnosis.[281]

The nomenclature of autoimmune hepatitis now recognizes the ambiguities associated with terms such as "chronic active hepatitis" and "chronic persistent hepatitis," which refer similarly to clinical and histologic diagnoses.[16] Accordingly, these terms have been deleted from the vocabulary. The clinical designation of autoimmune hepatitis should not be modified by the histologic manifestations, which may range from cirrhosis, portal hepatitis, interface hepatitis, and panacinar hepatitis to normal.

PATHOGENIC MECHANISMS

Autoimmune hepatitis is a disease of unknown cause. The presence of immunologic features does not establish its autoimmune nature, and the autoimmunity of autoimmune hepatitis has been more difficult to prove than to presume. Such proof requires the regular association of a specific autoantibody with the disease, demonstration of a similar autoimmune response in animals immunized with the autoantigen, production of histologic changes identical to the human disease in immunized animals, and transfer of the disease to non-immunized animals by the administration of antibodies or lymphocytes.[361] Failure to satisfy these criteria for autoimmunity have underscored the multi-faceted nature of autoimmune hepatitis and highlighted its various immunologic and genetic components. To develop a tenable hypothesis of pathogenesis, each of the components influencing disease occurrence and expression must be defined and interwoven.

Triggering Factors

Multiple triggering factors have been proposed, and they include infectious agents (hepatitis A, HBV, HCV, measles virus), drugs (minocycline), and toxins. There can be a long lag time between exposure to the trigger and onset of the disease, and the triggering factor may not be needed for perpetuation of the disorder. The multiplicity of triggering agents suggests that autoimmune hepatitis is caused by a commonly shared epitope.[156,157]

Molecular Mimicry

Molecular mimicry between a foreign antigen and a self-antigen is the most common explanation for the loss of self-tolerance. Cross-reactions, however, have only been described between non-pathogenic autoantibodies, not tissue-infiltrating immunocytes.[362] Furthermore, molecular mimicry has not yet been proven to be a cause of human autoimmune disease.[363]

Sequestered epitopes may be freshly recognized by uncommitted immunocytes; cryptic epitopes may be differentiated by exogenous factors.[156,157] Neo-epitopes may develop from the degradation of viruses, drugs, or toxins; superantigens, associated with an infectious process, may generate an exuberant and diverse immunocyte response. Each of these factors can lead to "autoantigenic overload" and impaired self-tolerance.

The autoreactive process can escalate because epitopes spread within the same molecule or between different molecules.[156,157] Extrinsic antigens can combine with autologous antigens and augment the immune reaction through adjuvant effects, and diverse antigens can be recruited into the inflammatory reaction by bystander effects. In this fashion, the primary immune reaction can be obscured by a plethora of secondary responses.

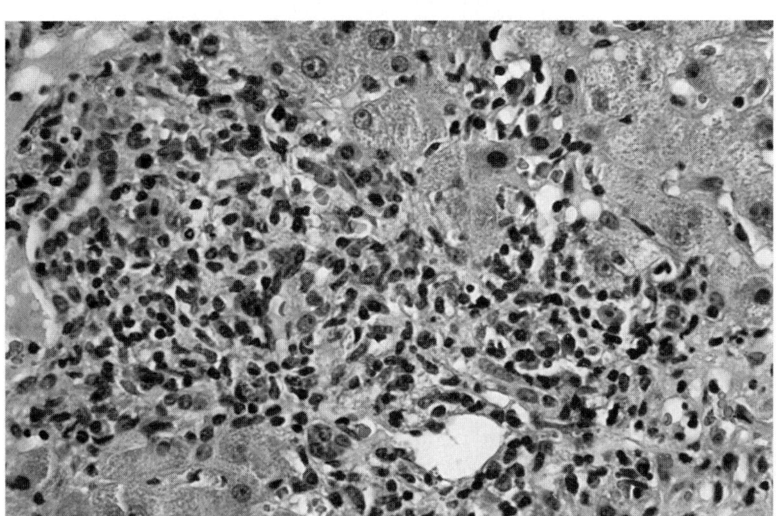

Figure 38-7 Plasma cell infiltration of the portal tract in autoimmune hepatitis (hematoxylin and eosin; ×400).

Autoimmune Synapse

The autoantigenic peptide must be processed by antigen-presenting cells and displayed within the antigen-binding groove of class II MHC molecules.[156,157] The peptide-MHC complex must then be recognized by the TCR of an uncommitted CD4 T helper cell. The interaction between the autoantigen, the class II MHC molecule, and the TCR constitutes the "autoimmune synapse," which initiates the autoreactive process. The CD4 T helper cell is the critical effector cell and its activation is required before differentiation can occur into a cytotoxic T cell or an antibody-producing cell. Autoantigen presentation and immunocyte activation are affected by genetic factors. In addition, differentiation of activated immunocytes into effectors of liver cell injury depends on the cytokine milieu.

Genetic Factors

The antigen-binding groove of the class II MHC molecule is encoded by alleles, which determine its configuration and its ability to activate immunocytes.[156,157] *DRB1*0301* and *DRB1*0401* encode the antigen-binding groove that can optimally present autoantigen to TCR in Caucasian Northern European or North American patients.[136,137] The antigen–class II MHC complex can then initiate a cascade of immune reactions that result in autoimmune hepatitis. The critical six amino acid sequence for antigen-positioning is encoded on the α-helix of the antigen binding groove in "hypervariable region 3." This region spans positions 67 to 72 on the DRβ polypeptide chain. Position DRβ71 is at the lip of the antigen-binding groove and at the contact point between the antigenic peptide, the class II MHC molecule, and the TCR of the CD4 T helper cell. Lysine at this position determines the steric and electrostatic properties that are necessary for optimal antigen presentation and immunocyte activation. Different ethnic groups have different susceptibility alleles, and the antigen-binding groove encoded by these alleles may accommodate indigenous antigens particular to their disease.

Autoantigen Selection

Antigenic peptides are selected for display by the nature of the amino acids that must interact with residues within the antigen-binding groove.[156,157] In type 1 autoimmune hepatitis, the six amino acid sequence in hypervariable region 3 restricts the range of peptides that can be accommodated within this groove. The ideal autoantigen of type 1 autoimmune hepatitis in Caucasian Northern European and North American patients must have a negatively charged aspartic acid or glutamic acid at position P4 from the N terminus. This residue can then link with a positively charged lysine or arginine at position DRβ71 by a salt bridge. Multiple self-antigens or foreign antigens may satisfy these minimum structural requirements and serve as immunogenic peptides.

Cytokine Milieu

Type 1 cytokines, such as interleukin (IL)-12 and IL-2, promote proliferation of cytotoxic T cells; this promotion may in part relate to the excess production of tumor necrosis factor (TNF)-α by a gene polymorphism.[156,157] Type 2 cytokines, such as IL-4 and IL-10, promote the proliferation of B cells and the production of immunoglobulin. This pathway may be favored by cytokine imbalances that are yet undefined. In autoimmune hepatitis, both pathways are active, and the predominant one may vary at different times in the same individual because the various cytokines counter-regulate each other.

Analyses of serum cytokine levels in type 1 autoimmune hepatitis indicate low or no concentrations of IL-2.[364] This cytokine profile favors a type 2 cytokine pathway that promotes autoantibody production and an antibody-dependent, cell-mediated form of cytotoxicity. Other studies of cell populations isolated from within the liver have also indicated a predominantly type 2 cytokine response in autoimmune hepatitis.

Autoimmune Promoter Genes

Autoimmune promoter genes inside and outside the MHC may also contribute to the occurrence, expression, and outcome of autoimmune hepatitis. These immunoregulatory proteins can affect autoantigen presentation, peptide processing, inflammation, fibrosis, apoptosis, immunocyte recruitment, and CD4 T helper cell activation. There may be synergy (epistasis) between primary and secondary susceptibility alleles; these genes may promote the expression and clinical severity of autoimmune hepatitis by acting in concert as a "permissive gene pool." Polymorphisms of the TNF-α promoter gene (*TNF-A*)[365,366] and the cytotoxic T lymphocyte antigen-4 gene (*CTLA-4*)[367] have been described in patients with type 1 autoimmune hepatitis and are prime examples of these non–disease-specific promoters.

The *TNFA*2* promoter polymorphism at position -308 involves substitution of an adenine for a guanine at position -308 of the *TNF-A* gene.[365,366] This substitution may influence *TNF-A* gene transcription and result in high constitutive and inducible levels of TNF-α. Increased levels of TNF-α may then alter the cytokine network regulating the CD4 T helper cell response and favor a type 1 cytokine response. Patients with *TNFA*2* present with disease at a younger age than patients without this substitution and enter remission less frequently during corticosteroid therapy, fail treatment more often—especially if they are homozygous for the adenine exchange, and progress to cirrhosis more commonly.[366] These patients also have *DRB1*0301* and the *A1-B8-DRB1*0301* phenotype more frequently than control subjects; this finding suggests a synergy between the principal susceptibility allele and the autoimmune promoter.[366]

The *CTLA-4* gene polymorphism involves a single base exchange of adenine for guanine at position 49 of the first exon of the *CTLA-4* gene on chromosome 2q33.[367] This substitution results in three genotypes associated with CTLA-4 production (adenine/adenine, guanine/guanine, and adenine/guanine). The guanine/guanine genotype is associated with higher serum levels of aspartate aminotransferase and a greater frequency of thyroid microsomal antibodies than other genotypes.[367] This polymorphism of the *CTLA-4* gene may result in a gene product that is less effective than the products of the other *CTLA-4* polymorphisms in preventing T lymphocyte activation. Because the *CTLA-4* and *DRB1* genes are encoded on different chromosomes and are not linked, their additive effect on disease expression is synergistic. Furthermore, the same *CTLA-4* polymorphism has been described in PBC, indicating that it is a nonspecific promoter of autoimmunity.[368]

Gender Effects

The female predilection for autoimmune hepatitis is well recognized but unexplained. An immunomodulatory gene on the X chromosome has been proposed, and the increased immunoreactivity in women may reflect a "double dose" of this gene.[369-371] Alternatively, estrogens and other gender-related hormones may influence the vigor of the immune response by facilitating antigen processing and recognition.[372] The heightened immunoreactivity in women is manifested by higher serum levels of immunoglobulin after exposure to a fixed antigen load, more common expression of natural autoantibodies, increased cell-mediated immunity after immunization, and greater occurrence of autoimmune phenomena and disease than men.[373]

Women develop a type 1 cytokine response after exposure to an infectious agent or antigen more commonly than men, and this heightened responsiveness to antigenic triggers may increase their propensity for autoimmune disease.[372] Estrogens affect the cytokine profile, and there are two estrogen receptors on immune cells sensitive to changes in estrogen concentration. High estrogen levels, as in pregnancy, inhibit the type 1 cytokine response and promote a type 2 cytokine response that favors antibody production and antibody-dependent pathogenic pathways. Low estrogen levels, as in normal non-pregnant women, favor a type 1 cytokine response and promote cell-mediated pathogenic pathways that have been implicated in autoimmune hepatitis. Pituitary hormones, such as prolactin and growth hormone, and sex hormones, such as progesterone and testosterone, counterregulate the immune response, probably by altering the cytokine milieu or estrogen receptor expression.[372]

Microchimerism may also affect self-tolerance.[372-376] Microchimerism can persist for years after pregnancy, and fetal cells in the maternal circulation have been associated with the initiation and exacerbation of autoimmune disease. Mechanisms by which microchimerism affects postpartum immunoreactivity are unknown, but it may compromise self-tolerance by promoting cross-reactivity.

Activation-induced Cell Death

The proliferation of activated immunocytes is modulated by "activation-induced cell death," and deficiencies in this braking mechanism may perpetuate the autoreactive response.[156,157] The binding of Fas and TNF receptor I with the complementary "death activators," Fas ligand and TNF-α, activates caspases within the cytoplasm of the cell. This activation leads to proteolysis of cytoplasmic contents and cell death (apoptosis). Bcl-2 is an antiapoptotic protein that is expressed on the outer membranes of mitochondria, nuclear envelope, and endoplasmic reticulum. Bcl-2 can bind caspase and reduce proteolysis, thereby protecting the cell against apoptosis. Up-regulation of Bcl-2 expression by interleukins such as IL-4, IL-7, and IL-15 can protect the immunocytes from cell death and enhance the immune reaction. Similarly, expression of a dysfunctional Fas ligand will also impair apoptosis and prolong the autoimmune response. None of these possible disturbances in the braking mechanisms of the immune response has yet been fully defined in autoimmune hepatitis and can only be postulated.

Mechanisms of Hepatocyte Injury

Liver cell destruction is accomplished by either cell-mediated cytotoxicity, antibody-dependent cell-mediated cytotoxicity, or a combination of both mechanisms.[156,157] Cell-mediated cytotoxicity depends on the clonal expansion of CD8 cytotoxic T cells that accomplish liver cell injury through the release of lymphokines. This mechanism is regulated by type 1 cytokines, and a genetic polymorphism that affects TNF-α production may facilitate this pathway. Antibody-dependent, cell-mediated cytotoxicity is regulated by type 2 cytokines; the natural killer cell accomplishes liver cell destruction by the binding of its Fc receptor with an antigen-antibody complex on the hepatocyte surface. The predominant mechanism depends on the phenotypic differentiation of the CD4 T helper cell that is in turn reflective of the cytokine milieu. The cytokine milieu may reflect polymorphisms of the cytokine genes that favor excess production of some modulators, such as TNF-α, or deficient production of others.

The most popular hypothesis of pathogenesis implicates a cell-mediated cytotoxicity in which autoantigen-sensitized liver-infiltrating CD8 T lymphocytes affect liver cell injury.[156,157] The most well-studied and scientifically supported hypothesis of pathogenesis implicates an antibody-dependent, cell-mediated form of cytotoxicity that accomplishes liver cell injury through natural killer cells that are directed against antigen-antibody complexes on the hepatocyte membrane.

Intrinsic to the hypothesis based on an antibody-dependent, cell-mediated form of cytotoxicity is a defect in the suppression of immunoglobulin production.[377,378] The unmodulated production of immunoglobulin G results in the formation of immunoglobulin aggregates that are attached to normal membrane constituents on the hepatocyte surface. These aggregates are then targeted by the natural killer cells, and cytolysis follows. The suppression defect has not been defined but it is presumably a result of cytokine interaction. Studies have indicated a defect in suppression function in patients[379,380] and in their first-degree relatives.[381,382] These family studies suggest that the suppression defect results from the inheritance of genetic factors linked to the MHC or other gene loci and not from chronic illness or hepatocellular inflammation. Because the suppression defect is most marked in relatives with the HLA A1-B8-DR3 phenotype, the abnormality in immunoregulatory function may well be inherited with the class II MHC alleles.[382]

Defects in the antibody-dependent, cell-mediated theory of cytotoxicity relate to the absence of antigen specificity for the suppression defect, detection of the suppression defect only in patients with active disease, and reversal of the defect when histologic remission is achieved during corticosteroid therapy.[383] Although this mechanism may amplify the clinical, biochemical, and histologic manifestations of autoimmune hepatitis, its lack of permanency suggests that there is another immunoregulatory defect of a more sustained nature that perpetuates the disease and accounts for its propensity for relapse after treatment. An antigen-specific suppression defect could perpetuate the autoimmune response, and a generalized non–antigen-specific suppression defect could enhance its clinical expression.[383]

Clarification of the pathogenic mechanisms of autoimmune hepatitis requires integration of the immunologic and genetic aspects of the disease. Triggering factors of a viral or environmental nature, genetic factors that affect immunoreactivity to intrinsic or extrinsic antigens, and immunologic mechanisms that fail to modulate or terminate the immunologic attack must be defined to improve therapeutic interventions and develop preventive strategies.

PROGNOSTIC FACTORS

The prognosis of autoimmune hepatitis relates to the severity of inflammatory activity at the time of presentation and the HLA phenotype. Sustained elevation of the serum aspartate aminotransferase level to at least tenfold normal or fivefold normal in conjunction with at least a twofold elevation of the γ-globulin level, histologic features of bridging necrosis or multi-acinar necrosis at presentation, or HLA DR3 augur a poor prognosis (see Figures 38-2 and 38-4).[60,79,125] Patients who develop cirrhosis during therapy invariably relapse after drug withdrawal.[384]

There are no features of autoimmune hepatitis before therapy that accurately predict prognosis. Endogenous hepatic encephalopathy has a dismal connotation but even these patients may be resurrected in an unpredictable fashion with corticosteroid therapy.[123] The risk of immediate mortality can only be assessed after institution of corticosteroid treatment. Patients who resolve at least one pretreatment laboratory abnormality, improve a pretreatment hyperbilirubinemia, or do not experience a biochemical deterioration after 2 weeks of corticosteroid therapy survive for at least 6 months in 98 percent of instances.[123] Alternatively, patients with multi-acinar necrosis at presentation who manifest at least one deficiency in their immediate biochemical response during a 2-week period of therapy have a poor prognosis. Death invariably occurs in patients with multi-acinar necrosis and unimproved hyperbilirubinemia after 2 weeks of treatment; these patients should be evaluated expeditiously for liver transplantation.[123]

Long-term survival in the absence of liver transplantation also depends on the response to corticosteroid therapy.[135] Inability to induce histologic remission after 4 years of continuous therapy or manifestations of deterioration during treatment, especially the development of ascites, identify a subpopulation of patients in whom liver transplantation is likely. Patients in this category are typically younger than their counterparts who do not warrant transplantation and commonly have HLA B8 or DR3.[135]

TREATMENT INDICATIONS

The indications for treatment are severe sustained abnormalities in the serum aminotransferase and γ-globulin levels or the presence of bridging necrosis or multi-acinar necrosis on histologic examination.[1-7] Relative indications for treatment are incapacitating symptoms attributable to inflammatory activity or relentless progression of the liver disease. All other patients can be followed closely, treated symptomatically, and managed with conventional regimens as the disease evolves.

TREATMENT REGIMENS

Prednisone, 10 mg daily, in combination with azathioprine, 50 mg daily, is the preferred treatment if azathioprine is not contraindicated by cytopenia, pregnancy, or malignancy (Table 38-10).[385,386] Prednisone, 20 mg daily, is equally effective but associated with a greater frequency of drug-related side effects. It is useful in patients in whom only a short trial of treatment is proposed (3 to 6 months) and in young fertile women who are contemplating pregnancy. In patients who have preexistent cytopenia or who develop cytopenia during therapy the thiopurine methyl transferase level should be determined before azathiopurine treatment.[387,388]

Treatment is continued until remission of the disease, deterioration despite compliance with the treatment regimen (treatment failure), development of drug toxicity, or failure to induce remission after protracted therapy.[389,390] Cosmetic changes (obesity, facial rounding, acne, or hirsutism) develop in 80 percent of patients after 2 years of therapy regardless of the regimen used. Severe, potentially debilitating complications (osteoporosis with vertebral compression, diabetes, cataracts, hypertension, and psychosis) usually develop only after 18 months of continuous therapy and at doses of prednisone that exceed 10 mg daily. Severe side effects occur less often with prednisone in combination with azathioprine (10 percent) than with a higher dose of prednisone alone (44 percent).[391]

Complications of azathioprine include cholestatic hepatitis, nausea, emesis, rash, and cytopenia.[385,386,389,390] Side effects develop in fewer than 10 percent of patients receiving 50 mg daily of azathioprine and all toxicities can be reversed by reduction of the dose or discontinuation of the drug. Importantly, the complications of the medication are frequently indistinguishable from the side effects of the liver disease. As a result, these complications may not resolve after drug withdrawal or be a reliable indication for the termination of therapy.

The long-term complications of immunosuppressive therapy include the theoretic possibilities of teratogenicity and oncogenicity.[385,386,389,390] Skeletal anomalies, cleft palate, reduction in thymic size, hydrops fetalis, anemia, and hematopoietic suppression have been described in

TABLE 38-10
Preferred Treatment Regimens at Diagnosis

Treatment interval	PREDNISONE AND AZATHIOPRINE		Prednisone only (mg daily)	Prime indications
	Prednisone (mg daily)	Azathioprine (mg daily)		
Week 1	30	50	60	**Prednisone and Azathioprine Therapy**
Week 2	20	50	40	Postmenopausal state, osteoporosis, brittle
Week 3	15	50	30	diabetes, labile hypertension, emotional
Week 4	15	50	30	lability, obesity
Week 5	10	50	20	**Prednisone Therapy Only**
Until end point	10	50	20	Cytopenia, thiopurine methyl transferase deficiency, pregnancy, malignancy, short trial ($\leq$6 months)

mice treated experimentally with higher than pharmacologic doses of azathioprine. Such effects undoubtedly reflect the experimental conditions, excessive dose schedules, and animal species tested but they generate sufficient concern to limit the use of azathioprine in pregnant women.

The oncogenicity of immunosuppressive therapy has been suggested mainly by the development of lymphomas in patients undergoing transplantation.[392] In the Mayo Clinic experience the frequency of extrahepatic malignancy is 5 percent in patients with a cumulative duration of treatment of 42 months.[393] The incidence of extrahepatic malignancy in corticosteroid-treated patients with autoimmune hepatitis is 1 per 194 patient-years of surveillance, and the probability of tumor occurrence is 3 percent after 10 years. The average duration to malignancy has been 116 months; the risk is 1.4-fold (range, 0.6 to 2.9) that of an age- and sex-matched normal population; no specific cell type has been encountered. At the Mayo Clinic, malignancies have involved the cervix, lymphatic tissue, breast, bladder, colon, kidneys, soft tissues, and unknown sites. The low but probably increased risk of extrahepatic malignancy in patients with autoimmune hepatitis does not contraindicate the use of immunosuppressive therapy but it does underscore the importance of carefully selecting patients for such treatment.

Only 13 percent of treated patients develop complications during therapy that necessitate dose reduction or premature drug withdrawal; patients with cirrhosis at presentation are most commonly afflicted (25 versus 8 percent), presumably because of increased serum levels of unbound prednisolone resulting from prolonged hypoalbuminemia or hyperbilirubinemia.[64] Postmenopausal patients and premenopausal counterparts tolerate initial therapy, and their outcomes after initial therapy are also similar.[394] Consequently, these patients can be treated as vigorously as others are at the time of presentation. Postmenopausal patients, however, tolerate relapse and retreatment less well than younger counterparts and the frequency of vertebral compression is higher in these patients.[394] Advanced age, postmenopausal status, and the presence of cirrhosis are a risk-laden combination[395]; patients with these features who relapse after initial conventional treatment are best managed empirically by low-dose, long-term corticosteroid therapy or azathioprine treatment rather than by readministration of conventional regimens.[396]

ADJUNCTIVE THERAPIES

Adjunctive therapies should include a regular exercise program that is tailored to individual tolerance (walking, swimming, or biking); vitamin supplementation, especially vitamin K as indicated (10 mg daily); calcium supplementation (1 g-1.5 g daily); and vitamin D (50,000 units once each week). Postmenopausal women should be considered for hormonal replacement therapy, and symptomatic osteoporosis should be treated with physical therapy and alendronate, 10 mg daily. Asymptomatic patients on long-term corticosteroid treatment should be monitored for bone disease by annual bone mineral densitometry of the lumbar spine and hip. Manifestations of osteopenia warrant therapeutic interventions identical to those used in patients with symptomatic osteoporosis.

INDICES OF RESPONSE

Treatment strategies are based on accurate determinations of response. The serum aspartate aminotransferase and γ-globulin levels are the most practical and useful indices.[63,397]

Laboratory Assessments

In patients with histologic features of moderate to severe interface hepatitis before therapy, an abnormal serum aspartate aminotransferase or γ-globulin level during treatment correctly predicts the presence of significant histologic activity in 91 percent to 98 percent of instances.[63] The absence of biochemical abnormality, however, predicts the absence of histologic disease in only 36 percent to 44 percent of instances; histologic examination is still required to confirm the disappearance of inflammatory activity.[63]

In monitoring patients after induction of remission and drug withdrawal an abnormal serum aspartate aminotransferase level predicts histologic recrudescence in 79 percent of instances; an abnormal γ-globulin concentration connotes histologic relapse in 93 percent.[63] Normal serum aspartate aminotransferase and γ-globulin levels after drug withdrawal indicate the absence of significant histologic disease in 81 percent of instances, and of those patients with active disease and normal laboratory findings only 7 percent have severe potentially aggressive histologic findings.[63] To date, no other laboratory tests have been as well studied or as successful in predicting histologic activity.

Histologic improvement can lag behind biochemical improvement by 3 to 6 months.[63] Continuation of therapy beyond biochemical resolution for at least 3 months will reduce the frequency of discordant laboratory and histologic findings and minimize the likelihood of premature drug withdrawal.

Histologic Assessments

Examinations of liver tissue define the degree and pattern of inflammatory activity with 90 percent consistency.[65,66] Reproducibility of the morphologic interpretation by the same observer is 94 percent and sampling error is trivial. The sampling error for cirrhosis may exceed 60 percent; intraobserver variability in diagnosing cirrhosis may approach 50 percent unless the definition of cirrhosis as fibrosis with a complete regenerative nodule is strictly enforced.[65] Liver biopsy examination, therefore, although excellent for evaluating inflammatory changes, cannot confidently exclude cirrhosis and cannot be used as a reliable monitoring mechanism to assess progression to cirrhosis or the effect of drugs on the prevention of cirrhosis. Strict criteria for the histologic diagnosis of cirrhosis undoubtedly reduce diagnostic sensitivity but the false diagnosis of cirrhosis is an error of greater consequence than is failure to make the diagnosis.

TREATMENT OUTCOMES

Remission

Prednisone alone or in combination with azathioprine induces clinical, biochemical, and histologic remission in 65 percent of patients within 18 months (average treatment duration, 22 months).[1,7] The 10-year life expectancy of treated patients is 93 percent, similar to that of an age- and sex-matched normal population.[398] Patients with histologic cirrhosis at presentation have the same 10-year survival expectation as those without this finding (89 percent and 90 percent, respectively) and respond similarly to initial therapy.[398,399] Complete and sustained resolution of the disease ("cure") is possible in 17 percent but its occurrence is unpredictable.[64] Only the therapies for Wilson's disease and hemochromatosis rival those of autoimmune hepatitis in overall efficacy.

Relapse

The major problem in treating severe autoimmune hepatitis is relapse after drug withdrawal. Recrudescence of inflammatory activity occurs in 50 percent of patients within 6 months after discontinuation of medication and 70 percent within 3 years.[384,400-402] Reinstitution of treatment consistently induces another remission but drug withdrawal is typically followed by another relapse.[384] The causes of relapse are unknown but premature discontinuation of medication may be an important factor.[64]

Continuation of treatment until reversion of the hepatic architecture to normal is associated with a 20 percent frequency of subsequent relapse, whereas treatment until the features of non-specific or portal hepatitis are achieved is associated with a 50 percent frequency of relapse.[62,64] Patients who develop cirrhosis during treatment have an 87 percent to 100 percent frequency of relapse despite treatment to inactive histologic disease.[64] Because histologic resolution cannot be deduced by the biochemical changes, a liver tissue examination is desirable before drug withdrawal. Failure to eliminate the risk of relapse even after reversion of the hepatic architecture to normal suggests that in many patients the pathogenic mechanisms perpetuating the disease cannot be permanently disrupted by corticosteroid therapy.

The major consequences of relapse and retreatment are drug-related side effects.[384] The frequency of side effects after initial therapy is 29 percent and similar to that after the first relapse and retreatment (33 percent). Subsequent relapses and retreatments, however, are associated with a complication frequency of 70 percent.[384] Patients who have relapsed multiple times are best managed by long-term, low-dose prednisone[396] or indefinite azathioprine therapy.[403,404]

Long-term, low-dose prednisone therapy implies that the dose of prednisone is reduced to the lowest level possible to control symptoms and maintain the serum aspartate aminotransferase level below fivefold normal (Table 38-11).[396] All patients who have relapsed multiple times can be managed in this fashion on lower than conventional doses (median dose of prednisone, 7.5 mg daily), and 87 percent can be treated with 10 mg daily or less. Side effects that had accrued during conventional treatment improve in 85 percent of patients, new side effects do not develop, and mortality is unaffected (9 percent versus 10 percent).

Indefinite azathioprine therapy (2 mg/kg daily) implies that azathioprine is used as the sole medication after clinical and biochemical remission has been achieved by conventional regimens (see Table 38-11).[403,404] Eighty-seven percent of patients managed by this strategy have remained in remission during a median observation interval of 67 months (range, 12 to 128 months). Follow-up liver biopsy assessments have shown inactive or minimal histologic disease in 94 percent of instances, corticosteroid-related side effects have improved or disappeared in most patients, and the drug has been well tolerated. The most common side effect has been withdrawal arthralgia (63 percent). Myelosuppression has developed in 7 percent of patients, lymphopenia in 57 percent, and diverse malignancies in 8 percent.

The long-term prednisone and azathioprine strategies for relapse have not been compared head to head, and there are no objective bases for preference. Selection of the appropriate strategy for an individual patient must reflect the presence or absence of complicating factors such as cytopenia, pregnancy, or active malignancy, and acceptance of the long-term uncertainties associated with each regimen.

TABLE 38-11
Preferred Treatment Regimens After Adverse Outcomes

Outcome	PREDNISONE AND AZATHIOPRINE Prednisone (daily)	Azathioprine (daily)	Prednisone only (daily)	Alternative empiric therapies
Treatment failure	30 mg × 1 month 10 mg reduction each month of improvement 10 mg maintenance until remission	150 mg × 1 month 50 mg reduction each month of improvement 50 mg maintenance until remission	60 mg × 1 month 10 mg reduction each month better 20 mg maintenance until remission	6-Mercaptopurine Cyclosporine Mycophenolate
Multiple relapses	30 mg reduced to 10 mg within 4 weeks 2.5 mg/month reductions to lowest level to keep AST ≤ × 5 normal	50 mg maintenance for 4 weeks Increase to 2 mg/kg (maximum, 150 mg) as steroid-sparing agent	60 mg reduced to 20 mg within 4 weeks 2.5 mg/month reductions to lowest level to keep AST ≤ × 5 normal	6-Mercaptopurine
Incomplete response	Same as for relapse	Same as for relapse	Same as for relapse	Cyclosporine 6-Mercaptopurine
Drug toxicity	Reduce dose of offending agent by 50% if minor Discontinue offending agent if major	Reduce dose of offending agent by 50% if minor Discontinue offending agent if major	Reduce dose by 50% if minor Discontinue if major	Cyclosporine 6-Mercaptopurine Ursodeoxycholic acid (13-15 mg/kg)

AST, Serum aspartate aminotransferase level.

Progression to Cirrhosis

Corticosteroid therapy does not preclude the development of cirrhosis. In the Mayo Clinic experience 40 percent of patients develop cirrhosis within 10 years.[398,399] Usually cirrhosis occurs early during the most active stages of the disease and its frequency diminishes after remission has been achieved. Patients who sustain their remission after drug withdrawal have only a 5 percent frequency of subsequent cirrhosis.[399] Ten-year survival after histologic cirrhosis is 89 percent; this finding suggests that prognosis is related to the stage of cirrhosis and degree of associated inflammatory activity.[398,399]

Esophageal varices can be demonstrated by barium contrast study in only 15 percent of patients with cirrhosis who are treated with corticosteroids.[405] The likelihood of developing varices within 5 years after institution of therapy is only 8 percent, and hemorrhage from varices is unusual. Indeed, bleeding from sites other than varices is more common than bleeding from varices in treated patients, and mortality is not increased by bleeding from any site. The probability of upper gastrointestinal bleeding is only 6 percent within 5 years of treatment, and the 5-year survival of patients who have bled is 93 percent.[405] These findings indicate that esophageal varices are an uncommon finding at presentation and that they do not develop quickly or hemorrhage early after institution of treatment. Because the consequences of esophageal varices in untreated patients are severe and common, the improved prognosis of treated patients suggests that corticosteroid therapy may slow or prevent progression of cirrhosis and portal hypertension.[405]

Treatment Failure

Deterioration despite therapy (treatment failure) occurs in 13 percent of patients.[4-7] High-dose prednisone alone (60 mg daily) or a lower dose (30 mg daily) in conjunction with azathioprine (150 mg daily) induces biochemical remission in more than 60 percent of patients within 2 years (see Table 38-11).[406] Histologic remission, however, is achieved in only 20 percent. Patients who fail conventional therapy may become candidates for liver transplantation.

The 5-year survival after liver transplantation is 86 percent.[135,407] Recurrence after transplantation does occur in as many as 17 percent after 4.6 ± 1 years, especially in individuals who are inadequately immunosuppressed.[407-409] Recurrent autoimmune hepatitis is typically managed satisfactorily by adjustments in the immunosuppressive regimen. Rarely, recurrent disease can progress to cirrhosis and result in graft failure.[410] HLA DR3 and DR4 are found more commonly in patients with recurrent disease than in those without recurrence (100 percent versus 40 percent, $P = 0.008$), but recurrent disease is unrelated to the HLA status of the donor.[407]

Incomplete Response

In 13 percent of patients corticosteroid therapy is unable to induce remission.[7] Failure to induce remission after 3 years of continuous therapy is associated with a diminishing benefit-risk ratio. Conventional therapy continued beyond 3 years has a 7 percent probability of inducing remission per year and an increasing probability of drug-related complications. These patients are candidates for low-dose, long-term corticosteroid or azathioprine (2 mg/kg daily) therapy (see Table 38-11).[396,403,404]

Drug Toxicity

Drug toxicity compels premature discontinuation of therapy in 13 percent of patients.[7] Most commonly, intolerable obesity or cosmetic changes (47 percent) justify this action. Osteoporosis with vertebral compression (27 percent), brittle diabetes (20 percent), and peptic ulceration (6 percent) limit therapy less frequently.[64,384] Cytopenia, hepatotoxicity, rash, and gastrointestinal upset associated with azathioprine therapy rarely justify a treatment change.

Drug-related side effects can improve with dose reduction—a 50 percent decrease in dose is the first course of action (see Table 38-11). Inability to reverse the complication within 1 month necessitates termination of treatment. Severe reactions, including psychosis, extreme cytopenia, and symptomatic osteopenia with or without vertebral compression, justify immediate discontinuation of the offending agent. In such instances, therapy with the tolerated agent can frequently be maintained with a change in dose to control disease activity. Treatment with azathioprine (2 mg/kg per day) is an option in patients who are intolerant of corticosteroids.

Hepatocellular Cancer

Hepatocellular cancer is a rare occurrence in autoimmune hepatitis, especially since the introduction of assays by which to exclude HBV and HCV infection.[301] The incidence of hepatocellular cancer in patients with cirrhosis is 1 per 1002 patient-years of follow-up, and the incidence in patients with cirrhosis of at least 5 years' duration is 1 per 965 patient-years of follow-up.[301] These findings indicate that hepatocellular cancer can develop in uninfected patients with autoimmune hepatitis but that its occurrence is rare and it occurs only in patients with long-standing cirrhosis. Cancer surveillance strategies that include regular determination of the serum alpha fetoprotein level and performance of hepatic ultrasonography must be reassessed in this context.

The serum alpha fetoprotein level may be elevated in 35 percent of patients with autoimmune hepatitis at the time of presentation in the absence of hepatocellular cancer.[411] Typically, in these patients, the alpha fetoprotein level returns to normal after institution of corticosteroid therapy. The late development of an elevated alpha fetoprotein level or an elevation in the absence of active hepatocellular necrosis and regeneration is worrisome for a true malignancy.

OTHER TREATMENT OPTIONS

Cyclosporine

Cyclosporine has mechanisms of action that make it an appealing drug in the treatment of autoimmune hepatitis (Table 38-12).[412] It acts specifically and reversibly on lymphocytes and can preferentially suppress the clonal expansion of activated T helper cells by inhibiting the release of soluble lymphokines. In this fashion, antibody production by B lymphocytes dependent on T helper cell interaction can be suppressed. Similarly, the clonal expansion of cytotoxic T cells can be inhibited by actions on IL-1 and IL-2.

Cyclosporine (5-6 mg/kg daily) has been used anecdotally in patients with autoimmune hepatitis who have recalcitrance to corticosteroids or had corticosteroid-related complications (see Table 38-8).[412,413] It has also been assessed as a front-line therapy in children with autoimmune hepatitis who are switched later to standard regimens.[415] Favorable results have been reported in all instances. Rigorous clinical trials, however, have not been undertaken, and cyclosporine has not been compared to conventional treatments in a randomized fashion. Its use in autoimmune hepatitis remains unestablished. Side effects include renal insufficiency, hypertension, and malignancy.

Tacrolimus

Tacrolimus is a immunosuppressive agent that has been extracted from a soil fungus (*Streptomyces tsukubaensis*) and found to have similar but more potent immunosuppressive actions than cyclosporine (see Table 38-12).[416] As with cyclosporine, tacrolimus prevents lymphokine production by T cells, inhibits expression of the IL-2 receptor, prevents proliferation of activated T lymphocytes, and inhibits generation of cytotoxic T cells. Furthermore, it may be 100-fold more potent than cyclosporine and less toxic.

Currently, tacrolimus is used mainly in the liver transplantation arena.[417] An open-label treatment trial in patients with autoimmune hepatitis has indicated improvement in the serum aminotransferase and bilirubin levels after 3 months of therapy at an oral dose of 4 mg twice daily.[418] Treatment, however, was not continued to clinical and biochemical remission, liver biopsy assessments were not performed to document drug-related improvements, and most patients developed abnormalities of the serum creatinine and blood urea nitrogen levels. Tacrolimus has promise but it must be assessed against prednisone in a prospective clinical trial to define its benefit-risk ratio and to establish its role in treating this disease.

6-Mercaptopurine

6-Mercaptopurine is a purine analog that inhibits nucleic acid synthesis and is the active metabolite of azathioprine (see Table 38-12).[419] It has a toxicity profile different from azathioprine and may have different immunosuppressive activity, possibly because of variations in intestinal absorption or metabolism. Administered in gradually increasing doses to a maximum level of 100 mg daily (1.5 mg/kg), the drug may induce improvement in some patients who are failing therapy with a conventional combination regimen. Experience with 6-mercaptopurine has been limited but it does offer an option in the patient experiencing treatment failure.

TABLE 38-12
Evolving Drug Therapies

Drug	Actions	Indications
6-Mercaptopurine (1.5 mg/kg daily)	Purine analog that inhibits nucleic acid synthesis Active metabolite of azathioprine	Drug intolerance Treatment failure
Cyclosporine (5-6 mg/kg daily)	Inhibits release of soluble lymphokines Suppresses clonal expansion of activated T helper cells	Drug intolerance Treatment failure
Tacrolimus (3 mg twice daily)	Macrolide antibiotic 10-200 times more immunosuppressive activity than cyclosporine Inhibits expression of IL-2 receptor Inhibits generation of cytotoxic T cells	Drug intolerance Treatment failure
Budesonide (3 mg three times daily)	Second-generation corticosteroid High first-pass clearance Low systemic availability Metabolites lack glucocorticoid activity Unsuccessful for steroid dependence	Mild disease Treatment-naive disease Osteopenia
Ursodeoxycholic acid (13-15 mg/kg daily)	Replaces hydrophobic bile acids Alters class I HLA expression Inhibits IL-2, IL-4, and IFN-γ Impairs nitric oxide production and apoptosis Unsuccessful in problematic patients	Mild disease Treatment-naive disease
Mycophenolate mofetil (1 g twice daily)	Inhibits inosine monophosphate dehydrogenase Restricts DNA synthesis and lymphocyte proliferation Lymphocyte-specific	Treatment intolerance Treatment failure Incomplete response
Rapamycin	Similar to tacrolimus Blocks IL-2, IL-4, and IL-6 signals Prevents effector cell expansion	Treatment failure

IL, Interleukin; *HLA,* human leukocyte antigen; *IFN,* interferon; *DNA,* deoxyribonucleic acid.

Mycophenolate Mofetil

Mycophenolate mofetil inhibits inosine monophosphate dehydrogenase, which in turn restricts DNA synthesis and lymphocyte proliferation (see Table 38-12).[420] Its actions are similar to those of azathioprine, but they are lymphocyte-specific. Mycophenolate mofetil was identified as an important drug to be evaluated in the management of autoimmune hepatitis at a recent Single Topic Conference sponsored by the American Association for the Study of Liver Diseases.[421] This recommendation has now been supported by the experience of British investigators who treated seven patients with mycophenolate mofetil, 1 g twice daily, after conventional therapies had been ineffective or poorly tolerated.[422] They demonstrated biochemical resolution in five patients, substantial reduction in the hepatic activity index after 7 months, and only one episode of leukopenia that required dose adjustment. The promise of this drug must be assessed in a formal scientific fashion.

Ursodeoxycholic Acid

Ursodeoxycholic acid is the 7β-hydroxy epimer of chenodeoxycholic acid that has been well tolerated as an oral agent in various animal species and humans (see Table 38-12).[423] It has been associated with improvements in hepatic dysfunction and is now a standard therapy for PBC. The therapeutic properties of ursodeoxycholic acid remain uncertain but they may relate to choleretic, cytoprotective, and immunomodulatory actions. Ursodeoxycholic acid has a greater stimulatory effect on bile flow than does the endogenous bile acids, producing choleresis not only by osmotic effects but also by stimulation of canalicular transport of inorganic ions. This choleretic effect may eliminate toxic hydrophobic bile acids from the liver that can perpetuate and extend hepatocyte injury.

Ursodeoxycholic acid may also exert a cytoprotective effect by associating with the hepatocyte membrane and creating a barrier to the toxic effects of these same hydrophobic bile acids.[424] It may also affect the immune response by reducing the expression of class I HLA on the hepatocyte membrane; suppressing immunoglobulin production by peripheral blood mononuclear cells; inhibiting IL-2, IL-4, and interferon-γ production; and improving lymphocyte function. Ursodeoxycholic acid also inhibits nitric oxide production—this action may, in turn, improve mitochondrial function and immune responsiveness. This drug may also inhibit apoptosis by modulating the production of reactive oxygen species.

Preliminary reports have suggested that ursodeoxycholic acid has efficacy in the treatment of autoimmune hepatitis. Studies in Japan have demonstrated clinical and biochemical improvement in eight patients who were treated with ursodeoxycholic acid, 600 mg daily, for 2 years.[425] Histologic features of inflammation, but not those of fibrosis, improved in each of four patients who underwent successive liver biopsy examinations. These findings have not yet been corroborated or extended.

In a randomized, placebo-controlled treatment trial, ursodeoxycholic acid (13-15 mg/kg daily) improved serum aspartate aminotransferase and alkaline phosphatase levels after 6 months in corticosteroid-treated, problematic patients with type 1 autoimmune hepatitis.[426] Such therapy, however, did not facilitate dose reduction or corticosteroid withdrawal, affect clinical outcome, or reduce histologic activity. These findings suggested that the role of ursodeoxycholic acid might be restricted to the treatment of naive patients with mild or uncomplicated autoimmune hepatitis. Future investigations must explore longer durations of treatment or higher doses of drug in treatment-naive patients before this drug can be incorporated into a management algorithm.

Budesonide

Budesonide is a second-generation corticosteroid that has a high first-pass clearance by the liver, low systemic availability, and metabolites that lack glucocorticoid activity (see Table 38-12).[427] It has been used safely and effectively in patients with asthma, allergic rhinitis, nasal polyposis, and inflammatory bowel disease. A small open-label study involving 13 patients with autoimmune hepatitis indicated that therapy with budesonide (usually 6 to 8 mg daily) for 9 months was well tolerated and improved laboratory indices.[428]

The initial success with budesonide was not extended when the drug was administered to patients with autoimmune hepatitis who were dependent on long-term corticosteroid therapy.[429] In a pilot study including 10 of these patients, laboratory indices did not improve significantly during 5 ± 1 months of therapy (range, 2-12 months) with budesonide, 3 mg three times daily. Only three patients entered clinical and biochemical remission; seven patients either relapsed after prednisone withdrawal, deteriorated during therapy, or became drug intolerant. Withdrawal symptoms complicated conversion from prednisone to budesonide treatment, and all patients developed at least one side effect. Mean bone densities actually increased slightly in the entire group, and preservation of bone density during this short treatment trial was the most beneficial effect of the drug.

EXPECTATIONS

Future investigations will focus on the identification, isolation, and cloning of the target autoantigens of autoimmune hepatitis. Only by continued efforts to sequence, clone, and map these molecules can the true targets of the autoimmune response be recognized and effective site-specific therapeutic interventions developed, such as blocking peptides, oral tolerance regimens, cytokine manipulations, T cell vaccination, and gene therapy.

By characterizing the epitopes responsible for the disease and the mechanisms by which they are recognized, the properties of an etiologic agent can be deduced and then studied in an animal model. The expression of autoreactive epitopes in transgenic animals has been a successful method of studying the bases for other autoimmune disorders, and it represents the next level of study in autoimmune hepatitis.

Genetic studies will fully define the HLA associations in patients with autoimmune hepatitis and the various autoimmune promoter genes that contribute to disease occurrence, clinical expression, and treatment outcome. In this fashion, susceptible populations will be recognized early and preventive strategies or monitoring programs developed. Poor responses to conventional treatments will be anticipated and countered by site-specific interventions or more powerful immunosuppressive medication.

Subclassifications will have a validity based on etiology or disease-specific pathogenic mechanisms. These insights into pathogenesis will in turn foster type-specific therapies. Autoantibodies will be identified that will have diagnostic precision and prognostic value and treatment end points will be refined to secure remission after drug withdrawal. The future of autoimmune hepatitis promises to be exciting as new technologies address the unresolved issues.

References

1. Czaja AJ: Natural history, clinical features, and treatment of autoimmune hepatitis. Semin Liver Dis 4:1, 1984.
2. Czaja AJ: Autoimmune chronic active hepatitis—a specific entity? The negative argument. J Gastroenterol Hepatol 5:343, 1990.
3. Czaja AJ: Autoimmune hepatitis: evolving concepts and treatment strategies. Dig Dis Sci 40:435, 1995.
4. Czaja AJ: Diagnosis and therapy of autoimmune liver disease. Med Clin North Am 80:973, 1996.
5. Czaja AJ: Current problems in the diagnosis and management of chronic active hepatitis. Mayo Clin Proc 56:311, 1981.
6. Czaja AJ: Diagnosis and treatment of chronic hepatitis. Compr Ther 10:58, 1984.
7. Czaja AJ: Diagnosis, prognosis, and treatment of classical autoimmune chronic active hepatitis. In Krawitt EL, Wiesner RH, eds: Autoimmune Liver Disease, New York, Raven Press, 1991:143-166.
8. Johnson PJ, McFarlane IG, Alvarez F, et al: Meeting report. International Autoimmune Hepatitis Group. Hepatology 18:998, 1993.
9. Alvarez F, Berg PA, Bianchi FB, et al: International Autoimmune Hepatitis Group report: review of criteria for diagnosis of autoimmune hepatitis. J Hepatol 31:929, 1999.
10. Czaja AJ, Carpenter HA: Autoimmune hepatitis. In MacSween RNM, Anthony PP, Scheuer PJ, et al, eds: Pathology of the Liver, ed 4, Edinburgh, Churchill Livingstone, 2002:415-433.
11. Baggenstoss AH, Soloway RD, Summerskill WHJ, et al: Chronic active liver disease. The range of histologic lesions, their response to treatment, and evolution. Hum Pathol 3:183, 1972.
12. Dienes HP, Popper H, Manns M, et al: Histologic features in autoimmune hepatitis. Z Gastroenterol 27:325, 1989.
13. Pratt DS, Fawaz KA, Rabson A, et al: A novel histological lesion in glucocorticoid-responsive chronic hepatitis. Gastroenterology 113:664, 1997.
14. Te HS, Koukoulis G, Ganger DR: Autoimmune hepatitis: a histological variant associated with prominent centrilobular necrosis. Gut 41:269, 1997.
15. Ludwig J, Czaja AJ, Dickson ER, et al: Manifestations of nonsuppurative cholangitis in chronic hepatobiliary disease: morphologic spectrum, clinical correlations and terminology. Liver 4:105, 1984.
16. Czaja AJ: Chronic active hepatitis: the challenge for a new nomenclature. Ann Intern Med 119:510, 1993.

17. Czaja AJ, Carpenter HA, Santrach PJ, et al: Autoimmune cholangitis within the spectrum of autoimmune liver disease. Hepatology 31:1231, 2000.
18. Czaja AJ: The variant forms of autoimmune hepatitis. Ann Intern Med 125:588, 1996.
19. Czaja AJ: Frequency and nature of the variant syndromes of autoimmune liver disease. Hepatology 28:360, 1998.
20. Czaja AJ: Variant forms of autoimmune hepatitis. Cur Gastroenterol Rep 1:63, 1999.
21. Czaja AJ, Carpenter HA: Validation of a scoring system for the diagnosis of autoimmune hepatitis. Dig Dis Sci 41:305, 1996.
22. Boberg KM, Fausa O, Haaland T, et al: Features of autoimmune hepatitis in primary sclerosing cholangitis: an evaluation of 114 primary sclerosing cholangitis patients according to a scoring system for the diagnosis of autoimmune hepatitis. Hepatology 23:1369, 1996.
23. Cullinan ER: Idiopathic jaundice (often recurrent) associated with subacute necrosis of the liver. St Barth Hosp Rep 69:55, 1936.
24. Amberg S: Hyperproteinemia associated with severe liver damage. Proc Staff Mayo Clin 17:360, 1942.
25. Waldenstrom J: Leber, Blutproteine und Nahrungseiweiss. Dtsch Gesellsch Verdau Stoffwechselkr 15:113, 1950.
26. Kunkel HG, Ahrens EH Jr, Eisenmenger WJ, et al: Extreme hypergammaglobulinemia in young women with liver disease of unknown etiology (abstract). J Clin Invest 30:654, 1951.
27. Bongiovanni AM, Eisenmenger WJ: Adrenal cortical metabolism in chronic liver disease. J Clin Endocrinol 11:152, 1951.
28. Bearn AG, Kunkel HG, Slater RJ: The problem of chronic liver disease in young women. Am J Med 21:3, 1956.
29. Saint EG, King WE, Joske RA, et al: The course of infectious hepatitis with special reference to prognosis and the chronic stage. Australas Ann Med 2:113, 1953.
30. Mackay JR, Taft LI, Cowling DC: Lupoid hepatitis. Lancet 2:1323, 1956.
31. Joske RA, King WE: The "LE cell" phenomenon in active chronic viral hepatitis. Lancet 2:477, 1955.
32. Taft LI, Mackay IR, Cowling DC: Autoclasia: a perpetuating mechanism in hepatitis. Gastroenterology 38:563, 1960.
33. Mackay IR: Immunological aspects of chronic active hepatitis. Hepatology 3:724, 1983.
34. Bartholomew LG, Hagedorn AB, Cain JC, et al: Hepatitis and cirrhosis in women with positive clot tests for lupus erythematosus. N Engl J Med 259:947, 1958.
35. Mackay IR, Taft LI, Cowling DC: Lupoid hepatitis and the hepatic lesions of systemic lupus erythematosus. Lancet 1:65, 1959.
36. Hall S, Czaja AJ, Kaufman DK, et al: How lupoid is lupoid hepatitis? J Rheumatol 13:95, 1986.
37. Gurian LE, Rogoff TM, Ware AJ, et al: The immunologic diagnosis of chronic active "autoimmune" hepatitis: distinction from systemic lupus erythematosus. Hepatology 5:397, 1985.
38. Wood JR, Czaja AJ, Beaver SJ, et al: Frequency and significance of antibody to double-stranded DNA in chronic active hepatitis. Hepatology 6:976, 1986.
39. Willcox RG, Isselbacher KJ: Chronic liver disease in young people. Clinical features and course of thirty-three patients. Am J Med 30:185, 1961.
40. Read AE, Sherlock S, Harrison CV: Active "juvenile" cirrhosis considered as part of a systemic disease and the effect of corticosteroid therapy. Gut 4:378, 1963
41. Schalm SW, Summerskill WHJ, Gitnick GL, et al: Contrasting features and responses to treatment of severe chronic active liver disease with and without hepatitis Bs antigen. Gut 17:781, 1976
42. Lam KC, Lai CL, Ng RP, et al: Deleterious effect of prednisolone in HBsAg-positive chronic active hepatitis. N Engl J Med 304:380, 1981
43. Mackay IR, Wood IJ: The course and treatment of lupoid hepatitis. Gastroenterology 45:4, 1963
44. Page AR, Condie RM, Good RA: Suppression of plasma cell hepatitis with 6-mercaptopurine. Am J Med 36:200, 1964.
45. Page AR, Good RA, Pollara B: Long-term results of therapy in patients with chronic liver disease associated with hypergammaglobulinemia. Am J Med 47:765, 1969.
46. Mistilis SP, Skyring AP, Blackburn CRB: Natural history of active chronic hepatitis. I. Clinical features, course, diagnostic criteria, morbidity, mortality, and survival. Australas Ann Med 17:214, 1968.
47. Copenhagen Study Group for Liver Diseases: Effect of prednisone on the survival of patients with cirrhosis of the liver. Lancet 1:119, 1969.
48. Cook GC, Mulligan R, Sherlock S: Controlled prospective trial of corticosteroid therapy in active chronic hepatitis. Q J Med 40:159, 1971.
49. Soloway RD, Summerskill WHJ, Baggenstoss AH, et al: Clinical, biochemical, and histological remission of severe chronic active liver disease: a controlled study of treatments and early prognosis. Gastroenterology 63:820, 1972.
50. Murray-Lyon IM, Stern RB, Williams R: Controlled trial of prednisone and azathioprine in active chronic hepatitis. Lancet 1:735, 1973.
51. Whittingham S, Irwin J, Mackay IR, et al: Smooth muscle autoantibody in "autoimmune" hepatitis. Gastroenterology 51:499, 1966.
52. Doniach D, Roitt IM, Walker JG, et al: Tissue antibodies in primary biliary cirrhosis, active chronic (lupoid) hepatitis, cryptogenic cirrhosis and other liver diseases and their clinical implications. Clin Exp Immunol 1:237, 1966.
53. Cohen S, Ohta G, Singer EJ, et al: Immunocytochemical study of gamma globulin in liver in hepatitis and postnecrotic cirrhosis. J Exp Med 11:285, 1960.
54. Paronetto F, Rubin E, Popper H: Local formation of gamma-globulin in the diseased liver and its relation to hepatic necrosis. Lab Invest 11:150, 1962.
55. Klatskin G: Subacute hepatic necrosis and postnecrotic cirrhosis due to anicteric infections with the hepatitis virus. Am J Med 25:333, 1958.
56. Boyer JL, Klatskin G: Pattern of necrosis in acute hepatitis. Prognostic value of bridging (subacute hepatic necrosis). N Engl J Med 283:1063, 1970.
57. Becker MD, Scheuer PJ, Baptista A, et al: Prognosis of chronic persistent hepatitis. Lancet 1:53, 1970.
58. Ware AJ, Eigenbrodt EH, Combes B: Prognostic significance of subacute hepatic necrosis in acute hepatitis. Gastroenterology 68:1063, 1975.
59. Boyer JL: Chronic hepatitis. A perspective on classification and determinants of prognosis. Gastroenterology 70:1161, 1976.
60. Schalm SW, Korman MG, Summerskill WHJ, et al: Severe chronic active liver disease. Prognostic significance of initial morphologic patterns. Am J Dig Dis 22:973, 1977.
61. Cooksley WGE, Bradbear RA, Robinson W, et al: The prognosis of chronic active hepatitis without cirrhosis in relation to bridging necrosis. Hepatology 6:345, 1986.
62. Czaja AJ, Ludwig J, Baggenstoss AH, et al: Corticosteroid-treated chronic active hepatitis in remission. Uncertain prognosis of chronic persistent hepatitis. N Engl J Med 304:5, 1981.
63. Czaja AJ, Wolf AM, Baggenstoss AH: Laboratory assessment of severe chronic active liver disease (CALD): correlation of serum transaminase and gamma globulin levels with histologic features. Gastroenterology 80:687, 1981.
64. Czaja AJ, Davis GL, Ludwig J, et al: Complete resolution of inflammatory activity following corticosteroid treatment of HBsAg-negative chronic active hepatitis. Hepatology 4:622, 1984.
65. Soloway RD, Baggenstoss AH, Schoenfield LJ, et al: Observer error and sampling variability tested in evaluation of hepatitis and cirrhosis by liver biopsy. Am J Dig Dis 20:1087, 1975.
66. Theodossi A, Skene AM, Portmann B, et al: Observer variation in assessment of liver biopsies including analysis by kappa statistics. Gastroenterology 79:232, 1980.
67. Czaja AJ, Steinberg AS, Saldana M, et al: Peritoneoscopy: its value in the diagnosis of liver disease. Gastrointest Endosc 20:23, 1973.
68. Redeker AG: Viral hepatitis: clinical aspects. Am J Med Sci 270:9, 1975.
69. Korman MG, Hofmann AF, Summerskill WHJ: Assessment of activity in chronic active liver disease: serum bile acids compared with conventional tests and histology. N Engl J Med 290:1399, 1974.
70. Hepner GW, Vesell ES: Assessment of aminopyrine metabolism in man by breath analysis after oral administration of ^{14}C-aminopyrine: effects of phenobarbital, disulfiram and portal cirrhosis. N Engl J Med 291:1384, 1974.
71. Mistilis SP, Blackburn CRB: Active chronic hepatitis. Am J Med 48:484, 1970.
72. Blumberg BS, Alter HJ, Visnich S: A "new" antigen in leukemia sera. JAMA 191:541, 1965.

73. Shulman NR, Hirschman RJ, Barker LF: Viral hepatitis. Ann Intern Med 72:257, 1970.
74. Czaja AJ: Serologic markers of hepatitis A and B in acute and chronic liver disease. Mayo Clin Proc 54:721, 1979.
75. Soloway RD, Summerskill WHJ, Baggenstoss AH, et al: "Lupoid" hepatitis, a nonentity in the spectrum of chronic active liver disease. Gastroenterology 63:458, 1972.
76. Goldstein GB, Lam KC, Mistilis SP: Drug-induced active chronic hepatitis. Am J Dig Dis 18:177, 1973.
77. Maddrey WC, Boitnott JK: Drug-induced chronic liver disease. Gastroenterology 72:1348, 1977.
78. Seeff LB: Drug-induced chronic liver disease, with emphasis on chronic active hepatitis. Semin Liver Dis 1:104, 1981.
79. Geall MG, Schoenfield LJ, Summerskill WHJ: Classification and treatment of chronic active liver disease. Gastroenterology 63:458, 1972.
80. Summerskill WHJ: Chronic active liver disease reexamined: prognosis hopeful. Gastroenterology 66:450, 1974.
81. Bulkey BH, Heizer WD, Goldfinger SE, et al: Distinctions in chronic active hepatitis based on circulating hepatitis-associated antigen. Lancet 2:1323, 1970.
82. Meyer zum Buschenfelde K-H, Kossling FK, Miescher PA: Experimental chronic active hepatitis in rabbits following immunization with human liver proteins. Clin Exp Immunol 10:99, 1972.
83. Meyer zum Buschenfelde K-H, Hopf U: Studies on the pathogenesis of experimental chronic active hepatitis in rabbits. I. Induction of the disease and protective effect on allogeneic liver specific proteins. Br J Exp Pathol 55:498, 1974.
84. Hopf U, Meyer zum Buschenfelde K-H, Arnold W: Detection of a liver-membrane autoantibody in HBsAg-negative chronic active hepatitis. N Engl J Med 294:578, 1976.
85. Eddleston ALWF, Williams R: The role of immunological mechanisms in chronic hepatitis. Ann Clin Res 8:162, 1976.
86. Williams R, Eddleston ALWF: Chronic active hepatitis: immunopathogenesis and immunotherapy. Isr J Med Sci 15:261, 1979.
87. Mackay IR, Morris PJ: Association of autoimmune active chronic hepatitis with HL-A1,8. Lancet 2:793, 1972.
88. Galbraith RM, Eddleston ALWF, Smith MGM, et al: Histocompatibility antigens in active chronic hepatitis and primary biliary cirrhosis. BMJ 3:604, 1974.
89. Page AR, Sharp HL, Greenberg LJ: Genetic analysis of patients with chronic active hepatitis. J Clin Invest 56:530, 1975.
90. Galbraith RM, Smith M, Mackenzie RM: High prevalence of seroimmunologic abnormalities in relatives of patients with chronic active hepatitis or primary biliary cirrhosis. N Engl J Med 190:63, 1974.
91. Manns M, Meyer zum Buschenfelde K-H: Fractionation of the liver membrane lipoprotein (LSP) and characterization of its antigenic determinants by autoantibodies and a heterologous antiserum. Gut 23:14, 1982.
92. Jensen DM, McFarlane IG, Portmann BS, et al: Detection of antibodies directed against a liver-specific membrane lipoprotein in patients with acute and chronic active hepatitis. N Engl J Med 299:1, 1978.
93. Miele Vergani G, Eddleston ALWF: Autoimmunity to liver membrane antigens in acute and chronic hepatitis. Clin Immunol Allergy 1:181, 1981.
94. Feighery C, McDonald GSA, Greally JF, et al: Histological and immunological investigation of liver-specific protein (LSP) immunized rabbits compared with patients with liver disease. Clin Exp Immunol 45:143, 1981.
95. Butler RC: Studies on experimental chronic active hepatitis in the rabbit. I. Induction of the disease by immunization with muscle as well as liver proteins. Br J Exp Pathol 65:499, 1984.
96. Frazer IH, Kronborg IJ, Mackay IR: Autoantibodies to liver membrane antigens in chronic active hepatitis. II. Specificity of high titers for autoimmune chronic active hepatitis. Clin Exp Immunol 54:213, 1983.
97. McFarlane BM, McSorley CG, McFarlane IG, et al: Serum autoantibodies reacting with the hepatic asialoglycoprotein receptor (hepatic lectin) in acute and chronic liver disorders. J Hepatol 3:196, 1986.
98. Choo Q-L, Kuo G, Weiner AJ, et al: Isolation of a cDNA clone from a blood-borne non-A,non-B viral hepatitis genome. Science 244:359, 1989.
99. Manns MP: Cytoplasmic autoantigens in autoimmune hepatitis: molecular analysis and clinical relevance. Semin Liver Dis 11:205, 1991.
100. Mackay IR: Autoimmune diseases of the liver: chronic active hepatitis and primary biliary cirrhosis. In Rose NR, Mackay IR, eds: The Autoimmune Diseases. Orlando, Fla, Academic Press, Inc., 1985:291-337.
101. Ryder LP, Andersen E, Svejgaard A: An HLA map of Europe. Hum Hered 28:171, 1978.
102. Lam KC, Lai CL, Wu PC, et al: Etiological spectrum of liver cirrhosis in the Chinese. J Chronic Dis 33:375, 1980.
103. Meyer zum Buschenfelde K-H, Hutteroth TH: Autoantibodies against liver membrane antigens in chronic active liver disease. In Eddleston ALWF, Weber JCP, Williams R, eds: Immune Reactions in Liver Disease. Kent, UK, Pitman Medical Publishing Co., 1979: 12-20.
104. Hodges JR, Millward-Sadler GH, Wright R: Chronic active hepatitis: the spectrum of disease. Lancet 1:550, 1982.
105. Boberg KM, Aadland E, Jahnsen J, et al: Incidence and prevalence of primary biliary cirrhosis, primary sclerosing cholangitis, and autoimmune hepatitis in a Norwegian population. Scand J Gastroenterol 33:99, 1998.
106. Wiesner RH, Demetris AJ, Belle SH, et al: Acute allograft rejection: incidence, risk factors, and impact on outcome. Hepatology 28:638, 1998.
107. Milkiewicz P, Hubscher SG, Skiba G, et al: Recurrence of autoimmune hepatitis after liver transplantation. Transplantation 68:253, 1999.
108. Rose NR: Fundamental concepts of autoimmunity and autoimmune disease. In Krawitt EL, Wiesner RH, Nishioka M, eds: Autoimmune Liver Diseases, ed 2. New York, Elsevier Science Publishers, 1998:1-20.
109. Hay JE, Czaja AJ, Rakela J, et al: The nature of unexplained chronic aminotransferase elevations of a mild to moderate degree in asymptomatic patients. Hepatology 9:193, 1989.
110. Maddrey WC: Subdivisions of idiopathic autoimmune chronic active hepatitis. Hepatology 7:1372, 1987.
111. Czaja AJ, Manns MP: The validity and importance of subtypes of autoimmune hepatitis: a point of view. Am J Gastroenterol 90:1206, 1995.
112. Czaja AJ: Special report. Autoimmune hepatitis. Curr Treatment Options Gastroenterol 2:423, 1999.
113. McFarlane IG: The relationship between autoimmune markers and different clinical syndromes in autoimmune hepatitis. Gut 42:599, 1998.
114. Czaja AJ, Davis GL, Ludwig J, et al: Autoimmune features as determinants of prognosis in steroid-treated chronic active hepatitis of uncertain etiology. Gastroenterology 85:713, 1983.
115. Lidman K, Biberfield G, Fagraeus A, et al: Anti-actin specificity of human smooth muscle antibodies in chronic active hepatitis. Clin Exp Immunol 24:266, 1976.
116. Toh B-H: Smooth muscle autoantibody and autoantigens. Clin Exp Immunol 38:621, 1979.
117. Homberg J-C, Abuaf N, Bernard O, et al: Chronic active hepatitis associated with antiliver/kidney microsome antibody type 1: a second type of "autoimmune" hepatitis. Hepatology 7:1333, 1987.
118. Amontree JS, Stuart TD, Bredfeldt JE: Autoimmune chronic active hepatitis masquerading as acute hepatitis. J Clin Gastroenterol 11:303, 1989.
119. Davis GL, Czaja AJ, Baggenstoss AH, et al: Prognostic and therapeutic implications of extreme serum aminotransferase elevation in chronic active hepatitis. Mayo Clin Proc 57:303, 1982.
120. Crapper RM, Bhathal PS, Mackay IR, et al: "Acute" autoimmune hepatitis. Digestion 34:216, 1986.
121. Nikias GA, Batts KP, Czaja AJ: The nature and prognostic implications of autoimmune hepatitis with an acute presentation. J Hepatol 21:866, 1994.
122. Burgart LJ, Batts KP, Ludwig J, et al: Recent onset autoimmune hepatitis: biopsy findings and clinical correlations. Am J Surg Path 19:699, 1995.
123. Czaja AJ, Rakela J, Ludwig J: Features reflective of early prognosis in corticosteroid-treated severe autoimmune chronic active hepatitis. Gastroenterology 95:448, 1988.
124. Czaja AJ, Carpenter HA, Santrach PJ, et al: Genetic predispositions for the immunological features of chronic active hepatitis. Hepatology 18:816, 1993.

125. Czaja AJ, Carpenter HA, Santrach PJ, et al: Significance of the human leukocyte antigen DR4 in type 1 autoimmune hepatitis. Gastroenterology 105:1502, 1993.
126. Czaja AJ, Carpenter HA, Santrach PJ, et al: Evidence against hepatitis viruses as important causes of severe autoimmune hepatitis in the United States. J Hepatol 18:342, 1993.
127. Czaja AJ, Dos Santos RM, Porto S, et al: Immune phenotype of chronic liver disease. Dig Dis Sci 43:2149, 1998.
128. Perdigoto R, Carpenter HA, Czaja AJ: Frequency and significance of chronic ulcerative colitis in severe corticosteroid-treated autoimmune hepatitis. J Hepatol 14:325, 1992.
129. Wiesner RH, LaRusso NF: Clinicopathologic features of the syndrome of primary sclerosing cholangitis. Gastroenterology 79:200, 1980.
130. Wee A, Ludwig J: Pericholangitis in chronic ulcerative colitis: primary sclerosing cholangitis of the small bile ducts? Ann Intern Med 102:581, 1985.
131. Rabinovitz M, Demetris AJ, Bou-Abboud CF, et al: Simultaneous occurrence of primary sclerosing cholangitis and autoimmune chronic active hepatitis in a patient with ulcerative colitis. Dig Dis Sci 37:1606, 1992.
132. Czaja AJ, Rakela J, Hay JE, et al: Clinical and prognostic implications of human leukocyte antigen B8 in corticosteroid-treated severe autoimmune chronic active hepatitis. Gastroenterology 98:1587, 1990.
133. Opelz G, Vogten AJM, Summerskill WHJ, et al: HLA determinants in chronic active liver disease: possible relation of HLA-Dw3 to prognosis. Tissue Antigens 9:36, 1977.
134. Donaldson PT, Doherty DG, Hayllar KM, et al: Susceptibility to autoimmune chronic active hepatitis: human leukocyte antigens DR4 and A1-B8-DR3 are independent risk factors. Hepatology 13:701, 1990.
135. Sanchez-Urdazpal L, Czaja AJ, van Hoek B, et al: Prognostic features and role of liver transplantation in severe corticosteroid-treated autoimmune chronic active hepatitis. Hepatology 15:215, 1992.
136. Doherty DG, Donaldson PT, Underhill JA, et al: Allelic sequence variation in the HLA class II genes and proteins in patients with autoimmune hepatitis. Hepatology 19:609, 1994.
137. Strettell MDJ, Donaldson PT, Thomson LJ, et al: Allelic basis for HLA-encoded susceptibility to type 1 autoimmune hepatitis. Gastroenterology 112:2028, 1997.
138. Vazquez-Garcia MN, Alaez C, Olivo A, et al: MHC class II sequences of susceptibility and protection in Mexicans with autoimmune hepatitis. J Hepatol 28:985, 1998.
139. Seki T, Kiyosawa K, Inoko H, et al: Association of autoimmune hepatitis with HLA-Bw54 and DR4 in Japanese patients. Hepatology 12:1300, 1990.
140. Seki T, Ota M, Furuta S, et al: HLA class II molecules and autoimmune hepatitis susceptibility in Japanese patients. Gastroenterology 103:1041, 1992.
141. Fainboim L, Marcos Y, Pando M, et al: Chronic active autoimmune hepatitis in children. Strong association with a particular HLA DR6 (DRB1*1301) haplotype. Hum Immunol 41:146, 1994.
142. Pando M, Larriba J, Fernandez GC, et al: Pediatric and adult forms of type 1 autoimmune hepatitis in Argentina: evidence for differential genetic predisposition. Hepatology 30:1374, 1999.
143. Bittencourt PL, Goldberg AC, Cancado ELR, et al: Genetic heterogeneity in susceptibility to autoimmune hepatitis types 1 and 2. Am J Gastroenterol 94:1906, 1999.
144. McFarlane BM, McSorley CG, McFarlane IG, et al: Serum autoantibodies reacting with the hepatic asialoglycoprotein receptor (hepatic lectin) in acute and chronic liver disorders. J Hepatol 3:196, 1986.
145. Poralla T, Treichel U, Lohr H, et al: The asialoglycoprotein receptor as target structure in autoimmune liver diseases. Semin Liver Dis 11:215, 1991.
146. Treichel U, Poralla T, Hess G, et al: Autoantibodies to human asialoglycoprotein receptor in autoimmune-type chronic hepatitis. Hepatology 11:606, 1990.
147. Treichel U, Gerken G, Rossol S, et al: Autoantibodies against the human asialoglycoprotein receptor: effects of therapy in autoimmune and virus-induced chronic active hepatitis. J Hepatol 19:55, 1993.
148. Wies I, Brunner S, Henninger J, et al: Identification of target antigen for SLA/LP autoantibodies in autoimmune hepatitis. Lancet 355:1510, 2000.
149. Costa M, Rodriques-Sanchez JL, Czaja AJ, et al: Isolation and characterization of cDNA encoding the antigenic protein of the human $tRNA^{(Ser)Sec}$ complex recognized by autoantibodies from patients with type 1 autoimmune hepatitis. Clin Exp Immunol 121:364, 2000.
150. Mackay IR: Genetic aspects of immunologically mediated liver disease. Semin Liver Dis 4:13, 1984.
151. Meyer zum Buschenfelde K-H, Lohse AW, Manns M, et al: Autoimmunity and liver disease. Hepatology 12:354, 1990.
152. McFarlane IG: Pathogenesis of autoimmune hepatitis. Biomed Pharmacother 53:255, 1999.
153. Krawitt EL, Kilby AE, Albertini RJ, et al: Immunogenetic studies of autoimmune chronic active hepatitis: HLA, immunoglobulin allotypes and autoantibodies. Hepatology 7:1305, 1987.
154. Czaja AJ: Autoimmune hepatitis and viral infection. Gastroenterol Clin North Am 23:547, 1994.
155. Czaja AJ: Overlap of chronic viral hepatitis and autoimmune hepatitis. In Willson RA, ed: Viral Hepatitis: Diagnosis, Treatment, Prevention. New York, Marcel Dekker, Inc., 1997:371-399.
156. Czaja AJ: Immunopathogenesis of autoimmune-mediated liver damage. In Moreno-Otero R, Clemente-Ricote G, Garcia-Monzon C, eds: Immunology and the liver: autoimmunity. Madrid, Aran Ediciones, SA, 2000:73-83.
157. Czaja AJ: Understanding the pathogenesis of autoimmune hepatitis. Am J Gastroenterol 96:1224-1231, 2001.
158. Laitinen O, Vaheri A: Very high measles and rubella virus antibody titers associated with hepatitis, systemic lupus erythematosus, and infectious mononucleosis. Lancet 1:194, 1974.
159. Robertson DAF, Zhang SL, Guy EC, et al: Persistent measles virus genome in autoimmune chronic active hepatitis. Lancet 2:9, 1987.
160. Vento S, Cainelli F, Ferraro T, Concia E: Autoimmune hepatitis type 1 after measles. Am J Gastroenterol 91:2618, 1996.
161. Vento S, Garofano T, Di Perri G, et al: Identification of hepatitis A virus as a trigger for autoimmune chronic hepatitis type 1 in susceptible individuals. Lancet 337:1183, 1991.
162. Huppertz H-K, Treichel U, Gassel AM, et al: Autoimmune hepatitis following hepatitis A virus infection. J Hepatol 23:204, 1995.
163. Laskus T, Slusarczyk J: Autoimmune chronic active hepatitis developing after acute type B hepatitis. Dig Dis Sci 34:1294, 1989.
164. Czaja AJ, Magrin S, Fabiano C, et al: Hepatitis C virus infection as a determinant of behavior in type 1 autoimmune hepatitis. Dig Dis Sci 40:33, 1995.
165. Vento S, Cainelli F, Renzini C, et al: Autoimmune hepatitis type 2 induced by HCV and persisting after viral clearance. Lancet 350:1298, 1997.
166. Agulo JM, Sigal LH, Espinoza LR: Coexistent minocycline-induced systemic lupus erythematosus and autoimmune hepatitis. Semin Arthritis Rheum 28:187, 1998.
167. Elkayam O, Yaron M, Caspi: Minocycline-induced autoimmune syndromes: an overview. Semin Arthritis Rheum 28:392, 1999.
168. Eichenfield AH: Minocycline and autoimmunity. Curr Opin Pediatr 11:447, 1999.
169. Esteban JI, Esteban R, Viladomiu L, et al: Hepatitis C virus antibodies among risk groups in Spain. Lancet 2:294, 1989.
170. McFarlane IG, Smith HM, Johnson PJ, et al: Hepatitis C virus antibodies in chronic active hepatitis: pathogenetic factor or false-positive result? Lancet 335:754, 1990.
171. Sanchez-Tapias JM, Barrera JM, Costa J, et al: Hepatitis C virus infection in patients with nonalcoholic chronic liver disease. Ann Intern Med 112:921, 1990.
172. Czaja AJ, Taswell HF, Rakela J, et al: Frequency and significance of antibody to hepatitis C virus in severe corticosteroid-treated autoimmune chronic active hepatitis. Mayo Clin Proc 66:572, 1991.
173. Czaja AJ, Taswell HF, Rakela J, et al: Duration and specificity of antibodies to hepatitis C virus in chronic active hepatitis. Gastroenterology 102:1675, 1992.
174. Nishiguchi S, Kuroki T, Ueda T, et al: Detection of hepatitis C virus antibody in the absence of viral RNA in patients with autoimmune hepatitis. Ann Intern Med 116:21, 1992.
175. Katkov WN, Dienstag JL, Cody H, et al: Role of hepatitis C virus in non-B chronic liver disease. Arch Intern Med 151:1548, 1991.
176. Brind AM, Codd AA, Cohen BJ, et al: Low prevalence of antibody to hepatitis C virus in north east England. J Med Virol 32:243, 1990.
177. Liddle C, Crewe EB, Swanson NR, et al: Does hepatitis C virus play a role in "non-viral" chronic liver disease? Med J Aust 153:265, 1990.

178. Magrin S, Craxi A, Fiorentino G, et al: Is autoimmune chronic active hepatitis a HCV-related disease? J Hepatol 13:56, 1991.
179. Magrin S, Craxi A, Fabiano C, et al: Hepatitis C virus replication in "autoimmune" chronic hepatitis. J Hepatol 13:364, 1991.
180. Cassani F, Muratori L, Manotti P, et al: Serum autoantibodies and the diagnosis of type-1 autoimmune hepatitis in Italy: a reappraisal at the light of hepatitis C virus infection. Gut 33:1260, 1992.
181. Saracco G, Touscoz A, Durazzo M, et al: Antibodies and response to alpha-interferon in patients with chronic viral hepatitis. J Hepatol 11:339, 1990.
182. Clifford BD, Donahue D, Smith L, et al: High prevalence of serological markers of autoimmunity in patients with chronic hepatitis C. Hepatology 21:613, 1995.
183. Noda K, Enomoto N, Arai K, et al: Induction of antinuclear antibody after interferon therapy in patients with type-C chronic hepatitis: its relation to the efficacy of therapy. Scand J Gastroenterol 31:716, 1996.
184. Gueguen M, Meunier-Rotival M, Bernard O, et al: Anti-liver kidney microsome antibody recognizes a cytochrome P450 from the IID subfamily. J Exp Med 168:801, 1988.
185. Zanger UM, Hauri H-P, Loeper J, et al: Antibodies against human cytochrome P-450db1 in autoimmune hepatitis type II. Proc Natl Acad Sci U S A 85:8256, 1988.
186. Manns MP, Johnson EF, Griffin KJ, et al: Major antigen of liver kidney microsomal autoantibodies in idiopathic autoimmune hepatitis is cytochrome P450db1. J Clin Invest 83:1066, 1989.
187. Manns M, Zanger U, Gerken G, et al: Patients with type II autoimmune hepatitis express functionally intact cytochrome P-450 db1 that is inhibited by LKM-1 autoantibodies in vitro but not in vivo. Hepatology 12:127, 1990.
188. Manns MP, Griffin KJ, Sullivan KF, et al: LKM-1 autoantibodies recognize a short linear sequence in P450IID6, a cytochrome P-450 monooxygenase. J Clin Invest 88:1370, 1991.
189. Czaja AJ, Manns MP, Homburger HA: Frequency and significance of antibodies to liver/kidney microsome type 1 in adults with chronic active hepatitis. Gastroenterology 103:1290, 1992.
190. Czaja AJ, Homburger HA: Autoantibodies in liver disease. Gastroenterology 120:239, 2001.
191. Czaja AJ, Carpenter HA, Manns MP: Antibodies to soluble liver antigen, P450 IID6 and mitochondrial complexes in chronic hepatitis. Gastroenterology 103:1290, 1992.
192. Ma Y, Peakman M, Lenzi M, et al: Case against subclassification of type II autoimmune chronic active hepatitis. Lancet 3411:60, 1993.
193. Vergani D, Mieli-Vergani G: Type II autoimmune hepatitis. What is the role of the hepatitis C virus? (editorial) Gastroenterology 104:1870, 1993.
194. Yamamoto AM, Cresteil D, Homberg JC, et al: Characterization of the anti-liver-kidney microsome antibody (anti-LKM1) from hepatitis C virus-positive and -negative sera. Gastroenterology 104:1762, 1993.
195. Gregorio GV, Portmann B, Reid F, et al: Autoimmune hepatitis in childhood. A 20 year survey. Hepatology 25:541, 1997.
196. Klein R, Zanger UM, Berg T, et al: Overlapping but distinct specificities of anti-liver-kidney microsome antibodies in autoimmune hepatitis type II and hepatitis C revealed by recombinant CYP2D6 and novel peptide epitopes. Clin Exp Immunol 118:290, 1999.
197. Loeper J, Descatoire V, Maurice M, et al: Presence of functional cytochrome P-450 on isolated rat hepatocyte plasma membrane. Hepatology 11:850, 1990.
198. Loeper J, Descatoire V, Maurice M, et al: Cytochromes P-450 in human hepatocyte plasma membrane: recognition by several autoantibodies. Gastroenterology 104:203, 1993.
199. Muratori L, Parola M, Ripalti A, et al: Liver/kidney microsomal antibody type 1 targets CYP2D6 on the hepatocyte plasma membrane. Gut 46:553, 2000.
200. Lohr H, Manns M, Kyriatsoulis A, et al: Clonal analysis of liver-infiltrating T cells in patients with LKM-1 antibody-positive autoimmune chronic active hepatitis. Clin Exp Immunol 84:297, 1991.
201. Czaja AJ, Kruger M, Santrach PJ, et al: Genetic distinctions between types 1 and 2 autoimmune hepatitis. Am J Gastroenterol 92:2197, 1997.
202. Manns M, Scheucher S, Jentsch M, et al: Genetics in autoimmune hepatitis type 2 (abstract). Hepatology 14:60A, 1991.
203. Aaltonen J, Borses P, Sandkuijl L, et al: An autosomal locus causing autoimmune disease: autoimmune polyglandular disease type 1 assigned to chromosome 21. Nat Genet 8:83, 1994.
204. Clemente MG, Obermayer-Straub P, Meloni A, et al: Cytochrome P450 1A2 is a hepatic autoantigen in autoimmune polyglandular syndrome type 1. J Clin Endocrinol Metab 82:1353, 1997.
205. Clemente MG, Meloni A, Obermayer-Staub P, et al: Two cytochromes P450 are major hepatocellular autoantigens in autoimmune polyglandular syndrome type 1. Gastroenterology 114:324, 1998.
206. Lenzi M, Ballardini G, Fusconi M, et al: Type 2 autoimmune hepatitis and hepatitis C virus infection. Lancet 335:258, 1990.
207. Todros L, Touscoz G, D'Urso N, et al: Hepatitis C virus-related chronic liver disease with autoantibodies to liver-kidney microsomes (LKM). Clinical characterization from idiopathic LKM-positive disorders. J Hepatol 13:128, 1991.
208. Giostra F, Manzin A, Lenzi M, et al: Low hepatitis C viremia in patients with anti-liver/kidney microsomal antibody type 1 positive chronic hepatitis. J Hepatol 25:433, 1996.
209. Garson JA, Lenzi M, Ring C, et al: Hepatitis C viraemia in adults with type 2 autoimmune hepatitis. J Med Virol 34:223, 1991.
210. Michel G, Ritter A, Gerken G, et al: Anti-GOR and hepatitis C virus in autoimmune liver diseases. Lancet 339:267, 1992.
211. Lunel F, Abuaf N, Frangeul L, et al: Liver/kidney microsome antibody type 1 and hepatitis C virus infection. Hepatology 16:630, 1992.
212. Reddy KR, Krawitt EL, Radick J, et al: Absence of LKM1 antibody in hepatitis C virus infection in the United States (abstract). Gastroenterology 18:173A, 1993.
213. Michitaka K, Durazzo M, Tillmann HL, et al: Analysis of hepatitis C virus genome in patients with autoimmune hepatitis type 2. Gastroenterology 106:1603, 1994.
214. Gerotto M, Pontisso P, Giostra F, et al: Analysis of the hepatitis C virus genome in patients with anti-LKM-1 autoantibodies. J Hepatol 21:273, 1994.
215. Desmet VJ, Gerber M, Hoofnagle JH, et al: Classification of chronic hepatitis: diagnosis, grading and staging. Hepatology 19:1513, 1994.
216. Manns M, Gerken G, Kyriatsoulis A, et al: Characterization of a new subgroup of autoimmune chronic active hepatitis by autoantibodies against a soluble liver antigen. Lancet 1:292, 1987.
217. Stechemesser E, Klein R, Berg PA: Characterization and clinical relevance of liver-pancreas antibodies in autoimmune hepatitis. Hepatology 18:1, 1993.
218. Wesierska-Gadek J, Grimm R, Hitchman E, et al: Members of the glutathione S-transferase gene family are antigens in autoimmune hepatitis. Gastroenterology 114:329, 1998.
219. Kanzler S, Weidemann C, Gerken G, et al: Clinical significance of autoantibodies to soluble liver antigen in autoimmune hepatitis. J Hepatol 31:635, 1999.
220. Ballo E, Homberg JC, Johanet C: Antibodies to soluble liver antigen: an additional marker in type 1 autoimmune hepatitis. J Hepatol 33:208, 2000.
221. Baeres M, Wies I, Kanzler S, et al: Establishment of a standardized SLA/LP immunoassay: SLA/LP positive autoimmune hepatitis occurs worldwide (abstract). Hepatology 32:166A, 2000.
222. Czaja AJ, Hay JE, Rakela J: Clinical features and prognostic implications of severe corticosteroid-treated cryptogenic chronic active hepatitis. Mayo Clin Proc 65:23, 1990.
223. Czaja AJ, Carpenter HA, Santrach PJ, et al: The nature and prognosis of severe cryptogenic chronic active hepatitis. Gastroenterology 104:1755, 1993.
224. Berg PA, Sayers T, Wiedmann KH, et al: Serological classification of chronic cholestatic liver disease by the use of two different types of antimitochondrial antibodies. Lancet 2:1329, 1980.
225. Kenny RP, Czaja AJ, Ludwig J, et al: Frequency and significance of antimitochondrial antibodies in severe chronic active hepatitis. Dig Dis Sci 31:705, 1986.
226. Chazouilleres O, Wendum D, Serfaty L, et al: Primary biliary cirrhosis-autoimmune hepatitis overlap syndrome: clinical features and response to therapy. Hepatology 28:296, 1998.
227. Cooksley WG, Powell LW, Kerr JF, et al: Cholestasis in active chronic hepatitis. Am J Dig Dis 17:495, 1972.

228. Christofferson P, Dietrichson O, Faber V, et al: The occurrence and significance of abnormal bile duct epithelium in chronic aggressive hepatitis. Acta Pathol Microbiol Scand 80:294, 1972.
229. Kloppel G, Seifert G, Lindner H, et al: Histopathological features in mixed types of chronic aggressive hepatitis and primary biliary cirrhosis. Virchows Arch A 373:143, 1977.
230. Geubel AP, Baggenstoss AH, Summerskill WHJ: Responses to treatment can differentiate chronic active liver disease with cholangitic features from the primary biliary cirrhosis syndrome. Gastroenterology 71:444, 1976.
231. Lohse AW, Meyer zum Buschenfelde K-H, Kanzler FB, et al: Characterization of the overlap syndrome of primary biliary cirrhosis (PBC) and autoimmune hepatitis: evidence for it being a hepatitic form of PBC in genetically susceptible individuals. Hepatology 29:1078, 1999.
232. Duclos-Vallee J-C, Hadengue A, Ganne-Carrie N, et al: Primary biliary cirrhosis-autoimmune hepatitis overlap syndrome: corticoresistance and effective treatment with cyclosporine A. Dig Dis Sci 40:1069, 1995.
233. Metcalf J, Mitchison HC, Palmer JM: Natural history of early primary biliary cirrhosis. Lancet 348:1399, 1996.
234. Fussey SPM, Guest JR, James OFW, et al: Identification and analysis of the major M2 autoantigens in primary biliary cirrhosis. Proc Natl Acad Sci U S A 85:8654, 1988.
235. Van de Water J, Cooper A, Surh CD, et al: Detection of autoantibodies to recombinant mitochondrial proteins in patients with primary biliary cirrhosis. N Engl J Med 320:1377, 1989.
236. Zurgil N, Konikoff F, Bakimer R, et al: Detection of antimitochondrial antibodies: characterization by enzyme immunoassay and immunoblotting. Autoimmunity 4:289, 1989.
237. Tsuruya T: Detection of anti-pyruvate dehydrogenase complex antibody in primary biliary cirrhosis by an enzyme-linked immunosorbent assay. Gastroenterologia Japonica 25:471, 1990.
238. Yoshida T, Bonkovsky H, Ansari A, et al: Antibodies against mitochondrial dehydrogenase complexes in primary biliary cirrhosis. Gastroenterology 99:187, 1990.
239. Zurgil N, Bakimer R, Kaplan M, et al: Anti-pyruvate dehydrogenase autoantibodies in primary biliary cirrhosis. J Clin Immunol 11:239, 1991.
240. Fregeau DR, Davis PA, Danner DJ, et al: Antimitochondrial antibodies of primary biliary cirrhosis recognize dihydrolipoamide acyltransferase and inhibit enzyme function of the branched chain alpha-ketoacid dehydrogenase complex. J Immunol 142:3815, 1989.
241. Mutimer DJ, Fussey SPM, Yeaman SJ, et al: Frequency of IgG and IgM autoantibodies to the four specific M2 mitochondrial autoantigens in primary biliary cirrhosis. Hepatology 10:403, 1989.
242. Heseltine L, Turner IB, Fussey SPM, et al: Primary biliary cirrhosis. Quantitation of autoantibodies to purified mitochondrial enzymes and correlation with disease progression. Gastroenterology 99:1786, 1990.
243. Chapman RW, Varghese Z, Gaul R, et al: Association of primary sclerosing cholangitis with HLA-B8. Gut 24:38, 1983.
244. Prochazka EJ, Terasaki PI, Park MS, et al: Association of primary sclerosing cholangitis with HLA-DRw52a. N Engl J Med 322:1842, 1990.
245. Donaldson PT, Farrant JM, Wilkinson ML, et al: Dual association of HLA DR2 and DR3 with primary sclerosing cholangitis. Hepatology 13:129, 1991.
246. Farrant JM, Doherty DG, Donaldson PT, et al: Amino acid substitutions at position 38 of the DRβ polypeptide confer susceptibility to and protection from primary sclerosing cholangitis. Hepatology 16:390, 1992.
247. Czaja AJ, Santrach PJ, Moore SB: Shared genetic risk factors in autoimmune liver disease. Dig Dis Sci 46:140-147, 2001.
248. Mieli-Vergani G, Vergani D: Immunological liver diseases in children. Semin Liver Dis 18:271, 1998.
249. Roberts EA: Primary sclerosing cholangitis in children. J Gastroenterol Hepatol 14:588, 1999.
250. Gregorio GV, Portmann B, Reid F, et al: Autoimmune hepatitis in childhood. A 20 year survey. Hepatology 25:541, 1997.
251. Mieli-Vergani G, Lobo-Yeo A, McFarlane BM, et al: Different immune mechanisms leading to autoimmunity in primary sclerosing cholangitis and autoimmune chronic active hepatitis of childhood. Hepatology 9:198, 1989.
252. Gohlke F, Lohse AW, Dienes HP, et al: Evidence for an overlap syndrome of autoimmune hepatitis and primary sclerosing cholangitis. J Hepatol 24:699, 1996.
253. McNair AN, Moloney M, Portmann BC, et al: Autoimmune hepatitis overlapping primary sclerosing cholangitis in five cases. Am J Gastroenterol 93:777, 1998.
254. Lindor KD: Ursodiol for primary sclerosing cholangitis. N Engl J Med 336:691, 1997.
255. Czaja AJ, Carpenter HA, Santrach PJ, et al: Genetic predispositions for immunological features in chronic liver diseases other than autoimmune hepatitis. J Hepatol 24:52, 1996.
256. Czaja AJ, Carpenter HA, Santrach PJ, et al: Immunologic features and HLA associations in chronic viral hepatitis. Gastroenterology 108:157, 1995.
257. Czaja AJ, Carpenter HA, Santrach PJ, et al: Significance of human leukocyte antigens DR3 and DR4 in chronic viral hepatitis. Dig Dis Sci 40:2098, 1995.
258. Vento S, DiPerri G, Garofano T, et al: Hazards of interferon therapy for HBV-seronegative chronic hepatitis. Lancet 2:926, 1989.
259. Papo T, Marcellin P, Bernuau J, et al: Autoimmune chronic hepatitis exacerbated by alpha-interferon. Ann Intern Med 116:51, 1992.
260. Shindo M, DiBisceglie AM, Hoofnagle JH: Acute exacerbation of liver disease during interferon alfa therapy for chronic hepatitis C. Gastroenterology 102:1406, 1992.
261. Garcia-Bury L, Garcia-Monzon C, Rodriguez S, et al: Latent autoimmune hepatitis triggered during interferon therapy in patients with chronic hepatitis C. Gastroenterology 108:1770, 1995.
262. Magrin S, Craxi A, Fabiano C, et al: Hepatitis C viremia in chronic liver disease: relationship to interferon-alpha or corticosteroid therapy. Hepatology 19:273, 1994.
263. Cassani F, Cataleta M, Valentini P, et al: Serum autoantibodies in chronic hepatitis C: comparison with autoimmune hepatitis and impact on the disease profile. Hepatology 26:561, 1997.
264. Durazzo M, Philipp T, van Pelt FNAM, et al: Heterogeneity of microsomal autoantibodies (LKM) in chronic hepatitis C and D virus infection. Gastroenterology 108:455, 1995.
265. Manns MP, Obermayer-Straub P: Cytochromes P450 and uridine triphosphate-glucuronosyltransferases: model autoantigens to study drug-induced, virus-induced, and autoimmune liver disease. Hepatology 26:1054, 1997.
266. Lunel F, Musset L, Cacoub P, et al: Cryoglobulinemia in chronic liver diseases: role of hepatitis C virus and liver damage. Gastroenterology 106:1291, 1994.
267. Pawlotsky J-M, Yahia MB, Andre C, et al: Immunological disorders in C virus chronic active hepatitis: a prospective case-control study. Hepatology 19:841, 1994.
268. Czaja AJ: Extrahepatic immunologic features of chronic viral hepatitis. Dig Dis 15:125, 1997.
269. Fong T-L, Valinluck B, Govindarajan S, et al: Short-term prednisone therapy affects aminotransferase activity and hepatitis C virus RNA levels in chronic hepatitis C. Gastroenterology 107:196, 1994.
270. Bellary S, Schiano T, Hartman G, et al: Chronic hepatitis with combined features of autoimmune chronic hepatitis and chronic hepatitis C: favorable response to prednisone and azathioprine. Ann Int Med 123:32, 1995.
271. Tran A, Benzaken S, Yang G, et al: Chronic hepatitis C and autoimmunity: good response to immunosuppressive therapy. Dig Dis Sci 42:778, 1997.
272. Yoshikawa M, Toyohara M, Yamane Y, et al: Disappearance of serum HCV-RNA after short-term prednisolone therapy in a patient with chronic hepatitis C associated with autoimmune hepatitis-like serological manifestations. J Gastroenterol 34:269, 1999.
273. Czaja AJ, Carpenter HA: Histological findings in chronic hepatitis C with autoimmune features. Hepatology 26:459, 1997.
274. Muratori L, Lenzi M, Cataleta M, et al: Interferon therapy in liver/kidney microsomal antibody type 1-positive patients with chronic hepatitis C. J Hepatol 21:199, 1994.
275. Todros L, Saracco G, Durazzo M, et al: Efficacy and safety of interferon alfa therapy in chronic hepatitis C with autoantibodies to liver-kidney microsomes. Hepatology 22:1374, 1995.
276. Jeffers LJ, Hasan F, De Medina M, et al: Prevalence of antibodies to hepatitis C virus among patients with cryptogenic chronic hepatitis and cirrhosis. Hepatology 15:187, 1992.

277. Brown J, Dourakis S, Karayiannis P, et al: Seroprevalence of hepatitis C virus nucleocapsid antibodies in patients with cryptogenic chronic liver disease. Hepatology 15:175, 1992.
278. Czaja AJ, Taswell HF, Rakela J, et al: Frequency and significance of antibody to hepatitis C virus in severe corticosteroid-treated cryptogenic chronic active hepatitis. Mayo Clin Proc 65:1303, 1990.
279. Czaja AJ, Taswell HF, Rakela J, et al: Frequency of antibody to hepatitis C virus in asymptomatic HBsAg negative chronic active hepatitis. J Hepatology 14:88, 1992.
280. Greeve M, Ferrell L, Kim M, et al: Cirrhosis of undefined pathogenesis: absence of evidence for unknown viruses or autoimmune processes. Hepatology 17:593, 1993.
281. Czaja AJ, Carpenter HA: Sensitivity, specificity and predictability of biopsy interpretations in chronic hepatitis. Gastroenterology 105:1824, 1993.
282. Goodman ZD, McNally PR, Davis DR, et al: Autoimmune cholangitis: a variant of primary biliary cirrhosis. Clinicopathologic and serologic correlations in 200 cases. Dig Dis Sci 40:1232, 1995.
283. Tsuneyama K, Van de Water J, Van Thiel D, et al: Abnormal expression of PDC-E2 on the apical surface of biliary epithelial cells in patients with antimitochondrial antibody-negative primary biliary cirrhosis. Hepatology 22:1440, 1995.
284. Omagari K, Ikuno N, Matsuo I, et al: Autoimmune cholangitis syndrome with a bias towards primary biliary cirrhosis. Pathology 28:255, 1996.
285. Nakanuma Y, Harada K, Kaji K, et al: Clinicopathological study of primary biliary cirrhosis negative for antimitochondrial antibodies. Liver 17:281, 1997.
286. Kinoshita H, Omagari K, Whittingham S, et al: Autoimmune cholangitis and primary biliary cirrhosis—an autoimmune enigma. Liver 19:122, 1999.
287. Gordon SC, Quattrociocchi-Longe TM, Khan BA, et al: Antibodies to carbonic anhydrase in patients with immune cholangiopathies. Gastroenterology 108:1802, 1995.
288. Akisawa N, Nishimori I, Miyaji E, et al: The ability of anti-carbonic anhydrase II antibody to distinguish autoimmune cholangitis from primary biliary cirrhosis in Japanese patients. J Gastroenterol 34:366, 1999.
289. Invernizzi P, Crosignani A, Battezzati PM, et al: Comparison of the clinical features and clinical course of antimitochondrial antibody-positive and -negative primary biliary cirrhosis. Hepatology 25:1090, 1997.
290. Lacerda MA, Ludwig J, Dickson ER, et al: Antimitochondrial antibody-negative primary biliary cirrhosis. Am J Gastroenterol 90:247, 1995.
291. Michieletti P, Wanless IR, Katz A, et al: Antimitochondrial antibody negative primary biliary cirrhosis: a distinct syndrome of autoimmune cholangitis. Gut 35:260, 1994.
292. Taylor SL, Dean PJ, Riely CA: Primary autoimmune cholangitis: an alternative to antimitochondrial antibody-negative primary biliary cirrhosis. Am J Clin Path 18:91, 1994.
293. Ben-Ari Z, Dhillon AP, Sherlock S: Autoimmune cholangiopathy: part of the spectrum of autoimmune chronic active hepatitis. Hepatology 18:10, 1993.
294. Muratori P, Muratori L, Lenzi M, et al: Antibodies to carbonic anhydrase in autoimmune cholangiopathy. Gastroenterology 112: 1053, 1997.
295. Geall MG, Schoenfield LJ, Summerskill WHJ: Classification and treatment of chronic active liver disease. Gastroenterology 63:458, 1972.
296. Kirk AP, Jain S, Pocock S, et al: Late results of the Royal Free Hospital prospective controlled trial of prednisolone therapy in hepatitis B surface antigen negative chronic active hepatitis. Gut 20:78, 1980.
297. Czaja AJ: Natural history of chronic active hepatitis. In Czaja AJ, Dickson ER, eds: Chronic Active Hepatitis. The Mayo Clinic Experience. New York, Marcel Dekker, Inc., 1986:9-224.
298. Burroughs AK, Bassendine MF, Thomas HC, et al: Primary liver cell cancer in autoimmune chronic liver disease. BMJ 282:273, 1981.
299. Jakobovits AW, Gibson PR, Dudley FJ: Primary liver cell carcinoma complicating autoimmune chronic active hepatitis. Dig Dis Sci 25:694, 1981.
300. Wang KK, Czaja AJ: Hepatocellular cancer in corticosteroid-treated severe autoimmune chronic active hepatitis. Hepatology 8:1679, 1988.
301. Park SZ, Nagorney DM, Czaja AJ: Hepatocellular carcinoma in autoimmune hepatitis. Dig Dis Sci 45:1944, 2000.
302. Ryder S, Koskinas J, Rizzi PM, et al: Hepatocellular carcinoma complicating autoimmune hepatitis: role of hepatitis C virus. Hepatology 22:718, 1995.
303. Thaler H: The natural history of chronic hepatitis. In Schaffner F, Sherlock S, Leevy CM, ed, The Liver and Its Diseases. New York, Stratton International Medical Books, 1974:207-215.
304. DeGroote J, Fevery J, Lepoutre L: Long-term follow-up of chronic active hepatitis of moderate severity. Gut 19:510, 1978.
305. Fevery J, Desmet VJ, DeGroote J: Long-term follow-up and management of asymptomatic chronic active hepatitis. In Cohen S, Soloway RD, eds: Chronic Active Liver Disease. New York, Churchill Livingstone, 1983:51-64.
306. Kemeny MJ, O'Hanlon G, Gregory PB: Asymptomatic chronic active hepatitis—prognosis and treatment (abstract). Gastroenterology 86:1325, 1984.
307. Porta G, Da Costa Gayotto LC, Alvarez F: Anti-liver-kidney microsome antibody-positive autoimmune hepatitis presenting as fulminant liver failure. J Ped Gastroenterol Nutr 11:138, 1990.
308. Galbraith RM, Smith M, Mackenzie RM, et al: High prevalence of seroimmunologic abnormalities in relatives of patients with active chronic hepatitis or primary biliary cirrhosis. N Engl J Med 290:63, 1974.
309. Whittingham S, Mackay IR, Kiss ZS: An interplay of genetic and environmental factors in familial hepatitis and myasthenia gravis. Gut 11:811, 1970.
310. Hilberg RW, Mulhern LM, Kenny JJ, et al: Chronic active hepatitis. Report of two sisters with positive lupus erythematosus preparations. Ann Intern Med 74:937, 1971.
311. Czaja AJ, Ammon HV, Summerskill WHJ: Clinical features and prognosis of severe chronic active liver disease (CALD) after corticosteroid-induced remission. Gastroenterology 78:518, 1980.
312. Czaja AJ, Wolf AM, Baggenstoss AH: Clinical assessment of cirrhosis in severe chronic active liver disease (CALD): specificity and sensitivity of physical and laboratory findings. Mayo Clin Proc 55:360, 1980.
313. Golding PL, Smith M, Williams R: Multisystemic involvement in chronic liver disease: studies on the incidence and pathogenesis. Am J Med 55:772, 1973.
314. Sabesin SM, Levinson MJ: Acute and chronic hepatitis: multisystemic involvement related to immunologic disease. Adv Intern Med 22:421, 1977.
315. Volta U, De Franceshi L, Molinaro N, et al: Frequency and significance of anti-gliadin and anti-endomysial antibodies in autoimmune hepatitis. Dig Dis Sci 43:2190, 1998.
316. Payami H, Khan MA, Grennan DM, et al: Analysis of genetic interrelationship among HLA-associated diseases. Am J Hum Genet 41:331, 1987.
317. Rakela J, Czaja AJ: Clinical, biochemical, and histologic features of HBsAg-negative chronic active hepatitis. In Czaja AJ, Dickson ER, eds: Chronic Active Hepatitis. The Mayo Clinic Experience. New York, Marcel Dekker, Inc., 1986:69-82.
318. Roux MEB, Florin-Christensen A, Arana RM, et al: Paraproteins with antibody activity in acute viral hepatitis and chronic autoimmune liver diseases. Gut 15:396, 1974.
319. Triger DR: Bacterial, viral and autoantibodies in acute and chronic liver disease. Ann Clin Res 8:174, 1976.
320. Laitinen O, Vaheri A: Very high measles and rubella virus antibody titers associated with hepatitis, systemic lupus erythematosus, and infectious mononucleosis. Lancet 1:194, 1974.
321. Lee WM, Lebwohl O, Chien S: Hyperviscosity syndrome attributable to hyperglobulinemia in chronic active hepatitis. Gastroenterology 74:918, 1978.
322. LaRusso NF, Summerskill WHJ, McCall JT: Abnormalities of chemical tests for copper metabolism in chronic active liver disease: differentiation from Wilson's disease. Gastroenterology 70:653, 1976.
323. Czaja AJ: Autoantibodies. Bailliere's Clin Gastroenterol 9:723, 1995.
324. Czaja AJ: Behavior and significance of autoantibodies in type 1 autoimmune hepatitis. J Hepatol 30:394, 1999.
325. Homburger HA, Cahen YD, Griffiths J, et al: Detection of antinuclear antibodies. Comparative evaluation of enzyme immunoassay and indirect immunofluorescence methods. Arch Pathol Lab Med 122:993, 1998.

326. Czaja AJ, Nishioka M, Morshed SA, et al: Patterns of nuclear immunofluorescence and reactivities to recombinant nuclear antigens in autoimmune hepatitis. Gastroenterology 107:200, 1994.
327. Parveen S, Morshed SA, Arima K, et al: Antibodies to Ro/La, Cenp-B, and snRNPs antigens in autoimmune hepatitis of North America versus Asia. Dig Dis Sci 43:1322, 1998.
328. Czaja AJ, Ming C, Shirai M, et al: Frequency and significance of antibodies to histones in autoimmune hepatitis. J Hepatol 23:32, 1995.
329. Chen M, Shirai M, Czaja AJ, et al: Characterization of anti-histone antibodies in patients with type 1 autoimmune hepatitis. J Gastroenterol Hepatol 13:483, 1998.
330. Czaja AJ, Morshed SA, Parveen S, et al: Antibodies to single-stranded and double-stranded DNA in antinuclear antibody positive type 1 autoimmune hepatitis. Hepatology 26:567, 1997.
331. Bottazzo GF, Florin-Christensen A, Fairfax A, et al: Classification of smooth muscle autoantibodies (SMA) detected by immunofluorescence. J Clin Path 29:403, 1976.
332. Lidman K, Biberfield G, Fagraeus A, et al: Anti-actin specificity of human smooth muscle antibodies in chronic active hepatitis. Clin Exp Immunol 24:266, 1976.
333. Dighiero G, Lymberi P, Monot C, et al: Sera with high levels of anti-smooth muscle and anti-mitochondrial antibodies frequently bind to cytoskeletal proteins. Clin Exp Immunol 82:52, 1990.
334. Pedersen JS, Toh BH, Mackay IR, et al: Segregation of autoantibody to cytoskeletal filaments, actin and intermediate filaments with two types of chronic active hepatitis. Clin Exp Immunol 48:527, 1982.
335. Cassani F, Fusconi M, Bianchi FB, et al: Precipitating antibodies to rabbit thymus extractable antigens in chronic liver disease: relationship with anti-actin antibodies. Clin Exp Immunol 68:588, 1987.
336. Reference deleted in proofs.
337. Cancado ELR, Vilas-Boas LS, Abrantes-Lemos CP, et al: Heat serum inactivation as a mandatory procedure for antiactin antibody detection in cell culture. Hepatology 23:1098, 1996.
338. Fusconi M, Cassani F, Zauli D, et al: Anti-actin antibodies: a new test for an old problem. J Immunol Methods 130:1, 1990.
339. Czaja AJ, Cassani F, Cataleta M, et al: Frequency and significance of antibodies to actin in type 1 autoimmune hepatitis. Hepatology 24:1068, 1996.
340. Martini E, Abuaf N, Cavalli F, et al: Antibody to liver cytosol (anti-LC1) in patients with autoimmune chronic active hepatitis type 2. Hepatology 8:1662, 1988.
341. Abuaf N, Johanet C, Chretien P, et al: Characterization of the liver cytosol antigen type 1 reacting with autoantibodies in chronic active hepatitis. Hepatology 16:892, 1992.
342. Han S, Tredger M, Gregorio GV, et al: Anti-liver cytosolic antigen type 1 (LC1) antibodies in childhood autoimmune liver disease. Hepatology 21:58, 1995.
343. Muratori L, Cataleta M, Muratori P, et al: Liver/kidney microsomal antibody type 1 and liver cytosol antibody type 1 concentrations in type 2 autoimmune hepatitis. Gut 42:721, 1998.
344. Lapierre P, Hajoui O, Homberg J-C, et al: Formiminotransferase cyclodeaminase is an organ-specific autoantigen recognized by sera of patients with autoimmune hepatitis. Gastroenterology 116:643, 1999.
345. Pelli N, Fensom AH, Slade C, et al: Argininosuccinate lyase: a new autoantigen in liver disease. Clin Exp Immunol 114:455, 1998.
346. Gelpi C, Sontheimer EJ, Rodriguez-Sanchez JL: Autoantibodies against a serine tRNA-protein complex implicated in cotranslational selenocysteine insertion. Proc Natl Acad Sci U S A 89:9739, 1992.
347. McFarlane IG, Hegarty JE, McSorley CG, et al: Antibodies to liver-specific protein predict outcome of treatment withdrawal in autoimune chronic active hepatitis. Lancet 2:954, 1984.
348. Czaja AJ, Pfeifer KD, Decker RH, et al: Frequency and significance of antibodies to asialoglycoprotein receptor in type 1 autoimmune hepatitis. Dig Dis Sci 41:1733, 1996.
349. Targan SR, Landers C, Vidrich A, et al: High-titer antineutrophil cytoplasmic antibodies in type 1 autoimmune hepatitis. Gastroenterology 108:1159, 1995.
350. Zauli D, Ghetti S, Grassi A, et al: Anti-neutrophil cytoplasmic antibodies in type 1 and type 2 autoimmune hepatitis. Hepatology 25:1105, 1997.
351. LaBrecque DR, Phillips MJP, Ippolito LA, et al: Antineutrophil cytoplasmic antibody and chronic liver disease (abstract). Hepatology 30:428A, 1999.
352. Orth T, Gerken G, Kellner R, et al: Actin is a target of anti-neutrophil cytoplasmic antibodies (ANCA) in autoimmune hepatitis type-1. J Hepatol 26:37, 1997.
353. Terjung B, Herzog V, Worman HJ, et al: Atypical antineutrophil cytoplasmic antibodies with perinuclear fluorescence in chronic inflammatory bowel diseases and hepatobiliary disorders colocalize with nuclear lamina proteins. Hepatology 28:332, 1998.
354. Bansi D, Chapman R, Fleming K: Antineutrophil cytoplasmic antibodies in chronic liver diseases: prevalence, titre, specificity and IgG subclass. J Hepatol 24:581, 1996.
355. Czaja AJ, Donaldson PT: Genetic susceptibilities for immune expression and liver cell injury in autoimmune hepatitis. Immunol Rev 174:250, 2000.
356. Czaja AJ, Strettell MDJ, Thomson LJ, et al: Associations between alleles of the major histocompatibility complex and type 1 autoimmune hepatitis. Hepatology 25:317, 1997.
357. Si L, Whiteside TL, Schade RR, et al: Studies of lymphocyte subpopulations in the liver tissue and blood of patients with chronic active hepatitis (CAH). J Clin Immunol 3:408, 1983.
358. Frazer IH, Mackay IR, Bell J, et al: The cellular infiltrate in the liver in autoimmune chronic active hepatitis: analysis with monoclonal antibodies. Liver 5:162, 1985.
359. Dienes HP, Popper H, Manns M, et al: Histologic features in autoimmune hepatitis. Z Gastroenterol 27:325, 1989.
360. Bach N, Thung SN, Schaffner F: The histological features of chronic hepatitis C and autoimmune chronic hepatitis: a comparative analysis. Hepatology 15:572, 1992.
361. Witebsky E, Rose NR, Terplan K, et al: Chronic thyroiditis and autoimmunization. JAMA 164:1439, 1957.
362. Choudhuri K, Gregorio GV, Mieli-Vergani G, et al: Immunological cross-reactivity to multiple autoantigens in patients with liver kidney microsomal type 1 autoimmune hepatitis. Hepatology 28:1177, 1998.
363. Albert LJ, Inman RD: Molecular mimicry and autoimmunity. N Engl J Med 341:2068, 1999.
364. Czaja AJ, Sievers C, Zein NN: Nature and behavior of serum cytokines in type 1 autoimmune hepatitis. Dig Dis Sci 45:1028, 2000.
365. Cookson S, Constantini PK, Clare M, et al: Frequency and nature of cytokine gene polymorphisms in type 1 autoimmune hepatitis. Hepatology 30:851, 1999.
366. Czaja AJ, Cookson S, Constantini PK, et al: Cytokine polymorphisms associated with clinical features and treatment outcome in type 1 autoimmune hepatitis. Gastroenterology 117:645, 1999.
367. Agarwal K, Czaja AJ, Jones DEJ, et al: CTLA-4 gene polymorphism and susceptibility to type 1 autoimmune hepatitis. Hepatology 31:49, 2000.
368. Agarwal K, Jones DE, Daly AK, et al: CTLA-4 gene polymorphism confers susceptibility to primary biliary cirrhosis. J Hepatol 32:538, 2000.
369. Blomberg G, Geckeler WR, Weigert M: Genetics of the antibody response to dextran in mice. Science 177:178, 1972.
370. Mackay IR, Whittingham S, Tait B: Genetic control of immune responsiveness in man. Vox Sang 32:10, 1977.
371. Chiovato L, Lapi P, Fiore E, et al: Thyroid autoimmunity and female gender. J Endocrinol Invest 16:384, 1993.
372. Whitacre CC, Reingold SC, O'Looney PA: A gender gap in autoimmunity. Science 283:1277, 1999.
373. Rowley MJ, Mackay IR: Measurement of antibody-producing capacity in man. I. The normal response to flagellin from *Salmonella adelaide.* Clin Exp Immunol 5:407, 1969.
374. Nelson JL: Microchimerism: implications for autoimmune disease. Lupus 8:370, 1999.
375. Tanaka A, Lindor K, Ansari A, et al: Fetal microchimerisms in the mother: immunologic implications. Liver Transpl 6:138, 2000.
376. Lambert NC, Evans PC, Hashizumi TL, et al: Cutting edge: persistent fetal microchimerism in T lymphocytes is associated with HLA-DQA1*0501: implications for autoimmunity. J Immunol 164:5545, 2000.
377. Vento S, Nouri-Aria KT, Eddleston ALWF: Immune mechanisms in autoimmune chronic active hepatitis. Scand J Gastroenterol 20(suppl 114):91, 1985.
378. Eddleston ALWF: Immunology of chronic active hepatitis. QJM 55:191, 1985.
379. Nouri-Aria KJ, Hegarty JE, Alexander GJM, et al: Effect of corticosteroids on suppressor-cell activity in "autoimmune" and viral chronic active hepatitis. N Engl J Med 307:1301, 1982.

380. Lobo-Yeo A, Mieli-Vergani G, Kenna G, et al: Evidence of impaired antigen non-specific but normal antigen specific suppressor cell function in children with autoimmune chronic active hepatitis. Clin Exp Immunol 70:411, 1987.
381. O'Brien CJ, Vento S, Donaldson PT, et al: Cell-mediated immunity and suppressor-T-cell defects to liver-derived antigens in families of patients with autoimmune chronic active hepatitis. Lancet 1:350, 1986.
382. Nouri-Aria KT, Donaldson PT, Hegarty JE, et al: HLA A1-B8-DR3 and suppressor cell function in first-degree relatives of patients with autoimmune chronic active hepatitis. J Hepatol 1:235, 1985.
383. Vento S, Hegarty JE, Bottazzo G, et al: Antigen specific suppressor cell function in autoimmune chronic active hepatitis. Lancet 1:1200, 1984.
384. Czaja AJ, Beaver SJ, Shiels MT: Sustained remission following corticosteroid therapy of severe HBsAg-negative chronic active hepatitis. Gastroenterology 92:215, 1987.
385. Czaja AJ: Autoimmune hepatitis: current therapeutic concepts. Clin Immunother 1:413, 1994.
386. Czaja AJ: Drug therapy in the management of type 1 autoimmune hepatitis. Drugs 57:49, 1999.
387. Lennard L, Van Loon JA, Weinshilboum RM: Pharmacokinetics of acute azathioprine toxicity: relationship to thiopurine methyltransferase genetic polymorphism. Clin Pharmacol Ther 46:149, 1989.
388. Ben Ari Z, Mehta A, Lennard L, et al: Azathioprine-induced myelosuppression due to thiopurine methyltransferase deficiency in a patient with autoimmune hepatitis. J Hepatol 23:351, 1995.
389. Czaja AJ: Autoimmune hepatitis. In Maddrey WC, ed: Gastroenterology and Hepatology. The Comprehensive Visual Reference, ed 2. Philadelphia, Current Medicine, 2000:3.1-3.22.
390. Czaja AJ: Treatment of autoimmune hepatitis. In Krawitt EL, Wiesner RH, Nishioka MM, eds: Autoimmune Liver Disease. Amsterdam, Elsevier Science Publishers, 1998:499-515.
391. Summerskill WHJ, Korman MG, Ammon HV, et al: Prednisone for chronic active liver disease: dose titration, standard dose, and combination with azathioprine compared. Gut 16:876, 1975.
392. Penn I: Tumor incidence in allograft recipients. Transplant Proc 11:1047, 1979.
393. Wang KK, Czaja AJ, Beaver SJ, et al: Extrahepatic malignancy following long-term immunosuppressive therapy of severe hepatitis B surface antigen-negative chronic active hepatitis. Hepatology 10:39, 1989.
394. Wang KK, Czaja AJ: Prognosis of corticosteroid-treated hepatitis B surface antigen-negative chronic active hepatitis in postmenopausal women: a retrospective analysis. Gastroenterology 97:1288, 1989.
395. Lebovics E, Schaffner F, Klion EM, et al: Autoimmune chronic active hepatitis in postmenopausal women. Dig Dis Sci 30:824, 1985.
396. Czaja AJ: Low dose corticosteroid therapy after multiple relapses of severe HBsAg-negative chronic active hepatitis. Hepatology 11:1044, 1990.
397. McCullough AJ: Laboratory assessment of liver function and inflammatory activity in chronic active hepatitis. In Czaja AJ, Dickson ER, eds: Chronic Active Hepatitis. The Mayo Clinic Experience. New York, Marcel Dekker, Inc., 1986:205-246.
398. Roberts SK, Therneau T, Czaja AJ: Prognosis of histological cirrhosis in type 1 autoimmune hepatitis. Gastroenterology 110:848, 1996.
399. Davis GL, Czaja AJ, Ludwig J: Development and prognosis of histologic cirrhosis in corticosteroid-treated HBsAg-negative chronic active hepatitis. Gastroenterology 87:1222, 1984.
400. Czaja AJ, Ammon HV, Summerskill WHJ: Clinical features and prognosis of severe chronic active liver disease (CALD) after corticosteroid-induced remission. Gastroenterology 78:518, 1980.
401. Davis GL, Czaja AJ: Immediate and long-term results of corticosteroid therapy for severe idiopathic chronic active hepatitis. In Czaja AJ, Dickson ER, eds: Chronic Active Hepatitis. The Mayo Clinic Experience. New York, Marcel Dekker, Inc., 1986:269-283.
402. Hegarty JE, Nouri-Aria KT, Portmann B, et al: Relapse following treatment withdrawal in patients with autoimmune chronic active hepatitis. Hepatology 3:685, 1983.
403. Stellon AJ, Keating JJ, Johnson PJ, et al: Maintenance of remission in autoimmune chronic active hepatitis with azathioprine after corticosteroid withdrawal. Hepatology 8:781, 1988.
404. Johnson PJ, McFarlane IG, Williams R: Azathioprine for long-term maintenance of remission in autoimmune hepatitis. N Engl J Med 333:958, 1995.
405. Czaja AJ, Wolf AM, Summerskill WHJ: Development and early prognosis of esophageal varices in severe chronic active liver disease (CALD) treated with prednisone. Gastroenterology 77:629, 1979.
406. Schalm SW, Ammon HV, Summerskill WHJ: Failure of customary treatment in chronic active liver disease: causes and management. Ann Clin Res 8:221, 1976.
407. Gonzalez-Koch A, Czaja AJ, Carpenter HA, et al: Recurrent autoimmune hepatitis after orthotopic liver transplantation. Liver Transplantation 4:302-310, 2001.
408. Neuberger J, Portmann B, Calne R, et al: Recurrence of autoimmune chronic active hepatitis following orthotopic liver grafting. Transplantation 37:363, 1984.
409. Wright HL, Bou-Abboud CF, Hassanein T, et al: Disease recurrence and rejection following liver transplantation for autoimmune chronic active liver disease. Transplantation 53:136, 1992.
410. Ratziu V, Samuel D, Sebagh M, et al: Long-term follow-up after liver transplantation for autoimmune hepatitis: evidence of recurrence of primary disease. J Hepatol 30:131, 1999.
411. Czaja AJ, Beaver SJ, Wood JR, et al: Frequency and significance of serum alpha-fetoprotein elevation in severe hepatitis B surface antigen-negative chronic active hepatitis. Gastroenterology 93:687, 1987.
412. Canafax DM, Ascher NL: Cyclosporine immunosuppression. Clin Pharm 2:515, 1983.
413. Mistilis SP, Vickers CR, Darroch MH, et al: Cyclosporin, a new treatment for autoimmune chronic active hepatitis. Med J Aust 143:463, 1985.
414. Hyams JS, Ballow M, Leichtner AM: Cyclosporine treatment of autoimmune chronic active hepatitis. Gastroenterology 93:890, 1987.
415. Alvarez F, Ciocca M, Canero-Velasco C, et al: Short-term cyclosporine induces a remission of autoimmune hepatitis in children. J Hepatol 30:222, 1999.
416. Thomson AW: FK-506: profile of an important new immunosuppressant. Transplant Rev 4:1, 1990.
417. Shaw BW Jr, Markin R, Strata R, et al: FK 506 rescue treatment of acute and chronic rejection in liver allograft recipients. Transplant Proc 23:2994, 1991.
418. Van Thiel DH, Wright H, Carroll P, et al: FK 506 in the treatment of autoimmune chronic active hepatitis: preliminary results (abstract). Am J Gastroenterol 87:1309, 1992.
419. Pratt DS, Flavin DP, Kaplan MM: The successful treatment of autoimmune hepatitis with 6-mercaptopurine after failure with azathioprine. Gastroenterology 110:271, 1996.
420. Allison AC, Eugui EM: Mycophenolate mofetil and its mechanisms of action. Immunopharmacology 47:85, 2000.
421. Czaja AJ, Manns MP, McFarlane IG, et al: Autoimmune hepatitis: the investigational and clinical challenges. Hepatology 31:1194, 2000.
422. Richardson PD, et al: Mycophenolate mofetil for maintenance of remission in autoimmune hepatitis patients resistant to or intolerant of azathioprine. J Hepatol 33:371, 2000.
423. Ward A, Brogden RN, Heel RC, et al: Ursodeoxycholic acid. A review of its pharmacological properties and therapeutic efficacy. Drugs 27:95, 1984.
424. Heuman DM, Mills AS, McCall J, et al: Conjugates of ursodeoxycholate protect against cholestasis and hepatocellular necrosis caused by more hydrophobic bile salts. In vivo studies in the rat. Gastroenterology 100:203, 1991.
425. Nakamura K, Yoneda M, Yokohama S, et al: Efficacy of ursodeoxycholic acid in Japanese patients with type 1 autoimmune hepatitis. J Gastroenterol Hepatol 13:490, 1998.
426. Czaja AJ, Carpenter HA, Lindor KD: Ursodeoxycholic acid as adjunctive therapy for problematic type 1 autoimmune hepatitis: a randomized placebo-controlled treatment trial. Hepatology 30:1381, 1999.
427. Clissold SP, Heel RC: Budesonide: a preliminary review of its pharmacodynamic properties and therapeutic efficacy in asthma and rhinitis. Drugs 28:485, 1984.
428. Danielsson A, Prytz H: Oral budesonide for treatment of autoimmune chronic active hepatitis. Aliment Pharmacol Ther 8:585, 1994.
429. Czaja AJ, Lindor KD: Failure of budesonide in a pilot study of treatment-dependent autoimmune hepatitis. Gastroenterology 119:1312, 2000.

CHAPTER

39

Primary Biliary Cirrhosis

Jayant A. Talwalkar, MD, MPH, and Keith D. Lindor, MD

INTRODUCTION

Primary biliary cirrhosis (PBC) is a chronic cholestatic liver disease of unknown etiology. The disease is characterized histologically by the presence of portal inflammation and necrosis of the interlobular and septal bile ducts. Progressive bile duct destruction is associated with the development of portal and periportal inflammation, subsequent fibrosis, and eventual cirrhosis associated with liver failure and the complications of portal hypertension. It remains one of the major indications for liver transplantation worldwide. The etiology of PBC remains unknown. Evidence suggests that immunologic factors, which include T cell activation directed at bile ducts, are involved. Highly specific autoantibodies reactive with biliary epithelial cell surface antigens and associated autoimmune disorders observed among patients with PBC have also been cited as further evidence for an immunologic cause. Patients affected by PBC are often middle-aged women who are commonly diagnosed after evaluation for asymptomatic elevations in serum hepatic biochemical parameters. Fatigue, pruritus, or unexplained hyperlipidemia may also be found at initial presentation and may suggest a diagnosis of PBC. Serum anti-mitochondrial antibody (AMA) positivity is nearly diagnostic of PBC when present. The identification of PBC is important because effective medical therapy with ursodeoxycholic acid (UDCA) has been demonstrated to halt disease progression and improve survival independent of liver transplantation. Therapeutic options for the medical complications of PBC such as fatigue and metabolic bone disease, however, are not available. Mathematical models have been developed that accurately characterize and predict the natural history of PBC and assist in determining the optimal timing for liver transplantation if indicated.

EPIDEMIOLOGY

PBC affects all races and has no specific geographic predilection. Women are primarily affected, with a female to male ratio of 9:1. The median age of disease onset is 50 years but varies between 20 and 90 years. Previously thought to be a rare condition, recent investigations have observed that PBC is not so uncommon (Table 39-1). Estimates of annual incidence have been reported between 2 and 24 cases per million population in PBC.[1,2] Prevalence estimates range from 19 to 240 cases per million population.[2,3] Recent data from Olmsted County, Minnesota,[4] suggest a stable incidence rate over the last 25 years but a higher prevalence than described in Canada.[5] Overall incidence and prevalence rates of 27 and 402 cases per million population,[4] respectively, are comparable to results from northern England.[2] Differences in study methodology and case definitions have made comparisons between investigations difficult.

The variation in disease prevalence worldwide suggests that environmental factors may also be required for the phenotypic expression of PBC. The selection of appropriate controls in determining the significance of putative risk factors for developing PBC has been recently addressed. From a population-based study of 100 PBC cases and 223 controls,[6] there were no significant associations found with various medical, surgical, and lifestyle factors other than tobacco use (odds ratio [OR] = 2.4, 95 percent confidence interval [CI] =1.4, 4.1), a protective effect from psoriasis (OR = 4.6, 95 percent CI = 1.2, 17.3), and a protective effect from eczema (OR = 0.13, 95 percent CI = 0.02, 1.0) among PBC cases compared to controls. The odds of having other autoimmune diseases (such as rheumatoid arthritis, thyroid disease, and celiac sprue) among first-degree relatives of PBC cases was twice as great when compared to controls, but was not considered statistically significant. A similar epidemiologic investigation[7] examined 241 PBC cases against contemporary control groups

TABLE 39-1
Prevalence of Primary Biliary Cirrhosis by Geographic Region

Region	Prevalence (per million population)
Australia[2]	19
Canada[5]	25
Northern England[3]	240
Olmsted County, USA[4]	402

(261 siblings and 225 friends, respectively). The prevalence rate of having at least one family member with PBC among identified cases was 6 percent. Mothers and sisters of PBC patients were more likely to have the disease than were brothers, daughters, and sons. Co-existing autoimmune diseases among PBC patients included Sjögren's syndrome (17.4 percent), Raynaud's phenomenon (12.5 percent), and autoimmune thyroid disease (11.5 percent), with significantly lower frequencies among siblings and friends. In comparison to siblings, PBC cases were more likely to be female (OR = 4.2, 95 percent CI = 2.2, 8.3), have one or more autoimmune diseases (OR = 2.3, 95 percent CI = 1.2, 4.4), a history of shingles (OR = 2.7, 95 percent CI = 1.1, 6.7), previous tonsillectomy (OR = 2.5, 95 percent CI = 1.5, 4.1), and previous cholecystectomy (OR = 2.3, 95 percent CI = 1.2, 4.6). Similar comparisons among friends revealed strong associations with a history of one or more autoimmune diseases (OR = 4.9, 95 percent CI = 2.4, 10.2), smoking (OR = 2.0, 95 percent CI = 1.1, 3.8), previous abdominal surgery (OR = 2.7, 95 percent CI = 1.4, 5.0), and previous tonsillectomy (OR = 1.9, 95 percent CI = 1.0, 3.4) among PBC cases. For women, a sixfold increase in risk of having one or more autoimmune diseases and twofold risk of smoking and/or urinary tract infections were seen among PBC cases versus siblings and friends, respectively. An increased rate of urinary tract infections among smokers with PBC has raised the possibility of an infectious etiology for PBC due to molecular mimicry.[8,9]

GENETICS

The genetic predisposition to autoimmunity in PBC has been associated with alleles from the major histocompatibility (MHC) loci. No association between class I MHC loci and PBC has been found. A number of class II MHC loci, including DR8, DQA1*0102 and DQ/β1*0402, have been observed among patients with PBC.[10] Class III complement antigens C4 null[11] and c4B2[12] alleles have also been described in association with PBC. The haplotypes DR3, DR8, and DR4 appear more prominent in Caucasian populations in contrast to DR2 and DR8 haplotypes among Japanese subjects.[13] The association between human leukocyte antigen (HLA) DR8 and PBC is most frequently observed but is present in less than 40 percent of reported cases.[14,15] Disease resistance, however, has been associated with the DQA1*0102 haplotype.[16] The use of linkage analysis methodologies to accurately identify susceptibility genes for PBC will ultimately require the prior identification of affected patients and families. The existence of mother-daughter cases of PBC suggests the involvement of non-MHC genes in PBC susceptibility.[17] Recently, a polymorphism involving exon 1 of the CTLA-4 gene has been identified as the first non-MHC susceptibility locus in PBC[18] that is observed among other autoimmune conditions (type 1 diabetes mellitus, autoimmune thyroid disease).

An increased familial risk for PBC is suggested as an indirect link to a genetic component for PBC susceptibility. Initial studies estimated the prevalence rate of PBC among first-degree relatives of index cases at 1.3 percent.[19] Using serum AMA as a screening test among family members of PBC patients, a 2 percent to 4 percent prevalence rate of seropositivity has been observed among asymptomatic individuals.[20,21] Criticisms regarding the generalizability of these results, however, have included the strict use of referred patients and absence of appropriate control groups from similar populations. From a recent population-based investigation among 157 patients with definite or probable PBC,[22] a positive family history was identified in 6.4 percent of instances. All familial cases were identified among women with PBC. An increased rate among first-degree relatives was due to a predominance of mother-daughter relationships. The overall prevalence rate among offspring of PBC patients was 1.2 percent, with a 2.3 percent rate among females. Given a population-based prevalence rate of 0.039 percent for PBC, the relative risk for PBC among siblings was calculated at 10.5. Similar relative risks for other autoimmune conditions among siblings have also been reported (Table 39-2). The relative risks (RR) for PBC among first-degree relatives (RR = 18), offspring (RR = 31), and daughters (RR = 59) of women with PBC have also been calculated. Among women greater than 40 years of age with PBC, the relative risk for PBC among their daughters was 15. Among six identified mother-daughter pairs, an earlier age of presentation (39.2 years for daughters versus 53.6 years for mothers, $P < .05$) was also observed.

TABLE 39-2

Sibling Relative Risks (RR) of Autoimmune Conditions, Including Primary Biliary Cirrhosis[22]

Autoimmune condition	Sibling RR
Rheumatoid arthritis	8
Primary biliary cirrhosis	10.5
Ulcerative colitis	12
Graves disease	15
Insulin-dependent diabetes mellitus	15
Crohn's disease	20
Systemic lupus erythematosus	20

From Jones DEJ, Watt FE, Metcalf JV, et al: Familial primary biliary cirrhosis reassessed: a geographically-based population study. J Hepatol 30:402, 1999.

PATHOGENESIS

Immune-mediated Mechanisms

Evidence to date strongly suggests that PBC is an immune-mediated process. The mechanisms that result in bile duct inflammation and fibrosis, however, remain incompletely understood. Both cellular and humoral abnormalities have been observed among patients affected by PBC. Aberrant expression of class II HLA phenotypes on bile duct epithelia has been reported but is nonspecific because similar findings occur in primary sclerosing cholangitis and, less often, biliary obstruction. Immunohistochemical staining of T lymphocytes located in areas of portal and periportal inflammation reveals a mixture of CD4- and CD8-positive T cells.[23] Damage within bile ducts is also mediated by direct cytotoxic reactions from CD4- and CD8-positive T cells.[24,25] Abnormal suppressor T cell activity has also been observed in asymptomatic first-degree relatives of PBC subjects.[26] B lymphocytes, however, are not commonly observed in areas of biliary injury. Specific lymphocyte subsets in peripheral blood including autoreactive T cells and abnormal concanavalin-A immunosuppression profiles have been identified.[27] Intracellular adhesion molecules (e.g., ICAM-1) are expressed in areas of epithelial cell damage by lymphocytes and may play a role in the pathogenesis of PBC.[28] Recent investigations have examined the role of serum cytokines in PBC, demonstrating the presence of increased levels of tumor necrosis factor alpha (TNF-α), interleukin (IL)-8, and IL-12 in advanced compared to early histologic stages.[29] The correlation between these findings and disease pathogenesis remains unknown.

The major finding associated with humoral immunity resides with recognition of the AMA.[30-32] These autoantibodies have been associated with the E2 subunit of the pyruvate dehydrogenase complex (PDC-E2), the E2 unit of the branched-chain ketoacid dehydrogenase complex, the E2 subunit of two oxaloglutaric dehydrogenase complexes, and E1 subunits of PDC and protein X.[33] AMA is directed against the PDC E2 subunit in greater than 95 percent of PBC patients.[34] The reasons for AMA development against proteins that lie in the inner surface of mitochondrial membranes are unknown. Recent data have demonstrated that these proteins share a common epitope with antigens in the cytoplasm of bile duct cells in PBC.[35,36] Of note, there have been similar findings observed in PBC patients without AMA seropositivity, which leaves the relationship between AMA and bile duct injury unclear.[37] Arguments against direct cytotoxic activity from AMA include (1) the persistence of antibody after liver transplantation without immediate disease recurrence; (2) the absence of correlation between serum antibody titer and hepatic involvement; (3) the absence of AMA in some patients with histologic confirmation of PBC; and (4) the induction of AMA after recombinant PDC-E2 protein administration in animal models without resulting PBC.[38]

The predominant immunoglobulin subtypes of AMA have been identified as immunoglobulin (Ig)G1 and IgG3, yet peripheral blood elevations of IgM appear most commonly in PBC. Errors in activating IgG synthesis[39] or abnormal T-cell suppressor activity[40] have been hypothesized as reasons for this discrepancy. An IgA-type AMA has recently been observed in the urine of female PBC patients.[41] The detection of circulating immune complexes in PBC is variable and not significantly correlated with disease severity.[42] Complement system activation has also been observed with abnormal serum C4 production.[43]

The recent identification of apoptosis in association with chronic liver disease has also been extended to PBC.[44] An increase in cholangiocyte Fas receptor expression[45] with reductions in Bcl-2 in small bile ducts[46] supports the involvement of apoptosis in disease pathogenesis. Evidence of anti-apoptotic effects from tauroursodeoxycholic acid in human hepatocytes includes mitochondrial membrane stabilization[47] and nuclear factor κ-b activation.[48]

Non–immune-mediated Mechanisms

The absence of self-tolerance to host antigens or proteins has suggested that infection may be a potential trigger for the development of PBC.[49] A number of infectious agents including *Escherichia coli*, *Helicobacter* organisms, and retroviruses have been implicated.[50] The concept of "molecular mimicry" by microbial antigens has been proposed as an underlying mechanism for PBC in which cross-reactivity with self-antigens occurs via the immune system.[8,9] The activation of T cell clones involved in PBC using peptides from *E. coli* analogous to sequences within the PDC-E2 subunit has been demonstrated.[51] In addition, serum antibodies to *E. coli* protease have been observed in 30 percent of PBC cases compared to 4 percent of controls.[52] *Helicobacter pylori* deoxyribonucleic acid (DNA) has also been identified more commonly within hepatic tissue from PBC patients when compared to controls.[53] Similar findings among patients with primary sclerosing cholangitis (PSC), ulcerative colitis, and other chronic liver diseases, however, limit the specificity of this observation. Colonization of biliary epithelium with *H. pylori* has not been observed in PBC.[54] The significance of an increased prevalence of gram-positive cocci DNA within the gallbladder bile of PBC subjects compared to controls (75 percent versus 5 percent) remains unknown.[55] Granulomas containing *Propionibacterium acnes* from liver biopsy specimens have not been consistently identified with PBC.[56] Initial descriptions of yeast antigen cross-reactivity to AMA among patients with PBC have not led to further developments.[57] Evidence for an underlying viral infection is supported by electron microscopy of cholangiocytes and the increased frequency of serum antibodies to retroviral antigens in PBC.[50] The triggering of abnormal PDC-E2 expression in cholangiocytes by an enveloped retrovirus has also recently been demonstrated.[58] Further investigations in this area are ongoing.

Fetal microchimerism, defined as the persistence of cells in the maternal circulation after delivery, has also been hypothesized to explain the increased association between female gender and autoimmune disease in general. In one study 42 percent of PBC patients showed evidence for fetal microchimerism within liver tissue without any microchimerism among control tissue.[59] However, the increased prevalence of fetal microchimerism discovered among PBC subjects with calcinosis, Raynaud's phenomenon, esophageal dysmotility, sclerodactyly, and telangiectasias (CREST) syndrome from this investigation is confounded by a similar association with scleroderma alone.[60]

Selenium deficiency[61] and impaired sulfoxidation of endogenous (bile acids) and exogenous (estrogen) compounds[62] are also mechanisms proposed for the development of PBC but have not been conclusively established to date.

CLINICAL FEATURES

Asymptomatic Primary Biliary Cirrhosis

Individuals with asymptomatic disease compose 20 percent to 25 percent of all PBC diagnoses, with prevalence rates as high as 60 percent based on the increased use of screening liver biochemistry profiles.[63] Asymptomatic patients have been reported to be older than symptomatic counterparts at the time of diagnosis.[5] The majority of asymptomatic patients with PBC, however, do appear to develop both symptoms and progression of hepatic disease over time.[2] No specific features that predict the development of symptomatic disease, however, have been identified.[64]

Symptomatic Primary Biliary Cirrhosis

Symptoms attributed to PBC are shown in Table 39-3, with fatigue and pruritus being the most commonly reported. Other symptoms include right upper quadrant abdominal pain, nausea, and anorexia. A greater prevalence of symptomatic PBC among female patients compared to male individuals has been observed without clear explanation.[65] Physical examination findings may include the presence of hyperpigmentation, hepatosplenomegaly, and xanthelasmas (excessive subcutaneous deposition of cholesterol-based material).[66] Though uncommon, the presence of steatorrhea in PBC is usually the result of bile salt malabsorption, pancreatic exocrine insufficiency, or concomitant celiac disease. Osteopenia resulting in bone pain or spontaneous fractures is associated with the metabolic bone disease that is common to PBC. Jaundice is usually a late symptom that heralds the onset of advanced histologic disease, but was seen in 20 percent of cases at the time of presentation in earlier series.[65] Complications from cirrhosis and portal hypertension such as ascites, variceal bleeding, and hepatic encephalopathy occur late in the course of disease.

Diagnosis

Biochemical Features

The most characteristic biochemical abnormality in PBC is an elevated serum alkaline phosphatase (usually 3 to 4 times the upper limit of normal). Subjects with a positive serum AMA and liver histology compatible with PBC may rarely have normal serum alkaline phosphatase levels.[67] No association exists between the degree of elevation of serum alkaline phosphatase and prognosis. Modestly increased values for alanine aminotransferase and aspartate aminotransferase are common. The finding of more significant elevations (greater than 200 U/L) requires the exclusion of superimposed virus- or drug-induced hepatic injury. Serum bilirubin levels often rise during disease progression but are commonly within normal limits at diagnosis. Levels reaching 20 mg/dl are unusual but can be associated with advanced hepatic disease. Elevations in serum bilirubin, hypoalbuminemia, and prolonged prothrombin time are associated with poor clinical outcomes and often justify consideration for liver transplantation. Hypercholesterolemia is observed in up to 85 percent of cases at diagnosis. Serum IgM levels and bile acids (cholic acid, chenodeoxycholic acid) are also elevated in patients with PBC.[68]

TABLE 39-3

Symptoms and Signs at Initial Presentation of Primary Biliary Cirrhosis

Feature	Prevalence (%)
Asymptomatic	25
Fatigue	65
Pruritus	55
Hepatomegaly	25
Hyperpigmentation	25
Splenomegaly	15
Jaundice	10
Xanthelasma	10

Serologic Features

Between 90 percent and 95 percent of patients testing positive for serum AMA in titers greater than or equal to 1:40 will have PBC.[69] The finding of AMA seropositivity is not organ-specific but remains highly sensitive (98 percent) as a diagnostic test. Of note, up to 25 percent of autoimmune hepatitis cases[70] and, less frequently, PSC or drug-induced hepatotoxicity, are AMA seropositive. Serum anti-centromere antibodies among PBC patients with CREST syndrome in the absence of scleroderma have also been noted between 10 percent and 15 percent of the time.[71] Other autoantibodies found in PBC include rheumatoid factor (70 percent) and anti-thyroid (anti-microsomal, anti-thyroglobulin) antibodies (40 percent).[33]

PBC patients may also exhibit elevated serum antinuclear antibody (ANA) or smooth muscle antibody (SMA) titres in 35 percent and 66 percent of cases, respectively.[33] The finding of a positive serum ANA and clinical features suggestive of PBC in the absence of a positive AMA has been termed autoimmune cholangitis or AMA-negative PBC.[72-74] No evidence for cross-reactivity between ANA and the anti-M2 subunit of AMA has been observed.[75]

Radiologic Features

Ultrasonography or cross-sectional imaging with computed tomography (CT) or magnetic resonance imaging (MRI) is useful in excluding biliary tract obstruction in patients suspected of having PBC. Increased hepatic echogenicity or features of portal hypertension (splenomegaly, intra-abdominal varices, reversal of portal vein flow) may also be observed but are generally absent at time of diagnosis. Non-progressive periportal adenopathy detected by all imaging modalities has been described in 15 percent of individuals with PBC.[76] The finding of large or bulky adenopathy warrants the exclusion of malignancy such as lymphoma or metastatic disease.

Histologic Features

Although a positive serum AMA is confirmatory for the diagnosis of PBC, a liver biopsy is needed for determining the stage of histologic disease. Wide variations in histology appear to exist despite the presence of mild elevations in serum bilirubin and alkaline phosphatase. The liver biopsy also provides prognostic information and helps to determine the need for surveillance of cirrhosis-related complications. Histologic classification schemes developed by Ludwig and colleagues[77]and by Scheuer and associates[78] are the most widely employed for staging PBC. Both systems describe the characteristic progression of liver injury in PBC that includes both focal and segmental destruction of intralobular bile ducts resulting in cholestasis and eventual biliary cirrhosis (Figure 39-1).

Stage I PBC is associated with portal tract inflammation by predominantly lymphoplasmacytic infiltrates resulting in the destruction of septal and interlobular bile ducts up to 100 μm in diameter. Focal duct obliteration with granuloma formation has been termed the "florid duct lesion" and is considered almost pathognomonic for PBC when present (Plate 39-1). Hepatic lobular involvement is uncommon at this stage of disease although rare microgranulomas are seen in some cases. Most subjects with stage I PBC are clinically asymptomatic.

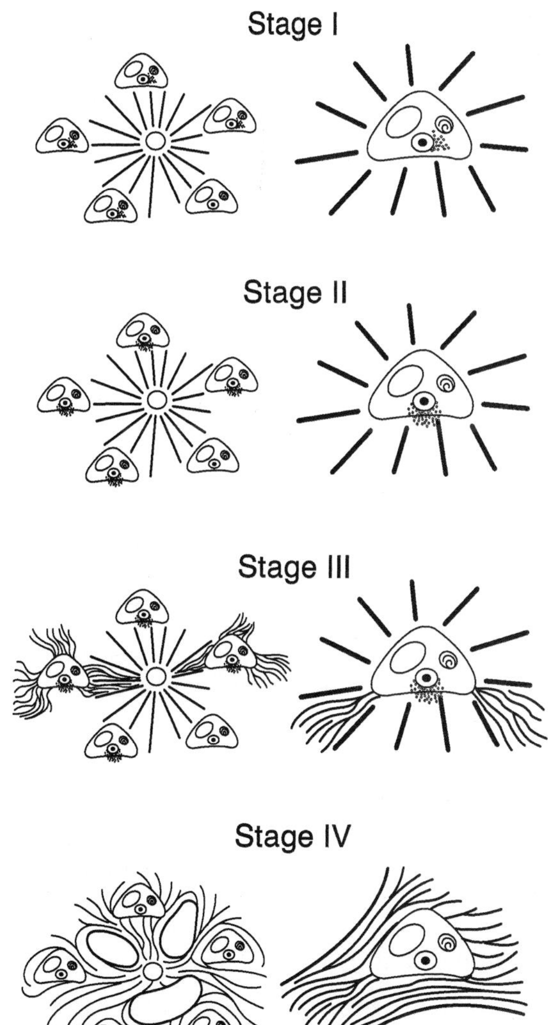

Figure 39-1 Schematic representation of the staging system of primary biliary cirrhosis (Ludwig's classification). Stage I is inflammation within the portal space, focused on the bile duct. Stage II is this inflammation extending into the hepatic parenchyma (interface hepatitis or piecemeal necrosis). Stage III is fibrosis; stage IV is cirrhosis with regenerative nodules. (From Lindor K: Primary biliary cirrhosis. In Feldman M, Scharschmidt BM, Sleisenger MH, eds: Sleisenger & Fordtran's GI and liver disease, ed 6, Philadelphia, WB Saunders, 1998:1277.)

Stage II PBC is consistent with the descriptions of periportal hepatitis by Ludwig and colleagues[77] or ductular proliferation by Scheuer and colleagues.[78] An extension of the portal infiltrates observed in stage I disease to periportal areas is most commonly observed with interface hepatitis (piecemeal necrosis). Eosinophils may also be present within the inflammatory reaction. The histologic findings of cholangitis, granulomas, and ductular proliferation are most commonly observed in stage II disease. Lobular involvement is similar to stage I disease. Individuals with stage II disease may be clinically asymptomatic but at a lower frequency when compared with stage I involvement.

Stage III PBC is dominated by the existence of septal or bridging fibrosis. The inflammatory features described with stage II disease are often seen in association with fibrosis spanning between portal tracts. Ductopenia (defined as the loss of more than 50 percent of interlobular bile ducts) becomes more common, resulting in cholestasis within periportal and paraseptal hepatocytes. Increased hepatic copper deposition that begins in stage II becomes more apparent. The majority of patients with stage III disease are symptomatic.

Stage IV disease in both classification systems is consistent with biliary cirrhosis. Nodular regeneration in association with features of stage III disease is observed with a "garland"-shaped appearance that is characteristic of advanced PBC. Portal tract involvement with cholangitis can also be seen in the remaining bile ducts. Cholestatic abnormalities involving the lobular parenchyma seen in stage III remain. Most subjects considered for liver transplantation have stage IV disease.

When histologic disease in PBC is staged, the most advanced finding must be used to determine the extent of involvement. The presence of both non-advanced and advanced histologic features in patients undergoing liver transplantation for PBC provides further evidence of the great sampling variability that is observed from liver biopsy.[79]

Differential Diagnosis

The patient who is diagnosed with PBC is typically a woman in the fifth or sixth decade of life with complaints of fatigue or pruritus. An increasing number of asymptomatic patients are diagnosed with PBC because of abnormal serum liver biochemistries. A number of other conditions, however, need to be excluded (Table 39-4).

Extrahepatic mechanical biliary obstruction is the primary alternative diagnosis that must be excluded. Potential etiologies include choledocholithiasis, strictures, and neoplasms. Ultrasonography and cross-sectional imaging (CT, MRI) have sufficient accuracy in detecting biliary obstruction such that invasive cholangiography is not required. The technique of magnetic resonance

TABLE 39-4

Differential Diagnosis of Primary Biliary Cirrhosis

Extrahepatic biliary tract obstruction
Choledocholithiasis
Strictures
Malignancy
Primary sclerosing cholangitis
Drug-induced cholestasis (e.g., estrogens, phenothiazines)
Granulomatous hepatitis
Autoimmune hepatitis
Chronic hepatitis C
Alcoholic hepatitis
Sarcoidosis
Celiac disease

TABLE 39-5

Systemic Conditions Associated with Primary Biliary Cirrhosis

Feature	Prevalence (%)
Keratoconjunctivitis sicca	75
Renal tubular acidosis	50
Gallstones	30
Arthritis	20
Thyroid disease	15
Scleroderma	15
Raynaud's phenomenon	10
CREST syndrome	5

CREST, Calcinosis, Raynaud's phenomenon, esophageal dysmotility, sclerodactyly, and telangiectasias.

cholangiopancreatography is 90 percent accurate for assessing bile duct patency.[80,81] Histologic findings of mechanical biliary obstruction including edema, ductular proliferation, and neutrophilic inflammation rather than lymphoplasmacytosis can help in identifying the patient with biliary obstruction.

In PSC the finding of a positive serum AMA is rare. The presence of inflammatory bowel disease (IBD) is also highly suggestive of PSC, although rare instances of IBD with PBC have been reported.[82,83] Histologic assessment is usually not specific enough to distinguish PSC from PBC. The finding of periductal fibrosis in PSC or granulomatous bile duct destruction in PBC, although pathognomic for both conditions when present, is found in only 10 percent of cases, respectively.[84] Cholangiography is required to confirm the existence of PSC and is considered the diagnostic gold standard. Small duct PSC is a variant of PSC and is found in 5 percent of affected patients with IBD and evidence of chronic cholestasis[85] (see Chap. 40).

Similar clinical and biochemical findings associated with PBC can be observed from drug-induced hepatotoxicity. Serum hepatic biochemical profiles are usually consistent with a cholestatic hepatitis. An idiosyncratic mechanism of action is the most common etiology for liver injury. Offending medications include estrogens, androgenic steroids, phenothiazines, amoxicillin-clavulanate, itraconazole, trimethoprim-sulfamethoxazole, and phenytoin.

In autoimmune hepatitis the presence of significant inflammatory changes that involve adjacent bile ducts has been reported in up to 20 percent of cases, which can mimic cholestatic liver disease.[86] Serum AMA detection, however, occurs in only 25 percent of cases of autoimmune hepatitis compared with 95 percent in PBC.[70] Approximately 5 percent to 10 percent of PBC patients will have features of true overlap with autoimmune hepatitis that is indistinguishable by accepted clinical parameters.[87,88] A significant treatment response to corticosteroids in this subset of individuals may be necessary but not sufficient for the diagnostic confirmation of overlap syndrome (see Chap. 38).

Hepatic sarcoidosis is associated with a similar cholestatic biochemical profile as is observed in PBC.[89] Occasionally, portal hypertension resulting from presinusoidal fibrosis has also been observed in patients with sarcoidosis. Histologic findings in hepatic sarcoidosis are characterized by extensive involvement with inflammatory granulomas in portal and periportal distributions. Chest radiograph abnormalities that suggest pulmonary involvement with sarcoidosis are found in 90 percent of cases.

In rare instances, the identification of granulomatous bile duct inflammation among patients with chronic hepatitis C is observed. This may occur in the absence of fibrosing cholestatic disease, which typically occurs after liver transplantation.[90] Serum AMA is usually negative.

Idiopathic adulthood ductopenia (IAD) is a cholestatic disease affecting men with normal cholangiograms and no evidence for IBD. Serum autoantibodies (ANA, SMA, or AMA) are rarely positive. In contrast to small duct PSC, IAD is associated with a more rapid course of disease progression.[91]

Autoimmune cholangitis (or AMA-negative PBC) is observed among patients with cholestatic biochemical profiles and liver histology compatible with PBC in the absence of detectable serum AMA.[72-74] Serum autoantibodies, including ANA, SMA, and anti-carbonic anhydrase,[92] are usually present. There appears to be no difference in natural history or responsiveness to UDCA therapy in autoimmune cholangitis when compared to AMA-positive patients with PBC.[93,94]

Associated Conditions

As many as 70 percent of individuals with PBC have coexistent extrahepatic autoimmune disease states (Table 39-5).[95] Keratoconjunctivitis sicca resulting in dry eyes and xerostomia (Sjögren's syndrome) is the most prevalent autoimmune disease and occurs in about 75 percent of cases.[96,97] Arthritis, including inflammatory joint disorders, has been observed in 10 percent to 40 percent of instances.[98,99] Scleroderma or any component of the CREST syndrome may be found in up to 10 percent of patients.[100]

Thyroid disease, which affects 15 percent to 20 percent of individuals, consists primarily of lymphocytic

(Hashimoto's) thyroiditis. The presence of detectable antithyroid antibodies (anti-microsomal, anti-thyrotropin) may not be associated with clinical disease.[101] Graves' disease and hyperthyroidism are uncommon.[102]

Proximal or distal renal tubular acidosis has been described in up to 50 percent of patients, yet is often without clinical significance. No specific cause has been identified but hypotheses include copper deposition as seen in Wilson's disease[103] and autoimmune-mediated injury.[104]

Cholelithiasis in up to 30 percent of PBC patients is also a common finding.[105] Idiopathic pulmonary fibrosis[106] and IBD[82,83] are observed in less than 5 percent of individuals, respectively.

TABLE 39-6
Complications from Primary Biliary Cirrhosis

Feature	Relative frequency (%)
Fatigue	75
Pruritus	50
Osteopenia	40
Osteoporosis	20
Hypercholesterolemia	85
Fat-soluble vitamin deficiency	20
Steatorrhea	10
Hepatocellular carcinoma	Fortyfold risk

DISEASE COMPLICATIONS

Several systemic complications associated with PBC have been documented, which represent disease progression and impaired health-related quality of life in some individuals (Table 39-6).

Fatigue

The prevalence of fatigue in PBC has been reported in between 65 percent and 85 percent of patients. Fatigue severity appears to be independent of hepatic disease extent, may spontaneously remit and reappear, and is not significantly improved with UDCA therapy.[107,108] There is no strong correlation between fatigue severity and hepatic disease as judged by the Mayo risk score.[109] Alterations in central neurotransmission[110] and impaired corticotrophin-releasing hormone response[111] have been hypothesized as mechanisms of fatigue in PBC. The use of validated measurement scales has allowed for the quantification of fatigue severity, which appears to correlate highly with verbally reported fatigue. PBC patients may also have problems with sleep disturbance[107] and depressed mood,[107,108] yet these conditions do not significantly contribute to fatigue in most patients. When fatigue is present, individuals are also likely to report mild symptoms of depressed mood when compared to PBC patients unaffected by fatigue.[107]

Pruritus

Pruritus is reported in 25 percent to 70 percent of patients affected by PBC.[112] The underlying pathogenesis remains unknown. Recent hypotheses include the accumulation of serum bile acids[113] and an increased release of endogenous opioids.[114] The severity of pruritus in PBC is independent of histologic stage and may be persistent or recurring. Most patients report more severe symptoms at night than in daylight hours. In most cases, pruritus gradually resolves with progression of hepatic disease.[115]

Symptoms can be adequately controlled in the majority of patients if appropriate therapeutic measures are applied. Initial attempts with antihistamines are often complicated by residual sedation and a 50 percent durable success rate.[115] Cholestyramine (a bile acid-binding resin) may decrease the intensity of pruritus but rarely leads to complete symptom resolution.[116] Among subjects with intact gallbladders, the use of 4 g of cholestyramine before or after breakfast is thought to maximize bile acid sequestration, resulting in symptom improvement. The use of divided doses over a 24-hour period postcholecystectomy is more effective than once or twice daily dosing. Administration of cholestyramine several hours apart from other medications (including UDCA) is recommended to prevent reductions in gastrointestinal absorption.

Hepatic enzyme inducers including phenobarbital and rifampin have been associated with improvements in bile acid flow experimentally and are used for the treatment of pruritus. Excessive sedation at higher doses has limited the clinical utility of phenobarbital.[117] Rifampin, in doses of 150 to 450 mg daily, is associated with a rapid onset of action and symptom relief.[118,119] Although well tolerated, this medication is also associated with liver injury in 15 percent of cases and bone marrow aplasia on rare occasions.[120] The drugs flumenicol[121] and stanazolol[122] have been reported to be of some benefit in limited numbers of PBC patients.

Parenteral naloxone[123,124] and oral nalmefene[125,126] have also been associated with the symptomatic improvement of pruritus in pilot and controlled trial settings. Intravenous propofol has also improved pruritus in selected patients.[127] Initial reports of symptom improvement with use of the $5HT_3$ antagonist ondansetron[128,129] await further confirmation. *S*-adenosylmethionine, an anti-oxidant compound involved with glutathione synthesis, has been suggested to impart anti-pruritic effects,[130] yet clinical testing in PBC has not occurred. Among patients with pruritus refractory to medical therapy, liver transplantation can be the most effective therapeutic option.

Hypercholesterolemia

Hypercholesterolemia is present in up to 85 percent of patients with PBC[131] and may be the initial serum biochemical abnormality in the asymptomatic patient. In early-stage disease lipoprotein abnormalities are commonly found,[132] including reduced lipoprotein (a) levels.[133] Initially, there is a marked elevation in high-density lipoprotein rather than low-density lipoprotein but this ratio is reversed with histologic disease progression. A reduction in serum cholesterol levels (specifically low-density lipoprotein) and improvement in xanthelasma formation have been associated with UDCA therapy.[134] There is no clear correlation between xanthelasma formation and serum cholesterol levels in PBC. When they do co-exist, it is among patients with advanced hepatic disease.[135] Nevertheless, there is often great concern expressed by patients about restricting fat intake, yet this is usually ineffective because the hypercholesterolemia is endogenous. Cosmetic surgery to remove unsightly xanthomata is not advised because they rapidly recur. There has been only one published investigation evaluating the risk of death from complications of hypercholesterolemia in 312 patients with PBC. Despite markedly altered serum lipid values, there was no evidence for an increased prevalence of atherosclerotic disease,[131] a finding only recently confirmed in abstract form.[136]

Metabolic Bone Disease

Metabolic bone disease in PBC is related to osteopenia rather than osteomalacia (defective bone mineralization) among North American patients. Although a number of chronic liver disease states have recently been associated with osteopenia, the greater involvement in PBC is likely due to cholestasis and its predilection for females who are independently at risk for metabolic bone disease.[33] Decreased bone formation rather than increased bone resorption is felt to be the most important cause of osteoporosis. In premenopausal women with PBC the defective formation of new bone (osteoblast activity) is also predominant.[137] Increased osteoclastic activity (bone resorption) can be present in premenopausal PBC patients and is accentuated by the postmenopausal state.[138] Calcium and vitamin D metabolism is often normal among anicteric patients with PBC.[139] The recent discovery of vitamin D polymorphisms and their potential association for an increased risk of osteoporosis in PBC has been described.[140] Cigarette smoking is also associated with reduced serum vitamin D levels and may explain the increased risk for osteopenia in these individuals.[141]

Approximately one third of patients with PBC have osteopenia and 11 percent have osteoporosis (i.e., a z score less than −2.5 by lumbar spine bone mineral densitometry).[142] Hence many patients are at an increased risk for osseous fractures. Hip fractures increase the morbidity and mortality of affected individuals, whereas vertebral body fractures are a cause of considerable pain and suffering. The asymptomatic nature of osteoporosis often means that this complication may not be identified at an optimal time. Failing to perform routine assessments of bone mineral density (BMD) in women with PBC is one reason. Among patients undergoing liver transplantation, a 20 percent worsening in BMD may occur up to 6 months after surgery, which can significantly increase the risk for osseous fractures (particularly involving vertebral bodies).[143] A gradual increase in BMD that approaches normal levels usually occurs over the next several years after transplant, especially in the context of reduced corticosteroid use for immunosuppression.

Ensuring adequate intake of calcium (1000 to 1200 mg daily) with weight-bearing activity is recommended as initial treatment for all patients. Measurement of serum vitamin D levels is also an essential part of the preventive management in PBC. The presence of vitamin D deficiency is variable among patients with metabolic bone disease but occurs because of fat-soluble vitamin malabsorption. Oral replacement therapy is indicated if measured serum levels are reduced compared to local normal values. The 25-hydroxylation of vitamin D is intact among PBC patients; therefore, vitamin D rather than 1,25-dihydroxyvitamin D or 25-hydroxyvitamin D can be used for replacement. Dosing is generally between 25,000 and 50,000 IU two to three times per week. The use of calcitonin, a drug that inhibits bone resorption, is not of proven benefit in PBC-related osteoporosis.[144,145]

Hormone replacement therapy (HRT) has been used for the prevention of osteoporosis in patients with PBC. Despite the cholestatic potential of higher dose estrogens, HRT was found to be safe and appeared effective in a small retrospective study of postmenopausal women with PBC.[146] The potential risk of worsening jaundice and liver failure was not observed. Repeat biochemical evaluation at 2-week intervals for 6 to 8 weeks is advised if treatment is to be initiated.

Sodium fluoride has been associated with improved lumbar spine BMD and increased bone formation in osteoporosis. Among subjects with PBC, the use of sodium fluoride in a placebo-controlled trial setting was not found to conclusively restore BMD or impede the progression of osteoporosis.[147] Use of higher doses is limited by gastrointestinal side effects, limiting its clinical usefulness.

The use of oral bisphosphonates (including alendronate and etidronate) has been successfully tolerated in patients with osteoporosis. Among PBC patients, the existence of slight improvements in lumbar spine BMD with etidronate have been reported[148] but not confirmed in a randomized trial.[149] Studies with oral alendronate in PBC are ongoing.

Steatorrhea

Steatorrhea is a common finding among patients with advanced hepatic disease from PBC. This finding has been attributed to a number of potential causes.[150] Impairment of bile acid delivery and insufficient critical micellar concentrations in the small intestine are the most common etiologies. The co-existence of untreated celiac disease has been reported as a cause of steatorrhea among PBC patients. Exocrine pancreatic insufficiency as a manifestation of overall glandular dysfunction may be seen in select individuals, causing diarrhea and fat malabsorption. Bacterial overgrowth syndrome is a potential cause of steatorrhea in PBC when associated with the presence of scleroderma and its variant forms.

Determining the exact cause of steatorrhea is important because a variety of specific therapeutic options can be employed for symptom relief. In patients with decreased bile acid concentrations, the oral replacement of medium-chain triglycerides for long-chain compounds coupled with an overall reduced fat intake is usually of benefit. Adherence to a gluten-free diet in celiac disease should improve symptoms as well. Pancreatic enzyme replacement therapy and rotating empiric antibiotics are also of benefit with pancreatic insufficiency and bacterial overgrowth, respectively.

Fat-soluble Vitamin Deficiency

Malabsorption of fat-soluble vitamins is common among PBC patients.[151] The cause is related to intrahepatic cholestasis and impaired bile acid delivery to the small intestine. Vitamin A deficiency, observed in 20 percent of cases, is often clinically asymptomatic. When symptomatic, the presence of night blindness is observed but can be subtle. Oral replacement therapy should be initiated with 25,000 IU to 50,000 IU two to three times a week. As discussed previously, vitamin D deficiency can also occur and is the next most common fat-soluble vitamin deficiency.

Vitamin E deficiency is rarely observed among individuals with PBC. When present, it may be associated with ataxia from abnormalities of the posterior vertebral columns of the spinal cord. The alleviation of neurologic symptoms with parenteral vitamin E replacement is not universal, however. Oral replacement therapy is indicated for asymptomatic patients.[152,153]

Prolongation of the serum prothrombin time is most commonly associated with vitamin K deficiency. Significant hepatic dysfunction resulting in coagulopathy is observed in end-stage PBC as well. The use of water-soluble oral vitamin K tablets (5 mg) with repeat measurement of serum prothrombin time is effective in determining the extent of malabsorption. If correction of prothrombin time is achieved, daily oral doses of between 5 mg and 10 mg should be initiated.

Cancer

An increased risk for hepatocellular carcinoma (HCC) in PBC remains controversial but is increasingly recognized in the late stages of disease.[154-156] The clinical effectiveness of HCC surveillance employing abdominal ultrasound with serum alpha-fetoprotein levels every 6 to 12 months among end-stage PBC patients, however, remains unknown. An increased risk of extrahepatic malignancy such as breast cancer is also controversial.[154,157,158]

DISEASE-MODIFYING THERAPIES

Limitations in knowledge about the pathogenesis underlying PBC have been associated with few therapies that reverse or prevent disease progression. Of all medical therapies attempted to date, only UDCA has been shown to be effective in patients with PBC, resulting in U.S. Food and Drug Administration approval for this indication in 1998.

Immunosuppressive Agents

Corticosteroids

Improvements in symptomatology, serum hepatic biochemistries, and histology occurred with the use of corticosteroids in 36 patients in a 1-year placebo-controlled trial.[159] No difference in mortality after 2 additional years, however, was observed.[160] A primary limitation of long-term use is worsening osteopenia leading to osteoporosis. The successful use of bisphosphonate agents in PBC may renew interest in systemic corticosteroid therapy. Larger randomized controlled trials will be required to determine treatment safety and efficacy.

Azathioprine

The successful use of azathioprine in autoimmune hepatitis has not been met with similar results in PBC. No improvements in symptoms, serum hepatic biochemistries, histology, or survival have been reported in two studies.[161,162] A suggestion of improved survival after statistical recalculation from one trial,[162] however, has not been met with widespread clinical use of this therapy.

Cyclosporine

Pilot investigations of cyclosporine in PBC showed improvements in symptoms and biochemical features. A randomized trial including 19 subjects receiving cyclosporine (4 mg/kg/day) and 10 subjects receiving placebo noted improved symptoms and hepatic biochemistries after 1 year in the treated patients.[163] Further examination in a large, randomized controlled trial of 346 patients with a median follow-up of 2.5 years,[164] however, failed to reveal any histologic benefit despite biochemical improvement. Significant renal toxicity and hypertension were noted in all studies.

Methotrexate

The initial use of oral methotrexate at 15 mg/week in two PBC patients was associated with symptomatic and biochemical improvement.[165] Subsequent experience among nine patients in an open-label investigation revealed histologic improvement in five subjects and stability in four others after 17 months of therapy.[166] One placebo-controlled trial has been reported involving a lower dose (7.5 mg/week), which resulted in biochemical improvement (not including total bilirubin) without an increase in survival. Of note, a significant number of patients with stage I or II histologic disease were enrolled in this study.[167] Interstitial pneumonitis has been observed in association with methotrexate in 15 percent of PBC patients (compared with 3 percent to 5 percent among patients with rheumatologic disease), raising safety concerns for long-term clinical use.[168] The risk of hepatic fibrosis commonly associated with cumulative doses of methotrexate in psoriatic arthritis has not been reported among PBC patients.

Anti-fibrotic Agents

D-penicillamine

Based on abnormalities in copper excretion and the presence of significant concentrations in hepatic tissue, a number of clinical trials using D-penicillamine for PBC have been performed.[169-175] No substantial benefits among 748 patients given the drug have been observed. In the largest study reported (312 subjects),[175] as many as 20 percent of patients developed serious drug-related side effects, including membranous glomerulonephritis.

Colchicine

A number of investigations have used colchicine in the treatment of PBC.[176-178] Improvements in hepatic biochemical parameters were noted at doses of 1.2 mg/day. An increase in liver-related survival was also observed at 4 years of follow-up in one study but only after all placebo-treated patients were crossed over to colchicine.[176] Improved hepatic biochemical parameters from two other trials have also been reported.[177,178] To date, no long-term benefits have been demonstrated with the use of colchicine in spite of minimal toxicity.

Ursodeoxycholic Acid

Complete Responders

Medical therapy with UDCA has been of most benefit and shown greatest safety in PBC patients. Five randomized controlled trials of adequate size and duration have provided extensive information regarding the effectiveness of UDCA in PBC.[179-183] Three studies employed doses of 13 to 15 mg/kg/day,[179-181] one study employed doses of 14 to 16 mg/kg/day,[182] and the remaining investigation used 10 to 12 mg/kg/day.[183] Improvements in hepatic biochemical parameters were demonstrated in all five studies. One investigation was able to demonstrate improvements in liver-related survival.[184] A combined analysis of three studies using UDCA at doses of 13 to 15 mg/kg/day revealed improvements in survival free of liver transplantation among patients receiving active drug.[185] Long-term (10-year) survival with UDCA has also been observed to exceed Mayo Clinic PBC model predictions in selected populations.[186] UDCA has also been shown to reduce the risk of developing esophageal varices and cirrhosis[187] and to be a cost-effective therapy.[188]

The mechanism of action for UDCA therapy in PBC is multi-factorial. In addition to promoting endogenous bile acid secretion, there is evidence to suggest that UDCA is associated with membrane stabilization,[189] reduced aberrant HLA type I expression on hepatocytes,[190] and decreased cytokine production.[191] UDCA also inhibits apoptosis and mitochondrial dysfunction caused by exposure to hydrophobic bile acids.[192] The possibility of increased benefit from dose escalation with UDCA was not confirmed by a recent three-dose clinical trial. Doses of UDCA ranging from 13 to 20 mg/kg/day, however, were associated with optimal bile enrichment.[193] The primary limitations associated with UDCA are its cost and need for long-term therapy.

The positive effects of UDCA on disease progression and survival free of liver transplantation have been questioned in a recent meta-analysis.[194] By combining eight placebo-controlled trials involving 1114 patients, no difference in overall death, liver-related death, or the need for liver transplantation between UDCA and placebo-treated patients was reported. The majority of identified studies, however, had follow-up periods of 2 years or less, limiting the ability of UDCA to demonstrate any effect over this time duration. A number of trials also used doses of UDCA at less than 13 mg/kg/day. With the exclusion of these investigations, the use of UDCA in PBC is associated with a 32 percent risk reduction in death or need for liver transplantation, which is consistent with results obtained from initial controlled studies (OR = 0.68, 95 percent CI 0.48-0.95).[195]

Incomplete Responders

An estimated 66 percent of patients with PBC have been described as incomplete responders to long-term UDCA monotherapy after an average treatment duration of 3 to 5 years at doses between 10 and 15 mg/kg/day.[196] Incomplete response is defined as the failure to normalize serum hepatic biochemistries or the development of cirrhosis on UDCA. Predictors of incomplete response include higher levels of serum alkaline phosphatase and gamma-glutamyltransferase at drug initiation when compared to complete responders. Incomplete response has been associated with histologic disease progression by one to three stages in 11 percent of patients in contrast to 4 percent of complete responders. The presence of histologic cirrhosis before UDCA therapy also reduces the chance for a successful response.

Among patients experiencing a suboptimal response to UDCA, a number of potential extrahepatic causes must be excluded. In addition to medication non-compliance or inappropriate dosing, the concomitant use of cholestyramine for pruritus may result in a lack of UDCA absorption resulting from binding to the resin. The diagnoses of autoimmune hypothyroidism and celiac disease must be eliminated as causes of elevated serum hepatic biochemistries. Finally, a lack of complete response to UDCA may suggest the presence of true overlap syndrome with autoimmune hepatitis. Subtle evidence of overlap includes unexplained increased elevations in serum aminotransferases and significant interface hepatitis on liver histology.[197]

Combination Therapies

UDCA and Corticosteroids

Reports from two randomized controlled trials showed reductions in serum hepatic biochemistry values and mixed results for histologic improvement.[198-201] Follow-up in both trials was short, ranging from 9 to 12 months. One study included the use of azathioprine at 50 mg/day.[199] The use of oral budesonide in combination with UDCA has been variably associated with biochemical improvement.[200,201] Conflicts between reported short-term histologic improvement[200] and significant worsening of osteopenia[201] with budesonide, however, may diminish interest in a long-term study of this medication.

UDCA and Colchicine

No significant benefit from combination therapy with UDCA and colchicine has been demonstrated.[202-204] Short durations of treatment (less than 2 years) and low doses of colchicine (approximately 1 mg/day) have been proposed as limitations. A recent investigation, however, reported reductions in the number of treatment failures, slower progression of Mayo risk score, and improvement in hepatic histology from UDCA with colchicine compared to patients receiving UDCA monotherapy.[205] Confirmation of these results is awaited.

UDCA and Methotrexate

A number of pilot investigations have examined UDCA with methotrexate in the treatment of PBC.[206-210] Despite improvements in biochemical parameters from an open-label investigation,[210] no overall benefit has been reported from other studies. Results of a long-term, multi-center North American trial involving UDCA and methotrexate are awaited.

Novel Agents

Malotilate

Malotilate is a compound associated with improved hepatic protein metabolism. In a randomized, multi-center trial of 101 PBC patients given malotilate (n = 52) or placebo (n = 49), improvements in serum hepatic biochemical parameters occurred in the active treatment arm compared to placebo.[211] No impact on disease progression or survival at the end of 2 years was noted, however.

Chlorambucil

In a randomized trial among 24 PBC patients using doses between 0.5 and 4 mg/day,[212] there was no significant improvement in biochemical or histologic parameters after 2 to 6 years of follow-up. Significant bone marrow suppression in four subjects required chlorambucil discontinuation.

Thalidomide

Thalidomide is a derivative of glutamic acid that selectively inhibits TNF-α production by monocytes. Among PBC patients given thalidomide (n = 10) or placebo (n = 8) in a small pilot trial,[213] no improvements in biochemical or histologic parameters were observed. Side effects including sedation and fatigue caused two patients to discontinue active treatment.

Silymarin

Silymarin is a drug that has been associated with hepatoprotective effects in experimental and clinical studies, especially among patients with chronic hepatitis C and alcoholic liver disease. Among patients with an incomplete response to UDCA monotherapy, the use of silymarin with UDCA was not associated with significant benefits in an open-label pilot investigation.[214]

Bezafibrate

Bezafibrate is a hypolipidemic medication that stimulates the canalicular phospholipid pump MDR3 via binding and activation of transcription factor peroxisome-proliferator–activated receptor-alpha. Activation of MDR3 results in an increased biliary secretion of phospholipids that are cytoprotective against bile salts. Bezafibrate used alone[215] or in combination with UDCA[216] in patients with PBC has been reported in association with improvements in serum hepatic biochemical parameters. Long-term studies, however, are required to confirm these early positive results.

NATURAL HISTORY AND PROGNOSIS

Histologic Progression

The natural history of histologic progression in PBC has been previously described. Among 916 liver biopsies performed on 222 PBC patients over 779 patient-years of follow-up,[217] a majority of individuals were estimated to undergo disease progression by one stage at 1- and 2-year intervals using a Markov simulation model (Table 39-7). The frequency of histologic progression was not associated with stage at initial liver biopsy. Treatment with UDCA has been observed to slow histologic disease progression and delay the onset of cirrhosis as well.[218,219]

Asymptomatic Primary Biliary Cirrhosis

The natural history of patients without symptoms of PBC has not been extensively reported. Twenty-nine subjects with AMA titers of more than or equal to 1:40, normal serum hepatic biochemistries, and no complaints were followed a median of 17.8 years (range, 11 to 24 years).[67] Initial liver histology at study entry was diagnostic or compatible with PBC in 24 patients (83 percent) and normal in 2 subjects. The development of abnormal serum hepatic biochemistries in 24 patients (83 percent) was observed during follow-up. Twenty-two patients (76 percent) developed symptoms associated with PBC, including fatigue, pruritus, and right upper quadrant abdominal pain. No subject died from liver-related causes despite a cohort mortality rate of 15 percent. A median time of 5.6 years from AMA positivity to persistent serum hepatic biochemistry elevations was observed (range, 1.9 to 19 years). Among 10 patients who underwent repeat liver biopsy, a 40 percent rate of histologic disease progression was observed over a median of 11.4 years (range, 1.3 to 14.3 years). Cirrhosis or portal hypertension was not identified among any individual at follow-up. Although a substantial proportion of asymptomatic

TABLE 39-7
Histologic Progression in Primary Biliary Cirrhosis[217]

	INITIAL HISTOLOGIC STAGE		
Rate of progression	1	2	3
1 year	41%	43%	35%
2 year	62%	62%	50%

From Locke GR III, Therneau TM, Ludwig J, et al: Time course of histologic progression in primary biliary cirrhosis. Hepatology 23:52, 1996.

patients will develop clinical disease from PBC, a subset of individuals will remain asymptomatic despite compatible histologic involvement. Asymptomatic patients have a greater overall median survival rate than symptomatic individuals with PBC. However, a lower overall median survival for asymptomatic PBC patients is observed when compared to an age- and sex-matched healthy population.[54]

Symptomatic Primary Biliary Cirrhosis

The development of cirrhosis and complications from portal hypertension occurs among symptomatic individuals with PBC. Prognostic indicators of poor outcome include older age, elevated serum bilirubin levels, depressed hepatic synthetic function, and advanced histologic stage. Stigmata of portal hypertension associated with end-stage PBC are similar to those found in other hepatic disease etiologies, including esophagogastric varices, portal hypertensive gastropathy, ascites, and portosystemic encephalopathy. Among PBC patients followed for a median of 3.4 years, there is a cumulative risk of 40 percent for developing esophageal varices.[220] Bleeding from esophageal varices occurs in 20 percent of cases and is associated with an increased risk of mortality. The development of portal hypertension in precirrhotic PBC patients results from portal hepatic fibrosis caused by granulomatous bile duct inflammation and portal edema.

PROGNOSTIC SURVIVAL MODELS

In the majority of patients with PBC a progressive clinical course resulting in fibrosis and eventual cirrhosis is observed. Estimates of overall median survival range between 10 and 15 years from the time of diagnosis, whereas advanced histologic disease (stage 3 or 4) imparts a median survival approaching 8 years.[221] Elevations in serum bilirubin above 8 to 10 mg/dl have been associated with median life expectancy of 2 years.[222] To account for these clinical variables as determinants of survival, a number of mathematical models simulating the natural history of PBC have been developed and refined for clinical use.

Among all developed models (Table 39-8)[223-226] the Mayo Clinic formula has undergone the most extensive cross-validation and is widely referred to for predicting long-term survival in PBC. This model is based on the serial follow-up of 312 PBC patients[223] and includes independent predictor variables such as patient age, serum bilirubin, albumin, prothrombin time, and the presence or absence of edema or ascites. The calculation of a risk score from these variables can be translated into a survival function to estimate mortality risk in an individual patient. Increases in risk score are associated with decreases in survival. The absence of histologic information for predicting survival offers the advantage of avoiding invasive procedures such as liver biopsy. Additional capabilities for the model include the monitoring of efficacy from experimental drug therapy in clinical trials and determining the optimal timing for liver transplantation. Subsequent model refinement using time-dependent methods based on serial assessments of clinical status has improved the accuracy for predicting short-term survival from PBC within 2 years from time of assessment.[227,228]

Initial concerns regarding the potential discrepancy between improvements in serum bilirubin and accuracy

TABLE 39-8
Prognostic Models in Primary Biliary Cirrhosis

Authors	Predictive variables	Formula	Extramural validation
Dickson et al[223]	Age	$R = 0.871 \log_e$ (bilirubin in mg/dl)	Yes
	Total bilirubin	$-2.53 \log_e$ (albumin in g/dl)	
	Serum albumin	$+0.039 \log_e$ (bilirubin in mg/dl)	
	Prothrombin time	$+2.38 \log_e$ (prothrombin time in seconds)	
	Edema score	$+0.859$ (edema)	
Rydning et al[224]	Bleeding varices	$\log_e R = 1.68$ (bleeding-0.25)	No
	Bilirubin	$+2.03 \log_e$ (bilirubin-30.3)	
Christensen et al[225]	Bilirubin	Calculated from pocket chart/tables	Yes
	Ascites		
	Albumin		
	Age		
	GI bleeding		
	Central cholestasis		
	Cirrhosis		
	IgM		
Poupon et al[226]	UDCA-treated	Not stated	No
	Bilirubin		
	Prothrombin time		
	Procollagen III		
	Hyaluronic acid		

GI, Gastrointestinal; *IgM,* immunoglobulin M; *UDCA,* ursodeoxycholic acid.

of survival prediction were raised after the approval of UDCA as medical therapy for PBC. Two independent studies[229,230] have subsequently shown that the Mayo Clinic PBC risk score retains its power to predict survival among UDCA-treated patients. The prolonged survival free of liver transplantation associated with UDCA therapy appears to continue for 10 years or more.

LIVER TRANSPLANTATION

The most effective therapeutic alternative for patients with end-stage PBC is liver transplantation. Indications for referral include accepted criteria required for all hepatic disease etiologies and refractory complications of portal hypertension (variceal bleeding, ascites requiring frequent large-volume paracentesis, hepatic encephalopathy, spontaneous bacterial peritonitis, hepatorenal syndrome, and hepatopulmonary syndrome). Severe fatigue, intractable pruritus, and severe pain from vertebral body compression fractures are also considered indications for liver transplantation. Increasing disparities in donor organ availability and recipient need, however, have significantly hampered the ability to perform liver transplantation for these symptoms.

PBC remains among the most frequent indications for liver transplantation in the United States. Patient and graft survival rates from liver transplantation are reported to approach 92 percent and 85 percent at 1-year and 5-year intervals, respectively.[231] Recent data examining the impact of liver transplantation among PBC patients showed an association between improved clinical and economic outcomes with a pretransplant Mayo Clinic risk score of less than 7.8.[232] Hepatic retransplantation occurs in less than 10 percent of PBC subjects. Survival after retransplantation is significantly reduced when performed more than 30 days after the initial transplant and is associated with increases in resource utilization.[233]

Previously considered a controversial topic, the recurrence of PBC after liver transplantation has now been demonstrated.[234-237] Initial reports of histologic features in the allograft consistent with stage I PBC were limited by the absence of explicit criteria for recurrent disease, including the exclusion of acute cellular rejection.[234] It has now been estimated that the rate of recurrent PBC may be as high as 15 percent at 3 years and 30 percent at 10 years.[238] Serum AMA status appears to be independent of recurrence risk. This antibody may disappear soon after transplantation only to return later with or without recurrent disease.[239] The tapering of corticosteroids from immunosuppression regimens after liver transplantation has been suggested to be a potential risk factor for recurrent PBC.[238] No information is available regarding the efficacy of UDCA therapy in halting disease progression from early-stage recurrent PBC.

CONCLUSIONS

PBC is an important hepatic disease that affects middle-aged women. Although data regarding the pathogenesis of PBC continue to emerge, much remains unknown about the interaction between host factors and immune system dysregulation that results in hepatic disease. The differential diagnosis is broad and PBC is often associated with other extrahepatic autoimmune conditions. Disease-specific complications including metabolic bone disease, fat-soluble vitamin deficiency, and steatorrhea are important to recognize and treat appropriately. Among various medical therapies intended to halt disease progression, only UDCA has been associated with an increase in transplant-free survival. Prognostic models are available to provide accurate predictions of survival even with UDCA therapy. The natural history of PBC is usually indolent but often accelerates after advanced histologic stages are reached. Liver transplantation is an effective therapeutic modality for patients with end-stage liver disease from PBC, with excellent patient and graft survival rates.

References

1. Remmel T, Remmel H, Uibo R, et al: Primary biliary cirrhosis in Estonia. With special reference to incidence, prevalence, clinical features, and outcome. Scand J Gastroenterol 30:367, 1995.
2. Metcalf JV, Bhopal RS, Gray J, et al: Incidence and prevalence of primary biliary cirrhosis in the city of Newcastle upon Tyne, England. Int J Epidemiol 26:830, 1997.
3. Watson RG, Angus PW, Dewar M, et al: Low prevalence of primary biliary cirrhosis in Victoria Australia. Melbourne Liver Group. Gut 36:927, 1985.
4. Kim WR, Lindor KD, Locke GR, et al: Epidemiology and natural history of primary biliary cirrhosis in a U.S. community. Gastroenterology 119:1631, 2000.
5. Witt-Sullivan H, Heathcote J, Cauch K, et al: The demography of primary biliary cirrhosis in Ontario, Canada. Hepatology 12:98, 1990.
6. Howel D, Fischbacher CM, Bhopal RS, et al: An exploratory population-based case-control study of primary biliary cirrhosis. Hepatology 31:1055, 2000.
7. Parikh-Patel A, Gold EB, Worman H, et al: Risk factors for primary biliary cirrhosis in a cohort of patients from the United States. Hepatology 33:16, 2001.
8. Shimoda S, Nakamura M, Ishibashi H, et al: HLA DRB4 0101-restricted immunodominant T cell autoepitope of pyruvate dehydrogenase complex in primary biliary cirrhosis: evidence of molecular mimicry in human autoimmune diseases. J Exp Med 181:1835, 1995.
9. Burroughs AK, Butler P, Sternberg MJE, et al: Molecular mimicry in liver disease. Nature 358:377, 1992.
10. Gershwin ME, Ansari A, Mackay IR, et al: Primary biliary cirrhosis: an orchestrated immune response against biliary epithelial cells. Immunol Rev 174:210, 2000.
11. Manns MP, Bremm A, Schneider PM, et al: HLA DRw 8 and complement C4 deficiency as risk factor in primary biliary cirrhosis. Gastroenterology 101:1367, 1991.
12. Briggs DC, Donaldson PR, Hayes P, et al: A major histocompatibility complex class III allotype (C4B2) associated with primary biliary cirrhosis (PBC). Tissue Antigens 29:141, 1987.
13. Mackay IR: Autoimmunity and primary biliary cirrhosis. Bailliere's Best Prac Res Clin Gastro 14:519, 2000.
14. Gores GJ, Moore SB, Fisher LD, et al: Primary biliary cirrhosis: association with class II major histocompatibility antigens. Hepatology 7:889, 1987.
15. Underhill J, Donaldson P, Bray G, et al: Susceptibility to primary biliary cirrhosis is associated with HLA-DR8-DQB1*0402 haplotype. Hepatology 16:1404, 1992.
16. Begovich AB, Klitz W, Moosamy PV, et al: Genes within the HLA class II region confer both predisposition and resistance to primary biliary cirrhosis. Tissue Antigens 43:71, 1994.
17. Neuberger J, Thomson R: PBC and AMA—what is the connection? Hepatology 29:271, 1996.
18. Agarwal K, Jones DE, Daly AK, et al: CTLA-4 polymorphism confers susceptibility to primary biliary cirrhosis. J Hepatol 32:538, 2000.
19. Bach N, Schaffner F: Familial primary biliary cirrhosis. J Hepatol 20:698, 1994.

20. Feizi T, Naccarato R, Sherlock S, et al: Mitochondrial and other tissue antibodies in relatives of patients with primary biliary cirrhosis. Clin Exp Immunol 10:609, 1972.
21. Caldwell SH, Leung PS, Spivey JR, et al: Antimitochondrial antibodies in all kindreds of patients with primary biliary cirrhosis: antimitochondrial antibodies are unique to clinical disease and are absent in asymptomatic family members. Hepatology 16:899, 1992.
22. Jones DEJ, Watt FE, Metcalf JV, et al: Familial primary biliary cirrhosis reassessed: a geographically-based population study. J Hepatol 30:402, 1999.
23. Krams SM, Van De Water J, Coppel RL, et al: Analysis of hepatic T lymphocyte and immunoglobulin deposits in patients with primary biliary cirrhosis. Hepatology 12:306, 1990.
24. Hashimoto E, Lindor KD, Homburger HA, et al: Immunohistochemical characterization of hepatic lymphocytes in primary biliary cirrhosis in comparison with primary sclerosing cholangitis and autoimmune chronic active hepatitis. Mayo Clin Proc 68:1049, 1993.
25. Yamada FG, Hyodo I, Tobe K, et al: Ultrastructural immunocytochemical analysis of lymphocytes infiltrating bile duct epithelia in primary biliary cirrhosis. Hepatology 6:385, 1986.
26. Miller KB, Sepersky RA, Brown KM, et al: Genetic abnormalities of immunoregulation in primary biliary cirrhosis. Am J Med 75:75, 1983.
27. Tsuji H, Murai K, Akagi K, Fujishima M: Familial primary biliary cirrhosis associated with impaired Concanavalin A-induced lymphocyte transformation in relatives. Two family studies. Dig Dis Sci 37:353, 1992.
28. Lim AG, Jazrawi RP, Ahmed HA, et al: Soluble intercellular adhesion molecule-1 in primary biliary cirrhosis: relationship with disease stage, immune activity, and cholestasis. Hepatology 20:882, 1994.
29. Angulo P, Neuman MG, Jorgensen RA, et al: Serum cytokines in patients with primary biliary cirrhosis: effect of treatment with ursodeoxycholic acid. Gastroenterology 116:A129, 1999.
30. Van De Water J, Ansari AA, Surh CD, et al: Evidence for the targeting by 2-oxo-dehydrogenase enzymes in the T cell response of primary biliary cirrhosis. J Immunol 146:89, 1991.
31. Leung PSC, Chuang DT, Wynn RM, et al: Autoantibodies to BCOADC-E2 in patients with primary biliary cirrhosis recognize a conformational epitope. Hepatology 22:505, 1995.
32. Maeda T, Loveland BE, Rowley MJ, et al: Autoantibody against dihydrolipoamide dehydrogenase, the E3 subunit of the 2-oxoacid dehydrogenase complexes: significance for primary biliary cirrhosis. Hepatology 14:994, 1991.
33. Angulo P, Lindor KD: Primary biliary cirrhosis and primary sclerosing cholangitis. Clin Liv Dis 3:529, 1999.
34. Gershwin ME, Rowley M, Davis PA, et al: Molecular biology of the 2-oxo-acid dehydrogenase complexes and anti-mitochondrial antibodies. In Boyer JL, Ockner RK, eds: Progress in Liver Diseases, Philadelphia, WB Saunders, 1992:47.
35. Tsuneyama K, Van De Water J, Leung PSC, et al: Abnormal expression of the E2 component of the pyruvate dehydrogenase complex on the luminal surface of biliary epithelium occurs before major histocompatibility complex class II and BB1-B7 expression. Hepatology 21:1031, 1995.
36. Joplin RE, Johnson GD, Matthews JB, et al: Distribution of pyruvate dehydrogenase dihydrolipoamide acetyltransferase (PDC-E2) and another mitochondrial marker in salivary gland and biliary epithelium from patients with primary biliary cirrhosis. Hepatology 19:1375, 1994.
37. Tsuneyama K, Van De Water J, Van Thiel DH, et al: Abnormal expression of PDC-E2 on the apical surface of biliary epithelial cells in patients with antimitochondrial antibody negative primary biliary cirrhosis. Hepatology 22:1440, 1995
38. Krams SM, Surh CD, Coppel RI, et al: Immunization of experimental animals with dehydrolipoamide acyltransferase, as a purified recombinant polypeptide, generates mitochondrial autoantibodies but not primary biliary cirrhosis. Hepatology 9:411, 1989.
39. Thomas HC, Holden R, Jones IV, et al: Immune response to $\phi\chi174$ in man. Primary and secondary antibody production in primary biliary cirrhosis. Gut 17:884, 1976.
40. Nouri-Aria KT, Hegarty JE, Neuberger JM, et al: In vitro studies on the mechanism of increased serum IgM levels in primary biliary cirrhosis. Clin Exp Immunol 61:297, 1985.
41. Tanaka A, Nalbandian G, Leung PS, et al: Mucosal immunity and primary biliary cirrhosis: presence of antimitochondrial antibodies in urine. Hepatology 32:910, 2000.
42. Ekdahl KN, Loof L, Nyberg A, et al: Defective Fc receptor-mediated clearance in patients with primary biliary cirrhosis. Gastroenterology 101:1076, 1991.
43. Potter EJ, Elias E, Thomas HC, et al: Complement metabolism in chronic liver disease: catabolism of C1q in chronic liver disease and primary biliary cirrhosis. Gastroenterology 78:1034, 1980.
44. Rust C, Gores GJ: Apoptosis and liver disease. Am J Med 108:567, 2000.
45. Matsunaga Y, Terada T: Mast cell subpopulations in chronic inflammatory hepatobiliary diseases. Liver 20:152, 2000.
46. Iwata M, Harada K, Kono N, et al: Expression of Bcl-2 familial proteins is reduced in small bile duct lesions of primary biliary cirrhosis. Hum Pathol 31:179, 2000.
47. Benz C, Angermuller S, Otto G, et al: Effect of tauroursodeoxycholic acid on bile acid-induced apoptosis in primary human hepatocytes. Eur J Clin Invest 30:203, 2000.
48. Rust C, Karnitz LM, Paya CV, et al: The bile acid taurochenodeoxycholate activates a phosphatidylinositol 3-kinase-dependent survival signaling cascade. J Biol Chem 275:20210, 2000.
49. Haydon GH, Neuberger J: PBC: an infectious disease? Gut 47:586, 2000.
50. Trauner M, Boyer JL: Cholestatic syndromes. Curr Opin Gastroenterol 17:242, 2001.
51. Shigematsu H, Shimoda S, Nakamura M, et al: Fine specificity of T cells reactive to human PDC-E2 163-176 peptide, the immunodominant autoantigen in primary biliary cirrhosis: implications for molecular mimicry and cross-recognition among mitochondrial autoantigens. Hepatology 32:901, 2000.
52. Nilsson I, Lindgren S, Eriksson S, et al: Serum autoantibodies to *Helicobacter hepaticus* and *Helicobacter pylori* in patients with chronic liver disease. Gut 46:410, 2000.
53. Nilsson HO, Taneera J, Castedal M, et al: Identification of *Helicobacter pylori* and other *Helicobacter* species by PCR, hybridization, and partial DNA sequencing in human liver samples from patients with primary sclerosing cholangitis or primary biliary cirrhosis. J Clin Microbiol 38:1072, 2000.
54. Myung SJ, Kim MH, Shim KN, et al: Detection of *Helicobacter pylori* DNA in human biliary tree and its association with hepaticolithiasis. Dig Dis Sci 45:1405, 2000.
55. Hiramatsu K, Harada K, Tsuneyama K, et al: Amplification and sequence analysis of partial bacterial 16S ribosomal RNA gene in gallbladder bile from patients with primary biliary cirrhosis. J Hepatol 33:9, 2000.
56. Harada K, Tsuneyama K, Sudo Y, et al: Molecular identification of bacterial 165 ribosomal RNA gene in liver tissue of primary biliary cirrhosis: is *Propionibacterium acnes* involved in granuloma formation? Hepatology 33:530, 2001.
57. Ghadiminejad I, Baum H: Evidence for the cell-surface localization of antigens cross-reacting with the "mitochondrial antibodies" of primary biliary cirrhosis. Hepatology 7:743, 1987.
58. Xu L, Guo L, Keogh A, et al: Isolation and characterization of a novel virus associated with primary biliary cirrhosis. Hepatology 32:297A, 2000.
59. Fanning PA, Jonsson JR, Clouston AD, et al: Detection of male DNA in the liver of female patients with primary biliary cirrhosis. J Hepatol 33:690, 2000.
60. Corpechot C, Barbu V, Chazouilleres O, et al: Fetal microchimerism in primary biliary cirrhosis. J Hepatol 32:528, 2000.
61. Thuluvath PJ, Triger DR: Selenium in primary biliary cirrhosis. Lancet 2:219, 1987.
62. Olomu AB, Vickers CR, Waring RH, et al: High incidence of poor sulfoxidation in patients with primary biliary cirrhosis. N Engl J Med 318:1089, 1988.
63. Inoue K, Hirohara J, Nakano T, et al: Prediction of prognosis of primary biliary cirrhosis in Japan. Liver 15:70, 1995.
64. Springer J, Cauch-Dudek K, O'Rourke K, et al: Asymptomatic primary biliary cirrhosis: a study of its natural history and prognosis. Am J Gastroenterol 94:47, 1999.
65. Rubel LR, Rabin L, Seef LB, et al: Does primary biliary cirrhosis in men differ from primary biliary cirrhosis in women? Hepatology 4:671, 1984.
66. Sherlock S, Scheuer PJ: The presentation and diagnosis of 100 patients with primary biliary cirrhosis. N Engl J Med 289:674, 1973.

67. Mitchison HC, Bassendine MF, Hendrick A, et al: Positive antimitochondrial antibody but normal alkaline phosphatase: is this primary biliary cirrhosis? Hepatology 6:1279, 1986.
68. Poupon RE, Chretien Y, Poupon R, et al: Serum bile acids in primary biliary cirrhosis: effect of ursodeoxycholic acid therapy. Hepatology 17:599, 1993.
69. Walker JG, Doniach D, Roitt IM, et al: Serologic tests in diagnosis of primary biliary cirrhosis. Lancet 1:827, 1965.
70. Kenny RP, Czaja AJ, Ludwig J, et al: Frequency and significance of antimitochondrial antibodies in severe chronic active hepatitis. Dig Dis Sci 31:705, 1986.
71. Bernstein RM, Callendar ME, Neuberger JM, et al: Anticentromere antibody in primary biliary cirrhosis. Ann Rheum Dis 41:612, 1982.
72. Goodman ZD, McNally PR, Davis KR, et al: Autoimmune cholangitis: a variant of primary biliary cirrhosis: clinicopathologic and serologic correlations in 200 cases. Dig Dis Sci 40:1232, 1995.
73. Ben-Ari Z, Dhillon AP, Sherlock S: Autoimmune cholangiopathy: part of the spectrum of autoimmune chronic active hepatitis. Hepatology 18:10, 1993.
74. Michieletti P, Wanless IR, Katz A, et al: Antimitochondrial antibody negative primary biliary cirrhosis: a distinct syndrome of autoimmune cholangitis. Gut 35:260, 1994.
75. Mackay IR, Rowley MJ, Whittingham S: Nuclear antibodies in primary biliary cirrhosis. In Meyer zum Buschenfelde K-H, Hoofnagle J, Manns M, eds: Immunology and Liver. Falk Symposium 70, Dordrecht, Kluwer, 1993:379-409.
76. Spivey JR, Silker BJ, Lindor KD: Prevalence and significance of perihepatic lymphadenopathy in cholestatic liver disease. Am J Gastroenterol 87:A1307, 1992.
77. Ludwig J, Dickson ER, McDonald GS: Staging of chronic non-suppurative destructive cholangitis (syndrome of primary biliary cirrhosis). Virchows Arch 379:103, 1978.
78. Scheuer PJ: Primary biliary cirrhosis: chronic non-suppurative destructive cholangitis. Am J Pathol 46:387, 1965.
79. Ludwig J: Pathology of PBC and autoimmune cholangitis. Baillieres Best Pract Res 14:601, 2000.
80. Angulo P, Pearce DH, Johnson CD, et al: Magnetic resonance cholangiography in patients with biliary disease: its role in primary sclerosing cholangitis. J Hepatol 33:520, 2000.
81. Fulcher AS, Turner MA, Franklin KJ, et al: Primary sclerosing cholangitis: evaluation with MR cholangiography—a case control study. Radiology 215:71, 2000.
82. Kato Y, Morimoto H, Unouri M, et al: Primary biliary cirrhosis and chronic pancreatitis in a patient with ulcerative colitis. J Clin Gastroenterol 7:425, 1985.
83. Bush A, Mitchison H, Walt R, et al: Primary biliary cirrhosis and ulcerative colitis. Gastroenterology 92:2009, 1987.
84. Ludwig J, Czaja AJ, Dickson ER, et al: Manifestations of nonsuppurative cholangitis in chronic hepatobiliary diseases: morphologic spectrum, clinical correlations, and terminology. Liver 4:105, 1984.
85. Boberg KM, Schrumpf E, Fausa O, et al: Hepatobiliary disease in ulcerative colitis. An analysis of 18 patients with hepatobiliary lesions classified as small-duct primary sclerosing cholangitis. Scand J Gastroenterol 29:744, 1994.
86. Czaja AJ, Carpenter HA: Autoimmune hepatitis with incidental histologic features of bile duct injury. Hepatology 34:659, 2001.
87. Czaja AJ: Frequency and nature of the variant syndromes of autoimmune liver disease. Hepatology 28:360, 1998.
88. Chazouilleres O, Wendum D, Serfaty L, et al: Primary biliary cirrhosis-autoimmune hepatitis overlap syndrome: clinical features and response to therapy. Hepatology 28:296, 1998.
89. Keeffe EB: Sarcoidosis and primary biliary cirrhosis. Am J Med 83:977, 1987.
90. Zafrani ES, Metreau JM, Douvin C, et al: Idiopathic biliary ductopenia in adults: a report of five cases. Gastroenterology 99:1823, 1990.
91. Davies SE, Portmann BC, O'Grady JG, et al: Hepatic histological findings after transplantation for chronic hepatitis B virus infection, including a unique pattern of fibrosing cholestatic hepatitis. Hepatology 13:150, 1991.
92. Gordon SC, Quattrociocchi-Longe TM, Khan BA, et al: Antibodies to carbonic anhydrase in patients with immune cholangiopathies. Gastroenterology 108:1802, 1995.
93. Inverizzi P, Crosignani A, Battezzati PM, et al: Comparison of the clinical features and clinical course of antimitochondrial antibody-positive and -negative primary biliary cirrhosis. Hepatology 25:1090, 1997.
94. Kim WR, Poterucha JJ, Jorgensen RA, et al: Does antimitochondrial antibody status affect response to treatment in patients with primary biliary cirrhosis? Outcomes of ursodeoxycholic acid therapy and liver transplantation. Hepatology 26:22, 1997.
95. Golding PL, Smith M, Williams R: Multisystem involvement in chronic liver disease: studies on the incidence and pathogenesis. Am J Med 55:772, 1973.
96. Alarcon-Segovia D, Diaz-Jouanen E, Fishbein E: Features of Sjogren's syndrome in primary biliary cirrhosis. Ann Intern Med 79:31, 1973.
97. Tsianos EV, Hoofnagle JH, Fox PC, et al: Sjogren's syndrome in patients with primary biliary cirrhosis. Hepatology 11:730, 1990.
98. Child DL, Mathews JA, Thompson RPH: Arthritis and primary biliary cirrhosis. BMJ 2:557, 1977.
99. Uddenfeldt P, Danielsson A: Evaluation of rheumatic disorders in patients with primary biliary cirrhosis. Ann Clin Res 18:148, 1986.
100. Murray-Lyon IM, Thompson RPH, Ansell ID, et al: Scleroderma and primary biliary cirrhosis. BMJ 3:258, 1970.
101. Crowe JP, Christensen E, Butler J, et al: Primary biliary cirrhosis and the prevalence of hypothyroidism and its relationship to thyroid autoantibodies and sicca syndrome. Gastroenterology 78:1437, 1980
102. Nieri S, Ricardo CG, Salvadori G, et al: Primary biliary cirrhosis and Grave's disease. J Clin Gastroenterol 7:434, 1985.
103. Pares A, Rimola A, Bruguera M, et al: Renal tubular acidosis in primary biliary cirrhosis. Gastroenterology 80:681, 1981.
104. Rai GS, Hamlyn AN, Dahl MGC, et al: Primary biliary cirrhosis, cutaneous capillaritis, and IgM-associated membranous glomerulonephritis. BMJ 1:817, 1977.
105. Summerfield JA, Elias E, Hungerford GD, et al: The biliary system in primary biliary cirrhosis: a study by endoscopic retrograde cholangiopancreatography. Gastroenterology 70:240, 1976.
106. Wallace JG Jr, Tong M, Ueki BH, et al: Pulmonary involvement in primary biliary cirrhosis. J Clin Gastroenterol 9:431, 1987.
107. Cauch-Dudek K, Abbey S, Stewart DE, et al: Fatigue in primary biliary cirrhosis. Gut 43:705, 1998.
108. Huet PM, Deslauriers J, Tran A, et al: Impact of fatigue on the quality of life of patients with primary biliary cirrhosis. Am J Gastroenterol 95:760, 2000.
109. Prince MI, James OF, Holland NP, et al: Validation of a fatigue impact score in primary biliary cirrhosis: towards a standard for clinical and trial use. J Hepatol 32:368, 2000.
110. Jones EA, Yurdaydin C: Is fatigue associated with cholestasis mediated by altered central neurotransmission? Hepatology 25:492, 1997.
111. Swain MG, Maric M: Defective corticotrophin-releasing hormone mediated neuroendocrine and behavioural responses in cholestatic rats: implications for cholestatic liver disease-related sickness behaviors. Hepatology 22:1560, 1995.
112. Bergasa NV, Mehlman JK, Jones EA: Pruritus and fatigue in primary biliary cirrhosis. Best Prac Res Clin Gastro 14:643, 2000.
113. Kirby J, Heaton KW, Burton JL: Pruritic effect of bile salts. BMJ 4:693, 1974.
114. Jones EA, Bergasa NV: The pruritus of cholestasis: from bile acids to opiate agonists. Hepatology 11:884, 1990.
115. Lloyd-Thomas HGL, Sherlock S: Testosterone therapy for the pruritus of obstructive jaundice. BMJ 2:1289, 1952.
116. Datta DV, Sherlock S: Cholestyramine for long term relief of the pruritus complicating intrahepatic cholestasis. Gastroenterology 50:323, 1966.
117. Bloomer JR, Boyer JL: Phenobarbital effects in cholestatic liver diseases. Ann Intern Med 82:310, 1975.
118. Ghent CN, Carruthers SG: Treatment of pruritus in primary biliary cirrhosis with rifampin. Results of a double-blind, crossover, randomized trial. Gastroenterology 94:488, 1988.
119. Bachs L, Pares A, Elena M, et al: Comparison of rifampicin with phenobarbitone for the treatment of pruritus in biliary cirrhosis. Lancet 1:574, 1989.
120. Bachs L, Pares A, Elena M, et al: Effects of long-term rifampicin administration in primary biliary cirrhosis. Gastroenterology 102:2077, 1992.
121. Turner IB, Rawlins MD, Wood P, et al: Flumenicol for the treatment of pruritus associated with primary biliary cirrhosis. Alim Pharm Ther 8:337, 1994.

122. Walt R, Daneshmend T, Fellows I: Effect of stanozolol on itching in primary biliary cirrhosis. BMJ 296:607, 1988.
123. Bergasa NV, Talbot TL, Alling DW, et al: A controlled trial of naloxone infusions for the pruritus of chronic cholestasis. Gastroenterology 102:544, 1992.
124. Bergasa NV, Alling DW, Talbot TL, et al: Naloxone ameliorates the pruritus of cholestasis: results of a double-blind, randomized placebo controlled trial. Ann Intern Med 123:161, 1995.
125. Bergasa NV, Talbot TL, Schmitt JP, et al: Open label trial of oral nalmefene therapy for the pruritus of cholestasis. Hepatology 27:679, 1998.
126. Bergasa NV, Alling DW, Talbot TL, et al: Oral nalmefene therapy reduces scratching activity due to the pruritus of cholestasis: a controlled study. J Am Acad Dermatol 41:431, 1999.
127. Borgeat A, Wilder-Smith OHG, Mentha G: Subhypnotic doses of propofol relieve pruritus associated with liver disease. Gastroenterology 104:244, 1993.
128. Schwoer H, Hartmann H, Ramadori G: Relief of cholestatic pruritus by a novel class of drugs: 5-hydroxytryptamine type 3 (5-HT3) receptor antagonists: effectiveness of ondansetron. Pain 61:33, 1995.
129. Muller C, Pngratz S, Pidlich J, et al: Treatment of pruritus of chronic liver disease with the 5-hydroxytryptamine type 3 receptor antagonist ondansetron: a randomized, placebo-controlled, double-blind cross-over trial. Eur J Gastro Hepatol 10:865, 1998.
130. Frezza M, Surrenti C, Manzillo G, et al: Oral S-adenosylmethionine in the symptomatic treatment of intrahepatic cholestasis. A double-blind, placebo-controlled study. Gastroenterology 99:211, 1990.
131. Crippin JS, Lindor KD, Jorgensen RA, et al: Hypercholesterolemia and atherosclerosis in primary biliary cirrhosis: what is the risk? Hepatology 15:858, 1992.
132. Jahn CE, Schaefer EJ, Taam LA, et al: Lipoprotein abnormalities in primary biliary cirrhosis: association with hepatic lipase inhibition as well as altered cholesterol esterification. Gastroenterology 89:1266, 1985.
133. Gregory WL, Game FL, Farrer M, et al: Reduced serum lipoprotein (a) levels in patients with primary biliary cirrhosis. Atherosclerosis 105:43, 1994.
134. Balan V, Dickson ER, Jorgensen RA, Lindor KD: Effects of ursodeoxycholic acid on serum lipids of patients with primary biliary cirrhosis. Mayo Clin Proc 69:923, 1994.
135. Michieletti P, Heathcote EJL: Xanthelasma and hypercholesterolemia in primary biliary cirrhosis. Clin Invest Med 15:A61, 1992.
136. Longo M, Crosignani A, Battezzati M, et al: Hyperlipidemic state and cardiovascular risk in primary biliary cirrhosis. Gastroenterology 118:A1008, 2000.
137. Hodgson SF, Dickson ER, Wahner HW, et al: Bone loss and reduced osteoblast function in primary biliary cirrhosis. Ann Intern Med 103:855, 1985.
138. Hodgson SF, Dickson ER, Eastell R, et al: Rates of cancellous bone remodeling and turnover in osteopenia associated with primary biliary cirrhosis. Bone 14:819, 1993.
139. Compston JE: Hepatic osteodystrophy: vitamin D metabolism in patients with liver disease. Gut 27:1073, 1986.
140. Springer JE, Cole DEC, Rubin LA, et al: Vitamin D-receptor genotypes as independent genetic predictors of decreased bone mineral density in primary biliary cirrhosis. Gastroenterology 118:145, 2000.
141. Brot C, Jorgensen NR, Sorensen OH: The influence of smoking on vitamin D status and calcium metabolism. Eur J Clin Nutr 53:920, 1999.
142. Hay JE: Bone disease in cholestatic liver disease. Gastroenterology 108:276, 1995.
143. Eastell R, Dickson ER, Hodgson SF, et al: Rates of vertebral bone loss before and after liver transplantation in women with primary biliary cirrhosis. Hepatology 14:296, 1991.
144. Floreani A, Zappala F, Fries W, et al: A 3-year pilot study with 1,25-dihydroxyvitamin D, calcium, and calcitonin for severe osteodystrophy in primary biliary cirrhosis. J Clin Gastroenterol 24:239, 1997.
145. Camisasca M, Crosignani A, Battezzati PM, et al: Parenteral calcitonin for metabolic bone disease associated with primary biliary cirrhosis. Hepatology 20:633, 1994.
146. Crippin JS, Jorgenson RA, Dickson ER, et al: Hepatic osteodystrophy in primary biliary cirrhosis: effects on medical treatment. Am J Gastroenterol 89:47, 1994.
147. Guanabens N, Pares A, del Rio L, et al: Sodium fluoride prevents bone loss in primary biliary cirrhosis. J Hepatol 15:345, 1992.
148. Guanabens N, Pares A, Monegal A, et al: Etidronate versus fluoride for treatment of osteopenia in primary biliary cirrhosis: preliminary results after 2 years. Gastroenterology 113:219, 1997.
149. Lindor KD, Jorgensen RA, Tiegs RD, et al: Etidronate for osteoporosis in primary biliary cirrhosis: a randomized trial. J Hepatol 33:878, 2000.
150. Lanspa SJ, Chan ATH, Bell S, et al: Pathogenesis of steatorrhea in primary biliary cirrhosis. Hepatology 5:837, 1985.
151. Kaplan MM, Elta GH, Furie B, et al: Fat-soluble vitamin nutriture in primary biliary cirrhosis. Gastroenterology 95:787, 1988.
152. Jeffrey GP, Muller DPR, Burroughs AK, et al: Vitamin E deficiency and its clinical significance in adults with primary biliary cirrhosis and other forms of chronic liver disease. J Hepatol 4:307, 1987.
153. Arria AM, Tarter RE, Warty J, et al: Vitamin E deficiency and psychomotor dysfunction in adults with primary biliary cirrhosis. Am J Clin Nutr 52:383, 1990.
154. Nijhawan PK, Therneau TM, Dickson ER, et al: Incidence of cancer in primary biliary cirrhosis: the Mayo experience. Hepatology 29:1396, 1999.
155. Loof L, Adami HO, Sparen P, et al: Cancer risk in primary biliary cirrhosis: a population-based study from Sweden. Hepatology 20:101, 1994.
156. Farinati F, Floreani A, DeMaria N, et al: Hepatocellular carcinoma in primary biliary cirrhosis. J Hepatol 21:315, 1994.
157. Goudie BM, Burt AD, Boyle P, et al: Breast cancer in women with primary biliary cirrhosis. BMJ 291:1597, 1985.
158. Wolke AM, Schaffner F, Kapleman B, et al: Malignancy in primary biliary cirrhosis: high incidence of breast cancer in affected women. Am J Med 76:1075, 1984.
159. Mitchison HC, Bassendine MF, Malcolm AJ, et al: A pilot, double-blind controlled 1-year trial of prednisolone treatment in primary biliary cirrhosis. Hepatic improvement but greater bone loss. Hepatology 10:420, 1989.
160. Mitchison HC, Palmer JM, Bassendine MF, et al: A controlled trial of prednisolone treatment in primary biliary cirrhosis: three-year results. J Hepatol 15:336, 1992.
161. Crowe J, Christensen E, Smith M, et al: Azathioprine in primary biliary cirrhosis: a preliminary report of an international trial. Gastroenterology 78:1005, 1980.
162. Christensen E, Neuberger J, Crowe J, et al: Beneficial effect of azathioprine and prediction of prognosis in primary biliary cirrhosis: final results of an international trial. Gastroenterology 89:1034, 1985.
163. Wiesner RH, Ludwig J, Lindor KD, et al: A controlled trial of cyclosporine in the treatment of primary biliary cirrhosis. N Engl J Med 322:1419, 1990.
164. Lombard M, Portmann B, Neuberger J, et al: Cyclosporin A treatment in primary biliary cirrhosis: results of a long-term placebo controlled trial. Gastroenterology 104:519, 1993.
165. Kaplan MM, Knox TA, Arora S: Primary biliary cirrhosis treated with low-dose oral pulse methotrexate. Ann Intern Med 109:429, 1988.
166. Kaplan MM, Knox TA: Treatment of primary biliary cirrhosis with low-dose weekly methotrexate. Gastroenterology 101:1332, 1991.
167. Hendrickse MT, Rigney E, Giaffer MH, et al: Low-dose of methotrexate is ineffective in primary biliary cirrhosis: long-term results of a placebo-controlled trial. Gastroenterology 117:400, 1999.
168. Sharma A, Provenzale D, McKusick A, et al: Interstitial pneumonitis after low-dose methotrexate therapy in primary biliary cirrhosis. Gastroenterology 107:266, 1994.
169. Epstein O, Jain S, Lee RG, et al: D-penicillamine treatment improves survival in primary biliary cirrhosis. Lancet 1:1275, 1981.
170. Matloff DS, Alpert E, Resnick RH, et al: A prospective trial of D-penicillamine in primary biliary cirrhosis. N Engl J Med 306:319, 1982.
171. James OFW: D-penicillamine for primary biliary cirrhosis. Gut 26:109, 1985.
172. Taal BG, Schlam SW, Ten Kate FWJ, et al: Low therapeutic value of D-penicillamine in a short-term prospective trial in primary biliary cirrhosis. Liver 3:345, 1983.

173. Neuberger J, Christensen E, Portmann B: Double-blind controlled trial of D-penicillamine in patients with primary biliary cirrhosis. Gut 26:114, 1985.
174. Bodenheimer HC, Schaffner F, Sternlieb I, et al: A prospective clinical trial of D-penicillamine in the treatment of primary biliary cirrhosis. Hepatology 5:1139, 1985.
175. Dickson ER, Fleming TR, Wiesner RH, et al: Trial of penicillamine in advanced primary biliary cirrhosis. N Engl J Med 312:1011, 1985.
176. Kaplan MM, Alling DW, Zimmerman HJ, et al: A prospective trial of colchicine for primary biliary cirrhosis. N Engl J Med 215:1448, 1986.
177. Bodenheimer H, Schaffner F, Pezzullo J: Evaluation of colchicine therapy in primary biliary cirrhosis. Gastroenterology 95:124, 1988.
178. Warnes TW: Colchicine in primary biliary cirrhosis. Alim Pharm Ther 5:321, 1991.
179. Lindor KD, Dickson ER, Baldus WP, et al: Ursodeoxycholic acid in the treatment of primary biliary cirrhosis. Gastroenterology 106:1284, 1994.
180. Poupon RE, Balkan B, Eschwege E, et al: A multicenter, controlled trial of Ursodiol for the treatment of primary biliary cirrhosis. N Engl J Med 324:1548, 1991.
181. Heathcote EJ, Cauch-Dudek K, Walker V, et al: The Canadian multicenter, double-blind, randomized controlled trial of ursodeoxycholic acid in primary biliary cirrhosis. Hepatology 19:1149, 1994.
182. Pares A, Caballeria L, Rodes J, et al: Long-term effects of ursodeoxycholic acid in primary biliary cirrhosis: results of a double-blind, controlled multicentric trial: the UDCA-Cooperative Group from the Spanish Association for the Study of the Liver. J Hepatol 32:561, 2000.
183. Combes B, Carithers RL, Maddrey WC, et al: A randomized, double-blind, placebo-controlled trial of ursodeoxycholic acid in primary biliary cirrhosis. Hepatology 22:759, 1995.
184. Poupon RE, Poupon R, Balkau B, and the UDCA-PBC Study Group: Ursodiol for the long-term treatment of primary biliary cirrhosis. N Engl J Med 330:1342, 1994.
185. Poupon RE, Lindor KD, Cauch-Dudek K, et al: Combined analysis of randomized controlled trials of ursodeoxycholic acid in primary biliary cirrhosis. Gastroenterology 113:884, 1997.
186. Poupon RE, Bonnand AM, Chretien Y, et al: Ten-year survival in ursodeoxycholic acid treated patients in primary biliary cirrhosis. Hepatology 29:1668, 1999.
187. Lindor KD, Jorgensen RA, Dickson ER: Ursodeoxycholic acid delays the onset of esophageal varices in primary biliary cirrhosis. Mayo Clin Proc 72:1137, 1997.
188. Pasha T, Heathcote J, Gabriel S, et al: Cost-effectiveness of ursodeoxycholic acid in patients with primary biliary cirrhosis. Hepatology 29:21, 1999.
189. Heuman DM, Bajaj R: Ursodeoxycholate conjugates protect against disruption of cholesterol-rich membranes by bile salts. Gastroenterology 106:1333, 1994.
190. Hillaire S, Boucher E, Calmus Y, et al: Effects of bile acids and cholestasis on major histocompatibility complex class I in human and rat hepatocytes. Gastroenterology 107:781, 1994.
191. Yoshikawa M, Tsujii T, Matsumura K, et al: Immunomodulatory effects of ursodeoxycholic acid on immune responses. Hepatology 16:358, 1992.
192. Rodrigues CM, Steer CJ: Mitochondrial membrane perturbations in cholestasis. J Hepatol 32:135, 2000.
193. Angulo P, Dickson ER, Therneau TM, et al: Comparison of three doses of ursodeoxycholic acid in the treatment of primary biliary cirrhosis: a randomized trial. J Hepatol 30:830, 1999.
194. Goulis J, Leandro G, Burroughs AK: Randomised controlled trials of ursodeoxycholic acid therapy for primary biliary cirrhosis: a meta-analysis. Lancet 354:1053, 1999.
195. Poupon RE: Ursodeoxycholic acid for primary biliary cirrhosis: lessons from the past—issues for the future. J Hepatol 32:689, 2000.
196. Leuschner M, Dietrich CF, You T, et al: Characterization of patients with primary biliary cirrhosis responding to long-term ursodeoxycholic acid treatment. Gut 46:121, 2000.
197. Poupon R, Poupon RE: Treatment of primary biliary cirrhosis. Best Prac Res Clin Gastro 14:615, 2000.
198. Leuschner M, Gultdutuna S, You T, et al: Ursodeoxycholic acid and prednisolone versus ursodeoxycholic acid and placebo in the treatment of early stages of primary biliary cirrhosis. J Hepatol 25:39, 1996.
199. Wolfhagen FHJ, van Hooganstraten HJF, van Buuren HR, et al: Triple therapy with ursodeoxycholic acid, prednisone, and azathioprine in primary biliary cirrhosis: a 1-year, randomized placebo-controlled study. J Hepatol 29:736, 1998.
200. Leuschner M, Maier K-M, Schlichting J, et al: Oral budesonide and ursodeoxycholic acid for the treatment of primary biliary cirrhosis: results of a prospective, double-blind trial. Gastroenterology 117:918, 1999.
201. Angulo P, Smith C, Jorgensen R, et al: Budesonide in the treatment of patients with primary biliary cirrhosis with suboptimal response to ursodeoxycholic acid. Hepatology 20:471, 1999.
202. Radesch R, Stiehl A, Walker S, et al: Effects of ursodeoxycholic acid and ursodeoxycholic acid plus colchicine in primary biliary cirrhosis: a double-blind pilot study. In Paumgartner G, Stiehl A, Gerok W, eds: Bile Acids as Therapeutic Agents: From Basic Science to Clinical Practice, Dordrecht, Kluwer Academic Publishers, 1991:301-304.
203. Ikeda T, Tozuka S, Noguchi O, et al: Effects of additional administration of colchicine in ursodeoxycholic acid-treated patients with primary biliary cirrhosis: a prospective randomized study. J Hepatol 24:88, 1996.
204. Poupon RE, Huet PM, Poupon R, et al: A randomized trial comparing colchicine and ursodeoxycholic acid combination to ursodeoxycholic acid in primary biliary cirrhosis. Hepatology 24:1098, 1994.
205. Almasio PL, Floreani A, Chiaramonte M, et al: Multicenter randomized placebo-controlled trial of ursodeoxycholic acid with or without colchicine in symptomatic primary biliary cirrhosis. Alim Pharm Ther 14:1645, 2000.
206. Buscher H-P, Zietzschmann Y, Gerok W: Positive responses to methotrexate and ursodeoxycholic acid in patients with primary biliary cirrhosis responding insufficiently to ursodeoxycholic acid alone. J Hepatol 18:19, 1993.
207. Lindor KD, Dickson ER, Jorgensen RA, et al: The combination of ursodeoxycholic acid and methotrexate for patients with primary biliary cirrhosis: the results of a pilot study. Hepatology 22:1158, 1995.
208. van Steenbergen W, Sciot R, vanEyken P, et al: Combined treatment with methotrexate and ursodeoxycholic acid in non-cirrhotic primary biliary cirrhosis. Acta Clin Belgica 51:8, 1996.
209. Gonzales-Koch A, Brahm J, Antezana C, et al: The combination of ursodeoxycholic acid and methotrexate for primary biliary cirrhosis is not better than ursodeoxycholic acid alone. J Hepatol 27:143, 1997.
210. Bonis PAL, Kaplan MM: Methotrexate improves biochemical tests in patients with primary biliary cirrhosis who respond incompletely to ursodiol. Gastroenterology 117:395, 1999.
211. European Muticentre Study Group: The results of a randomized double blind controlled trial evaluating malotilate in primary biliary cirrhosis. J Hepatol 17:227, 1993.
212. Hoofnagle JH, Davis GL, Schafer DF, et al: Randomized trial of chlorambucil for primary biliary cirrhosis. Gastroenterology 91:1327, 1986.
213. McCormick PA, Scott F, Epstein O, et al: Thalidomide as therapy for primary biliary cirrhosis: a double-blind placebo controlled pilot study. J Hepatol 21:496, 1994.
214. Angulo P, Patel T, Jorgensen RA, et al: Silymarin in the treatment of patients with primary biliary cirrhosis with a suboptimal response to ursodeoxycholic acid. Hepatology 32:897, 2000.
215. Kunihara T, NimiA, Maeda A, et al: Bezafibrate in the treatment of primary biliary cirrhosis: comparison with ursodeoxycholic acid. Am J Gastroenterol 95:2990, 2000.
216. Miyaguchi S, Ebinuma H, Imaeda H, et al: A novel treatment for refractory primary biliary cirrhosis? Hepatogastroenterology 47: 1518, 2000.
217. Locke GR III, Therneau TM, Ludwig J, et al: Time course of histologic progression in primary biliary cirrhosis. Hepatology 23:52, 1996.
218. Angulo P, Batts KP, Therneau T, et al: Long-term ursodeoxycholic acid delays histologic progression in primary biliary cirrhosis. Hepatology 1999:29, 644.

219. Corpechot C, Carrat F, Bonnand AM, et al: The effect of ursodeoxycholic acid therapy on liver fibrosis progression in primary biliary cirrhosis. Hepatology 32:1196, 2000.
220. Gores GJ, Wiesner RH, Dickson ER, et al: A prospective evaluation of esophageal varices in primary biliary cirrhosis. Development, natural history, and influence on survival. Gastroenterology 95;1552, 1989.
221. Christensen E, Crowe J, Doniach D, et al: Clinical pattern and course of disease in primary biliary cirrhosis based on an analysis of 236 patients. Gastroenterology 78:236, 1980.
222. Shapiro JM, Smith H, Schaffner F: Serum bilirubin: a prognostic factor in primary biliary cirrhosis. Gut 20:137, 1979.
223. Dickson E, Grambsch PM, Fleming TR, et al: Prognosis in primary biliary cirrhosis: model for decision making. Hepatology 10:1, 1989.
224. Rydning A, Schrumpf E, Abdelnoor M, et al: Factors of prognostic importance in primary biliary cirrhosis. Scand J Gastroenterol 25:119, 1990.
225. Christensen E, Altman DG, Neuberger J, et al: Updating prognosis in primary biliary cirrhosis using a time-dependent Cox regression model. Gastroenterology 105:1865, 1993.
226. Poupon RE, Balkau, B, Guechot J, et al: Predictive factors in ursodeoxycholic acid treated patients with primary biliary cirrhosis: role of serum markers of connective tissue. Hepatology 19:635, 1994.
227. Klion FM, Fabry TL, Palmer M, et al: Prediction of survival of patients with primary biliary cirrhosis: examination of the Mayo Clinic model on a group of patients with known endpoint. Gastroenterology 102:310, 1992.
228. Murtaugh PA, Dickson ER, van Dam GM, et al: Primary biliary cirrhosis: prediction of short-term survival based on repeated patient visits. Hepatology 20:126, 1994.
229. Angulo P, Lindor KD, Therneau TM, et al: Utilization of the Mayo risk score in patients with primary biliary cirrhosis receiving ursodeoxycholic acid. Liver 19:115, 1999.
230. Kilmurry M, Heathcote EJ, Cauch-Dudek K, et al: Is the Mayo model for predicting survival useful after the introduction of ursodeoxycholic acid treatment for primary biliary cirrhosis? Hepatology 23:1148, 1994.
231. 1999 Annual Report of the U.S. Scientific Registry of Transplant Recipients and the Organ Procurement and Transplantation Network: Transplant Data 1989-1998. (2000, February 21). Rockville, Md., and Richmond, Va.: HHS/HRSA/OSP/DOT and UNOS.
232. Kim WR, Wiesner RH, Therneau TM, et al: Optimal timing of liver transplantation for primary biliary cirrhosis. Hepatology 28:33, 1998.
233. Kim WR, Wiesner RH, Poterucha JJ, et al: Hepatic retransplantation in cholestatic liver disease: impact of the interval to retransplantation on survival and resource utilization. Hepatology 30:395, 1999.
234. Neuberger JM, Portmann B, MacDougall B, et al: Recurrence of primary biliary cirrhosis after liver transplantation. N Engl J Med 306:1, 1982.
235. Polson RJ, Portmann B, Neuberger J, et al: Evidence for disease recurrence after liver transplantation for primary biliary cirrhosis: clinical and histologic follow-up studies. Gastroenterology 97:715, 1989.
236. Hubscher SG, Elias E, Buckels JAC, et al: Primary biliary cirrhosis: histological evidence of disease recurrence after liver transplantation. J Hepatol 18:173, 1993.
237. Balan V, Batts KP, Porayko MK, et al: Histological evidence for recurrence of primary biliary cirrhosis after liver transplantation. Hepatology 18:1392, 1993.
238. Neuberger JM: Recurrent primary biliary cirrhosis. Best Prac Res Clin Gastro 14:669, 2000.
239. Dubel L, Gorges O, Bismuth H, et al: Kinetics of anti-M2 antibodies after liver transplantation for PBC. J Hepatol 23:674, 1995.

C H A P T E R

40

Hepatobiliary Complications of Ulcerative Colitis and Crohn's Disease

John M. Vierling, MD

Extraintestinal complications of inflammatory bowel disease (IBD), including diseases of the liver and biliary tract, affect a large number of patients with ulcerative colitis (UC) or Crohn's disease.[1] Indeed, hepatobiliary complications may affect as many as 5 percent to 10 percent of patients with IBD. The occurrences of specific hepatobiliary diseases associated with IBD (Table 40-1), however, vary widely; some disorders occur commonly and others rarely. The clinical significances of individual hepatobiliary disorders also vary, ranging from inconsequential to life-threatening. Current data indicate that primary sclerosing cholangitis (PSC) is the most common disease associated with either UC or Crohn's disease.[1] The purpose of this chapter is to review the spectrum, diagnosis, management, and concepts of pathogenesis of the hepatobiliary diseases associated with UC and Crohn's disease.

OVERVIEW AND CRITICAL COMMENTS

The association between UC and liver disease was first described in the late nineteenth century.[2,3] The number of patients reported before 1950, however, was small and reflected the biases of autopsy studies. During this period several studies of large numbers of patients with UC showed either no hepatobiliary complications[4,5] or the infrequent occurrence of hepatic abscess,[6,7] hepatitis,[8,9] or cirrhosis.[9]

From 1950 to the present numerous reports have verified an association between IBD and hepatobiliary complications. Such reports originally suggested that hepatobiliary disorders were more frequent in UC than in Crohn's disease. This misconception was due, in part, to the fact that patients with Crohn's disease mistakenly were reported as having UC[10] before the comprehensive description of the colitis of Crohn's disease in 1960.[11] In addition, there was little evidence initially that Crohn's disease of the small intestine was complicated by hepatobiliary disease. Subsequent studies have shown that hepatobiliary complications occur in patients with Crohn's disease of the small intestine, colon, or intestine and colon.[1,15-22] It is now recognized that hepatobiliary complications occur with comparable frequencies in male and female patients with UC and those with Crohn's disease,[1,10,15,19,20] although PSC predominantly afflicts males. The relationship between hepatobiliary complications and other extraintestinal complications in IBD remains unclear.[1] Patients who have hepatobiliary complications of UC and Crohn's disease, however, commonly have other concurrent extraintestinal complications.[10,19,23]

Because each of the disorders listed in Table 40-1 also occurs in patients without IBD, it is important to define the relationship between IBD and specific hepatobiliary diseases. To verify a true association between hepatobiliary disease and IBD requires comparison of the prevalences and incidences of the hepatobiliary disease in patients with and without IBD. Unfortunately, neither the prevalence nor the incidence of hepatobiliary complications in UC or Crohn's disease has been defined. The data from both retrospective and prospective studies do suggest, however, that hepatobiliary diseases occur more often in patients with IBD than in the general population.[24-37] The most common reported disorders are PSC,

TABLE 40-1
Hepatobiliary Complications of Ulcerative Colitis and Crohn's Disease

Hepatobiliary complication	Frequency
Primary sclerosing cholangitis	++++
Pericholangitis	++
Autoimmune hepatitis	++
Fatty liver	++
Hepatic fibrosis and cirrhosis	++
Amyloidosis	+
Hepatic granulomas	+
Carcinoma of the biliary tract	++
Cholelithiasis	++

"pericholangitis," autoimmune hepatitis (AIH), and cryptogenic cirrhosis.[1,24,37]

Perrett and associates found that 45 of 300 patients with UC had abnormal results in one or more liver tests (aspartate aminotransferase [AST], alkaline phosphatase, and bromsulphalein retention).[10] However, biopsies of the livers of these 45 patients showed abnormalities in only 65 percent. Thus the finding of abnormal liver tests could overestimate the frequency of histologic liver disease in patients with UC[20,38-40] and Crohn's disease.[14,18-20] Liver tests were performed in 396 patients with UC and 125 patients with Crohn's disease to determine the prevalence of hepatobiliary diseases.[14] In the UC group 17 percent (95 percent confidence interval [CI] 14 percent to 22 percent) had at least one abnormal test. Alkaline phosphatase was elevated in 8 percent, alanine aminotransferase (ALT) in 8 percent, bilirubin in 5 percent, and AST in 4 percent. Coagulopathy and hypoalbuminemia were found in 2 percent. Six patients (1 percent) who had abnormal tests more than twice the upper limit of normal on at least two occasions were assessed with ultrasonography, liver biopsy, and endoscopic retrograde cholangiography. Three patients had PSC, one had cholangiocarcinoma, and two had alcoholic liver disease. Among 125 patients with Crohn's disease, 30 percent (95 percent CI 23 percent to 38 percent) had at least one abnormal test. Alkaline phosphatase was elevated in 18 percent, ALT in 10 percent, AST in 3 percent, and bilirubin in 2 percent. Coagulopathy and hypoalbuminemia occurred in 1 percent. Three patients (2 percent) met criteria for extensive evaluation; one refused testing, one had hepatic granulomas, and one had alcoholic liver disease. A study of the prevalence of hepatobiliary dysfunction in a region of Denmark showed abnormal liver biochemical tests in 69 of 396 (17 percent with 95 percent CI 14 percent to 22 percent) patients with UC and 38 of 125 (30 percent, 95 percent CI 23 percent to 38 percent) of patients with Crohn's disease.[14] In UC patients with confirmed abnormalities more than twofold elevated, three had PSC, one had cholangiocarcinoma, and two had alcoholic liver disease. In the Crohn's disease group one patient had hepatic granulomas and one had alcoholic liver disease. Conversely, liver biopsies performed in patients with normal liver tests have shown an appreciable frequency of histologic abnormalities in patients with UC[10,20,41,42] or Crohn's disease.[14,18,19] In a study of patients with UC by Perrett and colleagues 54 percent of patients with normal liver tests had abnormal biopsy findings.[10] A retrospective study indicates that up to 55 percent of patients with UC have abnormal liver tests, but in 30 percent of this group the abnormalities are mild and transient.[32]

Overall, the data suggest that the severity, duration, and extent of the IBD correlate poorly with the type or severity of the hepatobiliary disease.* However, a contemporary retrospective study of 202 patients with UC indicated that pancolitis was significantly more frequent in patients with marked abnormalities in liver tests than in patients whose test results were normal or mildly abnormal.[32] Duration, unlike severity, was unrelated to liver test abnormalities.[32] More modern studies evaluated all patients for biochemical abnormalities and more frequently employed liver biopsy and cholangiography.[1,24]

*References 1, 18, 22, 24, 38, 41-47.

PERICHOLANGITIS

Prospective and retrospective studies have shown that patients with IBD frequently have chronic inflammatory lesions of the portal tracts.* Such lesions represent the most common hepatobiliary abnormality in biopsy specimens from living patients with IBD. Currently, the appropriate terminology for these lesions remains controversial.[37,44,51,52] Reports of cholangiographic studies challenge the original concept that the process is primarily a disease of the liver† rather than of the biliary tract by demonstrating the presence of sclerosing lesions of the bile ducts in many patients.[30-37,48,42-54] Morphologically, lesions are characterized by infiltration of the portal tracts with lymphocytes, plasma cells, macrophages, up to 15 percent neutrophils, and a variable but small number of eosinophils.[22,27] The involved portal tracts are expanded and edematous. Proliferation of bile ductules often is present. Most often, the bile duct epithelium is normal, even in chronic lesions when periductular fibrosis is present.[41] In the series reported by Mistilis abnormalities of the bile ducts such as swelling, edema, inflammatory infiltration of the bile ductules, and occasional desquamation of the epithelium were common.[27] Mistilis, a proponent of the concept that the bile duct is the focus of the inflammatory infiltrate, acknowledges that inflammation of both the portal venules and lymphatics is a common feature of pericholangitis.[27] The problems of nomenclature are compounded further by features of pericholangitis that overlap the morphologic features of chronic viral and AIH.[55] Furthermore, it also should be noted that the term *pericholangitis* has been used to describe histologic features in patients with chronic obstruction of the extrahepatic biliary tract, pancreatitis, diverticulitis, typhoid fever, septicemia, chronic hepatitis, primary biliary cirrhosis (PBC), benign recurrent intrahepatic cholestasis, drug-induced hepatitis, and PSC.[56] Only rarely did early investigators specify that their criteria for the diagnosis of pericholangitis include a normal biliary tract.[25,41,52] Using modern techniques of cholangiography, the intrahepatic and extrahepatic portions of the biliary tract have been studied in patients with typical pericholangitis.‡ These studies demonstrate sclerosing lesions of the biliary tract in a substantial proportion of patients with pericholangitis. Cholangiographic evidence of PSC also has been found in other patients with IBD, whose histologic diagnosis was pericholangitis.§ Based on these findings, it is clear that pericholangitis is

*References 1, 10, 15-22, 24, 25, 27, 30-37, 39, 40, 42, 48-50.
†References 21, 22, 37, 44, 49, 52.
‡References 34, 35, 37, 39, 43, 48, 52, 53, 57, 58.
§References 30, 31, 34, 35, 37, 52, 59.

the histologic consequence of PSC[37,52,60] (see the section on Primary Sclerosing Cholangitis).

Wee and Ludwig proposed the term *primary sclerosing cholangitis of the small bile ducts* to replace the term *pericholangitis*.[37,52] In their retrospective study of 107 patients with UC and hepatobiliary disease PSC of the small bile ducts was diagnosed in 37 patients whose disease was previously labeled pericholangitis but whose histopathologic features were similar to those of patients with classic PSC involving the extrahepatic ducts.[37] Only 11 of the 37 patients had exclusion of large-duct sclerosis. Six of 18 patients who ultimately developed large-duct sclerosing cholangitis had biopsy evidence of small-duct disease 1 to 12 years earlier and negative *intravenous* cholangiograms 1 to 4 years earlier. This observation suggests (but does not prove) that small-duct disease may evolve into classic PSC. Intravenous cholangiography is too insensitive a test, however, to exclude the possibility that these patients had early lesions of PSC when the biopsies were performed. The finding that 10 of the 37 patients with small-duct disease had no evidence of macroscopic PSC 7 to 31 years after diagnosis clearly indicates that progression does not occur in all such patients. Further support for a relationship between pericholangitis, small-duct PSC, and classic PSC with cholangiographic evidence of strictures will require prospective study of patients serially evaluated by both liver biopsy and retrograde cholangiography. Histopathology alone cannot discriminate between the conditions.[34,35,37,52,59]

Many biopsied patients have had cholangiographic evidence of PSC. Blackstone and Nemchausky performed endoscopic retrograde cholangiography in eight patients with UC complicated by pericholangitis.[53] Five of the eight were asymptomatic, two had pruritus for more than a year, and one was jaundiced. Sclerosing cholangitis was found in seven patients in whom the intrahepatic and extrahepatic bile ducts were visualized. All seven patients had abnormalities of the intrahepatic ducts; two had involvement of the common bile duct. In the remaining patient only the common bile duct was visualized, and it was normal. In another study using endoscopic retrograde cholangiography to assess patients with UC and biopsy-proven liver disease, Schrumpf and co-workers demonstrated sclerosing cholangitis in 5 of 18 patients with pericholangitis, 4 of 13 patients with portal inflammation and fibrosis, 1 of 8 patients with non-specific reactive changes, and 2 of 4 patients with cirrhosis.[48] Among 21 patients with abnormal liver tests in a group of 681 patients followed for UC, 17 were found to have sclerosing cholangitis.[34] In 6 of the 17 a histologic diagnosis of either chronic hepatitis or pericholangitis had been made before cholangiography. A recent study evaluated the natural history of 34 patients with small duct PSC.[61] The mean age was 38 years among 19 males and 15 females who had a mean follow-up of 103 months. Twenty of the 34 had IBD: 56 percent UC and 36 percent Crohn's disease. Liver biopsies showed stage 1 lesions in 80 percent and stages 2 or 3 in 20 percent (see Primary Sclerosing Cholangitis Pathology). Symptoms were present in 10 of 34 at diagnosis and subsequently developed in 8 of 24 who were asymptomatic. Ten of the 34 were treated with ursodeoxycholic acid. During serial evaluation with endoscopic retrograde cholangiopancreatography (ERCP) only 4 of 34 (12 percent) developed cholangiographic evidence of PSC and 2 required liver transplantation. In the 30 with persistently normal cholangiograms, 1 developed portal hypertension, 1 died of a liver-related cause, and another from cardiac disease. These findings suggest that a minority of patients with small-duct disease progress to macroscopic strictures, despite evidence of progressive hepatic dysfunction resulting from ductopenia.

The previous information supports the decision to abandon the term *pericholangitis* from the nomenclature because of its lack of disease specificity. Currently, it appears that the majority of patients previously reported to have pericholangitis have PSC involving either the small ducts alone (microscopic disease) or both small and larger ducts (macroscopic disease with strictures on cholangiography). Because the histopathologic features observed on liver biopsies of patients with PSC are mostly compatible with the diagnosis rather than pathognomonic, a comprehensive differential diagnosis, including viral hepatitis, AIH, hepatotoxic drug injury, and genetic and metabolic diseases is warranted for IBD patients with biopsies showing portal inflammation.

To determine the characteristics of patients with concomitant liver disease and UC in the absence of cholangiographic evidence of PSC, Boberg and colleagues retrospectively assessed 69 patients.[62] ERCP demonstrated extrahepatic biliary sclerosis in 51 of 69 (80 percent), whereas 13 of the remaining 18 had PSC of the intrahepatic ducts. Thus 5 of 69 (7 percent) patients exclusively had pericholangitis or small-duct PSC. They were indistinguishable from those with macroscopic strictures with respect to extent of UC, biochemical, or histopathologic features.

Hepatotoxicity of Medications

The possibility that abnormalities of liver tests are due to hepatotoxicity of medications must be considered in every patient. Hypersensitivity reactions to sulfonamides, especially sulfasalazine, are rare, but can be fatal.[10,19,54] Azathioprine therapy of IBD can cause hepatocellular injury through three mechanisms—hypersensitivity, idiosyncratic reactions, and an endothelial toxicity manifested as peliosis hepatis or venoocclusive disease. Intravenous azathioprine for severe UC caused hepatotoxicity in one of nine patients[63] and facilitated development of cytomegalovirus hepatitis in two patients with Crohn's disease.[64] The hepatic effects of long-term methotrexate treatment of IBD were evaluated in 32 patients with cumulative doses of 1.5 to 5.4 g. Nineteen of 20 patients (95 percent) who had liver biopsies had mild histologic abnormalities and the other patient had hepatic fibrosis.[65] Fourteen of the 20 patients, including the one with fibrosis, had normal liver biochemical tests. Cyclosporine, used for aggressive treatment of refractory IBD, can also cause hepatotoxicity, especially in patients with preexisting abnormal liver tests or those receiving total parenteral nutrition.[66] Intravenous cyclosporine caused ALT elevation in 6 of 24 patients with severe UC, including 5 of the 8 (62.5 percent) receiving total parenteral nutrition.[67] This contrasts with the 37 percent incidence of abnormal livers tests induced by total parenteral nutrition alone in UC patients. Nonsteroidal anti-inflammatory drugs (NSAIDs) also cause hepatotoxicity through idiosyncratic reactions or hypersensitivity.[68] Hepatoxicity is more frequent with aspirin, diclofenac, and sulindac than with other NSAIDs. Hepatic lesions in patients with IBD that are compatible with sulfonamide toxicity include hepatocellular necrosis, focal necrosis, granulomatous hepatitis, and chronic hepatitis.

FATTY LIVER

Fatty liver is defined as an acquired disorder of metabolism resulting in accumulation of triglycerides within hepatocytes in quantities sufficient to be visible by light microscopy.[56] Many processes may lead to such accumulations[37] and several are associated with progressive hepatic disease. The accumulation of fat within hepatocytes does not necessarily result in necrosis, inflammation, fibrosis, or cirrhosis and is potentially reversible. In contrast, hepatocytic fat associated with hepatocellular necrosis, inflammation, Mallory hyaline or perisinusoidal fibrosis in the absence of alcohol (non-alcoholic steatohepatitis [NASH]) can progress to cirrhosis (see Chap. 30). The biochemical features and pathophysiology of fatty liver disease are discussed in Chap. 3. Fatty liver occurs in patients with both UC and Crohn's disease (Table 40-2). Typically, diffuse macrovesicular fat is observed, although some report preferential distribution in the centrolobular or periportal areas.[10,19,21,49] Fat often is present concurrently with other histologic lesions, which makes interpretation of the clinical and biochemical significance of fatty liver more difficult.[18,22,27,49,69]

Fatty liver has been described in most reports of large series of patients. Reported frequencies range from 0 percent to 80 percent, with a mean of 33 percent (see Table 40-2). Analysis of the individual studies is complicated by variations in the diagnostic criteria. These range from the inclusion of all patients with any evidence of fat in the biopsy specimen to inclusion of only patients considered to have "severe" fatty changes. Based on autopsy studies, fatty liver is the hepatobiliary disorder most frequently associated with IBD. This impression probably is erroneous, because the frequency of fatty liver often is much lower in liver biopsy specimens from living patients as compared with liver obtained at autopsy.[27,52]

Individual investigators debate the relationship between fatty liver and the severity, duration, or extent of UC or Crohn's disease. Many reported patients have been chronically ill and often severely malnourished. This is especially true for patients in whom the fatty change is most extensive and for patients in autopsy series. The possibility that terminal illness and malnutrition contribute to the production of fatty liver led to a comparison of the frequency of fatty liver in patients dying from UC and those dying from other causes.[25,26] In one study 15 percent of autopsies in the UC group showed fatty liver, as compared with only 1.4 percent of 1000 unselected autopsies.[25] In the other study the frequency of fatty liver was 54 percent in patients with UC, 26 percent in unselected control patients, and 41 percent in patients dying from "debilitating causes."[26] These studies suggest that factors other than malnutrition are important in the development of fatty liver in patients with IBD.

In general, most patients with fatty liver are asymptomatic with respect to symptoms of liver disease. Examples to the contrary often represent patients in whom fatty liver occurs concomitantly with other hepatic lesions.[27] It is not possible to ascribe clinical or biochemical abnormalities to the presence of fat alone in such patients. The physical examination usually shows no abnormality but hepatomegaly may be present. Results of laboratory investigations of patients with fatty liver tend to be normal, but abnormal tests have been reported, especially for patients with histologic evidence of additional diseases. The specific patterns of laboratory abnormalities in such patients are those associated with the additional diseases.

The fatty infiltration may subside in seriously ill patients who respond to therapy for their IBD and malnutrition.[10,18,27] Persistence of fat, however, has been documented in several instances when repeat biopsies have been obtained.[10,18] The presence of fat alone is not associated with progressive hepatic damage in patients with IBD, but progression to fibrosis and cirrhosis can occur with NASH.

The pathogenesis of fatty liver in IBD is not known, but circumstantial evidence suggests that it is multi-factorial. Patients who have severe, debilitating illness and malnutrition may have protein-calorie malnutrition, a known cause of fatty liver.[55] A possible relationship between malnutrition and fatty liver is suggested by the finding that patients with UC or Crohn's disease and fatty livers have lower serum levels of carotene than do patients with either pericholangitis or cirrhosis.[18] Corticosteroids may contribute to the production of fatty liver[70,71] and have been used in the treatment of most reported patients with severe IBD. Fatty liver occurs, however, in a substantial number of patients not receiving corticosteroids. The possible role of unrecognized alcohol abuse is undefined. Several studies have attempted to exclude patients with alcoholism, but these have relied solely on a negative history. The possibility that some bacterial metabolite or chemical toxin induces fatty change in patients with IBD remains speculative. It is most likely that the same metabolic and dietary factors that cause fatty liver and NASH in the general population are involved in patients with IBD.

Treatment should be directed toward the IBD itself and restoration of protein-calorie nutrition. Resection of the bowel is neither beneficial nor indicated for the hepatic lesion. Eade and associates showed that the frequency of fatty liver was the same 3 to 7 years after colectomy for UC as it had been at the time of the bowel resection.[72] Comparable data have not been reported in Crohn's disease.

TABLE 40-2

Fatty Liver in Selected Series of Patients with IBD

Series	Type of IBD	Number of patients with liver biopsy	Frequency (%)	FEATURES OF HEPATIC DISEASE		
				Clinical	Laboratory	Comments
Kimmelstiel et al[25]	UC	93	15		—	Reports only *severe* fat accumulation
Kleckner et al[42]	UC	32	28	No physical findings of hepatic disease	Abnormal BSP retention	Reports all instances of fat accumulation
Boden et al[43]	UC	10	0	Jaundice, hepatosplenomegaly frequent	↑ AP, bili, abnormal BSP	—
Ross et al[100]	UC	17	0	Hepatosplenomegaly frequent	—	—
Eade[49]	UC	132	45	—	↑ AP	Reports all instances of fat accumulation; fat present with other lesions; severe fatty liver present in 14%
Palmer et al[26]	UC	51	54	—	—	Fat present with other lesions
Mistilis[27]	UC	49 living	12	—	—	Fat frequently associated with pericholangitis
Mistilis and Goulston[46]	34 autopsy	47	—	—	Frequency in autopsy groups may reflect effects of terminal illness	Vinnik et al[44]
	UC	8	0	—	—	—
de Dombal et al[69]	UC	58	83	—	—	Fat associated with portal tract inflammation
Stauffer et al[50]	UC	30	0	—	—	—
Perrett et al[10]	UC	50	38	—	↑ AP, abnormal BSP retention	Most severe fat accumulation in patients requiring emergency colectomy
Chapin et al[15]	CD of small bowel	39	51	—	—	Patients severely debilitated with high frequency of terminal infections; reports all instances of fat accumulation
Palmer et al[17]	CD of small bowel	8	25	Hepatosplenomegaly	—	Patients severely malnourished
Cohen et al[455]	CD of small bowel	19	37	—	—	Fat accumulation focal in 66%; fat present with other lesions
Kleckner[457]	CD of small bowel	20	15	Asymptomatic, no physical signs	Abnormal BSP retention in 1 patient	—
Perrett et al[19]	CD	39	21	—	—	Fat present with other lesions
Eade et al[22]	CD of small bowel, colon, or small bowel and colon	49	38	—	—	Reports all instances of fat accumulation
Eade et al[21]	CD of colon	20	40	—	—	—

IBD, Inflammatory bowel disease; *UC,* ulcerative colitis; *BSP,* bromsulphalein (sulfobromophthalein); *AP,* alkaline phosphatase; *bili,* bilirubin; —, not available; *CD,* Crohn's disease;.

Continued

TABLE 40-2
Fatty Liver in Selected Series of Patients with IBD

				FEATURES OF HEPATIC DISEASE		
Series	Type of IBD	Number of patients with liver biopsy	Frequency (%)	Clinical	Laboratory	Comments
Dordal et al[18]	CD of small bowel or small bowel and colon	27	26	—	↑AP; abnormal BSP retention in some, rare: ↑ bili	Fat present with other lesions
	UC	76	20	—	—	—
Dew et al[20]	CD	~32	0	—	↑AP (criterion for selection)	—
	UC	~51	0			
Monto[16]	UC	100	80	—	—	Clinical and laboratory data not matched to histology
	CD of small bowel	4	75	—	—	—
Perold et al[33]	UC	10	20	—	↑AST or BSP retention	Prospective study; mild fat deposition in centrolobular areas without other histopathologic lesions
Wee and Ludwig[37]	UC	107	24	—	↑AP, AST	Retrospective study; inconspicuous fat present in 43% of patients with small- or large-duct sclerosis; 2 other patients had true steatohepatitis
Ludwig et al[52]	UC	42	10	—	↑AP, AST	Retrospective study; of 23 patients with PSC, 9% had fat; of 19 patients with abnormal liver tests and normal bile ducts, 11% had fat

AUTOIMMUNE HEPATITIS

AIH is associated with IBD, but our current knowledge is limited by historic confusion about diagnostic nomenclature and failure to appreciate that histopathologic features of AIH are commonly observed in PSC.[32-35,37,52,55] Chronic hepatitis with interface hepatitis (piecemeal necrosis) was referred to historically as chronic active hepatitis.[34] Before diagnostic tests for hepatitis B and C, chronic active hepatitis was believed by many to be diagnostic of AIH and potentially responsive to immunosuppressive therapy. Thus many patients with PSC were incorrectly diagnosed as having AIH by liver biopsy.[34] Currently, two types of AIH are recognized on the basis of their autoantibody profiles. Type 1 is associated with antinuclear antibody (ANA) or smooth muscle antibody (SMA) autoantibodies and 50 percent to 96 percent of patients have anti-neutrophil cytoplasmic antibodies (pANCA).[73] The prevalence of pANCA in UC is 60 percent to 87 percent, which can create diagnostic uncertainty.[74] Type 2 is characterized by autoantibodies recognizing LKM1, and CYP 2D6 is the principal target epitope. Patients with PSC also have high prevalences of type 1 autoantibodies: 7 percent to 77 percent for ANA and 13 percent to 20 percent for SMA.[74] Type 2 AIH does not appear to be associated with IBD. One patient has been reported with autoantibodies against SLA,[75] which is now recognized as being specific for AIH but not representative of a distinctly different type of disease (see Chap. 38).

A recent study of patients with severe autoimmune hepatitis assessed the prevalence and impact of UC and the frequency of cholangiographic or histologic features of PSC in those found to have colitis.[76] Seventeen of 105 patients (16 percent) who had a screening colonoscopy had evidence of UC, and 5 of 12 of these patients who had cholangiograms had PSC. The patients with and without abnormal cholangiograms were indistinguishable with respect to clinical, biochemical, serologic, and histologic features. Obliterative fibrous cholangitis was found in two patients, one of whom had a normal cholangiogram. Patients with autoimmune hepatitis and UC responded well to immunosuppressive therapy. Thus autoimmune hepatitis and UC appear to be associated diseases, and concurrent colitis does not alter the response to therapy. In addition, cholangiography is required to differentiate autoimmune hepatitis from PSC in all patients with associated IBD (see section on Primary Sclerosing Cholangitis).

PSC patients not only may have features resembling type 1 AIH, but both diseases occur as an overlap syndrome in a minority of patients.[77-84] Application of the original version of an international diagnostic scoring system for AIH to 114 patients with unequivocal PSC resulted in 2 percent being classified as definite and 33 percent as probable for AIH.[85] Using the newest revision of the diagnostic scoring system for AIH to assess 211 PSC patients showed that only 1.4 percent were classified as definite and 6 percent as probable.[80] Distinction may be particularly difficult in PSC patients with only small-duct pathology and a normal cholangiogram.[86] Thus a diagnosis of PSC, AIH, and an overlap syndrome should be considered in all patients with IBD, abnormal liver tests, and autoantibodies.[60,64,76,87,88]

This differential diagnosis is particularly germane to children, who may exhibit both AIH and PSC sequentially or as an overlap syndrome. A 16-year prospective study of 55 children with hepatobiliary disease and ANA, SMA, or LKM1 autoantibodies showed that 27 of 55 (49 percent) had cholangiographic evidence of PSC.[82] IBD was strongly associated with presence of the overlap syndrome. Twenty-six of the 27 with overlap syndrome had ANA or SMA, whereas 1 had LKM1 autoantibodies. Both patients with overlap and AIH alone responded to immunosuppression, but cholangiographic progression occurred in the majority. One child with UC and AIH developed PSC after 8 years of follow-up.

Frequency

The frequency of histologic chronic hepatitis in association with IBD varies. In several early series of patients with UC and Crohn's disease chronic hepatitis was either absent or rare.[10,18-22,49] In contrast, Mistilis reported that 16 percent of patients receiving biopsies had chronic hepatitis.[27] One prospective study of patients with UC showed active hepatitis in 1 percent,[48] whereas another prospective study of UC showed a frequency of 20 percent.[33] Estimates of the frequency of chronic hepatitis associated with IBD have also been made by determining the prevalence of IBD in groups of patients selected because of the presence of liver disease.[28,89-93] These estimates, ranging from 4 percent to 28 percent, are biased by the selection of patients with moderate to severe symptomatic liver disease. Similar studies of the prevalence of IBD have not been made in patients with chronic active hepatitis who are asymptomatic or who have only moderately abnormal liver tests.

Wilcox and Isselbacher found UC in 7 of 33 patients less than 40 years old with chronic hepatitis,[28] but in none of 143 patients more than 40 years old with chronic hepatitis. Gray and co-workers reported eight patients with chronic hepatitis and IBD with concurrent evidence of autoimmune phenomenon.[92] MacKay and Wood reported that 5 of 22 patients with ""lupoid hepatitis"" (autoimmune hepatitis) had UC.[91] Read and associates reported 5 instances of UC among 81 patients with cirrhosis presumed to be secondary to chronic hepatitis.[89] Holdsworth and colleagues reported 22 patients with UC and chronic hepatitis seen over a 4-year period, 20 of whom had cirrhosis.[90] In keeping with the observation of Wilcox and Isselbacher these cirrhotic patients were significantly younger than those in a group of 200 patients with cirrhosis not related to alcohol abuse, who did not have UC. Olsson and Hulten reported 25 patients with chronic hepatitis, 7 of whom had coexisting UC.[93] Mistilis, in the description of 14 patients with chronic pericholangitis, noted piecemeal necrosis in 11 and bridging necrosis in 7.[27] In his series chronic hepatitis was diagnosed on the initial biopsy in an additional 8 of 49 patients.

In a retrospective analysis from the Johns Hopkins Hospital 8 patients with postnecrotic cirrhosis attributed to chronic hepatitis were identified among 202 patients with UC (4 percent).[32] In each patient PSC was excluded during laparotomy for portal-systemic shunting or colectomy. In a prospective study of 10 consecutive patients with UC and abnormal liver tests 2 (20 percent) had histologic chronic hepatitis, but cholangiography was not performed to exclude PSC.[33] Continued observation of patients with UC at Oxford revealed that 23 percent of patients with PSC had been incorrectly diagnosed as having chronic hepatitis.[34] One patient (6 percent of the population with persistently abnormal liver tests) had steroid-responsive AIH, and two additional patients were found to have heterozygous α_1-antitrypsin deficiency. In a comprehensive retrospective analysis of UC patients at the Mayo Clinic 14 of 107 patients (13 percent) with concurrent hepatobiliary disease had chronic hepatitis.[37] One patient had hepatitis B and three had changes suggestive of post-transfusion hepatitis C. In the remaining 9 patients the chronic hepatitis was considered idiopathic.

To date, the majority of reported patients with IBD and chronic hepatitis have had UC. Chronic hepatitis has not been reported in most studies of patients with Crohn's disease.[15,17,18,21,22] Perrett and associates described a single such patient with chronic hepatitis,[19] whereas Dew and co-workers omitted chronic hepatitis as a diagnostic category in their study.[20] The complex effects of changing nomenclature, morphologic overlap with the definition of pericholangitis, and biases in patient selection make it impossible to define the true incidence of chronic hepatitis in association with IBD. It appears, however, that chronic hepatitis is associated with UC more frequently than would be expected by chance. The data for Crohn's disease do not support a similar conclusion.

Clinical Features

The duration of IBD before recognition of chronic hepatitis is variable. In most reports there are examples of patients with documented UC preceding chronic hepatitis, instances of concurrent onset, and examples of chronic hepatitis preceding the onset of UC. Crohn's disease (sites of involvement unspecified) preceded symptoms leading to the diagnosis of chronic hepatitis in the patient reported by Perrett and associates.[19]

The majority of reported patients have had symptomatic liver disease, which reflects the use of outdated diagnostic criteria emphasizing symptoms. Specific autoimmune features have included polyarthritis,[92] thyroiditis,[94] glomerulonephritis,[90,92] thrombocytopenic purpura,[92] non-thrombocytopenic purpura,[95] and pericarditis.[92] Physical findings generally include hepatomegaly, cutaneous stigmata of chronic liver disease, and occasionally splenomegaly, ascites, and edema. This again reflects the severity of the hepatic disease in these selected patients, many of whom had "active cirrhosis"" at the time of biopsy.

Reporting of laboratory tests has not been uniform. The abnormalities, as expected, include moderate to marked elevations of aminotransferase activity and variable elevations of total bilirubin and alkaline phosphatase. The majority of reported patients had elevated gamma globulins, and tests for lupus erythematosus cells or anti-nuclear antibodies were frequently positive for patients with associated autoimmune features. Tests for hepatitis B surface antigen, performed in only a minority of patients in early studies, were most often negative.[93-95] Positive tests for antibodies against nuclear and SMAs were common, whereas there were no positive tests for anti-mitochondrial antibodies (AMAs).[48,93] These autoantibodies suggest an autoimmune pathogenesis. However, a minority of patients with chronic hepatitis C (see Chap. 33) also has anti-nuclear and anti-smooth muscle antibodies, and patients with UC alone may have ANA, SMA, and pANCA.[96-98]

Natural History and Prognosis

The activity and progression of autoimmune hepatitis do not correlate with the extent of involvement or severity of the IBD.[48,89,95] Indeed, the activities of the liver and bowel diseases vary independently.[93] Chronic hepatitis associated with IBD progresses to cirrhosis* in accordance with the natural history of autoimmune hepatitis alone.

Pathogenesis

The pathogenesis of type 1 AIH has not been elucidated. The autoantibodies present in patients with AIH are not organ-specific, and there is no evidence that they contribute to hepatic inflammation. The immunopathology of AIH suggests a direct role for the cellular immune system, presumably generated by a triggering event leading to a loss of tolerance to hepatic self-antigens in an immunogenetically predisposed individual. Other causes of chronic hepatitis can result in histopathology indistinguishable from autoimmune hepatitis including hepatitis B and C infections, hepatotoxic reactions to medications, and PSC.

Therapy

Corticosteroids have been used in symptomatic patients with presumed AIH associated with IBD. Gray and associates reported responses to steroids that were moderate to excellent in five and poor in three of eight patients with UC and chronic hepatitis with autoimmune features.[92] In the report of Read and co-workers 43 of 81 patients with chronic hepatitis and "active" cirrhosis were treated with corticosteroids.[89] It is difficult to determine whether all five of the patients with UC in this series were treated; however, one patient developed UC while receiving corticosteroids for chronic hepatitis. Overall, corticosteroids reduced symptoms in the treated patients, but did not prevent progression of the liver disease or prolong life. Harris and Neugarten described an excellent response to corticosteroids in a woman with chronic hepatitis, non-thrombocytopenic purpura, hypergammaglobulinemia, and positive tests for rheumatoid factor and Venereal Disease Research Laboratory (VDRL).[95] Czaja and Wolf compared the results of corticosteroid therapy in 8 patients with chronic hepatitis and UC with the results in 141 patients, including 25 patients who had associated immunopathic diseases.[96] Although corticosteroids alleviated the UC in each patient, their effect on the chronic hepatitis was consistently unsatisfactory. Indeed, a statis-

*References 28, 37, 89, 90, 92, 93.

tically significant decrease in remissions of chronic hepatitis and an increase in treatment failures were found in these patients. The possibility that UC adversely affects the responsiveness of AIH to corticosteroids is controversial. A larger study concluded that patients with AIH and UC responded well to immunosuppression.[76]

The effect of colectomy on putative AIH has been assessed in patients with severe UC.[28,93] In one series six patients had received corticosteroids or azathioprine for durations of more than a year before surgery.[93] Colectomy was performed on five patients because of exacerbations of colitis and was needed in one case because of colonic carcinoma. The activity of liver disease was assessed as mild to moderate at the time of surgery. After colectomy spontaneous improvement in abnormal results of liver tests was found for four of the six patients. Further studies of larger numbers of patients are needed to assess the role of colectomy in the treatment of chronic hepatitis associated with IBD.

FIBROSIS AND CIRRHOSIS

Conspicuous fibrosis and cirrhosis have been found in most large series of patients with IBD (Table 40-3). As discussed previously, "pericholangitis," chronic hepatitis, and PSC have been associated with progression to fibrosis and cirrhosis.

Pathology

Cirrhosis is characterized by extensive fibrosis and the presence of regenerative parenchymal nodules.[55] Regenerative nodules may contain hepatocytes from one or more than one lobule and are separated from adjacent nodules by fibrous tissue. The diagnosis of cirrhosis remains problematic, especially with percutaneous needle biopsy specimens, which may be too small to permit differentiation between fibrosis and cirrhosis. Thus the potential exists for either underestimating or overestimating the presence of cirrhosis in such specimens. Because of problems in distinguishing fibrosis and cirrhosis in many reports, the data for fibrosis and cirrhosis have been combined in Table 40-3.

Morphologic classification of cirrhosis is based on the sizes of regenerative nodules (micronodular, macronodular, and mixed macronodular and micronodular).[55] These terms replace most of the terms employed in the series summarized in Table 40-3 but offer no heuristic advantage. For clarity, both the current terms and those used in the individual reports have been tabulated. Cirrhosis in the majority of patients has been described as "postnecrotic" (macronodular),* with occasional examples of "portal or Laennec's" (micronodular) cirrhosis,† and "biliary cirrhosis,"[17,18,26,97,102] including "primary biliary cirrhosis."[26,39,50] In addition, Dordal and co-workers and Eade and associates use the term *bridging portal hepatofibrosis* to describe cirrhosis characterized by fibrosis extending between adjacent portal areas, distorted lobular architecture, regenerative nodules, and proliferation of bile ducts.[18,49]

*References 10, 17, 26, 27, 32, 34, 35, 37, 42, 47, 52, 69, 100, 101.

†References 19, 20, 26, 47, 50, 101.

Frequency and Clinical Features

The reported frequency of cirrhosis among patients with IBD varies widely (see Table 40-3). The range in UC is 0 percent to 45 percent, with an average of 12 percent. The range in Crohn's disease is 0 percent to 29 percent, with an average of 12 percent. Overall, the prevalence of cirrhosis appears to be between 1 percent and 5 percent in both UC and Crohn's disease. The prevalence was 1.2 percent in a prospective study of patients with UC.[48] The prevalence of cirrhosis in patients with IBD appears to exceed that expected in the general population. In one study by Kimmelstiel and colleagues the prevalence of cirrhosis was identical for patients with UC and control patients.[25] On the other hand, the autopsy study of Palmer and associates showed that the frequency of cirrhosis in patients with UC was increased twelvefold over that in the control group.[26] In patients selected solely on the basis of cirrhosis the prevalence of UC is five to six times greater than that in the general population.[89,90] Cirrhosis associated with Crohn's disease limited to the small bowel was absent in some studies,[16,22] but was present in others[15,17] In general, cirrhosis occurs more commonly in patients with extensive UC[10,20,32] or Crohn's colitis.[20,21] The frequency of cirrhosis appears to be comparable for patients with UC and those with Crohn's colitis, although fewer of the latter patients have been reported.[21]

Clinical features attributable to fibrosis alone are minimal in patients with IBD. The fibrosis primarily involves the portal tract and rarely is associated with portal venous hypertension (see section on Pericholangitis). The clinical features of the lesions associated with fibrosis, pericholangitis, and chronic hepatitis have been discussed previously. The clinical and laboratory features of patients with IBD and cirrhosis vary. Some patients are asymptomatic and have minimal abnormalities of liver tests.[20] Other patients have overt symptoms and signs of decompensated liver disease and marked abnormalities in liver tests. The clinical and laboratory features in symptomatic patients are similar to those seen in patients with chronic pericholangitis or chronic hepatitis (discussed previously). In more advanced cases complications of portal venous hypertension[20,32,103] may occur.

Natural History

The presence of IBD does not appear to influence the course of patients with cirrhosis as compared with that of cirrhotic patients without IBD. Hemorrhage from esophageal varices may occur in the former group, and recurrence can be prevented by portal-systemic shunting.[32,103] In patients with cirrhosis and UC or Crohn's colitis bleeding can occur from varices of the ileal stoma after colectomy.* In severe cases portal-systemic shunt surgery or liver transplantation has controlled the ileal bleeding.[109-111] Risk factors for the development of

*References 20, 91-93, 95, 99, 101, 104-111.

TABLE 40-3

Fibrosis and Cirrhosis in Selected Series of Patients with IBD

Series	Type of IBD	Number of patients with liver biopsy	Histologic term	Frequency (%)	FEATURES OF HEPATIC DISEASE: Clinical	FEATURES OF HEPATIC DISEASE: Laboratory	Comments*
Kimmelstiel et al[25]	UC	93	Fibrosis	1	Hepatomegaly	—	Fibrosis described as pseudolobulation: possibly true cirrhosis
			Cirrhosis	1	Jaundiced terminally	—	
Kleckner et al[42]	UC	32	Portal cirrhosis (micronodular); postnecrotic cirrhosis (macronodular); biliary cirrhosis	19	Hepatosplenomegaly; occasional jaundice, edema, ascites	Abnormal BSP retention, ↑ bili normal cholesterol	—
Boden et al[39]	UC	10	Biliary cirrhosis	20	Jaundice, hepatosplenomegaly, ascites	↑ AP, bili, abnormal BSP retention	One patient with pericholangitis progressing to cirrhosis
Ross et al[100]	UC	17	Portal cirrhosis (micronodular); postnecrotic cirrhosis (macronodular); biliary cirrhosis	76	Jaundice, hepatosplenomegaly	—	—
Eade[49]	UC	132	Fibrosis; cirrhosis	51	—	↑ AP, ↑ globulin, ↑ alb	Inflammatory infiltrates frequently present with fibrosis
			Fibrosis	4.5			
Palmer et al[26]	UC	51	Portal cirrhosis (micronodular); postnecrotic cirrhosis (macronodular); biliary cirrhosis	8	—	—	Two patients with cirrhosis secondary to biliary obstruction; 1 with choledocolithiasis, 1 with benign cholangioma
				12	Jaundice, hepatosplenomegaly, portal venous hypertension	↑ AP, bili, abnormal BSP retention	
Mistilis[27]	UC	49 living; 34 autopsy	Fibrosis	29	—	—	Fibrosis associated with subacute and chronic pericholangitis; cirrhosis preceded by pericholangitis in 50%
			Postnecrotic cirrhosis (macronodular)	12	—	—	
			Fibrosis	24			Fibrosis associated with chronic pericholangitis
de Dombal et al[69]	UC	58	Portal cirrhosis (micronodular)	2	—	—	Cirrhosis associated with fatty liver
Stauffer et al[50]	UC	30	Fibrosis	3	Jaundice, hepatosplenomegaly, portal venous hypertension	↑ AP, bili, AST, abnormal BSP retention	Patient with "primary biliary cirrhosis" had sclerosis of the common bile duct at surgery
			Portal cirrhosis (micronodular); postnecrotic cirrhosis (macronodular); primary biliary cirrhosis	20			

IBD, Inflammatory bowel disease; *UC,* ulcerative colitis; —, not available; *BSP,* bromsulphaleim (sulfobromophthalein); *bili,* bilirubin; *AP,* alkaline phosphatase; *AST,* aspartate aminotransferase (SGOT); *CD,* Crohn's disease.

*See Table 40-2 for general comments regarding each study.

Perrett et al[10]	UC	50	Postnecrotic cirrhosis (macronodular)	6	Jaundice	↑ AP, bili, ALT, abnormal BSP retention	—
Chapin et al[15]	CD of small bowel	39	Portal cirrhosis (micronodular)	8	—	—	66% with cirrhosis had a medical history of alcohol abuse
Palmer et al[17]	CD of small bowel	8	Portal cirrhosis (micronodular) Biliary cirrhosis	43	—	—	Hepatosplenomegaly
Cohen et al[455]	CD of small bowel	19	Fibrosis	26	—	—	All fibrosis associated with chronic pericholangitis; cirrhotic liver contained hemosiderin
Perrett et al[19]	CD	39	Fibrosis Portal cirrhosis (micronodular)	16 5	—	—	
Eade et al[22]	CD of small bowel, colon of small bowel and colon	49	Fibrosis	54	—	—	Fibrosis frequently associated with inflammatory infiltration of portal tracts; cirrhosis not present
Eade et al[21]	CD of colon	20	Fibrosis Micronodular cirrhosis	35 10	Jaundice in 1 cirrhotic	—	—
Dordal et al[18]	CD of small bowel of small bowel and colon	27	Cirrhosis of "bridging portal hepatofibrosis"	19	—	—	—
	UC	76	Same as above	20	—	—	One cirrhotic patient developed a cholangiocarcinoma
Dew et al[20]	CD	~32	Cirrhosis	9	Portal venous hypertension	↑ AP (criterion for selection)	—
	UC	~51	Cirrhosis	22	Portal venous hypertension	↑ AP (criterion for selection)	
Monto[16]	UC	100	Fibrosis "Early" cirrhosis	7 1	—	—	Fibrosis frequently associated with bile duct proliferation and fatty infiltration
	CD of small bowel	4	Fibrosis	75	—	—	
Lupinetti et al[32]	UC	Unstated	Cirrhosis	?	Moderate-to-severe portal hypertension	—	Retrospective study; 5 of 8 required portal-systemic shunts
Shepard et al[34]	UC	21	Cirrhosis	5	—	—	Prospective study; 1 cirrhotic
Steckman et al[35]	UC	6	Fibrosis	100	Jaundice, hepatomegaly	↑ AP, AST	Prospective study; 3 with progressive fibrosis, 3 with cirrhosis; all patients had liver disease before onset of UC

Continued

TABLE 40-3

Fibrosis and Cirrhosis in Selected Series of Patients with IBD—cont'd

					FEATURES OF HEPATIC DISEASE		
Series	Type of IBD	Number of patients with liver biopsy	Histologic term	Frequency (%)	Clinical	Laboratory	Comments*
Wee and Ludwig[37]		107				↑ AP, AST	Retrospective study of referred patients; 10 patients had small- or large-duct sclerosing cholangitis; 11 had chronic active hepatitis; 12 had cryptogenic cirrhosis
	UC		Cirrhosis	31	—		
Ludwig et al[52]		23				↑ AP, AST	Retrospective study; cirrhosis in 22% of 23 patients with PSC
	UC	20	Cirrhosis	22	—	↑ AP, AST	Cirrhosis in 45% of 20 patients with PSC in the absence of UC
	—		Cirrhosis	45	—		
		19				↑ AP, AST	Cirrhosis in 42% of 19 patients with UC in the absence of PSC
	UC		Cirrhosis	42	—		

peristomal bleeding after colectomy in patients with hepatobiliary disease include cirrhosis, splenomegaly, esophageal varices, low serum albumin, prolonged prothrombin time, and thrombocytopenia.[111] In such patients a proctocolectomy with ileoanal anastomosis should be considered because perirectal bleeding has not been observed.[111] Hepatocellular carcinoma has been reported to occur in patients with UC as a late complication of cirrhosis.[20,49,112]

Pathogenesis

The majority of cases of cirrhosis in patients with IBD result from PSC, AIH, or an overlap syndrome. The contribution of other etiologies, such as chronic hepatitis B or C and NASH, has not been defined. Cholangiography or surgery was performed in only a small proportion of patients with cirrhosis in early series to assess the presence of mechanical biliary obstruction or sclerosing cholangitis.[30,48,50]

In recent series employing cholangiography and liver biopsy for the diagnosis of PSC, cirrhosis has been very common.[35,37,52,113] The series of Steckman and co-workers is notable because five patients were evaluated for hepatobiliary disease before the clinical onset of UC.[35] Each of the five had PSC; one had cirrhosis at initial presentation, one developed cirrhosis during follow-up, and in two patients their disease progressed to severe fibrosis. Eight of 18 patients (44 percent) with classic large-duct sclerosing cholangitis studied at the Mayo Clinic had cirrhosis.[37] Among an additional group of patients with PSC and UC at the same institution, 5 of 23 (22 percent) had cirrhosis.[52] Over a period of 2 to 8 years Schrumpf and associates noted progression of disease in 14 patients with PSC and UC.[113] Thus PSC is the most important disease causing cirrhosis in patients with IBD.

As mentioned in the discussion of pericholangitis, the histologic features of mechanical obstruction and sclerosing cholangitis can be indistinguishable from those of pericholangitis, and both can progress to cirrhosis. The diagnosis of PBC in early reports of patients with IBD is probably erroneous.[27] There is no evidence that PBC contributes to the incidence of cirrhosis in patients with IBD, although coincidental occurrence of PBC has been reported.[114,115]

Therapy

There is no effective treatment for established fibrosis or cirrhosis. Therapy should be directed instead against the process(es) responsible for continued hepatocellular necrosis and fibrogenesis (see the sections on Pericholangitis, Chronic Hepatitis, and Primary Sclerosing Cholangitis). Colectomy is not appropriate therapy because its effectiveness is unproved.[20,21,32,49]

AMYLOIDOSIS

Amyloid infiltration of the liver has been reported to occur in patients with both UC and Crohn's disease (see Chap. 52).* Amyloidosis has been suspected generally on the basis of extrahepatic manifestations such as nephropathy, although in several reports amyloidosis was disclosed by liver biopsy in the absence of any previous clinical suspicion.

*References 10, 15, 17, 18, 21, 22, 49, 107, 116-118.

Pathology

Hepatic amyloid has been detected in patients with IBD on the basis of its affinity for Congo red. The distribution of the amyloid includes the media of vessels in the portal tract and the reticulin framework of the hepatic cords. Atrophy of hepatocytes may occur as a secondary consequence of compression. It is now recognized that the major protein components of amyloid fibrils vary in different organs, and that specific protein components are related to distinct clinicopathologic conditions.[119] *Reactive systemic amyloidosis* is preferred over the older term *secondary amyloidosis*[119] to describe the type of amyloidosis seen in patients with IBD. The major fibrillar protein in reactive systemic amyloidosis is AA, and the characteristic sites of deposition are the liver, spleen, and kidney.

Frequency and Clinical Features

Amyloidosis of the liver or other organs is rare among patients with IBD and occurs more often in patients with Crohn's disease.* Shorvon, in a review of the association between amyloidosis and IBD, summarized the findings in 41 patients reported since 1936.[118] He excluded nine patients because of inadequate diagnostic information. Of the remaining 33 patients, 18 had Crohn's disease and 15 were reported to have UC. The majority of the 15 cases of UC, however, were diagnosed before the clinical recognition of Crohn's colitis and 14 had features suggesting the diagnosis of Crohn's colitis. These features included jejunal or ileal disease, fistulae, perianal disease, rectal sparing, and inflammation of the full thickness of the colon. Eade, using pathologic changes in colectomy specimens as the diagnostic criterion for UC, found 1 case of hepatic amyloidosis among 132 consecutive patients with UC undergoing colectomy and liver biopsy.[49] Others have also noted that reactive systemic amyloidosis is rare in UC.[117] Amyloidosis occurs in patients with Crohn's disease regardless of the site of anatomic involvement. For example, amyloidosis was found in 1 of 62 patients with Crohn's colitis, 3 of 223 with ileocolitis, and 1 of 213 with exclusive small bowel involvement[107]—all five of these patients had renal involvement. Hepatic involvement, although anticipated, was not mentioned. The incidence of amyloidosis in Crohn's disease in a large longitudinal study was 15 of 1709 (0.9 percent) patients with an anatomic distribution of 706 with ileocolitis, 310 with colitis, and 693 with small bowel disease.[120] Thus colitis was associated with amyloidosis 4.4 times more often than with disease limited to the small bowel. In contrast, only 1 of 1341 (0.07 percent) patients with UC developed amyloidosis. Multiple organs were affected, resulting in hepatosplenomegaly, nephropathy, cardiomyopathy, and enteropathy.

*References 10, 15, 17, 18, 21, 22, 49, 118.

Clinical features have not been reported in most articles describing amyloidosis in IBD, except for the frequent occurrence of proteinuria. It is important to note, however, that the majority of patients with amyloidosis also have foci of chronic suppuration as extraintestinal complications of their IBD.[118] In addition, some patients have connective tissue diseases such as rheumatoid arthritis or ankylosing spondylitis.[116,117] The results of laboratory tests of patients with amyloidosis and IBD have not been reported. Based on the general experience with hepatic amyloidosis, evidence of hepatocellular necrosis is rare even with extensive deposition. Slight elevations of alkaline phosphatase, and, rarely, of bilirubin may occur.

Pathogenesis

Amyloid deposition in the liver is presumed to be secondary to chronic inflammation analogous to the amyloidoses associated with other chronic suppurative processes. The mechanism is unknown. The rare occurrence of amyloidosis in patients without extraintestinal foci of chronic suppuration or rheumatic disease suggests that inflammation of the bowel alone generally is insufficient to produce amyloidosis.

Prognosis and Treatment

Progressive amyloidosis is fatal if untreated. In reactive systemic amyloidosis the nature of the underlying disease and the rate of amyloid deposition determine the prognosis. Control of the underlying disease, in certain circumstances, has led to clinical recovery[119] but the applicability of this observation to patients with IBD remains undefined. In experimental models of reactive systemic amyloidosis, deposition can be increased by corticosteroids.[119] Despite these data, it seems unreasonable to withhold the use of corticosteroids if they are needed for the management of the IBD. There is no information concerning the possible usefulness of either colchicine or dimethyl sulfoxide in the treatment of hepatic amyloidosis associated with IBD.[119] Attempts to control extraintestinal foci of inflammation are rational, but may be difficult to accomplish.

HEPATIC GRANULOMAS

Hepatic granulomas (see Chap. 43) have been reported in several series.* The majority have been found in patients with Crohn's disease, although they also are seen in association with UC.[33,37,49] Frequencies in reported series range from 0 percent to 15 percent. The reports of Eade and colleagues describing patients with UC or Crohn's disease of either the small bowel or the colon suggest a frequency of approximately 8 percent.[21,22,49] In the series of Wee and Ludwig granulomas were present in 4 percent and were most frequently attributed to sarcoidosis.[37]

*References 14, 15, 18, 20-22, 26, 108, 109.

Pathology

The term *hepatic granulomatosis* describes the pathologic features more accurately than the term *granulomatous hepatitis*. The granulomas are non-caseating and are located in both the portal tracts and the parenchyma. Multi-nucleated giant cells have been present occasionally. In several instances aggregates of lymphocytes and histiocytes have been described as "granuloma-like."[21,22] Granulomas may be found alone or in association with fibrosis, fatty liver, pericholangitis, or cirrhosis.[18] One patient reported as having PBC in association with IBD had hepatic granulomas.[115]

Clinical Features and Prognosis

Available clinical detail is insufficient to assess whether patients with hepatic granulomatosis and IBD have any pathognomonic features. The majority is asymptomatic, and the abnormality found most commonly on laboratory testing is elevation of alkaline phosphatase. The prognosis for patients with hepatic granulomas and IBD is good. Such patients have not developed progressive liver disease or cirrhosis. One cirrhotic patient with UC, however, was found to have granulomas on repeat biopsy 2 years after the diagnosis of cirrhosis.[26] Another patient with hepatic granulomas and mild pericholangitis at the time of colectomy for UC subsequently developed a cholangiocarcinoma of the common bile duct.[58] Granulomas also were noted in a patient with chronic hepatitis associated with UC.[33]

Pathogenesis

The cause of hepatic granulomas in association with IBD remains unknown, and may be multi-factorial. Infectious agents do not appear to be the cause of the granulomas, and four patients in one series were thought to have sarcoidosis.[20,37] It is plausible that granulomas result from infrequent immune reactions to substances in portal venous blood or from deposits of immune complexes. The possibility of a drug-related pathogenesis is intriguing because hepatic granulomas occur as a consequence of sulfonamide hepatotoxicity.[121] Callen and Soderstrom reported one case of documented sulfasalazine-induced hepatic granulomas in a patient with UC.[123] Mesalamine was also reported to cause hepatic granulomas, fever, and cholestatic biochemical abnormalities in a patient with UC.[123]

Therapy

No specific therapy has been proposed for hepatic granulomas in patients with IBD. Treatment should be directed toward the IBD itself. The role of colectomy in the management of hepatic granulomas in patients with colitis is unknown. Eade and colleagues reported the results of repeat liver biopsies of two patients with hepatic granulomas 3 and 6 years after colectomy for Crohn's colitis.[21] Granulomas were decreased in number in one biopsy specimen and absent in the other.

MISCELLANEOUS DISORDERS

Several hepatic disorders have been reported to occur in only a few patients with IBD. The associations between most of these disorders and the IBD, therefore, appear to be coincidental. Pyogenic hepatic abscess represents a specific exception.

Hepatic Abscess

Before the availability of broad-spectrum anti-microbial therapy, pylephlebitis and pyogenic liver abscess were associated frequently with severe IBD. Today, hepatic abscesses in patients with IBD are rare.

Portal Vein Thrombosis

Chapin and co-workers reported four patients with Crohn's disease who developed thrombosis of the portal vein,[15] and Stauffer and associates found this complication in a patient with UC.[45]

Hepatic Infarction

Two patients dying of Crohn's disease had evidence of acute hepatic infarction and portal vein thrombosis at autopsy.[15]

Hepatic Venous Occlusion

Hepatic venous occlusion has been reported to occur in several patients with UC.[124] In one patient acute Budd-Chiari syndrome was the result of extrinsic compression of the hepatic veins by an anaplastic carcinoma of the bile duct.

Hepatic Sinusoidal Dilation

Sinusoidal dilation has been found rarely in patients with Crohn's disease.[125,126] Two reported patients were using oral contraceptives, which have been implicated in the pathogenesis of this lesion.[127]

Hepatoma

Hepatoma has been reported to occur in patients with cirrhosis and UC.[20,49,112]

Hemosiderosis

Perrett and associates reported that hemosiderosis was present in one patient with UC[10] and two patients with Crohn's disease.[19] Iron was present both in the hepatocytes and in the Kupffer cells in the patient with UC, who had a history of anemia and repeated transfusions. One of the patients with Crohn's disease had cirrhosis.

Sarcoidosis

Sarcoidosis of the liver has been reported in four patients with UC.[20,37]

Benign Neoplasia of the Bile Ducts

Palmer and colleagues reported one patient with UC and secondary biliary cirrhosis who had a benign cholangioma.[26]

Primary Biliary Cirrhosis

Early reports of PBC in association with IBD were probably erroneous because rigorous diagnostic criteria were unavailable and PSC was not excluded.[27] However, patients with unequivocal PBC and UC have been described.[114,115]

α_1-Antitrypsin Deficiency

Two patients with heterozygous α_1-antitrypsin deficiency were identified among 681 patients followed for UC in Oxford.[34] Both had persistently abnormal liver tests and low serum concentrations of α_1-antitrypsin. Each had the PiM_1Z phenotype, and immunoreactive granules of α_1-antitrypsin were identified in both biopsy specimens. Typical periodic acid–Schiff–positive, diastase-resistant granules, however, were present in only one patient.

PRIMARY SCLEROSING CHOLANGITIS

PSC is a chronic cholestatic liver disease afflicting children and adults that is characterized by segmental fibrosing inflammation of the intrahepatic or extrahepatic bile ducts.[60,128-133] Inflammation of small bile ducts produces microscopic disease, whereas that of medium to large intrahepatic or extrahepatic ducts produces a macroscopic disease detectable by cholangiography. Both microscopic and macroscopic disease lead to progressive narrowing or obliteration of bile duct lumens, biochemical and clinical features of cholestasis, and ultimately secondary biliary cirrhosis.[134] Cirrhotic patients are at risk for complications of portal hypertension and hepatic failure.[135-142] Patients with PSC, with or without cirrhosis, are at risk for cholangiocarcinoma,[143-147] indicating that PSC should be regarded as a premalignant condition. Introduction of endoscopic retrograde cholangiography in the early 1970s resulted in a marked increase in the frequency of diagnosis[148] and greatly contributed to the understanding of the clinical, radiologic, and histologic features of the disease. Despite these advances, the etiology and pathogenesis remain unknown, and no curative therapy has been identified. An immunopathogenesis of PSC is likely, based on strong associations with human leukocyte antigen (HLA) haptotypes, the presence of autoantibodies, and multiple immunologic abnormalities.[1,24,149-151]

Disease Associations

IBD

IBD occurs in 50 percent to 75 percent of patients with PSC.[30,31,148-151] The majority (87 percent to 98 percent) have UC; a minority (1.3 percent to 18 percent) have

Crohn's disease involving the colon (colitis or ileocolitis). PSC has been rarely reported with Crohn's disease restricted to the small bowel.[60,130]

AIH. As discussed previously, AIH is associated with IBD.* Clinical, laboratory, and histopathologic features of AIH[30,31,152] appear to co-exist in some patients.[77,82-85,87,154] Application of the original version of an international diagnostic scoring system for AIH in 114 patients with PSC showed that 2 percent could be classified as "definite" and 33 percent as "probable" AIH.[85] All five patients (four male) in another report met "definite" criteria for AIH and responded to therapy with corticosteroid and azathioprine.[84] Scoring of 211 patients with PSC showed that 4 (2 percent) met definite and 40 (19 percent) met probable criteria for AIH.[80] When a recently revised international diagnostic scoring system for AIH was used to assess these same 211 patients with PSC, 3 patients (1.4 percent) were classified as definitely having, 13 (6 percent) as probably having, and 195 (93 percent) as not having AIH. Significant differences between PSC patients with and without AIH were noted for total globulins, immunoglobulin (Ig)G levels, titers of autoantibodies, and histologic scores. These findings underscore the importance of endoscopic retrograde cholangiography (ERC) in diagnosing PSC and suggest that the prevalence of a PSC-AIH overlap syndrome is low. Distinction between AIH and PSC with only small-duct pathology and normal cholangiogram[86] is particularly difficult. In addition to IBD, secondary sclerosing cholangitis is associated with a variety of conditions (Table 40-4). The majority of secondary disease associations may be coincidental.

Twenty-five percent to 50 percent of cases of PSC occur in the absence of other diseases. Despite the legitimate question of whether PSC in association with IBD differs from that without IBD, no compelling evidence indicates that the processes are different. Clinical, biochemical, histologic, and cholangiographic features of PSC appear to be identical in patients with or without IBD.[148,155]

Diagnostic Criteria

Classic criteria for the diagnosis of PSC include (1) absence of previous biliary tract surgery, (2) absence of cholelithiasis, (3) diffuse involvement of the extrahepatic biliary tract, and (4) exclusion of cholangiocarcinoma. Warren argued that strict adherence to these criteria would lead to a correct diagnosis in most cases of PSC, but that indiscriminate application of the first three would exclude some cases of true PSC and hence underestimate both the frequency and the clinicopathologic spectrum of the disease.[156] Diagnostic criteria (Table 40-5) have been modified to include patients with cholelithiasis confined to the gallbladder[30,37,52,148-151] and involvement of the intrahepatic ducts alone.[24,149-151] Cholangiographic features are often diagnostic (Figure 40-1) and typically show diffuse, multi-focal strictures of the biliary tract and multiple areas of ectasia, resulting in a "beading" pattern. The small-duct sclerosing cholangitis variant of Wee and Ludwig[37,86] involves proximal bile ducts of such small calibers that cholangiography is normal. The high prevalence of autoantibodies (ANA and perinuclear pattern of reactivity of pANCA) suggests that they may become more useful as diagnostic tests in the future, especially as antigens specific for PSC are identified.[157] PSC must be distinguished from secondary sclerosing cholangitis, which may occur as a consequence of biliary surgery, choledocholithiasis, or cholangiocarcinoma. Differentiating benign strictures of PSC from sclerosis resulting from cholangiocarcinoma is not always possible and represents the major diagnostic difficulty. Using prolonged follow-up to exclude cholangiocarcinoma is inappropriate because cholangiocarcinoma develops de novo in patients with PSC.[158] Cholangiographic features suggestive of cholangiocarcinoma include (1) excessive dilation of ducts, (2) polypoid masses, (3) progression of ductular dilation or stricturing, and (4) a short dominant stricture of the extrahepatic ducts.

The lack of standardized nomenclature contributes to continued confusion regarding the relationship between pericholangitis, AIH, and PSC. As discussed previously, the term *pericholangitis* has been omitted from standardized nomenclature even though its spectrum of features is poorly encompassed by the designation "AIH associated with IBD."[55] In PSC, cholangiographic diagnostic criteria are well established,[149-151] but nomenclature for the hepatic histopathology has not been universally adopted.[52] In early studies some investigators describe pericholangitis concurrently with sclerosing cholangitis,[59,159] whereas others accept the diagnosis of pericholangitis only in the presence of normal bile ducts.[41] It is now well established that many patients with IBD diagnosed as having pericholangitis actually had PSC.* Cholangiography of additional patients with pericholangitis demonstrated sclerosis of the intrahepatic bile ducts without involvement of the extrahepatic bile ducts.[34,53] Thorpe and colleagues suggested that pericholangitis may reflect the intrahepatic component of a syndrome in which typical PSC represents the extrahepatic component,[50,59] whereas Wee and Ludwig reported that intrahepatic ("small-duct") sclerosing cholangitis may progress to large-duct sclerosing cholangitis.[52] Thus investigators now doubt whether pericholangitis exists as a clinical entity distinct from PSC.[31,52] It is important to note, however, that the frequency of PSC in patients with IBD remains substantially less than the reported frequency of pericholangitis. Moreover, the bile ducts have been reported to be normal in several well-studied patients with pericholangitis,[39,102] and serial evaluations showed that the majority of such patients do not progress to PSC.[52] These findings suggested either that PSC is a distinct entity or that, if it is a consequence of pericholangitis, it develops in only a fraction of patients with pericholangitis. Thus all IBD patients with liver biopsies consistent with the diagnosis of pericholangitis or AIH should have endoscopic retrograde cholangiogra-

*References 60, 64, 75, 76, 82-85, 87.

*References 34, 37, 48, 50, 52, 53, 59.

TABLE 40-4
Disease Associations in Primary and Secondary Sclerosing Cholangitis

Primary sclerosing cholangitis	Secondary sclerosing cholangitis
Ulcerative colitis	Choledocholithiasis
Crohn's colitis or ileocolitis	Infections in immunocompromised patients: *Cryptosporidium, Trichosporon,* and *Cytomegalovirus, Cryptococcus* organisms, visceral protothecosis
Type 1 autoimmune hepatitis	HTLV-1-associated myelopathy
Type 3 autoimmune hepatitis	Ischemic injury to hepatic artery or arterioles
	Trauma
	Neoplasm
	Toxic injury
	Floxuridine (hepatic artery injury)
	Formalin injection of ecchinococcal cysts
	Congenital abnormalities
	Celiac sprue
	Miscellaneous Conditions
	Alopecia universalis
	Angioblastic lymphadenopathy
	Autoimmune hemolytic anemia
	Biliary atresia
	Bronchiectasis
	Cavernous transformation of portal vein
	Cystic fibrosis
	Dermatitis herpetiformis
	Diabetes mellitus
	Focal nodular hyperplasia
	Glomerulonephritis
	Graves' disease
	Histiocytosis X
	Hodgkin's disease
	Hypereosinophilia
	Hyperimmunoglobulin M immunodeficiency
	Hypogammaglobulinemia
	IgA deficiency
	Immune thrombocytopenic purpura
	Inflammatory pseudotumor
	Intra-abdominal adenopathy
	Mast cell cholangiopathy
	Mediastinal fibrosis
	Metastatic prostate carcinoma
	Pancreatitis (acute or chronic)
	Perforating folliculitis
	Peyronie's disease
	Polymyositis
	Porphyria cutanea tarda
	Pseudotumor of orbit
	Pulmonary infiltrates
	Pyoderma gangrenosum
	Retroperitoneal fibrosis
	Rheumatoid arthritis
	Sarcoidosis
	Sclerosing sialadenitis
	Sjögren's syndrome
	Systemic lupus erythematosus
	Systemic sclerosis
	T-cell lymphoma of intestine
	Thymoma
	Trisomy 21
	Thyroiditis (Riedel's struma)
	Vasculitis

HTLV-1, Human T-cell leukemia virus; *IgA,* immunoglobulin A.

A

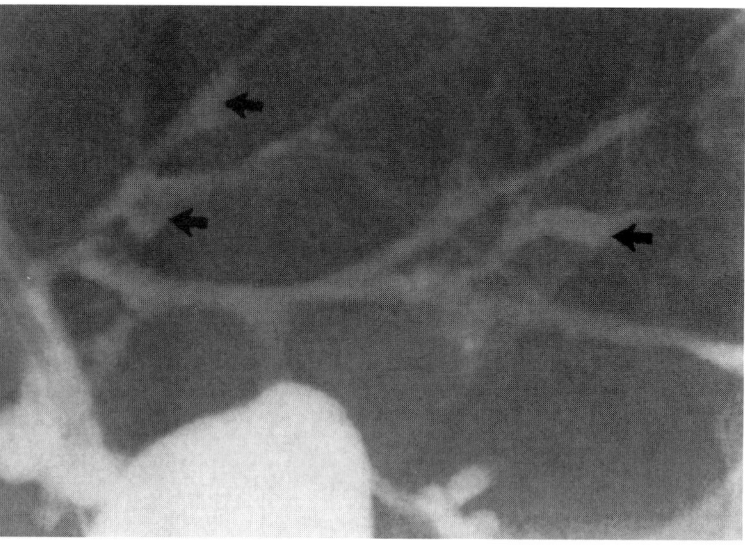

B

Figure 40-1 Cholangiogram from a patient with ulcerative colitis complicated by sclerosing cholangitis. **A,** The common bile duct *(straight arrow)* is narrowed and irregular. The cystic duct *(curved arrow)* is normal. **B,** Intrahepatic bile ducts are irregular, with stenotic areas alternating with areas of saccular dilation *(arrows)*. (**A** and **B** courtesy of Dr. Thomas Boyer.)

TABLE 40-5

Criteria for the Diagnosis of Primary Sclerosing Cholangitis

Feature	Inclusion criteria	Exclusion criteria
Clinical	History of IBD Cholestasis Hepatomegaly	Immunodeficiency syndrome Trauma or ischemia
Laboratory	↑ alkaline phosphatase ↑ aminotransferases Normal or ↑ bilirubin	Floxuridine Formalin Injection of hydatid cyst
Cholangiographic	Diffuse sclerosis of extrahepatic bile ducts with or without involvement of intrahepatic ducts Normal in small-duct variant	Choledocholithiasis Congenital abnormalities Normal cholangiogram and incompatible biopsy
Histopathologic	Bile ductular proliferation, periductal inflammation, periductal fibrosis, ductopenia, obliterative fibrous cholangitis	Viral hepatitis B or C Granulomas Non-suppurative destructing cholangitis
Serologic	pANCA ANA	AMA

IBD, Inflammatory bowel disease; *pANCA,* perinuclear staining pattern of anti-neutrophil cytoplasmic antibodies observed with indirect immunofluorescence of fixed neutrophils; *ANA,* anti-nuclear antibodies; *AMA,* anti-mitochondrial antibodies.

phy to evaluate the extrahepatic and intrahepatic bile ducts for features of PSC.

Pathology

Fibrosing inflammation of the common bile duct, hepatic ducts, and intrahepatic ducts results in stenosis, reduction of the luminal diameter, and thickening of the walls without dilation.[149-151] Stenosis may be present throughout the course of the common bile duct or only in isolated segments. Involvement of the intrahepatic ducts is characterized most commonly by segmental stenosis. Involved segments of bile ducts in strictured areas show diffuse fibrotic thickening and infiltration of the submucosal and subserosal areas with mononuclear inflammatory cells. The mucosal surface appears relatively normal by light microscopy. Electron microscopy of ductular epithelial cells in interlobular bile ducts has shown decreases in the numbers of organelles, fibrils, and intercellular junctions. Moreover, reduplication of the basement membrane has been present,[160] and finger-like projections have been observed on the basal surface of the bile ducts.[160] Point contacts between lymphocytes and biliary epithelial cells occasionally have been seen. Involvement of intrahepatic ducts culminates in ductopenia, principally of small- to medium-caliber ducts.[24]

Semiautomatic image analysis was used to calculate the intrahepatic bile duct volume from surgical biopsies from four patients with PSC. Both bile duct volumes in the liver and in portal tracts were decreased, and ductopenia was confirmed to affect the small- and medium-caliber bile ducts.[161]

The histologic appearances of the liver in PSC may be quite variable in specimens obtained by percutaneous needle biopsy, depending on the presence or absence of involvement of the intrahepatic bile ducts, the duration of the disease, and the number of sections examined.* The range of findings includes relatively normal-appearing interlobular ducts, portal tract inflammation with a predominantly periductular distribution, sclerosis of the bile ducts, formation of bile lakes, periportal fibrosis, intrahepatic cholestasis, bile ductopenia, and periportal (piecemeal) necrosis.† The quantity of Kupffer cells was increased threefold in PSC compared to PBC or controls with normal histology.[164] Thus the histologic findings may encompass features of "pericholangitis," extrahepatic biliary obstruction, chronic active hepatitis, or rarely, PBC.[30,31] In cases of long-standing biliary obstruction secondary biliary cirrhosis is common.[37,52,149-151,163] Accumulation of hepatic copper in PSC results from biliary obstruction.[30,31,52,149-163] The copper is confined primarily within lipolysosomes.[52]

Given the wide spectrum of histopathologic abnormalities and the absence of defined nomenclature, it is not surprising that liver biopsies are often not diagnostic for PSC. The most characteristic histopathologic features observed in PSC (in order of frequency) are (1) bile duct proliferation, (2) periductal fibrosis, (3) periductal inflammation, and (4) loss of bile ducts.[52] The presence of chronic nonsuppurative fibrous obliterative cholangitis is the most diagnostic lesion, but is observed infrequently in needle biopsy specimens (see the following section).[52,149-151,165,166] In the absence of diagnostic features Ludwig and associates have proposed a histologic classification subdividing the disease into four stages (Figure 40-2).[52] Stage I is characterized by changes confined to the portal tract such as portal inflammation, connective tissue expansion, and cholangitis. Stage II is characterized by extension of the fibrosis and inflammation into the periportal parenchyma, resulting in piecemeal necrosis and periportal fibrosis. Stage III is characterized by the formation of fibrous septa extending from the portal tract or bridging necrosis. Stage IV is characterized by biliary cirrhosis. The kinetics of histologic progression was assessed in 307 liver biopsies performed in 107 patients with PSC.[167] Progression in stage I disease could not be determined because of inadequate numbers of patients. Progression in patients with stage II disease occurred in 42 percent by year 1, 66 percent by year 2, and 93 percent by year 5. Progression from stage III occurred in 14 percent by year 1, 25 percent by year 2, and 52 percent by year 5. Regression was also observed, indicating sampling variability in serial biopsies in PSC. Despite prolonged necroinflammatory disease of the liver and the development of cirrhosis, hepatocellular carcinoma is rare.[30,37,138,168] The risk of cholangiocarcinoma is not confined to patients with advanced disease of long duration but can also occur in earlier stages. The tumor most often infiltrates the lamina propria of the bile ducts, resulting in strictures that are cholangiographically indistinguishable from PSC. Thus some patients with cholangiocarcinoma

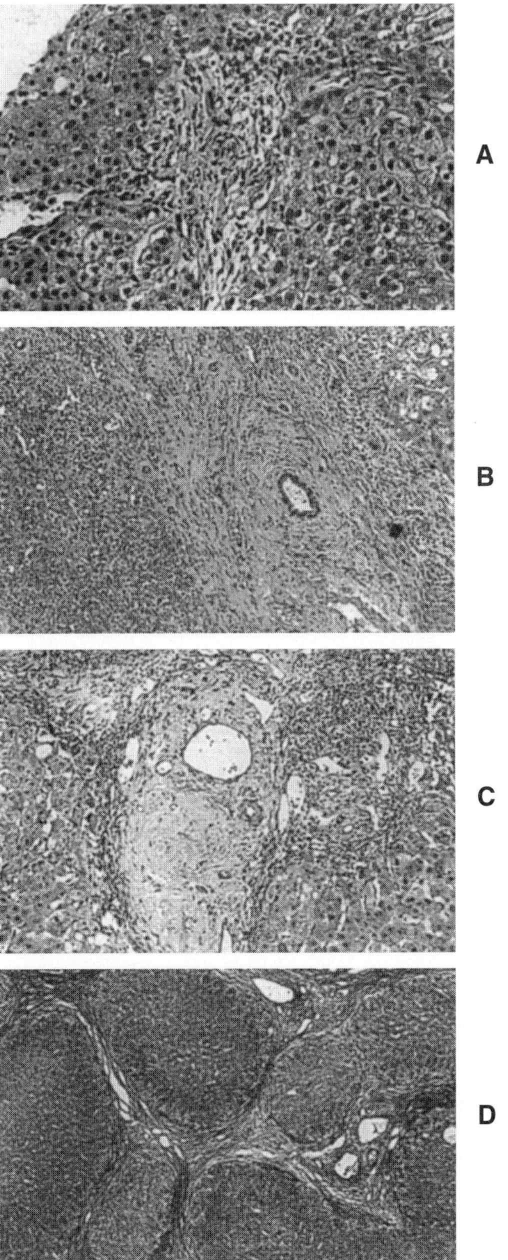

Figure 40-2 Histopathology of primary sclerosing cholangitis. **A,** Small-duct lesion with mild inflammation of portal tract and abnormal biliary epithelium. **B,** Portal inflammation with periductular, concentric fibrosis, and atrophy of the biliary epithelium. **C,** Ductopenia with fibrous scar at site of bile duct (inferior to portal vein). **D,** Biliary cirrhosis. (Photomicrographs courtesy of Lydia Petrovic, MD. From Vierling JM, and Amankonah TD: Primary sclerosing cholangitis. In Afdhal NH, ed: Gallbladder and Biliary Tract Diseases. New York, Marcel Dekker, Inc, 2000:659-703.)

*References 37, 52, 159-151, 160, 162, 163.

†References 30, 31, 37, 52, 149-151, 162, 163.

may not have PSC. Rarely, the tumor forms a nodular mass.[137,169]

A recent study of PSC livers obtained at the time of orthotopic liver transplantation showed that the histopathologic features of PSC varied with respect to the size of the bile ducts.[166] Ductopenia was the most common feature of small interlobular bile ducts and concentric peribiliary fibrosis of small ducts was inconspicuous. In contrast, concentric, periductal fibrosis and chronic non-suppurative fibrous obliterative cholangitis were exclusively observed in bile ducts of medium caliber. Large intrahepatic and extrahepatic bile ducts exhibited inflammation, ulceration of the epithelia, and cholangiectasia.

Gallstones are present infrequently in the gallbladders of patients with PSC,[149-151,170] although histologic changes of chronic cholecystitis have been found in more than 20 percent of such patients.[59,170,171] Occasionally choledocholithiasis is found in the absence of stones in the gallbladder[170]; this may occur as a secondary consequence of bile stasis caused by the sclerosing process.

The pancreatic duct may also be involved with sclerosis,[172,173] and chronic pancreatitis has been reported.[174,175] Involvement of the pancreatic duct indicates that the pathogenic mechanisms can involve all ducts derived from the embryonic foregut. The frequency of pancreatic duct involvement is unknown but appears to be rare. In a recent study of 38 patients with PSC evaluated by retrograde pancreatography none had abnormalities of the pancreatic duct.[173]

Epidemiology and Prevalence

PSC occurs in all races[60,130] but may be less common in people of African origin compared to those of European origin.[176] One prospective study of women with UC, however, showed that PSC developed more often (odds ratio [OR] 119, $P = .0002$) in those with African or Caribbean genetic origin than in patients of European or Asian descent.[176]

PSC is predominantly associated with UC.[30,37,47,59,148-151] It has also been found in a minority of patients with Crohn's disease.[20,30,177] In patients with Crohn's disease PSC has been associated almost exclusively with either colitis or ileocolitis.[20,30,149-151] An association with Crohn's disease limited to the small bowel has been reported.[177]

The most consistent epidemiologic feature of PSC is its association with IBD.[178] In early series the prevalence of IBD in patients with PSC was reported to be 30 percent.[156] The prevalence of PSC is inexactly known. Only approximately 100 cases had been reported before 1980,[179] but more cases were rapidly identified after the advent of diagnostic ERCP. Geographic variation in the prevalence of UC in PSC ranges from 21 percent to 23 percent in Japan,[180-182] 36 percent in Italy,[183] 44 percent in Spain,[184] 50 percent in India,[185] 71 percent in the United States,[186] to 98 percent in Norway.[187] To determine the true prevalence of IBD in PSC requires that all patients undergo colonoscopy with biopsy. One such Norwegian study showed that 98 percent of PSC patients had colitis,[187] whereas an American study found colitis in 71 percent.[186] Among patients with IBD and persistently abnormal liver tests, the prevalence of PSC ranges from 2.4 percent to 7.5 percent.[135] The prevalence of small-duct sclerosing cholangitis[86] is unknown, but a recent epidemiologic study in Sweden reported small-duct PSC in 7 percent of patients.[188] The mean frequency of PSC in prospective studies of several hundred patients with UC was 3.7 percent (range 2.4 to 5.6 percent).[24] Based on the prevalence of UC and the assumption that 3.7 percent of patients have PSC, the prevalence of PSC may approximate 4 per 100,000 population. Because PSC disproportionately afflicts males, this represents an underestimate in the population at greatest risk.

PSC occurs more frequently in non-smokers, and smokers with UC have a decreased risk of PSC.[189,190] However, a recent case control study showed that PSC patients who smoked had an increased risk of cholangiocarcinoma.[147]

Age and Gender

PSC can affect any age group, having been reported in infancy,[191] in childhood,[151,192,193] and throughout adult life.[1,24,149-151] Sixty percent to 70 percent of patients are male and two thirds are younger than 45 years of age at the time of diagnosis.[30,149-151] The age of clinical onset may also vary by gender. One large, longitudinal study noted that adult women developed UC between 30 and 40 years of age and PSC between 50 and 60 years of age.[194] Both ages of onset were approximately 10 years later than those observed in men.

Clinical Features

Despite the strong association between IBD and PSC, IBD is absent in a variable proportion of patients. Although two comparative studies found no histopathologic[52] or cholangiographic[195] differences among PSC patients with and without IBD, another study of 66 patients with mostly advanced PSC reported differences in gender ratios, symptoms, and cholangiographic findings.[196] IBD was present in 47 (71 percent); 39 (59 percent) had UC and 8 (12 percent) had Crohn's colitis. Nineteen patients (29 percent) did not have IBD. The male to female ratio was 2.9:1 for PSC with UC, 1:1 for PSC with Crohn's colitis, and 0.72:1 for PSC without IBD. At presentation, a significantly increased proportion (72 percent) of patients without IBD had jaundice, pruritus, or fatigue, compared with the proportion of symptomatic patients (41 percent) with IBD. Thus 59 percent of patients with IBD presented asymptomatically with only abnormal laboratory tests as the first manifestation of PSC. Strictures of both intrahepatic and extrahepatic ducts were more frequent in patients with IBD (86 percent) than in those without IBD (46 percent). Conversely, strictures confined solely to the extrahepatic ducts were less frequent in patients with IBD (7 percent) than in patients without IBD (38 percent). Despite these intriguing findings, it is unwarranted to conclude that PSC in association with IBD is an entity distinct from PSC occurring without IBD.

IBD is most often diagnosed years before PSC; however, PSC can also precede IBD or occur late in the course of IBD.[194,197-199] Asymptomatic IBD may be detected by colonoscopy and biopsy after PSC is diagnosed, and some of these biopsies showed dysplasia.[198] IBD became symptomatic 1 to 7 years after the diagnosis of PSC. PSC may occur after proctocolectomy for UC.[30,31,130,194] Similarly, IBD may develop after liver transplantation for PSC.[140,200] No correlation exists between the severity of UC and PSC.[30,19,130,194]

Several aspects of IBD differ among patients with and without PSC. For example, PSC is significantly less prevalent in distal colitis (0.05 percent) compared to more extensive colitis (5.5 percent).[201] Indeed, extensive colitis was present in more than 95 percent of PSC patients with UC, whereas only 5 percent had distal colitis. PSC was associated with a more quiescent course of UC than observed in patients with UC alone during a 20-year case-controlled study.[202] Colonoscopy with biopsies should be performed to diagnose UC in patients with PSC and to evaluate for dysplasia. Colonoscopy is preferred over flexible sigmoidoscopy because one study reported rectal sparing in 23 percent of patients with PSC and UC.[76] PSC has been diagnosed in children with and without IBD, but no striking differences have been reported.[151,192,193]

Patients with PSC may be either asymptomatic or symptomatic at the time of diagnosis.* Table 40-6 summarizes the symptoms and signs of PSC at the time of diagnosis. Common presenting features noted in early reports included intermittent or fluctuating jaundice, pruritus, nausea, abdominal pain, vomiting, and fever.[30,31,156] These occur with fatigue, malaise, diminished appetite, and, usually, weight loss. Symptoms of cholangitis usually are not found when the patients are first examined[30,31,148-151] because bacterial cholangitis before surgical exploration is rare.[1,24,196,205,206] Symptoms may be present for periods ranging from weeks to more than 10 years before the diagnosis[1,24,150]; the majority of patients have had symptoms for 2 years before diagnosis.

*References 60, 136, 183, 184, 186, 203, 204.

TABLE 40-6

Symptoms and Physical Examination Findings at the Time of Diagnosis of Primary Sclerosing Cholangitis

Clinical presentation	Frequency
Asymptomatic	15%-44%
Symptomatic	
Fatigue	75%
Abdominal pain	16%-37%
Pruritus	70%
Ascending cholangitis	5%-28%
Ascites	2%-10%
Hyperpigmentation	25%
Jaundice	30%-69%
Weight loss	10%-34%
Variceal bleeding	2%-14%
Splenomegaly	30%
Hepatomegaly*	34%-62%

Data from references 130, 136, 183, 184, 186, 203, 204, 228.
*Hepatomegaly presents in either asymptomatic or symptomatic patients.

Between 15 percent and 45 percent of recently diagnosed patients are asymptomatic,[183,186] whereas in the 1980s only 7 percent to 10 percent were asymptomatic.[30,31,207] Asymptomatic patients are more frequently diagnosed because of increasing awareness of PSC, screening with serum liver tests, and use of diagnostic ERCP. Patients may remain asymptomatic despite advancing disease, and up to 17 percent of asymptomatic patients have cirrhosis, compared to 50 percent of symptomatic patients.[136] In a longitudinal study recording daily symptoms in 84 PSC patients enrolled in a therapeutic trial of colchicine, symptoms (primarily pruritus and abdominal pain) were intermittent, usually lasting for a few days.[208] Other patients had symptoms for months or years before spontaneous resolution. Only pruritus was significantly correlated with serum alkaline phosphatase levels. Rarely, patients with PSC initially present with signs of decompensated cirrhosis such as ascites or variceal bleeding.[31,60,148,204,209] Recently, instruments have been validated to assess the quality of life in patients with PSC and PBC and showed that cholestatic liver disease impairs the quality of life and the impairment worsens with progression of disease severity.[210,211]

Results of initial physical examinations are normal in approximately 50 percent of patients.[1,24] At diagnosis, hepatomegaly is present in 55 percent of patients, jaundice in 50 percent, splenomegaly in 30 percent, cutaneous hyperpigmentation in 25 percent, and xanthomata in 4 percent. Fewer than 50 percent show tenderness to palpation of the right upper quadrant.[156] Vascular spiders, ascites, and clubbing are observed in advanced disease. Hyperpigmentation, xanthelasma, and xanthomata are less frequent in PSC than in PBC, despite progressive cholestatis.[212]

Laboratory Tests

The results of laboratory tests in PSC are variable.[30,31,48,148-151,156] During clinical episodes of cholestasis or cholangitis, leukocytosis may be present. Eosinophilia is rare in PSC, but hypereosinophilic syndrome has been reported.[213,214] Alkaline phosphatase is usually elevated, often to very high levels, but it can be normal even in advanced histologic stages of disease.[215] Indeed, 8.5 percent and 10 percent of patients with PSC in two series had normal alkaline phosphatase levels at diagnosis.[136,201] Thus an elevated alkaline phosphatase is not mandatory for diagnosis.[216] In the study by Schrumpf and colleagues alkaline phosphatase activity was found to be significantly greater in patients with PSC than in patients with other hepatobiliary diseases complicating UC.[48] Alkaline phosphatase levels may also fluctuate from normal to abnormal during the course of disease. Total bilirubin is normal in 60 percent at diagnosis but gradually increases with progression of disease.[60,135,183,148] Bilirubin may fluctuate with passage of sludge or calculi or during ascending cholangitis.[60] Aminotransferase levels may be normal or moderately elevated; mild elevations occur in more than 90 percent of patients.[24] Hypoalbuminemia and abnormal prothrombin times are infrequently present at diagnosis, having been found in 17 percent and 6 percent of patients, respectively, in one study.[30] Hypergammaglobulinemia occurs in approximately 30 percent of patients, and IgG concentrations were elevated in 44 percent[85]—20 percent to 45 percent had increased levels of IgM.[31,110]

Autoantibodies are frequent in patients with PSC.[24,150] In one report ANAs and anti-SMAs occurred in 55 percent and 35 percent of adult patients, respectively. In another series ANAs or anti-SMAs were present in 22 percent.[85] The titers, however, are often lower than those observed in patients with AIH type 1. AMAs are rarely detected, and the antigenic epitopes differ from those specifically recognized by AMAs in patients with PBC (pyruvate dehydrogenase complex–E2). Anti-neutrophil cytoplasmic antibodies binding in a perinuclear pattern (pANCA) are associated with both UC and PSC.[157,217-221] Approximately 80 percent of patients with PSC (with and without IBD) have pANCA. pANCA are also prevalent among relatives (25 percent positivity) of patients with PSC, indicating that they are linked to familial immunogenetics.[220] A pANCA is neither specific nor sensitive for the diagnosis of PSC, having been detected in UC without PSC,[214,218] PBC,[222] and type 1 AIH.[73,222] In one study the prevalence of pANCA was 87 percent in PSC, 17 percent in UC without PSC, 13 percent in PBC, and 16 percent in AIH.[222] In other series pANCA was present in 65 percent to 83 percent of patients with UC without PSC[218,220] and in 92 percent of patients with type 1 AIH.[73] However, the pANCA in PSC were composed of both IgG1 and IgG3 subclasses, whereas those in AIH had an IgG1 predominance. More importantly, the antigens recognized by the pANCA in PSC and AIH appeared to be different. For example, after treatment of neutrophils with deoxyribonuclease (DNase-I), the pANCA staining pattern with PSC sera is diffusely cytoplasmic, whereas that of AIH sera is granular.

PSC is associated with secondary abnormalities similar to those accompanying other syndromes of obstructive cholestasis. These include increased levels of unesterified cholesterol and phospholipid, abnormal low-density lipoproteins, liability for the formation of pigmented gallstones, changes in the proportions of primary bile acids and the urinary excretion of sulfated bile acid, and malabsorption of fat and fat-soluble vitamins. Hepatic copper retention and elevated urinary excretion of copper occur in 90 percent of patients as a result of decreased excretion of copper.[223]

Diagnostic Criteria

Warren's original diagnostic criteria for PSC[156] required: (1) absence of prior biliary surgery; (2) absence of cholelithiasis; (3) diffuse stricturing of the extrahepatic biliary tree; and (4) exclusion of structuring resulting from cholangiocarcinoma. Diagnostic criteria were subsequently modified after the advent of ERCP, recognition that biliary tract calculi can be caused by PSC,[170,224,225] and that cholangiocarcinoma is a complication of PSC.[143] Current diagnostic criteria rely on a combination of clinical, laboratory, cholangiographic, histopathologic, and serologic findings (Table 40-7). Secondary causes of sclerosing cholangitis that must be considered include prior

TABLE 40-7

Inclusion and Exclusion Criteria for the Diagnosis of Primary Sclerosing Cholangitis

Feature	Inclusion criteria	Exclusion criteria
History	Asymptomatic or symptomatic Presence of ulcerative colitis or Crohn's disease	Genetic or acquired immunodeficiency syndromes with infection Biliary tract trauma Hepatic arterial ischemia Floxuridine chemotherapy Formalin injections of ecchinococcal cysts
Physical findings	Hepatomegaly	
Laboratory tests	Normal or ↑ alkaline phosphatase ↑ Aminotransferases Normal or ↑ bilirubin	Markers of active viral hepatitis B or C
Histopathology	Portal inflammation Periductular inflammation/fibrosis Ductopenia Obliterative fibrous cholangitis Biliary cirrhosis	Histopathology incompatible with PSC Non-suppurative destructive cholangitis
Serology	ANA* pANCA*	AMA
Cholangiography	Normal (small duct histopathology) or Sclerosis of extrahepatic biliary tract with or without sclerosis of intrahepatic ducts	Normal Choledocholithiasis Congenital abnormalities

ANA, Anti-nuclear antibodies; *pANCA*, perinuclear staining of anti-neutrophil cytoplasmic antibodies; *AMA*, anti-mitochondrial antibodies; *NSDC*, non-suppurative destructive cholangitis.
*Neither autoantibody sensitive nor specific for diagnosis of PSC.

surgery of the biliary tract, trauma, biliary calculi, ischemic injury of hepatic artery or arterioles, arterial injury caused by floxuridine treatment, formalin injection of echinococcal cysts communicating with the biliary tract, congenital abnormalities of the biliary tract, and infectious cholangiopathies associated with genetic and acquired immunodeficiency syndromes.

ERCP is the single most important diagnostic procedure. Typical cholangiographic findings of PSC on ERCP or percutaneous transhepatic cholangiography[128,195,226] are multi-focal strictures separated by segments of ducts with normal or ectatic caliber (see Figure 40-1). Strictures are usually short and annular, but longer confluent strictures may occur in the common bile duct or with advanced disease. Large ectasias may appear to be diverticula.[195] Stricturing of both intrahepatic and extrahepatic ducts is most often observed, but strictures of the intrahepatic ducts or extrahepatic ducts alone occur in up to 20 percent[148] and 10 percent of patients,[31] respectively. The proximal intrahepatic ducts often appear tortuous, stretched, or attenuated in cirrhotic livers.[195] The gallbladder and cystic duct are involved in up to 15 percent of patients,[128] but abnormalities of the pancreatic duct are rare.[172] Although magnetic resonance cholangiography has been used as a substitute for ERC to detect strictures in distal intrahepatic and extrahepatic ducts,[227] the quality of detail remains inferior.

Sclerosis of the bile ducts also may occur in cholangiocarcinoma, and differentiation between carcinoma and sclerosing cholangitis can be difficult.[86] It is especially important to consider the possibility of cholangiocarcinoma in patients with IBD because the incidences of malignancies of the bile ducts and gallbladder are increased in these patients (discussed in the following section). Other diseases such as metastatic carcinoma, lymphoma, cirrhosis, and polycystic liver disease may cause narrowing and deformity of bile ducts; however, they do not usually cause the characteristic beaded appearance of PSC.

It is important to note that PSC may be manifested only by inflammatory changes of the small bile ducts without cholangiographic evidence of large duct disease.[86] In such cases the clinical diagnosis of small duct PSC should be based on (1) typical liver biopsy findings, (2) cholestatic liver tests similar to those found in large duct PSC, and (3) the presence of IBD. However, liver biopsy may not be diagnostic in PSC (see previous section on Pathology). The disease is segmental and the histologic features overlap those seen in pericholangitis, extrahepatic biliary obstruction, chronic hepatitis, and PBC.[30-32,37,52] A liver biopsy is useful to establish the histologic stage of disease.

Natural History

The natural history of PSC is incompletely understood and variability in the location of sclerotic lesions results in a wide spectrum of clinical disease. This is especially true for asymptomatic patients and the subgroup of patients with disease confined to the small intrahepatic ducts.[130,228] Thus some patients with PSC have exacerbations and remissions, whereas others have a rapid progression and some have non-progressive disease for decades.[60,136,186] The typical clinical course, however, is characterized by complications of progressive cholestasis, cirrhosis, portal venous hypertension, hepatic failure, or cholangiocarcinoma.[136,141,228] Recognition of patients without elevations of alkaline phosphatase[215] and large groups of asymptomatic patients suggests that the disease may evolve through four sequential phases.

The earliest, or preclinical, phase occurs in the absence of hepatobiliary symptoms or cholestatic abnormalities of standard liver tests. Patients in this phase of disease would be virtually undetectable unless evaluated for non-specific complaints. Indeed, patients reported by the Mayo Clinic had cholangiography primarily to evaluate chronic abdominal pain.[215] The patients evaluated were five men and five women with a mean age of 46 years. Cholangiographic evidence of extrahepatic and intrahepatic duct sclerosis was present in each group, and 8 of the 10 patients had IBD. Serial evaluation confirmed that the alkaline phosphatase and bilirubin remained normal, and causes of alkaline phosphatase reduction were excluded (e.g., hypophosphatasia, pernicious anemia, hypothyroidism, substances that can interfere with the assay). Similarly, causes of secondary sclerosing cholangitis were also excluded. Despite the absence of hepatobiliary symptoms or elevated alkaline phosphatase, the disease in 3 of the 10 patients was in advanced histologic stages on liver biopsy: two had stage III lesions and one had biliary cirrhosis. Further follow-up is required to assess the duration of this phase.

The second sequential phase is characterized by asymptomatic cholestatic abnormalities of liver tests with elevation of alkaline phosphatase. Asymptomatic patients constitute 15 percent to 25 percent in many series,[141] but a study of 305 patients recently reported that more than 40 percent were asymptomatic.[136] Differences in the use of the term *asymptomatic* have undoubtedly contributed to variation in the reported proportions of asymptomatic patients.[141] For example, in some reports 30 percent of "asymptomatic" patients have had fatigue, 24 percent have had weight loss, and some have had jaundice.[148,186,203] Regardless, modest elevations of aminotransferases also may occur, but the bilirubin is usually normal. Physical examination may be normal; however, up to 45 percent of patients have hepatomegaly and occasional patients have stigmata of advanced disease. Because progression of hepatic fibrosis and stricturing of ducts can occur without development of symptoms or signs,[31] up to 17 percent of asymptomatic patients may have cirrhosis.[136] PSC is being diagnosed with increasing frequency in this phase.* It remains unclear whether this primarily reflects increased physician awareness, use of screening laboratory tests, and application of ERC or an increase in incidence. Most clinical investigators favor the former explanation. This phase can be quite prolonged. In one retrospective analysis asymptomatic patients did not develop symptomatic disease during an average of 4.7 years of observation.[148] Actuarial analysis of another series (Figure 40-3) showed that approximately 45 percent of asymptomatic patients had developed symptoms after 7 years.[229]

*References 30,34, 113, 148-151, 218, 219.

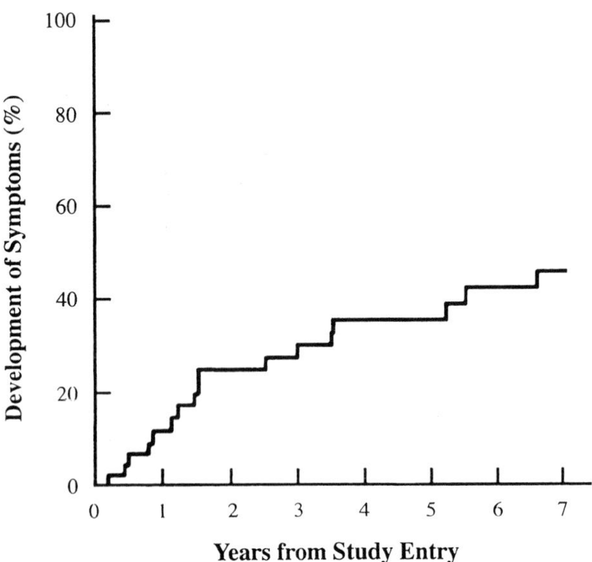

Figure 40-3 Kaplan-Meier estimate of the time to onset of symptoms in asymptomatic patients with primary sclerosing cholangitis. Time of diagnosis is used as the starting point. (From Porayko MK, Wiesner RH, LaRusso NF, et al: Patients with asymptomatic primary sclerosing cholangitis frequently have a progressive disease. Gastroenterology 98:151594-151602, 1990.)

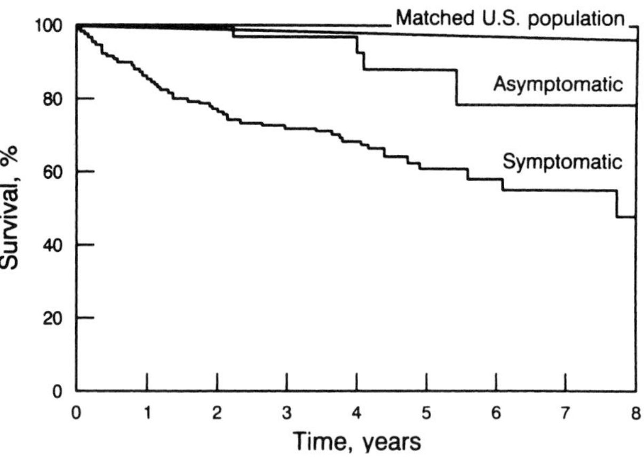

Figure 40-4 Comparison of Kaplan-Meier estimated survivals for asymptomatic and symptomatic patients with primary sclerosing cholangitis with age- and gender-matched controls from the United States. (From Wiesner RH, Grambsch PM, Dickson ER, et al: Natural history, prognostic factors, and survival analysis. Hepatology 10:430-436, 1989.)

The third, or symptomatic, phase refers to that period when patients exhibit a variety of hepatobiliary symptoms. The most frequent symptoms are fatigue, pruritus, jaundice, dark urine, and light stools. Fever, abdominal pain, episodic jaundice, and acute ascending cholangitis occur in a minority of patients. Physical examination frequently reveals jaundice, hepatomegaly, and splenomegaly. The clinical features in patients with associated IBD do not differ from those in patients without IBD. In addition, the pattern of bile duct involvement does not differ in symptomatic and asymptomatic patients with PSC.[30,148-151] Prospective and retrospective analyses indicate that symptoms and biochemical abnormalities progress with time.[30,148-151] Up to 50 percent of symptomatic patients have cirrhosis.[136]

The fourth, or terminal, phase of the disease is characterized by decompensated cirrhosis, complications of portal hypertension, hepatic failure, or development of cholangiocarcinoma. In adults partial biliary obstruction leads to cirrhosis over variable periods of time, generally taking 5 to 11 years. In the classic study by Warren and co-workers 7 of 12 patients had clinical evidence of portal venous hypertension at the time of laparotomy for jaundice. Nine of 12 patients progressed to cirrhosis in an average follow-up period of 4.5 years.[156] Secondary biliary cirrhosis may develop or progress despite apparent surgical relief of biliary strictures.

Prognosis

The prognosis of patients with PSC differs in reported series, depending on the proportion of symptomatic patients within the study group.*

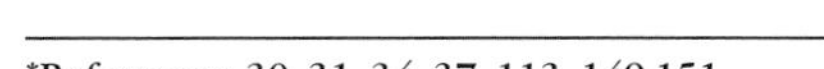

*References 30, 31, 34, 37, 113, 149-151.

Overall, the median duration of survival from diagnosis to either death or transplantation is 12 years, but the range extends to 21 years.[136,141,188,228] The wide range undoubtedly reflects the variable duration of disease before diagnosis and the increasing application of liver transplantation. Actuarial survival is significantly greater for asymptomatic patients than for symptomatic patients (Figure 40-4); at 10 years, survival is 80 percent for asymptomatic patients and only 50 percent for symptomatic patients.[136] Pregnancy does not affect the progression of PSC, but pruritus may become so intense that it results in premature delivery.[113]

Of 39 symptomatic patients 13 (33 percent) died between 5 and 108 months after diagnosis.[30] Ten of the 13 patients had portal venous hypertension, and 6 of the 13 had cirrhosis. Of interest, 7 of these 13 patients had IBD. Liver failure was the most common cause of death and occurred in 11 of the 13 patients. Of 26 survivors followed for 6 to 110 months after diagnosis, 12 had clinical evidence of portal venous hypertension and cirrhosis. Chapman and associates reported a similarly high mortality rate in symptomatic patients with PSC and IBD.[31] In their series 10 of the 11 patients who died had UC. A retrospective study of 38 patients (29 symptomatic at presentation) showed a poor prognosis in 45 percent during a mean follow-up period of 6.3 ± 4.9 years.[218] During this period 11 patients (29 percent) died and 6 (16 percent) developed variceal hemorrhage or encephalopathy or required hepatic transplantation. It is noteworthy that a poor outcome was not confined to symptomatic patients; five of nine asymptomatic patients had a similar outcome.

Two large series indicate that PSC progresses more rapidly among symptomatic patients. Among 174 patients reported by the Mayo Clinic, the combined rate of liver failure, need for transplantation, and cholangiocarcinoma was 41 percent over 6.25 years of observation.[186] The median survival for symptomatic patients was approximately 8.5 years compared to 11.9 years for the entire group of patients. Among 126 patients from Kings

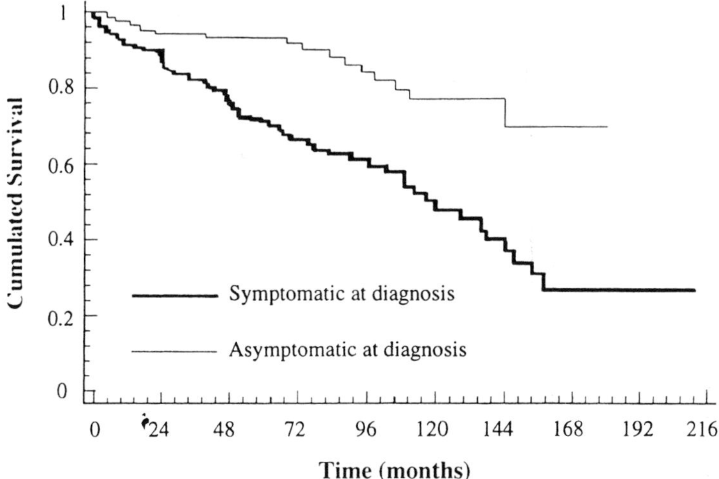

Figure 40-5 Kaplan-Meier estimates of survival for asymptomatic and symptomatic patients with primary sclerosing cholangitis. Note the highly significant difference in survival ($P < .001$). (From Broome U, Olsson R, Loof L, Bodemar G, et al: Natural history and prognostic factors in 305 Swedish patients with primary sclerosing cholangitis. Gut 38:610-615, 1996.)

College only 12.6 percent were asymptomatic and the median survival for the whole group was 12 years.[203]

In contrast, studies of asymptomatic patients suggest a much better prognosis. During prolonged observation Schrumpf and associates observed only 2 deaths in 18 asymptomatic patients with PSC—1 died of cholangiocarcinoma, the other from non-hepatic causes.[113] The remaining 16 were observed for an average of 6 years (range 3 to 13 years). Ten remained asymptomatic, four had intermittent symptoms, and two developed signs and symptoms of advanced disease. The majority of laboratory tests were stable, but bilirubin elevation progressed in four patients. Progressive worsening of cholangiographic findings was observed, but was unassociated with worsening of clinical, biochemical, or histopathologic features. During a mean follow-up of 6.8 years, asymptomatic patients had a significantly better prognosis than symptomatic patients.[231] Among 136 symptomatic patients, death occurred in 31 (23 percent) compared to a single death among 38 asymptomatic patients (2.6 percent). Ten-year actuarial survival was calculated to be 93 percent in asymptomatic patients and 47 percent in symptomatic patients. Helzberg and colleagues reported a retrospective analysis of 53 patients, indicating an improved survival among both symptomatic and asymptomatic patients.[148] During a mean follow-up of 4.7 years, most patients did not progress symptomatically. Calculation of actuarial survival indicated that 75 percent of patients survived for 9 years. Multi-variate analysis showed that elevated bilirubin (greater than 1.5 mg/dl) and hepatomegaly at presentation independently correlated with a poor prognosis, although the cholangiographic pattern of duct involvement, the presence or absence of IBD, advanced histologic stages, and age did not. Unique features of this population included a higher percentage of older, asymptomatic females and a substantial number of patients with disease confined to the intrahepatic ducts. Among asymptomatic patients without cirrhosis, actuarial estimates indicated that 45 percent developed symptoms by 7 years (Figure 40-5). Moreover, 31 percent died or had liver transplants.[229] Initial cholangiographic findings may also predict symptoms and signs: short, tight extrahepatic strictures were associated with pruritus, abdominal pain, and fever,[232] whereas jaundice was more common with tight intrahepatic strictures. Cholangiocarcinoma has the greatest negative impact on prognosis of any complication.[143]

The natural history and prognosis of PSC in pediatric patients are incompletely characterized.[233-235] In a study of 52 pediatric patients with PSC 43 (84 percent) had IBD and 36 of them were reviewed in detail.[233] UC and Crohn's disease were present in 89 percent and 11 percent, respectively. The majority had pancolitis, but rectal sparing was present in 27 percent. In 11 percent the IBD was asymptomatic. Proctocolectomy was performed for dysplasia in 17 percent and pouchitis developed in four of five patients with ileal pouch–anal anastomoses. Mieli-Vergani points out that sclerosing cholangitis in children is a heterogeneous collection of diseases, including inherited neonatal sclerosing cholangitis, AIH with sclerosing cholangitis, secondary sclerosing cholangitis, and true PSC, which is rare.[234] Thus the natural history, response to therapy, and prognosis depend on the etiology of biliary sclerosis. A comparison of pediatric PSC patients with mean follow-up 5.2 years and adult patients with mean follow-up of 6.9 years showed that only adults died or needed liver transplantation.[235]

Four prognostic models for PSC, based on the results of multi-variate analyses, have been published by the Mayo Clinic,[231]

Mayo Clinic Index = 0.06 × age (years) + 0.85 × $\log_e$ (minimum of bilirubin mg/dl or maximum of 10) − 4.49 × logze (minimum hemoglobin g/dl or maximum 12) + 0.51 × histologic stage + 1.59 (if IBD present)

King's College Hospital,[203]

King's College Index = 1.81 (if hepatomegaly present) + 0.88 (if splenomegaly present) + 2.66 $\times \log_{10}$ (alkaline phosphatase IU/L) + 0.58 $\times$ histologic stage + 0.04 $\times$ age (years)

a Multicenter Study Group that refined the original Mayo Clinic Index,[209]

Multicenter Study Group = (0.535 $\times \log_e$ bilirubin mg/dl) + 0.486 $\times$ histologic stage + 0.041 $\times$ age (years) + 0.705 (if splenomegaly present)

and the revised Mayo PSC Risk Score.[141,236]

Revised Mayo PSC Risk Score: R = 0.03 (age in years) + 0.54 $\times \log_e$ (bilirubin mg/dl) + 0.54 $\times \log_e$ (AST in U/L) + 1.24 (for history of variceal bleeding) − 0.84 $\times$ (albumin in g/dl)

These equations relate the independent variables for each prognostic model. The third revision excluded need for a current liver biopsy without compromising the accuracy of the survival estimate.[141,236] The second refinement was made by collaboration with four international centers (Multicenter Study Group) to create a database on 426 PSC patients that included clinical, laboratory, serologic, and histologic detail collected during a 20 year follow-up. The new model was created by randomly assigning half of the 426 PSC patients in the Multicenter Study Group to develop the model and using the other half to validate it. Because no therapy had been proven to alter the natural history of PSC, all patients were considered as untreated. The revised Mayo PSC Risk Score included the independent variables of age, total serum bilirubin, serum albumin, AST, and the presence or absence of prior variceal bleeding. The new Mayo model closely correlated with the earlier model and accurately predicted survival free of transplant across the disease spectrum in PSC.

The Child-Turcotte-Pugh (CTP) classification also predicted differences in survival over 7 years among patients with CTP class A (89.8 percent), B (68 percent), and C (24.9 percent) scores.[204] When 140 PSC patients with liver histology were analyzed using the Multicenter Group PSC score, the individual values of its four independent variables, and the CTP score, only patient age and CTP classification were found to be independent predictors of survival. Because the addition of the Multicenter Group PSC score did not improve prediction of survival, the CTP classification appeared to be a simpler alternative. However, when the revised Mayo PSC Risk Score was compared with the CTP scores of another 147 PSC patients, overlapping survival curves were observed between CTP class B and C patients, indicating an inability of the CTP to predict differences in survival.[236] In contrast, the revised Mayo PSC Risk Score discriminated survival among low-, medium-, and high-risk patients. A model testing the three variables of age, CTP class, and revised Mayo PSC Risk Score found that only age and the Mayo PSC Risk Score were significant, independent predictors of survival. Thus the revised Mayo PSC Risk Score appears to be the best available method to calculate a survival estimate for an individual patient.

It is important to note several limitations of all PSC Survival models and the CTP. None of the prognostic systems have been tested prospectively. None address the risk of developing either cholangiocarcinoma or variceal bleeding, factors known to increase mortality. Fluctuations of bilirubin levels are also problematic because serum bilirubin is the most heavily weighted independent variable. Thus calculations of risk scores or CTP class during reversible episodes of increased biliary obstruction or ascending cholangitis can significantly underestimate survival. Finally, estimates of long-term survival are imprecise because the confidence intervals for identical scores widen substantially over time.

Retrospective analysis of 216 patients transplanted for PSC between 1981 and 1990 demonstrated significantly increased 5-year survivals with transplantation (73 percent) compared with those predicted (28 percent) by the Mayo PSC model.[237] Long-term survival after liver transplantation was similar for PSC patients with low, intermediate, or high risk of death based on the Mayo Risk Score.

Pretransplant clinical variables identified in a cohort of 118 PSC patients were found to predict survival after liver transplantation.[237] Independent predictors of inferior survival included prior abdominal surgery, history of IBD, history of cholangiocarcinoma, serum creatinine level, and ascites. Subsequently, the model accurately predicted post-transplant survival in 30 PSC patients. However, validation will require independent testing, and wide confidence intervals limit application for individual patients.

Complications

Cholangiocarcinoma

The natural history of PSC is associated with multiple complications (Table 40-8). Hepatic failure and compli-

TABLE 40-8

Complications of Primary Sclerosing Cholangitis

Complication	Relative frequency
Cholangiocarcinoma	+++
Dominant strictures	+++
Ascending cholangitis	++
Cholelithiasis or choledocholithiasis	++
Hepatic failure	++++
Portal venous hypertension	++++
Hepatocellular carcinoma	+
Hepatic osteodystrophy	+++
Steatorrhea and fat-soluble vitamin deficiency	
Hyperlipidemia	+++
Pancreatitis	++
Peristomal varices after ileostomy	+
Pruritus	+
Colorectal carcinoma with ulcerative colitis	++

cations of portal venous hypertension are the primary indications for orthotopic liver transplantation in PSC.

The most serious and specific complication of PSC is cholangiocarcinoma, which has a reported prevalence of 7.1 percent to 13.8 percent in large series.[143,144,188] Autopsies of patients in these same series revealed a substantially higher prevalence, ranging from 27.3 percent to 41.7 percent. The prevalence of unsuspected or undetected cholangiocarcinomas found during laparotomy or in livers of PSC patients undergoing OLT averaged 17.8 percent (range 2.9 percent to 36.4 percent) in 10 reported series, corroborating the autopsy data. In one longitudinal study the cumulative actuarial incidence of cholangiocarcinoma was 30 percent between 8 and 15 years of disease.[238] These data clearly indicate that PSC is a premalignant disease and that occult cholangiocarcinomas are common in progressive PSC. A case-controlled study of 32 patients with PSC and cholangiocarcinoma at time of liver transplantation was performed using PSC patients without cholangiocarcinoma who were also referred for transplantation.[168] Interestingly, patients with cholangiocarcinoma had a shorter median duration of PSC (1 year) compared to controls (7 years) and varices were found in only 12 percent of patients with tumor compared with 56 percent of controls. Thus cholangiocarcinoma should not be regarded as a complication of only end-stage PSC. Cholangiocarcinoma occurs in the fifth decade of life in PSC, which is 20 years earlier than observed in patients without PSC.[144,147]

The dismal median survival after diagnosis of cholangiocarcinoma was only 5 months, and 63 percent had metastases, most often involving regional lymph nodes.[239] Virtually all cholangiocarcinomas identified before transplant recur lethally.[240] Among 305 patients with PSC, 26 percent died of cholangiocarcinomas.[136] Diagnosis of cholangiocarcinoma was made an average of 32.5 months after the diagnosis of PSC. One study indicated that cholangiocarcinoma developed more frequently in PSC patients with colonic dysplasia or carcinoma, suggesting that colonic biopsies may be useful in identifying patients at high risk.[198]

Early detection of cholangiocarcinoma remains difficult because tumor infiltration of the lamina propria of bile ducts causes fibrous stricturing that is often indistinguishable from progressive PSC.[143] Cholangiographic features suggestive of cholangiocarcinoma include[169] (1) excessive bile duct dilation; (2) polypoid masses; (3) a short, dominant stricture of the extrahepatic ducts; and (4) rapid progression of dilation or stricturing on serial cholangiograms. Although serial ERCP[169,241] may aid in detection of cholangiocarcinoma, suspicious findings are often absent.[241-243] Clinical features of fever, jaundice, weight loss, abdominal pain, pruritus, hepatosplenomegaly, and ascites did not differ significantly between PSC patients with and without cholangiocarcinoma.[31,239,244,245] Laboratory tests are also similar in patients with or without cholangiocarcinoma.[128]

Sensitivities of standard diagnostic tests are poor: ultrasonography (7 percent), computerized tomography (29 percent), and ERCP (58.3 percent).[242] Positron emission tomography (PET) may prove useful in detecting cholangiocarcinoma.[247,248] In one series of 26 patients with cholangiocarcinoma 24 were detected using PET with 18F fluoro-2-deoxy-D-glucose, and the scans were negative in 18 of 20 controls and all 8 patients with benign biliary lesions. Despite a specificity and accuracy of 92.9 percent, PET detected metastases in lymph nodes in only 2 of 15 and in peritoneum or lung in 7 of 10. Studies should be performed to compare diagnostic sensitivity of PET, magnetic resonance imaging, and magnetic resonance cholangiography.[227,248] Cholangiocarcinomas rarely occur as mass lesions.[137]

Cytology of aspirated bile or mucosal brushings has demonstrated high specificities and positive predictive values for cholangiocarcinomas in patients *without* PSC.[249,250] However, low sensitivities for bile (11 percent to 30 percent), brushings (50 percent to 56 percent), and poor negative predictive values do not permit exclusion of cholangiocarcinoma on the basis of negative cytology. Similarly, one series showed that brushings for cytologic diagnosis of cholangiocarcinoma in PSC had a sensitivity of 56 percent, specificity of 100 percent, and positive predictive value of 100 percent but a negative predictive value of only 51 percent and accuracy of 70 percent.[251] Diagnostic accuracy was increased when repeated samples were tested in another series that included patients with PSC.[252] Unfortunately cytology on multiple samples of bile, brushings, and washings from occluded biliary stents showed a combined sensitivity of only 75 percent,[253] indicating that cytologic examination of PSC strictures rarely detects cholangiocarcinoma but is quite accurate when positive. Biliary dysplasia in liver biopsies indicated the presence of cholangiocarcinoma in patients with PSC with low sensitivity but high specificity and accuracy.[254]

The diagnostic utility of carbohydrate antigen (CA) 19-9 and carcinoembryonic antigen (CEA) has been investigated.[143] CA-19-9 is a marker of pancreatic adenocarcinoma, with a sensitivity of nearly 70 percent and a specificity of up to 90 percent.[255,256] The monoclonal antibody used in the test reacts with a carbohydrate determinant, sialosylfucosyl-lactotetraose, found on the sialylated blood group antigen Lewis. Biliary epithelial cells in PSC aberrantly express ABO blood group antigens, including the Lewis antigen.[256] Immunohistochemistry of cholangiocarcinomas showed that 71 percent and 91 percent expressed CA-19-9 and CEA, respectively.[242] Thus both antigens were markers of the tumor rather than the epithelial cells lining strictures. Elevated levels of CA-19-9 have been observed in patients with cholangiocarcinoma, but levels overlapped with those observed in patients with cirrhosis or bacterial cholangitis and the sensitivity and specificity were 75 percent and 80 percent, respectively.[257,258] Because levels of both tumor markers alone were not sufficiently sensitive or specific, a combined index was developed. The formula CA-19-9 + (CEA × 40) was used to evaluate cholangiocarcinoma in three groups of PSC patients: (1) 15 patients with histologically confirmed tumor; (2) 22 transplanted patients without tumor in the explants; and (3) 37 patients with stable disease not requiring transplant and no clinical evidence of tumor.[242] With a value greater than 400 as a cutoff, both specificity and positive predictive values were 100 percent. Sensitivity was only

66 percent because of the occurrence of values of lower than 400 in the tumor group. None of the transplanted patients without tumor had values greater than 400, but the index was positive in only 54 percent of transplanted patients with occult tumors in the explant. Clearly, more reliable and accurate tests are needed to detect early cholangiocarcinoma.

Dominant Strictures

Dominant strictures, defined as focal, high-grade narrowings of the intrahepatic or extrahepatic ducts, cause mechanical biliary obstruction with intensified cholestasis manifested by jaundice, pruritus, ascending cholangitis, and malabsorption. Dominant strictures develop in 15 percent to 20 percent of PSC patients during the course of disease.[195] They must be differentiated from cholangiocarcinomas,[143,241] but such distinction may be difficult or impossible with currently available methods (see previous discussion).

Ascending Cholangitis

Ascending cholangitis is rare without surgical manipulation of the extrahepatic bile ducts or development of dominant, distal strictures.[259] After it is established it tends to recur and may be associated with both septicemia and hepatic abscesses. Recurrent episodes may be difficult to treat because of the emergence of antimicrobial-resistant bacteria.

Cholelithiasis and Cholecystitis

Cholelithiasis occurs in approximately 20 percent of patients with PSC,[59,170,171] which is more prevalent than the age- and sex-matched prevalence in the general population. Approximately 33 percent of patients with PSC undergo cholecystectomy. Bacteria are present in the bile in up to 80 percent of PSC patients with cholelithiasis.[259] The risk of choledocholithiasis is correspondingly increased and should be considered during episodes of worsening cholestasis. Chronic cholestasis predisposes to the formation of lithogenic bile and cholesterol gallstones, whereas bile stasis, recurrent ascending cholangitis, and biliary cirrhosis increase the risk of pigmented calcium bilirubinate stones. Calculi of the biliary tract should not be considered an exclusion criterion for the diagnosis of PSC. In a recent study 23 of 61 (38 percent) patients with PSC had calculi.[170] These patients did not differ from a group of 38 PSC patients without calculi with respect to age, incidence of IBD, extent of cholangiographic abnormalities, prevalence of HLA B8, DR3 haplotype, frequency of cholangiocarcinoma, or need for liver transplantation. Lymphoplasmacytic acalculous cholecystitis has been considered a distinctive form of chronic cholecystitis in PSC.[260]

Hepatic Failure

Progression of PSC leads to biliary cirrhosis and ultimately hepatic failure manifested by jaundice, decreased hepatocellular synthetic function, and wasting of the musculature.[142] Such patients most often also have portal venous hypertension.

Portal Venous Hypertension

Biliary cirrhosis causes portal venous hypertension, manifested by complications including ascites, edema, esophageal or gastric varices (with or without bleeding), hepatic encephalopathy, hypoalbuminemia, coagulopathy, hypersplenism, and spontaneous bacterial peritonitis.[204] In cirrhotics a platelet count of lower than 88,000 is associated with the presence of esophagogastric varices (OR 5.5).[261]

Hepatocellular Carcinoma

Hepatocellular carcinoma occurs infrequently in patients with PSC and is more common in patients with varices.[168] At the time of transplantation, the prevalence of hepatocellular carcinoma was 2 percent in 134 PSC patients compared to 6 percent in 386 patients without PSC.[138]

Hepatic Osteodystrophy

PSC is frequently complicated by significant hepatic osteodystrophy, primarily resulting from osteoporosis. In the series from the Mayo Clinic 50 percent of patients had vertebral bone mineral densities below the threshold for spontaneous fractures.[262] PSC patients in a randomized trial of ursodeoxycholic acid (UDCA) had significantly lower bone mineral densities than control values adjusted for age, gender, and ethnicity.[263] However, only 8.6 percent had bone mineral densities below the fracture threshold, and the rate of bone loss was similar for both PSC patients and controls. Risks for bone mineral densities beneath the fracture threshold included older age, longer duration of IBD, and advanced PSC. Bone mineral densitometry of the lumbar spine should be performed in patients at risk to detect osteoporosis.

Steatorrhea and Fat-soluble Vitamin Deficiency

Chronic cholestasis results in decreased concentrations of intestinal bile acids required for absorption of fat and fat-soluble vitamins. Steatorrhea, which may be clinically inapparent, results in malnutrition and deficiencies of vitamins A, D, E, and K.[264] Levels of lipids and fat-soluble vitamins were measured in 56 PSC patients with compensated disease and 87 with advanced disease undergoing transplant evaluation.[265] Vitamin deficiencies were present in a minority of compensated patients: 40 percent for vitamin A, 14 percent for vitamin D, and 2 percent for vitamin E. In contrast, the majority of patients with advanced disease had vitamin deficiencies: 82 percent for vitamin A, 57 percent for vitamin D, and 43 percent for vitamin E.

Hyperlipidemia

Chronic cholestasis is associated with hypercholesterolemia.[266] Lipoprotein-X, an abnormal low-density lipoprotein, is a sensitive and specific marker for the presence of intrahepatic or extrahepatic cholestasis. It is elevated in patients with PSC and other cholestatic diseases. It contributes to the development of hypercholesterolemia by its failure to inhibit hepatic cholesterol synthesis. Hyperlipidemia is common in PSC. Among 56 PSC patients with compensated disease, 41 percent had hypercholesterolemia, 20 percent had elevated high-density lipoprotein cholesterol, and 2 percent had hypertriglyceridemia.[265] Cholesterol levels correlated directly with both bilirubin levels and histologic stage. Among transplant candidates with PSC, hypercholesterolemia was found in only 29 percent, and 17 percent had hypertriglyceridemia. Cholesterol levels were inversely correlated with bilirubin in this group.

Pancreatitis

Chronic pancreatitis resulting from sclerosing lesions of the pancreatic duct is a rare complication of PSC.[174,175,267,268] Pancreatitis should be considered in patients with chronic abdominal pain or abnormalities on imaging.

Peristomal Varices

In patients with PSC and portal hypertension who undergo colectomy for UC, bleeding varices may develop at the stoma.[108,111,269,270]

Pruritus

Cholestatic pruritus can occur in PSC patients with elevated alkaline phosphatase regardless of serum bilirubin levels.[271] Abrupt onset or worsening resulting from intensified cholestasis can be associated with cholelithiasis, dominant strictures, ascending cholangitis, or cholangiocarcinoma.

Colorectal Carcinoma with UC

In addition to extensive duration of UC and pancolitis, PSC is also a risk factor for colorectal carcinoma.[272-279] In one large study the cumulative risk of colorectal carcinoma in patients with both PSC and UC was 9 percent after 10 years, 31 percent after 20 years, and 50 percent after 25 years of disease.[198] In contrast, the cumulative risk for patients with UC alone at the same time points was significantly lower: 2 percent, 5 percent, and 10 percent, respectively. A case-control study substantiated these results by showing a cumulative incidence of colorectal carcinoma in UC patients with PSC of 11 percent after 10 years and 31 percent after 20 years compared with 3 percent at 10 years and 8 percent at 20 years in patients with UC alone.[280] Among 178 patients with PSC[277] there was no increased risk of colorectal carcinoma compared to patients with UC (some of whom also had PSC). However, for patients with both PSC and UC, the cumulative incidence of colorectal carcinoma or dysplasia was 20 percent at 20 years and 67 percent at 30 years after diagnosis of UC.[280] PSC patients remain at risk even after successful liver transplant.[281,282]

Surveillance colonoscopy with multiple biopsies should be performed to screen for dysplasia. In 16 patients with PSC and UC 56 percent had aneuploidy and 25 percent had dysplasia in surveillance biopsies of the colon.[283] In another study 59 patients with PSC and UC underwent surveillance colonic biopsies.[284] Interestingly, UDCA therapy was significantly associated with decreased dysplasia (OR 0.18).

Differential Diagnosis

The differential diagnosis of PSC includes common hepatobiliary diseases associated with cholestasis, diseases with cholangiographic features resembling PSC, and chronic hepatitis. Because PSC and UC are so strongly associated, differential diagnosis should be considered in any UC patient with abnormal liver tests. Classic diseases that must be differentiated from PSC include extrahepatic biliary obstruction, secondary sclerosing cholangitis, idiopathic cholangiohepatitis, PBC, drug-induced cholestasis, and chronic hepatitis (viral, drug-induced, and autoimmune).

PSC patients may have features resembling type 1 AIH,[30,31,85] and both occur as an overlap syndrome in a minority of patients.[75,77,82-84,152] Application of the newest revision of the international diagnostic scoring system for AIH to 211 PSC patients classified 1.4 percent as definitely having and 6 percent as probably having AIH.[80] Distinction may be particularly difficult in PSC patients with only small-duct pathology and a normal cholangiogram.[86] Because type 1 AIH also occurs in patients with IBD, both PSC and AIH must be considered in all patients with IBD and abnormal liver tests.[76,87]

Several immunodeficiency states are also associated with PSC-like lesions of the biliary tract (see Chap. 51).[285] These include familial combined immunodeficiency, X-linked immunodeficiency, angioimmunoblastic lymphadenopathy, agammaglobulinemia, and acquired immunodeficiency syndrome. Biliary sclerosis on cholangiography is also caused by infections with cryptosporidium,[286] trichosporon,[287] cytomegalovirus,[288-290] and cryptococcus.[291]

Etiology and Pathogenesis

Autoimmune and Non-autoimmune Mechanisms

Neither the etiology nor the pathogenesis of PSC is known. Immunopathogenesis has been hypothesized on the basis of associations with HLA haplotypes, multiple autoantibodies, and IBD.[292-294] The hypothesis that PSC is an autoimmune disease[295,296] fails to explain important differences between PSC and autoimmunity that include (1) absence of female predilection, (2) absence of disease-specific autoantibodies, and (3) poor response to immunosuppressive medications. The strong association of PSC and IBD, especially UC, provides circumstantial support for an autoimmunopathogenesis in PSC.

A variety of immunologic abnormalities have been reported in PSC, but their involvement in pathogenesis remains speculative. Indeed, it is likely that many may be epiphenomena.[292] The diversity of abnormalities suggests that the pathogenesis of PSC causes or is facilitated by the presence of immunologic dysregulation. Immunologic abnormalities in PSC include (1) decreased proportions of circulating T cells and CD8 T cells[297,298] and increased proportions of circulating B cells,[299] (2) decreased in vitro T suppressor cell functions,[300] (3) increased autologous mixed lymphocyte reactivity,[301] (4) immune complex–like materials in blood and bile,[302] (5) inappropriate expression of blood group antigens on biliary and colonic epithelia,[256] (6) complement activation and increased levels of C3b and C4d,[303] (7) C3d deposits on hepatic arteries but not bile ducts,[304] and (8) decreased in vivo clearance of artificial immune complexes by the hepatic macrophages.[305]

Non-immune factors such as infection, toxicity, ischemia, and neoplasia also provoke pathogenetic mechanisms resulting in secondary PSC.[285] It is important to note that PSC in the minority of PSC patients who never develop IBD is indistinguishable from that in patients with IBD. Although this might result from distinctly different etiologies and pathogenetic mechanisms of PSC in patients with and without IBD, it is more plausible that a common pathogenetic mechanism exists that is facilitated by the presence of immunogenetic susceptibility and IBD but does not absolutely require either. After bile duct obstruction results in cholestasis, additional mechanisms common to all forms of biliary obstruction promote inflammation, fibrosis, and, ultimately, secondary biliary cirrhosis.[134]

Bacterial products may play a key role in the etiology and pathogenesis of UC and possibly in PSC. For example, in "knockout" mice with T-cell receptor α-deficiency, the immune response to intestinal bacterial antigens drives both the pathogenesis of colitis and development of pANCA.[306] In interleukin (IL)-10 (-/-) knockout mice, spontaneous onset of colitis was accompanied by production of pANCA, and perinuclear staining was decreased by absorption of sera with bacterial antigens.[307] Similarly, specific perinuclear staining of pANCA from patients with PSC was also decreased or abolished after absorption with bacterial antigens.[307] These observations strongly indicate that immune responses to bacterial antigens are involved in the generation of colitis and pANCA. Immune reactions to bacterial cell-wall elements in genetically susceptible rats also result in PSC lesions.[308] Reactions of immunogenetically susceptible individuals to bacterial antigens, possibly acting as molecular mimics for autoantigens, are an attractive explanation that unifies autoimmune and non-autoimmune pathogenetic mechanisms.[309]

Reovirus and Portal Bacteremia

Infection of biliary epithelial cells or hepatocytes by unidentified viruses also has been postulated. Reports that Reovirus type 3 can induce cholangitis and biliary atresia in weanling mice,[310,311] primates, and possibly human neonates[312] led to its proposal as an etiologic agent in PSC. Despite evidence that it can induce experimental fibrosis and obliterative cholangitis, infection of human liver has not been substantiated. Moreover, recent data show that neither the prevalence nor the titer of antibodies to Reovirus type 3 differ between normal adults and patients with PSC.[313] The possibility that hepatitis viruses are involved in the pathogenesis remains unsupported. Although cytomegalovirus infection affects intrahepatic bile ducts, the histopathology is distinct from that of PSC.[314]

Portal Bacteremia

Portal venous blood and the liver parenchyma are sterile in normal humans.[315] Uncontrolled studies by Brooke and colleagues supported the possibility that bacteremia of the portal vein resulting from disruption of mucosal barriers in the bowel could produce pericholangitis.[316-318] Eade and Brooke cultured, aerobically and anaerobically, portal venous blood obtained at the time of colectomy from 100 patients with UC.[318] Biopsy specimens of the livers were cultured in the same manner. The culture of portal venous blood was positive for 24 patients, and the culture of the liver specimen was positive for 11. These results exclude cultures positive for *Staphylococcus albus,* a contaminant in an additional nine specimens of either portal venous blood or liver. Organisms of potential pathogenic significance included fecal aerobes and, in four instances, anaerobes. Although results of liver tests were not reported, the frequencies of histologic lesions (fatty infiltration, inflammatory cell infiltration, fibrosis, bile duct proliferation, and hepatocellular necrosis) were similar in patients with and without positive cultures.

In contrast to these results, Perrett and associates cultured aerobically 45 liver biopsy specimens from 42 patients with UC and found 41 negative and 4 positive cultures.[10] Each positive culture was ascribed to contamination. An unsuccessful attempt was made to culture L forms in specimens from 20 patients. Dordal and colleagues obtained similar results of aerobic and anaerobic cultures with 69 needle biopsy specimens obtained from a group of 103 patients with either UC or Crohn's disease.[18] Fifty-two cultures were negative, 15 were considered contaminated, and the remaining 2 grew *Paracolobactrum aerogenoides* and non-hemolytic anaerobic streptococci, respectively. Cultures of a second biopsy specimen from one of the last two patients were negative. The types of IBD were not specified for the patients whose biopsy specimens were cultured; thus the specific numbers of patients with UC and Crohn's disease are unknown. At the time of colectomy for Crohn's disease, Eade and colleagues cultured portal venous blood before handling the bowel in 9 of 21 cases.[21] *Proteus vulgaris* was present in a single specimen. Perrett and co-workers aerobically cultured needle biopsy specimens of liver from 34 patients with Crohn's disease.[19] Cultures of 30 of the specimens were negative, and the remainder were considered to be contaminated.

Based on the above results, the role of portal bacteremia in the pathogenesis of PSC remains moot. One interpretation of these studies is that the prevalence of positive cultures is too low to suggest that portal bacteremia is a factor in pathogenesis. Alternatively, portal bacteremia could have injurious effects, but by occurring only intermittently, may not be detected readily by a single culture. The question of the possible role of anaerobic bacteria has not been settled.

Experimental evidence for hepatic injury induced by portal venous bacteremia is scant but intriguing. Hektoen found inflammation, bile duct proliferation, and fibrosis of portal tracts in guinea pigs after a single intraperitoneal injection of pseudodiphtheriae.[319] Weaver produced identical lesions in guinea pigs by injecting *Escherichia coli.*[320] MacMahon and Mallory showed that a single injection of hemolytic streptococci into the mesenteric vein of rabbits produced acute inflammation of the portal triads, bile duct proliferation, and focal necrosis.[321] Wachstein and associates produced focal degenerative changes and Kupffer cell proliferation by intraperitoneal injection of *Salmonella typhimurium* into rats.[322] Vinnik and coworkers evaluated the effect of chronic portal venous bacteremia in calves.[323] In three of six animals the researchers found edema of the portal tract with inflammation, focal necrosis, bile duct proliferation, and Kupffer cell hyperplasia in association with elevated aspartate aminotransferase, alkaline phosphatase, and 5′-nucleotidase. Results of similarly designed studies to evaluate chronic portal bacteremia have not been reported.

Immunogenetics of Susceptibility and Disease Progression

The human major histocompatibility complex (MHC), designated HLA, is divided into three regions: class I, II, and III.[292] Class I and II molecules are expressed on the surface of cells and mediate different functions. HLA class I A, B, and Cw molecules bind antigenic 8-9mer peptides within cells and transport them to the surface for presentation to CD8 T cells. HLA class II molecules (DR, DQ, DP) are expressed on antigen-presenting cells and present processed 13-23mer peptides to CD4 T cells. The antigen binding sites of the HLA class I and II molecules determine which peptides are bound and presented. Genetic polymorphisms result in differences among amino acid residues in the antigen binding sites of HLA class I and II molecules that can either increase or reduce the risk of autoimmunity. The HLA class III region contains genes for other polymorphic peptides involved in the immune response, including tumor necrosis factor (TNF)-α and TNFβ; complement proteins C4, C2, and Bf; and MHC class I chain-related (MIC) molecules encoded by MICA and MICB genes. HLA genes are inherited in a codominant manner with a single haplotype being contributed by each parent to the offspring. The degree of association of alleles or haplotypes with disease is most often presented as an OR or etiologic fraction (EF). The latter indicates the relative contribution of the allele or haplotype to susceptibility or resistance.

The immunogenetics of PSC patients has been extensively investigated, and currently five distinct HLA haplotypes have been associated with PSC.[324] Initial serologic typing indicated that PSC was associated with HLA B8 and DR3 and with a secondary association with DR2 in DR3-negative patients. Conversely, DR4 was associated with a decreased risk of PSC. Subsequent molecular genotyping showed that three extended haplotypes were associated with susceptibility to PSC:

1. B8-TNF*2-DRB3*0101-DRB1*0301-DQA1*0501-DQB1*0201
2. DRB3*0101-DRB1*1301-DQA1*0103-DQB1*0603
3. DRB5*0101-DRB1*1501-DQA1*0102-DQB1*0602

Susceptibility was strongest for the first two and weaker for the third. Shared amino acid motifs indicated that susceptibility was associated with leucine at position 38 of the DRβ polypeptide (OR for homozygosity 5.84; EF 0.27). It is noteworthy that UC is not associated with these HLA haplotypes. In contrast, two haplotypes were strongly associated with resistance to developing PSC:

1. DRB4*0103-DRB1*0401-DQA1*03-DQB1*0302
2. MICA*002

The strongest positive associations in recent analyses were with HLA B8 in haplotype 1 (OR 3.0; EF 0.34), but its absence in the other two haplotypes associated with susceptibility suggested that the B8 association was due to linkage dysequilibrium between HLA B8 and the true susceptibility alleles in HLA class III region: TNFα promoter (TNFA*2) and MICA*008. Because the greatest susceptibility is associated with homozygosity for MICA*008 (OR 4.89; EF 0.47), this is either the major susceptibility allele or it is closely linked to the true susceptibility allele. The presence of DRB1 alleles in all three susceptibility haplotypes led to analysis of position 86 on the DR-β peptide that encodes either valine or glycine. Valine at position 86 was associated with DRB1*0301, DRB1*1301, and DRB1*1501 (OR 3.01; EF 0.62). Conversely, glycine at position 86 was associated with protective alleles DRB1*0401 and DRB1*04 (OR 0.17). Another model, developed to assess susceptibility with haplotypes 2 and 3 or resistance with haplotype 1, suggested that leucine in position 87 and proline in position 55 of the DQB explained these associations (OR 2.78 versus 0.28). Currently, HLA associations account for less than 50 percent of PSC cases based on any one allele, leucine at position 38 of DR-β or homozygosity for MICA*008. Thus attempts to formulate and validate a unified hypothesis for HLA susceptibility and resistance continue.

HLA alleles and haplotypes may also be associated with risk of progression and clinical features in PSC. In a study of HLA class II alleles in 265 PSC patients from five European countries[325] heterozygous haplotype DRB1*03-DQA1*0501-DQB1*02 (HLA DR3, DR2) was associated with increased risk of liver transplantation or death (hazard ratio 1.63, 95 percent CI 1.06-2.52). In patients without HLA DR3, DR2 the presence of a DQ6 encoding DQB1*0603 or DQB1*0602 was associated with a reduced risk of transplantation or death (hazard ratio 0.57, 95 percent CI 0.36-0.88). HLA DR4, DQ8 exhibited a trend for an increased risk of cholangiocarcinoma, but this did not reach statistical significance.

As with other autoimmune diseases immunoregulatory genes encoded outside of the MHC probably contribute to susceptibility, severity, or progression of PSC. Cytokines are particularly attractive for study because they are polymorphic and regulate the type and extent of immunologic reactions. Neither IL-1 nor IL-10 gene polymorphisms were found to be associated with PSC. Because the CTLA4 G allele at position 49 of exon 1 is associated with increased susceptibility to most organ-specific autoimmune diseases, including type 1 AIH and

PBC, it was investigated by two groups. The first found a positive association, whereas the second did not, raising the question of whether PSC is truly an autoimmune disease. Studies of chemokine receptor 5 of *TNFSF6,* the gene encoding Fas, showed that neither was associated with PSC. The dynamic process of fibrosis involves an excess production of matrix and reduced degradation that is regulated by the balance between metalloproteinases (MMPs) and the tissue inhibitors of metalloproteinases (TIMPs). Homozygosity for the 5A polymorphism of the gene encoding MMP3 (stromelysin) was significantly associated with portal hypertension, presumed to result from hepatic fibrosis. Single nucleotide polymorphisms in the TGFB1 gene encoding the profibrotic cytokine TGFβ were not associated with PSC. More extensive testing of other non-MHC genes may detect polymorphisms associated with PSC.

Autoantibodies

Indirect immunofluorescent microscopy has identified three distinct staining patterns of anti-neutrophil cytoplasmic antibodies (ANCA): diffuse cytoplasmic, pANCA, and atypical pANCA in which there is broad band of staining at the edge of the nuclear membrane and staining of intranuclear spots, believed to be invaginations of the nuclear membrane.[74] Between 26 percent and 88 percent of PSC patients, with or without UC, have atypical pANCA. It is important to recognize that typical pANCA are not specific for PSC but are also found with a prevalence of 60 percent to 87 percent in UC,[326] 5 percent to 25 percent in Crohn's disease, 50 percent to 96 percent in type 1 AIH, and 5 percent in PBC.[74] Because atypical pANCA react with antigens localized to the periphery of the nucleus, Worman has proposed the more accurate term *peripheral anti-neutrophil nuclear antibodies* (pANNA).[74] The molecular identity of the nuclear antigens recognized by pANNA is unknown. One study that supports the presence of nuclear antigens showed that DNase digestion of neutrophils resulted in conversion of the pANCA pattern to cANCA pattern in the majority of patients with PSC and type 1 AIH.[327] Another study used phage cloning techniques to show that the pANCA antigens in UC are unique.[328] Although the role of pANNA in the immunopathogenesis of PSC remains speculative, some studies suggest that either the presence or titers of pANNA are correlated with clinical features of PSC. For example, the presence of pANNA correlated with biliary complications,[329] intrahepatic, rather than extrahepatic, strictures[330] and higher titers were characteristic of cirrhosis.[331]

Reactivity to the cytoplasmic antigen recognized by classical pANCA (actin, catalase, and enolase) is rarely detected in sera from patients with PSC, IBD, or AIH.[74] Evidence that bacterial antigens are essential for development of colitis and pANCA from the T-cell receptor α "knockout" mice[306] suggests that bacteria may also induce pANNA in PSC. The possibility that pANCA are cross-reactive with enteric bacterial antigens was supported by evidence that absorption of pANCA-positive sera with bacteria reduced or abolished perinuclear staining of ANCA.[307] Cross-reactivity of pANCA with bacterial antigens is also consistent with the finding that 81 percent of PSC patients have antibodies against enterobacterial proteins.[332] A recent report showed that bacterial/permeability-increasing protein (BPI), an endotoxin binding neutrophil leukocyte-granular protein with anti-bacterial and anti-endotoxin activity, is a target antigen of ANCA in PSC, IBD, cystic fibrosis, and vasculitis.[333] The titer of BPI-ANCA was associated with greater inflammation and organ damage, suggesting that BPI-ANCA may promote inflammation by interfering with the clearance of gram-negative bacteria and endotoxin.

Multiple other autoantibodies have been detected in PSC but their role in pathogenesis is unknown. As with pANNA, none of these autoantibodies is specific for PSC. In PSC the prevalences of non-specific autoantibodies are 7 percent to 77 percent for ANA, 13 percent to 20 percent for SMA, 0 percent to 9 percent for AMA, 4 percent to 66 percent for anti-cardiolipin antibodies, 7 percent to 16 percent for thyroperoxidase, 4 percent for thyroglobulin, and 15 percent for rheumatoid factor.[74,98] Autoantibodies against an epitope of human tropomycin were identified in patients with UC or PSC that do not cross-react with HLA DPw9 but cause antibody-dependent cellular cytotoxicity of cells expressing this allele.[334] Anti-colon autoantibodies, which cross-react with hepatobiliary tissues, were detected in 62 percent of patients with PSC and UC, but only 17 percent of patients with UC alone.[335] In contrast, another anti-colon autoantibody reacted with a 40-kd molecule expressed by colonic epithelial cells and cross-reacted with undefined antigens in skin and biliary epithelia.[336,337] This finding suggests, but does not prove, that immune responses may be directed against shared antigens in colonic and biliary epithelia.

Biliary Epithelial and Endothelial Cells as Immunologic Targets

Although biliary epithelial cells (BEC) are assumed to be immunologic targets in vanishing bile-duct syndromes,[292] several observations suggest that they are not primary targets in PSC. Even though BEC express class I HLA, aberrant class II HLA, and intercellular adhesion molecule-1 (ICAM-1), the phenotype of antigen presenting cells (APC) and target cells for either CD4 or CD8 CTLs, T-cell inflammation of the biliary epithelia (non-suppurative destructive cholangitis), is rare in PSC,[134] and peribiliary CD8 CTLs are infrequently observed in pre-cirrhotic biopsies when BEC destruction would be expected to be prominent.[298] Instead, portal infiltrates in PSC are composed primarily of neutrophils and CD4 T cells with increased proportions of monocytes/macrophages and decreased proportions of natural killer (NK) cells compared with blood.[298,338,329] Although expression of B7 co-stimulatory molecules in PBC[338,340,341] suggested that BEC could activate CD4 T cells, BEC expression of CD58 (LFA-3), co-stimulatory B7, and Fas (CD95) in PSC was scant and intermittent.[338] Moreover, BEC in patients with PSC did not concomitantly express both class II HLA and ICAM-1, indicating that only a minority of cells might present antigen or be targets of CTLs.[342] The observation that both BEC and colonocytes inappropriately expressed ABO blood group antigens in PSC suggested that they might be immunologic targets in PSC and colitis.[256] However, a pathogenetic role for ABO antigens appears unlikely because neither antibody-mediated bile duct injury nor T-cell reactions against ABO blood group antigens have been observed in PSC. Expression of ABO antigens instead may be an epiphenomenon induced by cytokines or an early marker of dysplasia.[256]

Recent reports indicate that direct injury to the peribiliary arteriolar plexus can result in injury to the biliary tract.[301,343] Intra-arterial infusion of floxuridine[344] produces diffuse, focal strictures of the extrahepatic and intrahepatic bile ducts and fibrous inflammation of the portal tracts. Lesions were indistinguishable from those in PSC. Interestingly, strictures most commonly occurred in both extrahepatic and intrahepatic ducts, but were also observed in either site exclusively. Experimental embolization of alcohol into the hepatic arteries of Rhesus monkeys resulted in diffuse, focal intrahepatic biliary strictures; mild dilation of the intervening segments of the bile ducts; and chronic inflammation and fibrosis of the portal tracts.[343] Again, the cholangiographic picture was similar to that seen in PSC. Therapeutic injection of formaldehyde into echinococcal cysts connecting with the biliary tract also caused sclerosing cholangitis. In addition, periarteritis nodosa of the hepatic artery has been associated with cholangiographic findings similar to those in PSC.[343] These data strongly suggest that a pathologic process with many features similar to PSC may be initiated by arterial injury. It is attractive to speculate that immunologic mechanisms may subsequently perpetuate the process. However, immunohistochemical studies showing that the peribiliary capillary plexi remain intact although being pushed away from the bile duct by concentric layers of peribiliary fibrosis[345] do not support this speculation. Thus endothelial cells are unlikely targets of the immune reaction in PSC, but direct injury to the arterioles or progressive separation of the capillary plexi from the bile ducts may cause ischemia of the biliary epithelia.

T Lymphocytes, Adhesion Molecules, Chemokines, Cytokines, and CD66a

Despite absence of immunopathologic features of T-cell–mediated bile duct destruction in PSC, recent studies suggest that portal tract T cells have been sensitized to epithelial antigens expressed by the gut. T-cell lines propagated from the common bile ducts of two PSC patients expressed oligoclonal T-cell–antigen receptors (TCR).[346] Identical oligoclonality was found in a second biopsy specimen taken more than a year later. These T-cell lines were cytotoxic for enterocyte cell lines and proliferated in response to enterocytes. T cells from PSC livers also preferentially expressed Vβ3 TCR,[347] indicating prior activation by a limited number of antigens. No correlation was noted between Vβ3 TCR expression and the histopathologic stage of disease. Together these findings indicate that T cells in hepatobiliary infiltrates may have been activated by limited antigens expressed by enterocytes. Interestingly, mucosal addressin cell adhesion molecule (MadCAM-1), an adhesion molecule important for the homing of T cells to the gut, is aberrantly expressed by hepatic endothelial cells in IBD and PSC.[348] MadCAM-1 expression in sections of PSC liver biopsies supported adhesion of gut-derived alpha4beta7 integrin-positive T cells. Thus aberrant expression of MadCAM-1 might explain recruitment of enterocyte-sensitized, gut-derived mucosal T cells to the liver in PSC. It is interesting to speculate that such T cells might react with antigens expressed by both enterocytes and BEC (derived from the embryonic foregut) and promote fibrous obliterative cholangitis through the secretion of cytokines. Lymphocytes isolated from the livers of patients with PSC contained reduced percentages of T cells, proliferated poorly to mitogens, exhibited intracytoplasmic IL-1β and TNFα, and secreted excessive amounts of IL-1β and TNFα and only low levels of IL-2, IL-10, or IFN-γ.[349] Neither hepatic T cells nor NK cells mediated cytotoxicity in vitro. These findings were unique to PSC and not observed with hepatic lymphocytes from patients with AIH or PBC. Anti–TNFα neutralizing antibodies partially restored the proliferative and cytotoxic functions of the PSC lymphocytes, suggesting that the local concentration of TNFα is a major determinant of immunologic function. Comparison of the quantities of Kupffer cells in PSC and other liver diseases showed that PSC patients had a threefold increase.[164] This increase would be expected to augment production of IL-1β and TNFα. Serum levels of the major profibrotic cytokine TGFβ were also significantly increased in PSC, presumably resulting from secretion by Kupffer cells chronically stimulated with proinflammatory cytokines.[164]

Chemokines (*chemo*attractant cyto*kines*) and cytokines are most likely important mediators of portal inflammation, periductular fibrosis, atrophy of the biliary epithelia, and portal fibrogenesis. BEC secrete multiple chemokines and cytokines (Table 40-9), and inflammation up-regulates their expression. Both normal human BEC and a cholangiocarcinoma cell line expressed mitochondrial ribonucleic acid (mRNA) for the chemokine IL-8 in response to recombinant IL-1β, TNFα, or endotoxin.[350,351] This strongly suggests that either proinflammatory cytokines or endotoxin in the portal venous blood could trigger events leading to peribiliary localization of inflammation in vivo. PSC and PBC are characterized by accumulation of endotoxin within BEC, and to a lesser extent in Kupffer cells and hepatocytes.[352] The finding that bile from PSC patients contained significantly increased levels of IL-8 compared to bile from patients with PBC, alcoholic cirrhosis, or fulminant hepatic failure, indicated a degree of disease specificity. This is supported by the findings that BEC from the PSC livers contained IL-8 mRNA, and that intracellular IL-8 is present in both isolated BEC and intact bile ducts. In addition, serum levels of IL-8 are also significantly elevated in PSC.[353] Concurrent secretion of other chemokines secreted by BEC (Table 40-9) could also attract and activate inflammatory cells in the peribiliary environment. It appears likely that chemokines expressed by BEC and peribiliary endothelial cells dictate the composition of portal inflammatory infiltrates, characterized by neutrophils,

CD4 T cells, increased monocyte/macrophages, and decreased NK cells.[298]

CD66a, also known as biliary glycoprotein, is present in human bile and may contribute to the pathogenesis of inflammation and fibrosis in PSC. CD66a, a member of the carcinoembryonic antigen family and the human homolog of rat cell CAM,[354] is expressed by neutrophils, monocytes, hepatocyte canaliculi, ductular epithelia, enterocytes, nonhepatic endothelial cells, and myoepithelial cells in the breast.[355] Specific binding of neutrophil CD66a with CD66b or with the non-specific cross-reacting CD66c increases β2 integrin-mediated adhesion and oxidant activity. It binds to E-selectin, galectin 3, and bacterial type-1 fimbriae. CD66a is also intensely expressed by myoepithelial cells within infiltrative scars and sclerosing adenosis of the breast, indicating a potential role in sclerosing fibrogenesis. Although CD66a expression has not been investigated in PSC, its role in neutrophil and myoepithelial cell functions suggests that it may contribute to inflammation and fibrogenesis in sclerotic lesions.

Animal Models of PSC

Experimental models of colitis and small bowel bacterial overgrowth support the hypothesis that immune responses to bacterial products of the gut by immunogenetically susceptible hosts play a primary role in pathogenesis of biliary sclerosis.[309] Models of muramylpeptide-induced colitis in rabbits[356] and *E. coli* chemotactic peptide-induced colitis in rats[357] are characterized by histopathologic lesions reminiscent of PSC. A rat model of small bowel bacterial overgrowth in genetically susceptible strains provides more compelling evidence.[358,359] In this model bacterial wall peptidoglycan-polysaccharide enters the portal vein and causes portal inflammation, bile ductular proliferation, and cholangiographic strictures of both intrahepatic and extrahepatic bile ducts. The extent of injury correlated significantly with production of TNFα by Kupffer cells. Ursodeoxycholic acid, polymyxin B (which binds intraluminal endotoxin), or immunosuppression with prednisone, methotrexate, or Cyclosporin A did not prevent lesions. In contrast, hepatobiliary inflammation and TNFα expression were prevented by treatment with (1) mutanolysin, which selectively cleaves peptidoglycan-polysaccharide; (2) palmitate, which blocks Kupffer cell phagocytosis; or (3) pentoxifylline, which inhibits Kupffer cell secretion of TNFα. Phagocytosis of bacterial cell wall components in portal venous blood is a critical event in this model of peribiliary inflammation and biliary sclerosis, strongly suggesting that bacterial products and stimulation of the innate immune response are involved in the pathogenesis of PSC (see Figure 40-6). These results are also in accord with immunogenetic studies showing that the class III HLA TNF A2 allele predisposes to PSC[324] and evidence that endotoxin, a marker

TABLE 40-9

Effect of Expression of Chemokines and Cytokines by Biliary Epithelial Cells

Secreted molecules	Target cells	Effects
Chemokines*		
IL-8	Neutrophils	Neutrophil chemotaxis
Monocyte chemotactic protein-1	Monocytes	Exocytosis of neutrophil granules
		Neutrophil integrin expression
	T-cell blasts	Monocyte activation, chemotaxis, and integrin expression
	CD4 T cells	Activation
	Fibroblasts	Activation
	Eosinophils	Activation
	Basophils	Activation
	BEC	Induction of cytokine secretion
Cytokines		
IFN-γ	BEC	Increased HLA class I expression
		Aberrant HLA class II expression
		Increased ICAM-1 expression
	T cells	Induction of CD4 Th1 subset
TGF-β	BEC?	Weak stimulus for apoptosis
	Stellate cells	Activation of stellate cells
		Fibrogenesis and matrix remodeling
	T cells	Suppression of T-cell toxicity
TNF-α*	BEC	Weak stimulus for apoptosis; stimulus increased when combined with IFN-γ
	Macrophages	Activation
IL-6*	Hepatocytes	Induction of acute phase reaction
	CD4 T cells	Increased IL-4 favoring development of CD4 Th2 subset

IL, Interleukin; *IFN,* interferon; *BEC,* biliary epithelial cells; *HLA,* human leukocyte antigen; *TGF,* transforming growth factor; *TNF,* tumor necrosis factor. *Chemokines are not constitutively expressed but inflammatory cytokines induce gene expression.

of bacterial cell wall products in portal venous blood, accumulates in the BEC of patients with PSC.[352]

Pathophysiology of Biliary Obstruction

Obstruction of the biliary tract, regardless of etiology, results in a deleterious sequence of events that undoubtedly play a role in PSC.[360] Obstruction leads to increased endotoxin levels in the portal space, innate immune activation of Kupffer cells, and portal tract macrophages by endotoxin and possibly other bacterial cell wall products; macrophage secretion of proinflammatory cytokines IL-1β, TNFα, IL-6, TGFα/β and leukotrienes; loss of BEC tight junctional integrity caused by TNF-α; and regurgitation of bile into the peribiliary space. Accumulation of endotoxin inhibits BEC production of HCO_3^- and interrupts cholehepatic cycling between BEC and peribiliary capillaries, leading to local retention of noxious molecules. This milieu containing proinflammatory cytokines and endotoxin stimulates BEC to secrete chemokines and cytokines that mediate recruitment and activation of neutrophils, monocytes, and T cells. This cholestatic inflammatory environment promotes enzymatic degradation of extracellular matrix and ductular proliferation. Interestingly, matrix metalloproteinase 3 polymorphisms appeared to influence susceptibility and progression in PSC.[361] Proliferating ductules secrete platelet-derived growth factor (PDGF),[362-363] a potent activator of adjacent hepatic stellate cells. This fibromuscular reaction leads to extension of fibrous septa into the parenchyma and, ultimately, secondary biliary cirrhosis. The fact that PDGF is also expressed by periductular mesenchymal cells suggests that it can also activate peribiliary fibroblasts. The BEC of both stenotic and dilated ducts in patients with either hepatolithiasis or PSC aberrantly express stem cell factor, which is a ligand for c-kit that is expressed by mast cells in the peribiliary area and around proliferating bile ductules.[364] These mast cells also expressed profibrotic TNFα and fibroblast growth factor. Thus BEC expression of stem cell factor may result in augmented fibrogenesis induced by mast cells. These pathogenetic mechanisms are pertinent to the pathogenesis of PSC because lesions of both small and larger ducts create partial biliary obstruction. Interruption of the mechanisms responsible for periductal inflammation and obliterative fibrosing cholangitis in PSC would be expected to retard or abort this cascade.

Postulated Mechanism of PSC Pathogenesis

PSC may be initiated by an innate immune reaction (see Figure 40-6) of Kupffer cells and portal tract macrophages

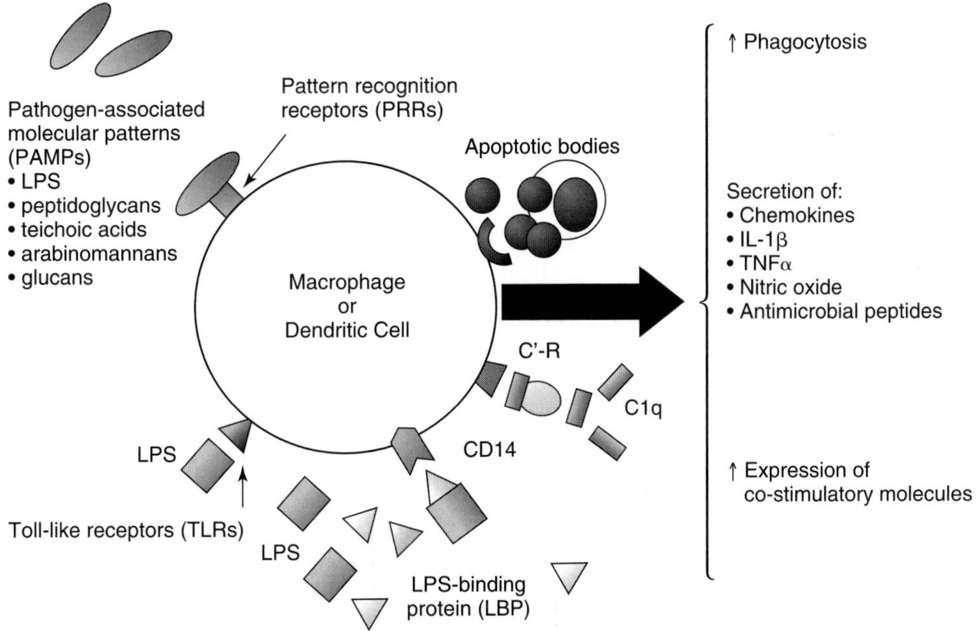

Figure 40-6 The innate immune response. Innate immunity is the capacity of phagocytes (macrophages, including Kupffer and dendritic cells) to react to pathogens by binding to specific molecules expressed by the pathogen or to complement molecules fixed to the pathogen. The innate immune response is not only the first defense against pathogens but also influences adaptive immune responses by modulating the activation thresholds of antigen-specific receptors and inducing co-stimulatory molecules and cytokines. Receptors on phagocytes, called pattern-recognition receptors, recognize invariant molecular structures called pathogen-associated molecular patterns (PAMPs). PAMPs include lipopolysaccharide (LPS, endotoxin), peptidoglycan, lipoteichoic acids, arabinomannans, glucans, and bacterial unmethylated CpG dinucleotides. In addition, the innate immune response also produces peptides with antimicrobial activity. (From Vierling JM: Animal models for primary sclerosing cholangitis. Best Pract Res Clin Gastroenterol 15:591-610, 2001.)

to bacterial cell wall products (e.g., endotoxin, peptidoglycans, lipoteichoic acid, arabinomannans, glucans, or unmethylated CpG) in an immunogenetically susceptible host (Figure 40-7). Increased permeability of the gut resulting from IBD or infectious enteritis and atypical flora resulting from subtle bacterial overgrowth would favor innate activation of hepatic macrophages and secretion of TNFα and other cytokines. The presence of TNFα and endotoxin in the peribiliary lymphatics draining the parenchyma would trigger a cascade of events, including induction of BEC secretion of chemokines and cytokines, increased permeability of BEC tight junctions with regurgitation of bile, inhibition of secretory functions of BEC, and disruption of the cholehepatic circulation. Chemokines and cytokines would attract and activate neutrophils, monocytes and macrophages, T cells, and fibroblasts in the peribiliary space. Sustained portal inflammation, abetted by high levels of TGFβ and PDGF, would activate peribiliary stellate cells, promote enzymatic digestion of extracellular matrix, and produce peribiliary fibrosis. New layers of concentric fibrosis would continuously displace the peribiliary capillary plexi away from the bile duct and produce a barrier to diffusion of gases and nutrients. This would interrupt the cholehepatic circulation, leading to retention of noxious substances, such as endotoxin. Focal ischemia would worsen as the distance between capillaries and bile ducts increased. The characteristic atrophy of BEC observed in PSC would result from these combined events. Inflammation and fibrosis would selectively destroy small bile ducts, and progressive stricturing of medium and large intrahepatic and extrahepatic ducts would accelerate biliary obstruction. Progressive cholestasis resulting from ductopenia and obliterative fibrous cholangitis of medium- to large-caliber ducts would activate additional pathophysiologic mechanisms common to all forms of mechanical biliary obstruction. Bile ductular proliferation at the margins of the portal tracts would initiate a fibroductular reaction resulting in interface hepatitis and bridging fibrous septa and, ultimately, secondary biliary cirrhosis. Prolonged ischemia, aberrant BEC gene expression, atrophy of BEC, exposure to chemokines and cytokines, and retention of noxious substances resulting from interruption of cholehepatic cycling may culminate in dysplasia and development of cholangiocarcinoma (see Figure 40-7).

Treatment

The treatment of PSC has three major goals: (1) prevention or retardation of complications, including those of chronic cholestasis, and (2) prevention or retardation of ductopenia and biliary obstruction that cause secondary cirrhosis. Despite major progress in the past decade, our ability to fulfill these goals remains limited, and a curative therapy for PSC has not been identified. Thus liver transplantation remains the only option for patients with advanced disease.

Management of Complications of Chronic Cholestasis

Pruritus

The benefit of anti-histamines for cholestatic pruritus is unpredictable and usually slight, but their soporific effect may promote sleep. Anion exchange resins

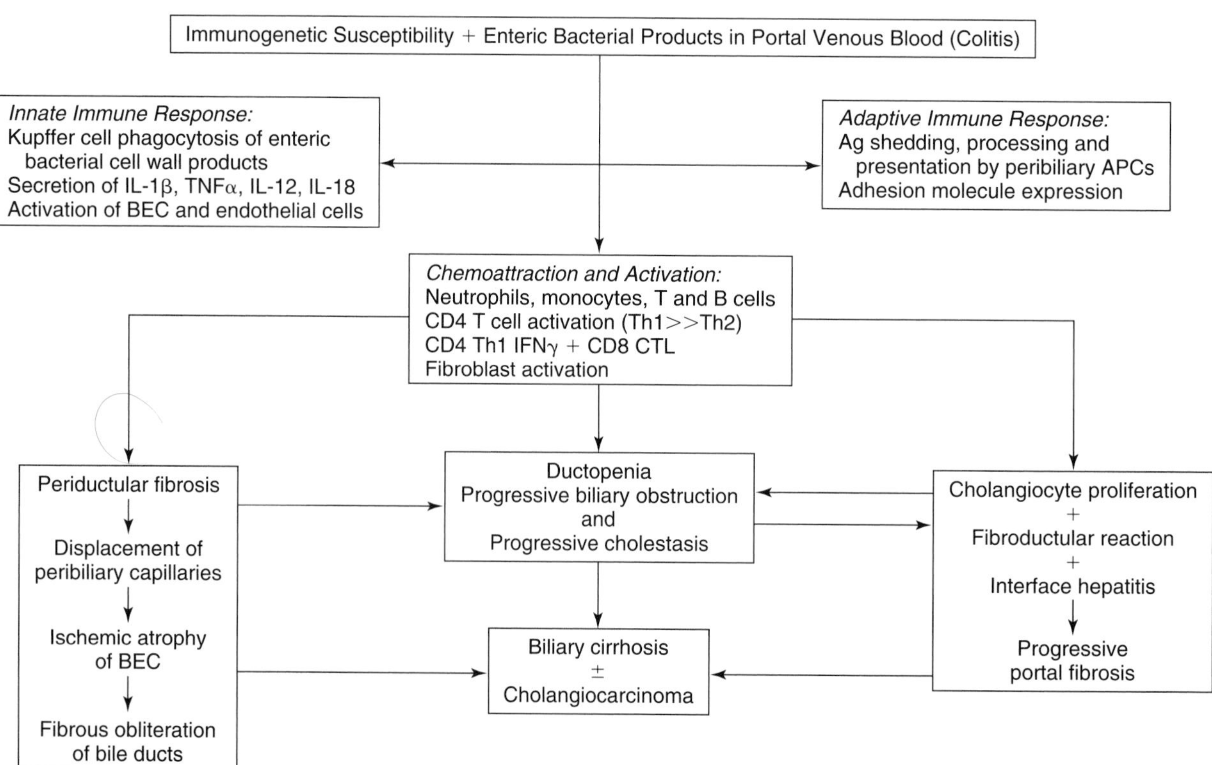

Figure 40-7 Postulated pathogenesis of primary sclerosing cholangitis.

(cholestyramine, colestipol, colesevelam) bind bile acids and putative pruritogens in the small intestine and prevent their absorption.[271] When pruritus is refractory to these measures, phenobarbital should be considered as a single dose at bedtime. Rifampicin improves pruritus in PBC[365,366] and malignant biliary obstruction,[367] and can be used empirically in PSC. Opiate antagonists for treatment of cholestatic pruritus are under investigation. For intractable pruritus with sleep deprivation or suicidal ideation, plasmapheresis, plasma exchange, or charcoal hemoperfusion has been anecdotally beneficial.[368-371]

Steatorrhea and Fat-soluble Vitamin Deficiency

All PSC patients are at risk for development of steatorrhea and secondary fat-soluble vitamin deficiencies; the risk increases with the duration and severity of cholestasis.[264] Steatorrhea in PSC can also occur as a result of celiac sprue,[372-374] chronic pancreatitis with pancreatic exocrine insufficiency,[267] and small bowel bacterial overgrowth.[375] Steatorrhea resulting from cholestasis results from inadequate concentrations of bile acids in the small bowel and can be improved by reducing dietary fat to less than 40 g/day. Patients should receive empirically vitamin D along with adequate dietary calcium and phosphorus. Vitamin E supplements of 400 IU/day are safe and effective in maintaining vitamin E levels. With severe fat malabsorption, water soluble d-α-tocopherol or tocopherol polyethylene glycol succinate are effective sources of vitamin E. Low serum levels of vitamin K can occur in the absence of coagulopathy but the clinical significance is unclear. Parenteral vitamin K1 is indicated for hypoprothrombinemia. Vitamin K2 (menadione-2 methyl-1, 4 naphthoquinone) should be avoided because of hepatotoxicity. Zinc deficiency should be treated before giving vitamin A supplements. Vitamin D deficiency can be assessed by testing serum levels of 25-hydroxy vitamin D. If levels are low, patients should take oral vitamin D derivatives, be advised to increase sun exposure to generate cutaneous vitamin D3, and to take supplemental calcium.[264,376] With severe malabsorption, tocopherol polyethylene glycol succinate not only provides vitamin E but can aid intestinal absorption of all fat-soluble vitamins.

Hyperlipidemia

Advancing cholestasis leads to hypercholesterolemia and, to a lesser degree, hypertriglyceridemia.[265,266] A fasting lipid panel should be obtained to evaluate the levels of low- and high-density lipoproteins. If low-density lipoproteins are significantly elevated sequential therapy with dietary fat restriction, colesevelam, or a statin should be considered.

Management of Complications of PSC

Ascending Cholangitis

Ascending cholangitis should be treated with intravenous antibiotics.[259] *E. coli, Klebsiella* species, and *Enterococcus faecalis* are the most common causes.[377] Broad-spectrum antibiotic treatment should be started empirically, recognizing that more than one organism is often identified in cultures of blood or bile.[377]

Cholangitis most commonly occurs after surgical manipulation of the bile ducts and less often as a spontaneous event.[24,30,31,35,149-151] Prompt treatment with antibiotics should be instituted to prevent hepatic abscesses and septicemia. Prophylactic antibiotics are of unproven benefit and may predispose to the development of resistant flora. Patients with recurrent episodes of cholangitis should have antibiotics (e.g., ciprofloxacin) available at home to initiate therapy at the onset of symptoms.

Dominant Strictures

Focal sclerosis of bile ducts may result in dominant strictures and acute or subacute worsening of clinical and biochemical cholestasis.[149-151,378] Dominant strictures should be dilated endoscopically or percutaneously. Stenting may be necessary to prevent rapid restructuring and the deleterious effects of biliary obstruction.[379-386] Although long-term stenting has been shown to be safe, others argue that it promotes ascending cholangitis.[385,387] Endoscopic sphincterotomy, dilation, and stenting of extrahepatic strictures were successful in 70 percent to 95 percent of patients, and patency was maintained in 50 percent to 70 percent after stent removal.[387] A retrospective review of prolonged stenting in 25 patients showed biochemical improvement in 84 percent who had stent replacement every 2 to 3 months.[384] Complications occurred in 14 percent of the 105 procedures. Among 15 PSC patients with dominant strictures, endoscopic therapy (dilation or stenting) alleviated the stricture in all. However, 5 of 15 (30 percent) developed cholangitis and 6 of 15 (40 percent) died, 5 of cholangiocarcinoma and 1 of colorectal carcinoma.[385] A retrospective study comparing the risks and benefits of balloon dilation alone versus dilation and stenting in 71 PSC patients showed that endoscopic stenting was associated with significantly greater incidence of acute cholangitis.[388] Stents provided no increased benefit over balloon dilation alone. Nasobiliary drainage and irrigation of the biliary tree was effective in improving symptoms in 8 of 12 (67 percent) patients during a mean follow-up period of 23 months.[389] Biliary diversion surgery should be avoided because of the risks of anastomotic strictures, increased incidence of bacterial ascending cholangitis,[206] and the adverse consequences of biliary surgery for liver transplantation.[139,238] However, in selected non-cirrhotic PSC patients with extrahepatic strictures, resection delayed the need for liver transplantation.[381]

Cholangiocarcinoma

No effective medical or surgical therapy for cholangiocarcinoma has been identified.[390,391] Long-term survival was dismal with radiation therapy or chemotherapy. Rare patients with localized tumor were candidates for resective surgery, whereas palliative stenting improved cholestasis resulting from obstructing lesions. Recently, photodynamic therapy was shown to relieve biliary obstruction in 6 patients with advanced cholangiocarcinoma.[392] Because nearly all recipients develop lethal recurrent tumor within 24 months after liver transplantation,[137,393,394] most transplant centers regard cholangiocarcinoma as an absolute contraindication. One large series indicated excellent long-term survival in transplanted patients with relatively rare nodular cholangiocarcinomas of smaller than 1 cm in diameter that were incidentally discovered in the explants.[137] A recent report indicated that a highly selected subgroup of patients with cholangiocarcinoma proximal to the cystic duct may be eligible for liver transplantation after treatment with a combination of radiation and chemotherapy and a laparotomy to exclude metastases.[395] All patients survived, and cholangiocarcinoma recurred in only one patient. Three patients had been followed for less than 12 months, whereas 8 had a median follow-up of 44 months, indicating acceptable long-term survival.

Cholelithiasis and Choledocholithiasis

Cholelithiasis and choledocholithiasis may occur in patients with chronic disease.[59,170,171] Cholecystitis should be considered in patients with PSC and right upper quadrant abdominal pain. Cholecystectomy is indicated only for symptomatic cholecystitis and cholelithiasis, not asymptomatic cholelithiasis. UDCA may prevent formation of or dissolve cholesterol gallstones in PSC. Pigmented stones composed of calcium bilirubinate may accumulate proximal to strictures and contribute to the degree of biliary obstruction. There is no specific therapy for pigmented stones. Impaction of intraductal stones may worsen cholestasis or precipitate cholangitis and should be excluded by retrograde cholangiography.[378] After the stones are identified, an endoscopic sphincterotomy should be performed and the stones removed.

Hepatic Osteodystrophy

There is no definitive therapy for osteoporosis. To minimize the rate of progression, patients with osteoporosis should maintain a diet high in calcium (1000-1500 mg/day of calcium carbonate), take bisphosphonates, and take supplemental vitamin D.[376]

Portal Venous Hypertension

Portal venous hypertension may result in hemorrhage from esophageal or gastric varices. Local measures such as injection of sclerosants or ligation should be performed to obliterate varices. If unsuccessful, a transjugular intrahepatic shunt or distal splenorenal shunt may be required for decompression.

MANAGEMENT OF PSC DISEASE

No specific therapy except for orthotopic liver transplantation (OLT) has been identified that is capable of curing or arresting the disease. Although some recent evidence indicated that progression can be retarded, these results require independent validation.[379] It remains difficult to assess therapeutic efficacy in PSC because of wide variation in the localization and severity of stricturing, a natural history characterized by exacerbations and remissions, and the impact of dominant strictures and cholangiocarcinoma.

Surgery to Alleviate Obstruction

In early reports surgery to relieve biliary obstruction did not retard the progress of disease,[30,31,196,203] and secondary biliary cirrhosis developed despite surgical relief of strictures.[171,381] Surgery of the bile ducts increases the risk of recurrent ascending cholangitis.[205] Both internal and external biliary drainage has been performed in uncontrolled reports but have not been shown to be beneficial. Currently, most surgeons advocate avoidance of hepatobiliary surgery in PSC.[380] A possible exception is resection of a dominant extrahepatic biliary stricture in a non-cirrhotic patient, which appeared to delay the need for transplantation.[381]

Proctocolectomy

The effect of proctocolectomy has been evaluated in uncontrolled series.[24,149-151] As discussed previously, there is no evidence that colectomy influences the course of PSC. Its lack of efficacy is best demonstrated by reports of PSC occurring in patients after colectomy.[206,396-398] Patients with PSC who require colectomy for UC have an increased risk of perioperative mortality.[397] The only clinical or biochemical factor that significantly predicted perioperative death was the presence of cirrhosis; 3 of 8 patients with cirrhosis died, whereas all 16 patients without cirrhosis survived. Peristomal varices may develop at the ileostomy site in PSC patients with portal hypertension.[108,269,270] As a result, ileoanal, ileorectal, or ileal pouch-anal anastomoses are preferred because they are unassociated with a risk of varices or bleeding.[399] However, the risk of chronic pouchitis is increased in PSC patients (60 percent) compared to UC patients without PSC (15 percent).[400] Pouchitis was unrelated to the severity of PSC, but was less common in patients with small-duct PSC. Interestingly, pouchitis may persist in patients after OLT, despite intense immunosuppression.[401] This observation suggests that anti-microbials, rather than immunosuppression, are the preferred treatment.

Medical Therapy

Varieties of medications have been used to treat PSC in open-label and controlled clinical trials. The principal categories include anti-microbial, immunosuppressive, anti-inflammatory, anti-fibrotic, and cytoprotective agents. Unfortunately, no medical therapy has been shown to be curative.

Antibiotics

Based on the concept that PSC was caused by portal bacteremia or bacterial toxins, uncontrolled trials with a variety of antibiotics were performed.[24,149,402,403] Antibiotics were ineffective. They should not be used for primary treatment but reserved for treatment of bacterial cholangitis.

D-penicillamine

Hepatic copper concentrations progressively increase in primary sclerosing cholangitis as a result of chronic cholestasis.[223,404] A randomized, double-blind, placebo-controlled therapeutic trial of D-penicillamine indicated that cupruresis occurred in the treatment group but was unassociated with improvement in clinical, biochemical, or histopathologic features or with increased survival.[405]

Corticosteroids and Azathioprine

A variety of therapies has been employed to suppress inflammation and immunologic reactions. Corticosteroids have been administered systemically and by nasobiliary lavage in PSC, but results are uninterpretable because of the small numbers of patients and lack of suitable controls.[24,149-151] However, occasionally benefit was observed.[406] A recent study of oral budesonide in 21 PSC patients showed a modest decrease in alkaline phosphatase and AST, significantly increased bilirubins, and lack of change in the Mayo PSC Risk Score.[407] Significant loss of bone mass occurred, contrary to the expectation that budesonide was a bone-sparing steroid. Azathioprine therapy has been reported in two patients: one improved and the other deteriorated.[408,409]

Colchicine

The efficacy of combined prednisone and colchicine was evaluated in 12 patients by comparing their natural history with that of concurrent historic controls.[410] Although significant improvements in liver tests were noted in the treatment group at both 6 and 12 months, there were no significant differences between groups after 24 months. Moreover, serial liver biopsies showed no differences. The results of a randomized, double-blind, placebo-controlled trial showed no effect of colchicine on clinical, laboratory, histopathology, or survival.[208]

Methotrexate

Improvement in the liver tests of two men with PSC treated with methotrexate led to larger therapeutic studies.[411] Initial reports of an open-label trial in 10 patients suggested a beneficial effect after 1 year of treatment.[412] However, the results of a randomized, placebo-controlled, double-blind trial of methotrexate in PSC from the same group did not confirm efficacy.[413] In the latter trial 24 patients were randomized to receive oral-pulse methotrexate or placebo for 2 years; 7 of 12 patients receiving methotrexate were cirrhotic, as were 5 of 12 receiving placebo. Despite a significant reduction of alkaline phosphatase in patients treated with methotrexate, there were no significant differences between the groups with respect to other liver tests, histologic progression, endoscopic retrograde cholangiography, or outcome. Although no significant toxicities were reported in these trials, one PSC patient treated with methotrexate developed severe *Pneumocystis carinii* infection.[414] Thus methotrexate should not be used empirically.

Cyclosporine

In a recent double-blind, placebo-controlled trial 35 precirrhotic patients with PSC were randomized to receive low-dose cyclosporine (4.1 mg/kg/day) or placebo for at least 1 year.[415] Thirty patients had UC and three had had previous colectomy. Although cyclosporine treatment significantly reduced alkaline phosphatase levels, it did not improve symptoms of cholestasis, prevent histologic progression, or retard development of complications of portal hypertension. Thus cyclosporine appears to be ineffective as a primary therapy. Two case reports, however, suggested that cyclosporine was beneficial. In the first a woman with PSC and UC was treated with cyclosporine 10 mg/kg/day for malignant pyoderma gangrenosum, and she experienced a remission of both PSC and UC.[416] In the second, cholangiographic features of PSC and pancreatic duct abnormalities significantly improved in a man treated with cyclosporine and methylprednisolone.[417]

During a double-blind, placebo-controlled therapeutic trial of cyclosporine in PSC, treatment significantly improved the UC.[418] At randomization there were no differences between the proportions of patients in the treatment and placebo groups with remission or mild colitis (88 percent versus 90 percent) or moderate colitis (12 percent versus 10 percent). During therapy the frequency of remission or mild colitis significantly increased in the cyclosporine-treated group and decreased in the placebo group. Similarly, the frequency of moderate colitis significantly decreased in the cyclosporine group and increased in the placebo group.

Tacrolimus

An open-label trial of 12 months of treatment with low-dose tacrolimus in 10 patients with PSC resulted in decreases of 75 percent for bilirubin, 70 percent for alkaline phosphatase, and 83 percent for aminotransferase.[419] Tacrolimus levels were maintained between 0.6 and 1.0 ng/ml, and no significant toxicities were noted. Controlled trials of tacrolimus therapy have not been reported.

Nicotine

Based on evidence that PSC occurs more frequently in non-smokers and that smoking reduces the risk of PSC in patients with UC,[189,190,420] a pilot study of oral nicotine was performed in eight patients with PSC.[421] Drug intolerance, manifested as reactivation of UC, dizziness, and palpitations, required discontinuation in three patients. Three of the five patients that completed 1 year of therapy temporarily decreased their dose because of adverse effects. No significant changes in liver tests were observed.

Pentoxifylline

Based on evidence that pentoxifylline inhibition of hepatic macrophage production of TNFα prevented PSC-like lesions in a rat model of small bowel bacterial overgrowth,[359] a pilot study was conducted in 20 patients with PSC.[422] Two were non-compliant and two others withdrew because of severe nausea. In the 16 who completed 1 year of therapy there were no significant changes in fatigue, pruritus, liver tests, serum TNFα, or TNF receptors.

Ursodeoxycholic Acid

Although safe, the efficacy of UDCA therapy in PSC remains controversial because of differences in doses, primary endpoints, and use of therapeutic endoscopy. Significantly improved laboratory tests have been reported in open-label and randomized, controlled trials of UDCA in PSC.[379] Whether UDCA retards long-term clinical and histologic progression or development of complications remains unclear. Randomized, placebo-controlled trials of UDCA therapy have shown significant improvement in laboratory tests, including bilirubin, and the degree of portal inflammation on biopsy.[423-425]

A prospective, randomized, double-blind, placebo-controlled trial of UDCA was conducted in 14 patients with PSC.[423] Eight patients received placebo and six UDCA; one patient from each group withdrew. UDCA treatment for 1 year significantly improved total bilirubin, alkaline phosphatase, gamma-glutamyl transpeptidase, and aminotransferases compared with values in the placebo group. Histology also improved significantly and the density of HLA class I antigen expression on hepatocytes was reduced in the treated patients. In contrast, results of another controlled trial using a lower dose of 600 mg/day were negative.[426]

In another trial 27 patients were treated with UDCA for 12 months before being enrolled in a controlled phase.[424,427] After 12 months of therapy 20 patients were enrolled in a double-blind, placebo-controlled trial. Statistically significant worsening of alkaline phosphatase, gamma-glutamyl transferase, and aminotransferases in patients treated with placebo led to discontinuation of the controlled trial and continuation as a prospective, open-label study in which new patients were enrolled. Unique features of this study were an annual surveillance, ERCP, and endoscopic dilation without stenting of all dominant strictures. In 65 patients treated with UDCA 750 mg/day (8.8-15.3 mg/kg/day; median 10.85 mg/kg/day) for up to 8 years 12 (18.4 percent) had dominant strictures at entry that responded to endoscopic dilation, whereas 11 (16.9 percent) developed dominant strictures requiring dilation. One patient died from cholangiocarcinoma and another required OLT. The Kaplan-Meier estimate of survival of the 65 patients was significantly greater than the predicted survival using the Mayo Risk Score model, but the relative contribution of UDCA and alleviation of dominant strictures cannot be assessed.[379] Thus UDCA does not prevent dominant strictures, but a combination of UDCA therapy and endoscopic dilation of dominant strictures may prolong survival.

Time to treatment failure was the primary endpoint in the Mayo Clinic's large, randomized, double-blind, placebo-controlled trial of UDCA (13-15 mg/kg/day) in 105 patients.[425] Treatment failures were defined as: (1) death or OLT; (2) progression of two histopathologic stages or development of cirrhosis; (3) occurrence of varices, ascites, or hepatic encephalopathy; (4) quadrupling of bilirubin; (5) significant worsening of fatigue or pruritus; (6) drug intolerance; or (7) withdrawal from the study. After a median follow-up of 2.2 years treatment failures were comparable in both UDCA (53 percent) and placebo groups (52 percent). As observed in prior studies, UDCA significantly improved alkaline phosphatase, AST, bilirubin, and albumin.

Results of a randomized, double-blind, placebo-controlled trial of the effect of higher dose UDCA (20 mg/kg/day) on clinical, biochemical, histologic, and cholangiographic endpoints in 26 PSC patients were recently reported.[428] Liver biopsies and cholangiography were performed at baseline and after 2 years of therapy. Two patients withdrew from the study: one in the UDCA group because of a dominant stricture requiring stenting and the other from the placebo group for variceal hemorrhage. One patient in the placebo group died of a non-hepatobiliary cause. Symptoms did not improve in either group, but significant improvements were found in patients treated with UDCA. As anticipated, liver biochemical tests significantly improved in the UDCA group. The hepatic activity index of biopsies was either stable or improved in 10 of 11 patients receiving UDCA but worsened in 7 of 10 patients receiving placebo. Similarly, histopathologic stage was either unchanged or decreased in 8 of 11 receiving UDCA, whereas it increased in 7 of 11 patients receiving placebo. Cholangiographic severity in 11 patients treated with UDCA was unchanged in 7, improved in 2, and worsened in 2. In contrast, cholangiography in 11 patients receiving placebo improved in 4 and worsened in 7. In an open-label, pilot study 30 PSC patients were treated with high-dose UDCA (25-30 mg/kg/day) for 1 year.[429] Changes in the Mayo Risk Score and the projected survival at 4 years in the treated patients were compared with those previously observed in the 105 patients randomized to treatment with 13 to 15 mg/kg/day or placebo.[425] After 1 year, the Mayo Risk Scores were significantly different among the three groups and the projected 4-year survival was significantly improved for patients treated with high-dose UDCA compared to placebo. In both trials high doses of UDCA were well tolerated without significant side effects. These encouraging results support the need for a large, multi-center, randomized, placebo-controlled trial of high-dose UDCA in PSC.

Ursodeoxycholic Acid and Corticosteroids

An 8-week, double-blind pilot study of the efficacy of budesonide (3 or 6 mg/day) or prednisone (10 mg/day) was conducted in 18 PSC patients who did not have biochemical remissions during UDCA treatment (mean dose 12 mg/kg/day) for at least 5 months.[430] No significant clinical or biochemical changes occurred in patients treated with budesonide, whereas prednisone treatment significantly reduced pruritus and alkaline phosphatase levels. Interestingly, one patient developed an AIH flare while being tapered off budesonide.

Ursodeoxycholic Acid and Methotrexate

A pilot study comparing the effect of combination therapy with UDCA (13-15 mg/kg/day) and methotrexate (0.25 mg/kg/wk) and UDCA alone did demonstrate significant differences.[431] Laboratory tests improved to a similar degree with both regimens. Methotrexate toxicities led to its withdrawal in several patients.

ORTHOTOPIC LIVER TRANSPLANTATION

OLT is the only life-sustaining and potentially curable therapy for PSC patients with decompensated cirrhosis and complications of portal venous hypertension or patients with debilitating complications of cholestasis, such as pruritus or hepatic osteodystrophy.[142,432] Because PSC frequently involves the extrahepatic bile ducts and is associated with the risk for cholangiocarcinoma in the recipient extrahepatic duct, OLT is performed exclusively with a choledochoenterostomy biliary anastomosis.

Optimal timing of OLT is difficult to predict because of the variability in the clinical progression in PSC, the impact of complications, and the inability to screen and detect cholangiocarcinoma. Most centers regard the diagnosis of cholangiocarcinoma as an absolute contraindication to OLT,[392] although patients with nodular tumors smaller than 1 cm in diameter discovered incidentally in the explant have an excellent survival. Further studies are required to assess the encouraging results of combined radiation and chemotherapy in selected patients with cholangiocarcinoma before OLT.[395] Guidelines for monitoring and selection of patients for OLT[142] include (1) biannual evaluations of asymptomatic patients; (2) close, individual monitoring of symptomatic patients with diffuse sclerotic lesions; (3) consideration as candidates for controlled therapeutic trials of medical therapy; (4) endoscopic balloon dilation of dominant strictures with brushings for cytology and biopsy to diagnose cholangiocarcinoma; (5) calculation of the Mayo Risk Score to predict survival; and (6) calculation of the Model of End-Stage Liver Disease score to determine eligibility and priority for OLT.

Recent retrospective analyses strongly indicate that OLT is effective therapy for advanced PSC.[142] Among 216 PSC patients who underwent OLT at either the University of Pittsburgh or the Mayo Clinic between 1981 and 1990, the mean age was 42 years and mean pretransplant bilirubin was 13 mg/dl.[237] Ninety-seven percent had cirrhosis. Survival of transplanted patients was compared with the survival predicted by the Mayo Multicenter Study Group calculation during a mean follow-up of 34 months (range 1-104 months). As early as 6 months, actual survival after OLT (89 percent) exceeded predicted survival (83 percent) by the end of 6 months, and the actual survival 5 years after OLT was 73 percent. This was significantly greater than the estimated survival of 28 percent without OLT. Another series reported the survival of 127 consecutive PSC patients transplanted during a 12-year period at UCLA.[137] IBD was present in 72 percent, and 62 percent had had previous biliary surgery. The actuarial 5-year graft survival was 72 percent and patient survival was 85 percent. Prior biliary surgery did not adversely affect graft or patient survival. All four transplant patients with cholangiocarcinoma had recurrent tumor within 6 months. In contrast, the 5-year survival was 83 percent for 10 patients with incidental nodular cholangiocarcinomas in the explants. Thus the outcome of OLT in patients with PSC is excellent in the absence of cholangiocarcinoma.

The effect of IBD on the outcome of PSC patients after OLT was assessed by comparing 31 patients with and 24 patients without IBD.[433] Patients with IBD had significantly more episodes of acute rejection, but the incidence of ductopenic rejection was comparable, as was the 5-year survival rate. Thus IBD does not adversely impact the success of OLT.

Recurrent Primary Sclerosing Cholangitis after Orthotopic Liver Transplantation

Intrahepatic biliary strictures, a common complication of OLT for any indication, occurred in 8.2 percent of 1590 allografts in one study[434] and in 15 percent of 687 allografts in another (see Chap. 56).[435] There were multiple strictures in 76 percent and single strictures in 24 percent of patients.[434,435] Statistically significant risk factors for postoperative strictures included hepatic artery occlusion, a diagnosis of PSC, choledochojejunostomy biliary anastomosis, use of Euro-Collins organ preservative solution, presence of cholangitis on liver biopsy, and young age.[434] The frequency of intrahepatic strictures was higher for PSC patients undergoing OLT (27 percent) than for patients with other liver diseases (13 percent), whereas the frequencies of anastomotic strictures (including choledochojejunostomy anastomoses) were similar.[435] Whether the higher incidence of intrahepatic biliary strictures in PSC patients after OLT is due to recurrent PSC remains debatable.[137,436-439] Comparison of post-OLT histopathology between 22 patients with PSC and 22 patients without PSC who had choledochojejunostomy biliary anastomoses[436] indicated that PSC can recur in the allograft. In the PSC group histologic cholangitis was found in 33 percent, and 14 percent had obliterative fibrous cholangitis. However, evidence of histologic cholangitis or obliterative fibrous cholangitis in 14 percent and 5 percent of the controls shows that neither feature is proof of recurrence. The prevalence of recurrent PSC, defined by strict criteria, was studied in 150 PSC patients transplanted at the Mayo Clinic.[440] Criteria for a probable recurrence included the presence of typical biliary strictures on cholangiography more than 90 days post-OLT or fibrous cholangitis on liver biopsy in the absence of exclusion criteria. Exclusion criteria included absence of hepatic artery thrombosis or stenosis, ductopenic rejection, solitary anastomotic stricture, nonanastomotic strictures occurring less than 90 days post-OLT, and ABO blood group incompatibility between donor and recipient. These criteria excluded 30 patients. The remaining 120 PSC patients were compared to 30 non-PSC patients with choledochojejunostomy biliary anastomoses and 434 patients with duct-to-duct anastomoses. Criteria for PSC recurrence were present in 24 patients (20 percent) after a mean post-OLT period of

421 days.Twenty-two (92 percent) met cholangiographic criteria, 11 (46 percent) had histopathologic criteria, and 9 (38 percent) fulfilled both. In contrast, strictures occurred in only 4 of 434 (1 percent) controls with duct-to-duct anastomoses and 1 of 26 (4 percent) controls with choledochojejunostomy biliary anastomoses. Recurrence is most often observed after withdrawal of corticosteroids from the immunosuppressive regimen.[441] Persistence of pANCA after OLT did not correlate with histologic evidence of recurrent PSC.[442] Overall, the data support the conclusion that PSC can recur after OLT, but distinction between recurrent disease, ischemic strictures, and histologic cholangitis unassociated with PSC remains difficult.

UC after Orthotopic Liver Transplantation

The impact of OLT and immunosuppression on the activity of UC varies widely.[200,393,443-446] Some patients have continued disease, some experience remission, others flare, and still others develop colitis for the first time. In one report 7 of 14 transplant patients with symptomatic UC continued to have active disease, and 3 of 13 with asymptomatic UC developed active disease.[443] Proctocolectomy was indicated for intractable UC in four patients. UC was also more severe after OLT in another 18 patients transplanted for PSC and active UC.[200] During a mean follow-up of 38 months, symptomatic UC continued in 50 percent and became worse in 50 percent. In contrast, 23 other PSC patients with asymptomatic UC were reported to remain asymptomatic after OLT, and 15 of 17 patients with symptomatic UC preoperatively improved dramatically after OLT.[444] Four of 12 patients with quiescent UC experienced flares after OLT. More importantly, UC developed for the first time after OLT in 3 of 12 patients. Among 25 patients transplanted for PSC and concomitant UC, 6 required proctocolectomy, 1 a subtotal colectomy, and 3 partial colectomies.[445] After a mean follow-up period of 37 months, 49 percent had quiescent disease, 14 percent had mild flares, and 6 percent had severe flares. Mild flares responded to treatment with 5′-aminosalicylates, whereas severe flares required increased doses of prednisone. PSC patients who required an ileal pouch–anal anastomosis for UC after OLT[446] experienced an increased frequency of complications, including bleeding and hepatic artery thrombosis. Thus even intense immunosuppression after OLT cannot prevent flares of UC or the de novo onset of disease in some patients. Post-OLT immunosuppression also may not improve pouchitis.[401]

Risk of Colon Cancer after Orthotopic Liver Transplantation

It is important to recognize that the risk of colorectal carcinoma in patients with PSC and UC is increased after OLT.[227,281,282,393,447] Among 33 patients with PSC and IBD (32 with UC and 1 with Crohn's colitis) undergoing OLT, 2 had had prior proctocolectomy and 4 died postoperatively.[281] Three of the remaining 27 patients (11 percent) developed colonic neoplasia within 9 to 13 months (2 had colon carcinoma and 1 had villous adenoma with dysplasia), despite negative screening colonoscopies before OLT. All had successful proctocolectomy. No differences in the mean duration of IBD among those with and without neoplasia were evident. In another series of 108 patients transplanted for PSC had IBD (80 with UC and 1 with Crohn's disease) 24 of 81 (30 percent) had had proctocolectomy.[277] The cumulative incidence of colonic dysplasia was 15 percent at 5 years and 21 percent at 8 years. Three of 57 patients developed colon carcinoma during a mean follow-up of 4.2 years, which represented a fourfold increased risk compared to that expected. Actuarial survival was comparable for those with and without proctocolectomy. Not all series have shown an increased risk of colon carcinoma. For example, no carcinomas occurred in 127 consecutive PSC patients transplanted over 12 years.[137,443,448] In conclusion the risk of colorectal dysplasia and carcinoma in transplanted patients transplanted with PSC and IBD warrants screening colonoscopy with multiple biopsies every 6 months for the first 2 years and every year thereafter to detect colonic dysplasia or carcinoma.

CARCINOMA OF THE BILIARY TRACT

Carcinoma of the biliary tract occurs in association with UC[29,158,449,450] with an estimated frequency of 0.4 percent, which is 10 times greater than in the general population.[29] In a comprehensive analysis of the association between carcinoma of the biliary tract and UC Ritchie and colleagues reviewed the cases of 67 patients.[29] The male-to-female ratio of 1.6:1 in patients with UC and carcinoma of the biliary tract is in accord with the observation of a male predominance in patients with cholangiocarcinoma who do not have UC.

Pathology

Most tumors are adenocarcinomas and are associated with an extensive desmoplastic reaction. An anaplastic tumor with a squamous cell component has been found in one patient.[124] The tumors occur most frequently in the extrahepatic ducts, but may involve the intrahepatic ducts or occur at the bifurcation of the hepatic ducts. Cholangiocarcinoma can develop in patients with long-standing PSC (discussed previously).[1,24,30,31,149-151] In 9 of 67 patients reviewed by Ritchie and colleagues tumors arose in the gallbladder.[29]

Clinical Features

Pancolitis was present in 87 percent of patients for whom the extent of colitis was reported.[29] The mean duration of UC before the diagnosis of carcinoma was 15 years, but the range was wide and included instances of carcinoma diagnosed within a year of the onset of symptoms of UC. In 19 patients carcinoma of the biliary tract occurred after colectomy for UC. In these patients the duration of illness before surgery ranged from 2 to 22 years, with a mean of 11 years. The operations included proctocolectomy performed as a one- or two-stage procedure in 18 and subtotal colectomy in 1 patient. Thus the complete excision of the inflamed bowel in the majority did not protect against the development of carcinoma 1 to 20 years after surgery (mean 8 years). Compared with an unselected patient population with carcinoma of the biliary tract, the tumors occur 20 or more years earlier in patients with UC.

Patients most often seek medical advice because of obstructive jaundice.[29] In 15 patients studied in detail 9 had no associated liver disease. In the remaining six patients the presence of cirrhosis in four and pericholangitis in two complicated the evaluation and interpretation of the jaundice. Cholangiocarcinoma is infrequently associated with cholelithiasis in patients with UC, in contradistinction to a 30 percent to 50 percent prevalence of cholelithiasis in patients without colitis who have cholangiocarcinoma. Tumors also have been found incidentally during colectomy or at autopsy.

As expected, the predominant abnormalities are increased total and direct-reacting bilirubin and alkaline phosphatase. Slight elevations of aminotransferases also may occur. Cholangiographic features suggestive of cholangiocarcinoma include (1) excessive dilation, (2) polypoid masses, (3) progressive ductular dilation or stricturing, and (4) a short, dominant stricture.

Pathogenesis

The nature of the association between carcinoma of the biliary tract and UC is unknown. Any hypothesis relating the occurrence to the extent, duration, or severity of the disease must be tempered because tumors can develop many years after proctocolectomy. The observation that patients with PSC are particularly predisposed to develop carcinoma of the biliary tract[1,24,30,31] suggests that chronic inflammation or bile stasis may contribute to the development of cholangiocarcinoma, possibly by increasing epithelial cell proliferation and the probability of mutation or failure of tumor suppressor gene expression.

Prognosis and Therapy

The prognosis is poor for carcinoma of the biliary tract. Small tumors of the bile ducts and tumors localized to the gallbladder may be excised surgically.[451] When resection is impossible, a biliary drainage procedure proximal to the tumor is recommended. This may involve a choledochoenterostomy, cholecystoenterostomy, or hepaticoenterostomy. In the latter case cholecystectomy is recommended to prevent obstruction of the cystic duct. When the extent of the tumor precludes a drainage procedure, operative or retrograde endoscopic dilation and placement of a stent may achieve palliative drainage. Percutaneous, transhepatic placement of stents can also be performed.[452] Chemotherapy[453] and radiotherapy[454] are ineffective.

CHOLELITHIASIS

In the United States an estimated 25 million individuals have gallstones, representing a prevalence of approximately 11 percent. It is not unexpected, therefore, that some patients with IBD will have cholelithiasis coincidentally. Indeed, patients with UC and Crohn's colitis appear to have gallstones with frequencies compatible with the age-related prevalence in the general population.[107,455] However, patients with extensive or long-standing Crohn's disease of the ileum and patients who have had ileal resection have significantly increased frequencies of cholelithiasis.[107,455-457] The prevalence of cholelithiasis in such patients was approximately 30 percent in three independent studies.[455-457] The increased frequency of cholelithiasis in patients with Crohn's disease is correlated directly with the duration and extent of the ileal disease or the interval after ileal resection.[455-457]

Pathogenesis

The stones reported in association with Crohn's disease of the ileum typically have been cholesterol gallstones.[455-457] This is the expected consequence of the physiologic derangement. In the presence of diffuse ileal disease or after ileal resection inadequate absorption of bile acids in the ileum results in their fecal loss. If the hepatic synthesis of bile acids is insufficient to solubilize cholesterol in bile acid–lecithin micelles, then lithogenic bile results. Subsequent precipitation of cholesterol crystals results in the formation of cholesterol gallstones (see Chap. 60).

Therapy

The therapy for symptomatic gallstones is laparoscopic or traditional cholecystectomy. The use of chenodeoxycholic acid or UDCA to prevent the production of lithogenic bile has not been evaluated in patients with Crohn's disease of the ileum.

References

1. Harmatz A: Hepatobiliary manifestations of inflammatory bowel disease. Med Clin North Am 78:1387, 1994.
2. Thomas GH: Ulceration of the colon with enlarged fatty liver. Trans Pathol Soc Philadelphia 4:87, 1874.
3. Lister TD: A specimen of diffuse ulcerative colitis with secondary diffuse hepatitis. Trans Pathol Soc London 50:130, 1899.
4. Jankelson IR, McClure CW, Sweetsir FN: Chronic ulcerative colitis. II. Complications outside the digestive tract. Rev Gastroenterol 9:99, 1942.
5. Banks BM, Korelitz BI, Zetsel L: The course of non-specific ulcerative colitis: review of 20 years experience and late results. Gastroenterology 32:983, 1957.
6. Bargen JA: The Management of Colitis. New York, National Medical Book Company, 1935.
7. Jackman RJ, Bargen JA, Helmholz HF: The life histories of 95 children with chronic ulcerative colitis. Am J Dis Child 59:459, 1940.
8. Comfort MW, Bargen JA, Morlock CG: The association of chronic ulcerative colitis (colitis gravis) with hepatic insufficiency: report of 4 cases. Med Clin North Am 22:1089, 1938.
9. Logan AH: Chronic ulcerative colitis. A review of 117 cases. Northwest Med 18:1, 1919.
10. Perrett AD, Higgins G, Johnston HH, et al: The liver in ulcerative colitis. QJM 40:211, 1971.
11. Lockhart-Mummery HE, Morson BC: Crohn's disease (regional enteritis) of the large intestine and its distinction from ulcerative colitis. Gut 1:87, 1960.
12. Van Patter WN, Bargen JA, Dockerty MB, et al: Regional enteritis. Gastroenterology 26:347, 1954.
13. Crohn BB: Regional Ileitis. New York, Grune & Stratton, 1949.
14. Wewer V, Gluud C, Schlichting P, et al: Prevalence of hepatobiliary dysfunction in a regional group of patients with chronic inflammatory bowel disease. Scand J Gastroenterol 26:97, 1991.

15. Chapin LE, Scudamore HH, Baggenstoss AH, et al: Regional enteritis: associated visceral changes. Gastroenterology 30:404, 1956.
16. Monto AS: The liver in ulcerative disease of the intestinal tract: functional and anatomic changes. Ann Intern Med 50:1385, 1959.
17. Palmer WL, Kirsner JB, Goldgraber MB, et al: Disease of the liver in regional enteritis. Am J Med Sci 246:663, 1963.
18. Dordal E, Glagov S, Kirsner JB: Hepatic lesions in chronic inflammatory bowel disease. I. Clinical correlations with liver biopsy diagnoses in 103 patients. Gastroenterology 52:239, 1967.
19. Perrett AD, Higgins G, Johnston HH, et al: The liver in Crohn's disease. QJM 40:187, 1971.
20. Dew MJ, Thompson H, Allain RN: The spectrum of hepatic dysfunction in inflammatory bowel disease. QJM 48:113, 1979.
21. Eade MN, Cooke WT, Brooke BN, et al: Liver disease in Crohn's colitis. A study of 21 consecutive patients having colectomy. Ann Intern Med 74:518, 1971.
22. Eade MN, Cooke WT, Williams JA: Liver disease in Crohn's disease. A study of 100 consecutive patients. Scand J Gastroenterol 6:199, 1971.
23. Rankin GB, Watts HD, Melnyk CS, et al: National cooperative Crohn's disease study: extraintestinal manifestations and perianal complications. Gastroenterology 77:914, 1979.
24. Vierling JM: Hepatobiliary diseases in patients with inflammatory bowel disease. In Targan S, Shanahan F, eds: Inflammatory Bowel Disease: From Bench to Bedside. Baltimore, Williams & Wilkins, 1994:654.
25. Kimmelstiel P, Large HL, Verner HD: Liver damage in ulcerative colitis. Am J Pathol 28:259, 1952.
26. Palmer WL, Kirsner JB, Goldgraber MB, et al: Disease of the liver in chronic ulcerative colitis. Am J Med 36:856, 1964.
27. Mistilis SP: Pericholangitis and ulcerative colitis. I. Pathology, etiology, and pathogenesis. Ann Intern Med 63:1, 1965.
28. Willcox RG, Isselbacher KJ: Chronic liver disease in young people. Am J Med 30:185, 1961.
29. Ritchie JK, Allan RN, Macartney J, et al: Biliary tract carcinoma associated with ulcerative colitis. QJM 43:263, 1974.
30. Wiesner RH, La Russo NF: Clinicopathologic features of the syndrome of primary sclerosing cholangitis. Gastroenterology 79:200, 1980.
31. Chapman RWG, Marborgh BA, Rhodes JM, et al: Primary sclerosing cholangitis: a review of its clinical features, cholangiography, and hepatic histology. Gut 21:870, 1980.
32. Lupinetti M, Mehigan D, Cameron JL: Hepatobiliary complications of ulcerative colitis. Am J Surg 139:113, 1980.
33. Perold JG, Bezuidenhout DJJ, Erasmus TD, et al: The association between ulcerative colitis and chronic liver disease at Tygerberg Hospital. S Afr Med J 61:186, 1982.
34. Shepard HA, Selby WS, Chapman RWG, et al: Ulcerative colitis and persistent liver dysfunction. QJM 208:503, 1983.
35. Steckman M, Drossman DA, Lesesne HR: Hepatobiliary disease that precedes ulcerative colitis. J Clin Gastroenterol 6:425, 1984.
36. Christophi C, Hughes ER: Hepatobiliary disorders in inflammatory bowel disease. Surg Gynecol Obstet 160:187, 1985.
37. Wee A, Ludwig J: Pericholangitis in chronic ulcerative colitis: primary sclerosing cholangitis of the small bile ducts? Ann Intern Med 102:581, 1985.
38. Kanin HJ, Levin JJ, Lindert MCF: The association of liver disease with ulcerative colitis. Am J Gastroenterol 25:172, 1956.
39. Boden RW, Rankin JG, Goulston SJM, et al: The liver in ulcerative colitis. The significance of raised serum-alkaline-phosphatase levels. Lancet 2:245, 1959.
40. Vinnik IE, Kern F, Corley WD: Serum 5-nucleotidase and pericholangitis in patients with chronic ulcerative colitis. Gastroenterology 45:492, 1963.
41. Vinnik IE, Kern F: Liver diseases in ulcerative colitis. Arch Intern Med 112:87, 1963.
42. Kleckner MS, Stauffer MH, Bargen JA, et al: Hepatic lesions in the living patient with chronic ulcerative colitis as demonstrated by needle biopsy. Gastroenterology 22:13, 1952.
43. Dyer NH, Dawson AM: The incidence and significance of liver dysfunction in Crohn's disease. Digestion 5:317, 1972.
44. Liver disease in ulcerative colitis. Lancet 2:402, 1970 (editorial).
45. Bargen JA: Disease of the liver associated with ulcerative colitis. Ann Intern Med 39:285, 1953.
46. Mistilis SP, Goulston SJM: Pericholangitis and ulcerative colitis. II. Clinical aspects. Ann Intern Med 63:17, 1965.
47. Olhagen L: Ulcerative colitis in cirrhosis of the liver. Acta Med Scand 162:143, 1958.
48. Schrumpf E, Elgjo K, Fausa D, et al: Sclerosing cholangitis in ulcerative colitis. Scand J Gastroenterol 15:689, 1980.
49. Eade MN: Liver disease in ulcerative colitis. I. Analysis of operative liver biopsy in 138 consecutive patients having colectomy. Ann Intern Med 72:475, 1970.
50. Stauffer MH, Sauer WG, Dearing WH, et al: The spectrum of cholestatic hepatic disease. JAMA 191:125, 1965.
51. Ludwig J: Some names hang on like leeches. Dig Dis Sci 24:967, 1979 (editorial).
52. Ludwig J, Barham SS, LaRusso NF, et al: Morphologic features of chronic hepatitis associated with primary sclerosing cholangitis and chronic ulcerative colitis. Hepatology 1:632, 1981.
53. Blackstone MO, Nemchausky BA: Cholangiographic abnormalities in ulcerative colitis associated pericholangitis which resemble sclerosing cholangitis. Dig Dis 23:579, 1978.
54. Geisse G, Melson GL, Tedesco FJ, et al: Stenosing lesions of the biliary tree. Am J Roentgenol 123:378, 1975.
55. Leevy CM, Popper H, Sherlock S: Diseases of the Liver and Biliary Tract. Standardization of Nomenclature, Diagnostic Criteria, and Diagnostic Methodology. Washington DC, US Government Printing Office, 1976.
56. Mistilis SP: Liver disease in bowel disorders. In Schiff L, ed: Diseases of the Liver, ed 4. Philadelphia, JB Lippincott, 1975: 1373.
57. Bendandi A: Liver function in ulcerative colitis. Gastroenterologia 86:658, 1956.
58. Elias E, Summerfield JA, Sherlock S: Endoscopic retrograde cholangiopancreatography in the diagnosis of jaundice associated with ulcerative colitis. Gastroenterology 67:907, 1974.
59. Thorpe MEC, Scheuer PJ, Sherlock S: Primary sclerosing cholangitis, the biliary tree, and ulcerative colitis. Gut 8:435, 1967.
60. Vierling JM, Amankonah TD: Primary sclerosing cholangitis. In Afdhal NH, ed: Gallbladder and Biliary Tract Diseases. New York, Marcel Dekker, Inc., 2000:659-703.
61. Bjornsson E, Boberg KM, Schrumpf E, et al: Patients with small duct primary sclerosing cholangitis have favorable long term prognosis. Hepatology 34:365A, 2002.
62. Boberg KM, Schrumpf E, Fausa O, et al: Hepatobiliary disease in ulcerative colitis. An analysis of 18 patients with hepatobiliary lesions classified as small-duct primary sclerosing cholangitis. Scand J Gastroenterol 29:744-752, 1994.
63. Mahadevan U, Tremaine WJ, Johnson T, et al: Intravenous azathioprine in severe ulcerative colitis: a pilot study. Am J Gastroenterol 95:3463-3468, 2000.
64. Castiglione F, Del Vecchio BG, Rispo A, et al: Hepatitis related to cytomegalovirus infection in two patients with Crohn's disease treated with azathioprine. Dig Liver Dis 32:626-629, 2000.
65. Te HS, Schiano TD, Kuan SF, Hanauer SB, et al: Hepatic effects of long-term methotrexate use in the treatment of inflammatory bowel disease. Am J Gastroenterol 95:3150-3156, 2000.
66. Moore RA, Greenberg E, Tangen L: Cyclosporine-induced worsening of hepatic dysfunction in a patient with Crohn's disease and enterocutaneous fistula. South Med J 88:843-844, 1995.
67. Actis GC, Debernardi-Venon W, Lagget M, et al: Hepatotoxicity of intravenous cyclosporin A in patients with acute ulcerative colitis on total parenteral nutrition. Liver 15:320-323, 1995.
68. Bjorkman D: Nonsteroidal anti-inflammatory drug-associated toxicity of the liver, lower gastrointestinal tract, and esophagus. Am J Med 105:17S-21S, 1998.
69. de Dombal FT, Goldie W, Watts J McK, et al: Hepatic histological changes in ulcerative colitis. A series of 58 consecutive operative liver biopsies. Scand J Gastroenterol 1:220, 1966.
70. Riegler G, D'Inca R, Sturniolo GC, et al: Hepatobiliary alterations in patients with inflammatory bowel disease: a multicenter study. Caprilli & Gruppo Italiano Studio Colon-Retto. Scand J Gastroenterol 33:93-98, 1998.
71. Hill RB, Droke WE, Harp AP: Hepatic lipid metabolism in the cortisone-treated rat. Exp Molec Pathol 4:320, 1965.
72. Eade MN, Cooke WT, Brooke BN: Liver disease in ulcerative colitis. II. The long-term effect of colectomy. Ann Intern Med 72:489, 1970.
73. Targan SR, Landers C, Vidrich A, Czaja AJ: High-titer antineutrophil cytoplasmic antibodies in type-1 autoimmune hepatitis (see comments). Gastroenterology 108:1159-1166, 1995.

74. Terjung B, Worman HJ: Anti-neutrophil antibodies in primary sclerosing cholangitis. Best Pract Res Clin Gastroenterol 15:629-642, 2001.
75. Domschke W, Klein R, Terracciano LM, et al: Sequential occurrence of primary sclerosing cholangitis and autoimmune hepatitis type III in a patient with ulcerative colitis: a follow up study over 14 years. Liver 20:340-345, 2000.
76. Perdigoto R, Carpenter HA, Czaja AJ: Frequency and significance of chronic ulcerative colitis in severe corticosteroid-treated autoimmune hepatitis. J Hepatol 14:325, 1992.
77. Gohlke F, Lohse AW, Dienes HP, et al: Evidence for an overlap syndrome of autoimmune hepatitis and primary sclerosing cholangitis. J Hepatol 24:699-705, 1996.
78. Hatzis GS, Vassiliou VA, Delladetsima JK: Overlap syndrome of primary sclerosing cholangitis and autoimmune hepatitis. Eur J Gastroenterol Hepatol 13:203-206, 2001.
79. Chazouilleres O: Diagnosis of primary sclerosing cholangitis—autoimmune hepatitis overlap syndrome: to score or not to score? J Hepatol 33:661-663, 2000.
80. Kaya M, Angulo P, Lindor KD: Overlap of autoimmune hepatitis and primary sclerosing cholangitis: an evaluation of a modified scoring system. J Hepatol 33:537-542, 2000.
81. Roberts EA: Re: McNair et al. Autoimmune hepatitis overlapping with primary sclerosing cholangitis. Am J Gastroenterol 94: 291-292, 1999 (letter).
82. Gregorio GV, Portmann B, Karani J, et al: Autoimmune hepatitis/sclerosing cholangitis overlap syndrome in childhood: a 16-year prospective study. Hepatology 33:544-553, 2001.
83. Griga T, Tromm A, Muller KM, May B: Overlap syndrome between autoimmune hepatitis and primary sclerosing cholangitis in two cases. Eur J Gastroenterol Hepatol 12:559-564, 2000.
84. McNair AN, Moloney M, Portmann BC, et al: Autoimmune hepatitis overlapping with primary sclerosing cholangitis in five cases. Am J Gastroenterol 93:777-784, 1998.
85. Boberg KM, Fausa O, Haaland T, et al: Features of autoimmune hepatitis in primary sclerosing cholangitis: an evaluation of 114 primary sclerosing cholangitis patients according to a scoring system for the diagnosis of autoimmune hepatitis. Hepatology 23:1369-1376, 1996.
86. Ludwig J: Small-duct primary sclerosing cholangitis. Semin Liver Dis 11:11-17, 1991.
87. Seibold F, Weber P, Jenss H, Scheurlen M: Autoimmune hepatitis in inflammatory bowel disease: report of two unusual cases. Z Gastroenterol 35:29-32, 1997.
88. Talwalkar JA, Larusso NF, Lindor KD: Defining the relationship between autoimmune disease and primary sclerosing cholangitis. Am J Gastroenterol 95:3024-3026, 2000.
89. Read AE, Sherlock S, Harrison CV: Active "juvenile" cirrhosis considered as part of a systemic disease and the effect of corticosteroid therapy. Gut 4:378, 1963.
90. Holdsworth CD, Hall EW, Dawson AM, et al: Ulcerative colitis in chronic liver disease. QJM 34:211, 1965.
91. MacKay IR, Wood IJ: Lupoid hepatitis: a comparison of 22 cases with other types of chronic liver disease. QJM 31:485, 1962.
92. Gray N, MacKay IR, Taft LI, et al: Hepatitis, colitis, and lupus manifestations. Am J Dig Dis 3:481, 1958.
93. Olsson R, Hulten L: Concurrence of ulcerative colitis and chronic active hepatitis. Clinical courses and results of colectomy. Scand J Gastroenterol 10:331, 1975.
94. Kane SP: Ulcerative colitis with chronic liver disease, eosinophilia and auto-immune thyroid disease. Postgrad Med J 53:105, 1977.
95. Harris AI, Neugarten J: Chronic active hepatitis and ulcerative colitis associated with eosinophilia, nonthrombocytopenic hypergammaglobulinemia purpura and serological abnormalities. Am J Gastroenterol 69:191, 1978.
96. Terjung B, Spengler U, Sauerbruch T, Worman HJ: "Atypical p-ANCA" in IBD and hepatobiliary disorders react with a 50-kilodalton nuclear envelope protein of neutrophils and myeloid cell lines. Gastroenterology 119:310-322, 2000.
97. Terjung B, Herzog V, Worman HJ, et al: Atypical antineutrophil cytoplasmic antibodies with perinuclear fluorescence in chronic inflammatory bowel diseases and hepatobiliary disorders colocalize with nuclear lamina proteins. Hepatology 28:332-340, 1998.
98. Angulo P, Peter JB, Gershwin ME, et al: Serum autoantibodies in patients with primary sclerosing cholangitis. J Hepatol 32:182-187, 2000.
99. Czaja AJ, Wolf AM: Immunopathic disease associated with severe chronic active liver disease: determinants of treatment response? Gastroenterology 78:1152, 1980 (abstract).
100. Ross JR, Nugent FW, Hajjar J-J, et al: Liver disease in chronic ulcerative colitis. Lahey Clin Found Bull 15:93, 1966.
101. Hoffbauer FW, McCartney JS, Dennis C, et al: The relationship of chronic ulcerative colitis and cirrhosis. Ann Intern Med 39:267, 1953.
102. Vinnik IE, Kern F: Biliary cirrhosis in a patient with chronic ulcerative colitis. Gastroenterology 45:529, 1963.
103. McCarthy CF, Read MD: Bleeding esophageal varices in ulcerative colitis. Gastroenterology 42:325, 1962.
104. Fiocchi C, Farmer RG: Autoimmunity in inflammatory bowel disease. Clin Aspects Autoimmunity 1:12, 1987.
105. Ronder M, Norday A, Elgjo K: Sulfonamide-induced chronic liver disease. Scand J Gastroenterol 9:93, 1974.
106. Edwards FC, Truelove SC: The course and prognosis of ulcerative colitis. Part III. Complications. Gut 5:1, 1964.
107. Greenstein AJ, Janowitz HD, Sachar DB: The extraintestinal complications of Crohn's disease and ulcerative colitis: a study of 700 patients. Medicine 55:401, 1976.
108. Eade MN, Williams JA, Cooke WT: Bleeding from an ileostomy caput medusae. Lancet 2:1166, 1969.
109. Cameron AD, Fone DJ: Portal hypertension and bleeding varices after colectomy and ileostomy for chronic ulcerative colitis. Gut 11:755, 1970.
110. Adson MA, Fulton RE: The ileal stoma and portal hypertension. An uncommon site of variceal bleeding. Arch Surg 112:501, 1977.
111. Wiesner RH, LaRusso NF, Dozois RR, et al: Peristomal varices after proctocolectomy in patients with primary sclerosing cholangitis. Gastroenterology 83:316, 1986.
112. Smith PM: Hepatoma associated with ulcerative colitis. Dis Colon Rectum 17:554, 1974.
113. Schrumpf E, Fausa O, Kolmannskog F, et al: Sclerosing cholangitis in ulcerative colitis. A follow-up study. Scand J Gastroenterol 17:33, 1982.
114. Kato Y, Morimoto H, Unoura M, et al: Primary biliary cirrhosis and chronic pancreatitis in a patient with ulcerative colitis. J Clin Gastroenterol 5:425, 1985.
115. Ludwig J, LaRusso NF: Primary biliary cirrhosis in a patient with chronic ulcerative colitis. In Ishak KG, ed: Hepatopathology 1985. Thorofare, NJ, American Association for the Study of Liver Diseases, 1985:197.
116. Werther JL, Schapira A, Rubenstein O, et al: Amyloidosis in regional enteritis: a report of five cases. Am J Med 29:416, 1960.
117. Benedek TG, Zawadzki ZA: Ankylosing spondylitis with ulcerative colitis and amyloidosis. Am J Med 40:431, 1966.
118. Shorvon PJ: Amyloidosis and inflammatory bowel disease. Dig Dis 22:209, 1977.
119. Glenner GG: Amyloid deposits and amyloidosis: the β-fibrilloses. N Engl J Med 302:1282, 1333, 1980.
120. Greenstein AJ, Sachar DB, Panday AK, et al: Amyloidosis and inflammatory bowel disease. A 50-year experience with 25 patients. Medicine (Baltimore) 71:261-270, 1992.
121. Espiritu CR, Kim TS, Levine RA: Granulomatous hepatitis associated with sulfadimethoxine hypersensitivity. JAMA 202:985, 1967.
122. Callen JP, Soderstrom RM: Granulomatous hepatitis associated with salicylazosulfapyridine therapy. South Med J 71:1159, 1978.
123. Braun M, Fraser GM, Kunin M, et al: Mesalamine-induced granulomatous hepatitis. Am J Gastroenterol 94:1973-1974, 1999.
124. Lytton DG, McCaughan G: Hepatic venous occlusion from carcinoma of bile duct in ulcerative colitis. Aust NZ J Med 7:404, 1977.
125. Bruguera M, Aranguibel F, Ros E, et al: Incidence and clinical significance of sinusoidal dilatation in liver biopsies. Gastroenterology 75:474, 1978.
126. Camilleri M, Schafler K, Chadwick VS, et al: Periportal sinusoidal dilatation, inflammatory bowel disease, and the contraceptive pill. Gastroenterology 80:810, 1981.
127. Winkler K, Poulsen H: Liver disease with periportal sinusoidal dilatation. A possible complication of contraceptive steroids. Scand J Gastroenterol 10:699, 1975.
128. Lee YM, Kaplan MM: Primary sclerosing cholangitis. N Engl J Med 332:924-933, 1995.
129. Martin M: Primary sclerosing cholangitis. Annu Rev Med 44:221-227, 1993.

130. Bergquist A, Broome U: Clinical features of primary sclerosing cholangitis. In Lindor KD, Dickson ER, eds: PBC, PSC, and Adult Cholangiopathies. Philadelphia, WB Saunders, 1998:283-301.
131. Ponsioen CI, Tytgat GN: Primary sclerosing cholangitis: a clinical review. Am J Gastroenterol 93:515-523, 1998.
132. Marotta PJ, Larusso NF, Wiesner RH: Sclerosing cholangitis. Baillieres Clin Gastroenterol 11:781-800, 1997.
133. Kunath T, Ordonez-Garcia C, Turbide C, Beauchemin N: Inhibition of colonic tumor cell growth by biliary glycoprotein. Oncogene 11:2375-2382, 1995.
134. Ludwig J: Histopathology of primary sclerosing cholangitis. In Manns MP, Chapman RW, Stiehl A, Wiesner RH, eds: Primary Sclerosing Cholangitis. Boston: Kluwer Academic Publishers, 14-21, 1998.
135. Aadland E, Schrumpf E, Fausa O, et al: Primary sclerosing cholangitis: a long-term follow-up study. Scand J Gastroenterol 22:655-664, 1987.
136. Broome U, Olsson R, Loof L, et al: Natural history and prognostic factors in 305 Swedish patients with primary sclerosing cholangitis. Gut 38:610-615, 1996.
137. Goss JA, Shackleton CR, Farmer DG, et al: Orthotopic liver transplantation for primary sclerosing cholangitis. A 12-year single center experience. Ann Surg 225:472-481, 1997.
138. Harnois DM, Gores GJ, Ludwig J, et al: Are patients with cirrhotic stage primary sclerosing cholangitis at risk for the development of hepatocellular cancer? J Hepatol 27:512-516, 1997.
139. Narumi S, Roberts JP, Emond JC, et al: Liver transplantation for sclerosing cholangitis. Hepatology 22:451-457, 1995.
140. Wiesner RH, Porayko MK, Hay JE, et al: Liver transplantation for primary sclerosing cholangitis: impact of risk factors on outcome. Liver Transpl Surg 2:99-108, 1996.
141. Talwalkar JA, Lindor KD: Natural history and prognostic models in primary sclerosing cholangitis. Best Pract Res Clin Gastroenterol 15:563-575, 2001.
142. Wiesner RH: Liver transplantation for primary sclerosing cholangitis: timing, outcome, impact of inflammatory bowel disease and recurrence of disease. Best Pract Res Clin Gastroenterol 15:667-680, 2001.
143. Riordan SM, Williams R: Risk of cholangiocarcinoma in primary sclerosing cholangitis. In Mann M, Stiehl A, Chapman R, Weisner RH, eds: Primary Sclerosis Cholangitis, vol 1. Freiburg, Kluwer Academic Publishers, 1998:69-85.
144. Bergquist A, Broome U: Hepatobiliary and extra-hepatic malignancies in primary sclerosing cholangitis. Best Pract Res Clin Gastroenterol 15:643-656, 2001.
145. Bergquist A, Glaumann H, Stal P, et al: Biliary dysplasia, cell proliferation and nuclear DNA-fragmentation in primary sclerosing cholangitis with and without cholangiocarcinoma. J Intern Med 249:69-75, 2001.
146. Bergquist A, Tribukait B, Glaumann H, Broome U: Can DNA cytometry be used for evaluation of malignancy and premalignancy in bile duct strictures in primary sclerosing cholangitis? J Hepatol 33:873-877, 2000.
147. Bergquist A, Glaumann H, Persson B, Broome U: Risk factors and clinical presentation of hepatobiliary carcinoma in patients with primary sclerosing cholangitis: a case-control study. Hepatology 27:311-316, 1998.
148. Helzberg JH, Petersen JM, Boyer JL: Improved survival with primary sclerosing cholangitis. A review of clinicopathologic features and comparison of symptomatic and asymptomatic patients. Gastroenterology 92:1869, 1987.
149. Martin FM, Braasch JW: Primary sclerosing cholangitis. Curr Probl Surg 29:133, 1992.
150. Wiesner RH: Current concepts in primary sclerosing cholangitis. Mayo Clin Proc 69:969, 1994.
151. Debray D, Pariente D, Urvoas E, et al: Sclerosing cholangitis in children. J Ped 124:49, 1994.
152. Rabinovitz M, Demetris AJ, Bou-Abboud CF, Van Thiel DH: Simultaneous occurrence of primary sclerosing cholangitis and autoimmune chronic active hepatitis in a patient with ulcerative colitis. Dig Dis Sci 37:1606-1611, 1992.
153. Chujo S, Sakamoto C, Ohno S, et al: Pericholangitis with ulcerative colitis following autoimmune hepatitis over 12 years. Intern Med 31:1228-1232, 1992.
154. Novelli A, Gambella GR, Anselmo E, Nanni G: [Experimental model of induction in the rat of rapidly developing biliary cirrhosis in peripartal nodular cirrhosis]. Pathologica 85:713-720, 1993.
155. Bartholomew LG, Cain JC, Woolner LB, et al: Sclerosing cholangitis: its possible association with Riedel's struma and fibrous retroperitonitis—report of two cases. N Engl J Med 269:8, 1963.
156. Warren KW, Athanassiades S, Monge JI: Primary sclerosing cholangitis. A study of forty-two cases. Am J Surg 111:23, 1966.
157. Freilich BL, Hu K-Q, Vierling JM: Immunopathogenesis of autoimmune hepatobiliary diseases. Curr Opin Gastroenterol 10:257, 1994.
158. Wee A, Ludwig J, Coffey RJ, et al: Hepatobiliary carcinoma associated with primary sclerosing cholangitis and chronic ulcerative colitis. Hum Pathol 16:719, 1985.
159. Smith MP, Loe RH: Sclerosing cholangitis: review of recent case reports and associated diseases and four new cases. Am J Surg 110:239, 1965.
160. Nakanuma Y, Hirai N, Kono N, et al: Histological and ultrastructural examination of the intrahepatic biliary tree in primary sclerosing cholangitis. Liver 6:317, 1986.
161. Casali AM, Carbone G, Cavalli G: Intrahepatic bile duct loss in primary sclerosing cholangitis: a quantitative study. Histopathology 32:449-453, 1998.
162. Mattila J, Pitkanen R, Halonen P, Matikainen M: Ultrastructural aspects of liver injury with special reference to small bile ducts in patients with ulcerative colitis. Liver 12:155, 1992.
163. Ludwig J: New concepts in biliary cirrhosis. Semin Liver Dis 7:293, 1987.
164. Cameron RG, Blendis LM, Neuman MG: Accumulation of macrophages in primary sclerosing cholangitis. Clin Biochem 34:195-201, 2001.
165. Ritland S, Elgio K, Johansen O, et al: Liver copper content in patients with inflammatory bowel disease and associated liver disorders. Scand J Gastroenterol 14:711, 1979.
166. Harrison RF, Hubscher SG: The spectrum of bile duct lesions in end-stage primary sclerosing cholangitis. Histopathology 19:321, 1991.
167. Angulo P, Larson DR, Therneau TM, et al: Time course of histological progression in primary sclerosing cholangitis. Am J Gastroenterol 94:3310-3313, 1999.
168. Leidenius M, Hockersted K, Broome U, et al: Hepatobiliary carcinoma in primary sclerosing cholangitis: a case control study. J Hepatol 34:792-798, 2001.
169. MacCarty RL, Larusso NF, May GR, et al: Cholangiocarcinoma complicating primary sclerosing cholangitis: cholangiographic appearances. Radiology 156:43-46, 1985.
170. Pokorny CS, McCaughan GW, Gallagher ND, Selby WS: Sclerosing cholangitis and biliary tract calculi—primary or secondary? Gut 33:1376, 1992.
171. Fraile G, Rodriguez-Garcia JL, Moreno A: Primary sclerosing cholangitis associated with systemic sclerosis. Postgrad Med J 67:189, 1991.
172. Epstein O, Chapman RWG, Lake-Bakaar G, et al: The pancreas in primary biliary cirrhosis and primary sclerosing cholangitis. Gastroenterology 83:1177, 1982.
173. Fausa O, Kolmannskog F, Ritland S: The pancreatic ducts in primary biliary cirrhosis and sclerosing cholangitis. Scand J Gastroenterol 20(suppl):32, 1985.
174. Montefusco PP, Geiss AC, Bronzo RL, et al: Sclerosing cholangitis, chronic pancreatitis, and Sjögren's syndrome: a syndrome complex. Am J Surg 147:822, 1984.
175. Waldram R, Kopelman H, Tsantoulas D, et al: Chronic pancreatitis, sclerosing cholangitis and sicca complex in two siblings. Lancet 1:550, 1975.
176. Kelly P, Patchett S, McCloskey D, et al: Sclerosing cholangitis, race and sex. Gut 41:688-689, 1997.
177. Atkinson AJ, Carroll WW: Sclerosing cholangitis, association with regional enteritis. JAMA 188:183, 1964.
178. Schrumpf E, Boberg KM: Epidemiology of primary sclerosing cholangitis. Best Pract Res Clin Gastroenterol 15:553-562, 2001.
179. Dickson ER, Larusso NF, Wiesner RH: Primary sclerosing cholangitis. Hepatology 4:33S-35S, 1984.
180. Takikawa H, Manabe T: Primary sclerosing cholangitis in Japan—analysis of 192 cases. J Gastroenterol 32:134-137, 1997.
181. Okada H, Mizuno M, Yamamoto K, Tsuji T: Primary sclerosing cholangitis in Japanese patients: association with inflammatory bowel disease. Acta Med Okayama 50:227-235, 1996.
182. Dillon P, Belchis D, Tracy T, et al: Increased expression of intercellular adhesion molecules in biliary atresia. Am J Pathol 145:263-267, 1994.

183. Okolicsanyi L, Fabris L, Viaggi S, et al: Primary sclerosing cholangitis: clinical presentation, natural history and prognostic variables: an Italian multicentre study. The Italian PSC Study Group. Eur J Gastroenterol Hepatol 8:685-691, 1996.
184. Escorsell A, Pares A, Rodes J, et al: Epidemiology of primary sclerosing cholangitis in Spain. Spanish Association for the Study of the Liver. J Hepatol 21:787-791, 1994.
185. Kochhar R, Goenka MK, Das K, et al: Primary sclerosing cholangitis: an experience from India. J Gastroenterol Hepatol 11:429-433, 1996.
186. Wiesner RH, Grambsch PM, Dickson ER, et al: Primary sclerosing cholangitis: natural history, prognostic factors and survival analysis. Hepatology 10:430-436, 1989.
187. Schrumpf E, Abdelnoor M, Fausa O, et al: Risk factors in primary sclerosing cholangitis. J Hepatol 21:1061-1066, 1994.
188. Broome U, Glaumann H, Hellers G, et al: Liver disease in ulcerative colitis: an epidemiological and follow up study in the county of Stockholm. Gut 35:84-89, 1994.
189. Loftus EVJ, Sandborn WJ, Tremaine WJ, et al: Primary sclerosing cholangitis is associated with nonsmoking: a case-control study (see comments). Gastroenterology 110:1496-1502, 1996.
190. van Erpecum KJ, Smits SJ, van de Meeberg PC, et al: Risk of primary sclerosing cholangitis is associated with nonsmoking behavior (see comments). Gastroenterology 110:1503-1506, 1996.
191. Amedee-Manesme O, Brunelle F, Hadchouel M, et al: Sclerosing cholangitis in infancy. Hepatology 4:786, 1984.
192. Ong JC, O'Loughlin EV, Kamath KR, et al: Sclerosing cholangitis in children with inflammatory bowel disease. Aust NZ J Med 24:149, 1994.
193. Classen M, Goetze H, Richter H-J, et al: Primary sclerosing cholangitis in children. J Ped Gastroenterol Nutr 6:197, 1987.
194. Fausa O, Schrumpf E, Elgjo K: Relationship of inflammatory bowel disease and primary sclerosing cholangitis. Semin Liver Dis 11:31, 1991.
195. MacCarty RL, Larusso NF, Wiesner RH, Ludwig J: Primary sclerosing cholangitis: findings on cholangiography and pancreatography. Radiology 149:39-44, 1983.
196. Rabinovitz M, Gavaler JS, Schade RR, et al: Does primary sclerosing cholangitis occurring in association with inflammatory bowel disease differ from that occurring in the absence of inflammatory bowel disease? A study of sixty-six subjects. Hepatology 11:7, 1990.
197. Broome U: Primary sclerosing cholangitis—relationship to inflammatory bowel disease. In Mann M, Stiehl A, Chapman R, Weisner RH, eds: Primary Sclerosis Cholangitis, vol 1. Freiburg, Kluwer Academic Publishers, 1998:60-68.
198. Broome U, Lofberg R, Lundqvist K, Veress B: Subclinical time span of inflammatory bowel disease in patients with primary sclerosing cholangitis. Dis Colon Rectum 38:1301-1305, 1995.
199. Vajro P, Cucchiara S, Vegnente A, et al: Primary sclerosing cholangitis preceding Crohn's disease in a child with Down's syndrome. Dig Dis Sci 43:166-169, 1998.
200. Papatheodoridis GV, Hamilton M, Mistry PK, et al: Ulcerative colitis has an aggressive course after orthotopic liver transplantation for primary sclerosing cholangitis (see comments). Gut 43:639-644, 1998.
201. Olsson R, Danielsson A, Jarnerot G, et al: Prevalence of primary sclerosing cholangitis in patients with ulcerative colitis. Gastroenterology 100:1319-1323, 1991.
202. Lundqvist K, Broome U: Differences in colonic disease activity in patients with ulcerative colitis with and without primary sclerosing cholangitis: a case control study. Dis Colon Rectum 40:451-456, 1997.
203. Farrant JM, Hayllar KM, Wilkinson ML, et al: Natural history and prognostic variables in primary sclerosing cholangitis. Gastroenterology 100:1710-1717, 1991.
204. Shetty K, Rybicki L, Carey WD: The Child-Pugh classification as a prognostic indicator for survival in primary sclerosing cholangitis. Hepatology 25:1049-1053, 1997.
205. Ismail T, Angrisani L, Powell JE, et al: Primary sclerosing cholangitis: surgical options, prognostic variables and outcome. Br J Surg 78:564, 1991.
206. Martin FM, Rossi RL, Nugent FW, et al: Surgical aspects of sclerosing cholangitis. Results in 178 patients. Ann Surg 212:551, 1990.
207. Boberg KM, Schrumpf E: Primary sclerosis cholangitis: diagnosis and differntial diagnosis. In Mann M, Stiehl A, Chapman R, Weisner RH, eds: Primary Sclerosis Cholangitis, vol 1. Freiburg, Kluwer Academic Publishers, 1998:3-13.
208. Olsson R, Broome U, Danielsson A, et al: Colchicine treatment of primary sclerosing cholangitis. Gastroenterology 108:1199-1203, 1995.
209. Dickson ER, Murtaugh PA, Wiesner RH, et al: Primary sclerosing cholangitis: refinement and validation of survival models. Gastroenterology 103:1893-1901, 1992.
210. Younossi ZM, Kiwi ML, Boparai N, et al: Cholestatic liver diseases and health-related quality of life. Am J Gastroenterol 95:497-502, 2000.
211. Kim WR, Lindor KD, Malinchoc M, et al: Reliability and validity of the NIDDK-QA instrument in the assessment of quality of life in ambulatory patients with cholestatic liver disease. Hepatology 32:924-929, 2000.
212. Wiesner RH, Larusso NF, Ludwig J, Dickson ER: Comparison of the clinicopathologic features of primary sclerosing cholangitis and primary biliary cirrhosis. Gastroenterology 88:108-114, 1985.
213. Mir-Madjlessi SH, Sivak MVJ, Farmer RG: Hypereosinophilia, ulcerative colitis, sclerosing cholangitis, and bile duct carcinoma. Am J Gastroenterol 81:483-485, 1986.
214. Seibold F, Weber P, Schoning A, et al: Neutrophil antibodies (pANCA) in chronic liver disease and inflammatory bowel disease: do they react with different antigens? Eur J Gastroenterol Hepatol 8:1095-1100, 1996.
215. Balasubramaniam K, Wiesner RH, LaRusso NF: Can serum alkaline phosphatase levels be normal in primary sclerosing cholangitis? Gastroenterology 92:1303, 1987 (abstract).
216. Balasubramaniam K, Wiesner RH, Larusso NF: Primary sclerosing cholangitis with normal serum alkaline phosphatase activity. Gastroenterology 95:1395-1398, 1988.
217. Snook JA, Chapman RW, Fleming K, et al: Anti-neutrophil nuclear antibody in ulcerative colitis, Crohn's disease and primary sclerosing cholangitis. Clin Exp Immunol 76:30, 1989.
218. Duerr RH, Targan SR, Landers CJ, et al: Neutrophil cytoplasmic antibodies: a link between primary sclerosing cholangitis and ulcerative colitis. Gastroenterology 100:1385, 1991.
219. Oudkerk Pool M, Ellerbroek PM, Ridwan BU, et al: Serum antineutrophil cytoplasmic autoantibodies in inflammatory bowel disease are mainly associated with ulcerative colitis. A correlation study between perinuclear antineutrophil cytoplasmic autoantibodies and clinical parameters, medical, and surgical treatment. Gut 34:46, 1993.
220. Seibold F, Weber P, Klein R, et al: Clinical significance of antibodies against neutrophils in patients with inflammatory bowel disease and primary sclerosing cholangitis. Gut 33:657, 1992.
221. Seibold F, Slametschka D, Gregor M, Weber P: Neutrophil autoantibodies: a genetic marker in primary sclerosing cholangitis and ulcerative colitis. Gastroenterology 107:532, 1994.
222. Klein R, Eisenburg J, Weber P, et al: Significance and specificity of antibodies to neutrophils detected by western blotting for the serological diagnosis of primary sclerosing cholangitis. Hepatology 14:1147-1152, 1991.
223. Gross JB, Ludwig J, Wiesner RH, et al: Abnormalities in tests of copper metabolism in primary sclerosing cholangitis. Gastroenterology 89:272, 1985.
224. Brandt DJ, MacCarty RL, Charboneau JW, et al: Gallbladder disease in patients with primary sclerosing cholangitis. AJR Am J Roentgenol 150:571-574, 1988.
225. Kaw M, Silverman WB, Rabinovitz M, Schade RR: Biliary tract calculi in primary sclerosing cholangitis (see comments). Am J Gastroenterol 90:72-75, 1995.
226. Prakash S, Robbins PW, Wyler DJ: Cloning and analysis of murine cDNA that encodes a fibrogenic lymphokine, fibrosin. Proc Natl Acad Sci U S A 92:2154-2158, 1995.
227. Ernst O, Asselah T, Sergent G, et al: MR cholangiography in primary sclerosing cholangitis. AJR Am J Roentgenol 171:1027-1030, 1998.
228. McMillan JS, Shaw T, Angus PW, Locarnini SA: Effect of immunosuppressive and antiviral agents on hepatitis B virus replication in vitro. Hepatology 22:36-43, 1995.
229. Porayko MK, Wiesner RH, Larusso NF, et al: Patients with asymptomatic primary sclerosing cholangitis frequently have progressive disease (see comments). Gastroenterology 98:1594-1602, 1990.
230. Janczewska I, Olsson R, Hultcrantz R, Broome U: Pregnancy in patients with primary sclerosing cholangitis. Liver 16:326-330, 1996.

231. Wiesner RH, Grambsch P, Dickson ER, et al: Primary sclerosing cholangitis: natural history, prognostic factors, and survival analysis. Hepatology 10:430, 1989.
232. Olsson RG, Asztely MS: Prognostic value of cholangiography in primary sclerosing cholangitis. Eur J Gastroenterol Hepatol 7:251-254, 1995.
233. Faubion Jr WA, Loftus EV, Sandborn WJ, et al: Pediatric "PSC": a descriptive report of associated inflammatory bowel disease among pediatric patients with PSC. J Pediatr Gastroenterol Nutr 33:296-300, 2001.
234. Mieli-Vergani G, Vergani D: Sclerosing cholangitis in the paediatric patient. Best Pract Res Clin Gastroenterol 15:681-690, 2001.
235. Floreani A, Zancan L, Melis A, et al: Primary sclerosing cholangitis (PSC): clinical, laboratory and survival analysis in children and adults. Liver 19:228-233, 1999.
236. Kim WR, Therneau TM, Wiesner RH, et al: A revised natural history model for primary sclerosing cholangitis. Mayo Clin Proc 75:688-694, 2000.
237. Abu-Elmagd KM, Malinchoc M, Dickson ER, et al: Efficacy of hepatic transplantation in patients with primary sclerosing cholangitis. Surg Gynecol Obstet 177:335-344, 1993.
238. Farges O, Malassagne B, Sebagh M, Bismuth H: Primary sclerosing cholangitis: liver transplantation or biliary surgery. Surgery 117:146-155, 1995.
239. Rosen CB, Nagorney DM, Wiesner RH, et al: Cholangiocarcinoma complicating primary sclerosing cholangitis. Ann Surg 213:21-25, 1991.
240. Marsh JWJ, Iwatsuki S, Makowka L, et al: Orthotopic liver transplantation for primary sclerosing cholangitis. Ann Surg 207:21-25, 1988.
241. Van Laethem JL, Deviere J, Bourgeois N, et al: Cholangiographic findings in deteriorating primary sclerosing cholangitis. Endoscopy 27:223-228, 1995.
242. Ramage JK, Donaghy A, Farrant JM, et al: Serum tumor markers for the diagnosis of cholangiocarcinoma in primary sclerosing cholangitis. Gastroenterology 108:865-869, 1995.
243. Martins EB, Fleming KA, Garrido MC, et al: Superficial thrombophlebitis, dysplasia, and cholangiocarcinoma in primary sclerosing cholangitis. Gastroenterology 107:537-542, 1994.
244. Broome U, Eriksson LS: Assessment for liver transplantation in patients with primary sclerosing cholangitis. J Hepatol 20:654-659, 1994.
245. Bismuth H: Comparison of FK 506- and cyclosporine-based immunosuppression: FK 506 therapy significantly reduces the incidence of acute, steroid-resistant, refractory, and chronic rejection whilst possessing a comparable safety profile. European FK 506 Multicenter Liver Study Group. Transplant Proc 27:45-49, 1995.
246. Adams DH, Hubscher S, Fear J, et al: Hepatic expression of macrophage inflammatory protein-1 alpha and macrophage inflammatory protein-1 beta after liver transplantation. Transplantation 61:817-825, 1996.
247. Keiding S, Hansen SB, Rasmussen HH, et al: Detection of cholangiocarcinoma in primary sclerosing cholangitis by positron emission tomography. Hepatology 28:700-706, 1998.
248. Kluge R, Schmidt F, Caca K, et al: Positron emission tomography with [(18)F]fluoro-2-deoxy-D-glucose for diagnosis and staging of bile duct cancer. Hepatology 33:1029-1035, 2001.
249. Desa LA, Akosa AB, Lazzara S, et al: Cytodiagnosis in the management of extrahepatic biliary stricture. Gut 32:1188-1191, 1991.
250. Kurzawinski T, Deery A, Dooley J, et al: A prospective controlled study comparing brush and bile exfoliative cytology for diagnosing bile duct strictures. Gut 33:1675-1677, 1992.
251. Ferrari Junior AP, Lichtenstein DR, Slivka A, et al: Brush cytology during ERCP for the diagnosis of biliary and pancreatic malignancies. Gastrointest Endosc 40:140, 1994.
252. Rabinovitz M, Zajko AB, Hassanein T, et al: Diagnostic value of brush cytology in the diagnosis of bile duct carcinoma: a study in 65 patients with bile duct strictures. Hepatology 12:747-752, 1990.
253. Mansfield JC, Griffin SM, Wadehra V, Matthewson K: A prospective evaluation of cytology from biliary strictures. Gut 40:671-677, 1997.
254. Fleming KA, Boberg KM, Glaumann H, et al: Biliary dysplasia as a marker of cholangiocarcinoma in primary sclerosing cholangitis. J Hepatol 34:360-365, 2001.
255. Nichols JC, Gores GJ, LaRusso NF, et al: Diagnostic role of serum CA-19-9 for cholangiocarcinoma in patients with primary sclerosing cholangitis. Mayo Clin Proc 68:874, 1993.
256. Bloom S, Heryet A, Fleming K, Chapman RW: Inappropriate expression of blood group antigens on biliary and colonic epithelia in primary sclerosing cholangitis. Gut 34:977, 1993.
257. Rogers SA, Poldolsky DK: Predicting cholangiocarcinoma in patients with primary sclerosing cholangitis: an analysis of the serological marker CA 19-9. Hepatology 19:543, 1994.
258. Patel AH, Harnois DM, Klee GG, et al: The utility of CA 19-9 in the diagnoses of cholangiocarcinoma in patients without primary sclerosing cholangitis. Am J Gastroenterol 95:204-207, 2000.
259. Ponsioen CIJ, Huibregtse K: Treatment of complications of primary sclerosing cholangitis. In Mann M, Stiehl A, Chapman R, Weisner RH, eds: Primary Sclerosis Cholangitis, vol 1. Freiburg, Kluwer Academic Publishers, 1998:115-123.
260. Jessurun J, Bolio-Solis A, Manivel JC: Diffuse lymphoplasmacytic acalculous cholecystitis: a distinctive form of chronic cholecystitis associated with primary sclerosing cholangitis. Hum Pathol 29:512-517, 1998.
261. Zaman A, Hapke R, Flora K, et al: Factors predicting the presence of esophageal or gastric varices in patients with advanced liver disease. Am J Gastroenterol 94:3292-3296, 1999.
262. Hay JE, Lindor KD, Wiesner RH, et al: The metabolic bone disease of primary sclerosing cholangitis. Hepatology 14:257, 1991.
263. Angulo P, Therneau TM, Jorgensen A, et al: Bone disease in patients with primary sclerosing cholangitis: prevalence, severity and prediction of progression. J Hepatol 29:729-735, 1998.
264. Kowdley KV: Lipids and lipid-activated vitamins in chronic cholestatic diseases. In Lindor KD, Dickson ER, eds: PBC, PSC, and Adult Cholangiopathies, vol 2. Philadelphia, WB Saunders, 1998:373-389.
265. Jorgensen RA, Lindor KD, Sartin JS, et al: Serum lipid and fat-soluble vitamin levels in primary sclerosing cholangitis. J Clin Gastroenterol 20:215-219, 1995.
266. Soros P, Bottcher J, Maschek H, et al: Lipoprotein-X in patients with cirrhosis: its relationship to cholestasis and hypercholesterolemia. Hepatology 28:1199-1205, 1998.
267. Borkje B, Vetvik K, Odegaard S, et al: Chronic pancreatitis in patients with sclerosing cholangitis and ulcerative colitis. Scand J Gastroenterol 20:539-542, 1985.
268. Imrie CW, Brombacher GD: Sclerosing cholangitis: a rare etiology for acute pancreatitis. Int J Pancreatol 23:71-75, 1998.
269. Fucini C, Wolff BG, Dozois RR: Bleeding from peristomal varices: perspectives on prevention and treatment. Dis Colon Rectum 34:1073-1078, 1991.
270. Peck JJ, Boyden AM: Exigent ileostomy hemorrhage. A complication of proctocolectomy in patients with chronic ulcerative colitis and primary sclerosing cholangitis. Am J Surg 150:153-158, 1985.
271. Bergassa NV, Jones EA: The pruritus of cholestasis. In Lindor KD, Dickson ER, eds: PBC, PSC, and Adult Cholangiopathies, vol 2. Philadelphia, WB Saunders, 1998:391-405.
272. Broome U, Lindberg G, Lofberg R: Primary sclerosing cholangitis in ulcerative colitis—a risk factor for the development of dysplasia and DNA aneuploidy? (see comments). Gastroenterology 102:1877-1880, 1992.
273. Brentnall TA, Haggitt RC, Rabinovitch PS, et al: Risk and natural history of colonic neoplasia in patients with primary sclerosing cholangitis and ulcerative colitis (see comments). Gastroenterology 110:331-338, 1996.
274. D'Haens GR, Lashner BA, Hanauer SB: Pericholangitis and sclerosing cholangitis are risk factors for dysplasia and cancer in ulcerative colitis (see comments). Am J Gastroenterol 88:1174-1178, 1993.
275. Kornfeld D, Ekbom A, Ihre T: Is there an excess risk for colorectal cancer in patients with ulcerative colitis and concomitant primary sclerosing cholangitis? A population based study (see comments). Gut 41:522-525, 1997.
276. Leidenius M: Ulcerative colitis—association with primary sclerosing cholangitis and colorectal neoplasia. Ann Chir Gynaecol 87:72-73, 1998.
277. Loftus EVJ, Aguilar HI, Sandborn WJ, et al: Risk of colorectal neoplasia in patients with primary sclerosing cholangitis and ulcerative colitis following orthotopic liver transplantation. Hepatology 27:685-690, 1998.

278. Marchesa P, Lashner BA, Lavery IC, et al:The risk of cancer and dysplasia among ulcerative colitis patients with primary sclerosing cholangitis. Am J Gastroenterol 92:1285-1288, 1997.
279. Nuako KW, Ahlquist DA, Sandborn WJ, et al: Primary sclerosing cholangitis and colorectal carcinoma in patients with chronic ulcerative colitis: a case-control study. Cancer 82:822-826, 1998.
280. Leidenius MH, Farkkila MA, Karkkainen P, et al: Colorectal dysplasia and carcinoma in patients with ulcerative colitis and primary sclerosing cholangitis. Scand J Gastroenterol 32:706-711, 1997.
281. Bleday R, Lee E, Jessurun J, et al: Increased risk of early colorectal neoplasms after hepatic transplant in patients with inflammatory bowel disease. Dis Colon Rectum 36:908-912, 1993.
282. Higashi H, Yanaga K, Marsh JW, et al: Development of colon cancer after liver transplantation for primary sclerosing cholangitis associated with ulcerative colitis. Hepatology 11:477-480, 1990.
283. Holzmann K, Klump B, Borchard F, et al: Flow cytometric and histologic evaluation in a large cohort of patients with ulcerative colitis: correlation with clinical characteristics and impact on surveillance. Dis Colon Rectum 44:1446-1455, 2001.
284. Tung BY, Emond MJ, Haggitt RC, et al: Ursodiol use is associated with lower prevalence of colonic neoplasia in patients with ulcerative colitis and primary sclerosing cholangitis. Ann Intern Med 134:89-95, 2001.
285. Sherlock S: Pathogenesis of sclerosing cholangitis: the role of nonimmune factors. Semin Liver Dis 11:5, 1991.
286. Hamour AA, Bonnington A, Hawthorne B, Wilkins EG: Successful treatment of AIDS-related cryptosporidial sclerosing cholangitis. AIDS 7:1449-1451, 1993.
287. Patel SA, Borges MC, Batt MD, Rosenblate HJ:Trichosporon cholangitis associated with hyperbilirubinemia, and findings suggesting primary sclerosing cholangitis on endoscopic retrograde cholangiopancreatography. Am J Gastroenterol 85:84-87, 1990;
288. Hayward AR, Levy J, Facchetti F, et al: Cholangiopathy and tumors of the pancreas, liver, and biliary tree in boys with X-linked immunodeficiency with hyper-IgM. J Immunol 158:977-983, 1997.
289. Mehal WZ, Hattersley AT, Chapman RW, Fleming KA: A survey of cytomegalovirus (CMV) DNA in primary sclerosing cholangitis (PSC) liver tissues using a sensitive polymerase chain reaction (PCR) based assay. J Hepatol 15:396-399, 1992.
290. Ferron GM, Mishina EV, Zimmerman JJ, Jusko WJ: Population pharmacokinetics of sirolimus in kidney transplant patients. Clin Pharmacol Ther 61:416-428, 1997.
291. Bucuvalas JC, Bove KE, Kaufman RA, et al: Cholangitis associated with *Cryptococcus neoformans*. Gastroenterology 88:1055-1059, 1985.
292. Vierling J, Hu K-Q: Immunologic mechanismof hepatobiliary injury. In Kaplowitz NE, ed: Liver and Biliary Disease, ed 2. Baltimore, Williams & Wilkins, 1996:55-87.
293. Vierling JM: Aetiopathogenesis of primary sclerosing cholangitis. In Manns MP, Chapman RW, Stiehl A, Wiesner RH, eds: Primary Sclerosing Cholangitis. Boston, Kluwer Academic Publishers, 1998:37-45.
294. Cullen S, Chapman R: Aetiopathogenesis of primary sclerosing cholangitis. Best Pract Res Clin Gastroenterol 15:577-589, 2001.
295. Chapman RWG, Jewell DP: Primary sclerosing cholangitis—An immunologically mediated disease? West J Med 143:193, 1985.
296. Chapman RW: Role of immune factors in the pathogenesis of primary sclerosing cholangitis. Semin Liver Dis 11:1, 1991.
297. Si L, Whiteside TL, Schade RR, et al: T-lymphocyte subsets in liver tissues of patients with primary biliary cirrhosis (PBC), patients with primary sclerosing cholangitis (PSC), and normal controls. J Clin Immunol 4:262-272, 1984.
298. Whiteside TL, Lasky S, Si L, Van Thiel DH: Immunologic analysis of mononuclear cells in liver tissues and blood of patients with primary sclerosing cholangitis. Hepatology 5:468-474, 1985.
299. Valenski WR, Herrod HG, Williams JW: In vitro evidence for B cell dysfunction in patients with chronic liver disease. J Clin Lab Immunol 28:169-172, 1989.
300. Kilby AE, Krawitt EL, Albertini RJ, et al: Suppressor T-cell deficiency in primary sclerosing cholangitis. Case and family study. Dig Dis Sci 36:1213-1216, 1991.
301. Lindor KD, Wiesner RH, LaRusso NF, et al: Enhanced autoreactivity of T-lymphocytes in primary sclerosing cholangitis. Hepatology 7:884, 1987.
302. Bodenheimer HCJ, Larusso NF, Thayer WRJ, et al: Elevated circulating immune complexes in primary sclerosing cholangitis. Hepatology 3:150-154, 1983.
303. Senaldi G, Donaldson PT, Magrin S, et al: Activation of the complement system in primary sclerosing cholangitis. Gastroenterology 97:1430-1434, 1989.
304. Garred P, Lyon H, Christoffersen P, et al: Deposition of C3, the terminal complement complex and vitronectin in primary biliary cirrhosis and primary sclerosing cholangitis. Liver 13:305-310, 1993.
305. Minuk GY, Angus M, Brickman CM, et al: Abnormal clearance of immune complexes from the circulation of patients with primary sclerosing cholangitis. Gastroenterology 88:166-170, 1985.
306. Mizoguchi E, Mizoguchi A, Chiba C, et al: Antineutrophil cytoplasmic antibodies in T-cell receptor alpha-deficient mice with chronic colitis. Gastroenterology 113:1828-1835, 1997.
307. Seibold F, Brandwein S, Simpson S, et al: pANCA represents a cross-reactivity to enteric bacterial antigens. J Clin Immunol 18:153-160, 1998.
308. Lichtman SN, Keku J, Clark RL, et al: Biliary tract disease in rats with experimental small bowel bacterial overgrowth. Hepatology 13:766-772, 1991.
309. Vierling JM: Animal models for primary sclerosing cholangitis. Best Pract Res Clin Gastroenterol 15:591-610, 2001.
310. Phillips PA, Keast D, Papadimitious JM, et al: Chronic obstructive jaundice induced by Reovirus type e in weanling mice. Pathology 1:193, 1969.
311. Bangaru B, Morecki R, Glaser JH, et al: Comparative studies of biliary atresia in the human newborn and reovirus-induced cholangitis in weanling mice. Lab Invest 43:456, 1980.
312. Morecki R, Glaser JH, Cho S, et al: Biliary atresia and reovirus type 3 infection. N Engl J Med 307:481, 1982.
313. Minuk GY, Paul RW, Lee PWK: The prevalence of antibodies to reovirus type 3 in adults with idiopathic cholestatic liver disease. J Med Virol 16:55, 1985.
314. Finegold MJ, Carpenter RJ: Obliterative cholangitis due to cytomegalovirus: a possible precursor of paucity of intrahepatic bile ducts. Hum Pathol 13:662, 1982.
315. Orloff MJ, Peskin GW, Ellis HL: A bacteriologic study of human portal blood: implications regarding hepatic ischemia in man. Ann Surg 148:738, 1958.
316. Brooke BN, Slaney G: Portal bacteremia in ulcerative colitis. Lancet 1:1206, 1958.
317. Brooke BN, Dykes PW, Walker FC: A study of liver disorders in ulcerative colitis. Postgrad Med J 37:245, 1961.
318. Eade MN, Brooke BN: Portal bacteremia in cases of ulcerative colitis submitted to colectomy. Lancet 1:1008, 1969.
319. Hektoen L: Experimental bacillary cirrhosis of the liver. J Pathol Bacteriol 7:214, 1901.
320. Weaver GH: Cirrhosis by injecting portal vein with *E. coli.* Johns Hopkins Hosp Rep 9:297, 1900.
321. MacMahon HE, Mallory FB: Streptococcus hepatitis. Am J Pathol 7:299, 1931.
322. Wachstein M, Meisel E, Falcon C: Enzymatic histochemistry in the experimentally damaged liver. Am J Pathol 40:219, 1962.
323. Vinnik IE, Kern F, Struthers JE, et al: Experimental chronic portal vein bacteremia. Proc Soc Exp Biol Med 115:311, 1964.
324. Donaldson PT, Norris S: Immunogenetics in PSC. Best Pract Res Clin Gastroenterol 15:611-627, 2001.
325. Boberg KM, Spurkland A, Rocca G, et al: The HLA-DR3,DQ2 heterozygous genotype is associated with an accelerated progression of primary sclerosing cholangitis. Scand J Gastroenterol 36:886-890, 2001.
326. Ruemmele FM, Targan SR, Levy G, et al: Diagnostic accuracy of serological assays in pediatric inflammatory bowel disease. Gastroenterology 115:822-829, 1998.
327. Vidrich A, Lee J, James E, et al: Segregation of pANCA antigenic recognition by DNase treatment of neutrophils: ulcerative colitis, type 1 autoimmune hepatitis, and primary sclerosing cholangitis. J Clin Immunol 15:293-299, 1995.
328. Eggena M, Targan SR, Iwanczyk L: Phage display cloning and characterization of an immunogenetic marker (perinuclear anti-neutrophil cytoplasmic antibody) in ulcerative colitis. J Immunol 156:4005-4011, 1996.
329. Pokorny CS, Norton ID, McCaughan GW, Selby WS: Anti-neutrophil cytoplasmic antibody: a prognostic indicator in primary sclerosing cholangitis. J Gastroenterol Hepatol 9:40-44, 1994.

330. Bansi DS, Bauducci M, Bergqvist A, et al: Detection of antineutrophil cytoplasmic antibodies in primary sclerosing cholangitis: a comparison of the alkaline phosphatase and immunofluorescent techniques. Eur J Gastroenterol Hepatol 9:575-580, 1997.
331. Mulder AH, Horst G, Haagsma EB, et al: Prevalence and characterization of neutrophil cytoplasmic antibodies in autoimmune liver diseases. Hepatology 17:411-417, 1993.
332. Hopf U, Berg T, Korber J, et al: Autoimmune markers in primary sclerosing cholangitis. In Mann M, Stiehl A, Chapman R, Weisner RH, eds: Primary Sclerosis Cholangitis, vol 1. Freiburg, Kluwer Academic Publishers, 1998:46-54.
333. Schultz H, Weiss J, Carroll SF, Gross WL: The endotoxin-binding bactericidal/permeability-increasing protein (BPI): a target antigen of autoantibodies. J Leukoc Biol 69:505-512, 2001.
334. Sakamaki S, Takayanagi N, Yoshizaki N, et al: Autoantibodies against the specific epitope of human tropomyosin(s) detected by a peptide based enzyme immunoassay in sera of patients with ulcerative colitis show antibody dependent cell mediated cytotoxicity against HLA-DPw9 transfected L cells. Gut 47:236-241, 2000.
335. Mandal A, Dasgupta A, Jeffers L, et al: Autoantibodies in sclerosing cholangitis against a shared peptide in biliary and colon epithelium. Gastroenterology 106:185-192, 1994.
336. Das KM: Relationship of extraintestinal involvements in inflammatory bowel disease: new insights into autoimmune pathogenesis. Dig Dis Sci 44:1-13, 1999.
337. Das KM, Vecchi M, Sakamaki S: A shared and unique epitope(s) on human colon, skin, and biliary epithelium detected by a monoclonal antibody. Gastroenterology 98:464-469, 1990.
338. Dienes HP, Lohse AW, Gerken G, et al: Bile duct epithelia as target cells in primary biliary cirrhosis and primary sclerosing cholangitis. Virchows Arch 431:119-124, 1997.
339. Hashimoto E, Lindor KD, Homburger HA, et al: Immunohistochemical characterization of hepatic lymphocytes in primary biliary cirrhosis in comparison with primary sclerosing cholangitis and autoimmune chronic active hepatitis (see comments). Mayo Clin Proc 68:1049-1055, 1993.
340. Tsuneyama K, Harada K, Yasoshima M, et al: Expression of co-stimulatory factor B7-2 on the intrahepatic bile ducts in primary biliary cirrhosis and primary sclerosing cholangitis: an immunohistochemical study. J Pathol 186:126-130, 1998.
341. Spengler U, Leifeld L, Braunschweiger I, et al: Anomalous expression of costimulatory molecules B7-1, B7-2 and CD28 in primary biliary cirrhosis. J Hepatol 26:31-36, 1997.
342. Broome U, Hultcrantz R, Scheynius A: Lack of concomitant expression of ICAM-1 and HLA-DR on bile duct cells from patients with primary sclerosing cholangitis and primary biliary cirrhosis. Scand J Gastroenterol 28:126-130, 1993.
343. Dikengil A, Siskind BN, Morse SS, et al: Sclerosing cholangitis from intra-arterial floxuridine. J Clin Gastroenterol 8:690, 1986.
344. Doppman JL, Girton ME: Bile duct scarring following ethanol embolization of the hepatic artery: an experimental study in monkeys. Radiology 152:621, 1984.
345. Washington K, Clavien PA, Killenberg P: Peribiliary vascular plexus in primary sclerosing cholangitis and primary biliary cirrhosis. Hum Pathol 28:791-795, 1997.
346. Probert CS, Christ AD, Saubermann LJ, et al: Analysis of human common bile duct-associated T cells: evidence for oligoclonality, T cell clonal persistence, and epithelial cell recognition. J Immunol 158:1941-1948, 1997.
347. Broome U, Grunewald J, Scheynius A, et al: Preferential V beta3 usage by hepatic T lymphocytes in patients with primary sclerosing cholangitis. J Hepatol 26:527-534, 1997.
348. Grant AJ, Lalor PF, Hubscher SG, et al: MAdCAM-1 expressed in chronic inflammatory liver disease supports mucosal lymphocyte adhesion to hepatic endothelium (MAdCAM-1 in chronic inflammatory liver disease). Hepatology 33:1065-1072, 2001.
349. Bo X, Broome U, Remberger M, Sumitran-Holgersson S: Tumour necrosis factor alpha impairs function of liver derived T lymphocytes and natural killer cells in patients with primary sclerosing cholangitis. Gut 49:131-141, 2001.
350. Yanagitani K, Kubota Y, Tsuji K, et al: Influence of biliary obstruction on neutrophil chemotaxis. J Gastroenterol 33:536-540, 1998.
351. Morland CM, Fear J, McNab G, et al: Promotion of leukocyte transendothelial cell migration by chemokines derived from human biliary epithelial cells in vitro. Proc Assoc Am Physicians 109:372-382, 1997.
352. Sasatomi K, Noguchi K, Sakisaka S, et al: Abnormal accumulation of endotoxin in biliary epithelial cells in primary biliary cirrhosis and primary sclerosing cholangitis. J Hepatol 29:409-416, 1998.
353. Bansal AS, Thomson A, Steadman C, et al: Serum levels of interleukins 8 and 10, interferon gamma, granulocyte-macrophage colony stimulating factor and soluble CD23 in patients with primary sclerosing cholangitis. Autoimmunity 26:223-229, 1997.
354. Stocks SC, Ruchaud-Sparagano MH, Kerr MA, et al: CD66: role in the regulation of neutrophil effector function. Eur J Immunol 26:2924-2932, 1996.
355. Riethdorf L, Lisboa BW, Henkel U, et al: Differential expression of CD66a (BGP), a cell adhesion molecule of the carcinoembryonic antigen family, in benign, premalignant, and malignant lesions of the human mammary gland. J Histochem Cytochem 45:957-963, 1997.
356. Kuroe K, Haga Y, Funakoshi O, et al: Extraintestinal manifestations of granulomatous enterocolitis induced in rabbits by long-term submucosal administration of muramyl dipeptide emulsified with Freund's incomplete adjuvant. J Gastroenterol 31:199-206, 1996.
357. Yamada S, Ishii M, Liang LS, et al: Small duct cholangitis induced by N-formyl L-methionine L-leucine L- tyrosine in rats. J Gastroenterol 29:631-636, 1994.
358. Lichtman SN, Bachmann S, Munoz SR, et al: Bacterial cell wall polymers (peptidoglycan-polysaccharide) cause reactivation of arthritis. Infect Immun 61:4645-4653, 1993.
359. Lichtman SN, Okoruwa EE, Keku J, et al: Degradation of endogenous bacterial cell wall polymers by the muralytic enzyme mutanolysin prevents hepatobiliary injury in genetically susceptible rats with experimental intestinal bacterial overgrowth. J Clin Invest 90:1313-1322, 1992.
360. Roskams T, Desmet V: Ductular reaction and its diagnostic significance. Semin Diagn Pathol 15:259-269, 1998.
361. Satsangi J, Chapman RW, Haldar N, et al: A functional polymorphism of the stromelysin gene (MMP-3) influences susceptibility to primary sclerosing cholangitis. Gastroenterology 121:124-130, 2001.
362. Pinzani M, Milani S, Grappone C, et al: Expression of platelet-derived growth factor in a model of acute liver injury. Hepatology 19:701-707, 1994.
363. Pinzani M, Milani S, Herbst H, et al: Expression of platelet-derived growth factor and its receptors in normal human liver and during active hepatic fibrogenesis. Am J Pathol 148:785-800, 1996.
364. Tsuneyama K, Kono N, Yamashiro M, et al: Aberrant expression of stem cell factor on biliary epithelial cells and peribiliary infiltration of c-kit-expressing mast cells in hepatolithiasis and primary sclerosing cholangitis: a possible contribution to bile duct fibrosis. J Pathol 189:609-614, 1999.
365. Ghent CN, Carruthers SG: Treatment of pruritus in primary biliary cirrhosis with rifampin. Results of a double-blind, crossover, randomized trial. Gastroenterology 94:488-493, 1988.
366. Podesta A, Lopez P, Terg R, et al: Treatment of pruritus of primary biliary cirrhosis with rifampin. Dig Dis Sci 36:216-220, 1991.
367. Price TJ, Patterson WK, Olver IN: Rifampicin as treatment for pruritus in malignant cholestasis. Support Care Cancer 6:533-535, 1998.
368. Lauterburg BH, Dickson ER, Pineda AA, et al: Removal of bile acids and bilirubin by plasmaperfusion of U.S.P. charcoal-coated glass beads. J Lab Clin Med 94:585-592, 1979.
369. Lauterburg BH, Pineda AA, Dickson ER, et al: Plasmaperfusion for the treatment of intractable pruritus of cholestasis. Mayo Clin Proc 53:403-407, 1978.
370. Gomez RL, Griffin JW, Squires JE: Prolonged relief of intractable pruritus in primary sclerosing cholangitis by plasmapheresis. J Clin Gastroenterol 8:301, 1986.
371. Lauterburg BH, Taswell HF, Pineda AA, et al: Treatment of pruritus of cholestasis by plasma perfusion through USP-charcoal-coated beads. Lancet 2:53, 1980.
372. Schrumpf E: Association of primary sclerosing cholangitis and celiac disease: fact or fancy? Hepatology 10:1020-1021, 1989.
373. Venturini I, Cosenza R, Miglioli L, et al: Adult celiac disease and primary sclerosing cholangitis: two case reports. Hepatogastroenterology 45:2344-2347, 1998.
374. Volta U, De Franceschi L, Molinaro N, et al: Frequency and significance of anti-gliadin and anti-endomysial antibodies in autoimmune hepatitis. Dig Dis Sci 43:2190-2195, 1998.
375. Drude RB Jr, Hines C Jr: The pathophysiology of intestinal bacterial overgrowth syndromes. Arch Intern Med 140:1349-1352, 1980.

376. Hay JE: Bone disease in cholestatic liver disease. Gastroenterology 108:276-283, 1995.
377. Csendes A, Mitru N, Maluenda F, et al: Counts of bacteria and pyocites of choledochal bile in controls and in patients with gallstones or common bile duct stones with or without acute cholangitis. Hepatogastroenterology 43:800-806, 1996.
378. Quinn PG, Binion DG, Connors PJ: The role of endoscopy in inflammatory bowel disease. Med Clin North Am 78:1331, 1994.
379. Stiehl A, Benz C, Sauer P, Theilmann L: Treatment of primary sclerosing cholangitis: the role of ursodeoxycholic acid and endoscopy. In Mann M, Stiehl A, Chapman R, Weisner RH, eds: Primary Sclerosis Cholangitis, vol 1. Freiburg, Kluwer Academic Publishers, 1998:99-102.
380. Eckhauser FE, Colleti LM, Knol JA: The changing role of surgery for sclerosing cholangitis. Dig Dis 14:180-191, 1996.
381. Ahrendt SA, Pitt HA, Kalloo AN, et al: Primary sclerosing cholangitis: resect, dilate, or transplant? Ann Surg 227:412-423, 1998.
382. Silvis SE, Nelson DB, Meier PB: Ten-year response to stenting in a patient with primary sclerosing cholangitis. Gastrointest Endosc 47:83-87, 1998.
383. van Milligen de Wit AW, Rauws EA, van Bracht J, et al: Lack of complications following short-term stent therapy for extrahepatic bile duct strictures in primary sclerosing cholangitis. Gastrointest Endosc 46:344-347, 1997.
384. van Milligen de Wit AW, van Bracht J, Rauws EA, et al: Endoscopic stent therapy for dominant extrahepatic bile duct strictures in primary sclerosing cholangitis. Gastrointest Endosc 44:293-299, 1996.
385. Linder S, Soderlund C: Endoscopic therapy in primary sclerosing cholangitis: outcome of treatment and risk of cancer. Hepatogastroenterology 48:387-392, 2001.
386. Springer DJ, Gaing AA, Siegel JH: Radiologic regression of primary sclerosing cholangitis following combination therapy with an endoprosthesis and ursodeoxycholic acid. Am J Gastroenterol 88:1957-1959, 1993.
387. Meier PN, Manns MP: Medical and endoscopic treatment in primary sclerosing cholangitis. Best Pract Res Clin Gastroenterol 15:657-666, 2001.
388. Kaya M, Petersen BT, Angulo P, et al: Balloon dilation compared to stenting of dominant strictures in primary sclerosing cholangitis. Am J Gastroenterol 96:1059-1066, 2001.
389. Wagner S, Gebel M, Meier P, et al: Endoscopic management of biliary tract strictures in primary sclerosing cholangitis (see comments). Endoscopy 28:546-551, 1996.
390. Torok N, Gores GJ: Cholangiocarcinoma. Semin Gastrointest Dis 12:125-132, 2001.
391. Kaya M, de Groen PC, Angulo P, et al: Treatment of cholangiocarcinoma complicating primary sclerosing cholangitis: the Mayo Clinic experience. Am J Gastroenterol 96:1164-1169, 2001.
392. Rumalla A, Baron TH, Wang KK, et al: Endoscopic application of photodynamic therapy for cholangiocarcinoma. Gastrointest Endosc 53:500-504, 2001.
393. Knechtle SJ, D'Alessandro AM, Harms BA, et al: Relationships between sclerosing cholangitis, inflammatory bowel disease, and cancer in patients undergoing liver transplantation. Surgery 118:615-619, 1995.
394. Cotton PB, Nickl N: Endoscopic and radiologic approaches to therapy in primary sclerosing cholangitis. Semin Liver Dis 11:40-48, 1991.
395. De VI, Steers JL, Burch PA, et al: Prolonged disease-free survival after orthotopic liver transplantation plus adjuvant chemoirradiation for cholangiocarcinoma. Liver Transpl 6:309-316, 2000.
396. Cangemi JR, Wiesner RH, Beaver SJ, et al: Effect of proctocolectomy for chronic ulcerative colitis on the natural history of primary sclerosing cholangitis. Gastroenterology 96:790-794, 1989.
397. Post AB, Bozdech JM, Lavery I, Barnes DS: Colectomy in patients with inflammatory bowel disease and primary sclerosing cholangitis. Dis Colon Rectum 37:175-178, 1994.
398. Mikkola K, Kiviluoto T, Riihela M, et al: Liver involvement and its course in patients operated on for ulcerative colitis. Hepatogastroenterology 42:68-72, 1995.
399. Kartheuser AH, Dozois RR, Larusso NF, et al: Comparison of surgical treatment of ulcerative colitis associated with primary sclerosing cholangitis: ileal pouch-anal anastomosis versus Brooke ileostomy. Mayo Clin Proc 71:748-756, 1996.
400. Penna C, Dozois R, Tremaine W, et al: Pouchitis after ileal pouch-anal anastomosis for ulcerative colitis occurs with increased frequency in patients with associated primary sclerosing cholangitis. Gut 38:234-239, 1996.
401. Zins BJ, Sandborn WJ, Penna CR, et al: Pouchitis disease course after orthotopic liver transplantation in patients with primary sclerosing cholangitis and an ileal pouch-anal anastomosis. Am J Gastroenterol 90:2177-2181, 1995.
402. Cox KL, Cox KM: Oral vancomycin: treatment of primary sclerosing cholangitis in children with inflammatory bowel disease. J Pediatr Gastroenterol Nutr 27:580-583, 1998.
403. Mistilis SP, Skyring AP, Goulston SJ: Effect of long-term tetracycline therapy, steroid therapy and colectomy in pericholangitis associated with ulcerative colitis. Australas Ann Med 14:286-294, 1965.
404. Munoz SJ, Heubi JE, Balistreri WF, et al: Vitamin E deficiency in primary biliary cirrhosis: mechanism and relation to deficiency in other lipid soluble vitamins. Gastroenterology 92:1758, 1987 (abstract).
405. LaRusso NF, Wiesner RH, Ludwig J, et al: Prospective trial of penicillamine in primary sclerosing cholangitis. Gastroenterology 95:1036, 1988.
406. Myers RN, Cooper JH, Padis N: Primary sclerosing cholangitis. Complete gross and histologic reversal after long-term steroid therapy. Am J Gastroenterol 53:527-538, 1970.
407. Angulo P, Batts KP, Jorgensen RA, et al: Oral budesonide in the treatment of primary sclerosing cholangitis. Am J Gastroenterol 95:2333-2337, 2000.
408. Javett SL: Azathioprine in primary sclerosing cholangitis. Lancet 1:810, 1971.
409. Wagner A: Azathioprine treatment in primary sclerosing cholangitis. Lancet 2:663, 1971.
410. Lindor KD, Wiesner RH, Colwell LJ, et al: The combination of prednisone and colchicine in patients with primary sclerosing cholangitis. Am J Gastroenterol 86:57, 1991.
411. Kaplan MM, Arora S, Pincus SH: Primary sclerosing cholangitis and low-dose oral pulse methotrexate therapy. Clinical and histologic response. Ann Intern Med 106:231, 1987.
412. Knox TA, Kaplan MM: Treatment of primary sclerosing cholangitis with oral methotrexate. Am J Gastroenterol 86:546, 1991.
413. Knox TA, Kaplan MM: A double-blind controlled trial of oral-pulse methotrexate therapy in the treatment of primary sclerosing cholangitis. Gastroenterology 106:494, 1994.
414. Duerksen DR, Blondel-Hill E, Bailey RJ: *Pneumocystis carinii* pneumonia complicating methotrexate treatment of primary sclerosing cholangitis. Am J Gastroenterol 90:1886-1887, 1995.
415. Wiesner RH, Steiner B, LaRusso NF, et al: A controlled clinical trial evaluating cyclosporine in the treatment of primary sclerosing cholangitis. Hepatology 14:63A, 1991.
416. Shelley ED, Shelley WB: Cyclosporine therapy for pyoderma gangrenosum associated with sclerosing cholangitis and ulcerative colitis. J Am Acad Dermatol 18:1084, 1988.
417. Kyokane K, Ichihara T, Horisawa M, et al: Successful treatment of primary sclerosing cholangitis with cyclosporine and corticosteroid. Hepatogastroenterology 41:449, 1994.
418. Sandborn WJ, Wiesner RH, et al: Ulcerative colitis disease activity following treatment of associated primary sclerosing cholangitis with cyclosporin. Gut 34:242, 1993.
419. Van Thiel DH, Carroll P, Abu-Elmagd K, et al: Tacrolimus (FK 506), a treatment for primary sclerosing cholangitis: results of an open-label preliminary trial. Am J Gastroenterol 90:455-459, 1995.
420. Sakamoto T, Kuwabara T, Tanaka Y, et al: Characterization of an HDV ribozyme which consists of three RNA oligomer strands. Nucleic Acids Symp Ser 34:131-132, 1995.
421. Angulo P, Bharucha AE, Jorgensen RA, et al: Oral nicotine in treatment of primary sclerosing cholangitis: a pilot study. Dig Dis Sci 44:602-607, 1999.
422. Bharucha AE, Jorgensen R, Lichtman SN, et al: A pilot study of pentoxifylline for the treatment of primary sclerosing cholangitis. Am J Gastroenterol 95:2338-2342, 2000.
423. Beuers U, Spengler U, Kruis W, et al: Ursodeoxycholic acid for treatment of primary sclerosing cholangitis: a placebo-controlled trial. Hepatology 16:707-714, 1992.
424. Stiehl A, Walker S, Stiehl L, et al: Effect of ursodeoxycholic acid on liver and bile duct disease in primary sclerosing cholangitis. A 3-year pilot study with a placebo-controlled study period. J Hepatol 20:57-64, 1994.

425. Lindor KD: Ursodiol for primary sclerosing cholangitis. Mayo Primary Sclerosing Cholangitis-Ursodeoxycholic Acid Study Group (see comments). N Engl J Med 336:691-695, 1997.
426. De Maria N, Colantoni A, Rosenbloom E, Van Thiel DH: Ursodeoxycholic acid does not improve the clinical course of primary sclerosing cholangitis over a 2-year period. Hepatogastroenterology 43:1472-1479, 1996.
427. Stiehl A, Rudolph G, Sauer P, et al: Efficacy of ursodeoxycholic acid treatment and endoscopic dilation of major duct stenoses in primary sclerosing cholangitis. An 8-year prospective study. J Hepatol 26:560-566, 1997.
428. Mitchell SA, Bansi DS, Hunt N, et al: A preliminary trial of high-dose ursodeoxycholic acid in primary sclerosing cholangitis. Gastroenterology 121:900-907, 2001.
429. Harnois DM, Angulo P, Jorgensen RA, et al: High-dose ursodeoxycholic acid as a therapy for patients with primary sclerosing cholangitis. Am J Gastroenterol 96:1558-1562, 2001.
430. van Hoogstraten HJ, Vleggaar FP, Boland GJ, et al: Budesonide or prednisone in combination with ursodeoxycholic acid in primary sclerosing cholangitis: a randomized double-blind pilot study. Belgian-Dutch PSC Study Group. Am J Gastroenterol 95:2015-2022, 2000.
431. Hay JE: Liver transplantation for primary biliary cirrhosis and primary sclerosing cholangitis: does medical treatment alter timing and selection? Liver Transpl Surg 4:S9-S17, 1998.
432. Wiesner RH, Porayko MK, Dickson ER, et al: Selection and timing of liver transplantation in primary biliary cirrhosis and primary sclerosing cholangitis. Hepatology 16:1290, 1992.
433. Sebagh M, Farges O, Kalil A, et al: Sclerosing cholangitis following human orthotopic liver transplantation. Am J Surg Pathol 19:81-90, 1995.
434. Campbell WL, Sheng R, Zajko AB, et al: Intrahepatic biliary strictures after liver transplantation. Radiology 191:735, 1994.
435. Sheng R, Zajko AB, Campbell WL, Abu-Elmagd K: Biliary strictures in hepatic transplants: prevalence and types in patients with primary sclerosing cholangitis vs those with other liver diseases. Am J Roentgenol 161:297, 1993.
436. Harrison RF, Davies MH, Neuberger JM, Hubscher SG: Fibrous and obliterative cholangitis in liver allografts: evidence of recurrent primary sclerosing cholangitis? Hepatology 20:356, 1994.
437. Boyer TD: Does primary sclerosing cholangitis recur after liver transplantation? No! Liver Transpl Surg 3:S24-S25, 1997.
438. Haagsma EB, Mulder AH, Gouw AS, et al: Neutrophil cytoplasmic autoantibodies after liver transplantation in patients with primary sclerosing cholangitis. J Hepatol 19:8, 1993.
439. Wojczys R: Liver involvement and its course in experimental colitis in rats. Hepatogastroenterology 44:1193-1195, 1997.
440. Graziadei IW, Wiesner RH, Batts KP, et al: Recurrence of primary sclerosing cholangitis following liver transplantation. Hepatology 29:1050-1056, 1999.
441. Jain A, Kashyap R, Marsh W, et al: Reasons for long-term use of steroid in primary adult liver transplantation under tacrolimus. Transplantation 71:1102-1106, 2001.
442. Sheng R, Campbell WL, Zajko AB, Baron RL: Cholangiographic features of biliary strictures after liver transplantation for primary sclerosing cholangitis: evidence of recurrent disease. AJR Am J Roentgenol 166:1109-1113, 1996.
443. Gavaler JS, Delemos B, Belle SH, et al: Ulcerative colitis disease activity as subjectively assessed by patient-completed questionnaires following orthotopic liver transplantation for sclerosing cholangitis. Dig Dis Sci 36:321, 1991.
444. Befeler AS, Lissoos TW, Schiano TD, et al: Clinical course and management of inflammatory bowel disease after liver transplantation. Transplantation 65:393-396, 1998.
445. Rowley S, Candinas D, Mayer AD, et al: Restorative proctocolectomy and pouch anal anastomosis for ulcerative colitis following orthotopic liver transplantation. Gut 37:845-847, 1995.
446. Stieber AC, Marino IR, Iwatsuki S, Starzl TE: Cholangiocarcinoma in sclerosing cholangitis. The role of liver transplantation. Int Surg 74:1-3, 1989.
447. Lesage G, Glaser SS, Gubba S, et al: Regrowth of the rat biliary tree after 70% partial hepatectomy is coupled to increased secretin-induced ductal secretion. Gastroenterology 111:1633-1644, 1996.
448. Shaked A, Colonna JO, Goldstein L, Busuttil RW: The interrelation between sclerosing cholangitis and ulcerative colitis in patients undergoing liver transplantation. Ann Surg 215:598, 1992.
449. Converse CF, Reagan JW, DeCosse JJ: Ulcerative colitis and carcinoma of the bile ducts. Am J Surg 121:39, 1971.
450. Ross AP, Braasch JW: Ulcerative colitis and carcinoma of the proximal bile ducts. Gut 14:94, 1973.
451. Black K, Hanna SS, Langer B, et al: Management of carcinoma of the extrahepatic bile ducts. Can J Surg 21:542, 1978.
452. Pereiras RV, Rheingold OJ, Hutson D, et al: Relief of malignant obstructive jaundice by percutaneous insertion of a permanent prosthesis in the biliary tree. Ann Intern Med 89:589, 1978.
453. Hall SW, Benjamin RS. Murphy WK, et al: Adriamycin, BCNU, FTORAFUR chemotherapy of pancreatic and biliary tract cancer. Cancer 44:2008, 1979.
454. Pilepich MV, Lambert PM: Radiotherapy of carcinomas of the extrahepatic biliary system. Radiology 127:767, 1978.
455. Baker AL, Kaplan MM, Norton RA, et al: Gallstones in inflammatory bowel disease. Dig Dis 19:109, 1974.
456. Cohen S, Kaplan M, Gottlieb L, et al: Liver disease and gallstones in regional enteritis. Gastroenterology 60:237, 1971.
457. Heaton KW, Read AE: Gallstones in patients with disorders of the terminal ileum and disturbed bile salt metabolism. BMJ 3:494, 1969.
458. Kleckner MS: The liver in regional enteritis. Gastroenterology 30:416, 1956.

CHAPTER

41

Wilson's Disease

Jonathan D. Gitlin, MD

Wilson's disease is an inherited disorder of copper metabolism resulting in hepatic cirrhosis and basal ganglia degeneration. Although clinical descriptions of individuals with hepatic cirrhosis and neurologic disease appear in the literature as early as 1850, Wilson's disease was not recognized as a distinct clinical entity until 1912. In this year the American-born, British-trained neurologist Samuel Alexander Kinnier Wilson published a monograph describing a familial syndrome of progressive lenticular degeneration invariably associated with cirrhosis of the liver at autopsy.[1] Wilson hypothesized the presence of a toxin in these patients, but a distinct role for copper in the organ pathology was not clearly recognized for another 35 years.[2] In 1952 Scheinberg and Gitlin demonstrated a deficiency of the copper-containing plasma protein ceruloplasmin in the serum of affected individuals, establishing a diagnostic test that is still in clinical use today.[3] Soon thereafter, Walshe introduced the use of D-penicillamine for systemic chelation, providing the first effective treatment in this disease.[4]

Autosomal-recessive inheritance of Wilson's disease was definitively demonstrated by Bearn in a series of comprehensive family studies,[5] and in 1985 Frydman and colleagues established linkage of the Wilson's disease locus with erythrocyte esterase D on chromosome 13.[6] Recognition of a genetic disorder resulting in aberrant hepatic copper homeostasis suggested that specific cellular mechanisms are involved in copper trafficking within hepatocytes. This concept was confirmed in 1993 when the Wilson's disease gene was cloned and shown to encode a novel copper-transporting P-type adenosine triphosphatase (ATPase) required for biliary copper excretion.[7-9] Characterization of the molecular defect in Wilson's disease has revealed a remarkable evolutionary conservation of the mechanisms of copper homeostasis and permitted fundamental insights into the cellular and molecular mechanisms of copper metabolism that may allow for the development of new approaches to the diagnosis and treatment of affected patients.

HEPATIC COPPER METABOLISM

Physiology

Copper is an essential trace element that plays a critical role in the biochemistry of aerobic organisms. The electron structure of this metal permits the facile transfer of electrons by specific cuproenzymes involved in neurotransmitter biosynthesis, pigment production, antioxidant defense, peptide amidation, connective tissue formation, iron homeostasis, and cellular respiration.[10] The signs and symptoms of copper deficiency result from the loss of activity of these essential enzymes. The useful chemical reactivity of copper in biologic systems also accounts for the toxicity of this metal in circumstances in which copper homeostasis is impaired. For these reasons, specific mechanisms have evolved that tightly regulate the absorption, transport, and excretion of copper, ensuring an adequate tissue supply while preventing cellular toxicity.

The daily adult diet contains approximately 5 mg of copper, about 40 percent of which is absorbed largely through the stomach and duodenum. There is no appreciable enterohepatic circulation of copper and thus each day an amount equivalent to that absorbed is excreted via the biliary tract (Figure 41-1).[11] This pathway of copper absorption and excretion is the only physiologically relevant mechanism for maintaining copper balance. Although copper is removed from the plasma by renal filtration 0this mechanism is significant only in the occurrence of marked copper excess. Metabolic studies indicate that a single oral dose of copper appears in the portal circulation bound to histidine and albumin that is then rapidly cleared by hepatic uptake.[12] Within 24 hours about 10 percent of this dose reappears in the plasma in newly synthesized ceruloplasmin, a finding that simply reflects the relative abundance of this cuproprotein because metabolic and genetic studies reveal no essential role for this protein in copper transport or distribution.[13,14] Copper is found in the plasma complexed to amino acids such as histidine; these complexes may be essential for uptake and utilization of this metal by multiple cell types.

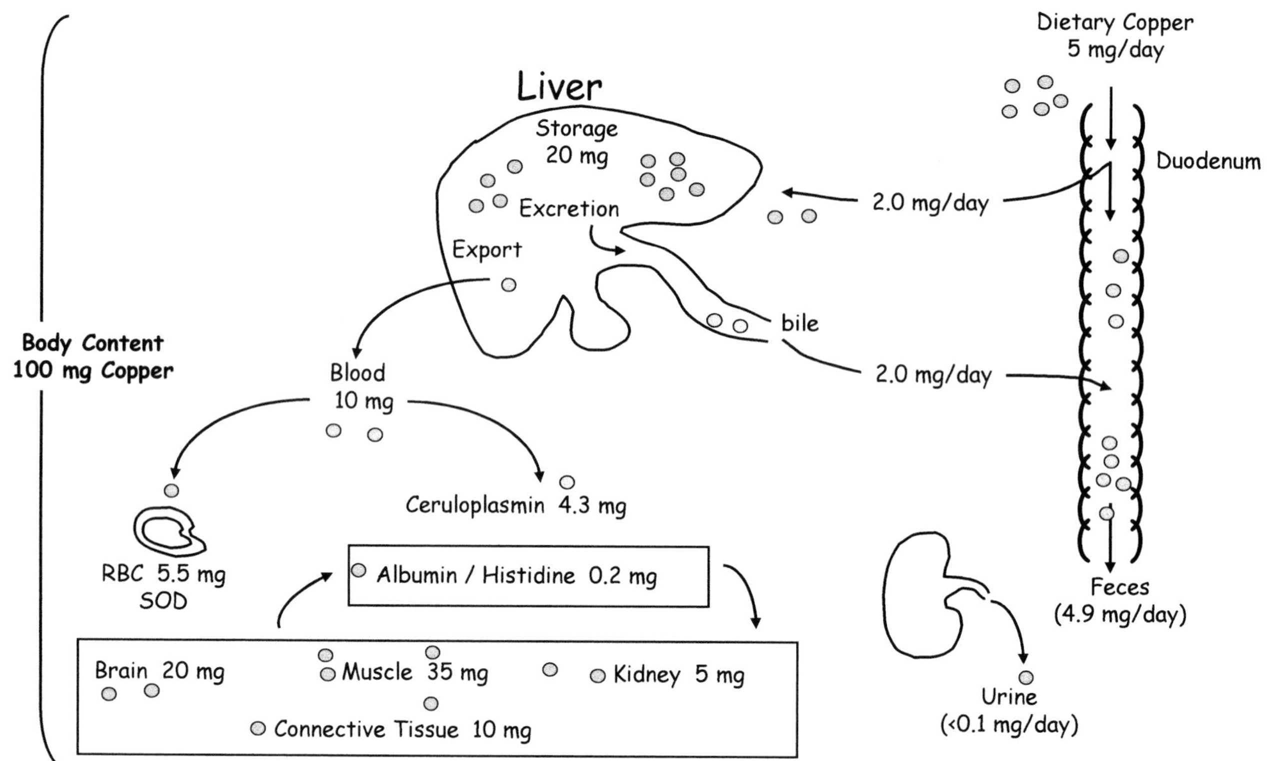

Figure 41-1 Physiology of human copper metabolism. The liver is the central organ of copper homeostasis. Copper balance is determined by biliary excretion, which is the only physiologic mechanism of excretion. There is no enterohepatic circulation of copper. (Modified from Harris ZL, Gitlin JD: Genetic and molecular basis for copper toxicity. Am J Clin Nutr 63:836S, 1996.)

Recent genetic experiments have begun to clarify the molecular mechanisms of copper uptake in mammalian cells.[15] The polytopic plasma membrane protein ctr1 is expressed in multiple cell types and tissues. Inactivation of the murine ctr1 gene by homologous recombination results in embryonic lethality in homozygous mutant embryos, revealing an essential role for this protein in copper homeostasis and embryonic development.[16,17] Biochemical studies of human ctr1 demonstrate that this protein transports copper with high affinity in a metal-specific and saturable manner.[18] Taken together, these studies suggest that ctr1 serves as the critical plasma membrane copper transport protein in enterocytes and hepatocytes.

The liver is the predominant organ of copper homeostasis with a considerable capacity for storage and excretion of this metal. Biliary excretion is the sole mechanism determining copper balance, and the amount of copper excreted in the bile is directly proportional to the size of the hepatic copper pool.[19] The form of copper appearing in the bile is unknown but radioisotope studies indicate that it exists as an unabsorbable macromolecular complex. Ceruloplasmin is not involved in biliary copper excretion; experimental studies of aceruloplasminemia reveal normal hepatic copper metabolism.[14] All plasma proteins are present in trace amounts in bile and the absence of ceruloplasmin in the bile of patients with Wilson's disease reflects the marked decrease in the serum concentration of this protein in affected patients. Given the capacity of the liver to increase biliary copper excretion, hepatic copper overload is a rare occurrence in the normal individual.

Hepatocytes are the predominant site of copper uptake and accumulation within the liver. Metallothionein is a small intracellular protein capable of chelating several metal ions, including copper.[20] Transgenic experiments propose a critical role for this protein in copper sequestration when the homeostasis of this metal is perturbed, suggesting that metallothionein mitigates the effects of copper accumulation in situations of hepatic copper excess.[21] The rate of biliary copper excretion is determined by the Wilson's disease ATPase, which is localized to the trans-Golgi network of hepatocytes (Plate 41-1).[22-24] With increasing intracellular copper concentration, this ATPase traffics to a cytoplasmic vesicular compartment near the canalicular membrane and accumulates copper for subsequent excretion into the bile. The decrease in cytoplasmic copper triggers relocalization of the ATPase, providing a rapid and efficient post-translational mechanism for maintaining intracellular copper homeostasis.

Ceruloplasmin is an essential serum ferroxidase that is synthesized in hepatocytes and secreted into the plasma after the incorporation of copper in the late secretory pathway.[25] Failure to incorporate copper during synthesis results in secretion of apoceruloplasmin, which is devoid of ferroxidase activity and rapidly degraded in the plasma.[26,27] Absence or dysfunction of the Wilson ATPase

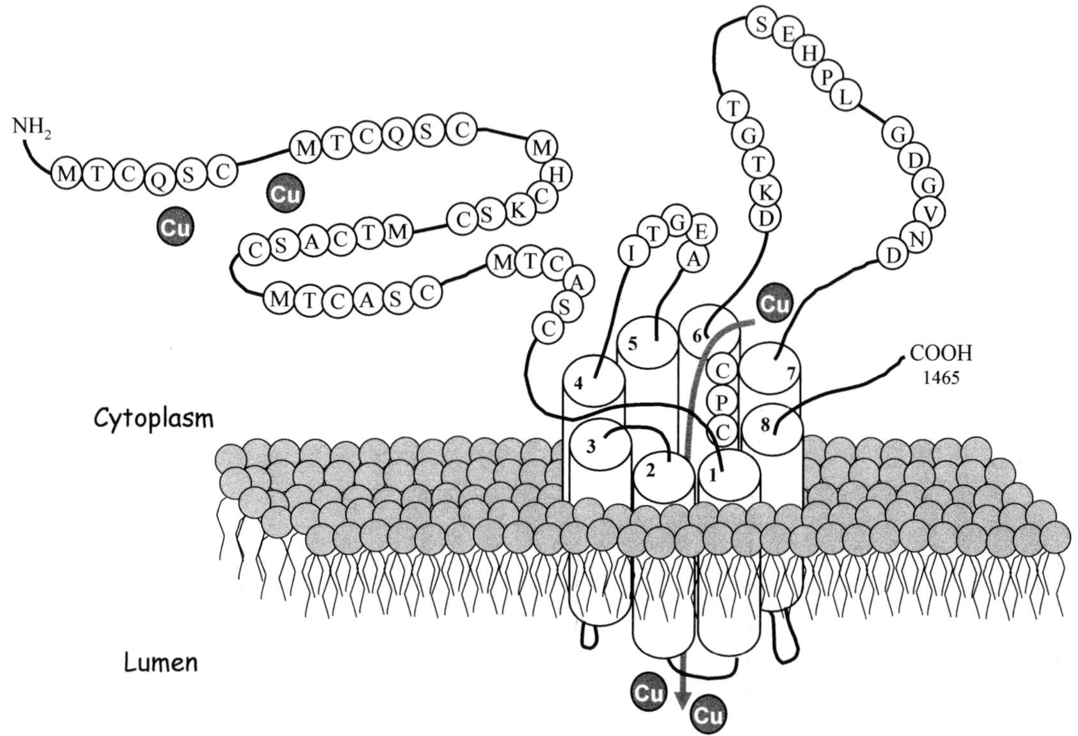

Figure 41-2 Topologic model of the Wilson's disease copper-transporting ATPase. Specific amino acids are noted in the conserved motifs discussed in the text. The proposed mechanism of energy-dependent ATP-driven cation transport across the membrane is illustrated. *ATP,* Adenosine triphosphate; *ATPase,* adenosine triphosphatase. (Modified from Payne A, Gitlin JD: Functional expression of the Menkes disease protein reveals common biochemical mechanisms among the copper-transporting P-type ATPases. J Biol Chem 273:3765, 1998.)

markedly impairs copper movement into the hepatocyte secretory pathway; this accounts for the decrease in serum ceruloplasmin observed in Wilson's disease. Biliary copper excretion is decreased in the fetus and newborn infant, resulting in an elevated hepatic copper content at birth. Consistent with this developmental difference in copper metabolism, the newborn liver synthesizes and secretes mostly apoceruloplasmin, abrogating use of this protein in newborn screening for Wilson's disease. The steady postnatal increase in biliary copper excretion is paralleled by a rise in serum ceruloplasmin, reflecting a maturation in the capacity of the hepatocyte for holoceruloplasmin biosynthesis.[28]

Cell Biology

Identification of the molecular defect in Wilson's disease has allowed for a detailed understanding of the cell biologic mechanisms of copper homeostasis in the liver. Wilson's disease results from the absence or dysfunction of a copper transporting ATPase (ATP7B) localized to the *trans*-Golgi network of hepatocytes (see Plate 41-1). This ATPase is required for the movement of copper into the secretory pathway where this metal is incorporated into ceruloplasmin and excreted into the bile. Sequence comparison and hydropathy plot analysis of the Wilson ATPase predicts a polytopic membrane protein positioned to transport copper across the lipid bilayer in an adenosine triphosphate (ATP)–dependent fashion (Figure 41-2). The homologous Menkes ATPase, which is encoded on the X chromosome, is localized to the trans-Golgi network of cells in the placenta, intestine, and blood-brain barrier and functions to transport copper across these tissues. As a result, infants with dysfunction of this ATPase present with the signs and symptoms of copper deficiency and neurodegeneration characteristic of Menkes disease.[10] Homologous copper transporting ATPases have now been identified in a variety of prokaryotic and eukaryotic species.[29]

The derived amino acid sequence of the Wilson ATPase reveals features characteristic of known P-type ATPases (see Figure 41-2). These proteins include the Ca^{2+} ATPase in the sarcoplasmic reticulum, the plasma membrane Na^+/K^+ ATPase, and the H^+ ATPase of the gastric mucosa. All P-type ATPases identified thus far contain an invariant aspartate residing within the consensus sequence DKTGT, which is reversibly phosphorylated to form a *β*-aspartyl phosphoryl intermediate required for the ATP-dependent transport of a specific ion across the membrane. Structural and biophysical studies indicate that this transport is accomplished using ATP reversibly bound to the consensus sequence GDGVND (see Figure 41-2). In these studies transport has been shown to be directly coupled to aspartyl phosphorylation, with ATP hydrolysis occurring only in the event of ion movement across the membrane.[30] Although the precise sequence of molecular events resulting in copper transport has not yet been identified for the copper P-type ATPases, studies with the Menkes ATPase indicate that this protein is transiently phosphorylated by ATP in a copper-specific and copper-dependent manner, undergoing conformational changes similar to what has been reported during the catalytic cycle of other P-type ATPases.[31] Recent experiments with the Wilson ATPase indicate that this protein also forms a phosphorylated intermediate and that mutation of the invariant aspartate residue abolishes phosphorylation in agreement with the proposed role of this residue as an acceptor of phosphate during the catalytic cycle.[32] Taken together these data suggest that the catalytic cycle of copper transport begins with the binding of copper to high-affinity binding sites in the transmembrane channel, followed by ATP binding and transient phosphorylation. Sequence comparison and site-directed mutagenesis suggest that the Wilson ATPase contains eight transmembrane domains, with both the amino and carboxyl terminus on the same side of the membrane within the cytoplasm of the cell (see Figure 41-2). The Wilson ATPase contains a cysteine-proline-cysteine (CPC) sequence within the sixth transmembrane domain that is highly conserved in all P-type ATPases known to play a role in heavy metal transport.[33] Mutational analysis has revealed that this motif is critical for copper transport, suggesting a direct role for copper binding by these cysteine residues during the catalytic cycle of transmembrane transport.[22,34]

The Wilson ATPase also contains domains that are unique to copper transporting ATPases. The amino terminus consists of six highly homologous domains, each of which contains the copper-binding motif MXCXXC (see Figure 41-2). These domains are essential for the copper transport and trafficking functions of both the Wilson and Menkes ATPases[35,36] and are the sites of protein-protein interaction with the copper chaperone atox1.[37,38] Structural analysis of one of these domains from the Menkes ATPase reveals a linear bicoordinate copper-binding environment dependent upon the conserved cysteine residues in the MXCXXC motif.[39] Although the precise function of the large cytoplasmic loop between transmembrane domains 6 and 7 (see Figure 41-2) is unknown, recent studies with purified fragments of the Wilson ATPase suggest that this region interacts specifically with the N-terminal copper-binding domains, perhaps regulating copper transfer from these domains to the CPC transport channel.[40] Interestingly, the histidine residue in the sequence SEHPL located within this same cytoplasmic loop is highly conserved in all known copper-transporting, P-type ATPases. This residue is the site of the most common mutation (H1069Q), in Northern European populations with Wilson's disease accounting for up to 40 percent of disease alleles. This mutation results in impaired trafficking of the Wilson protein, suggesting a potential role for the cytoplasmic loop and in particular the SEHPL motif in intracellular localization of the ATPase.[41] Thus far only one additional isoform of the Wilson ATPase has been identified, a truncated species generated through tissue-specific alternative promoter usage in the retina and pineal gland.[42] Although this pineal ATPase (PINA) lacks the entire amino-terminal copper-binding domains, recent studies suggest that these domains may not be critical for the catalytic activity of the ATPase.[31] Consistent with this concept, functional expression of PINA in yeast does result in demonstrable copper transport into the secretory pathway.[42] PINA exhibits a dramatic nocturnal increase in expression that is under control of the suprachiasmatic nucleus clock, suggesting a potential role for copper metabolism in circadian function.[42]

The intracellular location of the Wilson ATPase is consistent with the hypothesis that mutations resulting in the absence or dysfunction of this protein will impair the transport of copper into the secretory pathway and thus interfere with holoceruloplasmin biosynthesis and biliary copper excretion (Figure 41-3). This is supported by studies demonstrating that expression of the Wilson protein in yeast deficient in the homologous copper-transporting ATPase CCC2 restores copper incorporation into the ceruloplasmin homolog Fet3.[22] Expression of specific Wilson's disease mutants in *ccc2Δ* yeast fails to restore holoFet3 biosynthesis or function, providing direct evidence for the copper transport function of the Wilson ATPase and a useful assay for potential disease mutations.[22,43] Despite the utility of this yeast assay, expression studies in mammalian cells reveal a greater complexity in Wilson ATPase function. Elevation of the intracellular copper content of hepatocytes results in the translocation of the Wilson ATPase to a cytoplasmic vesicular compartment (see Plate 41-1). As copper is transported into these vesicles by the ATPase, the cytoplasmic copper concentration decreases and the ATPase traffics back to the trans-Golgi network (see Figure 41-3). This process, which is rapid and independent of new protein synthesis, provides a mechanism for the immediate response of the cell to changes in the steady-state intracellular copper concentration. Although the molecular determinants for recycling of the Wilson ATPase have not been well characterized, the Menkes ATPase has been shown to undergo a similar copper-induced trafficking pathway. Studies of this ATPase suggest that copper stimulates exocytic movement of the ATPase from the trans-Golgi network and that specific dileucine motifs within the carboxyl terminus are required for this trafficking response.[44,45]

The nature of the hepatocyte cytoplasmic vesicle into which copper is transported by the Wilson ATPase has not been well characterized. Genetic experiments in yeast indicate an essential role for both the H^+-transporting V-type ATPase[46] and a chloride channel Gef1[47,48] in ATPase-dependent copper transport into the homologous vesicular compartment in this organism. Presumably these proteins provide for both the acidic milieu and the necessary electrogenic shunt required to maintain active vesicular copper uptake. Interestingly, recent studies also suggest that this chloride channel may assure the chloride content within the vesicle required for the allosteric assembly of copper into Fet3.[49] The cellular mechanisms involved in subsequent movement of the copper-loaded vesicles to the canalicular membrane for biliary copper excretion are unknown, although one recent study suggests that the Wilson ATPase may also localize to this membrane during biliary copper excretion.[50]

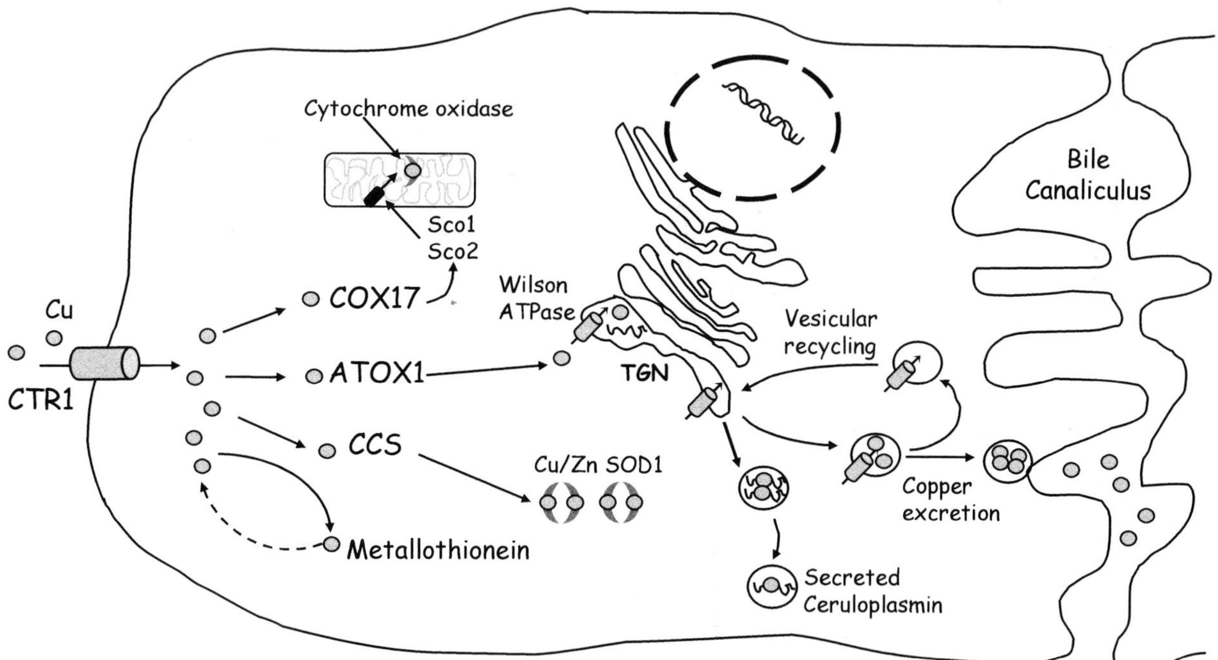

Figure 41-3 Model of the proposed pathways of intracellular copper trafficking within the human hepatocyte. The copper chaperones, recycling of the Wilson ATPase, and pathway of copper excretion into bile are illustrated. In this model copper movement to the canalicular membrane is predicted to be a final stage, which may be altered in cholestasis or idiopathic copper toxicosis. *ATP,* Adenosine triphosphate. (Modified from Harris ZL, Gitlin JD: Genetic and molecular basis for copper toxicity. Am J Clin Nutr 63:836S, 1996.)

Recent experiments in yeast have revealed that under physiologic circumstances intracellular copper availability is extraordinarily restricted.[51] As a result, the delivery of copper to specific pathways within the cell is mediated by a family of proteins termed *copper chaperones* that function to provide copper directly to target pathways while protecting this metal from intracellular scavenging (see Figure 41-3).[52-54] The cytoplasmic protein cox17 and two additional mitochondrial proteins, sco1 and sco2, are involved in the pathway of copper delivery to cytochrome oxidase; recent studies reveal that inherited mutations in both sco1 and sco2 can result in metabolic disease secondary to impaired respiratory chain assembly.[55-57] Similarly, the copper chaperone for superoxide dismutase (ccs) is essential for the delivery of copper to cytosolic copper/zinc superoxide dismutase (sod1).[58,59] The small cytoplasmic copper chaperone atox1 is required for copper delivery to the Wilson ATPase in the secretory pathway.[38,60] Atox1 contains a single copy of the MXCXXC copper-binding motif present in the amino-terminus of the copper-transporting ATPases; in vitro and in vivo studies indicate that these cysteines are required for copper binding and transport to both the Wilson and Menkes ATPases.[37,38] Structural studies of ccs and atox1 reveal that copper transfer between these chaperones and their target proteins is mediated by direct protein-protein interaction.[61,62]

WILSON'S DISEASE

Pathogenesis

Wilson's disease is an autosomal-recessive disorder found in all ethnic groups with a worldwide prevalence of 1:30,000. The heterozygous carrier rate is approximately 1:100, which gives an incidence of Wilson's disease of 15 to 25 per million.[63,64] In consanguineous populations this gene frequency is increased. The gene encoding the Wilson ATPase encompasses 65 kilobases and consists of 21 exons on chromosome 13q14.3. Analysis of deoxyribonucleic acid (DNA) from affected patients and families over the past 5 years has detected more than 200 distinct mutations in the Wilson's disease gene, the majority of which are catalogued in a database available through the Department of Medical Genetics at the University of Alberta (see the web site http://www.medgen.med.ualberta.ca). An overview of the published population genetics of these mutations indicates a small number of common mutations in specific populations and a greater number of rare individual alleles.[65-80] Molecular analysis reveals that about half of all reported mutations are missense and that the vast majority of these are confined to either well-defined consensus motifs or predicted transmembrane domains (see Figure 41-3). The remainder of mutations consists of small deletions, insertions, splice site errors, and nonsense mutations.

In populations of Northern European descent the H1069Q missense mutation accounts for about 40 percent of the identified disease alleles, whereas in most Asian populations an A778L missense mutation residing within the proposed fourth transmembrane domain has been identified in up to 30 percent of affected individuals. In specific populations in Sardinia and the Canary Islands haplotype studies and mutational analysis provide strong evidence for a founder effect.[81,82] Given the degree of allelic heterogeneity of the Wilson gene, analysis of mutations in most affected individuals will reveal compound heterozygotes, a finding that complicates phenotype genotype correlation. Nevertheless, recent studies in patients and families homozygous for specific alleles—including H1069Q—reveal little correlation between a specific mutation and the age of onset, clinical features, biochemical parameters, or disease activity in any given patient with Wilson's disease.[83] These data are consistent with the marked clinical variability often observed between affected siblings and even identical twins with Wilson's disease. Taken together these findings indicate that additional genetic and environmental factors significantly influence the outcome of a specific mutation in any given patient with Wilson's disease.[83]

Analysis of specific patient mutations has helped clarify the molecular pathogenesis of Wilson's disease and allows for the development of a model based upon our understanding of the cell biology of the Wilson ATPase (Figure 41-4). This model predicts that loss of function of this ATPase in the hepatocyte will result in a marked decrease in both holoceruloplasmin biosynthesis and biliary copper excretion with continuous intracellular copper accumulation, impaired copper homeostasis, and eventual copper overload in most tissues. Although the Wilson ATPase is expressed in multiple tissues, including the brain, the widespread copper accumulation clinically apparent in most affected patients is almost entirely the result of impaired ATPase function in hepatocytes because this copper accumulation will completely reverse upon hepatic transplantation (vide infra). Detailed biochemical studies of individual missense mutations are consistent with this model and reveal specific abnormalities in chaperone interaction, copper transport, subcellular localization, and copper-induced trafficking.[22,38,41,84] These studies have revealed that the common H1069Q mutation causes a temperature-sensitive defect in folding of the Wilson ATPase with resultant mislocalization to the endoplasmic reticulum. Analysis of this mutant ATPase at a temperature permissive for folding reveals that this conserved histidine residue is also required for copper-induced localization, suggesting a possible role for the SEHPL motif in vesicular trafficking.[41] The metallochaperone atox1 directly interacts with the Wilson ATPase in a copper-dependent fashion. Analysis of three disease mutations within the amino-terminal, copper-binding domains of the Wilson ATPase revealed a marked reduction in atox1 binding, indicating that impaired copper delivery by this chaperone constitutes the molecular

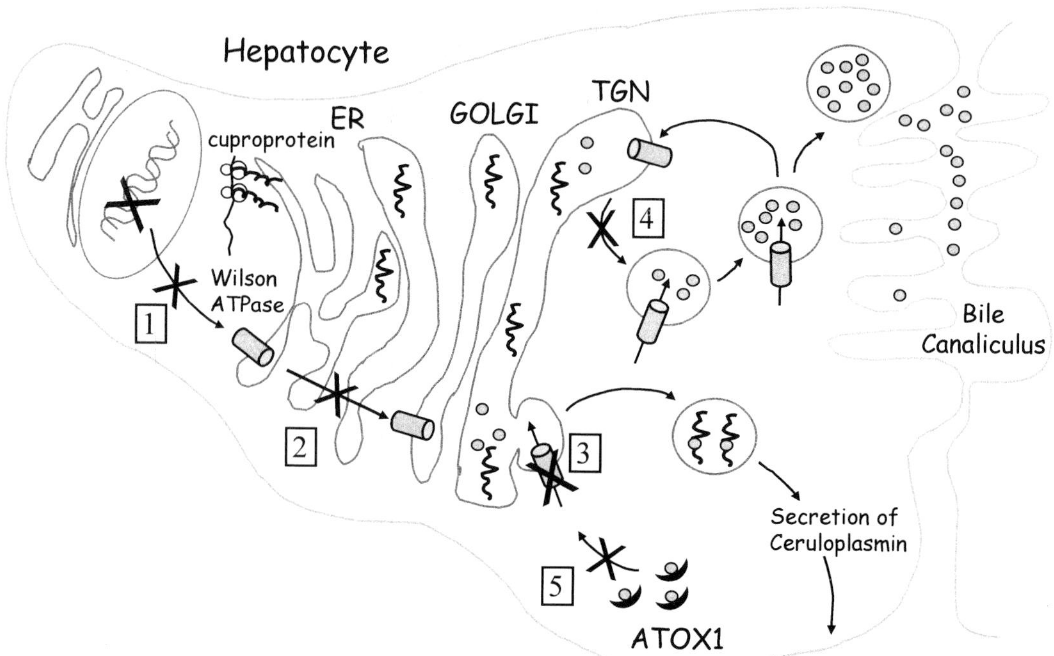

Figure 41-4 The molecular pathogenesis of Wilson's disease. Mutations in the Wilson ATPase result in specific cellular mechanisms of disease that include (1) gene interruption or impaired transcription, (2) defective protein folding and processing, (3) diminished copper transport function, (4) impaired recycling to and from the trans-Golgi network, and (5) defective interaction with the copper chaperone atox1. *ATPase,* Adenosine triphosphatase. (Modified from Hamza I, Gitlin JD: Copper metabolism and the liver. In Arias IM, Boyer JL, Chisari FV, et al, ed: The Liver: Biology and Pathology. Philadelphia, Lippincott Williams & Wilkins, 2001:331.)

basis of Wilson's disease in patients harboring these mutations.[38]

The model of cellular pathogenesis shown in Figure 41-4 also provides a starting point for defining additional genetic and environmental factors that may contribute to the enormous clinical heterogeneity observed among affected patients. Likely candidates in such a study include proteins that might influence the rate of copper delivery to the secretory pathway, such as atox1,[38,85] and proteins affecting the rate of vesicular copper accumulation and subsequent excretion such as homologues of the V-ATPase and chloride channel shown to play a role in this process in yeast.[46-49] As noted previously, metallothionein is essential for copper sequestration when copper's homeostasis is impaired, suggesting that allelic variability at this locus might also contribute to disease outcome in any given patient. The mechanisms of hepatocyte injury from copper accumulation are unknown although studies in rodents have implicated oxidant-mediated injury.[86] Copper treatment of hepatocytes in vitro results in activation of the CD95 system with subsequent induction of cellular apoptosis, suggesting that this mechanism may play a role in cell injury during the course of hepatic failure in Wilson's disease.[87] Although individuals heterozygous for mutations at the Wilson locus are asymptomatic, the paradigm illustrated previously also allows for the intriguing possibility that the presence of a single mutant Wilson allele might serve as a risk factor promoting copper-associated hepatic toxicity in circumstances of liver dysfunction from more common disorders such as alcoholic cirrhosis.[88]

There are currently three animal models that provide additional insight into the pathogenesis of Wilson's disease. The Long Evans Cinnamon (LEC) rat arose by spontaneous deletion of an extensive region of the rat ortholog of the Wilson ATPase.[89,90] LEC rats demonstrate marked impairment in biliary copper excretion with resulting hepatitis and liver failure preventable with copper chelation.[91] Consistent with the proposed role for the Wilson ATPase in copper homeostasis, hepatic copper accumulation is reversed in LEC rats after adenoviral-mediated expression of this protein in the liver.[92] Despite these similarities, LEC rats develop hepatocellular carcinoma and associated disturbances in hepatic iron metabolism not observed in humans with Wilson's disease, a finding that may limit the utility of these animals in elucidating the mechanisms of hepatic copper toxicity in affected patients.[93] The toxic milk mouse contains a spontaneous missense mutation (M1356V) in the murine ortholog of the Wilson ATPase, which results in a defect in copper-induced trafficking.[94] Newborn mice suckled by their affected mother develop severe copper deficiency, indicating a critical role for the Wilson ATPase in perinatal copper transport across the placenta and mammary gland in mice.[95] Although adult toxic milk mice demonstrate significant hepatic copper overload, these animals do not develop significant cirrhosis or neurologic disease, limiting their usefulness in pathogenesis studies. More recently a second spontaneously arising allele of the toxic milk mouse (*tx^J*) with identical phenotypic features has been analyzed and shown to contain a missense mutation (G712D) within the second transmembrane domain of the ATPase.[96] Deletion of a portion of the murine Wilson gene by homologous recombination has been used to create a second murine model of Wilson's disease.[97] These mice also demonstrate copper deficiency at birth with copper retention in the placenta, significant hepatic copper overload by 8 weeks of age, and evidence of brain copper accumulation. Similar to what has been observed in the toxic milk mouse, these animals do not develop hepatic cirrhosis or neurologic disease, a finding that, along with the observations in the LEC rat, suggests species-specific differences in the genetic and environmental factors that determine the outcome of copper-mediated hepatocyte injury. Bedlington terriers and North Ronaldsay sheep also accumulate significant amounts of hepatic copper with concomitant liver injury.[98-100] However, molecular genetic analysis has not revealed evidence of mutations in the Wilson ATPase in either species and the phenotypic features of these affected animals are more typical of those observed in children with idiopathic copper toxicosis (vide infra).

Clinical Presentation

Copper will eventually accumulate in almost every organ in a patient with Wilson's disease and may result in tissue injury and protean clinical manifestations. As such the physician must remain alert to the possibility of a variety of presenting signs and symptoms in any given patient, especially in the context of biochemical evidence of hepatic dysfunction.[101] Nevertheless, most individuals with Wilson's disease will have evidence of liver or neurologic disease early in the course of their illness. Wilson's disease rarely presents before the age of 5 years, a clinical finding that presumably reflects the minimum capacity of the hepatocyte to sequester excess cytoplasmic copper before injury results. Liver disease is the most common presenting feature in childhood, with an average age of presentation of 10 to 13 years, at least a decade younger than that observed in individuals presenting with neurologic dysfunction.[102] Although unusual, the initial diagnosis of Wilson's disease has been reported in individuals as late as the fifth or sixth decade.[101] Population studies indicate that liver disease accounts for the initial presentation in about 45 percent of affected individuals, with 35 percent presenting with neurologic disease and 10 percent with psychiatric problems. Of the remaining 10 percent, most are detected with hemolytic anemia and jaundice. Numerous endocrine and cardiac presentations, though rare, have also been recorded.

Liver Disease

Hepatic involvement in Wilson's disease is non-specific and the signs and symptoms often mimic the features of a number of acute and chronic liver diseases of childhood. Nevertheless, this liver disease usually occurs with one of four major clinical patterns that include mild elevation of the serum transaminases, often detected in an asymptomatic individual; cirrhosis; chronic active hepatitis; and fulminant hepatic failure.[103] In the earliest phases of liver disease or in the case of inactive cirrhosis many tests of hepatic function will be normal or only slightly disturbed. In such patients a course of progressive cirrhosis will develop slowly, with associated fatigue, anorexia, jaundice, and, eventually, ascites and splenomegaly. If this process is not recognized early the initial presentation may be that of hemorrhagic esophageal varices or hepatic encephalopathy. Chronic active hepatitis is a well recognized but less common outcome of liver involvement in Wilson's disease, occurring in up to 30 percent of all patients. Although Wilson's disease accounts for 5 percent to 8 percent of all cases of chronic active hepatitis in childhood, this diagnosis may not be initially considered because affected individuals often have no other overt evidence of copper accumulation.[104] Despite the mild elevation of serum transaminases observed in such cases, liver biopsy most frequently reveals significant evidence of hepatocellular injury with inflammatory changes. In certain circumstances the initial presentation may be that of acute liver failure with massive hepatocyte necrosis and release of copper into the systemic circulation. This process of acute hepatic deterioration is frequently accompanied by hemolytic anemia secondary to a rapid rise in free copper in the plasma.[105] Such individuals are often indistinguishable from those with fulminant hepatic failure from viral hepatitis or other causes, creating diagnostic difficulty and suggesting that in some patients with Wilson's disease infection or other external factors may precipitate sudden and massive hepatic necrosis in the copper-loaded liver. Patients with acute liver failure from Wilson's disease are usually young and will have a fulminant course with a very poor prognosis unless expeditious liver transplantation can be undertaken (vide infra).

Irrespective of the initial presentation all patients with hepatic involvement will have evidence of histologic changes on liver biopsy reflecting the cellular response to copper accumulation.[106,107] Early on such changes may include glycogen deposition and fatty infiltration but eventually will progress to micronodular cirrhosis with evidence of copper deposition variably distributed throughout the liver lobules. The heterogeneity of copper deposition and the insensitivity of staining techniques preclude the use of histochemical copper staining in diagnosis. In the case of chronic active hepatitis the biopsy is characterized by mononuclear cell infiltration with piecemeal necrosis and fibrosis. The development of cirrhosis may also occur in the absence of any inflammation; in such circumstances, the histologic picture will often reveal nodular regeneration with periportal fibrosis. Although hepatocellular carcinoma is a common finding in the LEC rat model, this diagnosis is rare in patients with Wilson's disease, a finding that may be due to species-specific differences in the response of hepatocytes to copper accumulation and injury or may reflect the fact that long-term survival is uncommon in untreated patients.[108]

Neurologic Disease

The neurologic signs and symptoms of Wilson's disease occur in up to 60 percent of patients at initial presentation. Such individuals are usually in the second or third decade of life; it is rare to find neurologic disease before adolescence.[109] Although patients may initially have more subtle evidence of neurologic dysfunction, including behavioral changes or deterioration in school performance, parkinsonian symptoms will come to predominate with diminution in facial expression, dystonia, tremor, and dysarthria.[110] Such features are consistent with the underlying neuropathology, which consists of cavitary degeneration in the basal ganglia with gliosis and neuronal loss in association with copper accumulation in these regions. These pathologic changes and accompanying copper accumulation are detectable at a relatively early stage in symptomatic individuals by magnetic resonance imaging (MRI); in addition, these radiologic findings have been observed to decrease with chelation therapy.[111] Although this increase in brain copper deposition presumably arises from elevated free plasma copper after hepatocyte injury, the mechanisms resulting in specific basal ganglia injury are unknown. Late manifestations of neurologic disease such as spasticity and seizures are increasingly rare as a result of early diagnosis and treatment. Some imaging studies have attempted to classify patients according to the neurologic signs and symptoms associated with specific MRI findings but it remains unclear if such classifications will be useful in evaluating therapeutic responses or determining prognosis.[112,113] Although neurologic deterioration will continue in untreated patients, in most cases the signs and symptoms of basal ganglia disease are reversible if chelation therapy is initiated before the onset of significant neurodegeneration.

Psychiatric Disease

Psychiatric disease may occur alone or in combination with other symptoms and will eventually develop in all patients if Wilson's disease is left untreated. Psychiatric illness is also more common in young adults and is rarely observed in children in the first decade of life. Psychiatric symptoms are the presenting disease manifestation in about 30 percent of all patients and may include abnormal behavior or personality changes, affective disorders, cognitive impairment, and schizophrenia.[114,115] Often such individuals may be improperly diagnosed with a progressive psychiatric illness; for this reason, it is recommended that all psychiatric patients with evidence of liver or neurologic disease be screened for Wilson's disease. Most frequently patients will exhibit personality changes with mood alterations and impulsive behavior that may reflect not only underlying changes secondary to brain copper deposition but also the reaction to progressive neurologic symptoms.[116] The incidence of schizophrenia and other delusional disorders is low but when present will also respond to chelation therapy if properly diagnosed at an early stage of illness.[117]

In addition to the more common hepatic and neurologic presentations, signs and symptoms may arise in Wilson's disease in any organ in which excess copper deposition results in impaired function or injury. With the marked elevation in plasma copper that occurs in affected patients, a fraction of this metal is removed from the plasma by renal filtration and excreted in the urine. As a result, renal tubular acidosis, nephrolithiasis, and Fanconi syndrome with aminoaciduria and glucosuria may occur after renal tubular cell injury from excess copper.[118] As noted previously, intravascular hemolysis is observed as the presenting sign in up to 10 percent of patients.[119] This is thought to occur after the rapid release of copper from hepatocytes with subsequent oxidative damage to the red blood cell membrane. Although hemolysis may often occur in association with acute hepatic failure, this process is also observed as a transient, self-limited manifestation that antedates the onset of hepatic or neurologic disease. For this reason it is imperative that all adolescents and young adults with Coombs-negative hemolytic anemia be screened for Wilson's disease. Cardiac dysrhythmias, pancreatitis, arthritis, osteomalacia, rhabdomyolysis, hypoparathyroidism, hypothyroidism, and secondary amenorrhea have all been reported in affected patients, most often in young adults and frequently with evidence of liver or neurologic disease.[120] Almost all these features are reversible with chelation therapy, supporting the concept that these signs and symptoms arise directly from copper accumulation rather than secondary to underlying liver disease.

Specific signs may also develop from asymptomatic deposition of copper in regions detectable by physical examination. Kayser-Fleischer rings are asymptomatic golden-brown discolorations arising from copper deposition in Descemet's membrane at the limbus of the cornea. These rings are present in the overwhelming majority of symptomatic patients and almost always occur in individuals with neurologic disease.[121] Kayser-Fleischer rings are often detectable on inspection of the cornea but may require slit-lamp ophthalmoscopic exam for detection in some cases. Although the presence of Kayser-Fleischer rings may be useful diagnostically this finding is not pathognomonic for Wilson's disease—such rings have been observed in a variety of hepatic diseases that result in excess liver copper, including biliary cirrhosis, intrahepatic cholestasis, and chronic active hepatitis (Plate 41-2).[122] Sunflower cataracts may also occur along with Kayser-Fleischer rings secondary to copper deposition in the anterior capsule of the lens (Plate 41-3). Azure lunulae occur secondary to copper deposition in the fingernails.

Diagnosis

Biochemical

The diagnosis of Wilson's disease is determined by the clinical signs and symptoms in correlation with laboratory studies indicating abnormal liver function and impaired copper homeostasis. Wilson's disease should be considered in any individual with an isolated elevation in serum transaminases, chronic active hepatitis of undetermined etiology, Kayser-Fleischer rings, or unexplained psychiatric or basal ganglia abnormalities. The absence or dysfunction of Wilson ATPase impairs the transfer of copper into the hepatocyte secretory pathway, resulting in a marked decrease in the serum ceruloplasmin concentration in most patients. Ceruloplasmin accounts for 95 percent of the copper present in the plasma; thus, the serum copper content will also be decreased in affected patients. Consistent with the release of copper into the serum from injured hepatocytes, many patients will have elevation in the non-ceruloplasmin bound or free serum copper, which is defined as the ceruloplasmin-bound copper (calculated as 0.05 μmol copper per mg of ceruloplasmin) minus the total serum copper concentration. Ceruloplasmin is an acute phase protein and in certain patients infection or inflammation, such as that observed in chronic active hepatitis, will result in elevation of the serum ceruloplasmin concentration to within the normal range. However, even in these circumstances the circulating ceruloplasmin will usually be devoid of oxidase activity, reflecting the absence of copper incorporation during biosynthesis.[123] Approximately 10 percent of obligate heterozygotes for Wilson's disease will have decreased serum ceruloplasmin but such individuals are healthy and do not present with any signs or symptoms of the disease.[124,125] Patients with aceruloplasminemia may also present with basal ganglia symptoms and absent serum ceruloplasmin but are distinguished by normal hepatic copper content and evidence of increased parenchymal iron accumulation.[126] Obligate heterozygotes for aceruloplasminemia are asymptomatic and show no evidence of iron overload. However, all such heterozygotes will have a 50 percent decrease in serum ceruloplasmin concentration; this will occasionally cause diagnostic confusion with Wilson's disease if hepatic or neurologic signs present secondarily to other causes. In such cases measurement of the serum ceruloplasmin concentration in the immediate family members will detect a 50 percent reduction in serum ceruloplasmin in an asymptomatic parent or sibling, confirming the inheritance of a mutant ceruloplasmin allele.

Despite these rare caveats noted above, the presence of Kayser-Fleischer rings on slit-lamp exam and a serum ceruloplasmin concentration below 20 mg/dl in an individual with neurologic or hepatic disease are sufficient in most cases to confirm the diagnosis of Wilson's disease. In all other diagnostic circumstances, where possible, a liver biopsy should be performed to quantitate the hepatic copper content, which will be increased even in presymptomatic individuals. The normal hepatic copper content varies from 20 to 60 μg/g dry weight, whereas untreated patients with Wilson's disease will have values greater than 250 μg/g dry weight and often in the 2500 μg range. Care must be taken to avoid contamination of the needle and biopsy container with copper, and an adequate size core (2 cm) must be obtained for quantitative analysis by atomic absorption spectrophotometry or a related methodology. The uneven distribution of hepatic copper accumulation observed in many patients must also be considered and will occasionally result in a false negative result because of a sampling error. Heterozygous carriers may have a small increase in hepatic copper content but, as noted previously, no evidence of hepatic dysfunction.[124,125,127] The finding of a normal hepatic copper concentration will exclude the diagnosis of Wilson's disease providing chelation therapy has not been initiated before biopsy. In contrast, an elevated copper concentration alone is not sufficient to make the diagnosis of Wilson's disease because this elevation may be observed in any patient with liver disease and impaired biliary excretion such as biliary cirrhosis or intrahepatic cholestasis. Although the normal urinary excretion of copper is less than 35 μg copper in 24 hours, in patients with Wilson's disease urinary copper concentration will often be elevated (more than 100 μg copper in 24 hours) as a result of the renal filtration of increased free copper in the plasma.[128] Indeed, in some circumstances such as fulminant hepatic failure, urinary copper excretion may exceed as much as 1000 μg copper 24 hours after the acute release of hepatic copper into the serum. Although inaccuracies in both urine collection and laboratory analysis can make this a difficult test, if performed with accuracy the quantitation of urinary copper excretion can be a useful addition to a cost effective approach to diagnosis and screening.

Molecular

An accurate diagnosis of Wilson's disease can be established in the majority of cases using history, physical exam, slit-lamp examination, serum transaminases, ceruloplasmin concentration, hepatic copper content, and urinary copper excretion. Unfortunately, the degree of allelic heterogeneity at the Wilson locus makes molecular genetic screening a difficult task in any given patient. The presence of more than 200 mutations, most compose single nucleotide changes or small deletions or insertions, has hampered the development of molecular screening methods that would encompass all possible mutations. Nevertheless, as pointed out previously, isolated populations will frequently contain private mutations; thus, directed analysis for these mutations in patients of defined ethnic origin can be an effective diagnostic approach in specific circumstances.[129] Furthermore, given the increasing ability of molecular screening methods to rapidly detect a multitude of mutations in any given sample, it is possible that broader approaches may become available for genetic diagnosis of Wilson's disease in any patient. In this regard, molecular screening of 26 selected patients, including 6 patients in which the diagnosis was uncertain using more traditional methods, demonstrated that 92 percent of disease alleles could be identified with such an approach.[130]

Screening

Wilson's disease is a treatable genetic disorder; a reliable test for newborn screening would be of enormous value for the early initiation of chelation therapy in asymptomatic individuals. Unfortunately, as discussed previously, the serum ceruloplasmin concentration is too low in the newborn period to be of value, and allelic heterogeneity at the Wilson locus makes molecular genetic screening impractical. Therefore screening is recommended only for siblings and first-degree relatives of affected patients. This process should follow the same diagnostic evaluation outlined previously, including history, physical examination, slit-lamp opthalmoscopy, serum trans-aminases, serum ceruloplasmin, and 24-hour urine copper excretion. If an unequivocal diagnosis is not possible from the results of this evaluation then a liver biopsy is warranted to quantitate hepatic copper content. Screening is especially important in the case of asymptomatic individuals because early treatment will be effective in preventing liver injury from hepatic copper overload. Screening evaluation will be normal in obligate heterozygotes, with the exception that 10 percent of such individuals will have a decreased serum ceruloplasmin in the absence of any other abnormalities.[124,125] When the proband mutation has been identified direct molecular analysis can offer a rapid and reliable approach to screening and diagnosis. Such a screening approach may prove especially useful in complicated cases in which chelation therapy has been initiated before a conclusive diagnosis.[130] In all circumstances reproductive and genetic counseling should be made available to any individual identified as a carrier for Wilson's disease.

Differential Diagnosis

Wilson's disease is the most common disorder resulting in hepatic copper overload. However, any process that impairs biliary excretion will eventually result in increased hepatocyte copper content. Consistent with this concept, elevated hepatic copper has been reported in biopsy samples from patients with several forms of cholestatic liver disease.[131] In most cases the associated signs and symptoms usually preclude diagnostic confusion with Wilson's disease. Furthermore, the serum ceruloplasmin is often elevated in cholestatic liver disease, reflecting a defect in the copper excretory pathway beyond the stage of copper incorporation into this protein (see Figure 41-3).[132] A severe form of rapidly progressive cirrhosis has been reported in young children in association with a marked elevation in the hepatic copper content. This disorder, which was originally described in children from rural, middle-class Hindu families, was termed *Indian childhood cirrhosis.*[133] Subsequent reports of identical findings in children from families without Hindu ancestry have made it apparent that this rare disease, now termed *idiopathic childhood cirrhosis,* occurs worldwide.[134] These children are diagnosed within the first 2 years of life with hepatosplenomegaly, elevation of serum aminotransferases, micronodular cirrhosis, and liver copper in excess of 2500 μg/g dry weight. Affected children have normal or elevated serum ceruloplasmin concentration, implying a specific defect in hepatic copper excretion late in the secretory pathway (see Figure 41-3). Consistent with the idea that these children have an intrinsic defect in hepatic copper excretion, early treatment with D-penicillamine is effective in many cases and hepatic transplantation is curative.[134,135] The normal serum ceruloplasmin and the early age of onset serve to distinguish children with idiopathic copper toxicosis from those with Wilson's disease.

Epidemiologic investigations of idiopathic childhood cirrhosis indicate that both genetic and environmental factors may play a role in this disease. Several studies have revealed an increase in the copper content of the diet of affected children whereas analysis of an affected pedigree in Austria indicates evidence of autosomal-recessive inheritance.[136] A similar form of copper-associated cirrhosis is observed as an autosomal-recessive disorder in inbred Bedlington terriers.[98,99] In these animals radioisotope studies reveal impaired biliary copper excretion but not holoceruloplasmin synthesis, suggesting a defect late in the pathway of biliary copper excretion. Genetic analysis has localized the affected gene to a region syntenic with human chromosome 2p13-16.[137,138]

Treatment

Chelation

The therapeutic goal in Wilson's disease is the restoration of hepatic copper homeostasis. This is accomplished by systemic chelation therapy with D-penicillamine, an amino acid derivative first detected in the urine of patients taking penicillin.[4] Oral D-penicillamine treatment will completely ameliorate the hepatic, neurologic, and psychiatric signs and symptoms in most patients with Wilson's disease and will prevent these features if initiated in asymptomatic individuals before the onset of any functional impairment.[139-142] D-penicillamine promotes urinary copper excretion in affected patients and prevents copper accumulation in presymptomatic individuals. Most patients will demonstrate a rapid and dramatic response within weeks of initiating treatment and will be asymptomatic within 4 months. Despite this response, the mechanism of action of D-penicillamine is not well established. The sulfhydryl moiety clearly binds copper and promotes urinary copper excretion, but long-term studies have suggested that the drug may serve more to detoxify rather than mobilize hepatic copper stores.[143] Consistent with this, life-long therapy is required and compliance is essential to prevent deterioration from copper mobilization within sequestered tissue sites. Acute deterioration may occur in patients with neurologic symptoms after the initiation of D-penicillamine.[144] Although this condition will require a decrease in the D-penicillamine dose, continued treatment is essential and most patients will demonstrate improvement within the first several months after these symptoms present. The mechanisms resulting in this deterioration in patients with neurologic disease are unknown but likely reflect acute changes in copper homeostasis within the brain and not a specific toxicity of D-penicillamine; similar problems have been observed in affected patients treated with other forms of chelation therapy.

Initially, D-penicillamine is given orally as 1 to 2 g daily divided in three or four doses, usually taken 30 minutes before eating. Excess hepatic copper will be mobilized in most patients within the first year of treatment; after symptoms have abated and a stable clinical course is achieved, the dose may be reduced to 1 g daily. Urinary copper excretion, initially markedly elevated with treatment, will return to normal during this period and may be useful as a therapeutic tool to follow compliance and initiate dosage changes.[140,141] Although D-penicillamine is a safe and effective treatment for patients with Wilson's disease, this drug is relatively toxic and a number of serious complications have been reported with both short- and long-term use.[120] Hypersensitivity reactions with fever, rash, and lymphadenopathy are initially common and may require concomitant use of steroids and dosage reduction if this therapy is to be continued.[145] Bone marrow suppression is less common but may result in life-threatening leukopenia or thrombocytopenia, prompting the immediate discontinuation of the drug and use of an alternative chelating agent. Long-term complications may include weakening and bruising of the skin and subcutaneous tissues, the development of autoimmune disease, and hepatotoxicity.[120] Urinalysis and blood counts should be followed closely in all patients treated with D-penicillamine and immediate discontinuation of the drug and substitution of a different chelating agent should be considered if complications persist. Despite these concerns, D-penicillamine has been used effectively for the treatment of Wilson's disease for more than 30 years and should be considered the first-line drug of choice for this disease.

Trientine (triethylene tetramine dihydrochloride) serves as a second choice for chelation therapy in those patients in whom D-penicillamine toxicity precludes further use of this drug.[146] One to two grams of oral trientine given daily in four divided doses will result in negative copper balance and improvement in clinical symptoms in most patients.[147] With the exception of the skin and subcutaneous tissue weakening, the side effects of D-penicillamine will resolve in patients switched to trientine therapy. Interestingly, the serum copper concentration wili rise during the period of trientine-induced cupriuresis, suggesting that the mechanism of action of this drug may differ from that of D-penicillamine.[148] Sideroblastic anemia is an apparent complication of long-term use of trientine in patients with Wilson's disease.[147] Although trientine has been shown to be an effective and safe chelating agent the long-term effectiveness of this drug remains less well studied, and current recommendations confine trientine use to patients in whom D-penicillamine is contraindicated. Ammonium tetrathiomolybdenate given orally as 100 mg per day in two divided doses has also been shown to be effective in lowering hepatic copper content in patients with Wilson's disease in whom D-penicillamine was poorly tolerated.[149] This drug works in part by chelating dietary copper in the gastrointestinal lumen and preventing absorption. Although molybdenate therapy may be needed in circumstances in which other drugs are not tolerated, bone marrow suppression has been reported in some patients and further studies are warranted before routine use of this agent is recommended for the treatment of Wilson's disease.[150]

Gastrointestinal absorption represents the only route for copper acquisition under normal circumstances. Unfortunately, the ubiquitous presence of copper in water and most foods makes dietary restriction an impractical approach for the treatment of Wilson's disease. Nevertheless it is not unreasonable to suggest that affected individuals avoid foods rich in copper such as chocolate, nuts, liver, and shellfish. Zinc inhibits copper absorption and if taken in large enough doses will result in copper deficiency in normal individuals.[151] Considerable clinical data now indicate that 50 to 75 mg of oral zinc sulfate in two or three divided doses between meals will effectively maintain neutral or negative copper balance in patients with Wilson's disease.[152,153] The effect of zinc is slow compared with chelation therapy and this drug should not be used for initial treatment of symptomatic patients. The role of zinc as the sole therapeutic agent in presymptomatic patients or for maintenance therapy in individuals previously stabilized with chelation therapy remains controversial.[154] Although there appears to be no effective synergy between zinc and chelation therapy some investigators do advocate the use of both drugs in the maintenance phase of treatment in symptomatic patients. Zinc is a relatively safe drug and the only short-term side effects are headache and mild gastrointestinal disturbance.[151] The long-term consequences of zinc therapy remain unknown and caution should be taken using this drug until such information is available. Although it has been suggested that zinc therapy may serve as a useful substitute in pregnant patients with Wilson's disease, D-penicillamine has been safely and successfully used in such circumstances for many years without convincing reports of an increased incidence of congenital malformations or other complications from this drug.[155]

Hepatic Transplantation

In patients with progressive liver failure unresponsive to chelation therapy or in the circumstance of acute liver failure from fulminant hepatitis, orthotoptic liver transplantation is the treatment of choice. The mortality of fulminant hepatitis in Wilson's disease is 100 percent without transplantation. It is estimated that Wilson's disease accounts for 5 percent of all hepatic transplants at major medical centers.[156,157] Indeed, the diagnosis of Wilson's disease must be considered in any child or young adult with fulminant hepatitis after hepatitis A and B and obvious toxin exposure have been ruled out as etiologies. Occasionally patients with Wilson's disease and fulminant hepatitis may present as late as the fourth or fifth decade of life; therefore, in all circumstances the transplant physician must be alert for a family history of cirrhosis or neuropsychiatric disease. In Wilson's disease patients with fulminant hepatitis the massive release of copper into the circulation increases the likelihood of renal failure secondary to copper-induced nephrotoxicity and in some cases plasmapheresis will be warranted to reduce the free copper content of the serum before transplantation. For unclear reasons the incidence of fulminant hepatitis in Wilson's disease is greater in females.[156,157] Although all patients will have increased hepatic copper, the degree of copper overload does not correlate with the occurrence or outcome of fulminant hepatitis.[156] Hepatic transplantation will normalize copper homeostasis within 6 months in most patients and results in sustained improvement in hepatic, neurologic, and psychiatric symptoms.[156-159] The 1-year survival rate in transplanted patients is 70 percent to 80 percent.[155,156] This outcome likely reflects the fact that hepatic transplantation will cure the basic defect in Wilson's disease by providing hepatocytes with a normal Wilson ATPase. Given the favorable outcome in most patients, living, related donor transplantation including from potential heterozygote family members has also been used and shown to be effective in specific patients.[160] Despite these outcomes the mortality from liver transplantation remains high and this treatment should only be considered under life-saving circumstances. In particular, caution must be observed in considering hepatic transplantation in patients with severe neuropsychiatric symptoms unresponsive to chelation therapy in whom the restoration of copper homeostasis would not be expected to reverse any neurodegeneration that has already occurred as a result of long-term copper toxicity.

ACKNOWLEDGMENTS

Work from the author's laboratory reported in this chapter was supported in part by National Institute of Health grants DK44464, DK61763, HL41536, and HD39952. The author is a recipient of a Burroughs-Welcome Scholar Award in Experimental Therapeutics.

References

1. Wilson SAK: Progressive lenticular degeneration: a familial nervous disease associated with cirrhosis of the liver. Brain 34:295, 1912.
2. Cummings JN: The copper and iron content of the liver and brain in the normal and hepatolenticular degeneration. Brain 71:410, 1948.
3. Scheinberg IH, Gitlin D: Deficiency of ceruloplasmin in patients with hepatolenticular degeneration. Science 116:484, 1952.
4. Walshe JM: Penicillamine, a new oral therapy for Wilson's disease. Am J Med 21:487, 1956.
5. Bearn A: A genetical analysis of 30 families with Wilson disease. Ann Hum Genet 24:33, 1960.
6. Frydman M, Bonne-Tamir B, Farrer LA, et al: Assignment of the gene for Wilson disease to chromosome 13: linkage to the esterase D locus. Proc Natl Acad Sci U S A 82:1819, 1985.
7. Bull PC, Thomas GR, Rommens JM, et al: The Wilson disease gene is a putative copper transporting P-type ATPase similar to the Menkes gene. Nat Genet 5:327, 1993.
8. Tanzi RE, Petrukhin K, Chernov I, et al: The Wilson disease gene is a copper transporting ATPase with homology to the Menkes disease gene. Nat Genet 5:344, 1993.
9. Yamaguchi Y, Heiny ME, Gitlin JD: Isolation and characterization of a human liver cDNA as a candidate gene for Wilson disease. Biochem Biophys Res Commun 197:271, 1993.
10. Culotta VC, Gitlin JD: Disorders of copper transport. In Scriver CR, Beaudet AL, Sly WS, Valle D, ed: The Molecular and Metabolic Basis of Inherited Disease. New York, McGraw-Hill, 2001:3105.
11. Hamza I, Gitlin JD: Copper metabolism and the liver. In Arias IM, Boyer JL, Chisari FV, et al, ed: The Liver: Biology and Pathology. Philadelphia, Lippincott Williams & Wilkins, 2001:331.
12. Harris ZL, Gitlin JD: Genetic and molecular basis for copper toxicity. Am J Clin Nutr 63:836S, 1996.
13. Harris ZL, Takahashi Y, Miyajima H, et al: Aceruloplasminemia: molecular characterization of this disorder of iron metabolism. Proc Natl Acad Sci U S A 92:2539, 1995.
14. Meyer LA, Durley AP, Prohaska JR, et al: Copper transport and metabolism are normal in aceruloplasminemic mice. J Biol Chem 276:36857, 2001.
15. Zhou B, Gitschier J: hCTR1: A human gene for copper uptake identified by complementation in yeast. Proc Natl Acad Sci U S A 94:7481, 1997.
16. Kuo YM, Zhou B, Cosco D, et al: The copper transporter CTR1 provides an essential function in mammalian embryonic development. Proc Natl Acad Sci U S A 98:6836, 2001.
17. Lee J, Prohaska JR, Thiele DJ: Essential role of mammalian copper transporter Ctr1 in copper homeostasis and embryonic development. Proc Natl Acad Sci U S A 98:6842, 2001.
18. Lee J, Pena MM, Nose Y, et al: Biochemical characterization of the human copper transporter Ctr1. J Biol Chem 277:4380, 2002.
19. Gollan JL, Gollan TJ: Wilson disease in 1998: genetic, diagnostic and therapeutic aspects. J Hepatol 28:28, 1998.
20. Palmiter RD: The elusive function of metallothioneins. Proc Natl Acad Sci U S A 95:8428, 1998.

21. Kelley EJ, Palmiter RJ: A murine model of menkus disease reveals a physiological function of metallothionein. Nat Genet 13:219, 1996.
22. Hung IH, Suzuki M, Yamaguchi Y, et al: Biochemical characterization of the Wilson disease protein and functional expression in the yeast Saccharomyces cerevisiae. J Biol Chem 272:21461, 1997.
23. Schaefer M, Hopkins R, Failla M, et al: Hepatocyte-specific localization and copper-dependent trafficking of the Wilson's disease protein in the liver. Am J Physiol 276:G639, 1999.
24. Schaefer M, Roelofsen H, Wolters H, et al: Localization of the Wilson's disease protein in human liver. Gastroenterology 117:1380, 1995.
25. Hellman NE, Kono S, Miyajima H, et al: Biochemical analysis of a missense mutation in aceruloplasminemia. J Biol Chem 277:1375, 2002.
26. Gitlin JD, Schroeder JJ, Lee-Ambrose LM, et al: Mechanisms of caeruloplasmin biosynthesis in normal and copper-deficient rats. Biochem J 282:835, 1992.
27. Sato M, Gitlin JD: Mechanisms of copper incorporation during the biosynthesis of human ceruloplasmin. J Biol Chem 266:5128, 1991.
28. Gitlin D, Biasucci A: Development of gamma G, gamma A, gamma M, beta 1C, beta 1A, Cl esterase inhibitor, ceruloplasmin, transferrin, hemopexin, haptoglobin, fibrinogen, plasminogen, alpha 1-antitrypsin, orosomucoid, beta-lipoprotein, alpha 2 macroglobulin and prealbumin in the human conceptus. J Clin Invest 48:1433, 1969.
29. Solioz M, Vulpe C: CPx-type ATPases: a class of P-type ATPases that pump heavy metals. Trends Biochem Sci 21:237, 1996.
30. Moller JV, Juul B, LeMaire M: Structural organization, ion transport, and energy transduction of P-type ATPases. Biochim Biophys Acta 1286:1, 1996.
31. Voskoboinik I, Mar J, Strausak D, et al: The regulation of catalytic activity of the Menkes copper-translocating P-type ATPase. Role of high affinity copper-binding sites. J Biol Chem 276:28620, 2001.
32. Tsivkovskii R, Eisses JF, Kaplan JH, et al: Functional properties of the copper-transporting ATPase ATP7B (the Wilson's disease protein) expressed in insect cells. J Biol Chem 277:976, 2002.
33. Lutsenko S, Kaplan JH: Organization of P-type ATPases—significance of structural diversity. Biochemistry 34:15607, 1995.
34. Payne A, Gitlin JD: Functional expression of the Menkes disease protein reveals common biochemical mechanisms among the copper-transporting P-type ATPases. J Biol Chem 273:3765, 1998.
35. Voskoboinik I, Strausak D, Greenough M, et al: Functional analysis of the N-terminal CXXC metal-binding motifs in the human Menkes copper-transporting P-type ATPase expressed in cultured mammalian cells J Biol Chem 274:22008, 1999.
36. Forbes J, Hsi G, Cox D: Role of the copper-binding domain in the copper transporter function of ATP7B, the P-type ATPase defective in Wilson disease. J Biol Chem 274:12408, 1999.
37. Larin D, Mekios C, Das K, et al: Characterization of the interaction between the Wilson and Menkes disease proteins and the cytoplasmic copper chaperone, HAH1p. J Biol Chem 274:28497, 1999.
38. Hamza I, Schaefer M, Klomp LW, et al: Interaction of the copper chaperone HAH1 with the Wilson disease protein is essential for copper homeostasis. Proc Natl Acad Sci U S A 96:13363, 1999.
39. Gitschier J, Moffat B, Reilly D, et al: Solution structure of the fourth metal-binding domain from the Menkes copper-transporting ATPase. Nat Struct Biol 5:47, 1998.
40. Tsivkovskii R, MacArthur BC, Lutsenko S: The Lys1010-Lys1325 fragment of the Wilson's disease protein binds nucleotides and interacts with the N-terminal domain of this protein in a copper-dependent manner. J Biol Chem 19:2234, 2001.
41. Payne AS, Kelly EJ, Gitlin JD: Functional expression of the Wilson disease protein reveals mislocalization and impaired copper-dependent trafficking of the common H1069Q mutation. Proc Natl Acad Sci U S A 95:10854, 1998.
42. Borjigin J, Payne AS, Deng J, et al: A novel pineal night-specific ATPase encoded by the Wilson disease gene. J Neurosci 19:1018, 1999.
43. Forbes JR, Cox DW: Functional characterization of missense mutations in ATP7B: Wilson disease mutation or normal variant? Am J Hum Genet 63:1663, 1998.
44. Francis M, Jones E, Levy E, et al: Identification of a di-leucine motif within the C terminus domain of the Menkes disease protein that mediates endocytosis from the plasma membrane. J Cell Sci 112:1721, 1999.
45. Petris MJ, Mercer JF: The Menkes protein (ATP7A; MNK) cycles via the plasma membrane both in basal and elevated extracellular copper using a C-terminal di-leucine endocytic signal. Hum Mol Genet 8:2107, 1999.
46. Eide D, Bridgham JT, Zhao Z, et al: The vacuolar H^+ ATPase of *Saccharomyces cerevisiae* is required for efficient copper detoxification, mitochondrial function and iron metabolism. Mol Genet 241:447, 1993.
47. Gaxiola RA, Yuan DS, Klausner RD, et al: The yeast CLC chloride channel functions in cation homeostasis. Proc Natl Acad Sci U S A 95:4046, 1998.
48. Schwappach B, Strobrawa S, Hechenberger M, et al: Golgi localization and functionally important domains in the NH_2 and COOH terminus of the yeast CLC putative chloride channel Geflp. J Biol Chem 273:15110, 1998.
49. Davis-Kaplan SR, Askwith CC, Bengtzen AC, et al: Chloride is an allosteric effector of copper assembly for the yeast multicopper oxidase fet3p: an unexpected role for intracellular chloride channels. Proc Natl Acad Sci U S A 95:13641, 1998.
50. Roelofsen H, Wolters H, Van Luyn MJ, et al: Copper-induced apical trafficking of ATP7B in polarized hepatoma cells provides a mechanism of biliary copper excretion. Gastroenterology 119:782, 2000.
51. Rae T, Schmidt P, Pufahl R, et al: Undetectable intracellular free copper: the requirement of a copper chaperone for superoxide dismutase. Science 284:805, 1999.
52. O'Halloran TV, Culotta VC: Metallochaperones: an intracellular shuttle service for metal ions. J Biol Chem 275:25057, 2000.
53. Rosenzweig AC: Copper delivery by metallochaperone proteins. Acc Chem Res 34:119, 2001.
54. Huffman DL, O'Halloran TV: Function, structure, and mechanism of intracellular copper trafficking proteins. Annu Rev Biochem 10:677, 2001.
55. Papadopoulou LC, Sue CM, Davidson MM, et al: Fatal infantile cardioencephalomyopathy with cox deficiency and mutations in sco2, a cox assembly gene. Nat Genet 23:333, 1999.
56. Jaksch M, Ogilvie J, Yao J, et al: Mutations in sco2 are associated with a distinct form of hypertrophic cardiomyopathy and cytochrome c oxidase deficiency. Hum Mol Genet 9:795, 2000.
57. Valnot I, Osmond S, Gigarel N, et al: Mutations of the SCO1 gene in mitochondrial cytochrome c oxidase deficiency with neonatal-onset hepatic failure and encephalopathy. Am J Hum Genet 67:1104, 2000.
58. Culotta VC, Klomp LWJ, Strain J, et al: The copper chaperone for superoxide dismutase. J Biol Chem 272:23469, 1997.
59. Wong PC, Waggoner D, Subramaniam JR, et al: Copper chaperone for superoxide dismutase is essential to activate mammalian Cu/Zn superoxide dismutase. Proc Natl Acad Sci U S A 97:2886, 2000.
60. Hamza I, Faisst A, Prohaska J, et al: The metallochaperone Atox1 plays a critical role in perinatal copper homeostasis. Proc Natl Acad Sci U S A 5:6848, 2001.
61. Wernimont AK, Huffman DL, Lamb AL, et al: Structural basis for copper transfer by the metallochaperone for Menkes/Wilson disease proteins. Nat Struct Biol 7:766, 2000.
62. Lamb AL, Torres AS, O'Halloran TV, et al: Heterodimeric structure of superoxide dismutase in complex with its metallochaperone. Nat Struct Biol 8:733, 2001.
63. Cuthbert JA: Wilson disease: update on a systemic disorder with protean manifestations. Gastroenterol Clin North Am 27:655, 1998.
64. Schilsky ML: Wilson disease: genetic basis of copper toxicity and natural history. Semin Liver Dis 16:83, 1996.
65. Curtis D, Durkie M, Balac P, et al: A study of Wilson disease mutations in Britain. Hum Mutat 14:304, 1999.
66. Haas R, Gutierrez-Rivero B, Knoche J, et al: Mutation analysis in patients with Wilson disease: identification of 4 novel mutations. Hum Mutat 14:88, 1999.
67. Kalinsky H, Funes A, Zeldin A, et al: Novel ATP7B mutations causing Wilson disease in several Israeli ethnic groups. Hum Mutat 11:145, 1998.
68. Kim EK, Yoo OJ, Song KY, et al: Identification of three novel mutations and a high frequency of the Arg778Leu mutation in Korean patients with Wilson disease. Hum Mutat 11:275, 1998.

69. Petrukhin K, Lutsenko S, Chernov L, et al: Characterization of the Wilson disease gene encoding a P-type copper transporting ATPase: genomic organization, alternative splicing, and structure/function predicting. Hum Mol Genet 3:1647, 1994.
70. Loudianos G, Dessi V, Angius A, et al: Wilson disease mutations associated with uncommon haplotypes in Mediterranean patients. Hum Genet 98:640, 1996.
71. Loudianos G, Dessi V, Lovicu M, et al: Haplotype and mutation analysis in Greek patients with Wilson disease. Eur J Hum Genet 6:487, 1998.
72. Loudianos G, Dessi V, Lovicu M, et al: Mutation analysis in patients of Mediterranean descent with Wilson disease: identification of 19 novel mutations. J Med Genet 36:833, 1999.
73. Nanji MS, Nguyen VT, Kawasoe JH, et al: Haplotype and mutation analysis in Japanese patients with Wilson disease. Am J Hum Genet 60:1423, 1997.
74. Shah AB, Chernov I, Zhang HT, et al: Identification and analysis of mutations in the Wilson disease gene (ATP7B): population frequencies, genotype-phenotype correlation, and functional analyses. Am J Hum Genet 61:317, 1997.
75. Shimizu N, Kawase C, Nakazono H, et al: A novel RNA splicing mutation in Japanese patients with Wilson disease. Biochem Biophys Res Commun 217:16, 1995.
76. Thomas GR, Forbes JR, Roberts EA, et al: The Wilson disease gene: spectrum of mutations and their consequences. Nat Genet 9:210, 1995.
77. Tsai CH, Tsai FJ, Wu JY, et al: Mutation analysis of Wilson disease in Taiwan and description of six new mutations. Hum Mutat 12:370, 1998.
78. Waldenstrom E, Lagerkvist A, Dahlman T, et al: Efficient detection of mutations in Wilson disease by manifold sequencing. Genomics 37:303, 1996.
79. Loudianos G, Lovicu M, Solinas P, et al: Delineation of the spectrum of Wilson disease mutations in the Greek population and the identification of six novel mutations. Genet Test 4:399, 2000.
80. Kusuda Y, Hamaguchi K, Mori T, et al: Novel mutations of the ATP7B gene in Japanese patients with Wilson disease. J Hum Genet 45:86, 2000.
81. Loudianos G, Dessi V, Lovicu M, et al: Molecular characterization of Wilson disease in the Sardinian population—evidence of a founder effect. Hum Mutat 14:294, 1999.
82. Garcia-Villarreal L, Daniels S, Shaw SH, et al: High prevalence of the very rare Wilson disease gene mutation Leu708Pro in the island of Gran Canaria (Canary Islands, Spain): a genetic and clinical study. Hepatology 32:1329, 2000.
83. Riordan SM, Williams R: The Wilson's disease gene and phenotypic diversity. J Hepatol 34:165, 2001.
84. Forbes JR, Cox DW: Copper-dependent trafficking of Wilson disease mutant ATP7B proteins. Human Mol Genet 13:1927, 2000.
85. Huffman DL, O'Halloran TV: Energetics of copper trafficking between the atx1 metallochaperone and the intracellular copper-transporter, Ccc2. J Biol Chem 275:18611, 2000.
86. Sokol RJ: Antioxidant defenses in metal-induced liver damage. Semin Liver Dis 16:39, 1996.
87. Strand S, Hofmann WJ, Grambihler A, et al: Hepatic failure and liver cell damage in acute Wilson's disease involve CD95 (APO-1/Fas) mediated apoptosis. Nat Med 4:588, 1998.
88. Pyeritz RE: Genetic heterogeneity in Wilson disease: lessons from rare alleles. Ann Intern Med 127:70, 1997.
89. Wu J, Forbes JR, Chen HS, et al: The LEC rat has a deletion in the copper transporting ATPase gene homologous to the Wilson disease gene. Nat Genet 7:541, 1994.
90. Li Y, Togahsi Y, Sato S, et al: Spontaneous hepatic copper accumulation in Long Evans Cinnamon rats with hereditary hepatitis. A model of Wilson's disease. J Clin Invest 87:1858, 1991.
91. Sone K, Maeda M, Wakabayashi K, et al: Inhibition of hereditary hepatitis and liver tumor development in Long-Evans cinnamon rats by the copper-chelating agent trientine dihydrochloride. Hepatology 23:764, 1996.
92. Terada K, Aiba N, Yang X, et al: Biliary excretion of copper in LEC rat after introduction of copper transporting P-type ATPase, ATP7B. FEBS Lett 448:53, 1999.
93. Kato J, Kobune M, Kohgo Y, et al: Hepatic iron deprivation prevents spontaneous development of fulminant hepatitis and liver cancer in Long Evans Cinnamon rats. J Clin Invest 98:923, 1996.
94. Theophanous MB, Cox DW, Mercer JF: The toxic milk mouse is a murine model of Wilson disease. Hum Mol Genet 5:1619, 1996.
95. Rauch H: The toxic milk, a new mutation affecting copper metabolism in the mouse. J Hered 74:141, 1983.
96. Coronado V, Nanji M, Cox DW: The Jackson toxic milk mouse as a model for copper loading. Mamm Genome 12:793, 2001.
97. Buiakova OI, Xu J, Lutsenko S, et al: Null mutation of the murine ATP7B (Wilson disease) gene results in intracellular copper accumulation and late-onset hepatic nodular transformation. Hum Mol Genet 8:1665, 1999.
98. Hultgren BD, Stevens JB, Hardy RM: Inherited, chronic progressive hepatic degeneration in Bedlington terriers with increased liver copper concentrations: clinical and pathologic observations and comparison with other copper-associated liver diseases. Am J Vet Res 47:365, 1986.
99. Stockman MJ: Copper toxicosis in the Bedlington terrier. Vet Rec 24:123, 1988.
100. Haywood S, Muller T, Muller W, et al: Copper-associated liver disease in North Ronaldsay sheep: a possible animal model for non-Wilsonian hepatic copper toxicosis on infancy and childhood. J Pathol 195:264, 2001.
101. Gow PJ, Smallwood RA, Angus PW, et al: Diagnosis of Wilson's disease: an experience over three decades. Gut 46:415, 2000.
102. Walshe JM: Wilson's disease presenting with features of hepatic dysfunction: a clinical analysis of eighty-seven patients. QJM 70:253, 1989.
103. Cuthbert JA: Wilson's disease: a new gene and an animal model for an old disease. J Invest Med 43:323, 1995.
104. Schilsky ML, Scheinberg IH, Sternlieb I: Prognosis of Wilsonian chronic active hepatitis. Gastroenterology 100:762, 1991.
105. McCullough AJ, Fleming R, Thistle JL, et al: Diagnosis of Wilson's disease presenting as fulminant hepatic failure. Gastroenterology 84:161, 1983.
106. Davies SE, Williams R, Portmann B: Hepatic morphology and histochemistry of Wilson's disease presenting as fulminant hepatic failure: a study of 11 cases. Histopathology 15:385, 1989.
107. Sternlieb I: Perspectives on Wilson's disease. Hepatology 12:1234, 1990.
108. Polio J, Enriquez RE, Chow A, et al: Hepatocellular carcinoma in Wilson's disease: case report and review of the literature. J Clin Gastroenterol 11:220, 1989.
109. Oder W, Grimm G, Kollegger H, et al: Neurologic and neuropsychiatric spectrum of Wilson's disease: a prospective study of 45 cases. J Neurol 238:281, 1991.
110. Cartwright GE: Diagnosis of treatable Wilson's disease. N Engl J Med 298:1347, 1978.
111. Takahashi W, Yoshii F, Shinohara Y: Reversible magnetic resonance imaging lesions in Wilson's disease: clinical-anatomical correlation. J Neuroimag 6:246, 1996.
112. Alanen A, Komu M, Penttinen M, et al: Magnetic resonance imaging and proton MR spectroscopy in Wilson's disease. Br J Radiol 72:749, 1999.
113. Aisen AM, Martel W, Gabrielsen TO, et al: Wilson's disease of the brain: MR imaging. Radiology 157:137, 1990.
114. Dening TR, Berrios GE: Wilson's disease: Psychiatric symptoms in 195 cases. Arch Gen Psychiatry 46:1126, 1989.
115. Stremmel W, Meyerrose K-W, Niederau C, et al: Wilson's disease: clinical presentation, treatment and survival. Ann Intern Med 115:720, 1991.
116. Dening TR, Berrios GE: Wilson disease: a prospective study of psychopathology in 31 cases. Br J Psychiatry 155:206, 1989.
117. Dening TR, Berrios GE: Wilson's disease: a longitudinal study of psychiatric symptoms. Biol Psychiatry 28:255, 1990.
118. Elias LJ, Hayslett JP, Spargo BH, et al: Wilson's disease with reversible renal tubular dysfunction. Ann Intern Med 75:427, 1971.
119. McIntyre N, Clink HM, Levi AJ, et al: Hemolytic anemia in Wilson's disease. N Engl J Med 276:439, 1967.
120. Brewer GJ, Yuzbasiyan-Gurkan V: Wilson's disease. Medicine 71:139, 1992.
121. Lau JYN, Lai CL, Wu PC, et al: Wilson's disease: 35 years experience. QJM 75:597, 1990.
122. Kaplinsky C, Sternlieb I, Javitt N, et al: Familial cholestatic cirrhosis associated with Kayser-Fleischer rings. Pediatrics 65:782, 1980.
123. Schilsky ML, Sternlieb I: Overcoming obstacles to the diagnosis of Wilson's disease. Gastroenterology 113:350, 1997.

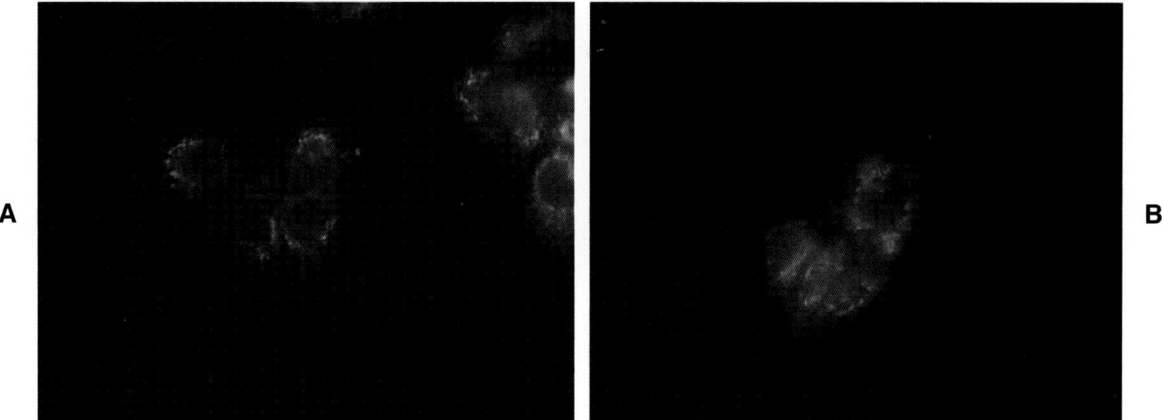

Plate 41-1 Intracellular localization of the Wilson's disease copper-transporting ATPase (ATP7B). Human hepatoblastoma-derived HepG2 cells were incubated with 40 μM bathocuproine disulfonate **(A)** or 10 μM copper **(B)**, and the Wilson ATPase was localized by immunofluorescence. In decreased intracellular copper **(A)** the ATPase is localized entirely to the trans-Golgi network, whereas in copper **(B)** some of the ATPase moving from this compartment is also localized to cytoplasmic vesicles. *ATPase,* Adenosine triphosphatase.

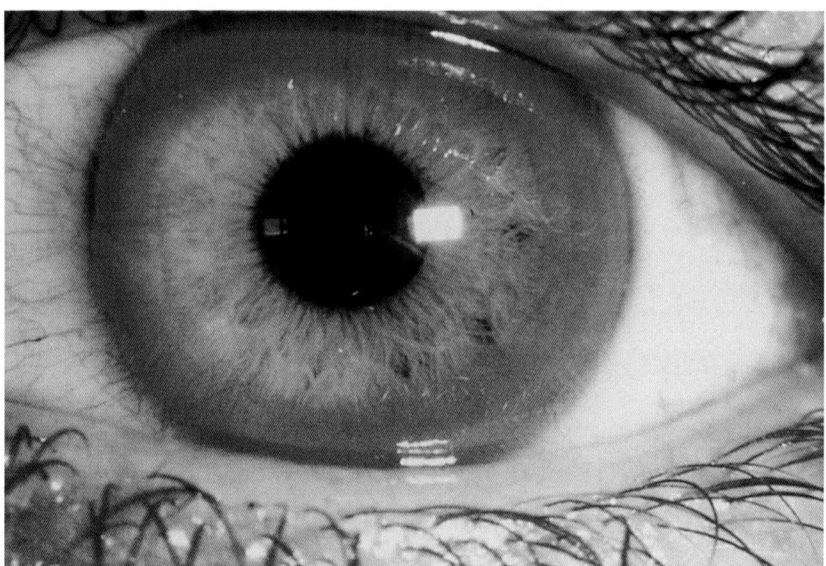

Plate 41-2 Kayser-Fleischer ring. (Courtesy of Professor Dame S. Sherlock, London.)

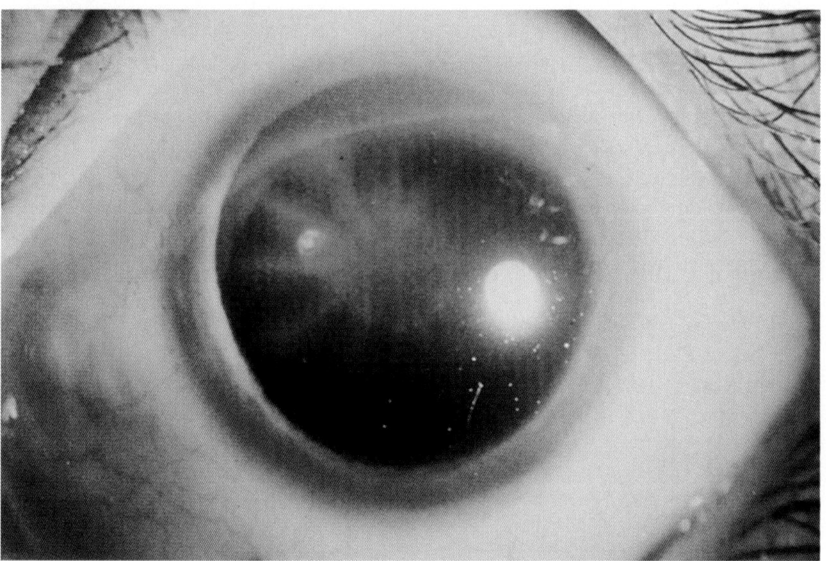

Plate 41-3 Sunflower cataract. (Courtesy of I. Sternlieb, New York.)

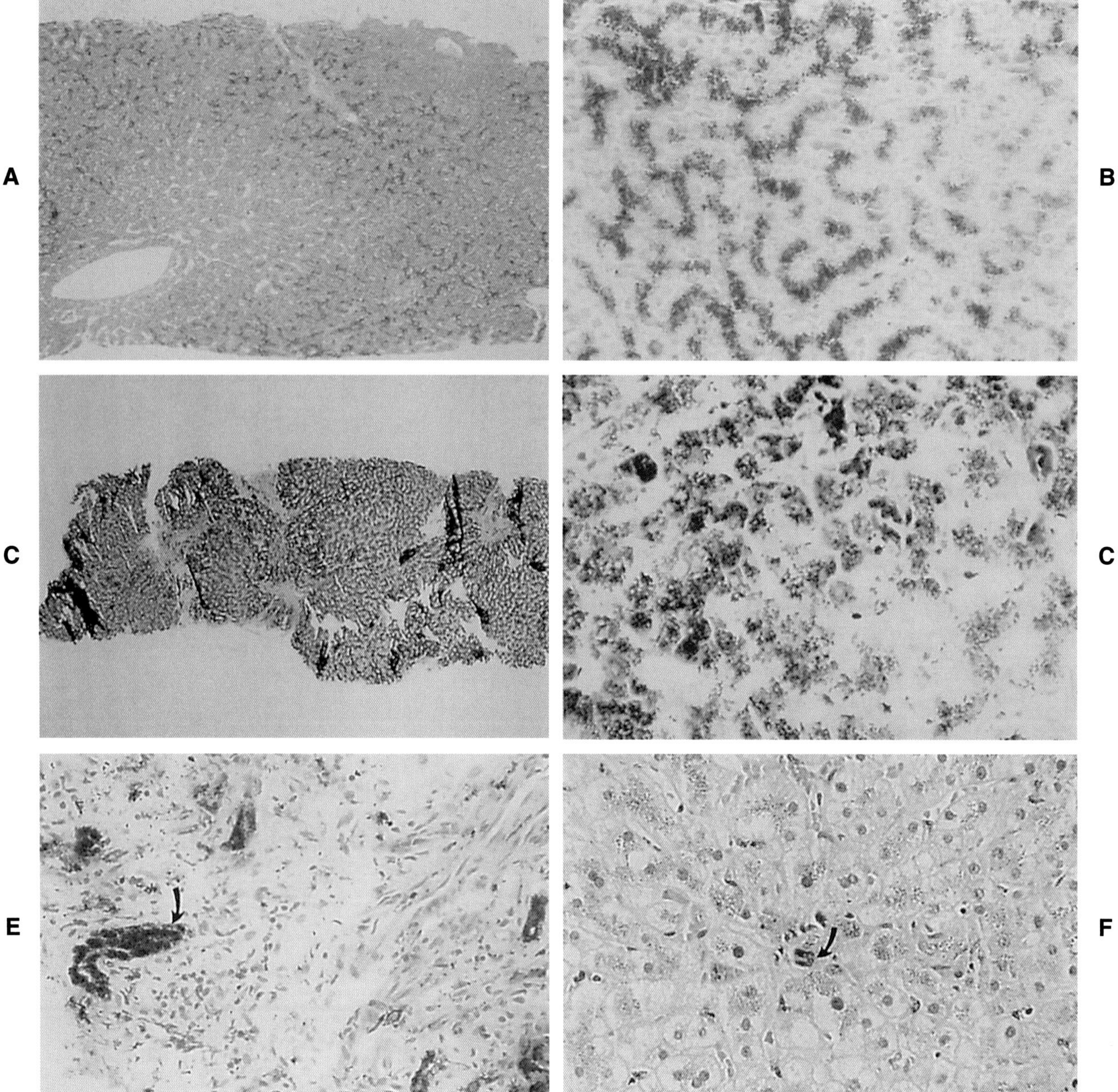

Plate 42-1 Hepatopathology of hereditary hemochromatosis. **A,** This liver biopsy specimen is from a young patient with early HH. Iron deposition is in a periportal distribution. (Perls' Prussian blue stain; ×100.) **B,** Higher power (×400) demonstrates hepatocellular iron deposition, with few or no iron deposits in Kupffer cells. **C,** Liver biopsy specimen from an older patient with late HH, complicated by cirrhosis. The periportal-to-central gradient is barely discerned. (Perls' Prussian blue stain; ×100.) **D,** At higher power (×400) iron deposits are still predominantly hepatocellular, but there is some Kupffer cell iron. **E,** Iron deposits in bile duct cells *(arrow)* are seen within a fibrous band in a patient with cirrhosis resulting from HH. (Perls' Prussian blue stain; ×300.) **F,** Sideronecrosis is identified as a necrotic hepatocyte (arrow in an area of heavy iron loading). (Hematoxylin and eosin; ×300). *HH,* Hereditary hemochromatosis.

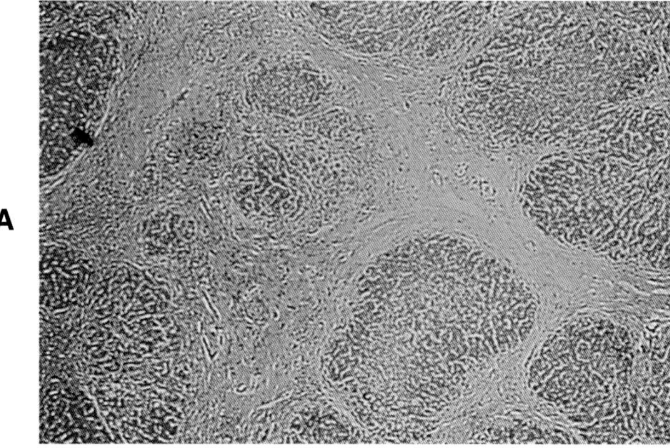

A

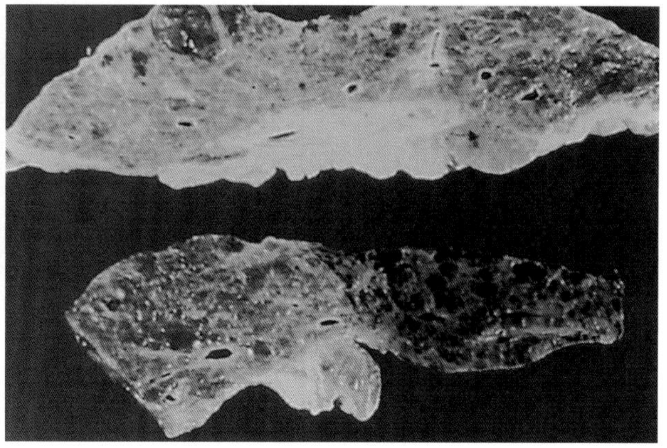

B

Plate 42-2 Cirrhosis and hepatocellular cancer in HH. **A,** Micronodular cirrhosis is seen in this explant liver from a patient with HH who received a successful orthotopic liver transplant. (Masson trichrome stain; ×50.) **B,** This gross specimen is from an autopsy of a patient who died from complications of HH. In the top section is a unicentric focus of hepatocellular carcinoma with two satellite lesions in the setting of micronodular cirrhosis. The lower section has been dipped in potassium ferrocyanide (Perls' Prussian blue) to stain storage ferric iron (Fe^{3+}) blue. *HH,* Hereditary hemochromatosis.

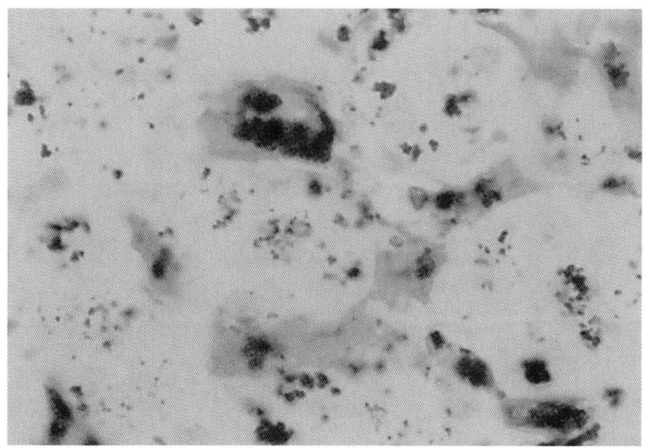

Plate 42-3 Parenteral iron overload. This liver biopsy is from a 22-year-old male with sickle cell disease who has received multiple red blood cell transfusions. Iron deposition is panlobular and predominantly in Kupffer cells. (Perls' Prussian blue stain; ×400.)

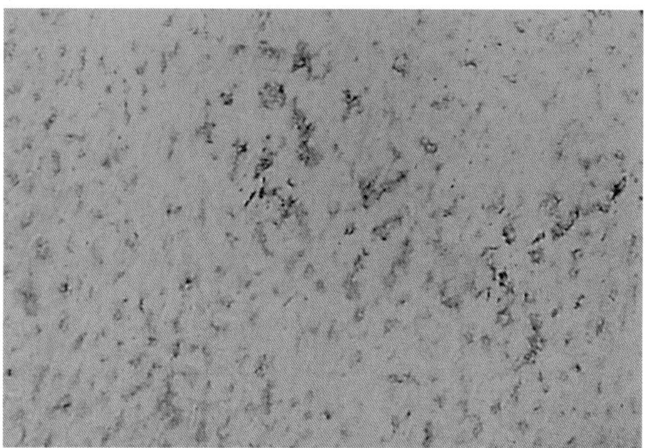

Plate 42-4 Secondary iron overload. This liver biopsy specimen is from a 45-year-old male with alcoholic liver disease and secondary iron overload. Iron deposition is panlobular with a slight periportal-to-central gradient with iron in both hepatocytes and Kupffer cells. (Perls' Prussian blue stain; ×200.)

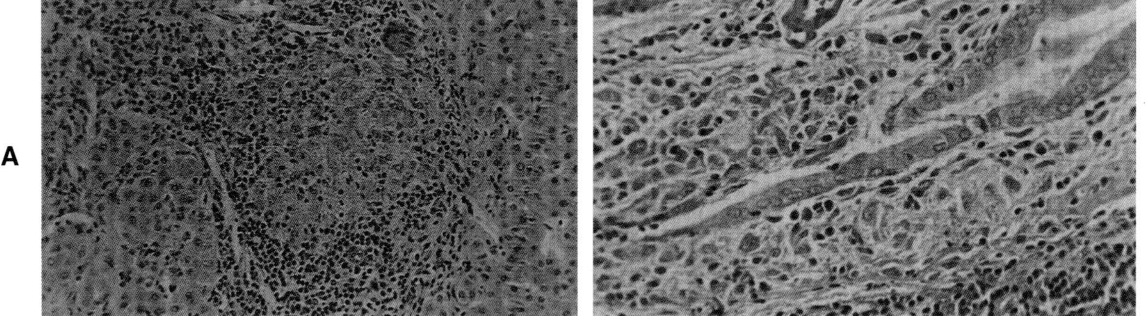

Plate 43-1 **A,** Portal granulomas in primary biliary cirrhosis. (Hematoxylin and eosin; ×55.) **B,** Granulomatous destruction of interlobular bile duct in primary biliary cirrhosis. (Hematoxylin and eosin; ×150.)

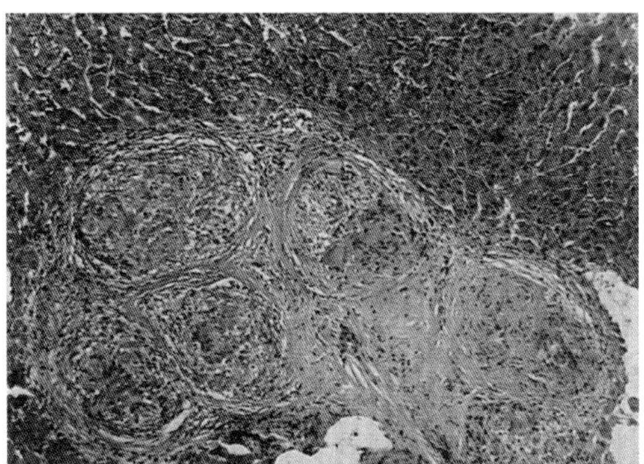

Plate 43-2 Compact non-necrotizing granuloma in sarcoidosis. Transection by fibrous bands is seen in larger granulomas. (Hematoxylin and eosin; ×55.)

124. Sternlieb I, Scheinberg IH: Prevention of Wilson's disease in asymptomatic patients. N Engl J Med 278:352, 1968.
125. Gibbs K, Walshe JM: A study of caeruloplasmin concentrations found in 75 patients with Wilson's disease, their kinships and various control groups. QJM 48:447, 1979.
126. Morita H, Ikeda S, Yamamoto K, et al: Hereditary ceruloplasmin deficiency with hemosiderosis: a clinicopathologic study of a Japanese family. Ann Neurol 37:646, 1995.
127. Levi AJ: Presymptomatic Wilson's disease. Lancet 2:575, 1967.
128. Cartwright GE, Hodges RE, Gubler CJ, et al: Studies on copper metabolism. XIII. Hepatolenticular degeneration. J Clin Invest 33:1487, 1954.
129. Maier-Dobersberger T, Ferenci P, Polli C, et al: Detection of the His1069Gln mutation in Wilson disease by rapid polymerase chain reaction. Ann Intern Med 127:21, 1997.
130. Butler P, McIntyre N, Mistry PK: Molecular diagnosis of Wilson disease. Mol Genet Metab 72:223, 2001.
131. Vierling JM: Copper metabolism in primary biliary cirrhosis. Semin Liver Dis 1:293, 1981.
132. Loudianos G, Gitlin JD: Wilson disease. Semin Liver Dis 20:353, 2000.
133. Pandit A, Bhave S: Present interpretation of the role of copper in Indian childhood cirrhosis. Am J Clin Nutr 63:830S, 1996.
134. Muller T, Muller W, Feichtinger H: Idiopathic copper toxicosis. Am J Clin Nutr 67:1082S, 1998.
135. Scheinberg IH, Sternlieb I: Wilson disease and idiopathic copper toxicosis. Am J Clin Nutr 63:842S, 1996.
136. Muller T, Feichtinger H, Berger H, et al: Endemic Tyrolean infantile cirrhosis: an ecogenetic disorder. Lancet 347:877, 1996.
137. Dagenais SL, Guevara-Fujita M, Loechel R, et al: The canine copper locus is not syntenic with ATP7B or ATX1 and maps to a region showing homology to human 2p21. Mamm Genome 10:753, 1999.
138. van de Sluis BJ, Breen M, Nanji M, et al: Genetic mapping of the copper toxicosis locus in Bedlington terriers to dog chromosome 10, in a region syntenic to human chromosome region 2p13- p16. Hum Mol Genet 8:501, 1999.
139. Deiss A, Lynch RE, Lee GR, et al: Long-term therapy of Wilson's disease. Ann Intern Med 75:57, 1971.
140. Sternlieb I, Scheinberg IH. Penicillamine therapy in hepatolenticular degeneration. JAMA 189:748, 1964.
141. Sass-Kortsak A: Wilson's disease: a treatable liver disease in children. Pediatr Clin North Am 22:963, 1975.
142. Arima M, Takeshita K, Yoshino K, et al: Prognosis of Wilson's disease in childhood. Eur J Pediatr 126:147, 1977.
143. Gibbs K, Walshe JM: Liver copper concentration in Wilson's disease: effect of treatment with "anti-copper" agents. J Gastroenterol Hepatol 5:420, 1990.
144. Glass JD, Reich SG, DeLong MR: Wilson's disease: development of neurologic disease after beginning penicillamine therapy. Arch Neurol 47:595, 1990.
145. Chan CY, Baker AL: Penicillamine hypersensitivity: successful desensitization of a patient with severe hepatic Wilson's disease. Am J Gastroenterol 89:442, 1994.
146. Scheinberg IH, Jaffe ME, Sternlieb I: The use of trientine in preventing the effects of interrupting penicillamine therapy in Wilson's disease. N Engl J Med 317:209, 1987.
147. Walshe JM: Treatment of Wilson's disease with trientine (triethylene tetramine). Lancet 1:643, 1982.
148. Walshe JM: Copper chelation in patients with Wilson's disease: a comparison of penicillamine with triethylene tetramine. QJM 42:441, 1973.
149. Brewer GJ, Dick RD, Johnson V, et al: Treatment of Wilson's disease with ammonium tetrathiomolybdenate. I. Initial therapy in 17 neurologically affected patients. Arch Neurol 51:545, 1994.
150. Harper PL, Walshe JM: Reversible pancytopenia secondary to treatment with tetrathiomolybdate. Br J Haematol 64:851, 1986.
151. Fosmire JM: Zinc toxicity. Am J Clin Nutr 51:225, 1990.
152. Brewer GJ, Hill GM, Prasad AS, et al: Oral zinc therapy for Wilson's disease. Ann Intern Med 99:314, 1983.
153. Brewer GJ, Yuzbasiyan-Gurkan V, Johnson V, et al: Treatment of Wilson's disease with zinc. XII. Dose regimen requirements. Am J Med Sci 305:199, 1993.
154. Rossaro L, Sturniolo GC, Giacon G, et al: Zinc therapy in Wilson's disease: observations in five patients. Am J Gastroenterol 86:665, 1990.
155. Sternlieb I: Wilson's disease and pregnancy. Hepatology 31:531, 2000.
156. Emre S, Atillasoy EO, Ozdemir S, et al: Orthotopic liver transplantation for Wilson's disease: a single-center experience. Transplantation 15:72, 2001.
157. Schilsky ML, Scheinberg IH, Sternlieb I: Liver transplantation for Wilson's disease: indications and outcome. Hepatology 19:583, 1994.
158. Bellary S, Hassanein T, Van Thiel DH: Liver transplantation for Wilson's disease. J Hepatol 23:373, 1995.
159. Schumacher G, Platz KP, Mueller AR, et al: Liver transplantation: treatment of choice for hepatic and neurological manifestation of Wilson's disease. Clin Transplant 11:217, 1997.
160. Asonuma K, Inomata Y, Kasahara M, et al: Living related liver transplantation from heterozygote genetic carriers to children with Wilson's disease. Pediatr Transplant 3:201, 1999.

CHAPTER 42

Hemochromatosis and the Iron Overload Syndromes

Anthony S. Tavill, MD, FACP, FRCP, and Bruce R. Bacon, MD

The association of diabetes, cirrhosis of the liver, fibrosis of the pancreas, and pigmentation of the skin was first described by Trousseau in 1865,[1] and 6 years later Troisier reported a case of "pigment cirrhosis in sugar diabetes."[2] In 1889 von Recklinghausen termed the association of these clinical features *hemochromatosis,* and although he established that the increased pigment in tissues was iron, he misplaced its source as the blood.[3] Thereafter, the favored synonyms for the syndrome were *bronze diabetes* or *pigment cirrhosis* (French literature) and *hemochromatosis* (German literature), although it was not at that time recognized that they could represent various stages of development of the same disease. Little new information was forthcoming on the natural history of hemochromatosis until Sheldon published his classic monograph in 1935.[4] With his detailed review of 311 published cases that he accepted as genuine examples of hemochromatosis, he established for the first time a unifying concept of the multiple organ involvement of a single disease and offered evidence for its familial occurrence. On the basis of his family studies Sheldon concluded that hemochromatosis was an inherited disease resulting from an inborn error of metabolism. The genetic basis of the disease was initially questioned by MacDonald,[5] who felt it was related to alcoholic liver disease (ALD), and it took another four decades after Sheldon's study before Simon and co-workers firmly established the genetic transmission of hemochromatosis based on the association between human leukocyte antigen (HLA) typing and the predisposition to the disease.[6] Likewise, the causal relationship between excessive iron deposition and tissue damage has been conclusively supported in the clinical setting by the demonstration that early diagnosis and treatment can prevent all of the long-term complications of the disease.[7,8] A new level of understanding of the pathogenesis of the disease's hereditary basis was reached with the discovery of the *HFE* gene and its predominant mutation in 1996[9] and subsequently the development of the *HFE* gene knockout model in the mouse (Table 42-1).[10]

CAUSES OF IRON OVERLOAD

Although Sheldon postulated the hereditary basis for so-called idiopathic or primary hemochromatosis in 1935, the use of this older nomenclature persisted in the medical literature until recently because of the lack of firm genetic markers of the disease (Table 42-2).[11] With the

TABLE 42-1
History of Hereditary Hemochromatosis

Year	Author	Event
1865	Trousseau[1]	First case described
1889	von Recklinghausen[3]	The term *hemochromatosis* first used
1935	Sheldon[4]	Description of 311 cases
1950	Davis[290]	First percutaneous liver biopsy in HH, followed by first phlebotomy therapy
1960	MacDonald[110]	Controversy over whether HH is an inherited or a nutritional disorder
1976	Bomford and Williams[129]	Benefit of phlebotomy described
1977	Simon[6]	HLA linkage first described
1985	Niederau[8,221]	Benefit of early diagnosis (confirmed 1996)
1988	Edwards[127]	High prevalence confirmed
1996	Feder[9]	Identification of gene mutation (termed *HFE*)
1998	Zhou[10]	*HFE* gene knockout model

HH, Hereditary hemochromatosis; *HLA,* human leukocyte antigen.

TABLE 42-2

Causes of Iron Overload

Iron Overload States: Classification
1. HH
• HH: *HFE*-related
- C282Y homozygosity
- C282Y/H63D compound heterozygosity
- Other mutations of *HFE*
• HH: non-*HFE* related; other gene mutations
• Juvenile hemochromatosis
• Autosomal-dominant hemochromatosis (Solomon Islands)
2. Secondary iron overload
• Iron loading anemias ± transfusion
- Thalassemia major
- Sideroblastic anemia
- Chronic hemolytic anemias
• Dietary iron overload
• Chronic liver diseases
- Hepatitis C
- Alcoholic liver disease
- Porphyria cutanea tarda
- Fatty liver disease
3. Miscellaneous causes of iron overload
• African iron overload
• Neonatal iron overload
• Aceruloplasminemia
• Congenital atransferrinemia

From Tavill AS: Diagnosis and management of hemochromatosis. AASLD Practice Guidelines. Hepatology 33:1321-1328, 2001.
HH, Hereditary hemochromatosis; *C282Y,* cysteine to tyrosine at amino acid position 282; *H63D,* histadine to aspartic acid at amino acid position 63.

advent of detailed pedigree analyses, HLA associations, and the discovery of the *HFE* gene mutations, idiopathic or primary hemochromatosis was renamed *hereditary* (or *genetic*) *hemochromatosis* (HH). Older terms such as idiopathic or primary hemochromatosis are rarely used.

Thus the term *hereditary hemochromatosis* is currently used to describe the *HFE*-related disease characterized by the inappropriately high absorption of iron by the intestinal mucosa and leading to the pathologic deposition of excessive iron in the parenchymal cells of the liver, heart, pancreas, and other organs, eventually resulting in cell and tissue damage, fibrosis, and functional insufficiency. The evidence of genetic mutations of genes other than the *HFE* gene on chromosome 6 may explain iron overload in certain families, and the term *HH* may also be applied to these other, rarer examples of hemochromatosis (see Table 42-2). *Hemosiderosis* is a term that continues to be used by some pathologists to indicate excessive stainable iron in tissues without regard to the specific target cell that is primarily involved or to the underlying pathogenesis of the iron deposition.

Because methods are now available for the detection of HH in asymptomatic probands, in presymptomatic relatives of patients with the disease, and in the general population, the diagnosis can be applied legitimately to individuals who have not yet developed any of the toxic consequences of iron overload in the tissues. It is no longer justified to confine the diagnosis only to those individuals who are either symptomatic or who manifest organ damage such as cirrhosis, diabetes, or skin pigmentation. Rather, all individuals who have inherited both alleles of the hemochromatosis gene and who have indirect or direct markers of iron overload should be regarded as homozygotes for hereditary hemochromatosis. This concept has heightened the awareness of the disease, leading to early diagnosis and treatment, and undoubtedly has already led to reduced morbidity and increased survival.

In disorders of ineffective erythropoiesis and in some patients with liver disease excessive iron absorption and tissue iron deposition can also occur (see Table 42-2).[12] These and other conditions associated with excessive iron absorption have been classified *secondary iron overload* because the increased absorption of intestinal iron is promoted by the underlying condition (other than the *HFE* gene or other gene mutations). In these syndromes pathologic and clinical consequences similar to those seen in HH can occur. In situations of ineffective erythropoiesis when transfusion is necessary, the iron burden may accumulate very rapidly because of these combined factors, and patients may present with the consequences of iron toxicity many years earlier than is commonly seen in HH.[13,14] In contrast, the iron burden observed in liver disease with secondary iron overload, whether it is acquired[7,15] or on the basis of another associated disorder such as porphyria cutanea tarda (PCT),[16,17] is considerably smaller and may play a lesser role in the pathogenesis of the liver damage seen in these conditions.

Both HH and the various causes of secondary iron overload should be distinguished from *parenteral iron overload,* which is virtually always iatrogenic and leads to iron deposition initially confined to the reticuloendothelial (RE) system.[13,18] When transfusion is required in disorders of erythropoiesis, a combination of parenchymal and RE iron overload will co-exist, and the total body iron burden may be very large. With long-term parenteral iron overload, parenchymal iron deposition occurs, presumably resulting from secondary uptake of iron released from RE cells. The degree of structural and functional damage to the organ largely parallels the extent of parenchymal cell involvement, regardless of the underlying etiology.

Two additional causes of iron overload that are distinctly different than those mentioned previously are *neonatal iron overload* and *African iron overload.* Neonatal (or perinatal) iron overload came to medical attention largely in the 1980s.[19] There have been at least 100 reported cases, and the disorder appears to have a familial occurrence in some cases.[20,21] Several studies have been unable to provide any relationship to HH[20] and the currently favored etiology is fetal liver disease (perhaps viral mediated) leading to abnormal fetal-placental handling of iron.[22] Secondary syndromes include African iron overload as a form of iron loading caused by the ingestion of large amounts of dietary iron.[23-26] This disorder was described in people living in sub-Saharan Africa in whom the increase in iron absorption was caused by the ingestion of large amounts of iron in beer brewed in steel drums.[25-27] Recently, it has been proposed that African iron overload is due to a genetic factor that is not *HFE*-related, in addition to the well-known dietary factor.[28,29]

PATHOPHYSIOLOGIC FACTORS IN IRON OVERLOAD

The initial step leading to phenotypic expression of the metabolic defect in HH, African iron overload, and to some degree, secondary iron overload, is the inappropriate absorption of iron from the proximal gastrointestinal tract. In the presence of expanded iron stores the continued absorption of iron together with decreased retention by reticuloendothelial cells results in an increase in circulating transferrin-bound iron. Both transferrin-bound iron and non–transferrin-bound iron can be taken up by parenchymal cells, particularly those in the liver, resulting in the progressive accumulation of hepatic storage iron in the form of ferritin and hemosiderin. Since the discovery of *HFE,* the gene found defective in 85 percent to 90 percent of typical HH patients, we have learned much about the mechanisms controlling normal intestinal iron absorption and the nature of the defect in these control mechanisms in HH.[30-32]

PATHOPHYSIOLOGY OF HEREDITARY HEMOCHROMATOSIS

Total body iron content is regulated by controlling the level of absorption of iron from the diet.[33,34] Normally, about 10 percent (about 1 mg per day) of dietary iron is absorbed. After uptake into the enterocyte, iron becomes part of an intracellular transit pool from which it may be incorporated and stored in ferritin or transported across the basolateral membrane of the enterocyte to be bound to apotransferrin in the portal circulation. Diferric transferrin is then available to bind to transferrin receptor (TfR) on cell membranes and the complex undergoes endocytosis, resulting in iron being provided for cellular needs. All cells require iron for incorporation into heme proteins and cytochromes that are involved in mitochondrial electron transport; iron in excess of these cellular needs is stored in ferritin.[35] Iron uptake into the body is regulated in the duodenum and proximal jejunum at both the apical and the basolateral plasma membrane of the enterocyte.[33,34] Both heme and ionic iron are transported across the apical membrane into the enterocyte using three different pathways. The best characterized pathway is the absorption of ferrous iron via divalent metal transporter 1 (DMT1), also known as DCT-1 or Nramp2.[36,37] Second, iron can be absorbed as heme iron as an intact heme moiety, which is then broken down by heme oxygenase within the enterocyte.[33,38] Third, absorption of ferric iron by the integrin/mobilferrin/paraferritin pathway has been described by Conrad and colleagues.[39] At the basolateral plasma membrane of the enterocyte, there are at least two proteins involved in iron export: an iron transporter called ferroportin 1[40-42] and a ferroxidase called hephaestin.[43] It appears that ferroportin 1 transports ferrous iron out of the enterocyte with hephaestin being involved in oxidizing ferrous iron to ferric iron, which then binds to circulating apotransferrin.

As mentioned previously, our knowledge of iron absorption has advanced considerably over the last several years as a direct consequence of the cloning of the *HFE* gene.[9] The *HFE* gene encodes a 343 amino acid protein consisting of a 22 amino acid signal peptide, a large extracellular domain, a single transmembrane domain, and a short cytoplasmic tail (Figure 42-1). The extracellular domain of HFE protein consists of three loops (alpha-1, alpha-2, and alpha-3), with intramolecular disulfide bonds within the second and third loops. The structure of HFE protein is similar to other major histocompatibility complex (MHC) class 1 proteins except that evidence provided by x-ray crystallographic studies suggests that HFE protein does not participate in antigen recognition or presentation.[44] However, as with other MHC class 1 proteins, HFE protein is physically associated with β2-microglobulin (β_2M). Two missense mutations were identified in *HFE* with the original cloning of the gene.[9] The major mutation responsible for HH results in the substitution of a tyrosine for a cysteine at amino acid position 282 (C282Y) in the alpha-3 loop. With the loss of the sulfur in cysteine, a disulfide bridge in the alpha-3 loop is no longer present, which interferes with the interaction of HFE protein with β_2M and also results in decreased presentation of the C282Y mutant protein at the cell surface.[45,46] There is increased retention of mutant HFE protein in the endoplasmic reticulum with enhanced protein degradation.[46] Initial suspicion that the protein involved in HH could be an MHC class 1–like protein came from work with the β_2M knockout mouse that clearly demonstrated an iron overload phenotype similar to that seen in HH.[47] Confirmation that HFE is the protein involved in human disease was provided by the development of the *HFE* knockout mouse, which has the characteristic phenotypic expression of HH with an elevated transferrin saturation and increased hepatic iron deposition in parenchymal cells in a periportal distribution.[10,48,49] The second mutation that was identified in

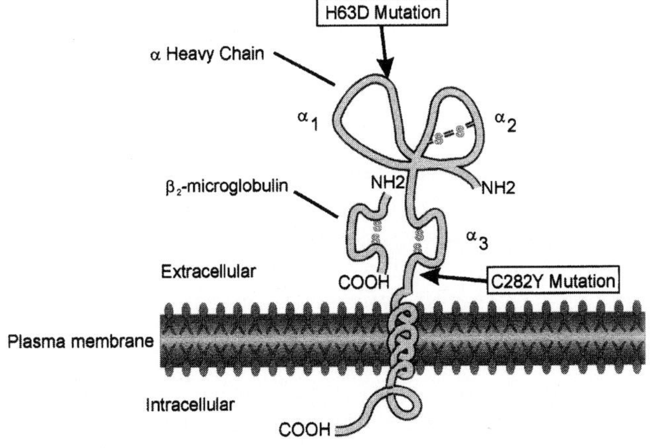

Figure 42-1 Proposed model of the HFE protein. (From Gastroenterology 116:193,1999).

HFE is the change of a histidine to an aspartate at amino acid position 63 (H63D) in the alpha-1 chain.[9] The functional consequences of this amino acid change on HFE protein are as yet unclear. Approximately 15 percent to 20 percent of the American population is heterozygous for H63D.[30]

Soon after the cloning of *HFE,* it was discovered that HFE protein along with β_2M forms a complex with TfR.[50-52] This physical association has been identified in cultured cells, in syncytiotrophoblasts of the placenta (a site of iron transport), and in duodenal crypt enterocytes, the site of regulation of dietary iron absorption. The stoichiometry of HFE protein, TfR, β_2M, and diferric transferrin at the cell membrane is unknown; however, crystallographic studies with soluble HFE protein suggest that the stoichiometry of the HFE protein-TfR complex in vitro is either a 1:2 or a 2:2 relationship.[53] With the knowledge that HFE and TfR bind to each other came numerous studies looking at the effect of HFE protein on TfR-mediated iron uptake.[32] This is an area of ongoing research, and conflicting results have been obtained because of methodologic differences related to various cell culture systems, the degree of HFE protein expression, and whether or not the cells express β_2M.

Nonetheless, putting these in vitro methodologic differences aside, it is clear that the primary disorder in HH is an increased rate of intestinal iron absorption relative to body iron stores.[33,34] Duodenal crypt enterocytes have long been thought to be the site of sensing the body iron stores. These cells influence the level of dietary iron absorption because they differentiate into absorptive enterocytes and migrate to the tip of the intestinal villus.[33,34] HFE protein and TfR are both highly expressed in crypt cells but not in villus cells of the duodenum.[54] Conversely, the DMT1 is expressed in the villus tip, which is the site of dietary iron absorption.[31,32] The expression of DMT1 messenger ribonucleic acid (mRNA), which has an iron regulatory element (IRE), is up-regulated in iron deficiency. These observations have led to the proposal that normal HFE protein facilitates the uptake of plasma iron by the TfR-mediated pathway in duodenal crypt cells and that mutant HFE protein lacks this facilitating effect.[52,54-58] In turn, this would lead to the reduction of the regulatory iron pool in crypt enterocytes, which would result in increased binding of iron regulatory protein to the IRE in DMT1 mRNA. There would subsequently be an up-regulation of DMT1 (and perhaps ferroportin 1), leading to an increase in dietary iron absorption. The validity of this hypothesis is supported by the observation that *HFE* knockout mice have increased duodenal expression of DMT1 mRNA[58] and protein,[59] whereas HH patients have elevated duodenal mRNA levels for DMT1[60,61] and ferroportin 1.[61]

MECHANISMS OF IRON TOXICITY

In HH the liver is the major recipient of excess absorbed iron, and after several years of high tissue iron concentration, fibrosis and eventually cirrhosis develop (Figure 42-2).[62-69] Accordingly, despite the adverse effects of iron on many organs of the body, virtually all of our understanding of the pathophysiologic effects of excess tissue iron is derived from clinical or experimental studies of the effects of iron on the liver, with a few studies in cultured myocytes. Clinical evidence for hepatic damage resulting from iron has been provided by studies of patients with HH, African iron overload, and secondary iron overload resulting from β-thalassemia in which correlation between hepatic iron concentration and the occurrence of liver damage has been demonstrated, or in

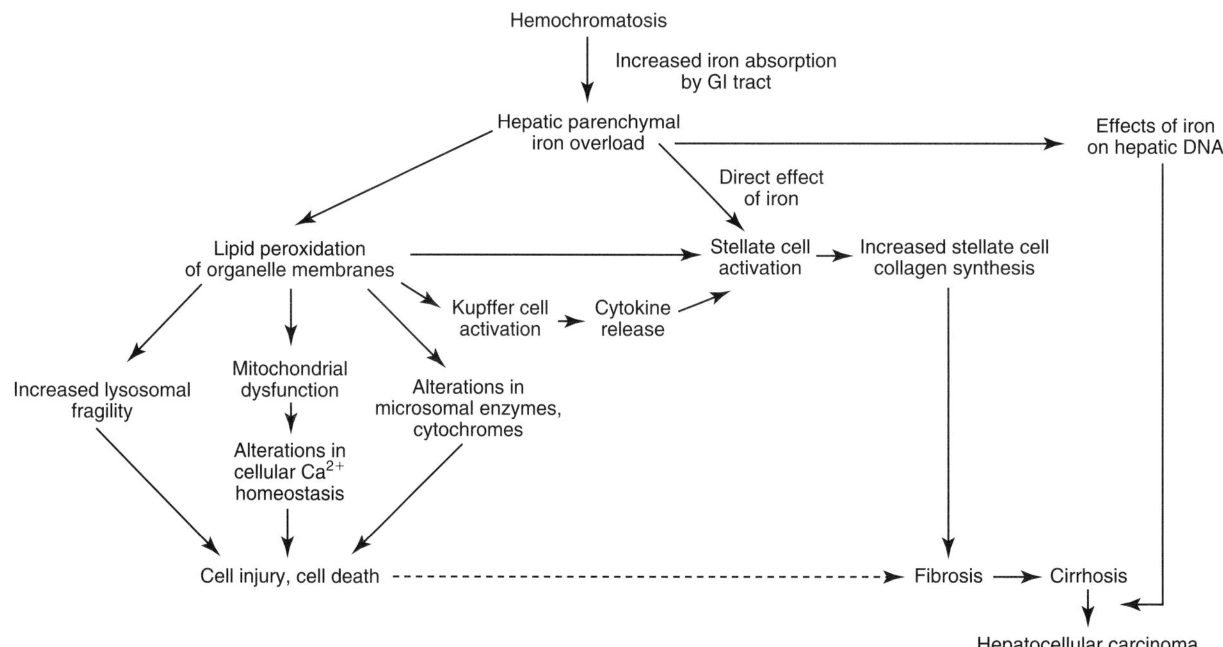

Figure 42-2 Proposed mechanisms of cellular injury (hepatocytes) and tissue damage (fibrogenesis) in chronic iron overload.

which therapeutic reduction of hepatic iron, either by phlebotomy or by chelation therapy, has resulted in clinical improvement. In the past a hepatic iron concentration "threshold" for the development of hepatic fibrosis was considered to be approximately 22,000 μg/g dry weight.[70] More recent studies, however, have shown that many of the earlier patients who had increased fibrosis at this iron concentration most likely had co-existing liver disease, such as ALD or hepatitis C. Recent results indicate that a relatively small proportion of HH patients with high levels of iron go on to develop cirrhosis in the absence of other co-existing liver disease.[71]

The mechanisms of tissue injury that occur in iron overload have been studied in several experimental models. Most work has been done using rats fed diets supplemented with carbonyl iron in which iron-induced lipid peroxidation has been identified in membrane fractions from hepatic mitochondria, microsomes, and lysosomes, and membrane-dependent functions are abnormal at iron concentrations at which oxidative damage occurs.[72,73] A relationship between iron-induced lipid peroxidation and hepatic fibrosis has also been demonstrated.[74,75] One hypothesis is that iron-induced lipid peroxidation occurs in hepatocytes causing liver cell injury or death. Kupffer cells may phagocytose damaged iron-loaded hepatocytes, resulting in their subsequent activation. These activated Kupffer cells, or the damaged hepatocytes themselves, may produce profibrogenic compounds that stimulate hepatic stellate cells to produce increased amounts of collagen leading to pathologic fibrosis.

PATHOLOGIC FINDINGS IN HEREDITARY HEMOCHROMATOSIS

The pathologic changes in HH in the various affected organs reflect both the primary evidence of excess storage iron and the secondary toxic consequences of the prolonged presence of the excess iron stores. The concept of a threshold for tissue damage encompasses both the level of accretion of tissue iron and the duration of exposure to toxic levels of iron. Marked differences exist in the concentrations of iron in the various organs and in the relative amount of iron in the different cell types within each organ. Furthermore, there appear to be markedly different susceptibilities to tissue damage among the vulnerable organs that do not relate necessarily to the storage iron concentration in the organ. Finally, there are distinct differences between the pathologic changes seen in HH when compared with those seen in certain other forms of iron overload. Both the different cellular distribution of iron and the forms of excess iron stores may have marked influences on the pathologic consequences of iron overload. When excessive alcohol intake accompanies HH or when HH patients have concomitant chronic hepatitis C or B, the pathologic features are significantly influenced, making the diagnosis more difficult. We have chosen to review the pathologic changes in HH first and then to contrast these with the changes in the various other syndromes of secondary and parenteral iron overload and in ALD with iron overload.

Liver

Because the liver is the primary storage organ for iron, it is usually the first organ damaged in HH. When a liver biopsy is obtained or the liver is examined at autopsy, the most striking abnormality is the presence of extensive hemosiderin granules in the hepatocytes, often with a predominant pericanalicular distribution, which stain positive with Perls' Prussian blue stain (potassium ferrocyanide) for ferric iron (Plate 42-1, *A-D*). The presence of excess ferritin iron deposition is reflected by a diffuse cytosolic bluish stain that is often dwarfed by the dense staining of the granular hemosiderin. The evolution of iron deposition from complete normality (absence or only 1+ staining) to uniform heavy deposition throughout all hepatocytes has been revealed by histopathologic studies of asymptomatic family members and by early diagnosis in young presymptomatic probands.[76-81] Initial deposition is in the periphery of the lobule in the periportal region, or Rappaport's acinar zone 1. With progressive increase in the iron burden, the cells in the central areas of the lobule (acinar zone 3) begin to show increased degrees of iron staining. Even with heavy iron deposition in fully established HH, a portal (zone 1) to central (zone 3) gradient can usually be identified. There is correlation between the concentration of ferritin/hemosiderin clusters seen on electron microscopy and the degree of Perls' Prussian blue staining.[76] Deposition of lipofuscin-like pigment can also be seen in association with iron accumulation, but it is often abundant in centrolobular cells and in a pericanalicular distribution.[76] This material is thought to be derived from free radical–induced, irreversible damage to lipids and other macromolecules.[82] In advanced hemochromatosis there is usually heavy iron deposition in bile ductular cells, in Kupffer cells, and in macrophages within fibrous tissue (Plate 42-1, *E*).[80] Associated pathologic changes of a nonspecific nature include steatosis and nuclear vacuolation, particularly in association with diabetes.

At an ultrastructural level there is evidence that both excessive quantities of crystalline ferritin and amorphous hemosiderin accumulate as a response to prolonged delivery of both transferrin-bound and non–transferrin-bound iron to the liver. In both experimental and clinical iron overload increased cytosolic ferritin becomes membrane-bound within so-called siderosomes. It is speculated that siderosome ferritin is a precursor of lysosomal ferritin that is subjected to degradative hydrolytic enzymes that denature the protein component, leading to progressive accumulation of amorphous hemosiderin.[82-87] In the complex spectrum of advanced hemochromatosis or experimental iron overload, ferritin iron may be found free in the cytosol or membrane-bound in siderosomes,[88-90] whereas hemosiderin, which is by far the predominant form of storage iron in moderate to heavy iron overload, is found largely within pericanalicular lysosomes.[91-93]

In symptomatic HH, fibrosis or cirrhosis is almost invariably present. Early fibrosis is confined to portal expansion with a subsequent periportal distribution surrounding partially preserved lobules or groups of lobules. The iron distribution is predominantly hepatocellular within nodules, with relative sparing of surrounding bands of fibrous tissue. Recent detailed histopathologic evaluation[94] has shown evidence of hepatocellular necrosis ("sideronecrosis") in areas of dense iron loading (Plate 42-1, *F*). These changes are often relatively mild and subtle. Increased fibrosis is seen in areas of most extensive iron deposition, lending credence to the hypothesis mentioned earlier wherein aldehydic products from damaged iron-loaded hepatocytes result in activation of stellate cells with subsequent stimulation of collagen production. It should be noted that although a correlation has been shown between the hepatic iron concentration and the presence of fibrosis and cirrhosis,[7,95,96] such a correlation has not been noted with the extent of stainable hepatic iron, illustrating the relative inaccuracy of qualitative iron staining.[76,97] Furthermore, fibrosis or cirrhosis can be seen at much lower hepatic iron concentrations when HH is accompanied by ALD or chronic viral hepatitis.[70,98]

Occasionally, in HH with cirrhosis nodules or areas within nodules contain less iron or maybe no iron relative to the surrounding parenchyma. This has suggested to some workers that nodules are formed predominantly by fibrous dissection of the parenchyma rather than from regenerative foci of surviving cells.[80] Alternatively, these "iron-free foci," described in a large series of patients with HH and hepatocellular carcinoma (HCC), were found to be accompanied by a high prevalence of proliferative (83 percent) and dysplastic (70 percent) areas in the non-tumorous liver of untreated patients.[99] Thus it has been suggested that these "iron-free foci" may be preneoplastic lesions from which HCC may arise.

Cirrhosis resulting from severe HH is micronodular (Plate 42-2, *A*). In patients with HH the incidence of HCC is increased approximately 100-fold above that found in the general population (see Plate 42-2, *B*).[8,100] HCC has been described predominantly in HH patients with cirrhosis and can develop after successful phlebotomy therapy and effective iron removal.[8,99-102] Several cases of HCC have now been described in HH patients without cirrhosis or after apparent reversal of cirrhosis.[99,103-105] In one series patients with HCC showed a higher prevalence of chronic alcoholism and tobacco smoking[99] than in controls, and others have suggested that concomitant hepatitis C virus (HCV) infection may predispose HH patients to develop HCC.[106] Primary liver cancers are typically unifocal, and with the advent of orthotopic liver transplantation have been identified incidentally (i.e., unknown at the time of transplant) in as many as 27 percent of patients.[107]

Pancreas

Both the exocrine (acinar) and endocrine (α and β cells in islets of Langerhans) secretory cells of the pancreas manifest excess storage iron, and by the time that homozygotes present symptomatically, there can be disorganization of acinar structure with fibrosis and a reduction in islet cells. Paradoxically, stainable iron is more prominent in acinar cells than in the islets of Langerhans, suggesting enhanced susceptibility of endocrine cells to the toxic effects of iron.[108,109] Iron can also be seen in duct epithelium and in the interstitium.

Other Endocrine Organs

Hemosiderin deposits can be seen in follicular and parafollicular cells of the thyroid, the zona glomerulosa of the adrenal cortex, the cells of the anterior pituitary with the exception of the acidophil cells, and the parathyroid glands.[108,110] In the thyroid, fibrosis with parenchymal atrophy has been described.[111] In the testes, there may be atrophy of the germinal epithelium with absent spermatogenesis and no Leydig cells in the presence of relatively low levels of iron loading.[112]

Heart

The majority of the early information on the cardiac pathology of iron overload resulted from studies in patients with refractory anemias who had received many blood transfusions over prolonged periods.[113] In individuals who received more than 100 units of blood, hemosiderin deposits have been observed predominantly in the ventricular myocardium, in the subepicardial regions, and in contractile cells. Iron deposits of a lesser degree were also found in conducting tissues, both the atrioventricular (AV) node and the sinus node. Iron deposition is also found in the perinuclear region of cardiomyocytes that undergo degeneration and necrosis and replacement by fibrous tissue.

Two recent studies have provided useful new information on cardiac iron deposition in HH.[114,115] In contrast to transfusional iron overload, iron deposits in HH were found consistently in the cytoplasm of cardiac muscle cells (rather than in the interstitium) and in the conducting fibers of the AV node. No iron deposition was found in the sinus node. The distribution was patchy and was more pronounced in the subepicardial region.[114,115] Thus it has been suggested that cardiac involvement in HH should be considered a storage disease rather than a degenerative process. Cardiac involvement in HH may be focal and patchy. Thus when HH is considered as an explanation for atypical cardiac disease, multiple endomyocardial biopsies may need to be performed for diagnosis.

Joints

In HH there may be heavy deposits of hemosiderin in the type B synovial lining cells that undergo proliferation and associated fibrosis.[116-118] Iron is confined to fibrocytic cells and chondrocytes in contrast to the macrophages, which contain relatively little iron. Secondarily, there are degenerative changes in the chondrocytes and surrounding cartilage with associated calcification and subchondral cyst formation.[116-118] Although excessive iron deposits may provide the initial stimulus to the deposition of calcium pyrophosphate crystals in the joint cartilage, the increase in calcium deposits may actually be the factor responsible for the arthropathy of HH (pseudogout).[118]

Skin

Most of the clinically visible pigmentation in HH is due to melanin deposition in the basal layers of the epidermis.[119] However, some of the grayish pigmentation is associated with hemosiderin deposition within macrophages, particularly around vascular endothelium in the basement membrane of the sweat glands, and in connective tissue of the dermis, which may be visible through the atrophic dermis and epidermis.[119] It has been proposed that iron may stimulate melanocytic activity through increased oxidative damage or by reacting with sulfhydryl groups in the epidermis.

Spleen and Bone Marrow

Even in the presence of massive hepatic iron overload in HH, the concentration of iron in the spleen and bone marrow is relatively low. In a semiquantitative analysis of the spleens of patients with symptomatic HH, there were only occasional fine granules of hemosiderin in some of the pulp macrophages,[120] with most of the iron confined to the capsule, trabeculae, and walls of blood vessels. Likewise, concentrations of iron from bone marrow biopsy samples were not significantly elevated.[121] For the most part, the pathology of the spleen reflects the extent of portal hypertension, rather than the effects of iron storage.

COMPARISONS AND CONTRASTS WITH SECONDARY IRON OVERLOAD AND ALCOHOLIC LIVER DISEASE WITH IRON OVERLOAD

Although many of the causes of secondary iron overload have in common with HH an increased delivery of transferrin-bound iron to parenchymal cells, there are useful distinguishing features that reflect differences in pathogenesis, in rates of accretion of storage iron, and in the role of associated parenteral iron overload. Because iron delivery through red blood cell transfusions is almost invariably associated with a concomitant refractory anemia with erythroid hyperplasia, the iron overload in this setting is usually due to both increased iron absorption and iron derived from effete red blood cells. In contrast, in hypoplastic anemias iron overload is almost exclusively derived from transfusions, and in this setting, iron-laden Kupffer cells predominate in the liver, and only later in the course of iron accumulation do hepatocytes share in the excessive iron storage (Plate 42-3).[122] Periportal fibrous tissue deposition occurs very late, and true cirrhosis is rare. Another contrasting feature in parenteral iron overload is the heavy deposition of iron in the macrophages of the spleen and bone marrow, emphasizing the important role of the reticuloendothelial system in processing the iron released from transfused red blood cells.

When ALD and secondary iron overload co-exist, the pathology of the liver relative to iron deposition may be confusing (Plate 42-4). This can arise as a result of the high frequency of stainable iron in alcoholic cirrhotic livers and the co-existence of excessive alcohol intake in patients with HH. In one series significant stainable iron was seen in 57 percent of liver biopsies from alcoholic patients; however, only 7 percent showed grade III or IV iron deposition.[123] The severity of the liver disease was not a factor in determining the overall prevalence of iron deposition because it was present in all stages of ALD and in as many non-cirrhotics as cirrhotics. In contrast, in the majority of alcoholics with HH the hepatic histopathology is indistinguishable from that of non-alcoholic HH patients[80]; however, the hepatic iron concentration at which fibrosis and cirrhosis occur may be much lower than that for non-alcoholic HH patients.[70,98] In these clinical settings it has been concluded that both iron and alcohol play a role in the pathogenesis of the liver disease. Currently, the principal methods for distinguishing HH with excessive alcohol use from ALD or other types of chronic liver disease with secondary iron overload are by measurement of the hepatic iron concentration and calculation of the hepatic iron index, a measure of the rate of hepatic iron accumulation and HFE gene mutation analysis.

CLINICAL FEATURES OF HEREDITARY HEMOCHROMATOSIS

General Systemic Symptoms

Clinically, HH evolves in stages: stage 1 (0-20 years of age, 0-5 g storage iron); stage 2 (approximately 20-40 years of age, 5-20 g storage iron); which, if untreated, progresses to stage 3 (usually in those older than 40 years of age and with more than 20 g storage iron).[124,125]

As early as 1935 Sheldon concluded that a total body iron burden of 25 to 50 g was required to establish symptomatic disease. He further determined that the net rate of iron accretion was slow and probably averaged no more than 1.5 mg/day to 2.5 mg/day throughout life. Although the classic triad of hepatomegaly, diabetes mellitus, and skin pigmentation formed the common clinical denominator of disease in the majority of patients reviewed by Sheldon, data that were accumulated on patients and their families in the next 20 years (1935 to 1955) indicated that the triad had to be expanded to include a number of other clinical features, several of which could antedate the triad by many years. For an in-depth review of these features, the reader is referred to several important publications that document the phenotypic expression of the disease in large groups of patients observed first-hand over many years.[8,79,81,126-131]

Currently, it is important to recognize that because of the advent of HLA typing and more recently *HFE* mutational analysis for the identification of homozygous relatives of probands with symptomatic disease and the use of iron studies on routine blood chemistry panels, the clinical picture of HH has taken on a much broader spectrum, ranging from totally asymptomatic individuals through precirrhotics and prediabetics with early manifestations of the disease to those patients with fully established end-organ toxicity who either have not sought medical help or have had their disease misdiagnosed or unrecognized. Several recent studies have included patients with early disease and have provided much-needed insights into the evolution of the clinical manifestations.[8,79,81] When groups of patients have been selected and analyzed based solely on pedigree analyses, HLA associations, and *HFE* mutations, fewer clinical features have been found compared with the studies of index cases in the earlier literature. When this method of detection is taken into account together with an increasing trend toward use of screening serum iron studies, it is not surprising that more patients are identified before the development of any significant pathology.[79,81,132-135] Now that the *HFE* gene has been identified and the genetic test for mutations is available, all affected individuals may be identified and treated for iron overload while asymptomatic. However, the question has been raised as to whether all, or even the majority, of genetic homozygotes will become phenotypically iron overloaded.

Analysis of studies of patients presenting with symptoms reveals that the mean age of presentation is typically about 50 years.[79,126,129] However, the mean age at diagnosis can often be delayed for 4 to 5 years because of failure to attribute the earliest symptoms and signs to hemochromatosis.[126] In a recent, large, long-term study 251 patients were followed for up to 44 years between 1947 and 1991.[8] The mean age and distribution by age at diagnosis were similar whether the individual was cirrhotic (46.2 years) or non-cirrhotic (45.1 years), diabetic (46.0 years) or non-diabetic (45.4 years). Of the 251 patients 89 percent were men and 11 percent women, a ratio of about 9:1, a figure that has been reported in other studies.[81] It is interesting that when probands, diagnosed initially on the basis of phenotypic features, were compared with individuals discovered by family studies, the ratio of male to female fell to almost 2:1, despite the similarity between age at diagnosis in the two groups.[136] This may well be a reflection of the parity of *HFE* gene mutations in the genders and confirms the earlier demonstration that the frequency of the disorder may be seriously underestimated when based solely on phenotypic expression.[81,137]

It is useful to compare the clinical features from the studies published in the last 20 years, which describe patients seen from the 1960s to the 1990s (Table 42-3). One study has selected 34 patients presenting to a single center over a 22-year period, in which diagnosis has been based purely on clinical and biochemical features.[126] The second has identified 35 homozygotes through pedigree studies using a baseline of 14 symptomatic probands.[79] Another has diagnosed patients early through indirect and direct screening techniques for iron overload, enabling the authors to put together a comprehensive evaluation of 251 patients, 109 of whom were shown to be in the precirrhotic phase of the disease and 131 of whom were non-diabetic.[8] This has allowed for comparison of the prevalence of the other features of HH, independent of the effects of liver disease.

In the large study by Niederau and colleagues[8] several symptoms and signs were more prevalent in patients with cirrhosis than in those who were non-cirrhotic: weakness and lethargy (88 percent and 73 percent, respectively), abdominal pain (68 percent and 39 percent), loss of libido or potency in males (43 percent and 27 percent), hepatomegaly (89 percent and 70 percent), splenomegaly (17 percent and 2 percent), edema (13 percent and 5 percent), ascites (9 percent and 0 percent), and jaundice (13 percent and 1 percent). Other features such as arthralgia, skin pigmentation, and gynecomastia occurred with similar frequency in both cirrhotics and non-cirrhotics. Overt diabetes mellitus occurred in 48 percent of all patients (both non–insulin-dependent and insulin-dependent) and was significantly more frequent in cirrhotics than non-cirrhotics (72 percent versus 17 percent). In the other two studies[79,126] there was a similar prevalence of the principal symp-

TABLE 42-3

Principal Clinical Features in Hereditary Hemochromatosis

Features	Niederau et al[8]	Milder et al[62]	Edwards et al[79]	Adams et al[81]
Number of subjects	251*	34†	35*	37‡
Symptoms (%)				
Weakness, lethargy	82	73	20	19
Abdominal pain	56	50	23	3
Arthralgias	44	47	57	40
Loss of libido, impotence	36	56	2	32
Cardiac failure symptoms	12	35	0*	3
Physical and Diagnostic Findings (%)				
Cirrhosis (biopsy)	57	94	57	3
Hepatomegaly	81	76	54	3
Splenomegaly	10	38	40	—
Loss of body hair	16	32	6	—
Gynecomastia	7	12	—	—
Testicular atrophy	—	50	14	—
Skin pigmentation	72	82	43	9
Clinical diabetes	48	53	6	11

*Patient selection occurred by both clinical features and family screening.
†Only symptomatic index cases were studied.
‡Discovered by family studies.

toms and signs in the probands as was observed in the patients with established cirrhosis in the series reported by Niederau and associates,[8] suggesting that the probands identified in other reported series have advanced disease with already established cirrhosis. In the study by Edwards and colleagues[79] in which some patients were identified by HLA typing, arthralgia was a prominent early symptom and usually preceded the diagnosis as determined by other clinical criteria.

Table 42-3 emphasizes the differences in the frequency of presenting symptoms and signs when groups of probands were compared with affected individuals discovered by pedigree analysis or by measurement of markers of iron overload. Finally, Adams and co-workers[81,136] have indicated that homozygous cases discovered by family studies and *HFE* mutation analysis have total body iron burdens that are on average considerably lower than index cases. Nevertheless, on direct questioning it was apparent that there were symptoms that had either been ignored or that had been attributed to other co-incidental illnesses. For example, abdominal pain and joint pain were commonly overlooked as probable presenting symptoms, whereas unexplained hepatomegaly and abnormal liver tests were often attributed by the physician to causes other than iron overload. Overall, both symptoms and signs, with the exception of arthropathy, were less prevalent in prospectively discovered cases than in index cases, and 46 percent of these individuals were totally asymptomatic. However, in spite of their relatively early diagnosis, 16 percent were already clinically diabetic and 5 percent (all males) had established cirrhosis. The level of symptomatic disease was related to the degree of iron overload; those with total body iron stores greater than 16 g were very likely to have evidence of organ damage.

Liver

Almost 57 percent of Niederau's 251 patients had cirrhosis at the time of diagnosis, whereas 81 percent of the group as a whole had clinical hepatomegaly.[8] It is evident, therefore, that hepatomegaly antedates the development of cirrhosis and is most likely related to the extent of iron overload. Its presence in 70 percent of non-cirrhotic patients with HH,[8] although significantly less than in those with established cirrhosis (89 percent), provides evidence that iron deposition per se plays a major role in its pathogenesis. Features of hepatocellular dysfunction and portal hypertension are most frequently observed when cirrhosis has become established. Similarly, in the laboratory evaluation of hepatic dysfunction, those tests that most closely reflect functional hepatocyte mass, such as serum albumin and prothrombin time, are not depressed until cirrhosis is established.[8,79] It is not uncommon to observe mild elevation in the serum aminotransferases in the absence of cirrhosis; usually twofold to fourfold elevations are evident and the degree of abnormality appears to be unrelated to the extent of hepatic iron accumulation.[8,79,138] These markers of hepatocellular necrosis usually return to normal with treatment. Other features such as loss of libido and potency or amenorrhea, presence of gynecomastia, and diabetes are also more common in the presence of cirrhosis. The increased prevalence of these features in cirrhotics may be a function of both the relationship of generalized tissue damage to the level and duration of iron deposition and the association with liver disease.

An evaluation of the relationship between hepatic iron concentration (HIC) and the prevalence of cirrhosis or fibrosis in the liver was made initially by Bassett and co-workers[7] and has been confirmed by others [95,96] In 30 homozygous relatives of 17 probands with hemochromatosis only those with HIC in excess of 22,000 μg/g dry weight had fibrosis or cirrhosis on liver biopsy. These tended to be older individuals than the prefibrotic homozygous individuals (41.7 years versus 26.5 years). Furthermore, only in HH homozygotes was there an age-related rise in HIC. The study by Bassett and colleagues[7] was the first to provide evidence that an iron concentration threshold may exist in the liver for the development of fibrosis and cirrhosis. This concept has also been shown in the study by Niederau and associates,[8] who found that those individuals whose cumulative iron stores were the greatest, averaging 25.7 g and 22,400 μg/g HIC, had the most frequent complications of cirrhosis and the worst prognosis. Conversely, no patients whose initial liver biopsy showed absence of cirrhosis developed cirrhosis in any subsequent biopsies, assuming appropriate phlebotomy treatment. In those with cirrhosis the two major causes of death were the complications of chronic liver disease (20 percent) and cancer of the liver (27.5 percent). In about 70 percent of the cirrhotics with signs of complications, death occurred before iron depletion could be completed. Although the prevalence of complications such as jaundice or ascites was relatively unusual at the time of diagnosis (only 13 percent of all patients) and was confined almost entirely to those with established cirrhosis (22 percent of cirrhotics), these were often the individuals who died before iron depletion could be completed. Liver cancers developed more than 119-fold more frequently than expected in the general population and were confined to cirrhotics. Death from liver cancer occurred in 19 patients between 3 and 19 years after documentation of iron depletion. The calculated iron stores in these patients were markedly higher than in those who survived or who died from other causes. In no case could hepatitis B or C be implicated. The majority of the cancers of the liver were primary HCC but some were intrahepatic cholangiocarcinomas (16 percent). In this large series the incidence of extrahepatic cancers was not increased in contrast to that reported in other studies.[129,139]

Finally, there is often unexplained epigastric or right upper quadrant pain, which is usually chronic. This has been attributed to associated hepatomegaly. Rare episodes of acute, severe abdominal pain, associated with circulatory shock, have been reported.[140] Several explanations have been offered, including bacterial peritonitis and gram-negative sepsis.

Pancreas, Diabetes

Again, the recent large study of Niederau and associates[8] provides an excellent source for data on the prevalence of diabetes mellitus. In the cirrhotic group (n = 142) 102 had overt diabetes (72 percent), of whom 44 (63 percent) were insulin-dependent. In contrast, in the non-cirrhotics ($n = 109$), only 18 (17 percent) were clinically diabetic, and of these, 12 (11 percent) were non–insulin-dependent. The overall prevalence of glucose intolerance (clinical and biochemical) was 61 percent, 85 percent in the cirrhotics, and 30 percent in the non-cirrhotics. Although this may simply reflect a similar degree of damage in the pancreas and the liver in untreated HH, it is likely that this is partly a feature of the glucose intolerance of cirrhosis. On the other hand, it has been shown that there is a higher prevalence of diabetes mellitus in the first-degree relatives of diabetic patients with HH than in those hemochromatotics who do not have diabetes.[141] Now that the diagnosis of HH is more frequently being made by detection of a homozygous relative to a proband, the frequency of diabetes in such individuals with discovered disease appears to be much lower, with 16 percent of men and 6 percent of women in the recent study of Adams and co-workers.[81] Although Sheldon[4] reported that vascular complications of diabetes were rare in HH, it is probable that prognosis was so limited by other complications of the disease that vascular complications had not yet had time to develop. In fact, as prognosis has improved, increased vascular complications typically seen in diabetes (retinopathy, nephropathy, neuropathy, peripheral vascular disease) have been observed,[141] and in the case of retinopathy, they occur with equal frequency to other long-standing diabetics without HH.[142] In more recent studies of patients with HH diagnosed early, diabetes is much less frequently observed.[81]

Other Endocrine Abnormalities

In the male with HH, loss of libido and impotence may occur relatively early in the course of the disease. Although these symptoms, accompanied by loss of secondary sexual characteristics and testicular atrophy, are often present with associated liver disease, they may, in many instances, antedate the development of cirrhosis. For example, although loss of libido or potency was present in 43 percent of cirrhotics, these symptoms were also present in 27 percent of non-cirrhotics.[8] When cases were identified by family studies the evidence of gonadal dysfunction was found in 32 percent of males.[81] Interestingly, amenorrhea in the female occurs with equal frequency in the presence or absence of established liver disease (13 percent versus 17 percent).[8] The majority of cases with gonadal failure are due to gonadotropin insufficiency with low levels of luteinizing hormone and follicle-stimulating hormone, and diminished responsiveness to gonadotropin-releasing hormone.[79,126,143-145] In contrast, pituitary-adrenal and pituitary-thyroid responsiveness are usually normal.[79,126] Gynecomastia is relatively less common in HH than in other causes of cirrhosis (only 8 percent in patients with hemochromatotic cirrhosis) and occurs in those without cirrhosis with almost equal frequency (5 percent).[8]

Cardiac Manifestations

Cardiomyopathy, cardiac dysrhythmia, and heart failure have been reported as the most common causes of death in young patients with secondary iron overload and associated parenteral iron overload.[146] The development of these complications carries a dire prediction of death within 3 months of onset.[147,148] Iron deposits in secondary and parenteral iron overload favor the ventricles rather than the atria, and contractile tissue rather than conducting tissue, with the development of cardiac failure rather than dysrhythmias.[149] Nevertheless, atrial tachyarrhythmias, ventricular ectopy, and tachycardia have been reported, which can aggravate the diminished systolic function produced by the iron-overload cardiomyopathy.[150] Although much of the information on cardiac involvement has been obtained in secondary iron overload, congestive heart failure resulting from a dilated cardiomyopathy has been well described in HH.[126] With the advent of effective phlebotomy therapy for HH, this complication has been shown to be relatively rare. Only 5 of 69 deaths in Niederau's series could be ascribed to cardiomyopathy[8]; however, this yielded a mortality ratio (observed/expected) of 13.8. Baseline non-invasive studies with echocardiography have shown abnormalities in approximately 35 percent of HH[8] and have indicated that ventricular enlargement is due principally to increased wall thickness. Later cavity dilation occurs with the advent of congestive failure. Based on studies in fetal rat myocardial cells in culture,[150a] it has been suggested that myocardial dysfunction is the consequence of iron-induced lipid peroxidation. Because of the sensitivity of myocardial tissue to iron-induced damage and the rapidity of fatal complications, the early detection of cardiac dysfunction is a clear indication for the use of iron chelators as an effective means for iron removal or detoxification.

Arthropathy

The overall prevalence of the arthropathy of HH is difficult to assess. The frequency of arthralgias at the time of diagnosis varies between 43 percent[8] and 57 percent[79] in reports from the 1980s derived from patients seen in the 1960s to the 1980s. The latter study included both probands and genotypic homozygotes discovered by HLA typing of first-degree relatives. Only 11 of 20 patients complaining of arthralgias had objective physical signs of arthropathy. However, several of those without painful joints or abnormal physical signs had radiologic evidence of joint disease. In the other study[8] comparing the frequency of arthralgia in those with and those without cirrhosis there was no difference in prevalence (44 percent versus 45 percent, respectively). This supports the notion that arthralgias may be an important first symptom, and in some cases arthritis may be the sole clinical manifestation of HH.[151] No correlation could be found between the mobilizable iron stores and the presence or absence of arthropathy.[8]

The polyarthropathy of HH tends to involve the metacarpophalangeal, proximal interphalangeal, knee, wrist, and vertebral joints. Although involvement is usually symmetric, it can be unilateral.[152] Pain and stiffness usually precede the objective evidence of enlargement, deformity, limitation of movement, and nodule formation, which are suggestive of osteoarthritis. Synovial thickening is not typically evident, and on radiologic evaluation several types of abnormalities can be detected. Characteristically, the arthropathy is manifested by subchondral cyst formation, osteopenia, squaring of the metacarpal joint heads, swelling of the metacarpophalangeal joints, and chondrocalcinosis.[79,151,152] The latter is present in about 50 percent of those with arthropathy. Less typically, non-specific radiologic evidence of degenerative joint disease is the only detectable radiologic abnormality.[79] Rarely, the arthritis progresses to devastating destruction of the smaller joints in spite of adequate iron removal. In others episodes of acute inflammatory synovitis are superimposed on the more chronic changes. These episodes of acute synovitis have been termed *pseudogout* and have been attributed to the precipitation of crystals of calcium pyrophosphate, possibly as a result of the inhibition of pyrophosphatase by iron deposited in synovial lining cells.[116,117,153,154] Although the foregoing description has resulted from studies exclusively in HH, arthropathy has been described in patients with parenteral iron overload also.[155]

Skin Pigmentation

In patients with overt HH excessive skin pigmentation is detectable almost invariably, particularly in exposed areas. However, it frequently eludes the patient's own attention or the attention of relatives because of its insidious development. The classic description of bronzed discoloration[4] has to be modified in some cases in favor of a slate-grey pigmentation. The former is due to predominant melanin pigmentation, whereas the latter is the result of iron deposition in the basal layers of the epidermis and the lining cells of the sweat glands. In advanced cases pigmentation also involves the conjunctivae, the lid margins, and the buccal mucosa.[119,156] In the study by Niederau and associates[8] the frequency of skin pigmentation at the time of diagnosis (overall 72 percent) was not significantly different in those with established cirrhosis (75 percent) than those without cirrhosis (69 percent). However, evaluation of homozygous relatives has shown a much lower prevalence of this physical sign (about 10 percent) than in index cases,[81] reflecting their younger age and lower iron stores.

Susceptibility to Infection

Patients with iron overload appear to have an increased susceptibility to infection; however, because the occurrences are uncommon, the association remains to be proved conclusively. Although occasional reports of infections have come from cases of HH, most have occurred in secondary iron overload. In some instances they have become manifest during the course of chelation therapy.[157,158] *Yersinia enterocolitica* septicemia and hepatic abscesses have been described in HH[159] and in secondary iron overload resulting from β-thalassemia with and without liver disease.[157] Other infections include those with *Pasteurella pseudotuberculosis,*[159a] *Vibrio vulnificus,*[159b] and *Listeria monocytogenes.*[160] Based on both experimental and clinical observations, it has been suggested that increased bioavailability of iron predisposes the host to infection[161,162]; the decrease in circulating apotransferrin leads to enhanced bacterial viability by making free iron available for bacterial growth and metabolism.[163,164] Alternatively, evidence has been presented to suggest that iron overload produces a defect in monocyte phagocytic capacity that is reversible by phlebotomy.[160] In either event the fundamental role of iron in bacterial metabolism and macrophage and neutrophil function in vivo requires further elucidation.

DIAGNOSIS OF HEMOCHROMATOSIS

The diagnosis of HH may be made in (1) symptomatic individuals with clinical features suggestive of the syndrome of HH, (2) asymptomatic relatives of patients with previously diagnosed HH (these are suspected homozygotes), and (3) asymptomatic individuals for whom suspicion of HH has been raised by abnormal liver enzymes or by the serendipitous discovery of a raised serum transferrin iron saturation or ferritin level. The last group is sometimes problematic because of the relative lack of specificity of such indirect markers (especially ferritin) and the frequency with which these markers can be increased in other diseases, particularly of the liver (e.g., ALD,[15] chronic viral hepatitis,[165] non-alcoholic steatohepatitis[166]). Because of the lack of appreciation of the diagnostic accuracy of these markers, there is a need to emphasize the cost-effectiveness of pursuing such clues with more specific and more invasive investigations. Nonetheless, with a gene frequency of approximately 5 percent and *HFE* gene mutation (C282Y) homozygous prevalence of about 1 in 250, it is agreed that HH is seriously underdiagnosed.

Unfortunately, many patients with HH are never diagnosed or the diagnosis is delayed by many years. This potentially fatal disease often escapes detection for several reasons. First, there is relatively little awareness of this disorder by the public or the medical profession. Physicians have been aware of the symptoms and physical findings of iron deficiency for many years; however, only in recent years have physicians become more aware of the prevalence of iron overload and its manifestations. Second, patients frequently do not develop symptoms until late adulthood, and when symptoms develop, they may mimic other common disorders in this age group, such as diabetes mellitus, arthritis, and congestive heart failure. Third, there is variability in the phenotypic expression of the disease, and, although it was earlier suggested that all homozygotes become iron loaded,[134] it is unclear why there is such variation in the degree of iron loading between probands, and it is now recognized that many C2824 homozygotes may manifest low or no penetrance to HFE gene mutation and may never become iron loaded.[167] Environmental factors such as the quantity of dietary iron, the ingestion of agents that can enhance iron absorption (e.g., ethanol, ascorbate), or factors such as gastrointestinal blood loss or blood donation can affect the expression of the disease. Variations in iron stores among homozygotes of approximately the same age can occur,[167] and although the degree of iron loading within a pedigree is not always constant, recent studies have shown reasonable concordance of iron storage in siblings with HH, suggesting that genetic factors are most important in determining the degree of iron loading.[168] However, it is not clear which patients with the genetic disease will go on to develop heavy iron loading and clinical symptoms.

Although it is generally agreed that homozygosity for the C282Y mutation has a high positive predictive accuracy for phenotypic HH, these are only two population studies to date that have evaluated the penetrance of this *HFE* gene mutation. In a comprehensive study from Western Australia the entire population of Busselton (more than 9000 individuals) were surveyed for phenotypic expression of the C282Y mutation. Although all C282Y homozygotes had elevated transferrin iron saturation (TS) (100 percent positive predictive accuracy) only 58 percent of these showed evidence of progressive hepatic iron overloading.[169] This issue of non-expression was also evaluated in a health appraisal clinic in the United States[170] but expression in this population was not assessed by evaluation of tissue iron levels (the ultimate gold standard). This correlation has relevance to both early diagnosis and the ultimate prognosis and need for treatment. It is under intensive scrutiny in North America with recruitment of 100,000 people to a large prospective study funded by the National Institutes of Health (NIH).[171]

The potential for early detection of homozygotes relies on the awareness of the significance of clinical markers such as asymptomatic hepatomegaly with normal or minimally abnormal aminotransferases, early onset sexual dysfunction, and unexplained atypical arthropathy or cardiac disease. Similarly, appropriate investigation of asymptomatic individuals with positive serum markers of iron overload can identify patients with early homozygous HH. Because timely removal of iron by phlebotomy can prevent long-term complications and will result in a normal life expectancy,[8] it is recommended that all clues to the presence of iron overload should be pursued, and if they are persistent, direct evidence of increased tissue iron should be sought. Currently, the minimum criteria for the diagnosis of HH are increased iron stores and compatible *HFE* gene mutations, both in the absence of a cause for secondary iron overload. A positive family history of iron overload is useful, but it is often lacking because of the inability to study a complete pedigree. Although a genetic diagnosis alone may supplant these combined criteria, and patients may be identified before they exhibit any phenotypic expression, the ultimate decision on the need for treatment will remain dependent on the assessment of the extent of the development of iron loading.

Data on diagnostic accuracy of phenotypic screening tests have been acquired by studies both in asymptomatic populations (e.g., healthy blood donors and large-scale screening of healthy populations) and in families of detected homozygotes.[137,171-173] As indicated previously, more recent studies are available for assessment of the correlation between genotypic mutations and phenotypic expression.[125,169,170,174]

Blood Studies

When HH is suspected for any of the reasons mentioned above, serum iron, total iron binding capacity (TIBC) or transferrin, and ferritin concentrations should be determined. Serum iron levels can vary both by diurnal variation[175] and after ingestion of meals[176]; therefore, iron studies should be obtained fasting in the morning. Serum transferrin has replaced total iron binding capacity in some laboratories and formulas exist for reliably calculating transferrin saturation regardless of whether TIBC or transferrin is used.[177] Normal values and those expected in HH are shown in Table 42-4. In iron overload the serum iron and ferritin are usually increased and the TIBC or transferrin may be normal or decreased. Transferrin saturation is typically increased. Elevations of serum iron in the absence of iron overload occur commonly; examples include determination in the nonfasting state, after ingestion of iron-containing multivitamin pills, in the presence of co-incidental hepatocellular necrosis in patients with other types of liver disease, and in some heterozygotes for HH without significant expansion of their iron stores.[130,178,179] The lack of sensitivity and specificity of the serum iron concentration makes it an unreliable test when used alone. The TS, calculated by dividing the serum iron by the total iron binding capacity, is far more sensitive and specific. The latter is determined from the sum of the iron and the unsaturated iron binding capacity. Significant elevations in iron stores are usually associated with a TS greater than 70 percent. However, a TS greater than 45 percent requires further investigation. In a recent study values for TS greater than 45 percent correctly identified 98 percent of homozygotes with no false positives in a control, normal population.[180] Although there are others who have pointed out exceptions to this rule in identified genetic homozygotes,[170] the Practice Guidelines Committee of the American Association for the Study of Liver Diseases has endorsed this blood test as the initial step in the algorithm for management of HH (Figure 42-3).[11]

Studies of large numbers of families with HH in several countries have shown that the serum ferritin level correlates well with the size of the body iron stores[172,181-184] and the liver iron concentration.[92,185] However, it fails to distinguish between parenchymal and reticuloendothelial iron and is not always specific for iron overload because tissue damage, inflammation, and certain neoplastic diseases can cause a nonspecific rise in serum ferritin.[15,165,166] Furthermore, it is recognized that young homozygotes may have normal or only slightly increased serum ferritin levels, but still have significantly elevated liver iron concentrations and total body iron stores.[92,172,181,183-188] Nevertheless, a serum ferritin level in the normal range shown in Table 42-4, taken in combination with a TS lower than 45 percent, has a negative predictive value of 97 percent and exceeds the accuracy of the indirect tests used in isolation.[172] Furthermore, in confirmed HH a level of serum ferritin greater than 1000 ng/ml is an accurate predictor of the degree of hepatic fibrosis and cirrhosis.[189]

Reconciliation of these dilemmas in interpreting serum iron studies requires careful evaluation of the clinical setting in which the iron studies are obtained. Thus when evaluating individuals who are asymptomatic, with no other co-existing inflammatory or neoplastic disease,

TABLE 42-4
Representative Iron Studies in Hemochromatosis

Determination	Normal range	Hemochromatosis
Serum		
Iron (μg/dl)	60-180	180-200
Total iron binding capacity (μg/dl)	250-410	200-300
Transferrin (mg/dl)	220-410	200-300
Transferrin saturation (%)	15-44	45-100
Ferritin (ng/ml)		
Men	20-200	300-6000
Women	15-150	250-6000
Hepatic		
Iron concentration		
(μg/g, dry weight)	300-1500	5000-30,000*
(μmol/g, dry weight)	5-27	89-550
Iron index†		
(μmol/g, dry weight per year)	<1.5	>1.9

*Some young homozygotes may have hepatic iron concentration < 5000 μg/g.
†Some homozygotes (~10%) will have hepatic iron index < 1.9.

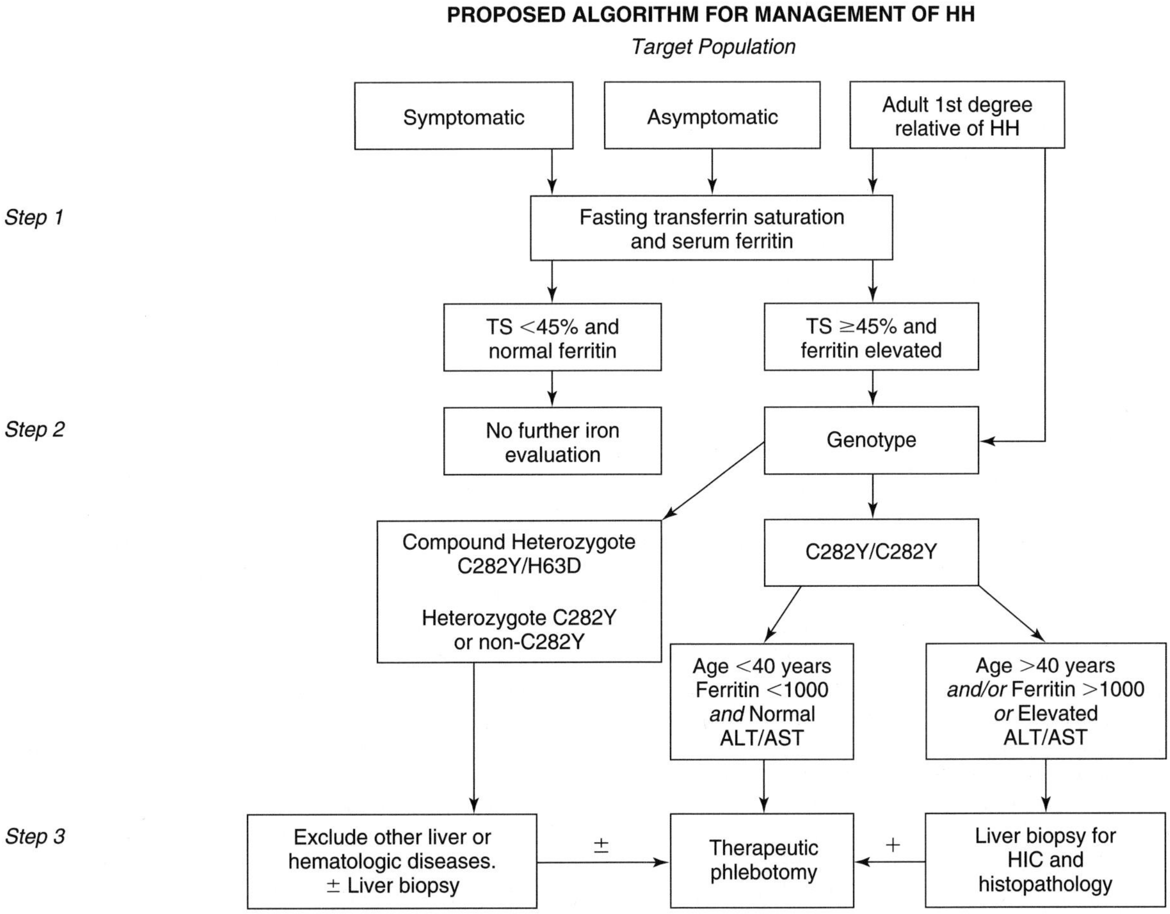

PROPOSED ALGORITHM FOR MANAGEMENT OF HH
Target Population
Symptomatic
Asymptomatic
Adult 1st degree relative of HH
Step 1
Fasting transferrin saturation and serum ferritin
TS <45% and normal ferritin
TS ≥45% and ferritin elevated
Step 2
No further iron evaluation
Genotype
Compound Heterozygote C282Y/H63D
Heterozygote C282Y or non-C282Y
C282Y/C282Y
Age <40 years Ferritin <1000 *and* Normal ALT/AST
Age >40 years *and/or* Ferritin >1000 *or* Elevated ALT/AST
Step 3
Exclude other liver or hematologic diseases. ± Liver biopsy
±
Therapeutic phlebotomy
+
Liver biopsy for HIC and histopathology

Figure 42-3 Proposed algorithm for management of HH. *HH,* Hereditary hemochromatosis. (From Hepatology 33:132, 2001.)

and with iron studies that are obtained in the fasting state, the results are quite reliable for either the presence or absence of HH.

A common clinical scenario is that in which serum iron studies are obtained in a patient who is hospitalized with some sort of acute or chronic illness or is an ambulatory outpatient with any one of a number of conditions known to affect serum iron tests. These include inflammatory disorders, various malignancies, and all types of necroinflammatory liver diseases.[15,165,166,190,191] For example, in patients with chronic viral hepatitis, serum ferritin can be elevated in up to 40 percent of individuals,[165] and in a study of patients with non-alcoholic steatohepatitis serum ferritin was increased in 50 percent of patients.[166] Iron studies are abnormal in up to 50 percent of ALD patients.[15,191] In certain of these clinical settings the only way to resolve the issue of whether abnormal iron studies represent HH or are merely related to another unrelated condition is to perform a liver biopsy for histochemical and biochemical evaluation of tissue iron stores.

Genotypic Testing: Mutation Analysis

The second step in the proposed diagnostic algorithm is to determine the presence of the *HFE* gene mutations C282Y and H63D (see Figure 42-3) in individuals with a TS equal to or greater than 45 percent and on a raised serum ferritin. These two missense mutations are responsible for 83 percent to 100 percent of phenotypic patients with this disorder,[30] and are most usually determined by restriction endonuclease digestion or oligonucleotide ligation assay of amplified deoxyribonucleic acid derived by polymerase chain reaction using the primers employed in the original cloning of the *HFE* gene.[9] This earlier anti-sense primer may overestimate these mutations because of a confounding single-nucleotide polymorphism in its binding region and may be replaced with new primers that exclude this polymorphism.[192]

C282Y homozygous individuals with serum indicators of iron overload who are unlikely to have significant hepatic injury may proceed to therapeutic phlebotomy without the need for a liver biopsy. These are likely to be individuals younger than 40 years of age without other risk factors for liver disease (e.g., alcohol or viral hepatitis), without evidence on physical examination or routine laboratory evaluation of necroinflammatory disease or established fibrosis and cirrhosis (raised alanine aminotransferase or clinical hepatomegaly), and usually with a serum ferritin that is less than 1000 ng/ml. The latter laboratory evaluation has been shown to be a useful discriminant function for the detection of fibrosis and cirrhosis.[189] Although it is recognized that the penetrance of the C282Y gene mutation is variable it is generally agreed that all first-degree relatives of a known proband older than age 20 years should be offered gene mutation analysis.[11] The use of mutation analysis in the spouse of a homozygote allows for determination of the genetic risk in children and may be a cost-effective way to avoid unnecessary testing of children when the spouse is found to be a non-carrier of the mutation.[136] The other mutation (H63D) has been associated as a cofactor in some cases of HH. In particular, compound heterozygosity (C282Y/H63D) accounts for 3 percent to 5 percent of phenotypic HH, which is a significantly higher genotypic frequency than in the general white population.[30] The value of an awareness of the genotypic constitution (C282Y/C282Y or C282Y/H63D) of a suspected proband is the additional evidence it offers that elevated indirect serum markers truly reflect iron overload resulting from HH. Likewise, in a first-degree relative of a homozygote, serum markers offer an indication of the need for careful monitoring of phenotypic markers and appropriate preventive phlebotomy when these become evident.

Although we continue to emphasize the predominant genotypic mutations responsible for the majority of HH in whites of Northern European origin, it is becoming increasingly recognized that there are almost certainly genes other than *HFE* that play a role in familial iron overload, particularly in Southern Europe.[193-195] Similar studies of hemochromatosis in Africa and juvenile hemochromatosis are lending credence to other genetic predispositions to iron overload. For this reason, this diagnostic algorithm emphasizes the importance of pursuing phenotypic clues on their own merits.[11,196] Even when previously unsuspected causes of secondary iron overload are excluded there remains a subgroup of patients who are homozygous wild-type at the 282 locus yet who meet all the criteria for iron overload seen in classic HH.[195]

Liver Biopsy

In uncomplicated patients with HH an elevated serum ferritin level indicates expansion of the total body iron stores, and a raised transferrin saturation points to their predominantly parenchymal localization; however, in the circumstances indicated previously, direct evidence is required for the accumulation of iron in the major storage organ, namely the liver, and for its pathologic effects in the form of fibrosis and cirrhosis. To achieve both of these aims a liver biopsy may be performed. A typical percutaneous needle biopsy yields sufficient tissue for histopathologic evaluation and for biochemical measurement of HIC. The Perls' Prussian blue stain (potassium ferrocyanide for ferric iron) is used for the determination and localization of storage iron. A semiquantitative grading system (grades 1-4) was initially established based on the extent of Prussian blue granule deposition,[76,80,198] so that grade 4 represents stainable iron in virtually 100 percent of hepatocytes, grade 3 in 75 percent, grade 2 in 50 percent, and grade 1 in 25 percent of hepatocytes. This approach seems logical in view of the initial periportal deposition of iron in HH with subsequent involvement of the entire lobule as iron accretion progresses. Numerous other grading methods have been proposed, but, unfortunately, there has typically been a poor correlation between qualitative evaluations of stainable iron and HIC.[76,97] Grades 1 and 2 Perls' Prussian blue staining can be seen in normal liver,[199,200] whereas grade 3 stainable iron is often observed in alcoholic cirrhosis, where it correlates poorly with HIC.[15,123] Although it is agreed that grade 4 deposition indicates a heavy iron burden, grades 2 and 3 are much more difficult to interpret. A more sophisticated grading system is that devised by Deugnier and associates, which, although tedious and complicated, allows for the most reliable estimation of hepatic iron stores short of biochemical measurement.[201]

Perls' Prussian blue staining is also important for determining the cellular and lobular distribution of the iron deposition, realizing that in HH iron deposits are predominantly in hepatocytes in a periportal distribution, whereas in parenteral iron overload, iron is predominantly in Kupffer cells in a panlobular distribution.

The biochemical determination of HIC is most often performed on fresh, untreated biopsy samples. At the time of biopsy, about 0.5 to 1.0 cm of the core is taken for determination of HIC. Samples should be transported dry and can be frozen if not assayed quickly.[202] Current methods employ colorimetric or atomic absorption spectrophotometric measurement of non-heme iron after appropriate chemical digestion of the tissue. In practice these analytical methods give very comparable results,[203] and the choice among them depends on whichever technique is available. The colorimetric method of Torrance and Bothwell[131,204] has proved to be very reproducible, relatively simple, and inexpensive to perform. If fresh liver is unavailable for measurement, tissue extracted from the paraffin block can be used. A recent study has shown an excellent correlation (r = 0.946) between HIC measured on fresh tissue and formalin-preserved tissue, providing that more than 0.4 mg of dry tissue (approximately 1.2 mg wet tissue) was available.[202]

Depending on the reference laboratory the upper limit of normal for HIC ranges from 900 to 1800 μg/g dry weight.[7,198] Virtually all patients with symptomatic HH have concentrations higher than10,000 μg/g and patients with established hepatic fibrosis and cirrhosis are typically higher than 22,000 μg/g dry weight, but may be as low as 12,000 to 14,000 μg/g even in the absence of associated excessive alcohol intake (see Table 42-4).[7,96] Patients with ALD and increased stainable iron usually fall in the range of 2000 to 5000 μg/g, but do not exceed 10,000 μg/g,[7,15,185] whereas those with HH and cirrhosis who drink excessive amounts of alcohol or have chronic viral hepatitis B or C can fall in the range of 8000 to 22,000 μg/g.[7,165,205] It should be emphasized that asymptomatic precirrhotic homozygotes almost always have an HIC above the normal range, but because iron accretion is age-related,[7] the actual level must be interpreted with the age factor in mind. This concept provided the basis for the development of the hepatic iron index (HII), which is the HIC (in μmol/g dry weight) divided by the age of the patient (in years),[7] as μmol/g per year (i.e., it expresses rate of accretion of iron).

Whereas the HIC with the calculated HII constitutes the "gold standard" by which iron overload is judged, the ultimate test of total body iron stores is the amount removed by phlebotomy. Each unit of blood removed is equivalent to about 250 mg of iron, depending on the hemoglobin. Most normal individuals, and those with spurious indirect markers of iron overload, will become iron deficient after removal of up to 2.5 g of iron. Patients with symptomatic HH will usually require at least 18 months of weekly phlebotomy (equivalent to 15-20 g of iron) before becoming iron depleted. Younger, prefibrotic patients will require significantly fewer phlebotomies.

The value of liver biopsy extends beyond the documentation of the HIC. Documentation of bridging fibrosis or cirrhosis may have an impact on the prognosis in HH. Reliance on aminotransferase levels in serum lacks predictive accuracy. For example, up to 50 percent of patients with cirrhotic HH have normal ALT levels.[174] Furthermore, cirrhosis and its complications, in particular HCC, account for 75 percent of HH related deaths[8]; therefore knowledge of the staging of fibrosis may be used as a guideline for future monitoring of an HH patient even after completion of iron removal. This recommendation is reinforced by the awareness that the majority of HCC in HH are diagnosed an average of 9 years after completion of phlebotomy.[8] As indicated previously there are circumstances in which liver biopsy may be considered unnecessary for diagnosis and the patient may proceed to therapeutic phlebotomy and ultimate confirmation of iron overload calculated from phlebotomy requirements. In particular, a very high serum ferritin (more than 1000 ng/ml), more likely to be found in homozygotes older than 40 years of age, or in those with an elevated ALT, hepatomegaly or other signs of chronic liver disease pointing to fibrosis or cirrhosis are indications for liver biopsy for the reasons given previously. Likewise, a similar approach should be taken in compound heterozygotes, C282Y heterozygotes, or non-*HFE* mutated individuals if they have elevated ALT or other evidence of liver disease.

The differentiation between patients with underlying liver disease (e.g., ALD, chronic viral hepatitis, nonalcoholic steatohepatitis) and associated abnormal serum iron studies with or without hepatic iron overload and the patient with HH who has abnormal liver function poses a diagnostic problem for the practicing internist and hepatologist. The problem is compounded by two factors: (1) the high prevalence of abnormal serum iron tests in patients with liver disease and the relatively low sensitivity and specificity of the indirect tests for assessment of iron overload in these patients with liver disease[15,165,166,185] and (2) the lack of correlation between stainable iron on liver biopsy and the HIC. Although the presence of increased iron deposition determined histologically is more common in alcoholics, very few have grade 3 to 4 stainable iron, and the latter most likely also have HH.[205]

In an earlier study determination of HIC in 60 ALD patients and 15 patients with HH showed that 29 percent of the alcoholic subjects had HIC that were elevated, ranging from 1400 μg/g to 7500 μg/g.[15] In contrast, HIC higher than 10,000 μg/g were found in all 15 patients with HH. Thus determination of HIC in this study clearly differentiated ALD with significant stainable iron from patients with HH. Because patients with HH are being identified at a younger age with lower HIC, there may be overlap in hepatic iron levels between these two groups. Delineation between these two groups and identification of heterozygotes with only trivial increases in HIC may be achieved by use of the HII, which adjusts for age. In the first study describing HII 30 homozygous relatives of HH probands were compared with 51 patients with ALD and 40 control subjects.[7] Use of the HII effectively discriminated between young HH homozygotes, HH heterozygotes, and patients with ALD and secondary iron overload. Since that first description of the HII, there have been at least five subsequent studies, all of which have shown that homozygotes with HH have an HII greater than 1.9 and that all patients with ALD and secondary iron overload and all HH heterozygotes had an index of less than 1.5 (Table 42-5).[95-97,201,206] For patients with an index between 1.5 and 1.8, additional clinical judgment is required and a conservative approach for these patients is to recommend phlebotomy treatment to determine their total body iron burden.

Although the application of the HII proved valuable in the differentiation of iron overload in HH from that in potentially other confounding clinical situations, with a rate in excess of 1.9 μmol/g per year providing strong support for the diagnosis of homozygous HH, recent data suggest that up to 15 percent of C282Y homozygotes have rates lower than this,[174,248] despite HIC that are significantly elevated, whereas end-stage liver disease patients without HH may have an HII in excess of 1.9.[207] The level of the HII has therefore lost some of its importance as an essential criterion of diagnosis.[124] Finally, it should be emphasized that the rate of accretion of iron in some causes of secondary iron overload, particularly those associated with dyserythropoiesis, is even higher than in HH, yielding very high HII values.

Non-invasive Imaging Modalities

Alternative, non-invasive techniques have been sought for those few individuals in whom liver biopsy is not possible. Such alternative techniques include (1) computed tomography (CT), (2) magnetic resonance imaging (MRI), and (3) magnetic susceptibility measurement. All exploit the physical properties of storage iron and depend on the calibration of that physical property with the HIC.

Computed Tomography

On CT scanning, the linear attenuation co-efficient (CT number) is increased by iron because of its high relative electron density compared with other cellular constituents (Figure 42-4).[208] In HH conventional single-energy CT scanning has not proved to be a very sensitive or specific test for iron overload, although it did appear in one study to be more specific than the serum ferritin concentration.[209] In addition, CT scanning has been shown to correlate well with the HIC in patients with iron overload resulting from thalassemia major.[210] Its sensitivity has been increased by the use of a dual-energy technique that yielded an excellent positive correlation between the attenuation co-efficient and the HIC in both the precirrhotic and cirrhotic stages of hemochromatosis.[211] However, this technique requires non-standard modifications of equipment and complicated calibration methodology, and the correlations have not been consistent at mild to moderate degrees of iron overload.[212]

Magnetic Resonance Imaging

MRI is currently being evaluated for application as a quantitative method for the assessment of HIC. Studies in experimental animals have shown decreased spin-echo image intensity in iron overload because of a marked decrease in the transverse (T2) relaxation time.[213-215] Use of tissue relaxation rates (l/Tl and l/T2) and optimized spin-echo sequences resulted in initial hopes for a reasonably

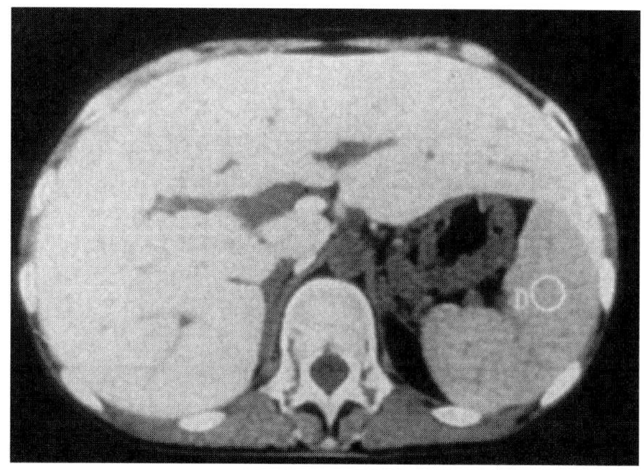

Figure 42-4 Computed tomography scan in HH. Massive iron overload results in increased density in the liver in HH. *HH,* Hereditary hemochromatosis.

TABLE 42-5

Hepatic Iron Index in Hereditary Hemochromatosis

				HEMOCHROMATOSIS	
Study	Country	Normal	Alcoholic liver disease	Heterozygotes	Homozygotes
Bassett et al[7]	Australia	<1.0	<1.4	<1.8	>2.0
Summers et al[45]	Australia	—	—	<1.5	>1.9
Olynyket al[97]	Australia	<1.1	<1.6	—	>2.1
Bonkovsky et al[206]	United States	<0.7	<1.1	<1.8	>2.0
Sallie et al[96]	Australia	—	<1.6	—	>2.0
Deugnier et al[201]	France, Australia	—	—	<1.5	>1.9

accurate assessment of hepatic iron overload in patients with HH.

Although these earlier studies using high Tesla MRI instruments showed promise in iron overload states, recent studies have indicated that the technology may give inaccurate and misleading results when there is very marked iron overload or hepatic fibrosis and cirrhosis.[216]

Magnetic Susceptibility

The paramagnetic properties of ferritin and hemosiderin have been exploited for the measurement of hepatic iron stores. Non-invasive human determinations became possible with the development of the superconducting quantum interference device. An induced magnetic field is amplified quantitatively by storage iron in the liver, and this enhancement can be specifically and reproducibly measured by the magnetic susceptometer. With appropriate calibration, measurements made in humans with iron overload have shown excellent correlation over a thirtyfold range of HIC, measured independently by the quantitative biochemical method.[217-219] Although an instrument is now available commercially it is expensive and can be used reliably only for the measurement of iron in the liver. As such, it has limited applicability, and is affordable only to specialized referral centers.

Abnormalities in Hereditary Hemochromatosis Heterozygotes

Earlier studies have shown that patients considered to be heterozygous for HH have mean HIC that are significantly higher than for controls but significantly lower than for HH homozygotes. It is likely that many of these heterozygotes were in fact compound heterozygotes with one allele containing the C282Y mutation and one allele containing the H63D mutation. In a study of patients with liver disease on whom HIC and *HFE* mutation analysis were performed, it has been shown that there is a significant increase in HIC for those patients who are compound heterozygotes (C282Y/H63D) but there was no difference in C282Y heterozygotes (C282Y/wt), H63D heterozygotes (H63D/wt), or H63D homozygotes (H63D/H63D), or in individuals without these mutations (wt/wt).[174] In fact the compound heterozygote genotype is found in about 1 percent to 2 percent of the general population, and this genotype accounts for about 4 percent to 5 percent of patients in series of typical HH patients. Thus some patients with the C282Y/H63D genotype can develop fairly significant degrees of hepatic iron loading but the vast majority of these patients are not heavily iron-loaded. In patients with heavy iron overload who are found to be C282Y heterozygotes (C282Y/wt), alternative causes of iron loading should be investigated. The diagnostic algorithm outlined previously provides for this pathway of evaluation.[11]

Approach to Population Screening

It seems reasonable to advocate routine population screening for HH, given the high prevalence of the disorder and the ease, safety, and success of phlebotomy therapy (Table 42-6). Population screening studies in Europe, North America, and Australia using an elevated transferrin saturation to assess phenotypic expression have shown that about 1 in 200 to 400 individuals have evidence of phenotypic expression of iron overload. Conversely, screening studies using *HFE* mutation analysis have shown many non-expressing C282Y homozygotes. Thus in a screening study in San Diego of 10,198 individuals, 43 were found to be C282Y homozygotes (i.e., 1 in 237 people).[170] Ten of these were already known and of the remaining 33 who were newly discovered, 36 percent had normal transferrin saturation levels (less than 45 percent). Thus the sensitivity of elevated transferrin saturation and elevated serum ferritin level for detecting C282Y homozygotes in this study was only 0.70. Currently, the NIH is sponsoring a large-scale screening study that will most likely result in policy decisions about population screening for HH. If a screening program is recommended it is anticipated that it will involve measuring transferrin saturation to assess phenotypic expression, followed by *HFE* mutation analysis in individuals with elevated transferrin saturation levels.[136,261] Also, this large NIH screening study will evaluate the significance of genetic discrimination and stigmatization resulting from *HFE* genotyping.

Family Screening and the Value of HFE Mutation Analysis

After an HH proband has been carefully identified and therapy is initiated, there is still a responsibility to the patient's family. For asymptomatic C282Y homozygotes and compound heterozygotes (C282Y/H63D), identified by *HFE* mutation analysis within a sibship, there is no

TABLE 42-6
Population Screening for Hereditary Hemochromatosis

Study	Country	Population	Prevalence
Velati et al[135]	Italy	Blood donors	1:500
Leggett et al[133]	Australia	General	1:300
Edwards et al[137]	United States	Blood donors	1:220
Borwein et al[173]	Canada	General	1:300
Olynyk et al[169]	Australia	General (large population with genotype correlation)	1:150
Beutler et al[170]	United States	General (large population with genotype correlation)	1:237

need for a liver biopsy. In this setting it is reasonable to proceed directly to therapeutic phlebotomy, reserving liver biopsy for those patients in whom there may be a question of other underlying liver disease.[11] For those individuals who are C282Y heterozygotes, there appears to be no risk for progressive iron overload. When a proband is identified questions often arise about the risk of their children having HH. In this setting the other parent of the children should be tested; if there are no mutations, then nothing further needs to be done for the children. On the other hand, if the other parent has either a C282Y or an H63D mutation, then the children are at risk of either being either a C282Y homozygote or a compound heterozygote (C282Y/H63D).[136] If children are identified as C282Y homozygotes or compound heterozygotes, then yearly ferritin levels should be performed and phlebotomy instituted when ferritin levels become elevated.

Whether or not genetic testing of children should be performed is controversial given the implications of a child having a "genetic disease." Obviously, appropriate recommendations could be made to ensure that no significant iron loading would ever occur because regular phlebotomy could be instituted early. With the complete characterization of the human genome, society will have to develop mechanisms for dealing with the genetic diagnoses that all individuals carry. Guarantees against insurance discrimination, job discrimination, and genetic stigmatization will have to be developed.

Treatment and Prognosis of Iron Overload

With the awareness of methods for the detection of presymptomatic homozygous cases, there has been a significant reduction in the morbidity and mortality of HH. Similarly, in secondary or parenteral iron overload resulting from inherited dyserythropoietic conditions with or without associated transfusions, early management with parenteral deferoxamine has proved effective in minimizing or delaying the toxic effects of iron accumulation.

Several studies have evaluated the benefits of iron depletion by phlebotomy.[62,132,220-222] Long ago, the outcome for patients with HH was determined by the course of the diabetes mellitus. With the availability of insulin the average expected survival after diagnosis improved from 2 to about 4 years.[62] In the first study to define the benefit of therapeutic phlebotomy, untreated patients experienced a 5-year survival of 18 percent and a 10-year survival of only 10 percent.[220] The survival with phlebotomy improved to 66 percent and 32 percent at 5 and 10 years, respectively. A later study demonstrated a survival rate with treatment of 70 percent at both 5 and 10 years after diagnosis.[62] However, a worsened prognosis was found when there was associated alcoholism. In the series of 163 patients first reported by Niederau and associates,[221] in the absence of diabetes or cirrhosis the life expectancy of treated patients with HH was virtually identical to that expected of age- and sex-matched controls. However, in the presence of established cirrhosis, 5- and 10-year survival rates were 90 percent and 70 percent, respectively; with diabetes, survival rates of 90 percent and 63 percent were observed at 5 and 10 years. Thus both complications were associated with significantly increased mortality compared with the control population. The primary factor in determining the presence of these two major complications was the extent of the iron burden. In the 77 patients depleted of iron within 18 months by regular phlebotomy, survival was normal, whereas in the 75 patients who could not be depleted in 18 months, only 60 percent were alive at 10 years. Furthermore, the patients who died after achieving iron depletion had iron stores larger than those who survived (32 g versus 21 g). Death rates from diabetes (sevenfold increase), cirrhosis (thirteenfold increase), primary liver cancer (220-fold increase), and cardiomyopathy (306-fold increase) were all significantly higher than those expected from these causes in a matched population. These conclusions were confirmed when the extended study was reported by this group 11 years later (Table 42-7).[8] Two other studies of long-term survival from Canada[132] and Italy[222] have yielded similar results wherein between 50 percent and 60 percent of the deaths occurred from causes that could be attributed directly to the effects of iron overload. These studies emphasize the importance of early diagnosis to improving survival.

Removal of iron by therapeutic phlebotomy is the mainstay of treatment of HH. Once weekly or twice weekly (if tolerated) removal of 500 ml of blood (equivalent to 250 mg of iron) should be continued until the storage iron pool is depleted. In practice this may take 2 to 3 years for those individuals with a very heavy body iron burden (more than 30 g). In the study by Edwards and colleagues[223] of 35 homozygotes the 20 treated males required an average of 68 phlebotomies to achieve depletion, whereas the 10 treated females required an av-

TABLE 42-7
Causes of Death in Hemochromatosis[8]

Cause of death*	Mortality ratio (observed/expected)	Proportion of all deaths (%)†
Cancer of liver	119	28
Cirrhosis	10	20
Diabetes mellitus	14	6
Cardiomyopathy	14	7

*These four causes of death among 69 patients who died in a series of 251 patients with hereditary hemochromatosis were shown to be significantly higher than the expected rates in a normal population.
†The remaining 39% of deaths occurred from causes that were not significantly more frequent than in the control population.

erage of 25 phlebotomies. The diagnosis of HH is now often made in presymptomatic homozygotes with genetic testing only, so phlebotomy requirements may be much lower. It is recommended that all individuals with HH who have evidence of iron overload indicated by an elevated ferritin above the upper limit of normal or an elevated transferrin saturation be offered treatment. With treatment the serum ferritin level can be expected to decline progressively during therapy,[62,223] with the greatest fall per mg of iron removed (about 1 ng/ml of ferritin per 2 mg of iron) occurring during the early phlebotomies (Figure 42-5). The serum iron and the transferrin saturation usually remain elevated until iron depletion has occurred. Usually, they do not fall until the serum ferritin falls below 30 to 50 ng/ml.[62,223] At this point the hematocrit also falls, which is an indication of the development of iron deficiency. Initial therapeutic phlebotomy should be continued until ferritin is less than 50 ng/ml and transferrin saturation is less than 50 percent. The frequency of phlebotomy can then be reduced to three to six per year to maintain transferrin saturation at 25 percent to 50 percent. During weekly phlebotomy therapy it is not necessary to repeat serum iron studies. Rather, the hematocrit, which should have returned to within 5 percent to 10 percent of its baseline value, can be used as a suitable safeguard to prevent the development of symptomatic anemia during therapy. Measurement of ferritin and transferrin saturation periodically (every 2 to 3 months) is useful to predict phlebotomy requirements and is helpful to encourage patients to continue with therapy, but it is not absolutely necessary.

Improvement in liver function and regression of hepatomegaly have been reported in about 50 percent of patients treated by phlebotomy.[220] Cirrhosis is usually not reversible; however, there have been occasional reports of regression of fibrosis and cirrhosis based on serial liver biopsies in treated patients.[224,225] Although the possibility of sampling error in these cases was not ruled out, the potential for reversibility supports the concept of phlebotomy treatment in all patients, even those with established cirrhosis. This is further supported by the improved survival of patients with cirrhosis treated by phlebotomy.[8,221] In contrast, fewer than one third of patients show improvement in diabetes, as evidenced by unchanged insulin requirements.[220] Although pigmentation is improved by removal of iron, hypogonadism and established arthropathy are not ameliorated. There is almost invariable relief of malaise, weakness, lethargy, and frequent right upper quadrant pain occurring in patients with heavy hepatic iron deposits.

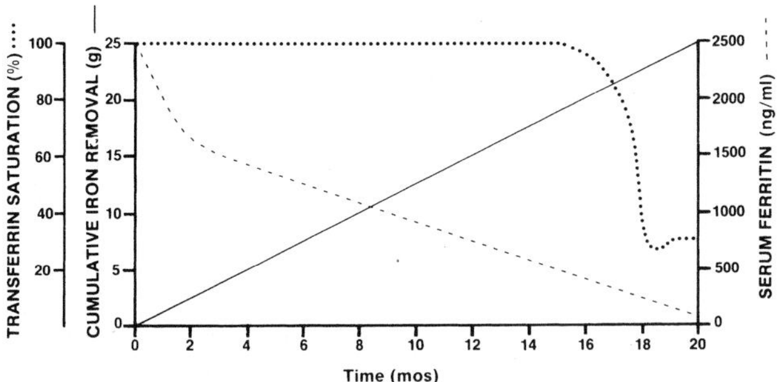

Figure 42-5 Response of indirect markers of iron overload to phlebotomy therapy. This figure illustrates the reciprocal relationship between the serum ferritin level and the removal of excess iron stores. The fall in transferrin iron saturation antedates the complete removal of storage iron (in this example, 25 g). At this time a fall in the hematocrit value can be expected, indicating a relative iron deficiency.

The single most common cause of acute death in HH and in secondary iron overload is cardiomyopathy and cardiac dysrhythmia (see Table 42-5).[8,62,221] This is regarded as a circumstance warranting accelerated removal of iron by a combination of phlebotomy and chelation therapy with deferoxamine.[226,227] Although it has been shown that ascorbic acid treatment can serve to maximize the chelatable iron pool, caution has been expressed regarding the adjuvant use of ascorbic acid with iron mobilization therapy because of deterioration in cardiac function.[228]

In HH, phlebotomy is the treatment of choice because of the rapidity with which storage iron can be mobilized. Although each unit of blood removed is equivalent to the loss of about 250 mg of iron, it should be remembered that iron absorption from the gastrointestinal tract is promoted by therapeutic reduction of iron stores, increasing from 1 to 4 mg/day to 4 to 8 mg/day during phlebotomy.[229] This increase is equivalent to an extra unit of blood every 2 months. Phlebotomy has been used in various forms of secondary iron overload, African iron overload,[230] and porphyria cutanea tarda (PCT)[231] with evidence of clinical benefit. However, in a preliminary study its use in patients with ALD and iron overload did not improve the outcome of the disease.[232] Although alcohol appears to have a synergistic effect with iron in producing liver damage in HH, adverse effects of smaller deposits (less than 10 g total) of iron in patients with ALD have not been demonstrated.

In those forms of secondary iron overload associated with anemia (e.g., the thalassemia syndromes) phlebotomy is not a feasible form of treatment. It is in these diseases that considerable effort has been devoted to the development of suitable chelation therapy. Deferoxamine, as first introduced 40 years ago, is still the only iron-chelating agent that is clinically useful. It is effective when delivered parenterally, either by subcutaneous or intravenous infusion. Although three major studies had demonstrated the efficacy of deferoxamine in increasing life expectancy and arresting the development of hepatic fibrosis in thalassemia,[233-235] the use of the drug did not become widespread until it was shown that continuous infusions were superior to bolus injections in enhancing urinary iron excretion.[236] The infusions are administered on 5 to 6 nights per week, for 8 to 12 hours, at a dose of 1 to 6 g depending on the age and weight of the patient and the degree of iron loading. With increasing dosage, fecal iron excretion is progressively enhanced and may exceed urinary excretion.[237] It is generally recommended that ascorbic acid in a small dose (100-200 mg) be given during the deferoxamine infusion to enhance urinary iron excretion.[227] This mode of administration (i.e., small doses in the presence of a chelator) has not been associated with enhanced cardiac toxicity. Because the rate of iron accumulation in dyserythropoietic anemias is more rapid than in HH, the potential for earlier tissue damage, particularly to the myocardium, is greater. The anticipated benefits of early chelation therapy in the prevention of cardiac, hepatic, and pancreatic injury have been realized in a number of trials supporting the efficacy and safety of such intervention.[226,233-235]

LIVER TRANSPLANTATION FOR HEREDITARY HEMOCHROMATOSIS

With the advent of successful and readily available orthotopic liver transplantation (OLT) in the early 1980s a significant number of patients with end-stage liver disease due to HH, either alone or in conjunction with other liver diseases (e.g., alcohol, chronic hepatitis C), have now received transplants. A number of important issues and observations have arisen from this experience. First, it has been recognized that patients who undergo transplantation for HH are frequently undiagnosed (relative to their HH) at the time of transplant, usually because of severe coagulopathy precluding pretransplant biopsy. Second, with the advent of *HFE* mutation analysis, studies of heavily iron-loaded patients coming to liver transplantation have shown that only about 10 percent of patients who have heavy degrees of iron overload in the explant liver actually were C282Y homozygotes.[238] The remaining patients had other causes of end-stage liver disease (e.g., hepatitis C, alcohol) and, in fact, were found to have severe secondary iron overload as a result of their underlying liver disease.

The 1-year survival after OLT in iron-loaded patients in several studies has been only about 50 percent,[238-242] which is much lower than that for all types of liver disease evaluated in the aggregate (approximately 80 percent to 90 percent). Usual reasons for decreased survival are infectious complications or those resulting from severe cardiac dysfunction in the peritransplant or immediate post-transplant period.[238,241,242] Deferoxamine given intravenously at the time of these cardiac events has occasionally resulted in significant improvement and ultimate long-term survival. In one study survival was not influenced by the presence of concomitant primary liver cancer, a finding that was unsuspected preoperatively in 70 percent of cases.[241] It is hoped that greater recognition of HH will lead to increased pretransplant diagnosis so that patients can be at least partially treated before OLT, with the expectation that this will reduce post-transplant iron-related complications.

At least four patients undergoing liver transplantation for non-HH liver disease have received livers from donors with previously undiagnosed HH.[239,243-245] In three of these four patients there was a rapid loss of iron over subsequent follow-up, suggesting that the liver was not the cause of the genetic defect in HH, but rather was just a "passive recipient" of the excess absorbed iron.[239,243,245] In the single patient in whom iron loading remained after transplant[244] a question was raised as to whether this patient might have been a heterozygote for HH who thus absorbed excess amounts of iron and maintained the high hepatic iron content that was present in the transplanted liver. This question was not answerable before the discovery of the *HFE* gene. Finally, for HH patients who have undergone transplantation successfully and for whom there has been a 3- to 4-year follow-up, there has been no significant reaccumulation of hepatic iron, suggesting that either a longer time of follow-up is necessary to document hepatic iron reaccumulation or the effects of multiple medications, including immunosuppressive agents, could affect iron absorption.[246,247] Additional long-term follow-up of this interesting group of patients will undoubtedly provide greater understanding of the pathophysiologic mechanisms present in HH.

SECONDARY IRON OVERLOAD

The foregoing account has been devoted largely to the clinical and pathologic consequences of iron overload in HH, and the pathologic features of the various forms of secondary iron overload have been briefly compared and contrasted with those of HH. The next section of this chapter will discuss certain aspects of secondary and parenteral iron overload.[249] The causes of secondary iron overload are listed in Table 42-1; certain of these will be selectively reviewed.

Iron-loading Anemias

The common theme in the iron-loading anemias is refractory anemia with a hypercellular bone marrow and ineffective erythropoiesis. These conditions include thalassemia major, the sideroblastic anemias, pyruvate kinase deficiency, and a variety of other anemias characterized by defective incorporation of iron into hemoglobin and chronic hemolytic anemias. Although the parenchymal distribution of the iron overload is in keeping with enhanced iron absorption, the extent of iron overload has not always been related to the level of the anemia.[250] Thus it has been postulated that either the level of marrow erythroid activity in some cases, or a linkage to the HH gene in others,[251,252] may be responsible for the variable degree of iron overload observed in the dyserythropoietic anemias. An association with HH has been disputed and the prevalence of HLA-A3 in a group of patients with idiopathic sideroblastic anemia in Brittany was equal to a control group.[253] Thus there has been no evidence linking the hemochromatosis gene to the pathogenesis of iron overload in idiopathic sideroblastic anemia.[249,253] Other studies have shown similar results for the presence of secondary iron overload in PCT[254] or ALD.[255]

In the dyserythropoietic anemias and, in particular, thalassemia major, the lifelong excessive gastrointestinal absorption of iron, compounded by the usual requirement for red blood cell transfusions, results in a pattern of organ damage with clinical and pathologic consequences that are often similar to those in HH.[146,256] Because the rate of iron accretion is so much more rapid in thalassemia, the major targets of damage, namely the liver, the pancreas, and the heart, are vulnerable at an earlier age than in HH, and the need for prophylactic therapy to prevent iron overload is therefore more urgent. Hence an aggressive approach to the use of chelation therapy with deferoxamine in young children has become the usual practice.[219,226,257] It should also be emphasized that, whereas it has been assumed that blood transfusion constitutes only an accessory source of iron in the secondary iron overload syndromes, there is evidence that hypertransfusion per se can result in pathologic and clinical sequelae. It is relevant that, in 15 non-thalassemic adults transfused with a mean of 120 units of blood, portal fibrosis was noted at a mean HIC of 22,000 μg/g,[258] which is in remarkably close agreement with that seen for liver damage in HH in some studies.[7]

Chronic Liver Diseases

Secondary iron overload associated with other types of liver disease is usually related to ALD, chronic viral hepatitis, non-alcoholic fatty liver disease or non-alcoholic steatohepatitis (NASH), and PCT. About 40 to 50 percent of patients with ALD,[15] chronic viral hepatitis,[165] or NASH[166] have abnormal serum iron tests, with an increase in ferritin being most commonly seen. Only a small proportion of these patients (about 5 percent to 10 percent) have a mild increase in HIC, which is less than that seen in homozygous HH.

Several factors have been suggested as contributing to iron accumulation in ALD in particular. These range from increased bioavailability of dietary iron to increased intestinal absorption and hepatic uptake. In other forms of liver disease, including viral hepatitis and NASH, varying but mild degrees of iron overload have been described,[174,259] and in some cases of NASH it has been suggested that this iron may be contributory to hepatic fibrosis.[260] In some cases of chronic liver disease with portal hypertension requiring decompression by portacaval anastomosis it was suggested that iron overload was pathogenetically related to the surgery. However, in prospective controlled evaluation this hypothesis was not borne out,[261] and it has not resurfaced since more selective decompressive shunts have been performed. Definitive differentiation from homozygous HH requires liver biopsy for histologic and biochemical iron determination. The hepatic iron deposition is usually found in both hepatocytes and Kupffer cells, but may have a periportal lobular distribution. Phlebotomy therapy has been shown to be unhelpful in ALD,[232] but has not been studied in NASH, although from recent studies, it may have an adjunctive role in the treatment of chronic hepatitis C.[262,263]

Porphyria Cutanea Tarda

PCT is the most common form of hepatic porphyria and results from variable degrees of deficiency in uroporphyrinogen decarboxylase normally expressed in the liver, leading to accumulation of intermediary porphyrins. The liver is the site of overproduction of these porphyrins, which lead to the cutaneous manifestations of the disease.[231] The disease occurs in two forms; the more common sporadic PCT syndrome and the rarer familial form. In both forms there is evidence to suggest that excessive storage iron plays a central role in promoting the biochemical and clinical manifestations of PCT. Rare cases of toxic PCT have been described that were due to exposure to the polyhalogenated hydrocarbon hexachlorobenzene. In sporadic PCT it has been suggested that heterozygosity for HH may be responsible for the associated iron overload and clinical expression of the disease.[264] However, Beaumont and coworkers[254] have performed HLA typing in 69 patients with PCT (42 sporadic and 27 familial) and the prevalence of the HLA-A3 haplotype (about 23 percent) was similar in both groups and no different than a control population. However, others have shown an allelic frequency considerably in excess of the *HFE* heterozygote prevalence in the general population.[265,266] In the latter study the availability of *HFE* mutation testing revealed a rate of C282Y heterozygosity in PCT of approximately 40 percent.

No correlation between the porphyria activity and the extent of liver damage has been demonstrated. Liver damage often has alcoholic characteristics, cirrhosis is present in about 30 percent of patients, and alcohol abuse has been documented in 25 percent to 100 percent of patients with clinical PCT in a number of studies.[267] In older studies the histopathologic changes of mild periportal hemosiderosis, focal lobular hepatocyte necrosis and steatosis, marked hepatocyte hyperplasia, and periductal lymphocytic aggregates have suggested that porphyrin deposition may be the basis for specific hepatotoxic manifestations. More recently, a high prevalence of anti-HCV positivity (70 percent) in patients with PCT has suggested that hepatitis C could be responsible for many, if not all, of these histologic changes.[268]

About 75 percent of patients with PCT have excessive hepatic iron on light microscopy that is distributed in both hepatocytes and Kupffer cells[267] and increased HIC.[17] It may be a consequence of increased intestinal iron absorption.[269,270] The degree of iron deposition is usually not severe and reflects total body iron stores of no more than 4 to 5 g. The role of this increased iron and its interaction with the enzyme uroporphyrinogen decarboxylase remain controversial. Whereas some workers have suggested that iron may play a role in the inhibition of uroporphyrinogen decarboxylase,[271,272] others have not been able to demonstrate inhibition of enzyme activity in vitro[273] or in vivo in experimental iron overload,[274,275] nor has removal of iron restored reduced hepatic uroporphyrinogen decarboxylase activity in patients with PCT.[276] In contrast, a role for iron has been supported by reports documenting the beneficial effects of phlebotomy[231,277,278] and the deleterious effects of iron administration.[279,280] It has been shown that the hepatic uroporphyrinogen decarboxylase activity may be restored to normal during remission.[281,282] Whereas iron may play a synergistic role in the inhibition of uroporphyrinogen decarboxylase, a more fundamental role has been postulated for an uncoupling of the cytochrome P450 reductase-cytochrome P450 system with the release of activated oxygen.[283,284] In the sporadic form of PCT, factors that rapidly induce the system without providing a rapid turnover of porphyrinogen substrate can serve to initiate porphyria. In these circumstances the formation of an active oxygen species oxidizes the porphyrinogen substrate to porphyrin, which, together with the active oxidant, inhibits the uroporphyrinogen decarboxylase activity. Iron released from ferritin may serve to catalyze the free radical-induced toxic sequence.

Treatment of PCT, as with HH, is the removal of iron by phlebotomy. Iron removal decreases the hepatic overproduction of porphyrins and improves both skin and the hepatic abnormalities even in the absence of evidence of excessive iron in the liver. Removal of as little as 2 to 4 g of iron will produce remission of the porphyria symptoms.[277,278] It remains to be demonstrated whether benefits for the associated liver disease also ensue. Where alcohol is incriminated, only abstinence offers an opportunity for potential reversal of hepatic damage.

NEONATAL IRON OVERLOAD

It has been emphasized by Knisely[285] that HIC in normal newborn infants are higher than in older children or adults, giving the appearance histopathologically of an abnormal degree of iron deposition. Likewise, markers of iron status in serum are also physiologically higher in the newborn, with levels of transferrin saturation up to 78 percent being recorded in normal infant cord serum, often in association with high serum ferritin concentrations. Despite these often misleading indicators of pathologic iron overload, there have been about 100 cases of so-called neonatal or perinatal hemochromatosis that compose a syndrome of severe liver disease characterized by parenchymal iron deposition, destruction of normal hepatic architecture, and relative sparing of the reticuloendothelial system.[19-22,285,286] Neonatal liver disease characterized by parenchymal iron overload is not a variant of *HFE*-associated HH, and the extent of iron loading in neonatal iron overload is no greater than that recorded in other neonatal liver diseases of known etiology.

Most infants with neonatal iron overload are the products of complicated pregnancies, with a high frequency of premature delivery and intrauterine growth retardation. Early signs of decompensated liver disease are seen at birth, and virtually all cases have had a fatal outcome.[20] Autopsy has revealed collapse of normal hepatic architecture and variable degrees of nodular regeneration, bile ductular proliferation, and giant cell transformation. Hepatocellular iron deposition has been graded 3+ to 4+, with minimal RE cell iron deposition. Quantitative liver iron has been higher than 2000 μg/g in most cases, a level that is not uncommon in normal neonatal livers and in other neonatal liver diseases. However, values as high as 38,000 μg/g have also been recorded. Attempts to remove iron by chelation with deferoxamine have been unsuccessful, although there have been several successful orthotopic liver transplants performed early in infancy.

With regard to pathogenesis it has been argued that neonatal iron overload is due to either abnormal transport of iron by the placental trophoblast or abnormal handling of iron by the fetal liver. To date no specific defect in the former has been identified,[20] whereas the latter still remains a feasible hypothesis in light of the quantitative similarities in liver iron concentration compared with other, more specific, neonatal liver diseases.[22] Whether there is a common role for high concentrations of non-transferrin-bound iron in the enhanced delivery of iron to the fetal liver in these circumstances remains unproven. It has been argued that the high iron stores normally present in fetal liver may potentiate other as yet unidentified noxious agents late in intrauterine development, or in the absence of normal cytoprotective mechanisms, have increased toxicity.

AFRICAN IRON OVERLOAD

African iron overload as a specific type of iron overload syndrome has only come about relatively recently. Although evidence suggests that iron is particularly well absorbed from fermented maize cooked in iron pots and the route of ingress, as in HH, is via the alimentary tract, there are marked differences in iron distribution between African iron overload and HH. Thus in African iron overload, there is proportionately more iron in the spleen at all levels of hepatic iron overload than is seen in HH.[24] The ratio of splenic:hepatic iron is approximately 2:1, and although concentrations of hepatic iron of up to 18,000 μg/g dry weight are seen by 40 to 50 years of age, this ratio is maintained. Kupffer cell and portal tract macrophage iron accumulation is far more prominent in African iron overload than in HH, sharing more equally with parenchymal cell deposition.[29,287] Nevertheless, the final common pathway of histopathology is characterized by portal fibrosis and cirrhosis that is indistinguishable from the pattern seen in HH, except for the persistence of hemosiderin granules in the portal tracts and fibrous tissue.[288] As in HH, there is good correlation between fibrosis and cirrhosis and the concentration of hepatic iron.[24-26] At levels in excess of 15,000 μg/g dry weight more than 70 percent of individuals with African iron overload have established fibrosis or cirrhosis,[287,288] but it must be remembered that this degree of iron loading is usually seen in association with significant alcohol ingestion.

Recent pedigree analysis of families of probands with African iron overload has identified iron-loaded family members who do not drink the iron-loaded alcoholic beverage.[28] These studies have suggested that African iron overload is a separate non-*HFE*-related iron overload disorder that can be enhanced by dietary iron loading.

SUMMARY AND FUTURE PERSPECTIVES

When Sheldon reviewed the literature on hemochromatosis available to him in 1935[4] he concluded that the two principal features of tissue damage, cirrhosis and diabetes mellitus, evolved concurrently in the course of iron accumulation resulting from a common inherited pathogenetic mechanism, concepts that have withstood the test of time. We now know that iron accumulation is usually, but not invariably, progressive throughout the life of patients with HH and that a relationship exists between HIC and fibrosis and cirrhosis. There is convincing evidence that these complications and many of the other manifestations of HH can be preempted by early diagnosis and timely initiation of phlebotomy therapy—an endorsement of the original observation of Davis and Arrowsmith in 1950.[289] Confirmation has been provided for the value of screening tests of iron overload in the homozygous relatives of patients with diagnosed hemochromatosis and for the value of *HFE* mutational analysis in the detection of those at risk for the disease. Careful observations of treated presymptomatic homozygotes should yield answers as to whether all phenotypic expression of the disease can be prevented and indeed whether phenotypic expression is inevitable in untreated genetic homozygotes. Although there is a gathering momentum for the adoption of combined phenotypic-genotypic screening of the general U.S. population,[11] other multi-national groups have been more hesitant in recommending this at the present time,[290] largely because they have reservations about cost-effectiveness and societal concerns that have yet to be resolved. There is agreement, however, regarding the need for further study of these important issues.

ACKNOWLEDGMENT

Part of the work reported was supported by grant R01-DK-41816 from the National Institutes of Health (BRB).

References

1. Trousseau A: Glycosurie, diabète sucré. In Clinique Medicale de l'Hotel-Dieu de Paris, vol 2, ed 2. Paris, Balliere, 1865:663.
2. Troisier M: Diabète sucré. Bull Soc Anat Paris 16:231, 1871.
3. Von Recklinghausen FD: Uber Haemochromatose. Tagebl Versamml Natur Arzte Heidelberg 62:324, 1889.
4. Sheldon JH: Haemochromatosis. London, Oxford University Press, 1935.
5. MacDonald RA: Hemochromatosis and Hemosiderosis. Springfield, Ill., Charles C Thomas, 1964.
6. Simon M, Bourel M, Genetet B, et al: Idiopathic hemochromatosis: demonstration of recessive transmission and early detection by family HLA typing. N Engl J Med 297:1017, 1977.
7. Bassett ML, Halliday JW, Powell LW: Value of hepatic iron measurements in early hemochromatosis and determination of the critical iron level associated with fibrosis. Hepatology 6:24, 1986.
8. Niederau C, Fischer R, Pürschel A, et al: Long-term survival in patients with hereditary hemochromatosis. Gastroenterology 110: 1107-1119, 1996.
9. Feder JN, Gnirke A, Thomas W, et al: A novel MHC class 1-like gene is mutated in patients with hereditary haemochromatosis. Nat Genet 13:339, 1996.
10. Zhou XY, Tomatsu S, Fleming RE, et al: *HFE* gene knockout produces mouse model of hereditary hemochromatosis. Proc Natl Acad Sci U S A 95:2492, 1998.
11. Tavill AS: Diagnosis and management of hemochromatosis. AASLD Practice Guidelines. Hepatology 33:1321-1328, 2001.
12. Pippard MJ: Secondary iron overload. In Brock JH, Halliday JW, Pippard MJ, et al, eds: Iron Metabolism in Health and Disease. London, WB Saunders Co., 1994:271.
13. Modell CB: Transfusional haemochromatosis. In Kief H, ed: Iron Metabolism and Its Disorders. Amsterdam, Excerpta Medica, 1975:230.
14. Modell CB: Advances in the use of iron-chelating agents for the treatment of iron overload. In Brown EB, ed: Progress in Hematology. New York, Grune and Stratton, 1979:267.
15. Chapman RW, Morgan MY, Laulicht M, et al: Hepatic iron stores and markers of iron overload in alcoholics and patients with idiopathic hemochromatosis. Dig Dis Sci 27:909, 1982.
16. Sauer GF, Funk DD: Iron overload in cutaneous porphyria. Arch Intern Med 124:190, 1969.
17. Lundvall O, Weinfeld A, Lundin P: Iron storage in porphyria cutanea tarda. Acta Med Scand 188:37, 1970.
18. Pechet GS: Parenteral iron overload. Organ and cell distribution in rats. Lab Invest 20:119, 1969.
19. Knisely AS, Magid MS, Dische MR, et al: Neonatal hemochromatosis. Birth Defects 23:75, 1989.
20. Knisely AS: Neonatal hemochromatosis. Adv Pediatr 39:383, 1992.
21. Silver MM, Beverley DW, Valberg LS, et al: Perinatal hemochromatosis: clinical, morphologic and quantitative iron studies. Am J Pathol 128:538, 1987.
22. Silver MM, Valberg LS, Cutz E, et al: Hepatic morphology and iron quantitation in perinatal hemochromatosis: comparison with a large perinatal control population, including cases with chronic liver disease. Am J Pathol 143:1312, 1993.
23. Charlton RW, Bothwell THE, Seftel HC: Dietary iron overload. In Callender ST, ed: Clinics in Haematology. London, WB Saunders Co., 1973:383.
24. MacPhail AP, Simon MO, Torrance JD, et al: Changing patterns of dietary iron overload in black South Africans. Am J Clin Nutr 32:1272, 1979.
25. Bothwell TH, Bradlow BA: Siderosis in the Bantu. A combined histopathological and chemical study. Arch Pathol 70:279, 1960.
26. Isaacson C, Seftel H, Keeley KJ, et al: Siderosis in the Bantu. The relationship between iron overload and cirrhosis. J Lab Clin Med 58:845, 1961.
27. Gordeuk VR, Boyd RD, Brittenham GM: Dietary iron overload persists in rural sub-Saharan Africa. Lancet 1:1310, 1986.
28. Gordeuk VR, Mukubi J, Hasstedt J, et al: Iron overload in Africa—interaction between a gene and dietary iron content. N Engl J Med 326:95, 1992.
29. Bacon BR: Causes of iron overload. N Engl J Med 326:126, 1992.
30. Bacon BR, Powell LW, Adams PC, et al: Molecular medicine and hemochromatosis: at the crossroads. Gastroenterology 116:193, 1999.
31. Andrews NC: Disorders of iron metabolism. N Engl J Med 341:1986, 1999.
32. Roy CN, Enns CA: Iron homeostasis: new tales from the crypt. Blood 96:4020, 2000.
33. Skikne B, Baynes RD: Iron absorption. In Brock JH, Halliday JW, Pippard MJ, et al, eds: Iron Metabolism in Health and Disease. London, WB Saunders Co., 1994:151.
34. Anderson GJ: Control of iron absorption. J Gastroenterol Hepatol 11:1030, 1996.
35. Chasteen ND, Harrison PM: Mineralization in ferritin: an efficient means of iron storage. J Struct Biol 126:182, 1999.
36. Gunshin H, Mackenzie B, Berger UV, et al: Cloning and characterization of a mammalian proton-coupled metal-ion transporter. Nature 388:482, 1997.
37. Fleming MD, Trenor CC 3rd, Su MA, et al: Microcytic anaemia mice have a mutation in Nramp2, a candidate iron transporter gene. Nat Genet 16:383, 1997.
38. Turnbull A, Cleton F, Finch CA: Iron absorption. IV. The absorption of hemoglobin iron. J Clin Invest 41:1894, 1962.
39. Umbreit JN, Conrad ME, Moore EG, Latour LF: Iron absorption and cellular transport: the mobilferrin/paraferritin paradigm. Semin Hematol 35:13, 1998.
40. Donovan A, Brownlie A, Zhou Y, et al: Positional cloning of zebrafish ferroportin1 identifies a conserved vertebrate iron exporter. Nature 403:776, 2000.
41. McKie AT, Marciani P, Rolfs A, et al: A novel duodenal iron-regulated transporter, IREG1, implicated in basolateral transfer of iron to the circulation. Mol Cell Biol 5:299, 2000.
42. Abboud S, Haile DJ: A novel mammalian iron-regulated protein involved in intracellular iron metabolism. J Biol Chem 275:19906, 2000.
43. Vulpe CD, Kuo YM, Murphy TL, et al: Hephaestin, a ceruloplasmin homologue implicated in intestinal iron transport, is defective in the sla mouse. Nat Genet 21:195-199, 1999.
44. Lebron JA, Bennett MJ, Vaughn DE, et al: Crystal structure of the hemochromatosis protein *HFE* and characterization of its interaction with transferrin receptor. Cell 93:111, 1998.
45. Feder JN, Tsuchihashi Z, Irrinki A, et al: The hemochromatosis founder mutation in HLA-H disrupts β2-microglobulin interaction and cell surface expression. J Biol Chem 272:14025, 1997.
46. Waheed A, Parkkila S, Zhou XY, et al: Hereditary hemochromatosis: effects of C282Y and H63D mutations on association with β2-microglobulin, intracellular processing, and cell surface expression of the *HFE* protein in COS-7 cells. Proc Natl Acad Sci U S A 94:12384, 1997.
47. de Sousa M, Reimao R, Lacerda R, et al: Iron overload in β2-microglobulin-deficient mice. Immunol Lett 39:105, 1994.
48. Bahram S, Gilfillan S, Kuhn LC, et al: Experimental hemochromatosis due to MHC class I *HFE* deficiency: immune status and iron metabolism. Proc Natl Acad Sci U S A 96:13312, 1999.

49. Levy JE, Montross LK, Cohen DE, et al: The C282Y mutation causing hereditary hemochromatosis does not produce a null allele. Blood 94:9, 1999.
50. Feder JN, Penny DM, Irrinki A, et al: The hemochromatosis gene product complexes with the transferrin receptor and lowers its affinity for ligand binding. Proc Natl Acad Sci U S A 95:1472, 1998.
51. Parkkila S, Waheed A, Britton RS, et al: Association of the transferrin receptor in human placenta with *HFE,* the protein defective in hereditary hemochromatosis. Proc Natl Acad Sci U S A 94:13198, 1997.
52. Waheed A, Parkkila S, Saarnio J, et al: Association of *HFE* protein with transferrin receptor in crypt enterocytes of human duodenum. Proc Natl Acad Sci U S A 96:1579, 1999.
53. Bennett MJ, Lebron JA, Bjorkman PJ: Crystal structure of the hereditary haemochromatosis protein *HFE* complexed with transferrin receptor. Nature 403:46, 2000.
54. Parkkila S, Waheed A, Britton RS, et al: Immunohistochemistry of HLA-H, the protein defective in patients with hereditary hemochromatosis, reveals unique pattern of expression in gastrointestinal tract. Proc Natl Acad Sci U S A 94:2534, 1997.
55. Cox TM, Kelly AL: Haemochromatosis: an inherited metal and toxicity syndrome. Curr Opin Genet Dev 8:274, 1998.
56. Kuhn LC: Iron overload: molecular clues to its cause. Trends Biochem Sci 24:164, 1999.
57. Rolfs A, Hediger MA: Metal ion transporters in mammals: structure, function and pathological implications. J Physiol 518:1, 1999.
58. Fleming RE, Migas MC, Zhou X, et al: Mechanism of increased iron absorption in murine model of hereditary hemochromatosis: Increased duodenal expression of the iron transporter DMT1. Proc Natl Acad Sci U S A 96:3143, 1999.
59. Griffiths WJ, Sly WS, Cox TM: Intestinal iron uptake determined by divalent metal transporter is enhanced in *HFE*-deficient mice with hemochromatosis. Gastroenterology 120:1420, 2001.
60. Zoller H, Pietrangelo A, Vogel W, Weiss G: Duodenal metal-transporter (DMT-1, NRAMP-2) expression in patients with hereditary haemochromatosis. Lancet 353:2120, 1999.
61. Zoller H, Koch RO, Theurl I, et al: Expression of the duodenal iron transporters divalent-metal transporter 1 and ferroportin 1 in iron deficiency and iron overload. Gastroenterology 120:1412, 2001.
62. Milder MS, Cook JD, Sunday S, et al: Idiopathic hemochromatosis, an interim report. Medicine 59:39, 1980.
63. McLaren GD, Muir WA, Kellermeyer RW: Iron overload disorders. Natural history, pathogenesis, diagnosis, and therapy. Crit Rev Clin Lab Sci 19:205, 1983.
64. Bassett ML, Halliday JW, Powell LW: Genetic hemochromatosis. Semin Liver Dis 4:217, 1984.
65. Gordeuk VR, Bacon BR, Brittenham GM: Iron overload: causes and consequences. Annu Rev Nutr 7:485, 1987.
66. Smith LH Jr: Overview of hemochromatosis. West J Med 153:296, 1990.
67. Edwards CQ, Griffen LM, Kushner JP: Southern Blood Club Symposium: an update on selected aspects of hemochromatosis. Am J Med Sci 300:245, 1990.
68. Adams PC: Hemochromatosis: new insights in pathogenesis and diagnosis following the discovery of the gene. Crit Rev Clin Lab Sci 35:239, 1998.
69. Powell LW: Hereditary hemochromatosis. Pathology 32:24, 2000.
70. Bassett ML, Halliday JW, Powell LW: Value of hepatic iron measurements in early hemochromatosis and determination of the critical iron level associated with fibrosis. Hepatology 6:24, 1986.
71. Fletcher LL, Dixon AL, Powell LW, Crawford DHG: Hepatic cirrhosis in hereditary hemochromatosis is seldom due solely to iron: Evidence for a synergistic effect of alcohol and iron. Hepatology 32:412A, 2000 (abstract).
72. Bacon BR, Britton RS: The pathology of hepatic iron overload: a free radical-mediated process? Hepatology 11:127, 1990.
73. Britton RS: Metal-induced hepatotoxicity. Semin Liver Dis 16:3, 1996.
74. Britton RS, Bacon BR: Role of free radicals in liver diseases and hepatic fibrosis. Hepatogastroenterology 41:343, 1994.
75. Pietrangelo A: Iron, oxidative stress and liver fibrogenesis. J Hepatol 28(suppl 1):8, 1998.
76. Scheuer PJ, Williams R, Muir AR: Hepatic pathology in relatives of patients with haemochromatosis. J Pathol 84:53, 1962.
77. Brick IB: Liver histology in six asymptomatic siblings in a family with hemochromatosis; genetic implications. Gastroenterology 40:210, 1961.
78. Bothwell THE, Cohen I, Abrahams OL, et al: A familial study in idiopathic hemochromatosis. Am J Med 27:730, 1959.
79. Edwards CO, Cartwright GE, Skolnick MH, et al: Homozygosity for hemochromatosis: clinical manifestations. Ann Intern Med 93:511, 1980.
80. Powell LW, Kerr JFR: The pathology of the liver in hemochromatosis. Pathobiol Ann 5:317, 1975.
81. Adams, PC, Kertesz AE, Valberg LS: Clinical presentation of hemochromatosis: a changing scene. Am J Med 90:445, 1991.
82. Sohal R, Brunk U: Lipofuscin an indicator of oxidative stress and aging. Adv Exp Med Biol 266:17, 1990.
83. Richter GW: The iron-loaded cell—the cytopathology of iron storage. Am J Pathol 91:363, 1978.
84. Richter GW: Studies of iron overload. Rat liver siderosome ferritin. Lab Invest 50:26, 1984.
85. Trump BF, Valigorsky JM, Arstila AA, et al: The relationship of intracellular pathways of iron metabolism to cellular iron overload and iron storage diseases. Am J Pathol 72:295, 1973.
86. Hoy TG, Jacobs A: Ferritin polymers and the formation of haemosiderin. Br J Haematol 49:593, 1981.
87. Hoy TG, Jacobs A: Changes in the characteristics and distribution of ferritin in iron loaded cell cultures. Biochem J 193:87, 1981.
88. Park CH, Bacon BR, Brittenham GM, et al: Pathology of dietary carbonyl iron overload in rats. Lab Invest 57:555, 1987.
89. Iancu TC, Rabinowitz H, Brissot P, et al: Iron overload of the liver in the baboon: an ultrastructural study. J Hepatol 1:261, 1985.
90. Weintraub LR, Goral A, Grasso J, et al: Pathogenesis of hepatic fibrosis in experimental iron overload. Br J Haematol 59:321, 1985.
91. Selden C, Owen M, Hopkins JMP, et al: Studies on the concentration and intracellular localization of iron proteins in liver biopsy specimens from patients with iron overload with special reference to their role in lysosomal disruption. Br J Haematol 44:593, 1980.
92. Beaumont C, Simon M, Smith PM, et al: Hepatic and serum ferritin concentration in patients with idiopathic hemochromatosis. Gastroenterology 79:877, 1980.
93. Seymour CA, Peters TJ: Organelle pathology in primary and secondary haemochromatosis with special reference to lysosomal changes. Br J Haematol 40:239, 1978.
94. Deugnier YM, Loreal O, Turlin B, et al: Liver pathology in genetic hemochromatosis: a review of 135 homozygous cases and their bioclinical correlations. Gastroenterology 102:2050, 1992.
95. Summers KM, Halliday JW, Powell LW: Identification of homozygous hemochromatosis subjects by measurement of hepatic iron index. Hepatology 12:20, 1990.
96. Sallie R, Reed WD, Shilkin KB: Confirmation of the efficacy of the hepatic iron index in differentiating genetic haemochromatosis from alcoholic liver disease complicated by alcoholic haemosiderosis. Gut 32:207, 1991.
97. Olynyk J, Hall P, Sallie R, et al: Computerized measurement of iron in liver biopsies: a comparison with biochemical iron measurement. Hepatology 12:26, 1990.
98. Loreal D, Deugnier YM, Moirand R, et al: Liver fibrosis in genetic hemochromatosis. Respective roles of iron and non-iron-related factors in 127 homozygous patients. J Hepatol 16:122, 1992.
99. Deugnier YM, Guyader D, Crantook L, et al: Primary liver cancer in genetic hemochromatosis: a clinical, pathological and pathogenetic study of 54 cases. Gastroenterology 104:228, 1992.
100. Bradbear RA, Bain C, Siskind V, et al: Cohort study of internal malignancy in genetic hemochromatosis and other chronic nonalcoholic liver diseases. J Natl Cancer Inst 75:81, 1985.
101. Berk JE, Lieber MM: Primary carcinoma of liver in hemochromatosis. Am J Med Sci 202:708, 1941.
102. Tiniakos G, Williams R: Cirrhotic process, liver cell carcinoma and extra hepatic malignant tumors in idiopathic hemochromatosis. Study of 71 patients treated with venesection therapy. Appl Pathol 6:128, 1988.
103. Blumberg RS, Chopra S, Ibrahim R, et al: Primary hepatocellular carcinoma in idopathic hemochromatosis after reversal of cirrhosis. Gastroenterology 95:1399, 1988.

104. Fellows IW, Stewart M, Jeffcoate WJ, et al: Hepatocellular carcinoma in primary hemochromatosis in the absence of cirrhosis. Gut 29:1603, 1988.
105. Kew MD: Pathogenesis of hepatocellular carcinoma in hereditary hemochromatosis: occurrence in noncirrhotic patients. Hepatology 11:1086, 1990.
106. Fargion S, Piperno A, Francanzani AL, et al: Iron in the pathogenesis of hepatocellular carcinoma. Ital J Gastroenterol 23:584, 1991.
107. Kowdley KV, Hassanein T, Kaur S, et al: Primary liver cancer and survival in patients undergoing liver transplantation for hemochromatosis. J Liver Transplant Surg 1:237, 1995.
108. Jacobs A: Iron overload—clinical and pathologic aspects. Semin Hematol 14:89, 1977.
109. Suda K: Hemosiderin deposition in the pancreas. Arch Pathol Lab Med 109:996, 1985.
110. MacDonald RA, Mallory GH: Hemochromatosis and hemosiderosis. Study of 211 autopsied cases. Arch Intern Med 105:686, 1960.
111. Edwards CQ, Kelly TM, Ellwein G, et al: Thyroid disease in hemochromatosis. Increased incidence in homozygous men. Arch Intern Med 143:1890, 1983.
112. Siemons AJ, Mahler CH: Hypogonadotropic hypogonadism in hemochromatosis: recovery of reproductive function after iron depletion. J Clin Endocrinol Metab 65:585, 1987.
113. Buja LM, Roberts WC: Iron in the heart. Etiology and clinical significance. Am J Med 51:209, 1971.
114. Olson LJ, Edwards WD, McCall JT, et al: Cardiac iron deposition in idiopathic hemochromatosis: histologic and analytic assessment of 14 hearts from autopsy. J Am Coll Cardiol 10:1239, 1987.
115. Olson LJ, Edwards WD, Holmes DR, et al: Endomyocardial biopsy in hemochromatosis: clinicopathologic correlates in six cases. J Am Coll Cardiol 13:116, 1989.
116. Atkins CJ, McIvor J, Smith RM, et al: Chondrocalcinosis and arthropathy: studies in haemochromatosis and in idiopathic chondrocalcinosis. QJM 39:71, 1970.
117. Shumacher HR: Hemochromatosis and arthritis. Arthritis Rheum 7:41, 1964.
118. Shumacher HR: Articular cartilage in the degenerative arthropathy of hemochromatosis. Arthritis Rheum 25:1460, 1982.
119. Chevrant-Breton J, Simon M, Bourel M, et al: Cutaneous manifestations of idiopathic hemochromatosis. A study of 100 cases. Arch Dermatol 113:161, 1977.
120. Bothwell TH, Abrahams C, Bradlow BA, et al: Idiopathic and Bantu haemochromatosis: comparative histological study. Arch Pathol 79:163, 1965.
121. Rink B, Disler P, Lynch S, et al: Patterns of iron storage in dietary iron overload and idiopathic hemochromatosis. J Lab Clin Med 88:725, 1976.
122. Oliver RAM: Siderosis following transfusions of blood. J Pathol 77:171, 1959.
123. Jakobovits AW, Morgan MY, Sherlock S: Hepatic siderosis in alcoholics. Dig Dis Sci 24:305, 1979.
124. Adams PC, Bradley C, Henderson AR: Evolution of the hepatic iron index as a diagnostic criterion for genetic hemochromatosis. J Lab Clin Med 130:509-514, 1997.
125. Crawford DHG, Jazwinska EC, Cullen LM, Powell LW: Expression of HLA-linked hemochromatosis in subjects homozygous for the C282Y mutation. Gastroenterology 114:1003-1008, 1998.
126. Milder MS, Cook JD, Sunday S, et al: Idiopathic hemochromatosis, an interim report. Medicine 59:39, 1980.
127. McLaren GD, Muir WA, Kellermeyer RW: Iron overload disorders. Natural history, pathogenesis, diagnosis, and therapy. Crit Rev Clin Lab Sci 19:205, 1983.
128. Edwards CQ, Griffen LM, Kushner JP: Southern Blood Club Symposium: an update on selected aspects of hemochromatosis. Am J Med Sci 300:245, 1990.
129. Bomford A, Williams R: Long-term results of venesection therapy in idiopathic haemochromatosis. QJM 45:611, 1976.
130. Cartwright GE, Edwards CQ, Kravitz K, et al: Hereditary hemochromatosis. Phenotypic expression of the disease. N Engl J Med 301:175, 1979.
131. Bothwell TH, Charlton RW, Cook JD, et al: Iron Metabolism in Man. Oxford, Blackwell, 1979.
132. Adams PC, Speechley M, Kertesz AE: Long-term survival analysis in hereditary hemochromatosis. Gastroenterology 101:368, 1991.
133. Leggett BA, Halliday JW, Brown NN, et al: Prevalence of haemochromatosis amongst asymptomatic Australians. Br J Haematol 74:525, 1990.
134. Powell LW, Summers KM, Board PG, et al: Expression of hemochromatosis in homozygous subjects: implications for early diagnosis and prevention. Gastroenterology 98:1625, 1990.
135. Velati C, Piperno A, Fargion S, et al: Prevalence of idiopathic hemochromatosis in Italy: study of 1,301 blood donors. Haematologica 75:309, 1990.
136. Adams PC, Chakrabarti S: Genotypic/phenotypic correlations in genetic hemochromatosis: evolution of diagnostic criteria. Gastroenterology 114:319-323, 1998.
137. Edwards CQ, Griffen LM, Goldgar D, et al: Prevalence of hemochromatosis among 11,065 presumably healthy blood donors. N Engl J Med 318:1355, 1988.
138. Lin E, Adams PC: Biochemical liver profile in hemochromatosis: a survey of 100 patients. J Clin Gastroenterol 13:316, 1991.
139. Ammann RW, Muller E, Bansky J, et al: High incidence of extrahepatic carcinomas in idiopathic hemochromatosis. Scand J Gastroenterol 15:733, 1980.
140. MacSween RN: Acute abdominal crisis, circulatory collapse and sudden death in haemochromatosis. QJM 35:589, 1966.
141. Dymock IW, Cassar J, Pyke DA, et al: Observations on the pathogenesis, complications and treatment of diabetes in 115 cases of haemochromatosis. Am J Med 52:203, 1972.
142. Griffiths JD, Dymock IW, Davies EWG, et al: Occurrence and prevalence of diabetic retinopathy in hemochromatosis. Diabetes 20:766, 1971.
143. Stocks AE, Martin FIR: Pituitary function in hemochromatosis. Am J Med 45:839, 1968.
144. Stocks AE, Powell LW: Pituitary function in idiopathic haemochromatosis and cirrhosis of the liver. Lancet 2:298, 1972.
145. Bezwoda WR, Bothwell THE, Van der Walt LA, et al: An investigation into gonadal function in patients with idiopathic haemochromatosis. Clin Endocrinol 6:377, 1977.
146. Modell B, Berdoukas V: Death and survival. In The Clinical Approach to Thalassemia. London, Grune and Stratton, 1984:151.
147. Engle MA: Cardiac involvement in Cooley's anemia. Ann N Y Acad Sci 9:694, 1964.
148. Ehlers KH, Levin AR, Markenson AL, et al: Longitudinal study of cardiac function in thalassemia major. Ann N Y Acad Sci 344:397, 1980.
149. Vigorita VJ, Hutchins GM: Cardiac conduction system in hemochromatosis: clinical and pathologic features of six patients. Am J Cardiol 44:418, 1979.
150. Candell-Riera J, Lu L, Seres L, et al: Cardiac hemochromatosis: beneficial effects of iron removal therapy. Am J Cardiol 52:824, 1983.
150a. Link G, Pinson A, Hershko C: Heart cells in culture: a model of myocardial iron-overload and chelation. J Lab Clin Med 106:147, 1985.
151. Hamilton E, Williams R, Barlow KA, et al: The arthropathy of idiopathic haemochromatosis. QJM 37:171, 1968.
152. Askari AD, Muir WA, Rosner IA, et al: Arthritis of hemochromatosis. Clinical spectrum, relation to histocompatibility antigens and effectiveness of early phlebotomy. Am J Med 75:957, 1983.
153. Alexander GM, Dieppe PA, Doherty M, et al: Pyrophosphate arthropathy: a study of metabolic associations and laboratory data. Ann Rheum Dis 41:377, 1982.
154. Utsinger PD, Zvaifler NJ, Resnick D: Calcium pyrophosphate dihydrate deposition disease without chondrocalcinosis. J Rheumatol 2:258, 1975.
155. Abbott DF, Gresham GA: Arthropathy in transfusional siderosis. BMJ 1:418, 1972.
156. Davies G, Dymock IW, Harry J, et al: Deposition of melanin and iron in ocular structures in haemochromatosis. Br J Ophthalmol 56:338, 1972.
157. Chiesa C, Pacifico L, Renzulli F, et al: *Yersinia* hepatic abscesses and iron overload. JAMA 257:3230, 1987.
158. Robins-Browne RM, Prpic JK: Desferrioxamine and systemic yersiniosis. Lancet 1:1372, 1984.
159. Capron JP, Capron-Chivrac D, Tosson H: Spontaneous *Yersinia enterocolitica* peritonitis in idiopathic hemochromatosis. Gastroenterology 87:1372, 1984.
159a. Yamaschiro KW, Goldman RH, Harris DR, et al: *Pasteurella pseudotuberculosis* acute sepsis with survival. Arch Intern Med 128:605, 1971.

159b. Blake PA, Merson MH, Weaver RE, et al: Disease caused by a marine vibrio. N Engl J Med 300:1, 1979.
160. Van Asbeck BS, Verbrugh HA, Van Oost BA, et al: *Listeria monocytogenes* meningitis and decreased phagocytosis associated with iron overload. BMJ 284:542, 1982.
161. Weinberg ED: Iron withholding: a defense against infection and neoplasm. Physiol Rev 64:65, 1984.
162. Weinberg ED: Iron, infection and neoplasia. Clin Physiol Biochem 4:50, 1986.
163. Wright AC, Simpson LM, Oliver JD: Role of iron in the pathogenesis of *Vibrio vulnificus* infections. Infect Immun 34:503, 1981.
164. Hegenauer J, Saltman P: Letter: iron and susceptibility to infectious disease. Science 188:1038, 1975.
165. DiBisceglie AM, Axiotis CA, Hoofnagle JH, et al: Measurements of iron status in patients with chronic hepatitis. Gastroenterology 102:2108, 1992.
166. Bacon BR, Farahvash MJ, Janney CG, et al: Nonalcoholic steatohepatitis: an expanded clinical entity. Gastroenterology 107:1103, 1994.
167. Adams PC: Intrafamilial variation in hereditary hemochromatosis. Dig Dis Sci 37:361, 1992.
168. Crawford DHG, Halliday JW, Summers KM, et al: Concordance of iron storage in siblings with genetic hemochromatosis: evidence for a predominantly genetic effect on iron storage. Hepatology 17:833, 1993.
169. Olynyk JK, Cullen DJ, Aquila S, et al: A population based study of the clinical expression of the hemochromatosis gene. N Engl J Med 341:718-724, 1999.
170. Beutler E, Felitti V, Gelbart T, Ho N: The effect of *HFE* genotypes on measurements of iron overload in patients attending a health appraisal clinic. Ann Int Med 133:321-327, 2000.
171. Adams PC: Nonexpressing homozygotes for C282Y hemochromatosis: minority or majority of cases? Minireview. Mol Genet Metab 71:81-86, 2000.
172. Bassett ML, Halliday JW, Ferris RA, et al: Diagnosis of hemochromatosis in young subjects: predictive accuracy of biochemical screening tests. Gastroenterology 87:628, 1984.
173. Borwein ST, Ghent CN, Flanagan PR, et al: Genetic and phenotypic expression of hemochromatosis in Canadians. Clin Invest Med 6:171, 1983.
174. Bacon BR, Olynyk JK, Brunt EM, et al: *HFE* genotype in patients with hemochromatosis and other liver diseases. Ann Int Med 130:953-962, 1999.
175. Wiltink WF, Kruithof J, Mol C, et al: Diurnal and nocturnal variations in the serum iron in normal subjects. Clin Chim Acta 49:99, 1973.
176. Bowie EJW, Tauxe WN, Sjoberg WE, et al: Daily variation in the concentration of iron in serum. Am J Clin Pathol 40:491, 1963.
177. Beilby J, Olynyk J, Ching S, et al: Transferrin index: an alternative method for calculating the iron saturation of transferrin. Clin Chem 38:2078, 1992.
178. Valberg LS, Lloyd DA, Ghent CN, et al: Clinical and biochemical expression of the genetic abnormality in idiopathic hemochromatosis. Gastroenterology 79:884, 1980.
179. Bassett ML, Halliday JW, Powell LW: HLA typing in idiopathic hemochromatosis: distinction between homozygotes and heterozygotes with biochemical expression. Hepatology 1:120, 1981.
180. McLaren CE, McLachlan GJ, Halliday JW, et al: Distribution of transferrin saturation in an Australian population: relevance to the early diagnosis of hemochromatosis. Gastroenterology 114:543-549, 1998.
181. Beaumont C, Simon M, Fauchet R, et al: Serum ferritin as a possible marker of the hemochromatosis allele. N Engl J Med 301:169, 1979.
182. Halliday JW, Cowlishaw JL, Russo AM, et al: Serum ferritin in diagnosis of haemochromatosis—a study of 43 families. Lancet 2:621, 1977.
183. Edwards CQ, Carroll M, Bray P, et al: Hereditary hemochromatosis: diagnosis in siblings and children. N Engl J Med 297:7, 1977.
184. Batey RG, Hussein S, Sherlock S, et al: The role of serum ferritin in the management of idiopathic haemochromatosis. Scand J Gastroenterol 13:953, 1978.
185. Brissot P, Bourel M, Henry D, et al: Assessment of liver iron content in 271 patients; a re-evaluation of direct and indirect methods. Gastroenterology 80:557, 1981.
186. Wands JR, Rowe JA, Mezey SE, et al: Normal serum ferritin concentrations in precirrhotic hemochromatosis. N Engl J Med 294:302, 1976.
187. Feller ER, Pont A, Wands JR, et al: Familial hemochromatosis: physiological studies in the precirrhotic stage of the disease. N Engl J Med 296:1422, 1977.
188. Bassett ML, Powell LW, Halliday JM, et al: Early detection of idiopathic haemochromatosis: relative value of serum ferritin and HLA typing. Lancet 2:4, 1979.
189. Guyader D, Jacquelinet C, Moirand R, et al: Non-invasive prediction of fibrosis in C282Y homozygous hemochromatosis. Gastroenterology 115:929-936, 1998.
190. Norwood M: Editorial review: serum ferritin. Clin Sci 70:215, 1986.
191. Prieto J, Barry M, Sherlock S: Serum ferritin in patients with iron overload and with acute and chronic liver diseases. Gastroenterology 68:525, 1975.
192. Jeffery CP, Chakrabarti S, Hegele RA, Adams PC: Polymorphism in intron 4 of *HFE* may cause overestimation of C282Y homozygote prevalence in haemochromatosis. Nat Genet 22:325-326, 1999.
193. Carella M, D'Ambrosio L, Totaro A, et al: Mutation analysis of the HLA-H gene in Italian hemochromatosis patients. Am J Hum Genet 60:828-832, 1997.
194. Camaschella C, Fargion S, Sampietro M, et al: Inherited *HFE*-unrelated hemochromatosis in Italian families. Hepatology 29:1563, 1999.
195. Pietrangelo A, Montosi G, Totaro A, et al: Hereditary hemochromatosis in adults without pathogenic mutations in the hemochromatosis gene. N Engl J Med 341:725-731, 1999.
196. Tavill AS: Clinical implications of the hemochromatosis gene. N Engl J Med 341:755-757, 1999 (editorial).
197. Jeffery CP, Chakrabarti S, Hegele RA, Adams PC. Polymorphism in intron 4 of *HFE* may cause overestimation of C282Y homozygote prevalence in haemochromatosis. Nat Genet 22:325-326, 1999.
198. Ludwig J, Batts KP, Moyer TP, et al: Liver biopsy diagnosis of homozygous hemochromatosis: a diagnostic algorithm. Mayo Clin Proc 68:263, 1993.
199. Weinfeld A, Lundin P, Lundvall O: Significance for the diagnosis of iron overload of histochemical and chemical iron in the liver of normal subjects. J Clin Pathol 21:35, 1968.
200. Walker RJ, Miller JPG, Dymock IW, et al: Relationship of hepatic iron concentration to histochemical grading and total chelatable iron in conditions associated with iron overload. Gut 12:1011, 1971.
201. Deugnier YM, Turlin B, Powell LW, et al: Differentiation between heterozygotes and homozygotes in genetic hemochromatosis by means of a histologic hepatic iron index: a study of 192 cases. Hepatology 17:30, 1993.
202. Olynyk JK, O'Neill R, Britton RS, et al: Determination of hepatic iron concentration in fresh and paraffin-embedded tissue: diagnostic implications. Gastroenterology 106:674, 1994.
203. Kreeftenberg HG, Koopman BJ, Huizenga JR, et al: Measurement of iron in liver biopsies—a comparison of three analytical methods. Clin Chim Acta 144:255, 1984.
204. Torrance JD, Bothwell TH: A simple technique for measuring storage iron concentrations in formalinized liver samples. S Afr J Med Sci 33:9, 1968.
205. LeSage GD, Baldus WP, Fairbanks VF, et al: Hemochromatosis: genetic or alcohol-induced? Gastroenterology 84:1471, 1983.
206. Bonkovsky HL, Slaker DP, Bills EB, et al: Usefulness and limitations of laboratory and hepatic imaging studies in iron-storage disease. Gastroenterology 99:1079, 1990.
207. Cotler SJ, Bronner MP, Press RD, et al: End-stage liver disease without hemochromatosis associated with elevated hepatic iron index. J Hepatol 29:257-262, 1998.
208. Mills SR, Doppman JL, Nienhuis AW: Computed tomography in the diagnosis of excessive iron storage of the liver. J Comput Assist Tomogr 1:101, 1977.
209. Howard JM, Ghent CN, Carey LS, et al: Diagnostic efficacy of hepatic computed tomography in the detection of body iron overload. Gastroenterology 84:209, 1983.
210. Houang MTW, Arozena X, Skalicka A, et al: Correlation between computed tomographic values and liver iron content in thalassemia major with iron overload. Lancet 1:1322, 1979.
211. Chapman RWG, Williams G, Bydder G, et al: Computed tomography for determining liver iron content in primary haemochromatosis. BMJ 280:440, 1980.

212. Guyader D, Gandon Y, Deugnier Y, et al: Evaluation of computed tomography in the assessment of liver iron overload. Gastroenterology 97:737, 1989
213. Stark DD, Moseley ME, Bacon BR, et al: Magnetic resonance imaging and spectroscopy of hepatic iron overload. Radiology 154:137, 1985.
214. Stark DD: Hepatic iron overload: paramagnetic pathology. Radiology 179:333, 1991.
215. Gomori JM, Horev G, Tamary H, et al: Hepatic iron overload: quantitative MR imaging. Radiology 179:367, 1991.
216. Angelucci E, Giovagnoni A, Valeri S, et al: Limitations of magnetic resonance imaging in measurement of hepatic iron. Blood 90:4736-4742, 1997
217. Brittenham GM, Danish EH, Harris JW: Assessment of bone marrow and body iron stores: old techniques and new technologies. Semin Hematol 18:194, 1981.
218. Brittenham GM, Farrell DE, Harris JW, et al: Magnetic-susceptibility measurement of human iron stores. N Engl J Med 307:1671, 1982.
219. Brittenham GM, Griffith PM, Nienhuis AW, et al: Efficacy of deferoxamine in preventing complications of iron overload in patients with thalassemia major. N Engl J Med 331:567, 1994.
220. Bomford A, Williams R: Long-term results of venesection therapy in idiopathic haemochromatosis. QJM 45:611, 1976.
221. Niederau C, Fischer R, Sonnenberg A, et al: Survival and causes of death in cirrhotic and noncirrhotic patients with primary hemochromatosis. N Engl J Med 313:1256, 1985.
222. Fargion S, Mandelli C, Piperno A, et al: Survival and prognostic factors in 212 Italian patients with genetic hemochromatosis. Hepatology 15:655, 1992.
223. Edwards CQ, Cartwright GE, Skolnick MH, et al: Homozygosity for hemochromatosis: clinical manifestations. Ann Intern Med 93:511, 1980.
224. Weintraub LR, Conrad ME, Crosby WH: The treatment of hemochromatosis by phlebotomy. Med Clin North Am 50:1533, 1966.
225. Powell LW, Kerr JFR: Reversal of "cirrhosis" in idiopathic haemochromatosis following long-term intensive venesection therapy. Aust Ann Med 1:54, 1970.
226. Cohen A, Martin M, Schwartz E: Depletion of excessive liver iron stores with desferrioxamine. Br J Haematol 58:369, 1984.
227. Pippard MJ, Callender ST: The management of iron chelation therapy. Br J Haematol 54:503, 1983.
228. Nienhuis AW: Vitamin C and iron. N Engl J Med 304:170, 1981.
229. Smith PM, Godfrey BE, Williams R: Iron absorption in idiopathic haemochromatosis and its measurement using a whole-body counter. Clin Sci 37:519, 1969.
230. Cliff JL, Speight ANP: Venesection in haemosiderosis. East Afr Med J 53:289, 1976.
231. Pimstone NR: Porphyria cutanea tarda. Semin Liver Dis 2:132, 1982.
232. Grace ND, Greenberg MS: Phlebotomy in the treatment of iron overload: a controlled trial (a preliminary report). Gastroenterology 60:744, 1971 (abstract).
233. Barry M, Flynn DM, Letsky EA, et al: Long-term chelation therapy in thalassemia major: effect on liver iron concentration, liver histology and clinical progress. BMJ 2:16, 1974.
234. Modell B, Letsky EA, Flynn DM, et al: Survival and desferrioxamine in thalassemia major. BMJ 284:1081, 1982.
235. Hoffbrand AV, Gorman A, Laulicht M, et al: Improvement in iron status and liver function in patients with transfusional iron overload with long-term subcutaneous desferrioxamine. Lancet 1:947, 1979.
236. Propper RD, Shurin SB, Nathan DG: Reassessment of the use of desferrioxamine B in iron overload. N Engl J Med 294:1421, 1976.
237. Pippard MJ, Callender ST, Finch CA: Ferrioxamine excretion in iron-loaded man. Blood 60:288, 1982.
238. Brandhagen DJ, Alvarez W, Therneau TM, et al: Iron overload in cirrhosis: *HFE* genotypes and outcome after liver transplantation. Hepatology 31:456, 2000.
239. Dietz O, Vogel W, Brausperger B, et al: Liver transplantation in idiopathic hemochromatosis. Transplant Proc 22:1512, 1990.
240. Farrell FJ, Nguyen M, Woodley S, et al: Outcome of liver transplantation in patients with hemochromatosis. Hepatology 20:404, 1994.
241. Kowdley KV, Hassanein T, Kaur S, et al: Primary liver cancer and survival in patients undergoing liver transplantation for hemochromatosis. J Liver Transplant Surg 1:237, 1995.
242. Tung BY, Farrell FJ, McCashland TM, et al: Long-term follow-up after liver transplantation in patients with hepatic iron overload. Liver Transpl Surg 5:369, 1999.
243. Adams PC, Ghent CN, Grant DR, et al: Transplantation of a donor liver with haemochromatosis: evidence against an inherited intrahepatic defect. Gut 32:1082, 1991.
244. Koskinas J, Portmann B, Lombard M, et al: Persistent iron overload four years after inadvertent transplantation of a haemochromatotic liver in a patient with primary biliary cirrhosis. J Hepatol 16:351, 1992.
245. Dabkowski PL, Angus PW, Smallwood RA, et al: Site of principal metabolic defect in idiopathic haemochromatosis: Insights from transplantation of an affected organ. BMJ 306:1726, 1993.
246. Kowdley KV, Tavill AS: An "ironic" case of mistaken identity. Hepatology 16:500, 1992.
247. Powell LW: Does transplantation of the liver cure genetic hemochromatosis? J Hepatol 16:259, 1992.
248. Kowdley KV, Trainer TD, Saltzman JR, et al: Utility of hepatic iron index in American patients with hereditary hemochromatosis: a multicenter study. Gastroenterology 113:1270-1277, 1997.
249. Bottomley SS: Secondary iron overload disorders. Semin Hematol 35:77-86, 1998.
250. Weatherall DJ, Clegg JB: The Thalassaemia Syndromes, ed 3. Oxford, Blackwell Scientific, 1981.
251. Cartwright GE, Edwards CQ, Skolnick MH, et al: Association of HLA-linked hemochromatosis with idiopathic refractory sideroblastic anemia. J Clin Invest 65:989, 1980.
252. Fargion S, Piperno A, Panaiotopoulos N, et al: Iron overload in subjects with beta-thalassemia trait: role of idiopathic haemochromatosis gene. Br J Haematol 61:487, 1985.
253. Simon M, Beaumont C, Briere J, et al: Is the HLA-linked hemochromatosis allele implicated in idiopathic refractory sideroblastic anaemia? Br J Haematol 60:75, 1985.
254. Beaumont C, Fauchet R, Nhu Phung L, et al: Porphyria cutanea tarda and HLA-linked hemochromatosis: evidence against a systematic association. Gastroenterology 92:1833, 1987.
255. Simon M, Bourel M, Genetet B, et al: Idiopathic hemochromatosis and iron overload in alcoholic liver disease: differentiation by HLA phenotype. Gastroenterology 73:655, 1977.
256. Risdon RA, Barry M, Flynn DM: Transfusional iron-overload: the relationship between tissue iron concentration and hepatic fibrosis in thalassemia. J Pathol 116:83, 1975.
257. Cohen A, Witzleben C, Schwartz E: Treatment of iron overload. Semin Liver Dis 4:228, 1984.
258. Schafer AI, Cheron RG, Oluhy R, et al: Clinical consequences of acquired transfusional iron overload in adults. N Engl J Med 304:319, 1981.
259. Bonkovsky HL, Banner BF, Lambrecht RW, et al: Iron in liver diseases other than hemochromatosis. Semin Liver Dis 16:65-82, 1996.
260. George DK, Goldwurm S, Macdonald GA, et al: Increased hepatic iron concentration in nonalcoholic steatohepatitis is associated with increased fibrosis. Gastroenterology 114:311-318, 1998.
261. Conn HO: Portacaval anastomosis and hepatic hemosiderin deposition: a prospective controlled investigation. Gastroenterology 62:61-72, 1972.
262. DiBisceglie AM, Bonkovsky HL, Chopra S, et al: Iron reduction as an adjuvant to interferon therapy in patients with chronic hepatitis C who have previously not responded to interferon. A prospective randomized controlled trial. Hepatology 32:135-138, 2000.
263. Fontana RJ, Israel J, LeClair P, et al: Iron reduction before and during interferon therapy of chronic hepatitis C: results of a multicenter, randomized, controlled trial. Hepatology 31:730-736, 2000.
264. Kushner JP, Edwards CQ, Dadone MM, et al: Heterozygosity for HLA-linked hemochromatosis as a likely cause of the hepatic siderosis associated with sporadic porphyria cutanea tarda. Gastroenterology 88:1232, 1985.
265. Edwards CQ, Griffen LM, Goldgar DE, et al: HLA-linked hemochromatosis alleles in sporadic porphyria cutanea tarda. Gastroenterology 97:972-981, 1989.
266. Roberts AG, Whatley DS, Morgan RR, et al: Increased frequency of the hemochromatosis Cys282Tyr mutation in sporadic porphyria cutanea tarda. Lancet 349:321-323, 1997.
267. Grossman ME, Bickers DR, Poh-Fitzpatrick MB, et al: Porphyria cutanea tarda. Clinical features and laboratory findings in 40 patients. Am J Med 67:277-286, 1979.

268. Fargion S, Piperno A, Cappellini MD, et al: Hepatitis C virus and porphyria cutanea tarda: evidence of a strong association. Hepatology 17:551, 1993
269. Reizenstein P, Hoglund S, Lauergren J, et al: Iron metabolism in porphyria cutanea tarda. Acta Med Scand 198:95-99, 1975.
270. Turnbull A, Baker H, Vernon-Roberts B, et al: Iron metabolism in porphyria cutanea tarda and in erythropoietic protoporphyria. QJM 42:341-355, 1973.
271. Mukerji SK, Pimstone NR, Burns M: Dual mechanism of inhibition of rat liver uroporphyrinogen decarboxylase activity by ferrous iron: its potential role in the genesis of porphyria cutanea tarda. Gastroenterology 87:1248, 1984.
272. Kushner JP, Steinmuller D, Lee GR: The role of iron in the pathogenesis of porphyria cutanea tarda II. Inhibition of uroporphyrinogen decarboxylase. J Clin Invest 56:661, 1975.
273. De Verneuil H, Sassa S, Kappas A: Effects of polychlorinated biphenyl compounds, 2,3,7,8-tetrachlorodibenzo-*p*-dioxin, phenobarbital and iron on hepatic uroporphyrinogen decarboxylase. Implications for the pathogenesis of porphyria. Biochem J 214:145, 1983.
274. Bonkovsky HL, Healey JF, Sinclair PR, et al: Iron and the liver: acute effects of iron-loading on hepatic heme synthesis of rats. Role of decreased activity of 5-amino-levulinate dehydrase. J Clin Invest 71:1175, 1983.
275. Bonkovsky HL, Healey JF, Lincoln B, et al: Hepatic heme synthesis in a new model of experimental hemochromatosis: studies in rats fed finely divided elemental iron. Hepatology 7:2295, 1987.
276. Felsher BF, Carpio NM, Engleking DW, et al: Decreased hepatic uroporphyrinogen decarboxylase activity in porphyria cutanea tarda. N Engl J Med 306:766, 1982.
277. Lundvall O: The effect of phlebotomy in porphyria cutanea tarda. Acta Med Scand 189:33, 1971.
278. Epstein JH, Redeker AG: Porphyria cutanea tarda: a study of the effect of phlebotomy. N Engl J Med 279:1301, 1968.
279. Lundvall O: The effect of replenishment of iron stores after phlebotomy therapy in porphyria cutanea tarda. Acta Med Scand 189:51, 1971.
280. Felsher BF, Jones ML, Redeker AG: Iron and hepatic uroporphyrin synthesis: relation in porphyria cutanea tarda. JAMA 226:663, 1973.
281. Elder GH, Tovey JA, Sheppard DM, et al: Immunoreactive uroporphyrinogen decarboxylase in porphyria cutanea tarda. Lancet 1:1301, 1983.
282. Elder GH, Urquhart AJ, DeSalamanca RE, et al: Immunoreactive uroporphyrin decarboxylase in the liver in porphyria cutanea tarda. Lancet 2:229, 1986.
283. Smith AG, Francis JE, Kay SJE, et al: Mechanistic studies of the inhibition of hepatic uroporphyrinogen decarboxylase in SBL10 mice by iron-hexachlorobenzene synergism. Biochem J 238:871, 1986.
284. Smith AG, Francis JE: Chemically-induced formation of an inhibitor of hepatic uroporphyrinogen decarboxylase in inbred mice with iron overload. Biochem J 246:221, 1987.
285. Knisely AS: Iron and pediatric liver disease. Semin Liver Dis 14:229, 1994.
286. Witzlebin CL, Uri A: Perinatal hemochromatosis: entity or end result? Hum Pathol 20:335, 1989.
287. Bothwell TH, Isaacson C: Siderosis in the Bantu. A comparison of the incidence in males and females. BMJ 1:522, 1962.
288. Isaacson C, Seftel H, Keeley KJ, et al: Siderosis in the Bantu. The relationship between iron overload and cirrhosis. J Lab Clin Med 58:845, 1961.
289. Davis WD, Arrowsmith WR: The effect of repeated bleeding in hemochromatosis. J Lab Clin Med 36:814, 1950.
290. EASL International Consensus Conference on Haemochromatosis: J Hepatol 33:485-504, 2000.

CHAPTER

43

Granulomatous Diseases of the Liver

Shobha Sharma, MD

The interpretation of hepatic granulomas is more difficult than is generally appreciated; first, because the etiology of such lesions can seldom be established on histologic grounds alone, and, second, because the presence of granulomas in the liver does not necessarily imply an underlying systemic granulomatous process. Unless these two points are borne in mind, the discovery of granulomas in the liver may prove to be misleading rather than diagnostic.[1]

DEFINITION

Granulomas (Figure 43-1) are composed of discrete aggregates of epithelioid cells, which are transformed macrophages that have abundant cytoplasm, are rich in endoplasmic reticulum, and have fewer phagolysosomes than macrophages. These characteristics are consistent with a secretory function. Macrophages, by contrast, are primarily phagocytic. It is possible to distinguish an epithelioid cell granuloma from an aggregate of macrophages using the PAS (periodic acid Schiff) stain. Epithelioid cell granulomas are PAS-negative. An aggregate of macrophages may contain PAS-positive debris. Aggregated macrophages are always separate from one another, whereas epithelioid cells fuse to form a syncytium and multi-nucleated giant cells. In addition to epithelioid cells a variable number of multi-nucleated giant cells and granulomas contain other inflammatory cells such as lymphocytes and macrophages.[2]

IMMUNOLOGY

The purpose of a granuloma is to destroy or contain an injurious agent that cannot be disposed of by the humoral limb of the immune system. The infectious agent may be intracellular as in mycobacterial infection, extracellular as in schistosomiasis, or unknown as in sarcoidosis. It is well recognized that intracellular pathogens elicit a cytokine response that is distinct and different from that induced by extracellular pathogens. In a type 1 or Th1 response, the cytokines secreted are interferon gamma (INF-γ), interleukin 2 (IL-2) and IL-12. The type 1 response develops against intracellular pathogens and typically is seen in mycobacterial and sarcoid granulomas.[3-5] The type 2 or Th2 response is characterized by secretion of IL-4, IL-5, IL-6, and IL-10[3,6,7] and

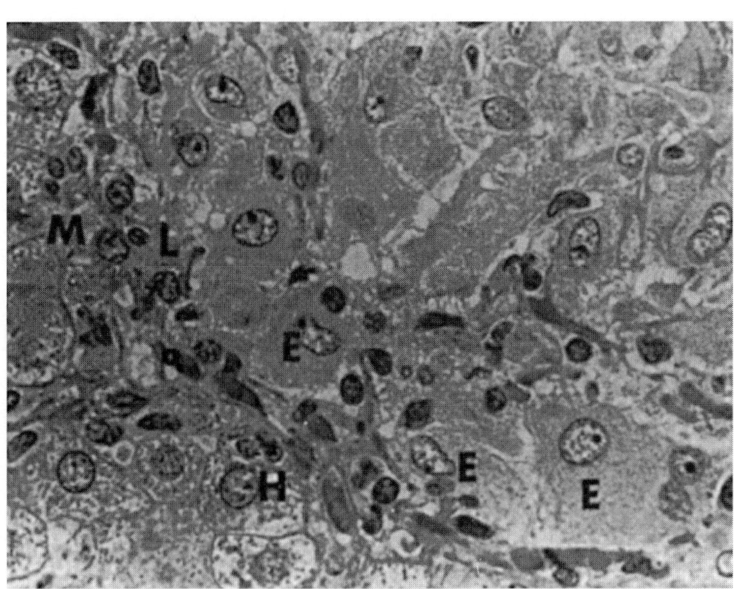

Figure 43-1 High-power photomicrograph of margin of epithelioid granuloma. Epithelioid cells have abundant cytoplasm and indistinct cytoplasmic borders. Other inflammatory cells such as lymphocytes are also present. (Hematoxylin and eosin; ×480.)

primarily is directed against extracellular antigens. Granulomas that develop under the influence of a Th1 response are larger, poorly formed, and more destructive than those in response to Th2 cytokines. Schistosomal ova induce a Th2 response against soluble egg antigens, contain prominent numbers of eosinophils, and may be associated with fibrosis—features that are attributed to IL-5 and IL-4, respectively.

Antigen-presenting cells such as macrophages and dendritic cells process antigens and present them to major histocompatibility complex class II-restricted helper T cells. These macrophages also secrete IL-12, which stimulates differentiation of CD4 lymphocytes. These in turn secrete INF-γ and IL-2 (Th1 response).[8] In a positive feedback loop, INF-γ and IL-2 amplify the immune response by stimulating proliferation of T cells and further production of INF-γ and IL-2. These cytokines then recruit monocytes and stimulate them to differentiate into macrophages that secrete tumor necrosis factor-alpha (TNF-α), which up-regulates expression of intercellular adhesion molecules (ICAMs). This last event allows inflammatory cells to adhere to endothelial cells and localize to the antigenic stimulus. TNF-α also stimulates T-cell proliferation and secretion of INF-γ.[9,10] In schistosomiasis an initial type 1 response usually evolves into a type 2 response.[9,11] This shift in cytokine profiles appears to be mediated by IL-10. Both IL-12 (Th1) and IL-10 (Th2) are cross-regulatory cytokines. For example, INF-γ and IL-12 secreted in a Th1 response can suppress the production of IL-4 and IL-10 associated with the Th2 response, and similarly IL-10 can suppress a Th1 response.[8,12] Which response predominates depends on the antigen and the timing of the cytokines secreted in relationship to the chronologic evolution of the granuloma. Thus the type 1 and type 2 responses are not mutually exclusive.[3,4] One response can evolve into another. This flexibility may provide protection to the host. This is illustrated in schistosomiasis in a nude mouse model in which an unabated Th1 response causes hepatotoxicity and death.[13] Type 1 and 2 cytokine responses are not restricted to T helper cells. Similar but not identical responses have been demonstrated in cytotoxic T cells, B cells, natural killer cells, and dendritic cells.[3,4]

In addition to immune induction a non-immune granulomatous reaction can be induced around indigestible foreign material such as talc. However, this material frequently accumulates in macrophages within the portal tract and Kupffer cells and does not form distinct granulomas. Talc crystals are birefringent and can be identified under polarized light.[14,15]

HISTOPATHOLOGY

The morphologic appearance of granulomas is variable. They may be distinct and well formed as in sarcoidosis, or they may be ill defined as in some drug reactions. They may be necrotizing in infections such as tuberculosis or non-necrotizing as in sarcoidosis. The location of granulomas within the liver (i.e., portal or acinar) is unlikely to be of diagnostic use unless primary biliary cirrhosis is the consideration. In general, granulomas in PBC are portal though they can be found in the acini.[1,2]

In the absence of acid-fast organisms, fungi, parasites, or foreign material, it is not possible to identify the etiology of a granuloma on morphologic grounds. An attempt should be made to examine granulomas for foreign material under polarized light and stain them for acid-fast bacilli and fungi even though the likelihood of finding them is low, particularly when the granulomas are found incidentally during the work-up of chronic hepatitis. Organisms are more likely to be found when the liver biopsy is performed in the investigation of pyrexia of unknown origin (PUO).[16-18]

Granulomas other than those associated with primary biliary cirrhosis, sarcoidosis, and schistosomiasis are rarely destructive and are not associated with consistent derangements of liver function tests (LFTs). Damage to bile ducts is seen in primary biliary cirrhosis and less frequently in sarcoidosis. Destruction of hepatic and portal veins with subsequent obliteration and scarring is implicated as a mechanism of portal hypertension in granulomatous hepatitis.

There is a discrepancy between the detection of granulomas in needle biopsies and autopsy samples.[19] This discrepancy reflects the amount of tissue sampled and selection of abnormal areas for sampling at autopsy. The likelihood of finding granulomas in a liver affected by granulomatous disease increases with the number of biopsies and increases from 50 percent to 100 percent from one core to three cores.[20,21]

LIPOGRANULOMAS

Lipogranulomas are distinctive but inconsequential granuloma in the liver (Figure 43-2). They are composed of lipid-laden histiocytes, lipid vacuoles, and a variable number of chronic inflammatory cells. They are well circumscribed and usually are located around the central vein. They may be present in the portal areas. The surrounding hepatic parenchyma may be normal or steatotic.[2,22] In non-fatty livers these granulomas appear to develop in response to exogenous mineral oils that are widely used in food processing. Using thin-layer and gas-liquid chromatography studies, lipids extracted from liver tissue, candies, and polished skins of apples and cucumbers show characteristics similar to mineral oil. The incidence of lipogranulomas has increased over the years, which is consistent with the wide use of mineral oils in the food industry.[22]

INCIDENCE AND CAUSES

The incidence of granulomas detected in liver biopsies varies from 0.8 percent to 15 percent.[1,19,23-30] The two major known causes of granulomas in liver biopsies are tuberculosis and sarcoidosis (Table 43-1). Sarcoidosis is more frequent in developed countries; tuberculosis is more common in underdeveloped nations. Fungal and schistosomal granulomas are seen in endemic areas.[19,28] After excluding a potpourri of diagnoses that include drugs, malignancies, and infections (listed in Table 43-2), there remains a category of granulomas of unknown significance. These may be incidental findings in patients being staged for chronic viral hepatitis.[1,24,31-33] There is a

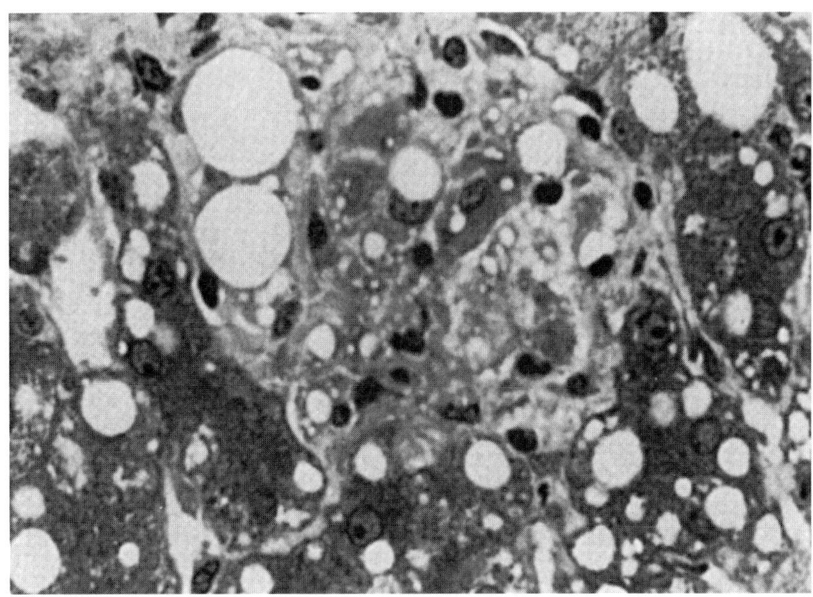

Figure 43-2 Lipogranuloma. Note small lipid droplets in histiocytes. (Hematoxylin and eosin; ×480.)

TABLE 43-1

Most Frequent Known Causes of Hepatic Granulomas

Ref	Year	City or Country	No. bx	Bx with gran	Sarcoidosis (%)	TB (%)	Unknown (%)	Miscellaneous*
23	1953	Cincinnati, Ohio	1100	54	11	24	18.5	
19	1966	Texas	1505	35	23	20	37	
24	1970	Scandinavia	2813	21	29	48		
25	1974	Cleveland, Ohio	2086	50	22	10	36	
1	1977	New York	6075	565	38	12	21	
26	1979	Washington, DC	N/A	73	55	12	3	
27	1988	Australia	N/A	59	12	4	17	
28	1990	Saudi Arabia	404	59	0	32	0	54% schistosomiasis
29	1994	Ireland	4124	163	18	18	11	55% PBC

Bx, Biopsy; *gran,* granuloma; *TB,* tuberculosis; *N/A,* not available; *PBC,* primary biliary cirrhosis.

*Miscellaneous causes of granulomas included syphilis,[23] lymphogranuloma venereum,[23] lymphoma,[19,23,25-27] brucellosis,[1,19,26,28] mycoses,[19,26] drugs,[26,27,29] Crohn's disease,[26,29] cytomegalovirus,[26,27] berylliosis,[1] temporal arteritis,[1] Q fever,[27] renal and hepatocellular carcinoma,[27] and typhoid.[28]

small group of patients, however, in whom idiopathic granulomatous hepatitis is the cause of symptoms and disordered LFTs. Thus the interpretation of hepatic granulomas is largely dependent on the clinical indication for the biopsy.

Granulomas may be found in liver biopsies performed for the following indications.

- Grading and staging in a patient with chronic viral hepatitis
- Investigation and staging of primary biliary cirrhosis
- Confirmation of diagnosis of sarcoidosis
- Investigation of portal hypertension
- Investigation of liver cell dysfunction of undetermined etiology
- Investigation of PUO

Incidental hepatic granulomas have been found in patients being investigated for documented hepatitis C infection. The reported incidence in this setting varies from 0.73 percent to 10 percent[31-33] but is probably closer to the former.

Granulomas are a pathognomonic feature of primary biliary cirrhosis. This disease predominantly affects middle-aged white women who may be diagnosed during the investigation of non-specific symptoms such as fatigue or in whom the diagnosis is suspected because of cholestatic symptoms (e.g. pruritus, jaundice). The granulomas are portal in location and may be intimately associated with damage to interlobular bile ducts (Plate 43-1).[34,35] Laboratory investigations show a twofold to fivefold increase in alkaline phosphatase and the presence of the diagnostic anti-mitochondrial antibodies.

Among the many causes of PUO in immunocompetent patients are intra-abdominal infections and neoplasms, which are diagnosed using increasingly sophisticated imaging modalities. Increasingly sensitive and specific serologic tests identify patients with a variety of collagen vascular disorders and infections. A thorough clinical history pertaining to medications and travel may be clues to a drug-induced hepatitis and a serologic search for unusual infections. For these

TABLE 43-2
Classification and Causes of Hepatic Granulomas

Found Incidentally in the Evaluation of Primary Liver Disease
Hepatitis C, incidental
Hepatitis B, incidental[27]

Primary Biliary Cirrhosis
Sarcoidosis: destruction of bile ducts and portal veins

Associated with Portal Hypertension
Schistosomiasis
Sarcoidosis

Associated with Pyrexia of Unknown Origin
Usual
Sarcoidosis
Tuberculosis, miliary and pulmonary
Atypical mycobacteria
Q fever[27]
Brucellosis[1,23,28]
Cat-scratch disease
Mycoses (e.g., histoplasmosis, *Coccidioides immitis,* South American blastomycosis, candidiasis)
Drugs
Idiopathic granulomatous hepatitis

Rare
Cytomegalovirus[26,27]
Temporal arteritis[1]
Listeriosis
Leprosy, reactional states

Miscellaneous
Lymphoma[23,26,27]
Hepatic adenomas
Hepatocellular carcinoma[27]
Renal carcinoma[27]
Leprosy
Syphilis[23]
Lymphogranuloma venereum[23]
Crohn's disease[26,29]
Berylliosis[1]

reasons, the diagnostic utility of a blind liver needle biopsy in the evaluation of PUO is arguable. In patients with PUO, hepatomegaly, and deranged LFTs, the diagnostic yield for informative granulomas such as mycobacterial or fungal infection in the liver biopsy varies from 0 percent to 17 percent.[16-18]

Hepatic granulomas are more likely to be found in 16 percent to 75 percent of patients[36,39-41] in the investigation of PUO, deranged LFTs, or hepatomegaly in patients infected with the human immunodeficiency virus (HIV), including those with acquired immunodeficiency disease.[36-38] The most likely cause for these granulomas is mycobacterial infection with *Mycobacterium tuberculosis* or *Mycobacterium avium intracellulare* (MAI). If the organisms are identified on acid-fast bacillus stains, a definitive diagnosis is quickly established. And even though these diseases are likely to be disseminated, early treatment can be instituted.[37] The role of blood and tissue culture is controversial but is useful to characterize the organism and identify patients with negative liver or bone marrow biopsies.[38]

In both immunocompetent and immunocompromised patients, the diagnostic yield for fungi and mycobacterial infections is greater in the liver biopsy compared with bone marrow biopsy.[37,42]

LIVER FUNCTION TESTS

LFT abnormalities are generally non-specific; but as noted previously, a selective elevation in alkaline phosphatase suggests primary biliary cirrhosis or sarcoidosis.

SARCOIDOSIS

Sarcoidosis is a systemic granulomatous disease characterized by a Th1 response against an unknown antigen. Clustering of patients suggests a temporal and spatial relationship that would be expected if the cause were a transmissible agent or shared environmental factor. Clustering is greater between relatives of patients than among their spouses, however, which suggests a genetic predisposition in addition to contact and shared environment.[43-46]

Sarcoid afflicts people 20 to 40 years of age. It affects whites and blacks, but Swedes, Danes, and blacks have the highest prevalence rates. The disease is indolent in most patients. In a small proportion patients may be severely symptomatic and the disease can result in death. The course tends to be more severe in blacks and Swedes. Poor prognostic features include black origin, age of more than 40 years, and involvement of three organ systems.[47-48]

Patients may present with PUO, non-productive cough and chest pain, malaise, and weight loss. The most commonly affected organs are lung (100 percent) and mediastinal lymph nodes (90 percent). The diagnosis is one of exclusion. The history must exclude occupational or environmental factors that could cause granulomas. Confirmation of the diagnosis is by biopsy, the preferred sites being the tracheobronchial tree and lung.[47,48] Hepatic involvement is usually silent, and liver dysfunction is an unusual manifestation of sarcoidosis. Presentation of the disease as either hepatitis or carditis is unusual and is seen in 4 percent to 7 percent of patients.[48] Symptoms and signs suggestive of hepatic involvement include abdominal pain, hepatomegaly, jaundice, and portal hypertension.[49-51] Patients may present with PUO. In a third of patients there is a disproportionate elevation in alkaline phosphatase in comparison to the transaminases.[49,52-54]

Non-necrotizing granulomas are identified in the liver in 24 percent to 75 percent of patients with sarcoidosis.[52,55,56] Sarcoidosis is one of the most common causes of hepatic granulomas associated with a known cause (see Table 43-1). The incidence is slightly higher in biopsy series than in autopsies, probably because a liver biopsy is more likely to be performed when there are symptoms and signs of liver involvement in a patient with established sarcoidosis.[52,55,57]

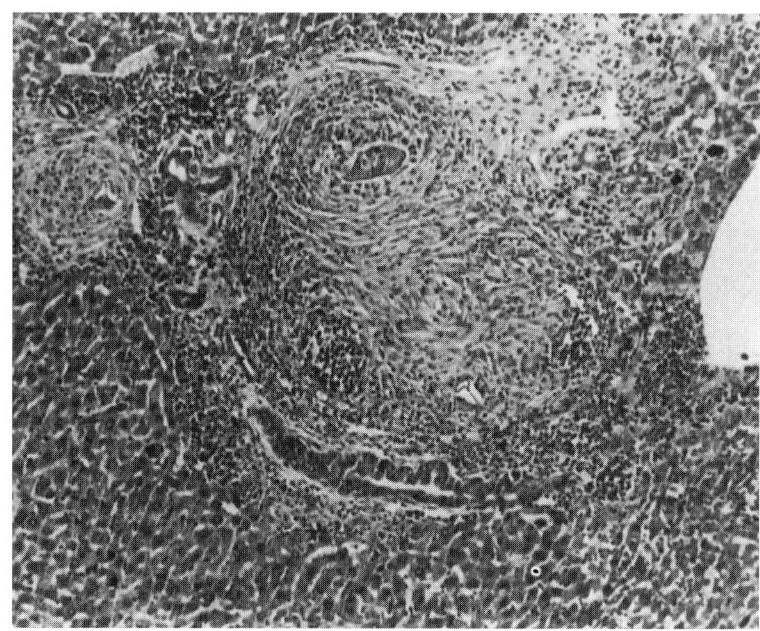

Figure 43-3 Portal granulomatous response and fibrosis around schistosome ova *(arrow)*. (Hematoxylin and eosin; ×55.)

The granulomas are characteristically tight, well formed, and non-necrotizing (Plate 43-2). They are uniformly distributed throughout the liver. They tend to be periportal but are seen in both periportal and lobular locations. A component of lobular hepatitis and portal triaditis may be present.[57] Most sarcoid granulomas resolve spontaneously. Some heal by fibrosis and scarring. Cirrhosis may result because of scarring of granulomas or a co-existent disease such as viral hepatitis. Portal hypertension can develop in the absence of cirrhosis. Explanations for this include presinusoidal portal hypertension secondary to scarring and obliteration of small portal and hepatic veins by portal granulomas and arteriovenous shunts within the granulomas.[49,53,58-60] Destruction of interlobular bile ducts produces a histologic picture that is indistinguishable from primary biliary cirrhosis.[50,51,54,57] Damaged bile ducts resembling sclerosing cholangitis have also been described.[54,61]

Patients with sarcoid and hepatic involvement may improve symptomatically and biochemically when placed on steroids but structural damage, particularly ductopenia, is irreversible.[62,63] Ursodeoxycholic acid has been used to alleviate cholestatic symptoms.[64-65] Recurrence of disease after liver transplantation has been documented but is unusual.[66-68]

SCHISTOSOMIASIS

Schistosomiasis (bilharziasis) is another example of a granulomatous hepatitis that can be associated with portal hypertension. It affects 200 million people worldwide, and the infestation is seen in a wide geographic belt that extends from South America, across the Caribbean islands, sub-Saharan Africa and the Middle East, South Africa, to the South Pacific and Southern China. As a result of travel and migration, 400,000 people with schistosomiasis live in the United States.[69-72]

Schistosomes are digenetic trematodes (sexual and asexual reproduction in alternating generations). The most common species are *Schistosoma haematobium* (Africa and Middle East), *Schistosoma mansoni* (South America, Caribbean, Africa, and Middle East), and *Schistosoma japonicum* (Far East). The adult worms reside in the mesenteric (*S. mansoni* and *S. japonicum*) and perivesical venous plexus (*S. haematobium*). The adult worm is not immunogenic, but the *Schistosoma* ova are highly antigenic.[73-75] They elicit a Th2 cytokine response resulting in the development of eosinophil-rich granulomas in the portal tracts (Figure 43-3). In mice with severe combined immunodeficiency, the inability to elicit a granulomatous response leads to severe hepatotoxicity and death resulting from the egg antigens.[13] Although the granulomatous response kills at least one third of eggs and protects the host from the toxicity of the egg antigens, it is also used by the parasite to protect the egg from further host damage and to permit egg migration.[13,73] Granulomas and fibrosis resulting from the release of fibrogenic cytokines such as IL-4 cause obliteration or compression of the portal veins, resulting in presinusoidal portal hypertension. In a small proportion of patients extensive fibrosis develops along the portal venous system. This is also known as the pipe stem fibrosis of Symmers. The fibrosis follows the distribution of the portal veins but does not transect the hepatic parenchyma. Therefore it is distinct from cirrhosis.[76-79]

Hepatic fibrosis does not develop in all patients. This complication is seen most often in young adults (5-15 years), who have had prolonged, intense infection (15-20 years). Using segregation and linkage analysis, a genetic locus controlling for intensity of infection was identified in a Brazilian cohort. This locus mapped to chromosome 5q31-q33. The genes for IL-4 and IL-5 are also located in this region.[80] Similar studies identify a locus controlling for fibrosis located on chromosome 6q22-q23. The gene on chromosome 6 is linked closely to the IFN-γ R1 (interferon gamma receptor) gene. The exact genes and their protein products have yet to be identified.[81] Patients with hepatosplenic schistosomiasis have high levels of INF-γ, TNF-α, and soluble TNF receptors, and low levels of IL-5 in their serum. This Th1 cytokine profile suggests that patients who do not develop a Th2 response are more likely to develop hepatic fibrosis.[82] Understanding how cytokines modulate the development of granulomas may allow therapeutic immunomodulation to achieve the balance between walling of the toxic egg antigens in a granulomatous response while controlling the development of fibrosis.[75]

A good clinical history that elicits origin or travel to endemic regions is perhaps the first clue to suspecting the diagnosis. Though most patients are asymptomatic in the early phase of the infection, there may be a local skin rash at the site of entry of schistosomal cercaria (cercarial dermatitis). Although people living in endemic regions are usually asymptomatic, visitors to endemic areas develop fever, chills, cough, diarrhea, malaise, and arthralgias 4 to 10 weeks after infection. The physical examination of acute schistosomiasis is characterized by hepatosplenomegaly. The blood shows peripheral eosinophilia. LFTs demonstrate a mild elevation of aminotransferases.[71,72]

In endemic areas the diagnosis is made on examination of the stool and urine for ova. However, when the infestation is light, this may be an insensitive tool. In this situation detection of antibodies using sensitive and specific enzyme-linked immunoassays developed against microsomal antigens of the adult worm can be performed. Antibody testing can only be performed 6 to 8 weeks after exposure.[83]

Treatment is with praziquantel, which can be given in doses of 20 mg three times in one day or a one time dose of 40 mg. Oxamniquine is an alternative in patients infected with *Schistosoma mansoni*[71-72] (see Chap. 35).

The following section examines a variety of infections that cause pyrexia and are associated with granulomas in the liver.

TUBERCULOSIS

Tuberculosis may manifest primarily as liver disease either because of hepatomegaly or abnormal LFTs. The majority of affected patients have miliary tuberculosis. Caseating granulomas are seen in more than 80 percent of these patients.[84] In one study of 36 patients with miliary tuberculosis, granulomas were present in 91 percent of the liver biopsies. Of these, 52 percent were caseating granulomas. Acid-fast bacilli are identified in only 9 percent of hepatic granulomas in miliary tuberculosis.[84] In contrast to liver biopsies, granulomas were noted in only 53 percent of bone marrow biopsies performed in the same patients. Moreover, hepatic granulomas were present in 78 percent of patients with negative bone marrow biopsies. The conclusion of this study was that though bone marrow biopsies are safer to perform, the diagnostic yield of the liver biopsy in miliary tuberculosis is higher.[42]

Non-necrotizing hepatic granulomas are seen in 25 percent of patients with pulmonary tuberculosis. It is unusual to find acid-fast organisms in these biopsies.[85] Therefore although acid-fast staining should be performed in all cases of granulomatous inflammation, the stain is insensitive in detecting acid-fast organisms. Similarly, culture of biopsies yields organisms in less than 10 percent of biopsies. Polymerase chain reaction (PCR) for *M. tuberculosis* has been performed on formalin-fixed, paraffin-embedded sections. This test has a specificity of 96 percent but the sensitivity is only 53 percent. On the other hand, PCR is a relatively rapid method of detection, with a 90 percent positive predictive value and a 76 percent negative predictive value.[86]

ATYPICAL MYCOBACTERIA

The characteristic appearance of MAI in immunocompromised patients is the presence of collections of foamy macrophages filled with acid-fast organisms. Infection with *Mycobacterium gevanese* also has been described in patients immunocompromised by HIV infection and has similar morphology.[87] The morphology of MAI is different in immunocompetent people, in whom well-formed granulomas have been described in the liver and spleen. In these patients it is unusual to demonstrate acid-fast organisms in the tissue sections. Confirmation is by culture.[89]

A hepatic presentation has been described in a patient infected with *Mycobacterium scrofulaceum*. Non-caseating granulomas were identified on liver biopsy, and the diagnosis was confirmed on tissue culture.[89]

Bacille Calmette-Guérin

Bacille Calmette-Guérin is an attenuated strain of *Mycobacterium bovis* used in the immunotherapy of superficial bladder carcinoma. Hepatic dysfunction and granulomatous hepatitis are very rare complications of intravesical therapy.[90] In a large series of 2602 patients, tuberculous hepatitis or pneumonia developed in 18 patients (0.7 percent). The frequency of hepatic granulomas in the absence of liver dysfunction was probably higher.[90,91] It is rare to culture or find acid-fast organism in the granulomas in these patients,[92,93] which makes it difficult to distinguish between a hypersensitivity reaction and systemic mycobacteremia. The goal of treatment in patients, who develop symptoms and signs of hepatic dysfunction, is to cover both possibilities—a 6-month course of rifampin and isoniazid accompanied by steroids, if indicated, and possibly cessation of immunotherapy.[90]

Q Fever

Q, or query, fever, was described in 1937 as an occupational disease among slaughter house workers and dairy farmers.[94] It became a notifiable disease in 1999. It is a zoonotic infection caused by the intracellular gram-negative rickettsial organism *Coxiella burnetii*. The primary but not exclusive reservoirs are cattle, goats, and sheep. The infection is maintained in ticks and other arthropods. The organisms are excreted into milk, urine, and feces of infected animals, and there is a high concentration of the organisms in the placenta and amniotic fluid. For this reason, the incidence rises during the lambing season in sheep-farming communities. The organisms are resistant to heat and drying, and the most common method of infection is inhalation of aerosolized bacteria. Ingestion of contaminated milk and tick bites are other sources of infection. The incubation period is between 2 and 3 weeks.[95]

Most infected patients are asymptomatic. Those who do develop symptoms have a self-limited illness characterized by high spiking fever (38.5°-40° C), malaise, bifrontal headache, and pneumonia.[96] In most patients there is resolution in 2 to 3 weeks, but in up to 16 percent of patients, chronic Q fever develops, characterized by endocarditis.[97]

Liver abnormalities are found in 11 percent to 65 percent of patients. In a study of 72 patients, 85 percent had abnormal LFTs and 65 percent had hepatomegaly.[98]

Liver biopsies may be performed in patients who present with PUO. Although non-specific granulomas may be seen in a background of non-specific reactive hepatitis and steatosis, a characteristic fibrin ring granuloma has been described. The granuloma surrounds a clear space felt to represent a lipid vacuole. A fibrin ring is present that either surrounds the lipid vacuole within the granuloma or is at the periphery of the entire granuloma.[99] Variations on this histology include a granuloma around a lipid vacuole without a fibrin ring or a granulomatous response around fragmented fibrin material.[100,101] The granulomas do not show a preferential lobular or periportal distribution. The recognition of the characteristic histology of the granuloma has led to serologic testing and confirmation of *C. burnetii* infection in some patients with PUO.[100,102] In patients who respond to treatment and are followed up with a repeat biopsy, there is resolution of the histologic findings in the liver. There are individual reports of fibrosis developing in these livers, based on sequential biopsies. These reports were made before the availability of hepatitis C testing, however. A definite association cannot be made between Q fever and the development of hepatic fibrosis.[103]

Although fibrin ring granulomas (Figure 43-4) are characteristic in acute Q fever and have led to serologic testing and confirmation of the diagnosis, they are not seen in all patients with Q fever[102] and are not specific for this disease. Isolated case reports have described similar granulomas in liver biopsies from patients with viral hepatitis A, temporal arteritis, Epstein-Barr virus, cytomegalovirus, systemic lupus erythematosus, leishmaniasis, and allopurinol-induced hepatitis. Q fever was considered in all these cases, but it was excluded by serologic testing.[104-110]

Confirmation of diagnosis is by identification of specific antibodies. The organism exists in two antigenic phases. Antibodies to phase II antigens are seen early in the disease. Chronicity should be suspected if there are rising titres of antibodies to phase I antigens with either constant or falling levels of phase II antibodies.[111,112]

Doxycycline 100 mg taken twice daily for 15 to 21 days is the treatment of choice.[94]

Brucellosis

Brucellosis is a zoonotic infection found in a variety of farm animals including goats, pigs, cattle, and dogs. Human infection is caused by *Brucella abortus* (cattle), *Brucella suis* (pigs), and *Brucella melitensis* (goats). *B. abortus* is most widely prevalent in the United States, but worldwide, the most clinically important species is *Brucella melitensis*.[113] Human infection occurs through contact with animals or animal products, such as cheese made from unpasteurized milk. Similar to Q fever, brucellosis enters the body through aerosols of the organisms, ingestion of foods, or contamination of wounds. Hence people who consume these products, workers in abattoirs, animal inspectors and handlers, and veterinarians are at greatest risk.

Based on information from the Centers for Disease Control and Prevention, brucellosis is not a common in-

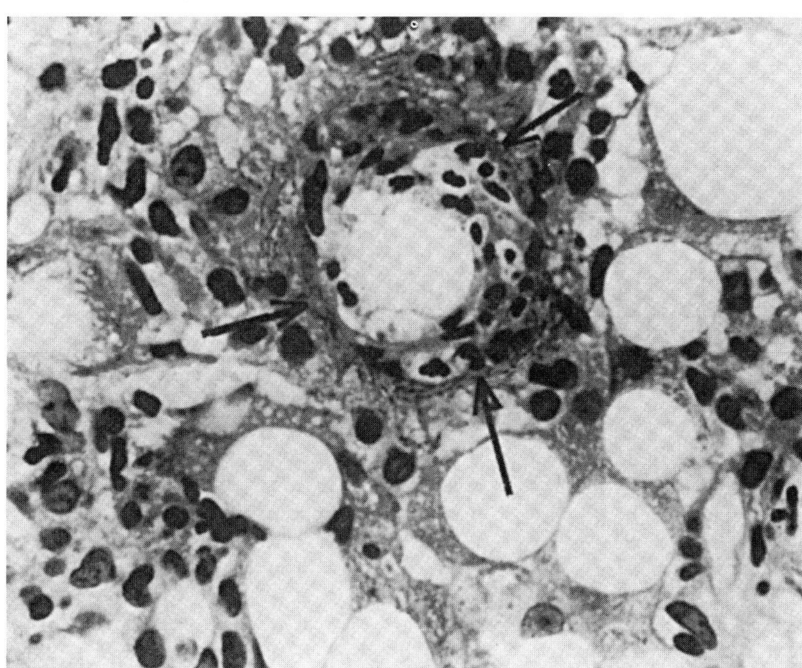

Figure 43-4 Fibrin ring granuloma in patient with Q fever. Note fibrinoid ring *(arrows)* around the central vacuole. (Hematoxylin and eosin; ×460.)

fection in the United States (fewer than 0.5 cases per 100,000), which reflects strict animal control regulations and vaccination programs. The majority of U.S. cases are reported from California, Florida, Texas, and Virginia. However, people in countries bordering the Mediterranean Basin (i.e., Portugal, Spain, Southern France, Italy, Greece, Turkey, North Africa, and South and Central America) and the Middle East are at high risk, particularly from unpasteurized cheeses.

In the acute phase patients present with recurrent episodes of high fever; drenching sweats; frontal and occipital headaches; body, chest, and abdominal pains; and anorexia. Physical examination reveals splenomegaly and variable hepatomegaly. Resolution is slow and may take weeks or months.[114,115]

Hepatic involvement is not a common presentation for brucellosis, but symptoms of liver disease were noted in 40 of 82 patients in one series.[116] The exact nature of the symptoms was not detailed, but patients had mild abnormalities in transaminases and alkaline phosphatase. In addition, 65 percent had hepatomegaly. The main finding on liver biopsy was a non-specific reactive hepatitis. Small non-necrotizing granulomas were noted in 28 patients (Figure 43-5). Development of granulomas appears to be an early event because only 3 of 28 patients with granulomas had symptoms for longer than 100 days. These granulomas of brucellosis are smaller than those usually associated with sarcoidosis or tuberculosis. Thus they may suggest the diagnosis of brucellosis in a patient being investigated for PUO.[116] A good history may also draw attention to this diagnosis. Confirmation of brucellosis is made by serologic testing, and exceptionally, through blood and bone marrow culture of the organism. Antibody testing performed 2 weeks apart shows increase in the antibody titers.[115]

Treatment is difficult. The World Health Organization recommends a combination of doxycycline 200 mg and rifampin 600 to 800 mg taken daily for 6 weeks; this has been substantiated in more recent studies.[117,118]

Cat-scratch Disease

Cat-scratch disease is caused by *Bartonella henselae.*[119] The classic presentation is lymphadenopathy associated with mild general symptoms such as malaise, aches and pains, and abdominal pain. On directed questioning, a history of contact with a kitten is elicited (an animal younger than 1 year old). The organism is introduced into the skin through a scratch or wound and produces a papule at the site of inoculation within 3 to 5 days. Lymphadenopathy develops in the region draining that location and is noted 2 weeks later.[120] On histopathologic examination, the lymph nodes show stellate, necrotizing granulomas. The organisms can be identified by a Warthin-Starry stain. The disease appears to be seasonal, preferentially occurring in the second half of the year.

Occasionally, the disease presents with hepatic involvement in the absence of peripheral lymphadenopathy.[121-125] This presentation has mainly been described in children, who present with fever, malaise, and abdominal pain. Blood tests show mild but non-specific abnormalities in LFTs. After an exhaustive search for the etiology, a computed tomography (CT) scan is performed that shows filling defects suspicious for a malignant neoplasm. However, on biopsy, necrotizing granulomas and the organism are identified. Retrospectively, a history of contact with a kitten and a positive cat-scratch skin test confirm the diagnosis.

The reason why only some children develop visceral manifestations is unclear. One child had a persistent deficiency of T lymphocytes, suggesting an underlying immunologic abnormality, but this was not further elucidated.[126]

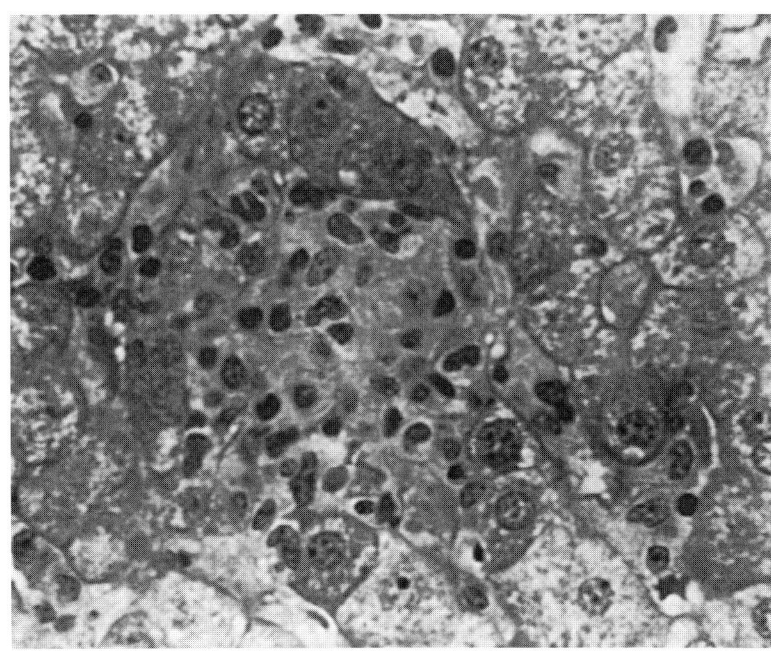

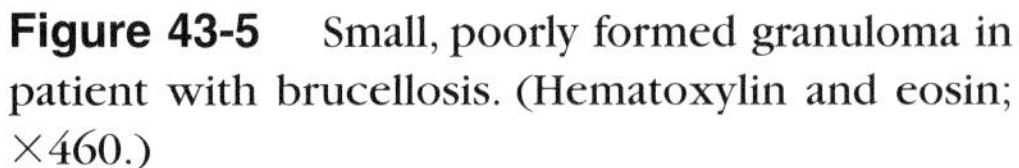

Figure 43-5 Small, poorly formed granuloma in patient with brucellosis. (Hematoxylin and eosin; ×460.)

The symptoms and findings in both scenarios resolve spontaneously. When severe, they can be treated with rifampicin, ciprofloxacillin, or gentamicin.[127]

DRUG-INDUCED HEPATITIS

A number of criteria need to be fulfilled for a drug to be considered responsible for hepatic granulomas. Other causes, such as those listed previously, should be excluded. A time course demonstrating that the symptoms leading to the liver biopsy developed after initiation of therapy must be established. Both symptoms and liver biopsy findings should resolve after stopping the drug and should return on rechallenge. Obviously, it is not always possible to establish cause and effect in this fashion, though it has been done for allopurinol,[129,130] carbamazepine,[132,133] chlorpropamide,[136] phenylbutazone,[137] methyldopa,[142] and quinidine.[138-140] Other drugs that have been implicated in the development of hepatic granulomas in the liver include hydralazine,[143] diltiazem,[144,145] phenytoin,[146] mebendazole,[147] gold,[148] quinine,[149,150] halothane,[151] amoxicillin-clavulanic acid,[152] aluminum,[153] pyrazinamide,[154] paracetamol,[155] glyburide,[156] and mesalamine[157] (Table 43-3). Both gold and aluminum have been demonstrated within granulomas using spectroscopic methods but were incidental findings. Gold was noted in patients with rheumatoid arthritis who were resistant to gold therapy and switched to methotrexate for which they underwent protocol liver biopsies. Excessive aluminum was present in the dialysate fluid in patients with chronic renal failure.

The granulomas are usually seen in a background of lobular hepatitis and or portal triaditis. Cholangitis is a more variable finding. Eosinophils may or may not be a prominent component of the inflammatory infiltrate.

Patients usually present with symptoms such as fever, arthralgias, nausea, and vomiting within a month of starting the new medication, but symptoms may develop a few months later. Physical examination may reveal jaundice and hepatomegaly; LFTs show abnormalities in transaminases and alkaline phosphatase or isolated elevations in alkaline phosphatase. Hyperbilirubinemia is an inconstant finding. Peripheral blood eosinophilia is not seen in all patients; but when present, it is suggestive of a drug-induced hepatitis.

TABLE 43-3

Some Drugs Associated with Granulomas in the Liver

Drug	Class
Allopurinol[129,130]	Anti-hyperuricemic
Carbamazepine[132,133]	Anti-convulsant
Glyburide[156]	Oral hypoglycemic
Chlorpropamide[136]	Oral hypoglycemic
Phenylbutazone[137]	Anti-inflammatory
Quinidine[138-140]	Anti-arrhythmic
Methyldopa[142]	Anti-hypertensive
Hydralazine[143]	Anti-hypertensive
Diltiazem[144,145]	Calcium channel blocker
Phenytoin[146]	Anti-convulsant
Mebendazole[147]	Anti-helminthic
Quinine[149,150]	Skeletal muscle relaxant
Halothane[151]	Anesthetic gas
Amoxicillin-clavulanic acid[152]	Antibacterial
Pyrazinamide[154]	Anti-tuberculous agent
Paracetamol[155]	Analgesic/antipyretic
Mesalamine[157]	Anti-inflammatory (sulfasalazine derivative)

GRANULOMATOUS HEPATITIS WITH NO OBVIOUS CAUSE

After all the more common causes of pyrexia or abnormalities in LFTs resulting in granulomatous inflammation in the liver are excluded, there remains a group of patients with granulomatous hepatitis of unknown etiology. Most of the literature does not specifically address the question of an autoimmune cause in these patients.[158-160,162-164]

Many of these patients present with spiking high fever that is often associated with chills and rigors and significant weight loss.[158-160,163] The duration of symptoms varies from months to years. Liver biopsy is performed in the work-up of PUO and abnormal LFTs.

These patients do not respond to empiric anti-tuberculous therapy. In some patients there is spontaneous resolution of symptoms. Others require treatment with steroids, to which they show a dramatic response. Some patients are cured with short-term steroids. Others must be maintained for long periods to prevent relapse off medication. The duration depends on the response to withdrawal and can vary from months to years. In patients who have undergone sequential liver biopsies, the granulomas disappear on therapy. They reappear when the patient relapses.[159,160]

Treatment consists of prednisone 0.75 to 1.0 mg/kg/day.[163] The mean duration of therapy in one study was approximately 1 year. A prophylactic course of antituberculous medication is advised, particularly if the Mantoux test is positive or there is an unexplained anergic response.[159,163] In one child who presented with high fever and a palpable liver, the ultrasound showed abnormal findings. A follow-up CT scan showed multiple focal lesions suspicious for malignancy. The biopsy showed necrotizing granulomatous inflammation that responded to indomethacin, after cultures and acid-fast stains ruled out other causes.[162] Methotrexate has been used in patients who are steroid-resistant.[165]

Granulomatous lesions of unknown significance describes patients who present with fever, abdominal pain, and weight loss and who are detected to have multiorgan granulomatous inflammation that appears to be primarily subdiaphragmatic, involving the liver, spleen, and lymph nodes. These granulomas differ from sarcoid granulomas in that they are rich in B rather than T lymphocytes. Because none of the other studies discussed under idiopathic granulomatous hepatitis have examined the phenotype of the inflammatory cells within the

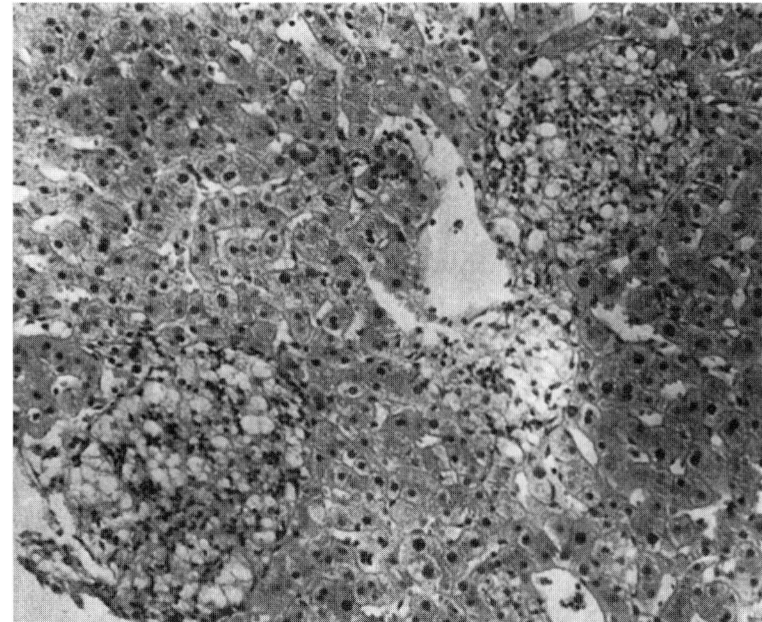

Figure 43-6 Granulomata composed of foam cells in patient with lepromatous leprosy. These foam cells would be filled with acid-fast bacilli on an acid-fast bacillus stain. (Hematoxylin and eosin; ×92.)

granulomas, it is possible that all these entities form a spectrum of granulomatous hepatitis of unknown etiology.[166]

The remaining sections deal with causes of granulomas that may be found in the investigation of liver cell dysfunction of undetermined etiology or as an incidental finding in the investigation of another disease.

LYMPHOMA

Hepatic granulomas have been identified in patients with both Hodgkin's and non-Hodgkin's lymphoma. They are usually discovered as part of the staging procedure and not because of liver dysfunction.[167-169] The presence of granulomas is not synonymous with involvement by lymphoma but warrants a careful examination of the lymphoid cells intermixed within the granuloma and within the adjacent parenchyma.

In one study more than half of the liver biopsies examined as a part of the staging protocol for Hodgkin's disease showed granulomas in the absence of hepatic involvement by Hodgkin's disease.[167] In another report a hypodense lesion was noted on a CT scan of the liver in a patient with Hodgkin's disease. The liver biopsy showed the lesion to be composed of a necrotizing, granulomatous reaction. An abnormal lymphoid infiltrate also was noted in the adjacent portal tracts within the biopsy. No microorganisms were identified, and the lesion resolved with treatment of the lymphoma.[168]

Examples of both B and T cell lymphomas have been described in which involvement of the liver by the non-Hodgkin's lymphoma has been associated with a granulomatous reaction either separate from[169] or intimately admixed with the abnormal lymphoid infiltrate.[170] It is hypothesized that this reaction may represent a host response to the lymphoma.

LEPROSY

Leprosy is rare in the United States but may be seen in immigrants.[171] After the nerves, skin, and lymph nodes, the liver is the organ most commonly involved in leprosy.[172,173] Granulomatous involvement of the liver occurs in all forms of leprosy (excluding neuritic) but is not associated with significant abnormalities of LFTs or clinical symptoms (Figure 43-6).[172] Epithelioid granulomas are seen in tuberculoid leprosy. These lesions contain few acid-fast organisms in contrast to lepromatous leprosy, in which granulomas are composed of foamy histiocytes laden with acid-fast bacilli.[171,173] This pattern of foamy macrophages laden with acid-fast bacilli is unusual in *M. tuberculosis*, but as noted, it may be seen in MAI infection.

Presentation with PUO is uncommon in leprosy except in reactional states. In this situation there is a high likelihood of misdiagnosis as tuberculosis unless clues (e.g., macular skin lesion, hair loss) lead to skin testing for acid-fast organisms.[171]

MISCELLANEOUS

Case reports and studies of miscellaneous causes and associations of granulomas in the liver include listeriosis,[174,175] candidiasis in leukemic patients,[176] histoplasmosis,[177] coccidioidomycosis (Figure 43-7),[178] cryptococcosis,[179] blastomycosis,[180] toxoplasmosis,[181] cytomegalovirus infection,[182] giant cell arteritis,[183] and hepatocellular neoplasms.[184] Listerial and candidal granulomas are necrotizing[174-176] and associated with a neutrophilic inflammatory infiltrate. Mycotic granulomas are usually part of disseminated infection and develop mainly in patients from endemic regions. They may be seen in both immunocompetent and immunocompro-

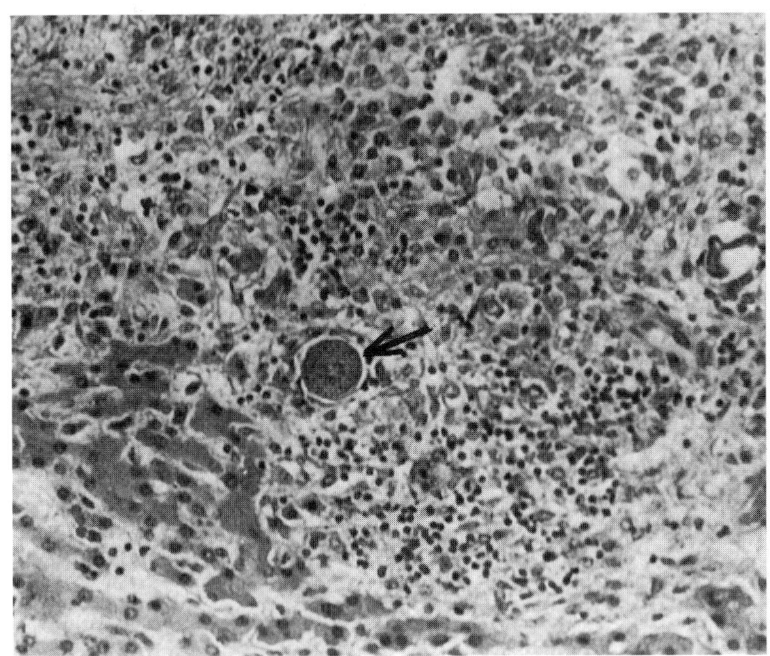

Figure 43-7 *Coccidioides* in hepatic granuloma. (Hematoxylin and eosin; ×92.)

mised patients. Hepatic histoplasmosis is associated with granulomas in only 19 percent of patients.[177] The different fungi and toxoplasmosis were identified within the lesions in contrast to listeriosis and cytomegalovirus infection in which the organisms were not noted either within the granulomas or the surrounding hepatic parenchyma.

References

1. Klatskin G: Hepatic granulomata; problems in interpretation. Mt Sinai J Med 44:798-812, 1977.
2. Denk H, Scheuer PJ, Baptista A, et al: Guidelines for the diagnosis and interpretation of hepatic granulomas. Histopathology 25:209-218, 1994.
3. Lucey DR, Clerici M, Shearer GM: Type 1 and type 2 cytokine disregulation in human infectious, neoplastic, and inflammatory diseases. Clin Microbiol Rev 9:532-562, 1996.
4. Baumer I, Zissel G, Schlaak M, et al: Th1/Th2 cell distribution in pulmonary sarcoidosis. Am J Resp Cell Molec Biol 16:171-177, 1997.
5. Agostini C, Basso U, Semenzato G: Cells and molecules involved in the development of sarcoid granuloma. J Clin Immunol 18:184-192, 1998.
6. Infante-Duarte C, Kamradt T: Th1/Th2 balance in infection. Springer Semin Immunopathol 21:317-338, 1999.
7. Mitchison NA, Schuhbauer D, Muller B: Natural and induced regulation of Th1/Th2 balance. Springer Semin Immunopathol 21:199-210, 1999.
8. Chensue SW, Ruth JH, Warmington K, et al: In vivo regulation of macrophage IL-12 production during type 1 and type 2 cytokine-mediated granuloma formation. J Immunol 155:3546-3551, 1995.
9. Chensue SW, Warmington K, Ruth J, et al: Cytokine responses during mycobacterial and schistosomal antigen-induced pulmonary granuloma formation. Production of Th1 and Th2 cytokines and relative contribution of tumor necrosis factor. Am J Pathol 145:1105-1113, 1994.
10. Wynn TA, Cheever AW: Cytokine regulation of granuloma formation in schistosomiasis. Curr Opin Immunol 7:505-511, 1995.
11. Chensue SW, Warmington KS, Hershey SD, et al: Evolving T cell responses in murine schistosomiasis. Th2 cells mediate secondary granulomatous hypersensitivity and are regulated by CD8+ T cells in vivo. J Immunol 151:1391-1400, 1993.
12. Chensue SW, Warmington K, Ruth JH, et al: Effect of slow release IL-12 and IL-10 on inflammation, local macrophage function and the regional lymphoid response during mycobacterial (Th1) and schistosomal (Th2) antigen-elicited pulmonary granuloma formation. Inflamm Res 46:86-92, 1997.
13. Amiri P, Locksley RM, Parslow TG, et al: Tumor necrosis factor α restores granulomas and induces parasite egg-laying in schistosome-infected SCID mice. Nature 356:604-607, 1992.
14. Molos MA, Litton N, Schubert TT: Talc liver. J Clin Gastroenterol 9:198-203, 1987.
15. Allaire GS, Goodman ZD, Ishak KG, et al: Talc in liver tissue of intravenous drug abusers with chronic hepatitis. A comparative study. Am J Clin Pathol 92:583-588, 1989.
16. Mitchell DP, Hanes TE, Hoyumpa AM, et al: Fever of unknown origin. Assessment of the value of percutaneous liver biopsy. Arch Intern Med 137:1001-1004, 1977.
17. Masana L, Guardia J, Clotet B, et al: Liver biopsy in fever of unknown origin. Gastroenterol Clin Biol 4:215-218, 1980.
18. Holtz T, Moseley RH, Scheiman JM: Liver biopsy in fever of unknown origin. A reappraisal. J Clin Gastroenterol 17:29-32, 1993.
19. Guckian JC, Perry JE: Granulomatous hepatitis. An analysis of 63 cases and review of the literature. Ann Intern Med 65:1081-1100, 1966.
20. Abdi WA, Millan JC, Mezey E: Sampling variability on percutaneous liver biopsy. Arch Intern Med 139:667-669, 1979.
21. Maharaj B, Maharaj RJ, Leary WP, et al: Sampling variability and its influence on the diagnostic yield of percutaneous needle biopsy of the liver. Lancet 8480:523-525, 1986.
22. Dincsoy HP, Weesner RE, MacGee J: Lipogranulomas in non-fatty human livers. A mineral oil induced environmental disease. Am J Clin Pathol 78: 35-41, 1982.
23. Wagoner GP, Anton AT, Gall EA, et al: Needle biopsy of the liver. VIII. Experiences with hepatic granulomas. Gastroenterology 25:487-494, 1953.
24. Iversen K, Christoffersen P, Poulsen H: Epithelioid cell granulomas in liver biopsies. Scand J Gastroenterol 7(suppl):61-67, 1970.
25. Mir-Madjilessi SH, Farmer RG, Hawk WA: Spectrum of hepatic manifestations of granulomatous hepatitis of unknown etiology. Am J Gastroenterol 62:221-229, 1974.
26. Irani SK, Dobbins WO III: Hepatic granulomas: a review of 73 patients from one hospital and a survey of the literature. J Clin Gastroenterol 1:131-143, 1979.
27. Anderson CS, Nicholls N, Rowland R, et al: Hepatic granulomas: a 15-year experience in the Royal Adelaide Hospital. Med J Aust 148:71-74, 1988.

28. Satti MB, Al-Freihi H, Ibrahim EM, et al: Hepatic granuloma in Saudi Arabia: a clinicopathological study of 59 cases. Am J Gastroenterol 85:669-674, 1990.
29. McCluggage WG, Sloan JM: Hepatic granulomas in Northern Ireland: a thirteen year review. Histopathology 25:219-228, 1994.
30. Sabharwal BD, Malhotra N, Garg R, et al: Granulomatous hepatitis: a retrospective study. Indian J Pathol Microbiol 38:413-416, 1995.
31. Barcena R, Sanroman AL, Del Campo S, et al: Posttransplant liver granulomatosis associated with hepatitis C? Transplantation 65:1494-1495, 1998.
32. Yamamoto S, Iguchi Y, Ohomoto K, et al: Epithelioid granuloma formation in type C chronic hepatitis: report of two cases. Hepatogastroenterology 42:291-293, 1995.
33. Emile JF, Sebagh M, Feray C, et al: The presence of epithelioid granulomas in hepatitis C virus related cirrhosis. Hum Pathol 24:1095-1097, 1993.
34. Kaplan MM: Primary biliary cirrhosis. N Engl J Med 335:1570-1580, 1996.
35. Portmann BC, MacSween RNM: Diseases of the intrahepatic bile ducts. In MacSween RNM, Antony PP, Scheuer PJ, et al, eds: Pathology of the Liver, ed 3. Edinburgh, Churchill Livingstone Co., 1994:477.
36. Comer GM, Mukherjee S, Scholes JV, et al: Liver biopsies in the acquired immune deficiency syndrome: influence of endemic disease and drug abuse. Am J Gastroenterol 84:1525-1531, 1989.
37. Prego V, Glatt AE, Roy V, et al: Comparative yield of blood culture for fungi and mycobacteria, liver biopsy, and bone marrow biopsy in the diagnosis of fevers of undetermined origin in human immunodeficiency virus-infected patients. Arch Intern Med 150:333-336, 1990.
38. Bach N, Theise ND, Schaffner F: Hepatic histopathology in the acquired immunodeficiency syndrome. Semin Liver Dis 12:205-212, 1992.
39. Wilkins MJ, Lindley R, Dourakis SP, et al: Surgical pathology of the liver in HIV infection. Histopathology 18:459-464, 1991.
40. Orenstein MS, Tavitian A, Yonk B, et al: Granulomatous involvement of the liver in patients with AIDS. Gut 26:1220-1225, 1985.
41. Lebovics E, Thung SN, Schaffner F, et al: The liver in the acquired immunodeficiency syndrome: a clinical and histologic study. Hepatology 5:293-298, 1985.
42. Cucin RL, Coleman M, Eckardt JJ, et al: The diagnosis of miliary tuberculosis: utility of peripheral blood abnormalities, bone marrow and liver needle biopsy. J Chronic Dis 26:355-361, 1973.
43. Parkes SA, Baker SB de C, Bourdillon RE, et al: Incidence of sarcoidosis in the Isle of Man. Thorax 40:284-287, 1985.
44. Parkes SA, Baker SB de C, Bourdillon RE, et al: Epidemiology of sarcoidosis in the Isle of Man-1: a case-controlled study. Thorax 42:420-426, 1987.
45. Hills SE, Parkes SA, Baker SB de C: Epidemiology of sarcoidosis in the Isle of Man-2: evidence for space time clustering. Thorax 42:427-430, 1987.
46. Mandel J, Weinberger SE: Clinical insights and basic science correlates in sarcoidosis. Am J Med Sci 1:99-107, 2001.
47. Newman LS, Rose CS, Maier LA: Sarcoidosis. N Engl J Med 336:1224-1234, 1997.
48. Statement on sarcoidosis. The joint statement of the American Thoracic Society (ATS), the European Respiratory Society (ERS) and the World Association of Sarcoidosis and other Granulomatous Disorders (WASOG). Am J Respir Crit Care Med 160:736-755, 1999.
49. Maddrey WC, Johns CJ, Boitnott JK, et al: Sarcoidosis and chronic hepatic disease: a clinical and pathologic study of 20 patients. Medicine 49:375-395, 1970.
50. Rudzki C, Ishak KG, Zimmerman HJ: Chronic intrahepatic cholestasis of sarcoidosis. Am J Med 59:373-387, 1975.
51. Nakanuma Y, Ohta G, Yamazaki Y, et al: Intrahepatic bile duct destruction in a patient with sarcoidosis and chronic intrahepatic cholestasis. Acta Pathol Japon 29:211-219, 1979.
52. Lehmuskallio E, Hannuksela M, Halme H: The liver in sarcoidosis. Acta Med Scand 202:289-293, 1977.
53. Valla D, Pessegueiro-Miranda H, Degott C, et al: Hepatic sarcoidosis with portal hypertension. A report of seven cases with a review of the literature. Q J Med 63:531-544, 1987.
54. Ishak KG: Sarcoidosis of the liver and bile ducts. Mayo Clin Proc 73:467-472, 1998.
55. Hercules HC, Bethlem NM: Value of liver biopsy in sarcoidosis. Arch Pathol Lab Med 108:831-834, 1984.
56. Rasmussen SM, Neukirch F: Sarcoidosis. A clinical study with special reference to the choice of biopsy procedure. Acta Med Scand 199:209-216, 1976.
57. Devaney K, Goodman ZC, Epstein MS, et al: Hepatic sarcoidosis. Clinicopathologic features in 100 patients. Am J Surg Pathol 17:1272-1280, 1993.
58. Tekeste H, Latour F, Levitt R: Portal hypertension complicating sarcoid liver disease: case report and review of the literature. Am J Gastroenterol 79:389-396, 1984.
59. Moreno-Merlo F, Wanless IR, Shimamatsu K, et al: The role of granulomatous phlebitis and thrombosis in the pathogenesis of cirrhosis and portal hypertension in sarcoidosis. Hepatology 26:554-560, 1997.
60. Nakanuma Y, Kouda W, Harada K, et al: Hepatic sarcoidosis with vanishing bile duct syndrome, cirrhosis, and portal phlebosclerosis. Report of an autopsy case. J Clin Gastroenterol 32:181-184, 2001.
61. Alam I, Levenson SD, Ferrell LD, et al: Diffuse intrahepatic biliary strictures in sarcoidosis resembling sclerosing cholangitis. Case report and review of the literature. Dig Dis Sci 42:1295-1301, 1997.
62. Israel HL, Goldstein RA: Hepatic granulomatosis and sarcoidosis. Ann Intern Med 79:669-678, 1973.
63. Murphy JR, Sjogren MH, Kikendall JW, et al: Small bile duct abnormalities in sarcoidosis. J Clin Gastroenterol 12:555-561, 1990.
64. Becheur H, Dall'Osto H, Chatellier G, et al: Effect of ursodeoxycholic acid on chronic intrahepatic cholestasis due to sarcoidosis. Dig Dis Sci 42:789-791, 1997.
65. Baratta L, Cascino A, Delfino M, et al: Ursodeoxycholic acid treatment in abdominal sarcoidosis. Dig Dis Sci 45:1559-1562, 2000.
66. Casavilla FA, Gordon R, Wright HI, et al: Clinical course after liver transplantation in patients with sarcoidosis. Ann Intern Med 118:865-866, 1993.
67. Fidler HM, Hadziyannis SJ, Dhillon AP, et al: Recurrent hepatic sarcoidosis following liver transplantation. Transplant Proc 29:2509-2510, 1997.
68. Hunt J, Gordon FD, Jenkins RL, et al: Sarcoidosis with selective involvement of a second liver allograft: report of a case and review of the literature. Modern Pathol 12:325-328, 1999.
69. Wiest PM, Olds GR: Clinical schistosomiasis. R I Med J 75:179-185, 1992.
70. Second Report of the WHO Expert Committee: The control of schistosomiasis. WHO Tech Rep Ser 830:1-87, 1993.
71. Elliot DE: Schistosomiasis. Pathophysiology, diagnosis and treatment (review). Gastroenterol Clin North Am 25:599-625, 1996.
72. Bica I, Hamer DH, Stadecker MJ: Hepatic schistosomiasis. Infect Dis Clin North Am 3:583-604, 2000.
73. McKerrow JH: Cytokine induction and exploitation in Schistosome infections. Parasitology 115:S107-S112, 1997.
74. Boros DL: T helper cell populations, cytokine dynamics, and pathology of the schistosome egg granuloma. Microb Infect 1:511-516, 1999.
75. Stadecker MJ: The development of granulomas in schistosomiasis: genetic backgrounds, regulatory pathways, and specific egg antigen responses that influence the magnitude of disease. Microb Infect 1:505-510, 1999.
76. Cheever AW, Andrade ZA: Pathological lesions associated with *Schistosoma mansoni* infection in man. Trans Roy Soc Trop Med Hyg 61:626-639, 1967.
77. Edington GM, von Lichtenberg F, Nwabuebo I, et al: Pathologic effects of schistosomiasis in Ibadan, Western State of Nigeria. I. Incidence and intensity of infection; distribution and severity of lesions. Am J Trop Med Hyg 19:982-995, 1970.
78. Cheever AW: Pipe-stem fibrosis of the liver. Trans Roy Soc Trop Med Hyg 66:947-948, 1972.
79. Bhagwandeen SB: Bilharzial pipe-stem portal fibrosis in Zambia. J Pathol 111:23-30, 1973.
80. Marquet S, Abel L, Hillaire D, et al: Genetic localization of a locus controlling the intensity of infection by *Schistosoma mansoni* on chromosome 5q31-q33. Nat Genet 14:181-184, 1996.
81. Dessein AJ, Hillaire D, Eldin N, et al: Severe hepatic fibrosis in *Schistosoma mansoni* infection is controlled by a major locus that is closely linked to the interferon-γ receptor gene. Am J Hum Genet 65:709-721, 1999.

82. Mwatha JK, Kimani G., Kamau T, et al: High levels of TNF, soluble TNF receptors, soluble ICAM-1 and IFN-γ, but low levels of IL-5, are associated with hepatosplenic disease in human *Schistosomiasis mansoni.* J Immunol 160:1992-1999, 1998.
83. Tsang VC, Wilkins PP: Immunodiagnosis of schistosomiasis. Immunol Invest 26:175-188, 1997.
84. Essop AR, Posen JA, Hodkinson JH, et al: Tuberculosis hepatitis: a clinical review of 96 cases. Q J Med 53:465-477, 1984.
85. Bowry S, Chan CH, Weiss H, et al: Hepatic involvement in pulmonary tuberculosis. Histologic and functional characteristics. Am Rev Resp Dis 101:941-948, 1970.
86. Diaz ML, Herrera T, Lopez-Vidal Y, et al: Polymerase chain reaction for the detection of *Mycobacterium tuberculosis* DNA in tissue and assessment of its utility in the diagnosis of hepatic granulomas. J Lab Clin Med 127:359-363, 1996.
87. Maschek H, Georgii A, Schmidt RE, et al: *Mycobacterium genavense*. Autopsy findings in three patients. Am J Clin Pathol 101:95-99, 1994.
88. Farhi DC, Mason UG III, Horsburgh CR Jr: Pathologic findings in disseminated *Mycobacterium avium-intracellulare* infection. A report of 11 cases. Am J Surg Pathol 85:67-72, 1986.
89. Patel KM: Granulomatous hepatitis due to *Mycobacterium scrofulaceum*: report of a case. Gastroenterology 81:156-158, 1981.
90. Lamm DL, Mander Meijden ADPM, Morales A, et al: Incidence and treatment of complications of Bacillus Calmette-Guerin intravesical therapy in superficial bladder cancer. J Urol 147:596-600, 1992.
91. Bodurtha A, Kim YH, Laucius JF, et al: Hepatic granulomas and other hepatic lesions associated with BCG immunotherapy for cancer. Am J Clin Pathol 61:747-752, 1974.
92. Proctor DD, Chopra S, Rubenstein SC, et al: Mycobacteremia and granulomatous hepatitis following initial intravesical Bacillus Calmette-Guerin instillation for bladder carcinoma. Am J Gastroenterol 88:1112-1115, 1993.
93. McParland C, Cotton DJ, Gowda KS, et al: Miliary *Mycobacterium bovis* induced by the intravesical Bacillus Calmette-Guerin immunotherapy. Am Rev Resp Dis 146:1330-1333, 1992.
94. Maurin M, Raoult D, Q fever. Clin Microbiol Rev 12:518-553, 1999.
95. Epidemiologic notes and reports. Q fever among slaughterhouse workers—California. CDC MMWR Weekly Report 35:223-226, 1986.
96. Hofmann CE, Heaton JW Jr: Q fever hepatitis: clinical manifestations and pathological findings. Gastroenterology 83:474-479, 1982.
97. Turck WPG, Howitt G, Turnberg LA, et al: Chronic Q fever. Q J Med 45:193-217, 1976.
98. Powell OW: Liver involvement in "Q" fever. Australasian Ann Med 10:52-58, 1961.
99. Pellegrin M, Delsol G, Auvergnat JC, et al: Granulomatous hepatitis in Q fever. Hum Pathol 11:51-57, 1980.
100. Qizilbash AH: The pathology of Q fever as seen on liver biopsy. Arch Pathol Lab Med 107:364-367, 1983.
101. Travis LB, Travis WD, Li CY, et al: Q fever. A clinicopathologic study of five cases. Arch Pathol Lab Med 110:1017-1020, 1986.
102. Westlake P, Price LM, Russell M, et al: The pathology of Q fever hepatitis. A case diagnosed by liver biopsy. J Clin Gastroenterol 9:357-363, 1987.
103. Atienza P, Ramond MJ, Degott C, et al: Chronic Q fever hepatitis complicated by extensive fibrosis. Gastroenterology 95:478-481, 1988.
104. Ruel M, Sevestre H, Henry-Biabaud E, et al: Fibrin ring granulomas in hepatitis A. Dig Dis Sci 37:1915-1917, 1992.
105. De Bayser L, Roblot P, Ramassamy A, et al: Hepatic fibrin-ring granulomas in giant cell arteritis. Gastroenterology 105:272-273, 1993.
106. Nenert M, Mavier P, Dubuc N, et al: Epstein-Barr virus infection and hepatic fibrin-ring granulomas. Hum Pathol 19:608-610, 1988.
107. Lobdell DH: 'Ring' granulomas in cytomegalovirus hepatitis. Arch Pathol Lab Med 9:357-363, 1987.
108. Murphy E, Griffiths MR, Hunter JA, et al: Fibrin-ring granulomas: a non-specific reaction to liver injury? Histopathology 19:91-93, 1991.
109. Moreno A, Marazuela M, Yebra M, et al: Hepatic fibrin-ring granulomas in visceral leishmaniasis. Gastroenterology 95:1123-1126, 1988.
110. Vanderstigel M, Zafrani ES, Lejonc JL, et al: Allopurinol hypersensitivity syndrome as a cause of hepatic fibrin-ring granulomas. Gastroenterology 90:188-190, 1986.
111. Hunt JG, Field PR, Murphy AM: Immunoglobulin responses to Coxiella burnetii (Q fever): single-serum diagnosis of acute infection using an immunofluorescence technique. Infect Immun 39:977-981, 1983.
112. Peter O, Dupuis G, Burgdorfer W, et al: Evaluation of the complement fixation and indirect immunofluorescence tests in the early diagnosis of primary Q fever. Eur J Clin Microbiol 4:394-396, 1985.
113. Corbel MJ: Brucellosis: an overview. Emerging Infect Dis 3:213-221, 1997.
114. Williams E: Brucellosis. BMJ 1:791-793, 1973.
115. Williams E: Brucellosis in humans: its diagnosis and treatment. APMIS 3(suppl):21-25, 1988.
116. Cervantes F, Bruguera M, Carbonell J, et al: Liver disease in brucellosis. A clinical and pathological study of 40 cases. Postgrad Med J 58:346-350, 1982.
117. Joint FAO/WHO Expert Committee on Brucellosis. 6th Report. WHO Tech Rep Ser 740:56-58, 1986.
118. Ariza J, Gudiol F, Pallares R, et al: Treatment of human brucellosis with doxycycline plus rifampin or doxycycline plus streptomycin. Ann Int Med 117:25-30, 1992.
119. Bass JW, Vincent JM, Person DA: The expanding spectrum of Bartonella infections: II. Cat-scratch disease. Pediatr Infect Dis J 16:163-179, 1997.
120. Carithers HA: Cat scratch disease. An overview based on a study of 1200 patients. Am J Dis Child 139:1124-1133, 1985.
121. Malatack JJ, Jaffe R: Granulomatous hepatitis in three children due to cat-scratch disease without peripheral adenopathy. An unrecognized cause of fever of unknown origin. Am J Dis Child 147:949-953, 1993.
122. Dangman BC, Albanese BA, Kacica MA, et al: Cat scratch disease in two children presenting with fever of unknown origin: imaging features and association with a new causative agent, *Rochalimaea henselae.* Pediatrics 95:767-771, 1995.
123. Destuynder O, Vanlemmans P, Mboyo A, et al: Systemic cat scratch disease: hepatic and splenic involvement about 3 pediatric cases. Eur J Pediatr Surg 5:365-368, 1995.
124. Lamp LW, Gray GF, Scott MA: The histologic spectrum of hepatic cat scratch disease. A series of six cases with confirmed *Bartonella henselae* infection. Am J Surg Pathol 20:1253-1259, 1996.
125. Rivera-Penera T, Nielsen K, Hall TR: Radiological case of the month. Granulomatous hepatitis in cat-scratch disease. Arch Pediatr Adolesc Med 152:87-88, 1998.
126. Kahr A, Kerbl R, Gschwandtner K, et al: Visceral manifestation of cat scratch disease in children. A consequence of altered immunological state? Infection 28:778-784, 2000.
127. Margileth AM: Antibiotic therapy for cat-scratch disease: clinical study of therapeutic outcome in 268 patients and a review of the literature. Pediatr Infect Dis J 11:474-478, 1992.
128. Simmons F, Feldman B, Gerety D: Granulomatous hepatitis in a patient receiving allopurinol. Gastroenterology 62:101-104, 1972.
129. Espiritu CR, Alalu J, Glueckauf LG, et al: Allopurinol-induced granulomatous hepatitis. Am J Dig Dis 21:804-806, 1976.
130. Swank LA, Chejfec G, Nemchausky BA: Allopurinol-induced granulomatous hepatitis with cholangitis and a sarcoid-like reaction. Arch Intern Med 138:997-998, 1978.
131. Vanderstigel M, Zafrani ES, Lejonc JL, et al: Allopurinol hypersensitivity syndrome as a cause of hepatic fibrin-ring granulomas. Gastroenterology 90:188-190, 1986.
132. Levander HG: Granulomatous hepatitis in a patient receiving carbamazepine. Acta Med Scand 208:333-335, 1980.
133. Levy M, Goodman MW, Van Dyne BJ, et al: Granulomatous hepatitis secondary to carbamazepine. Ann Intern Med 95:64-65, 1981.
134. Mitchell MC, Boitnott JK, Arregui A, et al: Granulomatous hepatitis associated with carbamazepine therapy. Am J Med 71:733-735, 1981.
135. Soffer EE, Taylor RJ, Bertram PD, et al: Carbamazepine-induced liver injury. South Med J 76:681-683, 1983.
136. Rigberg LA, Robinson MJ, Espiritu CR: Chlorpropamide-induced granulomas. A probable hypersensitivity reaction in liver and bone marrow. JAMA 235:409-410, 1976.
137. Ishak KG, Kirchner JP, Dhar JK: Granulomas and cholestatic-hepatocellular injury associated with phenylbutazone. Report of two cases. Am J Dig Dis 22:611-617, 1977.
138. Chajek T, Lehrer B, Geltner D, et al: Quinidine-induced granulomatous hepatitis. Ann Intern Med 81:774-776, 1974.

139. Geltner D, Chajek T, Rubinger D, et al: Quinidine hypersensitivity and liver involvement. A survey of 32 patients. Gastroenterology 70:650-652, 1976.
140. Bramlet DA, Posalaky Z, Olson R: Granulomatous hepatitis as a manifestation of quinidine hypersensitivity. Arch Intern Med 140:395-397, 1980.
141. Knobler H, Levij IS, Gavish D, et al: Quinidine-induced hepatitis. A common and reversible hypersensitivity reaction. Arch Intern Med 146:526-528, 1986.
142. Miller AC Jr, Reid WM: Methyldopa-induced granulomatous hepatitis. JAMA 235:2001-2002, 1976.
143. Jori GP, Peschile C: Hydralazine disease associated with transient granulomas in the liver. A case report. Gastroenterology 64:1163-1167, 1973.
144. Sarachek NS, London RL, Matulewicz TJ: Diltiazem and granulomatous hepatitis. Gastroenterology 88:1260-1262, 1985.
145. Toft E, Vyberg M, Therkelsen K: Diltiazem-induced granulomatous hepatitis. Histopathology 18:474-475, 1991.
146. Cook IF, Shilkin KB, Reed WD: Phenytoin induced granulomatous hepatitis. Aust N Z J Med 11:539-541, 1981.
147. Colle I, Naegels S, Hoorens A, et al: Granulomatous hepatitis due to mebendazole. J Clin Gastroenterol 28:44-45, 1999.
148. Landas SK, Mitros FA, Furst DE, et al: Lipogranulomas and gold in the liver in rheumatoid arthritis. Am J Surg Pathol 16:171-174, 1992.
149. Katz B, Weetch M, Chopra S: Quinine-induced granulomatous hepatitis. BMJ 286:264-265, 1983.
150. Mathur S, Dooley J, Scheuer PJ: Quinine induced granulomatous hepatitis and vasculitis. BMJ 300(6724):613, 1990.
151. Shah IA, Brandt H: Halothane-associated granulomatous hepatitis. Digestion 28:245-249, 1983.
152. Silvain C, Fort E, Levillain P, et al: Granulomatous hepatitis due to a combination of amoxicillin and clavulanic acid. Dig Dis Sci 37:150-152, 1992.
153. Kurumaya H, Kono N, Nakanuma Y, et al: Hepatic granulomata in long-term hemodialysis patients with hyperaluminumemia. Arch Pathol Lab Med 113:1132-1134, 1989.
154. Knobel B, Buyanowsky G, Dan M, et al: Pyrazinamide-induced granulomatous hepatitis. J Clin Gastro 24:264-266, 1997.
155. Lindgren A, Aldenborg F, Norkrans G, et al: Paracetamol-induced cholestatic and granulomatous liver injuries. J Intern Med 241:435-439, 1997.
156. Saw D, Pitman E, Maung M, et al: Granulomatous hepatitis associated with gliburide. Dig Dis Sci 41:322-325, 1996.
157. Braun M, Fraser GM, Kunin M, et al: Mesalamine-induced granulomatous hepatitis. Am J Gastroenterol 94:1973, 1999.
158. Eliakim M, Eisenberg S, Levij IS, et al: Granulomatous hepatitis accompanying a self-limited febrile disease. Lancet 1:1348-1352, 1968.
159. Simon HB, Wolff SM: Granulomatous hepatitis and prolonged fever of unknown origin: a study of 13 cases. Medicine 52:1-21, 1973.
160. Penchas S, Ligumski M, Eliakim M: Idiopathic granulomatous hepatitis with a prolonged course: effect of corticosteroid therapy. Digestion 17:46-55, 1978.
161. Shee CD, Creamer B: Idiopathic granulomatous hepatitis and abdominal pain. Postgrad Med J 56:342-343, 1980.
162. Berlin CM Jr, Boal DK, Zaino RJ, et al: Hepatic granulomata presenting with prolonged fever. Resolution with anti-inflammatory treatment. Clin Pediatr 29:339-342, 1990.
163. Zoutman DE, Ralph ED, Frei JV: Granulomatous hepatitis and fever of unknown origin. An 11-year experience of 23 cases with three years' follow-up. J Clin Gastroenterol 13:69-75, 1991.
164. Sartin JS, Walker RC: Granulomatous hepatitis: a retrospective review of 88 cases at the Mayo Clin Proc 66:914-918, 1991.
165. Knox TA, Kaplan MM, Gelfand JA, et al: Methotrexate treatment of idiopathic granulomatous hepatitis. Ann Intern Med 122:592-595, 1995.
166. Brincker H: Granulomatous lesions of unknown significance: the GLUS syndrome. In James DG, ed: Sarcoidosis and Other Granulomatous Disorders. New York, Marcel Dekker, 1994:69-86.
167. Kadin ME, Donaldson SS, Dorfman RF: Granulomas in Hodgkin's disease. N Engl J Med 283:859-861, 1970.
168. Johnson LN, Iseri O, Knodell RG: Caseating hepatic granulomas in Hodgkin's lymphoma. Gastroenterology 99:1837-1840, 1990.
169. Braylan RC, Long JC, Jaffe ES, et al: Malignant lymphoma obscured by concomitant extensive epithelioid granulomas: report of three cases with similar clinicopathologic features. Cancer 39:1146-1155, 1977.
170. Saito K, Nakanuma Y, Ogawa S, et al: Extensive hepatic granulomas associated with peripheral T cell lymphoma. Am J Gastroenterol 86:1243-1246, 1991.
171. Weissman JB, Neu HC: Lepromatous leprosy masquerading as disseminated tuberculosis. Am J Med 67:113-116, 1979.
172. Karat ABA, Job CK, Rao PSS: Liver in leprosy. Histologic and biochemical findings. BMJ 1:307-310, 1971.
173. Chen TS, Drutz DJ, Whelan GE: Hepatic granulomas in leprosy. Their relation to bacteremia. Arch Pathol Lab Med 100:182-185, 1976.
174. De Vega T, Echevarria S, Crespo J, et al: Acute hepatitis by *Listeria monocytogenes* in an HIV patient with chronic HBV hepatitis. J Clin Gastroenterol 15: 251-255, 1992.
175. Henderson JR, Ramsey CA: Miliary granulomata in a fatal adult case of listerial meningitis. Postgrad Med J 43:794-796, 1967.
176. Jones JM: Granulomatous hepatitis due to *Candida albicans* in patients with acute leukemia. Ann Intern Med 94:475-477, 1981.
177. Lamps LW, Molina CP, West AB, et al: The pathologic spectrum of gastrointestinal and hepatic histoplasmosis. Am J Clin Pathol 113:64-72, 2000.
178. Howard PF, Swith JW: Diagnosis of disseminated coccidiomycosis by liver biopsy. Arch Intern Med 143: 1335-1338, 1983.
179. Lefton HB, Farmer RG, Buchwald R, et al: Cryptococcal hepatitis mimicking primary sclerosing cholangitis. A case report. Gastroenterology 67:511-515, 1974.
180. Teixeira F, Gayotto LC, De Brito T: Morphological patterns of the liver in South American blastomycosis. Histopathology 2:231-237, 1978.
181. Weitberg AB, Alper JC, Diamond I, et al: Acute granulomatous hepatitis in the course of acquired toxoplasmosis. N Engl J Med 300:1093-1096, 1979.
182. Clarke J, Craig RM, Saffro R, et al: Cytomegalovirus granulomatous hepatitis. Am J Med 66:264-269, 1979.
183. Litwack KD, Bohan A, Silverman L: Granulomatous liver disease and giant cell arteritis. Case report and literature review. J Rheumatol 4:307-312, 1977.
184. Malatjalian DA, Graham CH: Liver adenoma with granulomas. The appearance of granulomas in oral contraceptive-related hepatocellular adenoma and in the surrounding nontumorous liver. Arch Pathol Lab Med 106:244-246, 1982.

SECTION

IV D

Tumors of the Liver

CHAPTER

44

Molecular Pathogenesis of Hepatocellular Carcinoma

Darius Moradpour, MD, and Jack R. Wands, MD

Hepatocellular carcinoma (HCC) is one of the most common malignant tumors worldwide.[1,2] The incidence ranges from 1 to 4 cases per 100,000 population in North America and western Europe to 50 to 150 cases per 100,000 population in parts of Africa and Asia, where HCC is responsible for a large proportion of cancer deaths.[3] A rise in the incidence of and mortality from HCC, most likely reflecting an increase in hepatitis C virus (HCV) infection, has recently been observed in different industrialized countries.[4-9]

The major risk factors for development of HCC are now well defined (Table 44-1), and some of the steps involved in its molecular pathogenesis have been elucidated. As with most types of cancer, hepatocarcinogenesis is a multi-step process involving different genetic alterations that ultimately lead to malignant transformation of the hepatocyte. However, although significant progress has been made in recognizing the sequence of events involved in other forms of cancer, notably colorectal cancer,[10,11] the molecular contribution of the multiple factors and their interactions in hepatocarcinogenesis are still poorly understood. In fact, a picture of HCCs as genetically very heterogenous tumors is emerging.[12] This is not unexpected given the heterogeneity of etiologic factors implicated in HCC development and the complexity of hepatocyte functions. As shown in Figure 44-1, malignant transformation of hepatocytes may occur regardless of the etiologic agent through a pathway of increased liver cell turnover, induced by chronic liver injury and regeneration in a context of inflammation and oxidative deoxyribonucleic acid (DNA) damage. This may result in genetic alterations—such as chromosomal rearrangements, activation of cellular oncogenes, or inactivation of tumor suppressor genes—possibly in cooperation with defective DNA mismatch repair, telomerase activation, and induction of growth and angiogenic factors. Chronic viral hepatitis, alcohol, and metabolic liver diseases such as hemochromatosis and α_1-antitrypsin deficiency may act predominantly through this pathway of chronic liver injury, regeneration, and cirrhosis. On the other hand, there is evidence that hepatitis B virus (HBV)—and possibly HCV—may under certain circumstances play an additional direct role in the molecular pathogenesis of HCC. Finally, aflatoxins have been shown to induce mutations of the p53 tumor suppressor gene, thus pointing to the contribution of environmental factors to tumor development at the molecular level.

TABLE 44-1
Risk Factors for Hepatocellular Carcinoma

Chronic viral hepatitis B, C, and D
Toxins and drugs (e.g., alcohol, aflatoxins, microcystin, anabolic steroids)
Metabolic liver diseases (e.g., hereditary hemochromatosis, α_1-antitrypsin deficiency)

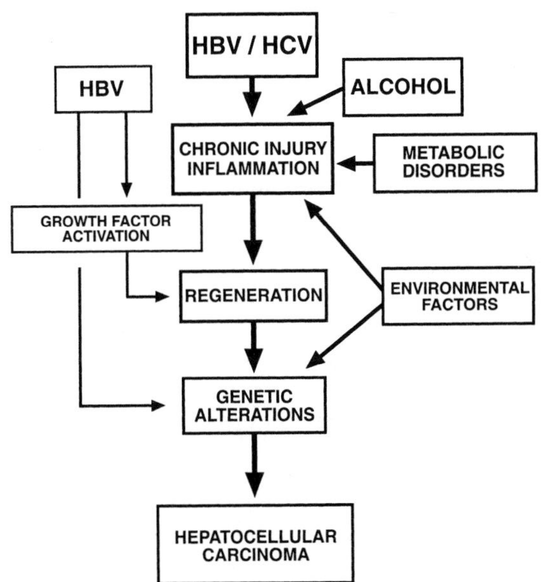

Figure 44-1 Factors involved in the pathogenesis of hepatocellular carcinoma.

CELLULAR ORIGIN OF HEPATOCELLULAR CARCINOMA

To understand the pathogenesis of HCC, it is of general interest to know which liver cells become transformed. However, the identification of cells that serve as precursors to HCCs has been difficult. Studies performed in rodent models of chemical carcinogenesis have led to the concept of clonal expansion of transformed, "dedifferentiated" mature hepatocytes as a cellular mechanism of hepatocellular carcinogenesis.[13] According to this view, liver cancer develops in a step-wise manner through initiation, promotion, and progression. During active growth, transformed hepatocytes become more basophilic and form nodules of altered hepatocytes. With malignant progression, additional foci of altered hepatocytes appear in these nodules ("nodules within nodules") and ultimately lead to HCC.

In contrast to this cellular pathway, a concept based on the aberrant differentiation and proliferation of pluripotent liver stem cells has been proposed.[14-16] The slow cell turnover and the capacity of differentiated hepatocytes to proliferate rapidly after both partial hepatectomy and chemical injury has made the need for a stem cell compartment theoretically less critical than, for example, in constantly self-renewing tissues such as the skin, intestinal mucosa, and bone marrow. In this context, recent experimental evidence indicates that some hepatocytes have a growth potential comparable to hematopoietic stem cells, at least in the mouse.[17,18] In addition, it has recently been shown that hematopoietic stem cells can differentiate into hepatocytes in vivo.[19-21] Nevertheless, there is increasing evidence for the existence of a hepatic stem cell compartment.[22] This compartment has been proposed to be the major source of new hepatocytes after severe or protracted liver damage in the context of an experimentally induced impaired regeneration capacity of normal hepatocytes and therefore has been referred to as the *facultative stem cell* compartment. Alternatively, according to the "streaming liver" hypothesis, an active stem cell population will continuously replenish mature cells that have lost the ability to divide.[23] According to this model, the degree of differentiation of HCC is a direct reflection of the state of differentiation of the precursor cell at the time of transformation ("maturation arrest"). That is, if the precursor cells are at an early stage of development, then the tumor that develops from such cells will be poorly differentiated, whereas transformation of cells at a later stage of hepatocyte development would produce more highly differentiated tumors. Studies using genetic labeling do not seem to support the streaming liver hypothesis.[24]

Most of the experimental evidence regarding a compartment of hepatic stem cells has been obtained from rodent models. In the early stages of chemical hepatocarcinogenesis the appearance of a rapidly growing population of small cells characterized by oval nuclei and dense cytoplasm, commonly referred to as *oval cells*, has been found.[25,26] Evidence now suggests that oval cells are the progeny of facultative hepatic stem cells that have the capacity to develop into hepatocytes and other cell lineages, such as bile, intestinal epithelial, and pancreatic cells.[15] Liver regeneration takes place via the hepatic stem cell compartment when proliferation of mature hepatocytes is inhibited by specific experimental regimens. For example, when rats are treated with 2-acetylaminofluorene, an agent that blocks hepatocyte proliferation, and the animals are subsequently subjected to partial hepatectomy, extensive proliferation of oval cells has been observed. Pulse-chase nuclear labeling studies show that labeled DNA in the nuclei of proliferating oval cells subsequently appears in the nuclei of hepatocytes in regenerative nodules,[27] indicating that oval cells may differentiate into hepatocytes. The precise anatomic location of the stem cell compartment within the liver has not been clarified. Available evidence indicates that cells located in or near the terminal bile ductules (canals of Hering)[15,28] constitute the hepatic stem cell compartment.

Evidence supporting the view that HCC may arise from oval cells is derived primarily from cell culture experiments. Oval cells or rat liver epithelial cells (cells that share common phenotypic features with oval cells and are regarded as their in vitro counterpart) have been transformed in vitro; when these transformed cells are injected into nude mice in vivo they will produce HCC-type tumors.[14,29] Oval cell proliferation has also been observed during hepatocarcinogenesis in woodchucks chronically infected with the woodchuck hepatitis virus (WHV).[30] Finally, putative human oval cells that appear structurally and antigenically similar to those observed in the early stages of chemical hepatocarcinogenesis in rats have been described in regenerating liver nodules associated with human HCC.[31]

HEPATITIS B VIRUS

An estimated 300 million individuals worldwide are chronically infected with HBV. Prevalence rates range from 0.1 percent to 1 percent of the general population in North America and western Europe to up to 20 percent in Southeast Asia and parts of Africa. Epidemiologic studies have convincingly shown that HCC is closely associated with chronic HBV infection.[32] The incidence of HCC in chronically HBV-infected individuals is approximately 100-fold higher than in the uninfected population, and the lifetime HCC risk of males infected at birth is estimated to approach 40 percent. Importantly, a recent study from Taiwan demonstrated a decline in the incidence of HCC in children after implementation of a universal hepatitis B vaccination program.[33]

A common molecular mechanism for HBV-induced hepatocarcinogenesis has not been discovered thus far, but both viral and host factors have been implicated in the process. Most cases of HCC occur after many years of chronic hepatitis, which could provide the mitogenic and mutagenic environment to precipitate random genetic and chromosomal damage and lead to the development of HCC. In this context Nakamoto and colleagues, using an elegant transgenic mouse model, recently showed that chronic immune-mediated liver cell injury is sufficient to cause HCC.[34] However, several lines of evidence support a more direct oncogenic contribution of HBV to development of HCC, as discussed in the following section.

Hepatitis B Virus DNA Integration

HBV and retroviruses share a replication strategy that includes the reverse transcription of a ribonucleic acid (RNA) intermediate.[35] Integration of provirus into the host cell genome is an integral feature of the retroviral life cycle. HBV DNA integration, however, is not part of the viral life cycle, but rather occurs as an epiphenomenon of HBV replication. Hepadnaviral DNA integration does not preserve the viral genome sequence, thereby rendering it impossible for the viral integrant to function as a template for virus replication. Integrated HBV sequences have been found by Southern blot analysis in HCC cell lines[36-39] and in the majority of HCCs that develop in patients with chronic HBV infection.[36,40-46] Expectations that there might be a common target sequence in the cellular DNA led investigators to examine the viral junction and flanking cellular DNA sequences of many different HBV integration sites. These studies have shown that integration is random within human chromosomes. HBV, therefore, may act as a non-selective insertional mutagenic agent. In addition, secondary chromosomal rearrangements associated with HBV DNA integration, such as duplications, translocations, and deletions, suggest that a major oncogenic effect of HBV DNA integration may be increased genomic instability.

There are multiple viral integrations (usually 3 to 4 but sometimes more than 10) into the cellular DNA in many tumors. Alexander's cell line PLC/PRF/5, for example, carries at least seven HBV integrants.[47-49] The presence of discrete Southern blot bands in individual tumors suggests clonal expansion of a single transformed hepatocyte, as shown in Figure 44-2. Molecular evidence for a monoclonal origin and subsequent expansion of a single transformed hepatocyte during tumor growth, intrahepatic spread, and metastasis has been provided by identical hybridization patterns from tumor tissue obtained at different locations in a given patient.[50,51] In contrast to HCC, DNA samples derived from acutely or chronically HBV-infected livers commonly show a hybridization profile that is consistent with multiple different integration sites. To date, no differences in the molecular structure of viral integrations found in HCC and in non-tumorous liver have been discovered.

The molecular structure of viral integrations has been found to be quite variable and to range from simple, non-rearranged stretches of viral DNA to highly complex rearranged patterns (Figure 44-3). Although the former integration pattern is believed to represent the result of the primary integration event, the more complex pattern may be a consequence of secondary rearrangements that evolve during either chronic infection or tumor progression. More than 50 percent of the integrated HBV sequences have at one viral-cellular junction the so-called cohesive end region that lies between the viral direct repeat 1 and 2 (DR1 and DR2) sequences of the HBV genome.[52-56] The second end of viral DNA joins cellular DNA at variable positions of the viral genome. Integration at the former site, together with associated viral deletions and rearrangements, commonly precludes the expression of viral core and polymerase open reading frames, although often leaving the envelope region, the enhancer I element, and the 5′ sequences of the viral X gene intact.

Inverted duplications are a common rearrangement found in HCCs associated with HBV infection. These duplications consist of inverted identical repeat sequences of viral and flanking cellular DNA (see Figure 44-3, *D*).[57-60] Chromosomal translocations have been found after HBV DNA integration. In these HBV DNA integration sites the two ends of the HBV DNA are joined by cellular DNA from different chromosomes (see Figure 44-3, *E* and *F*).[59,61,62] Integration of HBV into hepatocyte DNA may also trigger large chromosome deletions.[63] It is apparent that large-scale deletions and translocations

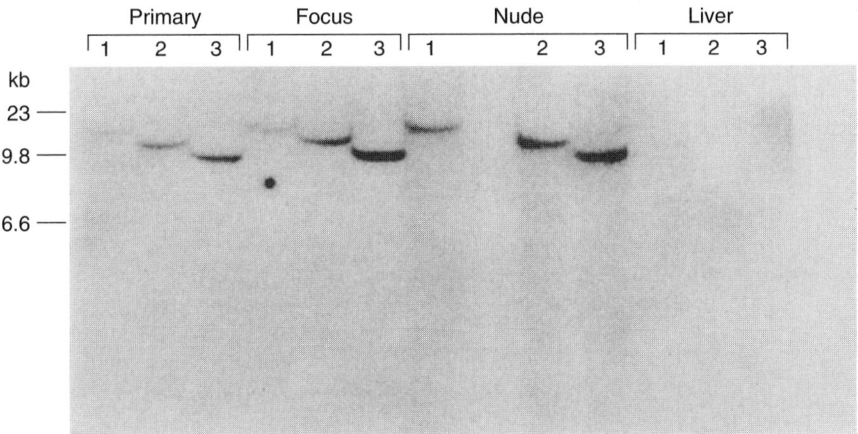

Figure 44-2 Southern blot analysis of DNA isolated from a HCC (PRIMARY), a cell line derived from the same tumor (FOCUS), and a FOCUS tumor grown in a nude mouse (NUDE). DNA was digested with three different restriction enzymes, electrophoresed through an agarose gel, transferred to a nylon membrane, and probed with ^{32}P-labeled HBV DNA. Note the stable integration pattern in the primary tumor, the derived cell line, and the nude mouse tumor. No HBV DNA integration was detectable in the non-tumorous liver (LIVER). *DNA,* Deoxyribonucleic acid; *HBV,* hepatitis B virus.

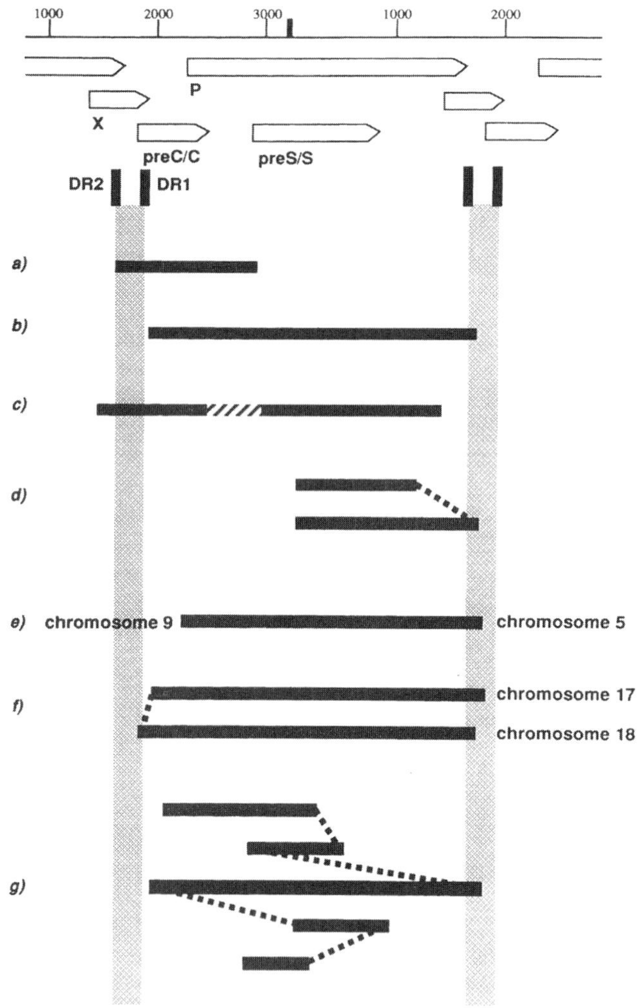

Figure 44-3 Structure of hepadnaviral integrants. The HBV genome is indicated on top as a tandemly arranged structure. Base pairs are numbered from the *Eco*RI site of subtype adw2. Open reading frames are shown by open arrows. Integrated HBV sequences are denoted by closed black bars. *a* and *b,* Simple integrants.[66,70] *c,* Integrant with deleted viral sequences.[49] *d,* Inverted duplication.[59] *e,* Chromosomal translocation.[59] *f,* Inverted duplication with chromosomal translocation.[61] *g,* Highly rearranged WHV integration from a woodchuck HCC.[137] *P,* Polymerase gene; *preC/C,* precore/core gene; *preS/S,* presurface/surface gene; *X,* X gene; *DR1 and DR2,* direct repeats 1 and 2; *HBV,* hepatitis B virus; *WHV,* woodchuck hepatitis virus; *HCC,* hepatocellular carcinoma. (Adapted from Matsubara K, Tokino T: Integration of hepatitis B virus DNA and its implications for hepatocarcinogenesis. Mol Biol Med 7:248, 1990.)

may result in the loss of tumor suppressor genes or other genes involved in growth control. In rare cases amplification of a chromosomal region has been found after HBV DNA integration.[64]

Several models have been proposed for the mechanism of HBV DNA integration, among them a strand invasion or "roll-in" mechanism involving the 3′ free end of the viral minus-strand[54] or an integration mechanism mediated by cellular topoisomerase I.[55,65]

Despite intensive study of numerous integration sites by several laboratories, only a few examples of HBV DNA integrations within or near known cellular genes have been documented. In this regard, characterization of a single HBV DNA integration site in an early HCC (see Figure 44-3, *A*) revealed insertion into an exon of the retinoic acid receptor (RAR)-β gene, resulting in overexpression of an aminoterminal-truncated RAR-β with altered functions.[66-69] Investigation of another HBV DNA integration site (see Figure 44-3, *B*) led to the identification of the human cyclin A gene.[70] The sequential activation and inactivation of cyclin-cyclin-dependent kinase (CDK) complexes is responsible for cell cycle control.[71] This integration had occurred within the second intron of the gene, resulting in the production of a spliced HBV-cyclin A fusion transcript. In the chimeric protein the aminoterminal domain of cyclin A, including the signals for regulated cyclin degradation, was replaced by viral pre-S2/S sequences, with transcription being initiated from the pre-S2/S promoter, although the carboxyterminal two thirds of cyclin A, including the evolutionary well-conserved cyclin box, were intact.[72] Therefore it is likely that the chimeric protein retained the ability to complex and activate kinases involved in cell-cycle regulation. Constitutive and strong expression of this stabilized cyclin A protein may have led to or contributed to increased cell proliferation. The HCC from which this integration had been derived had developed in a histologically normal liver, which further supports a direct carcinogenic role of HBV in the absence of cirrhosis. These and a few additional well-characterized cases[73-77] are notable exceptions, however, because HBV has not been found to integrate commonly into specific domains of known cellular genes.

Transactivation of Cellular Genes by Hepatitis B Virus

Mammalian hepadnaviruses contain a gene that can function as a transcriptional transactivator. It is called the X gene because its role during acute and chronic virus infection is not yet known. The X gene was found not to be essential for viral replication in vitro[78] but appears to be necessary for the establishment of productive infection in vivo.[79,80] The X gene product of HBV, referred to as HBx, can function as a transcriptional transactivator of various cellular genes associated with growth control. This observation has led to the hypothesis that HBx may be involved in the development of HBV-associated HCC.[81-84] HBx appears to be expressed in a significant proportion of HBV-associated HCCs.[85-87] The X gene spans the cohesive end region, which is the preferred viral site for joining cellular DNA after viral integration. Thus 3′ truncated X coding sequences are often retained in viral integration sites within the cellular DNA. In this context, it has been demonstrated experimentally that HBx can retain its transactivating function despite truncation or fusion with cellular-encoded sequences.[88-90] The failure of HBx to directly bind to any defined DNA sequences suggests, however, that the transactivation mechanism does not involve a known, direct DNA sequence-specific interaction. The biologic role of HBx may be mediated through an effect on cellular transcription factors.[91] For example, it has been reported that HBx transactivates via a signal transduction pathway comprising 1,2-diacylglycerol, protein kinase C (PKC), and the transcription factors AP-1 (Jun-Fos), AP-2, and NF-κB.[92] This mechanism of gene regulation is reminiscent of Ras and Src proteins with respect to cell growth. Moreover, by activating through the PKC signal transduction pathway, HBx could achieve pleiotropic effects and mimic the activity of known tumor promoters such as phorbol esters. Alternatively, it was postulated that HBx may promote hepatocarcinogenesis through activation of the Ras-Raf-MAP kinase pathway.[93-95] In addition, malignant transformation of certain rodent cells,[96] deregulation of cell cycle control,[97,98] and interference with cellular DNA repair[99-102] and apoptosis[103,104] have, among numerous other interactions with host cell functions, been described in different experimental systems. A role of HBx in HBV-associated hepatocarcinogenesis was further supported by the observation that transgenic mice carrying the X gene under control of its own regulatory elements develop HCC.[105,106] However, other investigators have not found tumors in HBx-transgenic mice.[107,108] This discrepancy may be explained by differences in the level and duration of X gene expression and the genetic background of the mouse strains used in these studies.

We note that the avian hepadnaviruses lack an X open reading frame and that HCCs do not arise in the context of chronic duck or heron HBV infection. These data support an oncogenic role of HBx in tumor development.

Recent studies suggested that HBx may, similar to gene products of other DNA tumor viruses, interact with p53 and thereby interfere with the known functions of p53.[100,109,110] However, it is presently unclear how such an interaction is significant at HBx levels expressed in hepatocytes during natural HBV infection. In this context, Puisieux and colleagues found that HBV replication in Hep G2.2.15 cells did not interfere with p53 functions.[111] Further studies are needed to clarify this intriguing issue.

Another HBV gene product that was reported to have transactivational properties is a truncated form of the pre-S2/S gene, referred to as truncated middle hepatitis B surface antigen.[112-114] It is unusual that a structural viral protein gains regulatory functions after truncation. Truncated pre-S2/S sequences are found frequently in HBV DNA integration sites in HCC, however.[115] A potential role of such sequences as a transactivator of cellular genes is an interesting observation that also warrants further investigation.[84]

Chronic Hepadnavirus Infection and Hepatocellular Carcinoma

HBV is a member of the *Hepadnaviridae* family. These hepatotropic DNA viruses share common features—such as a similar genomic organization, virion structure, replication cycle, and pattern of gene expression.[116,117] Hepadnaviruses are divided into the mammalian and avian branches. Mammalian hepadnaviruses include HBV; WHV, which infects woodchucks *(Marmota monax)* in the mid-Atlantic states of North America[118]; the ground squirrel hepatitis virus (GSHV)[119]; and the woolly monkey hepatitis B virus.[120] Both woodchucks and ground squirrels belong to the *Sciuridae* family of rodents. Avian hepadnaviruses include the duck hepatitis B virus (DHBV),[121] the heron hepatitis B virus (HHBV),[122] and the snow goose hepatitis B virus (SGHBV).[123] The discovery of HBV-related viruses with similar biologic characteristics and the capability to study them in their natural host have contributed significantly to our understanding of the hepadnaviral life cycle and have allowed the investigation of various aspects of hepadnavirus-associated hepatocarcinogenesis. Indeed, although the evidence for a role of HBV in the pathogenesis of human HCC is convincing, the association of woodchuck HCC with chronic WHV infection is even stronger.

Hepatic tumors have been known for many years to occur at a high rate in woodchucks.[45,124,125] Six of 10 captive woodchucks with chronic WHV infection were found by Popper and colleagues to have HCC.[126] Tumor development was associated with acute and chronic hepatic inflammation in the absence of liver cirrhosis. The absence of cirrhosis allowed the recognition of a gradual transition from normal hepatocytes to neoplastic nodules to HCC. Further studies revealed that 6 of 6 woodchucks experimentally infected with WHV at birth and 2 of 2 carriers infected as adults developed HCC after 1.5 to 3 years.[127] The absence of any known external carcinogenic agents in these well-monitored woodchucks provided strong biologic evidence for the carcinogenicity of chronic WHV infection. Of the 63 experimentally infected chronic WHV carriers followed under controlled conditions at Cornell University, all developed HCC by 3 years after experimental infection, compared to none of the uninfected controls. Tumors appeared as early as 12 months, and by 30 months more than 50 percent of the animals had developed HCC.[128] Of considerable interest was the observation that HCC also occurred in 17 of 63 woodchucks that had serologically recovered from experimental WHV infection (negative WHsAg and positive anti-WHc and anti-WHs antibodies). WHV DNA was detected in a substantial number of such tumors by Southern blot analysis.[129] It is noteworthy that an increased incidence of HCC in hepatitis B surface antigen (HBsAg)-negative individuals with serologic evidence of past HBV infection (positive anti-HBc and anti-HBs antibodies) has also been documented. With the use of highly sensitive immunoassays and the polymerase chain reaction (PCR), HBV has been shown to persist at low levels in a number of these subjects.[130-134]

Investigation of hepadnaviral integration sites to identify cellular oncogenes involved in HCC development was particularly rewarding in the case of HCCs associated with chronic WHV infection.[45,135] Activation of *myc* family oncogenes, presumably resulting from *cis-* and *trans*-acting effects of integrated WHV regulatory elements, was found in the majority of these tumors.[136,137] Analysis of WHV DNA integration sites in woodchuck HCCs has led to the identification of a second, intronless N-*myc* gene.[138] One N-*myc* locus was homologous to the known mammalian N-*myc* genes (N-*myc*1); the other had a structure typical of a retroposon (N-*myc*2). WHV DNA integration, either upstream of N-*myc*2 or in the 3′

non-coding region of N-*myc*2, was observed in 27 of 66 (41 percent) woodchuck HCCs investigated in three studies (Figure 44-4).[138-140] Interestingly, in a significant proportion of tumors in which N-*myc*2 expression was up-regulated in the absence of a nearby viral integration WHV DNA, integration was found in a common chromosomal site located at about 200 Kb downstream of N-*myc*2, suggesting long-range proto-oncogene activation by the WHV enhancer.[141]

The high oncogenic potential of insertionally activated *myc* family genes in this animal model was underscored by the observation that transgenic mice carrying a mutated c-*myc* gene and adjacent WHV DNA cloned in original configuration from a woodchuck HCC integration site[142] or transgenic mice harboring the woodchuck N-*myc*2 gene controlled by WHV regulatory elements[143] develop liver tumors. Finally, anti-sense down-regulation of N-*myc*1 in woodchuck hepatoma cells has been shown to reverse the malignant phenotype.[144]

In contrast to the findings in woodchucks, evidence for an association between persistent GSHV infection and HCC development has been obtained only after long-term observation of captive ground squirrels, demonstrating that HCCs occur at a lower rate and after a longer latency period in this animal model.[145] These differences in the incidence and onset of HCC may be due to either viral or host factors. Because GSHV can infect woodchucks, the oncogenic potential of the two viruses could be experimentally studied in the same host. Interestingly, although WHV and GSHV established a similar rate of chronic infection, had comparable viremia levels, and produced a similar degree of chronic hepatitis in woodchucks, hepatic neoplasms were observed in 50 percent of chronic WHV carriers within 32 months after infection whereas only 1 of 14 (7 percent) chronic GSHV carriers developed HCC during this interval.[146] The oncogenic behavior of GSHV and WHV in a common host suggests that hepadnaviruses use different mechanisms to produce hepatocyte transformation. In this context, activation of the *myc* proto-oncogenes also occurs in GSHV-infected ground squirrels. However, in contrast to WHV-induced tumors, integrated GSHV DNA was detected in only a few ground squirrel HCCs and activation of N-*myc* genes occurred only rarely. However, c-*myc* activation was much more common. It was attributable in many tumors to amplification of the c-*myc* genomic locus.[140,147]

Taken together, activation of *myc* genes by integration of WHV DNA is an important event in the pathogenesis of HCC in woodchucks. In the woodchuck, however, there is an earlier onset of tumor development than in man, and the absence of associated cirrhosis suggests that WHV may act more directly as a carcinogenic agent than HBV. On the other hand, the absence of cirrhosis could reflect an intrinsic difference between rodents and man with respect to the liver reaction to chronic injury. Deregulated expression of *myc* family genes has been associated with many human neoplasms but only occasionally with HCC. HBV DNA integration near *myc* genes or other currently known proto-oncogenes has not been observed thus far.

Chronic DHBV infection is not associated with HCC in Pekin ducks. Indeed, HCC has been observed only in DHBV-infected ducks originating from Qidong County in China,[148-150] but not in Pekin ducks infected by DHBV in Western countries. Experimental data support the idea that aflatoxins may be the hepatic carcinogen for ducks in the former region of China and that persistent DHBV infection does not contribute significantly to the emer-

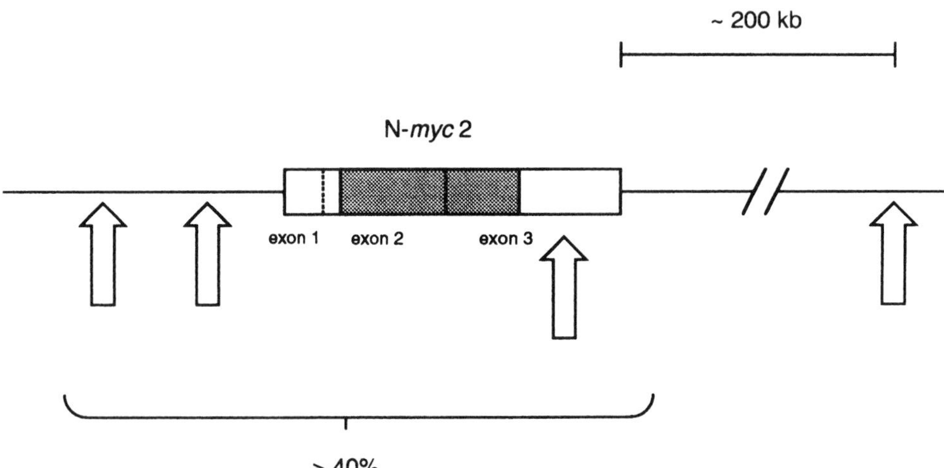

Figure 44-4 WHV integration sites within or near the N-*myc*2 gene. In about 50 percent of woodchuck HCCs, WHV DNA has been found integrated within or near *myc* family genes. Of these, the majority are found at the N-*myc*2 gene, which is specific to the *Sciuridae* family of rodents. Coding regions are shaded and untranslated regions open. The arrows indicate common WHV integration sites. *WHV,* Woodchuck hepatitis virus; *HCC,* hepatocellular carcinoma; *DNA,* deoxyribonucleic acid. (Adapted from Fourel G, Trepo C, Bougueleret L, et al: Frequent activation of N-myc genes by hepadnavirus insertion in woodchuck liver tumours. Nature 347:295, 1990; Wei Y, Fourel G, Ponzetto A, et al: Hepadnavirus integration: mechanism of activation of the N-*myc*2 retrotransposon in woodchuck liver tumors. J Virol 66:5270, 1992.)

gence of hepatic tumors in such animals.[151-154] Finally, hepatic neoplasms have not been reported in association with chronic HHBV or SGHBV infection.

Interestingly, chronic HBV infection has been associated with the development of HCC in tree shrews *(Tupaia belangeri chinensis)*,[155,156] which are being explored as a small-animal model of HBV infection.[157,158]

HEPATITIS C VIRUS

HCV infection is a leading cause of chronic hepatitis, liver cirrhosis, and HCC.[159] It is estimated that about 170 million people worldwide are chronically infected with HCV.[160] The seroprevalence rate is about 1 percent in North America and Western Europe, 3 percent to 4 percent in some Mediterranean and Asian countries, and up to 10 percent to 20 percent in parts of Central Africa and Egypt.[161,162] HCV has been classified in the *Hepacivirus* genus within the *Flaviviridae* family of viruses, which includes the classical flaviviruses such as yellow fever virus and the animal pestiviruses.[163] HCV contains a single-stranded RNA genome of positive polarity and an approximately 9600 nucleotide length. As in flaviviruses and pestiviruses, the viral genome is composed of a 5′ noncoding region (NCR), a long open reading frame encoding a polyprotein precursor of about 3000 amino acids, and a 3′ NCR.[164,165] The HCV polyprotein precursor is co- and posttranslationally processed by cellular and viral proteases to yield the mature structural and non-structural proteins. The structural proteins include the core protein, which forms the viral nucleocapsid, and the envelope glycoproteins E1 and E2. These are released from the polyprotein precursor by the endoplasmic reticulum signal peptidase. The non-structural proteins NS2 through NS5 include the NS2-3 autoprotease and the NS3 serine protease, which are essential for processing the polyprotein precursor, an RNA helicase located in the carboxy-terminal region of NS3, the NS4A polypeptide, the NS4B and NS5A proteins, and an RNA-dependent RNA polymerase represented by NS5B. NS4A is a co-factor for the NS3 serine protease. The functions of NS4B and NS5A, a serine phosphoprotein, remain to be established.

Epidemiologic surveys have revealed the presence of anti-HCV antibodies as a marker of chronic hepatitis C in 15 percent to 80 percent of patients with HCC depending upon the patient population studied.[166-175] It is apparent that the percentage of patients with HCC infected by HCV will vary from population to population and will depend in part on the exposure of the general population to this virus and on the number of HCC cases attributable to chronic HBV infection. For example, HCV is now the major cause of HCC in Japan and Europe, whereas it may play a less important role in South Africa and Taiwan.

Similar to HBV, HCC associated with HCV infection evolves after many years of chronic infection and is generally preceded by the development of cirrhosis.[176-178] HCV infection, therefore, offers a paradigm for the role of chronic liver injury followed by regeneration, cirrhosis, and the development of HCC as shown in Figure 44-1. Kiyosawa and colleagues have demonstrated that after exposure to HCV via blood transfusion, as depicted in Figure 44-5, there is a sequence of events that takes place over 20 to 40 years; this process is characterized by the development of chronic hepatitis 10 to 15 years after exposure, cirrhosis 20 years later, and the emergence of HCC 20 to 40 years after the onset of chronic infection.[176]

Recent clinical and experimental evidence raises the possibility that HCV might operate also through other pathways in promoting malignant transformation of hepatocytes. HCCs have been found in chronically HCV-infected patients without liver cirrhosis.[179] A transforming potential of the aminoterminal portion of the NS3 protein,[180] the core protein,[181-185] NS4B,[186] and NS5A[187-189] has been described. In this context, the core protein has been reported to interact with a variety of cellular proteins and to influence various host cell functions.[190] These include, among others, enhancement[191] or inhibition[192] of apoptosis, repression of p53[183] and p21^{WAF1} promoter activity,[185] and immunosuppression.[193] NS5A has been reported, in biochemical, transfection, and yeast functional assays, to interact with the interferon-induced, double-stranded, RNA-activated protein kinase (PKR) and to inhibit its catalytic activity.[194,195] In addition, disruption of PKR-dependent translational control and apoptotic programs by NS5A have been suggested to confer oncogenic potential on HCV.[187] Finally, a recent study has provided evidence for a src homology 3 domain-dependent interaction of NS5A with growth factor receptor-bound protein 2 (Grb2) adaptor protein that could interfere with mitogenic signal transduction pathways.[188] All of these studies, however, were performed in heterologous overexpression systems, and their relevance to natural HCV infection will need to be further addressed.

METABOLIC LIVER DISEASES

The importance of the pathway of chronic liver cell injury, regeneration, and cirrhosis in the pathogenesis of HCC is best illustrated by the development of HCC in association with metabolic diseases of the liver. Metabolic

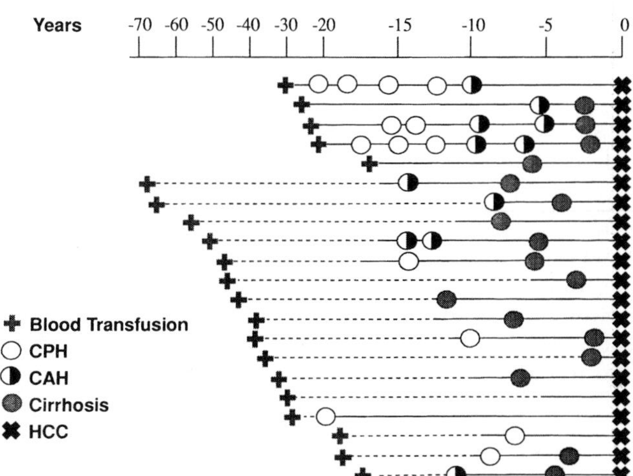

Figure 44-5 Role of chronic HCV infection in the sequence of clinical events leading to the development of HCC. *CPH,* Chronic persistent hepatitis; *CAH,* chronic active hepatitis; *HCV,* hepatitis C virus; *HCC,* hepatocellular carcinoma. (Adapted from Kiyosawa K et al: Hepatology 12:671-675, 1990.)

diseases such as acute intermittent and variegate porphyria, hypercitrullinemia, and hereditary fructose intolerance have no associated cirrhosis, and HCC has been found to be rare in these clinical conditions.[196,197] In contrast, there are metabolic liver diseases associated with cirrhosis, such as hereditary hemochromatosis, α_1-antitrypsin deficiency, porphyria cutanea tarda, and hereditary tyrosinemia; in the clinical setting of cirrhosis a greatly increased risk of HCC over the lifetime of the individual has been observed.[198-203] Particularly noteworthy in this regard is hemochromatosis, in which the risk of HCC is extraordinarily high after liver cirrhosis is established.[204] Indeed, there are only a few reported cases of HCC occurring in precirrhotic hemochromatosis.[201] A notable exception is Wilson's disease in which the risk of HCC is low even in the setting of cirrhosis and suggests that copper may have a cytoprotective function.[205]

ONCOGENES

Activated cellular oncogenes, particularly those of the *ras* family, have been found in spontaneous and chemically induced rodent hepatocarcinogenesis models.[206-214] In human hepatocarcinogenesis, however, no consistent pattern of protooncogene activation has emerged for HCC.[215-219] It is also of interest that no structural or functional changes of a large panel of oncogenes have been found in a transgenic mouse model, which is believed to resemble the process of human hepatocarcinogenesis.[220] Taken together, in contrast to other human tumors, activation of cellular oncogenes has been found to be infrequent in human HCC.[12,135] Cyclin D1, however, has been found to be amplified in 10 percent to 20 percent of HCCs.[221,222]

TUMOR SUPPRESSOR GENES

Several investigations have demonstrated chromosomal allelic losses in HCC tissues, suggesting the deletion or alteration of tumor suppressor genes, which may play a role in the development and progression of HCC. The use of the restriction fragment length polymorphism (RFLP) technique combined with Southern hybridization with a repertoire of DNA markers scattered throughout the genome has been particularly informative for assessing whether a region of a chromosome has been deleted. Loss of one copy of a defined region of the genome is termed allelic deletion or loss of heterozygosity (LOH),[223] as shown in Figure 44-6. The second copy of the tumor suppressor gene on the other allele may develop loss of function by a point mutation ("second hit"). By this mechanism, there is a complete loss of the function of a tumor suppressor gene product such as p53.

RFLP studies of paired HCC and non-tumorous liver samples have revealed relatively frequent LOH in HCC on chromosomes 1, 2q, 4, 5q, 6q, 8, 9, 10q, 11p, 13q, 14q, 16, 17, and 22q,[12,135] suggesting that these sites may harbor tumor suppressor genes involved in the pathogenesis of HCC. More recently, large genome-wide scans using microsatellite markers, which can be typed by PCR, or comparative genomic hybridization, have confirmed and extended these findings.[135,224-227] At present, however, only few tumor suppressor genes located in these deleted regions have been clearly involved in a significant subset of HCC. In general, these genetic alterations appear to occur at later stages of HCC development.[228-230] HBV DNA integrants have been described on the short arm of chromosome 17, which includes the *p53* gene.[59-62] However, the significance, if any, of HBV infection and HBV DNA integration in the development of *p53* alterations remains to be determined. There is no direct evidence yet to link HBV DNA integration to the loss of a tumor suppressor gene.[231]

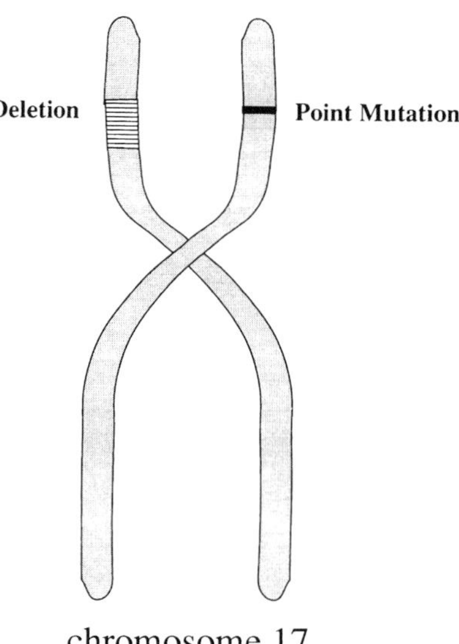

Figure 44-6 Diagram demonstrating loss of heterozygosity on the short arm of chromosome 17 by a deletional event. A tumor suppresser gene such as *p53* becomes inactivated by a point mutation on the second allele.

The *p53* gene is mutated in about 30 percent of HCCs worldwide.[12] All reported *p53* mutations in HCC are somatic. Both the frequency and the type of *p53* mutations are different depending on geographic location and suspected etiology of these tumors, as discussed in the following section.

Involvement of the retinoblastoma gene in the molecular pathogenesis of HCC was initially suggested by studies showing LOH at the *RB1* locus on chromosome 13q.[229,230,232] Besides the retinoblastoma protein, $p16^{INK4A}$ and cyclin D are involved in the regulation of the G1 phase of the cell cycle. Cyclin D forms active complexes with CDK4, whereas $p16^{INK4A}$ is an inhibitor of CDK4 activity. The retinoblastoma protein is the main substrate of CDK4. Upon phosphorylation by CDK4, E2F transcription factors are released from a complex with the retinoblastoma protein and promote cell cycle progression. Loss of the retinoblastoma protein or its increased phosphorylation by an excess of cyclin D or a deficit in $p16^{INK4A}$, therefore, will lead to a loss of growth control at the G1 phase of the cell cycle. Recent studies demonstrated that all three genes, namely *RB1*, $p16^{INK4A}$, and cyclin D, may be altered in HCC.[12] LOH at the *RB1* locus has quite frequently been observed in HCC, and mutations of the *RB1* gene were found in about 15 percent of

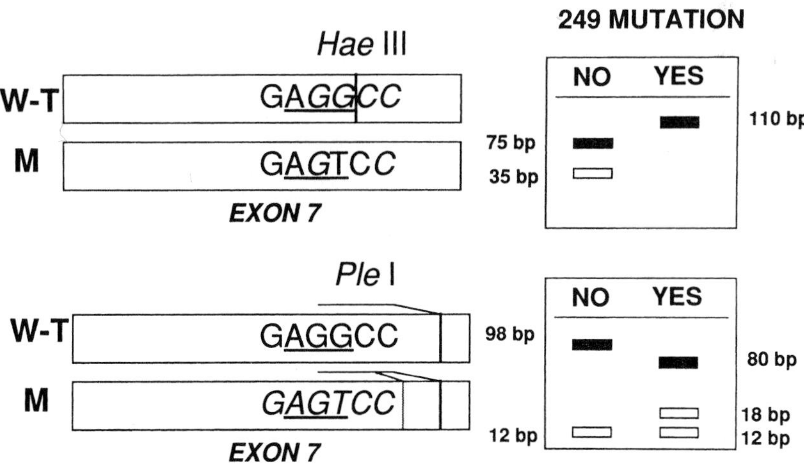

Figure 44-7 Identification of the G to T mutation at the third base of codon 249 of the *p53* gene by restriction enzyme analysis of PCR-amplified exon 7 sequences with *Hae*III (top) and *Ple*I (bottom). Digestion of the wild-type *p53* gene with *Hae*III results in two fragments of 75-bp and 35-bp lengths. In the presence of a mutation the *Hae*III recognition site at codon 249 is lost and only one 110-bp fragment is detected after *Hae*III digestion. The same mutation creates a new *Ple*I recognition site and digestion with this enzyme yields three fragments of 80 bp, 18 bp, and 12 bp. In the absence of a codon 249 mutation *Ple*I digestion yields only two fragments of 98 bp and 12 bp. *PCR,* Polymerase chain reaction.

these tumors.[12,229,230,233,234] Mutations of the $p16^{INK4A}$ gene or inactivation of the gene by methylation have also been found.[235-237] As mentioned previously, cyclin D was found to be amplified in 10 percent to 20 percent of HCCs. Even if *RB1*, $p16^{INK4A}$, and cyclin D are mutated individually in only 10 percent to 20 percent of HCCs, their involvement in control of the same cell cycle checkpoint implies that when combined, these mutations will lead to a loss of growth control in more than 30 percent of HCCs.[12] Recently, a protein consisting of six ankyrin repeats, termed gankyrin, was found to be overexpressed in all HCCs examined.[238] Gankyrin bound to the retinoblastoma protein and increased its phosphorylation. More important, gankyrin was found to accelerate the degradation of the retinoblastoma protein and was identical to or interacted with a subunit of the 26S proteasome. It was speculated, therefore, that gankyrin overexpression contributes to hepatocarcinogenesis by destabilizing the retinoblastoma protein.

The adenomatous polyposis coli *(APC)* gene was identified originally in the familial adenomatous polyposis coli syndrome.[239,240] APC and β-catenin are central molecules in a recently discovered signal transduction pathway mediated by Wnt/wingless ligands. β-Catenin functions as a cell-adhesion component with E-cadherin. In addition, β-catenin can bind members of the TCF/LEF family of transcription factors and activate transcription of genes associated with cell migration and growth.[241] Regulation of the level of free cytoplasmic β-catenin is, at least in part, through the opposing actions of APC and Wnt signals. APC cooperates with the glycogen synthase kinase-3β (GSK-3β) to regulate β-catenin via phosphorylation on serine and threonine residues and targeting for degradation by the ubiquitin-proteasome pathway. By contrast, the presence of a Wnt signal leads to inactivation of GSK-3β, accumulation of β-catenin in the cytoplasm, and passage into the nucleus where it acts as a transcription factor with TCF/LEF family members.

In colorectal cancer β-catenin acquires oncogenic activity when it is mutated or when it is up-regulated as a result of inactivation of APC.[242] Somatic *APC* gene mutations appear to be rare in HCC, but may be more frequent in hepatoblastomas.[243] Activating mutations of β-catenin were reported in 18 percent to 41 percent of HCCs[244-246] and were found to correlate with nuclear β-catenin staining.[247] It has been noted that β-catenin mutations in HCC correlate with a low rate of LOH, suggesting that a mechanism of hepatocarcinogenesis involving β-catenin mutations overrides the need for multiple genetic events and loss of tumor suppressor genes in the multi-step process of hepatocarcinogenesis and may lead more directly to the malignant phenotype.[248] Interestingly, mutations of AXIN1, another factor in the Wnt signaling pathway, have been found recently in a substantial proportion of HCCs with β-catenin accumulation in the absence of mutation of the β-catenin gene.[249] Taken together, deregulated expression of β-catenin, resulting from APC defects, β-catenin gene mutations, or alterations of Wnt signaling pathway, appears to be important in more than 30 percent of HCCs.[12] With the identification of *c-myc* and cyclin D1 as downstream target genes of β-catenin signaling,[250] new molecular clues to HCC pathogenesis are emerging. Finally, the E-cadherin gene was found to display frequent LOH and methylation in HCC.[251]

The *p53* Tumor Suppressor Gene and Aflatoxins

Mutations and allelic deletions of the *p53* gene are the most common genetic alterations found in human tumors[252]; *p53* abnormalities were described initially in a number of HCC cell lines.[253,254] Interestingly, a G to T mutation at the third base position of codon 249 of the *p53* gene, leading to an arginine to serine substitution (R249S), was found in a significant number of HCCs in patients from southern Africa and the Qidong area in China (Figures 44-7 and 44-8).[255,256] This "hot spot" mutation was suggested to be associated with high aflatoxin B1 (AFB1) intake in food and may have contributed to the high incidence of HCC in these areas. This finding was supported by studies in vitro indicating that the third base of codon 249 of *p53* was preferentially targeted to form adducts with AFB1.[257,258] When one compares the frequency of the *p53* R249S mutation in more than 500 HCCs analyzed to date, there are mainly two regions, namely southern China and southern Africa

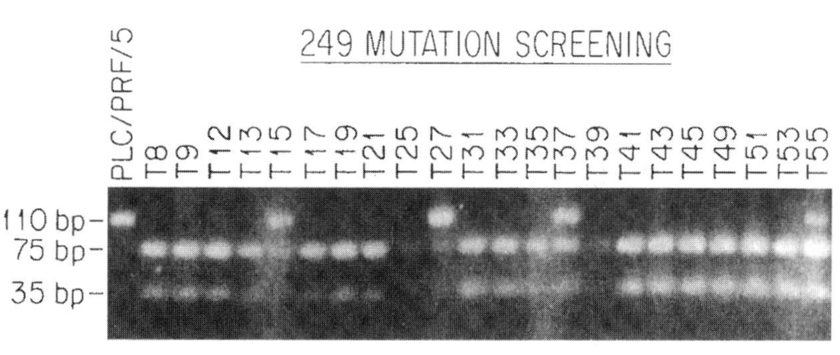

Figure 44-8 Identification of the G to T mutation at the third base of codon 249 of the *p53* gene by restriction enzyme analysis of PCR-amplified exon 7 sequences with *Hae*III (top) and *Ple*I (bottom). Exon 7 of the *p53* gene from different HCCs was amplified and digested with *Hae*III or *Ple*I, electrophoresed through an agarose gel, and visualized by ethidium bromide staining. Four tumors (15, 27, 37, and 55) carry the specific G to T mutation at codon 249. *PCR,* Polymerase chain reaction; *HCC,* hepatocellular carcinoma. (Courtesy of Dr. Mehmet Ozturk.)

TABLE 44-2

Incidence of *p53* Tumor Suppressor Gene Mutations in Various Geographic Locations

Reference	Geographic location	AFB1 exposure	LOH *17p13*	*p53* mutations	*p53* mutations at codon 249
Bressac et al, 1991	Southern Africa	High	3/5	5/10	3/10
Hsu et al, 1991	Qidong (China)	High	NA	8/16	8/16
Ozturk et al, 1991	South Africa and southeast coast of China	High	NA	NA	12/72
Patel et al, 1992	Africa and others	High	NA	NA	2/8
Scorsone et al, 1992	Qidong (China)	High	22/36	NA	21/36
Li et al, 1993	Qidong (China)	High	2/12	9/20	9/20
Ozturk et al, 1991	Various locations	Low	NA	NA	0/95
Murakami et al, 1991	Japan	Low	NA	7/43	0/43
Hayward et al, 1991	Australia	Low	NA	NA	0/16
Oda et al, 1992	Japan	Low	55/80	49/169	7/169
Patel et al, 1992	UK and others	Low	NA	NA	2/64
Challen et al, 1992	UK	Low	NA	2/19	0/19
Kress et al, 1992	Germany	Low	3/8	2/13	0/13
Hosono et al, 1993	Taiwan	Low	3/20	3/29	0/29
Hollstein et al, 1993	Thailand	Low	NA	2/15	1/15
Kar et al, 1993	North America	Low	NA	NA	0/47
Li et al, 1993	Shanghai (China)	Low	6/18	3/18	1/18*
Nishida et al, 1993	Japan	Low	24/49	17/53	0/53
Nose et al, 1993	Japan	Low	5/14	3/20	0/20

AFB1, Aflatoxin B1; *LOH,* loss of heterozygosity (cases with LOH/informative cases); *NA,* not available.
*This patient had previously resided in Nantong, an area of high AFB1 exposure.

(particularly Mozambique), where clustering of this specific mutation (up to 50 percent-70 percent of HCCs) has been found (Table 44-2).[12,259-262] These are two areas of highest aflatoxin exposure in the world. In other regions where aflatoxin levels in food are low or undetectable, including North America,[259,263] Europe,[259,264-266] the Middle East,[259] Japan,[229,259,267-269] Taiwan,[270] Thailand,[271] and Australia,[272] no such mutational specificity of the *p53* gene has been detected (less than 4 percent of HCCs). More recent studies were aimed at the functional characterization of the codon 249 *p53* mutant or of the equivalent mutation at codon 246 of the mouse *p53* gene. It was found that this particular mutation may confer a growth advantage specifically on liver-derived cell lines. This mutation, however, does not appear to result in a loss of apoptotic function and is not—consistent with the multi-stage process of hepatocarcinogenesis and the identification in apparently normal liver of AFB1-exposed individuals—sufficient to transform hepatocytes.[273-278]

Aflatoxins are mycotoxins produced by the molds *Aspergillus flavus* and *Aspergillus parasiticus* and contaminate inappropriately processed and stored food such as corn, peanuts, and rice in some areas of the world.[279-285] Epidemiologic investigations have revealed that there is a linear relationship between the content of AFB1 in the diet and the risk of HCC.[282,286] The use of experimental models[287,288] and specific biomarkers for aflatoxin exposure, such as urinary metabolites or aflatoxin adducts, have validated these epidemiologic observations.[283-285] Importantly, AFB1 contamination of food and co-existing HBV infection are associated with even higher rates of HCC within a given population. Therefore the effects of these two carcinogenic agents may be synergistic.[283,289,290] Consistent with these epidemiologic observations, HCCs appear earlier and at a higher incidence in chronically WHV-infected woodchucks exposed to AFB1, whereas AFB1 does not induce HCCs in uninfected woodchucks.[291] Of note, the *p53* R249S mutation has

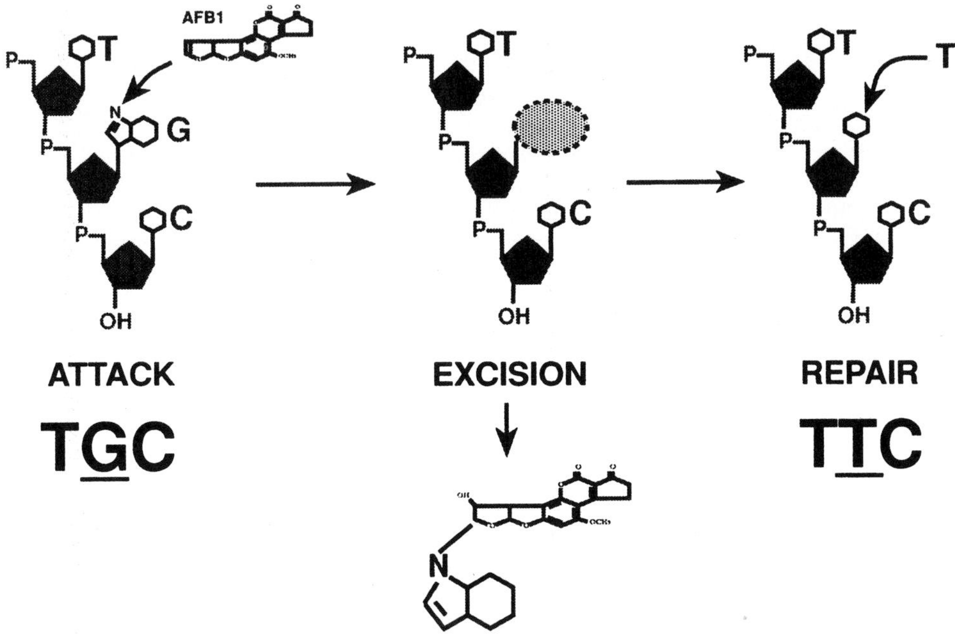

Figure 44-9 AFB1 binding to guanine residues in DNA leads to an excisional event and subsequent repair by replacement with a thymidine residue. The genetic code is changed from TGC to TTC in this example. *AFB1,* Aflatoxin B1; *DNA,* deoxyribonucleic acid.

been identified primarily in patients who were also infected with HBV. It is possible, therefore, that HBV-induced chronic hepatitis contributes to the frequency of this mutation in high aflatoxin areas of the world. Increased cellular proliferation in the context of chronic inflammation could allow fixation of the G to T mutation at codon 249 and selective clonal expansion of cells containing this mutant *p53*.

AFB1 is metabolized by the liver microsomal system to a very reactive epoxide intermediate, which binds selectively to guanine residues in cellular DNA to form AFB1-N7 guanine adducts.[285,292,293] This binding is followed by an excisional event that removes the AFB1 guanine adduct from the DNA. This product is excreted and can be detected in the urine.[289,294-296] By unclear molecular mechanisms there is a preferential replacement of the guanine by a thymidine residue during the DNA repair process. AFB1 DNA adduct formation, therefore, preferentially induces G to T mutations in chromosomal DNA, as shown in Figure 44-9.

The blue algal hepatotoxin microcystin was identified as another environmental carcinogen accounting for the high incidence of HCC among ditch-water drinkers in Haimen City, Jian-Su Province, and Fusui County in the Guangxi Province of China.[297] Importantly, the transition from stagnant ditch or pond water to deep well water consumption has led to a decline in the incidence of HCC in these areas.[298]

DNA MISMATCH REPAIR

In addition to oncogenes and tumor suppressor genes DNA mismatch repair genes have been identified as a class of susceptibility genes involved in the pathogenesis of inherited and sporadic human tumors, notably hereditary nonpolyposis colorectal cancer (HNPCC).[10] Defective DNA mismatch repair can lead to the accumulation of mutations and microsatellite instability in the cellular genome, thus increasing the chance of malignant transformation. DNA mismatch repair gene defects appear to play a role in a subset of HCCs[299,300] but the frequency of such defects is currently debatable.[301,302] In one study microsatellite instability (MSI) as a manifestation of defective DNA mismatch repair was found in one third of HCCs examined.[299] MSI was often associated with LOH at the *hMSH2* and *hMLH1* gene loci. In some cases MSI was also found in the cirrhotic liver adjacent to the tumor, an observation that underscores the importance of liver cirrhosis as a premalignant condition. Interestingly, experimental data suggest that HBx may interfere with components of the DNA repair machinery.[99-102]

TELOMERASE ACTIVATION

The progressive shortening of chromosome ends, or telomeres, accompanies normal cell division and may contribute to cellular aging and serve as a control mechanism against unregulated cellular proliferation.[303] A remarkable correlation between certain types of cancer and the expression of telomerase, a ribonucleoprotein enzyme preventing the shortening of telomeres, has been found.[304] Indeed, expression of telomerase may be a common pathway leading to cancer. In this regard, telomerase activation was found in a high proportion of HCC tissues.[305-307] Of interest, telomerase activity was relatively low in well-differentiated compared to poorly or moderately differentiated HCCs.[308-310]

GROWTH FACTORS

As in most forms of cancer the unregulated expression of growth factors and of components of their signaling pathways may be important for hepatocarcinogenesis.[311] Knowledge regarding growth factor activation during hepatic proliferation and transformation is incomplete. Some of the growth factors that may be involved in one or more steps in the development of HCC are insulin-like growth factor II (IGF-II), transforming growth factor (TGF)-α, TGF-β, hepatocyte growth factor (HGF), and insulin receptor substrate 1 (hIRS-1).

Insulin-like Growth Factor II

IGF-II is a polypeptide hormone produced during fetal development and is structurally and functionally related to insulin and IGF-I.[312] The expression of IGF-II messenger RNAs is regulated through the activation of different promoters and alternative splicing of 5′ non-translated sequences during development. IGF-II is expressed at high levels in fetal liver; however, IGF-II transcription rates decline after birth. IGF-II is expressed at very low levels in the normal adult liver. Re-expression of IGF-II at high levels has been found in chemically induced hepatocarcinogenesis,[313] transgenic mouse models of hepatocarcinogenesis,[314,315] WHV-related liver carcinogenesis,[30,316,317] and human HCCs.[318,319] These observations demonstrate that IGF-II reactivation is a common molecular event in hepatocarcinogenesis regardless of mammalian species and may confer a selective growth advantage on premalignant or malignant hepatocytes via an autocrine mechanism.

Transforming Growth Factor Alpha

TGF-α is a member of a family of structurally related polypeptide growth factors, of which epidermal growth factor (EGF) was the first member to be isolated and biochemically characterized.[320] TGF-α and EGF signal through a common cell surface receptor tyrosine kinase, referred to as the EGF receptor.[321] Based on experiments on TGF-α expression during liver regeneration after partial hepatectomy, it has been proposed that TGF-α acts in an autocrine fashion as a direct stimulator of hepatocyte DNA synthesis during liver regeneration.[322] Increased production of TGF-α and its receptor has frequently been found in human tumors and malignantly transformed cells in culture, including HCC cell lines.[323,324] Sixty-five percent of transgenic mice bearing a human TGF-α complementary DNA under the control of the mouse metallothionein promoter have been shown to develop HCC at age 10 to 15 months.[325] Although the molecular mechanisms by which TGF-α induces liver neoplasia in these animals remain to be elucidated, the long latency period between the expression of the transgene and the development of HCC suggests a promoting effect in the multistep process of tumor development. In accordance with this notion, HBsAg–TGF-α double-transgenic mice had a dramatically accelerated appearance of HCCs, compared to single transgenic HBsAg or TGF-α littermates.[326] With respect to clinical observations, 65 percent of HCC patients had elevated TGF-α levels in the urine,[327] and TGF-α was found to be overexpressed in the majority of HCCs.[31,328]

Transforming Growth Factor Beta

TGF-β is the prototype member of a family of structurally and functionally related multi-functional polypeptides, which includes various forms of TGF-β, the bone morphogenic proteins, the nodals, the activins, the anti-Müllerian hormone, and many structurally related factors.[329] Produced by diverse cell types, these factors regulate cell migration, adhesion, proliferation, differentiation, and death. TGF-β assembles two different transmembrane receptor protein kinases, known as receptor types I and II, that activate SMADs, which assemble multi-subunit complexes that regulate transcription.

The tissue effects of TGF-β are complex. TGF-β is believed to exert an action on various cell and tissue types by counteracting the growth-promoting effects of other growth factors, such as TGF-α, under physiologic conditions. There also is interest in TGF-β because it may be important in liver fibrogenesis.[330-332] TGF-β is a potent inhibitor of proliferation of HCC cell lines.[333] Several studies have demonstrated an increase in the expression of TGF-β in HCC tissue[323] and elevated serum levels of TGF-β in patients with HCC.[334] Non-parenchymal, mesenchymal cells are the principal source of TGF-β in normal and pathologic states of the liver.[330,335] Thus TGF-β is believed to act in a paracrine fashion. Based on observations from chemical hepatocarcinogenesis models it has been suggested that a close interaction between non-parenchymal cells and carcinoma cells may be necessary for the activation of TGF-β expression.[336] The activation of TGF-β may represent a physiologic attempt by the liver to inhibit the growth of transformed hepatocytes under these conditions.

LOH at the mannose-6-phosphate/IGF-II receptor (M6P/IGFIIR) locus on chromosome 6q25-27 has been found in about 30 percent of HCCs.[227,337] The M6P/IGFIIR has been implicated in tumor growth. Furthermore, binding of latent TGF-β to the M6P/IGFIIR stimulates the production of active TGF-β, leading to growth inhibition. Loss of function of the M6P/IGFIIR gene, therefore, may deregulate growth through different mechanisms. In this context mutations of the M6P/IGFIIR gene were found in 25 percent of HCCs harboring LOH at chromosome 6q25-27.[338,339] The *Smad2* and *Smad4* genes appear to be rarely mutated in HCCs.[340] Taken together, the TGF-β system appears to be involved in the pathogenesis of about 25 percent of HCCs.[12]

Hepatocyte Growth Factor

HGF is a heterodimer comprising a high-molecular-weight α chain and a lower-molecular-weight β chain.[341,342] The heavy chain has four kringle domains, which are double-loop polypeptide structures consisting of a smaller loop held together with disulfide bonds within a larger loop. This structure is reminiscent of the kringle domains in plasminogen and several other fibrinolytic and coagulation-related proteins. HGF is a potent stimulator of DNA synthesis in cultured hepatocytes and has been shown to act on a variety of cell types with respect to mitogenic activity. In addition to its mitogenic action on a wide spectrum of cell types, HGF can transmit information that determines the spatial organization of epithelial cells in tissues.[343] It also has been shown to be identical to "scatter factor," which can induce dissociation and increased migration of a variety of epithelial cells and is believed, therefore, to be important in tumor metastasis.[344] The receptor for HGF is the *c-met* protooncogene product, a member of the protein tyrosine kinase receptor family.[345,346]

Surprisingly, HGF inhibits the growth of a number of hepatoma cell lines in vitro,[347,348] and no neoplasms develop in transgenic mice expressing HGF in the liver under control of the albumin promoter.[349] Moreover, *c-myc*-HGF double transgenics show markedly reduced neoplastic changes, compared to *c-myc* single transgenics. Thus although HGF is mitogenic for normal hepatocytes, it appears to display an inhibitory action on HCC cells and other malignant cells through unknown mechanisms and illustrates that the regulation of hepatocyte proliferation versus transformation is complex.

Insulin Receptor Substrate 1

Investigators have identified activation of the hIRS-1 signal transduction cascade in the majority of HCCs (Figure 44-10)[350,351]; additional pancreatic and breast studies implicate hIRS-1 in tumor cell growth.[352-354] The hIRS-1 is phosphorylated on tyrosine residues after cellular stimulation by ligands (i.e., insulin; IGF-I; interleukin-4 and interleukin-13; interferon α, β, ω, and γ; growth hormone; leukemia inhibitory factor; and TGFs).[355] The hIRS-1 protein is the main intracellular substrate for receptor tyrosine kinase activity of the insulin/IGF-I receptor, emitting downstream signals through interaction with SH2 domain–containing molecules at specific motifs located in the C-terminal region. Such protein-protein interaction leads to Ras/Raf/MAPKK/MAPK cascade activation involved in cell growth regulation. There is experimental evidence to suggest that HBV and HCV proteins, namely HBx and NS5A, interact with Ras and Grb2, perhaps modulating the growth factor signal transduction cascade.[93-95,188] These investigations provide a link between viral and cellular proteins, emphasizing the potential importance of the hIRS-1 pathway in the pathogenesis of HCC.

Several lines of transgenic mice have been established to study hIRS-1 overexpression with liver-specific synthesis controlled by an albumin enhancer promoter; it was hypothesized that overexpression of this critical protein, high in the signal transduction cascade, might drive hepatocytic proliferation and transformation. The overexpressed hIRS-1 protein was tyrosyl phosphorylated and interacted with downstream SH2 domain–containing molecules such as the p85 subunit of

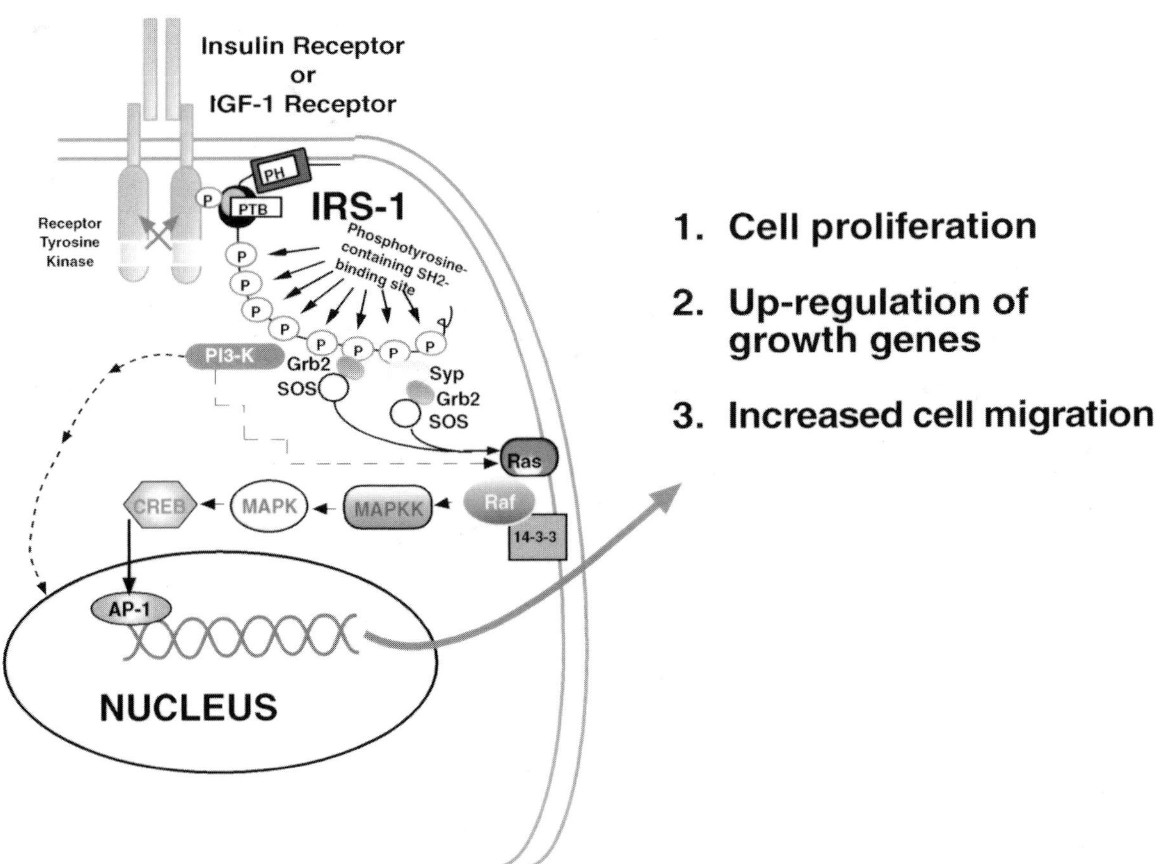

Figure 44-10 Diagram depicting the major features and proposed role(s) of the IRS-1 signal transduction pathway during hepatocyte growth and transformation.

phosphatidylinositol-3 kinase PI3K, Grb2 adaptor, and SHP2 phosphatase proteins.[356] The functional consequences of hIRS-1 overexpression were reflected by constitutive activation of both the MAPK and PI3K signal transduction cascades. More important, hIRS-1 overexpression in the transgenic liver led to increased hepatocyte DNA synthesis and induced molecular downstream signaling associated with hepatocyte growth.[356] Interestingly, expression of a dominant negative mutant of hIRS-1 was found to reverse the malignant phenotype in HCC cell lines, thus underscoring the central significance of this pathway.[357]

ANGIOGENESIS

Angiogenesis is central to the development and progression of solid tumors. It may be particularly important in hepatocarcinogenesis because HCC is often a highly vascular tumor. Overexpression of vascular endothelial growth factor, one of the most important angiogenic factors, has been documented in HCC,[358-360] and additional factors, such as basic fibroblast growth factor[358] and angiopoetin-2,[361] seem to be involved as well.

TRANSGENIC MOUSE MODELS OF HEPATOCARCINOGENESIS

A variety of transgenic mouse models of hepatocarcinogenesis have contributed to the understanding of mechanisms involved in HCC development.[362-364] Examples include mice carrying the simian virus 40 large-tumor antigen (SV40 T Ag), activated *c-Ha-ras* or *c-myc*, or TGF-α driven by the regulatory elements of liver-specific genes (e.g., mouse metallothionein, albumin, α_1-antitrypsin).[325,365-368] Liver cancer develops within a few months after birth after sequential stages of hyperplasia and diffuse liver cell dysplasia in transgenic mouse lines harboring the SV40 T Ag gene under the control of liver-specific regulatory elements.[365-369] Expression of an activated *c-Ha-ras*, *c-myc*, and SV40 T Ag directed to the liver by the albumin enhancer or promoter was associated with progressive transformation of hepatocytes. Crossbreeding of animals to obtain dual transgenics resulted in acceleration of tumor development, suggesting that these oncogenes may cooperate with one another during transformation of hepatocytes to the malignant phenotype.[366] Expression of TGF-α produces hyperplasia and dysplasia in the liver,[370] with hepatomas seen in one mouse lineage.[325]

The mouse model developed by Chisari and colleagues is particularly noteworthy in the context of hepatocarcinogenesis. In these transgenic mice the HBV pre-S1 and pre-S2, S, and X, and most of the P coding region are under the transcriptional control of the mouse albumin promoter.[371-373] Normally, the HBV pre-S1 promoter directs expression of the large envelope polypeptide, and an internal promoter in the pre-S1 region directs expression of the middle and small polypeptides. In this construct, however, the internal promoter was still present but the pre-S1 promoter was replaced by the albumin promoter, which led to constitutive dysbalanced expression in the hepatocyte. Dysregulated expression of large envelope polypeptides prevents the formation of small spherical HBsAg particles and causes the formation of long, branching HBsAg filaments that become trapped in the endoplasmic reticulum of the hepatocyte, thereby inhibiting secretion of HBsAg from the cell.[371,372] Progressive accumulation of large amounts of these filamentous particles led to a dramatic expansion of the endoplasmic reticulum of the hepatocyte that eventually caused the changes characteristic of "ground-glass" hepatocytes characteristic of patients with chronic HBV infection. In the transgenic mouse line 50-4, accumulation of these aberrant particles initiated a process characterized by chronic hepatocellular injury, inflammation, and regenerative hyperplasia, followed sequentially by the development of regenerative nodules, liver adenomas, hepatocyte dysplasia, and ultimately HCC by 12 months of age.[373,374] One hundred percent of mice of this lineage develop HCC by 20 months of age, whereas no histopathologic changes were observed in non-transgenic litter mates. Thus prolonged hepatocellular injury followed by regenerative hyperplasia was sufficient in this model to set in motion a complex series of events leading ultimately to or contributing to malignant transformation. This, therefore, is similar to the sequence of cellular events often observed in human hepatocarcinogenesis. In the transgenic mouse lineage 50-4 exposure to AFB1 and diethylnitrosamine produced more rapid and extensive tumor development than was seen in transgenic mice not exposed to such carcinogens.[375] This last observation suggests that increased cellular turnover in the context of chronic liver injury and repair increases the chance for mutational events and predisposes to the carcinogenic effects of exogenous agents. Indeed, hepatocellular turnover in these mice, relative to non-transgenic controls, was increased nearly 100-fold for at least a year before the onset of HCC.[376] In addition, extensive hepatic oxidative DNA damage was found in these mice in the setting of chronic necroinflammatory liver disease.[377] This model and the observation that HCC does not develop in a number of other HBV transgenic mice in which no hepatocellular injury is observed[363,378] provide considerable evidence for the indirect role of chronic hepatocyte injury and regeneration in hepatocarcinogenesis, as shown in Figure 44-1.

An interesting sequence of events was observed in a transgenic mouse model with extensive hepatic injury and regeneration shortly after birth secondary to expression of the murine urokinase-type plasminogen-activator transgene. In mice that survived to adulthood the entire liver was repopulated by regenerative nodules containing clonally expanded cells that no longer expressed the transgene. Apparently, chromosomal rearrangements occurred.[379] Several months after a period of intensive hyperplasia, these mice developed HCCs that were derived from the transgene-deficient cells. Because tumors arose only from a particular subclass of transgene-deficient cells, in which the entire transgene array had been deleted, it was proposed that chromosomal rearrangements may have extended into flanking cellular DNA and caused the loss of genomic DNA with important regulatory functions. Thus loss of genomic DNA, and not increased cellular turnover per se, was an important determinant for neoplastic transformation in this model.[380]

SUMMARY AND PERSPECTIVES

Hepatocyte transformation occurs in the setting of chronic liver injury, regeneration, and cirrhosis. Increased cell turnover in this context of inflammation and oxidative DNA damage may result in genetic alterations, such as chromosomal rearrangements, oncogene activation, or inactivation of tumor suppressor genes, possibly in cooperation with defective DNA mismatch repair, telomerase activation, and induction of growth and angiogenic factors. Chronic viral hepatitis, alcohol, and certain metabolic liver diseases may act predominantly through this pathway. On the other hand, experimental evidence suggests that HBV and HCV may, under certain circumstances, have a direct role in the molecular pathogenesis of HCC. Finally, aflatoxins induce mutations of the p53 tumor suppressor gene, thus pointing to the contribution of environmental factors to tumor development at the molecular level. Understanding hepatocyte growth regulation at the molecular level may lead eventually not only to a better understanding of the cellular events involved in hepatocyte transformation, but in all likelihood also to improved preventive measures and innovative therapies for one of the most devastating human malignancies in the world today. Preventive measures are of greatest importance and include, among others, systematic HBV immunization, blood screening, and needle-exchange programs to reduce transmission of hepatic viruses, anti-viral treatment of patients with chronic hepatitis B and C,[381] timely diagnosis and treatment of metabolic diseases such as hemochromatosis and α_1-antitrypsin deficiency, improved storage of staple foods to control aflatoxin exposure, and possibly chemoprevention programs.[382] Finally, novel therapeutic strategies, including gene therapy[383] and immunotherapy,[384,385] are being explored based on an improved understanding of the molecular pathogenesis of HCC.

References

1. Wands JR, Blum HE: Primary hepatocellular carcinoma. N Engl J Med 325:729, 1991.
2. Okuda K: Hepatocellular carcinoma. J Hepatol 32(suppl 1):225, 2000.
3. Bosch FX, Ribes J, Borras J: Epidemiology of primary liver cancer. Semin Liver Dis 19:271, 1999.
4. Okuda K, Fujimoto I, Hanai A, et al: Changing incidence of hepatocellular carcinoma in Japan. Cancer Res 47:4967, 1987.
5. Taylor-Robinson SD, Foster GR, Arora S, et al: Increase in primary liver cancer in the UK, 1979-94. Lancet 350:1142, 1997.
6. Deuffic S, Poynard T, Buffat L, et al: Trends in primary liver cancer. Lancet 351:214, 1998.
7. Stroffolini T, Andreone P, Andriulli A, et al: Characteristics of hepatocellular carcinoma in Italy. J Hepatol 29:944, 1998.
8. El-Serag HB, Mason AC: Rising incidence of hepatocellular carcinoma in the United States. N Engl J Med 340:745, 1999.
9. El-Serag HB, Mason AC: Risk factors for the rising rates of primary liver cancer in the United States. Arch Intern Med 160:3227, 2000.
10. Kinzler KW, Vogelstein B: Lessons from hereditary colorectal cancer. Cell 87:159, 1996.
11. Hanahan D, Weinberg RA: The hallmarks of cancer. Cell 100:57, 2000.
12. Ozturk M: Genetic aspects of hepatocellular carcinogenesis. Semin Liver Dis 19:235, 1999.
13. Farber E: On cells of origin in liver cell cancer. In Sirica AE, ed: The Role of Cell Types in Hepatocarcinogenesis. Boca Raton, Fla., CRC Press, 1992.
14. Fausto N, Lemire JM, Shiojiri N: Oval cells in liver carcinogenesis: cell lineages in hepatic development and the identification of facultative stem cells in normal liver. In Sirica AE, ed: The Role of Cell Types in Hepatocarcinogenesis. Boca Raton, Fla., CRC Press, 1992.
15. Thorgeirsson SS, Evarts RP: Growth and differentiation of stem cells in adult rat liver. In Sirica AE, ed: The Role of Cell Types in Hepatocarcinogenesis. Boca Raton, Fla., CRC Press, 1992.
16. Alison M, Sarraf C: Hepatic stem cells. J Hepatol 29:676, 1998.
17. Overturf K, Al-Dhalimy M, Tanguay R, et al: Hepatocytes corrected by gene therapy are selected in vivo in a murine model of hereditary tyrosinaemia type I. Nat Genet 12:266, 1996.
18. Overturf K, al-Dhalimy M, Ou CN, et al: Serial transplantation reveals the stem-cell-like regenerative potential of adult mouse hepatocytes. Am J Pathol 151:1273, 1997.
19. Petersen BE, Bowen WC, Patrene KD, et al: Bone marrow as a potential source of hepatic oval cells. Science 284:1168, 1999.
20. Lagasse E, Connors H, Al-Dhalimy M, et al: Purified hematopoietic stem cells can differentiate into hepatocytes in vivo. Nat Med 6:1229, 2000.
21. Theise ND, Nimmakayalu M, Gardner R, et al: Liver from bone marrow in humans. Hepatology 32:11, 2000.
22. Sell S: Heterogeneity and plasticity of hepatocyte lineage cells. Hepatology 33:738, 2001.
23. Sigal SH, Brill S, Fiorino AS, et al: The liver as a stem cell and lineage system. Am J Physiol 263:G139, 1992.
24. Bralet MP, Branchereau S, Bréchot C, et al: Cell lineage study in the liver using retroviral mediated gene transfer. Evidence against the streaming of hepatocytes in normal liver. Am J Pathol 144:896, 1994.
25. Sell S, Hunt JM, Knoll BJ, et al: Cellular events during hepatocarcinogenesis in rats and the question of premalignancy. Adv Cancer Res 48:37, 1987.
26. Evarts RP, Nakatsukasa H, Marsden ER, et al: Cellular and molecular changes in the early stages of chemical hepatocarcinogenesis in the rat. Cancer Res 50:3439, 1990.
27. Evarts RP, Nagy P, Marsden E, et al: A precursor-product relationship exists between oval cells and hepatocytes in rat liver. Carcinogenesis 8:1737, 1987.
28. Theise ND, Saxena R, Portmann BC, et al: The canals of Hering and hepatic stem cells in humans. Hepatology 30:1425, 1999.
29. Marceau M, Blouin M-J, Noël M, et al: The role of bipotential progenitor cells in liver ontogenesis and neoplasia. In Sirica AE, ed: The Role of Cell Types in Hepatocarcinogenesis. Boca Raton, Fla., CRC Press, 1992.
30. Fu X-X, Su CY, Lee Y, et al: Insulinlike growth factor II expression and oval cell proliferation associated with hepatocarcinogenesis in woodchuck hepatitis virus carriers. J Virol 62:3422, 1988.
31. Hsia CC, Axiotis CA, Di Bisceglie AM, et al: Transforming growth factor-alpha in human hepatocellular carcinoma and coexpression with hepatitis B surface antigen in adjacent liver. Cancer 70:1049, 1992.
32. Beasley RP, Hwang L-Y, Lin C-C, et al: Hepatocellular carcinoma and hepatitis B virus—a prospective study of 22707 men in Taiwan. Lancet ii:1129, 1981.
33. Chang M-H, Chen C-J, Lai M-S, et al: Universal hepatitis B vaccination in Taiwan and the incidence of hepatocellular carcinoma in children. N Engl J Med 336:1855, 1997.
34. Nakamoto Y, Guidotti LC, Kuhlen CV, et al: Immune pathogenesis of hepatocellular carcinoma. J Exp Med 188:341, 1998.
35. Summers J, Mason WS: Replication of the genome of a hepatitis B-like virus by reverse transcription of an RNA intermediate. Cell 29:403, 1982.
36. Bréchot C, Pourcel C, Louise A, et al: Presence of integrated hepatitis B virus DNA sequences in cellular DNA of human hepatocellular carcinoma. Nature 286:533, 1980.
37. Chakraborty PR, Ruiz-Opazo N, Shouval D, et al: Identification of integrated hepatitis B virus DNA and expression of viral RNA in an HBsAg-producing human hepatocellular carcinoma cell line. Nature 286:531, 1980.

38. Edman JC, Gray P, Valenzuela P, et al: Integration of hepatitis B virus sequences and their expression in a human hepatoma cell. Nature 286:535, 1980.
39. Marion PL, Salazar FH, Alexander JJ, et al: State of hepatitis B viral DNA in a human hepatoma cell line. J Virol 33:795, 1980.
40. Bréchot C, Hadchouel M, Scotto J, et al: State of hepatitis B virus DNA in hepatocytes of patients with hepatitis B surface antigen-positive and -negative liver diseases. Proc Natl Acad Sci U S A 78:3906, 1981.
41. Koshy R, Maupas P, Müller R, et al: Detection of hepatitis B virus-specific DNA in the genomes of human hepatocellular carcinoma and liver cirrhosis tissues. J Gen Virol 57:95, 1981.
42. Shafritz DA, Shouval D, Sherman HI, et al: Integration of hepatitis B virus DNA into the genome of liver cells in chronic liver disease and hepatocellular carcinoma. Studies in percutaneous liver biopsies and post-mortem tissue specimens. N Engl J Med 305:1067, 1981.
43. Dejean A, Bréchot C, Tiollais P, et al: Characterization of integrated hepatitis B viral DNA cloned from a human hepatoma and the hepatoma-derived cell line PLC/PRF/5. Proc Natl Acad Sci U S A 80:2505, 1983.
44. Matsubara K, Tokino T: Integration of hepatitis B virus DNA and its implications for hepatocarcinogenesis. Mol Biol Med 7:243, 1990.
45. Buendia MA: Hepatitis B viruses and hepatocellular carcinoma. Adv Cancer Res 59:167, 1992.
46. Koike K: HBV DNA integration and insertional mutagenesis. In Caselmann WH, Koshy R, eds: Hepatitis B Virus, ed 1. London, Imperial College Press, 1998.
47. Koch S, Freytag von Loringhoven A, Kahmann R, et al: The genetic organization of integrated hepatitis B virus DNA in the human hepatoma cell line PLC/PRF/5. Nucl Acids Res 12:6871, 1984.
48. Shaul Y, Ziemer M, Garcia PD, et al: Cloning and analysis of integrated hepatitis virus sequences from a human hepatoma cell line. J Virol 51:776, 1984.
49. Ziemer M, Garcia P, Shaul Y, et al: Sequence of hepatitis B virus DNA incorporated into the genome of a human hepatoma cell line. J Virol 53:885, 1985.
50. Esumi M, Aritaka T, Arii M, et al: Clonal origin of human hepatoma determined by integration of hepatitis B virus DNA. Cancer Res 46:5767, 1986.
51. Blum HE, Offensperger W-B, Walter E, et al: Hepatocellular carcinoma and hepatitis B virus infection: molecular evidence for monoclonal origin and expansion of malignantly transformed hepatocytes. J Cancer Res Clin Oncol 113:466, 1987.
52. Dejean A, Sonigo P, Wain-Hobson S, et al: Specific hepatitis B virus integration in hepatocellular carcinoma DNA through a viral 11-base-pair direct repeat. Proc Natl Acad Sci U S A 81:5350, 1984.
53. Nagaya T, Nakamura T, Tokino T, et al: The mode of hepatitis B virus DNA integration in chromosomes of human hepatocellular carcinoma. Genes Dev 1:773, 1987.
54. Shih C, Burke K, Chou M-J, et al: Tight clustering of human hepatitis B virus integration sites in hepatomas near a triple-stranded region. J Virol 61:3491, 1987.
55. Hino O, Ohtake K, Rogler CE: Features of two hepatitis B virus (HBV) DNA integrations suggest mechanism of HBV integration. J Virol 63:2638, 1989.
56. Tokino T, Matsubara K: Chromosomal sites for hepatitis B virus integration in human hepatocellular carcinoma. J Virol 65:6761, 1991.
57. Mizusawa H, Taira M, Yaginuma K, et al: Inversely repeating integrated hepatitis B virus DNA and cellular flanking sequences in the human hepatoma-derived cell line huSP. Proc Natl Acad Sci U S A 82:208, 1985.
58. Yaginuma K, Kobayashi M, Yoshida E, et al: Hepatitis B virus integration in hepatocellular carcinoma DNA: duplication of cellular flanking sequences at the integration site. Proc Natl Acad Sci U S A 82:4458, 1985.
59. Tokino T, Fukushige S, Nakamura T, et al: Chromosomal translocation and inverted duplication associated with integrated hepatitis B virus in hepatocellular carcinomas. J Virol 61:3848, 1987.
60. Zhou Y-Z, Slagle BL, Donehower LA, et al: Structural analysis of a hepatitis B virus genome integrated into chromosome 17p of a human hepatocellular carcinoma. J Virol 62:4224, 1988.
61. Hino O, Shows TB, Rogler CE: Hepatitis B virus integration site in hepatocellular carcinoma at chromosome 17:18 translocation. Proc Natl Acad Sci U S A 83:8338, 1986.
62. Meyer M, Wiedorn KH, Hofschneider PH, et al: A chromosome 17:7 translocation is associated with a hepatitis B virus DNA integration in human hepatocellular carcinoma DNA. Hepatology 15:665, 1992.
63. Rogler CE, Sherman M, Su CY, et al: Deletion in chromosome 11p associated with a hepatitis B integration site in hepatocellular carcinoma. Science 230:319, 1985.
64. Hatada I, Tokino T, Ochiya T, et al: Co-amplification of integrated hepatitis B virus DNA and transforming gene hst-1 in a hepatocellular carcinoma. Oncogene 3:537, 1988.
65. Wang H-P, Rogler CE: Topoisomerase I-mediated integration of hepadnavirus DNA in vitro. J Virol 65:2381, 1991.
66. Dejean A, Bougueleret L, Grzeschik K-H, et al: Hepatitis B virus DNA integration in a sequence homologous to v-erb-A and steroid receptor genes in a hepatocellular carcinoma. Nature 322:70, 1986.
67. de Thé H, Marchio A, Tiollais P, et al: A novel steroid thyroid hormone receptor-related gene inappropriately expressed in human hepatocellular carcinoma. Nature 330:667, 1987.
68. Brand N, Petkovich M, Krust A, et al: Identification of a second human retinoic acid receptor. Nature 332:850, 1988.
69. Dejean A, de Thé H: Hepatitis B virus as an insertional mutagene in a human hepatocellular carcinoma. Mol Biol Med 7:213, 1990.
70. Wang J, Chenivesse X, Henglein B, et al: Hepatitis B virus integration in a cyclin A gene in a hepatocellular carcinoma. Nature 343:555, 1990.
71. Nurse P: A long twentieth century of the cell cycle and beyond. Cell 100:71, 2000.
72. Wang J, Zindy F, Chenivesse X, et al: Modification of cyclin A expression by hepatitis B virus DNA integration in a hepatocellular carcinoma. Oncogene 7:1653, 1992.
73. Zhang X-K, Egan JO, Huang D-P, et al: Hepatitis B virus DNA integration and expression of an erb B-like gene in human hepatocellular carcinoma. Biochem Biophys Res Commun 188:344, 1992.
74. Graef E, Caselmann WH, Koshy R: Differential splicing of overexpressed hepatitis B viral-mevalonate kinase fusion transcripts in human hepatoma cells. Hepatology 18:184A, 1993.
75. Graef E, Caselmann WH, Wells J, et al: Insertional activation of mevalonate kinase by hepatitis B virus DNA in a human hepatoma cell line. Oncogene 9:81, 1994.
76. Graef E, Caselmann WH, Hofschneider PH, et al: Enzymatic properties of overexpressed HBV-mevalonate kinase fusion proteins and mevalonate kinase proteins in the human hepatoma cell line PLC/PRF/5. Virology 208:696, 1995.
77. Pineau P, Marchio A, Terris B, et al: A t(3;8) chromosomal translocation associated with hepatitis B virus integration involves the carboxypeptidase N locus. J Virol 70:7280, 1996.
78. Blum HE, Zhang Z-S, Galun E, et al: Hepatitis B virus X protein is not central to the viral life cycle in vitro. J Virol 66:1223, 1992.
79. Chen H-S, Kaneko S, Girones R, et al: The woodchuck hepatitis virus X gene is important for establishment of virus infection in woodchucks. J Virol 67:1218, 1993.
80. Zoulim F, Saputelli J, Seeger C: Woodchuck hepatitis virus X protein is required for viral infection in vivo. J Virol 68:2026, 1994.
81. Twu JS, Schloemer RH: Transcriptional transactivating function of hepatitis B virus. J Virol 61:3448, 1987.
82. Zahm P, Hofschneider PH, Koshy R: The HBV X-ORF encodes a transactivator: a potential factor in viral hepatocarcinogenesis. Oncogene 3:169, 1988.
83. Colgrove R, Simon G, Ganem D: Transcriptional activation of homologous and heterologous genes by the hepatitis B virus X gene product in cells permissive for viral replication. J Virol 63:4019, 1989.
84. Caselmann WH, Koshy R: Transactivators of HBV, signal transduction and tumorigenesis. In Caselmann WH, Koshy R, eds: Hepatitis B Virus, ed 1. London, Imperial College Press, 1998.
85. Wang W, London WT, Feitelson MA: Hepatitis B x antigen in hepatitis B virus carrier patients with liver cancer. Cancer Res 51:4971, 1991.
86. Diamantis I, McGandy CE, Chen T-J, et al: Hepatitis B X-gene expression in hepatocellular carcinoma. J Hepatol 15:400, 1992.
87. Paterlini P, Poussin K, Kew M, et al: Selective accumulation of the X transcript of hepatitis B virus in patients negative for hepatitis B surface antigen with hepatocellular carcinoma. Hepatology 21:313, 1995.
88. Wollersheim M, Debelka U, Hofschneider PH: A transactivating function encoded by the hepatitis B virus X gene is conserved in the integrated state. Oncogene 3:545, 1988.

89. Takada S, Koike K: Trans-activation function of a 3? truncated X gene-cell fusion product from integrated hepatitis B virus DNA in chronic hepatitis tissues. Proc Natl Acad Sci U S A 87:5628, 1990.
90. Balsano C, Avantaggiati ML, Natoli G, et al: Full-length and truncated versions of the hepatitis B virus X protein transactivate the c-myc protooncogene at the transcriptional level. Biochem Biophys Res Commun 176:985, 1991.
91. Seto E, Mitchell PJ, Zen TSB: Transactivation by the hepatitis B virus X protein depends on AP-2 and other transcription factors. Nature 344:72, 1990.
92. Kekulé AS, Lauer U, Weiss L, et al: Hepatitis B virus transactivator HBx uses a tumour promoter signalling pathway. Nature 361:742, 1993.
93. Benn J, Schneider RJ: Hepatitis B virus X protein activates Ras-GTP complex formation and establishes a Ras, Raf, MAP kinase signaling cascade. Proc Natl Acad Sci U S A 91:10350, 1994.
94. Natoli G, Avantaggiati ML, Chirillo P, et al: Ras- and Raf-dependent activation of c-jun transcriptional activity by the hepatitis B virus transactivator pX. Oncogene 9:2837, 1994.
95. Doria M, Klein N, Lucito R, et al: The hepatitis B virus HBx protein is a dual specificity cytoplasmic activator of Ras and nuclear activator of transcription factors. EMBO J 14:4747, 1995.
96. Höhne M, Schaefer S, Seifer M, et al: Malignant transformation of immortalized transgenic hepatocytes after transfection with hepatitis B virus DNA. EMBO J 9:1137, 1990.
97. Koike K, Moriya K, Yotsuyanagi H, et al: Induction of cell cycle progression by hepatitis B virus HBx gene expression in quiescent mouse fibroblasts. J Clin Invest 94:44, 1994.
98. Benn J, Schneider RJ: Hepatitis B virus HBx protein deregulates cell cycle checkpoint controls. Proc Natl Acad Sci U S A 92:11215, 1995.
99. Lee T-H, Elledge SJ, Butel JS: Hepatitis B virus X protein interacts with a probable cellular DNA repair protein. J Virol 69:1107, 1995.
100. Wang XW, Forrester K, Yeh H, et al: Hepatitis B virus X protein inhibits p53 sequence-specific DNA binding, transcriptional activity, and association with transcription factor ERCC3. Proc Natl Acad Sci U S A 91:2230, 1994.
101. Becker SA, Lee T-H, Butel JS, et al: Hepatitis B virus X protein interferes with cellular DNA repair. J Virol 72:266, 1998.
102. Jia L, Wang XW, Harris CC: Hepatitis B virus X protein inhibits nucleotide excision repair. Int J Cancer 80:875, 1999.
103. Su F, Schneider RJ: Hepatitis B virus HBx protein sensitizes cells to apoptotic killing by tumor necrosis factor alpha. Proc Natl Acad Sci U S A 94:8744, 1997.
104. Terradillos O, Pollicino T, Lecoeur H, et al: p53-independent apoptotic effects of the hepatitis B virus HBx protein in vivo and in vitro. Oncogene 17:2115, 1998.
105. Kim C-M, Koike R, Saito I, et al: HBx gene of hepatitis B virus induces liver cancer in transgenic mice. Nature 351:317, 1991.
106. Koike K, Moriya K, Iino S, et al: High-level expression of hepatitis B virus HBx gene and hepatocarcinogenesis in transgenic mice. Hepatology 19:810, 1994.
107. Lee T-H, Finegold MJ, Shen R-F, et al: Hepatitis B virus transactivator X protein is not tumorigenic in transgenic mice. J Virol 64:5939, 1990.
108. Reifenberg K, Lohler J, Pudollek HP, et al: Long-term expression of the hepatitis B virus core-e- and X-proteins does not cause pathologic changes in transgenic mice. J Hepatol 26:119, 1997.
109. Feitelson MA, Zhu M, Duan L-X, et al: Hepatitis B x antigen and p53 are associated in vitro and in liver tissues from patients with primary hepatocellular carcinoma. Oncogene 8:1109, 1993.
110. Ueda H, Ullrich SJ, Gangemi JD, et al: Functional inactivation but not structural mutation of p53 causes liver cancer. Nat Genet 9:41, 1995.
111. Puisieux A, Ji J, Guillot C, et al: p53-mediated cellular response to DNA damage in cells with replicative hepatitis B virus. Proc Natl Acad Sci U S A 92:1342, 1995.
112. Kekulé AS, Lauer U, Meyer M, et al: The preS2/S region of integrated hepatitis B virus DNA encodes a transcriptional transactivator. Nature 343:457, 1990.
113. Caselmann WH, Meyer M, Kekulé AS, et al: A trans-activator function is generated by integration of hepatitis B virus preS/S sequences in human hepatocellular carcinoma DNA. Proc Natl Acad Sci U S A 87:2970, 1990.
114. Lauer U, Weiss L, Hofschneider PH, et al: The hepatitis B virus pre-S/St transactivator is generated by 3? truncations within a defined region of the S gene. J Virol 66:5284, 1992.
115. Schlüter V, Meyer M, Hofschneider PH, et al: Integrated hepatitis B virus X and 3? truncated preS/S sequences derived from human hepatomas encode functionally active transactivators. Oncogene 9:3335, 1994.
116. Nassal M: Hepatitis B virus replication: novel roles for virus-host interactions. Intervirology 42:100, 1999.
117. Seeger C, Mason WS: Hepatitis B virus biology. Microbiol Mol Biol Rev 64:51, 2000.
118. Summers J, Smolec JM, Snyder R: A virus similar to human hepatitis B virus associated with hepatitis and hepatoma in woodchucks. Proc Natl Acad Sci U S A 75:4533, 1978.
119. Marion PL, Oshiro LS, Regnery DC, et al: A virus in Beechey ground squirrels that is related to hepatitis B virus of humans. Proc Natl Acad Sci U S A 77:2941, 1980.
120. Lanford RE, Chavez D, Brasky KM, et al: Isolation of a hepadnavirus from the woolly monkey, a New World primate. Proc Natl Acad Sci U S A 95:5757, 1988.
121. Mason WS, Seal G, Summers J: Virus of Pekin ducks with structural and biological relatedness to human hepatitis B virus. J Virol 36:829, 1980.
122. Sprengel R, Kaleta EF, Will H: Isolation and characterization of a hepatitis B virus endemic in herons. J Virol 62:3832, 1988.
123. Chang SF, Netter HJ, Bruns M, et al: A new avian hepadnavirus infecting snow geese (*Anser caerulescens*) produces a significant fraction of virions containing single-stranded DNA. Virology 262:39, 1999.
124. Tennant BC: Hepatocarcinogenesis in experimental woodchuck hepatitis virus infection. In Sirica AE, ed: The Role of Cell Types in Hepatocarcinogenesis. Boca Raton, Fla., CRC Press, 1992.
125. Radaeva S, Li Y, Hacker HJ, et al: Hepadnaviral hepatocarcinogenesis: in situ visualization of viral antigens, cytoplasmic compartmentation, enzymic patterns, and cellular proliferation in preneoplastic hepatocellular lineages in woodchucks. J Hepatol 33:580, 2000.
126. Popper H, Shih J-K, Gerin JL, et al: Woodchuck hepatitis and hepatocellular carcinoma: correlation of histologic with virologic observations. Hepatology 1:91, 1981.
127. Popper H, Roth L, Purcell RH, et al: Hepatocarcinogenicity of the woodchuck hepatitis virus. Proc Natl Acad Sci U S A 84:866, 1987.
128. Gerin JL, Cote PJ, Korba BE, et al: Hepatitis B virus and liver cancer: the woodchuck as an experimental model of hepadnavirus-induced liver cancer. In Hollinger FB, Lemon SM, Margolis H, eds: Viral Hepatitis and Liver Disease. Baltimore, Williams & Wilkins, 1991.
129. Korba BE, Wells FV, Baldwin B, et al: Hepatocellular carcinoma in woodchuck hepatitis virus-infected woodchucks: presence of viral DNA in tumor tissue from chronic carriers and animals serologically recovered from acute infection. Hepatology 9:461, 1989.
130. Bréchot C, Degos F, Lugassy C, et al: Hepatitis B virus DNA in patients with chronic liver disease and negative tests for hepatitis B surface antigen. N Engl J Med 312:270, 1985.
131. Paterlini P, Gerken G, Nakajima E, et al: Polymerase chain reaction to detect hepatitis B virus DNA and RNA sequences in primary liver cancers from patients negative for hepatitis B surface antigen. N Engl J Med 323:80, 1990.
132. Wands JR, Liang TJ, Blum HE, et al: Molecular pathogenesis of liver disease during persistent hepatitis B virus infection. Semin Liver Dis 12:252, 1992.
133. Paterlini P, Driss F, Nalpas B, et al: Persistence of hepatitis B and hepatitis C viral genomes in primary liver cancers from HBsAg-negative patients: a study of a low-endemic area. Hepatology 17:20, 1993.
134. Rehermann B, Ferrari C, Pasquinelli C, et al: The hepatitis B virus persists for decades after patients' recovery from acute viral hepatitis despite active maintenance of a cytotoxic T-lymphocyte response. Nat Med 2:1104, 1996.
135. Nagai H, Buendia MA: Oncogenes, tumor suppressors and co-factors in hepatocellular carcinoma. In Caselmann WH, Koshy R, eds: Hepatitis B virus, ed 1. London, Imperial College Press, 1998.
136. Möröy T, Marchio A, Etiemble J, et al: Rearrangement and enhanced expression of c-myc in hepatocellular carcinoma of hepatitis virus infected woodchucks. Nature 324:276, 1986.
137. Hsu T-Y, Möröy T, Etiemble T, et al: Activation of c-myc by woodchuck hepatitis virus insertion in hepatocellular carcinoma. Cell 55:627, 1988.

138. Fourel G, Trepo C, Bougueleret L, et al: Frequent activation of N-myc genes by hepadnavirus insertion in woodchuck liver tumors. Nature 347:294, 1990.
139. Wei Y, Fourel G, Ponzetto A, et al: Hepadnavirus integration: mechanisms of activation of the N-myc2 retrotransposon in woodchuck liver tumors. J Virol 66:5265, 1992.
140. Hansen LJ, Tennant BC, Seeger C, et al: Differential activation of myc gene family members in hepatic carcinogenesis by closely related hepatitis B viruses. Mol Cell Biol 13:659, 1993.
141. Fourel G, Couturier J, Wei Y, et al: Evidence for long-range oncogene activation by hepadnavirus insertion. EMBO J 13:2526, 1994.
142. Etiemble J, Degott C, Renard CA, et al: Liver-specific expression and high oncogenic efficiency of a c-myc transgene activated by woodchuck hepatitis virus insertion. Oncogene 9:727, 1994.
143. Renard CA, Fourel G, Bralet MP, et al: Hepatocellular carcinoma in WHV/N-myc2 transgenic mice: oncogenic mutations of beta-catenin and synergistic effect of p53 null alleles. Oncogene 19:2678, 2000.
144. Wang H-P, Zhang L, Dandri M, et al: Antisense downregulation of N-myc1 in woodchuck hepatoma cells reverses the malignant phenotype. J Virol 72:2192, 1998.
145. Marion PL, van Davelaar MJ, Knight SS, et al: Hepatocellular carcinoma in ground squirrels persistently infected with ground squirrel hepatitis virus. Proc Natl Acad Sci U S A 83:4543, 1986.
146. Seeger C, Baldwin B, Hornbuckle WE, et al: Woodchuck hepatitis virus is a more efficient oncogenic agent than ground squirrel hepatitis virus in a common host. J Virol 65:1673, 1991.
147. Transy C, Fourel G, Robinson WS, et al: Frequent amplification of c-myc in ground squirrel liver tumors associated with past or ongoing infection with a hepadnavirus. Proc Natl Acad Sci U S A 89:3874, 1992.
148. Omata M, Uchiumi K, Ito Y, et al: Duck hepatitis B virus and liver disease. Gastroenterology 85:260, 1983.
149. Yokosuka O, Omata M, Zhou Y-Z, et al: Duck hepatitis B virus DNA in liver and serum of Chinese ducks: integration of viral DNA in a hepatocellular carcinoma. Proc Natl Acad Sci U S A 82:5180, 1985.
150. Imazeki F, Yaginuma K, Omata M, et al: Integrated structures of duck hepatitis B virus DNA in hepatocellular carcinoma. J Virol 62:861, 1988.
151. Uchida T, Suzuki K, Esumi M, et al: Influence of aflatoxin B1 intoxication on duck livers with duck hepatitis B virus infection. Cancer Res 48:1559, 1988.
152. Cullen JM, Marion PL, Sherman GJ, et al: Hepatic neoplasms in aflatoxin B1-treated, congenital duck hepatitis B virus-infected, and virus-free Pekin ducks. Cancer Res 50:4072, 1990.
153. Cova L, Wild CP, Mehrotra R, et al: Contribution of aflatoxin B1 and hepatitis B virus infection in the induction of liver tumors in ducks. Cancer Res 50:2156, 1990.
154. Seawright AA, Snowden RT, Olubuyide IO, et al: A comparison of the effects of aflatoxin B1 on the livers of rats and duck hepatitis virus-infected and noninfected ducks. Hepatology 18:188, 1993.
155. Yan RQ, Su JJ, Huang DR, et al: Human hepatitis B virus and hepatocellular carcinoma. I. Experimental infection of tree shrews with hepatitis B virus. J Cancer Res Clin Oncol 122:283, 1996.
156. Park US, Su JJ, Ban KC, et al: Mutations in the p53 tumor suppressor gene in tree shrew hepatocellular carcinoma associated with hepatitis B virus infection and intake of aflatoxin B1. Gene 251:73, 2000.
157. Walter E, Keist R, Niederöst B, et al: Hepatitis B virus infection of tupaia hepatocytes in vitro and in vivo. Hepatology 24:1, 1996.
158. Ren S, Nassal M: Hepatitis B virus (HBV) virion and covalently closed circular DNA formation in primary tupaia hepatocytes and human hepatoma cell lines upon HBV genome transduction with replication-defective adenovirus vectors. J Virol 75:1104, 2001.
159. Moradpour D, Cerny A, Heim MH, et al: Hepatitis C: an update. Swiss Med Wkly 131:291, 2001.
160. Global surveillance and control of hepatitis C. Report of a WHO Consultation organized in collaboration with the Viral Hepatitis Prevention Board, Antwerp, Belgium. J Viral Hepat 6:35, 1999.
161. Wasley A, Alter MJ: Epidemiology of hepatitis C: geographic differences and temporal trends. Semin Liver Dis 20:1, 2000.
162. WHO: Hepatitis C—global prevalence (update). Wkly Epidemiol Rec 75:18, 2000.
163. van Regenmortel MHV, Fauquet CM, Bishop DHL, et al, eds: Virus Taxonomy. The VIIth Report of the International Committee on Taxonomy of Viruses. San Diego, Academic Press, 2000.
164. Bartenschlager R, Lohmann V: Replication of hepatitis C virus. J Gen Virol 81:1631, 2000.
165. Reed KE, Rice CM: Overview of hepatitis C virus genome structure, polyprotein processing, and protein properties. Curr Top Microbiol Immunol 242:55, 2000.
166. Colombo M, Kuo G, Choo QL, et al: Prevalence of antibodies to hepatitis C virus in Italian patients with hepatocellular carcinoma. Lancet ii:1006, 1989.
167. Saito I, Miyamura T, Ohbayashi A, et al: Hepatitis C virus infection is associated with the development of hepatocellular carcinoma. Proc Natl Acad Sci U S A 87:6547, 1990.
168. Hasan F, Jeffers LJ, De Medina M, et al: Hepatitis C-associated hepatocellular carcinoma. Hepatology 12:589, 1990.
169. Kew MC, Houghton M, Choo QL, et al: Hepatitis C virus antibodies in southern African blacks with hepatocellular carcinoma. Lancet 335:873, 1990.
170. Chen DS, Kuo GC, Sung JL, et al: Hepatitis C virus infection in an area hyperendemic for hepatitis B and chronic liver disease: the Taiwan experience. J Infect Dis 162:817, 1990.
171. Tanaka K, Hirohata T, Koga S, et al: Hepatitis C and hepatitis C in the etiology of hepatocellular carcinoma in the Japanese population. Cancer Res 51:2842, 1991.
172. Lee S-D, Lee F-Y, Wu J-C, et al: The prevalence of anti-hepatitis C virus among Chinese patients with hepatocellular carcinoma. Cancer 69:342, 1992.
173. Simonetti R, Cammà C, Fiorello F, et al: Hepatitis C virus infection as a risk factor for hepatocellular carcinoma in patients with cirrhosis. Ann Intern Med 116:97, 1992.
174. Blum HE: Does hepatitis C virus cause hepatocellular carcinoma? Hepatology 19:251, 1994.
175. Di Bisceglie AM: Hepatitis C and hepatocellular carcinoma. Hepatology 26(suppl 1):34S, 1997.
176. Kiyosawa K, Sodeyama T, Tanaka E, et al: Interrelationship of blood transfusion, non-A, non-B hepatitis and hepatocellular carcinoma: analysis by detection of antibody to hepatitis C virus. Hepatology 12:671, 1990.
177. Seeff LB: Natural history of hepatitis C. Hepatology 26(suppl 1):21S, 1997.
178. Di Bisceglie AM: Natural history of hepatitis C: its impact on clinical management. Hepatology 31:1014, 2000.
179. De Mitri MS, Poussin K, Baccarini P, et al: HCV-associated liver cancer without cirrhosis. Lancet 345:413, 1995.
180. Sakamuro D, Furukawa T, Takegami T: Hepatitis C virus nonstructural protein NS3 transforms NIH 3T3 cells. J Virol 69:3893, 1995.
181. Ray RB, Lagging LM, Meyer K, et al: Hepatitis C virus core protein cooperates with ras and transforms primary rat embryo fibroblasts to tumorigenic phenotype. J Virol 70:4438, 1996.
182. Moriya K, Fujie H, Shintani Y, et al: The core protein of hepatitis C virus induces hepatocellular carcinoma in transgenic mice. Nat Med 4:1065, 1998.
183. Ray RB, Steele R, Meyer K, et al: Transcriptional repression of p53 promoter by hepatitis C virus core protein. J Biol Chem 272:10983, 1997.
184. Chang J, Yang S-H, Cho Y-G, et al: Hepatitis C virus core from two different genotypes has an oncogenic potential but is not sufficient for transforming primary rat embryo fibroblasts in cooperation with the H-ras oncogene. J Virol 72:3060, 1998.
185. Ray RB, Steele R, Meyer K, et al: Hepatitis C virus core protein represses p21WAF1/Cip1/Sid1 promoter activity. Gene 208:331, 1998.
186. Park JS, Yang JM, Min MK: Hepatitis C virus nonstructural protein NS4B transforms NIH3T3 cells in cooperation with the Ha-ras oncogene. Biochem Biophys Res Commun 267:581, 2000.
187. Gale M Jr, Kwieciszewski B, Dossett M, et al: Antiapoptotic and oncogenic potentials of hepatitis C virus are linked to interferon resistance by viral repression of the PKR protein kinase. J Virol 73:6506, 1999.
188. Tan SL, Nakao H, He Y, et al: NS5A, a nonstructural protein of hepatitis C virus, binds growth factor receptor-bound protein 2 adaptor protein in a Src homology 3 domain/ligand-dependent manner and perturbs mitogenic signaling. Proc Natl Acad Sci U S A 96:5533, 1999.
189. Majumder M, Ghosh AK, Steele R, et al: Hepatitis C virus NS5A physically associates with p53 and regulates p21/waf1 gene expression in a p53-dependent manner. J Virol 75:1401, 2001.

190. McLauchlan J: Properties of the hepatitis C virus core protein: a structural protein that modulates cellular processes. J Viral Hepat 7:2, 2000.
191. Ruggieri A, Harada T, Matsuura Y, et al: Sensitization to Fas-mediated apoptosis by hepatitis C virus core protein. Virology 229:68, 1997.
192. Ray RB, Meyer K, Ray R: Suppression of apoptotic cell death by hepatitis C virus core protein. Virology 226:176, 1996.
193. Kittlesen DJ, Chianese-Bullock KA, Yao ZQ, et al: Interaction between complement receptor gC1qR and hepatitis C virus core protein inhibits T-lymphocyte proliferation. J Clin Invest 106:1239, 2000.
194. Gale M Jr, Korth MJ, Tang NM, et al: Evidence that hepatitis C virus resistance to interferon is mediated through repression of the PKR protein kinase by the nonstructural 5A protein. Virology 230:217, 1997.
195. Gale M Jr, Blakely CM, Kwieciszewski B, et al: Control of PKR protein kinase by hepatitis C virus nonstructural 5A protein: molecular mechanisms of kinase regulation. Mol Cell Biol 18:5208, 1998.
196. Kauppinen R, Mustajoki P: Acute hepatic porphyria and hepatocellular carcinoma. Br J Cancer 57:117, 1988.
197. Nakayama M, Okamoto Y, Morita T, et al: Promoting effect of citrulline in hepatocarcinogenesis: possible mechanism in hypercitrullinemia. Hepatology 11:819, 1990.
198. Weinberg AG, Mize CE, Worthen HG: The occurrence of hepatoma in the chronic form of hereditary tyrosinemia. J Pediatr 88:434, 1976;
199. Bradbear RA, Bain C, Siskind V, et al: Cohort study of internal malignancy in genetic hemochromatosis and other chronic nonalcoholic liver diseases. J Natl Cancer Inst 75:81, 1985.
200. Eriksson S, Carlson J, Velez R: Risk of cirrhosis and primary liver cancer in a1-antitrypsin deficiency. N Engl J Med 314:736, 1986.
201. Niederau C, Fischer R, Sonnenberg A, et al: Survival and causes of death in cirrhotic and in noncirrhotic patients with primary hemochromatosis. N Engl J Med 313:1256, 1985.
202. Packe GE, Clarke CW: Is porphyria cutanea tarda a risk factor in the development of hepatocellular carcinoma? A case report and review of the literature. Oncology 42:44, 1985.
203. Salata H, Cortes JM, Enriquez de Salamanca R, et al: Porphyria cutanea tarda and hepatocellular carcinoma. Frequency of occurrence and related factors. J Hepatol 1:477, 1985.
204. Fracanzani AL, Conte D, Fraquelli M, et al: Increased cancer risk in a cohort of 230 patients with hereditary hemochromatosis in comparison to matched control patients with non-iron-related chronic liver disease. Hepatology 33:647, 2001.
205. Wilkinson ML, Portmann B, Williams R: Wilson's disease and hepatocellular carcinoma: possible protective role of copper. Gut 24:767, 1983;
206. Fox TR, Watanabe PG: Detection of a cellular oncogene in spontaneous liver tumors of B6C3F1 mice. Science 228:596, 1985.
207. Reynolds SH, Stowers SJ, Maronpot RR, et al: Detection and identification of activated oncogenes in spontaneously occurring benign and malignant hepatocellular tumors of the B6C3F1 mouse. Proc Natl Acad Sci U S A 83:33, 1986.
208. Reynolds SH, Stowers SJ, Patterson RM, et al: Activated oncogenes in B6C3F1 mouse liver tumors: implications for risk assessment. Science 237:1309, 1987.
209. Sinha S, Webber C, Marshall CJ, et al: Activation of ras oncogene in aflatoxin-induced rat liver carcinogenesis. Proc Natl Acad Sci U S A 85:3673, 1988.
210. Chandar N, Lombardi B, Locker J: c-myc Gene amplification during hepatocarcinogenesis by a choline-devoid diet. Proc Natl Acad Sci U S A 86:2703, 1989.
211. Fox TR, Schumann AM, Watanabe PG, et al: Mutational analysis of the H-ras oncogene in spontaneous C57BL/6 x C3H/He mouse liver tumors and tumors induced with genotoxic and nongenotoxic hepatocarcinogens. Cancer Res 50:4014, 1990.
212. McMahon G, Davis EF, Huber LJ, et al: Characterization of c-Ki-ras and N-ras oncogenes in aflatoxin B1-induced rat liver tumors. Proc Natl Acad Sci U S A 87:1104, 1990.
213. Buchmann A, Bauer-Hofmann R, Mahr J, et al: Mutational activation of the c-Ha-ras gene in liver tumors of different rodent strains: correlation with susceptibility to hepatocarcinogenesis. Proc Natl Acad Sci U S A 88:911, 1991.
214. Dragani TA, Manenti G, Colombo BM, et al: Incidence of mutations at codon 61 of the Ha-ras gene in liver tumors of mice genetically susceptible and resistant to hepatocarcinogenesis. Oncogene 6:333, 1991.
215. Lee H-S, Rajagopalan MS, Vyas GN: A lack of direct role of hepatitis B virus in the activation of ras and c-myc oncogenes in human hepatocellular carcinogenesis. Hepatology 8:1116, 1988.
216. Takada S, Koike K: Activated N-ras gene was found in human hepatoma tissue but only in a small fraction of the tumor cells. Oncogene 4:189, 1989.
217. Tada M, Omata M, Ohto M: Analysis of ras gene mutations in human hepatic malignant tumors by polymerase chain reaction and direct sequencing. Cancer Res 50:1121, 1990.
218. Ogata N, Kamimura T, Asakura H: Point mutation, allelic loss and increased methylation of c-Ha-Ras gene in human hepatocellular carcinoma. Hepatology 13:31, 1991.
219. Collier JD, Guo K, Mathew J, et al: c-erbB-2 oncogene expression in hepatocellular carcinoma and cholangiocarcinoma. J Hepatol 14:377, 1992.
220. Pasquinelli C, Bhavani K, Chisari FV: Multiple oncogenes and tumor suppressor genes are structurally and functionally intact during hepatocarcinogenesis in hepatitis B virus transgenic mice. Cancer Res 52:2823, 1992.
221. Zhang Y-J, Jiang W, Chen CJ, et al: Amplification and overexpression of cyclin D1 in human hepatocellular carcinoma. Biochem Biophys Res Commun 196:1010, 1993.
222. Nishida N, Fukuda Y, Komeda T, et al: Amplification and overexpression of the cyclin D1 gene in aggressive human hepatocellular carcinoma. Cancer Res 54:3107, 1994.
223. Lasko D, Cavanee W, Nordenskjold M: Loss of constitutional heterozygosity in human cancer. Annu Rev Genet 25:281, 1991.
224. Boige V, Laurent-Puig P, Fouchet P, et al: Concerted nonsyntenic allelic losses in hyperploid hepatocellular carcinoma as determined by a high-resolution allelotype. Cancer Res 57:1986, 1997.
225. Marchio A, Meddeb M, Pineau P, et al: Recurrent chromosomal abnormalities in hepatocellular carcinoma detected by comparative genomic hybridization. Genes Chromosomes Cancer 18:59, 1997.
226. Nagai H, Pineau P, Tiollai P, et al: Comprehensive allelotyping of human hepatocellular carcinoma. Oncogene 14:2927, 1997.
227. Pineau P, Buendia MA: Studies of genetic defects in hepatocellular carcinoma. J Hepatol 33:152, 2000.
228. Tsuda H, Zhang W, Shimosato Y, et al: Allele loss on chromosome 16 associated with progression of human hepatocellular carcinoma. Proc Natl Acad Sci U S A 87:6791, 1990.
229. Murakami Y, Hayashi K, Hirohashi S, et al: Aberrations of the tumor suppressor p53 and retinoblastoma genes in human hepatocellular carcinomas. Cancer Res 51:5520, 1991.
230. Nishida N, Fukuda Y, Kokuryu H, et al: Accumulation of allelic loss on arms of chromosomes 16q and 17p in the advanced stages of human hepatocellular carcinoma. Int J Cancer 51:862, 1992.
231. Fujimori M, Tokino T, Hino O, et al: Allelotype study of primary hepatocellular carcinoma. Cancer Res 51:89, 1991.
232. Walker GJ, Hayward NK, Falvey S, et al: Loss of somatic heterozygosity in hepatocellular carcinoma. Cancer Res 51:4367, 1991.
233. Fujimoto Y, Hampton LL, Wirth PJ, et al: Alterations of tumor suppressor genes and allelic losses in human hepatocellular carcinomas in China. Cancer Res 54:281, 1994.
234. Zhang X, Xu H-J, Murakami Y, et al: Deletions of chromosome 13q, mutations in RB1 and RB protein state in human hepatocellular carcinoma. Cancer Res 54:4177, 1994.
235. Kita R, Nishida N, Fukuda Y, et al: Infrequent alterations of the p16INK4A gene in liver cancer. Int J Cancer 67:176, 1996.
236. Chaubert P, Gayer R, Zimmermann A, et al: Germ-line mutations of the p16INK4(MTS1) gene occur in a subset of patients with hepatocellular carcinoma. Hepatology 25:1376, 1997.
237. Liew CT, Li HM, Lo KW, et al: High frequency of p16INK4A gene alterations in hepatocellular carcinoma. Oncogene 18:789, 1999.
238. Higashitsuji H, Itoh K, Nagao T, et al: Reduced stability of retinoblastoma protein by gankyrin, an oncogenic ankyrin-repeat protein overexpressed in hepatomas. Nat Med 6:96, 2000.
239. Groden J, Thliveris A, Samowitz W, et al: Identification and characterization of the familial adenomatous polyposis coli gene. Cell 66:589, 1991.

240. Joslyn G, Carlson M, Thliveris A, et al: Identification of deletion mutations and three new genes at the familial polyposis locus. Cell 66:601, 1991.
241. Willert K, Nusse R: Beta-catenin: a key mediater of Wnt signaling. Curr Opin Genet Dev 8:95, 1998.
242. Morin PJ, Sparks AB, Korinek V, et al: Activation of beta-catenin-Tcf signaling in colon cancer by mutations in beta-catenin or APC. Science 275:1787, 1997.
243. Oda H, Imai Y, Nakatsuru Y, et al: Somatic mutations of the APC gene in sporadic hepatoblastomas. Cancer Res 56:3320, 1996.
244. de La Coste A, Romagnolo B, Billuart P, et al: Somatic mutations of the beta-catenin gene are frequent in mouse and human hepatocellular carcinomas. Proc Natl Acad Sci U S A 95:8847, 1998.
245. Miyoshi Y, Iwao K, Nagasawa Y, et al: Activation of the beta-catenin gene in primary hepatocellular carcinomas by somatic alterations involving exon 3. Cancer Res 58:2524, 1998.
246. Huang H, Fujii H, Sankila A, et al: Beta-catenin mutations are frequent in human hepatocellular carcinomas associated with hepatitis C virus infection. Am J Pathol 155:1795, 1999.
247. Terris B, Pineau P, Bregeaud L, et al: Close correlation between beta-catenin gene alterations and nuclear accumulation of the protein in human hepatocellular carcinomas. Oncogene 18:6583, 1999.
248. Legoix P, Bluteau O, Bayer J, et al: Beta-catenin mutations in hepatocellular carcinoma correlate with a low rate of loss of heterozygosity. Oncogene 18:4044, 1999.
249. Satoh S, Daigo Y, Furukawa Y, et al: AXIN1 mutations in hepatocellular carcinomas, and growth suppression in cancer cells by virus-mediated transfer of AXIN1. Nat Genet 24:245, 2000.
250. He TC, Sparks AB, Rago C, et al: Identification of c-MYC as a target of the APC pathway. Science 281:1509, 1998.
251. Slagle B, Zhou Y-Z, Birchmeier W, et al: Deletion of the E-cadherin gene in hepatitis B virus-positive Chinese hepatocellular carcinomas. Hepatology 18:757, 1993.
252. Hollstein M, Sidransky D, Vogelstein B, et al: p53 mutations in human cancers. Science 253:49, 1991.
253. Bressac B, Galvin KM, Liang TJ, et al: Abnormal structure and expression of p53 gene in human hepatocellular carcinoma. Proc Natl Acad Sci U S A 87:1973, 1990.
254. Hsu IC, Tokiwa T, Bennet W, et al: p53 gene mutation and integrated hepatitis B viral DNA sequences in human liver cancer cell lines. Carcinogenesis 14:987, 1993.
255. Bressac B, Kew M, Wands J, et al: Selective G to T mutations of p53 gene in hepatocellular carcinoma from southern Africa. Nature 350:429, 1991.
256. Hsu IC, Metcalf RA, Sun T, et al: Mutational hotspot in the p53 gene in human hepatocellular carcinomas. Nature 350:427, 1991.
257. Puisieux A, Lim S, Groopman J, et al: Selective targeting of p53 gene mutational hotspots in human cancers by etiologically defined carcinogens. Cancer Res 51:6185, 1991.
258. Aguilar F, Hussain SP, Cerutti P: Aflatoxin B1 induces the transversion of G -> T in codon 249 of the p53 tumor suppressor gene in human hepatocytes. Proc Natl Acad Sci U S A 90:8586, 1993.
259. Ozturk M and collaborators: p53 mutation in hepatocellular carcinoma after aflatoxin exposure. Lancet 338:1356, 1991.
260. Scorsone KA, Zhou Y-Z, Butel JS, et al: p53 mutations cluster at codon 249 in hepatitis B virus-positive hepatocellular carcinomas from China. Cancer Res 52:1635, 1992.
261. Li D, Cao Y, He L, et al: Aberrations of p53 gene in human hepatocellular carcinoma from China. Carcinogenesis 14:169, 1993.
262. Ozturk M: Chromosomal rearrangements and tumor suppressor genes in primary liver cancer. In Bréchot C, ed: Primary liver cancer: etiological and progression factors. Boca Raton, Fla., CRC Press, 1994.
263. Kar S, Jaffe R, Carr BI: Mutation at codon 249 of p53 gene in a human hepatoblastoma. Hepatology 18:566, 1993.
264. Patel P, Stephenson J, Scheuer PJ, et al: p53 codon 249ser mutations in hepatocellular carcinoma in patients with low aflatoxin exposure. Lancet 339:881, 1992.
265. Challen C, Lunec J, Warren W, et al: Analysis of the p53 tumor-suppressor gene in hepatocellular carcinomas from Britain. Hepatology 16:1362, 1992.
266. Kress S, Jahn U-R, Buchmann A, et al: p53 mutations in human hepatocellular carcinomas from Germany. Cancer Res 52:3220, 1992.
267. Oda T, Tsuda H, Scarpa A, et al: p53 gene mutation spectrum in hepatocellular carcinoma. Cancer Res 52:6358, 1992.
268. Nishida N, Fukuda Y, Kokuryu H, et al: Role and mutational heterogeneity of the p53 gene in hepatocellular carcinoma. Cancer Res 53:368, 1993.
269. Nose H, Imazeki F, Ohto M, et al: p53 gene mutations and 17p allelic deletions in hepatocellular carcinoma from Japan. Cancer 72:355, 1993.
270. Hosono S, Chou M-J, Lee C-S, et al: Infrequent mutation of p53 gene in hepatitis B virus positive primary hepatocellular carcinomas. Oncogene 8:491, 1993.
271. Hollstein MC, Wild CP, Bleicher F, et al: p53 mutations and aflatoxin B1 exposure in hepatocellular carinoma patients from Thailand. Int J Cancer 53:51, 1993.
272. Hayward NK, Walker GJ, Graham W, et al: Hepatocellular carcinoma mutation. Nature 352:764, 1991.
273. Aguilar F, Harris CC, Sun T, et al: Geographic variation of p53 mutational profile in nonmalignant human liver. Science 264:1317, 1994.
274. Ponchel F, Puisieux A, Tabone E, et al: Hepatocarcinoma-specific mutant p53-249ser induces mitotic activity but has no effect on transforming growth factor β1-mediated apoptosis. Cancer Res 54:2064, 1994.
275. Dumenco L, Ougey D, Wu J, et al: Introduction of a murine p53 mutation corresponding to human codon 249 into a murine hepatocyte cell line results in growth advantage, but not in transformation. Hepatology 22:1279, 1995.
276. Ghebranious N, Sell S: The mouse equivalent of the human p53ser249 mutation p53ser246 enhances aflatoxin hepatocarcinogenesis in hepatitis B surface antigen transgenic and p53 heterozygous null mice. Hepatology 27:967, 1998.
277. Yin L, Ghebranious N, Chakraborty S, et al: Control of mouse hepatocyte proliferation and ploidy by p53 and p53ser246 mutation in vivo. Hepatology 27:73, 1998.
278. Schleger C, Becker R, Oesch F, et al: The human p53 gene mutated at position 249 per se is not sufficient to immortalize human liver cells. Hepatology 29:834, 1999.
279. Alpert ME, Hutt MS, Wogan GN, et al: Association between aflatoxin content of food and hepatoma frequency in Uganda. Cancer 28:253, 1971.
280. Peers FG, Linsell CA: Dietary aflatoxins and liver cancer: a population based study in Kenya. Br J Cancer 27:473, 1973.
281. van Rensburg SJ, van der Watt JJ, Purchase IFH, et al: Primary liver cancer rate and aflatoxin intake in a high cancer area. S Afr Med J 48:2508A, 1974.
282. van Rensburg SJ, Cook-Mozaffari P, van Schalkwyk DJ, et al: Hepatocellular carcinoma and dietary aflatoxin in Mozambique and Transkei. Br J Cancer 51:713, 1985.
283. Henry SH, Bosch FX, Troxell TC, et al: Reducing liver cancer—global control of aflatoxin. Science 286:2453, 1999.
284. Jackson PE, Groopman JD: Aflatoxin and liver cancer. Baillieres Best Pract Res Clin Gastroenterol 13:545, 1999.
285. Wogan GN: Aflatoxin as human carcinogen. Hepatology 30:573, 1999.
286. Yeh FS, Yu MC, Mo CC, et al: Hepatitis B virus, aflatoxins, and hepatocellular carcinoma in southern Guangxi, China. Cancer Res 49:2506, 1989.
287. Adamson RH, Correa P, Dalgard DW: Brief communication: occurrence of a primary liver carcinoma in a Rhesus monkey fed aflatoxin B1. J Natl Cancer Inst 50:594, 1973.
288. Sieber SM, Correa P, Dalgard DW, et al: Induction of osteogenic sarcomas and tumors of the hepatobiliary system in non-human primates with aflatoxin B1. Cancer Res 39:4545, 1979.
289. Autrup H, Seremet T, Wakhisi J, et al: Aflatoxin exposure measured by urinary excretion of aflatoxin B1-guanine adduct and hepatitis B virus infection in areas with different liver cancer incidence in Kenya. Cancer Res 47:3430, 1987.
290. Sun Z, Lu P, Gail MH, et al: Increased risk of hepatocellular carcinoma in male hepatitis B surface antigen carriers with chronic hepatitis who have detectable urinary aflatoxin metabolite M1. Hepatology 30:379, 1999.
291. Bannasch P, Imain Khoshkhou N, Hacker HJ, et al: Synergistic hepatocarcinogenic effect of hepadnaviral infection and dietary aflatoxin B1 in woodchucks. Cancer Res 55:3318, 1995.

292. Groopman JD, Busby WFJ, Wogan GN: Nuclear distribution of aflatoxin B1 and its interaction with histones in rat liver in vivo. Cancer Res 40:4343, 1980.
293. Groopman JD, Donahue PR, Zhu J, et al: Aflatoxin metabolism in humans: detection of metabolites and nucleic acid adducts in urine by affinity chromatography. Proc Natl Acad Sci U S A 82:6492, 1985.
294. Groopman JD, Roebuck BD, Kensler TW: Molecular dosimetry of aflatoxin DNA adducts in humans and experimental rat models. Prog Clin Biol Res 374:139, 1992.
295. Groopman JD, Zhu JQ, Donahue PR, et al: Molecular dosimetry of urinary aflatoxin-DNA adducts in people living in Guangxi Autonomous Region, People's Republic of China. Cancer Res 52:45, 1992.
296. Ross RK, Yuan JM, Yu MC, et al: Urinary aflatoxin biomarkers and risk of hepatocellular carcinoma. Lancet 339:943, 1992.
297. Ueno Y, Nagata S, Tsutsumi T, et al: Detection of microcystins, a blue-green algal hepatotoxin, in drinking water sampled in Haimen and Fusui, endemic areas of primary liver cancer in China, by highly sensitive immunoassay. Carcinogenesis 17:1317, 1996.
298. Yu SZ: Primary prevention of hepatocellular carcinoma. J Gastroenterol Hepatol 10:674, 1995.
299. Macdonald GA, Greenson JK, Saito K, et al: Microsatellite instability and loss of heterozygosity at DNA mismatch repair gene loci occurs during hepatic carcinogenesis. Hepatology 28:90, 1998.
300. Kondo Y, Kanai Y, Sakamoto M, et al: Microsatellite instability associated with hepatocarcinogenesis. J Hepatol 31:529, 1999.
301. Piao Z, Kim H, Malkhosyan S, et al: Frequent chromosomal instability but no microsatellite instability in hepatocellular carcinoma. Int J Oncol 17:507, 2000.
302. Yamamoto H, Itoh F, Fukushima H, et al: Infrequent widespread microsatellite instability in hepatocellular carcinoma. Int J Oncol 16:543, 2000.
303. Erlitzki R, Minuk GY: Telomeres, telomerase and HCC: the long and the short of it. J Hepatol 31:939, 1999.
304. Kim NW, Piatyszek MA, Prowse KR, et al: Specific association of human telomerase activity with immortal cells and cancer. Science 266:2011, 1994.
305. Tahara H, Nakanishi T, Kitamoto M, et al: Telomerase activity in human liver tissues: comparison between chronic liver disease and hepatocellular carcinomas. Cancer Res 55:2734, 1995.
306. Kojima H, Yokosuka O, Imazeki F, et al: Telomerase activity and telomere length in hepatocellular carcinoma and chronic liver disease. Gastroenterology 112:493, 1997.
307. Kojima H, Yokosuka O, Kato N, et al: Quantitative evaluation of telomerase activity in small liver tumors: analysis of ultrasonography-guided liver biopsy specimens. J Hepatol 31:514, 1999.
308. Nakashio R, Kitamoto M, Tahara H, et al: Significance of telomerase activity in the diagnosis of small differentiated hepatocellular carcinoma. Int J Cancer 74:141, 1997.
309. Miura N, Horikawa I, Nishimoto A, et al: Progressive telomere shortening and telomerase reactivation during hepatocellular carcinogenesis. Cancer Genet Cytogenet 93:56, 1997.
310. Hytiroglou P, Kotoula V, Thung SN, et al: Telomerase activity in precancerous hepatic nodules. Cancer 82:1831, 1998.
311. Cross M, Dexter TM: Growth factors in development, transformation, and tumorigenesis. Cell 64:271, 1991.
312. Frösch ER, Schmid C, Schwander J, et al: Actions of insulin-like growth factors. Ann Rev Physiol 47:443, 1985.
313. Ueno T, Takahashi K, Matsuguchi T, et al: Reactivation of rat insulin-like growth factor II gene during hepatocarcinogenesis. Carcinogenesis 9:1779, 1988.
314. Cariani E, Dubois N, Lasserre C, et al: Insulin-like growth factor II (IGF-II) mRNA expression during hepatocarcinogenesis in transgenic mice. J Hepatol 13:220, 1991.
315. Schirmacher P, Held WA, Yang D, et al: Reactivation of insulin-like growth factor II during hepatocarcinogenesis in transgenic mice suggests a role in malignant growth. Cancer Res 52:2549, 1992.
316. Yang D, Rogler CE: Analysis of insulin-like growth factor II expression in neoplastic nodules and hepatocellular carcinomas of woodchucks utilizing in situ hybridization and immunocytochemistry. Carcinogenesis 12:1893, 1991.
317. Yang D, Alt E, Rogler CE: Coordinate expression of N-myc 2 and insulin-like growth factor II in precancerous altered hepatic foci in woodchuck hepatitis virus carriers. Cancer Res 53:2020, 1993.
318. Cariani E, Lasserre C, Seurin D, et al: Differential expression of insulin-like growth factor II mRNA in human primary liver cancers, benign liver tumors, and liver cirrhosis. Cancer Res 48:6844, 1988.
319. Cariani E, Lasserre C, Kemeny F, et al: Expression of insulin-like growth factor II, α-fetoprotein, and hepatitis B virus transcripts in human primary liver cancer. Hepatology 13:644, 1991.
320. Derynck R: The physiology of transforming growth factor-α. Adv Cancer Res 58:27, 1992.
321. Massagué J: Epidermal growth factor-like transforming growth factor. II. Interaction with epidermal growth factor receptors in human placenta membranes and A431 cells. J Biol Chem 258:13614, 1983.
322. Mead JE, Fausto N: Transforming growth factor α may be a physiological regulator of liver regeneration by means of an autocrine mechanism. Proc Natl Acad Sci U S A 86:1558, 1989.
323. Derynck R, Goeddel DV, Ullrich A, et al: Synthesis of messenger RNAs for transforming growth factors alpha and beta and the epidermal growth factor receptor by human tumors. Cancer Res 47:707, 1987.
324. Hisaka T, Yano H, Haramaki M, et al: Expressions of epidermal growth factor family and its receptor in hepatocellular carcinoma cell lines: relationship to cell proliferation. Int J Oncol 14:453, 1999.
325. Jhappan C, Stahle C, Harkins RN, et al: TGFα overexpression in transgenic mice induces liver neoplasia and abnormal development of the mammary gland and pancreas. Cell 61:1137, 1990.
326. Jakubczak JL, Chisari FV, Merlino G: Synergy between transforming growth factor alpha and hepatitis B virus surface antigen in hepatocellular proliferation and carcinogenesis. Cancer Res 57:3606, 1997.
327. Yeh Y-C, Tsai J-F, Chuang L-Y, et al: Elevation of transforming growth factor α and its relationship to the epidermal growth factor and α-fetoprotein levels in patients with hepatocellular carcinoma. Cancer Res 47:896, 1987.
328. Chung YH, Kim JA, Song BC, et al: Expression of transforming growth factor-alpha mRNA in livers of patients with chronic viral hepatitis and hepatocellular carcinoma. Cancer 89:977, 2000.
329. Massagué J, Wotton D: Transcriptional control by the TGF-β/Smad signaling system. EMBO J 19:1745, 2000.
330. Nakatsukasa H, Nagy P, Evarts RP, et al: Cellular distribution of transforming growth factor-β1 and procollagen types I, III, and IV transcripts in carbon tetrachloride-induced rat liver fibrosis. J Clin Invest 85:1833, 1990.
331. Nagy P, Schaff Z, Lapis K: Immunohistochemical detection of transforming growth factor-β1 in fibrotic liver diseases. Hepatology 14:269, 1991.
332. Castilla A, Prieto J, Fausto N: Transforming growth factors β1 and a in chronic liver disease—effects of interferon alfa therapy. N Engl J Med 324:933, 1991.
333. Inagaki M, Moustakas A, Lin HY, et al: Growth inhibition by transforming growth factor β (TGF-β) type I is restored in TGF-β-resistant hepatoma cells after expression of TGF-β receptor type II cDNA. Proc Natl Acad Sci U S A 90:5359, 1993.
334. Shirai Y, Kawata S, Ito N, et al: Elevated levels of plasma transforming growth factor-β in patients with hepatocellular carcinoma. Jpn J Cancer Res 83:676, 1992.
335. Nagy P, Evarts RP, McMahon JB, et al: Role of TGF-β in normal differentiation and oncogenesis in rat liver. Mol Carcinog 2:345, 1989.
336. Nakatsukasa H, Evarts RP, Hsia C-C, et al: Expression of transforming growth factor-b1 during chemical hepatocarcinogenesis in the rat. Lab Invest 65:511, 1991.
337. Koyama M, Nagai H, Bando K, et al: New target region of allelic loss in hepatocellular carcinomas within a 1-cM interval on chromosome 6q23. J Hepatol 33:85, 2000.
338. De Souza AT, Hankins GR, Washington MK, et al: M6P/IGF2R gene is mutated in human hepatocellular carcinomas with loss of heterozygosity. Nat Genet 11:447, 1995.
339. Yamada T, De Souza AT, Finkelstein S, et al: Loss of the gene encoding mannose 6-phosphate/insulin-like growth factor II receptor is an early event in liver carcinogenesis. Proc Natl Acad Sci U S A 94:10351, 1997.

340. Yakicier MC, Irmak MB, Romano A, et al: Smad2 and Smad4 gene mutations in hepatocellular carcinoma. Oncogene 18:4879, 1999.
341. LaBrecque DR: Hepatocyte growth factor—how do I know thee? Let me count the ways. Gastroenterology 103:1686, 1992.
342. Michalopoulos GK, Zarnegar R: Hepatocyte growth factor. Hepatology 15:149, 1992.
343. Montesano R, Matsumoto K, Nakamura T, et al: Identification of a fibroblast-derived epithelial morphogen as hepatocyte growth factor. Cell 67:901, 1991.
344. Weidner M, Arakaki N, Hartmann G, et al: Evidence for the identity of human scatter factor and human hepatocyte growth factor. Proc Natl Acad Sci U S A 88:7001, 1991.
345. Bottaro DP, Rubin JS, Faletto DL, et al: Identification of the hepatocyte growth factor receptor as the c-met proto-oncogene product. Science 251:802, 1991.
346. Naldini L, Vigna E, Narsimhan RP, et al: Hepatocyte growth factor stimulates the tyrosine kinase activity of the receptor encoded by the proto-oncogene c-met. Oncogene 6:501, 1991.
347. Tajima H, Matsumoto K, Nakamura T: Hepatocyte growth factor has potent anti-proliferative activity in various tumor cell lines. FEBS Lett 291:229, 1991.
348. Shiota G, Rhoads DB, Wang TC, et al: Hepatocyte growth factor inhibits growth of hepatocellular carcinoma cells. Proc Natl Acad Sci U S A 89:373, 1992.
349. Shiota G, Wang TC, Nakamura T, et al: Hepatic growth factor in transgenic mice: effect on hepatocyte growth, liver regeneration and gene expression. Hepatology 19:962, 1994.
350. Nishiyama M, Wands JR: Cloning and increased expression of an insulin receptor substrate-1-like gene in human hepatocellular carcinoma. Biochem Biophys Res Commun 183:280, 1992.
351. Ito T, Sasaki Y, Wands JR: Overexpression of human insulin receptor substrate 1 induces cellular transformation with activation of mitogen-activated protein kinases. Mol Cell Biol 16:943, 1996.
352. Bergmann U, Funatomi H, Yokoyama M, et al: Insulin-like growth factor I overexpression in human pancreatic cancer: evidence for autocrine and paracrine roles. Cancer Res 55:2007, 1995.
353. Jackson JG, White MF, Yee D: Insulin receptor substrate-1 is the predominant signaling molecule activated by insulin-like growth factor-I, insulin, and interleukin-4 in estrogen receptor-positive human breast cancer cells. J Biol Chem 273:9994, 1998.
354. Lee AV, Jackson JG, Gooch JL, et al: Enhancement of insulin-like growth factor signaling in human breast cancer: estrogen regulation of insulin receptor substrate-1 expression in vitro and in vivo. Mol Endocrinol 13:787, 1999.
355. Myers MG, White MF: Insulin signal transduction and the IRS proteins. Annu Rev Pharmacol Toxicol 36:615, 1996.
356. Tanaka S, Mohr L, Schmidt EV, et al: Biological effects of human insulin-receptor substrate-1 overexpression in hepatocytes. Hepatology 27:598, 1997.
357. Tanaka S, Wands JR: A carboxy-terminal truncated insulin receptor substrate-1 dominant negative protein reverses the human hepatocellular carcinoma malignant phenotype. J Clin Invest 98:2100, 1996.
358. Mise M, Arii S, Higashituji H, et al: Clinical significance of vascular endothelial growth factor and basic fibroblast growth factor gene expression in liver tumor. Hepatology 23:455, 1996.
359. Torimura T, Sata M, Ueno T, et al: Increased expression of vascular endothelial growth factor is associated with tumor progression in hepatocellular carcinoma. Hum Pathol 29:986, 1998.
360. Yamaguchi R, Yano H, Iemura A, et al: Expression of vascular endothelial growth factor in human hepatocellular carcinoma. Hepatology 28:68, 1998.
361. Tanaka S, Mori M, Sakamoto Y, et al: Biologic significance of angiopoietin-2 expression in human hepatocellular carcinoma. J Clin Invest 103:341, 1999.
362. Sell S, Knoll B: Transgenic mouse models of hepatocarcinogenesis. In Sirica AE, ed: The Role of Cell Types in Hepatocarcinogenesis. Boca Raton, Fla., CRC Press, 1992.
363. Chisari FV: Hepatitis B virus transgenic mice: insights into the virus and the disease. Hepatology 22:1316, 1995.
364. Sandgren E: Transgenic models of hepatic growth regulation and hepatocarcinogenesis. In: Jirtle RL, ed: Liver Regeneration and Carcinogenesis—Molecular and Cellular Mechanisms. San Diego, Academic Press, 1995.
365. Messing A, Chen HY, Palmiter RD, et al: Peripheral neuropathies, hepatocellular carcinomas and islet cell adenomas in transgenic mice. Nature 316:461, 1985.
366. Sandgren EP, Quaife CJ, Pinkert CA, et al: Oncogene-induced liver neoplasia in transgenic mice. Oncogene 4:715, 1989.
367. Sepulveda AR, Finegold MJ, Smith B, et al: Development of a transgenic mouse system for the analysis of stages in liver carcinogenesis using tissue-specific expression of SV40 large T-antigen controlled by regulatory elements of the human a-1-antitrypsin gene. Cancer Res 49:6108, 1989.
368. Hino O, Kitagawa T, Nomura K, et al: Hepatocarcinogenesis in transgenic mice carrying albumin-promoted SV40 T antigen gene. Jpn J Cancer Res 82:1226, 1991.
369. Held WA, Mullins JJ, Kuhn NJ, et al: T antigen expression and tumorigenesis in transgenic mice containing a mouse major urinary protein/SV40 T antigen hybrid gene. EMBO J 8:183, 1989.
370. Sandgren EP, Luetteke NC, Palmiter RD, et al: Overexpression of TGF a in transgenic mice: induction of epithelial hyperplasia, pancreatic metaplasia, and carcinoma of the breast. Cell 61:1121, 1990.
371. Chisari FV, Filippi P, McLachlan A, et al: Expression of hepatitis B virus large envelope polypeptide inhibits hepatitis B surface antigen secretion in transgenic mice. J Virol 60:880, 1986.
372. Chisari FV, Filippi P, Buras J, et al: Structural and pathological effects of synthesis of hepatitis B virus large envelope polypeptide in transgenic mice. Proc Natl Acad Sci U S A 84:6909, 1987.
373. Chisari FV, Klopchin K, Moriyama T, et al: Molecular pathogenesis of hepatocellular carcinoma in hepatitis B virus transgenic mice. Cell 59:1145, 1989.
374. Dunsford HA, Sell S, Chisari FV: Hepatocarcinogenesis due to chronic liver cell injury in hepatitis B virus transgenic mice. Cancer Res 50:3400, 1990.
375. Sell S, Hunt JM, Dunsford HA, et al: Synergy between hepatitis B virus expression and chemical hepatocarcinogens in transgenic mice. Cancer Res 51:1278, 1991.
376. Huang SN, Chisari FV: Strong, sustained hepatocellular proliferation precedes hepatocarcinogenesis in hepatitis B surface antigen transgenic mice. Hepatology 21:620, 1995.
377. Hagen TM, Wehr C, Huang S-N, et al: Extensive oxidative DNA damage in hepatocytes of transgenic mice with chronic active hepatitis destined to develop hepatocellular carcinoma. Proc Natl Acad Sci U S A 91:12808, 1994.
378. Pourcel C: Hepatitis B virus transgenic mouse model. In McLachlan A, ed: Molecular Biology of the Hepatitis B Virus. Boca Raton, Fla., CRC Press, 1991.
379. Sandgren EP, Palmiter RD, Heckel JL, et al: Complete hepatic regeneration after somatic deletion of an albumin-plasminogen activator transgene. Cell 66:245, 1991.
380. Sandgren EP, Palmiter RD, Heckel JL, et al: DNA rearrangement causes hepatocarcinogenesis in albumin-plasminogen activator transgenic mice. Proc Natl Acad Sci U S A 89:11523, 1992.
381. Nishiguchi S, Shiomi S, Nakatani S, et al: Prevention of hepatocellular carcinoma in patients with chronic active hepatitis C and cirrhosis. Lancet 357:196, 2001.
382. Wang JS, Shen X, He X, et al: Protective alterations in phase 1 and 2 metabolism of aflatoxin B1 by oltipraz in residents of Qidong, People's Republic of China. J Natl Cancer Inst 91:347, 1999.
383. Qian C, Drozdzik M, Caselmann WH, et al: The potential of gene therapy in the treatment of hepatocellular carcinoma. J Hepatol 32:344, 2000.
384. Vollmer CM Jr, Eilber FC, Butterfield LH, et al: Alpha-fetoprotein-specific genetic immunotherapy for hepatocellular carcinoma. Cancer Res 59:3064, 1999.
385. Takayama T, Sekine T, Makuuchi M, et al: Adoptive immunotherapy to lower postsurgical recurrence rates of hepatocellular carcinoma: a randomised trial. Lancet 356:802, 2000.

CHAPTER

45

Tumors of the Liver

John R. Craig, MD, PhD

CLASSIFICATION, CLINICAL FEATURES, AND DIAGNOSIS

Hepatic tumors are common, and primary liver cancer (predominately hepatocellular carcinoma) is the fifth leading cause of death on a worldwide basis. Nearly 85 percent of primary malignant tumors of the liver are hepatocellular carcinoma (HCC), but in northern Thailand cholangiocarcinoma (CC) accounts for most of the primary malignant hepatic tumors (90 percent). In Western European countries and North America metastatic carcinoma is the most common malignant hepatic tumor.

Metastatic carcinoma in the liver is 40 times more frequent than primary liver cancer in North America and Europe.[1] Many metastatic carcinomas to liver have no apparent source. Clinical symptoms caused by ductal obstruction or massive involvement by tumor (e.g., jaundice, pruritus) are more likely with carcinoma arising in nearby organs including the pancreas, stomach, and gallbladder (Table 45-1). In Western populations the primary sites of metastatic carcinomas are reflected in the general incidence of such tumors and include colon, lung, breast, esophagus, and genitourinary organs. Metastatic lymphoma and sarcoma to the liver are less common. In an English survey of 1500 liver biopsies, 38 percent of the biopsies were performed because of suspected malignancy, which was advanced in many patients.[2] The primary site was unknown in the majority of these patients. Only 3 percent of the biopsies (50 patients) were performed for suspected primary hepatic tumor, which was confirmed in 32 percent of these 50 patients. Two patients had HCC on biopsy without prior clinical suspicion of malignant tumor.

TABLE 45-1

Metastatic Adenocarcinoma Producing Clinical Liver Disease: Jaundice in 100 Consecutive Autopsies at LAC and USC MC

Site	No.	%
Gallbladder	6/6	100
Pancreas	11/21	52
Stomach	5/13	38
Colon-rectum	4/20	25
Breast	3/15	20
Lung	0/9	0

LAC, Los Angeles County; *USC MC,* University of Southern California Medical Center.

Metastatic carcinoma to the liver produces clinically apparent effects in about two thirds of patients. These manifestations include ascites, hepatomegaly, hepatic pain, jaundice, weight loss, and anorexia. Rapid liver failure is rarely encountered, and extensive replacement of the liver occurs before liver symptoms develop. Carcinoid tumors may produce dramatic clinical symptoms after liver metastasis occurs; the volume of this tumor may be enormous before clinical detection. Laboratory studies are non-specific for most tumors. Radiographic studies identify hepatic defects or lesions that may require needle biopsy. Ultrasound can identify tumors 1 cm or larger and can distinguish cystic lesions from solid ones. Computed tomography (CT) scan with contrast is helpful because most metastatic lesions have diminished blood flow. Lesions as small as 0.5 cm may be detected. Metastatic tumors associated with hypervascular flow include melanoma, carcinoid tumor, and breast carcinoma.

The gross appearance of hepatic metastasis (which may be appreciated at surgery as an incidental finding during elective procedures) varies from a single large umbilicated lesion to numerous small lesions. The umbilication is due to central necrosis or fibrosis and is typical of carcinoma from stomach, pancreas, and colon. Pseudocyst formation is noted in metastatic carcinoid tumors.[3] Hemorrhage is associated with renal cell carcinoma, thyroid carcinoma, neuroendocrine carcinoma, and angiosarcoma. Metastatic breast cancer may produce a "cirrhotic" appearance because of the numerous small metastatic lesions with fibrosis. Diffuse, metastatic breast carcinoma can be associated with splenomegaly, esophageal varices, and ascites.[4] Distinction of a (benign) Meyenburg complex from metastatic adenocarcinoma can be challenging. Frozen section of one of many small lesions (Meyenburg complex) has surprised many surgeons because the gross appearance is typical of widespread metastatic adenocarcinoma—even the histologic appearance simulates carcinoma. In addition, the radiographic appearance simulates metastatic lesions although there are some distinctive features.[5] Tumor cells with no prior clinical (or histologic) diagnosis require selected staining procedures to help identify a likely source. HCC is recognizable in the majority of patients, but when poorly differentiated (usually late in development) can be mistaken for metastatic lesions. Special stains include the hepatocyte paraffin 1 (HepPar 1) antigen* and carcinoembryonic antigen (CEA).[6] Melanoma provides great difficulty by routine microscopy but positive staining for HMB45 and S-100 is diagnostic. Clear cell carcinoma (CC) may arise in the liver and be histologically identical to primary tumors arising in the adrenal gland and the kidney. There is no diagnostic staining reaction in widespread use. The distinction of CC from metastatic adenocarcinoma can be very difficult. The expression of cytokeratin 7 and 19 but not 20 is typical for primary hepatic adenocarcinoma (i.e., CC). Metastatic primary gastrointestinal (GI) tumors are usually positive for cytokeratin 20 and negative for cytokeratin 7.[7] Lung carcinoma (especially small cell carcinoma) commonly presents with an occult primary lesion and abundant hepatic metastasis. Spindle cell lesions include sclerosing and sarcomatous HCC and primary lesions from gallbladder and gastrointestinal stromal tumors such as leiomyosarcoma. The c-kit and CD34 are diagnostic of GI stromal tumors; various keratin stains are needed to recognize sclerosing HCC or CC. There are specific markers for a few metastatic tumors such as prostatic carcinoma, thyroid carcinoma, and gonadal tumors (alpha fetoprotein [AFP] and beta HCG positive). Accurate identification of metastatic tumor and the number of lesions may present an opportunity for selected treatment (ablation therapy, chemo-infusion, or surgical resection or various combinations of treatment [see Chap. 46]). A large, single institution series of 1001 patients with colorectal metastasis to liver demonstrated a 5-year survival of 44 percent for patients with a solitary lesion and 28 percent for multiple lesions.[8] In a separate multi-variate analysis of 155 patients with four or more metastatic lesions, significant prognostic factors were the presence of a positive resection margin and increasing number of lesions.[9]

Classification of *primary hepatic tumors* is based on the cell of origin (hepatocellular, cholangiolar, or mesenchymal cell origin). Benign liver tumors are common. They can be found in at least 5 percent to 20 percent of adults by a thorough autopsy. In one small series of 95 consecutive necropsies, 49 patients had some form of liver tumor including bile duct tumor in 26 patients (adenomas and Meyenburg complex); cavernous hemangioma was found in 19 patients, focal nodular hyperplasia occurred in 3 patients, and other tumors in 4 patients.[10] Table 45-2 presents the authors' experience and a large autopsy compilation of the relatively common varieties of benign and malignant hepatic tumors. In clinical practice many hepatic tumors are identified and staged by radiographic techniques to elucidate treatment options.

Radiographic Evaluation of Liver Lesions

The widespread use of CT scanning has led to discovery of many incidental lesions that result in additional procedures. Ultrasonography is a common investigational procedure for abdominal pain that incidentally detects hepatic lesions. Additionally, many patients with chronic liver disease (primarily hepatitis B virus [HBV] and C virus [HCV]) are screened with ultrasound and serum AFP. CT scan (especially helical CT) is useful for finding colorectal metastasis to liver.[11] Because of interest in hepatic resection of isolated metastasis, the preoperative evaluation for multiple lesions is critical. Helical CT has improved the detection of small lesions over conventional CT, but lesions 4 to 15 mm still may be missed. Lesions smaller than 10 mm are often missed with helical CT. False-positive lesions are identified that may result from hemorrhage. The addition of multiple phases after contrast has enhanced the detection rate. Whereas most metastatic lesions are hypovascular, HCC is typically well

*HepPar 1 antigen is a commercial name of antibody from Clone OCH 1E5.2.10 that is specific for hepatocytes and is widely utilized.

TABLE 45-2
Classification of Hepatic Tumors

Benign Epithelial		**Malignant Epithelial**	
Focal nodular hyperplasia	Common	None	
Hepatocellular adenoma	Rare	Hepatocellular carcinoma	Common in cirrhosis
Bile duct adenoma; Meyenburg complex	Common	Cholangiocarcinoma	Uncommon
Biliary cystadenoma	Rare	Biliary cystadenocarcinoma	Rare
		Hepatoblastoma (mixed also)	Pediatric only
Benign Mesenchymal		**Malignant Mesenchymal**	
Cavernous hemangioma	Very common		
Infantile hemangioendothelioma	Rare	Angiosarcoma	Rare
		Epithelioid hemangioendothelioma	Rare
Mesenchymal hamartoma	Rare	None	
Solitary fibrous tumor	Rare	None	
		Embryonal sarcoma	Rare

supplied by the arterial phase and is hypervascular on scan.[12]

Introduction of helical CT scan requires more attention to detail and careful selection of protocol. The radiologist must determine the ideal collimation, table increment, scanning time, and intravenous injection dynamics to optimize interpretation.[13] In the non-enhanced CT scan the liver has the highest attenuation of all abdominal organs; metastases, which lack hepatocytes, appear hypoattenuated. With helical CT scan a bolus injection allows a rapid scan in a single phase. Magnetic resonance imaging (MRI) may detect more lesions and smaller lesions than CT scan. Development of new contrast agents for MRI is in progress. These are either reticuloendothelial agents (RE) or hepatocellular agents. RE agents are small, superparamagnetic, iron oxide particles that are taken up by the RE system in the liver and spleen. Hepatocellular agents (e.g., mangafodipir trisodium, gadobenate dimeglumine) are absorbed by hepatocytes and excreted at differing rates. Metastatic tumors do not match hepatocytes for uptake and excretion; therefore defects or anomalies are noted by MRI. Fusion scanning techniques are developing that allow synchronized interpretation of various combinations of scans including positron emission tomography (PET), which uses metabolic activity by infusion of a radiolabeled glucose analog. In one prospective study, dynamic arterial-phase MRI was superior to helical CT for detecting HCC smaller than 3 cm in diameter.[14] MRI can discriminate focal fatty liver change. CT scan is less accurate with fatty liver.

Hepatocellular Carcinoma

HCC is the most common primary malignant hepatic neoplasm but has a variable worldwide incidence. High-incidence regions include Asia and Africa, with reported incidence rates of 150 cases per 100,000. Low incidence occurs in the United States, with 3 to 7 cases per 100,000. This variation in incidence is attributed to chronic hepatitis B infection and aflatoxin exposure in developing countries (mostly Asian countries and various African regions). HCC in regions of low-incidence, including North and South America, Northern Europe, Australia, and New Zealand, is related to several hepatitis viruses (HBV and HCV), alcohol use, and smoking.[15] In Osaka, Japan, approximately 70 percent of HCC is related to chronic HCV infection.[16] An increase in HCV-related HCC is projected for the United States in the next decades.[17]

Factors predisposing to HCC include cirrhosis (of many types and often related to chronic viral hepatitis but primarily resulting from HBV and HCV), hemochromatosis, and some genetic conditions such as tyrosinemia and glycogen storage disease.[18] The etiology of the cirrhosis influences evolution to HCC (Table 45-3). HCV has a higher frequency of progression to HCC than does HBV.[19] In one large series the 5-year cumulative incidence of HCC (in chronic hepatitis C infection) was 9 percent; at 15 years, the incidence was 42 percent. Furthermore, the activity of chronic hepatitis (as measured by serum transaminase levels) influences the rate of progression.[20] Co-infection with human immunodeficiency virus may accelerate the development of HCC in chronic hepatitis C.[21] Approximately 70 percent of HCC evolves in a cirrhotic liver, and many affected patients have decades of asymptomatic liver disease. Alcohol ingestion aggravates the progression of chronic HCV infection to HCC. The presence of both HBV and HCV increases the risk of HCC more than 22 times, and these two viruses account for 55 percent of HCC arising in non-Asians of Los Angeles County.[22]

Clinical Features

The clinical presentation of HCC is dramatically different in different parts of the world. Many patients with HCC related to chronic HBV and HCV in high-incidence locations present with severe decompensation with jaundice and massive enlargement of the liver as an initial clinical episode. These patients may have weight loss and abdominal pain. The common presentation in the United States follows routine laboratory screening for HCC in an early stage before symptoms are prominent. The typical age for detection of HCC is the third or fourth decades of life in high-incidence regions. In the United States many patients with HCC are identified in their seventh or eighth decades of life. The male:female ratio is also related to geographic origin and is 8:1 in the high-incidence regions and only 2.5:1 in the low-incidence areas (such as in the United States). In the United States many patients are identified with chronic hepatitis C infection after screening and then referred for treatment.

Paraneoplastic syndromes including erythrocytosis, hypoglycemia, hypercholesterolemia, and porphyria cutanea tarda are reported but are uncommon in North American patients. Unusual presentation also results

TABLE 45-3

Incidence of Hepatocellular Carcinomas: Complication of Cirrhosis

Cirrhosis: High incidence of HCC (>15%)
Hemochromatosis
HCV-related
HBV-related
Alcoholic cirrhosis with HCV
Cirrhosis: Intermediate incidence of HCC (5%-15%)
Alcoholic cirrhosis without HCV
Cryptogenic cirrhosis
Cirrhosis: Low incidence of HCC (<5%)
Primary biliary cirrhosis
Wilson disease cirrhosis
Autoimmune hepatitis

Adapted from Craig JR, Klatt EC, Yu M: Role of cirrhosis and the development of HCC: evidence from histologic studies and large population studies. In Tabor E, DiBisceglie AM, Purcell RH, eds: Etiology, Pathology, and Treatment of Hepatocellular Carcinoma in North America, vol 13, Advances in Applied Biotechnology Series, Gulf Publishing Co, Houston, 1991:177-189, and based on autopsy study. *HCC,* Hepatocellular carcinoma; *HCV,* hepatitis C virus; *HBV,* hepatitis B virus.

from tumor spread into the biliary tree (jaundice), the right atrium, and distant metastasis to the spine or soft tissue. Unexplained deterioration of chronic liver disease (or cirrhosis) is also a clue to the presence of HCC.

Physical findings associated with HCC depend on the geographic location of the patient and stage at discovery. In developing countries a large abdominal mass is typical and reflects an enlarged liver with HCC replacing most of the organ. Hepatic tenderness may be noted and an arterial bruit is recognized up to 25 percent of the time. But an arterial bruit over the upper abdomen may be transmitted from a source other than liver; therefore, additional signs are useful. Ascites may be present, especially if HCC has developed in a cirrhotic liver. The signs of portal hypertension may be accentuated because of expansion of the veins by HCC tumor spread. Jaundice is a late sign but may occur early with tumor spread to common duct. Fever occurs in up to 50 percent of patients; an occasional patient may present with fever (without recognized cause). Routine liver tests are not specific for HCC but reflect underlying chronic liver disease. However, in patients with stable chronic liver disease (normal to minimal serum enzyme elevation), a rising serum alkaline phosphatase may be a clue to infiltrative disease, including HCC. Routine screening for HCC in patients with chronic liver disease depends upon regular serum marker and radiographic studies (usually ultrasound). The timing of these tests for North American patients is not established. Performance of serum AFP at 6-month intervals in a high-risk group of Alaskan natives with chronic hepatitis allowed early detection of HCC and improved survival compared with a historic control group.[23] In high-incidence areas for HCC, routine screening is associated with better survival after treatment versus non-screened patients.[24] Although screening intervals of 3 to 6 months have been studied, there is no proof that such screening improves curability in North American patients.[25] Therefore attempts to time liver transplantation in patients with advanced cirrhosis before evolution to HCC is a goal; guidelines for this have been proposed on the basis of several laboratory and clinical features.[26] A serum albumin below 4.1 g/dl and hepatic decompensation of a cirrhotic patient with chronic hepatitis C indicate high risk for evolution of HCC.

Laboratory Features: Serum Markers

AFP, a widely used HCC screening test, is an alpha 1 globulin produced by fetal liver cells and yolk sac cells and is normally present in high concentration during gestation. Its presence in adults is associated with HCC, metastatic carcinoma to the liver, and a few other malignant tumors—most notably germ cell tumors such as embryonal carcinoma of the testis. Although AFP is often increased in HCC and is easily measured, it has limited usefulness for screening. Mild-to-moderate elevations (20-400 ng/ml) occur in cirrhosis, and up to 35 percent of patients with small HCC (smaller than 3 cm) do not have elevated AFP in serum. Refinement of the assay and assay of molecular variants may enhance the value of screening with AFP. The tumor makes normal AFP and variants that are fucosylated or species that agglutinate lectin. Measurement of these variants is common in Japan, but not well established or evaluated in the United States. Des-gamma-carboxyprothrombin (DCP), also called "protein induced by vitamin K absence," or antagonist II and L3 (a variant form of AFP) have been used as screening tests for HCC.[27] Many patients with HCC are negative for AFP but positive by DCP.[28] Administration of vitamin K produces a rapid reduction of elevated levels of serum DCP. For screening purposes the normal cut-off levels for AFP and DCP (with an improved detection method) were 20 ng/ml and 40 mAU/ml, respectively, in a large series of Japanese patients with HCC and chronic liver disease. Using the two tests together, 87 percent of the HCC patients had at least one abnormal value, and many of the tumors were less than 3 cm.[29] Many authorities recommend quarterly and semiannual serum AFP (and DCP) testing (with or without ultrasound) for high-risk patients. Monthly serum testing has been reported not to be of better value.[30] Elevation of a serum marker usually appears several months before ultrasonographic change is detectable. An abnormal value for DCP is associated with portal venous invasion, which is important information for selecting treatment modalities.[31] Future application of highly sensitive markers such as AFP messenger ribonucleic acid (mRNA) may assist in monitoring for recurrence.[32] The level of this marker is higher in poorly differentiated HCC compared with well-differentiated tumors. Elevated mRNA (AFP) is associated with distant metastasis; however, overall survival is not different between groups with and without mRNA AFP at diagnosis. However, for patients with HCC and an elevated mRNA AFP at diagnosis, overall survival was better for patients who became mRNA AFP negative after treatment versus (embolization or ethanol injection) non-responders. In a series of 88 HCC patients, two thirds had elevated serum AFP mRNA before treatment. Treatment produced a loss of this marker in patients with a small tumor.

Radiologic Evaluation

Routine imaging with ultrasound, CT (helical with various phases), MRI, and sometimes PET follows abnormal blood studies (e.g., elevated AFP or other marker). Nevertheless, some benign lesions are resected because of a preoperative diagnosis of malignant tumor. Focal nodular hyperplasia and hepatocellular adenoma are the lesions most often confused with carcinoma.[33] Ultrasound imaging is improved markedly by injection of carbon dioxide microbubbles, via catheter, into the hepatic artery. This technique is sensitive enough to localize lesions as small as 1 cm. After peripheral injection, 2- to 4-μm microbubbles pass through the lung capillaries to reach the liver and produce an atypical ultrasonic wave pattern (galactose-based ultrasound contrast agent).[34] Study of macroregenerative nodules may identify areas of likely dysplastic "nodule in nodule" patterns of growth.

Liver Biopsy and Pathology

After an isolated nodule or lesion is identified (usually by radiographic study or incidental finding at laparoscopic surgery) a needle aspiration or core biopsy may be performed. Because HCC is often a friable tumor, tumor seeding is a concern after needle biopsy. A second aspiration or needle core biopsy of "non-lesional" tissue taken at the same setting may improve diagnostic interpretation because many slightly enlarged cirrhotic nodules may demonstrate some atypia. Comparison of "control" tissue from the same liver may resolve interpretative confusion.

Although the majority of HCCs have a trabecular growth pattern composed of eosinophilic polygonal tumor cells, a wide variety of histologic patterns have been described. These include microtrabecular, macrotrabecular, adenoid (pseudoglandular), clear cell, spindle cell, pleomorphic, and giant cell type. Histologic features of HCC include bile production (within acini), sinusoidal lining cells at margins of clusters, and alcoholic hyaline.[35] Immunohistochemical reactions that help to confirm the diagnosis include the polyclonal CEA canalicular reactivity pattern and a positive reaction with HepPAR antibody. Metastatic carcinoma, melanoma, and neuroendocrine carcinoma provide histologic similarities to HCC. Immunohistochemical reaction to AFP is reported in approximately 50 percent of HCC. But because this stain is rarely positive in difficult cases, its routine use is not helpful. Small tumors (smaller than 2 cm in diameter) are usually well differentiated whereas larger lesions have multiple grades within a single nodule. Approximately 40 percent of nodules 1 to 3 cm in diameter contain two histologic grades.[36] The well-differentiated component may be at the edge; the less-differentiated tumor is usually in the center. As the nodule enlarges the less-differentiated component expands and can replace the entire mass. All cells in HCC nodules may be from a single clone or from multiple clones with dedifferentiation of an initial clone.[37] Despite the sampling problems of a needle core biopsy of HCC, there is a general correlation with prognosis and histologic grade of such biopsy samples.[38]

The gross appearance of HCC usually correlates with the radiographic appearance (Plates 45-1, *A* and *B*). Furthermore, there are geographic variations in the gross patterns of HCC.[39] The gross pattern also may be influenced by the time of detection and examination. In the large autopsy series from the USC Liver Unit the cirrhotomimetic spreading pattern was the most common. This autopsy series was based on HCC arising in late stage cirrhosis, not by detecting HCC through routine screening in chronic hepatitis clinics. Small HCC (smaller than 2 cm diameter) is either nodular or indistinct. Large HCC usually has several growth patterns, including massive (often without cirrhosis), nodular (single or multiple), diffuse, and encapsulated (common in Japan). The most common gross pattern in Japan is the nodular form arising in cirrhosis. The surface is bulging (not umbilicated as in CC or metastatic carcinoma). The massive form that arises in a non-cirrhotic liver is the most prone to rupture and may cause hemoperitoneum. Diffuse intrahepatic spread of HCC may not be readily apparent by gross examination. The cut surface of small nodules may be light brown. Larger lesions include regions of hemorrhage and necrosis and variation in color. Anaplastic tumors often are yellow to white on cut surface. Sclerosis is firm and white (so-called sarcomatoid HCC). Bile production produces a green color of the individual nodules.

The surgical pathology report may enhance the staging process by addressing numerous issues as recommended by the College of American Pathologists Cancer Protocol Manual for Liver Cancer. Factors to include in the evaluation of specimens include the number and size of tumor nodules, surgical margins (width), gross growth pattern, vessel invasion, histologic grade, histologic pattern (trabecular, solid, etc.), condition of adjacent noninvolved liver, and evaluation of submitted lymph nodes. A synoptic report form has been proposed to simplify communication of staging information.[40]

Prognosis of HCC is related to the stage at diagnosis and histologic grade. There are several staging systems including the tumor lymph node metastasis system (TNM) and modifications that add liver tests as prognostic variable. The TNM system uses the number and size of nodules, lymph node status, and presence of metastatic disease. Okuda proposed a staging system that includes components of the Child-Pugh stage.[41] Based on a retrospective review of HCC evaluated at multiple Italian liver centers, a multi-variate analysis indicated other important factors, such as AFP level, portal vein invasion, and gross morphology of tumor.[42] Prospective validation indicated the discriminating power of the variables in a series of 150 patients.[43] A large series from the AFIP confirmed that prognosis is related to histologic grade.[44] Microscopic appearance is graded from well-differentiated (good acinar production with modest size of cells and nuclei) to intermediate (moderate) grade to pleomorphic and undifferentiated forms (Plates 45-1, *C, D,* and *E*). Portal vein invasion is correlated with poor prognosis and is associated with larger tumors. In a large review of 403 HCC patients studied at a single referral institution the most common sites for extrahepatic spread of HCC were lung (39 percent), perihepatic and abdominal lymph nodes (41 percent), and bone (28 percent).[45]

The data in Table 45-4 reveal the surprise experience with hepatic tumors at a single center and reject that the problem of hepatic tumors are highly heterogeneous.

Fibrolamellar Hepatocellular Carcinoma

This distinctive histologic variant of HCC arises in noncirrhotic liver, has equal sex incidence, occurs typically in young adults (average age, 23 years), and is rare in Asian and African countries.[46] Most patients with fibrolamellar hepatocellular carcinoma (FLHCC) have mild symptoms that are non-specific, delaying discovery from 3 to 12 months. Pain, hepatomegaly, and right upper quadrant mass are common. Tumor markers in serum are different from what is found in HCC. AFP is elevated in only 25 percent of patients, but the serum DCP, serum neurotensin, and vitamin B_{12} binding globulin are commonly increased. These markers are useful in monitoring the disease and detecting recurrence. Radiographic procedures identify a large liver microcalcification. Ultrasound reveals mixed echogenicity, and a central scar is visualized as hyperechoic in 50 percent of tumors with a scar.[47] CT and MRI are more useful than ultrasound (US). Preoperative staging of FLHCC is best accomplished by CT scan. Lymphadenopathy is noted in 50 percent of patients, and some patients have pulmonary metastasis, direct organ invasion, or peritoneal implants. The MRI identifies the central scar in most cases (hypointense). The Tc99m sulfur colloid exam shows a photopenic defect because there is no uptake within the tumor, which correlates with the lack of sinusoidal lining cells in the tumor. The lesion most confused with FLHCC by radiographic studies is focal nodular hyperplasia. Needle biopsy of FLHCC is usually diagnostic, especially if the marginal tissue is included rather than cores of the central fibrous scar. The tumor is typically a large mass (average diameter in some series is 13-20 cm). There may be satellite lesions as well (Plates 45-2, *A*, *B*, and *C*). The left lobe is the common site of origin (60 to 70 percent) in most large series. Cyst-like areas or necrosis are common (65 percent of 31 cases).[48] At surgical excision the massive tumor usually has a bulging contour, a central scar region (simulating focal nodular hyperplasia), and no capsule. The adjacent liver is compressed. The cut surface is variegated because of hemorrhage and necrosis and pale because of fibrosis. The prognosis of this tumor has been debated, but several large series (including from a single center) indicate a better 5- and 10-year survival compared with HCC arising in non-cirrhotic liver.[49] Aggressive pursuit and resection of recurrent tumor, metastatic tumor, and multiple lesions are warranted. Routine CT scanning in search of recurrence is useful, especially in the early postoperative period (i.e., first few years).[50]

Cholangiocarcinoma

CC is an adenocarcinoma derived from biliary epithelium that is distributed from the small biliary radicles to larger ducts and to the major bile ducts within the liver. The tumor also will arise within the common bile duct (so called extrahepatic CC). By convention the term CC is applied only to intrahepatic and hilar (intrahepatic or near hepatic) tumors. The same histologic type of tumor occurring in more distal ducts is termed extrahepatic bile duct cancer. This general classification is based on the location of the major lesion.[51] The intrahepatic lesions are peripheral (derived from small interlobular bile ducts), and the major intrahepatic bile duct tumors may form a hilar mass (Plates 45-7, *A* and *B*). The term peripheral is not physiologic but is applied because the tumor is in the periphery of the liver rather than hilar (central). Klatskin described a series of CC arising in the hilum that caused jaundice. This specific clinical presentation of CC is commonly referred to as "Klatskin tumor."[52] Although the need for histologic confirmation previously led to surgical exploration, improved radiographic studies including endoscopy indicate that only 50 percent of patients require histologic confirmation for accurate diagnosis.[53] There is a group of intraductal papillary neoplasms that may have a prolonged course. These tumors vary from a solitary lesion (papilloma) to multi-focal (papillomatosis) to overt papillary adenocarcinoma.[54]

Geographic variation in CC is related to fluke infestation, with high incidence of CC in northern Thailand and Laos. CC accounts for 90 percent of liver cancer in one region of Thailand (Khon Kaen) and is related to *Opisthorchis viverrini* infection.[55] *Clonorchis sinensis* is endemic in Korea, and CC is more common in this area as well. CC accounts for approximately 10 percent of primary hepatic malignancies in most Western populations.

The clinical presentation of CC varies with the location of the primary lesion. Occlusion of the major bile ducts by hilar CC produces symptoms (jaundice) early, before widespread dissemination. A peripheral tumor can grow to considerable size and form multiple intrahepatic nodules before the tumor burden induces symptoms, including weight loss and abdominal pain.[56] Primary sclerosing cholangitis is associated with CC that often is occult and detected only after liver transplantation for the cholangitis. Nearly 25 percent of these transplant candidates prove to develop CC.[57,58] Cirrhosis occurs in only a small number of patients with CC. In some referral series the association of chronic liver disease represents a minority of cases (less than 20 percent). Intrahepatic calculi (and recurrent pyogenic cholangitis) are common in the Far East and are associated with CC. Mucosal dysplasia occurs with intrahepatic calculi and is a precursor to peripheral CC.[59] Thorotrast was associated with CC but is no longer used. Some biliary malformations, such as unilocular or multiple cysts, Caroli's disease, congenital hepatic fibrosis, and von Meyenburg complex, are also related to CC.

The age of presentation is broad (usually 20 to 80 years; average, 60 years). The tumor is equally frequent in males and females. As alluded to previously, jaundice is the presenting problem for 90 percent of perihilar and distal bile duct–related tumors. Fever is noted in less than 5 percent of patients. Laboratory tests used to help detect CC include the serum marker Ca 19-9.[60] However,

TABLE 45-4

Hepatic Resection in Major Tertiary Referral Center: Distribution of Types of Liver Tumors, 411 Hepatic Resections 1964-1987[141]

Benign liver tumor	182 patients (44%)	Malignant liver tumor	106 patients (26%)	Metastatic liver tumor	123 patients (30%)
Hemangioma	100	Hepatocellular cancer	55	Colorectal cancer	90
Hepatocellular adenoma	22	Fibrolamellar cancer	12	Intestinal-carcinoid	6
Focal nodular hyperplasia	17	Cholangiocarcinoma	14	Renal cancer	5
Congenital cystic disease	16	Bile duct cancer	6	Adrenal cancer	5
Others	27	Others	19	Others	17

Data from Iwatsuki S, Starzl T: Personal experience with 411 hepatic resections. Ann Surg 208:411-434, 1988.

this marker is not specific and may be elevated in other conditions such as biliary cystadenoma.[61] The CEA is increased in about 50 percent of patients with CC. An index using both Ca 19-9 and the CEA has been proposed to detect occult CC in primary sclerosing cholangitis.[62] Serum AFP is increased in 20 percent of patients, with a broad range from slightly increased to markedly elevated.

PET scans may be helpful, but further studies with comparison of explant liver are necessary to document the sensitivity of this staging procedure.[63] The CT radiographic appearance is highly variable, from hypervascular to hypovascular. Although tissue confirmation of adenocarcinoma is reassuring, the image may replace the biopsy in some patients.[64] The central area is often sclerotic; consequently, the central area shows delayed filling. The precise site of origin of intrahepatic perihilar tumors has been classified by Bismuth into four types to assist in analysis of surgical resection technique.[65]

Peripheral CC is gray to gray-white, solid, firm, and may be solitary or occur as multiple nodules. A few tumors have easily recognized intraductal growth (polypoid or not). Large lesions (greater than 2 cm) have central necrosis. A slimy surface is noted if there is abundant mucin production. The mucin may produce a powdery appearance on CT scan, which corresponds to a microcystic change.[66] In CC related to disorders such as primary sclerosing cholangitis, the underlying liver disease may be grossly apparent. Recurrent pyogenic cholangitis produces left lobe atrophy with massive intrabiliary calculi, and there may be superimposed sclerosing carcinoma near the hilum. Metastasis to adjacent perihilar lymph nodes is noted in many hilar tumors; frozen section of these nodes may dictate the course of surgery. For intrahepatic CC in the left lobe, some patients have no evidence of tumor spread in the lymph nodes of the hepatoduodenal ligament. It is necessary in these patients to sample lymph nodes around the cardiac portion of the stomach or common hepatic artery.[67]

The histologic appearance of CC varies with site of origin. The degree of gland formation varies from well differentiated (gland forming) to poorly differentiated (solid sheets) tumor. The degree of sclerosis varies as well. Many tumors are fibrogenic and produce profound sclerosis of the surrounding duct (which enhances bile duct obstruction). Intrahepatic, peripheral CC is usually marked by sclerotic masses and is large (average size, 7 cm; range, 1 to 15 cm). Perihilar tumors are also typically sclerotic (90 percent) but papillary variants are also encountered. Spindle cells may produce a sarcomatoid appearance that also occurs with HCC. Therefore a needle biopsy of a sarcomatoid primary liver cancer may be either CC or HCC and special studies must be considered.[68] Search for keratin-positive cells and numerous sections may help classify this pattern and exclude metastatic sarcoma. In some patients squamous differentiation may be noted and mixed with glandular elements (so-called adenosquamous carcinoma). Abundant mucin production appears as lakes of mucin. Such patients may have a rapid downhill course.[69]

Histologic distinction of CC from metastatic colorectal adenocarcinoma remains challenging, and immunohistochemical staining patterns are useful. CC is almost always cytokeratin-7 positive. Cytokeratin-20 staining occurs in 70 percent of cases and is less commonly positive in peripheral compared to hilar CC.[70] Distinction between sclerosing cholangitis and a small CC can be difficult and may require multiple biopsies and study over time. CC also arises with HCC and is thus termed *combined HCC-CC.* If the two tumors are separate masses and grow together, this may be a collision tumor instead of a single tumor mass with bidirectional differentiation (more common).[71]

Bile duct adenoma is a small (usually less than 1.5 cm), often solitary white lesion noted during elective surgery and is removed and often submitted for frozen section. In a large series from a referral center the average size of bile duct adenoma was 6 mm in 152 cases.[72] The histologic appearance was similar to metastatic adenocarcinoma and CC. The smallest CC may be indistinguishable from bile duct adenoma, but key features of the latter are the uniform mixture of sclerosis and glands throughout the lesion and a lack of sinusoidal invasion (which occurs in carcinoma). Although there is variation in the ratio of fibrous stromal and glandular proliferation in the different nodules, within each nodule the ratio is constant. No mitotic figures are noted. Surgical excision is common, although 10 percent of the patients have numerous nodules.

Congenital hepatic fibrosis can be confused with metastatic carcinoma and is an incidental finding at surgery or discovered by CT scan or US study.[73] The numerous von Meyenburg complexes of congenital hepatic fibrosis will produce numerous surface defects noted by external examination (such as laparoscopic surgery) or US examination. Typically the surface is depressed rather than expanded and pushing up from the surrounding liver. The clinician (surgeon or laparoscopist) may insist that the lesion is metastatic carcinoma and obtain a small biopsy, which also may be difficult to interpret and be miscalled adenocarcinoma. The key histologic findings in Von Meyenburg complexes are the presence of uniform small ducts with no invasion of the adjacent sinusoids and the lack of variation in the admixture of fibrosis and glands. The ductular structures have thin cuboidal, nearly atrophic, epithelium.

Combined Hepatocellular Cholangiocarcinoma

This tumor has both HCC and CC areas that are distinct and yet connected and intermingled (in contrast to the collision of two separate tumors). The general clinical features are similar to those of HCC alone. This entity occurs in 1 percent to 3 percent of all HCC cases (Plate 45-1, *E*). Abundant sampling of large tumors is necessary to document this condition.[74] The hepatocellular component may be identified with hepatocyte stain and by the canalicular staining pattern with the CEA immunostain. Cytokeratins 8 and 18 are present. The CC component is negative for these cytokeratins but positive for cytokeratins 7 and 19. Several histologic growth patterns of this combined tumor have been correlated with the CT appearance.[75] Cirrhosis occurs in many of these patients (60 percent). AFP is increased in nearly 50 percent. The fibrolamellar variant was a form of the combined tumor in 8 of the original 24 cases reported as combined HCC-CC tumors. The dilated glandular component had a mucin component and thus is related to CC. Because the prognosis is different in the fibrolamellar variant, this combined variant (with FLHCC) should be considered a separate category.

Hepatocellular Adenoma

Hepatocytes may form a solitary nodule and be arranged in broad sheets with portal areas at the margins. Prominent vascular structures are contained within the hepatocellular masses. The clinical setting is typically a large hepatic mass that is identified by a radiographic procedure performed because of vague abdominal pain. Associated clinical features include long-term oral contraceptive use (longer than 5 years), anabolic steroid use, and a metabolic disorder such as glycogen storage disease. The widespread use of anabolic steroids among athletes has increased awareness of this hormone-related tumor (Plates 45-5, *A* and *B*). Such tumors may be large or multiple and are prone to hemorrhage with minimal trauma.[76]

Preoperative diagnosis based on radiographic studies is about 90 percent accurate. Biopsy or resection may be required for diagnosis in atypical cases (see Chap. 46).[77] Bleeding within the tumor can account for pain. Rupture can produce a sudden demise. Histologic identification of tumor can be difficult in small samples of tissue in which key features of the tumor may not be apparent. These include sheets of hepatocytes with variable vascular structures and the absence of portal regions (with major interlobular bile ducts, hepatic arterioles, and portal vein radicles). Acinar formation, cytologic atypia, and thick cell plates (more than 3 cells) point to the diagnosis of HCC.

Focal Nodular Hyperplasia

Focal nodular hyperplasia (FNH) is a mixture of benign hepatocytes in masses separated by fibrous bands. There also is prominent cholangiolar proliferation and vascular structures (Plates 45-4, *C* and *D*). Patients, who are usually asymptomatic, are recognized by radiographic review or incidental findings at surgery (laparoscopic or open abdominal surgery). Most lesions border on the liver surface and may bulge or protrude. Rupture is unusual but more likely for pedunculated tumors. Women are affected more often than men (5:1), and the most likely age for diagnosis is the third or fourth decade. Whereas most of the tumors are smaller than 5 cm and asymptomatic, larger tumors are associated with a mass effect or pain (10 percent-15 percent). And although most lesions are solitary, approximately 10 percent are multiple. Some are associated with other non-hepatic lesions, including meningioma.[78] The characteristic radiographic appearance of FNH is a lesion of moderate size (3-5 cm) that is homogenous by US and CT scan. The lesions have both hepatocellular and reticuloendothelial functions. A central hypoattenuating scar is visualized in one third of cases. The tumor has a rich arterial supply (and may be a congenital vascular anomaly), which enhances dramatically during contrast-enhanced CT scanning.[79] In one series of 12 patients with FNH, helical CT had typical features in only 2 patients.[80] Therefore diagnosis typically depends on needle biopsy or resection.

In general, radiographic features of FNH may mimic HCC, hepatocellular adenoma, metastatic tumor, and fibrolamellar carcinoma. Therefore needle biopsy may be performed. The differential diagnosis of FNH for the radiologist includes several focal lesions: fibrolamellar carcinoma, metastatic tumor, and even hepatocellular adenoma. FLHCC has similarities by radiographic study because it also has a central scar. One half of tumors have distinctive uptake of sulfur colloid. Hepatocellular adenoma also may have colloid uptake (10 percent). If resected, the gross appearance of FNH is homogenous brown to orange firm tissue with no capsule at the margin. The lesion is well demarcated from the surrounding normal liver. The cut surface reveals septation by thin fibrous strands and often a large, central scar with prominent vessels. Microscopic features are sheets of benign hepatocytes with prominent cholangiolar proliferation and admixed vascular structures. No major intralobular bile duct is noted, which distinguishes the fibrous areas from portal regions ("triads"). By contrast, the cut surface of FLHCC has hemorrhage, necrosis, and evidence of bile staining (i.e., green color). The histologic feature required for diagnosis of FNH is marked cholangiolar proliferation with benign hepatocytes. Unfortunately, small biopsy samples may not have sufficient tissue to reveal all these histologic features. In a recent series of 29 patients with surgical resection for benign hepatic tumor (hepatic adenoma in 16; FNH in 13), one third had no symptoms and 3 had a lesion in the setting of prior malignancy.[81] The mean size of the resected FNH lesions was 8.8 cm, which is slightly larger than the mean for the hepatocellular adenomas (8.1 cm).

Nodular Regenerative Hyperplasia

The term *nodular regenerative hyperplasia* is applied to the condition displaying numerous and diffuse small (1-2 mm diameter) regenerative nodules in a normal liver.[82] Occasionally, clusters of nodules several centimeters in diameter are noted, which are pale compared to the adjacent brown liver parenchyma. Associated conditions include rheumatoid arthritis and Felty's syndrome. The histologic diagnosis is difficult to make on small biopsies. Sometimes, extensive necrosis (i.e., submassive hepatic necrosis) produces a dramatic regenerative response with formation of large nodules that simulate cirrhosis.

Macroregenerative Nodules (in Cirrhotic Liver)

In the last several decades there has been a flurry of activity in classifying and documenting enlarging hepatocellular nodules in the cirrhotic liver. Improvement in radiographic sensitivity has allowed recognition of smaller nodules, some of which are HCC and others that are benign cirrhotic nodules with various degrees of atypia. The latter have been called macroregenerative nodules (MRN) or adenomatous hyperplasia. An international committee suggested the term *dysplastic nodule* to describe these lesions.[83-85] Screening of cirrhotic patients has led to diagnostic pursuit of many nodules. Some needle aspirations of these nodules are easily classified as benign, but other nodules demonstrate varying degrees of atypia and even overt HCC. After review of a series of "nodules" by a panel of expert hepatopathologists, diagnostic criteria were revised[86] because of the panel's difficulty in making a histologic diagnosis. A macroregenerative nodule must be at least 0.8 cm in diameter to distinguish it from the numerous nodules in the advanced, cirrhotic liver. The histologic features are normal: thin cell plates (two cells thick) and a lack of cytologic atypia defended by the nuclear/cytoplasmic ratio. Large cell dysplasia (i.e., normal nuclear/cytoplasmic ratio but enlarged hepatocytes) is acceptable. A macroregenerative nodule includes multiple portal areas distributed within the lesion that are grossly distinctive compared to the surrounding nodules. The MRN arises in many types of chronic liver disease including cirrhosis related to hepatitis B and C but also in cirrhosis related to autoimmune hepatitis and hemochromatosis. Many livers contain multiple MRNs (rarely more than 10); careful search of cirrhotic liver reveals MRNs in 14 percent to 21 percent of patients.[87]

The clonality of adenomatous nodules suggests that they are neoplastic and possibly premalignant. The clonality of atypical adenomatous hyperplasia was demonstrated first in HBV-related HCC.[88] In one large study of 30 large regenerative nodules, 12 adenomatous hyperplastic nodules, 2 atypical adenomatous nodules, and 5 adenomatous nodules with HCC, 40 percent of adenomatous hyperplastic nodules became malignant.[89] The transition of macroregenerative nodule to dysplastic nodule to small HCC is associated with changes in the vascular pattern of the nodule that may produce a change in the radiographic appearance.[90]

Hepatic Cysts: Biliary Cystadenoma and Carcinoma

Hepatic cysts are not common and usually do not provoke symptoms that lead to resection (see Chap. 49). Many cysts are small and found incidentally during radiologic staging procedures or elective surgery (Plate 45-3, *D*). Precise classification (by radiographic study) is not easy, as reflected in the change in the preoperative diagnosis after resection.[91] In a major tertiary referral center, cystic lesions accounted for 6 percent of hepatic resections, with most of the lesions classified as congenital cysts (19 of 44).[92]

Some cystic lesions are derived from biliary epithelium and may have prominent, densely cellular stroma. These lesions have been classified as biliary cystadenoma with mesenchymal stroma.[93] Malignant transformation may occur, accounting for an enlarging cyst.[94] The age range in the largest series of biliary cystadenoma (52 patients) was 2 to 87 years with a mean of 45 years.[95] All of these cysts were multi-locular with benign cuboidal and columnar epithelial lining; 85 percent had recognizable mesenchymal (ovarian-like) stroma. Females predominated (96 percent) in contrast to the nearly even sex incidence in the 18 patients with biliary cystadenocarcinoma. Six of the malignant lesions had areas of benign epithelium, indicating that malignant transformation had occurred. Males with cystadenocarcinoma do not have ovarian-like stroma and have a more aggressive clinical course than females. The size of these cystic lesions ranged from 2.5 cm to 28 cm (mean, 15 cm) in the large AFIP series. Cystadenocarcinoma arising within the liver resembles metastatic tumor from a similar tumor arising in the pancreas or ovary. Interestingly, primary carcinoma of the gallbladder or bile ducts may metastasize to the ovary and mimic a primary tumor in that organ.[96]

Hepatoblastoma

Hepatoblastoma (HB) is a common primary hepatic tumor occurring in childhood. It accounts for 25 percent of all primary hepatic tumors arising before age 20 and for nearly 50 percent of the malignant hepatic tumors in the first 2 years of life.[97] Indeed, most HBs are identified before the age of 2 years (nearly 70 percent). None of the adult risk factors for HCC are associated with HB. However, there is a variety of clinical syndromes associated with this tumor, including congenital anomalies.

Abdominal enlargement is typically the presenting problem. Other findings include anorexia and weight loss. Occasionally hormone production (HCG) in young boys provokes genital enlargement, deepening voice, and pubic hair. Laboratory studies may reveal anemia and thrombocytosis. Only one quarter of patients have elevated liver enzymes or bilirubin. Serum AFP is usually elevated and sometimes is very high. Keep in mind, however, that elevation is normal in young infants until 6 months of age. Radiographic study shows a hepatic mass that is solitary. Calcification occurs in 50 percent of patients. MRI usually discriminates other hepatic tumors of this age group, including mesenchymal hamartoma, infantile hemangioendothelioma, and HCC. The mixed form of HB has a heterogenous MRI pattern in contrast to the pure epithelial form that is homogenous. US shows a mass lesion with heterogeneity, punctate calcification, and occasionally cystic changes.

The gross pathology of HB is typically a large, solitary hepatic mass of the right lobe (60 percent of patients). The tumors can be massive: more than 22 cm in diameter and up to 1400 g.[98] Necrosis and hemorrhage are usually apparent, and soft and gelatinous large nodules occur within the large multi-lobated mass. Six histologic patterns have been proposed: four epithelial categories (fetal type, fetal and embryonal type, macrotrabecular type, and small cell undifferentiated type) and two types with mesenchymal elements (with and without teratoid features). The embryonal type is composed of small, polygonal, hepatoid cells in thin cell plates with some variation in the cytoplasm (clear and solid). The macrotrabecular pattern is characterized by cell plates more than 10 cells in width. The small, undifferentiated pattern is typified by cells that resemble neuroblastoma cells with scanty cytoplasm and hyperchromatic nuclei. The mixed epithelial and mesenchymal type contains fetal and embryonal hepatocytes admixed with a mesenchymal component that resembles osteoid and cartilage. Some of these mixed HBs contain other heterologous elements, including squamous epithelium, melanin, mucinous epithelium, and striated muscle. Hematopoietic tissue is also present. These latter features characterize the teratoid form of HB. The most common histologic variant has both the epithelial and mesenchymal mixtures. Eighty percent of tumors have mesenchymal stroma resembling osteoid and cartilage. Fine needle aspiration provides considerable diagnostic challenge. Other small cell tumors of childhood may be aspirated from metastases to liver.

Treatment is surgical resection, often preceded by chemotherapy to reduce the tumor size. Nearly 85 percent of the tumors are resectable after chemotherapy. Prognosis is related to staging that is accomplished at the initial surgery. Survival appears to be independent of histologic subtype, but extent of tumor at diagnosis is important. Pulmonary metastases occur in 10 percent to 20 percent of patients at initial diagnosis. Metastases to other sites include bone, brain, ovary, and orbit. With combined surgery and chemotherapy, 65 percent to 70 percent of patients are cured.

Benign Mesenchymal Hepatic Tumors—Cavernous Hemangioma

The most frequently encountered benign hepatic tumor, cavernous hemangioma, is estimated to be present in at least 5 percent to 7 percent of adults (and even in 20 percent in one autopsy series).[99] The lesion comprises endothelium-lined channels with a thin fibrous stroma and a sharp demarcation from the surrounding normal liver (Plates 45-3, *A*, *B*, and *C*). Although more frequent in females (2 to 5 times more than in men) and occurring in all age groups, only a small number of cavernous hemangiomas become massive, produce clinical symptoms, or require attention. Whereas many hepatic hemangiomas are "classic" by radiographic study, the presence of low blood flow, perhaps secondary to variable sclerosis or thrombosis, can reduce the accuracy of diagnosis. But 90 percent of hemangiomas have radiographic images that are reasonably diagnostic. Additional studies are indicated in the remaining patients. The presence of marked fatty liver, adjacent lesions (such as FNH), known cancer, and unusual radiographic features should stimulate persistent evaluation.

The presence of cavernous hemangiomas complicates the staging of patients with known carcinoma (such as colon cancer) or other hepatic lesions. Doppler ultrasound, tagged red blood cell studies, MRI, and CT scan all may be helpful. The imaging features depend on the size of the hemangioma. Small lesions, less than 3 cm in diameter, are usually classic. Confusion with angiosarcoma can occur even with red blood cell scintigraphy.[100] Recent study with color and power Doppler sonography indicates that this test modality is not definitive either.[101] Fine needle aspiration or needle biopsy may reveal the lesion and may be performed because of atypical radiographic findings that suggest the focal lesion is not a hemangioma. The hemangioma is an arterial-fed lesion but has slow flow compared with surrounding liver. The classic pattern of hemangioma on contrast CT scan is slow filling of the lesion during the arterial, then portal, and delayed phases. Some hemangiomas lack contrast filling because of sclerosis. Atypical patterns for hemangioma include an echogenic border detected by US, large hemangiomas with irregular filling that fill rapidly, calcified hemangiomas and hyalinized hemangiomas, cystic and multi-locular hemangiomas, and pedunculated hemangiomas.[102] Rapid-filling hemangiomas tend to be small (42 percent smaller than 1 cm).[103]

Giant hemangiomas, defined as ranging from 4 or 6 to 12 cm in diameter, often appear heterogenous. Such large lesions may produce hepatomegaly and symptoms like abdominal pain and nausea. There also can be mild elevation in liver enzyme tests.[104]

A sclerotic, cavernous hemangioma may be noted at surgery as a retracted well-rounded sunken nodule (Plate 45-3, *B*). These hyalinized nodules may mimic metastasis in patients with known cancer. Thus surgical excision (elective perhaps at the time of colon cancer resection) or needle biopsy is often performed. Capsular retraction is a feature of sclerotic hemangiomas; similar retraction may be noted in malignant tumors, including CC, epithelioid hemangioendothelioma, and metastatic carcinoma.

Multiple hemangiomas occur in 10 percent of patients with hemangiomas; some patients have diffuse hemangiomatosis (multi-organ). A rare, clinically important complication is consumption coagulopathy within the hemangioma and is termed Kasabach-Merritt syndrome.[105] Spontaneous rupture is unusual; therefore most hemangiomas do not require resection. The rare pedunculated hemangioma is resected to preclude torsion and rupture. FNH is commonly associated with hemangioma; 23 percent of patients with FNH have hemangioma as well. This association is stronger when there is multiple FNH (up to 33 percent).

Liver biopsy is performed for focal hepatic lesions (not expected to be hemangioma), and a small number prove to be hemangiomas. In one series of 14 patients with hemangiomas confirmed by biopsy, 6 patients had extrahepatic cancer. The attending physicians requested exclusion of metastatic cancer in these patients despite strong radiographic findings indicating a diagnosis of hemangioma.[106] The remaining eight patients did not have classic radiographic findings of hemangioma, and biopsy demonstrated various degrees of fibrosis and recent thrombosis. One patient had calcifications. The size of hemangiomas in this series was 1 to 10.9 cm. There was an inverse relationship of the T2 relaxation time and the endothelial content. This observation correlates with those hemangiomas that have small vascular spaces rather than giant dilated channels, which would have more endothelial cells relative to size of vascular space. Follow-up of hemangiomas indicates that they are stable. An increase in size suggests the need for further evaluation.[107] Needle biopsy may be performed safely.[108] Surgical resection of symptomatic patients (i.e., those with pain) provides excellent long-term results.[109]

Mesenchymal Hamartoma

Mesenchymal hemartoma is a "malformation" that begins in utero and accounts for nearly 10 percent of pediatric liver tumors. Arising early in life, it is discovered within the first 2 years and involves the right lobe in 75 percent of patients. Abdominal swelling is noted, and there is rapid fluid accumulation within the tumor. These tumors may be massive (up to 30 cm in diameter). Resection is usually curative.

Laboratory studies are normal. A large tumor with central cystic change and septation is noted by various radiographic studies (US and CT scan).[110] The cut surface shows multiple cysts separated by solid, pink-tan areas. Abundant myxoid and edematous tissue forms large sheets of with portal areas (with residual bile ducts) "trapped" at the margins. There is a proliferation of cholangiolar units. Numerous vascular structures are present, as is hematopoiesis.

Infantile Hemangioendothelioma

Infantile hemangioendothelioma is a vascular tumor derived from endothelial cells that proliferate and form numerous small channels. The tumor may be solitary or multi-focal within the liver and other organs, such as skin, lung, lymph nodes, and bone. These tumors account for about 12 percent of all childhood hepatic tumors. More than 90 percent are recognized before the age of 6 months. They occur more often in females (63 percent). As the lesions expand and grow in size, vascular flow increases and the young patient may have congestive heart failure. Thrombocytopenia may be pronounced. Hepatic nodules may rupture to produce hemoperitoneum. The presence of cutaneous hemangiomas is a clinical clue to this diagnosis.

Radiographic studies reflect heart failure and hepatomegaly. US may be helpful in tracking the course of these lesions because they usually involute in time. Diffuse or multiple hepatic lesions are common (45 percent). Solitary lesions (55 percent) may be very large (up to 14 cm in diameter), and the right lobe is favored.[111] If multiple nodules are present, their size varies from 5 mm to more than 30 mm. The larger lesions are umbilicated.

Cavernous areas are present in half of the patients, which correlates with the "puddling" noted on angiogram. The unenhanced CT scan shows the lesion as a solitary, well-defined hypoattenuating mass, and some may have calcification. After contrast, the lesion may resemble a hemangioma. The multi-focal type may mimic metastatic tumor and appear as scattered small nodules.[112] The lesions are cold by scintigraphy because no Kupffer cells are present in the nodules. The round, sharply defined nodules may have a red-brown surface or be white-gray in color. A central fibrotic area develops, as does calcification, hemorrhage, and even infarction. The histologic pattern is an orderly proliferation of small vascular channels with no cytologic atypia. Limited tissue examination may provide a challenge to discriminate from mesenchymal hamartoma (for the isolated large lesions).[113] Small bile ducts may be trapped between some of the vascular structures, and hematopoiesis is present. Prognosis of this condition is good if heart failure is managed successfully. In a large series the 6-month survival was 70 percent.[114] Single, large tumors may be resected, and some lesions undergo spontaneous regression. Hepatic artery ligation and embolization are used to promote involution. A rare case may appear to become malignant (angiosarcoma).

Angiomyolipoma

Angiomyolipoma (AML) is a benign tumor comprising a variable mixture of mesenchymal components including adipose tissue (fat), smooth muscle (spindle or epithelioid type) and numerous blood vessels, and sometimes other components such as hematopoietic elements (Plates 45-4, *A* and *B*). These lesions provide considerable confusion with HCC and focal fatty change. First described in the liver by Ishak in 1976, numerous reports of AML followed.[115,116] The tumor is usually solitary, with 60 percent in the right lobe, 30 percent in the left lobe, 20 percent in both lobes, and 8 percent in the caudate lobe.[117] These tumors occur with equal sex incidence and a broad age range (27 to 76 years).[118] This tumor was once considered relatively rare but is discovered more often now because of numerous radiographic procedures of screening. Symptoms include a hepatic mass. Radiographic study reveals a hypervascular lesion. Liver tests often reveal mild elevation in transaminases. Fine needle aspiration may provide limited tissue, including the large epithelioid cells that are readily confused with the plump cells of HCC. Additional tissue may be helpful and demonstrate large, thick-walled vessels and adipose tissue. The tumor is sharply demarcated from the surrounding normal liver and is fleshy and firm with a golden yellow color or firm tan texture. The size range is wide; reported tumors may be small (0.3 to 5 cm) or very large and more than 10 to 36 cm in diameter.[119] These tumors are clonal and belong to a family of lesions characterized by proliferation of a perivascular cell.[120] The multiple histologic components provide a variable pattern from easily classified fatty tumors to complex mixtures with epithelioid large cells that are HMB45 positive.[121]

Solitary Fibrous Tumor

A solitary fibrous tumor is typically found in the pleura, but also occurs in other sites including liver.[122] The tumor is an incidental finding in some; others may experience abdominal fullness related to the large size. There is an equal sex incidence in some series. Others reveal a female predominance. The age range is 16 to 83 years, with an average of about 40 years. Hypoglycemia has been associated with this tumor. Liver tests may be abnormal (such as alkaline phosphatase). The CT scan may reveal a large, solitary tumor. The size range is broad (from 2 to 27 cm in diameter); the weight may be high (up to 3700 g).[123] The tumor is usually on the liver surface. Rarely it is pedunculated. The cut surface is firm white tissue. Adjacent liver is normal. A needle biopsy may be diagnostic, but the highly cellular areas may suggest a sarcoma or malignant change.[124] Although the central portion is densely fibrotic, the periphery has high cellularity. Sarcomatoid carcinoma is considered in the differential diagnosis. Numerous histologic sections and special stains may be necessary to clarify the proper diagnosis. The prognosis is good. Resection is the usual treatment.

Inflammatory Pseudotumor

Many benign, inflammatory conditions produce an inflammatory mass lesion that may lead to biopsy or resection. Furthermore, numerous benign and malignant tumors mimic this condition.[125] In some patients pseudotumors may be the healing phase of hepatic abscess or traumatic injury, but commonly the initiating injury is obscure. These "tumors" are often incidental findings, but they may cause profound symptoms including weight loss, fever, abdominal distension, fatigue, or jaundice. The clinical course can have a long duration (even a few years).[126] The reported patients have a male predominance (3:1) with a broad age range from 10 months to more than 80 years. Confusion with malignant tumors, especially HCC, is noted based on US and angiographic studies. The lesions are typically solitary, and although many are small (2-4 cm), some are as large as 25 cm in diameter. Jaundice may occur if the process is in the porta hepatis. Splenomegaly is reported as well. The histologic appearance is of marked spindle cell proliferation that simulates sarcoma (including leiomyosarcoma), malignant fibrous histiocytoma, and angiosarcoma. Treatment can be with steroids or resection.

Malignant Mesenchymal Hepatic Tumors—Embryonal Sarcoma

Embryonal sarcoma (ES), also called undifferentiated sarcoma and malignant mesenchymoma, accounts for 6 percent to 13 percent of primary hepatic tumors in the pediatric age group. More than 50 percent occur in the age range 6 to 10 years. Patients have been reported from 19 months up to 44 years, but adult patients are rare. Abdominal swelling (and mass) and pain are the usual clinical findings. Extension of tumor into the vena cava and heart occurs. Liver tests are abnormal in less than half of patients. Radiography reveals a large liver mass with cystic areas. A large, well-defined, mixed echogenic mass with multiple small anechoic spaces may be identified by US.[127] The gross appearance is a large multi-cystic and hemorrhagic mass with variable firm white regions at the margins (Plate 45-6, *E*). The microscopic pattern varies considerably, with some edematous regions containing small spindle cells and other highly cellular areas with large pleomorphic multi-nucleated cells. Scattered hyaline globules (PAS positive) within the cytoplasm are a hallmark of this tumor. The adjacent liver is normal and free of chronic liver disease. ES can be resected or subjected to chemotherapy to reduce the size and allow resection. The prognosis has been poor until recently, but chemotherapy and surgery have produced cures.[128]

Angiosarcoma

Angiosarcoma is rare (appearing in less than 1 percent of primary hepatic malignant tumors) but rapidly lethal. This tumor is derived from the sinusoidal lining cells or spindle cells of the small vascular spaces. Associated prior conditions include exposure to vinyl chloride or Thorotrast, but the majority of patients have no known risk factor. Most patients with angiosarcoma have symptoms related to liver involvement because the tumor is large. Some patients have splenomegaly. Rupture of the liver occurs in up to 15 percent of patients. Examination demonstrates a diffuse tumor involving the entire liver and multiple dense nodules (with hemorrhage). Atypical spindle cells line the sinusoids in the surrounding cords of atrophic hepatocytes at the margins of the tumor nodules. Papillary growth is prominent, with large, blood-filled channels. Survival is usually less than 6 months.[129]

Epithelioid Hemangioendothelioma

Epithelioid hemangioendothelioma (EHE), an uncommon (but not rare) tumor, was first described in soft tissue and recently recognized as often arising or metastasizing to the liver. It is easily confused with CC and other hepatic tumors. EHE is derived from an endothelial cell but grows with abundant fibrosis. It usually produces some degree of hepatic impairment. Ishak and colleagues reported 32 patients with hepatic involvement; consequently, so many series have been summarized that by 1996 there were 129 cases in the literature.[130] A single large series of 137 patients was reported in 1998.[131] The tumor produces a spectrum of clinical symptoms. Usually, there is a slowly progressive course that can cause liver failure resulting from gradual replacement of the liver. The age range is broad (12 to 86 years with a mean of 47 years), and there is a mild female predominance. The highest tumor prevalence is in the 30- to 40-year age group. Clinical symptoms are often vague and include weakness, malaise, upper abdominal pain, and hepatosplenomegaly. Some patients develop jaundice, ascites, and the Budd-Chiari syndrome.[132] However, the hepatic tumor is an incidental finding in nearly 40 percent of patients. Laboratory tests reveal elevated transaminases in approximately one third of the patients. Radiographic studies commonly show multiple hepatic calcifications. The CT scan reveals multiple nonhomogenous, hypodense lesions in both lobes (Plate 45-6, *B*). A target lesion may be noted, as may diffuse nodules or isolated surface changes.[133] Occasionally, as the tumor grows and "strangles" the liver, the caudate lobe may hypertrophy.[134] Angiographic studies indicate hypovascular lesions in some patients. The liver has multiple tumor nodules in 80 percent of patients and may be a single large nodule in 20 percent (Plate 45-6, *A*). The portal areas remain intact the longest, with the perivenular (centrolobular regions) undergoing gradual sclerosis. The neoplastic cells are a minor component of the process and are prominent at the edges of the lesions. The neoplastic cells have been classified as epithelioid, dendritic, and intermediate cells. The epithelioid cells are separated by fibrous tissue; the residual bile ducts and cholangiolar proliferation add to the histologic resemblance to CC. The epithelioid cells are also vacuolated and are dramatically CD34-positive (Plates 45-6, *C* and *D*). The histologic diagnosis is challenging because of the high degree of variation in fibrosis and cellularity. The correct histologic diagnosis was submitted with only 25 percent of the cases referred to the AFIP for consultation. CC and angiosarcoma are the main mistaken diagnoses. More than half of the patients have metastatic disease at first diagnosis.[135] The prognosis of the hepatic lesions is difficult to predict. Overall survival is much better, however, than with angiosarcoma. In the large AFIP series, 43 percent of patients survived more than 5 years and one patient remained alive after 27 years even though she had presented with a large liver. The tumor in this one patient seemed to regress spontaneously. Other patients have been well served by hepatic transplantation, even with recognized metastatic disease.[136,137]

LYMPHOMA OF THE LIVER

Lymphoma may be a primary hepatic tumor or metastasize to the liver. Clinical features of primary hepatic lymphoma include mass effect, pain, discomfort, weight loss, and fever. There may be an absence of lymph node enlargement in the rest of the body. The hepatic tumor may be a large solitary mass or multiple masses, especially with a B-cell lymphoma.[138] Diffuse, large B cells account for nearly 60 percent of hepatic lymphoma. Overall, however, secondary involvement of the liver is more common than primary hepatic lymphoma. The presence of hepatic disease is important for staging processes, and two histologic subtypes are associated with hepatic spread: T-cell–rich B-cell lymphoma and histiocyte-rich B-cell lymphoma.[139] Large numbers of non-neoplastic cells, including reactive small T cells and histiocytes, are recruited so that the underlying malignant component of B cells is obscured and challenging to recognize. Confusion with Hodgkin's disease may occur. Another type of hepatic lymphoma is the peripheral T-cell lymphoma with sinusoidal infiltration. This tumor is especially difficult to recognize without special studies and is very aggressive and resistant to therapy.[140]

References

1. Anthony PP, DeMatos P: Secondary tumours of the liver in pathology and genetics of tumours of the digestive system. In Hamilton SR, Aaltonen LA, eds: WHO IARC Lyon 2000.199-202.
2. Jenkins D, Gilmore IT, Doel C, et al: Liver biopsy in the diagnosis of malignancy. Q J Med 88:819-825, 1995.
3. Dent GA, Feldman JM: Pseudocyst liver metastases in patients with carcinoid tumors: report of three cases. Am J Clin Path 82:275-279, 1984.
4. Borja ER, Hori JM, Pugh RP: Metastatic carcinomatosis of the liver mimicking cirrhosis: case report and review of the literature. Cancer 35:445-449, 1975.
5. Luo T, Itai Y, Eguchi N, et al: Von Meyenburg complexes of the liver: imaging findings. J Comp Assoc Tomog 22:372-378, 1998.
6. Leong AS, Sormunen RT, Tsui WM, et al: HepPar 1 and selected antibodies in the immunohistological distinction of hepatocellular carcinoma from cholangiocarcinoma, combined tumours and metastatic carcinoma. Histopathology 33:318-324, 1998.
7. Maeda T, Kajiyama K, Adachi E, et al: The expression of cytokeratins 7, 19 and 20 in primary and metastatic carcinomas of the liver. Mod Pathol 9:901-909, 1998.
8. Fong Y, Fortner J, Sun RL, et al: Clinical score for predicting recurrence after hepatic resection for metastatic colorectal cancer: analysis of 1001 consecutive cases. Ann Surg 230:309-321, 1999.
9. Weber SM, Jarnagin WR, DeMatteo RP, et al: Survival after resection of multiple hepatic colorectal metastases. Ann Surg Oncol 7:643-650, 2000.
10. Karhunen PJ: Benign hepatic tumours and tumour like conditions in men. J Clin Pathol 39:183-188, 1986.
11. Valls C, Lopez E, Guma A, et al: Helical CT versus CT arterial portography in the detection of hepatic metastasis of colorectal carcinoma. AJR 170:1341-1347, 1998.
12. Tsao JI, DeSanctis J, Rossi RL, et al: Hepatic malignancies. Surg Clin North Am 80:603-632, 2000.
13. Paley MR, Ros PR: Hepatic metastasis. Rad Clin North Am 36:349-363, 1998.
14. Yamashita Y, Mitsuzaki K, Yi T, et al: Small hepatocellular carcinoma in patients with chronic liver damage: prospective comparison of detection with dynamic MR imaging and helical CT of the whole liver. Radiology 200:79, 1996.
15. Hiroshashi S, et al: Hepatocellular carcinoma in pathology and genetics of tumours of the digestive system. In Hamilton SR, Aaltonen LA, eds: Lyon, France, IARC, 2000:159-172.
16. Okuda K: Hepatitis C virus and hepatocellular carcinoma. In Okuda K, Tabor E, eds: Liver Cancer. New York, Churchill Livingstone, 1997.
17. El-Serag HB, Mason AC: Rising incidence of hepatocellular carcinoma in the United States. N Engl J Med 340:745-750, 1999.
18. Craig JR, Klatt EC, Yu M: Role of cirrhosis and the development of HCC: evidence from histologic studies and large population studies. In Tabor E, DiBisceglie AM, Purcell RH, eds: Etiology, Pathology, and Treatment of Hepatocellular Carcinoma in North America, vol 13, Advances in Applied Biotechnology Series, Gulf Publishing Co, Houston, 1991:177-189.
19. Aizawa Y, Shibamoto Y, Takagi I, et al: Analysis of factors affecting the appearance of hepatocellular carcinoma in patients with chronic hepatitis c. A long term follow-up study after histologic diagnosis. Cancer 89:53-59, 2000.
20. Tarao K, Rino Y, Ohkawa S, et al: Association between high serum alanine aminotransferase levels and more rapid development and higher rate of incidence of hepatocellular carcinoma in patients with hepatitis c virus-associated cirrhosis. Cancer 86:589-595, 1999.
21. Garcia-Samaniego J, Rodriiquez M, Berenguer J, et al: Hepatocellular carcinoma in HIV-infected patients with chronic hepatitis C. Amer J Gastro 96:179-183, 2001.
22. Yu MC, Yuan J, Ross R, et al: Presence of antibodies to the hepatitis B surface antigen is associated with an excess risk for hepatocellular carcinoma among non-Asians in Los Angeles County, California. Hepatology 25:226-228, 1997.
23. McMahon BJ, Bulkow L, Harpster A, et al: Screening for hepatocellular carcinoma in Alaska Native infected with chronic hepatitis B: a 16 year populated-based study. Hepatology 32:842-846, 2000.
24. Yuen M, Cheng C, Lauder IJ, et al: Early detection of hepatocellular carcinoma increases the chance of treatment: Hong Kong experience. Hepatology 31:330-335, 2000.
25. Zoli M, Magalotti D, Bianchi G, et al: Efficacy of a surveillance program for early detection of hepatocellular carcinoma. Cancer 78:977-985, 1996.
26. Bonis PA, Tong MJ, Blatt LM., et al: A predictive model for the development of hepatocellular carcinoma, liver failure, or liver transplantation for patients presenting to clinic with chronic hepatitis C. Amer J Gastroenterol 94:1605-1612, 1999.
27. Rimal N, Ikeda S, Taketa K, et al: Mass screening for early detection of hepatocellular carcinoma by setting a high-risk population with alpha-fetoprotein and its glycoforms. Hepatol Res 19:9-19, 1997.
28. Okuda H, Obata H, Nakanishi T, et al: Production of abnormal prothrombin (des-gamma-carboxy prothrombin) by hepatocellular carcinoma: a clinical study. J Hepatol 4:347-363, 1987.
29. Okuda H, Nakanishi T, Takatsu K, et al: Measurement of serum levels of des-γ-carboxy prothrombin in patients with hepatocellular carcinoma by a revised immunoassay kit with increased sensitivity. Cancer 85:812-818, 1999.
30. Ishii M, Gama H, Chida N, et al: Simultaneous measurements of serum α-fetoprotein and protein induced by vitamin k absence for detecting hepatocellular carcinoma. Amer J Gastroenterol 95:1036-1040, 2000.
31. Koike Y, Shiratori Y, Sato S., et al: Des-λ-carboxy prothrombin as a useful predisposing factor for the development of portal venous invasion in patients with hepatocellular carcinoma. Cancer 91:561-560, 2001.
32. Matsumura M, Shiratori Y, Niwa Y, et al: Presence of α-fetoprotein mRNA in blood correlates with outcome in patients with hepatocellular carcinoma. J Hepatol 31:332-339, 1999.
33. Shimizu S, Takayama T, Kosuge T, et al: Benign tumors of the liver resected because of a diagnosis of malignancy. Surg Gynecol Obstet 174:403-407, 1992.

34. Kudo M: Ultrasound. In Okuda K, Tabor E, eds: Liver Cancer. New York, Churchill Livingstone, 1997:331-346.
35. Craig JR, Peters RL, Edmondson HA: Hepatocellular carcinoma. In Atlas of Tumor Pathology, second series, fascicle 26, Tumor of the Liver and Intrahepatic Bile Ducts. Washington, DC, AFIP, 1989: 123-189.
36. Kenmochi K, Sugihara S, Kojiro M: Relationship of histologic grade of hepatocellular carcinoma (HCC) to tumor size, and demonstration of tumor cells of multiple different grades in single small HCC. Liver 7:18-26, 1987.
37. Sakamoto M, Hirohashi S, Tsuda H, et al: Multicentric independent development of hepatocellular carcinoma revealed by analysis of hepatitis virus integration pattern. Am J Surg Pathol 13:1064-1067, 1989.
38. Chapel F, Guettier C, Chastang C, et al: Needle biopsy of hepatocellular carcinoma. Assessment of prognostic contribution of histologic parameters including proliferating cell nuclear antigen labeling and correlations with clinical outcomes. Cancer 77:864-871, 1996.
39. Okuda K, Peters RL, Simson IW: Gross Anatomic features of hepatocellular carcinoma from three disparate geographic areas: proposal of a new classification. Cancer 54:2165-2173, 1984.
40. Ruby SG: Protocol for examination of specimens from patients with hepatocellular carcinoma, and cholangiocarcinoma, including intrahepatic bile ducts. Cancer Committee of the College of American Pathologists Arch Pathol Lab Med 124:41-45, 2000.
41. Okuda K, Ohtsuki T, Obata H, et al: Natural history of hepatocellular carcinoma and prognosis in relation to treatment. Cancer 56:918-928, 1985.
42. Cancer of the Liver Italian Program (CLIP) Investigators: a new prognostic system for hepatocellular carcinoma: a retrospective study of 435 patients. Hepatology 28:751-755, 1998.
43. Cancer of the Liver Italian Program (CLIP) Investigators: Prospective validation of the CLIP score: a new prognostic system for patients with cirrhosis and hepatocellular carcinoma. Hepatology 31:840-845, 2000.
44. Nzeako U, Goodman ZG, Ishak KG: Hepatocellular carcinoma in cirrhotic and noncirrhotic livers. A clinico-histopathologic study of 804 North American patients. Am J Clin Pathol 105:65-75, 1996.
45. Katyal S, Oliver JH, Peterson MS, et al: Extrahepatic metastases of hepatocellular carcinoma. Radiology 216:698-703, 2000.
46. Craig JR: Fibrolamellar carcinoma. In Okuda K, Tabor E, eds: Liver Cancer. New York, Churchill Livingstone, 1997:255-262.
47. McLarney JK, Rucker PT, Bender GN, et al: Fibrolamellar carcinoma of the liver: radiologic-pathologic correlation. Radiographics 19:453-471, 1999.
48. Ichikawa T, Federle MP, Grazioli L, et al: Fibrolamellar hepatocellular carcinoma: imaging and pathologic findings in 31 recent cases. Radiology 213:352-361, 1999.
49. Pinna AD, Iwatsuki S, Lee RG, et al: Treatment of fibrolamellar hepatoma with subtotal hepatectomy or transplantation. Hepatology 26:877-883, 1997.
50. Stevens WR, Johnson CD, Stephens DH, et al: Fibrolamellar hepatocellular carcinoma: stage at presentation and results of aggressive surgical management. AJR 164:1153-1158, 1995.
51. Nakeeb A, Pitt HA, Sohn TA, et al: Cholangiocarcinoma: a spectrum of intrahepatic, perihilar, and distal tumors. Ann Surg 224:463-475, 1996.
52. Klatskin G: Adenocarcinoma of the hepatic duct at its bifurctation within the porta hepatis: an unusual tumor with distinctive clinical and pathological features. Am J Med 38:241-256, 1965.
53. Van Leeuwen DJ, Huibregtse K, Tytgat GNJ: Carcinoma of the hepatic confluence 25 years after Klatskin's description: diagnosis and endoscopic management. Semin Liver Dis 10:102-113, 1990.
54. Yoon KH, Ha HK, Kim CG, et al: Malignant papillary neoplasms of the intrahepatic bile ducts: CT and histologic features. AJR 175:1135-1139, 2000.
55. Parkin DM, Ohshima H, Srivatanakul P, et al: Cholangiocarcinoma: epidemiology, mechanisms of carcinogenesis and prevention. Cancer Epidemiol Biomarkers Prev 2:537-544, 1993.
56. Chu K, Lai ECS, Al-Hadeedi S, et al: Intrahepatic cholangiocarcinoma. World J Surg 21:301-306, 1997.
57. Nashan B, Schlitt HJ, Tusch G, et al: Biliary malignancies in primary sclerosing cholangitis: timing for liver transplantation. Hepatology 23:1105-1111, 1996.
58. Bergquist A, Glaumann H, Persson B, et al: Risk factors and clinical presentation of hepatobiliary carcinoma in patients with primary sclerosing cholangitis: a case-control study. Hepatology 27:311-316, 1998.
59. Ohta T, Nagakawa T, Ueda N, et al: Mucosal dysplasia of the liver and the intraductal variant of peripheral cholangiocarcinoma in hepatolithiasis. Cancer 68:2217-2223, 1991.
60. Nichols JC, Gores GJ, LaRusso NF, et al: Diagnostic role of serum CA 19-9 for cholangiocarcinoma in patients with primary sclerosing cholangitis. Mayo Clin Proc 68:874-879, 1993.
61. Kim K, Choi J, Park Y, et al: Biliary cystadenoma of the liver. J Hepatol Pancreat Surg 5:348-352, 1998.
62. Ramage J, Donaghy A, Farrant JM, et al: Serum tumor markers for the diagnosis of cholangiocarcinoma in primary sclerosing cholangitis. Gastroenterology 108:865-869, 1995.
63. Keiding S, Hansen S, Rasmussen HH, et al: Detection of cholangiocarcinoma in primary sclerosing cholangitis by positron emission tomography. Hepatology 28:700-706, 1998.
64. Van Leeuwen DJ: The imager replacing the pathologist in the diagnosis of hepatobiliary and pancreatic disease. Ann Diagn Pathol 5:57-66, 2001.
65. Bismuth H, Corlette MB: Intrahepatic cholangioenteric anastomosis in carcinoma of the hilus of the liver. Surg Obstet Gynecol 140:170-176, 1995.
66. Choi BE, Park JH, Kim YI, et al: Peripheral cholangiocarcinoma and clonorchiasis: CT findings. Radiology 169:149-153, 1988.
67. Nozaki Y, Yamamoto M, Ikai I, et al: Reconsideration of the lymph node metastasis pattern (n factor) from intrahepatic cholangiocarcinoma using the international union against cancer TNM staging system for primary liver carcinoma. Cancer 83:1923-1929, 1998.
68. Nakajima T, Tajima Y, Sugano I, et al: Intrahepatic cholangiocarcinoma with sarcomatous change. Clinicopathologic and immunohistochemical evaluation of seven cases. Cancer 72:1872-1877, 1993.
69. Sasaki M, Nakanuma Y, Shimizu K, et al: Pathological and immunohistochemical findings in a case of mucinous cholangiocarcinoma. Pathol Int 45:781-786, 1995.
70. Rullier A, LeBail B, Fawaz R, et al: Cytokeratin 7 and 20 expression in cholangiocarcinomas varies along the biliary tract but still differs from that in colorectal carcinoma metastasis. Am J Surg Pathol 24:870-876, 2000.
71. Haratake J, Hashimoto H: An immunohistochemical analysis of 13 cases with combined hepatocellular and cholangiocellular carcinoma. Liver 15:9-15, 1995.
72. Allaire GS, Rabin L, Ishak KG, et al: Bile duct adenoma. A study of 152 cases. Am J Surg Pathol 12:708-715, 1977.
73. Eisenberg D, Hurwitz L, Yu AC: CT and sonography of multiple bile duct hamartomas simulating malignant liver disease (case report). AJR 147:279-280, 1986.
74. Goodman ZD, Ishak KG, Langloss JM, et al: Combined hepatocellular-cholangiocarcinoma. A histologic and immunohistochemical study. Cancer 55:124-135, 1985.
75. Aoki K, Takayasu K, Kawano T, et al: Combined hepatocellular carcinoma and cholangiocarcinoma: clinical features and computed tomographic findings. Hepatology 18:1090-1095, 1993.
76. Bagia S, Hewitt PM, Morris DL: Anabolic steroid-induced hepatic adenomas with spontaneous haemorrhage in a bodybuilder. Aust NZ J Surg 70:686-687, 2000.
77. Herman P, Pugliese V, Machado MAC, et al: Hepatic adenoma and focal nodular hyperplasia: differential diagnosis and treatment. World J Surg 24:372-376, 2000.
78. Wanless IR, Albrecht S, Bilbao J, et al: Multiple focal nodular hyperplasia of the liver associated with vascular malformations of various organs and neoplasia of the brain: a new syndrome. Mod Pathol 2:456-462, 1989.
79. Buetow PC, Pantongrag-Brown L, Buck JL, et al: Focal nodular hyperplasia of the liver: radiologic-pathologic correlation. Radiographics 16:369-388, 1996.
80. Choi CS, Freeny PC: Triphasic helical CT of hepatic focal nodular hyperplasia: incidence of atypical findings. AJR 170:391-395, 1998.
81. Closset J, Veys I, Peny MO, et al: Retrospective analysis of 29 patients surgically treated for hepatocellular adenoma or focal nodular hyperplasia. Hepatogastroenterology 47:1382-1384, 2000.
82. Wanless IR: Micronodular transformation (nodular regenerative hyperplasia) of the liver: a report of 64 cases among 2,500 autop-

sies and a new classification of benign hepatocellular nodules. Hepatology 11:787-797, 1990.
83. Rabinowitz J, Kinkabwala M, Ulreich S: Macro-regenerating nodule in the cirrhotic liver. Am J Roentgenol Radium Ther Nucl Med 121:401-411, 1974.
84. Anonymous: Terminology of nodular hepatocellular lesions. International Working Party. Hepatology 22:983-993, 1995.
85. Arawaki M, Kage M, Sugihara S, et al: Emergence of malignant lesions within an adenomatous hyperplastic nodule in a cirrhotic liver. Observations in five cases. Gastroenterology 91:198-208, 1986.
86. Ferrell LD, Crawford JM, Dhillon AP, et al: Proposal for standardized criteria for the diagnosis of benign, borderline, and malignant hepatocellular lesions arising in chronic advanced liver disease. Am J Surg Pathol 17:1113-1123, 1993.
87. Theise ND: Macroregenerative (dysplastic) nodules and hepatocarcinogenesis: theoretical and clinical considerations. Semin Liver Dis 15:360-371, 1995.
88. Tsuda H, Hirohashi S, Shimosato Y, et al: Clonal origin of atypical adenomatous hyperplasia of the liver and clonal identity with hepatocellular carcinoma. Gastroenterology 95:1664-1666, 1988.
89. Eguchi A, Nakashima O, Okudaira S, et al: Adenomatous hyperplasia in the vicinity of small hepatocellular carcinoma. Hepatology 15:843-848, 1992.
90. Kudo M: Imaging diagnosis of hepatocellular carcinoma and premalignant/borderline lesions. Semin Liver Dis 19:297-309, 1999.
91. Shimada M, Takenaka K, Gion T, et al: Treatment strategy for patients with cystic lesions mimicking a liver tumor. Arch Surg 133:643-646, 1998.
92. Madariaga JR, Iwatsuki S, Starzl TE, et al: Hepatic resection for cystic lesions of the liver. Ann Surg 218:610-614, 1993.
93. Wheeler DA, Edmondson HA: Cystadenoma with mesenchymal stroma (CMS) in the liver and bile ducts. Cancer 56:1434-1445, 1985.
94. Joseph J, Martinet O, Prella M, et al: Malignant Transformation of a liver cystadenoma. Surg Rounds 23:522-526, 2000.
95. Devaney K, Goodman ZD, Ishak KG: Hepatobiliary cystadenoma and cystadenocarcinoma. A light microscopic and immunohistochemical study of 70 patients. Am J Surg Pathol 18:1078-1091, 1994.
96. Young RH, Scully RE: Ovarian metastases from carcinoma of the gallbladder and extrahepatic bile ducts simulating primary tumors of the ovary. A report of 6 cases. Int J Gynecol Pathol 9:60-72, 1990.
97. Stocker JT, Conran RM: Hepatoblastoma. In Okuda K, Tabor E, eds: Liver Cancer. New York, Churchill Livingstone, 1997:263-278.
98. Stocker JT, Schmidt D: Hepatoblastoma in pathology and genetics of tumours of the digestive system. In Hamilton SR, Aaltonen LA, eds: Lyon, France, IARC Press, 2000:184-189.
99. Karhunen PJ: Benign hepatic tumors and tumor-like conditions in men. J Clin Pathol 39:183-188, 1986.
100. Ginsberg F, Slavin JD, Spencer RP: Hepatic angiosarcoma: mimicking of angioma on three-phase technetium-99 red blood cell scintigraphy. J Nucl Med 27:1861-1863, 1986.
101. Perkins AB, Iman K, Smith WJ, et al: Color and power doppler sonography of liver hemangiomas: a dream unfulfilled? J Clin Ultrasound 28:159-165, 2000.
102. Vilgran V, Boulos L, Vullierme MP, et al: Imaging of atypical hemangiomas of the liver with pathologic correlation. Radiographics 20:379-397, 2000.
103. Hanafusa K, Ohashi I, Himeno Y, et al: Hepatic hemangioma: findings with two-phase CT. Radiology 196:465-469, 1995.
104. Avva R, Shah HR, Angtuaco TL: US case of the day. Radiographics 19:1689-1691, 1999.
105. About I, Capdeville J, Bernard P, et al: Hémangiome hépatique géant non-résectable et syndrome de Kasabach-Merritt. Rev Med Interne 15:846-850, 1994.
106. Tung GA, Vaccaro JP, Cronan JJ, et al: Cavernous hemangioma of the liver: pathologic correlation with high field MR imaging. AJR 162:1113-1117, 1994.
107. Mungovan JA, Cronan JJ, Vacarro J: Hepatic cavernous hemangiomas: lack of enlargement over time. Radiology 191:111-113, 1994.
108. Cronan JJ, Esparza AR, Dorfman GS, et al: Cavernous hemangioma of the liver: role of percutaneous biopsy. Radiology 166:135-138, 1988.
109. Ozden J, Emre A, Alper A, et al: Long-term results of surgery for liver hemangiomas. Arch Surg 135:978-981, 2000.
110. DeMaioribus CA, Lally KP, Sim K, et al: Mesenchymal hamartoma of the liver. A 35 year review. Arch Surg 125:598-600, 1990.
111. Ishak KG, Anthony PP, Niederau C, et al: Mesenchymal tumours of the liver. In Hamilton SR, Aaltonen LA, eds: Pathology and Genetics of Tumors of the Digestive System. Lyon, France, IARC, 2000:191-198.
112. Keslar P, Buck J, Selby D: Infantile hemangioendothelioma of the liver revisited. Radiographics 13:657-670, 1993.
113. Craig JR, Peters RL, Edmondson HA: Infantile hemangioendothelioma. In Hartmann WH, ed: Tumors of the Liver and Intrahepatic Bile Ducts. Atlas of Tumor Pathology, second series, vol 26. Washington, DC, AFIP, 1989:75-82.
114. Selby DM, Stocker JT, Waclawiw MA, et al: Infantile hemangioendothelioma of the liver. Hepatology 20:39-45, 1994.
115. Ishak KG: Mesenchymal tumor of the liver. In Okuda K, Peters RL, eds: Hepatocellular Carcinoma. New York, John Wiley & Sons, 1976:247-304.
116. Pounder DJ: Hepatic angiomyolipoma. Am J Surg Pathol 6:677-681, 1982;
117. Nonomura A, Mizukami Y, Kodaya N: Angiomyolipoma of the liver. J Gastroenterol 29:95-105, 1994.
118. Sajima S, Kinoshite H, Okuda K, et al: Angiomyolipoma of the liver. A case report and review of 48 cases reported in Japan. Kurume Med J 46:127-131, 1999.
119. Hoffman AL, Emre S, Verham RP, et al: Hepatic angiomyolipoma: two case reports of caudate based lesions and review of the literature. Liver Transplant Surg 3:16-53, 1997.
120. Zamboni G, Pea M, Martignoni G, et al: Clear cell "sugar" tumor of the pancreas. a novel member of the family of lesions characterized by the presence of perivascular epithelioid cells. Am J Surg Pathol 20:722-730, 1996.
121. Tsui WMS, Yuen AKT, Ma KF, et al: Hepatic angiomyolipomas with a deceptive trabecular pattern and HMB 45 reactivity. Histopathology 21:569-573, 1992.
122. Moran CA, Ishak KG, Goodman ZD: Solitary fibrous tumor of the liver: a clinicopathologic and immunohistochemical study of nine cases. Ann Diagn Pathol 2:19-24, 1998.
123. Bejarno PA, Blanco R, Hanto DW: Solitary fibrous tumor of the liver. a case report, review of the literature and differential diagnosis of spindle cells lesions of the liver. Intern J Surg Pathol 6:93-100, 1998.
124. Fuksbrunner MS, Klimstra D, Panicek DM: Solitary fibrous tumor of the liver: imaging findings. AJR 175:1683-1687, 2000.
125. Craig JR: Pseudoneoplastic lesions of the liver and biliary tree. In Wick MR, Humphrey PA, Ritter JH, eds: Pathology of Pseudoneoplastic Lesions. Philadelphia, Lippincott-Raven, 1997:151-174.
126. Shek TWH, Ng IOL, Chan KW: Inflammatory pseudotumor of the liver. Report of four cases and review of the literature. Am J Surg Pathol 17:231-238, 1993.
127. Moon WK, Kim WS, Kim IO, et al: Undifferentiated embryonal sarcoma of the liver: US and CT findings. Pediatr Radiol 24:500-503, 1994.
128. Urban CE, Mache CJ, Schwinger W, et al: Undifferentiated (embryonal) sarcoma of the liver in childhood. Successful combined modality therapy in four patients. Cancer 72:2511-2516, 1993.
129. Ishak KG: Malignant mesenchymal tumors and some other nonhepatocellular tumors of the liver. In Okuda K, Tabor E, eds: Liver Cancer. New York, Churchill Livingstone, 1997:291-314.
130. Ishak KG, Sesterhenn IA, Goodman ZD, et al: Epithelioid hemangioendothelioma of the liver; a clinicopathologic and follow-up study of 32 cases. Human Pathol 15:839-852, 1984.
131. Makhlouf HR, Ishak KG, Goodman ZD: Epithelioid hemangioendothelioma of the liver. a clinicopathologic study of 137 cases. Cancer 85:562-582, 1999.
132. Walsh MM, Hytiroglou P, Thung SN, et al: Epithelioid hemangioendothelioma of the liver mimicking Budd-Chiari syndrome. Arch Pathol Lab Med 122:846-848, 1998.
133. Ros LH, Fernandez L, Villacampa VM, et al: Epithelioid hemangioendothelioma of the liver—characteristics on magnetic resonance imaging: case report. Can Assoc Radiol J 50:387-389, 1999.
134. Radin GR, Craig JR, Colletti PM, et al: Hepatic epithelioid hemangioendothelioma. Radiology 169:145-148, 1988.

135. Ben-Haim M, Roayaie S, Ye MQ, et al: Hepatic epithelioid hemangioendothelioma: resection or transplantation, which and when? Liver Transplant Surg 5:526-531, 1999.
136. Marino IR, Todo S, Tzakis AG, et al: Treatment of hepatic epithelioid hemangioendothelioma with liver transplantation. Cancer 62: 2079-2084, 1988.
137. Madariaga JR, Marino IR, Karavias DD, et al: Long-term results after liver transplantation for primary hepatic epithelioid hemangioendothelioma. Ann Surg Oncol 2:483-487, 1995.
138. Lei KI: Primary non-Hodgkin's lymphoma of the liver. Leuk Lymphoma 29:293-299, 1998.
139. Dargent JL, De Wolf-Peeters C: Liver involvement by lymphoma: identification of a distinctive pattern of infiltration related to T-cell/histiocyte-rich B-cell lymphoma. Ann Diagn Pathol 2:363-369, 1998.
140. Farcet JP, Gaulard P, Marolleau JP, et al: Hepatosplenic T cell lymphoma: sinusal/sinusoidal localization of malignant cells expressing the T cell receptor gammadelta. Blood 75:2213-2219, 1990.
141. Iwatsuki S, Starzl T: Personal experience with 411 hepatic resections. Ann Surg 208:411-434, 1988.

CHAPTER

46

Surgical Therapy of Hepatic Tumors

Charles A. Staley, MD

BENIGN LIVER TUMORS

Cavernous Hemangioma

Hepatic hemangiomas are the most common benign liver tumor, with an overall autopsy incidence of approximately 7 percent. They have a uniform geographic distribution worldwide and are seen predominantly in women in their third, fourth, and fifth decades of life. Most of these tumors are found incidentally at laparotomy or on sophisticated diagnostic imaging studies during evaluations for other intra-abdominal pathology. Because of the increasing use of these imaging studies, more hemangiomas are being identified. During the period from 1960 to 1980, 122 patients were found with cavernous hemangiomas of the liver, whereas from 1980 to 1986, 245 patients were found to have hemangiomas.[1]

There are no clearly defined risk factors for the development of a hepatic hemangioma. There are reports of cavernous hemangiomas enlarging during pregnancy.[2-4] Although these reports are anecdotal the possibility of an undefined role of female sex hormones in the development of hepatic hemangiomas must be considered. There are no well-documented reports of malignant transformation.

Most patients with cavernous hepatic hemangiomas are asymptomatic, and their lesions are found during a work-up for unrelated abdominal complaints or at the time of laparotomy. The majority of patients are females ranging in age from 30 to 50 years old. The hemangiomas are usually solitary lesions, but can be multiple in 10 percent of cases. There is no predilection for either lobe of the liver. Most hemangiomas are less than 2 cm; however, in some cases they can replace one entire lobe and occasionally occupy the greater part of the liver.[5] Symptoms from a hemangioma are generally associated with larger lesions. In a study from the Mayo Clinic, patients with a hemangioma smaller than 4 cm or 4 to 10 cm had symptoms in 14 percent and 15 percent of cases, respectively.[1] However, patients with lesions larger than 10 cm had symptoms 90 percent of the time.[1] Symptoms, when present, are often non-specific but can include right upper quadrant abdominal pain, abdominal fullness, early satiety, nausea, vomiting, fever, or right-sided flank or back pain. Pain is most likely related to stretching and inflammation of Glisson's capsule. Physical examination is usually unremarkable unless a palpable liver mass is encountered. Thrombocytopenia and hypofibrinogenemia are occasionally associated with hemangiomas of the liver, probably related to the consumption of coagulation factors by active thrombosis.[6] Natural history studies have demonstrated that most hemangiomas do not change their size over time. Trastek and colleagues from the Mayo Clinic followed 36 patients with large cavernous hemangiomas for a mean of 5.5 years.[4] During this period there were no instances of death or progression of symptomatic hemangioma. Furthermore, no patient required surgical resection. Spontaneous rupture of cavernous hemangiomas is very rare. In multiple studies after large asymptomatic hemangiomas, the incidence of spontaneous rupture was 1.2 percent.[7] Most cases of hemorrhage from hemangiomas are iatrogenic from ill-advised attempts at needle biopsy.

Hemangiomas on an unenhanced computed tomography (CT) scan appear as a hypodense, well-marginated mass that may have central areas of markedly decreased attenuation that correspond to the areas of fibrosis and cystic change seen grossly.[8] CT imaging with rapid-sequence bolus contrast injection shows characteristic early peripheral enhancement with homogenous filling of the entire lesion on delayed scans. This classic appearance is well seen in larger hemangiomas (larger than 3 cm), but may be non-diagnostic or only suggestive of a hemangioma in lesions less than 3 cm.[6] In these cases, magnetic resonance imaging (MRI) or radionuclide scanning with technetium (Tc)-labeled red blood cells can provide confirmatory information.[6] At MRI, hemangiomas usually appear hypodense and well defined on T1-weighted images and demonstrate a marked hyperintensity that increases with echo time on T2-weighted images. After injection of intravenous gadopentetate dimeglumine, a hemangioma demonstrates the same characteristic enhancement as is seen on CT imaging.[9] Published series have reported a sensitivity of 90 percent to 100 percent with a specificity approaching 90 percent in the diagnosis of hemangioma with MRI.[6] A ^{99}Tc pertechnetate-labeled red blood cell scan demonstrates a characteristic appearance of a hemangioma. The hemangioma appears as a defect in early phases of scanning and produces a late accumulation of the radionuclide. These findings differ from those in other liver lesions such as a hepatocellular adenoma, focal nodular hyperplasia, hepatoma, and hypervascular liver metastases, all of which usually have early accumulation of radionuclide. Because of the limitations of planar nuclear radiology, a red blood cell scan may have difficulty imaging small hemangiomas (<3 cm) similar to CT imaging, though the specificity is nearly 100 percent.[6] The addition of single-photon emission computed tomography (SPECT) to traditional planar nuclear radiology imaging increases the sensitivity for detecting smaller hemangiomas. SPECT is able to detect lesions as small as 1.3 cm.[10]

Because most hepatic hemangiomas (1) are asymptomatic, (2) rarely enlarge in size or rupture, and (3) have no malignant potential, operative intervention is rarely indicated. However, it is important to confirm the diagnosis through diagnostic studies such as CT scan, MRI, or blood pool studies with erythrocytes labeled with ^{99}Tc. After the diagnosis is confirmed, no further follow-up studies are needed unless the patient develops symptoms. Metastatic or primary liver tumors must be excluded. In typical appearing lesions, biopsy is not warranted because of the risk of bleeding. For those patients with symptoms attributable to large hemangiomas, segmental resection, formal lobectomy, or enucleation should be performed. Because hemangiomas are expansive and not invasive, there is a fibrous cleavage plane of compressed liver between the tumor and normal liver parenchyma that can be used to facilitate tumor enucleation.[6] This technique allows for sparing of normal liver parenchyma and major vessels, thereby decreasing operative blood loss.

Focal Nodular Hyperplasia

Focal nodular hyperplasia (FNH) is the second most common benign neoplasm of the liver after hemangioma and appears in all ages and in both sexes. More than 90 percent of patients with FNH are women in their second through fourth decades of life. Patients with FNH on oral contraceptives have had relatively larger and more symptomatic tumors compared with those not taking oral contraceptives.[11] This observation would support a trophic effect of oral contraceptives, but these are not thought to be a risk factor for the development of FNH.

The etiology of FNH is unknown but may develop from a vascular malformation in the liver. This theory is supported by a study showing that there is a single artery supplying the tumor in FNH but no associated portal vein or bile duct. There is also an association of FNH with other vascular anomalies. Twenty-three percent of patients with FNH have an associated hepatic hemangioma.[12]

Similar to patients with hemangiomas, the majority of patients with FNH are asymptomatic and are found incidentally at the time of laparotomy or on diagnostic imaging studies looking for other pathology. In approximately 10 percent to 20 percent of cases FNH may produce symptoms ranging from frank abdominal pain to mild discomfort.[8] In most cases FNH is a single tumor of variable size but usually less than 5 cm in diameter. A large palpable mass representing FNH can occasionally be seen clinically. FNH appears more often in the right lobe of the liver and classically is found as a pedunculated mass on the surface.[13] Although FNH is highly vascular, spontaneous hemorrhage is extremely rare. There have been no reports of malignant transformation in FNH.[9] Although there does not appear to be a direct correlation between oral contraceptives and FNH, there is a relative increase in associated symptoms in women on hormone therapy.[6] The most characteristic feature of FNH is the central, stellate fibrovascular zone representing a central scar, which is seen on CT scan imaging in the majority of cases.[13]

On unenhanced CT scans, FNH frequently appears as a hypodense lesion that then becomes isodense with the rest of the liver when intravenous contrast is administered.[8] This emphasizes the importance of performing both a contrast and non-contrast scan. If only a contrast scan is done, a mass may not be detected because the area of FNH will appear isodense with the surrounding normal liver. Classically, a central, hypodense, irregular zone can be seen that corresponds to the central fibrotic scar typical for FNH in about 60 percent of patients.[14] At MRI, FNH tumors usually appear isodense in T1-weighted and T2-weighted images with a hyperintense central scar on high T2 sequences.[15] After injection of intravenous gadopentetate dimeglumine, FNH demonstrates early arterial enhancement in the mass followed by late enhancement within the scar. Cherqui and colleagues found that MRI detected a central scar better than CT imaging (78 percent versus 60 percent).[14] However, Vilgrain and colleagues found a typical MRI appearance in only 43 percent of patients with FNH.[16] Furthermore, the typical central scar seen in FNH has also been seen in 60 percent of primary hepatocellular tumors, thereby challenging the role of MRI in the accurate diagnosis of FNH.[17] ^{99}Tc sulfur colloid scintigraphy is indicated as a confirmatory study after a CT scan or MRI suspects a FNH but does not have the classic CT/MRI characteristics. Despite the presence of Kupffer cells within these lesions, only about 60 percent to 70 percent of FNH lesions will demonstrate increased uptake on a sulfur colloid scan. However, when present, this increased uptake is diagnostic of FNH.[6] Weimann and colleagues reported that the combination of a sulfur colloid scan and a CT scan made the correct diagnosis of FNH in 82 of 92 (89.1 percent) patients.[17]

Because most FNH tumors are asymptomatic and rarely enlarge in size, operative intervention is rarely indicated. However, it is important to confirm the diagnosis through diagnostic studies such as CT scan, MRI, or ^{99}Tc sulfur colloid scintigraphy. After the diagnosis is confirmed, no further follow-up studies are needed unless the patient develops symptoms. Metastatic or primary liver tumors must be excluded. Biopsy is not warranted for lesions that have a typical appearance because of the risk of bleeding. For those patients with symptoms attributable to large FNH tumors, segmental resection or formal lobectomy should be performed. Atypical or equivocal lesions should have a laparoscopic or surgical biopsy when lesions are large or wedge excisional biopsy for smaller lesions. Because FNH tumors tend to be small (less than 5 cm), many can be resected with a wedge or segmental excision.

Most important, the clinician must be confident about the diagnosis of FNH. The combination of ultrasound, CT scan, and scintigraphy has been able to diagnose FNH with an accuracy of 90 percent.[17]

Hepatic Adenoma

Hepatic adenomas were extremely rare tumors before 1960. With the widespread use of oral contraceptives, however, the incidence of hepatic adenomas has increased dramatically.[1] Not surprisingly, therefore, the majority of these tumors occur in young women taking oral contraceptives. The use of oral contraceptives has been clearly linked to the increased incidence of hepatic adenomas. The incidence of hepatic adenomas seems to be proportional to the duration of oral contraceptive usage, drug dosage, and age over 30.[1] For example, the risk of developing a hepatic adenoma increases steadily with the duration of oral contraceptive use to about 500-fold for 85 or more months of consumption.[8] Approximately 60 percent of patients with type Ia glycogen storage disease develop hepatic adenoma.[12] Males taking androgenic steroids are also at risk for development of hepatic adenomas.

Hepatic adenomas are characterized by hepatocellular proliferation in the appearance of a well-circumscribed and encapsulated tumor.[15] Interestingly, compared with normal liver, hepatic adenomas do not contain a portal tract or bile ducts. It seems as if hepatic adenomas are a relatively pure growth of hepatocytes to the near exclusion of other cellular elements.[1]

Unlike hemangiomas and FNH tumors, the majority of patients with hepatic adenomas are symptomatic and more specifically complain of right upper quadrant pain. A smaller percentage of adenomas are found incidentally at the time of laparotomy or on diagnostic radiology studies looking for other pathology. Approximately one third of patients present with acute onset of abdominal pain or hepatomegaly resulting from spontaneous hemorrhage.[8] Multiple adenomas are found in 10 percent to 20 percent of patients. Adenoma regression with the discontinuation of oral contraceptives has been described; however, this is unpredictable and progression in some patients may still occur. Unlike other benign liver tumors, adenomas can undergo malignant transformation.[19]

On unenhanced CT scans, hepatic adenomas frequently appear as well-defined focal areas of low attenuation.[8] Areas of intratumoral hemorrhage will appear as high-density areas. With intravenous contrast the adenomas appear as complex lesions with areas of normal, increased, and decreased density within them. These typical findings occur in 75 percent of patients with hepatic adenomas.[20] ^{99}Tc sulfur colloid scintigraphy is indicated as a confirming study after a CT scan is suspicious for hepatic adenoma but does not have the classic CT imaging characteristics. Because hepatic adenomas consist of pure hepatocytes and no Kupffer cells, sulfur colloid scans will usually show no uptake of radioactive ^{99}Tc.[18] This differentiates adenomas from FNH, which usually shows normal or increased uptake. On MRI, hepatic adenomas appear as hyperintense heterogenous masses. A peripheral rim is seen in 30 percent of patients.[20] Overall, MRI of hepatic adenomas has a sensitivity of 75 percent and a specificity of 100 percent.

In typical appearing adenomas, biopsy is not warranted because of the risk of bleeding and sample error for detecting malignant transformation. For atypical lesions open surgical biopsy with frozen section analysis can accurately distinguish adenoma from FNH.[14] Because most hepatic adenomas are symptomatic and have the propensity to bleed acutely or transform into a malignant cancer, operative resection is indicated for all solitary adenomas. This recommendation is based on the significant risk of bleeding (30 to 50 percent) and malignant transformation.[18] Discontinuation of oral contraceptives can cause regression of the adenoma, but this clinical course is fairly unpredictable. Patients with multiple adenomas that would require a risky liver resection should undergo careful observation with follow-up imaging scans and alpha-fetoprotein (AFP) levels. Patients with intraperitoneal bleeding from a hepatic adenoma pose a difficult management issue. Preoperative hepatic artery embolization can be helpful, followed by resection when hemodynamically stable. Patients with acute exsanguination, who are too unstable for hepatic resection, may benefit from appropriate temporizing measures that include hepatic artery ligation or packing.

Biliary Cystic Tumors

Biliary cystadenomas are rare cystic, multi-loculated, benign tumors of biliary origin. They are extremely rare and make up less than 5 percent of intrahepatic cysts.[21] They occur predominantly in females, with a peak incidence in the fifth decade. There are no known risk factors. No association with oral contraceptives has been documented.[22]

The histologic similarity to embryonic gallbladder and large bile ducts, derivatives of the foregut, suggests that biliary cystadenomas develop from ectopic rests of this primitive tissue. Cystadenomas have a well-defined thick capsule and microscopically have cuboidal epithelium.[21]

Many patients are asymptomatic, except for an increase in abdominal girth or the presence of a palpable mass.[21] Symptomatic patients can present with right upper quadrant pain, nausea, early satiety, or jaundice. Cystadenomas range in size from 1 to 35 cm. Eighty-seven percent are intrahepatic in location.[21] Of the intrahepatic cystadenomas 50 percent are in the right lobe, 29 percent in the left lobe, and 16 percent in both lobes.[22] Differential diagnosis includes congenital hepatic cysts, hydatid cyst, hepatic abscess, cystic hamartomas, hepatoma, metastatic cancers, cystadenocarcinoma, Caroli's disease, and polycystic disease (see Chap. 49).

Ultrasound evaluation of a cystadenoma usually reveals an anechoic cystic mass with internal echoes representing papillary infoldings or a hypoechoic mass with echogenic septations.[21] CT scans of cystadenomas demonstrate a hypodense, well-defined mass with internal septations. Solid nodular masses or coarse mural or septal calcifications may indicate a cystadenocarcinoma. The complementary role of CT imaging and ultrasound in the diagnosis of cystic liver lesions has been well described.[22]

The major challenge in assessing cystic lesions is differentiating a simple cyst from a cystadenoma or cystadenocarcinoma. Imaging studies showing internal septations are suspicious for cystadenoma or cystadenocarcinoma. Patients with inconclusive imaging studies may benefit from laparoscopic or open exploration with intraoperative ultrasound. Because of complications such as bleeding, inflammation, infection, and malignant transformation, cystadenomas should be resected. The treatment of choice for cystadenomas or cystadenocarcinomas is complete excision, either as a segmental resection or anatomic lobectomy depending on the size and location of the lesion. When the lesion is completely resected, the prognosis is excellent.[21]

HEPATOCELLULAR CARCINOMA

Hepatocellular carcinoma (HCC) is the most common solid cancer in the world, with an annual incidence estimated to be at least 1 million new patients. Unfortunately, because of underlying cirrhosis and lack of effective treatment, HCC is responsible for a significant amount of morbidity and mortality throughout the world. Ninety-four percent of patients diagnosed with HCC die of their disease.[23] Countries like South Africa have traditionally had endemic high rates of HCC; however, recently there has been a dramatic increase in the United States, currently about 2500 cases per year. The rising incidence in the United States is largely attributed to increasing incidence of hepatitis C-related liver disease. The incidence of hepatitis B infection has remained stable.[24] In Japan 80 percent of HCC is now associated with chronic hepatitis infection.[25] Individuals with persistent hepatitis B and C virus infections have 100 times the relative risk of developing HCC as do uninfected patients.[26] Other risk factors include alcoholic cirrhosis, aflatoxin exposure, and a variety of inherited metabolic disorders.

Diagnosis and Staging

Patients with HCC can present with non-specific complaints of vague abdominal pain, weakness, jaundice, abdominal fullness resulting from ascites, or weight loss. High-risk patients with chronic hepatitis or cirrhosis routinely undergo screening with serum AFP and transabdominal ultrasound to detect occult HCC. The sensitivity of ultrasound for the detection of HCC, however, is only 50 percent in the end-stage cirrhotic liver.[27] A normal level of AFP is less than 20 ng/ml. A level of more than 500 ng/ml is considered diagnostic for HCC. However, AFP is often elevated to equivocally high levels (20-400 ng/ml) in serum of cirrhotic patients, posing a diagnostic dilemma.[28] Furthermore, 35 percent of HCCs smaller than 3 cm have normal levels of AFP.

On unenhanced CT scans, HCC appears as a hypodense mass. Calcifications can be seen in 7.5 percent of HCC tumors.[24] Because of their vascularity, some HCCs become isodense to normal liver during the portal venous phase of a contrast-enhanced CT. One study using dual-phase helical CT scan showed that 11 percent of HCCs were only seen on the arterial phase images. Thus a dual-phase CT scan has become an important imaging modality for the diagnosis of HCC. CT scans after intra-arterial lipiodol administration and CT arterial portography are more sensitive tests for the detection of small HCCs; however, these tests are invasive and should not be used for routine screening. Recent advances in MRI technology, including faster protocols, breath-hold imaging, and the use of organ-specific contrast agents such as ferumoxide particles (Feridex I.V.) allow for better characterization of hepatic lesions. In well-controlled studies comparing helical CT and MRI for detection of HCC, MRI detected more lesions, and the average size of the lesions detected by MRI was significantly smaller than those detected by helical CT.[28] Compared with ultrasound, MRI had a much better sensitivity for detection of HCC (68 percent versus 43 percent).[26] However, MRI is still relatively insensitive for discrimination between small HCC and regenerative nodules.[30] In addition to finding lesions, it is important to identify major portal vein invasion, which usually precludes resection because of its poor prognostic significance.

Even in cirrhotic livers the sensitivity of intraoperative ultrasound is 98 percent for HCC lesions 1 to 3 cm in size and 86 percent for lesions smaller than 1 cm.[31] Therefore, intraoperative ultrasound remains an important imaging modality for determining resectability of HCC. Recently, encouraging results for staging liver malignancies by laparoscopy with laparoscopic ultrasound have been reported.[32] In particular, laparoscopy with laparoscopic ultrasound may avoid unnecessary laparotomy in certain patients with HCC.

Preoperative fine needle biopsy is usually not indicated in patients with resectable lesions on imaging studies and elevated AFP (>500 ng/ml). Percutaneous biopsy may be helpful in patients with unresectable tumors undergoing palliative procedures such as chemoembolization or radiofrequency ablation and also in those being considered for liver transplantation.

Assessment of hepatic functional reserve is vitally important for deciding whether surgical resection, liver transplantation, chemoembolization, or other treatment modality should be undertaken. Prognostically useful data for both surgical and medical patients may be obtained from staging using the Child-Pugh classification system. A CT or MRI can identify loss of liver volume associated with cirrhosis. Unilateral atrophy can indicate portal vein thrombosis. Varices, splenomegaly, and ascites usually indicate more advanced liver dysfunction. Functional studies measuring indocyanine green retention and galactose elimination can provide an estimate of underlying liver function; however, these tests should be interpreted within the clinical situation. Other than good clinical judgment, there are no specific guidelines for evaluating hepatic function before treatment of HCC.

After a clinical diagnosis has been established, the staging of HCC is based on tumor size, multiplicity, vascular invasion, and the presence of regional lymph nodes, or distant metastases (Table 46-1).[33] Accurate clinical staging along with consideration of performance status, co-morbid factors, and liver function, will greatly influence which treatment options are available to a patient with HCC.

TABLE 46-1

Tumor Node Metastasis Classification for Hepatocellular Carcinoma

Primary Tumor (T)			
TX	Cannot be assessed		
TO	No evidence of primary tumor		
T1	Solitary tumor < 2 cm without vascular invasion		
T2	Solitary tumor < 2 cm with vascular invasion, or Multiple tumors < 2 cm limited to one lobe without vascular invasion, or Solitary tumor > 2 cm without vascular invasion		
T3	Solitary tumor > 2 cm with vascular invasion, or Multiple tumors < 2 cm limited to one lobe with vascular invasion, or Multiple tumors > 2 cm limited to one lobe with or without vascular invasion		
T4	Multiple tumors in more than one lobe, or Tumor invasion of a major branch of the portal or hepatic vein, or Tumor invasion of adjacent organs other than the gallbladder, or Perforation of the visceral peritoneum		
Regional Lymph Nodes (N)			
NX	Cannot be assessed		
NO	No regional lymph node metastasis		
N1	Regional lymph node metastasis		
Distant Metastasis (M)			
MX	Cannot be assessed		
MO	No distant metastasis		
M1	Distant metastasis		
Stage Grouping			
I	T1	NO	MO
II	T2	NO	MO
IIIA	T3	NO	MO
IIIB	T1-3	NO	MO
IVA	T4	Any N	MO
IVB	Any T	Any N	M1

Adapted from Fleming I, Cooper J, Henson D, et al (eds): AJCC Cancer Staging Manual, ed 5, Philadelphia, Lippincott Williams & Wilkins, 1997:97-101.

Surgical Resection

The optimal treatment for HCC is surgical excision with a curative intent. Unfortunately, only 5 percent to 15 percent of newly diagnosed patients with HCC undergo a potentially curative resection. Important factors that are contraindications to resection include multi-focal tumors, extrahepatic disease, main portal vein thrombosis, inadequate hepatic reserve as a result of underlying cirrhosis, or proximity to key vascular or bile ducts that preclude a margin-negative resection. For patients without cirrhosis, margin-negative surgical resection is the treatment of choice. Patients with well-compensated mild cirrhosis (Child's class A-B) should be considered for partial hepatic resection. Tumor size, underlying cirrhosis, and extent of resection are the main determinants of a margin-negative resection.

Recent advances in patient selection, screening programs, surgical technique, and perioperative care have lowered operative mortality from 27 percent to less than 10 percent, but the morbidity rate remains high, ranging from 24 percent to 57 percent.[34] Several studies now show no significant difference in operative mortality, morbidity, and overall survival between patients with or without cirrhosis.[34] After partial hepatectomy the overall 5-year survival rates are reported between 35 percent and 50 percent (Table 46-2).[35] Favorable prognostic factors include single tumors, presence of a capsule, absence of vascular invasion, and small size. However, even after a margin-negative resection, intrahepatic recurrence develops in 70 percent of patients.[36] Most of these recurrences are not at the resection margin and represent either multi-focal disease or new primary cancers. This unacceptably high rate of recurrence has prompted recent studies examining the role of liver transplantation in HCC.

Liver Transplantation

In the United States where HCC typically develops in the setting of well-established cirrhosis, fewer than 5 percent to 10 percent of patients are eligible for hepatic resection. Even when resection is possible 70 percent of these patients will develop intrahepatic recurrence. Because so few patients with HCC are candidates for resection and their survival is limited because of intrahepatic recurrence, many physicians favor orthotopic liver transplantation (OLT) for early HCC.[37] The disappointing survival and tumor recurrence rates reported in early trials of OLT were associated with inappropriate criteria for patient selection. More recently, OLT has been limited to patients with a single tumor less than 5 cm in diameter or with three tumors less than 3 cm each.[38] With these selection criteria, 5-year survival rates have improved to 60 percent to 70 percent.[37,39] Furthermore, the rate of intrahepatic recurrence has decreased to between 4 percent and 11 percent. Stage by stage, comparable or superior 5-year survival rates can be obtained with liver transplantation compared to partial hepatic resection in selected cases (Table 46-3).[35] Contraindications to liver transplantation include extrahepatic disease and comorbid factors. Other relative contraindications include presence of vascular invasion or a poorly differentiated tumor.[38] For patients with end-stage cirrhosis and tumor characteristics meeting the selection criteria, OLT appears to be the best treatment. However, as the waiting time for transplantation in the United States grows longer, disease progression may disqualify many patients. Given this concern, several institutions have begun pretransplant treatments with chemoembolization, percutaneous ethanol ablation, or percutaneous radiofrequency ablation (RFA). Preliminary results using these modalities report improvement in the probability of transplantation and in overall survival.[39] No specific recommendation of preoperative or adjuvant chemotherapy can be endorsed until results of ongoing multi-center randomized clinical trials are known. OLT is still limited by a shortage of

TABLE 46-2
Liver Resection for Hepatocellular Carcinoma

Study	No. of patients	Incidence of cirrhosis	30-day mortality	ACTUARIAL SURVIVAL RATE 1 yr	3 yr	5 yr	Recurrence rate
Bismuth, 1993	60	100%	10%*	52%	73%		
Nagasue, 1993	229	77%	7%	80%	51%	26%	28%†
Nagashima, 1996	50	82%	12%	90%	75%	53%	70%
Takenaka, 1996	280	52%	2%	50%	71%		
Tani, 1997	90	70%	4%	64%	38%	74%	
Lise, 1998	100	78%	4%	70%	48%	38%	50%
Fan, 1999	211	46%	9.5%‡	67%	50%	37%	68%
Fong, 1999	154	65%	4.5%	81%	54%	37%	56%,† 77%§
Llovet, 1999	77	100%	3%‡	85%	62%	51%	26%

From Nakakura E, Choti M: Management of hepatocellular carcinoma. Oncology 14(7):1089, 2000.
*2-Month mortality.
†3-Month mortality.
‡Hospital mortality.
§HCC > 5 cm.

TABLE 46-3
Total Hepatectomy with Orthotopic Liver Transplantation for Hepatocellular Carcinoma

Study	Number of patients	30-day mortality	ACTUARIAL SURVIVAL RATE 1 yr	3 yr	5 yr	Recurrence rate
Bismuth, 1993	60	5%*		49%		54%
Iwatsuki, 1993	105		66%	39%	36%	43%
Olthoff, 1995†	25		77%	46%		5%
Mazzaferro, 1996†	48	6%		75%‡		8%
Colella, 1997†	71	25%§	96%	81%	81%	11%
Figueras, 1997	84		83%	77%		4%
Loinaz, 1998†	26		60%		40%	
Klintmalm, 1998‖	422	5%	72%		44%	26%
Llovet, 1999	87	2%§	82%	69%	69%	2%
Neuhaus, 1999	73				74%	

From Nakakura E, Choti M: Management of hepatocellular carcinoma. Oncology 14(7):1090, 2000.
*2-Month mortality.
†4-Year actuarial survival.
‡3-Month mortality.
§Adjuvant chemotherapy.
‖International Registry of Hepatic Tumors in Liver Transplantation.

donated organs. The increasing use of living donor transplantation may improve availability of organs for cancer patients.

Ablative Techniques

Percutaneous Ethanol Injection

Percutaneous ethanol injection (PEI) has been widely performed and is accepted as an attractive alternative to surgery in patients with small HCCs. Although the indication criteria vary somewhat, it is generally accepted that patients with HCCs less than 3 cm in size and 3 or fewer in number are suitable for PEI.[41] Patients with tumor recurrence or residual tumor after successful chemoembolization are also good candidates for PEI. In PEI, absolute ethanol is injected into the lesion under ultrasound or CT guidance. The amount of ethanol injected is determined by the volume of the tumor. The injections are repeated once or twice per week for up to four or six sessions, depending on the tumor size. The majority of these treatments can be done under local anesthesia. Uneven distribution of ethanol restricts this technique mostly to lesions less than 3 cm in size. PEI is contraindicated in patients with gross ascites, severe coagulopathy, obstructive jaundice, extrahepatic disease, and main portal vein thrombosis. The most common side effects of PEI are pain, fever, and elevated transaminases. Procedure-related mortality is rare.[42,43] Recurrence rates after PEI range from 50 percent to 75 percent, which is almost the same as after curative resection.[42,43] Reported overall survival rates after PEI for small HCCs have been encouraging, with 5-year rates of 28 percent to 51 percent in various series.[35] However, no randomized trials have compared PEI to surgical resection. Liver resection should still be the treatment of choice for resectable HCC. The minimal invasiveness, simplicity, safety, repeatability, and low cost of PEI make it an attractive form of therapy for patients with HCC, who are not candidates for partial hepatectomy.

Cryosurgery

Hepatic cryosurgery has had limited application in the United States for patients with HCC. In general, cryosurgery uses in situ destruction of the tumor and surrounding margin carried out by liquid nitrogen probes placed into the tumor under ultrasound guidance. Unfortunately, compared with other techniques of ablation, cryosurgery usually requires an open laparotomy. Indications for this technique are unresectable lesions in patients healthy enough to undergo general anesthesia. In the United States there are limited studies with small numbers of patients documenting the safety and efficacy of cryoablation in HCC. Zhou and colleagues reported their experience in China with 235 patients with HCC.[44] The overall 5-year survival was 39.8 percent for all HCC patients treated with cryosurgery alone.[44] There were no operative or severe complications. Studies comparing resection to cryosurgery have not been done. Morbidity is not insignificant and can include fever, liver cracking, renal failure, and elevated transaminases. Because bile ducts do not tolerate cryosurgery, central lesions near the biliary bifurcation should not be treated. Because of the expense and necessity for an operative approach under general anesthesia, the role of cryosurgery in the treatment of HCC is limited.

Radiofrequency Ablation

RFA produces thermal destruction with an electric current that passes to the tumor via an electrode tip, resulting in heat generation and coagulative necrosis.[45] Compared with other modes of ablation, RFA can be performed by either a percutaneous, laparoscopic, or open technique. Compared with cryosurgery, RFA is less expensive and has fewer complications and fewer local tumor recurrences.[46] Compared with PEI, percutaneous RFA requires fewer treatment sessions and may achieve superior tumor necrosis of small (less than 3 cm) HCCs.[47] In a large series of 110 cirrhotic patients undergoing RFA, there was no mortality. Complications occurred in 12.7 percent of patients.[48] Seventy percent of patients were treated percutaneously, and more than 50 percent were Child class B or C. Local recurrence at the RFA site occurred in only 3.5 percent of patients treated. However, similar to surgical resection, 50 percent of RFA patients developed new hepatic lesions or extrahepatic disease.[48] With improving technology, larger tumors up to 5 cm can be treated in one application. Although RFA appears safe and minimally invasive, further clinical trials with long-term follow-up are needed.

Chemoembolization

Transcatheter arterial chemoembolization (TACE) has become one of the most popular and effective treatments for patients with unresectable HCC. The rationale for this treatment is the observation that hepatic tumors derive their blood supply from the hepatic artery, as opposed to normal hepatic tissue that is supplied from the portal vein. During TACE, interventional radiology is used to embolize the hepatic arterial blood supply to the tumor with an emulsion of lipiodol, gelatin-sponge particles, and chemotherapeutic agents. Institutional chemotherapy protocols vary but may include doxorubicin hydrochloride, epirubicin hydrochloride, mitomycin C, cisplatin, or floxuridine used in either single or combination therapy.[49] Before TACE is performed a visceral angiogram is mandatory to document portal vein patency. TACE is contraindicated in a patient with portal vein occlusion because of the high risk of hepatic failure. Complications of TACE include abdominal pain, nausea, fever, elevated transaminases, and rarely a liver abscess or liver failure. The initial response is a greater than 50 percent tumor reduction in 12 percent to 30 percent of patients.[49] The median survival is about 20 months.[49] Overall cumulative survival rates are 69 percent at 1 year, 42 percent at 2 years, 22 percent at 3 years, 13 percent at 4 years, and 10 percent at 5 years.[49] In a non-randomized trial of intra-arterial chemotherapy or a combination of embolization and intra-arterial chemotherapy, a survival advantage was seen in the chemoembolization arm (22 percent versus 4 percent).[50] Thus the effect of vascular occlusion may potentiate the effects of chemotherapy, but further controlled trials are needed. Despite retrospective studies demonstrating a benefit of TACE, several randomized clinical trials have found that TACE offers no improvement in survival compared with supportive therapy alone.[51-53] Nevertheless, in some patients, TACE will induce significant tumor reduction and subjective improvements in symptoms such as abdominal pain.[54,55] With all the varied chemotherapy agents used with or without embolization, no definitive superior treatment protocol exists. Future randomized controlled trials may better define the role of TACE in HCC patients.

METASTATIC LIVER TUMORS

About 150,000 patients are diagnosed each year with colorectal cancer in the United States.[56] Despite a margin-negative colorectal resection and appropriate adjuvant therapy, 50 percent of patients will develop recurrence of their colorectal cancer. Ten percent to 15 percent will have synchronous liver metastases at the time of original diagnosis. It is estimated that from 5 percent to 10 percent of all patients with colorectal cancer will develop liver metastases that may be suitable for potentially curative resection. Disease metastatic to the liver is the primary determinant of patient survival in the natural history of colorectal cancer.[57]

Staging and Diagnosis

Most patients with recurrent colorectal disease metastatic to the liver are asymptomatic. Those patients with abdominal pain or abnormal liver function studies tend to have extensive recurrence. Thus to diagnose recurrent disease early, aggressive surveillance with serial carcinoembryonic antigen (CEA) assays and, with some debate, serial CT scans is vitally important. Surveillance should be most intensive early because recurrent disease develops within the first 2 years after primary resection in about 80 percent of patients destined to have a recurrence and in less than 5 percent of patients after 5 years.[57] Prospective studies indicate that serial CEA assays are the most effective screening mechanism for the detection of subsequent hepatic metastases.[58] Eighty-five percent to 90 percent of patients with hepatic metastases have an elevated CEA, which remains superior to all tumor markers.

When recurrent disease is suspected or detected by any screening test, a complete restaging work-up is mandatory. This work-up should include a detailed history and physical exam, a chest x-ray to rule out pulmonary metastasis, a colonoscopy to rule out a metachronous colorectal cancer (if not done in the last 6 months), and a helical CT of the abdomen and pelvis. Several advances in CT and MRI technology have improved our ability to carefully image the liver. Dual-phase contrast-enhanced CT provides images obtained during the hepatic-arterial phase of liver perfusion, followed by a second set of images obtained during the portal-venous phase. Although most metastases are best detected as a hypoattenuated liver mass during the portal-venous phase, some will be better seen on the arterial phase.[59] The dual-phase technique offers advantages for both detection and characterization of lesions over single-phase studies.[59] The development of fast MRI sequences has reduced acquisition times to the point that the entire liver can be imaged in 15 to 30 seconds. Using this technique, multiple sets of gadolinium-enhanced, T1-weighted images can be acquired in a manner similar to the dual-phase CT technique. Because of its wide availability, dual-phase CT scan is being considered for most patients undergoing hepatic resection. The sensitivity of lesion detection ranges from 75 percent to 80 percent.[59] Comparative studies between dual-phase CT and MRI have concluded that MRI has a better sensitivity (80 percent-95 percent), better specificity (88 percent), and is superior at detecting small lesions less than 2 cm.[59] MRI is helpful in cases of inconclusive CT scans before operative resection. For years CT angiography had been considered the gold standard and the most sensitive exam for liver metastases. Recent studies have shown that dual-phase CT and MRI are equal to the invasive CT angiography.

Positron emission tomography (PET) has evolved rapidly in the last few years as a useful staging modality for lung, lymphoma, melanoma, and colorectal cancer. In a comparative trial with CT scans, PET scans had superior sensitivity, specificity, and accuracy. The potential benefits of a PET scan include avoiding surgery in patients with extrahepatic disease and detecting early small resectable disease before it is detected by CT. In one study with PET and CT, 21 percent of patients had their surgery canceled because of previously undiagnosed extrahepatic metastases.[60] Another 21 percent of patients had negative CT scans and underwent surgery on the basis of their PET images; all had histologically proven disease.[60] PET scans seem to be an ideal imaging modality to detect both intra- and extrahepatic metastases from colorectal cancer; however, long-term follow-up is needed.

Despite the improvements in preoperative imaging, intraoperative ultrasound (IOUS) still discovers new lesions at the time of surgery in 20 percent to 35 percent of patients.[61] Based on these intraoperative findings the planned surgery was changed in 20 percent to 49 percent of the patients.[61] IOUS is also helpful in confirming the preoperative impression and evaluating the relationship of the tumor to the hepatic vascular structures and major bile ducts.

Surgical Resection

To evaluate the benefit of surgical resection of liver metastases, it is important to understand the natural history of the disease. Wagner and colleagues reviewed 252 patients with hepatic metastases, who did not undergo surgical resection and can be considered historic controls.[62] As shown in Figure 46-1, the 3-year survival rate for widespread or multiple metastases was 4 percent and 6 percent, respectively.[62] Twenty-one percent of patients with solitary metastasis were alive at 3 years.[62]

The goals of a preoperative assessment for resection of metastatic colon cancer are to determine the location and number of liver metastases and to rule out extrahepatic disease. Advances in understanding liver anatomy, resection techniques, anesthesia care, and defined centers with excellence in hepatic surgery have translated into low mortality (0 percent-5 percent) and morbidity(20 percent).[58] Complications include bleeding, abdominal abscess, bile leak, and right pleural effusion. The most ominous complication is liver failure, occurring in approximately 4 percent of all major resections.[58] In a multi-center retrospective review of 859 patients treated by potentially curative liver resection between 1948 and 1985, Hughes and colleagues reported the actuarial 5-year survival to be 33 percent (Figure 46-2).[63] Improvements in preoperative imaging and

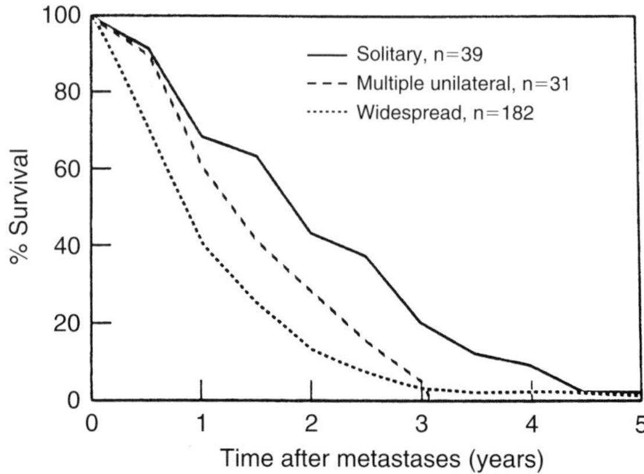

Figure 46-1 Survival rates of patients who had unresected hepatic metastases without evidence of other residual disease.

intraoperative staging including IOUS, assessment of porta hepatis lymph nodes, and attention to an adequate 1-cm surgical margin have resulted in 5-year survival rates of 43 percent to 47 percent.[64-66] Further analysis of surgical studies identified poor prognostic factors that included extrahepatic disease, the presence of satellite nodules, and more than four tumors. Thus patients with resectable tumors, four or fewer metastases, and no extrahepatic disease are considered for potentially curative hepatic resection. One particular subset of patients with extrahepatic disease that may be worthy of consideration for resection are highly selected young patients with limited resectable pulmonary and hepatic metastases. In selected patients who had staged resection of pulmonary and hepatic metastases, the 5-year survival rate was 31 percent.[67] After surgical resection 65 percent to 70 percent of patients will develop recurrence of colorectal cancer.[68]

The liver is the most common site of recurrence and was the only site of recurrence in 54 percent of patients. Despite several studies addressing the role of adjuvant chemotherapy after liver resection, no improvement in survival was demonstrated.[58] Because the liver is the most common site of recurrence, regional hepatic chemotherapy is a theoretically attractive mode of adjuvant therapy. A recent study by Kemeny and colleagues compared combined hepatic arterial infusion (HAI) and systemic 5-FU adjuvant therapy to systemic adjuvant chemotherapy alone after resection of hepatic metastases.[69] The actuarial rate of overall survival at 2 years was 86 percent in the group with HAI therapy and 72 percent in the group given systemic chemotherapy alone (p = .03).[69] This study demonstrated the benefit of HAI chemotherapy in the adjuvant setting after liver resections for colorectal metastases.

The role of hepatic resection in non-colorectal hepatic metastases is much less clear. Careful patient selection and consideration of tumor biology may define a small subgroup of patients with metastatic neuroendocrine, breast, malignant melanoma, sarcoma, or renal cancer who may benefit from hepatic resection. The overall 5-year survival rate after resection of non-colorectal hepatic metastases is about 20 percent.[70]

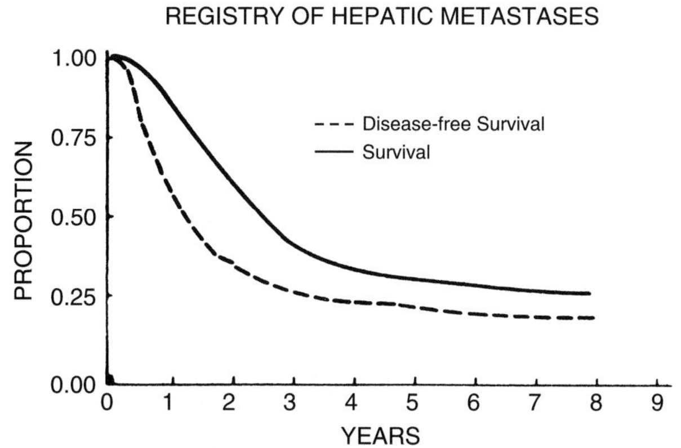

Figure 46-2 Survival and disease-free survival for 859 patients who have undergone hepatic resection for colorectal carcinoma metastases to the liver.

Cryoablation

In the United States there has been a more extensive experience with cryosurgery for liver metastases than for HCC. The development of vacuum-insulated cryoprobes and high-quality IOUS has allowed for precise, rapid, controlled freezing of liver tumors. The indications for cryosurgery are treatment of unresectable disease such as bilobar tumors with no extrahepatic disease. Cryosurgery can be used alone or in combination with surgical resection. Several studies have shown that cryosurgery is safe, with operative mortality from 0 percent to 4 percent and complication rates of 8 percent to 15 percent.[71,72] Potential complications include right pleural effusion, renal failure, liver cracking, bleeding, hepatic abscess, and bile duct injuries. The number of lesions treated has ranged from 1 to 12, but most have treated 1 to 5 lesions. Ravikumar and colleagues reported long-term results in a small group of treated patients.[71] After a median follow-up of 2 years, 62 percent of patients were alive, 28 percent without evidence of recurrence.[71] The majority of recurrences are seen in the liver with or without extrahepatic disease. No trials exist comparing surgical resection and cryosurgery. Resectable lesions should still undergo hepatic resection. RFA, which characteristically is less expensive, can be done percutaneously, is easier to use, and has fewer complications; as a result, cryosurgery has fallen out of favor in many institutions.

Radiofrequency Ablation

Pathologic studies have demonstrated coagulative necrosis in the area of tumor ablation.[73] Two recent studies have demonstrated that RFA is a safe and effective treatment for unresectable colorectal metastases.[74,75] RFA-related mortality ranged from 0 percent to 4 percent and complications occurred in 2.4 percent to 8 percent of patients.[74,75] Reported complications included skin burn, bleeding, hepatic abscess, and heat-necrosis injury to the diaphragm. Lesions near the diaphragm should not be treated percutaneously. The median size of tumors treated was 3.4 cm. With a short follow-up, local recurrence at the RFA site was only 1.8 percent to 18 percent. Longer follow-up is needed, but it appears that RFA is an effective treatment for unresectable colorectal metastases confined to the liver. The only limitation of RFA is the small size of lesions that can be treated—generally less 4 cm. The laparoscopic or open technique is preferred because IOUS detects 30 to 35 percent more lesions than do preoperative imaging studies. With the recent data showing a benefit of adjuvant HAI after liver resection, studies evaluating adjuvant HAI after RFA are ongoing.

Hepatic Artery Chemotherapy

The rationale for the use of HAI is that metastatic tumors like HCC obtain most of their blood from the hepatic artery.[76] Optimal agents for this regional treatment would be drugs extracted by the liver during the first pass, thereby reducing systemic drug levels and toxicity. Ensminger and Gyves demonstrated that hepatic extraction of floxuridine (FUDR) was fourfold higher after

TABLE 46-4

Randomized Studies of Hepatic Arterial Infusion versus Systemic Chemotherapy for Hepatic Metastases from Colorectal Carcinoma

		RESPONSE RATE (%)		% ALIVE (HAI/SYSTEMIC)	
Study	No. patients	HAI	Systemic	1 yr	2 yr
Memorial Sloan-Kettering Cancer Center	163	52	20	60/50	35/18
Northern California Oncology Group	142	42	10	60/42	30/30
National Cancer Institute	64	62	17	85/60	44/13
Mayo Clinic	74	48	21	60/42	18/10
France	168	49	14	61/44	22/10

HAI, Hepatic arterial infusion.

hepatic arterial injection compared with systemic injection.[77] The ability to administer a higher dose locally exposes tumors to a higher drug concentration than can be achieved with systemic therapy. The indications for HAI are patients with diffuse unresectable liver metastases, but no extrahepatic disease, who have failed systemic chemotherapy. The first trials with HAI used external pumps with percutaneously placed catheters that required hospitalization. With the development of implantable pumps placed during a laparotomy into the gastroduodenal artery, outpatient therapy could be accomplished. From 1980 to 1990 five randomized studies were done comparing HAI to systemic chemotherapy for unresectable colorectal hepatic metastases (Table 46-4).[58] Overall, these trials showed a significantly better response rate with HAI compared with systemic therapy. However, survival between the two groups was similar. The criticism of the lack of survival difference was that cross-over to the other treatment occurred in the majority of patients, thereby making it difficult to interpret the survival data. More recently Kemeny and colleagues have added leucovorin, a potent modulator of FUDR, and dexamethasone to reduce the risk of biliary sclerosis.[78] Response rates of 70 percent can now be achieved with low toxicity and a median survival that approaches 2 years.[78] Phase I/II trials studying the effects of systemic Camptosar and oxaliplatin used in combination with FUDR are currently being done.[79]

References

1. Nichols FC, van Heerden J, Weiland LH: Benign liver tumors. Surg Clin North Am 69:297, 1989.
2. Schwartz SI, Husser WC: Cavernous hemangioma of the liver: a single institution report of 16 resections. Ann Surg 205:456, 1987.
3. Sewell JH, Weis K: Spontaneous rupture of hemangioma of the liver. Arch Surg 83:105, 1961.
4. Trastek VF, van Heerden JA, Sheedy PF, et al: Cavernous hemangiomas of the liver: Resect or observe? Am J Surg 145:49, 1983.
5. Ishak KG, Rabin L: Benign tumors of the liver. Med Clin North Am 59:995, 1975.
6. Jenkins RL, Johnson LB, Lewis DW: Surgical approach to benign liver tumors. Semin Liver Dis 14:178, 1994.
7. Hobbs KE: Hepatic hemangiomas. World J Surg 14:468, 1990.
8. Benign liver tumors. Curr Probl Diagn Radiol May/June:127, 1989.
9. Horton KM, Bluemke DA, Hruban RH, et al: CT and MR imaging of benign hepatic and biliary tumors. Radiographics 19:431, 1999.
10. Tumeh SS, Benson C, Nagel JS, et al: Cavernous hemangioma of the liver: detection with single-photon emission computed tomography. Radiology 164:353, 1987.
11. Ishak KG: Hepatic neoplasms associated with contraceptive and anabolic steroids. In Lingeman CH, ed: Carcinogenic Hormones. New York, Springer-Verlag Inc., 1979:73-128.
12. Buetow PC, Pantongrag-Brown L, Buck JL, et al: Focal nodular hyperplasia of the liver: radiologic-pathologic correlation. Radiographics 16:369, 1996.
13. Petrovic M: Benign hepatocellular tumors and tumor-like lesions. Pathology 3:119, 1994.
14. Cherqui D, Rahmouni A, Charlotte F, et al: Management of focal nodular hyperplasia and hepatocellular adenoma in young women: a series of 41 patients with clinical, radiological, and pathological correlations. Hepatology 22:1674, 1995.
15. Vauthey JN: Liver imaging: a surgeon's perspective. Radiol Clin North Am 36:445, 1998.
16. Vilgrain V, Flejou JF, Arrive L, et al: Focal nodular hyperplasia of the liver: MR imaging and pathologic correlation in 37 patients. Radiology 184:699, 1992.
17. Weimann A, Ringe B, Klempnauer J, et al: Benign liver tumors: differential diagnosis and indications for surgery. World J Surg 21:983, 1997.
18. Shortell CK, Schwartz SI: Hepatic adenoma and focal nodular hyperplasia. SGO 173:426, 1991.
19. Foster JH, Berman MM: The malignant transformation of liver cell adenoma. Arch Surg 129:712, 1994.
20. Herman P, Pugliese V, Machado MA, et al: Hepatic adenoma and focal nodular hyperplasia: differential diagnosis and treatment. World J Surg 24:372, 2000.
21. Tsiftsis D, Christodoulakis M, Bree E, et al: Primary intrahepatic biliary cystadenomatous tumors. J Surg Oncol 64:341, 1997.
22. Palacios E, Shannon M, Solomon C, et al: Biliary cystadenoma: ultrasound, CT, and MRI. Gastrointest Radiol 15:313, 1990.
23. Curley S, Izzo F, Delrio P et al: Radiofrequency ablation of unresectable primary and metastatic malignancies. Ann Surg 230:1, 1999.
24. Fernandez M, Redvanly R: Primary hepatic malignant neoplasms. Radiol Clin North Am 36:333-348, 1998.
25. Okuda K: Hepatocellular carcinoma. J Hepatol 32:225, 2000.
26. Gogel B, Goldstein R, Kuhn J, et al: Diagnostic evaluation of hepatocellular carcinoma in the cirrhotic liver. Oncology 14:15, 2000.
27. Dodd G, Miller W, Baron R, et al: Detection of malignant tumors in end-stage cirrhotic liver: efficacy of sonography as a screening technique. Am J Roentgenol 159:727, 1992.
28. Okuda K: Clinical aspects of hepatocellular carcinoma—analysis of 134 cases. In Okuda K, Peters RL, eds: Hepatocellular carcinoma. New York, Wiley, 1976:387-436.
29. Schultz J, McCarty T: Hepatic imaging with iron oxide magnetic resonance imaging. Oncology 14:29-36, 2000.
30. Krinsky G, Lee V, Theise N, et al: Hepatocellular carcinoma and dysplastic nodules in patients with cirrhosis: prospective diagnosis with MR imaging and explantation correlation. Radiology 219:445, 2001.

31. Takayasu K, Moriyama N, Muramatsu Y, et al: The diagnosis of small hepatocellular carcinoma: efficacy of various imaging procedures in 100 patients. AJR Am J Roentgenol 155:49, 1990.
32. John T, Greig J, Crosbie J, et al: Superior staging of liver tumors with laparoscopy and laparoscopic ultrasound. Ann Surg 220:711, 1994.
33. Fleming I, Cooper J, Henson D, et al, eds: AJCC Cancer Staging Manual, ed 5, Philadelphia, Lippincott-Raven, 1997:97-101.
34. Hsia C, Lui W, Chau G, et al: Perioperative safety and prognosis in hepatocellular carcinoma patients with impaired liver function. J Am Coll Surg 190:574, 2000.
35. Nakakura E, Choti M: Management of hepatocellular carcinoma. Oncology 14:1085, 2000.
36. Poon R, Fan S, Ng I, et al: Significance of resection margin in hepatectomy for hepatocellular carcinoma. Ann Surg 231(4):544, 2000.
37. Figueras J, Jaurrieta E, Valls C, et al: Resection or transplantation for hepatocellular carcinoma in cirrhotic patients: outcomes based on indicated treatment strategy. J Am Coll Surg 190:580, 2000.
38. Bismuth H, Chiche L, Adam R, et al: Liver resection versus transplantation for hepatocellular carcinoma in cirrhotic patients. Ann Surg 218(2):145, 1993.
39. Llovet J, Mas X, Aponte J, et al: Radical treatment of hepatocellular carcinoma during the waiting list for orthotopic liver transplantation: a cost effective analysis on an intention to treat basis. Hepatology 30:223A, 1999.
40. Klintmalm G: Liver transplantation for hepatocellular carcinoma: a registry report of the impact of tumor characteristics on outcome. Ann Surg 228:479, 1998.
41. Okada S: Local ablation therapy for hepatocellular carcinoma. Semin Liver Disease 19(3):323, 1999.
42. Livraghi T, Lazzaroni S, Meloni F, et al: Intralesional ethanol in the treatment of unresectable liver cancer. World J Surg 19:801, 1995.
43. Lencioni R, Bartolozzi C, Caramella D, et al: Treatment of small hepatocellular carcinoma with percutaneous ethanol injection: analysis of prognostic factors in 105 western patients. Cancer 76:1737, 1995.
44. Zhou XD, Tang ZH: Cryotherapy for primary liver cancer. Semin Surg Oncol 14:171, 1998.
45. Rossi S, Buscarini E, Garbagnati F, et al: Percutaneous treatment of small hepatic tumors by an expandable RF needle electrode. AJR Am J Roentgenol 170:1015, 1998.
46. Pearson A, Izzo F, Fleming R, et al: Intraoperative radiofrequency ablation or cryoablation for hepatic malignancies. Am J Surg 178:592, 1999.
47. Livraghi T, Goldberg SN, Lazzaroni S, et al: Small hepatocellular carcinoma: Treatment with radio-frequency ablation vs. ethanol injection. Radiology 210:655, 1999.
48. Curley S, Izzo F, Ellis L, et al: Radiofrequency ablation of hepatocellular cancer in 110 patients with cirrhosis. Ann Surg 232(2):381, 2000.
49. Ueno K, Miyazono N, Inoue H, et al: Transcatheter arterial chemoembolization therapy using iodized oil for patients with unresectable hepatocellular carcinoma. Cancer 88:1574, 2000.
50. Hirai K, Kawazoe Y, Yamashita K, et al: Arterial chemotherapy and transcatheter arterial embolization therapy for non-resectable hepatocellular carcinoma. Cancer Chemother Pharmacol 23:537, 1989.
51. Pelletier G, Roche A, Ink O, et al: A randomized trial of hepatic arterial chemoembolization in patients with unresectable hepatocellular carcinoma. J Hepatol 11:181, 1990.
52. Groupe d'Etude et de Traitement du Carcinomae Hepatocellulaire: A comparison of lipiodol chemoembolization and conservative treatment for unresectable hepatocellular carcinoma. N Engl J Med 332(19):1256, 1995.
53. Madden M, Krige J, Bailey S, et al: Randomised trial of targeted chemotherapy with lipiodol and 5-epidoxorubicin compared with symptomatic treatment for hepatoma. Gut 34:1598, 1993.
54. Rose D, Chapman W, Brockenbrough A, et al: Transcatheter arterial chemoembolization as primary treatment for hepatocellular carcinoma. Am J Surg 177(5):405, 1999.
55. Huang Y, Wu J, Chau G, et al: Supportive treatment, resection and transcatheter arterial chemoembolization in resectable hepatocellular carcinoma: an analysis of survival in 419 patients. Eur J Gastroenterol Hepatol 11(3):315, 1999.
56. Parker SL, Tong T, Bolder S, Wings PA: Cancer statistics. Cancer J Clin 46:5, 1997.
57. Asbun H, Hughes K: Management of recurrent and metastatic colorectal carcinoma. Surg Clin North Am 73:145, 1993.
58. Fong Y, Kemeny N, Paty P et al: Treatment of colorectal cancer: hepatic metastasis. Semin Surg Oncol 12:219, 1996.
59. Earls J, Morgan R: Comparison studies of CT and MRI in patients with hepatic metastases. Oncology 14:21, 2000.
60. Boykin K, Zibari G, McMillan, et al: The use of FDG-positron emission tomography for the evaluation of colorectal metastases of the liver. Am Surg 65(12):1183, 1999.
61. Jarnagin W, Bach A, Winston C, et al: What is the yield of intraoperative ultrasonography during partial hepatectomy for malignant disease? J Am Coll Surg 192:577, 2001.
62. Wagner J, Adson M, Van Heerden J: The natural history of hepatic metastases from colorectal cancer. Ann Surg 199:502, 1984.
63. Hughes KS, Rosenstein RB, Songhorabodi S, et al: Resection of the liver for colorectal carcinoma metastases: a multi-institutional study of indications fore resection. Surgery 103:278, 1988.
64. Fuhrman GM, Curley SA, Hohn DC, Roh MS: Improved survival after resection of colorectal liver metastases. Ann Surg Oncol 2(6):537, 1995.
65. Taylor M, Forster J, Langer B, et al: A study of prognostic factors for hepatic resection for colorectal metastases. Am J Surg 173:467, 1997.
66. Harmon K, Ryan J, Biehl T, et al: Benefits and safety of hepatic resection for colorectal metastases. Am J Surg 177:402, 1999.
67. Kobayashi K, Kawamura M, Ishihara T: Surgical treatment for both pulmonary and hepatic metastases from colorectal cancer. J Thorac Cardiovasc Surg 118:1090, 1999.
68. Holm A, Bradley E, Aldrete J: Hepatic resection of metastasis from colorectal carcinoma. Ann Surg 209:428, 1989.
69. Kemeny N, Huang Y, Cohen A, et al: Hepatic arterial infusion of chemotherapy after resection of hepatic metastases from colorectal cancer. N Engl J Med 341:2039, 1999.
70. Wolf R, Goodnight J, Krag D, et al: Results of resection and proposed guidelines for patient selection in instances of noncolorectal hepatic metastases. SGO 173:454, 1991.
71. Ravikumar TS, Kane R, Cady B, et al: A 5-year study of cryosurgery in the treatment of liver tumors. Arch Surg 126:1520, 1991.
72. Weaver M, Ashton J, Zemel R: Treatment of colorectal liver metastases by cryosurgery. Semin Surg Oncol 14(2):163, 1998.
73. Goldberg S, Gazelle G, Compton C, et al: Treatment of intrahepatic malignancy with radiofrequency ablation. Cancer 88:2452, 2000.
74. Curley S, Izzo F, Delrio P et al: Radiofrequency ablation of unresectable primary and metastatic malignancies. Ann Surg 230:1, 1999.
75. Wood T, Rose M, Chung M, et al: Radiofrequency ablation of 231 unresectable hepatic tumors: indications, limitations, complications. Ann Surg Oncol 7(8):593, 2000.
76. Breedis C, Young C: The blood supply of neoplasms in the liver. Am J Pathol 30:969, 1954.
77. Ensminger WD, Gyves JW: Clinical pharmacology of hepatic arterial chemotherapy. Semin Oncol 10:176, 1983.
78. Kemeny N, Seiter K, Conti J, et al: Hepatic arterial floxuridine and leucovorin for unresectable liver metastases from colorectal carcinoma: new dose. Improved response rate schedules and survival update. Cancer 73:1134, 1994.
79. Kemeny N, Gonen M, Sullivan D, et al: Phase I study of hepatic arterial infusion of floxuridine and dexamethasone with systemic irinotecan for unresectable hepatic metastases from colorectal cancer. J Clin Oncol 19(10):2687, 2001.

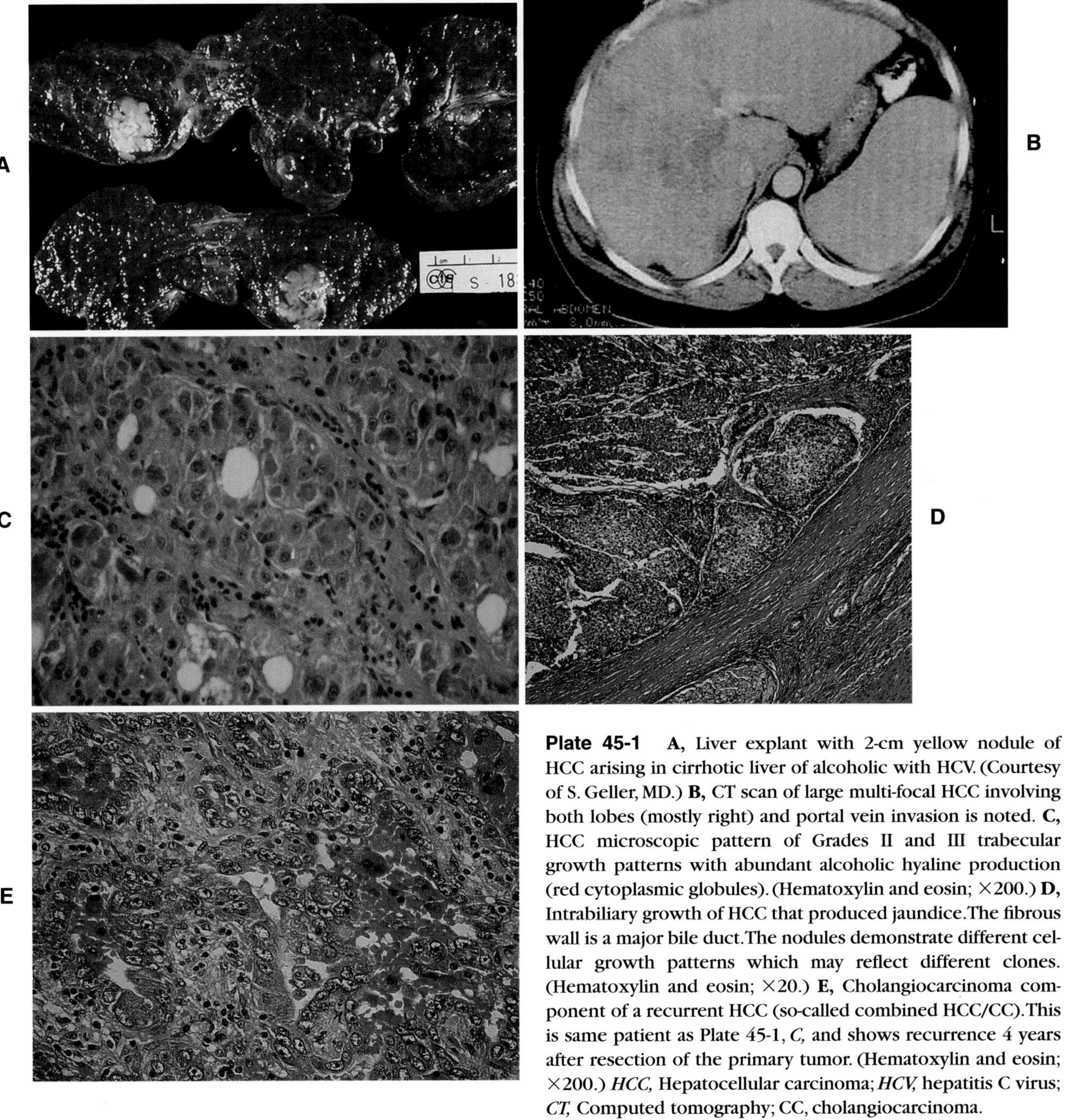

Plate 45-1 **A,** Liver explant with 2-cm yellow nodule of HCC arising in cirrhotic liver of alcoholic with HCV. (Courtesy of S. Geller, MD.) **B,** CT scan of large multi-focal HCC involving both lobes (mostly right) and portal vein invasion is noted. **C,** HCC microscopic pattern of Grades II and III trabecular growth patterns with abundant alcoholic hyaline production (red cytoplasmic globules). (Hematoxylin and eosin; ×200.) **D,** Intrabiliary growth of HCC that produced jaundice. The fibrous wall is a major bile duct. The nodules demonstrate different cellular growth patterns which may reflect different clones. (Hematoxylin and eosin; ×20.) **E,** Cholangiocarcinoma component of a recurrent HCC (so-called combined HCC/CC). This is same patient as Plate 45-1, *C,* and shows recurrence 4 years after resection of the primary tumor. (Hematoxylin and eosin; ×200.) *HCC,* Hepatocellular carcinoma; *HCV,* hepatitis C virus; *CT,* Computed tomography; CC, cholangiocarcinoma.

A

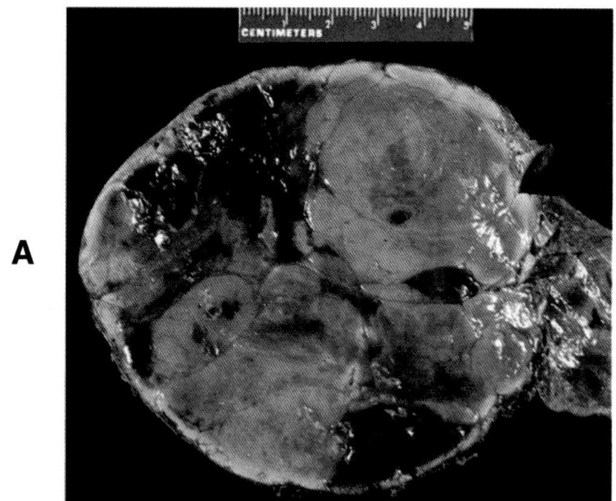

B

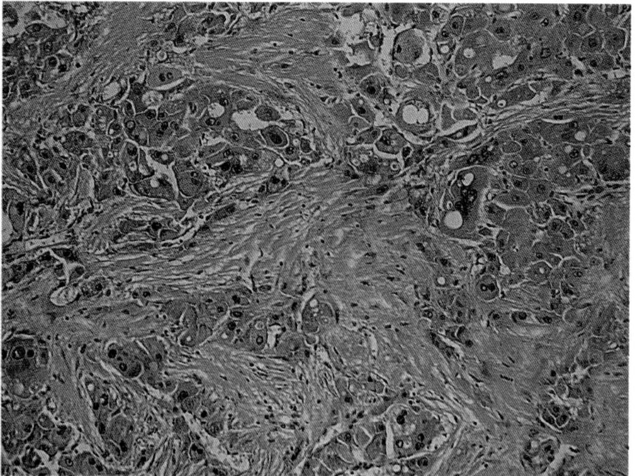

C

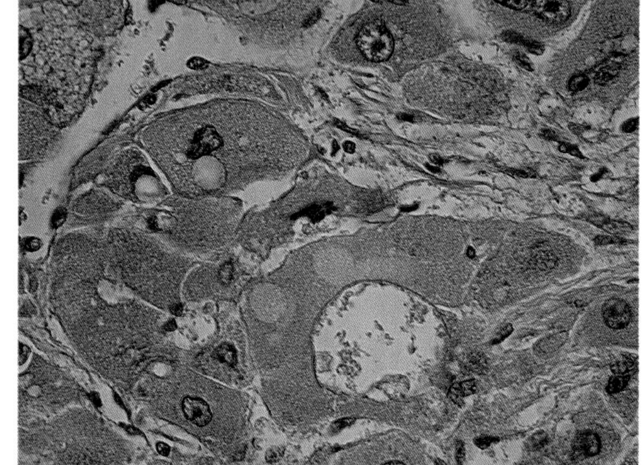

Plate 45-2 **A,** Fibrolamellar HCC (gross appearance) with a large, solitary tumor with areas of hemorrhage and necrosis. Some areas may be slightly green because of bile retention. Adjacent rim of liver is brown and not cirrhotic. **B,** Fibrolamellar HCC with mixture of lamellar fibrosis and large, polygonal, eosinophilic epithelial cells. (Hematoxylin and eosin; ×100.) **C,** Fibrolamellar HCC epithelial component may have "pale bodies" and acinar formation. Large nucleoli are typical. (Hematoxylin and eosin; ×400.) *HCC,* Hepatocellular carcinoma.

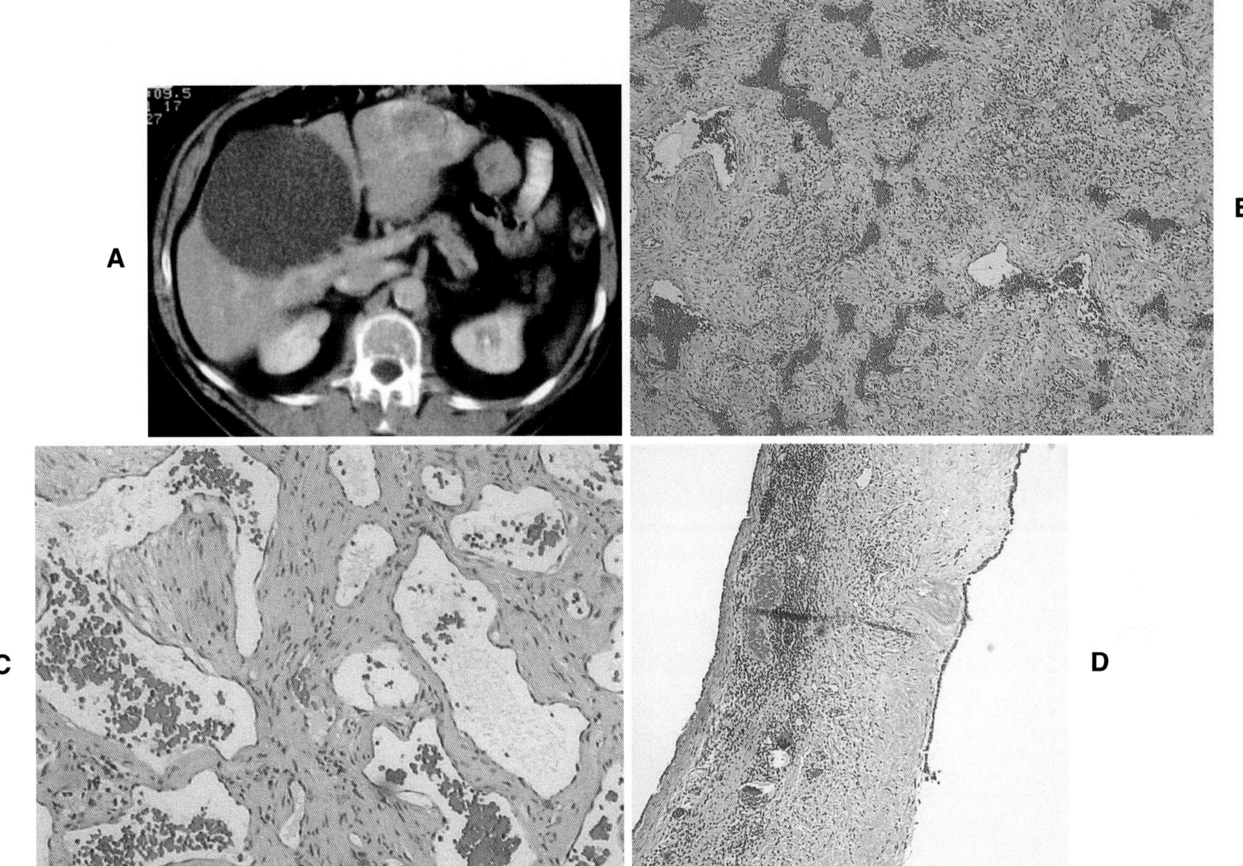

Plate 45-3 **A,** CT scan of large biliary cystadenoma (right lobe), which was drained but recurred and was painful. After 5 years it was resected. Left lobe contains 3 to 4 cm cavernous hemangioma. **B,** Sclerotic hemangioma: the marked fibrosis may progress to solid fibrosis and the blood flow is markedly diminished. (Hematoxylin and eosin; ×50.) **C,** Cavernous hemangioma with open vascular channels that allow pooling of blood and slow flow compared to adjacent intact liver. (Hematoxylin and eosin; ×200.) **D,** Biliary cystadenoma with thin walls resulting from cyst expansion and atrophy of surrounding tissue (including liver parenchyma). The wall includes thin, atrophic hepatic cords, lymphocytes, bile ducts, and small vessels. (Hematoxylin and eosin; ×50.) *CT,* Computed tomography.

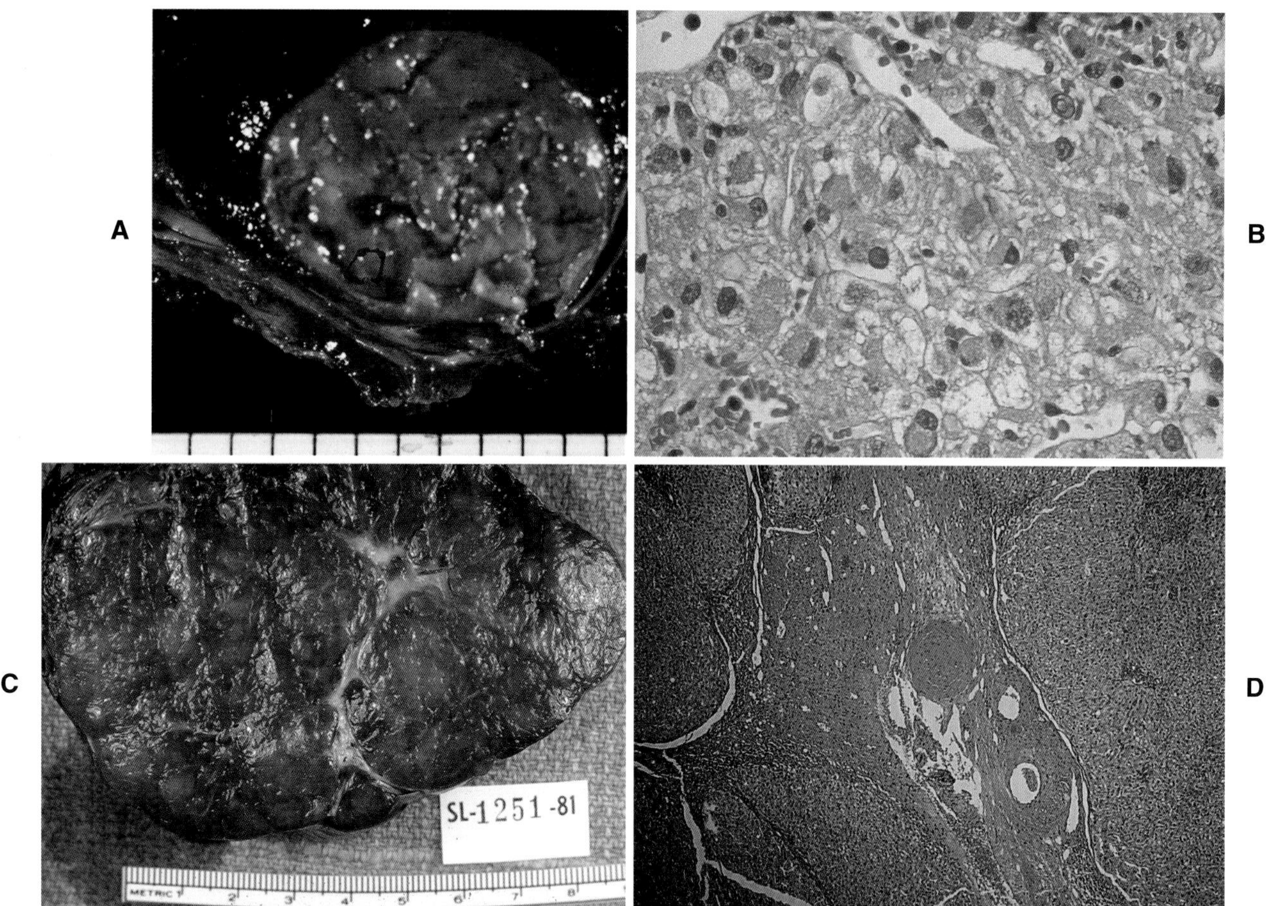

Plate 45-4 **A,** Angiomyolipoma with bright yellow color distinct from adjacent brown liver. **B,** Needle biopsy of 5-cm lesion composed of large epithelioid cells that mimic carcinoma. (Hematoxylin and eosin; ×400.) **C,** Focal nodular hyperplasia (gross appearance) with bulging nodules of brown-orange tissue; the white bands are fibrosis. **D,** Central sclerosis of focal nodular hyperplasia. Major arterial branches are prominent, as are small aggregates of cholangiolar units. (Hematoxylin and eosin; ×20.)

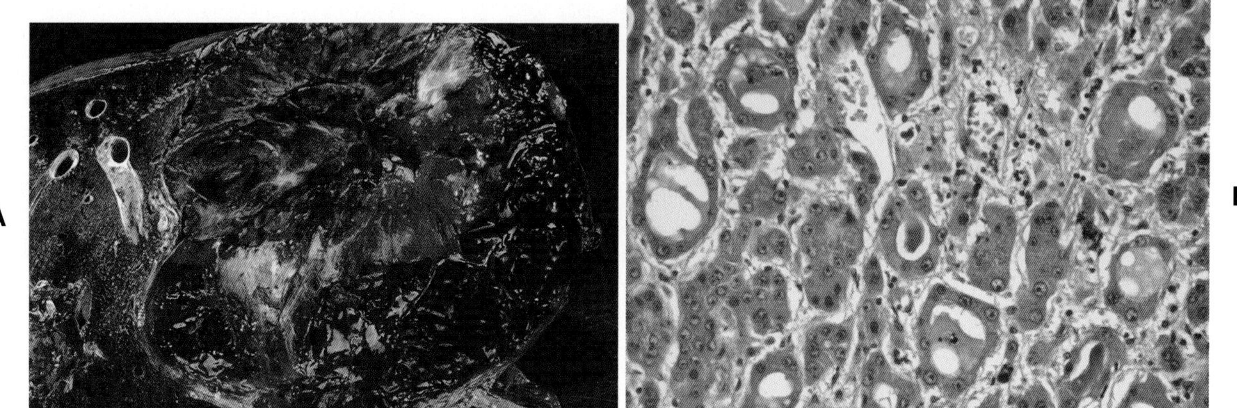

Plate 45-5 **A,** Hepatocellular adenoma arising in young man on anabolic steroids for 3 years. There is hemorrhage and near-rupture. **B,** Anabolic steroid–related hepatocellular adenoma. Abundant benign hepatocytes form large acinar structures that suggest HCC. These form large sheets of tumor, but note the normal nuclear/cytoplasmic ratio. (Hematoxylin and eosin; ×300.) *HCC,* Hepatocellular carcinoma.

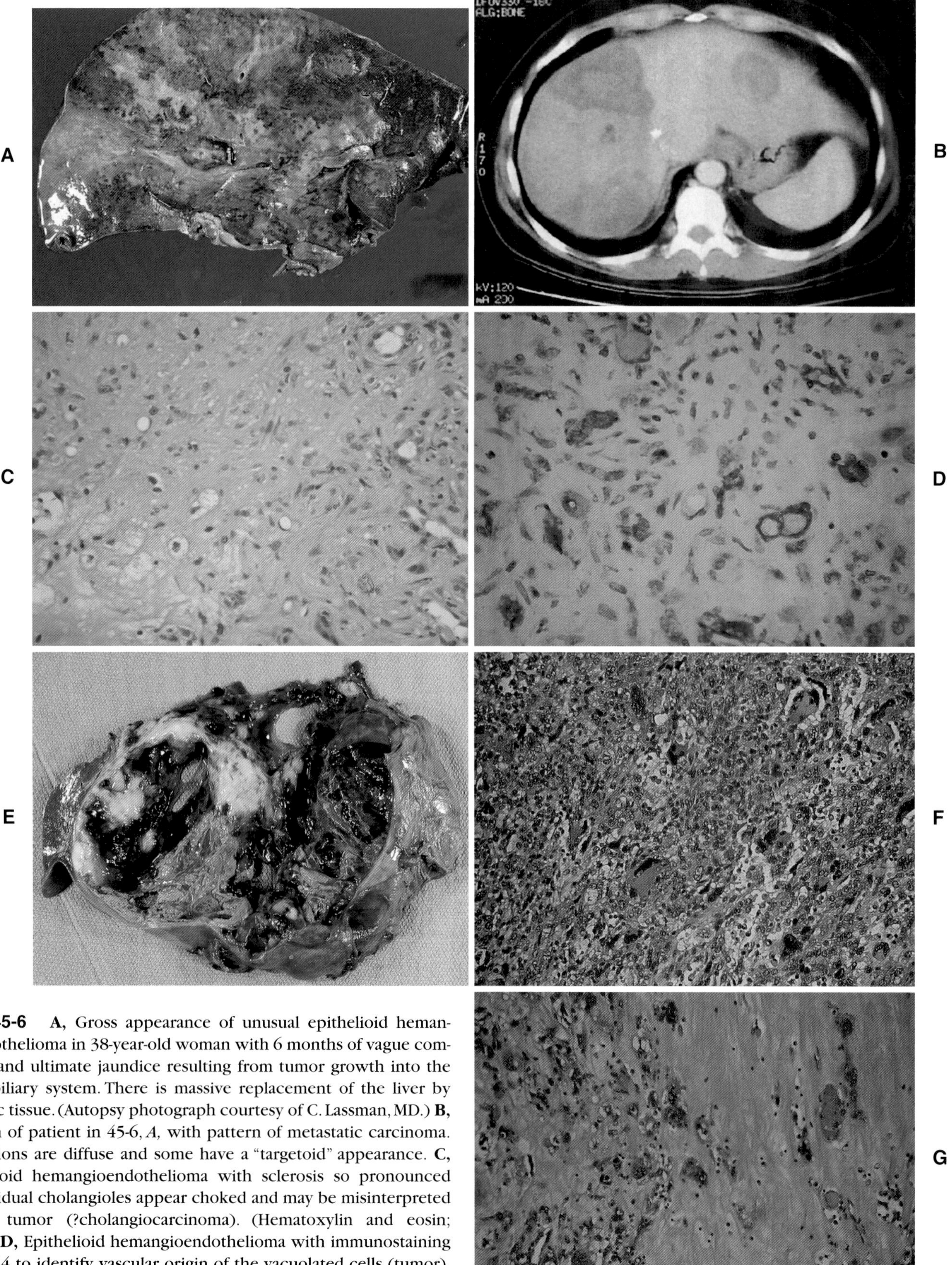

Plate 45-6 **A,** Gross appearance of unusual epithelioid hemangioendothelioma in 38-year-old woman with 6 months of vague complaints and ultimate jaundice resulting from tumor growth into the major biliary system. There is massive replacement of the liver by sclerotic tissue. (Autopsy photograph courtesy of C. Lassman, MD.) **B,** CT scan of patient in 45-6, *A,* with pattern of metastatic carcinoma. The lesions are diffuse and some have a "targetoid" appearance. **C,** Epithelioid hemangioendothelioma with sclerosis so pronounced that residual cholangioles appear choked and may be misinterpreted as the tumor (?cholangiocarcinoma). (Hematoxylin and eosin; ×200.) **D,** Epithelioid hemangioendothelioma with immunostaining for CD34 to identify vascular origin of the vacuolated cells (tumor). Rare positive staining cells are noted in the abundant sclerosis. (Hematoxylin and eosin; ×300.) **E,** Embryonal sarcoma gross appearance in 12-year-old male with abundant sclerosis, hemorrhage, and "cyst" formation (surgical resection). (Courtesy of P. Chu, MD.) **F,** Embryonal sarcoma has a mixed mesenchymal pattern with fibrosis and extremely pleomorphic sarcomatous component. (Hematoxylin and eosin; ×180.) **G,** Epithelioid hemangioendothelioma with sarcomatous growth pattern including numerous multi-nucleated giant tumor cells. (Hematoxylin and eosin; ×100.) *CT,* Computed tomography.

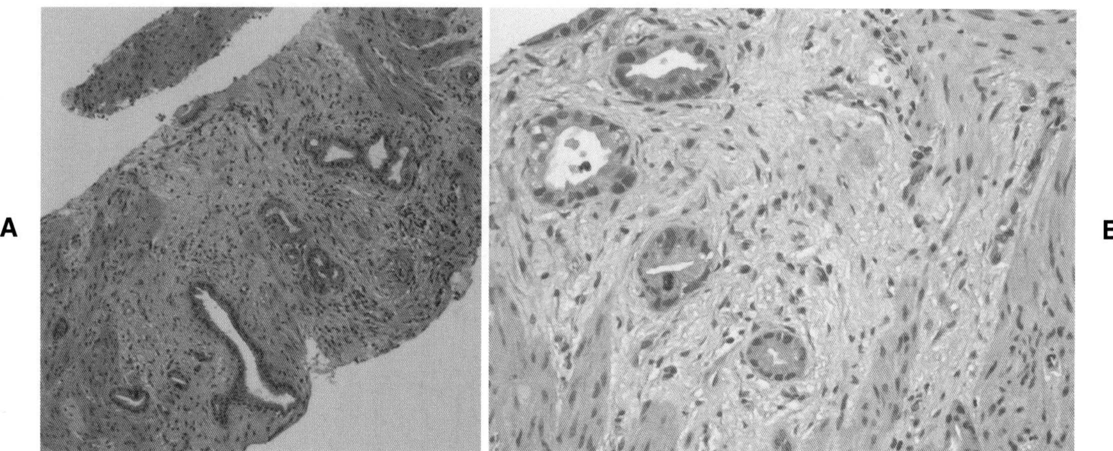

Plate 45-7 **A,** Cholangiocarcinoma identified by needle biopsy of a hilar mass in an 87-year-old woman with jaundice. Many normal major bile ducts are present; careful search allows identification of the few malignant glands. (Hematoxylin and eosin; ×100.) **B,** Cholangiocarcinoma (Klatskin type) from patient in **A** of few malignant glands (mitosis present). (Hematoxylin and eosin; ×300.)

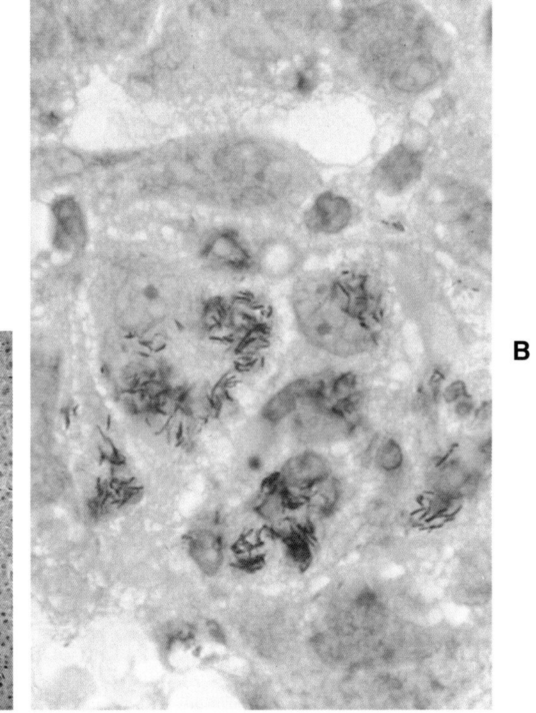

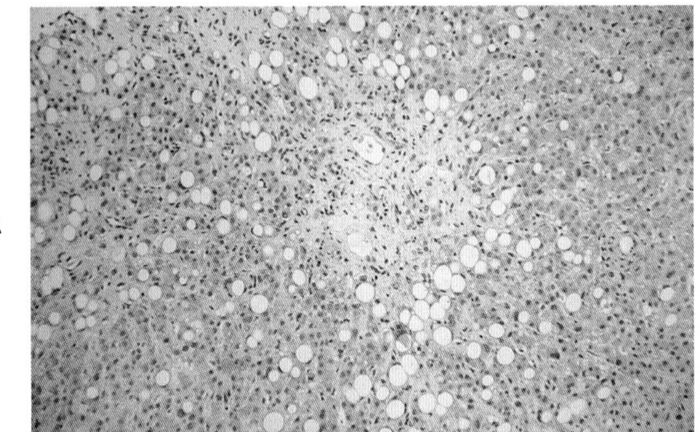

Plate 51-1 Hepatic granuloma caused by *Mycobacterium avium* complex. **A,** Well-formed granuloma with normal surrounding hepatic architecture. **B,** Acid-fast staining demonstrates multiple organisms. Cultures of the biopsy grew *M. avium* complex.

SECTION IV E

Liver Disease Primarily of Children

CHAPTER

47

α_1-Antitrypsin Deficiency

Fayez K. Ghishan, MD

ABBREVIATIONS

PAS periodic acid-Schiff
Pi protease inhibitor

In 1963 Laurell and Eriksson discovered a genetically determined deficiency in a major serum protease inhibitor, α_1-antitrypsin. This deficiency was associated with the early onset of emphysema in adults.[1] In 1969 Sharp and co-workers reported the association of α_1-antitrypsin deficiency and hepatic cirrhosis in children. Since then several reports from different parts of the world have included histories of neonatal hepatitis.[2] Soon it became apparent from several published reports that approximately 15 percent to 30 percent of neonates with conjugated hyperbilirubinemia have α_1-antitrypsin deficiencies.[3,4]

CHARACTERISTICS OF α_1-ANTITRYPSIN

α_1-Antitrypsin derived its name from its identification as α_1-globulin and from the original method used for measuring its activity. α_1-Antitrypsin is a glycoprotein synthesized in the liver and, to a minor extent, in macrophages.[5] It has a relatively short half-life of 4 to 5 days.[6] Ninety percent of the serum's ability to inhibit trypsin is due to this glycoprotein, which also inhibits chymotrypsin, pancreatic elastase, skin collagenase, renin, urokinase, Hageman factor co-factor, and the neutral proteases of polymorphonuclear leukocytes.[7] α_1-Antitrypsin belongs to a large gene family of serine protease inhibitors referred to as serpins.[8] The serpin family includes some of the best-characterized proteins involved in a group of disorders termed *conformation disorders* in which a protein undergoes a change in topology that leads to self-association, tissue deposition, and disease state.[9,10] The best characterized serpin is α_1-antitrypsin, which is composed of 394 amino acids arranged into three β-sheets (A, β, and C), nine α-helices (A through I), and a mobile inhibitory reactive center loop.[11] Protease inhibition occurs by the formation of a 1:1 complex between α_1-antitrypsin and the target protease. The reactive site in the α_1-antitrypsin protein is a methionine residue at position 358-, close to the C terminus of the molecule.[12] The reactive site of many of the serine protease inhibitors is similar. The specificity of the methionine at position 358 has been proven by the discovery of α_1-antitrypsin$_{\text{Pittsburgh}}$ variant, in which methionine 358 is substituted by arginine 358. This mutant does not inhibit pancreatic elastase. It is a highly effective inhibitor of thrombin, however, and leads to a severe bleeding diathesis.[13] α_1-Antitrypsin is present in tears, duodenal fluid, saliva, nasal secretions, cerebrospinal fluid, pulmonary secretions, and mother's milk. Its level in normal amniotic fluid is approximately 10 percent of the normal serum level. Inflammation, neoplastic disease, pregnancy, or estrogen therapy increases the serum level of α_1-antitrypsin twofold to threefold. Such a stimulus has little inductive effect, however, in a patient deficient in α_1-antitrypsin.[7]

MEASUREMENT AND TYPING OF PROTEASE INHIBITOR

Approximately 2 mg of α_1-antitrypsin is present in 1 ml of serum. α_1-Antitrypsin function can be quantitated by measuring the ability of serum samples to inhibit the action of trypsin.[14] The production of anti-serum to the α_1-globulin fraction has made possible the use of radial immunodiffusion plates for measuring the concentration of this protein. In general, the results of this inhibitor function correlate well with the electroimmunodiffusion assay.[15] Protein electrophoresis on starch gel has contributed greatly to our understanding of variations in α_1-antitrypsin.[16] α_1-Globulins appear in this system as a series of characteristic bands of variable intensity. A system of labeling based on the letters of the alphabet has been adopted. Faster-moving protein complexes are identified by earlier letters in the alphabet and the slowest-moving protein is labeled Z. Variants exhibiting similar electrophoretic properties are further classified by the geographic location of the proband. The system itself is titled Pi (protease inhibitor). The technique of isoelectric focusing on polyacrylamide gel has considerably improved the separation of the protein bands.[17]

Fagerhol and Laurell have demonstrated that the serum α_1-antitrypsin is inherited via a series of co-dominant alleles that appear to control the electrophoretic mobility of the α_1-antitrypsin.[18,19] There are at least 75 different alleles for this gene.[19] Restriction fragment length polymorphism (RFLP) of genomic deoxyribonucleic acid (DNA)[20,21] and nucleotide sequencing of various cloned human α_1-antitrypsin alleles[22] led to the identification of numerous variants. The normal allele is the PiM type with overall allelic frequency of 0.95. There are three forms of the normal PiM allele—designated M_1, M_2, and M_3—that exhibit identical electrophoretic properties but differ from each other by one or two amino acid substitutions.[23] Each person inherits a maximum of two different alleles. Different allelic forms of α_1-antitrypsin have different capacities for inhibiting trypsin. The activities of different phenotypes are listed in Table 47-1. The P and S alleles have a 12.5 percent and 30 percent activity of α_1-antitrypsin, respectively. Thus a PiPS individual—that is, a person found to have protease inhibitor PS—would have 42.5 percent of maximum activity of α_1-antitrypsin. Children and adults who have hepatic cirrhosis secondary to deficiencies of α_1-antitrypsin are termed *PiZZ.* The association of hepatic cirrhosis with heterozygotic expressions such as PiSZ or PiFZ is uncertain because only a few reports of such associations have been published. A rare "null" phenotype has been described with no detectable immunoreactive protein in the serum.[24-26] Several null alleles have been identified, such as Pi $Null_{Granite\ Falls}$,[25] Pi $Null_{Hong\ Kong}$,[27] Pi $Null_{Mattawa}$,[28] and Pi $Null_{Bellingham}$.[29] These alleles show single-base deletions or insertions causing frameshift mutations and premature translational termination of the protein.[29] The null type patients are prone to development of emphysema but not liver disease. Several other rare variant alleles have been reported and include PiM_{Malton},[30] PiM_{Duarte},[31] $PiM_{Heerlen}$,[32] and $PiM_{Procida}$.[33] These variants code for full-length proteins that exhibit deletions or substitution of an amino acid residue. Table 47-2 depicts the amino acid substitutions in several α_1-antitrypsin variants.

TABLE 47-1

Relationship Between Pi Phenotypes and Serum Concentrations of α_1-Antitrypsin

Phenotype	Serum concentration (%)
MM	100
MZ	60
SS	60
FZ	60
M—	50
PS	40
SZ	42.5
ZZ	15
Z—	10
—	0

PATHOPHYSIOLOGIC BASIS OF THE DEFECT

Microscopic examinations of livers from patients who are PiZZ almost uniformly disclose globules of an amorphous material within the hepatocytes, particularly in the periportal area.[34] These globules, which enlarge as the infant matures, are most easily discerned by positive periodic acid-Schiff (PAS) staining after treatment of the liver biopsy specimen with diastase. These globules are also detected in the livers of patients who are PiZZ but have no liver disease and in those of healthy heterozygotes.

A basic difference between PiZ and PiM molecules has been demonstrated by peptide mapping. A glutamic

TABLE 47-2

Amino Acid Substitutions in α_1-Antitrypsin Alleles

Pi type	Amino acid number	Normal amino acid	Variant amino acid
Normal Variants			
M_1	213	Valine	Alanine
M_2	376	Glutamic acid	Asparagine
	101	Arginine	Histidine
M_3	376	Glutamic acid	Asparagine
Deficient Variants			
Z	342	Glutamic acid	Lysine
S	264	Glutamic acid	Valine
P	256	Asparagine	Valine
Null Variants			
$Null_{Hong\ Kong}$	318	Leucine	Deletion
$Null_{Matawa}$	353	Phenylalanine	Deletion
$Null_{Granite\ Falls}$	160	Tyrosine	Deletion
$Null_{Bellingham}$	217	Lysine	Deletion
Dysfunctional Variants			
Pittsburgh	358	Methionine	Arginine

acid in a peptide fragment from normal α_1-antitrypsin is replaced by a lysine in the abnormal form.[35,36] Accumulation of α_1-antitrypsin also occurs in the endoplasmic reticulum of transgenic mouse hepatocytes as detected by immunoelectromicroscopy.[37,38] Several studies suggest that proper folding or assembly of polypeptides is prerequisite for their exit from the endoplasmic reticulum.[39] Misfolding of α_1-antitrypsin variants may cause them to be retained. The retained α_1-antitrypsin variants have mutations in the protein that cause misfolding.[40] The rate of the protein folding is much slower in the Z variant as compared to that of the M variant.[41,42] Evidence of misfolding is the observation that the secreted fraction of α_1-antitrypsin in PiZZ patients shows a decreased anti-elastase activity, suggesting that its conformation is abnormal.[43] The retained α_1-antitrypsin of the PiZZ variant forms an insoluble aggregate, which undergoes degradation in dense ribosome-bearing vesicles in the liver.[44]

The substitution for Glu 342 of lysine in the α_1-antitrypsin Z variant results in reducing the stability of the molecule in its monomeric form to a polymeric form by way of a mechanism termed *loop-sheet insertion* by Lomas' laboratory.[45] Indeed, Lomas' group has shown that the site of the amino acid substitution in the Z variant was the base of the reactive center loop. A change in the charge at this residue prevents the insertion of the reactive site loop into the gap in the A-sheet. The A-sheet is the dominant structure of the five-stranded β-pleated sheet representing the internal domain of α_1-antitrypsin molecule as depicted by radiographic crystallography. Thus in the Z variant, the reactive center loop of one α_1-antitrypsin molecule inserts into a gap in the β-pleated A-sheet of another α_1-antitrypsin molecule. This causes polymerization, which occurs spontaneously and to a greater extent during a systemic inflammation with a rise in temperature. Recently it has been shown that the Z variant causes an expansion of the β-sheet A and partial insertion of the reactive center loop. This opening of β-sheet A then allows the reactive center loop of another molecule to insert and cause polymerization.[46]

The current evidence suggests that polymerization of α_1-antitrypsin results in its retention within the endoplasmic reticulum. However, it is not known whether the degradation process of these polymeric molecules is altered or less efficient compared to the normal monomeric α_1-antitrypsin.[47] The retention of α_1-antitrypsin in polymeric form in the liver could be responsible for the liver disease (the accumulation theory); however, why only 10 percent to 15 percent of patients with α_1-antitrypsin Z variant develop liver disease is not known. It is possible that environmental factors or other genetic factors may act in concert with the Z variant to produce liver disease. Certainly the etiologic puzzle of liver disease with PiZZ needs further study.

MOLECULAR BASIS OF THE DEFECT IN α_1-ANTITRYPSIN DEFICIENCY

The gene encoding the α_1-antitrypsin protein is 15 Kb in length[48,49] and has been localized to chromosome 14q31-32.2.[50,51] The human gene consists of seven exons, designated I_A, I_B, I_C, II, III, IV, and V. Exons II through V are translated into protein.[52] The first three exons (I_A, I_B, I_C) and a short 5′ segment of exon II code for 5′ untranslated regions of the α_1-antitrypsin messenger ribonucleic acid (mRNA). α_1-Antitrypsin is mainly synthesized in the liver and, to a minor extent, in macrophages.[13,52] The same gene is responsible for α_1-antitrypsin production in the liver and macrophages. The first two exons (I_A, I_B) and a short 5′ segment of I_C are included in the primary transcript in macrophages but not in hepatocytes.[52] The α_1-antitrypsin protein of baboons and humans consists of a single polypeptide of 394 amino acids[48,53] with a molecular mass of 56 Kd. The protein has three asparagine-linked branched oligosaccharide moieties (Figure 47-1). As indicated previously, the basis of the defect in the PiZZ type of α_1-antitrypsin deficiency is the substitution of lysine for glutamic acid at position 342 from the carboxyl terminus in the Z-type protein.

Sequencing of human cDNA indicated that the codon for the glutamic acid residue at position 342 of the protein is GAG. It is believed that the α_1-antitrypsin deficiency is caused by a point mutation involving the G to A position—that is, nucleic acid GAG in the M type is changed to AAG in the Z type. This mutation occurs in exon V region of the human α_1-antitrypsin gene. The structure of the gene has been established by electron microscopy of hybrid molecules formed between the cloned chromosomal DNA and baboon α_1-antitrypsin mRNA. The chromosomal α_1-antitrypsin gene contains five exon-coding regions and four introns that do not code for protein sequence. Further studies have indicated that two more exons exist in upstream DNA regions that are used in the expression of α_1-antitrypsin in macrophages.[52] The molecular defect in the S type of protein appears to be a substitution of glutamic acid by valine.[49] In the null type (absence of detectable serum levels of α_1-antitrypsin), however, the defect appears to be an inability of the gene to direct the synthesis of a detectable mRNA transcript.[24]

Genetics

The most common allele is PiM, which has a frequency distribution of 0.86 to 0.99, depending on the population studied.[54] In Americans the frequency is about 0.95, with a frequency of 0.98 in blacks.[55] The next two most common alleles in the United States are PiS at 0.03 and PiZ at 0.01. Blacks have lower frequencies of these alleles.[54,55] In Sweden the frequency of PiZ is 0.026.[56] Calculations from allelic frequencies predict that in the United States PiZZ will occur in about 1 in 3630 subjects and PiSZ in 1 in 830.

Levels of circulating α_1-antitrypsin are unreliable in identification of the heterozygous state. Thus members of families containing a patient with PiZZ should be phenotyped.[57] Prenatal diagnosis is now available to detect the ZZ α_1-antitrypsin deficiency. The Z mutation, as with many single-base substitutions, does not occur within a restriction recognition site; however, it can be detected by using a mutation-specific oligonucleotide. This method has been successfully used to detect the ZZ type using amniotic cells.[58,59] Identification of human α_1-antitrypsin

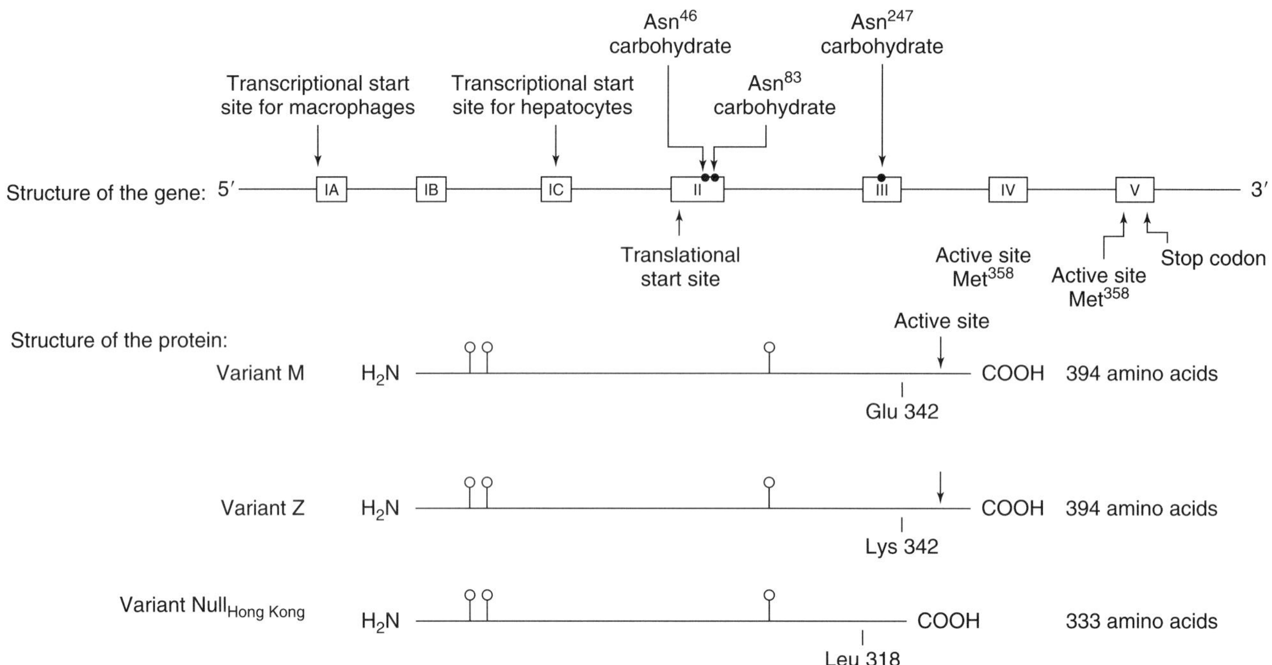

Figure 47-1 Structure of human α_1-antitrypsin gene and protein. (Adapted from Perlmutter D: Pediatric Gastrointestinal Disease. Philadelphia, BC Decker, 1991; from Sifers RN, et al: Semin Liver Dis 12:301, 1992, Thieme Medical Publishers, Inc.)

variants has also been achieved by amplification of human genomic DNA using the polymerase chain reaction.[60,61] Carrier detection can be accomplished by polymerase chain reaction–mediated, site-directed mutagenesis in which a base substitution near the mutation site can be introduced, such that the restriction enzyme (TaqI) is used to differentiate normal subjects, carriers, and affected patients.[62,63]

Clinical Features

Although α_1-antitrypsin deficiency was originally described in association with pulmonary emphysema in early adulthood,[1] this chapter discusses only the hepatic manifestations. Extrahepatic manifestations, such as pancreatic fibrosis,[64] membranoproliferative glomerulonephritis,[65] and panniculitis,[66] are not dealt with here.

Liver Disease in Children

The association of PiZZ and neonatal cholestasis is now well established.[3] Early reports indicated that by the second decade of life most patients had developed overt cirrhosis and that the clinical outlook for these patients was grave.[7] However, it is clear that many patients with PiZZ do not develop neonatal cholestasis.[67,68]

In a prospective study of 200,000 Swedish newborns 125 were found to have the phenotype PiZZ. Eleven percent of these infants developed neonatal cholestatic jaundice; at 2 years of age only three of them had cirrhosis. About 50 percent of the asymptomatic PiZZ subjects had occasional elevations of alanine aminotransferase (ALT). In 15 percent of the asymptomatic PiZZ subjects the level of ALT was probably permanently elevated. In the same study 48 infants with the phenotype PiSZ were identified. None of these infants had significant liver disease and only two had elevated ALT levels.[56,67] At 12 years of age a follow-up study of 14 children with neonatal cholestatic jaundice showed that 3 children died of liver disease, 1 died from an unrelated cause, and 5 had abnormal liver tests. Of the children who presented originally with abnormal liver tests, 15 percent had abnormal liver tests and the remainder of the children were normal.[69] In screening 107,038 newborns in the United States 21 infants were found to have the phenotype PiZZ. Of the 18 infants followed, only one had neonatal cholestatic jaundice. Five had hepatomegaly, biochemical abnormalities, or both. At 3 to 6 years of age, none of the children had evidence of hepatic cirrhosis.[68] In contrast, another report suggests that infants with PiZZ who present with neonatal cholestasis are more likely to develop serious liver disease in the future compared with those without a history of neonatal cholestasis.[70]

The cholestatic jaundice may appear during the first week of life. Acholic stools and dark urine may be seen. On physical examination hepatomegaly is usually detected. The biochemical signs of obstructive jaundice are found. The jaundice usually disappears during the second to fourth months of life.[67] Histologic studies of liver biopsies from those infants with cholestatic jaundice may be helpful in predicting the course of liver disease. Details of such histologic studies of livers of infants with cholestatic jaundice are provided in the section describing the pathology of α_1-antitrypsin deficiency. Hepatic cirrhosis may develop during the second year of life or later in childhood.[67,71] The long-term consequences of the PiZZ phenotype in patients without neonatal cholestatic jaundice remain to be determined by following such infants to adulthood.

Liver Disease in Adults

Ganrot and co-workers initially reported two cases of cirrhosis and one case of primary hepatic carcinoma in adults with the PiZZ phenotype.[72] Subsequently, several case reports of hepatic cirrhosis in adults with the PiZZ phenotype were published.[73,74] One study of 13 autopsied patients from Sweden revealed cirrhosis or hepatic fibrosis in 8 of these patients, 3 of whom also had hepatomas.[75] However, the patients were selected from an unspecified number of autopsies. In another study 9 patients with hepatic cirrhosis were discovered among a group of 200 adult patients who had the PiZZ phenotype. None of these patients had a history of neonatal cholestasis. Most of these patients experienced the fairly acute onset of portal hypertension without prior histories of alcoholic liver disease. Coma or bleeding from varices or both was the most common cause of death.[71] Emphysema was common in this group. It is estimated that the risk of developing hepatic cirrhosis in adults with α_1-antitrypsin deficiency is about 10 percent.[75] Eriksson and colleagues assessed the risk of developing liver cirrhosis and primary liver cancer in a retrospective study based on 17 autopsied cases of α_1-antitrypsin deficiency identified in the city of Malmö, Sweden, from 1963 to 1982. Each autopsied case was matched with four controls selected from the same autopsy register. The results indicated a strong relation between α_1-antitrypsin deficiency, cirrhosis, and primary liver cancer. However, when the data were analyzed according to sex, these associations were significant only for male patients. This study suggests clearly that male patients are at higher risk for the development of cirrhosis and hepatoma with α_1-antitrypsin deficiency. The reason for male selectivity is not clear; however, it could be secondary to a small sample size or to a true lower risk for women.[76]

The relationship between cirrhosis and partial deficiency or heterozygotic phenotypes of α_1-antitrypsin is not well defined. Campra and associates reported a case of a patient with adult-onset cirrhosis associated with the phenotype PiSZ.[77] Similar case reports followed, with an association between FZ and MZ phenotypes and hepatic cirrhosis.[78,79] However, in a prospective study the heterozygous state occurred with approximately equal frequencies in patients with and without hepatobiliary disease.[80] Another study showed an increased prevalence of phenotype MZ in patients with cryptogenic cirrhosis and with non-B chronic hepatitis.[81] The possibility remains that patients with partially deficient states are at greater risk for the development of chronic liver disease when exposed to certain unspecified stimuli. This possibility needs to be explored by long-term prospective follow-up studies of patients with heterozygous phenotypes who do not have liver disease.

Cirrhotic patients with α_1-antitrypsin deficiencies have an exceedingly high incidence of hepatomas. Thus Eriksson found six hepatomas in the nine cirrhotic adults who were phenotypically PiZZ. Four of these tumors were hepatocellular carcinomas and two were cholangiocarcinomas. The hepatoma cells did not contain α_1-antitrypsin globules.[75]

Pathology

Sharp found distinctive, sharply defined, round-to-oval deposits 1 to 40 μm in diameter in the periportal hepatocytes of individuals who were PiZZ, regardless of whether they had liver disease or not.[32] These globules, which enlarge with increasing age, become increasingly easy to detect as the infant matures. They are seen with hematoxylin-eosin staining as slightly eosinophilic deposits in the cytoplasm of the hepatocytes. They are discerned most easily by positive PAS staining after diastase treatment (Figures 47-2 and 47-3).

Immunofluorescent and immunocytochemical studies have shown that the inclusions consist of material antigenically related to α_1-antitrypsin. These globules have also been observed in heterozygous individuals. There appears to be no definite relationship between the intensity and extent of involvement with the globules and the occurrence of liver disease.[7] However, the absence of liver disease in the few Pi null individuals who have no deposits of these globules suggests that the deposits may have a role in the pathogenesis of liver disease.[82,83] Hepatic steatosis has been a non-specific finding in some patients with α_1-antitrypsin deficiencies.[3]

Electron microscopy shows that the hepatocyte contains characteristic amorphous deposits, primarily within dilated rough endoplasmic reticulum,[7,45] although one study demonstrated the deposits to be in the smooth endoplasmic reticulum.[84] Such deposits were not present in Golgi apparatus. The amounts of material in the deposits vary from one patient to another and are not limited to the hepatocytes but may also be seen in biliary duct cells. Glycogen, clear vacuoles, and heterogeneous electron-dense bodies (lipofuscin) may be seen in the cytoplasm of the hepatocytes.[84] Bile stasis may be present in some hepatocytes.

In neonates of the PiZZ phenotype with cholestatic jaundice secondary to α_1-antitrypsin deficiencies, three morphologic patterns of hepatic alterations can be distinguished.[85]

1. Hepatocellular damage. Features in this group include giant cell transformation and relatively little infiltration with chronic inflammatory cells. The bile ducts are normal, with either no or minimal fibrosis. Bile stasis is present; however, bile plugs are not seen in the portal area.
2. Portal fibrosis with biliary duct proliferation. Extensive portal fibrosis, sometimes sufficiently advanced to give a picture of cirrhosis, is usually seen. Marked ductular proliferation is present and bile plugs are occasionally seen in the ducts. In five such infants jaundice disappeared before the age of 6 months, but the liver and spleen became progressively larger and harder. Portal hypertension was later found in two of these infants. Four of the five infants underwent exploratory surgery for presumed extrahepatic biliary atresia. A normal, patent extrahepatic biliary tree was found in each.

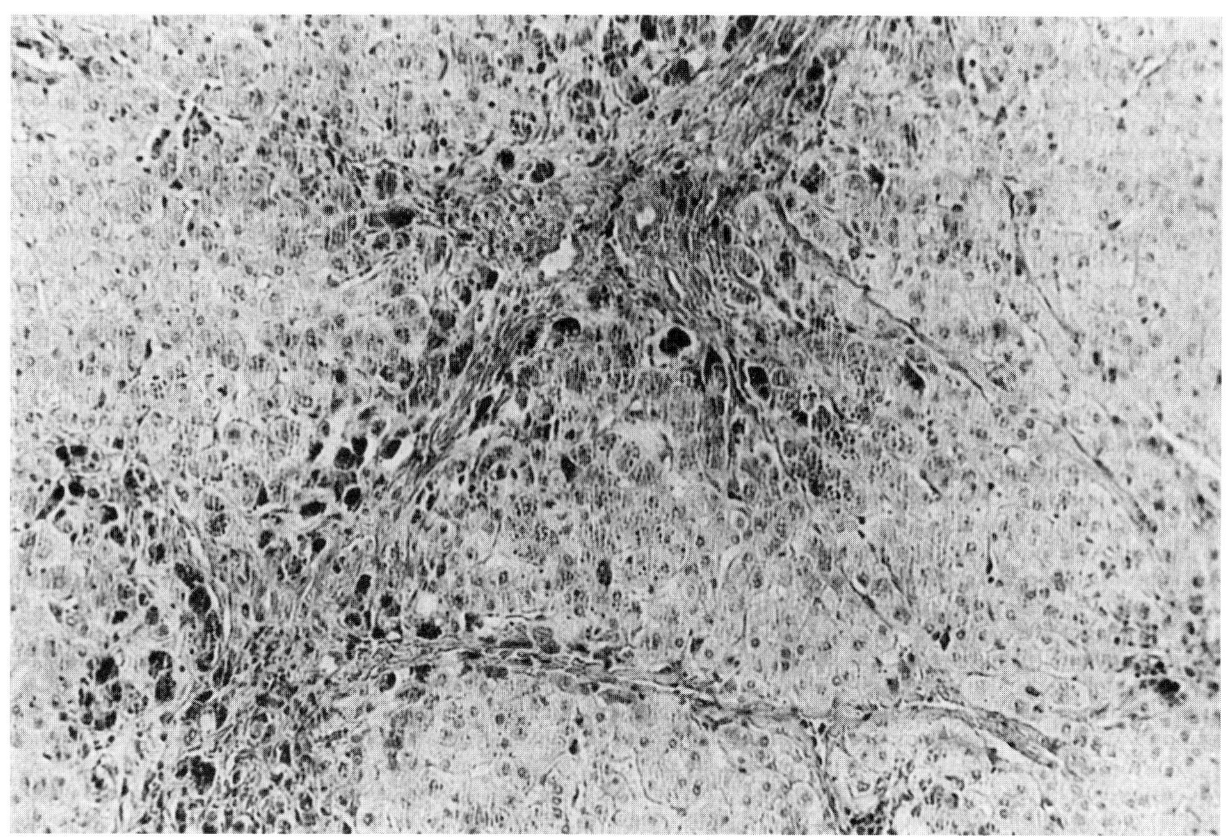

Figure 47-2 Wedge biopsy of the liver, showing cirrhosis. The hepatocytes contain deposits of typical α_1-antitrypsin. (PAS staining with diastase, ×80.) *PAS,* Periodic acid-Schiff.

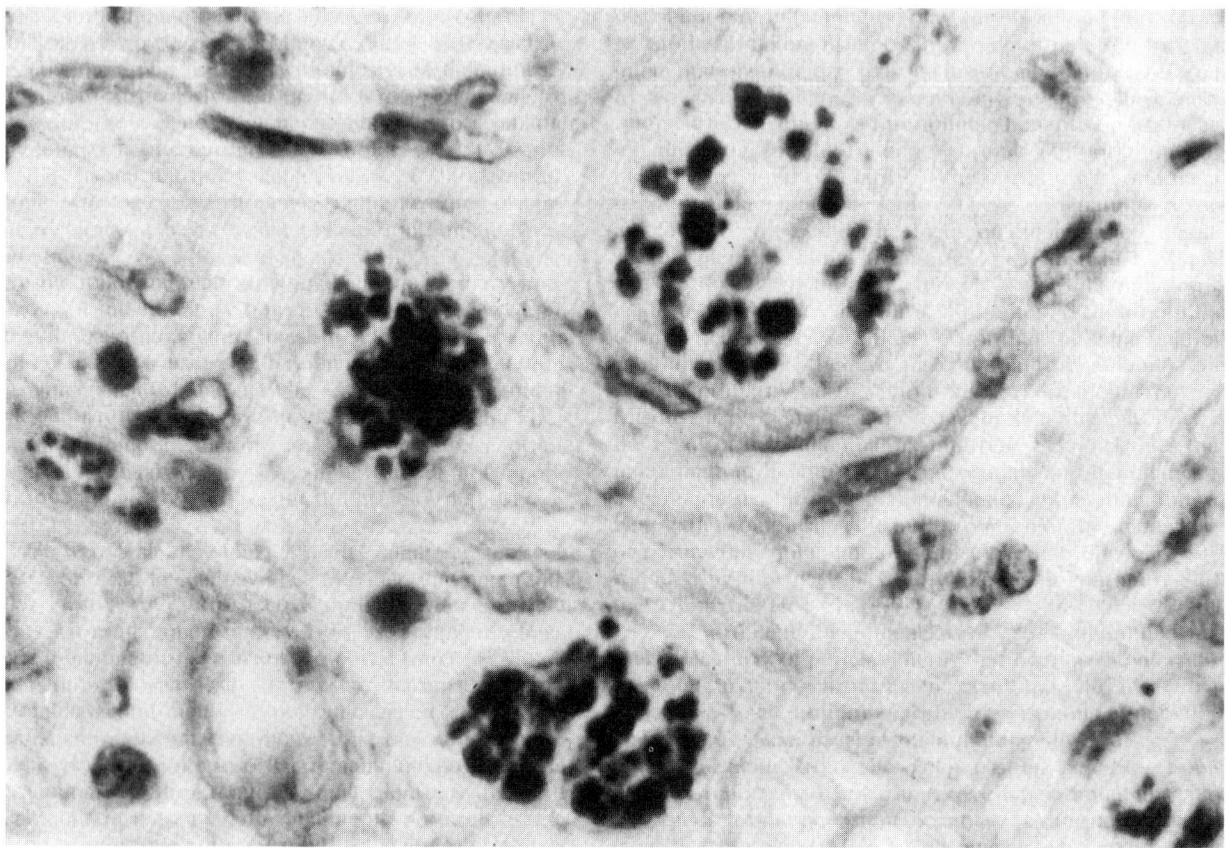

Figure 47-3 Hepatocytes containing deposits of α_1-antitrypsin. (PAS staining with diastase, ×400.) *PAS,* Periodic acid-Schiff.

3. Ductular hypoplasia. The hepatic architecture is intact with minimal hepatocellular damage. The portal areas show minimal fibrosis, but there is a marked diminution of the number of biliary ducts. In one such infant no biliary duct could be detected in 11 portal areas. Bile stasis, randomly distributed in the hepatic lobules, is always present. The clinical course in these infants is one of continued jaundice with pruritus and high levels of serum cholesterol.

These three categories may be useful in predicting the course of liver disease, but exceptions will occur. Longer follow-up is necessary to determine the long-term outcome in infants with neonatal cholestatic jaundice secondary to severe α_1-antitrypsin deficiency.

Therapy

α_1-Antitrypsin deficiency results in two important clinical problems. The first is emphysema and the second is liver disease leading to cirrhosis. Avoidance of smoking is the most important preventive therapy in the development of emphysema because smoking accelerates the destructive lung disease.[86,87] Efforts to induce α_1-antitrypsin using danazol (isoxazole derivative of 17-ethinyl testosterone) are hampered by liver toxicity and the potential for increase in the accumulation of α_1-antitrypsin deposition in the liver.[88] Replacement of α_1-antitrypsin in patients with emphysema has been carried out and found to be effective in raising the concentration of α_1-antitrypsin in serum and in the lung.[89] Of importance is the observation that the diffused α_1-antitrypsin in the lung was active as an inhibitor of neutrophil elastase. No significant adverse reactions were noted in more than 800 weekly infusions of α_1-antitrypsin.[90] A recombinant α_1-antitrypsin has been produced in *Escherichia coli*[91,92] and in yeast[93] and was found to be functionally active as an elastase inhibitor. Unfortunately it lacks the carbohydrate side chains, thus making the recombinant product unstable with a short half-life.[94] Gene therapy appears to be theoretically possible and likely to be a reality in the future.[95,96]

In the case of liver disease associated with α_1-antitrypsin deficiency, orthotopic liver transplantation appears to be the only available form of therapy.[97,98] In a study of 39 patients (29 children and 10 adults) who underwent orthotopic liver transplantation for liver disease associated with α_1-antitrypsin deficiency from March 1980 to March 1986 20 percent died during the first 3 months. The 5-year actuarial survival was 83 percent and 60 percent in pediatric and adult recipients, respectively; 76 percent of the recipients are alive, with follow-ups of 8 to 64 months.[98] In selected patients with mild hepatic dysfunction and portal hypertension a splenorenal shunt can be considered, as the progression of liver disease in α_1-antitrypsin deficiency can be slow.

SUMMARY

Various metabolic disorders may permanently injure the liver. Most of these disorders carry enzymatic defects that have been identified; others remain speculative. Most of the diseases that are associated with enzymatic defects in carbohydrate metabolism are treatable, with good to excellent results. However, most defects in lipid and bile acid metabolism are poorly responsive to dietary or drug therapy. Table 47-3 summarizes the disorders discussed in this and the following chapter.

References

1. Laurell CB, Eriksson S: The electrophoretic α_1-globulin pattern of serum in α_1-antitrypsin deficiency. Scand J Clin Lab Invest 15:132, 1963.
2. Sharp HL, Bridges RA, Krivit W, et al: Cirrhosis associated with α_1-antitrypsin deficiency: a previously unrecognized inherited disorder. J Lab Clin Med 73:934, 1969.
3. Porter CA, Mowat AP, Cook PJK, et al: α_1-Antitrypsin deficiency and neonatal hepatitis. BMJ 3:435, 1972.
4. Mowat AP, Psacharopoulos HT, Williams R: Extrahepatic biliary atresia versus neonatal hepatitis. Arch Dis Child 51:763, 1976.
5. Perlmutter DH, Cole FS, Kilbridge P, et al: Expression of the α_1-proteinase inhibitor gene in human monocytes and macrophages. Proc Natl Acad Sci U S A 82:795, 1985.
6. Makino S, Reed CE: Distribution and elimination of exogenous α_1-antitrypsin. J Lab Clin Med 75:742, 1970.
7. Sharp HL: The current status of α_1-antitrypsin, a protease inhibitor, in gastrointestinal disease. Gastroenterology 70:611, 1976.
8. Holmes WE, Nelles L, Lijnen HR, et al: Primary structure of human α_2-antiplasmin, a serine protease inhibitor. J Biol Chem 262:1659, 1987.
9. Carrell RW, Gooptu B: Conformational changes and disease serpins, prions and Alzheimer's. Curr Opin Struct Biol 8:799-809, 1998.
10. Carrell RW, Lomas DA: Conformational disease. Lancet 350:134-138, 1997.
11. Elliott PR, Lomas DA, Carrell RW, et al: Inhibitory conformation of the reactive loop of α_1-antitrypsin. Nat Struct Biol 3:676-681, 1996.
12. Loebermann H, Tokuoka R, Deisenhofer J, et al: Human α1-antiproteinase inhibitor. Crystal structure analysis of two crystal modifications: molecular model and preliminary analysis of the implications for function. J Mol Biol 177:531, 1984.
13. Owen MC, Brennan SO, Lewis JH, et al: Mutation of antitrypsin to antithrombin: α_1-antitrypsin Pittsburgh (358 Met-Arg), a fatal bleeding disorder. N Engl J Med 309:694, 1983.
14. Greene L, Lieberman J: Statement of methods for selecting α_1-antitrypsin abnormalities. In Mittman C, ed: Pulmonary Emphysema and Proteolysis. New York, Academic Press, 1972:141.
15. Talamo RC, Langley CE, Hyslop JR: A comparison of functional and immunochemical measurement of serum α_1-antitrypsin. In Mittman C, ed: Pulmonary Emphysema and Proteolysis. New York, Academic Press, 1972:167.
16. Fagerhol MK: Quantitative studies on the inherited variants of serum α_1-antitrypsin. Scand J Clin Lab Invest 23:97, 1967.
17. Allen RC, Harley RA, Talamo RC: A new method for determination of α_1 AT phenotypes using isoelectric focusing on polyacrylamide gel slabs. Am J Clin Pathol 62:732, 1974.
18. Fagerhol MK, Laurell CB: The polymorphism of "prealbumins" and α_1-antitrypsin in human sera. Clin Chim Acta 16:199, 1967.
19. Fagerhol MK: Pi typing techniques. In Peters H, ed: Twenty-second Colloquium on Peptides of Biological Fluids. Amsterdam, Elsevier, 1975:493.
20. Cox DW, Woo SLC, Mansfield T: DNA restriction fragments associated with α_1-antitrypsin indicate a single origin of deficiency allele PiZ. Nature 316:79, 1985.
21. Kueppers F, Christopherson MJ: α_1-Antitrypsin: further genetic heterogeneity revealed by isoelectric focusing. Am J Hum Genet 30:359, 1978.
22. Nukiwa T, Brantly M, Ogushi F, et al: Characterization of the MI(ala^{213}) type of α_1-antitrypsin, a newly recognized, common "normal" α_1-antitrypsin haplotype. Biochemistry 26:5259, 1987.
23. Brantly M, Nukiwa Y, Crystal RG: Molecular basis of α_1-antitrypsin deficiency. Am J Med 84:13, 1988.
24. Garver RI, Mornex JF, Nukiwa T, et al: α_1-Antitrypsin deficiency and emphysema caused by homozygous inheritance of non-expressing α_1-antitrypsin genes. N Engl J Med 314:762, 1986.

TABLE 47-3
Metabolic Liver Diseases that Lead to Permanent Injury

Inborn errors of metabolism	Enzyme deficiency	Common clinical manifestations	Laboratory data	Treatment
Carbohydrate Metabolism				
Hereditary fructose intolerance	Fructose-1-phosphate aldolase	Hepatomegaly Jaundice Vomiting	↓Glucose ↑PO_4 ↑Uric acid ↑SGOT Renal tubular dysfunction	Fructose-free, sucrose-free diet
Galactosemia	Galactose-1-phosphate uridyl transferase	Failure to thrive Hepatomegaly Jaundice Vomiting	↓Glucose Reducing substances in the urine Abnormal liver function tests Renal tubular dysfunction	Lactose-free diet
Glycogen storage disease, type I	Glucose-6-phosphatase	Growth failure Hepatomegaly	Hypoglycemia Hyperlipemia Acidosis ↑Uric acid	Nocturnal nasogastric feedings Uncooked cornstarch during the day
Glycogen storage disease, type III	Amylo-1,6-glucosidase (debrancher enzyme)	Growth failure Hepatomegaly Muscle weakness	Hypoglycemia Hyperlipemia	Frequent feedings of high-protein diet
Glycogen storage disease, type IV	α-1,4-Glucan6-glycosyl transferase (brancher)	Diarrhea Failure to thrive Hepatosplenomegaly Vomiting	Abnormal liver function tests Acidosis	Frequent feedings of high-protein diet
Protein Metabolism				
Hereditary tyrosinemia	Fumarylacetoacetase	Failure to thrive Hepatosplenomegaly Jaundice Rickets	Abnormal liver function tests Renal tubular dysfunction	Low-phenylalanine, low-tyrosine diet NTBC
Lipid Metabolism				
Wolman's disease	Acid lipase	Diarrhea Failure to thrive Hepatosplenomegaly Vomiting	Symmetrical calcification of adrenals Anemia Vacuolation of lymphocytes Deposition of triglycerides and cholesterol ester in various organs	None
Cholesterol ester	Acid lipase	Hepatosplenomegaly	Deposition of triglyceride and cholesterol ester in various organs Portal hypertension	None

Bile Acid Metabolism				
PFIC1 (Byler's disease)	Mutations in canalicular P-type ATPase chromosome 18q21-22	Jaundice Severe pruritus	Normal γ-GT Low primary bile salts	Biliary diversion Liver transplant ? Ursodeoxycholic acid
PFIC2 (BSEP deficiency)	Mutations in SPGP (BSEP) canalicular transporter chromosome 2q24	Jaundice Severe pruritus	Low γ-GT Low primary bile acids	Biliary diversion Liver transplant ? Ursodeoxycholic acid
PFIC3 (MDR3 deficiency)	Mutations in MDR3 chromosome 7q21	Jaundice Moderate pruritus	High γ-GT Low phospholipid concentration	Biliary diversion Liver transplant ? Ursodeoxycholic acid
Arteriohepatic dysplasia	Mutations in the JAGGED-1 gene, a ligand for the Notch gene	Characteristic facies Hepatomegaly Jaundice Posterior embryotoxon Pruritus Pulmonary stenosis Vertebral anomalies	↑Bilirubin ↑Cholesterol ↑Alkaline phosphatase ↑Bile acids	Nutritional management Pancreatic enzymes Ursodeoxycholic acid
Zellweger's syndrome	Mutations in peroxisomal PEX gene	Characteristic facies Hepatomegaly Hypotonia Jaundice	↑Precursors of cholic and chenodeoxycholic acid ↑Serum iron	None
Hereditary lymphedema with recurrent cholestasis	? Impaired bile acid secretion ? Abnormalities of liver lymphatics	Jaundice Lymphedema of the lower extremities Pruritus	↑Bilirubin ↑Cholesterol ↑Alkaline phosphatase Abnormal lymphangiograms	None
THCA (3α-, 7α-, 12α-trihydroxy-5β-cholestane-26-oic acid) syndrome	Block in conversion of ? THCA → variant acid	Hepatosplenomegaly Jaundice	↑THCA in serum and bile	? Phenobarbital ? Cholestyramine
Unclassified				
α_1-Antitrypsin deficiency	Missense mutations	Hepatomegaly Neonatal cholestatic jaundice Portal hypertension	↓Serum α_1-antitrypsin phenotype→PiZZ	Liver transplant None medically
Cystic fibrosis	Deletions, mutations in the cystic fibrosis gene leading to defective cystic fibrosis transmembrane conductor regulator	Hepatomegaly Neonatal cholestatic jaundice Pancreatic insufficiency Portal hypertension Pulmonary infection	↑Sweat Cl Steatorrhea Possibly abnormal liver function tests	Antibiotics for pulmonary complications Pancreatic enzymes Ursodeoxycholic acid ? Gene therapy

PO4, Phosphate; *SGOT,* serum glutamic-oxaloacetic transaminase; *PFIC,* progressive familial intrahepatic cholestasis; *ATPase,* adenosine triphosphatases; *γ-GT,* gamma-glutamyltransferase; *BSEP,* bile salt export pump; *SPGP,* sister of P-glycoprotein; *MDR,* multidrug resistant; *PEX,* peroxin gene; *THCA,* 11-nor-9-carboxy-Δ^9-tetrahydrocannabinal.

25. Nukiwa T, Takahashi H, Brantly M, et al: α1-AntitrypsinNull$_{Granite\ Falls}$, a nonexpressing α_1-antitrypsin gene associated with a frameshift stop mutation in a coding exon. J Biol Chem 262:11999, 1987.
26. Muensch H, Gaidulis L, Kueppers F, et al: Complete absence of serum α_1-antitrypsin in conjugation with an apparently normal gene structure. Am J Hum Genet 38:898, 1986.
27. Sifers RN, Brashears-Macatee S, Kidd VJ, et al: A frameshift mutation results in a truncated α_1-antitrypsin that is retained within the rough endoplasmic reticulum. J Biol Chem 263:7330, 1988.
28. Curiel D, Brantly M, Cureil E, et al: α_1-Antitrypsin deficiency caused by the α_1-antitrypsin Null$_{Mattawa}$ gene. An insertion mutation rendering the α_1-antitrypsin gene incapable of producing α_1-antitrypsin. J Clin Invest 83:1144, 1989.
29. Satoh K, Nukiwa T, Brantly M, et al: Emphysema associated with a complete absence of α_1-antitrypsin gene incapable of producing α_1-antitrypsin. J Clin Invest 83:1144, 1989.
30. Curiel DT, Holmes MD, Okayama H, et al: Molecular basis of liver and lung disease associated with the α_1-antitrypsin deficiency allele M$_{Malton}$. J Biol Chem 264:15528, 1988.
31. Lieberman J, Gaidulis L, Klotz SD: A new deficient variant of α_1-antitrypsin (M$_{Duarte}$). Inability to detect the heterozygous state by α_1-antitrypsin phenotyping. Am Rev Respir Dis 113:31, 1976.
32. Hofker MH, Nukiwa T, van Paassen HMB, et al: A pro→leu substitution in codon 369 of the α_1-antitrypsin deficiency variant PiMHeerlen. Am J Hum Genet 41:A220, 1987.
33. Takahashi H, Nukiwa T, Satoh K, et al: Characterization of the gene and protein of the α_1-antitrypsin "deficiency" allele M$_{Procida}$. J Biol Chem 264:15528, 1988.
34. Sharp HL: α_1-Antitrypsin deficiency. Hosp Pract 6:83, 1971.
35. Jeppson JO: Amino acid substitution Glu→Lys in α_1-antitrypsin PiZ. FEBS Lett 65:195, 1976.
36. Yoshida A, Lieberman J, Giadulis L, et al: Molecular abnormality of human α_1-antitrypsin variant (PiZZ) associated with plasma activity deficiency. Proc Natl Acad Sci U S A 73:1324, 1976.
37. Dyaico MJ, Grant SGN, Fells K, et al: Neonatal hepatitis induced by α_1-antitrypsin: a transgenic mouse model. Science 242:1409, 1988.
38. Carlson JA, Rogers BB, Sifers RN, et al: The accumulation of PiZ α_1-antitrypsin causes liver damage in transgenic mice. J Clin Invest 83:1183, 1989.
39. Rothman JE: Protein sorting by selective retention in the endoplasmic reticulum and Golgi stack. Cell 50:521, 1987.
40. Le A, Graham KS, Sifers RN: Intracellular degradation of the transport-impaired human PiZ α_1-antitrypsin variant. Biochemical mapping of the degradative event among compartments of the secretory pathway. J Biol Chem 265:14001, 1990.
41. Yu MH, Lee KH, Kim J: The Z type variation of human α_1-antitrypsin causes a protein-folding defect. Nat Struct Biol 2:363-367, 1995.
42. Kang HA, Lee KH, Yu MH: Folding and stability of the Z and S(iiyama) genetic variants of human α_1-antitrypsin. J Biol Chem 272:510-516, 1997.
43. Ogushi F, Fells GA, Hubbard RC, et al: Z-type α_1-antitrypsin is less competent than Ml-type α_1-antitrypsin as an inhibitor of neutrophil elastase. J Clin Invest 89:1366, 1987.
44. Le A, Ferrell GA, Dishon DS, et al: Soluble aggregates of the human PiZ α_1-antitrypsin variant are degraded within the endoplasmic reticulum by a mechanism sensitive to inhibitors of protein synthesis. J Biol Chem 267:1072, 1992.
45. Lomas DA, Evans DL, Finch JJ, et al: The mechanism of Z α_1-antitrypsin accumulation in the liver. Nature 357:605-607, 1992.
46. Gooptu B, Hazes B, Chang WS, et al: Inactive conformation of the serpin α_1-antichymotrypsin indicates two-stage insertion of the reactive loop: implications for inhibitory function and conformational disease. Proc Natl Acad Sci U S A 97:67-72, 2000.
47. Burrows JAJ, Willis LK, Perlmutter DH: Chemical chaperones mediate increased secretion of mutant α_1-antitrypsin (α_1-AT) Z: a potential pharmacological strategy for prevention of liver injury and emphysema in α_1-AT deficiency. Proc Natl Acad Sci U S A 97:1796-1801, 2000.
48. Kyrachi K, Chandra T, Friezneo SJ, et al: Cloning and sequence of cDNA coding for α_1-antitrypsin. Proc Natl Acad Sci U S A 78:6826, 1981.
49. Long G, Chandra T, Woo S, et al: Complete sequence of cDNA for human α_1-antitrypsin and the gene for the S variant. Biochemistry 23:4878, 1984.
50. Schroeder WT, Miller MF, Woo SLC, et al: Chromosomal localization of the human α_1-antitrypsin gene (Pi) to 14q31-32. Am J Hum Genet 37:868, 1985.
51. Rabin M, Watson M, Kidd V, et al: Regional localization of α_1-antichymotrypsin and α_1-antitrypsin genes on human chromosome 14. Somat Cell Mol Genet 12:209, 1986.
52. Perlino E, Cortese R, Ciliberto G: The human α1-antitrypsin gene is transcribed from two different promoters in macrophages and hepatocytes. EMBO J 6:2767, 1987.
53. Wu Y, Whitman I, Molmenti E, et al: A lag in intracellular degradation of mutant α_1-antitrypsin correlates with the liver disease phenotype in homozygous PiZZ α_1-antitrypsin deficiency. Proc Natl Acad Sci U S A 91:9014-9018, 1994.
54. Kueppers F: α_1-Antitrypsin: physiology, genetics and pathology. Hum Genet 11:177, 1971.
55. Pierce JA, Eradio B, Dew TA: Antitrypsin phenotypes in St. Louis. JAMA 231:609, 1975.
56. Sverger T: Liver disease in α_1-antitrypsin deficiency detected by screening of 200,000 infants. N Engl J Med 294:1316, 1976.
57. Talamo RC, Langley CE, Levine BW, et al: Genetic vs. quantitative analysis of serum α_1 antitrypsin. N Engl J Med 287:1067, 1972.
58. Kidd V, Wallace RB, Itakura K, et al: α_1-Antitrypsin deficiency detection by direct analysis of the mutation in the gene. Nature 304:230, 1983.
59. Kidd V, Golbus MS, Wallace RB, et al: Prenatal diagnosis of α_1-antitrypsin deficiency by direct analysis of the mutation site in the gene. N Engl J Med 310:639, 1984.
60. Dermer SJ, Johnson EM: Methods in laboratory investigation: rapid DNA analysis of α_1-antitrypsin deficiency. Lab Invest 59:403, 1988.
61. Petersen KB, Kolvroa S, Bolund L, et al: Detection of α_1-antitrypsin genotypes by analysis of amplified DNA sequences. Nucleic Acids Res 16:352, 1988.
62. Tazelaar JP, Friedman KJ, Kline RS, et al: Detection of α_1-antitrypsin Z and S mutations by polymerase chain reaction-mediated site-directed mutagenesis. Clin Chem 38(8):1486, 1992.
63. Dry PJ: Rapid detection of α_1-antitrypsin deficiency by analysis of a PCR-induced TaqI restriction site. Hum Genet 87:742, 1991.
64. Freeman HJ, Weinstein WM, Shnitka TK, et al: α_1-Antitrypsin deficiency and pancreatic fibrosis. Ann Intern Med 85:73, 1976.
65. Moroz SP, Cutz E, Balfe JW, et al: Membranoproliferative glomerulonephritis in childhood cirrhosis associated with α_1-antitrypsin deficiency. Pediatrics 57:232, 1976.
66. Smith KC, Su WP, Pittelkow MR, et al: Clinical and pathologic correlations in 96 patients with panniculitis, including 15 patients with deficient levels of α_1-antitrypsin. J Am Acad Dermatol 21(6):1192, 1989.
67. Sveger T: α_1-Antitrypsin deficiency in early childhood. Pediatrics 62:22, 1978.
68. O'Brien ML, Buist NRM, Murphey H: Neonatal screening for α_1-antitrypsin deficiency. J Pediatr 92:1006, 1978.
69. Sveger T: The natural history of liver disease in α_1-antitrypsin deficient children. Acta Paediatr Scand 77:847, 1988.
70. Ghishan FK, Greene HL: Liver disease in children with PiZZ α_1-antitrypsin deficiency. Hepatology 8:307, 1988.
71. Odievre M, Martin JP, Hadchouel M, et al: α_1-Antitrypsin deficiency and liver disease in children: phenotypes, manifestations and prognosis. Pediatrics 57:226, 1976.
72. Ganrot PO, Laurell CB, Eriksson S: Obstructive lung disease and trypsin inhibitors in α_1-antitrypsin deficiency. Scand J Clin Lab Invest 19:205, 1967.
73. Ishak KG, Jenas EH, Marshall ML, et al: Cirrhosis of the liver associated with α_1-antitrypsin deficiency. Arch Pathol 94:445, 1972.
74. Berg NO, Eriksson S: Liver disease in adults with α_1-antitrypsin deficiency. N Engl J Med 287:1264, 1972.
75. Eriksson S, Hagerstrand I: Cirrhosis and malignant hepatoma in α_1-antitrypsin deficiency. Acta Med Scand 195:451, 1974.
76. Eriksson S, Carlson J, Velez R: Risk of cirrhosis and primary liver cancer in α_1-antitrypsin deficiency. N Engl J Med 314:736, 1986.
77. Campra JL, Craig JP, Peters RL, et al: Cirrhosis associated with partial deficiency of α_1-antitrypsin in adults. Ann Intern Med 78:233, 1973.
78. Brand B, Bezahler GH, Gould R: Cirrhosis and heterozygous FZ α_1-antitrypsin deficiency in an adult. Case report and review of the literature. Gastroenterology 66:264, 1974.
79. Rawlings W, Moss J, Cooper HS, et al: Hepatocellular carcinoma and partial deficiency of α_1-antitrypsin (MZ). Ann Intern Med 81:771, 1974.
80. Fisher RL, Taylor L, Sherlock S: α_1-Antitrypsin deficiency in liver disease: the extent of the problem. Gastroenterology 71:646, 1976.

81. Hodges JR, Millwand-Sadler GH, Barbatis C, et al: Heterozygous MZ α_1-antitrypsin deficiency in adults with chronic active hepatitis and cryptogenic cirrhosis. N Engl J Med 304:557, 1981.
82. Talamo RC, Langley CE, Reed CE, et al: α_1-Antitrypsin deficiency: a variant with no detectable α_1-antitrypsin. Science 181:70, 1973.
83. Martin JP: Further examples confirming the existence of Pi null (Pi-). Pathol Biol 23:521, 1975.
84. Yunis EJ, Agostini RM, Glen RH: Fine structural observations of the liver in α_1-antitrypsin deficiency. Am J Pathol 82:265, 1976.
85. Hadchouel M, Goutier M: Histopathologic study of the liver in the early cholestatic phase of α_1-antitrypsin deficiency. J Pediatr 89:211, 1976.
86. Larsson C: Natural history and life expectancy in severe α_1-antitrypsin deficiency, PiZ. Acta Med Scand 204:345, 1978.
87. Janus ED, Phillips NT, Carrell RW: Smoking, lung function and α_1-antitrypsin deficiency. Lancet i:152, 1985.
88. Wewers MD, Gadek JE, Keogh BA, et al: Evaluation of danazol therapy for patients with PiZZ α_1-antitrypsin deficiency. Am Rev Respir Dis 134:476, 1986.
89. Wewers MD, Casolaro MA, Sellers SE, et al: Replacement therapy for α_1-antitrypsin deficiency associated with emphysema. N Engl J Med 316:1055, 1987.
90. Schmidt EW, Rasche B, Ulmer WT, et al: Replacement therapy for α_1-protease inhibitor deficiency in PiZ subjects with chronic obstructive lung disease. Am J Med 84(6A):63, 1988.
91. Courtney M, Jallat S, Tessier L-H, et al: Synthesis in *E. coli* of α_1-antitrypsin variants of therapeutic potential for emphysema and thrombosis. Nature 313:149, 1985.
92. Courtney M, Buchwalder A, Tessier L-H, et al: High-level production of biologically active human α_1-antitrypsin in *Escherichia coli.* Proc Natl Acad Sci U S A 81:669, 1984.
93. Rosenberg S, Barr PJ, Najarian RC, et al: Synthesis in yeast of a functional oxidation-resistant mutant of human α_1-antitrypsin. Nature 312:77, 1984.
94. Travis J, Owen MC, George P, et al: Isolation and properties of recombinant DNA produced variants of human α_1-proteinase inhibitor. J Biol Chem 260:4384, 1985.
95. Ledley FD: Somatic gene therapy for human disease. J Pediatr 110:167, 1987.
96. Ledley FD, Woo SLC: Molecular basis of α_1-antitrypsin deficiency and its potential therapy by gene transfer. J Inherit Metab Dis 9(suppl 1):85, 1986.
97. Hood JM, Koep LJ, Peters RL, et al: Liver transplantation for advanced liver disease with α1-antitrypsin deficiency. N Engl J Med 302:272, 1980.
98. Esquivel CO, Vicente E, van Thiel D, et al: Orthotopic liver transplantation for α_1-antitrypsin deficiency: an experience in 29 children and 10 adults. Transplant Proc 19(5):3798, 1987.

CHAPTER

48

Inborn Errors of Metabolism that Lead to Permanent Hepatic Injury

Fayez K. Ghishan, MD

ABBREVIATIONS

ADP	adenosine diphosphate
ATP	adenosine triphosphate
BSP	sulfobromophthalein
FDPase	fructose-1,6-diphosphatase
GSD	glycogen storage disease
HFI	hereditary fructose intolerance
PAS	periodic acid–Schiff
P_i	inorganic phosphate
PRPP	phosphoribosyl pyrophosphate
THCA	$3\alpha,7\alpha,12\alpha$-trihydroxy-5β-cholestan-26-oic acid
TPN	total parenteral nutrition
UDP	uridine diphosphate

The liver is often affected by inborn errors of metabolism, but only a few of these injure it severely enough to cause permanent damage. Because the use of the Menghini needle for percutaneous liver biopsy has proved safe in infants and children, histologic and biochemical evaluations of liver specimens from living patients have provided the means for major advances in the study of metabolic diseases during the past few years. Advances in molecular genetics promise greater advances in diagnosis and treatment of metabolic illnesses as our understanding of the pathophysiology of such disorders improves. Table 48-1 lists the major metabolic diseases that involve the liver. Those marked with asterisks may lead to progressive disease and are discussed here or elsewhere in this book.

TABLE 48-1

Inborn Errors of Metabolism Resulting in Injury to the Liver

Inborn errors of carbohydrate metabolism:
- Glycogen storage disease, types I-XII*
- Galactosemia*
  - Fructose-1-phosphate aldolase deficiency
  - Fructose-1,6-diphosphatase deficiency

Inborn errors of protein metabolism:
- Tyrosinemia*
- Urea cycle enzymic defects (see Chaps. 4 and 15)

Inborn errors of lipid metabolism:
- Gaucher's disease
- Niemann-Pick disease
- Gangliosidosis
- Acid cholesterol ester hydrolase deficiency*
  - Wolman's disease
  - Cholesterol ester storage disease
- Lipodystrophy

Inborn errors of mucopolysaccharide metabolism

Inborn errors of porphyrin metabolism:
- Protoporphyria (see Chap. 11)*

Inborn errors of bile acid metabolism:
- Progressive familial intrahepatic cholestasis*
- Type I (Byler's disease)*
- Type II (Byler's syndrome)*
- Type III*
- Hereditary lymphedema with recurrent cholestasis (Aagenaes's syndrome)
- THCA syndrome

Disorders of peroxisome biogenesis:
- Zellweger's syndrome*
- Alagille's syndrome (arteriohepatic dysplasia)*

Inborn errors of copper metabolism:
- Wilson's disease (see Chap. 41)*

Unclassified:
- α_1-Antitrypsin deficiency*
- Cystic fibrosis*

*Diseases that lead to progressive disease and are discussed in this chapter or other sections of this book.

EVALUATION OF HEPATIC METABOLIC DISORDERS

The clinical history and physical examination are the first essentials in evaluating infants and children with metabolic liver disorders. Of particular importance is a family history of any metabolic liver disease. Symptoms that may be associated with metabolic liver disorders are usually non-specific and include vomiting, diarrhea, jaundice, seizures, and abnormal urinary odor. Clinical findings include hepatosplenomegaly, hypotonicity or hypertonicity, coarse facial features, and respiratory distress. The physical examination should include adequate ophthalmologic examination by slit lamp for corneal, lenticular, and retinal alterations. Psychomotor evaluation to detect developmental delays is important in identifying those diseases that may involve the central nervous system. Initial laboratory screening tests such as analysis of the urine for reducing substances may help in early diagnosis of galactosemia. The peripheral blood smear may reveal vacuolation of the lymphocytic cytoplasm, which signifies deposition of storage material. Skeletal x-rays may reveal changes consistent with certain storage diseases, as in the case of mucopolysaccharidosis. In general, storage diseases usually cause marked hepatomegaly. By contrast, disorders resulting in hepatocellular damage cause only modest hepatomegaly. Confirmatory tests depend on assays of appropriate enzymes in tissues such as leukocytes, skin fibroblasts, intestine, and liver, and deoxyribonucleic acid (DNA) analysis for mutations in those disorders with known genetic defects.

DISORDERS OF CARBOHYDRATE METABOLISM

Inborn errors resulting from abnormal metabolism of lipids are mostly untreatable at present, and most of the errors in protein metabolism that respond to treatment require relatively stringent dietary restrictions. In contrast, most errors in carbohydrate metabolism, which respond favorably to treatment, do so with relatively modest dietary restrictions. Liver diseases that occur in untreated patients with inborn errors of carbohydrate metabolism, such as fructose intolerance and galactosemia, are usually preventable. Although these particular conditions are relatively rare (about 1:30,000 live births for fructose intolerance and 1:20,000 live births for galactosemia), their combined incidence is similar to that of phenylketonuria (about 1:14,000 births in the United States). Considering the outcome in untreated patients and the simplicity of either measuring urinary reducing sugar or assaying the blood sample that is obtained to screen for phenylketonuria, it seems reasonable to implement the practice of routine screening of all newborn infants for both galactosemia and fructose intolerance.

Three inborn errors in carbohydrate metabolism that may result in permanent liver damage are disorders of fructose metabolism, disorders of galactose metabolism, and certain of the glycogen storage diseases (Figure 48-1). These three abnormalities are discussed separately.

DISORDERS OF FRUCTOSE METABOLISM

Fructose Phosphate Aldolase Deficiency (Hereditary Fructose Intolerance) and Fructose-1,6-diphosphatase Deficiency

Until the mid-1950s the only identified defect in fructose metabolism was the benign disorder essential fructosuria, identified because of the large amounts of fructose in the urine after oral fructose.[1] It was recognized in 1956, in some patients, that ingestion of fructose was followed by vomiting, severe hypoglycemia, and liver disease.[2] A year later this illness was characterized and named hereditary fructose intolerance (HFI).[3] A third dis-

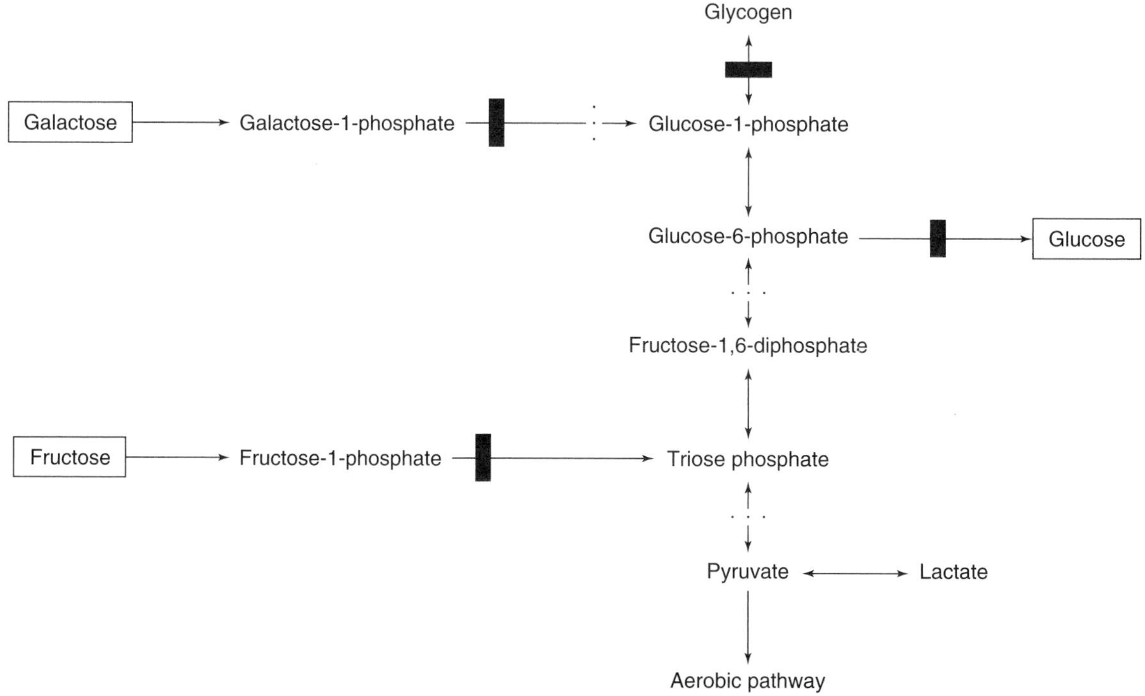

Figure 48-1 Metabolic relationship between disorders in glycogen, galactose, glucose, and fructose metabolism. Solid rectangle indicates site of metabolic block; "..." indicates omission in the metabolic sequence.

order of fructose metabolism was identified in 1970. It was associated with fasting-induced and diet-induced hypoglycemia, but more strikingly, both fasting and dietary fructose caused lactic acidosis.[4] Each of these three disorders is distinct from the others both clinically and biochemically. Essential fructosuria is due to deficient activity of hepatic fructokinase; HFI is due to deficiency of fructose-1-phosphate aldolase; and the third condition results from deficiency of fructose-1,6-diphosphatase (FDPase). Essential fructosuria does not cause liver injury. Patients with FDPase deficiency may show transient fatty infiltration of the liver. However, liver injury may be a permanent feature of HFI. For this reason, only HFI is discussed in detail.

Hereditary Fructose Intolerance

In 1957 Froesch and colleagues described the typical syndrome of HFI in two siblings and two relatives.[3] They recognized that the disorder, as with essential fructosuria, was inherited and was associated with urinary excretion of fructose, but they also realized it was due to a different enzymatic defect and had different prognostic implications.

Molecular Basis of Hereditary Fructose Intolerance

HFI occurs in 1:20,000 individuals. It has a recessive mode of inheritance. HFI is caused by a deficiency of fructose-1-phosphate aldolase (aldolase B), which is present normally in the liver, kidneys, and small intestine. The enzymatic activities of the two other aldolase isoenzymes, aldolase A in muscle and aldolase C in the brain, are normal. The three isoenzymes are related and are derived from a single ancestral gene.

The aldolase B gene has been sequenced and is mapped to human chromosome 9q13→q32.[5] The gene has nine exons encoding 364 amino acids.[5,6] The first exon is untranslated. The gene consists of 14,500 base pairs. The first mutation described was a G→C transversion in exon 5, which resulted in an amino acid substitution (alanine→proline) at position 149 of the protein within a region critical for substrate binding (A149P). The G→C transversion created a new recognition site for the restriction enzyme Aha II.[7] The alanine at position 149 is a conserved amino acid because it is present in the aldolase B gene of humans, rats, and chickens.[8] The substitution of proline is likely to disrupt the spatial configuration of juxtaposed residues in aldolase B and adversely affect its catalytic activity. The mutation alanine→proline was found in 67 percent of 50 patients studied by Cross and colleagues.[9] This mutation is encountered more frequently in patients from Northern than from Southern Europe. Several other mutations have been described, such as alanine 174→aspartic acid (A174D) and asparagine 334→lysine (N334K).[10] Tolan and Brooks characterized the molecular defects in the aldolase B gene in 31 North Americans with HFI. Fifty-nine percent of mutant North American alleles were alanine 149→proline. Alanine 174→aspartic acid and asparagine 334→lysine represented 11 percent and 2 percent of North American alleles, respectively. Nine subjects (32 percent) had HFI alleles that were not of these common, missense mutations.[11] The missense mutations could be classified into two groups: catalytic mutants with retained tetrameric structure but altered kinetic properties (W147R, R303W, and A337V) and structural mutations in which heterotetramers dissociate into subunits with impaired enzymatic activity (A149P, A174D, and N334K).[12]

Clinical Features

Patients with HFI may be extremely ill and may die after continuous exposure to fructose. However, affected patients are generally healthy and symptom-free so long as they do not ingest fructose or fructose-containing foods.[13,14] For this reason, symptoms do not arise until breast milk or cow's milk formulas are supplemented with fructose-containing foods. In fortunate cases fructose is not introduced until after an affected infant is 5 to 6 months of age. By this time, the child is likely to associate nausea, vomiting, and symptoms of hypoglycemia with sweet-tasting food. In such cases aversion to sweets is probably life-saving, and the diagnosis may go undetected until adulthood.[15] When this occurs, the diagnosis may be suspected on the basis of a careful history that recognizes the extreme aversion to dietary "sweets."

The largest single collection of patients consists of 55 patients diagnosed between 1961 and 1977 as having HFI.[16] Fifty of the patients had become symptomatic because of dietary fructose, and five were diagnosed shortly after birth because an older sibling of each infant was known to have HFI. Fourteen patients received fructose in their first feedings, and symptoms usually appeared within a few days. The remaining patients received a fructose-free diet (breast milk or cow's milk formula). Their symptoms began immediately after introduction of dietary fructose or sucrose. Thirty-two (64 percent) were diagnosed as having HFI at less than 6 months of age, 12 (24 percent) between 6 and 12 months of age, and 6 (12 percent) after 1 year of age.

The younger patients were usually admitted to the hospital on an emergency basis with acute liver impairment, sepsis, bleeding diathesis, shock, or dehydration. Patients less than 6 months old developed a triad of jaundice, edema, and bleeding tendency. Older patients were admitted more often because of liver enlargement, ascites, or both.

Vomiting and hepatomegaly were observed in all patients. Half had anorexia, weight retardation, and bleeding tendency. About a third had jaundice; diarrhea; edema, ascites, or both; and growth retardation. Thirteen of the 50 had developed an aversion to sweet foods. This aversion had developed as early as 3 months of age and in two patients had resulted in continued breast-feeding until 9 months of age. Vomiting and diarrhea in the young children were sometimes severe enough to cause dehydration.

The laboratory findings were variable, but liver function was severely deranged in the younger patients. Deficiency of clotting factors and elevated alanine aminotransferase (ALT) were present in all but one of the patients less than 6 months old. Two patients also had serum albumin levels of 2.8 g/dl. Fifteen patients had aminoaciduria; the predominant amino acids were tyrosine and methionine in 3 of the 15. All patients showed complete resolution of laboratory abnormalities in response to removal of fructose from the diet during a succeeding 2-week period.

Histologic abnormalities were found in the livers of all patients. Fibrosis without inflammation was present in either periportal or intralobular areas in most; all but three patients had some steatosis. These three patients were older and had voluntarily restricted themselves to diets with small amounts of fructose.

Treatment of the symptomatic patients consisted of immediate cessation of fructose intake. Those with normal liver function were given fructose-free diets normal in protein content. Infants who had acute liver dysfunction were given a glucose-electrolyte mixture intravenously and were given exchange transfusion when they had a serious bleeding tendency. Thereafter, a fructose-free, low-protein diet was fed; when the liver dysfunction had been corrected, a diet normal in protein was begun.

Clinical and biochemical improvement was dramatic after exchange transfusion. Vomiting ceased immediately. The bleeding tendency disappeared in less than 24 hours, and renal tubular dysfunction disappeared within 3 days. All patients showed resolution of symptoms and normalization of laboratory findings within 2 weeks. Catch-up growth occurred within 2 to 3 years. The only persistent abnormality was hepatomegaly with steatosis, which was present from birth in the five patients restricted in dietary fructose.

Although there were no deaths in the series reported by Odievre and co-workers,[16] the continuous intake of fructose may cause death resulting from hypoglycemic seizures or progressive liver failure and inanition. The second child of such a family may profit from experience with the first child by more rapid recognition of the illness.

With greater awareness, more cases of HFI in children are being diagnosed, and the condition is arrested by feeding fructose-restricted diets. One cautionary note is that a number of proprietary milks, primarily the soy-based formulas, contain sucrose as a significant source of the carbohydrate calories. The remaining carbohydrate is usually a glucose oligosaccharide. Hypoglycemia and seizures may not be a problem in affected infants fed these formulas because the remaining carbohydrate is glucose. The liver disease resulting from fructose ingestion may be progressive, however, and infants fed these formulas may simply fail to thrive, have hepatomegaly and vomiting, or progress to chronic liver failure and death. Acute liver failure from fructose intolerance is exceedingly unusual, and the absence of hepatomegaly in an infant who has severe liver disease and has reducing sugar in the urine should make one doubt the diagnosis of HFI. Follow-up studies of infants and recognition of older patients with HFI indicate a normal life expectancy. Patients retain their sensitivity to dietary fructose as adults, but the hypoglycemic response to fructose may be somewhat more delayed in adults than in infants (45 to 60 minutes in infants; 60 to 90 minutes in adults).[14] The sensitivity to fructose may be life-threatening for adult patients. For example, patients with known HFI have been given sorbitol intravenously after surgery. Because sorbitol is metabolized to fructose, the patients died of complications from the sorbitol infusion.[17,18]

Biochemical Characteristics

The clinical and biochemical abnormalities seen in patients with HFI result from deficient activity of hepatic fructose-1-phosphate aldolase (aldolase B). This enzyme is present normally in the liver, renal tubular cells, and intestinal mucosa.[19] It catalyzes the conversion of fructose-1-phosphate to D-glyceraldehyde and dihydroxyacetone phosphate (Reaction [1]).

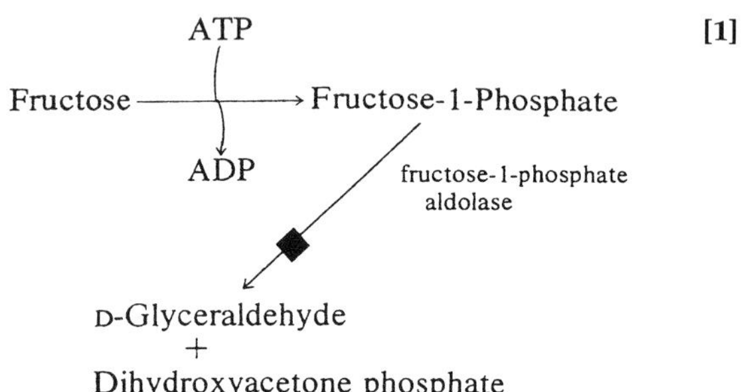

[1]

The metabolic consequences of this enzymatic deficiency are accumulation of large amounts of fructose-1-phosphate in the liver and depletion of inorganic phosphate (P_i) and adenosine triphosphate (ATP). The inability to metabolize fructose-1-phosphate in cells of affected patients leads to sequestration of large amounts of P_i. One of the many effects secondary to this is an inability to regenerate ATP, a process that depends on the presence of P_i. The clinical and laboratory features of HFI can be understood on the basis of this simple scheme (Figure 48-2).

Patients with HFI have been shown to have levels of activity of fructose-1-phosphate aldolase ranging from 0 percent to 12 percent of normal.[14,20,21] In addition, most patients have reduced levels of activity of hepatic fructose-1,6-diphosphate aldolase ranging from 25 percent to 85 percent of normal.[20,22] The differential between the activities of the two aldolase enzymes suggests that they are separate protein moieties. However, Gurtler and Leuthardt have crystallized human liver aldolase and have shown that both enzymatic activities are attributable to a single liver aldolase.[23] In addition, slight alterations of the aldolase molecule, such as splitting off an end-terminal residue, may change the ratio of its affinity for fructose-1-phosphate or fructose-1,6-diphosphate.[24,25]

Patients with HFI produce a protein that has the immunologic properties of fructose-1-phosphate aldolase but is biologically inactive.[26] On the basis of these findings, it seems probable that a mutation of the structural gene is responsible for the enzyme defect in HFI. More recent studies suggest that the mutation in HFI is not homogeneous.[27]

Accumulation of fructose-1-phosphate apparently causes the major manifestations of the disease through inhibition of other enzymatic reactions. Two metabolic pathways studied most extensively are gluconeogenesis

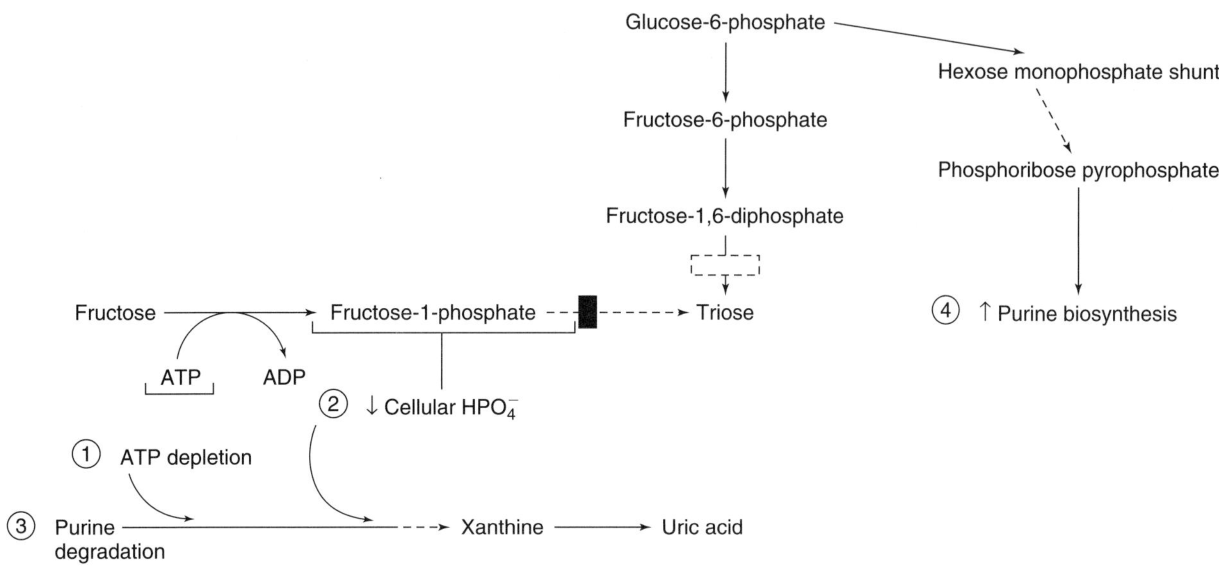

Figure 48-2 Mechanism of hyperuricemia and hypophosphatemia in hereditary fructose intolerance. After fructose intake there is rapid phosphorylation to fructose-1-phosphate, causing ATP depletion 1 because of the aldolase block. The accumulated fructose-1-phosphate inhibits the aldolase step, preventing ATP generation from anaerobic glycolysis. Phosphate is not released from the sugar, causing depletion of intracellular phosphate 2. Low ATP and HPO_4 levels favor degradation of preformed purines to uric acid 3. There is compensatory increase in purine biosynthesis 4. Solid rectangle indicates site of metabolic block. *ATP,* Adenosine triphosphate; *HPO_4^-,* phosphate.

and glycogenolysis (see also Chap. 3). Their inhibition by fructose-1-phosphate explains fructose-induced hypoglycemia. Concentrations of fructose-1-phosphate in excess of 10 mm completely inhibit fructose-1,6-diphosphate aldolase activity in vitro.[28] This finding suggests that fructose-1-phosphate inhibits gluconeogenesis at this enzymatic step. Inhibition at this site is further supported by the finding that fructose-induced hypoglycemia is not prevented by simultaneous infusions of gluconeogenic precursors such as dihydroxyacetone or glycerol. In addition, liver specimens from patients with HFI do not form glucose from ^{14}C-glycerol when fructose

Glucose-6-phosphate → glucose **[2]**

Fructose-1,6-diphosphate

Fructose → Fructose-1-phosphate → ■ fructose-1,6-diphosphate aldolase

Dihydroxyacetone phosphate + Glyceraldehyde-3-phosphate

CO_2 ← Pyruvate ← Glycerol

is present, whereas oxidation of ^{14}C-glycerol is apparently unaffected by fructose (Reaction [2]).[29]

Patients with HFI apparently also have inhibition of glycogenolysis after fructose intake. This inhibition occurs above the level of phosphoglucomutase. In support of this, it was shown that when galactose is administered together with fructose, hypoglycemia is less pronounced and does not last as long as when fructose is given alone (Reaction [3]).[13] Thus a defect in the phosphorylation of glycogen to glucose-1-phosphate is incriminated. Several studies of normal liver indicate that depletion of P_i and accumulation of fructose-1-phosphate may contribute to an almost complete failure of glycogen mobilization.[30-32] In addition, depletion of intracellular ATP levels may contribute to the lack of glycogen degradation to glucose-1-phosphate.[32-34]

A variant of fructose intolerance has been described in which the red cell galactose-1-phosphate uridyl transferase activity was normal but galactose and fructose caused hypoglycemia.[35] The nature of this finding is unclear, because a reevaluation of these patients 12 years later showed normal blood glucose responses to fructose and galactose.[36]

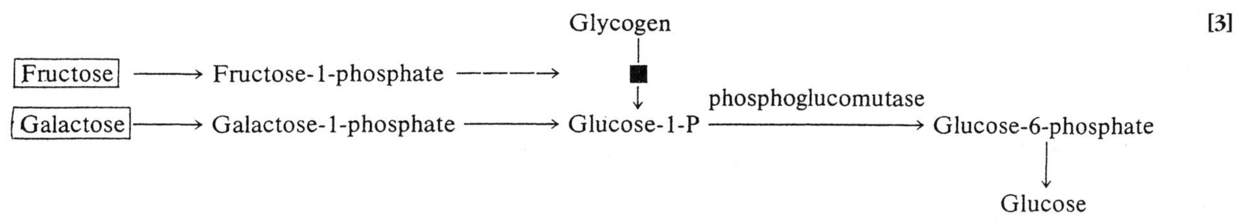

Results of studies by Schwartz and colleagues suggest that newborn infants delivered at term have less capacity for fructose metabolism in the first few days of life as compared with later in life.[37] This is believed to be caused by the immaturity of the enzymes for handling fructose. In these studies a rapid infusion of fructose caused a prompt but transient decrease in blood glucose and suppressed the glucagon-induced elevation of blood glucose. Although hepatic aldolase was not measured, the findings suggest that until further studies are completed, the use of fructose or sorbitol as a calorie source (as in total parenteral nutrition) for term infants in the first few days of life may not be justified. Enzymatic maturation may take longer in premature infants, although definitive studies have not been reported.

Laboratory Features

The primary laboratory features of HFI are fructose-induced hypoglycemia and hypophosphatemia or chronic liver disease. In addition, serum and urinary urate levels may be increased.

Hypoglycemia. Hypoglycemia induced by dietary or intravenous fructose is a characteristic of the illness. The hypoglycemia is not due to excess circulating insulin.[28,38] That sorbitol provokes hypoglycemia before substantial amounts of fructose are released into the circulation is evidence against a direct effect of fructose on blood glucose levels.[14] More likely, the adverse effects of fructose result from intracellular accumulation of a fructose metabolite, such as fructose-1-phosphate.[28,39] The metabolite impairs both gluconeogenesis and glycogenolysis (Reactions [2] and [3]). Studies with ^{14}C-glucose indicate a complete cessation of hepatic glucose release after fructose infusion.[38] Also, glucagon does not increase blood glucose after fructose-induced hypoglycemia, even in the presence of normal to slightly elevated hepatic glycogen content.[40]

Hypophosphatemia. This is the second prominent feature of fructose-induced hypoglycemia. The reduction of inorganic phosphorus precedes that of glucose and may be the only abnormal finding when a small dose of fructose is administered.[14] Hypophosphatemia appears to be a consequence of binding and sequestration of phosphorus in the form of fructose-1-phosphate within the hepatocytes.[39,41] The first step in fructose metabolism is phosphorylation by ATP. With large doses of fructose, ATP is depleted rapidly. With deficient activity of aldolase, as occurs in HFI, P_i is not released back into the cell. To compensate, phosphate from the serum is sequestered by the liver, with a resulting reduction in available circulating phosphate levels.[14] Phosphorylation of fructose decreases intracellular phosphate in normal individuals, but the phosphate sequestered in normal liver is made available by further metabolism of fructose-1-phosphate. Thus changes in serum levels of phosphate are extremely transient in a normal individual and depend on the amount of fructose ingested.

Hepatic Enzyme Elevation. This appears to be the direct effect of increased hepatic fructose-1-phosphate levels. Within 1.5 hours of a large dose of fructose, aminotransferase levels may increase more than twofold.[42] The mechanism of liver cell damage is not clear, but it may result from a combination of depletion of ATP and a direct toxic effect of elevated levels of the phosphorylated hexose.

Hyperuricemia and Increased Urate Excretion. These conditions appear to result from depletion of intracellular ATP and P_i increases the rate of purine degradation to uric acid (see Figure 48-2).[32,33]

Other laboratory findings are less consistent. Some patients show substantial decreases in serum potassium and increases in serum magnesium after fructose intake.[14,40] Some have increases in serum lactate and pyruvate.[13,14,20] These changes appear to be related to the extent of liver damage and the severity of hypoglycemia. Granulocytosis may be noted with chronic fructose ingestion. A galactose infusion may relieve the hypoglycemia, but this also is an inconsistent finding. As blood glucose declines after fructose ingestion, insulin and insulin-like activity decrease. Levels of glucagon, epinephrine, and growth hormone increase. In response to these hormonal changes the non-esterified fatty acids in plasma increase more than twofold, a response not observed in normal subjects.[13,20,43,44]

Renal tubular acidosis and a Fanconi-like syndrome with renal tubular reabsorptive defects have been reported.[16,45,46] In one patient renal tubular acidosis persisted despite restriction of dietary fructose.[15] The renal tubular acidosis is normalized in most patients as soon as fructose intake ceases.[47,48] Fructose-1-phosphate aldolase normally is present in the renal tubules. It is absent in patients with HFI. Hence the transient renal disturbance in affected patients may be due to accumulation of fructose-1-phosphate in renal tubular cells after fructose intake.[19]

Pathology

The changes in hepatic ultrastructure within 1.5 to 2 hours after a single dose of fructose are "glycogen-associated membrane arrays" and cytolysosomes in various stages of development. These may represent lysosomes ingesting the accumulated fructose-1-phosphate in an attempt to get rid of it by acid hydrolysis. With chronic ingestion of fructose, the primary histologic changes are lipid accumulation and varying stages of hepatocellular necrosis and bile duct proliferation. Liver disease may progress to cirrhosis with impairment of liver-dependent coagulation factors.[49]

Despite extremely severe hepatic disease, the liver shows a remarkable ability to regenerate after dietary fructose is excluded. For example, a 3-month-old child who had cirrhosis, hypoalbuminemia, hypoprothrombinemia, and ascites had normal liver function and disappearance of ascitic fluid after 3 weeks of a fructose-free diet. Except for slight fibrosis, the hepatic architecture was normal 3 years later.[40]

The pathogenesis of acute and chronic liver cell injury after fructose intake has not been studied in detail. By analogy with galactosemia, a six-carbon sugar phosphorylated at carbon 1 may have a direct cytotoxic effect, whereas phosphorylation of the carbon 6 position apparently has no obvious toxicity. In addition, the severe alterations in energy metabolism may have a role in derangement of liver cell function and may thereby result in the pathologic changes observed after ingestion of dietary fructose. The reason for lipid accumulation is also unclear, but it may represent only general cellular dysfunction seen in a number of unrelated conditions.[13,20,44]

Although renal function may be severely impaired, little histologic change occurs in the kidneys other than some increase in medullary lipid.

The teeth of patients who have HFI are unusually free of caries. This has been taken to indicate that fructose and sucrose are important cariogenic substrates.[50]

Despite the recurrent episodes of hypoglycemia and seizures that are common in undiagnosed cases, the brain is remarkably free of abnormalities. In contrast to patients with galactosemia, who commonly show psychomotor retardation, HFI patients surviving even the most severe forms of liver disease appear to have normal intelligence after being given fructose-free diets.

Genetics

The genetic findings are compatible with an autosomal-recessive trait. Levels of hepatic fructose-1-phosphate aldolase activity in five parents of patients with HFI were normal.[51] In addition, carriers usually metabolize substantial fructose loads without difficulty. This is in contradistinction to carriers of galactosemia, who metabolize galactose at slower rates than normal and who may develop lenticular opacification with chronic galactose ingestion.

As mentioned previously, the molecular basis of HFI is missense mutations in the gene. Testing for these mutations in amplified DNAs by the polymerase chain reaction with a limited panel of allele-specific oligonucleotides identifies more than 95 percent of patients. A reverse-dot blot screening method is available as a screening tool, which can detect the two most common mutations (A149P and A174D).[52]

Differential Diagnosis

During infancy various conditions may be associated with hypoglycemia,[53,54] but most of them are associated with fasting. Hypoglycemia after eating should be a clue to the possibility of HFI, particularly in the presence of urinary reducing sugar. Other diseases in which hypoglycemia follows ingestion of food are deficiency of fructose diphosphatase, galactosemia, and leucine intolerance. In addition, premature infants may have transient fructose intolerance resulting from immaturity of hepatic aldolase activity.[37] Some patients with Tay-Sachs disease have deficient levels of fructose-1-phosphate aldolase.[55,56] Three such patients were given fructose loads but did not develop the hypoglycemia, hypophosphatemia, or hypermagnesemia that affects patients with HFI. The relationship of the decreased enzymatic activity to the pathogenesis of Tay-Sachs disease is unknown, although measurement of fructose-1-phosphate aldolase activity has been used as a marker to detect the carrier state of Tay-Sachs disease.[56,57]

The diagnosis of HFI can be made by an intravenous fructose tolerance test. The smallest dose that produces the typical symptoms without causing nausea and vomiting is 0.25 g/kg of body weight.[14] A dose of 0.25 g/kg of body weight or 3 g/m^2 surface area is given as a single, rapid injection. Marked, prolonged reductions of blood glucose and phosphate levels occur regularly with this dose. However, at least one infant with marked hepatomegaly and severely deranged hepatic function did not have the typical changes in blood glucose and phosphate until the intravenous dose was doubled. Thus with severe liver disease, blood and urinary levels of fructose are inconsistently elevated with the lesser fructose load. The lower dose of fructose may be a valuable aid as an initial screen for HFI during use of an unrestricted diet, but a negative result, as described previously, should not be used to rule out the diagnosis of HFI. Because the fructose load may cause symptomatic hypoglycemia, vomiting, and derangement of liver function, measurement of intestinal aldolase activity may be preferable in patients strongly suspected of having HFI.[58] The presumptive diagnosis made from tolerance tests should be confirmed by assay of enzyme activity in percutaneous liver biopsy specimens.

Treatment

A diet containing no fructose alleviates all the symptoms and liver dysfunction associated with HFI.[3,11-15] It is important that children and their parents receive detailed dietary counseling about which foods contain fructose. Older children commonly may associate discomfort with specific foods and regularly avoid them; however, infants are completely dependent on dietary selections made by the parents.

The common practice of adding small amounts of sugar to processed foods demands almost constant attention to avoid substantial fructose intake. One patient with HFI who continued to consume small amounts of fructose had chronic slight elevations in aspartate aminotransferase (AST) levels and hepatic fat accumulation. Because pharmacologic doses of folate are known to cause non-specific increases in both aldolase activities, the patient was treated with 5 mg folate daily, with a resultant 53 percent increase in hepatic fructose-1-phosphate aldolase activity. With no change in dietary intake there were decreases in AST and hepatic lipid contents. Tolerance tests, however, showed that folate treatment did not increase this patient's ability to handle a large dietary intake of fructose.[58]

Prognosis

Patients maintained on fructose-free diets have developed entirely normally, with normal life spans, although most continue to have slight hepatomegaly with hepatic steatosis.[16] Even infants with severely deranged liver function and substantial hepatic fibrosis can achieve remarkable recoveries after fructose is removed from their diets.

Fructose-diphosphatase Deficiency

In 1970 Baker and Winegrad described a patient who had a third type of genetic defect in fructose metabolism.[4] The predominant clinical findings were hepatomegaly and fasting-induced hypoglycemia with lactic acidosis. The patient was shown later to have deficient hepatic FDPase activity. Other cases with similar clinical and laboratory findings have subsequently been reported.[59] The primary difference between patients with FDPase deficiency and patients with HFI is that fasting and dietary fructose induces symptoms in patients with deficiencies of FDPase. As a result, an occasional patient with FDPase deficiency has been diagnosed incorrectly as having type IB glycogen storage disease (GSD). Several patients have been found to have "partial" FDPase deficiencies. These patients do not have lactic acidosis but develop hypoglycemia during fasting or secondary to dietary intake of fructose or glycerol. One such patient had many of the characteristics of the syndrome ketotic hypoglycemia.[60] Others have been erroneously diagnosed during infancy as having acute tyrosinosis. The deficiency of FDPase is inherited as an autosomal-recessive trait.

DISORDERS OF GALACTOSE METABOLISM

In 1935 Mason and Turner provided the first detailed description of a patient intolerant of galactose.[61] Since then numerous case reports have described the constellation of nutritional failure, liver disease, cataracts, and mental retardation that results from a deficiency of hepatic galactose-1-phosphate uridyl transferase activity.[62-64] The defect in galactosemia was initially though, to be a lack of synthesis of transferase protein.[65] Advances in molecular cloning have shown, however, that there are missense mutations in the gene coding for the transferase enzyme in the majority of patients with galactosemia (discussed in the following section). Subsequently, Gitzelmann described the case of a 44-year-old patient with galactosuria and early-onset cataracts.[66] Later reports indicated that this patient represented a second defect in galactose metabolism, which was a deficiency of galactokinase.[67,68] This defect apparently does not result in progressive liver disease and mental retardation. In 1972 Gitzelmann discovered a third type of galactosemia, caused by uridine diphosphate galactose-4-epimerase deficiency.[69] This condition has been considered benign to the extent that the deficiency is limited to leukocytes and erythrocytes and that affected individuals show no other laboratory or clinical abnormalities.[70] More recently, generalized epimerase deficiency has been described.[71-75] These patients show signs and symptoms identical to those of transferase-deficiency galactosemia. Because each of these conditions results in milk-induced galactosemia but represents three distinct biochemical entities, it has been suggested that the term *galactosemia* be supplemented by the specific enzymatic defect—that is, transferase-deficiency galactosemia, galactokinase-deficiency galactosemia, and epimerase-deficiency galactosemia.

Transferase-deficiency Galactosemia

Human beings are capable of metabolizing large quantities of galactose, as demonstrated by the rapid elimination of galactose from blood.[76,77] An elevation of the level of plasma glucose occurs shortly after galactose infusion as a result of conversion of galactose to glucose. Tracer studies indicate that as much as 50 percent of galactose may be found in body glucose pools within 30 minutes of injection.[77] Under normal circumstances plasma galactose is removed so rapidly by the liver that the rate of galactose clearance has been used as an index of hepatic blood flow[78] and liver function.[79] The removal mechanism is saturated at plasma levels of about 50 mg/dl, a level corresponding to the limits of the ability of galactokinase to phosphorylate the sugar. With a load of galactose that increases blood levels by 30 to 40 mg/dl, urinary losses may be substantial because the kidney threshold is at plasma levels of 10 to 20 mg/dl.[80]

Almost half of the calorie source in most mammalian milks is from hydrolysis of lactose to its two monosaccharides, glucose and galactose. Consequently, the series of enzymatic steps involved in conversion of galactose to glucose are most stressed during infancy. As a consequence, enzymatic defects of this pathway are most likely to produce clinical signs and symptoms and marked elevations of blood and urinary galactose levels during this crucial period of development.

The first described defect resulting in galactosemia results from deficient activity of the enzyme required for the second of four steps in galactose metabolism (Figure 48-3). The consequences of this defect are much more severe than are those of the other defects in galactose metabolism, galactokinase deficiency and uridine diphosphate (UDP)-galactose-4-epimerase deficiency.

Molecular Basis of Transferase-deficiency Galactosemia

Transferase deficiency is an autosomal-recessive disorder. The sequence of the homologous protein from *Escherichia coli,*[81] from *Saccharomyces cerevisiae,*[82] and from humans shows overall sequence identity of 35 percent. The complementary DNA (cDNA) coding for the human transferase enzyme is 1295 nucleotide bases in length and predicts a 43-kd protein.[83] The gene has been mapped to chromosome 9p18 and spans 4 Kb with 11 exons. The amino acids histidine (164)-proline-histidine (166) form an active site sequence that is essential for activity of the enzyme.[84] Southern, Northern, and Western blotting experiments suggest that the majority of galactosemia mutations are missense mutations that result in low or undetectable enzyme activity. The two most commonly characterized mutations are glutamine 188→arginine (Q188R) and arginine 333→tryptophan (R333W). The arginine 188 mutation is the most common galactosemia mutation, accounting for one fourth of the galactosemia alleles studied.[85] The second mutation, arginine 333→tryptophan, occurs at a highly conserved domain in the homologous enzymes from *E. coli,* yeast, and humans. Several other mutations have been described, such as valine 44→methionine (M) and methionine 142→lysine (k). Mutation S135L involving leucine substitution by serine occurs mostly in blacks. Mutation N314D involves asparagine to aspartate change as the basis for the Duarte variant. This variant is benign and expresses diminished enzyme activity.[86] The

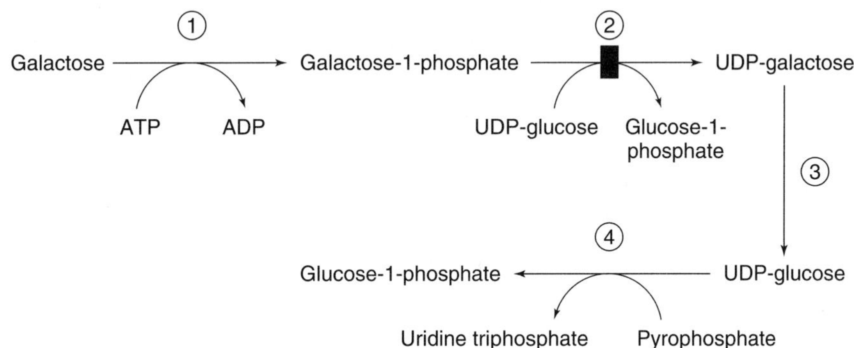

Figure 48-3 Reactions in the conversion of galactose to glucose. *1,* Galactokinase; *2,* galactose-1-phosphate uridyltransferase; *3,* uridine diphosphate (UDP) galactose-4-epimerase; *4,* UDP glucose pyrophosphorylase.

TABLE 48-2

Common Clinical Findings in 43 Symptomatic Galactosemic Patients

	Number of patients	% Incidence
Anorexia and weight loss	23	53
Hepatomegaly	39	91
Jaundice	34	79
Ascites or edema	7	16
Vomiting	17	40
Abdominal distention	9	21
Cataracts	21	49
Infection	10	23
Sepsis	5	12

From Koch R, Donnell GN, Fishler K, et al: Galactosemia. In Kelley VC, ed: Practice of Pediatrics. Hagerstown, MD, Harper & Row, 1979:4.

other mutations result in low or total loss of activity of the transferase. Therefore it appears that transferase-deficiency galactosemia results from missense mutations that tend to occur in regions that are highly conserved throughout evolution.[87] So far more than 150 mutations have been described.[88]

Clinical Features

Since transferase-deficiency galactosemia was first described in 1935, numerous patients with the disorder have been monitored for long periods. In 1970 Komrower and Lee reported the results of long-term follow-up of the 60 known cases of galactosemia in Great Britain.[89] Long-term follow-up studies of 47 families have been reported from Los Angeles.[90]

Transferase-deficiency galactosemia varies in severity. Some patients may present with an acute, fulminant illness after the first milk feedings or, more commonly, as a subacute illness with gastrointestinal symptoms (i.e., jaundice and failure to thrive). In milder cases moderate intestinal upset after galactose ingestion may be the only manifestation. In severe cases anorexia, abdominal distention, diarrhea, vomiting, and hypoglycemic attacks may occur shortly after birth. The most common initial symptoms are failure to thrive and vomiting, usually starting within the first few days of milk ingestion. Table 48-2 lists the more common findings in 43 symptomatic patients.[74] Within the first week of life, hepatomegaly and jaundice are usually noted. In fact, prolonged obstructive jaundice in a neonate is a common presenting feature, and examination of urine for reducing sugar should be done in all infants with clinical jaundice. The jaundice from intrinsic liver disease may be accentuated in some infants with galactosemia by severe hemolysis and erythroblastosis. With continued galactose ingestion, ascites may develop as early as 2 to 5 weeks after birth. Cataracts may be seen within a few days after birth or, if the mother has consumed large amounts of milk late in gestation, they may be present at delivery. The cataracts, consisting of punctate lesions in the nucleus of the fetal lens, may be so small that they can be seen only with slit-lamp examination. Retardation of mental development may be apparent after the first several months. A few patients homozygous for the disorder have been entirely asymptomatic while ingesting milk. These patients, who are usually of African decent, may be capable of metabolizing moderate amounts of galactose.[75,91]

Because milk-substitute formulas have become easily accessible, infants who have recurrent vomiting and poor weight gain during the first few weeks of life are often given trials of one of the lactose-free formulas. An occasional infant with galactosemia may be unwittingly changed to such a formula with resulting improvement without any awareness of the child's underlying defect. In such instances the patient may have the disease undetected until months or years later when they may have motor retardation, hepatomegaly, and cataracts.[92]

An important clinical observation about galactosemia is that of Levy and associates, who showed the strong association between galactosemia and *E. coli* sepsis.[93] In routine screening of more than 700,000 infants during a 12-year period 8 infants with classic transferase-deficiency galactosemia were identified. Four of these infants had septicemia at the time galactosemia was detected (second week of life), and three of the four died. A review of results from eight other states that routinely screen newborns for galactosemia indicates that in screening more than 2.5 million newborns, 35 such patients were identified. Of the 35 patients 10 are known to have had systemic infection, and 9 of the 10 died of bacteremia despite therapy. Infections usually seem to develop at the end of the first week or during the second week of life, and their incidence appears to correlate directly with continued intake of galactose. These findings suggest that infants with *E. coli* sepsis should be considered possibly galactosemic and that infants recently diagnosed as galactosemic should be considered possibly infected with *E. coli*.

With initiation of a galactose elimination diet, all acute manifestations of the disease usually improve within 72 hours, and hepatic dysfunction begins to normalize within 1 week. During the first year of life small amounts of dietary galactose may cause symptoms; however, around puberty, most patients show an improved tolerance to dietary galactose. To account for this improved tolerance, an alternative metabolic pathway for galactose has been postulated to develop around the time of puberty. This pathway is thought to bypass the deficient transferase step by forming UDP-galactose from the interaction of galactose-1-phosphate and uridine triphosphate (Figure 48-4).[94] This reaction in liver and brain would reduce the concentration of galactose-1-phosphate to normal levels and would thus protect against the effects of the defective pathway. Although this hypothesis represents an attractive explanation for the increased ability to tolerate galactose later in life, tracer studies do not support an increased rate of galactose metabolism. A third pathway involving the formation of xylulose is unimportant in normal humans but may permit survival of some patients who continue to ingest galactose (Figure 48-4).

Laboratory Findings

Routine laboratory findings may be varied but include elevated blood and urinary levels of galactose, hyperchloremic acidosis, albuminuria, aminoaciduria, hypoglycemia, and blood changes reflecting deranged liver function. Occasionally, infants may have severe and prolonged hypoglycemia. The galactosuria may be intermittent because of poor food intake or may disappear within 3 or 4 days of intravenous feeding. Thus if the urine is not tested for reducing sugar during a period of galactosuria, the diagnosis may not be suspected. The finding of a urinary reducing substance that does not react with the glucose oxidase test should alert one to the possibility of galactosemia. This finding does not establish the diagnosis, because several other conditions such as fructosuria, lactosuria (from deficient intestinal lactase), and severe liver disease of any origin may impair the clearance of blood galactose and result in the presence of urinary reducing sugar that is not glucose.[92]

Biochemical Characteristics and Pathogenesis of Galactose Toxicity

The hepatic manifestations of transferase-deficiency galactosemia are due entirely to the abnormal metabolism of galactose, and patients never exposed to galactose should have no abnormality. Toxicity apparently results from accumulation of the metabolic products of galactose rather than from galactose itself. The two compounds that have been studied most extensively are galactose-1-phosphate and galactitol, the product of an alternate pathway (see Figure 48-4). The biochemical causes of toxicity in individual organs may differ, depending on the metabolic patterns and functions of the involved organs. For example, cataracts are apparently caused by galactitol accumulation, whereas this compound appears to have little, if any, relation to the renal abnormalities or hepatic dysfunction.

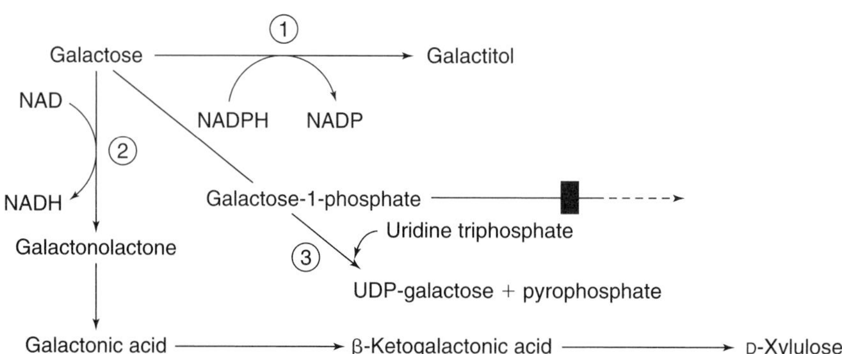

Figure 48-4 Alternate pathways of galactose metabolism. *1,* Aldose reductase or L-hexonate dehydrogenase; *2,* galactose dehydrogenase; *3,* uridine diphosphate galactose pyrophosphorylase.

Hypoglycemia. Hypoglycemia that may occur after galactose ingestion is apparently caused by inhibition of glucose release from glycogen. The mechanism responsible is postulated to be high levels of galactose-1-phosphate that interfere with phosphoglucomutase, the enzyme that catalyzes the conversion of glucose-1-phosphate to glucose-6-phosphate.[95] In addition, there is an inhibition of glucose formation through gluconeogenesis.[96] The galactose-1-phosphate may be toxic in other ways as well, although investigations aimed at answering this question depended primarily on changes induced in normal animals fed high-galactose diets and do not necessarily reflect the changes that occur in patients who have deficiencies of enzymatic activity.

The organs primarily involved in galactosemia are the lens of the eye, the liver, the brain, and the kidney. The mechanism by which galactose feeding causes these pathologic changes is not understood for all tissues.

Lenticular Changes. Changes in the lens appear to result primarily from accumulation of galactitol. Van Heyningen showed galactitol accumulation, and Kinoshita and associates showed that an increase in galactitol concentration caused a concomitant increase in water content secondary to the oncotic pressure from the galactitol.[97-99] The poor diffusion of the alcohol from the lens makes this organ particularly susceptible. Reversing the osmotic effect of the galactitol accumulation with an osmotically balanced incubation medium prevents the lenticular opacification.[98] Many biochemical alterations occur concurrently in the lens as it undergoes cataract formation. These include decreases in amino acid transport, protein synthesis, several enzymatic activities, and alteration of ion fluxes.[99-104] Glycolysis and respiration of the lens are reduced by about 30 percent after about 2 days of galactose feeding and remain at this level until cataracts occur.[103] It is not surprising, then, that nutrient supplements can alter the rate of cataract formation in galactose-fed animals.[105] Thus nutrient imbalances and alterations in lenticular water content from galactitol formation together are prime initiators of lenticular opacification. The causes of cellular damage in other organs are less clear.

Liver. The concentration in liver of both galactose-1-phosphate and galactitol is elevated in patients fed galactose.[106,107] However, the liver damage in patients with transferase deficiencies does not occur in normal animals fed high-galactose diets despite high hepatic levels of galactose-1-phosphate in rats[108] and high hepatic galactitol levels in chicks.[109] In addition, patients with galactokinase deficiencies form large amounts of galactitol but show no liver damage. This suggests that some other metabolite or metabolites may accumulate to act singly or in concert to cause cellular toxicity. In this respect, galactosamine, which was increased in the liver of one patient, is known to induce hepatocellular changes in animals.[109]

Kidneys. Kidneys of transferase-deficient patients develop renal tubular dysfunction after galactose ingestion. They accumulate both galactose-1-phosphate and galactitol.[106,107] However, accumulation of galactitol alone does not appear to be toxic; patients with galactokinase deficiencies do not develop renal dysfunction but do excrete large amounts of galactitol. This suggests that the alcohol is not the primary renal insult in patients with transferase deficiency. Aminoaciduria can be induced in both normal humans and rats by large amounts of galactose.[110,111] This could be because of an accumulation of galactose-1-phosphate that secondarily impairs amino acid accumulation by the tubules.[112] If analogous to that in the human intestine, the inhibition is non-competitive.[113]

Brain. Changes in the brains of patients with transferase-deficiency galactosemia may not be entirely reversible after galactose restriction. For this reason, substantial efforts have been made to delineate the pathogenesis of galactose-induced brain damage. In the brains of patients and those of rats fed galactose, galactitol accumulates in higher concentrations than in any other tissue except the lens.[108,114] This suggests that galactitol accumulation may be important in the pathogenesis of the brain abnormality. However, in patients with galactokinase deficiencies, galactitol accumulation does not appear to damage tissues other than the lens.

Studies in a chick brain showed that galactose administration diminished ATP, reduced brain glucose and glycolytic intermediates, redistributed hexokinase, enhanced fragility of neural lysosomes, and decreased fast axoplasmic transport.[115-119] The effects could be temporarily reversed by glucose.[120] Changes in the chick brain appear to be related to several factors such as hyperosmolality,[119] an alteration in energy metabolism,[116] abnormal serotonin levels,[121] and interference with active uptake of glucose into the neurons. Whether these changes in chicks are similar to galactose-induced abnormalities in patients with transferase deficiencies remains to be determined.

Although intestinal epithelium of patients with galactosemia is also deficient in its activity of the transferase enzyme, it does not appear to alter intestinal transport of galactose. Many infants develop intestinal symptoms of vomiting and diarrhea after galactose ingestion, but it is unclear whether this is a direct effect on the intestine or secondary to the effects on the central nervous system.

Gonads. The majority of galactosemic females have ovarian failure as manifested clinically by infertility and biochemically by hypergonadotropic hypogonadism.[122] Males with galactosemia have normal testicular function. The mechanism underlying ovarian failure in galactosemic women is not known, although galactose toxicity has been implicated. It is interesting to note that tissues with the highest specific activity of transferase and messenger ribonucleic acid (mRNA) level are target organs for the dysfunction and are affected to the greatest extent in galactosemia. In this regard, the ovary has five times more transferase activity and transferase mRNA than the testis.[123]

Pathology

Early hepatic lesions, present in the first weeks of life, consist of cholestasis and diffuse fatty vacuolation with little or no inflammatory reaction. The fatty changes are extensive and generalized throughout the lobule. Later, disorganization of the liver cells with pseudoductular and pseudoglandular orientation occurs. This tendency toward pseudoglandular orientation of cells has been described as characteristic of galactosemia but is relatively non-specific. As the disease progresses delicate fibrosis appears, first in the periportal regions, then eventually extending to bridge adjacent portal tracts. Regenerating nodules and hepatic fibrosis are late features that, with continued galactose ingestion, progress to cirrhosis similar in many respects to the cirrhosis of ethanol abuse. Death usually occurs in the first year of life unless galactose intake is decreased or curtailed. Frank cellular necrosis is unusual but may occur with large amounts of dietary galactose. Despite the severity of the hepatic lesion there is a remarkable lack of inflammatory infiltration.[124]

Except for cataract formation in the lens, the tissues show only minor changes. Kidneys show dilation of tubules at the corticomedullary junction. The spleen enlarges as a result of portal hypertension. Lesions in the brain are subtle, with minor loss of nerve cells and gliosis in the dentate nucleus and gliosis in the cerebral cortex and gray matter.[125]

Genetics

Investigations of red blood cell and leukocytic transferase activities in family members indicate that the disorder is transmitted as an autosomal-recessive trait.[126] Heterozygotes have about 50 percent of normal activity, and genotype detection is more accurate when the transferase to galactokinase ratio is determined.[127] Population studies indicate that the incidence of heterozygosity for galactosemia is between 0.9 percent and 1.25 percent and that between 8 percent and 13 percent carry the Duarte gene.[128] Incidences of transferase-deficiency galactosemia derived from large-scale screening in neonatal nurseries have been between 1:10,000 and 1:70,000 live births.[129,130] At least one patient with transferase-deficiency galactosemia has delivered a normal heterozygous infant.[90]

Diagnostic Screening for Galactosemia

The rationale for genetic screening is threefold: (1) to detect disease at its incipient stage and thereby offset harmful expression of the mutant gene through appropriate medical treatment, (2) to identify a variant genotype for which reproductive options (family planning) may be provided, and (3) to identify gene frequency or biologic significance and natural history of variant phenotypes.

Various screening methods for galactosemia have been used.[131] The original Guthrie test used filter paper blood samples from which a microbiologic assay detected elevated galactose levels. The newer Beutler test assays the erythrocyte transferase activity directly from dried filter paper, and the Paigen assay is an improved bacteriologic method that includes detection of elevated galactose and galactose-1-phosphate. Measurements of elevated galactose require that the infant receive sufficient dietary galactose or a false-negative test will result. Conversely, the normal enzyme may become inactive in a hot or humid climate, and a false-positive (negative enzyme activity) may be reported.

The relatively common inaccuracies of the screening tests for galactosemia and the low prevalence of the illness, coupled with the observation that infants born into families without a known history of galactosemia may be affected at birth, have prompted some screening centers not to screen for galactosemia. For example, in Quebec, the spaces on the blood sample filter paper assigned to galactosemia were given over to screening for congenital hypothyroidism, with a striking increase in cost effectiveness.

In utero assay for galactosemia is indicated in pregnant women with a family history of galactosemia. Cultured fibroblasts from amniotic fluid can be assayed for transferase activity. Additionally, the technique of chorionic villus sampling has been used to detect galactosemia during the tenth week of gestation.[132]

More recently, cloning of the cDNA encoding for the transferase enzyme and the finding that the majority of galactosemic patients have missense mutations have allowed for rapid molecular approaches using the polymerase chain reaction to detect common mutations.

Diagnosis

The presumptive diagnosis of galactosemia in an infant with vomiting and failure to thrive on milk feedings may be made by identification of a urinary reducing sugar that does not react with glucose oxidase reagents. It should be remembered that lactose, fructose, and pentose may give similar results, but if the formula is milk-based and there is no other dietary sugar, galactosemia is the presumed diagnosis, and restriction of dietary galactose should be initiated immediately. Identification of the sugar can be made by paper or gas-liquid chromatography. Paper impregnated with galactose oxidase makes screening for galactosuria easier. Normal premature and some normal-term infants may excrete as much as 60 mg/dl urinary galactose during the first week or two of life.

Unlike suspected fructose intolerance, which may be diagnosed by use of a fructose tolerance test, demonstration of galactosuria or galactosemia by a galactose tolerance test should never be used. Although not clearly documented, it has been suggested that a single, large exposure to galactose may result in severe and prolonged hypoglycemia, with possible resulting brain damage. For this reason, the definitive diagnosis should be made on the basis of direct measurement of transferase activity and not by tolerance test.[74,76]

The red cell UDP-glucose consumption test has been used extensively as a screening test for the past decade.[92,129,130,133] It is based on the assay of UDP-glucose before and after incubation of galactose-1-phosphate with red cell hemolysate as the source of transferase. Conversion of UDP-glucose to UDP-glucuronic acid by UDP-glucose dehydrogenase forms nicotinamide adenine dinucleotide (NAD) from the reduced form of nicotinamide adenine dinucleotide (NADH), which is measured spectrophotometrically. With this procedure, a complete absence of red cell transferase activity is found in homozygous patients; intermediate levels characterize heterozygous carriers. Infants identified as having 50 percent of normal activity should have further tests to rule out other variants that may be homozygous at 50 percent activity (discussed in the following section).

With the advent of screening for galactosemia, multiple variants of this disease have become apparent, the variants being more prevalent than classic transferase-deficiency galactosemia.[134] There are three homozygotic types.

1. "Classic" galactosemia is autosomal-recessive, and there is no transferase activity in erythrocytes, fibroblasts, liver, and presumably in any other tissue. In heterozygotic, unaffected carriers activity is 50 percent of normal.
2. The Duarte variant is the most common form of galactosemia and is detected only by enzyme screening because these infants are asymptomatic. Red cell activity is 50 percent of normal, and on starch gel electrophoresis the enzyme migrates faster than normal. Red cells of patients who have this variant produce two distinct bands rather than the single normal band. In addition, red cells of a parent of a Duarte-homozygous patient have three bands for the variant enzyme. Homozygotic Duarte erythrocytes have 50 percent of normal enzyme activity; heterozygous Duarte erythrocytes, 75 percent of normal. Ten percent to 15 percent of the population may have Duarte-variant galactosemia. The Duarte gene is apparently allelic with the normal and galactosemic genes because the most frequently detected abnormality on neonatal screening tests is the compound heterozygous state, consisting of classic galactosemia with the Duarte variant. Two protein bands are present on protein electrophoresis, and erythrocyte transferase activity is 25 percent. Although some of these infants appear asymptomatic at birth and remain so during infancy, others have systemic symptoms with metabolic manifestations of galactosemia.
3. In the "Negro" variant, erythrocytic transferase activity is absent, but 10 percent of normal activity is present in liver and intestine. The Duarte and the Negro variants may be asymptomatic despite galactose ingestion, although patients with the variant may develop a galactose toxicity syndrome in the neonatal period.

In addition to the homozygotic variants, several heterozygotic variants have been identified: (1) an Indiana variant, in which erythrocytic transferase activity is approximately 35 percent of normal and is highly unstable (mobility on starch gel electrophoresis is slower than normal); (2) a Rennes variant, which has about 7 to 10 percent of normal transferase activity (this variant also travels more slowly than normal by electrophoresis); and (3) a Los Angeles variant, which has erythrocytic transferase activity higher than normal (about 140 percent). The latter variant has been detected in six families. Electrophoretic mobility of this variant of the enzyme is similar to that of the Duarte variant. West German and Chicago variants have also been identified by screening procedures.

Treatment

Although the cause of the entire toxicity syndrome in transferase deficiency is uncertain, there is no disagreement that elimination of galactose intake reverses the biochemical manifestations of transferase-deficiency galactosemia. Some patients seem to have increasing tolerance to galactose with advancing age; however, studies using ^{14}C-galactose do not support the clinical impression that alternate pathways of galactose metabolism develop at puberty,[90-92] nor is there any indication that any drug will increase galactose oxidation, although some patients with variant forms of transferase deficiencies can oxidize limited amounts of galactose.

The only acceptable treatment at present is elimination of dietary galactose. Permissible diets are described in at least two publications.[77,90] Preparations used in treating infants are Pregestimil, Nutramigen, and the soybean milk preparations. Both Pregestimil and Nutramigen are prepared from casein and may contain small amounts of lactose, but these do not appear to be sufficient to impair therapeutic efficacy. The soybean formulas contain small amounts of galactose in raffinose and stachyose, and other dietary constituents contain small amounts of galactosides, but these carbohydrates are not digested by human intestinal enzymes and should not affect the efficacy of treatment.[90] Because of the frequent addition of milk to a number of proprietary food items, strict attention must be given to the diet during and after weaning. Concern has been raised regarding the presence of galactose in grains, fruits, and vegetables.[135] These foods contain significant amounts of soluble galactose, although newer information related to substantial endogenous productivity of galactose has minimized this concern.[136]

It is important to be aware that asymptomatic heterozygotic mothers may have elevated serum galactose levels after ingestion of diets high in milk. Infants delivered of such mothers may have the galactosemic syndrome at birth. For this reason, restriction of galactose during the pregnancies of women who have previously borne children with galactosemia is recommended.[90-92] The use of uridine and aldose reductase inhibitors in galactosemic patients has not been shown to be effective despite their theoretical advantage.[137,138]

Prognosis

When untreated, galactosemia results in early deaths of many affected children and is attended by the prospect of mental retardation of those who survive. In a series of 43 galactosemic patients described by Koch and colleagues there were 13 neonatal deaths.[90] The deaths, occurring at an average age of 6 weeks, were usually attributed to infection. Levy and co-workers noted that 9 of 35 patients died of *E. coli* infections and strongly recommended early cultures and institution of antibiotics effective against *E. coli* in any infant with galactosemia who appears ill.[93]

Treatment of galactosemic patients with a galactose-free diet results in survival with reversal of the acute symptoms, normal growth, and complete recovery of liver function; however, the long-term outcome (particularly for intellectual development) is not entirely certain. Experience gained in the long-term follow-up of 59 patients in the Los Angeles area indicates that many patients have developed well and have attained college-level educations.[90] Others who were equally well treated with galactose restriction have had various intellectual deficiencies, including verbal dyspraxia, reduced intelligence, learning disabilities, and neurologic deficits.[139] The causes of the variability in the responses to treatment need further exploration.

Hypergonadotropic hypogonadism is another long-term disorder observed in galactosemic women.[140,141] Although successful pregnancy is possible, 65 percent of galactosemic women develop ovarian failure with atrophic gonads. The mechanism is believed to be related to excess galactose exposure during fetal and childhood development[142] or to galactose restriction and a specific galactose need during ovarian development. The male gonads, however, appear more resistant to the effects of galactosemia.[143]

Osteoporosis is a frequent complication among females with galactosemia. The mechanisms underlying this complication may relate to low calcium intake, lack of sex hormones associated with ovarian failure, and an independent defect in collagen synthesis resulting in disturbances in bone mineralization.[144,145] Renner and coworkers have shown that treatment with hormone replacement and vitamin D therapy (1000 IU/day) resulted in the onset of menarche and increased bone density in two 28-year-old galactosemic twins when treatment was started at 25 years of age.[145]

Although genetic and social factors may influence results of intelligence tests, such factors do not explain all the differences observed. The association of thyroid dysfunction with galactosemia may have some role in the outcome.[146,147] A factor that definitely affects outcome is the age of the patient at diagnosis. Evidence supports the previous impression that a more favorable outcome can be expected when a patient is treated at an early age. For example, the mean intelligence quotient of 16 patients treated before 7 days of age was 99.5, whereas that of patients treated between 4 and 6 months of age was 62. It is generally desirable to institute treatment at the earliest possible age, and neonatal screening is an important step in this direction.

Although diagnosis and treatment at birth are desirable objectives, it is also possible that homozygotic galactosemic infants may have experienced unfavorable intrauterine exposure to galactose or its metabolites. Even with maternal dietary restriction of lactose during pregnancy, levels of erythrocytic galactose-1-phosphate in samples of cord blood from 12 homozygotic infants still averaged 11.3 mg/dl. Thus it appears that the intrauterine environment is not ideal for a homozygotic galactosemic fetus.[90]

Galactokinase-deficiency Galactosemia

Galactokinase deficiency is less common than classic transferase deficiency, with an incidence of about 1:10,000.[148] It does not result in progressive liver disease and mental retardation, but galactose exposure may result in cataract formation.[66-68] It is appropriate to compare this entity with transferase deficiency because it affects the first reaction (kinase) and the second reaction of the galactose pathway (transferase) (see Figure 48-3). Comparison of patients with these two defects and the defect involving the third reaction (epimerase) has helped to determine some of the mechanisms of toxicity in several organs, including the development of cataracts. With galactokinase deficiency there is no accumulation of galactose-1-phosphate, no systemic manifestations, and no mental retardation. Cataract formation is related to synthesis of galactitol in the lens and osmotic disruption of lens fiber architecture, as discussed in the previous section. Maternal galactokinase deficiency may result in fetal cataract formation.[148] Because of the potential for cataract formation, lifelong elimination of galactose is suggested.

Uridine Diphosphate Galactose-4-epimerase-deficiency Galactosemia

Galactose epimerase catalyzes the third reaction of galactose metabolism (see Figure 48-3). Epimerase deficiency was discovered incidentally while screening for galactosemia and has an incidence of about 1:46,000 in Switzerland. Patients have normal erythrocyte transferase activity but elevated levels of galactose-1-phosphate.[69,70] One form of this condition is apparently caused by a decreased stability of epimerase and leads to enzyme deficiency in those cells in which its turnover is slow or absent, such as erythrocytes.[149] It is therefore considered to be a benign illness inasmuch as the enzyme deficiency is limited to leukocytes and red blood cells. Affected people have no symptoms, but patients with generalized epimerase deficiency have been described.[71,75] The latter patients have signs and symptoms identical to transferase-deficiency galactosemia.

By contrast with transferase deficiency, in which uridine diphosphogalactose can be formed from uridine diphosphoglucose, one patient with generalized epimerase deficiency was unable to synthesize the galactose precursor necessary for synthesis of glycoproteins and glycolipids. These glycosylated compounds are necessary for cell membrane integrity, especially in the central nervous system. Thus in contrast to patients with transferase deficiency, the rare patient with systemic epimerase deficiency may require small quantities of galactose for normal growth and development. One patient with epimerase deficiency continued to show slightly elevated levels of galactose-1-phosphate in red cells even with dietary restriction of galactose. Appropriate treatment of this disorder therefore requires frequent monitoring of erythrocyte galactose-1-phosphate levels to best determine the optimal dietary level of galactose.

Glycogen Storage Diseases

Clinical and pathologic recognition of GSD affecting the liver and kidneys was described by von Gierke in 1929.[150] Three years later Pompe recognized another type of GSD that involved not only the liver and kidneys but most other organs as well.[151] In 1952 Cori and Cori showed that hepatic glucose-6-phosphatase activity was deficient in patients with von Gierke's disease.[152] This marked the beginning of a classification of glycogenoses by the types of enzymatic defects and the primary organs of involvement. In most types of GSD the glycogen content of liver or muscle or both is excessive. In unusual cases the glycogen content may be less than normal, the molecular structure of glycogen may be abnormal, or both may occur. Despite differences in the specific enzymatic defects, most of the syndromes are not readily distinguishable on clinical grounds alone, and tissue analyses for glycogen content and enzymatic activity are necessary to confirm the diagnoses.[153,154] Deficiencies of enzymes involving almost every step of glycogen synthesis and degradation have been identified. Their locations in the sequence of glycogen synthesis and degradation are illustrated in Figure 48-5.

Most enzymatic defects giving rise to hepatic glycogenosis involve degradation of glycogen to glucose-6-phosphate or, in rare instances, the synthesis of glycogen from glucose-6-phosphate.[153-156] On the other hand, patients with von Gierke's disease are deficient in the activity of glucose-6-phosphatase, a gluconeogenic enzyme. As a consequence of this enzymatic difference, many of the clinical and chemical features of von Gierke's disease, or type I GSD (GSD-I), are unique among the GSDs. For example, the tetrad of a bleeding tendency from thrombasthenia, urate stones from hyperuricemia, hyperlipidemia, and lactic acidosis accompanies GSD-I and is not part of the aberrations seen with other glycogenoses.

Despite the number of enzymatic deficiencies leading to the glycogenoses, only types 0 (glycogen synthetase deficiency) and IV (α-1,4-glucan:α-1,4-glucan 6-glycosyl transferase deficiency) invariably lead to cirrhosis and liver failure. Patients who have type I (glucose-6-phosphatase deficiency) may develop benign hepatic adenomas and hepatic adenocarcinomas, and patients with type III (amylo-1,6-glucosidase deficiency; debrancher enzyme deficiency) may develop hepatic fibrosis or cirrhosis. Because only a few patients have been reported with type 0 GSD, only types I, III, and IV are discussed in detail here.

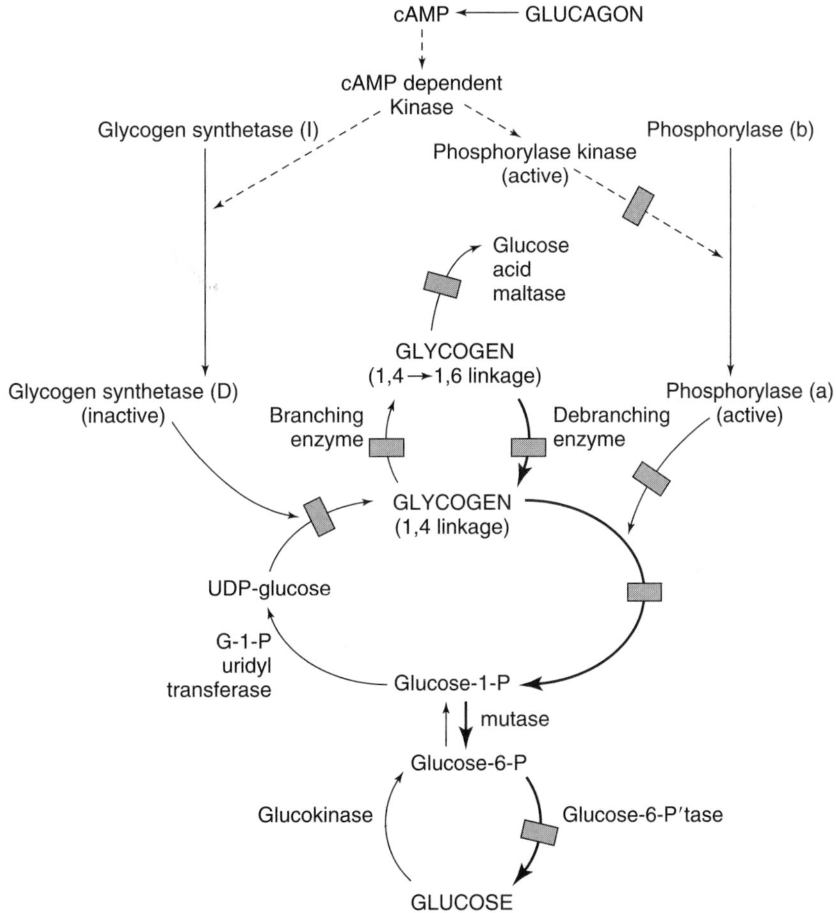

Figure 48-5 Pathway for glycogen synthesis and degradation to glucose. Broken lines indicate enzymic activation after glucagon stimulation, heavy arrows indicate glycogen degradation from glucagon infusion, and hatched boxes indicate points in the metabolic sequence in which enzymic defects have been identified.

Type I Glycogenosis (Glucose-6-phosphatase Deficiency)

Classification of Type I Glycogenosis

Type I glycogenosis represents a deficiency of glucose-6-phosphatase. This enzyme is alleged to be a multicomponent system consisting of three transport proteins—T_1, T_2 and T_3—which transport glucose-6-phosphate, phosphate/pyrophosphate, and glucose, respectively, across the endoplasmic reticulum membrane. Two other components of this enzyme system include the catalytic subunit and a regulatory, calcium-stabilizing protein (SP).[157] A schematic representation of the glucose-6-phosphatase enzyme system is shown in Figure 48-6. Although this is the generally accepted concept for glucose-6-phosphatase, there is no proof for its existence; and other interpretations of the relevant data are possible.

Several subtypes of GSD-I have been identified. Type Ia is the classic type and represents a complete absence of glucose-6-phosphatase activity. The catalytic subunit of the enzyme is a polypeptide doublet with molecular mass of 36.5.[158] Type IaSP subtype describes patients with clinically classic type Ia with normal activity of the enzyme but lacking a 21-kd stabilizing polypeptide protein (SP).[159] Type IIb has a clinical picture similar to type Ia; however, in these patients, the activity of glucose-6-phosphatase in fully disrupted microsomes is completely normal, whereas the activity in intact microsomes and in vivo is lacking. The patients have a putative defect in the transport protein T_1.[160] Clinically, patients with type Ib are similar to those with type Ia, except for the presence of neutropenia. Type Ic is characterized by a putative deficiency of T_2, the microsomal phosphate/pyrophosphate transport protein.[161] Some patients with type Ic have impaired insulin release in response to glucose[162]; others have a normal response. Type Id is limited to defects in the putative T_3 transport protein; however, there are no reports of a deficiency in T_3.

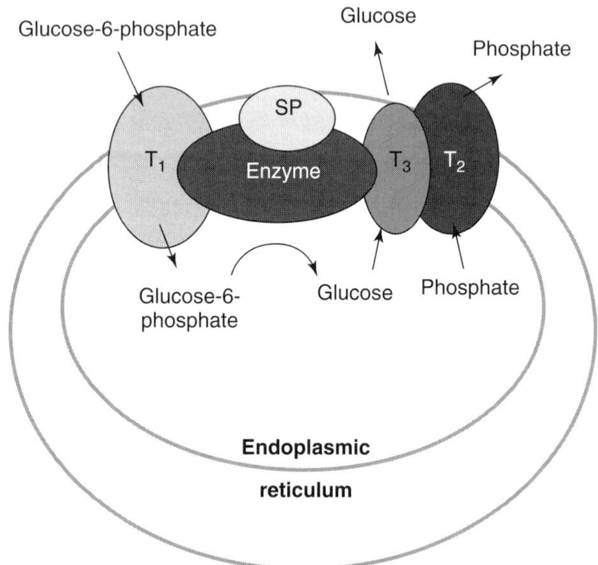

Figure 48-6 Schematic model of hepatic microsomal glucose-6-phosphatase. Glucose-6-phosphate entry into the endoplasmic reticulum is via a transport protein (T1). Hydrolysis occurs by the catalytic subunit of the glucose-6-phosphatase. SP is a stabilizing protein. Phosphate is returned to the cytosol via a transport protein (T2). Glucose is returned via T3. *SP,* Stabilizing protein. (Modified from Burchell A: Molecular pathology of glucose-6-phosphatase. FASEB J 4:2978, 1990.)

Molecular Basis of Glycogen Storage Disease Type I

The cDNA encoding the murine glucose-6-phosphatase enzyme was cloned by screening a mouse liver cDNA library differentially with mRNA populations representing the normal and the albino deletion mouse known to express markedly reduced level of glucose-6-phosphatase enzyme.[163] This discovery allowed the cloning of the human glucose-6-phosphatase cDNA by homology screening. The human gene spans 12 Kb, is composed of fine exons, and encodes for a 357-amino acid protein.[164-166] The gene has been localized to chromosome 17q21. The glucose-6-phosphatase mRNA is expressed in the liver, kidney, and intestine. However, it is not expressed in human neutrophils and monocytes.[167] To date, more than 60 mutations have been identified in the glucose-6-phosphatase gene of patients with type Ia.[166-173] The two most common mutations are R83C and Q347X, which account for more than 70 percent of mutations in Caucasian populations.[174] The common mutation Q347X causes a protein truncation of the last 10 carboxyterminal amino acids that contain the signal for retention in the endoplasmic reticulum.

Clinical Characteristics

This form of glycogenosis, the most commonly diagnosed type, represents one fourth of all cases diagnosed. A general discussion of type Ia (designated GSD-I) is presented followed by a brief discussion of type IB. The clinical picture is one of severe hepatomegaly, which may be apparent within the first 2 weeks of life. Profound hypoglycemia may develop shortly after birth or may not be prominent for several weeks, depending on frequency of feeding, the presence of intercurrent infection, and the severity of the disease. Because glucose-6-phosphatase activity is also deficient in the kidneys, patients have substantial enlargement of the kidneys. Serum transaminase levels may be slightly elevated but become normal with effective treatment that maintains blood glucose between 75 and 110 mg/dl at all times. Neither the liver nor the kidneys show functional abnormalities other than the inability to release free glucose into the circulation. In this regard, patients who receive a renal transplant remain unable to maintain normal fasting blood glucose levels.[175] Consanguinity of parents is common, and the disease is transmitted as an autosomal-recessive trait. During the past decade, major improvements in therapy have been documented.[176-179] The study of mechanisms whereby deficiencies of glucose-6-phosphatase activity can cause striking abnormalities in lipid, purine, and carbohydrate metabolism has been instrumental in these therapeutic advances. To place GSD-I in metabolic perspective, the mechanisms by which this single enzyme deficiency can have such profound effects on other metabolic pathways are reviewed.

Biochemical Characteristics

Blood Glucose Changes. The most consistent and life-threatening feature of GSD-I is the low blood glucose levels that result from relatively short periods of fasting. Fasting for as short a time as 2 to 4 hours is almost always associated with decreases in blood glucose to less than 70 mg/dl, and it is not uncommon to observe 6- to 8-hour fasting levels of 5 to 10 mg/dl. In normal individuals blood glucose levels are maintained within a relatively narrow range by hepatotropic agents such as glucagon, which release glucose either from stored glycogen or by gluconeogenesis.[180] In GSD-I, degradation of glycogen can occur or lactate or other gluconeogenic precursors can be converted to glucose-6-phosphate, but in the absence of glucose-6-phosphatase, glucose is not released, and blood glucose levels continue to decline. Blood hormone measurements indicate that during periods of hypoglycemia, insulin levels are appropriately low and glucagon levels are high. After a glucose load, there is a substantial—although somewhat delayed—insulin release, with concomitant decreases in glucagon and alanine levels.[154,176,181] Thus the hormonal response to changes in the blood glucose concentrations appears appropriate.

Lactic Acid Changes. Under normal circumstances most circulating lactate is generated by muscle glycolysis during exercise. Removal and metabolism of this lactate are efficiently performed by the liver.[180] On the other hand, much of the circulating lactate in patients with GSD-I is generated by hepatic glycolysis.[182] This phenomenon apparently is the result of hepatic stimulation to release glucose from glycogen in combination with inefficient gluconeogenesis. Excess glucose-6-phosphate formed during glycogenolysis cannot be hydrolyzed to free glucose because of the lack of glucose-6-phosphatase activity. Instead, glucose-6-phosphate is diverted through the glycolytic pathway. This metabolic diversion appears to be the basis for enhancement of lactate formation, as illustrated in Figure 48-7.

Hyperlipidemia. Elevation of plasma lipids is a consistent and striking abnormality.[183,184] Levels of triglyceride may reach 6000 mg/dl, with associated cholesterol levels of 400 to 600 mg/dl. Free fatty acid levels are also usually elevated. Around puberty, xanthomas can appear over extensor surfaces, but they may also appear in childhood, with involvement of the nasal septum. Those located on the septum may contribute to the frequency of prolonged nosebleeds seen in some patients.

As with lacticemia, elevated levels of triglyceride and cholesterol appear to be a consequence of increased rates of glycogenolysis and glycolysis. Observations by Sadeghi-Nejad and co-workers suggest that excess hepatic glycolysis increases hepatic NADH, nicotinamide adenine dinucleotide phosphate, and acetyl co-enzyme A (CoA), three compounds important in fatty acid and cholesterol synthesis.[182] Thus increases in glycerol-3-phosphate and acetyl CoA generated by the glycolytic pathway, together with high levels of reduced co-factors, could sustain an increased rate of triglyceride and

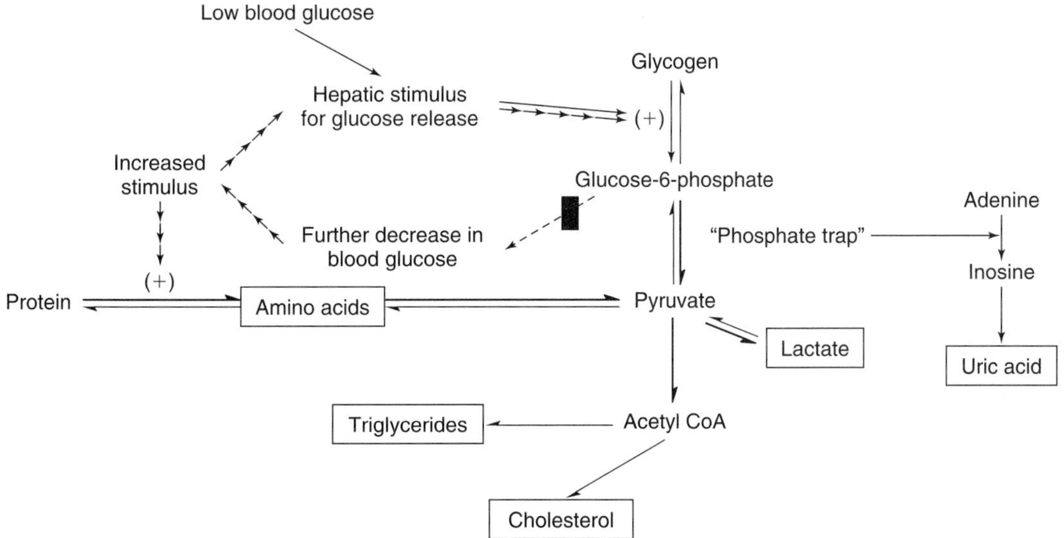

Figure 48-7 Biochemical basis for the primary laboratory findings in patients with glucose-6-phosphatase deficiency (indicated by the solid rectangle). The increased production of glucose-6-phosphate that results from continuous stimulation of glycogen breakdown apparently increases glycolysis, which in turn results in a net increase (indicated by dark arrows) in the production of lactate, triglyceride, cholesterol, and uric acid. Both glycogenolysis and gluconeogenesis are involved in the overproduction of substrate.

cholesterol synthesis.[185,186] In addition to this apparent increased rate of lipid synthesis, an event concomitant with hypoglycemia is lipolysis from peripheral lipid stores. This further augments the tendency for hyperlipidemia and hepatic steatosis to occur by increasing circulating free fatty acids.[183,187]

Hyperuricemia. Although blood levels of uric acid and the tendency to develop gouty arthritis and nephropathy vary in different patients, those who survive puberty often have gouty complications.[188,189] Hyperuricemia was originally attributed to the increased levels of serum lactate and lipid, which competitively inhibit urate excretion.[184] However, the high level of urate excretion together with the rate of incorporation of ^{14}C-L-glycine into plasma and urinary urate indicates that an increased rate of purine synthesis de novo is probably more important in the genesis of hyperuricemia than is a decrease in urate excretion.[190,191] The rate of purine synthesis can be influenced by at least two mechanisms: (1) alteration of the substrate (precursor) concentration (i.e., phosphoribosyl pyrophosphate [PRPP] and glutamine levels) and (2) alteration of the end-product, or purine concentration (i.e., low intracellular purine levels increase purine synthesis).[192-194] In support of the former, two substrates, PRPP and glutamine, are necessary for the first committed reaction. This reaction transfers the amine from L-glutamine to PRPP to form 5-phosphoribosyl-1-amine and is apparently rate limiting for the entire sequence of purine synthesis (Reaction [4]). Although tissue glutamate and glutamine levels have not been measured, blood levels of the two substrates obtained from hyperuricemic patients with GSD-I are threefold to eightfold higher than are values obtained after urate is normalized by glucose infusion.[186] In addition to the possibility of increased availability of glutamine, the high levels of glucose-6-phosphate produced during periods of hypoglycemia and excessive glycogenolysis may increase synthesis of the second important substrate in purine synthesis, ribose-5-phosphate.[184,188,195] This suggests that an apparent increased availability of purine precursors, glutamine, and ribose-5-phosphate may cause a secondary increase in PRPP and thus increase the rate of purine synthesis. Studies using human leukocytes indicate, however, that an increase in availability of glutamine and ribose-5-phosphate alone will not increase the generation of PRPP.[196] Assuming this is true in liver, the second mechanism, alteration of end-product concentration, should be more important in modulating the increased rate of purine synthesis in patients with GSD-I.

In support of the second mechanism for hyperuricemia a decreased concentration of purine ribonucleotides would favor an increase in the rate of purine biosynthesis by releasing the glutamine pyrophosphate-ribose-phosphate aminotransferase from end-product inhibition.[197] Although hepatic nucleotide levels during hypoglycemic episodes have not been determined directly, indirect evidence suggests that in patients with GSD-I, hypoglycemia can reduce adenyl ribonucleotide levels. Such a conclusion is based on measured values of hepatic ATP before and after simulating the effects of hypoglycemia with intravenous glucagon administration.[198] Seven patients had a threefold decrease in hepatic ATP levels with concomitant 1.3-fold decreases in adenosine diphosphate (ADP). Such a reduction in ATP has been shown to favor the rapid degradation of adenyl or guanyl ribonucleotides to xanthine and uric acid. The latter set of reactions is also favored by low intracellular phos-

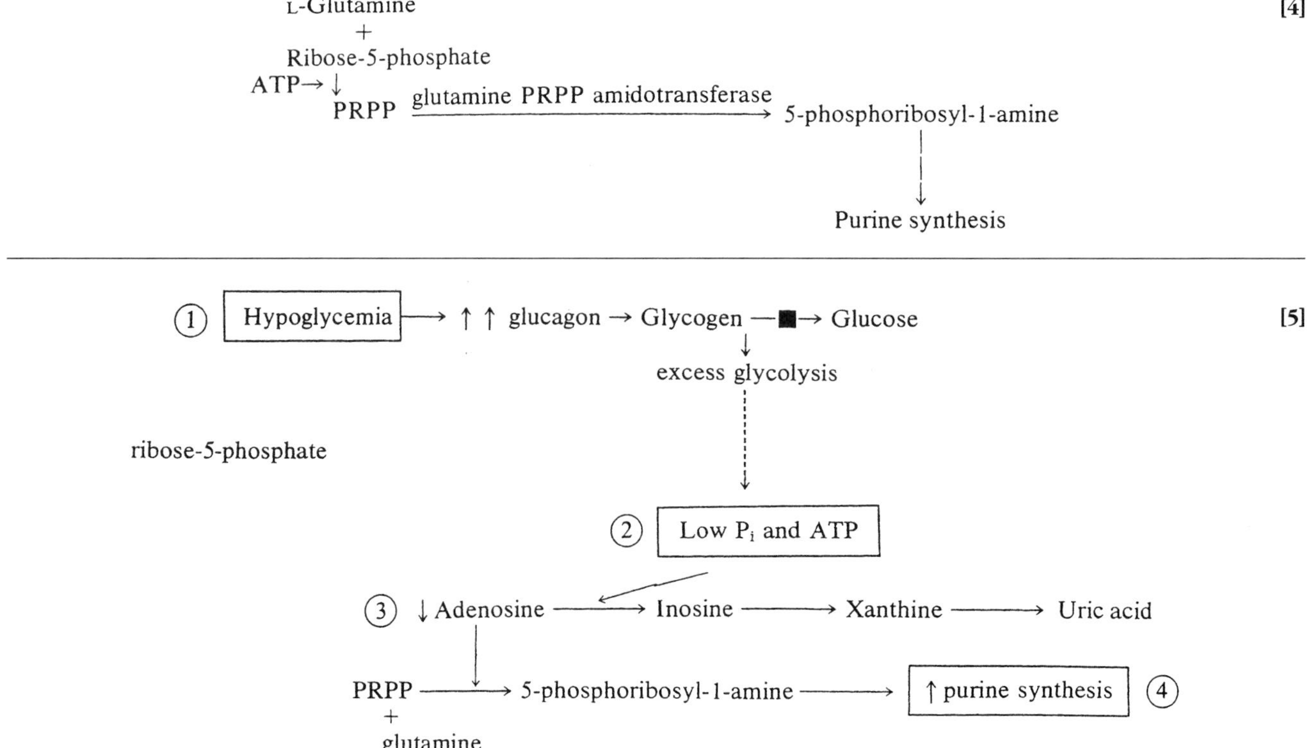

phate levels, which apparently occur through phosphate trapping of the phosphorylated sugar. Normally, this accumulation of glucose-6-phosphate is prevented by the action of glucose-6-phosphatase.[199,200]

These observations suggest that the increase in urate production is secondary to recurrent episodes of hypoglycemia (Reaction [5]), which result in compensatory glucagon release. This hepatotropic agent stimulates glycogen degradation to glucose-6-phosphate. The absence of phosphatase activity results in a phosphate-trapping effect and lowering of ATP levels, which in turn promotes degradation of preformed purines to uric acid (Reaction [5]).[25,200,201] Finally, the decrease in end-product (purine) concentration promotes a high rate of purine biosynthesis (Reaction [5]).

Hypophosphatemia. Low serum phosphate levels are not an invariable finding but are more likely to be present during periods of hypoglycemia and acidosis. It has been noted that a glucagon injection is followed by an acute decrease in serum phosphate that spontaneously reverts to the preinjection level within 3 hours. This suggests that cellular [P_i] levels are rapidly depleted by the glucagon effects and that there is a compensatory shift of phosphate out of the circulating pool. A well-demonstrated corollary occurs after fructose ingestion in patients with hereditary fructose intolerance. This has been shown to result from phosphate trapping on the fructose moiety because of blockage of the aldolase step.[14,25,200,201] As a result of the inability to release P_i from the sugar, the liver cell must take up phosphorus from serum (Reaction [6]). For example, when 6.6 mmol of fructose is administered to an 8.8-kg infant, the fructose load exceeds the amount of P_i mole per mole, in the entire extracellular fluid.[14]

A phenomenon analogous to that in hereditary fructose intolerance apparently occurs because of the phosphate trap created as a result of glucose-6-phosphatase deficiency. A relative metabolic block at the aldolase step would also be expected because of the progressive increase in NADH formed during the initial phase of the reaction cascade from glucose-6-phosphate to pyruvate. The demonstrated decrease in hepatic glycogen content by a mean of 2.3 percent after a glucagon injection provides a large amount of glucose-6-phosphate that cannot be hydrolyzed to release the bound P_i (Reaction [7]).[198] The series of reactions (Reaction [7]) reflects the phosphate trapping by the accumulated sugars of the anaerobic pathway, thus causing an acute shift of circulating phosphate to the intracellular pool. As the phosphate is lost from the sugars, there is a compensatory shift of phosphate back into the circulation.

Recurrent Fever. A few patients have recurrent fever in association with acidosis and hypoglycemia. In these patients the fever can be reproduced by intravenous injection of glucagon if the patient is already slightly hypoglycemic (blood glucose 35 to 55 mg/dl) and acidotic (arterial blood pH 7.28 to 7.36). The febrile response begins 8 to 12 minutes after glucagon injection (0.1 mg/kg given over 3 minutes) and usually peaks 12 to 16 minutes later. If the low blood glucose level is corrected by intravenous administration of glucose and the acidosis is corrected by sodium bicarbonate, the temperature usually returns to normal within 45 minutes after glucagon infusion.

If the explanation for hypophosphatemia just postulated is correct, the febrile response may represent an uncoupling of oxidative phosphorylation secondary to lack of P_i. For example, the glucagon results in the excessive formation of glucose-6-phosphate from glycogen. Because of the glucose-6-phosphatase deficiency, a burst of glycolysis results in excess production of reduced cofactors, which normally produce high-energy phosphates. Because of low intracellular phosphate levels, oxidative phosphorylation, were it to occur, would have to be uncoupled, leading to production of heat rather than chemical energy in the form of ATP (Reaction [8]).

Platelet Dysfunction. Patients with GSD-I usually have prolonged bleeding times secondary to abnormal platelet aggregation. Corby and co-workers examined platelet function in 13 patients, each with deficient hepatic activity of one of the following enzymes: glucose-6-phosphatase, debrancher enzyme, phosphorylase, or phosphorylase kinase.[201] Only the seven patients with glucose-6-phosphatase deficiencies had abnormal platelet aggregation, and four of these also had abnormal platelet adhesiveness. The defect appears to be intrinsic, because crossover and resuspension studies using patients' platelets in normal plasma and normal platelets in patients' plasma did not alter in vitro platelet function. Two such patients had the ADP content of affected

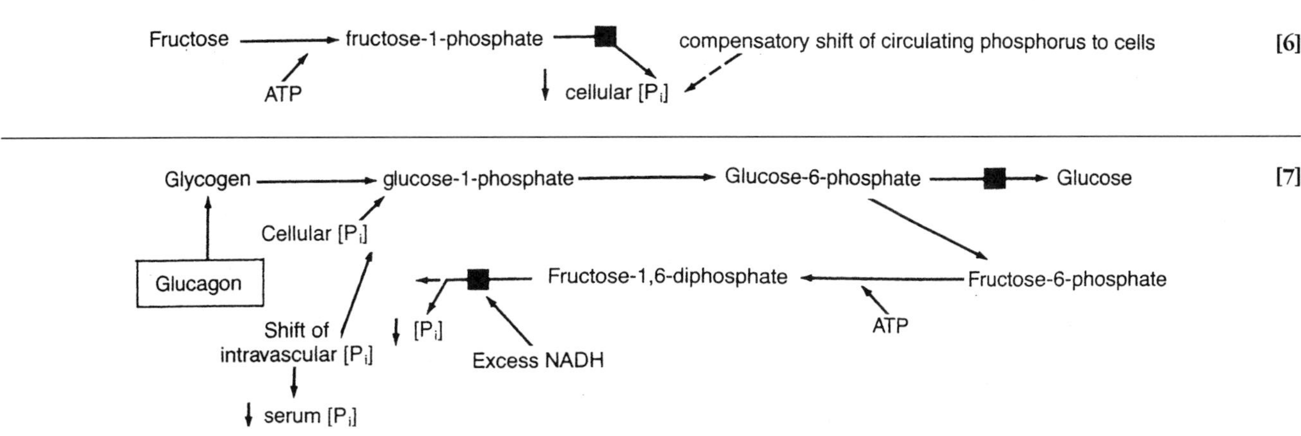

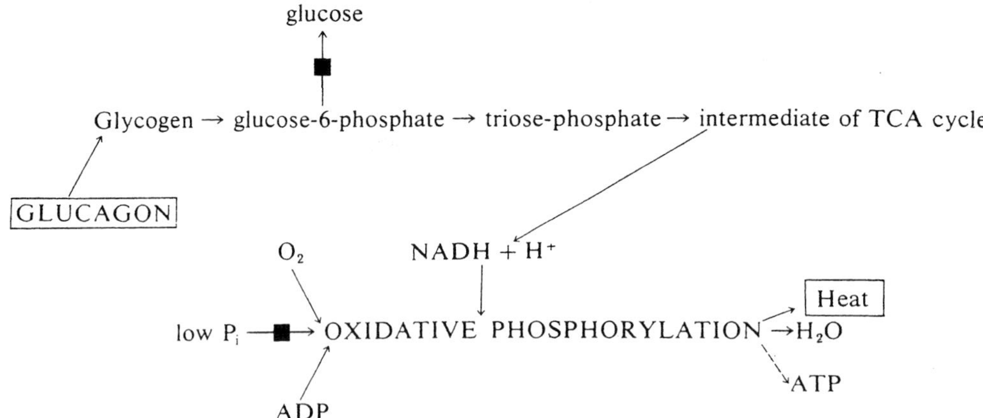

[8]

platelets measured, and in both instances it was normal. Nevertheless, the release of ADP from platelets in response to added collagen and epinephrine was markedly impaired. These observations suggest that the functional defect is an impairment of the ability of the platelet membrane to release ADP. Cooper has shown a similar defect in ADP release from platelets with elevated cholesterol content.[202] The elevated cholesterol content impaired fluidity of the membrane, causing secondary impairment of ADP and epinephrine-induced aggregation. Although platelet cholesterol levels of patients with GSD-I have not been measured, the elevated serum cholesterol content might reflect elevated platelet cholesterol content and therefore may contribute to the abnormality of platelet function in patients with GSD-I. If this postulate is correct, then treatment that lowers blood and platelet cholesterol levels should also normalize platelet function. One of the author's patients was found to have abnormal platelet function but had normal serum cholesterol and triglyceride levels. This finding does not support the hypothesis.

Growth Impairment. Children who have GSD-I are of short stature but without disproportionate head sizes or limb or trunk lengths. The abdomen is usually massively enlarged as a result of hepatomegaly. Bones may be osteoporotic, and some patients have delayed bone age. The mechanism leading to these changes is not clear. Growth hormone and thyroid hormone levels are normal or increased.[154,176] Measurements of calorie-protein intake in three patients for 2 weeks indicated adequate caloric consumption. Observations suggest that chronic lactic acidosis and concomitant reversal of the insulin to glucagon ratio may be more important factors in preventing normal growth.

Hepatic Adenomas and Carcinomas. The development of adenomatous nodules within hepatic parenchyma once was an infrequent finding. Most patients with GSD-I who are more than 15 years old are now found to develop adenomas. This is at variance with the previously held view that they occur only infrequently. Adenomas develop in most patients during the second decade of life, but they may be found in 3-year-old children. The nodules, which are best demonstrated by ultrasonography and radioisotopic scanning, show increased echodensity and decreased isotope uptake. At laparotomy, they appear as discrete, pale nodules that range in number from one to many and in size from 1 to 5 cm. A number of patients have been found to have solitary hepatocellular adenocarcinomas in individual nodules.[20-206] The mechanism causing the adenomas or their malignant degeneration is unknown, but treatment with portacaval shunting does not prevent their development. The author now has two patients who had adenomas before nocturnal feedings, but after 3 years of treatment, nodules were no longer detectable by scanning (Figure 48-8). A subsequent older patient (age 16 years) developed adenomas during treatment with nocturnal feedings; the feedings were later found to be inadequate to maintain blood glucose above 75 mg/dl. After readjustment of therapy, the nodules decreased in size but did not show complete resolution. This suggests that chronic stimulation of the liver by hepatotropic agents (glucagon and others) that increase blood glucose levels may be important in the genesis of the adenomas.

The tendency for adenoma formation and malignant transformation is highest in young adult patients and appears to be a consequence of supportive therapy, which currently ensures survival into childhood and young adulthood. The mechanism leading to hepatic malignancy is unknown, although review of case histories suggests that the adenomatous cells rather than the non-adenomatous cells are transformed. A similar progression has been observed in experimental hepatocarcinogenesis from exposure to N-nitrosomorpholine. The progression from normal hepatocytes to malignancy appears to be as follows. First, multi-focal areas of cells containing excessive glycogen develop. The cells in these areas also show decreased glucose-6-phosphatase activity. Second, the focal cluster of cells develops a gradual reduction in glycogen content and a concomitant increase in ribosomes, reflected as basophilia by hematoxylin and eosin staining. Finally, the foci enlarge and acquire the phenotypic markers of hepatocellular carcinoma. These experimental observations, coupled with the findings in patients with GSD-I, have led Bannasch and associates to postulate that the metabolic disturbance leading to hepatocellular glycogenesis is fixed at the genetic level in both the experimental animals and the patients and is causally related to the neoplastic transformation.[207]

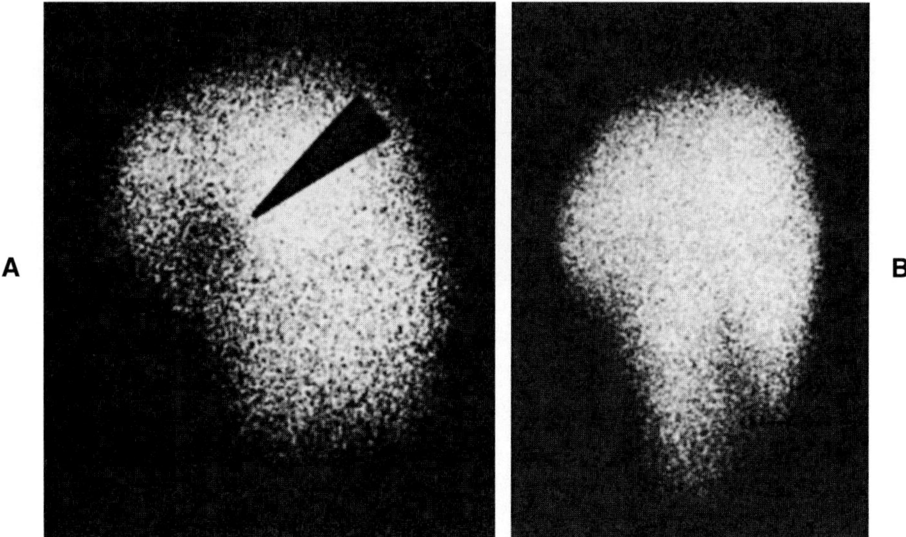

Figure 48-8 Technetium scan of the liver showing regression of hepatic filling defect in response to dietary therapy. The arrow in **A** indicates a hepatic adenoma before therapy; **B** shows its disappearance, with reduction in the size of the liver after 4 years of dietary therapy.

Severity of Illness. Despite the fact that there is no difference in activities of the phosphatase enzyme between patients, the expression of symptoms and of chemical anomalies varies substantially from one patient to another without detectable differences in management. Some patients may have only moderate abnormalities in blood chemistry and slightly decreased growth rates, whereas others may have marked alterations in blood lipids, require frequent hospitalizations for fever and lactic acidosis, or even die in infancy or early childhood. In addition, hypoglycemia seems to abate somewhat, after patients have reached adulthood. In fact, a few patients who had had moderately severe symptoms during childhood improved so dramatically during adulthood that they were able to have successful pregnancies.[208,209]

Glucose Production. In 1967 Havel and colleagues reported that two adult patients with GSD-I showed near normal basal rates of glucose production using ^{14}C-glucose as a marker.[210] This observation has been confirmed in patients of all ages by several investigators who used dideuteroglucose as the isotopic marker.[211-214] These studies also indicate several features of the illness that have important therapeutic implications.

1. Patients with GSD-I can release glucose into the circulation at close to normal basal rates.
2. Patients cannot increase glucose release during hypoglycemia or after a pharmacologic dose of glucagon; therefore, their basal rates of glucose production are also their maximal rates of production.
3. Maximal glucose production is variable between patients but is not related to residual activity of hepatic glucose-6-phosphatase. However, the tendency for fasting-induced hypoglycemia and severity of the clinical illness are directly related to maximal rates of glucose production.
4. Endogenous glucose production is not inhibited unless an exogenous source of glucose is provided at a rate of 8 mg/kg/minute, an amount that maintains blood glucose levels at about 90 mg/dl.
5. The improvement in ability to fast for a longer time after the second decade of life appears to result from a decrease in glucose utilization rather than an increase in glucose production.

Diagnosis

Characteristically, these patients have no increase in blood glucose levels after administration of glucagon or epinephrine, and usually they show substantial decreases in blood glucose within 20 minutes after intravenous glucagon administration. As mentioned in the previous section, a major product of glycogenolysis is lactate rather than glucose. In some patients who are already slightly acidotic glucagon stimulation may cause severe acidosis. Aside from the glucagon tolerance test, other tolerance tests have been used as an aid in diagnosing the type of glycogenosis. For example, neither galactose nor fructose is converted to free glucose in patients with GSD-I, and a tolerance test with either of these sugars results in a flat blood glucose curve. These tolerance tests have the advantage of avoiding liver biopsy. On the other hand, a substantial volume of blood is required to complete all the tolerance testing and, not infrequently, the results are inconclusive. For example, the author has had several patients referred with erroneous diagnoses based on tolerance tests. Thus for accurate diagnosis, the author feels that measurement of hepatic enzyme activity is necessary. To provide a basis for some selectivity in the enzymatic analyses of biopsy specimens, the author's practice is to determine serial blood glucose and lactate measurements during a 4- to 6-hour fast, followed by the maximum glucose response to glucagon before liver biopsy. For example, a rise in glucose of more than 30 mg/dl generally indicates a defect in phosphorylase kinase, which is not routinely measured from needle biopsy material.

Before an effective form of treatment was available, the need for accurate diagnosis was less important than it is today. Because of the effectiveness of treatment of patients with glucose-6-phosphatase deficiency, the suspected diagnosis of GSD should be confirmed by enzymatic assay of hepatic tissue. A diagnosis can be confirmed by examination of needle biopsy material, which avoids potential complications of surgery and general anesthesia.[215]

Pathology

In GSD-I the liver cells are distended with glycogen and often contain medium-sized to large lipid vacuoles. The lipid content in the liver of an untreated patient is substantially greater than that in the liver of a patient who has been treated, but in either instance, hepatic steatosis is a prominent morphologic feature. The liver cells are pale staining and have prominent plasma membranes. Three notable features differentiate GSD-I from other glycogenoses: (1) the presence of substantial steatosis, (2) a lack of associated fibrosis, and (3) nuclear hyperglycogenosis. Nuclear glycogenosis is commonly noted in hepatocytes of normal children, but in GSD-I (and GSD-III), the nuclei are grotesquely enlarged—that is, hyperglycogenosis is present.

It is not possible to distinguish between normal and elevated levels of cytoplasmic glycogen in the liver in any of the forms of glycogenosis through the use of periodic acid–Schiff (PAS) stain.[216] Thus to make a diagnosis of excessive glycogen content, a quantitative determination is necessary. It is also important to note that the livers of normal individuals and those of patients with glucose-6-phosphatase deficiencies can degrade glycogen. Thus postmortem analyses of surgical specimens that are not frozen promptly may give inappropriately low (e.g., "normal") levels.

Treatment

Patients with some glycogenoses—for example, those who have deficiencies of hepatic phosphorylase kinase activity and some patients with GSD-III (debrancher deficiency)—have excellent prognoses without specific treatment. In fact, with the exception of those who have defects in glycogen synthesis, generalized glycogenosis (acid maltase deficiency; GSD-II; Pompe's disease), or glucose-6-phosphatase deficiencies, most patients who have hepatic glycogenoses have favorable prognoses and are successfully treated with attention to frequencies of food intake. This, however, has not been true of most patients who have GSD-I.

Recommendations for treatment of GSD-I stem primarily from the studies by Folkman and associates,[217] who first illustrated the reversal of most biochemical abnormalities after total parenteral nutrition (TPN). Their observation that both TPN and portacaval shunting[218,219] delivered nutrients primarily into the systemic circulation suggested that hepatic exposure to nutrients was important in the pathogenesis of many biochemical abnormalities. Nevertheless, it was later demonstrated that the same beneficial effect seen with TPN or portacaval shunting could be achieved with an intragastric infusion of a nutrient solution similar in content to that used for TPN.[220] This suggested that bypassing the liver with nutrients was not the most important factor in reversing the abnormalities. The similarity in the three types of treatment (i.e., portacaval shunting, TPN, continuous intragastric infusion of glucose) was that a hormonal stimulus to the liver to produce glucose was decreased or averted. Specifically, both TPN and continuous intragastric feeding prevented a hepatic stimulus for glucose release by maintaining blood glucose levels in the range of 90 to 150 mg/dl, whereas the portacaval shunt prevented such a stimulus by diverting pancreatic and enteric blood into systemic circulation. On this basis, the hypothesis for treatment illustrated in Figure 48-9 was formulated.

The hypothesis states that as blood glucose falls below a critical level, compensatory mechanisms cause

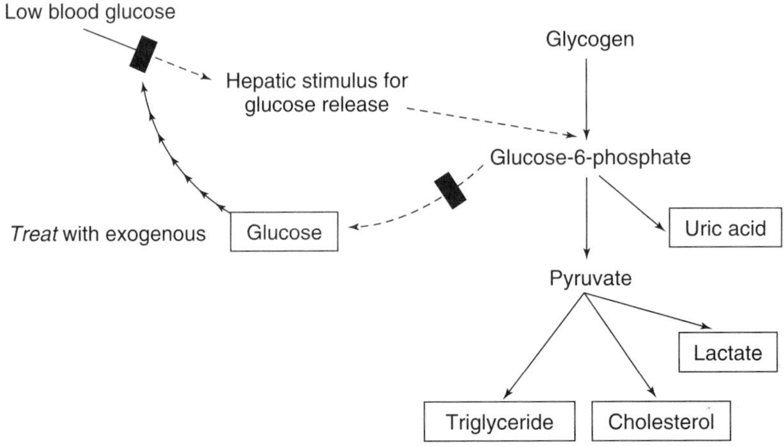

Figure 48-9 A biochemical basis for management of patients with glucose-6-phosphatase deficiency (indicated by solid rectangle). By preventing the decrease in blood glucose with an exogenous supply of glucose, excessive glycolysis and glyconeogenesis are prevented. This results in a net decrease in production of circulating triglyceride, cholesterol, lactate, and uric acid.

glycogen degradation to glucose-6-phosphate. In the absence of glucose-6-phosphatase, glucose-6-phosphate is not hydrolyzed to release free glucose; the hepatic stimulus for glycogenolysis results in formation of other intermediates such as lactate, triglycerides, and cholesterol. To interrupt the stimulus treatment with an exogenous source of glucose inhibits the release of hepatotropic stimuli and thus the excess glycogenolysis. If this postulate is correct any method of treatment that maintains blood glucose above a critical level should also prevent or at least alleviate biochemical manifestations of the illness. In addition, the hypothesis suggests that diversion of portal vein blood flow should dilute hepatotropic agents in the systemic circulation. This dilution should result in less stimulation of glycogenolysis.

Theoretically, either portacaval shunting or continuous infusion of a high-glucose diet should be effective in reversing most manifestations of the illness, with the exception that portacaval shunting should have little or no beneficial effect on hypoglycemia. Thus portacaval shunting is not recommended as a sole form of treatment for those patients who are expected to have frequent episodes of very low blood glucose levels or for small children, in whom shunts may be more likely to close spontaneously.

Although TPN and continuous intragastric infusion of glucose are effective treatment modalities for GSD-I, they are impractical on a long-term basis. A more practical method was devised to maintain blood glucose at physiologic concentrations or at levels that would prevent stimulation of excess glycogenolysis and glycolysis. This treatment consisted of a high-glucose diet given to simulate TPN. Thus it was given enterally either by nasogastric tube or by gastrostomy during nighttime sleep, along with a high-starch diet, which was consumed at frequent intervals while the patient was awake. Such a regimen has successfully maintained a large number of patients relatively symptom-free for more than 10 years and has provided normal or near normal growth and development.[221,222]

Chen and colleagues found that a number of patients can maintain normal blood glucose levels by taking cold, uncooked cornstarch (2 g/kg) at 6-hour intervals.[223] This regimen has been used by a number of patients to avoid the continuous nocturnal feedings. A number of the younger children have not been able to maintain normal glucose and lactate levels with the cornstarch regimen as well as they had with the continuous nocturnal feeding regimen.[224,225] In the author's experience growth rates were less with the raw starch regimen than with continuous feedings, and one patient consumed such large quantities of cornstarch that protein intake was insufficient to maintain normal secretory proteins (albumin, transferrin, and retinol-binding protein). Thus although the cornstarch feedings can be beneficial as a time-release form of glucose in some patients, a dose response to the starch preparation and careful monitoring of blood glucose levels should be carried out to ensure that treatment is appropriate for individual patients. The author believes that many patients require an intensive feeding regimen at least until they have stopped growing. This consists of high starch feedings at 2- to 3-hour intervals during the day, continuous nocturnal feeding of a complete, low lipid-containing (less than 5 percent calories) formula, and periodic monitoring to ensure normal blood glucose and lactate levels throughout the day and night. As patients become fully grown and have a relatively lower requirement for glucose, the uncooked cornstarch regimen may allow discontinuation of the nighttime nasogastric feedings.

Prognosis

Until the use of nocturnal feedings, the first few years of life were usually marked by frequent hospitalizations for treatment of hypoglycemia and acidosis, with a high rate of death or permanent central nervous system impairment from recurrent and prolonged episodes of hypoglycemia. Patients who survived puberty appeared to have fewer problems than they had when younger. Patients with persistent hyperuricemia had gouty complications during the second and third decades of life, and many patients had complications of hyperlipemia, with xanthomas, and higher rates of cardiovascular disease and pancreatitis than those in the general population.[153-155,180,226] Recognition of hepatic adenomas has been relatively recent, and the incidence of complications from benign hepatic adenomas is unclear, although several patients have developed malignant hepatomas.[203,205]

Long-term follow-up of the results of portacaval shunting or nocturnal feedings is not complete. Ten-year follow-up of patients treated with nocturnal feedings indicates that infants so treated have many fewer problems than they had before treatment and that some patients with hepatic adenomas may show resolution after a few years of treatment. Too few patients have been monitored into the third decade of life to permit conclusions, but early observations indicate that for optimal treatment, the nocturnal feedings are necessary for most young patients, whereas raw cornstarch administration may suffice for older patients. On the other hand, patients generally have a lower tendency to hypoglycemia after the age of 20. A 22-year-old patient who was severely affected at the age of 15 years had been treated with nocturnal feedings for 6.5 years, with complete resolution of all chemical manifestations of the illness except hypoglycemia (blood glucose 62 mg/dl) and lactate elevation (7 mEq/L) after a 9-hour fast. She was weaned off nocturnal feedings by gradually decreasing the hourly feeding over a period of a month. After 2.5 years of no nocturnal feedings, she continues to have completely normal blood chemistry results after an 8-hour fast. There is still no hepatic glucose-6-phosphatase activity, however.

As long as blood glucose is consistently maintained between 70 and 120 mg/dl, most children appear to lead fairly normal, healthy lives, with normal growth and development, although in at least one patient the disease has been unresponsive to this type of management.[227] One report indicates that a blood level of 90 mg/dl (achieved by a glucose infusion of 8 mg/kg/minute) is necessary to completely inhibit endogenous glucose production. However, this dose provides additional calories, and unless the lower infusion rate does not correct the metabolic abnormalities, the greater tendency for obesity can be avoided by the lower rate of infusion.

Chen and colleagues observed that older patients (more than 18 years of age) with suboptimal treatment have a high incidence of progressive renal disease. The affected individuals show progressive glomerular sclerosis with proteinuria as an early manifestation.[228] Renal involvement appears initially with microalbuminuria and hyperfiltration progressing to frank proteinuria and hypertension.[229] Although the cause of the lesion is unclear, it appears that the incidence is lowered by maintenance of good control of blood glucose and other blood abnormalities, because none of the author's nine patients ages 25 to 34 show renal abnormalities.

GSD Type IB

In 1968 Senior and Loridan described a patient with clinical and laboratory features identical to GSD-I except that no enzyme defect was identified from frozen liver.[230] Subsequently, a number of similar patients have been identified.[231-240] In addition to the hepatic abnormality, patients have repeated infections because of neutropenia and abnormal leukocyte migration,[234-238] and some show decreased neutrophil phagocytosis-stimulated oxygen consumption, decreased nitroblue tetrazolium (NBT) reduction,[237] defective bactericidal activity, defective hexose monophosphate shunt activity, and increased incidence of inflammatory bowel disease.[238,241] These patients have been diagnosed as having GSD-IB. There has been little mention of a familial occurrence in the reports of GSD-IB. This is curious because a number of patients with GSD-I have affected siblings. One of the author's patients with GSD-IB has seven unaffected siblings. The number of reported cases is small, however, and the mode of inheritance is presumed to be autosomal recessive.

The reason for the discrepancy between the in vitro and in vivo activity of glucose-6-phosphatase in patients with GSD-IB is not known. Steady-state kinetic measurements led Arion and associates to conclude that the normal microsomal glucose-6-phosphatase enzyme is a two-compartment system consisting of a specific glucose-6-phosphate carrier on the outer half (side) of the membrane of the endoplasmic reticulum and a catalytic phosphorylase component located on the inner half of the membrane.[238] Because disruption of isolated microsomes of patients with GSD-IB with cholate or freeze-thawing results in a marked increase in activity, the general assumption has been that the defect in GSD-IB is a deficiency of the translocase or carrier portion of the enzyme system,[231,232,239,240] although the putative translocase has never been identified in microsomes from normal liver. Zakim and Edmonson, using methods to measure presteady-state kinetics,[242] have shown that the limiting step in the reaction is not glucose release from the enzyme but the release of phosphate. These findings in normal liver microsomes are similar in the liver of a patient with GSD-IB, although the presteady-state kinetics are blunted. These findings question the general concept of a translocase and suggest that patients with GSD-IB may have a configurational abnormality in the enzyme-membrane interaction that can be overcome by alteration of the membrane lipid rather than by an opening of the microsomal vesicle.[242,243]

Molecular Basis of GSD Type IB

GSD-Ib is caused by mutation in the gene encoding microsomal glucose-6-phosphate transporter.[244] The gene has been mapped to chromosome 11q23 and is composed of nine exons spanning a genomic region of 4 Kb. The gene is expressed in the liver, kidney, and leukocytes.[245] More than 15 mutations have been described in the gene, resulting in functional deficiency of glucose-6-phosphate transporter, which explains the neutropenia and neutrophil-monocyte dysfunction characteristic of GSD-Ib.[244] No genotype-phenotype correlations have been described for type Ia or Ib disorders.[246]

Treatment of GSD-IB is identical to that of GSD-IA, with the possible exception that prophylactic antibiotics may lessen the tendency for frequent infection.[234-238,247] Improvement in neutrophil function with treatment has been reported by some investigators.[237,238] However, the authors' experience was that the neutropenia and abnormal migration persisted even after 3 months of management that normalized all parameters of disease in the blood, and even after subsequent portacaval shunting.[247,248] The lack of improvement in neutrophil function in some of the well-treated patients suggests that the defect in GSD-IB is intrinsic to both the liver and leukocytes. Because glucose-6-phosphatase is not known to have any importance for normal neutrophil function, the relationship between the hepatic enzyme defect and leukocyte dysfunction is not known. Improvement of neutropenia and neutrophil dysfunction occurs in response to granulocyte colony-stimulating factor.[249]

GSD-III

GSD-III (amylo-1,6-glucosidase [debrancher] deficiency) accumulates a polysaccharide that has a structure of a limit dextrin produced by degradation of glycogen with phosphorylase and oligo-1,4-1,4 glucanotransferase but no debrancher activity (Reaction [9]).[250]

As depicted, the terminal α-1,4-glucosyl units are hydrolyzed by the combined activity of oligo-1,4-1,4 glucanotransferase and phosphorylase, but the inner

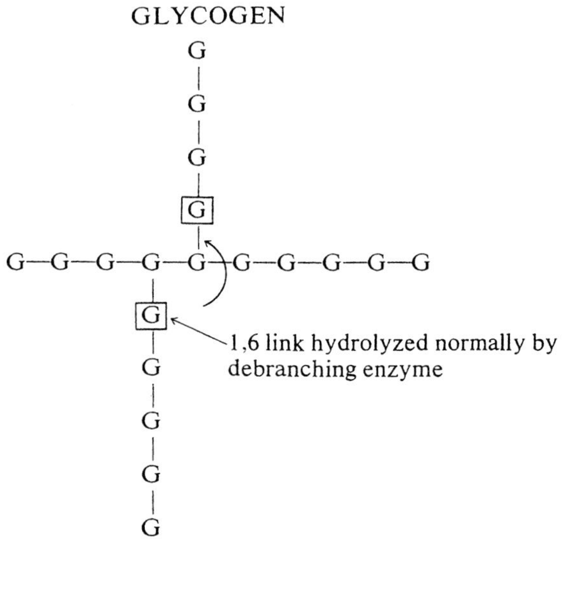

```
                GLYCOGEN                         [9]
                    G
                    |
                    G
                    |
                    G
                    |
                   [G]
                    |
G—G—G—G—G—G—G—G—G—G
            |
           [G] <— 1,6 link hydrolyzed normally by
            |      debranching enzyme
            G
            |
            G
            |
            G
            |
            G
```

branch points of α-1,6 linkages are not hydrolyzed by debranching enzyme. Thus the glycogen molecule is abnormal, with an excessive number of branch points (1,6 linkages). The debrancher enzyme contains two catalytic subunits on a single polypeptide chain. The two activities are oligo-1,4-1,4-glucantransferase and amylo-1,6-glucosidase.

Molecular Basis of Type II GSD

The human gene encoding for glycogen debranching enzyme is 85 Kb is length and consists of 35 exons.[251] The gene has been localized to chromosome 1p21.[252] The cDNA includes a 454 bp of encoding region and 2371 bp of 3'-untranslated region. The predicted protein is ≈172 Kd, consistent with the estimated size of the purified protein.[253] Six mRNA isoforms have been identified.[254] Isoform 1 is expressed in the liver; isoforms 2, 3, and 4 are muscle specific; and isoforms 5 and 6 are minor isoforms. Mutations in the glycogen debranching gene have been described in patients with type IIIa and IIIb. These mutations include missense, nonsense, splicing, and deletion insertion lesions.[255] Specific mutations in exon 3 such as 17delAG and Q6x are seen only in type IIIb.[256]

Depending on the tissue(s) involved and enzymatic characteristics, subtypes of GSD-III have been described (e.g., GSD-IIIA, GSD-IIIB). Type IIIA describes patients who exhibit complete absence of debrancher enzyme activity in hepatic and muscle tissue. Type IIIB describes patients with liver involvement only.

Clinical Characteristics

By physical examination alone, these patients cannot be readily distinguished from patients who have GSD-I. Early in life, hepatomegaly and growth failure may be striking. However, a few patients may develop splenomegaly at 4 to 6 years of age.[257] These patients usually have evidence of hepatic fibrosis but do not necessarily develop cirrhosis and liver failure.

In addition to hepatic involvement, a number of patients with GSD-III have muscle weakness. Rapid walking and climbing result in increased weakness without cramps.[258] Some patients may have a progressive myopathy. Glycogen may also accumulate in the heart, and moderate cardiomegaly with non-specific electrocardiographic changes is sometimes present.[222] However, congestive heart failure and cardiac arrhythmias are not reported. There is no renal enlargement in GSD-III, in contradistinction to GSD-I.

The clinical course in GSD-III is generally much milder than that of GSD-I, in that severe hypoglycemia is not a problem except with prolonged fasting. Some patients have shown relative decreases in liver size around puberty,[250,259] but rare patients have shown evidence of progressive fibrosis and liver failure.[153,260,261] The latter patients may have an additional phosphorylase or phosphorylase kinase deficiency.[153]

In a study of 41 patients with type III GSD 31 patients had involvement of the liver and muscle (type IIIA), 4 patients had liver involvement only (type IIIB), 3 patients had unknown muscle status, and 3 patients had isolated deficiency of transferase activity with retention of glucosidase activity.[262]

Biochemical Characteristics and Laboratory Findings

Lipid levels in plasma are variably elevated and to some extent appear to be related to the individual tendency toward fasting-induced hypoglycemia.[259] That is, the patients who develop lower glucose levels with 6- to 8-hour fasts tend to have higher blood lipid levels. However, none of the patients approach the severe elevations of 4000 to 6000 mg/dl seen with GSD-I. Uric acid levels are generally normal, but rare patients reportedly have slight elevations. Serum transaminase levels are consistently moderately elevated (300 to 600 IU; normal is less than 40 IU),[63] although some patients show elevations of 900 to 2000 IU.

Galactose and fructose are readily converted to glucose by these patients; similarly, protein and amino acid mixtures induce small and prolonged increases in blood glucose levels.[181,259] Both glucagon and epinephrine increase blood glucose when given between 1.5 and 3 hours after a meal but elicit little response after a 14-hour fast ("double glucagon tolerance test").[263] This result is interpreted to indicate available 1,4 glucosyl linkages that can be degraded by phosphorylase shortly after a meal. The glycogen in this case is degraded only until 1,6 linkages are encountered. Access to 1,4 linkages is blocked by terminal 1,6 glycosyl linkages that would be present after a prolonged fast, and these would prevent glucose increase after glucagon administration. Unfortunately, the glucose response to the double glucagon tolerance test is not a consistent finding, and it should not be used as a definitive diagnostic test. Because glucagon also stimulates gluconeogenesis, the inconsistency of the test results is possibly the result of glucose formation via this pathway.

The liver content of glycogen is often markedly increased (to as much as 17.4 g/100 g tissue) in GSD-III.[250] By various techniques, the glycogen is found to have abnormally short outer branch points. Many patients also show some depression of glucose-6-phosphatase activity. Hug has found several patients with combined defects in phosphorylase and phosphorylase kinase. These patients are generally more severely affected and tend to develop cirrhosis.[153]

A series of techniques is available for measuring debrancher activity: (1) liberation of glucose from phosphorylase-treated limit dextrin, (2) incorporation of ^{14}C-glucose into glycogen, (3) 1,4→1,4 transfer of an oligoglucan (glucan transferase activity), and (4) hydrolysis of singly branched oligosaccharides. Using these various techniques, Hers and associates have identified a series of biochemical subtypes of GSD-III. These subtypes are also divided according to types of muscle glycogen.[250,264,265]

Pathology

The liver in GSD-III is very similar in appearance to that in GSD-I, with two notable exceptions: (1) the presence of fibrous septa or frank cirrhosis and (2) the paucity of fat (Figure 48-10). Progression of the fibrosis to cirrhosis

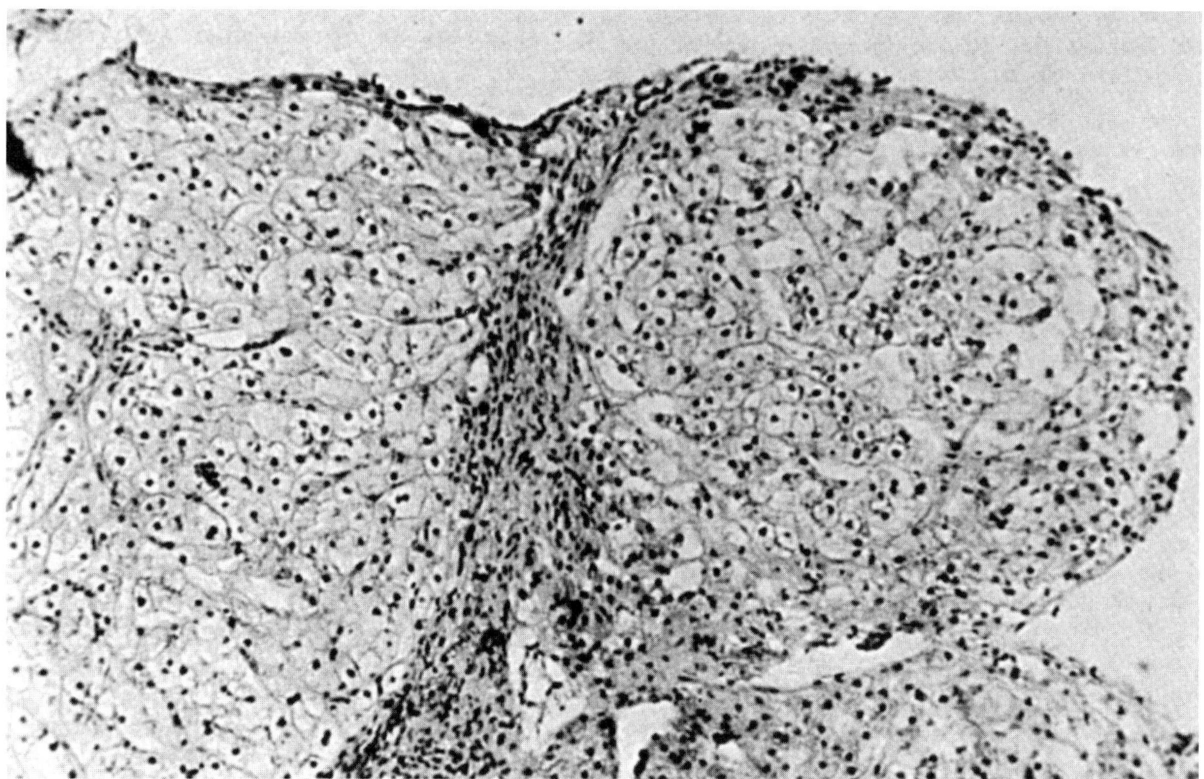

Figure 48-10 Percutaneous liver biopsy specimen from a patient with glycogen storage disease type III, showing increased fibrosis. The hepatocytes do not contain fat deposition (×80).

has been demonstrated. Hug reports that progression to cirrhosis is more likely to occur in patients who have combined enzymatic defects.[153,265] The ultrastructural appearance of the liver is not distinguishable from that in GSD-I, except that in GSD-III lipid vacuoles are small and are less frequent.[265]

If muscle is affected, excessive glycogen is readily demonstrable in ethanol-fixed specimens by the PAS method. Glycogen accumulates between intact myofibrils and in the subsarcolemmal position,[266] locations in which glycogen usually occurs but not in abundance. The diagnosis depends on demonstration of deficient activity of amylo-1,6-glucosidase (debrancher enzyme).

Treatment

Treatment of this disorder remains investigative. It should be restricted to patients who have obvious muscle involvement, progressive fibrotic changes in the liver, or both. An accurate correlation between the type of glycogen accumulation and progression of liver disease, so that a clear-cut prognosis could be assigned to each patient, would be helpful in showing a positive therapeutic response.

Present investigative efforts combine the technique of nocturnal feedings with the known responses to protein and amino acids.[181,259,267] Slonim and co-workers have shown improved growth and increased muscle strength in a patient given a high-protein diet during the day and continuous nocturnal intragastric feedings of a high-protein liquid formula (Sustacal) at night.[268] Borowitz and Greene[269] have found that growth and transaminase and blood glucose levels were more positively influenced by a high-starch diet with a standard (recommended dietary allowance) protein intake. This therapy is therefore virtually identical to that for GSD-I. This outcome is encouraging, but more extensive follow-up evaluation over a longer period of treatment is needed.

Type IV Glycogenosis

Type IV GSD (α-1,4 glucan-6-glycosyl transferase deficiency; GSD-IV), a rare form of glycogenosis, was first described clinically and pathologically in 1952 by Anderson.[270] Illingsworth and Cori showed that the glycogen possessed abnormally long outer and inner chains of glucose units.[271] Ten years later Brown and Brown demonstrated the absence of branching enzyme activity in this disorder.[272] The few descriptions of the disorder (about 20 documented cases) have illustrated its unusual clinical, biochemical, and pathologic aspects.[273-279]

Clinical Characteristics

Infants with GSD-IV are normal at birth and for some months thereafter. The onset of symptoms during the first year of life is insidious. Symptoms may manifest as early as 3 months or as late as 15 months of age. The disorder is usually diagnosed because of hepatosplenomegaly, abdominal distention, signs and symptoms referable to hepatic dysfunction, non-specific gastrointestinal symptoms, and failure to thrive. Muscle hypotonia and wasting may be present. Superficial veins over the distended abdomen are prominent as the disease progresses. Patients who live beyond infancy develop hepatic cirrhosis with accompanying portal hypertension, ascites, and esophageal varices. The terminal course is usually the result of chronic hepatic failure and jaundice with bleeding esophageal varices, although a few patients develop cardiac failure, apparently from myofibrillar damage caused by polysaccharide deposits within myocardial cells. Intercurrent infection is a common terminal complication. The duration of survival after diagnosis is usually 2 to 37 months, although an occasional patient may survive 3 to 4 years.

Mental development is normal in some instances, although it is now clear that GSD-IV may involve the neuromuscular axis at all levels—skeletal muscle, peripheral nervous system, and central nervous system. The level and extent of the neuromuscular lesions appear to vary from patient to patient, and at least one patient showed signs of involvement of all levels simultaneously.[279]

A 59-year-old man with GSD-IV had deficient branching enzyme in skeletal muscle with normal muscle glycogen and low normal enzyme activity in leukocytes.[280] The man had a 30-year history of progressive, asymmetric limb-girdle weakness and a vacuolar myopathy. The vacuoles contained glycogen, which was partially resistant to diastase. Ultrastructural changes resembled the amylopectin polysaccharide deposits encountered in childhood GSD-IV. Three other adult patients have been reported with an amylopectin-like storage myopathy; two of these later developed involvement of the heart and brain, but none showed hepatic involvement.[281-283]

Approximately 50 percent of infants with GSD-IV have signs suggestive of involvement of the neuromuscular system and abnormal deposits of polysaccharide in skeletal muscle.[284-287] The pathologic changes can occur in the absence of clinical changes.[287] Because the majority of these patients have not had comparative measurements of branching enzyme activity in fibroblasts, liver, muscle, and leukocytes, it is not possible to correlate apparent clinical and pathologic findings with enzymatic changes. It has been suggested that two branching enzymes may be acting at different sites[288,289] and that the clinical expression of this disease depends on deficiency of organ-specific brancher isoenzymes.

The author has had experience in managing two unusual patients with deficient branching enzyme measured in both the liver and skin fibroblasts (by Dr. Barbara Brown, St. Louis, Missouri). The first patient, a male, showed the usual progression to cirrhosis and liver failure by 18 months of age.[290] At age 2 years, he underwent liver transplantation and standard treatment with immunosuppressants. He is now 6 years post-transplant with normal liver function and shows no evidence of nerve, muscle, or cardiac abnormalities. Thus despite the generalized nature of the defect, transplantation of a normal liver has not been associated with obvious progression in other organs. The second patient, a 6-year-old boy, was noted at 3 years of age to have hepatomegaly and chronically elevated serum aminotransferases.[291] Open liver biopsy showed moderate, generalized micronodular fibrosis and typical PAS-positive, diastase-resistant deposits in about 25 percent of the hepatocytes. Electron microscopy showed accumulation of Drochman fibrils characteristic of GSD-IV, but these fibrils were not present in all cells. During the succeeding 3 years, the boy showed normal growth and development with spontaneous normalization of liver tests. Liver biopsy at the age of 6 years showed minimal periportal fibrosis with no PAS-positive, diastase-resistant deposits present in any hepatocytes and normal-appearing glycogen by electron microscopic analysis. Assays of hepatocytes and skin fibroblasts showed no detectable branching enzyme activity. These two patients plus previous reports of GSD-IV indicate that branching enzyme deficiency may present in various ways, with the classic infantile variety primarily affecting the liver. As more patients have the opportunity for transplantation, it is anticipated that a more accurate classification system can be found for the various subgroups of this unusual disorder.

Laboratory Findings

Blood electrolytes are usually within normal limits except in patients with renal tubular defects, who have low bicarbonate concentrations. Serum transaminase and alkaline phosphatase levels are usually elevated to three to six times normal. Except with malnutrition, late in the disease, serum cholesterol is often slightly elevated. Until liver failure develops, serum albumin, globulin, bilirubin, and ammonia are normal. All liver test results become abnormal as liver failure becomes severe. Glucagon and epinephrine tolerance tests cause a positive glucose response, with levels of 15 to 23 mg/dl, with the maximum response occurring about 30 minutes after hormone injection and 2 hours after a meal.[274] Both hormones may allow detection of urinary ketone bodies. Hypoglycemia is not a characteristic feature of the illness until terminal liver failure occurs. Chronic and severe acidosis may occur secondary to a renal tubular defect in hydrogen ion excretion.[275-277] Oral glucose and fructose tolerance tests show no abnormality, and serum lactate and pyruvate levels are normal.[274]

Biochemical Characteristics

The stored polysaccharide in GSD-IV is a glucose polymer whose properties differ from those of normal mammalian glycogen. The normal level of liver glycogen in a child in the fed state is roughly 6 percent of the hepatic wet weight.[292,293] Normal glycogen has the following characteristics: (1) at least 36 percent of the glucose units are susceptible to phosphorylase-catalyzed degradation; (2) chain lengths are 8 to 12 glycosyl units; (3) branch points (1,6 linkages) make up 8 percent of the glycogen; and (4) the $KI:I_2$ absorption band is at 460 nm.[21]

Patients with GSD-IV usually have hepatic glycogen levels slightly lower than normal (3.5 to 5 percent), although one patient had a level of 10.7 percent. Hepatic glycogen in these patients is unusually susceptible to phosphorylase-induced hydrolysis (more than 40 percent phosphorylase degradation), suggesting that it has longer outer chain lengths and fewer branch points (about 6 percent) than does normal glycogen. The polysaccharide is highly chromogenic, with a maximal $KI:I_2$ absorption band at about 525 nm.[294] About half of the extracted polysaccharide may be insoluble and poorly characterized. Muscle glycogen appears normal; leukocytic glycogen is abnormal, as is brancher enzyme activity in these cells.

Although the deficiency of branching enzyme explains the formation of an amylopectin-like polysaccharide, it does not account for the presence of an appreciable proportion of branch points in the abnormal glycogen. Brown and Brown suggest that normal liver contains two enzymes with branching activities of different specificities, only one of which is measured by the methods used.[272] Another possibility is that the mutant gene in this disorder has produced a protein with substantially modified enzymatic specificity such that branching occurs mainly with long outer chains.[273]

The liver glycosyl deposits and myocardial deposits are believed to be biochemically the same, because they appear similar histochemically and are both resistant to digestion by α-amylase. This resistance to digestion by amylase is difficult to explain, because there is no other evidence for the existence of an α-amylase-resistant glycogen.

Pathology

Examination of the liver shows a uniform micronodular cirrhosis with broad bands of fibrous tissue extending around and into the lobules. Portal veins, lymphatic channels, and hepatic arteries are normal with slight portal biliary duct proliferation. Liver cell plates are distorted, and as the disease progresses, the lobules develop prominent sinusoidal channels with fibrous walls coursing between thick liver plates.

Pale amphophilic or basophilic deposits occur in liver cells, cardiac and skeletal muscle, and brain.[273,276,279] The deposits in cardiac muscle resemble cardiac colloid, and those in brain resemble Lafora's bodies.[218,221]

Liver cell nuclei are frequently eccentric in position. They appear (with hematoxylin and eosin stain) to be displaced by pale, slightly eosinophilic or colorless inclusions deposited in the cytoplasm. This is the most striking and characteristic finding and is generally limited to the periphery of the lobule. The inclusions vary from hyaline to reticulate and are usually sharply demarcated from normal cytoplasm. Clear halos may surround the contents of the inclusions. In the late stages of the disease nodular accumulations of a slightly different hyaline, fibrillar material are scattered throughout the hepatic lobules. This material is birefringent, appearing in polarized light as sheaths of crystals that cannot be easily distinguished from deposits that typify α_1-antitrypsin deficiency, except perhaps on the basis of their greater frequency and larger size in GSD-IV. In both conditions, the peripheral lobular deposits are PAS-positive and diastase-resistant.[292]

Examination of myocardial tissue shows hypertrophied muscle fibers with large rectangular nuclei. Within the fibers, colorless discrete deposits similar to those in the liver are found. These deposits are uniformly distributed, with only a slight predilection for subendocardial regions. The epicardium and vessels are normal, without significant myocardial fibrosis, endocardial sclerosis, necrosis, or calcification.

PAS-positive material may be present within foamy macrophages of the spleen and lymph nodes, smooth muscle of the gastrointestinal tract and large blood vessels, and skeletal muscle around the larynx, diaphragm, tongue, and esophagus. Peripheral skeletal muscle is usually free of any abnormality except for scant amounts of abnormal polysaccharide.

Central nervous system abnormalities have been found in only 6 of 20 reported cases. In these instances discrete, spherical PAS-positive globules were widely scattered throughout the neuraxis. They were usually most prominent in white matter and in subependymal and subapical regions but were also numerous in gray matter. Peripheral nerves also contain PAS-positive globules in the endoneurium. The PAS-positive deposits in neuronal tissue are also resistant to amylase digestion.[279]

Electron microscopic studies show a decrease in cytoplasmic organelles. The organelles are found in tongues of cytoplasm extending between large, irregular aggregates of low electron density. The contents of these aggregates are variable and may include two or three components: glycogen rosettes or the alpha particles of Drochman fibrils and granular material. Some areas, which contain primarily glycogen, frequently fail to stain well despite the use of lead citrate. The fibrils are straight or curved and are about 65-nm wide.[278]

Myocardial fibers are distended by zones of material with low electron density, similar to those seen in the liver. Unlike liver cells, cardiac cells rarely contain material thought to be glycogen. Electron microscopic examination of skeletal muscle reveals granulofibrillar deposits similar to those in the viscera but less conspicuous; beta glycogen is more prominent in these deposits. Ultrastructural studies of the central nervous system tissue show the presence of large numbers of globules with a granulofibrillar appearance and of medium electron density. In some deposits the fibrils are oriented radially; in others they assume a whorled appearance. The material is mostly restricted to astrocytic processes. It is not found within neuronal perikaryons or processes.[274,279]

Histochemical stains of the liver deposits indicate that the material is an abnormal glycogen with fewer branch points than usual. The deposits also have properties unusual for a glucose polymer: a positive colloidal iron stain and resistance to α-amylase digestion of conventional duration. Only pectinase was able to reduce the PAS and colloidal iron reactions significantly.

Genetics

Because a branching enzyme deficiency has been reported to occur in siblings, the condition is inherited, presumably as a recessive trait.[293] Although an autosomal inheritance is most likely, the preponderance of males reported suggests that X-linked inheritance cannot be ruled out. Most of the other glycogenoses are autosomal recessive. Examination of leukocytes from parents could not detect the heterozygotic state. Prenatal diagnosis is possible by enzymatic assay of fibroblasts from amniotic fluid cultures.

Treatment

Three types of treatment, without decided improvement, were used for one patient.[294] First, a high-protein, low-carbohydrate diet with corn oil added to the milk fat caused no change in weight gain or in the progression of cirrhosis. Second, with progression of the disease, treatment with purified α-glucosidase from *Aspergillus niger* was given for 6 days. This treatment resulted in a striking decrease in hepatic glycogen content—from a 10 percent to a 20 percent decrease. Although no unfavorable reaction occurred, liver size did not decrease. Glycogen content was maintained at 3 percent by a third treatment—intramuscular injection of zinc-glucagon, 1 mg three times a day for 24 days. Any positive effect of these treatments remains doubtful. On the other hand, the poor clinical results after the treatments might have been related to the advanced state of cirrhosis before their initiation.

Other than supportive nutritional management[290] for terminal cirrhosis, no specific treatment appears to be beneficial. The finding that the *Aspergillus* extract caused a striking decrease in hepatic glycogen suggests that if the accumulation of abnormal glycogen is in some way hepatotoxic, this form of treatment might be studied in patients before the onset of severe cirrhosis.

A recent study by Starzl's group suggests that liver transplantation in GSD-IV results in resorption of extrahepatic deposits of amylopectin, possibly by systemic microchimerism (i.e., cells of the host organs became mixed with cells with the donor genomes that had migrated from the allograft into the recipient tissues and presumably serve as enzyme carriers).[295]

INBORN ERRORS OF AMINO ACID METABOLISM

Hereditary tyrosinemia is the only inborn error of amino acid metabolism that results in permanent liver injury. This section summarizes the normal metabolic pathway of tyrosine, and then discusses the disorders associated with abnormal tyrosine metabolism.

Tyrosine Metabolism

The principal hepatic pathway for degradation of tyrosine is shown in Figure 48-11. These reactions normally catabolize 99 percent of tyrosine. The steady-state plasma concentration of tyrosine is determined by two primary factors: (1) gastrointestinal uptake, which is regulated by an active transport system, and (2) the rate of production of tyrosine from phenylalanine and its subsequent catabolism to carbon dioxide and water. Most of the ingested phenylalanine is catabolized via tyrosine. The rate-limiting reaction in the tyrosine oxidation pathway is that catabolized by tyrosine aminotransferase (Figure 48-11, Reaction [1]).[296,297] Pyridoxal phosphate is the co-enzyme. Tyrosine aminotransferase is found mainly in the cytosol of the liver. Its activity shows a circadian rhythm. Also, the activity of tyrosine aminotransferase is induced by various compounds, including corticosteroids.[298-300]

p-Hydroxyphenylpyruvic hydroxylase is the second enzyme involved in tyrosine catabolism. This enzyme is found in the cytosol of the human liver and kidney.[301,302] It catalyzes the conversion of p-hydroxyphenylpyruvic acid to homogentisic acid (see Figure 48-11, Reaction [2]) and converts phenylpyruvic acid to p-hydroxyphenylacetic acid.[303] The enzyme requires a reducing agent. Ascorbic acid can serve both in vivo and in vitro in this capacity.[304] p-Hydroxyphenylpyruvic acid is not normally found in the urine. When its normal catabolism to homogentisic acid is blocked, the levels of both the α-keto acid and tyrosine in the plasma may be increased. At the same time, p-hydroxyphenyl lactic acid is formed through the action of lactic dehydrogenase. p-Hydroxyphenylacetic acid also can be formed from decarboxylation of p-hydroxyphenylpyruvic acid. Homogentisic acid oxidase catalyzes the conversion of homogentisic acid to maleylacetoacetic acid. This reaction also requires vitamin C for maximum activity in vivo. Fumaryl acetoacetase acts on maleylacetoacetic acid to yield fumaric acid and acetoacetic acid.

Disorders of Tyrosine Metabolism

Several conditions associated with abnormalities in tyrosine metabolism have been described; however, only hereditary tyrosinemia (hepatorenal type) is associated with permanent injury to the liver. Other abnormalities in tyrosine metabolism, summarized in Table 48-3, are discussed briefly.

Tyrosinosis

The first known case of abnormal excretion of a tyrosine metabolite was described by Medes and colleagues in 1927.[305] The patient, a 49-year-old Russian Jew who had myasthenia gravis, was found to have an unusual reducing substance in the urine. The reducing compound was later isolated and identified as p-hydroxyphenylpyruvic acid, the α-keto acid of tyrosine. The condition was named tyrosinosis by Medes.[306] When the patient was fasting, the urine contained 1.6 g p-hydroxyphenylpyruvic acid in a 24-hour period. This quantity was considered to represent endogenous production from the catabolism of endogenous protein. When the patient was fed a regular diet, the amount of urinary p-hydroxyphenylpyruvic acid doubled, and tyrosine also could be isolated from his urine. One of the interesting findings was that feeding large amounts of tyrosine also led to the excretion of 3,4-dihydroxyphenylalanine (dopa), a product of the minor pathway of tyrosine metabolism. Medes postulated a defect in the conversion of p-hydroxyphenylpyruvic acid to homogentisic acid. No other case of tyrosinosis has been described.

Transitory Tyrosinemia of the Newborn

This condition affects approximately 30 percent of premature infants and as many as 10 percent of full-term infants.[307-309] It is assumed that the hepatic enzymes

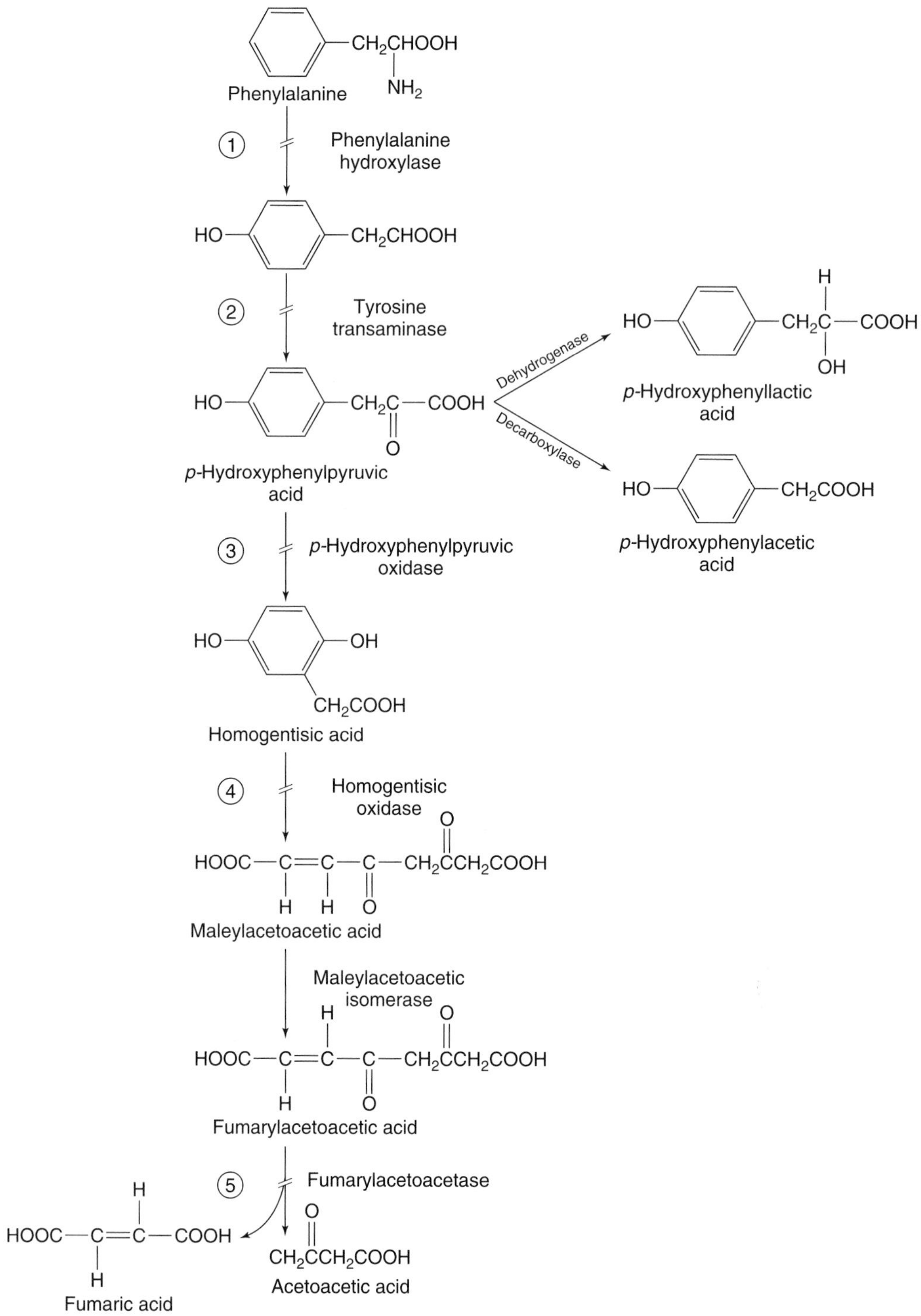

Phenylalanine
① Phenylalanine hydroxylase
② Tyrosine transaminase
p-Hydroxyphenylpyruvic acid
Dehydrogenase
p-Hydroxyphenyllactic acid
Decarboxylase
p-Hydroxyphenylacetic acid
③ p-Hydroxyphenylpyruvic oxidase
Homogentisic acid
④ Homogentisic oxidase
Maleylacetoacetic acid
Maleylacetoacetic isomerase
Fumarylacetoacetic acid
⑤ Fumarylacetoacetase
Fumaric acid
Acetoacetic acid

Figure 48-11 Metabolic pathway of phenylalanine and tyrosine. *//,* Block in the metabolic pathway; *1,* block in phenylketonuria; *2,* block in persistent hypertyrosinemia; *3,* block in Medes's tyrosinemia patient; *4,* block in alkaptonuria; *5,* block in hereditary tyrosinemia.

catalyzing the early steps of tyrosine metabolism are not well developed in these infants.[310,311] Administration of vitamin C, which is known to protect p-hydroxyphenylpyruvic oxidase from unphysiologic levels of its own substrate, usually corrects the transitory tyrosinemia.[312] The transitory tyrosinemia in infants usually disappears within a few weeks but occasionally persists for several months. A reduction in protein intake to 1.5 to 2 g/kg/day with administration of vitamin C should correct the condition. Although it is generally assumed that transitory tyrosinemia is harmless, this may not be true, because persistent hypertyrosinemia (discussed in the following section) is regularly associated with mental retardation. There is a definite need for prospective studies of infants, specifically, premature infants with transitory hypertyrosinemia.

TABLE 48-3
Conditions Associated with Hypertyrosinemia

	Enzyme deficiency	Clinical features
Transitory tyrosinemia of the newborn	p-Hydroxyphenylpyruvic acid oxidase	None
Tyrosinosis (Medes's patient)	p-Hydroxyphenylpyruvic acid oxidase	Mental retardation Skin and eye lesions
Persistent tyrosinemia	Cytosol tyrosine transaminase in one case	No hepatic or renal disease
Hereditary tyrosinemia (hepatorenal type)	Fumaryl acetoacetase	Cirrhosis, hepatomas Renal tubular defects
Hypertyrosinemia secondary to liver disease	Generalized partial defects of tyrosine transaminase, p-hydroxyphenylpyruvic acid oxidase, and homogentisic acid oxidase	

Persistent Hypertyrosinemia (Tyrosinemia II, Richner-Hanhart Syndrome)

Several patients with persistent tyrosinemia without associated hepatic or renal disease have been described.[313-318] The patients were reported to have cataracts, corneal ulcers, keratotic skin lesions, and neuropsychiatric abnormalities. Enzymatic studies were carried out in four patients. A total deficiency of cytosolic tyrosine transaminase was found in two[315]; however, the activity was only reduced in two others.[319] The keratotic lesions abated in response to low-phenylalanine, low-tyrosine diets in two cases.[317,320] Large doses of vitamin C had no effect on the tyrosinemia in those patients.

Hypertyrosinemia Secondary to Liver Disease

Patients with hepatic cirrhosis have a reduced capacity to metabolize tyrosine and other amino acids.[321] Cirrhotic patients have significantly increased fasting levels of plasma tyrosine and basal levels of p-hydroxyphenylpyruvic acid. They have impaired tolerance to oral loading doses of tyrosine, p-hydroxyphenylpyruvic acid, and homogentisic acid.[322] These findings suggest generalized partial defects in tyrosine transaminase, p-hydroxyphenylpyruvic acid oxidase, and homogentisic acid oxidase enzymes in patients with cirrhosis. Levels of tyrosine are also slightly elevated in other diseases, including cystic fibrosis,[323] hypoxia with respiratory failure,[324] and rheumatoid arthritis.[325]

Hereditary Tyrosinemia (Hepatorenal Tyrosinemia)

In 1965 Baber reported the case of a 9-month-old infant with failure to thrive, abdominal distention, and diarrhea. The child was found to have cirrhosis of the liver, a renal tubular defect with gross aminoaciduria of a distinct type, and vitamin D-resistant rickets.[326]

From 1957 to 1959 Sakai and co-workers reported the case of another patient with a similar clinical picture and marked p-hydroxyphenyl lactic aciduria. They drew attention to the abnormal metabolism of tyrosine in this patient and named the condition atypical tyrosinosis.[327-329] Since then many cases have been reported from Norway,[330] Canada,[331,332] Sweden,[333] and the United States.[334,335] Although many names have been given to the disorder in these cases, hereditary tyrosinemia is generally accepted.

Clinical Features

Hereditary tyrosinemia may be either acute or chronic.[331,336] Symptoms appear in the first month with acute disease, and the patient usually dies with hepatic failure within the first 3 to 9 months.[331] In the chronic form of the disease the symptoms appear later. The life spans of these patients are longer than those of patients who have the acute form.[331-336] Both forms can occur within the same family. The main symptoms are failure to thrive, vomiting, diarrhea, anorexia, hepatosplenomegaly, ascites, edema, jaundice, bruising, and rickets.[330] Some patients have slight mental deficiencies.

In the chronic form of the disease hepatoma may develop. A review of the literature by Weinberg and colleagues in 1976 disclosed 16 cases of hepatoma in 43 patients surviving beyond 2 years of age. This incidence is higher than that in adults with macronodular cirrhosis.[337]

Laboratory Findings

Biochemical evidence of hepatocellular damage is found in elevated serum levels of AST and ALT. Total and direct bilirubin were elevated in 19 of 20 patients so tested.[330] However, total serum bilirubin levels were usually less than 10 mg/dl until the appearance of signs of liver failure, at which time they became markedly elevated. Synthetic function of the liver is also disturbed, as evidenced by low levels of serum albumin and vitamin K-dependent clotting factors. Hematologic studies show mild anemia, elevated reticulocyte counts, and normal serum iron levels. Bone marrow aspirates show erythroid hyperplasia. These findings suggest a hemolytic anemia, which may be related to an intracorpuscular defect secondary to abnormal accumulation of tyrosine metabolites.[338] In the chronic form of the disease anemia, leukopenia, and thrombocytopenia are present secondary to hypersplenism.

A tendency to develop hypoglycemia has been found in association with hereditary tyrosinemia.[338,339] Marked hyperplasia of the islets of Langerhans is a rather constant finding, but insulin levels are reported to be normal. The responses to epinephrine and glucagon of two patients thus examined showed flat curves.[338] These findings suggest a disturbance in the release of glucose from glycogen; however, hepatic glycogen content and structure and glycogenolytic enzymes are normal. The glycolytic enzymes are also normal.

The laboratory findings related to the renal tubular defects include hyperphosphaturia, glucosuria, proteinuria, and gross aminoaciduria. Biochemical evidence of rickets secondary to hypophosphatemia is seen in almost all cases.[331] The urinary excretion of amino acids follows a distinctive pattern.[340] The aminoaciduria is more pronounced in the acute disease. The pattern of urinary excretion of tyrosine and phenolic acids (p-hydroxyphenyl lactic, p-hydroxyphenylpyruvic, and p-hydroxyphenylacetic acids) by tyrosinemic patients is similar to that described for premature infants with transitory tyrosinemia.[341]

Chromatography of the serum amino acids reveals slight hypertyrosinemia and, frequently, hypermethioninemia. Other amino acids, including phenylalanine, occasionally are slightly elevated. Some of these results must be interpreted with caution because liver damage may cause modest elevations of these amino acids.

In six patients with hereditary tyrosinemia urinary δ-aminolevulinic acid levels were elevated to as much as 100-fold above control values. In two of these cases attacks of abdominal pain and paresis of a peripheral type, resembling acute intermittent porphyria, prompted investigation for porphyrins. The amounts of porphobilinogen and porphyrins excreted were normal or slightly elevated, but δ-aminolevulinic acid levels were markedly elevated.[342] Similar abnormal pyrrole metabolism was found by Kang and Gerald in a patient with hereditary tyrosinemia. δ-Aminolevulinic acid synthetase activity in liver tissue was increased.[335] It was believed that the abnormality of pyrrole metabolism is a secondary process related to induction of δ-aminolevulinic acid synthetase activity by one of the accumulated metabolites of tyrosine. However, Lindblad and colleagues[343] and Melancon and associates[344] have shown that accumulation of succinyl acetoacetate inhibits porphobilinogen synthetase (δ-aminolevulinic acid dehydratase), leading to increased excretion of δ-aminolevulinic acid. This observation has been confirmed by Berger and co-workers.[345]

Biochemical Features

The clinical and biochemical improvements in the renal tubular condition and synthesis of proteins in the liver in response to introduction of a diet low in phenylalanine and tyrosine suggest that the aromatic amino acid derivatives exert a toxic effect on the kidneys and liver. The failure to correct all the liver disease has been attributed to extensive, only partly reversible, pathologic changes.

Patients with hereditary tyrosinemia are reported to lack or to have markedly reduced activity of p-hydroxyphenylpyruvic acid oxidase in liver and kidneys.[346,347] There is reason to question whether deficiency of this enzyme can account for the clinical manifestations in patients with hereditary tyrosinemia. Thus activity of p-hydroxyphenylpyruvic acid oxidase is reduced in 30 percent of premature infants, 10 percent of full-term infants, and patients with persistent hypertyrosinemia (but these patients have no derangement of function of the liver or kidneys). Perry and colleagues induced experimental hypertyrosinemia in vitamin C–deficient newborn guinea pigs fed diets containing large amounts of tyrosine. There was no evidence of a liver or kidney disturbance.[348] Gaull and associates therefore proposed that deficiency of p-hydroxyphenylpyruvic acid oxidase is not the primary defect in patients with hereditary tyrosinemia. These researchers believe that there are deficiencies in methionine-activating enzyme and cystathionine synthetase in affected patients and that the signs and symptoms of the disease reflect these deficiencies.[349,350]

Feeding large amounts of methionine to guinea pigs in fact produced a syndrome similar to that in infants with hereditary tyrosinemia. The animals showed hypertyrosinemia, hypermethioninemia, generalized aminoaciduria, hypoglycemia, and pancreatic islet cell degeneration.[348] Hence some metabolite of methionine may be the toxic factor responsible for the pathologic and biochemical changes in hereditary tyrosinemia. Some findings, however, do not support this idea: (1) hypertyrosinemia usually precedes hypermethioninemia in infants with hereditary tyrosinemia, (2) transient neonatal hypermethioninemia is an apparently benign condition unassociated with tyrosinemia, and (3) weanling rats fed high-methionine diets have increases of methionine, taurine, and alanine, but not tyrosine, in the serum.[351]

An apparently identical clinical and biochemical picture resembling hereditary tyrosinemia has occasionally been found in patients with hereditary fructosemia[352-354] but not in galactosemia, although severe liver damage is noted in both conditions. Plasma levels of tyrosine and methionine and the excretion of phenolic acid decreased markedly with the exclusion of fructose from the diets of patients with hereditary fructosemia.[353]

Lindblad and associates[343] reported increased excretion of succinyl acetone and succinyl acetoacetate in the urine of patients with hereditary tyrosinemia. These compounds presumably originate from maleylacetoacetate or fumarylacetoacetate or both. Their accumulation indicates a block in metabolism of tyrosine at the fumarylacetoacetase reaction (see Figure 48-11). These observations have been confirmed by Melancon and colleagues.[344] Since then several groups have confirmed the defect in fumarylacetoacetase in liver tissues from patients with hereditary tyrosinemia.[355-359] Additionally, the activity of fumarylacetoacetase was found to be markedly decreased in patients with the acute form of hereditary tyrosinemia. It is reasonable to conclude that severe liver and kidney damage in hereditary tyrosinemia is secondary to accumulation of succinyl acetone and succinyl acetoacetate, which can bind to the sulfahydryl (SH) group of proteins, thereby destroying their function. The liver and kidneys would be the organs affected principally by these metabolites, because these tissues are the only ones with p-hydroxyphenylpyruvate hydroxylase activity—that is, metabolism of tyrosine to potentially toxic metabolites depends on the presence of this enzyme. Of interest in this regard are the findings of Lindblad, which indicate that patients with the more benign form of hereditary tyrosinemia have lower levels of activity of p-hydroxyphenylpyruvate hydroxylase in their livers than do patients who have more serious forms of the illness. The cause of the low activity of p-hydroxyphenylpyruvic hydroxylase in hereditary tyrosinemia remains to be determined. The possibility of a defect in a regulatory gene common to p-hydroxyphenylpyruvic hydroxylase and fumarylacetoacetase can be considered. Continued search for other possible biochemical defects that may be responsible for all the clinical and biochemical features is needed.

Molecular Basis of Hereditary Tyrosinemia

The gene responsible for hereditary tyrosinemia fumaryl acetoacetate hydrolyase (FAH) has been cloned and mapped to chromosome 15q23-25. The cDNA encodes for a 419-amino acid cytosolic homodimer protein, which is present in the liver, kidney, lymphocytes, erythrocytes, fibroblast, and chorionic villi.[360] Several mutations in the fumaryl acetoacetate hydrolyase have been described. The IVS12+4G-A → an allele accounts for more than 94 percent of mutant FAH allele in the Saguenay-Lac St-Jean area of Quebec.[361,362] Certain populations have specific mutations including W262X in Finns[363,364] and Q64H in Pakistanis.[365]

Pathology

The major pathologic findings are in the liver and kidneys.[366-368] Macroscopically, the liver is enlarged, firm, and nodular. The kidneys are enlarged, with poor architectural demarcations. Microscopically, the architecture of the liver is distorted by extensive fibrosis, with infiltration by lymphocytes and plasma cells in the portal areas. The liver cell cords have a pseudoglandular appearance. The hepatocytes show fatty metamorphosis, and some may undergo acidophilic degeneration and, occasionally, giant cell transformation. Glycogen is either lacking or markedly decreased. Pancreatic islet cell hyperplasia has been found in the majority of cases.[366-368]

Genetics

Tyrosinemia has been found with increased frequency in French Canadians. Inheritance is autosomal recessive. The carrier rate in northeastern Quebec is 1:14, for an estimated frequency of 14.6 cases per 10,000 population.[369] An automated fluorometric test for hypertyrosinemia has been described.[370] In the province of Quebec a neonatal screening program has been developed. The association of increased serum levels of alphafetoprotein with hypertyrosinemia distinguishes patients with hereditary tyrosinemia from patients with transient hypertyrosinemia of the newborn.[371] Prenatal diagnosis has been accomplished by measurement of fumarylacetoacetase in cultured amniotic fluid cells.[372]

Treatment

A diet low in phenylalanine and tyrosine has been used in management of the acute and chronic forms of the disease by several groups of investigators.[330,373-376] This diet decreases serum tyrosine. It increases serum phosphorus secondary to enhanced renal tubular reabsorption of phosphorus.[330] Similar beneficial effects on renal function are reflected by reductions of glycosuria, hyperaminoaciduria, and proteinuria. The effect of diet on hepatic dysfunction is uncertain. In only one acute case of tyrosinemia were reductions of fibrosis and infiltration of the liver by inflammatory cells found.[377] Other patients did not respond to the diet in this manner.[332,375,378] The available evidence suggests that a diet low in phenylalanine and tyrosine should be given to patients with the acute and chronic forms of the disease. Signs of deficiency of phenylalanine and tyrosine should be monitored in patients receiving this diet. The amounts of phenylalanine and tyrosine used in such diets are approximately 25 mg/kg/day of each; however, there is some variation in the optimal minimum requirements for individual patients.

In one case dietary treatment returned the elevated levels of phenylalanine and tyrosine to normal in the serum of a patient with hereditary tyrosinemia. However, the patient continued to have hypermethioninemia and clinical evidence of liver disease. Strict control of his dietary intake of methionine, phenylalanine, and tyrosine returned all serum amino acid levels to normal and eliminated the hepatic abnormalities.[379] Large doses of vitamin D (10,000 to 15,000 U/day), together with dietary restrictions of phenylalanine and tyrosine, are necessary to correct the rickets of hereditary tyrosinemia.

Other recent treatment modalities pioneered by the Quebec investigators include utilization of NTBC [2-(2-nitro-4-trifluoro-methylbenzoyl)-1,3-cyclohexanedione. NTBC appears to block the conversion of 4-hydroxyphenylpyruvate to homogentisate and to maleylaceto-acetate. The treatment protocol includes maintenance of plasma tyrosine level below 400 μM by dietary phenylalanine and tyrosine restriction. NTBC is given at a starting dose of 1 mg/kg/day in two divided doses and adjusted to achieve plasma NTBC of greater than 50 μM and no detectable urinary and blood succinylacetone. In asymptomatic patients diagnosed by neonatal screening, none developed hepatic nodules and no acute liver crises have been seen. However, in patients who present with liver disease, progression to cirrhosis was noted requiring transplantation.[380] The major complications of NTBC treatment have been corneal crystals, photophobia, and ocular inflammation. Hepatocellular carcinoma has developed in FAH-deficient mice despite NTBC treatment.[381]

Liver transplantation has been carried out in four patients with chronic hereditary tyrosinemia and hepatoma. All were reported to be alive and well 3 months to 3 years after transplantation. Therefore this modality of therapy needs to be considered in patients who develop hepatoma as a complication from their chronic hereditary tyrosinemia.[382] A follow-up of 10 patients who underwent liver transplantation for tyrosinemia suggests the feasibility of this therapy.[383] The indications for liver transplantation were hepatoma in three, acute liver failure in two, and progressive chronic liver disease in five. One patient died during surgery. Of the remaining nine, seven patients are alive 6 months to 6.5 years after transplantation. Two died of complications.

Prognosis

Patients who have acute hereditary tyrosinemia die in the first few months of life. Unfortunately, this is the most common form of the disease.[331,336] In patients with the chronic form the disease progresses slowly, with the eventual development of cirrhosis. Hepatoma has been reported to occur in 37 percent of patients with chronic hereditary tyrosinemia.[337]

INBORN ERRORS OF LIPID METABOLISM

Intracellular Metabolism of Cholesterol

Metabolism of cholesterol and cholesterol esters has been studied primarily in cultured human fibroblasts (see Chap. 5). Study of patients with inborn errors of lipid metabolism has provided information that tends to support most of the general hypotheses developed from growing fibroblasts in cultures. A brief discussion of the origin, transport, and degradation of free cholesterol and cholesterol esters is included to provide a basis for understanding the metabolic consequences of a deficiency of lysosomal acid lipase.

Peripheral cells can synthesize free cholesterol and cholesterol esters, but they derive most cholesterol from exogenous sterols circulating in the serum as low-density lipoproteins (LDLs). Intracellular levels of cholesterol are the primary regulators of the rate of synthesis of cholesterol and of uptake from LDLs. The metabolism of cholesterol esters is illustrated schematically in Figure 48-12. The origin of lipoproteins enriched in cholesterol and cholesterol esters, which are the main sources of cholesterol for tissues, is discussed in Chapter 5.

As discussed in Chapter 5, the initial event in the intracellular metabolism of LDLs (i.e., particles enriched in cholesterol esters) is binding to receptors on the cell surface. LDL receptors bind only those human plasma lipoproteins that contain apolipoproteins B and E (e.g., LDL and very low-density lipoprotein). After LDL is bound to its specific receptor site, the lipoprotein remains metabolically inactive until the endosomes fuse with lysosomes (see Chap. 5). At this point, the protein component is hydrolyzed by lysosomal enzymes to products that consist mostly of free amino acids and small peptides (molecular mass less than 1000). The cholesterol ester component of LDL is hydrolyzed by a lysosomal acid lipase. The liberated cholesterol is then available for metabolic use by the cell.[384] A consequence of the uptake and storage of LDL cholesterol is that the synthesis of cholesterol in non-hepatic tissues is maintained at a low level.

Patients with isolated deficiencies of acid hydrolase activity (Wolman's disease) should develop predictable changes in tissue lipids. For example, cholesterol ester as cholesterol linoleate should accumulate in lysosomes of affected individuals. This has been shown to occur.[314,315] Because of a reduced rate of generation of free cholesterol within cells, there also should be decreased suppression of the activity of 3-hydroxy-3-methylglutaryl CoA reductase and reduced activation of endogenous cholesterol acyltransferase. These two events result in increased cholesterol synthesis by the cell and decreased cholesterol esterified with oleic acid, respectively. These abnormalities have been shown to occur in patients with cholesterol ester storage disease.[385,386] However, patients with Wolman's disease have additional abnormalities such as accumulation of oxygenated steryl esters, which are difficult to explain solely on the basis of an isolated deficiency of acid hydrolase.[387] Similarly, patients with

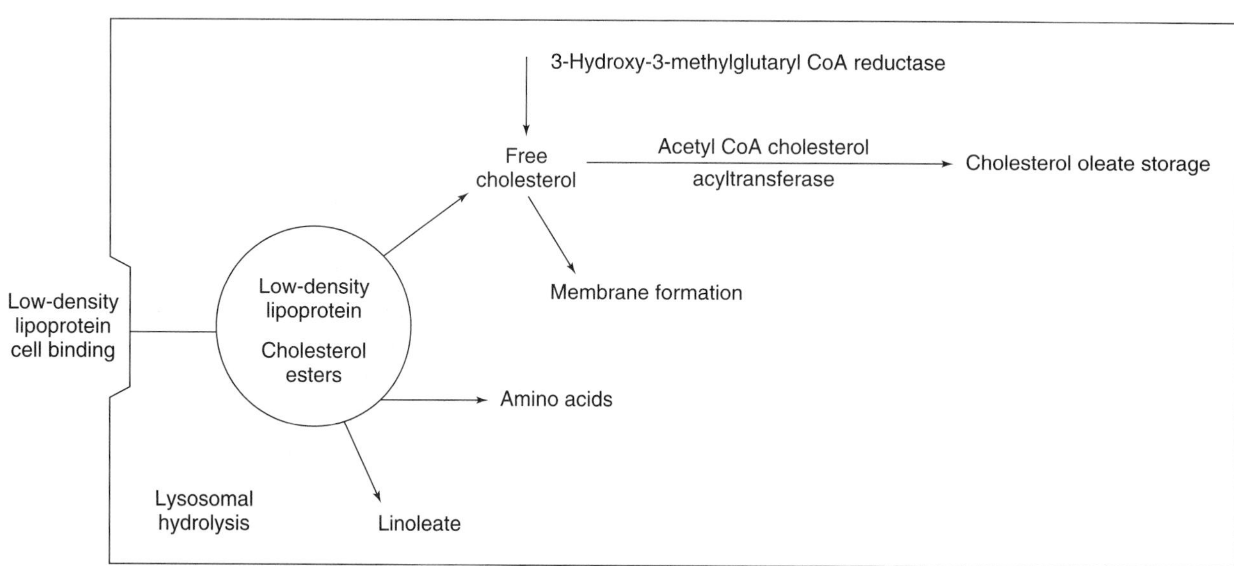

Figure 48-12 Metabolism of cholesterol esters.

Wolman's disease have unexplained steatorrhea, which may be secondary to defects in the metabolism of bile acids.

Molecular Basis of Lysosomal Acid Lipase Disorders (Wolman's Disease and Cholesterol Ester Storage Disease)

Deficiency of lysosomal acid lipase leads to either Wolman's disease or the more benign cholesterol ester storage disease. Both disorders are inherited as autosomal-recessive diseases and are associated with reduced activity and genetic defects of lysosomal acid lipase. The gene for lysosomal acid lipase has been cloned and mapped to chromosome 10q24-q25. The gene is expressed in most tissues with high expression in the hepatocytes, splenic and thymic cells, small intestinal villus cells, and adrenal cortex.[388] Homozygotes for exon-8 splice junction mutation resulting in incomplete exon skipping have been described in many Wolman's disease patients.[389] Cholesterol ester storage disease is distinct from Wolman's disease in that at least one mutant allele has the potential to produce some residual enzymatic activity to ameliorate the phenotype. Thus in the majority of cholesterol ester storage disease cases, a single splicing mutation occurs in one allele.[390] A knockout mouse model of Wolman's disease has been produced by targeted disruption of the lysosomal acid lipase gene.[391]

Wolman's Disease

Enzymatic Abnormalities

In 1956 Abramov and colleagues reported an infant who died at 2 months of age after a short illness characterized by abdominal distention, severe vomiting, diarrhea, hepatosplenomegaly, and radiographic evidence of calcification of the adrenal glands.[392] In 1961 Wolman and co-workers reported the cases of two siblings of their first patients who were found to have the same illness.[318] Accumulations of cholesterol esters and triglycerides were found in the liver, spleen, lymph nodes, and adrenal glands. The disorder was reported under the title generalized xanthomatosis with calcified adrenals.[393] In 1965 Crocker and associates described three patients with this disorder as having Wolman's disease; since then, the latter term has been widely accepted.[394] In 1969 Patrick and Lake confirmed that the accumulated cholesterol was esterified and demonstrated an acid hydrolase deficiency in the livers and spleens of those patients.[395] The activity of acid hydrolase was also deficient in cultured fibroblasts of patients with Wolman's disease.[396]

Deficiency of acid hydrolase or acid esterase manifests in two phenotypic forms. Wolman's disease represents the clinically acute and severe form. Affected patients die in the first year of life. Cholesterol ester storage disease represents a chronic form of deficiency of acid hydrolase. Patients who have this latter disorder do not have adrenal calcifications, and they live to adulthood.[385] Forty patients with Wolman's disease and more than 20 patients with cholesterol ester storage disease have been described so far.

Clinical Features

The majority of patients have similar clinical courses. Projectile vomiting, diarrhea, abdominal distention, and failure to thrive—the first noticeable symptoms—appear in about the second week of life.[392,393] Some patients are jaundiced.[394,397] Neurologic development of these infants is not normal. A decrease in activity may be noticed in the second month of life. It is not clear whether these symptoms are related to severe malnutrition or reflect neurologic defects. Konno and Fujii reported the case of an infant who had exaggerated tendon reflexes, ankle clonus, and opisthotonos.[397] Electroencephalography was reported to show no abnormality in this patient or several others.[386,398] On physical examination a patient is usually slightly feverish, irritable, and wasted. Non-specific skin eruptions may be observed. Abdominal distention with hepatosplenomegaly is noted in all patients; lymphadenopathy is detected in some. Subsequently progressive hepatosplenomegaly and abdominal distention, fever, and vomiting and diarrhea occur, persisting until the death of the patient, usually in the first 6 months of life.[392,393]

Laboratory Findings

Anemia usually appears early in the course of the disease, and hemoglobin levels progressively decrease to as low as 5 g/dl. Peripheral blood lymphocytes show intracytoplasmic and intranuclear vacuolation.[394,397,398] Acanthocytosis was found in a Japanese infant.[397] Lipid-laden histiocytes or foam cells are seen in bone marrow aspirates and in the peripheral blood.[392]

Total serum bilirubin and the conjugated fraction are elevated in some patients.[393,394,397] Some have elevated serum levels of AST and ALT.[394,397] Steatorrhea is present, evidenced by a high fecal fat content[394,397,398] and an abnormal ^{156}I-triolein absorption test.[398] The most consistent diagnostic finding, present in all reported cases of Wolman's disease, is calcification of the adrenal glands. The adrenal glands are symmetrically enlarged and show extensive punctate calcifications (Figure 48-13).[392,393] This is the only disease that causes such calcification of the adrenal glands. In all other conditions the calcifications are scattered. In most patients the responses of the adrenal glands to adrenocorticotropic hormone stimulation are depressed. Plasma cholesterol and triglycerides are usually normal in patients with Wolman's disease.[393,394,398-400] Triglycerides and very low-density lipoproteins were elevated in two patients.[399] It is expected that LDL levels should be high, because the acid hydrolase deficiency decreases cellular metabolism of LDLs. Some patients, however, had hypolipoproteinemia.[398] The severe inanition and reduced production of lipoproteins by the liver probably offset the tendency toward hyperlipoproteinemia.

Biochemical Characteristics

Most of the enzymes that hydrolyze fatty acid esters are active at neutral or alkaline pH. An ester hydrolase active

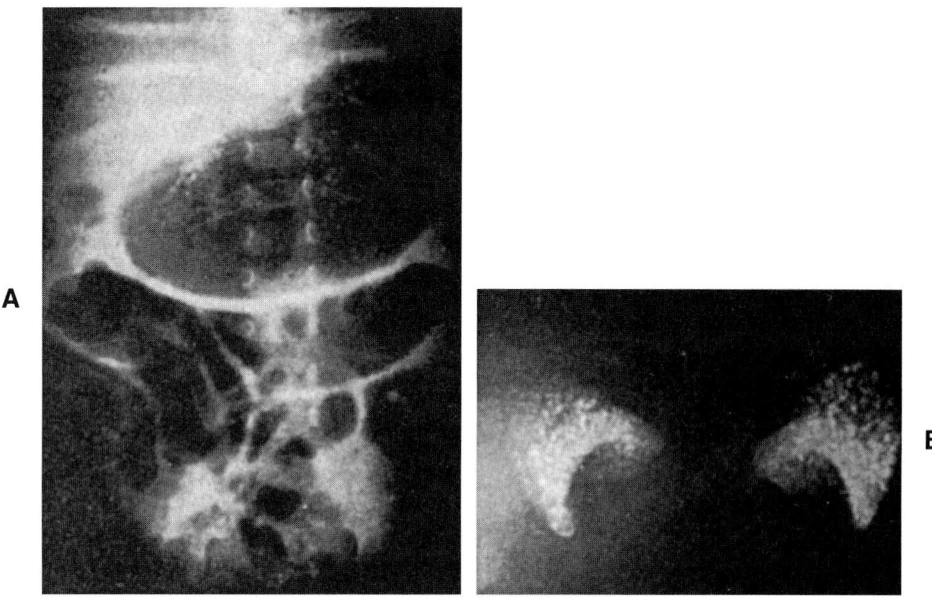

Figure 48-13 Radiograms showing calcification of the enlarged adrenal glands in a patient with Wolman's disease. **A,** Patient in the supine position. **B,** The adrenals after removal at autopsy. (From Crocker AC, Vawter GF, Neuhauser EBD, et al: Wolman's disease: three new patients with a recently described lipidosis. Pediatrics 35:627, 1965.)

TABLE 48-4

Tissue Lipid Analysis in Patients with Wolman's Disease

	Triglyceride	Total cholesterol	Free	Esterified	Reference no.
Liver, wet weight (mg/g)	137	97	38	59	322
	61	170	9	161	320
	44	32	14	18	316
Upper limit of normal	20	5	4	1	316
Spleen, weight (mg/g)	8	26	10	16	322
	99	35	8	27	320
	29	8	4	4	324
Upper limit of normal	1	5	4	<1	343-345

at acidic pH (4.0 to 5.6) has been found in lysosomes and cell membranes.[395] This enzyme requires no co-factors and uses triglycerides and cholesterol ester as substrates. Lysosomal acid lipase/cholesteryl ester hydrolyase has been purified,[401] and the cDNA encoding the human enzyme has been cloned and expressed.[402] Accumulation of cholesterol esters apparently results from the deficiency of cholesterol ester hydrolase activity.[403] Accumulations of triglycerides and other lipid products in large quantities are more difficult to explain. These biochemical abnormalities are discussed in more detail in the section on cholesterol ester storage disease. Table 48-4 shows the results of analyses of lipids in various tissues in Wolman's disease.

The triglyceride content is several-fold greater in the liver and as much as 100-fold greater in the spleen of a patient with Wolman's disease than in comparable tissues of controls.[395] The total cholesterol in liver and spleen is elevated in every case of Wolman's disease. The majority of the increase is in the cholesterol ester fraction. Similar accumulations of triglycerides and cholesterol esters have been found in the bone marrow, thymus, and lymph nodes. Slight increases were also detected in the lungs and kidneys.[399] Cholesterol and triglyceride contents of the brain were reported to be elevated in some patients[394,399]; however, they were normal in others.[397]

That severe malabsorption is seen in Wolman's disease but not in cholesterol ester storage disease could be explained by the differences in bile acid metabolism in these two diseases. Total serum bile acid levels were either normal or increased in patients with cholesterol ester storage disease.[386] Assmann and colleagues found oxygenated steryl esters in Wolman's disease but not in cholesterol ester storage disease. The accumulation of these oxygenated esters would suggest a defect in bile acid synthesis in Wolman's disease.[387] Boyd suggested that cholesterol linoleate may be the precursor in 7α-hydroxycholesterol formation.[404] If the pathway from 7α-hydroxycholesterol to bile acids were blocked, an accumulation of oxygenated steryl esters would occur. These speculations await confirmation by the study of bile acid metabolism in Wolman's disease. Such a defect in bile acid synthesis in Wolman's disease would explain the steatorrhea.

Pathology

Liver. Enlargement of the liver is a constant finding. It is firm and appears yellow. The hepatic architecture is usually distorted. The hepatic parenchymal cells show marked steatosis. Sinusoids are plugged by swollen histiocytes with foamy, vacuolated cytoplasm. Kupffer cells are distended and vacuolated. The portal areas are enlarged, with increased fibrosis that extends to the periportal areas. The fibrosis may be extensive, and a classic picture of hepatic cirrhosis may be seen.[392,393,399,400]

Electron microscopic examination of the liver shows that parenchymal organelles are distorted by the accumulation of large osmiophilic lipid droplets, which are identified as neutral lipids. These droplets are seen mostly in the lysosomes. The smooth endoplasmic reticulum and rough endoplasmic reticulum appear distended but are usually empty. The Kupffer cells are so distended that they almost obstruct the sinusoids.[400]

Spleen and Lymph Nodes. The spleen is greatly enlarged, firm, and mottled with yellowish flecks. Microscopic section shows that the reticular cells are transformed into large foam cells. The lymphatic follicles are atrophied and compressed. The lymph nodes are enlarged, firm, and yellowish. Microscopically, the lymph nodes are similar to the spleen. The same changes are seen also in the bone marrow and thymus.[394,399]

Intestines. The small intestine is usually thickened and has a yellowish serosal surface. The mucosa is greasy, yellowish, and granular. Microscopic sections show thick, flattened villi with numerous foamy, lipid-filled histiocytes in the lamina propria. Some of the foam cells extend into the muscularis mucosa. These changes are most evident in the proximal intestine or occasionally in the colon.[394,399]

Adrenal Glands. Both glands are symmetrically enlarged, firm, and difficult to cut. The cortex on cut sections is yellowish. Medially, the tissue is whitish. Microscopic sections of the glands show preservation of the architecture of the cortex. Many of the cells are swollen and vacuolated and contain sudanophilic lipid. Some of the foam cells are necrotic and appear as lipid cysts. Most of the calcium deposition occurs in a finely granular pattern; however, in some regions it may be condensed to form crystalline bumps.[399] Extensive fibrosis is found in the inner cortical areas. The medullary cells are normal.

Electron microscopic sections show that the innermost part of the adrenal cortex is necrotic, with calcification. The histiocytes are filled with large amounts of both crystalline and droplet lipid. Histochemical analysis of the lipid indicates the presence of cholesterol esters and triglycerides.[399,400]

Other Organs. The vascular endothelium shows lipid deposition, but frank atherosclerosis is not seen. Foam cells have been observed in the intestinal tissue and in the lungs, thyroid, testes, ovaries, leptomeninges, Purkinje cells, Auerbach's plexus, and Meissner's plexus.

Genetics

Wolman's disease is inherited as an autosomal-recessive trait. Seven of the patients reported so far have been Jews of Iraqi or Iranian origin. The other patients have been from Japan, Western Europe, and North America. Young and Patrick reported that the enzyme acid hydrolase in the leukocytes of the parents and a sibling of one patient had half the normal activity.[403] Kyriakides and associates reported similar findings in skin fibroblasts from the parents of a patient.[396] A prenatal diagnosis using cultured amniotic fluid cells has been described.[405]

Differential Diagnosis

Calcifications of the adrenal glands, invariably present in Wolman's disease, can be seen in conditions such as Addison's disease, adrenal hemorrhage, neuroblastoma, ganglioneuroma, adrenal cysts, pheochromocytoma, cortical carcinoma, and adrenal teratoma.[392,406] However, the calcifications in Wolman's disease characteristically outline the shape of the adrenal gland. Niemann-Pick disease may result in gastrointestinal symptoms, hepatosplenomegaly, and failure to thrive in early infancy, but adrenal calcifications are absent. The definitive diagnosis of Wolman's disease depends on the clinical picture and assay of acid hydrolase in cultured leukocytes or skin fibroblasts, using p-nitrophenyllaurate as a substrate.[407] Acid hydrolase activity that is less than 5 percent of normal confirms the diagnosis.

Treatment and Prognosis

Several therapeutic approaches have been tried, including TPN[408] and bone marrow transplantation.[409] A diet free of hydrophobic esters in which cholesterol and the essential fatty acids are bound to protein has been proposed by Wolman.[410]

Cholesterol Ester Storage Disease

Clinical Picture

In 1963 Fredrickson reported the first known case of hepatic cholesterol ester storage disease. The patient was a child with hepatomegaly and hyperlipidemia.[411] In 1967 Lageron and co-workers reported the case of a French adult with the same disease.[412,413] In 1968 Schiff and associates reported the cases of a brother and sister with the disease. Mild cirrhosis was evident in liver biopsy specimens, along with marked increases in fat content. Four of five younger siblings were found to have hepatomegaly. Liver biopsy specimens from three of the siblings showed vacuoles in their hepatocytes similar to those seen in the hepatocytes of the original patients.[386] Partin and Schubert found deposits of cholesterol esters in the lamina propria and mucosal smooth muscle and vascular pericytes[414] in jejunal tissue from two of the severely affected children in the family described by Schiff.

The majority of patients come to medical attention early in childhood, but one patient sought treatment at the age of 23. Hepatomegaly has been present in all patients reported.[386,411-419] In one patient hepatomegaly was present at birth. Hepatomegaly is progressive; eventually, hepatic fibrosis develops. Splenomegaly was found in 54 percent of patients. Esophageal varices secondary to portal hypertension were present in 27 percent of the patients. One patient had recurrent episodes of abdominal pain without known cause.[413,416] Two of the patients were reported to have had delays in sexual maturation.[412,414]

Laboratory Findings

Results of liver tests are usually normal. Jaundice has not been found, except in two patients who may have developed hepatitis with lethal complications.[403,417] Schiff and colleagues studied the serum bile acid profiles of two patients and those of five siblings, both parents, an uncle, and a grandfather of these patients. Total serum bile acids were markedly elevated in one patient and in all but three relatives. The ratio of cholic acid to chenodeoxycholic acid was decreased in duodenal bile obtained from one of the two patients.[386] Plasma lipoprotein patterns show hypercholesterolemia and some hypertriglyceridemia. The majority of the patients have increased levels of LDL. Two patients had low levels of high-density lipoprotein.

Biochemical Characteristics

Results of lipid analyses of liver tissue obtained from three patients with cholesterol ester storage disease are shown in Table 48-5. The major abnormality was the marked increase in cholesterol esters. The fatty acid composition of the cholesterol esters showed a predominance of oleic and linoleic acids.[386,392] The stored esters contained less than the expected amount of cholesterol linoleate.

Increased levels of LDLs in serum are routinely found in cholesterol ester storage disease. The presence of atherosclerosis in two patients with cholesterol ester storage disease is of interest because current speculation about the role of acid hydrolase in arterial intima predicts that accelerated atherosclerosis will be a consequence of the enzymatic deficiency.

The reason for the different clinical courses of Wolman's disease and cholesterol ester storage disease is unclear. It may be that there is a small but critical difference between the levels of residual acid hydrolase in the two groups of patients. A slightly greater deficiency of acid hydrolase in tissues has been recorded for patients with Wolman's disease.[415] Another possibility is that the two diseases are different at the levels of the enzymatic defects. For example, liver tissue from a patient with Wolman's disease did not hydrolyze DL-hexadecanyl-1,2-dioleate, whereas liver tissue from a patient with cholesterol ester storage disease hydrolyzed this substrate at a normal rate.[420] There could be isoforms of acid hydrolase with deficiency of different isoenzymes in Wolman's disease and cholesterol ester storage disease. Alternatively, it may be that the nature of the defect in a single type of acid hydrolase differs in these disorders.

Burton and co-workers reported that the intracellular acid hydrolase activity in cultured cells from Wolman's patients was 10 to 20 percent of control hydrolytic activity, whereas cholesterol ester storage disease cells exhibited 30 percent to 45 percent of control activity. These differences were found only when intracellular rather than cell lysate activity of the enzyme was measured.[421]

Pathology

The pathologic changes are secondary to the intralysosomal deposition of cholesterol esters and triglycerides.

Liver. Macroscopically, the liver is greatly enlarged and appears orange. On microscopic examination, the hepatic parenchymal cells and Kupffer cells show deposition of lipid droplets (Figure 48-14). In frozen sections the lipid droplets in the hepatocytes are birefringent but not autofluorescent. Those in Kupffer cells are not birefringent but show yellow autofluorescence. The differences are thought to be due to peroxidation of the fatty acids of cholesterol esters in macrophages but not in parenchymal cells. Electron microscopic studies show the lipid deposits to be limited by a single trilaminar membrane. The deposits in the hepatocytes are electron

TABLE 48-5

Lipid Concentrations in Liver Tissue of Patients with Cholesterol Ester Storage Disease

	Total lipids	Triglycerides	Total cholesterol	Free	Esterified	Reference no.
Lipids, wet weight (mg/g)	280	64	121	9	187	344
	244	36	112	11	174	333
Upper limit of normal		19	4	3	1	345

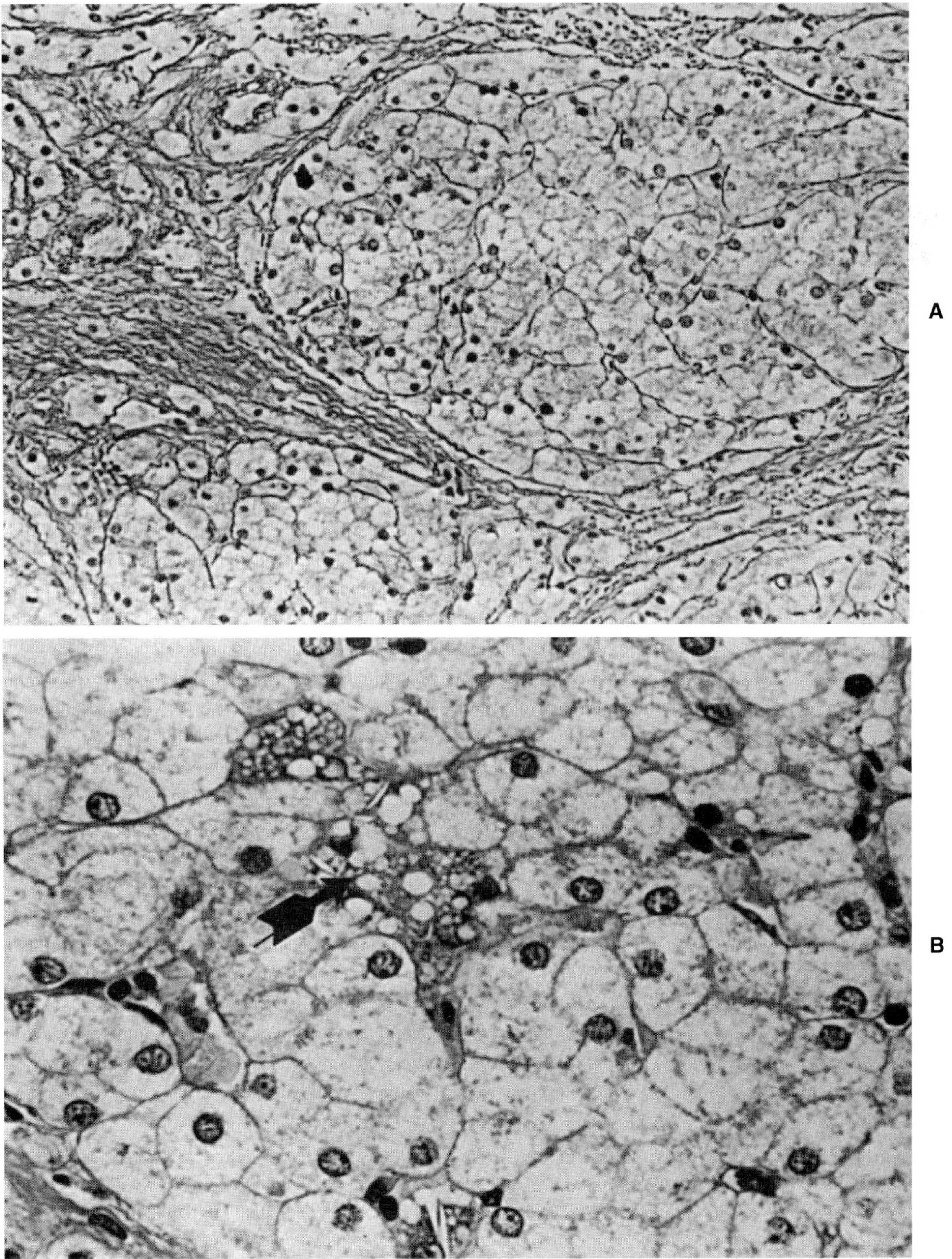

Figure 48-14 Biopsy specimens from a patient with cholesterol ester storage disease. **A,** Liver, showing dense bands of connective tissue extending through the liver, forming nodules (Wilder's reticulum stain; ×200). **B,** The individual foam vacuoles of different sizes plus acinar clefts interpreted as cholesterol, indicated by arrow (Gomori's trichrome; ×500).

Continued

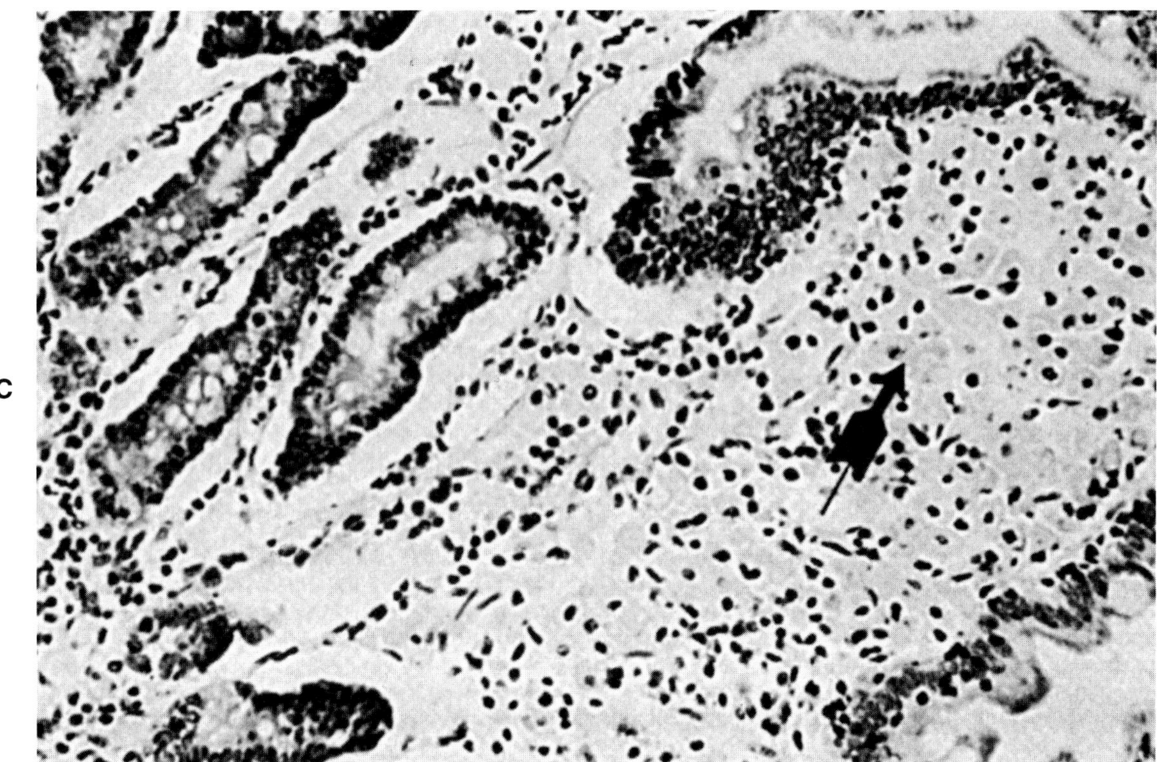

Figure 48-14, cont'd C, The lamina propria of the small intestine, containing foam cells, indicated by arrow, in dense nodules distorting the involved villus (Gomori's trichrome; ×200). (From Beaudet AL, Ferry GD, Nichols BL Jr, et al: Cholesterol ester storage disease: clinical, biochemical, and pathological studies. J Pediatr 90:910, 1977.)

lucent; however, those in the Kupffer cells are interspersed with electron-dense material. In the majority of patients dense bands of fibrous tissue extend through the liver, forming lobules of different sizes. Fibrosis may progress in some patients to give a classic picture of cirrhosis, with the development of portal hypertension and esophageal varices.[417]

Other Tissues. Partin and Schubert studied small intestinal biopsy specimens from two patients. The biopsy specimens had an orange tinge. In contradistinction to Tangier disease, which features storage of cholesterol esters, abnormal coloration of the colonic mucosa or the tonsils has not been found in cholesterol ester storage disease. Histologic sections of the small bowel show that the epithelial cells are normal; however, foam cells were found in the lacteal area and were especially abundant in the villus tips. Free droplets of fat were present in the extracellular spaces of the lamina propria.[415]

Electron microscopic studies of small intestine show foam cells in clusters beneath the basement membrane of the epithelial cells surrounding the lacteals. The cytoplasm of the lacteal endothelium is distended by numerous large osmiophilic lipid vacuoles. Smooth muscle fiber cells, vascular pericytes, fibrocytes, and Schwann cells of nerve fibers contain lucent lipid droplets. Deposits of lipids, similar to those seen in Wolman's disease, were found in other tissues. Although clinically there was no evidence of atherosclerosis in patients with cholesterol ester storage disease, two of three patients examined by necropsy had atherosclerosis.[417]

Genetics

Cholesterol ester storage disease is probably inherited as an autosomal-recessive trait.[415] There is a preponderance of females among the patients reported. It is possible to detect heterozygotes by quantitation of acid hydrolase activity in leukocytes or cultured fibroblasts. Heterozygotes have 40 percent to 50 percent of the reported normal enzymatic activity.[417] Prenatal diagnosis can be established using cultured amniotic fluid cells.

Treatment and Prognosis

Cholesterol ester storage disease is relatively benign. Death in childhood from hepatic complications has been reported.[417] Two patients died at 43 years of age.[412,422]

Two reports suggested the utility of inhibitors of 3-hydroxy-3-methylglutaryl-CoA reductase as a safe and effective treatment for children with acid lipase deficiency. A significant decrease in hepatomegaly and the levels of cholesterol and triglycerides was observed in the treated patients.[423,424]

INBORN ERRORS OF BILE ACID METABOLISM

Inborn errors of bile acid include disorders involving molecular defects in the genes encoding canalicular transport proteins, peroxisomal disorders, and a heterogeneous group of disorders including Alagille's syndrome with mutations in the Jagged-1 gene (JAG1) and cystic fibrosis with mutations in the cystic fibrosis transconductor regulator (CFTR) (see Chap. 10).

Progressive Familial Intrahepatic Cholestasis

Progressive familial intrahepatic cholestasis (PFIC) is a heterogeneous group of autosomal-recessive disorders in which hepatocellular cholestasis often presents in the neonatal period or the first year of life leading to death from liver failure during the childhood to adolescent periods. The clinical, biochemical, and histologic features and the advances in the understanding of the canalicular membrane transport proteins in the liver have provided evidence for the heterogeneity of this clinical entity and suggested defects in bile secretion and/or bile acid metabolism. Three types of PFIC have been described based on the recent molecular and genetic studies, which allowed identification of the molecular basis of these three types.

PFIC-I (Byler's Disease)

PFIC-1 is also known as Byler's disease and was described originally in 1965 by Clayton and associates, who described a syndrome of progressive intrahepatic cholestasis in an extensive study of Amish descendants from Jacob Byler, who was born in the United States in 1799. Six members of four interrelated, inbred Amish sibships were described in Clayton's original abstract.[425] The disease was characterized by onset of pruritus, jaundice, steatorrhea, and hepatosplenomegaly early in infancy. Four of the six patients died between 17 months and 8 years of age. Similar cases have been reported from France and Japan.[426-428] Biochemically, all Clayton's patients had conjugated hyperbilirubinemia and elevated serum alkaline phosphatase with normal serum cholesterol levels. Subsequently, Byler's disease patients are characterized as having low serum γ-glutamyl transferase concentrations, high serum bile-salt concentrations, and low biliary chenodeoxycholic bile-salt concentrations. This form of progressive familial intrahepatic cholestasis has been mapped by positional cloning to chromosome 18q21-22.[429,430]

Clinical Features. Progressive intrahepatic cholestasis usually manifests between the ages of 1 and 10 months.[429,431] In four of the reported cases onset of the disease occurred in the first week of life.[429] Pruritus and jaundice are the earliest symptoms. In infants pruritus may be severe enough to interfere with sleep. The jaundice is usually accompanied by dark urine and pale stools that may become totally acholic. The stools are loose, foul-smelling, and greasy because of steatorrhea.[429,432] The level of jaundice usually fluctuates. Recurrent cholestatic episodes alternate with periods of remission. The cholestatic episodes have been reported to be triggered by upper respiratory tract infections.[429] After several months remissions are less frequent. Rickets is seen in some patients.[429,433] Most have growth retardation[433]; developmental retardation was found in 30 percent of the reported patients. Bleeding episodes secondary to hypoprothrombinemia have been reported for approximately half the patients. Some patients have clubbing of the fingers.[434] Xanthomatosis of the skin does not occur. Hepatomegaly has been present in all patients reported so far, but splenomegaly has been found in only half of the patients. Liver enlargement persists during remissions, and with the progression of disease, the liver becomes hard, irregular, and nodular. The majority of patients die between the ages of 2 and 15 years, but occasionally a patient has survived until the age of 25 years.[428] Dahms reported the cases of twin brothers with Byler's disease, both of whom developed hepatocellular carcinomas. The two brothers died at 13 and 17 years of age of liver failure.[435]

Laboratory Findings. All reported patients have had elevations of total serum bilirubin. Levels of 40 to 50 mg/dl are not unusual during the cholestatic episodes.[432] The direct fraction is usually half of the total bilirubin.[426-428] The serum AST and ALT levels are elevated. Serum cholesterol is usually normal or low.[426] Serum γ-glutamyl transpeptidase (GGTP) levels are normal, despite the elevation of serum alkaline phosphatase levels.[436] Levels of GGTP in the liver are reported to be elevated.[437] Serum GGTP could be used as a marker for Byler's disease because normal values were found in 22 of 28 patients with the disease.[438] Prothrombin time and thromboplastin time are increased secondary to malabsorption of vitamin K. Malabsorption studies reveal severe steatorrhea, excretion of fat amounting to 50 percent to 80 percent of intake.[427] Both transport maximum (T_m) and storage capacity for sulfobromophthalein (BSP) are markedly reduced. A parent heterozygotic for the trait is clinically normal but may have an abnormally decreased BSP T_m.[426]

Total serum bile acids have been elevated in the patients studied. Total bile acids in duodenal aspirates of one patient studied by Linarelli and associates were 0.07 to 0.5 mm, which is below the critical micellar concentration of 2 mm.[439,440] The clearance of labeled cholic acid and chenodeoxycholic acid was normal at 20 minutes and slightly impaired at 60 minutes. The half-life of the labeled bile acid was prolonged. The major loss of the isotopes was in urine rather than feces. Serum lithocholic acid was reported to be high in Linarelli's patient.

Radiographic examination of the biliary tree by operative cholangiography showed patency of the biliary tree in the patients studied. In the series reported from France cholelithiasis and intrapancreatic calcification were found in some patients.[428]

The biochemical findings suggest a defect in the excretion of bile acids across the canalicular membrane of the liver cell. The gene for PFIC-1 is called FIC1, which encodes for a P-type adenosine triphosphatase that is expressed predominantly in the small intestine and the liver and likely to be important in the transfer of amino phospholipids from the outer to the inner leaflet of the plasma membrane bilayer.[430] Although the exact function of FIC-1 has not been characterized it is likely to be involved in bile acid transport.

Pathology. Light microscopy of liver biopsy specimens early in the disease shows normal hepatic architecture. Hepatocellular and canalicular cholestasis with pseudoacinar transformation is commonly seen. Bile duct damage leading to ductal paucity is seen in 70 percent of older patients. The striking feature of all liver biopsy specimens is the marked cholestasis in the parenchymal cells and in canaliculi, especially in the lumina of the tubular formations and around the veins. As the disease progresses, the classic picture of biliary cirrhosis develops.[441]

Electron microscopic studies show markedly abnormal biliary duct canaliculi. The pericanalicular ectoplasm is greatly thickened, and the microvilli are swollen, fused, or blunted. The canalicular lumina are filled with coarsely particulate and amorphous granular material.[441]

Prognosis. Death usually occurs between the ages of 17 months and 8 years of hepatic complications such as liver failure, bleeding, and malnutrition. An occasional patient has survived to 25 years of age.

Therapy. Oral ursodeoxycholic acid appears effective in all types of progressive familial intrahepatic cholestasis for improving the clinical status of some children.[442] Alagille and Odievre reported rapid relief of cholestasis in four patients in whom cholecystojejunostomy was performed; however, the long-term benefit from such a major surgical procedure is unknown.[428] Similarly, Whittington and colleagues have shown improvement in cholestasis with external biliary drainage.[443] The researchers' experience suggests heterogeneity in the response to biliary diversion. Some patients improved markedly; others showed no improvement. The latter patients had liver transplantation, and favorable experience with liver transplantation in patients with Byler's disease has been reported.[444]

PFIC Type II

Patients with initial typical findings of PFIC type I, and those unrelated to the Byler family, has been designated as having Byler syndrome. Cases have been described in isolated populations, the Middle East, Greenland, and Sweden.[445-448] Homozygosity mapping and linkage analysis in six consanguineous patients of Middle Eastern origin have resulted in identification of a gene location on chromosome on q24.[448] Patients with type II familial progressive intrahepatic cholestasis present with severe pruritus, normal serum γ-glutamyl transferase activity and cholesterol levels, high concentration of serum primary bile acids, and low biliary primary bile acid concentrations. Clinically these patients present with more severe and permanent jaundice with the onset of rapid liver failure. Liver histology shows absence of ductular proliferation with canalicular cholestasis and periportal biliary metaplasia of hepatocytes.[435,449] However, the liver architecture is more severely altered with lobular and portal fibrosis and inflammation and giant cell proliferation compared to PFIC-1. More recent studies suggest that the defect may reside in the canalicular bile-salt export pump (BSEP). At least 10 BSEP mutations in PFIC-2 patients from several different populations have been determined.[450] Moreover, the human BSEP gene has been mapped to the 2q24 locus, which is the gene locus for PFIC-2. The findings of mutations in BSEP are consistent with the decrease in canalicular excretion of bile acids described in these patients. Indeed, patients with PFIC-2 were found to have a close correlation between BSEP gene mutations and canalicular BSEP expression resulting in a decrease in the concentration of biliary bile acids in these deficient patients.[451]

PFIC Type III

Patients with PFIC-3 usually present later in life with significant potential for biliary cirrhosis and liver failure at a later age. These patients can be distinguished from the other types of progressive intrahepatic cholestasis by the finding of very high serum γ-glutamyl transferase activity and liver histology that show portal fibrosis with bile duct proliferation and inflammatory infiltrate in the early stages despite the fact that their intrahepatic and extrahepatic bile ducts are patent.[433] The genetic basis of PFIC-3 has been shown to be related to mutations in the human multi-drug resistant 3 (MDR-3) P-glycoprotein, which transports phospholipids into the biliary system.[452,453] The finding of mutation on MDR-3 was based on analysis of bile in these patients, which showed very low concentration of phospholipid and the phenotype of the analogous MDR-2 knockout mouse.[454] MDR-3 belongs to the family of ABC transporter and is expressed in the canalicular membrane of the hepatocytes. Immunohistochemistry revealed the lack of canalicular staining for MDR-3 in the liver tissue of patients with PFIC-3. Mutations in the MDR-3 gene have been described in patients with PFIC-3. Some of these mutations lead to a truncated MDR-3 protein, which lacks at least one ABC motif. Additional nonsense mutations and missense mutations associated with low biliary phospholipid levels have been identified in patients with PFIC-3. The liver pathology may be related to the toxic effects of bile acids on bile canaliculi and the biliary epithelium in the absence of phospholipids. Recent studies have also suggested that heterozygous state for a MDR-3 gene defect may represent a genetic predisposition in families with cholestasis, noted during pregnancy.[455,456] The MDR-3 has been mapped to 7q21-36. A recent study has identified 16 different mutations in 17 different patients. These mutations include frameshifts, nonsense, and missense. Gallstones or episodes of cholestasis of pregnancy were found in patients or parents. Children with missense mutations had a less severe disease and more often a beneficial effect of ursodeoxycholic acid therapy was noted.[454]

Hereditary Lymphedema with Recurrent Cholestasis (Norwegian Cholestasis; Aagenaes's Syndrome)

In 1968 Aagenaes and associates reported the cases of 16 patients from Norway in whom hereditary recurrent intrahepatic cholestasis appeared during the neonatal period.[457] In 1971 Sharp and Krivit reported two sisters of Norwegian extraction with a similar syndrome.[458] Consanguinity was present in six of the seven parental couples in the series reported by Aagenaes and co-workers, suggesting an autosomal-recessive inheritance. In 1974 Aagenaes described two additional families with a similar syndrome.[459] All patients had early onset of intrahepatic cholestasis with elevated levels of total and direct serum bilirubin. Lymphedema of the lower extremities appeared late in childhood in all of Aagenaes's patients. It appeared early and at the onset of cholestatic jaundice in the patients of Sharp and Krivit.

Clinical Features

All reported patients became jaundiced during the first month of life.[458-460] The jaundice lasted about 1 to 6 years, and during this period, the patients had severe pruritus. Growth retardation with complications of malabsorption such as rickets, anemia, and bleeding tendency was evident during the period of cholestasis. When the cholestasis resolved, catch-up growth occurred, so the patients' adult heights were normal. One or more further episodes of cholestasis have occurred in all adult patients. Lymphedema, once present, persists throughout life.

Laboratory Findings

Total serum bilirubin is elevated, with the direct fraction 50 percent to 80 percent of the total. Especially during periods of cholestasis and in the first year of life, serum AST and ALT levels are increased.[458-461] Serum alkaline phosphatase is always increased. Results of the BSP excretion test are abnormal, with retention of 25 percent to 40 percent at 45 minutes. Serum cholesterol and triglycerides are elevated. Lipoprotein electrophoresis shows increases in prebeta and beta lipoproteins. Protein electrophoresis shows elevation of the α_2-globulin fraction with low serum albumin. Prothrombin time and thromboplastin time are elevated secondary to malabsorption of vitamin K. Fecal fat measurements show excretion of about 30 percent to 50 percent of ingested fat. Fecal nitrogen excretion is normal.

Lymphangiography with visualization of the deep lymphatics was attempted in only one case. The lymphatics were found to be abnormally tortuous. Injection of blue dye into the interdigital spaces in another patient resulted in a chicken-wire pattern, indicative of an absence of deep lymphatics.[459]

Pathology

Examination of liver biopsy specimens reveals intact architecture with marked bile stasis, giant cell transformation, and minimal hepatic cell necrosis. The portal areas show a slight increase in fibrosis, and in most instances biliary ducts are difficult to find. In one patient repeat liver biopsies at 10 years of age showed progression to cirrhosis.

Biochemical Characteristics

The elevated total serum bile acids and retention of BSP suggest deterioration of the excretory function of the liver. However, the nature of the defect is not known. The association of lymphedema of both lower extremities and cholestasis raises the possibility of abnormal lymphatic drainage from the liver. Aagenaes and colleagues injected colloidal gold into the liver capsule of one of their patients. Instead of normal excretion by lymphatic vessels, there was puddling of the isotope in the liver, which suggests a defect in the hepatic lymphatic system.[460] The close functional relationship between lymphatic and biliary drainage systems of the liver was shown experimentally in animals. After experimental obstruction of the common bile duct, bilirubin and bile acids rapidly appeared in the lymphatic system before elevation in the serum.[461-464] Conversely, an increased biliary flow with increased excretion of bilirubin and bile acids occurred after interruption of the hepatic lymphatics in cats.[460] Thus it is possible that abnormalities of the lymphatics of the liver contribute to the pathogenesis of this entity. More recently, the locus for Aagenaes's syndrome has been mapped to a 6.6-cm interval on chromosome 15q.[465]

Prognosis

Initially, the syndrome was thought to carry a favorable prognosis[458]; however, a subsequent report indicated that one of the earlier reported patients had died of liver failure. As previously mentioned, in another patient, a repeat liver biopsy at 10 years of age showed evidence of cirrhosis.[459]

Therapy

No effective therapy is available. Cholestyramine has been used to alleviate pruritus during the cholestatic episodes. Because of the cholestasis, fat-soluble vitamins and fats in the form of medium-chain triglycerides should be given.

Alagille's Syndrome (Arteriohepatic Dysplasia)

Although reports of biliary duct hypoplasia and chronic liver disease appeared in the early 1950s,[466-468] it was not until 1973 that Watson and Miller described the cases of nine patients who had neonatal liver disease and familial pulmonary dysplasia.[469] A full description of the syndrome was provided by Alagille and co-workers. These investigators emphasized the characteristic facial appearance and vertebral and cardiovascular anomalies.[470] The syndrome is not rare; investigators were able to report large groups of patients.[470-474] The recent identification of JAG1 gene mutations in patients with Alagille's syndrome made it possible to understand the mechanism of the disease and explain the various clinical manifestations.[475,476]

Clinical Features

The major features of Alagille's syndrome are chronic liver disease, characteristic facies, cardiovascular and vertebral anomalies, and ophthalmologic abnormalities. Minor features include central nervous system, renal, endocrine, pancreas, gut, systemic vascular system, ear, lung, and larynx abnormalities. Table 48-6 summarizes the major and minor abnormalities.

Chronic Liver Disease

Alagille's syndrome is associated with cholestasis, which may develop during the neonatal period and usually becomes apparent in the first 2 years of life.[477-479] Pruritus develops early in infancy and persists despite the disappearance of jaundice. The liver is usually enlarged, firm, smooth, and not tender. The spleen may be enlarged even in the absence of portal hypertension. The stools may be clay colored and the urine dark yellow. Xanthomas may be seen on the extensor surfaces of the fingers and in creases of the palms, anal folds, and popliteal and vaginal areas. These xanthomas represent long-standing severe intrahepatic cholestasis. With the progression of the disease about the beginning of the second year of life, jaundice may subside or disappear, but cholestasis persists. The long-term outlook for the liver disease is variable, with 10 percent to 50 percent of the patients developing cirrhosis and portal hypertension. In one study only 3 of 36 patients monitored by the Alagille group developed hepatic cirrhosis.[428]

Characteristic Facies

The face is small with a prominent, broad forehead. The eyes are set widely and deeply (hypertelorism). The mandible is small and pointed, giving the appearance of a triangular face.[477-479] The peculiar facies become more prominent with increasing age.

Cardiovascular Abnormalities

All patients with Alagille's syndrome have cardiac murmurs as infants. Most have peripheral pulmonary stenosis, which is usually mild and does not necessitate surgery.[478] Other cardiac lesions, including ventricular septal defects, coarctation of the aorta, and cyanotic heart disease, have also been reported (see Table 48-6).

Osseous Abnormalities

The hands show various degrees of shortening of the distal phalanges, stiffening, swelling, and limitation of motion at the proximal interphalangeal joints. Radiographs of the spine show either frank or incomplete butterfly vertebrae and decreased interpediculate distances in the lumbar spine.[471]

Ocular Findings

Posterior embryotoxon (prominent Schwalbe's ring) visible to the unaided eye, by slit-lamp examination, or on

TABLE 48-6
Clinical Features of Alagille's Syndrome

Major Features	
Liver	Paucity of intrahepatic ducts
Heart	Peripheral pulmonary stenosis
Eye	Posterior embryotoxon
Facies	Prominent forehead; deep-set eyes; mild hypertelorism; small, pointed chin
Vertebra	Butterfly vertebrae
Minor Features	
Congenital heart disease	Coarctation of the aorta, tetralogy of Fallot, ventricular and atrial septal defects, patent ductus arteriosus, truncus arteriosus, abnormal venous return, right ventricular hypoplasia
Systemic vascular malformations	Arterial hypoplasia, renal artery stenosis, carotid artery aneurysm, intracranial hemorrhage
Skeletal anomalies	Spina bifida, short distal phalanges and metacarpal bones, clinodactyly, short distal ulna and radius
Eye abnormalities	Retinal pigmentation, iris strands, cataract myopia, strabismus, glaucoma
Renal abnormalities	Cystic disease, renal agenesis, horseshoe kidney, renal hypoplasia, mesangiolipidosis, tubular dysfunction
Pancreas abnormalities	Exocrine pancreatic dysfunction, diabetes mellitus
Lung abnormalities	Tracheal and bronchial stenosis
Ear abnormalities	Deafness, chronic otitis media
Gut abnormalities	Small bowel atresia

gonioscopy, is the most important ocular abnormality and occurs in 56 percent to 95 percent of patients. In addition, retinal pigmentary changes are usually found. Nischal and co-workers reported ultrasound evidence of optic disc drusen in a large percentage of Alagille's patients.[480] Other abnormalities include microcornea keratoconus exotropia, iris hypoplasia, and abnormalities of the optic disc.[481-484]

Central Peripheral Nervous System Findings

Gross motor delays and mental retardation were reported in a small number of patients.[473] Intracranial bleeding is the most significant neurologic complication. It occurs in approximately 15 percent of the patients,[472,481] and in 30 percent to 50 percent the bleeding is fatal. It is of note that many of the patients with bleeding did not have coagulopathy, raising the issue of cerebrovascular malformation.[472] Moyamoya disease (progressive arterial occlusion of the distal intracranial carotids) has been reported in patients with Alagille's syndrome.[485,486] In support of the involvement of the central nervous system is the observation that the autosomal-dominant cerebral arteriopathy with subcortical infarct and leukoencephalopathy is also caused by a mutation in Notch 3.[487]

Pancreatic Abnormalities

Chong and associates described pancreatic insufficiency in some patients with Alagille's syndrome.[488] Other investigators have shown that 41 percent of their patients had pancreatic insufficiency, some of whom also developed diabetes mellitus.[489]

Other Abnormalities

Growth retardation, which decreased with age, was documented in the majority of cases of children. Slight to moderate mental retardation was documented in some of these cases. Renal function is impaired, with hyperuricemia and decreased creatinine clearance in some patients. Hypogonadism was suspected to be present in six male patients reported by Alagille and colleagues. Testicular biopsy showed no abnormality in two; in two others, fibrous tissue proliferation was present. In the remaining two patients spermatogenic cells were almost completely lacking.[470]

Laboratory Findings

Total serum bilirubin is elevated during infancy, with levels between 4 and 14 mg/dl. The direct fraction is 30 percent to 50 percent of the total. Serum bilirubin usually returns to normal after the second year of life.[470] Some patients remain deeply jaundiced with bilirubin levels greater than 20 mg/dl. Serum cholesterol levels may be as high as 2000 mg/dl. Serum triglyceride levels range from 500 to 1000 mg/dl. Serum alkaline phosphatase and glutamyl transferase levels are very high. Serum AST and ALT are slightly elevated. Despite the return of serum bilirubin to normal, biochemical evidence of severe cholestasis is usually found. Total serum bile acids have been markedly elevated in the patients so studied, with increases in both cholic acid and chenodeoxycholic acid. No major unidentified chromatographic peak was present in the serum or duodenal bile of the patients so studied.[477]

Retention of BSP at 45 minutes is abnormal; however, storage capacity for BSP is normal. Prothrombin time and partial thromboplastin time are abnormal secondary to malabsorption of fats. Both values return to normal in response to intramuscular administration of vitamin K.

Pathology

Exploratory laparotomy of a patient who has arteriohepatic dysplasia shows uniformly patent extrahepatic biliary ducts. In the neonatal period liver biopsy shows intact hepatic architecture with marked cholestasis. The hepatocytes may be swollen with balloon degeneration and minimal giant cell transformation. The most dramatic changes are in the portal areas, where a decrease in the number of biliary ducts is observed, with a slight increase in connective tissue. However, Ghishan and colleagues reported finding biliary duct proliferation in two patients with arteriohepatic dysplasia whose livers were sampled when they were 5 and 49 days old, respectively. Subsequent liver biopsies, when the patients were 2 and 27 months old, respectively,[490] showed a paucity of biliary ducts in the portal areas. Biopsies of the livers of adult patients with arteriohepatic dysplasia have shown no biliary ducts in the portal areas with variable progression to biliary cirrhosis. Indeed, 3 of 26 patients followed by the Alagille group developed hepatic cirrhosis. Other investigators reported the finding of cirrhosis in as many as 50 percent of patients.[472,473]

Genetics

Alagille's syndrome is inherited as an autosomal-dominant trait with reduced penetrance and variable expression when both parents are clinically normal; the percentage of sporadic cases is 45 percent to 50 percent. Bryne and colleagues first noted deletions of the short arm of chromosome 20.[491] Since then, several investigators mapped the gene for Alagille's syndrome to chromosome 20p12.[492-496] The gene was eventually identified as the gene JAG1, which is a ligand for the NOTCH-1 receptor by physical, genetic, and gene mapping covering the 20p12 region.[497,498] Mutations in JAG1 genes have been have been demonstrated in 60 percent to 75 percent of patients with Alagille's syndrome. Analysis of 233 cases revealed that 72 percent of the reported mutations lead to frameshifts that cause a premature termination codon.[499] The spectrum of mutations identified is consistent, with haploinsufficiency for JAG1 being a mechanism for Alagille's syndrome. The JAG1 gene encodes a protein, which belongs to the family of NOTCH ligands. The NOTCH signaling pathway is important for control of cell fate during embryogenesis. JAG1 is expressed ubiquitously in tissues of humans including liver biliary epithelia, heart, kidney, eye, and brain.[500] The role of JAG1 in remodeling embryonic vasculature has been delineated by a null mouse model. Mice homozygous for JAG1 mutations die from bleeding during early embryogenesis. Heterozygotic mice show eye malformations.

Biochemical Characteristics

The majority of the patients with Alagille's syndrome have elevated conjugated hyperbilirubinemia. Serum bile acids and γ-glutamyl transferase levels are elevated. Liver enzymes are modestly elevated.

Therapy

Phenobarbital and cholestyramine have not been shown to be effective in the treatment of Alagille's syndrome; however, Alagille and colleagues reported alleviation of pruritus and reductions of serum cholesterol, triglyceride, and bilirubin levels in response to very high doses of cholestyramine—12 to 15 g/day.[428] Anti-histamines, rifampin, and naltrexone have been used to relieve pruritus.[501] Some patients were subjected to biliary drainage.[502] Improved nutrition via gastrostomy with supplements of fat-soluble vitamins has been used. Pancreatic enzyme replacement for patients with pancreatic insufficiency is indicated.

Prognosis

Data from early studies suggest that the long-term prognosis is good. Three of Alagille's 26 patients developed cirrhosis,[428] but recent reports suggest that 10 percent to 50 percent of patients develop liver cirrhosis and portal hypertension. Hepatocellular carcinoma has been reported. Liver transplant is eventually necessary in 21 percent to 31 percent of patients.[473,474] Hoffenberg and colleagues have estimated that 50 percent of patients will eventually require liver transplants.[472]

INBORN ERRORS OF PEROXISOME BIOGENESIS

Zellweger's Syndrome (Cerebrohepatorenal Syndrome)

In 1964 Bowen and associates described an autosomal-recessive disease occurring in two siblings. It was characterized by severe hypotonia, growth and mental retardation, renal cortical cysts, and hepatic dysfunction. Both patients died before the age of 5 months.[503] Patients with a similar clinical syndrome were described by Smith and co-workers[504] and by Passarge and McAdams.[505] In 1969 Opitz and colleagues described four new patients and identified iron deposition in the liver. Because the original two patients were Professor Hans Zellweger's patients, his name was used by Opitz's group as an eponymic designation for this condition.[506] In 1972 Goldfischer and co-workers described mitochondrial abnormalities and lack of peroxisomes in electron microscopic studies of liver biopsy specimens from patients with Zellweger's syndrome.[507] In 1975 Danks and associates reported finding pipecolic acid in the urine of four patients.[508] In 1979 Hanson and colleagues described a defect in bile acid synthesis found in three patients with Zellweger's syndrome.[509]

Studies conducted in the 1980s confirmed that Zellweger's syndrome belongs to a group of disorders of peroxisome biogenesis.[510] This group includes neonatal adrenoleukodystrophy, infantile Refsum's disease, and hyperpipecolic acidemia. Affected patients have reduced or absent peroxisomes with multiple enzyme defects that are normally present within peroxisomes. The peroxisomal functions include beta oxidation of long-chain fatty acids, ether-phospholipid biosynthesis, glyoxylate metabolism, degradation of pipecolic acid, and oxidation of phytanic acid.

Clinical Features

Severe hypotonia with simian creases is common, together with camptodactyly, which may involve several fingers. There may be some ulnar deviation of hands and fingers. Partial flexion of the knees with various degrees of equinovarus deformities of the feet is often seen. All patients have high foreheads with shallow supraorbital ridges and flat facies. Sucking and swallowing difficulties, generalized seizures, and delays in psychomotor developmental maturation are common. Patent ductus arteriosus and septal defects are present in approximately 40 percent of the patients. Hepatomegaly is common; splenomegaly occasionally is found. Jaundice is evident in 30 percent to 50 percent of the patients.[508]

Laboratory Findings

Hematologic investigations have shown elevated serum iron and nearly total saturation of the serum iron-binding protein in more than half the cases reported.[511] The true incidences of these abnormalities may be higher because iron status has not been determined in many cases. Tissue concentrations of iron in the liver, spleen, kidneys, and lungs are increased. In one reported case tissue iron in the liver was 50 mg/100 g wet weight (normal values for the same age group range from 7 to 21 mg/100 g). Ferrokinetic studies in this case demonstrated a rapid disappearance of iron and a markedly increased plasma iron turnover.[511] Ferrokinetic incorporation into circulating red cells was significantly impaired, with abnormal accumulation of the radiolabeled iron in the liver. Intestinal absorption of iron was normal. Desferrioxamine induced a marked increase in urinary iron excretion. However, ferrokinetic studies of a second patient done by the same investigator showed no abnormality.[511]

Prothrombin time and thromboplastin time are usually prolonged, secondary to hepatic dysfunction. Serum AST and ALT levels are moderately elevated. Conjugated hyperbilirubinemia may be detected. Aminoaciduria was present in four cases. Urinary excretion of pipecolic acid, a minor breakdown product of lysine, was found to be markedly increased in four infants in whom adequate qualitative tests were made.[508] Hanson and colleagues showed that three infants excreted excessive $3\alpha,7\alpha$-dihydroxy-5β-cholestan-26-oic acid; 3α,7α,12α-trihydroxy-5β-cholestan-26-oic acid (THCA); and 3α,7α,12α,24gj-tetrahydroxy-5β-cholestan-26-oic acid (varanic acid). These compounds are precursors of chenodeoxycholic acid and cholic acid that have undergone only partial side chain oxidation.[509] These findings were confirmed in two other cases of Zellweger's syndrome.[512] Increased accumulation of very long-chain fatty acids in tissues, blood cells, and plasma is present in these patients secondary to defective beta oxidation of long-chain fatty acids.[513] Accumulation of phytanic acid also occurs secondary to defective oxidation.[514] Tissue levels of plasmalogens are reduced secondary to defective synthesis.[515] These abnormalities reflect defective peroxisomal function.[516]

Radiographic studies of patients with Zellweger's syndrome reveal certain characteristic findings, mainly the presence of patches of calcification in cartilage. These have a dense cortex and a reticular central region and characteristically are present in the triradiate cartilage in the acetabulum, the patellae, the sternum, and the scapulae.[517]

Pathology

Liver. Macroscopically, the liver grossly appears unremarkable. Histologic sections of biopsy and autopsy specimens of the liver show changes that may vary from minimal to severe diffuse fibrosis with cirrhosis.[508] The original patients were described as having biliary dysgenesis; however, recent reports show normal biliary ducts in the portal areas, with various degrees of portal fibrosis. The hepatic lobules may contain foci of liver cell necrosis and loss. Prussian blue staining for iron shows a marked increase in iron deposition, mainly in the reticuloendothelial cells.[506] Some patients have minimal or no deposition of iron.[508,518] There is no correlation between the extent of liver damage and iron deposition.[508] Electron microscopic studies show swollen hepatocytes filled with glycogen. The mitochondria are often extremely dense and reduced in number; their cristae are twisted and irregular, with dilation of the intracristate spaces. Typical arrays of rough endoplasmic reticulum are sparse. No peroxisomes can be found in the hepatocytes.[507]

Kidneys. Macroscopically, the surface is studded with small (less than 3 mm in diameter), fluid-filled cysts. Microscopically, the cysts contain dysplastic glomerular and tubular elements and are lined by cuboidal or flattened epithelium. Cysts of glomerular origin and others that appear to be dilated tubular structures are also present. Ultrastructural studies demonstrate a lack of peroxisomes in the proximal tubules.[506,507]

Central Nervous System. Severe cerebral gliosis, subependymal cyst formation, macrogyria, and polymicrogyria were noted. Myelinization was incomplete or lacking.[506] Prussian blue staining shows deposition of iron. Ultrastructurally, the mitochondria of the cortical astrocytes are abnormally dense and often appear degenerate.[507]

Biochemical Features

The mitochondria in the livers, kidneys, and brains of patients with Zellweger's syndrome are structurally abnormal. Functionally, oxygen consumption of mitochondrial fractions prepared from the livers and brains of two patients was diminished by 70 percent. Addition of ADP to the mitochondrial fractions failed to stimulate respiration, although this response was elicited in the control mitochondria.[507]

In vitro studies suggest that the formation of C24 bile acids (chenodeoxycholic acid and cholic acid) from cholesterol is defective in affected patients. It seems that mitochondrial defects are the cause of the abnormalities in bile acid synthesis (see Chap. 10). Because cholic acid and chenodeoxycholic acid are present in these patients, the defect in synthesis is not a complete one. It is possible that in Zellweger's syndrome, chenodeoxycholic and cholic acids are synthesized via an alternate pathway requiring only microsomal enzymes.[519,520]

Molecular Basis of Zellweger's Syndrome

The primary defect in Zellweger's syndrome is impaired assembly of peroxisomes.[521] A rat cDNA encoding the peroxisome assembly factor-1 (PAF-1) was cloned.[522] This cDNA encodes for a 35-kd protein that restores the assembly of peroxisomes in peroxisome-deficient Chinese hamster ovary cell.[523] A human cDNA has been cloned that complements the disease symptoms, including defective peroxisome assembly in fibroblasts from a patient with Zellweger's syndrome.[522] A point mutation in the cDNA of a patient with Zellweger's syndrome resulted in premature termination of PAF-1.[524] These observations were extended to show that at least 23 proteins are required for proper peroxisome assembly.[525-527] Complementation analysis indicated that 12 different complementation groups are defective in patients with peroxisomal disorder. The genes involved in protein assembly of peroxisomes (peroxins) are termed *PEX genes.* Mutations in 10 different PEX genes have been described.[527-537]

Zellweger's syndrome is caused by mutations in any of several different genes involved in peroxisome biogenesis including PEX1, PEX2, PEX5, PEX6, PEX10, PEX12, PEX13, PEX16, and PEX19.[525] The gene affected in complementation group 1 is PEX1. Approximately 65 percent of patients with peroxisomal biogenesis disorders harbor mutations in PEX1. A complete lack of PEX1 protein was found to be associated with Zellweger's syndrome; however, residual amounts of PEX1 protein were found in milder phenotype (neonatal adrenoleukodystrophy) and infantile Refsum's disease. The most common mutation described is G843D. This missense mutation results in misfolded protein.[538]

Prognosis

Patients who have Zellweger's syndrome die in the first year of life of malnutrition, liver failure, and intercurrent infections.[506,508] Desferrioxamine enhances urinary excretion of iron but unfortunately does not influence ultimate outcome.

Genetics

An autosomal recessive inheritance is suggested by family studies. A prenatal diagnosis based on detection of elevated levels of a very long-chain fatty acid, hexacosanoic acid (C26:0) in cultured amniotic fluid cells has been described.[539] The impaired oxidation of very long-chain fatty acids is secondary to the absence of the peroxisomes seen in Zellweger's patients. Determination of mutations in PEX genes will eventually replace the biochemical analysis of urine in these patients.

The THCA Syndrome

In 1972 Eyssen and co-workers described two children with neonatal cholestatic liver disease and markedly elevated levels of THCA in the duodenal fluid. In normal individuals THCA is not present in either serum or bile. The patients had other congenital abnormalities such as frontal bossing, epicanthal folds, and simian creases.[540] In 1975 Hanson and associates described two siblings with a rapidly progressive form of intrahepatic cholestasis that was associated with very high levels of THCA in bile and serum.[541] Hanson's patients differed from those described by Eyssen and colleagues in that no other congenital abnormality was present in the former group. However, all four patients had a paucity of bile ducts, and all died before the age of 2 years.

Clinical Features

The two patients reported by Eyssen's group had cholestatic jaundice at 2 to 3 months of age. Jaundice remitted in both between 4 and 5 months of age. The first patient died at the age of 8 months of severe malnutrition.[540] The two patients reported by Hanson's group had jaundice. Hepatosplenomegaly was present at birth in one and at 4 months of age in the other. Pruritus was not observed. Both patients failed to gain weight and died with progressive liver disease before the age of 2 years.[541]

Laboratory Findings

Both patients reported by Hanson and co-workers had elevated total and direct serum bilirubin. Serum alkaline phosphatase was markedly elevated; however, cholesterol and triglycerides were normal in one patient. Both patients had radiographic evidence of rickets. Results of bile acid analyses of the duodenal fluids of the patients of Eyssen and associates are shown in Table 48-7. In the two cases reported by Hanson THCA amounted to 72 percent and 65 percent of total bile acids in the sera. Cholic acid was not detectable in the serum of the first patient and constituted only 6 percent of serum bile acids in the second. Chenodeoxycholic acid amounted to 28 percent and 22 percent of the total bile acids, respectively. Normally, THCA is not detectable in human bile or serum.

Biochemical Features

All four patients had very high levels of THCA in their sera. The metabolism of THCA was studied in one patient after an intravenous injection of [^{3}H]THCA, and the cause of the increase in THCA was found to be a metabolic defect in the conversion of THCA to cholic acid.[541] Because varanic acid, a metabolite of THCA, could not be identified in the serum of either of the two patients reported by Hanson's group, it is reasonable to assume that the defect is due to a deficiency of the 24-hydroxylating enzyme system required to convert THCA to varanic acid.[541] The toxicity of THCA has not been investigated thoroughly, although Lee and Whitehouse demonstrated that THCA is a potent uncoupler of oxidative phosphorylation.[542] Thus it is possible that the destruction of the intrahepatic biliary ducts might be due to an accumulation of THCA.

Pathology

Liver biopsy specimens show a paucity of ductular structures with an increase in connective tissue in the portal areas. Subsequent liver biopsy specimens show rapid progression to cirrhosis.

Prognosis

All four patients whose cases were reported died before the age of 2 years with hepatic cirrhosis.

Genetics

The disease appears to be inherited as an autosomal-recessive trait.

TABLE 48-7
Results of Duodenal Bile Acid Analysis in THCA Syndrome*

			RELATIVE CONCENTRATION (%)		
	Age (months)	Total bile salt (mg/100 ml)	Chenodeoxycholic acid	Cholic acid	THCA
Patient 1	4.5	26	23	58	19
Patient 2	3.5	61	18	37	45
Control 1	3	251	51	49	0
Control 2	4	424	39	61	0

THCA, $3\alpha,7\alpha,12\alpha$-trihydroxy-5β-cholestan-26-oic acid.
*Patients of Eyssen H, Parmentier G, Compernolle F, et al: Trihydroxycoprostanic acid in the duodenal fluid of two children with intrahepatic bile duct anomalies. Biochim Biophys Acta 273:212, 1972.

Therapy

Cholestyramine therapy was not effective in preventing the development of hepatic cirrhosis.[541]

CYSTIC FIBROSIS

Cystic fibrosis is the most common cause of chronic obstructive pulmonary disease and of pancreatic insufficiency in the first three decades of life in the United States. Today, as more patients with cystic fibrosis reach reproductive age, the hepatic complications of cystic fibrosis are encountered with increasing frequency. In her first review of cystic fibrosis of the pancreas Anderson found three patients with hepatic cirrhosis already reported and added one of her own.[543] Farber provided an excellent description of an unfamiliar type of cirrhosis with gross lobulation of the liver, which he found in a few of his 87 patients with cystic fibrosis. Early histologic changes in the liver included enlargement of the portal areas with biliary duct proliferation and accumulation of eosinophilic material within the lumens of the biliary ducts. The cirrhotic change was attributed to obstruction of the biliary ductules by inspissated secretions.[544] Bodian described focal cirrhotic lesions found in one fourth of 62 patients with cystic fibrosis examined at necropsy. These findings were present in virtually all patients older than 1 year. Bodian proposed the descriptive term *focal biliary cirrhosis.* This lesion had been asymptomatic in all of Bodian's patients.[545]

Craig and associates found 7 patients with cirrhosis of the liver among 150 patients with cystic fibrosis examined at necropsy. Microscopically, the investigators found obstruction of biliary ductules by eosinophilic amorphous material surrounded by areas marked by fibrosis and biliary duct proliferation. The focal character of the extensive hepatic damage was emphasized.[546]

di Sant'Agnese and Blanc described cystic fibrosis and multi-lobular hepatic cirrhosis in seven patients 4 to 10 years old. To establish the evolution of the hepatic lesions, di Sant'Agnese and Blanc reviewed the autopsy material of 116 patients with cystic fibrosis. Of 25 patients who had cirrhotic lesions, 16 had single or multiple lesions of focal biliary cirrhosis. The changes were more extensive in nine. A multi-lobular biliary cirrhosis was found in six of these. Younger patients had focal biliary cirrhosis; older patients had multi-lobular cirrhosis.[547]

Clinical Features

Liver Disease in Infancy

Cystic fibrosis may manifest in the newborn period with obstructive jaundice.[548-554] In all of 10 such infants the onset of jaundice was before 3 weeks of age, and it occurred before 10 days of age in 8 patients.[544] Jaundice persisted from 20 days to 6 months. Meconium ileus with or without small intestinal atresia or combined with volvulus was found in approximately half of these patients. In three patients subjected to laparotomy accumulation of thick, viscid bile was thought to have caused extrahepatic obstruction.[552-555] Biliary duct proliferation without plugging by inspissated material was detected in the livers of five of nine patients with meconium ileus and intestinal atresia whose livers were examined. However, the authors do not rule out that the obstruction might have occurred in more central ducts.[549] Neonatal hepatitis with marked giant cell transformation of the hepatocytes was documented in a 2-month-old patient with cystic fibrosis and obstructive jaundice.[555] Some infants may make a complete recovery, and some may die of liver failure and other complications of cystic fibrosis. The diagnosis is suspected on the basis of a history of meconium ileus.

Liver Disease in Childhood and Adolescence

Symptomatic liver disease was noted in 2.2 percent[556,557] to 16 percent[554] of patients with cystic fibrosis in two series. In the largest reported series from Boston 48 of 2500 patients with cystic fibrosis developed portal hypertension. The incidence of portal hypertension increases more than tenfold for patients who are adolescent or older.[558,559] Interestingly, several members of the same family developed cirrhosis and its complications. A similar observation was reported by Stern and colleagues. Initial symptoms of hepatic complications begin between 9 and 19 years of age. Of 693 patients with cystic fibrosis observed during a period of 18 years, 15 developed clinical hepatic disease, an incidence of 2.2 percent. In 13 of these 15 patients all symptoms were related to portal hypertension, such as gastrointestinal bleeding or hypersplenism. Hepatocellular dysfunction was the principal feature in one of the remaining two cases, and massive hepatomegaly and failure to thrive were dominant in the other.[556] A similar experience was reported from Switzerland. Of 204 unselected patients with cystic fibrosis 7 were found to have hepatic cirrhosis, an incidence of 3.4 percent. Two of the seven patients came to medical attention because of hematemesis. The hepatic abnormality in the others was detected because of hepatosplenomegaly and failure to thrive.[560] In two further studies 24 percent of 233 adults with cystic fibrosis in Britain had abnormal results of liver tests.[561] Similarly, 35 percent of 31 Swedish teenagers with cystic fibrosis had hepatosplenomegaly.[562]

To assess the evolution of liver disease in cystic fibrosis patients, Ling and co-workers prospectively followed 124 children with cystic fibrosis for 4 years. At the initial assessment 42% had hepatic biochemical abnormalities, 35 percent had ultrasound abnormalities, and 6 percent had clinical abnormalities of the liver. In cross sectional analysis, abnormal biochemistry was present in 40 percent of children with ultrasound and clinical abnormalities. Sixty-eight percent of the children showed ultrasound or clinical evidence of liver abnormality at some point during the 4-year follow-up. However, no association between liver disease and nutritional status was found.[563]

Documentation of mild hepatic involvement is often difficult, because clinical manifestations, including jaundice, may be lacking. Results of liver tests may be normal. The BSP excretion test may be of help in detecting early hepatic involvement.[564] The best early indication of hepatic involvement is an elevated level of the hepatic isoenzyme of alkaline phosphatase.[565,566] Total serum alkaline phosphatase activity is not reliable in the evaluation of hepatic involvement in children with cystic fibrosis because age-related normal values for alkaline phosphatase are hard to establish. Also, puberty is often delayed in patients with cystic fibrosis; hence total alkaline phosphatase may appear to be normal in the presence of liver disease.[560]

It is important to emphasize that hepatic disease, including portal hypertension, may be present in patients with cystic fibrosis even when results of liver tests are normal or only slightly abnormal. In fact, the first manifestation of cystic fibrosis may be portal hypertension in a previously asymptomatic patient. Thus children and young adults with unexplained portal hypertension or other hepatic abnormalities should be tested by pilocarpine iontophoresis and by chemical determination of the chloride level in sweat.

Gallbladder Disease

Clinical symptoms of cholelithiasis and cholecystitis have been found in some patients with cystic fibrosis. Microgallbladder has been reported to be present in approximately 15 percent of cases and poor or non-visualization of the gallbladder in another 25 percent.[567] Gallbladder stones are found in as many as 8 percent of patients.[568] The gallbladder disease in these patients may be related to occlusion of the cystic duct by precipitation of abnormal secretions and to abnormal biliary lipid composition.[569]

The pathogenesis of the increased incidence of gallbladder stones in cystic fibrosis was investigated by analysis of biliary lipid in 26 patients with cystic fibrosis, 7 children with cholelithiasis without cystic fibrosis, and 13 controls. For 14 patients with cystic fibrosis who had stopped taking pancreatic enzymes a week earlier, the molar percentage of lipid composition accounted for by cholesterol (mean ± standard error 16.3 ± 2.9) and the saturation index (2.0 ± 0.3) were comparable to values obtained for the group with cholelithiasis but no cystic fibrosis. For 12 patients with cystic fibrosis taking pancreatic enzymes, the molar percentage of cholesterol (8.6 ± 1.7) and the saturation index (1.0 ± 0.1) did not differ from those of controls. Bile salt analysis revealed a striking preponderance of cholic acid over chenodeoxycholic acid, and the glycine to taurine ratio of conjugated bile acids was lower in enzyme-treated patients with cystic fibrosis than in those not currently receiving treatment. The high ratio of cholic acid to chenodeoxycholic acid is a well-known response to malabsorption of bile acids. The decrease of this ratio and the concomitant normalization of biliary lipids during treatment of patients with cystic fibrosis suggest that the lithogenic bile in cystic fibrosis is secondary to bile acid malabsorption.[569]

Biochemical Characteristics

Cystic fibrosis is related to an abnormality in secretions of the exocrine glands. These secretions contain high concentrations of sodium chloride. Defective chloride secretion is the hallmark of the disease.[570-572]

The biochemical characteristics of the liver disorder are not well understood. Intrahepatic obstruction by eosinophilic concentrations of mucus occurs early in the disease and has been proposed as the cause of cirrhosis in cystic fibrosis.[547] Shwachman found that cirrhosis did not develop in patients with cystic fibrosis who had pulmonary involvement without pancreatic involvement. Thus defects in digestion and absorption appear to be prerequisites for liver disease, except possibly during the neonatal period.[573] Patients with cystic fibrosis and pancreatic insufficiency have markedly elevated fecal bile acid excretion compared with age-matched controls.[574]

Bile acid kinetics were investigated by double-isotope dilution technique in six children with previously untreated cystic fibrosis. All six children had pancreatic insufficiency. The bile acid pool sizes were small and turned over rapidly in untreated patients. When fat excretion was reduced by therapy, the turnover rate of the pool decreased, with twofold enlargement of the pool size. These findings suggest an interruption of enterohepatic circulation.[575] The pathophysiologic mechanism of the interruption of the enterohepatic circulation and its relation to hepatobiliary disease have not been defined.

Molecular Basis of Cystic Fibrosis

The cystic fibrosis gene has been cloned and mapped to chromosome 7.[576] The gene spans 250,000 base pairs and encodes a membrane protein of 1480 amino acids termed *CFTR*.[577] CFTR is believed to be a cyclic adenosine monophosphate (AMP)–regulated chloride channel.[578] CFTR is predicted to have five domains: two membrane-spanning domains, two nucleotide-binding domains, and one unique regulatory (R) domain. The membrane-spanning domains appear to contribute to the organization of the chloride channel, because mutations of specific amino acid residues within the first membrane-spanning domain alter the anion selectivity of the channel. Phosphorylation of the (R) domain, generally by cyclic AMP–dependent protein kinase, is essential for opening of the channel.[579] More than 750 mutations within the cystic fibrosis gene have been reported.[580] The most common mutation is a three base pair–deletion removing a phenylalanine residue at amino acid position 508 (δ508). The 508 mutation accounts for approximately 70 percent of cystic fibrosis cases in the United States.[581] There are four mechanisms by which mutations disrupt the function of CFTR (Figure 48-15).[579] Class I mutations (defective protein products) result in production of little or no full-length protein, with loss of CFTR chloride channel function. These mutations produce premature termination signals because of frameshifts resulting from insertions, deletions, or nonsense mutations.[582] Class II mutations (defective protein processing) result in failure to traffic the CFTR to the correct cellular location.[583] This class includes the most common mutation (δF508). Class III mutations (defective regulation) result from mutations in the nucleotide-binding proteins.[583] Class IV mutations lead to defective chloride conduction. Several mutations in the first membrane-spanning domain affect arginine residues located in putative membrane-spanning sequences. These mutations result in markedly reduced rates of ion flow through single, open channels in inside-out membrane patches. The develop-

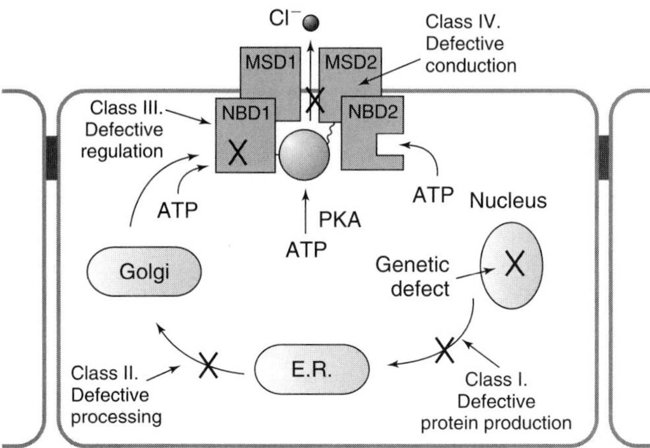

Figure 48-15 Biosynthesis and function of CFTR. *CFTR,* Cystic fibrosis transconductor regulator; *ER,* endoplasmic reticulum; *MSD,* membrane-spanning domain; *NBD,* nuclear-binding domain. (Modified from Welsh MJ, Smith AE: Molecular mechanisms of CFTR chloride channel dysfunction in cystic fibrosis. Cell 73:1251, 1993.)

ment of liver disease in patients with cystic fibrosis was not found to be related to specific mutations in the gene; other environmental or genetic factors may influence the development of liver disease. In this regard a recent study showed that the presence of liver cirrhosis in cystic fibrosis patients is significantly associated with the presence of mutated mannose binding lectin variants.[584] Mannose lectin binding is an important protein of the immune system and has been shown to be a modulating protein in the respiratory involvement of cystic fibrosis.

Laboratory Findings

Sweat chloride levels are elevated in all patients with cystic fibrosis. Total pancreatic exocrine dysfunction is found in 80 percent to 85 percent of the patients. Five percent to 10 percent of the patients have partial insufficiency. The remainder has normal exocrine function. Steatorrhea and azotorrhea are the major consequences of the pancreatic insufficiency. Malabsorption of fat-soluble vitamins A, D, E, and K is the result of pancreatic insufficiency and the use of antibiotics, which alter the bacterial flora of the intestinal tract. Vitamin K deficiency may occur in the first year of life and produce overt hemorrhage.[585] Vitamin A levels are low in the serum but normal or elevated in the liver. A defect in the transport of vitamin A out of the liver is probable. Night blindness and benign increases in intracranial pressure secondary to low vitamin A levels in blood have been reported.[586,587] Vitamin D is poorly absorbed; however, overt rickets is rare. Serum levels of 25-OH vitamin D are reported to be similar to values obtained for normal controls.[588] Two other studies demonstrated low serum levels of 25-OH vitamin D in 4 of 17 patients in one series[589] and in all 21 patients in another.[590] Differences in serum levels reflect different assays and the times of the year during which the patients were studied, because 85 percent of circulating 25-OH vitamin D is of endogenous origin.[588] When patients were studied in winter and early spring, values of serum 25-OH vitamin D were low[589]; however, the other studies were conducted in the summer and early fall.[588,590] These observations suggest a subtle deficiency of vitamin D in patients who have cystic fibrosis and are deprived of sunlight and endogenous vitamin D production.

Liver tests usually show no abnormality. Conjugated hyperbilirubinemia and elevations of serum AST, ALT, and alkaline phosphatase are noted in neonates with obstructive jaundice secondary to cystic fibrosis. Some infants with cystic fibrosis have hypoproteinemia and edema as a result of protein malabsorption, particularly infants who have been breast-fed or fed soybean-based formulas. Breast milk contains only 1.1 percent protein; although adequate for normal infants, it is suboptimal for those who have cystic fibrosis. Soybean-based formula contains small amounts of anti-tryptic activity, which may potentiate the existing malabsorption.

Detecting mild liver involvement in cystic fibrosis is often difficult. The best early indication is elevated alkaline phosphatase of hepatic origin. Measurement of total serum alkaline phosphatase is not helpful (see the previous discussion). The kinetics of BSP excretion show a decrease in hepatic removal rate and biliary secretion and an increase in hepatic-to-plasma reflux as liver disease progresses.[564] In patients with cystic fibrosis and biliary cirrhosis, abnormal liver function and hematologic abnormalities or hypersplenism usually are detected. Abnormalities related to the gallbladder are found in approximately 20 percent of the patients. Oral cholecystography may result in non-visualization of the gallbladder, or microgallbladder or cholesterol stones may be detected.[567]

Pathology

Focal biliary cirrhosis is found in approximately 25 percent of patients with cystic fibrosis examined by necropsy.[547] Progression to a multi-lobular cirrhosis occurs in about 5 percent of surviving children and adolescents. Three histologic types of lesions were identified by Oppenheimer and Esterly[591] in young infants with cystic fibrosis.

1. Focal biliary cirrhosis, characterized by biliary duct proliferation, inspissated granular eosinophilic material filling the biliary ducts, chronic inflammatory infiltration, and variable degrees of fibrosis. The lesions are focal in distribution and vary in number and severity. The incidence of focal biliary cirrhosis increases with age.
2. Excess mucus in biliary duct radicles or in the linings of epithelial cells with periportal changes. The distribution of the biliary mucus is variable and focal, but it is found most often in the large intrahepatic ducts. Biliary duct proliferation and, less commonly, metaplasia of the ductal epithelium are observed. The periportal changes include edema and inflammatory infiltrate. This type of lesion is commonly seen in infants younger than 1 year.
3. Periportal changes without biliary mucus. These changes are common in infants younger than 3 months but are not observed in older children.

It appears that the periportal changes are non-specific and transitory. The accumulation of biliary mucus appears to be related to cystic fibrosis, and because its frequency decreases with age, this indicates that biliary mucus is only one factor in the pathogenesis of focal biliary cirrhosis. Why such a small percentage of the patients (5 percent) develop multi-lobular biliary cirrhosis remains uncertain. Shwachman noted a familial tendency to develop hepatic complications.[573] Nutritional deficiencies and intercurrent infection do not explain the progression to multi-lobular cirrhosis. The relationship in cystic fibrosis between the abnormalities in bile salt metabolism and hepatobiliary disease awaits further investigation.

Hemosiderosis and fatty infiltration of the liver are two other pathologic features of the liver in cystic fibrosis. The increased intestinal absorption of iron that occurs in untreated patients with pancreatic insufficiency may produce hepatic hemosiderosis. The early institution of supplemental enzymes reduces the increased absorption of iron.[592] Hepatic infiltration with fat secondary to chronic malnutrition is frequently observed with cystic fibrosis.[573]

Genetics

Cystic fibrosis is inherited as an autosomal-recessive trait.[593] The highest reported incidence of cystic fibrosis is in Caucasians, primarily those of European origin. The incidence in the Caucasian population in the United States is approximately 1:2000.[594] The disease is less frequent in blacks and Asians.[595] No good incidence figures are available for non-whites with the exception of Hawaiians, for whom the incidence has been reported to be 1:90,000.[596]

Prenatal diagnosis was initially accomplished using a DNA probe (DOCRI-917) that detects restriction fragment length polymorphisms after DNA digestion with Hind III and Hind II. The location of this probe was shown to be about 15 centimorgans from the cystic fibrosis locus.[597] The DOCRI-917 locus was mapped to chromosome 7. Other DNA markers such as met oncogene and PJ3.11, which are known to be on chromosome 7, are also close to the cystic fibrosis locus and have been used by Beaudet and co-workers for prenatal diagnosis.[598] The new development in cloning the cystic fibrosis gene has allowed accurate prenatal diagnosis by analysis of specific mutations in the gene.

Therapy

Hepatic complications of cystic fibrosis that need treatment include those of newborns with obstructive jaundice and those of patients first seen for treatment as adolescents with multi-lobular biliary cirrhosis and portal hypertension. Jaundiced neonates may escape severe hepatic involvement later. Drugs that stimulate bile flow are not helpful. Flushing of the extrahepatic biliary tree with normal saline has been successful in two cases.[552,554] In some cases spontaneous relief of the jaundice has occurred without treatment.[554] The hydrophilic bile acid, ursodeoxycholic acid has been recommended by the U.S. Cystic Fibrosis Foundation Hepatobiliary Disease Census group[599] for patients with established liver disease. However, the Cochrane collaboration concluded that there was insufficient evidence to justify the use of ursodeoxycholic acid.[600] Vitamin supplementation with ADEK preparation appears to reduce the incidence of vitamin K deficiency.[601] More recently Nathanson and coworkers showed that ursodeoxycholic acid stimulates ATP secretion by isolated hepatocytes thus promoting bile flow.[602] The decision to perform portal-systemic shunting in an older patient with portal hypertension depends largely on pulmonary status of the patient. Patients who have severe pulmonary disease are poor candidates for surgery. The long-term survival of these patients is poor, and the complication rate for such a major operation is very high. Those patients who have had single episodes of hemorrhaging or have esophageal varices with good pulmonary function are considered candidates for the shunting procedure.[558,559] Liver, lung, and heart transplantation has been performed in few patients with cystic fibrosis.

References

1. Sachs B, Sternfeld L, Kraus G: Essential fructosuria: its pathophysiology. Am J Dis Child 63:252, 1974.
2. Chalmers RA, Pratt RTC: Idiosyncrasy to fructose. Lancet 2:340, 1956.
3. Froesch ER, Prader A, Labhart A, et al: Die hereditäre Fructose intoleranz, ein bisher nicht bekannte kongenitale Stoff wechselstorung. Schweiz Med Wochenschr 87:1168, 1957.
4. Baker L, Winegrad AI: Fasting hypoglycemia and metabolic acidosis associated with deficiency of hepatic fructose-1,6-diphosphatase activity. Lancet 2:13, 1970.
5. Henry I, Gallano P, Besmond C, et al: The structural gene for aldose B (ALDB) maps to 9q13→32. Ann Hum Genet 49:173, 1985.
6. Mukai T, Yatsuki H, Arai Y, et al: Human aldolase B gene: characterization of the genomic aldolase B gene and analysis of sequences required for multiple polyadenylations. J Biochem 102:1043, 1987.
7. Tolan DR, Penhoet EE: Characterization of the human aldolase B gene. Mol Biol Med 3:245, 1986.
8. Cross NCP, Tolan DR, Cox TM: Catalytic deficiency of human aldolase B in hereditary fructose intolerance caused by a common missense mutation. Cell 53:881, 1988.
9. Cross NCP, Franchis RD, Sebastio G, et al: Molecular analysis of aldolase B genes in hereditary fructose intolerance. Lancet 335:306, 1990.
10. Sebastio G, de Franchis R, Strisciuglio P, et al: Aldolase B mutations in Italian families affected by hereditary fructose intolerance. J Med Genet 28:241, 1991.
11. Tolan DR, Brooks CC: Molecular analysis of common aldolase B alleles for hereditary fructose intolerance in North Americans. Biochem Med Metab Biol 48:19, 1992.
12. Rellos P, Sygusch J, Cox TM: Expression, purification and characterization of natural mutants of human aldolase B. Role of quaternary structure in catalysis. J Biol Chem 275:1145-1151, 2000.
13. Cornblath M, Rosenthal IM, Reisner SH, et al: Hereditary fructose intolerance. N Engl J Med 269:1271, 1963.
14. Froesch ER, Wolf HP, Baitsch H, et al: Hereditary fructose intolerance: an inborn defect of hepatic fructose-1-phosphate splitting aldolase. Am J Med 34:151, 1963.
15. Swales JD, Smith ADM: Adult fructose intolerance. QJM 35:455, 1966.
16. Odievre M, Gentil C, Gautier M, et al: Hereditary fructose intolerance in childhood. Am J Dis Child 132:605, 1978.
17. Mass RE, Smith WR, Welsh JR: The association of hereditary fructose intolerance and renal tubular acidosis. Am J Med Sci 251:516, 1966.
18. Schulte MJ, Widukind L: Fatal sorbitol infusion in a patient with fructose-sorbitol intolerance. Lancet 2:188, 1977.

19. Morris RC Jr, Ueki I, Loh D, et al: Absence of renal fructose-1-phosphate aldolase activity in hereditary fructose intolerance. Nature 214:920, 1967.
20. Perheentupa JE, Pitkanen E, Nikkila EA, et al: Hereditary fructose intolerance: a clinical study of four cases. Ann Paediatr Fenn 8:221, 1962.
21. Shapira F, Dreyfus JC: L'aldolase hépatique dans intolerance au fructose. Rev Fr Etud Clin Biol 12:486, 1967.
22. Hers HG, Joassin G: Anomalie de l'aldolase hépatique dans l'intolérance au fructose. Enzymol Biol Clin 1:4, 1961.
23. Gurtler B, Leuthardt F: Ueber die Heterogeniatat der Aldolase. Helv Chir Acta 53:654, 1970.
24. Rutter JW, Richards OC, Woodfin BM: Comparative studies of liver and muscle aldolase. I. Effects of carboxypeptidase on catalytic activity. J Biol Chem 236:3193, 1961.
25. Drechler ER, Boyer PD, Kowalesky AG: The catalytic activity of carboxypeptidase-degraded aldolase. J Biol Chem 234:2627, 1959.
26. Nordmann Y, Shapira F, Dreyfus JC: A structurally modified aldolase in fructose intolerance: immunologic and kinetic evidence. Biochem Biophys Res Commun 31:884, 1968.
27. Gitzelmann R, Steinmann B, Bally C, et al: Antibody activation of mutant human fructose-diphosphate aldolase B in liver extracts of patients with hereditary fructose intolerance. Biochem Biophys Res Commun 59:1270, 1974.
28. Froesch ER, Prader A, Wolf HP, et al: Die hereditäre Fructose intoleranz. Helv Paediatr Acta 14:99, 1959.
29. Froesch ER: Essential fructosuria, hereditary fructose intolerance, and fructose-1,6-diphosphatase deficiency. In Stanbury JB, Wyngaarden JB, Fredrickson DS, eds: The Metabolic Basis of Inherited Disease, ed 4. New York, McGraw-Hill, 1978:131.
30. van Den Berg G, Hue L, Hers HG: Effect of administration of fructose on glycolytic action of glucagon. An investigation of the pathogeny of hereditary fructose intolerance. Biochem J 134:637, 1973.
31. Kaufmann U, Froesch ER: Inhibition of phosphorylase-a by fructose-1-phosphate, α-glycerophosphate and fructose-1,6-diphosphate: explanation for fructose-induced hypoglycemia and fructose-1,6-diphosphatase deficiency. Eur J Clin Invest 3:407, 1973.
32. Woods HF, Eggleston LV, Krebs HA: The cause of hepatic accumulation of fructose-1-phosphate on fructose loading. Biochem J 119:501, 1970.
33. Raivio KO, Kekomaki MP, Maenpaa PH: Depletion of liver adenine nucleotides induced by D-fructose: dose dependency and specificity of the fructose effect. Biochem Pharmacol 18:2615, 1969.
34. Levin B, Snodgrass GJAI, Oberholzer VG, et al: Fructosemia: observations on seven cases. Am J Med 45:826, 1968.
35. Dormandy TL, Porter RJ: Familial fructose and galactose intolerance. Lancet 1:1189, 1961.
36. Turner RC, Spathis GS, Nabarro JDN, et al: Familial fructose and galactose intolerance. Lancet 2:872, 1972.
37. Schwartz R, Gamsu H, Mulligan PB, et al: Transient intolerance to exogenous fructose in the newborn. J Clin Invest 43:333, 1964.
38. Dubois R, Loeb H, Ooms HA, et al: Etude d'un cas d'hypoglycémie fonctionell par intolérance au fructose. Helv Paediatr Acta 16:90, 1961.
39. Milhaud G: Téchnique nouvelle de misc en evidence d'erreurs congénitales du métabolism chez l'homme. Argent Bras Endocr 13:49, 1964.
40. Levin B, Oberholzer VG, Snodgrass GJAI, et al: Fructosemia: an inborn error of fructose metabolism. Arch Dis Child 38:220, 1963.
41. Lelong M, Alagille D, Gentil C, et al: Cirrhose hépatique et tubulopathie par absence congenitale de l'aldolase hépatique: intolérance héréditare au fructose. Bull Soc Med Hop (Paris) 113:58, 1962.
42. Levin B, Snodgrass GJAI, Oberholzer VG, et al: Fructosemia: observation of seven cases. Am J Med 45:826, 1968.
43. Gentil C, Colin J, Valette AM, et al: Investigation of carbohydrate metabolism in hereditary intolerance to fructose: attempt at interpretation of hypoglycemia. Rev Fr Etud Clin Biol 9:596, 1964.
44. Nikkila EA, Perheentupa J: Non-esterified fatty acids and fatty liver in hereditary fructose intolerance. Lancet 2:1280, 1962.
45. Morris RC: Fructose-induced disruption of renal acidification in patients with hereditary fructose intolerance. J Clin Invest 44:1076, 1965.
46. Morris RC: Evidence for an acidification defect of the proximal renal tubule in experimental and clinical renal disease. J Clin Invest 45:1048, 1966.
47. Morris RC Jr: An experimental renal acidification defect in patients with hereditary fructose intolerance. I. Its resemblance to renal tubular acidosis. J Clin Invest 47:1389, 1968.
48. Morris RC Jr: An experimental renal acidification defect in patients with hereditary fructose intolerance. II. Its distinction from classical renal tubular acidosis: its resemblance to the renal acidification defect associated with the Fanconi syndrome of children with cystinosis. J Clin Invest 47:1648, 1968.
49. Phillips MJ, Path MC, Little JA, et al: Subcellular pathology of hereditary fructose intolerance. Am J Med 44:910, 1968.
50. Marthaler TM, Froesch ER: Hereditary fructose intolerance: dental status of eight patients. Br Dent J 132:597, 1967.
51. Raivio K, Perheentupa J, Nikkila EA: Aldolase activities in the liver of patients with hereditary fructose intolerance. Clin Chim Acta 17:275, 1967.
52. Ian J, Tolan DR: Screening for hereditary fructose intolerance mutations by reverse dot blot. Mol Cell Probes 13:35, 1999.
53. Cornblath M, Schwartz R: Carbohydrate Metabolism in the Neonate. Philadelphia, WB Saunders, 1966.
54. Greenberg RE, Christiansen O: The critically ill child: hypoglycemia. Pediatrics 46:915, 1970.
55. Aronson SM, Perle G, Saifer A, et al: Biochemical identification of the carrier state in Tay-Sachs disease. Proc Soc Exp Biol Med 64:4, 1962.
56. Schneck LG, Perle G, Volk BW: Fructose intolerance in Tay-Sachs disease. Pediatrics 36:273, 1965.
57. Volk BD, Aronson SM, Saifer A: Fructose-1-phosphate aldolase deficiency in Tay-Sachs disease. Am J Med 36:481, 1964.
58. Greene HL, Stifel FB, Herman RH: Hereditary fructose intolerance: treatment with pharmacologic doses of folic acid. Clin Res 20:274, 1972.
59. Melancon SB, Khachadurian AK, Nadler HL: Metabolic and biochemical studies in fructose-1,6-diphosphatase deficiency. J Pediatr 82:650, 1973.
60. Greene HL, Stifel FB, Herman RH: "Ketotic hypoglycemia" due to fructose diphosphatase deficiency and treatment with folic acid. Am J Dis Child 124:415, 1972.
61. Mason HH, Turner ME: Chronic galactosemia. Am J Dis Child 50:359, 1935.
62. Komrower GM, Schwartz V, Holzel A, et al: A clinical and biochemical study of galactosemia. Arch Dis Child 31:254, 1956.
63. Isselbacher KJ, Anderson EP, Kurahashi K, et al: Congenital galactosemia, a single enzymatic block in galactose metabolism. Science 123:635, 1956.
64. Donnell GN, Bergren WR, Cleland RS: Galactosemia. Pediatr Clin North Am 7:315, 1960.
65. Anderson MW, Williams VP, Helmer GR Jr, et al: Transferase-deficiency galactosemia: evidence for the lack of a transferase protein in galactosemic red cells. Arch Biochem Biophys 222:326, 1983.
66. Gitzelmann R: Hereditary galactokinase deficiency, a newly recognized cause of juvenile cataracts. Pediatr Res 1:14, 1967.
67. Chacko CM, McCrone L, Nadler HL: A study of galactokinase and glucose-4-epimerase from normal and galactosemic skin fibroblasts. Biochim Biophys Acta 284:552, 1972.
68. Dahlqvist A, Gamstrup I, Madsden H: A patient with hereditary galactokinase deficiency. Acta Pediatr Scand 29:669, 1970.
69. Gitzelmann R: Deficiency of uridine diphosphate galactose-4-epimerase in blood cells of an apparently healthy infant. Helv Paediatr Acta 27:125, 1972.
70. Gitzelmann R, Steinmann B, Mitchell B: Uridine diphosphate galactose-4-epimerase deficiency. IV. Report of eight cases in three families. Helv Paediatr Acta 31:44, 1976.
71. Holton JB, Gillett MG, MacFaul R, et al: Galactosemia: a new variant due to uridine diphosphate galactose-4-epimerase deficiency. Arch Dis Child 56:885, 1981.
72. Henderson MJ, Holton JB, MacFaul R: Further observations in a case of uridine diphosphate galactose-4-epimerase deficiency with a severe clinical presentation. J Inherit Metab Dis 6:17, 1983.
73. Marchese N, Borrore C: Galactosemia caused by generalized uridine diphosphate galactose-4-epimerase deficiency. J Pediatr 103:927, 1983.

74. Bowling FG, Fraser DK, Clague AE, et al: A case of uridine diphosphate galactose-4-epimerase deficiency detected by neonatal screening for galactosemia. Med J Aust 144:150, 1986.
75. Garibaldi LR, Canine S, Supert-Furga A, et al: Galactosemia caused by generalized uridine diphosphate galactose-4-epimerase deficiency. J Pediatr 103:927, 1983.
76. Stenstam T: Peroral and intravenous galactose tests: comparative study of their significance in different conditions. Acta Med Scand Suppl 177, 1946.
77. Segal S, Blair A: Some observations on the metabolism of D-galactose in normal man. J Clin Invest 40:2016, 1961.
78. Tygstrup N, Winkler K: Galactose blood clearance as a measure of hepatic blood flow. Clin Sci 17:1, 1958.
79. Colcher H, Patek AJ, Kendall FE: Galactose disappearance from the blood stream: calculation of a galactose removal constraint and its application as a test of liver function. J Clin Invest 25:768, 1946.
80. Tygstrup N: Determination of the hepatic elimination capacity (Lm) of galactose by single injection. Scand J Clin Lab Invest 18(suppl 92):118, 1966.
81. Lemaire HG, Mueller-Hill B: Nucleotide sequences of the galE gene and the galT gene of *E. coli*. Nucleic Acids Res 14:7705, 1986.
82. Tajima J, Nogi Y, Fukasawa T: Primary structure of the Saccharomyces cerevisiae GAL7 gene. Yeast 1:67, 1985.
83. Flach JE, Reichardt TKV, Elsas LJ: Sequence of a cDNA encoding human galactose-1-phosphate uridyl transferase. Mol Biol Med 7:365, 1990.
84. Field TL, Reznikoff WS, Frey PA: Galactose-1-phosphate uridyl transferase: identification of histidine-164 and histidine-166 as critical residues by site directed mutagenesis. Biochemistry 28:2094, 1989.
85. Reichardt JKV, Packman S, Woo SLC: Molecular characterization of two galactosemic mutations: correlation of mutations with highly conserved domains in galactose-1-phosphate uridyl transferase. Am J Hum Genet 49:860, 1991.
86. Wang B, Xu Y, Ng WG, et al: Molecular and biochemical basis of galactosemia. Mol Genet Metab 63:263, 1998.
87. Reichardt JKV, Levy HL, Woo SL: Molecular characterizations of two galactosemic mutations and one polymorphism: implications for structure-function analysis of human galactose-1-phosphate uridyl transferase. Biochemistry 311:5430, 1992.
88. Tyfield L, Reichardt J, Fridovich-Keil, et al: Classical galactosemia and mutations at the galactose-1-phosphate uridyl transferase (GALT) enzyme. Hum Mutat 13(6): 417, 1999.
89. Komrower GM, Lee DH: Long-term follow-up of galactosemia. Arch Dis Child 45:367, 1970.
90. Koch R, Donnell GN, Fishler K, et al: Galactosemia. In Kelley VC, ed: Practice of Pediatrics. Hagerstown, MD, Harper & Row, 1979:14.
91. Segal S, Blair A, Roth H: The metabolism of galactose by patients with congenital galactosemia. Am J Med 38:62, 1965.
92. Segal S: Disorders of galactose metabolism. In Stanbury JB, Wyngaarden JB, Fredrickson DS, eds: The Metabolic Basis of Inherited Disease. New York, McGraw-Hill, 1978:164.
93. Levy HL, Sepe SJ, Shih VE, et al: Sepsis due to *Escherichia coli* in neonates with galactosemia. N Engl J Med 297:823, 1977.
94. Segal S, Cuatrecasas P: The oxidation of ^{14}C galactose by patients with congenital galactosemia. Evidence for a direct oxidative pathway. Am J Med 44:340, 1968.
95. Sidbury JB Jr: The role of galactose-1-phosphate in the pathogenesis of galactosemia. In Gardner LE, ed: Molecular Genetics and Human Disease. Springfield, IL, Charles C Thomas, 1960:61.
96. Tada K: Glycogenesis and glycolysis in the liver from congenital galactosemia. Tohoku J Exp Med 82:168, 1964.
97. van Heyningen R: Formation of polyols by the lens of the rat with "sugar" cataracts. Nature 184:194, 1959.
98. Kinoshita JH, Dvornik D, Krami M, et al: The effect of aldose reductase inhibition on the galactose exposed rabbit lens. Biochim Biophys Acta 158:472, 1968.
99. Kinoshita JH, Barber GW, Merola LO, et al: Changes in levels of free amino acids and myo-inositol in the galactose-exposed lens. Invest Ophthalmol 8:625, 1969.
100. Dische Z, Zelmenis G, Youlous J: Studies on protein and protein synthesis—during the development of galactose cataract. Am J Ophthalmol 44:332, 1957.
101. Sippel TO: Enzymes of carbohydrate metabolism in developing galactose cataracts of rats. Invest Ophthalmol 6:59, 1967.
102. Korc I: Biochemical studies on cataracts in galactose fed rats. Arch Biochem 94:196, 1961.
103. Sippel TO: Energy metabolism in the lens during development of galactose cataract in rats. Invest Ophthalmol 5:576, 1966.
104. Kinoshita JH, Merola LO, Tung B: Changes in cation permeability in the galactose-exposed rabbit lens. Exp Eye Res 7:80, 1968.
105. Heffley JD, Williams RJ: The nutritional teamwork approach. Prevention and regression of cataracts in rats. Proc Natl Acad Sci U S A 71:4164, 1974.
106. Schwarz V: The value of galactose phosphate determination in the treatment of galactosemia. Arch Dis Child 35:428, 1960.
107. Quan-Ma R, Wells H, Wells W, et al: Galactitol in the tissues of a galactosemic child. Am J Dis Child 112:477, 1966.
108. Quan-Ma R, Wells W: The distribution of galactitol in tissues of rats fed galactose. Biochem Biophys Res Commun 20:486, 1965.
109. Keppler D, Decker K: Studies on the mechanisms of galactosamine hepatitis. Eur J Biochem 10:219, 1969.
110. Fox M, Thier S, Rosenberg L, et al: Impaired renal tubular function induced by sugar infusion in man. J Clin Endocrinol 24:1318, 1964.
111. Rosenberg L, Weinberg A, Segal S: The effect of high galactose diets on urinary excretion of amino acids in the rat. Biochim Biophys Acta 48:500, 1961.
112. Thier S, Fox M, Rosenberg L, et al: Hexose inhibition of amino acid uptake in the rat kidney cortex slice. Biochim Biophys Acta 93:106, 1964.
113. Saunders S, Isselbacher KJ: Inhibition of intestinal amino acid transport by hexoses. Biochim Biophys Acta 102:397, 1965.
114. Wells W, Pittman T, Wells H, et al: The isolation and identification of galactitol from the brains of galactosemia patients. J Biol Chem 240:1002, 1965.
115. Wells HJ, Gordon M, Segal S: Galactose toxicity in the chick: oxidation of radioactive galactose. Biochim Biophys Acta 222:327, 1970.
116. Granett SE, Kozak LP, McIntyre JP, et al: Studies on cerebral energy metabolism during the course of galactose neurotoxicity in chicks. J Neurochem 19:1659, 1972.
117. Knull HR, Lobert PF, Wells WW: Galactose neurotoxicity in chicks. Effects on fast axoplasmic transport. Brain Res 79:524, 1974.
118. Malone J, Wells H, Segal S: Decreased uptake of glucose by brain of the galactose toxic chick. Brain Res 43:700, 1972.
119. Malone JI, Wells HJ, Segal S: Galactose toxicity in the chick: hyperosmolality. Science 174:952, 1971.
120. Knull HR, Wells WW: Recovery from galactose-induced neurotoxicity in the chick by the administration of glucose. J Neurochem 20:415, 1973.
121. Wooly DW, Gommi BW: Serotonin receptors. IV. Specific deficiency of receptors in galactose toxicity and its possible relationship to the idiocy of galactosemia. Proc Natl Acad Sci U S A 52:14, 1964.
122. Fraser IS, Russell P, Greco S, et al: Resistant ovary syndrome and premature ovarian failure in young women with galactosemia. Clin Reprod Fertil 4:133, 1986.
123. Heidenreich RA, Mallee J, Rogers S, et al: Developmental and tissue specific modulation of rat galactose-1-phosphate uridyl transferase steady state mRNA and specific activity levels. Pediatr Res 34:416, 1993.
124. Robbins SL, Cotran RS: Diseases of infancy and childhood. In Robbins SL, Cotran RS, eds: Pathologic Basis of Disease, ed 2. Philadelphia, WB Saunders, 1979:582.
125. Smetana HF, Olen E: Hereditary galactose disease. Am J Clin Pathol 38:3, 1962.
126. Walker FA, Hsia DYY, Slatis HM, et al: Galactosemia: a study of 27 kindreds in North America. Ann Hum Genet 25:287, 1962.
127. Kirkman HN, Bynum E: Enzymatic evidence of a galactosemic trait in parents and galactosemic children. Ann Hum Genet 23:117, 1959.
128. Mellman WJ, Tedesco TA, Feige P: Estimation of the gene frequency of the Duarte variant of galactose-1-phosphate uridyl transferase. Ann Hum Genet 32:1, 1968.
129. Brandt MJ: Frequency of heterozygotes for hereditary galactosemia in a normal population. Acta Genet (Basel) 17:289, 1967.
130. Tedesco TA, Miller KL, Rawnsley BE, et al: Human erythrocyte galactokinase and galactose-1-phosphate uridyltransferase: a population survey. Am J Hum Genet 27:737, 1975.

131. Scriver CR: Population screening: report of a workshop. Prog Clin Biol Res 163B:89, 1985.
132. Kleijer WJ, Janse HC, van Diggelen OP, et al: First trimester diagnosis of galactosemia. Lancet 1:748, 1986.
133. Anderson EP, Kalckar HM, Kurahashi K, et al: A specific enzymatic assay for the diagnosis of congenital galactosemia. J Lab Clin Med 50:569, 1957.
134. Kliegman RM, Sparks JM: Perinatal galactose metabolism. J Pediatr 107:831, 1985.
135. Gross KC, Acosta PB: Fruits and vegetables are a source of galactose: implications in planning the diets of patients with galactosemia. J Inherit Metab Dis 14:253, 1991.
136. Walter JH, Collins JE, Leonard JV (UK Galactosemia Steering Committee): Recommendations for the management of galactosemia. Arch Dis Child 80:93, 1999.
137. Manis FR, Cohn LB, McBride-Change C, et al: A longitudinal study of cognitive functioning in patients with classic galactosemia, including a cohort on uridine. J Inherit Metab Dis 20:549, 1997.
138. Berry GT: The role of polyols in the pathophysiology of galactosemia. Eur J Pediatr 154(suppl 2):40, 1995.
139. Schweitzer S, Shin Y, Jakobs C, et al: Long-term outcome in 134 patients with galactosemia. Eur J Pediatr 152:36, 1993.
140. Kaufman F, Kogut M, Donnell G, et al: Hypergonadotropic hypogonadism in female patients with galactosemia. N Engl J Med 304:994, 1981.
141. Steinmann B, Gitzelmann R, Zachmann M: Hypogonadism and galactosemia. N Engl J Med 304:995, 1981.
142. Chen YT, Mattison DR, Feigenbaum L, et al: Reduction in oocyte number following prenatal exposure to a diet high in galactose. Science 214:1145, 1981.
143. Chen YT, Mattison DR, Bercu BB, et al: Resistance of the male gonad to a high galactose diet. Pediatr Res 18:345, 1984.
144. Kaufmann FR, Loro ML, Azen C, et al: Effect of hypogonadism and deficient calcium intake on bone density in patients with galactosemia. J Pediatr 123:365, 1993.
145. Renner C, Razeghi S, Uberall MA, et al: Hormone replacement therapy in galactosemic twins with ovarian failure and severe osteoporosis. J Inherit Metab Dis 22:194, 1999.
146. Campbell S, Kulin HE: Transient thyroid-binding globulin deficiency with classic galactosemia. J Pediatr 105:335, 1984.
147. Holtzman NA: Pitfalls of newborn screening (with special attention to hypothyroidism): when will we ever learn? Birth Defects 19:111, 1983.
148. Segal S: Disorders of galactose metabolism. In Stanbury J, Wyngaarden J, Fredrickson D, et al, eds: The Metabolic Basis of Inherited Disease, ed 5. New York, McGraw-Hill, 1983:167.
149. Gitzelmann R, Haigis E: Appearance of active UPD-galactose-4-epimerase in cells cultured from epimerase-deficient persons. J Inherit Metab Dis 1:41, 1978.
150. von Gierke E: Hepato-nephromegalia glykogenia (Glykogenspeicherkrankheiten Leber und Nieren). Beitr Pathol Anat 82:497, 1929.
151. Pompe JC: Over idiopatische hypertrophie van het hart. Ned Tijdschr Geneeskd 76:304, 1932.
152. Cori GT, Cori DF: Glucose-6-phosphatase of the liver in glycogen storage disease. J Biol Chem 199:661, 1952.
153. Hug G: Glycogen storage disease. Birth Defects 12:145, 1976.
154. Howell RR: The glycogen storage diseases. In Stanbury JB, Wyngaarden JB, Fredrickson DS, eds: The Metabolic Basis of Inherited Disease, ed 4. New York McGraw-Hill, 1977:137.
155. Senior B: The glycogenoses. Clin Perinatol 3:79, 1976.
156. Tarui S, Okuno G, Ikuka Y, et al: Phosphofructokinase deficiency in skeletal muscle: a new type of glycogenosis. Biochem Biophys Res Commun 19:517, 1965.
157. Burchell A: Molecular pathology of glucose-6-phosphatase. FASEB J 4:2978, 1990.
158. Countaway JL, Waddell ID, Burchell A, et al: The phosphohydrolase component of the hepatic microsomal glucose-6-phosphatase system is a 36.5 kilodalton polypeptide. J Biol Chem 263:2673, 1988.
159. Waddell ID, Zomerschoe AG, Burchell A: Isolation of a cDNA coding for the glucose-6-phosphatase activity stabilizing protein. Biochem Soc Trans 18:583, 1990.
160. Nordlie R-C, Sukalski KA: Multiple forms of type 1 glucogen storage disease. Trends Biochem Sci 11:88, 1986.
161. Burchell A, Waddell ID, Stewart L, et al: Perinatal diagnosis of type 1 c glycogen storage disease. J Inherit Metab Dis 12:315, 1989.
162. Burchell A, Jung RT, Lang CC, et al: Diagnosis of type Ia and Ic glycogen storage disease in adults. Lancet 1:1059, 1987.
163. Shelly LL, Lei K-J, Pan C-J, et al: Isolation of the gene for murine glucose-6-phosphatase, the enzyme deficient in glycogen storage disease type Ia. J Biol Chem 268:21482, 1993.
164. Brody LC, Abel JK, Castill a LH, et al: Construction of a transcription map surrounding the CRCA1 locus of human chromosome 17. Genomics 25:238, 1995.
165. Lei JK, Shelly LL, Pan CJ, et al: Mutations in the glucose-6-phosphatase gene that cause glycogen storage disease type Ia. Science 262:850, 1993.
166. Lei KJ, Pan CJ, Shelly LL, et al: Identification of mutations in the gene for glucose-6-phosphatase, the enzyme deficient in glycogen storage disease type Ia. J Clin Invest 93:1994–1999, 1994.
167. Brody LC, Abel KJ, Castilla LH, et al: Construction of transcription map surrounding the BRCA1 locus of human chromosome 17. Genomics 25:238, 1995.
168. Hemrika W, Wever R: A new model for the membrane topology of glucose-6-phosphatase: the enzyme involved in von Gierke disease. FEBS Lett 409:317, 1997.
169. Pan CJ, Lei KJ, Annabi B, et al: Transmembrane topology of glucose-6-phosphatase. J Biol Chem. 273:6144, 1998.
170. Lei JK, Chen YT, Chen H, et al: Genetic basis of glycogen storage disease type Ia: prevalent mutations at glucose-6-phosphatase locus. Am J Hum Genet 57:766, 1995.
171. Parvari R, Lei KJ, Bashan N, et al: Glycogen storage disease type Ia in Israel: biochemical, clinical and mutational studies. Am J Med Genet 72:286, 1997.
172. Lei KJ, Pan CJ, Liu, et al: Structure-function analysis of human glucose-6-phosphatase, the enzyme deficient in glycogen storage disease type Ia. J Biol Chem 270:11882, 1995.
173. Kajihara S, Matsuhashi S, Yamamotto K, et al: Exon redefinition by a point mutation within exon 5 of the glucose-6-phosphatase gene is the major cause of glycogen storage disease type Ia in Japan. Am J Hum Genet 57:549, 1995.
174. Stroppian M, Regis S, DiRocco M, et al: Mutations in the glucose-6-phosphatase gene of 53 Italian patients with glycogen storage disease type Ia. J Inherit Metab Dis 22:43, 1999.
175. Emmett M, Narins RG: Renal transplantation in type I glycogenosis: failure to improve glucose metabolism. JAMA 239:1642, 1942.
176. Greene HL, Slonim AE, O'Neill JA Jr, et al: Continuous nocturnal intragastric feeding for management of type I glycogen storage disease. N Engl J Med 294:423, 1976.
177. Roe TF, Kogu MD: Chronic effects of oral glucose alimentation and portacaval shunt in patients with glycogen storage disease type I. Pediatr Res 10:414, 1976 (abstract).
178. Baker L, Mills JL: Long-term treatment of glycogen storage disease type I: clinical improvement but persistent abnormalities of lactate and triglyceride concentration. Pediatr Res 12:502, 1978 (abstract).
179. Crigler JR Jr, Folkman J: Glycogen storage disease: new approaches to therapy. In Porter R, Whelan J, eds: Hepatotrophic Factors. Amsterdam, Ciba Foundation Symposium, 1978:331.
180. Coleman JE: Metabolic interrelationships between carbohydrates, lipids, and proteins. In Bondy PK, Rosenberg LE, eds: Diseases of Metabolism, ed 7. Philadelphia, WB Saunders, 1974:107.
181. Slonim AE, Lacy WW, Terry AB, et al: Nocturnal intragastric therapy in type I glycogen storage disease: effect on hormonal and amino acid metabolism. Metabolism 28:707, 1979.
182. Sadeghi-Nejad A, Presente E, Binkiewicz A, et al: Studies in type I glycogenosis of the liver. The genesis and deposition of lactate. J Pediatr 85:49, 1974.
183. Jakovcic S, Khachadurian AK, Hsia DYY: The hyperlipidemia in glycogen storage disease. J Lab Clin Med 68:769, 1966.
184. Howell RR, Ashton DM, Wyngaarden JB: Glucose-6-phosphatase deficiency glycogen storage disease. Studies on the interrelationships of carbohydrate, lipid and purine abnormalities. Pediatrics 29:553, 1962.
185. Ockerman PA: Glucose, glycerol and free fatty acids in glycogen storage disease type I blood levels in the fasting and nonfasting state: effect of glucose and adrenalin administration. Clin Chim Acta 12:370, 1965.
186. Forget PP, Fernandes J, Begemann PH: Triglyceride clearing in glycogen storage disease. Pediatr Res 8:114, 1974.
187. Hulsmann WD, Eijenboom WHM, Koster JF, et al: Glucose-6-phosphatase deficiency and hyperlipaemia. Clin Chim Acta 30:775, 1970.

188. Fine RN, Strauss J, Connel GN: Hyperuricemia in glycogen storage disease type I. Am J Dis Child 112:572, 1966.
189. Howell RR: The interrelationship of glycogen storage disease and gout. Arthritis Rheum 8:780, 1965.
190. Alepa FP, Howell RR, Klineberg JR, et al: Relationships between glycogen storage disease and tophaceous gout. Am J Med 42:58, 1967.
191. Jakovcic S, Sorensen LB: Studies of uric acid metabolism in glycogen storage disease associated with gouty arthritis. Arthritis Rheum 10:129, 1967.
192. Henderson JF, Khoo KY: Synthesis of 5-phosphoribosyl-1-pyrophosphate from glucose in Ehrlich ascites tumor cells in vitro. J Biol Chem 240:2349, 1965.
193. Greene ML, Seegmiller JE: Elevated erythrocyte phosphoribosylpyrophosphate in X-linked uric aciduria: importance of PRPP concentration in regulation of human purine biosynthesis. J Clin Invest 48:32a, 1969.
194. Raivio KO, Seegmiller JE: Role of glutamine in purine synthesis and in guanine nucleotide formation in normal fibroblasts and in fibroblasts deficient in hypoxanthine phosphoribosyltransferase activity. Biochim Biophys Acta 299:282, 1973.
195. Howell RR: Hyperuricemia in childhood. Fed Proc 27:1078, 1968.
196. Brosh S, Boer P, Jupfer J, et al: De novo synthesis of purine nucleotides in human peripheral blood leukocytes: excessive activity of the pathway in hypoxanthine-guanine phosphoribosyl-transferase deficiency. J Clin Invest 58:289, 1976.
197. Holmes EW, McDonald JA, McCord JM, et al: Human glutamine phosphoribosyl-pyrophosphate amidotransferase: kinetic and regulatory properties. J Biol Chem 248:143, 1973.
198. Greene HL, Wilson FA, Hefferan P, et al: ATP depletion a possible role in the pathogenesis of hyperuricemia in glycogen storage disease type I. J Clin Invest 62:321, 1978.
199. Bode JC, Zelder O, Rumpelt HJ, et al: Depletion of liver adenosine phosphates and metabolic effects of intravenous infusion of fructose or sorbitol in man and in the rat. Eur J Clin Invest 3:436, 1973.
200. Roe TF, Kogut MD: The pathogenesis of hyperuricemia in glycogen storage disease type I. Pediatr Res 11:664, 1977.
201. Corby DG, Putnam CW, Greene HL: Impaired platelet function in glucose-6-phosphate deficiency. J Pediatr 85:71, 1974.
202. Cooper RA: Abnormalities of cell-membrane fluidity in the pathogenesis of disease. N Engl J Med 297:371, 1977.
203. Howell RR, Stevenson RE, Ben-Menachem Y, et al: Hepatic adenomata with type I glycogen-storage disease. JAMA 236:1481, 1976.
204. Roe TF, Kogut MD, Buckingham BA, et al: Hepatic tumors in glycogen-storage disease type I. Pediatr Res 13:931, 1979.
205. Levine G, Mierau G, Favara BE: Hepatic glycogenosis, renal glomerular cysts and hepatocarcinoma. Am J Pathol 82:PPC-37, 1976.
206. Maruyama Y, Kida E, Takagi M: An autopsy case of glycogen storage disease in female adults. J Osaka Med College 25:207, 1962.
207. Bannasch P, Hacker HJ, Klimek, Mayer D: Hepatocellular glycogenosis and related pattern of enzymatic changes during hepatocarcinogenesis. Adv Enzyme Regul 22:97, 1983.
208. Sidbury JB: The genetics of the glycogen storage diseases. Progr Med Genet 4:32, 1965.
209. Farber M, Knuppel RA, Binkiewicz A, et al: Pregnancy and von Gierke's disease. Obstet Gynecol 47:226, 1976.
210. Havel RJ, Blasse EO, Williams HE, et al: Splanchnic metabolism in von Gierke's disease (glycogenosis type I). Tran Assoc Am Physicians 82:302, 1969.
211. Tsalikian E, Simmons P, Gerich JE, et al: Glucose production and utilization in children with glycogen storage disease type I. Am J Physiol 247:E513, 1984.
212. Kalhan SC, Gilfillan C, Tserng K-Y, et al: Glucose production in type I glycogen storage disease. J Pediatr 101:159, 1982.
213. Powell RC, Wentworth SM, Brandt IK: Endogenous glucose production of type I glycogen storage disease. Metabolism 30:443, 1981.
214. Schwenk WF, Haymond MW: Optimal rate of enteral glucose administration in children with glycogen storage disease type I. N Engl J Med 314:682, 1986.
215. Edelstein G, Hirschman CA: Hyperthermia and ketoacidosis during anesthesia in a child with glycogen storage disease. Anesthesiology 52:90, 1980.
216. McAdams AJ, Hug G, Bove KE: Glycogen storage disease types I to X. Criteria for morphologic diagnosis. Hum Pathol 5:463, 1974.
217. Folkman J, Philippart A, Tze WJ, et al: Portacaval shunt for glycogen storage disease: value of prolonged intravenous hyperalimentation before surgery. Surgery 72:306, 1972.
218. Starzl TE, Marchioro TL, Secton AW, et al: The effect of portacaval transposition on carbohydrate metabolism: experimental and clinical observations. Surgery 57:687, 1965.
219. Riddell RG, Davies RP, Clark AD: Portacaval transposition in the treatment of glycogen storage disease. Lancet 2:1205, 1966.
220. Burr IM, O'Neill JA, Karzon DT, et al: Comparison of the effects of total parenteral nutrition, continuous intragastric feeding, and portacaval shunt on a patient with type I glycogen storage disease. J Pediatr 85:792, 1974.
221. Greene HL, Slonim AE, Burr IM: Type I glycogen storage disease: advances in treatment. Adv Pediatr 26:63, 1979.
222. Levin S, Moses SW, Chayoth R, et al: Glycogen storage diseases in Israel. Isr J Med Sci 3:397, 1967.
223. Chen YT, Cornblath M, Sidbury JB: Cornstarch therapy in type I glycogen storage disease. N Engl J Med 310:171, 1984.
224. Collins JE, Leonard JV: The dietary management of inborn errors of metabolism. Hum Nutr Appl Nutr 39:255, 1985.
225. Leonard JV, Dunger DB: Hypoglycemia complicating feeding regimens for glycogen storage disease. Lancet 2:1203, 1978.
226. Greene HL, Slonim AE, Burr IM, et al: Type I glycogen storage disease: five years of management with nocturnal intragastric feeding. J Pediatr 96:590, 1980.
227. Michels VV, Beaudet AL, Pott VE, et al: Glycogen storage disease: long-term follow-up of nocturnal intragastric feeding. Clin Genet 17:220, 1980.
228. Chen Y-T, Coleman RA, Sheinman JI, et al: Renal disease in type I glycogen storage disease. N Engl J Med 318:7, 1988.
229. Baker L, Dahlem S, Goldfarb S, et al: Hyperfiltration and renal disease in glycogen storage disease type I. Kidney Int 35:1345, 1989.
230. Senior B, Loridan L: Studies of liver glycogenosis with particular reference to the metabolism of intravenously administered glycerol. N Engl J Med 279:958, 1968.
231. Bialek DS, Sharp HL, Kane WJ, et al: Latency of glucose-6-phosphatase in type IB glycogen storage disease. J Pediatr 91:938, 1977 (abstract).
232. Harisawa K, Igarashi Y, Otomo H, et al: A new variant of glycogen storage disease type I, probably due to a defect in the glucose-6-phosphatase transport system. Biochem Biophys Res Commun 83:1360, 1978.
233. Lange AJ, Arion WJ, Beaudet AL: Type Ib glycogen storage disease is caused by a defect in the glucose-6-phosphate translocase of the microsomal glucose-6-phosphatase system. J Biol Chem 255:8381, 1980.
234. Anderson DC, Mace ML, Brinkley BR, et al: Recurrent infection in glycogenosis type IB: abnormal neutrophil motility related to impaired redistribution of adhesion sites. J Infect Dis 143:447, 1981.
235. Beaudet AL, Anderson DC, Michels VV, et al: Neutropenia and impaired neutrophil migration in type Ib glycogen storage disease. J Pediatr 97:906, 1980.
236. Heyne K, Gahr M: Phagocytotic extra-respiration: differences between cases of glycogenosis type Ia and Ib. Eur J Pediatr 133:186, 1980.
237. Seger R, Steinmann B, Tiefenauer L, et al: Glycogenosis Ib: neutrophil microbicidal defects due to impaired monophosphate shunt. Pediatr Res 18:297, 1984.
238. Arion WJ, Wallen BK, Lange AJ, et al: On the involvement of a glucose-6-phosphate transport system in the function of microsomal glucose-6-phosphatase. Mol Cell Biochem 6:75, 1975.
239. Skaug WA, Warford LL, Figueroa JM, et al: Glycogenosis type IB: possible membrane transport defect. South Med J 74:761, 1981.
240. Lange AJ, Arion WJ, Beaudet L: Type IB glycogen storage disease is caused by a defect in the glucose-6-phosphatase system. J Biol Chem 255:8381, 1980.
241. Visser G, Rake JP, Fernandes J, et al: Neutropenia, neutrophil dysfunction and inflammatory bowel disease in glycogen storage disease type Ib: results of the European study on glycogen storage disease type Ib. J Pediatr 137(2):187, 2000.
242. Zakim D, Edmonson DE: The role of the membrane in regulation of activity of microsomal glucose-6-phosphatase. J Biol Chem 257:1145, 1982.

243. Greene HL, Zakim D, Edmonson D: Measurement of hepatic steady state and pre-steady state kinetic of glucose-6-phosphatase in a patient with type Ib glycogen storage disease. Pediatr Res 1986.
244. Hiraiwa H, Pan CJ, Ling B, et al: Inactivation of the glucose-6-phosphatase transporter causes glycogen storage disease Ib. J Biol Chem 274:5532, 1999.
245. Hershkovitz E, Mandel H, Fryman M, et al: The gene for glycogen storage disease Ib maps to chromosome 11q23. Am J Hum Genet 62:400, 1998.
246. Elpeleg ON: The molecular background of glycogen metabolism disorders. J Pediatr Endoc Metab 12:363, 1999.
247. Ambruso DR, McCabe ERB, Anderson D, et al: Infectious and bleeding complications in patients with glycogenosis type Ib. Am J Dis Child 139:691, 1985.
248. Corbeel L, Boogaerts M, Van den Berghe G, et al: Clinical and biochemical findings before and after portal-caval shunt in a girl with type Ib glycogen storage disease. Pediatr Res 15:58, 1981.
249. Ishiguro A, Nakahata T, Shimbo T, et al: Improvement of neutropenia and neutrophil dysfunction by granulocyte colony-stimulating factor in a patient with glycogen storage disease type Ib. Eur J Pediatr 152:18, 1993.
250. Brown B, Brown DH: The glycogen storage diseases: types I, III, IV, V, VII, and unclassified glycogenoses. In Whelan WJ, ed: Carbohydrate Metabolism and Its Disorders, vol 2. New York, Academic Press, 1968:123.
251. Bao Y, Dawson TL Jr, Chen YT: Human glycogen debranching enzyme gene (AGL): complete structural organization and characterization of the 5′ flanking region. Genomics 38:155, 1996.
252. Kang-Feng TL, Zheng K, Yu J, et al: Assignment of the human glycogen debrancher gene to chromosome 1p21. Genomics 13:131, 1992.
253. Yang B-Z, Ding J-H, Enghild JJ, et al: Molecular cloning and nucleotide sequence of cDNA encoding human muscle glycogen debranching enyzme. J Biol Chem 267:9294, 1992.
254. Bao Y, Yang BZ, Dawson TL, et al: Isolation and nucleotide sequence of human liver glycogen debranching enzyme mRNA: identification of multiple tissue-specific isoforms. Gene 197:389, 1997.
255. Okubo M, Kanda F, Horinishi A, et al: Glycogen storage disease type IIIa: first reports of a causative missense mutation (G1448R) of the glycogen storage disease type III found in homozygous patients. Hum Mutat 14:542, 1999.
256. Shen J, Bao Y, Liu HM, et al: Mutation in exon 3 of the glycogen debranching enzyme associated with glycogen storage disease that is differentially expressed in the liver and muscle. J Clin Invest 98:252, 1996.
257. Brandt IK, DeLuca VA Jr: Type III glycogenosis: a family with an unusual tissue distribution of the enzyme lesion. Am J Med 40:779, 1966.
258. Murase T, Ikeda H, Muro T, et al: Myopathy associated with type III glycogenosis. J Neurol Sci 20:287, 1973.
259. Van Creveld S, Huijing F: Glycogen storage disease. Am J Med 38:554, 1965.
260. Starzl TE, Putnam CW, Porter KA, et al: Portal diversion for the treatment of glycogen storage disease in humans. Ann Surg 178:525, 1973.
261. Alagille D, Odievre M: Inborn errors of metabolism. In Alagille D, Odievre M, eds: Liver and Biliary Tract Disease in Children. New York, John Wiley & Sons, 1979:217.
262. Ding J-H, de Barsy T, Brown BI, et al: Immunoblot analyses of glycogen debranching enzyme in different subtypes of glycogen storage disease type III. J Pediatr 116:95, 1990.
263. Hug G, Krill CE Jr, Perrin EV, et al: Cori's disease (amylo-1,6-glucosidase deficiency). N Engl J Med 268:113, 1963.
264. Hers HG: Amylo-1,6-glucosidase activity in tissues of children with glycogen storage disease. Biochem J 76:69, 1960.
265. van Hoof F, Hers HG: The subgroups of type III glycogenosis. Eur J Biochem 2:265, 1967.
266. McAdams AJ, Hug G, Bove KE: Glycogen storage disease, types I to X. Criteria for morphologic diagnosis. Hum Pathol 5:463, 1974.
267. Garancis JS, Panares RR, Good TA, et al: Type III glycogenosis: a biochemical and electron microscopic study. Lab Invest 22:468, 1970.
268. Slonim AE, Terry AB, Moran R, et al: Differing food consumption for nocturnal intragastric therapy in types I and III glycogen storage disease. Pediatr Res 12:512/894, 1978 (abstract).
269. Borowitz SM, Greene HL: Cornstarch therapy in a patient with type III glycogen storage disease. J Pediatr Gastroenterol Nutr 6:631, 1987.
270. Anderson DH: Studies on glycogen disease with report of a case in which the glycogen was abnormal. In Ajjar VA, ed: Carbohydrate Metabolism. Baltimore, Johns Hopkins Press, 1952:28.
271. Illingworth B, Cori GT: Structure of glycogens and amylopectins. III. Normal and abnormal human glycogen. J Biol Chem 199:653, 1952.
272. Brown BI, Brown D: Lack of an α-1,4-glucan: α-1,4 glucan 6-glycosyl transferase in a case of type IV glycogenosis. Proc Natl Acad Sci U S A 56:725, 1966.
273. Reed GB Jr, Dixon JFP, Neustein HB, et al: Type IV glycogenosis. Patient with absence of a branching enzyme α-1, 4-glucan: α-1,4-glucan 6-glycosyl transferase. Lab Invest 19:546, 1968.
274. Levin B, Burgess EA, Mortimer PE: Glycogen storage disease type IV, amylopectinosis. Arch Dis Child 43:548, 1968.
275. Motoi J, Sonobe H, Ogawa K: Two autopsy cases of glycogen storage disease-cirrhotic type. Acta Pathol Jpn 23:211, 1973.
276. Brass K: Zur histologischen diagnose der glykogenose type IV (amylopektinose). A Kinkerheilk 117:187, 1974.
277. Ishihara T, Uchino F, Adachi H: Type IV glycogenosis: a study of two cases. Acta Pathol Jpn 25:613, 1975.
278. Bannayan GA, Dean WJ, Howell RR: Type IV glycogen storage disease. Am J Clin Pathol 66:702, 1976.
279. McMaster KR, Powers JM, Hennigar GR Jr, et al: Nervous system involvement in type IV glycogenosis. Arch Pathol Lab Med 103:105, 1979.
280. Ferguson IT, Mahon M, Cumming WJK: An adult case of Anderson's disease-type IV glycogenosis. J Neurol Sci 60:337, 1983.
281. Holmes JM, Houghton CR, Woolf AL: A myopathy presenting in adult life with features suggestive of glycogen storage disease. J Neurol Neurosurg Psychiatr 23:302, 1960.
282. Torvik A, Dietrichson P, Svaar H, et al: Myopathy with tremor and dementia—a metabolic disorder? Case report with post-mortem study. J Neurol Sci 21:181, 1974.
283. Pelissier JF, DeBarsy T, Bille J, et al: Polysaccharide (amylopectin-like) storage myopathy—histochemical, ultrastructural and biochemical studies. Acta Neuropathol 7(suppl):292, 1970.
284. Schochet SS, McCormick WF, Zellweger H: Type IV glycogenosis (amylopectinosis)—light and electron microscopic observations. Arch Pathol 90:354, 1970.
285. Howell RR, Kaback MM, Brown BI: Type IV glycogen storage disease—branching enzyme deficiency in skin fibroblasts and possible heterozygote detection. J Pediatr 78:638, 1971.
286. McMaster KR, Powers JM, Hennigan GR, et al: Nervous system involvement in type IV glycogenosis. Arch Pathol Lab Med 103:105, 1979.
287. Ishihara TF, Uchino H, Adachi M, et al: Type IV glycogenosis—a study of 2 cases. Acta Path Jpn 25:613, 1975.
288. Brown BI, Brown DH: Lack of α-1,4 glucan-α-1,4 glucan 6 glucosyl transferase in a case of type IV glycogenosis. Proc Natl Acad Sci U S A 56:725, 1966.
289. Reed GB, Dixon JFP, Neustein HB, et al: Type IV glycogenosis—patient with absence of a branching enzyme α-1,4 glucan-α-1,4 glucan 6-glucosyltransferase. Lab Invest 19:546, 1968.
290. Greene HL, Ghishan FK, Brown B, et al: Hypoglycemia in type IV glycogenosis: hepatic improvement in patients treated to normalize blood glucose concentrations. J Pediatr 112:55, 1988.
291. Greene HL, Brown B, McClanathan DI: A new variant of type IV glycogenosis: deficiency of branching enzyme activity without apparent progressive liver disease. Hepatology 8:302, 1988.
292. Hers HG: Glycogen storage disease. In Levine R, Luft R, eds: Advances in Metabolic Disorders, vol 1. New York, Academic Press, 1964:1.
293. Ockerman PA: Glycogen storage disease in Sweden. Acta Paediatr Scand Suppl 160, 1965.
294. Fernandes J, Huijing F: Branching enzyme deficiency glycogenosis: studies in therapy. Arch Dis Child 43:347, 1968.
295. Starzl TE, Demetris A, Trucco M, et al: Chimerism after liver transplantation for type IV glycogen storage disease and type I Gaucher disease. N Engl J Med 328:745, 1993.

296. Lin ECC, Knox WE: Specificity of the adaptive response of tyrosine-α-ketoglutarate transaminase in the rat. J Biol Chem 233:1186, 1958.
297. La Du BN, Zannoni VG, Laster L, et al: The nature of the defect in tyrosine metabolism in alcaptonuria. J Biol Chem 230:251, 1958.
298. Shambaugh GE, Warner DA, Biesel WR: Hormonal factors altering rhythmicity of tyrosine-α-ketoglutarate transaminase in rat liver. Endocrinology 81:811, 1967.
299. Gelehrter TD, Tomkins GM: Control of tyrosine aminotransferase synthesis in tissue culture by a factor in serum. Proc Natl Acad Sci U S A 64:723, 1969.
300. Granner D, Chase LR, Auerbach GD, et al: Tyrosine aminotransferase: enzyme induction independent of adenosine 3,5′-monophosphate. Science 162:1018, 1968.
301. Goswami MND, Knox WE: Developmental changes of p-hydroxyphenylpyruvate oxidase activity in mammalian liver. Biochim Biophys Acta 50:35, 1961.
302. Fellman JH, Fujita TS, Roth ES: Assay, properties and tissue distribution of p-hydroxyphenylpyruvate hydroxylase. Biochim Biophys Acta 284:90, 1972.
303. Taniguchi K, Armstrong MD: The enzymatic formation of α-hydroxyphenylacetic acid. J Biol Chem 238:4091, 1963.
304. Goswami MND, Knox WE: An evaluation of the role of ascorbic acid in the regulation of tyrosine metabolism. J Chronic Dis 16:363, 1963.
305. Medes G, Berglund H, Lohmann A: An unknown reducing urinary substance in myasthenia gravis. Proc Soc Exp Biol Med 25:210, 1927.
306. Medes G: A new error of tyrosine metabolism: tyrosinosis. The intermediary metabolism of tyrosine and phenylalanine. Biochem J 26:917, 1932.
307. Mathews J, Partington MW: The plasma tyrosine levels of premature babies. Arch Dis Child 39:371, 1964.
308. Avery ME, Clow CI, Menkes JH, et al: Treatment of tyrosinemia of the newborn: dietary and clinical aspects. Pediatrics 39:371, 1964.
309. Levy HI, Shih VE, Madigan PM, et al: Transient tyrosinemia in full-term infants. JAMA 209:249, 1969.
310. Constantsas NS, Nicolopoulos DA, Agathopoulos AS, et al: Properties and developmental changes of human hepatic and pyruvate enzymes. Biochim Biophys Acta 192:545, 1969.
311. Rizzardini M, Abeliuk P: Tyrosinemia and tyrosyluria in low birthweight infants. A new criterion to assess maturity at birth. Am J Dis Child 121:182, 1971.
312. Bakker HD, Wadman SK, Van Sprang FJ, et al: Tyrosinemia and tyrosyluria in healthy prematures. Time courses not vitamin C-dependent. Clin Chim Acta 6:73, 1975.
313. Wadman SK, Van Sprang FJ, Mass JW, et al: An exceptional case of tyrosinosis. J Ment Defic Res 12:269, 1968.
314. Holston JL Jr, Levy HL, Tomlin GA, et al: Tyrosinosis: a patient without liver or renal disease but with mental retardation. Pediatr Res 48:393, 1971.
315. Kennaway NG, Buist NRM: Metabolic studies in a patient with hepatic cytosol tyrosine aminotransferase deficiency. Pediatr Res 5:287, 1971.
316. Zaleski WA, Hill A: Tyrosinosis: a new variant. Can Med Assoc J 108:477, 1973.
317. Goldsmith LA, Kang E, Beinfang DC, et al: Tyrosinemia with plantar and palmar keratosis and keratitis. J Pediatr 83:798, 1973.
318. Louis WJ, Pitt DD, Davies H: Biochemical studies in a patient with tyrosinosis. Aust N Z J Med 4:281, 1974.
319. Goldsmith LA, Thorpe JM, Roe CR: Hepatic enzymes of tyrosine metabolism in tyrosinemia II. J Invest Dermatol 73:530, 1979.
320. Zaleski WA, Hill A, Kushniruk W: Skin lesions in tyrosinosis. Response to dietary treatment. Br J Dermatol 88:335, 1973.
321. Levine RJ, Conn HO: Tyrosine metabolism in patients with liver disease. J Clin Invest 46:2012, 1967.
322. Norlinger BM, Fulenwider JT, Ivey GL, et al: Tyrosine metabolism in cirrhosis. J Lab Clin Med 94:833, 1979.
323. Van Der Heiden C, Wauters EAK, Ketting D, et al: Gas chromatographic analysis of urinary tyrosine and phenylalanine metabolites in patients with gastrointestinal disorders. Clin Chim Acta 34:289, 1971.
324. Newberry PD, Rohrer JW, Cherian G, et al: Degree and duration of hypoxia needed to produce tyrosyluria. Lancet 1:750, 1972.
325. Kallimaki JL, Lehtonen A, Seppala P: Oral tyrosine tolerance test in rheumatoid arthritis. Ann Rheum Dis 25:469, 1966.
326. Baber MA: A case of congenital cirrhosis of the liver with renal tubular defects akin to those in the Fanconi syndrome. Arch Dis Child 31:335, 1956.
327. Sakai K, Kitagawa T: An atypical case of tyrosinosis. I. Clinical and laboratory findings. Jikeikai Med J 4:1, 1957.
328. Sakai K, Kitagawa T: An atypical case of tyrosinosis. II. A research on the metabolic bloc. Jikeikai Med J 4:11, 1957.
329. Sakai K, Kitagawa T: An atypical case of tyrosinosis. III. The outcome of the patient: pathological and biochemical observations on the organ tissues. Jikeikai Med J 6:15, 1959.
330. Halvorsen S, Gjessing LR: Studies on tyrosinosis: 1, effect of low-tyrosine and low-phenylalanine diet. BMJ 2:1171, 1964.
331. Larochelle J, Mortezai A, Belanger M, et al: Experience with 37 infants with tyrosinemia. Can Med Assoc J 97:1051, 1967.
332. Scriver CR, Larochelle J, Silverberg M: Hereditary tyrosinemia and tyrosyluria in a French Canadian geographic isolate. Am J Dis Child 113:41, 1967.
333. Gentz J, Jagenburg R, Zetterstrom R: Tyrosinemia: an inborn error of tyrosine metabolism with cirrhosis of the liver and multiple renal tubular defects (de Toni-Debre-Fanconi syndrome). J Pediatr 660:670, 1965.
334. Kogut MD, Shaw KN, Donnell GN: Tyrosinosis. Am J Dis Child 113:47, 1967.
335. Kang ES, Gerald PS: Hereditary tyrosinemia and abnormal pyrrole metabolism. J Pediatr 77:397, 1970.
336. Halvorsen S, Pande H, Loken AC, et al: Tyrosinosis: a study of 6 cases. Arch Dis Child 41:238, 1966.
337. Weinburg AG, Mize CE, Worthen HG: The occurrence of hepatoma in the chronic form of hereditary tyrosinemia. J Pediatr 88:434, 1976.
338. Sass-Kortsak A, Ficici S, Paunier L, et al: Secondary metabolic derangements in patients with tyrosyluria. Can Med Assoc J 97:1079, 1967.
339. Scriver CR, Silverberg M, Clow CL: Hereditary tyrosinemia and tyrosyluria: clinical report of four patients. Can Med Assoc J 97:1047, 1967.
340. La Du BN, Gjessing LR: Tyrosinosis and tyrosinemia. In Stanbury JB, Wyngaarden JB, Fredrickson DS, eds: The Metabolic Basis of Inherited Disease, ed 4. New York, McGraw-Hill, 1978:256.
341. Coward RF, Smith P: Urinary excretion of 4-hydroxyphenyllactic acids and related compounds in man, including a screening test for tyrosyluria. Biochem Med 2:216, 1968.
342. Gentz J, Johansson S, Lindblad B, et al: Excretion of δ-aminolevulinic acid in hereditary tyrosinemia. Clin Chim Acta 23:257, 1969.
343. Lindblad B, Lindstedt S, Steen G: On the enzymic defects in hereditary tyrosinemia. Proc Natl Acad Sci U S A 74:4641, 1977.
344. Melancon SB, Gagne R, Grenier A, et al: Deficiency of fumarylacetoacetase in the acute form of hereditary tyrosinemia with reference to prenatal diagnosis. In Fisher MM, Roy CC, eds: Pediatric Liver Disease. New York, Plenum Press, 1983:223.
345. Berger R, Van Farssen H, Smith GPA: Biochemical studies on the enzymatic deficiencies in hereditary tyrosinemia. Clin Chim Acta 134:129, 1983.
346. Taniguchi K, Gjessing LR: Studies on tyrosinosis: 2, activity of the transaminase, parahydroxyphenylpyruvate oxidase, and homogentisic acid oxidase. BMJ 1:969, 1965.
347. Gentz J, Lindblad B: p-Hydroxyphenylpyruvate hydroxylase activity in fine-needle aspiration liver biopsies in hereditary tyrosinemia. Scand J Clin Lab Invest 29:115, 1972.
348. Perry TL, Hardwick DF, Hansen S, et al: Methionine induction of experimental tyrosinaemia. J Ment Defic Res 11:246, 1967.
349. Gaull GE, Rassin DK, Solomon GE, et al: Biochemical observations on so-called hereditary tyrosinemia. Pediatr Res 4:337, 1970.
350. Gaull GE, Rassin DK, Sturman JA: Significance of hypermethioninaemia in acute tyrosmosis. Lancet 1:1318, 1968.
351. Daniel RG, Waisman HA: The influence of excess methionine on the free amino acids of brain and liver of the weanling rat. J Neurochem 16:787, 1969.
352. Lindemann R, Gjessing LR, Merton B, et al: Fructosaemia/"acute tyrosinosis." Lancet 1:891, 1969.
353. Grant DB, Alexander FW, Seakins JWT: Abnormal tyrosine metabolism in hereditary fructose intolerance. Acta Paediatr Scand 59:432, 1970.
354. Bakker HD, De Bree PK, Ketting D, et al: Fructose-1,6-diphosphatase deficiency: another enzyme defect which can present it-

self with the clinical features of "tyrosinosis." Clin Chim Acta 55:41, 1974.
355. Berger R, Smith GPA, Stoker-de Vries SA, et al: Deficiency of fumarylacetoacetate in a patient with hereditary tyrosinemia. Clin Chim Acta 114:37, 1981.
356. Kvittingen EA, Jellum E, Stokke O: Assay of fumarylacetoacetate fumarylhydroxylase in human liver-deficient activity in a case of hereditary tyrosinemia. Clin Chim Acta 115:311, 1981.
357. Furukawa N, Kinugasa A, Seo T, et al: Enzyme defect in a case of tyrosinemia type I acute form. Pediatr Res 18:463, 1984.
358. Kvittingen EA, Brodtkorb E: The pre-and post-natal diagnosis of tyrosinemia type I and the detection of the carrier state by assay of fumarylacetoacetase. Scand J Clin Lab Invest Suppl 184:35-40:1986.
359. Mitchell GA, Grompe M, Lambert M, et al: Hypertyrosinemia. In Scriver CR, Beaudet AL, Sly WS, et al, eds: The Metabolic and Molecular Bases of Inherited Disease. New York: McGraw-Hill, 1998.
360. Phaneuf D, Labelle Y, Bérubé D, et al: Cloning and expression of the cDNA encoding human fumarylacetoacetate hydrolase, the enzyme deficient in hereditary tyrosinemia: assignment of the gene to chromosome 15. Am J Hum Genet 48:525-535, 1991.
361. Grompe M, St-Louis M, Demers SI, et al: A single mutation of the fumarylacetoacetate hydrolase gene in French Canadians with hereditary tyrosinemia type I. N Engl J Med 331:353-357, 1994.
362. Poudrier J, St-Louis M, Lettre F, et al: Frequency of the IVS12+4G-A splice mutation of the fumarylacetoacetate hydrolase gene in carriers of hereditary tyrosinaemia in the French-Canadian population of Saguenay-Lac-St-Jean. Prenat Diagn 16:59-64, 1996.
363. St-Louis M, Leclerc B, Lain J, et al: Identification of a stop mutation in five Finnish patients suffering from hereditary tyrosinemia type I. Hum Mol Genet 3:69-72, 1994.
364. Rootwelt H, Hoie K, Berger R, et al: Fumarylacetoacetate mutations in tyrosinaemia type I. Hum Mutat 7:239-243, 1996.
365. Rootwelt H, Berger R, Gray G, et al: Novel splice, missense, and nonsense mutations in the fumarylacetoacetase gene causing tyrosinemia type I. Am J Hum Genet 55:653-658, 1994.
366. Prive L: Pathological findings in patients with tyrosinemia. Can Med Assoc J 97:1054, 1967.
367. Partington MW, Haust MD: A patient with tyrosinemia and hypermethioninemia. Can Med Assoc J 97:1059, 1967.
368. Perry TL: Tyrosinemia associated with hypermethioninemia and islet cell hyperplasia. Can Med Assoc J 97:1067, 1967.
369. Bergeron P, Laberge C, Grenier A: Hereditary tyrosinemia in the province of Quebec. Prevalence at birth and geographic distribution. Clin Genet 5:157, 1974.
370. Grenier A, Laberge C: A modified automated fluorometric method for tyrosine determination in blood spotted on paper. A mass screening procedure for tyrosinemia. Clin Chim Acta 57:71, 1974.
371. Grenier A, Belanger L, Laberge G: Alpha-1-fetoprotein measurement. Clin Chem 22:1011, 1976.
372. Kvittingen EA, Steinmann B, Gitzelmann R, et al: Prenatal diagnosis of hereditary tyrosinemia by determination of fumarylacetoacetase in cultured amniotic fluid cells. Pediatr Res 19:334, 1985.
373. Gentz J, Lindblad B, Lindstedt S, et al: Dietary treatment in tyrosinemia (tyrosinosis) with a note on the possible recognition of a carrier state. Am J Dis Child 113:31, 1967.
374. Halvorsen S: Dietary treatment of tyrosinosis. Am J Dis Child 113:38, 1967.
375. Sass-Kortsak A, Ficici S, Paunier L, et al: Observations on treatment in patients with tyrosyluria. Can Med Assoc J 97:1089, 1967.
376. Kogut MS, Shaw KN, Donnell GN: Tyrosinosis. Am J Dis Child 113:54, 1976.
377. Tada K, Wada Y, Yazaki N, et al: Dietary treatment of infantile tyrosinemia. Tohoku J Exp Med 95:337, 1968.
378. Bodegard G, Gentz J, Lindblad B, et al: Hereditary tyrosinemia. III. On the differential diagnosis and the lack of effect of early dietary treatment. Acta Paediatr Scand 58:37, 1969.
379. Michals K, Matalon R, Wong PWK: Dietary treatment of tyrosinemia type I. J Am Diet Assoc 73:507, 1978.
380. Mitchell GA, Russo PA, Dubois J, et al: Tyrosinemia. In Suchy FJ, Sokol RJ, Balistreri WF, eds: Liver Disease in Children, ed 2. Philadelphia, Lippincott, Williams & Williams, 2001: 667-685.
381. Grompe M, Lindstedt S, Al-Dhalimy M, et al: Pharmacological correction neonatal lethal hepatic dysfunction in a murine model of hereditary tyrosinaemia type I. Nat Genet 10:453-460, 1995.
382. Starzl TE, Zitelli BJ, Shavv B Jr, et al: Changing concepts: liver replacement for hereditary tyrosinemia and hepatoma. J Pediatr 106:604, 1985.
383. Mieles LA, Esquivel CO, Thiel V, et al: Liver transplantation for tyrosinemia: a review of 10 cases from the University of Pittsburgh. Dig Dis Sci 35:153, 1990.
384. Goldstein JD, Dana SE, Faust JR, et al: Role of lysosomal acid lipase in the metabolism of plasma low density lipoprotein: observations in cultured fibroblasts from a patient with cholesteryl ester storage disease. J Biol Chem 250:8487, 1975.
385. Sloan HR, Fredrickson DS: Enzyme deficiency in cholesteryl ester storage disease. J Clin Invest 51:1923, 1972.
386. Schiff L, Schubert WK, McAdams AJ, et al: Hepatic cholesterol ester storage disease, a familial disorder. I. Clinical aspects. Am J Med 44:538, 1968.
387. Assmann G, Fredrickson DS, Sloan HR, et al: Accumulation of oxygenated steryl esters in Wolman's disease. J Lipid Res 16:28, 1975.
388. Du H, Witte DP, Grabowski GA: Tissue and cellular specific expression of murine lysosomal acid lipase mRNA and protein. J Lipid Res 37:937-949, 1996.
389. Lohse P, Maas S, Lohse P, et al: Compound heterozygosity for a Wolman mutation is frequent among patients with cholesteryl ester storage disease. J Lipid Res 41:23-31, 2000.
390. Anderson RA, Bryson GM, Parks JS: Lysosomal acid lipase mutations that determine phenotype in Wolman and cholesterol ester storage disease. Mol Genet Metab 68:333-345, 1999.
391. Du H, Duanmu M, Witte D, Grabowski GA: Targeted disruption of the mouse lysosomal acid lipase gene: long-term survival with massive cholesteryl ester and triglyceride storage. Hum Mol Genet 7:1347-1354, 1998.
392. Abramov S, Schorr S, Wolman M: Generalized xanthomatosis with calcified adrenals. J Dis Child 91:282, 1956.
393. Wolman M, Sterk VV, Gatt S, et al: Primary familial xanthomatosis with involvement and calcification of the adrenals. Report of two more cases in siblings of a previously described infant. Pediatrics 28:742, 1961.
394. Crocker AC, Vawter GF, Neuhauser EBD, et al: Wolman's disease: three new patients with a recently described lipidosis. Pediatrics 35:627, 1965.
395. Patrick AD, Lake BD: Deficiency of an acid lipase in Wolman's disease. Nature 222:1067, 1969.
396. Kyriakides EC, Paul B, Balint JA: Lipid accumulation and acid lipase deficiency in fibroblasts from a family with Wolman's disease, and their apparent correction in vitro. J Lab Clin Med 80:810, 1972.
397. Konno T, Fujii M: Wolman's disease: the first case in Japan. Tohoku J Exp Med 90:375, 1966.
398. Eto Y, Kitagawa T: Wolman's disease with hypolipoproteinemia and acanthocytosis: clinical and biochemical observations. J Pediatr 77:862, 1970.
399. Marshall WC, Ockenden BG, Fosbrooke AS, et al: Wolman's disease: a rare lipidosis with adrenal calcification. Arch Dis Child 44:331, 1969.
400. Lough J, Fawcett J, Wiegensberg B: Wolman's disease. An electron microscopic, histochemical and biochemical study. Arch Pathol 89:103, 1970.
401. Sando GN, Rosenbaum LM: Human lysosomal acid lipase/cholesteryl ester hydrolase. J Biol Chem 260:15186, 1985.
402. Anderson RA, Sando GN: Cloning and expression of cDNA encoding human lysosomal acid lipase/cholesteryl ester hydrolase. J Biol Chem 266:22479, 1991.
403. Young EP, Patrick ND: Deficiency of acid esterase activity in Wolman's disease. Arch Dis Child 45:664, 1970.
404. Boyd GS: Effect of linoleate and estrogen on cholesterol metabolism. Fed Proc 21(suppl 11):86, 1962.
405. Coates PM, Cortner J: Acid lipase in cultured amniotic fluid cells. Implications for the prenatal diagnosis of Wolman's disease. Pediatr Res 12:450, 1978.
406. Meyers MA: Diseases of the Adrenal Glands in Radiologic Diagnosis. Springfield, IL, Charles C Thomas, 1963.
407. Beaudet AL, Lipson MH, Ferry GD, et al: Acid lipase in cultured fibroblasts. Cholesterol ester storage disease. J Lab Clin Med 84:54, 1974.
408. Meyers WF, Hoeg JM, Demosky SJ, et al: The use of parenteral nutrition and elemental formula feeding in the treatment of Wolman's disease. Nutr Res 5:423, 1985.

409. Krivit W, Freese D, Chan KW, et al: Wolman's disease: a review of treatment with bone marrow transplantation and considerations for the future. Bone Marrow Transplant 10(suppl 1):97, 1992.
410. Wolman M: Proposed treatment for infants with Wolman's disease. Pediatrics 83:1074, 1989.
411. Fredrickson DS: Newly recognized disorders of cholesterol metabolism. Ann Intern Med 58:718, 1963.
412. Lageron A, Caroli J, Stralin H, et al: Polycorie cholésterolique de l'adulte. I. Etude clinique, électronique, histochinique. Press Med (Paris) 75:2785, 1967.
413. Infante R, Polonovski J, Caroli J: Polycorie cholésterolique de l'adulte. II. Etude biochimique. Press Med 75:2829, 1967.
414. Partin JC, Schubert WK: Small intestinal mucosa in cholesterol ester storage disease: a light and electron microscope study. Gastroenterology 57:524, 1969.
415. Sloan HR, Fredrickson DS: Enzyme deficiency in cholesterol ester storage disease. J Clin Invest 51:1923, 1973.
416. Burke JA, Schubert WK: Deficient activity of hepatic acid lipase in cholesterol ester storage disease. Science 176:309, 1972.
417. Beaudet AL, Ferry GD, Nichols BL Jr, et al: Cholesterol ester storage disease: clinical, biochemical, and pathological studies. J Pediatr 90:910, 1977.
418. Wolf H, Hug G, Michaelis R, et al: Seltene angeborene Erkraukung mit Cholesterinester Speicherung in der Leber. Helv Paediatr Acta 29:195, 1974.
419. Lageron A, Lichtenstein H, Bodin F, et al: Polycorie cholesterolique de l'adulte: Aspects cliniques et histochimiques. Med Chir Dig 4:9, 1975.
420. Fredrickson DS, Sloan HF, Ferrans VJ, et al: Cholesterol ester storage disease: a most unusual manifestation of deficiency of two lysosomal enzyme activity. Trans Assoc Am Physicians 85:109, 1972.
421. Burton BK, Remy WT, Rayman L: Cholesterol ester and triglyceride metabolism in intact fibroblasts from patients with Wolman's disease and cholesterol ester storage disease. Pediatr Res 18:1242, 1984.
422. Lageron A, Lichtenstein H, Bodin F, et al: Polycorie cholesterolique de l'adulte: ápropos d'une nouvelle observation. Nouv Presse Med 3:1233, 1974.
423. Jain L, Vidyasagar D: Use of simvastatin plus cholestyramine in the treatment of lysosomal acid lipase deficiency. J Pediatr 119:1008, 1991.
424. Tarantino MD, McNamara DJ, Granstrom P, et al: Lovastatin therapy for cholesterol ester storage disease in two sisters. J Pediatr 118:131, 1991.
425. Clayton RJ, Iber FL, Ruebner BH, et al: Byler's disease: fatal familial intrahepatic cholestasis in an Amish kindred. J Pediatr 67:1025, 1965 (abstract).
426. Hirooka M, Ohno T: A case of familial intrahepatic cholestasis. Thohku J Exp Med 94:293, 1968. 1968.
427. Clayton RJ, Iber FL, Ruebner BH, et al: Byler disease: fatal familial intrahepatic cholestasis in an Amish kindred. Am J Dis Child 117:112, 1969.
428. Alagille D, Odievre M: Liver and Biliary Tract Disease in Children. New York, John Wiley & Sons, 1978.
429. Carlton VEH, Kinsely AS, Freimer NB: Mapping of a locus for progressive familial intrahepatic cholestasis (Byler's disease) to 18q21-22. Human Mol Genet 4:1049, 1995.
430. Bull LN, Van Eijik MJT, Pawlikowska L, et al: A gene encoding a P-type ATPase mutated in two forms of hereditary cholestasis. Nat Genet 18:219, 1998.
431. Gray OP, Saunders RA: Familial intrahepatic cholestatic jaundice in infancy. Arch Dis Child 41:320, 1966.
432. Odievre M, Gautier M, Hadchouel M, et al: Severe familial intrahepatic cholestasis. Arch Dis Child 48:806, 1973.
433. Whittington PE, Freese DK, Sharp HL, et al: Clinical and biochemical findings in progressive familial intrahepatic cholestasis. J Pediatr Gastroenterol Nutr 18:134, 1994.
434. Ballow M, Margolis CZ, Schachtel B, et al: Progressive familial intrahepatic cholestasis. Pediatrics 51:998, 1973.
435. Dahms BB: Hepatoma in familial cholestatic cirrhosis of childhood: its occurrence in twin brothers. Arch Pathol Lab Med 103:30, 1979.
436. Maggiore G, Bernard O, Riley CA, et al: Normal serum gammaglutamyltransferase activity identifies groups of infants with idiopathic cholestasis with poor prognosis. J Pediatr 111:251, 1987.
437. Chobert MN, Bernard O, Bulle F, et al: High hepatic gammaglutamyltransferase activity with normal serum gamma GT in children with progressive idiopathic cholestasis. J Hepatol 8:22, 1989.
438. Maggiore G, Bernard O, Hadchonel M, et al: Diagnostic value of serum gamma-glutamyl transpeptidase activity in liver disease in children. J Pediatr Gastroenterol Nutr 12:21, 1991.
439. Watkins JB, Perman JA: Bile acid metabolism in infants and children. Clin Gastroenterol 6, 1977.
440. Linarelli LG, Williams CN, Phillips MJ: Byler's disease: fatal intrahepatic cholestasis. J Pediatr 81:484, 1972.
441. Alonso EM, Snover DC, Montag A, et al: Histologic pathology of the liver in progressive familial intrahepatic cholestasis. J Pediatr Gastronenterol Nutr 18:128, 1994.
442. Jacquemin E, Hermans D, Myara A, et al: Ursodeoxycholic acid therapy in pediatric patients with progressive familial intrahepatic cholestasis. Hepatology 25:519, 1997.
443. Whitington PF, Whitington GL: Partial external diversion of bile for the treatment of intractable pruritus associated with intrahepatic cholestasis. Gastroenterology 95:130, 1988.
444. Soubrane O, Gauthier F, DeVictor D, et al: Orthotopic liver transplantation for Byler disease. Transplantation 50:804, 1990.
445. Arnell A, Nometh A, Anneren G, et al: Progressive familial intrahepatic cholestasis (PFIC): evidence for genetic heterogeneity by exclusion of linkage to chromosome 18q21-22. Hum Genet 100:378, 1997.
446. Bourke B, Goggin N, Walsh D, et al: Byler-like familial cholestasis in an extended kindred. Arch Dis Child 75:223, 1996.
447. Bull LN, Carlton VEH, Stricker NL, et al: Genetic and morphological findings in progressive familial intrahepatic cholestasis (Byler disease [PFIC-1] and Byler syndrome): evidence for heterogeneity. Hepatology 26:155, 1997.
448. Strautnieks SS, Kagalwalla AF, Tanner MS, et al: Identification of a locus for progressive familial intrahepatic cholestasis (PFIC2) on chromosome 2q24. Am J Hum Genet 61:630, 1997.
449. Estella MA, Snover DC, Montag A, et al: Histologic pathology of the liver in progressive familial intrahepatic cholestasis. J Pediatr Gastroenterol Nutr 18:128, 1994.
450. Strautnieks SS, Bull LN, Knisely AS, et al: A gene encoding a liver specific ABC transporter is mutated in progressive familial intrahepatic cholestasis. Nat Genet 20:233, 1998.
451. Jansen PLM, Strautnieks SS, Jacquemin E, et al: Hepatocanalicular bile SaH export pump deficiency in patients with progressive familial intrahepatic cholestasis. Gastroenterology 117:1370, 1999.
452. de Vree JML, Jacquemin E, Strom E, et al: Mutations in MDR3 gene cause progressive familial intrahepatic cholestasis. Proc Natl Acad Sci U S A 95:282, 1998.
453. Jacquemin E, de Vree JML, Cresteil D, et al: The wide spectrum of multidrug resistance 3 deficiency: from neonatal cholestasis to cirrhosis of adulthood. Gastroenterology 120:1448, 2001.
454. Smit JJM, Shinkel AH, Oude Elferink RPJ, et al: Homozygous disruption of the murine MDR2 P-glycoprotein gene leads to a complete absence of phospholipid from bile and to liver disease. Cell 75:451, 1993.
455. Jacquemin E, Cresteil D, Manouvrier S, et al: Heterozygous nonsense mutation of the MDR3 gene in familial intrahepatic cholestasis of pregnancy. Lancet 353:210, 1999.
456. Dixon PH, Weerasekera N, Linton KJ, et al: Heterozygous MDR3 missense mutation associated with intrahepatic cholestasis of pregnancy: evidence for a defect in protein trafficking. Hum Mol Genet 9:1209, 2000.
457. Aagenaes Ö, Van Der Hagen CB, Refsum S: Hereditary recurrent intrahepatic cholestasis from birth. Arch Dis Child 43:646, 1968.
458. Sharp HL, Krivit W: Hereditary lymphedema and obstructive jaundice. J Pediatr 78:491, 1971.
459. Aagenaes Ö: Hereditary recurrent cholestasis with lymphoedema—two new families. Acta Paediatr Scand 63:465, 1974.
460. Aagenaes Ö, Cudeman B, Sigstad H, et al: Clinical and experimental relationships between cholestasis and abnormal hepatic lymphatics. Pediatr Res 4:377, 1970.
461. Bloom W: The role of the lymphatics in the absorption of bile pigment from the liver in early obstructive jaundice. Bull Johns Hopkins Hosp 34:316, 1923.
462. Shafiroff BG, Doubilet H, Ruggiero W: Bilirubin resorption in obstructive jaundice. Proc Soc Exp Biol Med 42:203, 1939.
463. Cain JC, Grindlay JH, Bollman JL, et al: Lymph from liver and thoracic duct. Surg Gynecol Obstet 85:559, 1947.

464. Friedman M, Byers SO, Omoto C: Some characteristics of hepatic lymphs in the intact rat. Am J Physiol 184:11, 1956.
465. Bull LN, Roche E, Song EJ, et al: Mapping of the locus for cholestasis-lymphedema syndrome (Aagenaes syndrome) to a 6.6-cM interval on chromosome 15q. Am J Hum Genet 67:994, 2000.
466. Ahrens EH Jr, Harris RC, MacMahon HE: Atresia of the intrahepatic bile ducts. Pediatrics 8:628, 1951.
467. MacMahon HE, Thannhauser SJ: Congenital dysplasia of the interlobular bile ducts with extensive skin xanthomata: congenital acholangic biliary cirrhosis. Gastroenterology 21:488, 1952.
468. Haas L, Dobbs RH: Congenital absence of the intrahepatic bile ducts. Arch Dis Child 33:396, 1958.
469. Watson GH, Miller V: Arteriohepatic dysplasia: familial pulmonary arterial stenosis with neonatal liver disease. Arch Dis Child 48:459, 1973.
470. Alagille D, Odievre M, Gautier M, et al: Hepatic ductular hypoplasia associated with characteristic facies, vertebral malformations, retarded physical, mental, and sexual development, and cardiac murmur. J Pediatr 86:63, 1975.
471. Berrocal T, Gamo E, Navalon J, et al: Syndrome of Alagille: radiological and sonographic findings: a review of 37 cases. Eur Radiol 7:115, 1997.
472. Hoffenberg EJ, Narkewicz MR, Sondheimer JM, et al: Outcome of syndromic paucity of interlobular bile ducts (Alagille syndrome) with onset of cholestasis in infancy. J Pediatr 127:220-224, 1995.
473. Emerick KM, Rand EB, Goldmuntz E, et al: Features of Alagille syndrome in 92 patients: frequency and relation to prognosis. Hepatology 29:822-829, 1999.
474. Quiros-Tejeira RE, Ament ME, Heyman MB, et al: Variable morbidity in Alagille syndrome: a review of 43 cases. J Pediatr Gastronterol Nutr 29:431, 1999.
475. Oda T, Elkahloun AG, Pike BL, et al: Mutations in the human Jagged1 gene are responsible for Alagille syndrome. Nat Genet 16:235, 1997.
476. Li L, Krantz ID, Deng Y, et al: Alagille syndrome is caused by mutations in human Jagged1, which encodes a ligand for Notch1. Nat Genet 16:243, 1997.
477. Riely CA, LaBrecque DR, Ghent C, et al: A father and son with cholestasis and peripheral pulmonic stenosis. J Pediatr 92:406, 1978.
478. Henriksen NT, Langmark F, Sorland SJ, et al: Hereditary cholestasis combined with peripheral pulmonary stenosis and other anomalies. Acta Paediatr Scand 66:7, 1977.
479. Greenwood RD, Rosenthal A, Crocker AC, et al: Syndrome of intrahepatic biliary dysgenesis and cardiovascular malformations. Pediatrics 58:243, 1976.
480. Nischal KK, Hingorani M, Bentley CR, et al: Ocular ultrasound in Alagille syndrome: a new sign. Ophthalmologoy 104:79-85, 1997.
481. Hingorani M, Nischal KK, Davies A, et al: Ocular abnormalities in Alagille syndrome. Ophthalmology 106:33-37, 1999.
482. Brodsky MC, Cunniff C: Ocular anomalies in the Alagille syndrome (arteriohepatic dysplasia). Ophthalmology 100:1767, 1993.
483. Romanchuk KG, Judisch GF, LaBrecque DR: Ocular findings in arteriohepatic dysplasia (Alagille's syndrome). Can J Ophthalmol 16:94-99, 1981.
484. Wells KK, Pulido JS, Judisch GF, et al: Ophthalmic features of Alagille syndrome (arteriohepatic dysplasia). J Pediatr Ophthalmol Strabismus 30:130-135, 1993.
485. Rachmel A, Zeharia A, Neuman-Levin M, et al: Alagille syndrome associated with moyamoya disease. Am J Med Genet 33:89-91, 1989.
486. Woolfenden AR, Albers GW, Steinberg GK, et al: Moyamoya syndrome in children with Alagille syndrome: additional evidence of a vasculopathy. Pediatrics 103:505, 1999.
487. Jouttel A, Corpechot C, Ducros A, et al: Notch3 mutations in CADASIL, a hereditary adult-onset condition causing stroke and dementia. Nature 383:707-710, 1996.
488. Chong SKF, Lindridge J, Moniz C, et al: Exocrine pancreatic insufficiency in syndromic paucity of interlobular bile ducts. J Pediatr Gatroenterol Nutr 9:445-449, 1989.
489. John HA, Loomes K, Weyler R, et al: A study of pancreatic function in 17 children with Alagille syndrome. Gastroenterology 114:A885, 1998.
490. Ghishan FK, LaBrecque DR, Mitros F, et al: The evolving course of infantile obstructive cholangiopathy. J Pediatr 97:27, 1980.
491. Byrne JLB, Harrod MJE, Friedmann JM, et al: Del(20p) with manifestations of arteriohepatic dysplasia. Am J Med Genet 24:673, 1986.
492. Spinner NB, Rand EB, Fortina P, et al: Cytologically balance t(2;20) in a two generation family with Alagille syndrome: cytogenetic and molecular studies. Am J Hum Genet 55:238, 1994.
493. Teebi AS, Krishna Murthy DS, Ismail EAR, et al: Alagille syndrome with de novo del(20)(p11.2). Am J Med Genet 42:35, 1994.
494. Anad F, Burn J, Matthews D, et al: Alagille syndrome and deletion of 20p. J Med Genet 27:729, 1990.
495. Deleuze JF, Hazan J, Dhorne-Pollet S, et al: Mapping of microsatellite markers in the Alagille region and screening of microdeletion by genotyping 23 patients. Eur J Hum Genet 2:185, 1994.
496. Desmaze C, Deleuze JF, Dutrillaux AM, et al: Screening of microdeletions of chromosome 20 in patients with Alagille syndrome. J Med Genet 29:233, 1992.
497. Oda T, Elkahloun AG, Meltzer PS, et al: Identification and cloning of the human homologue (JAG1) of the rat Jagged1 gene from the Alagille syndrome critical region at 20p12. Genomics 43:376, 1997.
498. Pollet N, Boccaccio C, Dhorne-Pollet S, et al: Construction of an integrated physical and gene map of human chromosome 20p12 providing candidate genes for Alagille syndrome. Genomics 42:489, 1997.
499. Spinner NB, Colliton RP, Crosnier C, et al: Jagged1 mutations in Alagille syndrome. Hum Mutat 17(1):18, 2001.
500. Louis AA, Van Eyken P, Haber BA, et al: Hepatic Jagged1 expression studies. Hepatology 30:269, 1999.
501. Yerushalmi B, Sokol RJ, Narkewicz MR, et al: Use of rifampin for severe pruritus in children with chronic cholestasis. J Pediatr Gastroenterol Nutr 29:442-447, 1999.
502. Gauderer MW, Boyle JT: Cholecystoappendicostomy in a child with Alagille syndrome. J Pediatr Surg 32:166, 1997.
503. Bowen P, Lee CSN, Zellweger H, et al: A familial syndrome of multiple congenital defects. Bull Johns Hopkins Hosp 114:402, 1964.
504. Smith DW, Opitz JM, Inhorn SL: A syndrome of multiple developmental defects including polycystic kidneys and intrahepatic biliary dysgenesis in two siblings. J Pediatr 67:617, 1965.
505. Passarge E, McAdams AJ: Cerebro-hepatorenal syndrome. J Pediatr 71:691, 1967.
506. Opitz JM, ZuRhein GM, Vitale L, et al: The Zellweger syndrome (cerebro-hepato-renal syndrome). Birth defects: Original Article Series. New York, Alan R Liss, Inc, 5:144, 1969.
507. Goldfischer S, Moore CL, Johnson AD, et al: Peroxisomal and mitochondrial defects in the cerebro-hepato-renal syndrome. Science 182:62, 1972.
508. Danks DM, Tippett P, Adams C, et al: Cerebro-hepato-renal syndrome of Zellweger: a report of eight cases with comments upon the incidence, the liver lesion and a fault in pipecolic acid metabolism. J Pediatr 86:382, 1975.
509. Hanson RF, Szczepanik-Vanleeuwen P, Williams GC, et al: Defects of bile acid synthesis in Zellweger's syndrome. Science 203:1107, 1979.
510. Moser HW, Bergin A, Cornblath D: Peroxisomal disorders. Biochem Cell Biol 69:463, 1991.
511. O'Brien RT: Iron overload. Pediatrics Semin Hematol 115:122, 1977.
512. Monnens L, Bakkeren J, Parmentier G, et al: Disturbances in bile acid metabolism of infants with the Zellweger (cerebro-hepatorenal) syndrome. Eur J Pediatr 133:31, 1980.
513. McGuinnes MC, Moser AB, Moser HW, Watkins IA: Peroxisomal disorders: complementation analysis using beta-oxidation of very long chain fatty acids. Biochem Biophys Res Commun 172:364, 1990.
514. Poll-The BT, Skjeldal OH, Stokke O, et al: Complementation analysis of peroxisomal disorders and classical Refsum. Fatty Acid Oxidation 321:537, 1990.
515. Brul S, Westerveld A, Strijland A, et al: Genetic heterogeneity in the cerebrohepatorenal (Zellweger) syndrome and other inherited disorders with a generalized impairment of peroxisomal functions. J Clin Invest 81:1710, 1988.
516. Wanders RJA, Schutgens RBH, Barth PG, et al: Postnatal diagnosis of peroxisomal disorders: a biochemical approach. Biochemie 75:269, 1993.
517. Williams JP, Secrist L, Fowler GW, et al: Roentgenographic features of the cerebrohepatorenal syndrome of Zellweger. Am J Roentgenol Radium Ther Nucl Med 115:607, 1972.
518. Patton RG, Christie DL, Smith DW, et al: Cerebro-hepato-renal syndrome of Zellweger: two patients with islet cell hyperplasia,

hypoglycemia, and thymic anomalies, and comments on iron metabolism. Am J Dis Child 124:840, 1972.
519. Setoguchi T, Salen G, Tint GS, et al: A biochemical abnormality in cerebrotendinous xanthomatosis: impairment of bile acid biosynthesis associated with incomplete degradation of the cholesterol side chain. J Clin Invest 53:1393, 1974.
520. Salen G, Shefer S, Setoguchi T, et al: Bile alcohol metabolism in man: conversion of 5β-cholestane-3α, 7α, 12α, 25-tetrol to cholic acid. J Clin Invest 56:226, 1975.
521. Santos MJ, Imanaka T, Shio H, et al: Peroxisomal membrane ghosts in Zellweger syndrome—aberrant organelle assembly. Science 239:1536, 1988.
522. Tsukamoto T, Mirua S, Fujiki Y: Restoration by a 35K membrane protein of peroxisome assembly in a peroxisome-deficient mammalian cell mutant. Nature 350:77, 1991.
523. Tsukamoto T, Yokota S, Fujiki Y: Isolation and characterization of Chinese hamster ovary cell mutants defective in assembly of peroxisomes. J Cell Biol 110:651, 1990.
524. Shimozawa N, Tsukamoto T, Suzuki Y, et al: A human gene responsible for Zellweger syndrome that affects peroxisome assembly. Science 255:1132, 1992.
525. Muntau AC, Mayerhofer PU, Paton BC, et al: Defective peroxisome membrane synthesis due to mutations in human PEX3 causes Zellweger syndrome, complementation group G. Am J Hum Genet 67(4):967-975, 2000.
526. Moser HW: Genotype-phenotype correlations in disorders of peroxisome biogenesis. Mol Genet Metab 68:316-327, 1999.
527. Wanders RJ: Peroxisomal disorders: clinical, biochemical and molecular aspects. Neurochem Res 24:565, 1999.
528. Reuber BE, Germain-Lee E, Collins CS, et al: Mutations in PEX1 are the most common cause of peroxisome biogenesis disorders. Nat Genet 17:445, 1997.
529. Portsteffen H, Beyer A, Becker E, et al: Human PEX1 is mutated in complementation group 1 of the peroxisome biogenesis disorders. Nat Genet 17:449, 1997.
530. Braverman N, Stell G, Obie C, et al: Human PEX7 encodes the peroxisomal PTS2 receptor and is responsible for rhizomelic chondrodysplasia punctata. Nat Genet 15:369, 1997.
531. Motley AM, Hettema EH, Hogenhout EM, et al: Rhizomelic chondrodysplasia punctata is a peroxisomal protein targeting disease caused by a non-functional PTS2 receptor. Nat Genet 15:377, 1997.
532. Purdue PE, Zhang JW, Skoneczny M, et al: Rhizomelic chondrodysplasia punctata is caused by deficiency of human PEX7, a homologue of the yeast PTS2 receptor. Nat Genet 15:381, 1997.
533. Dodt G, Braverman N, Wong C, et al: Mutations in the PTS1 receptor gene, PXR1, define complementation group 2 of the peroxisome biogenesis disorders. Nat Genet 9:115-125, 1995.
534. Chang CC, Lee WH, Moser H, et al: Isolation of the human PEX12 gene, mutated in group 3 of the peroxisome biogenesis disorders. Nat Genet 15:385-388, 1997.
535. Okumoto K, Itoh R, Shimozawa N, et al: Mutations in PEX10 is the cause of Zellweger peroxisome deficiency syndrome of complementation group B. Hum Mol Genet 7:1399-1405, 1998.
536. South ST, Gould SJ: Peroxisome synthesis in the absence of preexisting peroxisomes. J Cell Biol 144:255-266, 1999.
537. Matsuzono Y, Kinoshita N, Tamura S, et al: Human PEX19: cDNA cloning by functional complementation, mutation analysis in a patient with Zellweger syndrome and potential role in peroxisomal membrane assembly. Proc Natl Acad Sci U S A 96:2116-2121, 1999.
538. Walter C, Gootjes J, Mooijer PA, et al: Disorders of peroxisome biogenesis due to mutations in PEX1: phenotypes and PEX1 protein levels. Am J Hum Genet 69:35-48, 2001.
539. Moser AB, Singh I, Brown FR, et al: The cerebro-hepato-renal (Zellweger) syndrome. Increased levels and impaired degradation of very long-chain fatty acids and their use in prenatal diagnosis. N Engl J Med 310:1141, 1984.
540. Eyssen H, Parmentier G, Compernolle F, et al: Trihydroxycoprostanic acid in the duodenal fluid of two children with intrahepatic bile duct anomalies. Biochim Biophys Acta 273:212, 1972.
541. Hanson RF, Isenberg JN, Williams GC, et al: The metabolism of 3α, 7α, 12α-trihydroxy-5β cholestan-26-oic acid in two siblings with cholestasis due to intrahepatic bile duct anomalies. J Clin Invest 56:577, 1975.
542. Lee MJ, Whitehouse MW: Inhibition of electron transport and coupled phosphorylation in liver mitochondria by cholenic (bile acids) and their conjugates. Biochim Biophys Acta 100:317, 1965.
543. Anderson DH: Cystic fibrosis of the pancreas and its relation to celiac disease. Am J Dis Child 56:344, 1938.
544. Farber S: Pancreatic function and disease in early life. V. Pathologic changes associated with pancreatic insufficiency in early life. Arch Pathol 37:238, 1944.
545. Bodian M, ed: Fibrocystic Disease of the Pancreas. London, Heinemann, 1952.
546. Craig JM, Gellis SS, Hsia DY: Cirrhosis of the liver in infants and children. Am J Dis Child 90:299, 1955.
547. di Sant'Agnese PA, Blanc WA: A distinctive type of biliary cirrhosis of the liver associated with cystic fibrosis of the pancreas. Pediatrics 18:387, 1956.
548. Gatzimos CD, Jowitt RH: Jaundice in mucoviscidosis. Am J Dis Child 89:182, 1955.
549. Bernstein J, Vawter G, Harris GBC, et al: The occurrence of intestinal atresia in newborns with meconium ileus. Am J Dis Child 99:804, 1960.
550. Sheir KJ, Horn RC Jr: The pathology of liver cirrhosis in patients with cystic fibrosis of the pancreas. Can Med Assoc J 89:645, 1963.
551. Talamo RC, Hendren WH: Prolonged obstructive jaundice. Am J Dis Child 115:74, 1968.
552. Kulczycki LL: Editorial note. In Quarterly Annotated References to Cystic Fibrosis, Vol. 6. New York, National Cystic Fibrosis Research Foundation, 1967:2.
553. Bachand JP: Un cas insuité de mucoviscidose: atteinte hépatique néonatale. Laval Med 38:371, 1967.
554. Valman HB, France NE, Wallis PG: Prolonged neonatal jaundice in cystic fibrosis. Arch Dis Child 46:805, 1971.
555. Rosenstein BJ, Oppenheimer EH: Prolonged obstructive jaundice and giant cell hepatitis in an infant with cystic fibrosis of pancreas. J Pediatr 91:1022, 1977.
556. Stern RC, Stevens DP, Boat TF, et al: Symptomatic hepatic disease in cystic fibrosis: incidence, course, and outcome of portal systemic shunting. Gastroenterology 70:645, 1976.
557. Feigelson J, Pecau Y, Cathelineau L, et al: Additional data on hepatic function tests in cystic fibrosis. Acta Paediatr Scand 64:337, 1975.
558. Tyson KRT, Schuster SR, Shwachman H: Portal hypertension in cystic fibrosis. J Pediatr Surg 3:271, 1968.
559. Schuster SR, Shwachman H, Toyama WM, et al: The management of portal hypertension in cystic fibrosis. J Pediatr Surg 12:201, 1977.
560. Schwarz HP, Kraemer R, Thurnheer U, et al: Liver involvement in cystic fibrosis. A report of 9 cases. Helv Paediatr Acta 33:351, 1978.
561. Nagel RA, Westerby D, Javaid A, et al: Liver disease and bile duct abnormalities in adults with cystic fibrosis. Lancet 2:1422, 1989.
562. Sinaasapel M: Hepatobiliary pathology in patients with cystic fibrosis. Acta Paediatr Scand 363:45, 1989.
563. Ling SC, Wilkinson JD, Hollman AS, et al: The evolution of liver disease in cystic fibrosis. Arch Dis Child 81:129-132, 1999.
564. Lebenthal E, Jacobson M, Kevy S, et al: Predictive value of BSP kinetics for early liver involvement in cystic fibrosis. Gastroenterology A-30:807, 1974.
565. Boat TF, Doershuk CF, Stern RC, et al: Serum alkaline phosphatase in cystic fibrosis. Interpretation of elevated values based on electrophoretic analysis. Clin Pediatr 13:505, 1974.
566. Kattwinkel J, Taussig LM, Statland BE, et al: The effects of age on alkaline phosphatase and other serologic liver function tests in normal subjects and patients with cystic fibrosis. J Pediatr 82:234, 1973.
567. Rovsing H, Sloth K: Micro-gallbladder and biliary calculi in mucoviscidosis. Acta Radiol 14:588, 1973.
568. Warwick WT, L'heurex PR, Sharp HL, et al: Gallstones in cystic fibrosis. Proceedings of VII International Cystic Fibrosis Congress, 1976:100.
569. Roy CC, Weber AM, Morin CL, et al: Abnormal biliary lipid composition in cystic fibrosis. Effect of pancreatic enzymes. N Engl J Med 297:1301, 1977.
570. Quinton PM: Chloride impermeability in cystic fibrosis. Nature 301:421, 1983.
571. Frizzell RA, Rechkemmer G, Shoemaker RL: Altered regulation of airway epithelial cell chloride channels in cystic fibrosis. Science 233:558, 1986.

572. Quinton PM: Missing Cl conductance in cystic fibrosis. Am J Physiol 251:C649, 1986.
573. Shwachman H: Gastrointestinal manifestation of cystic fibrosis. Pediatr Clin North Am 22:787, 1975.
574. Weber AM, Roy CC, Chartrand L, et al: Relationship between bile acid malabsorption and pancreatic insufficiency in cystic fibrosis. Gut 17:295, 1976.
575. Watkins JB, Tercyak S, Klein PD: Bile salt kinetics in cystic fibrosis: influence of pancreatic enzyme replacement. Gastroenterology 73:1023, 1977.
576. Rommens JM, Iannuzzi MC, Kerem B-S, et al: Identification of the cystic fibrosis gene: chromosome walking and jumping. Science 245:1059, 1989.
577. Riordan JR, Rommens JM, Kerem B-S, et al: Identification of the cystic fibrosis gene: cloning and characterization of complementary DNA. Science 245:1066, 1989.
578. Rich DP, Anderson MP, Gregory RJ, et al: Expression of cystic fibrosis transmembrane conductance regulator corrects defective chloride channel regulation in cystic fibrosis airway epithelial cells. Nature 347:358, 1990.
579. Welsh MJ, Smith AE: Molecular mechanisms of CFTR chloride channel dysfunction in cystic fibrosis. Cell 73:1251, 1993.
580. Tsui L-C, Buchwald M: Biochemical and molecular genetics of cystic fibrosis. In Harris H, Hirschorn K, eds: Advances in Human Genetics. New York, Plenum Press, 1991:153-266.
581. Kerem B-S, Rommens JM, Buchanan JA, et al: Identification of the cystic fibrosis gene: genetic analysis. Science 245:1073, 1989.
582. Tsui L-C: Mutations and sequence variations detected in the cystic fibrosis transmembrane conductance regulator (CFTR) gene: a report from the Cystic Fibrosis Genetic Analysis Consortium. Hum Mutat 1:197, 1992.
583. Cheng SH, Gregory RJ, Marshall J, et al: Defective intracellular transport and processing of CFTR is the molecular basis of most cystic fibrosis. Cell 63:827, 1990.
584. Gabolde M, Hubert D, Guilloud-Bataille M, et al: The mannose binding lectin gene influences the severity of chronic liver disease in cystic fibrosis. J Med Genet 38:310-311, 2001.
585. Walters TJ, Koch HF: Hemorrhagic diathesis and cystic fibrosis in infancy. Am J Dis Child 124:641, 1972.
586. Underwood BA, Denning CR: Blood and liver concentrations of vitamins A and E in children with cystic fibrosis of the pancreas. Pediatr Res 6:26, 1972.
587. Keating J, Feigin RD: Increased intracranial pressure associated with probable vitamin A deficiency in cystic fibrosis. Pediatrics 41:46, 1970.
588. Weisman Y, Reiter E, Stern RC, et al: Serum concentrations of 25-hydroxyvitamin D and in patients with cystic fibrosis. J Pediatr 95:416, 1979.
589. Hubbard VS, Farrell PM, di Sant'Agnese PA: 25-Hydroxycholecalciferol levels in patients with cystic fibrosis. J Pediatr 94:84, 1979.
590. Hahn TJ, Squires AE, Halstead LR, et al: Reduced serum 25-hydroxyvitamin D concentration and disordered mineral metabolism in patients with cystic fibrosis. J Pediatr 94:38, 1979.
591. Oppenheimer EH, Esterly TR: Hepatic changes in young infants with cystic fibrosis: possible relation to focal biliary cirrhosis. J Pediatr 86:683, 1975.
592. Caplan A, Gross S: Hematologic and serologic studies in cystic fibrosis. J Pediatr 73:540, 1968.
593. Danks DM, Allan J, Anderson CM: A genetic study of fibrocystic disease of the pancreas. Ann Hum Genet 28:323, 1965.
594. Merritt AD, Hanna BL, Todd CW, et al: The incidence and mode of inheritance of cystic fibrosis. J Lab Clin Med 60:998, 1962.
595. Oppenheimer EH, Esterly JR: Cystic fibrosis in non-Caucasian patients. Pediatrics 42:547, 1968.
596. Wright SW, Morton NE: Genetic studies on cystic fibrosis in Hawaii. Am J Hum Genet 20:157, 1968.
597. Tsui LC, Buchwald M, Barker D, et al: Cystic fibrosis locus defined by a genetically linked polymorphic DNA marker. Science 230:1054, 1985.
598. Beaudet AL, Rosenbloom C, Spece JE, et al: Linkage of cystic fibrosis and the met oncogene. Pediatr Res 20:470A, 1986.
599. Sokol RJ, Durie PR for the Cystic Fibrosis Foundation Hepatobiliary Disease Consensus Group: Recommendations for management of liver and biliary tract disease in cystic fibrosis. J Pediatr Gastoenterol Nutr 28:S1-S13, 1999.
600. Cheng K, Ashby D, Smyth R: Ursodeoxycholic acid for cystic fibrosis-related liver disease (Cochrane Review). In The Cochrane Library, Issue 2. Oxford: Update Software, 1999:1-11.
601. Wilson DC, Rashid M, Durie PR, et al: Treatment of vitamin K deficiency in cystic fibrosis: Effectiveness of a daily fat-soluble vitamin combination. J Pediatr 138:851, 2001.
602. Nathanson MH, Burgstahler AD, Masyuk A, et al: Stimulation of ATP secretion in the liver by therapeutic bile acids. Biochem J 358(Pt 1):1-5, 2001.

CHAPTER

49

Cystic Diseases of the Liver

C.L. Witzleben, BS, MD, and Eduardo Ruchelli, MD

ABBREVIATIONS

ADPKD	autosomal-dominant polycystic kidney disease
ARPKD	autosomal-recessive polycystic kidney disease
CHF	congenital hepatic fibrosis
DPM	ductal plate malformation

The most interesting advances since the last edition of the book have been in hereditary disorders. A biochemical disorder has been clearly elucidated that provides a possible pathogenesis for ductal plate malformation (DPM) and thus for some hepatic cysts. Molecular biologic studies in renal disease have provided pathogeneses for other hepatic cysts and offer potential avenues for therapy and prevention. In addition, a chromosomal marker has apparently now been established for a previously suspected heritable hepatic cystic disease without renal cysts. Each of these will be described in detail in this chapter.

In this chapter a cyst is defined as a tissue-enclosed space that is abnormal in location or size. The space or cyst may contain only air or it may be filled wholly or partially with liquid or solids. So defined, a cyst may be a normal structure that has become dilated (e.g., a biliary duct) or it may be an abnormal structure with a discrete wall. The latter can be fibrous or composed of various tissues, including those in which it has formed. Abscesses, which are a variety of cyst as defined here, are not discussed in this chapter (see Chaps. 35 and 36). Table 49-1 presents a proposed classification of hepatic cysts. It includes several types (e.g., parasitic, neoplastic) that are discussed more extensively in Chapters 35 and 45.

The classification in Table 49-1 differs somewhat from those usually presented. In our opinion most classifications of hepatic cysts make capricious (and in some respects clinically insignificant) distinctions between congenital and acquired cysts and use the terms Caroli's disease and polycystic disease in an imprecise (or at least inadequately defined) way. In this chapter the definitions used for the classification in Table 49-1 are discussed in detail.

SOLITARY CYSTS

Solitary cysts have no consistent association with cysts in other viscera. They do not have an obvious vascular or lymphatic origin, nor are they components or complications of a discernible tumor. Not all so-called solitary cysts are truly solitary, however, as discussed later. Also there is enough variation among the cysts included in this group to leave open the possibility of diverse origins and types of solitary cysts. On occasion solitary cysts are congenital, in the sense of being present at birth. They are not hereditary, however. Whether or not all solitary cysts deserve to be considered congenital (as indicated in some classifications) is uncertain. A few of the reported cases of solitary cysts (especially when multiple) may have been unrecognized examples of one of the polycystic diseases.

The origins of the cysts included in the group of solitary cysts are not known. The age range of the patients and the variability in the types of cells lining the cyst, and the numbers and sizes of the cysts, raise the possibility that more than one type of cystic disease is represented in this group. There is no convincing evidence for teratomatous origin or for other neoplastic origin (e.g., cystadenoma). The typical lack of bile argues against a duct retention origin in most cases. Some solitary cysts that have no epithelial lining possibly have a traumatic origin. The frequent presence of columnar epithelium in solitary cysts suggests that many have a ductal origin, but their precise genesis is unclear.

The incidence of solitary cysts in the population at large has not been defined, but solitary cysts are uncommon. Henson and co-workers found only 38 cases in a 47-year period at the Mayo Clinic.[1] Increasing numbers of solitary cysts are being discovered, however, with increased use of hepatic sonography. The ratio of symptomatic to asymptomatic solitary cysts was approximately 1:2 in the Mayo Clinic series.[1] Thus the majority of solitary cysts are asymptomatic.

Solitary cysts occur at all ages, from before birth to the ninth decade of life,[2,3] but symptomatic solitary cysts occur predominantly in the fourth and fifth decades of life. In adults there is a clear predominance in women, perhaps in the range of 4:1.[4] This ratio is less well established in children.[5]

TABLE 49-1

Proposed Classification of Hepatic Cysts

I. Parasitic
II. Non-parasitic
  A. Solitary (sporadic; occasionally multiple, possibly multiple origin)
  B. Heritable hepatic cysts
    1. Non-communicating ductal cysts, with cysts and lesions in viscera (ADPKD1, ADPKD2, ?ADPKD3)
    2. With DPM (communicating cysts)
      a. CHF
      b. ARPKD
      c. Phosphomannoseisomerase deficiency (no lesions known in other viscera)
      d. Malformation syndromes
        Meckel-Gruber syndrome
        Other (i.e., Ivemark syndrome)
      e. CHF-nephronophthisis†
    3. "Isolated" hepatic (PLD) (no lesions known in other viscera; cholangiography not done; hepatic histopathology not examined)
  C. Systemic biliary dilatation (not heritable, no DPM, no lesions known in other viscera)
    1. Without choledochal cyst ("simple Caroli's Disease?)
    2. With choledochal cyst
  D. Other
    1. Traumatic
    2. Infarcts
    3. Duodenal duplication
    4. Neoplastic
      a. Cystadenoma and cystadenocarcinoma
      b. Mesenchymal hamartoma
      c. Giant cavernous hemangioma
      d. Teratoma
      e. Other
    5. Peliosis

ADPKD, Autosomal-dominant polycystic kidney disease; *DPM,* ductal plate malformation; *CHF,* congenital hepatic fibrosis; *PLD,* polycystic disease.
*A percentage of cases may have DPM.
†May be unrelated to B-2-a, but is heritable (see text).

Increased abdominal girth is perhaps the most common presenting complaint or finding in patients with solitary cysts. This is nearly always accompanied by a palpable but poorly delineated abdominal mass in the right upper quadrant. Patients also may complain of fullness, flatulence, diarrhea, vomiting, or pain. Nausea, weakness, dysphagia, and weight loss have been reported. Pain, when present, can be either dull, with some aggravation resulting from changes in position, or sharp and intermittent. The latter seems to correlate with pathologic evidence of hemorrhage into the cyst and may be accompanied by chills and fever.[1] Other complications include inflammation, with or without infection, and perforation, which may occur either spontaneously or after trauma.[2] Laboratory findings are typically normal when infection is not present. Occasionally, however, the pressure of a large cyst, usually against the extrahepatic biliary system, causes obstructive jaundice.

The diaphragm may be elevated on the right side, and a mass or density may be evident in the right upper quadrant. Calcification occurs but much less frequently than in hydatid cysts. Other abdominal viscera may be displaced. Sonography is accurate in evaluating cystic masses of the liver (Figure 49-1), and in selected cases, it may be combined with needle aspiration, culture, and microscopic examination of the aspirate.[6] The fluid in a typical solitary cyst is clear, sterile, and cytologically negative. Bleeding into the cyst may occasionally occur, however, or the cyst may communicate with the biliary system. Hydatid disease should be ruled out before aspirating the cyst or cysts (see Chap. 35).[7] Scans may be useful in determining the size, number, and location of cysts and, if appropriate, can be combined with excretory radiography (see Figure 49-1). As mentioned, so-called solitary cysts are not always solitary; not uncommonly, three or four cysts may be present close to one another. There may be multiple cysts throughout one lobe, or on occasion, there may be cysts in both lobes.[4] In all cases of cysts of the liver but particularly in cases of multiple cysts, a careful search should be made for cysts or other abnormalities in other viscera, especially the kidneys. This search must include a careful family history. Extrahepatic cysts, a positive family history, or the presence of the DPM suggests that the patient has one of

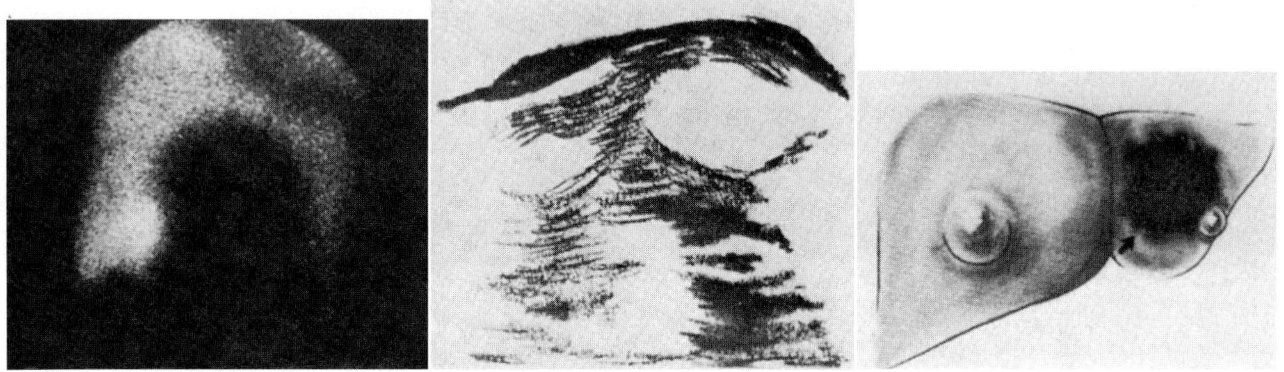

Figure 49-1 Two solitary cysts demonstrated by scan **(A)** and ultrasonography **(B)** and as seen at operation **(C).** (From Hadad AR, et al: Am J Surg 134:739, 1977.)

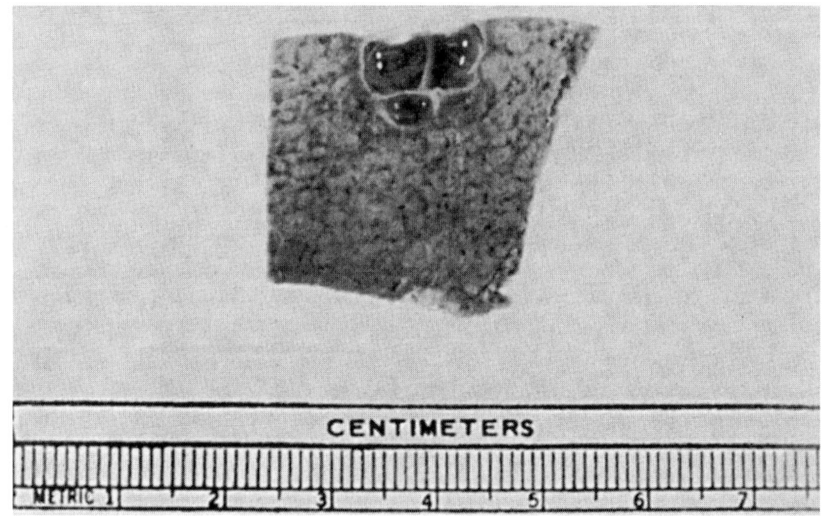

Figure 49-2 Gross photograph of asymptomatic solitary cyst found incidentally at autopsy. The cyst is multilocular, and cyst walls are translucent.

the polycystic diseases (discussed in the section on Hereditary Hepatic Cystic Disease).

Solitary cysts are present in the right lobe of the liver more frequently than in the left. The most common locus is on the anterior-inferior surface. Solitary cysts (Figure 49-2) may be completely intrahepatic or pedunculated. They can vary in diameter from a few millimeters to many centimeters. One of the largest reported cysts contained 17 L of fluid.[2] In general the cysts in symptomatic cases are larger than those in asymptomatic cases.[1]

The external surface of the cyst is smooth and usually translucent; the wall thickness is usually 1 cm or less. Although they are usually unilocular, solitary multilocular cysts have been described (see Figure 49-2). The lining is usually described as smooth. The contents vary from pale yellow, serous fluid to viscid material to semisolid, brownish-black material. Among the contents that have been identified are blood, mucin, cellular debris, albumin, cholesterol, and rarely, bile. The pH is said to be alkaline.[2,4] Usually there are no connections with the biliary system, vasculature, or lymphatics. As mentioned, connections with the biliary system may be present in rare cases.

Microscopically, the wall of the cyst has three layers. The outermost layer consists of moderately dense fibrous tissue with abundant blood vessels, biliary ducts, and hepatic parenchymal cells; muscle cells may occasionally be present.[6] The middle layer consists of dense fibrous tissue of variable vascularity. The inner layer consists of less dense fibrous tissue. The inner layer often but not always has an epithelial lining. A number of lining epithelia have been described. A single layer of columnar epithelium is most common. Ciliated columnar epithelium has been observed,[1] and in at least one case, stratified squamous epithelium was present.[1] Some of the contents of the cyst may adhere to the inner layer. Inflammation can be present in any of the layers; when present, it usually is modest in amount and interpreted as a secondary phenomenon. Carcinoma has been observed rarely to arise in a solitary cyst.[8] Benign common duct tumors have been associated sufficiently often that this additional lesion should be considered, especially in jaundiced patients.[9]

In considering the treatment of solitary cysts, two principles should be kept in mind. First is the essentially benign character of these lesions. Second, surgery is most often the treatment of choice when therapy is required.[10,11] The advisability of aspirating asymptomatic cysts with a typical sonographic appearance is debatable and aspiration is generally ineffective as therapy.[12] Surgical treatment is indicated when symptoms and complications develop, such as pain, weight loss, jaundice, infection, hemorrhage into the cyst, rupture of the cyst, torsion and strangulation of a pedunculated cyst, or malignancy. The appropriate surgical procedure depends on a number of factors, including the overall condition of the patient. Removing fluid too rapidly from a large cyst has resulted in death.[3] External drainage of infected cysts has been recommended, although prolonged sinus formation may develop after external drainage.[3] Excision should be carried out whenever possible. If excision is not feasible, subtotal resection is recommended, with removal of at least one third of the cyst wall to allow drainage into the peritoneal cavity. There is some disagreement about the advisability of the latter approach when there is bile in the cyst.[10,13] Some researchers suggest[13] that radiopaque material be injected intraoperatively to rule out communication of the cyst with the biliary tree. If the cyst or cysts are multilocular, establishment of drainage requires extensive removal of the septa. The wall of the cyst should be examined grossly and microscopically as extensively as possible to diagnose rare instances of malignancy. If the cyst cannot be excised completely and the wall is uniform, random sections may be taken. Focal areas of abnormality should be sampled if present. If the cyst contains bile or if bile radicles can be observed to enter the cyst, peritoneal drainage is contraindicated. Cystojejunostomy is recommended in this instance.[14] Both alcohol sclerotherapy[15] and instillation of minocycline chloride[16] have been effective in only a few cases; such approaches may not be definitive invariably.[15]

The prognosis for patients with solitary cysts is generally excellent if ill-advised surgical procedures and complications of surgery are avoided. As far as can be determined, only one patient who was not treated surgically has died with apparent cyst-related problems.[1] This patient had prolonged diarrhea and vomiting and may have died of inadequate replacement therapy. Despite the occasional occurrence of hemorrhage into a cyst, there are no reported fatalities from this complication.

TRAUMATIC CYSTS

Traumatic cysts are uncommon.[17] They probably are sequelae to intrahepatic hemorrhage. The blood is resorbed and bile leaks into the space.[18] Presumably because of this pathogenesis, traumatic or posttraumatic cysts often are not manifested for some time after the initial trauma.

The symptoms and signs of a traumatic cyst may include abdominal distention, pain, and anorexia. On occasion obstructive jaundice may be present.[17] Perforation and its symptoms may lead to recognition of such cysts. Rarely, the cyst becomes infected secondarily, and the patient has signs of infection.[17] A history of trauma usually can be obtained because the initiating trauma often is severe. Also, a history of trauma usually is the basis for concluding that the cyst is posttraumatic. An abdominal mass is often palpable. Serum bilirubin levels may be elevated. Routine x-ray films may show elevation of the diaphragm or displacement of other abdominal viscera. Posttraumatic cysts occur predominantly in the right lobe of the liver and vary considerably in size. They may contain as much as several liters of fluid. As indicated previously, most of these cysts are filled with bile unless they are infected, in which case they contain pus. The wall of the cyst is composed of fibrous tissue with variable amounts of inflammation, which is typically chronic. An epithelial lining is not present. Various surgical treatments have been used with success, including incision and packing, incision and drainage, and partial excision and marsupialization to the abdominal wall. Simple drainage seems to be adequate treatment in most cases.[17]

CYSTS SECONDARY TO INFARCTION

Cysts can develop after apparent focal arterial insufficiency of the liver. Clinically, this is a rare occurrence. In one patient in whom hepatic cysts were observed to develop on the basis of vascular insufficiency,[19] the cysts were apparently asymptomatic. They were discovered during a computed tomographic scan and were found to be avascular on angiography. Microscopically, the cysts had fibrous walls, were lined by endothelium, and contained bile. Exuberant formation of bile ducts was noted in the area adjacent to the cyst. Cysts that are secondary to infarction may become infected.[19] Similar lesions have been created in monkeys by introducing emboli into the hepatic arterial tree.[19] Experimentally induced cystic lesions are presumed to develop secondary to focal hepatic infarction. They contain bile and therefore seem to connect with the biliary tree. The role of vascular lesions in the genesis of hepatic cysts of undetermined origin—for example, bile-containing solitary cysts—remains to be elucidated.

CYSTS OF MISCELLANEOUS ORIGIN

Duodenal duplication is an uncommon anomaly of the gastrointestinal tract. Imamoglu and Walt described an extraordinary case in which such a duplication, which had luminal continuity with the normal duodenum, lay within the liver.[20] The patient had a 5-year history of recurrent epigastric distress. The duplication, identified by barium examination of the upper gastrointestinal tract, was found at laparotomy to be located within the liver as a large cystic mass. External drainage failed to reduce its size. At a second operation, a loop of jejunum was anastomosed to the cyst wall at the hepatic surface by a Roux-en-Y anastomosis, which appeared to be successful. This particular case seemed to be a unique occurrence.

Periductal glands on occasion give rise to hepatic cysts and can even cause obstructive jaundice.[21,22]

Ciliated hepatic foregut cyst is a rare, benign, solitary, unilocular cyst lined by ciliated, pseudostratified columnar epithelium. The cyst's wall also includes subepithelial connective tissue, a smooth muscle layer, and an outer fibrous capsule.[23] Ciliated hepatic foregut cyst may result from a process of ciliation in an anomalous detached primordium of the hepatic diverticulum or in an independent bud from the nearby enteric foregut.[24] The cyst occurs most often in men of approximately 50 years of age and is found most commonly in the medial segment of the left hepatic lobe. The cyst typically is discovered incidentally on radiologic imaging or during surgical exploration. It does not appear to be associated with any other developmental lesion. This type of cyst is considered benign; however, one instance of squamous cell carcinoma arising in a ciliated, hepatic foregut cyst was reported in a 51-year-old man.[25]

CYSTS ASSOCIATED WITH NEOPLASMS

Virtually any hepatic neoplasm, whether primary or metastatic, can be cystic, at least by virtue of the occurrence of central necrosis. Other tumors involving the liver may be considered cystic on the basis of their fundamental structure. This discussion is limited to primary hepatic tumors for which a cystic component is a frequent or constant feature that is not related to central necrosis.

Cystadenoma and Cystadenocarcinoma

Cystadenomas and cystadenocarcinomas are among the most consistently cystic tumors involving the liver. Cystadenomas may involve either the liver or the extrahepatic biliary tree (including the gallbladder), but predominantly the former. In comparison, cystadenocarcinomas have been found thus far only within the liver.[26] Cystadenomas are more common in females than in males. Approximately two thirds occur when the patient is 40 years old or older. They are extremely rare in children.[26,27] The most common presenting symptoms of cystadenomas are right upper quadrant or epigastric pain, increasing abdominal girth, and a palpable abdominal mass.[26,27] Less commonly, biliary obstruction may be a presenting complaint. On occasion, the obstruction may be episodic. In one patient, the tumor was discovered after perforation into the peritoneal cavity. Sometimes the tumor is found incidentally during abdominal surgery or at autopsy.[26] Rarely, the wall of the tumor may be calcified. With modern imaging techniques, it is often possible to diagnose cystadenocarcinoma, but differentiation from cystadenoma may not be possible.[28] On occasion, cystadenocarcinomas have been identified preoperatively by aspiration and examination of the contents of the cyst, but this procedure carries the risk of peritoneal seeding of the tumor.[29] The lesions most frequently involve the right lobe only but may involve the left lobe or both lobes. In one case, a patient had a concomitant pancreatic cystadenoma.[30]

Cystadenomas vary markedly in size, ranging from 1.5 to 15 cm in diameter and weighing as much as 6000 g.[26,27] Grossly, the lesions usually have a smooth external surface and characteristically are multilocular. Rarely, they may be unilocular. The contents are liquid and variable in appearance and composition. Cholesterol crystals or bile may be present.[26] The lining of the cyst may be smooth or rough, and papillary projections may be evident. Microscopically, cystadenomas are lined by mucus-secreting cuboidal or columnar epithelium, often in papillary folds. Ultrastructural studies may reveal absorptive, argentaffin, and mucus-secreting cells.[31] Ulcerations may be present. The stroma immediately beneath the epithelium is typically quite cellular, resembling ovary, but may be simply fibrotic. Wheeler and Edmondson have suggested that cysts with a cellular stroma (mesenchyme) are an entity distinct from cysts without this feature, that these cysts occur predominantly in females, and that they have an incidence of malignancy.[32] Rarely, however, the stroma has been sarcomatous.[33] A few smooth muscle fibers and inflammatory cells may be present in the wall; lipofuscin-laden macrophages also are common. The outer layers of the wall may contain arteries, veins, nerve fibers, and bile ducts. On occasion apparent bile duct hamartomas (von Meyenburg complexes) may be adjacent.

The histologic features of the tumor and its occurrence both in the liver and in the extrahepatic tree indicate that it is derived from the biliary ducts, although it has been suggested that the intrahepatic lesions may arise from solitary cysts. Bile is present in some of these tumors; in one case, an aberrant duct connected the tumor to the extrahepatic biliary system.[26] Cystadenomas can be created experimentally.[34]

Treatment of these tumors is surgical. Because of the thick capsule, the lesions often can be excised. If the tumor is sufficiently large, lobectomy may be indicated. Because of the apparent potential for malignant transformation of cystadenomas, complete excision is the treatment of choice,[35] and lesser procedures, such as drainage or marsupialization, should be considered only if excision is contraindicated in an individual case. Recurrence is uncommon, but it has been reported in tumors involving the extrahepatic biliary tree.[26]

Cystadenocarcinomas are said to arise by malignant change in cystadenomas. The malignant change may be focal.[26] Wheeler and Edmonson argue, as mentioned previously, that most cystadenocarcinomas do not arise from the group of cystadenomas with cellular stroma.[32] Cystadenocarcinomas are less common than are cystadenomas, in a ratio of 27:64.[36] As previously mentioned, cystadenocarcinomas have not been reported to arise in the extrahepatic biliary tree. Female predominance may be less marked than with cystadenoma.[26] The tumor has occurred as early as the third decade of life. If the tumor has not spread, the gross features are those of cystadenoma. The tumor is an adenocarcinoma that may involve the entire lining or be focal. The lesion is capable of extrahepatic spread and distant metastasis, but it can be cured by complete excision. It may be biologically less aggressive than cholangiocarcinoma.[26] The effect of non-surgical therapy (e.g., radiation or chemotherapy) for the tumor is unknown.

Mesenchymal Hamartoma

So-called mesenchymal hamartomas are uncommon primary hepatic neoplasms in children, usually occurring before the age of 1 year. On occasion they may be predominantly cystic.[37-39] They have a predilection for occurrence in males. The tumor characteristically presents as a painless abdominal mass. Routine x-ray films show no distinctive features. Calcification is typically absent. Imaging techniques reveal a multiloculated mass with variation in the size of septa and cystic spaces.[40] Angiography may reveal hypovascular or avascular foci, which probably represent the cystic areas of the tumor. More than half of the tumors occur in the right lobe, but a small proportion may involve both lobes. The tumors usually are quite large at the time of diagnosis—some have exceeded 1000 g. Their gross appearances vary considerably. They are typically solitary. A tumor may be nearly solid with only scattered small cystic areas, have a large number of cysts, or be predominantly cystic. The cysts typically contain gelatinous or mucoid material and their lining is smooth. The tissue intervening between the cystic structures is solid but gelatinous. Histologically (Figure 49-3), the lesions are heterogeneous, with clusters of normal-appearing hepatocytes entrapped in a poorly cellular mesenchyme that contains variable numbers of lymphatic-like spaces. The latter typically are the cysts, but dilated biliary lined channels may be present or even predominate.[39,41] It is not clear whether the latter represent an epithelialization of the more typical cysts or whether they arise primarily from elements of the bile ducts. Bands of collagen may be present in the mesenchyme, and clusters of bile ducts are typically scattered throughout. Islands of hematopoiesis and scattered blood vessels are common features. No significant atypical features are present in any of the elements. Electron microscopic studies indicate a derivation from both mesenchyme and bile ducts.[37] Chromosomal analysis has been reported in three instances of mesenchymal hamartoma. In all, there was a single abnormality consisting of a balanced translocation involving a common breakpoint 19q13.4.[42] Although most lesions show no predisposition to malignant transformation, a histiogenic relationship between mesenchymal hamartoma and embryonal sarcoma of the liver has been suggested.[42-44] Embryonal sarcoma arising in conjunction with mesenchymal hamartoma has been described,[43,44] and in one instance cytogenetic analysis of the embryonal sarcoma demonstrated a complex karyotype.[44]

Cavernous Hemangiomas

Hemangiomas of the liver are essentially of two types, hemangioendotheliomas and cavernous hemangiomas. The former are encountered principally in childhood, usually in the first year of life.[45] They tend to be solid or at least relatively so. Cavernous hemangiomas, the more common of the two types, are more consistently cystic.

Cavernous hemangiomas are the most common benign hepatic tumors in all age groups.[46] They have no significant capacity for invasion of tissue and none for

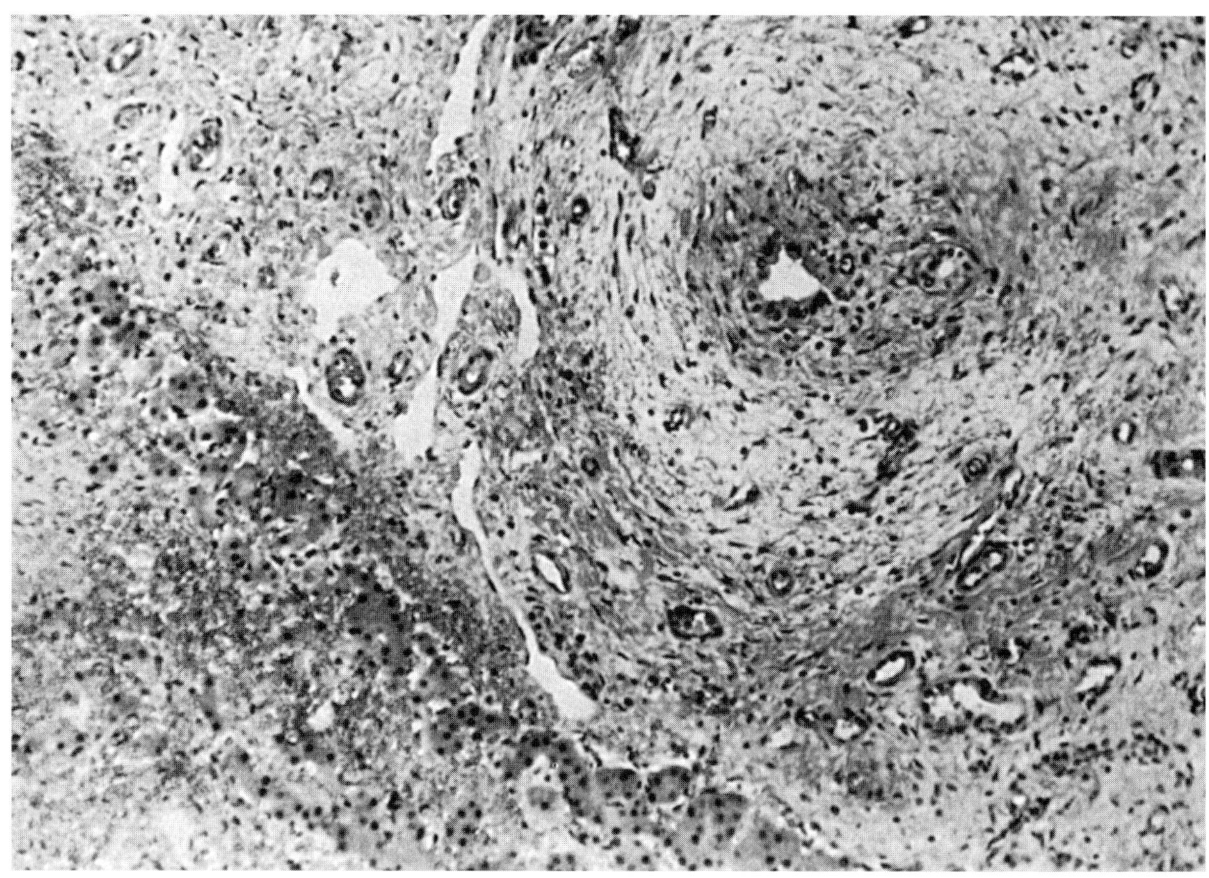

Figure 49-3 Light micrograph of a mesenchymal hamartoma, illustrating several duct elements in the mesenchyme *(upper right),* lymphatic-like spaces *(center),* and adjacent entrapped hepatocytes *(lower left)* (hematoxylin and eosin, ×10).

metastasis. Probably fewer than 20 percent become symptomatic.[46] By convention, lesions larger than 4 cm in diameter have been designated giant cavernous hemangiomas.[47,48] In one series of 122 cases, 49 of these tumors were giant; of those, 40 percent were symptomatic.[49] It appears from autopsy series that the incidence in males and females is approximately equal, but surgical series (which deal largely with symptomatic patients) have had a striking female predominance. Symptoms of these tumors generally become more common with increasing age. There is reason to suspect that hormones, especially estrogenic ones, enhance their growth, an effect that probably increases the probability of symptoms. Symptoms may arise from the effects of a mass in the abdomen and may include fullness, belching, weight loss, abdominal distention, vomiting, and pain. Anemia (caused by sequestration of the red blood cells in the tumor), hemorrhage (caused by extensive clotting within the tumor), or rupture of the tumor may also occur. Rupture usually is secondary to blunt abdominal trauma, but it may follow either percutaneous or operative attempts at biopsy. It also may develop spontaneously.

An upper abdominal mass may be palpable. Routine x-ray films of the abdomen can show elevation of the diaphragm. Calcification of the tumor or phleboliths may be evident. Scans or ultrasonography may show a defect. The most valuable diagnostic test, however, is angiography, which shows distinctive features in typical cases. The angiographic features include large feeding vessels displaced and curled at the margins of the lesions, varix-like spaces that fill rapidly and remain opacified throughout the examination, and a tendency for the vascular spaces to be arranged in rings or to be C-shaped.[50]

The tumors are usually single. There appears to be a slight predilection for occurrence in the right lobe. In approximately 20 percent of patients with giant hemangiomas, both lobes are involved.[48] Reported tumors have a great range of diameters, from a few millimeters to 45 cm.[47] A few have been pedunculated.[46] Typically, they are reddish blue or purple, cystic, and quite clearly vascular. Some may appear solid. The cut surfaces are honeycombed, with various degrees of fibrosis, thrombosis, and calcification. Microscopically the lesions consist of large, dilated, blood-filled channels lined by epithelium. A variable inflammatory reaction is present in the underlying fibromuscular wall. Thrombosis and calcification are common. Biopsy of hepatic hemangiomas is contraindicated.

Unless the tumor is symptomatic, there appears to be minimal risk in observing the patient.[49] If treatment is necessary, the treatment of choice is surgical. The precise procedure depends on the size of the tumor, the number of lesions, and the general condition of the patient. Because of the possibility of rupture, the operating room staff must be prepared to rapidly provide clotting factors, large amounts of blood, or both. The lesions should be removed by a wedge resection through normal liver or by lobectomy when necessary and feasible. Lesser procedures are likely to result in significant hemorrhage; even operative biopsy and aspiration have precipitated life-threatening hemorrhage.[47] Rarely, when a tumor is unresectable, it may be possible to selectively ligate the arteries supplying it.[48] More commonly irradiation is used in these circumstances. Radiation therapy may relieve symptoms, but it does not eradicate the tumor.[47] Administering steroids is associated with shrinkage of the lesion in some cases in children. The extent of an inoperable tumor can be delineated by placing clips along its margins during laparotomy. Rupture of the tumor, either preoperatively or intraoperatively, is associated with a high mortality rate. When rupture does not occur, mortality is very low and the prognosis is favorable.

Teratomas

Primary hepatic teratomas are rare; approximately a dozen cases have been reported to date.[51-53] These tumors occur predominantly in children and, as with teratomas elsewhere, may have a significant cystic component. The great majority of teratomas are noted within the first year of life. One patient was anencephalic, and another had trisomy 13.[53] The symptoms are those of an enlarging hepatic mass. Routine x-ray films may show calcification, representing either teeth or bits of bone arising as components of the tumor. Angiograms and scans of the liver show an avascular defect within it. The majority of reported tumors have been in the right lobe of the liver. The tumor characteristically has both solid and cystic regions. Such tumors are relatively large, and lobectomy may be necessary for complete excision. The histologic features are typical of a teratoma, with well-differentiated tissues (some of which may be immature) derived from multiple germ layers. The cystic areas contain keratinized debris with strands of hair. The cystic structures are a component of the tumor and are not related to the biliary duct system. In several of the reported cases, the tumors have had histologically malignant areas, one in the form of squamous cell carcinoma and another in the form of hepatoblastoma. Pulmonary metastases developed in both of these patients. All but three of the nine patients with malignant changes in the tumor died, with or without resection of the tumor. Nevertheless, resection appears to be the treatment of choice. Subsequent therapy, if any, depends on the presence and character of any malignant element.

Other Cystic Neoplasms

A single case of a malignant cystic hepatic neoplasm, possibly of mesothelial origin, has been reported in a 6-month-old girl.[54] On occasion von Meyenburg complexes have been seen as cystic by sonography[55] (although their inclusion with neoplasms may be inappropriate).

PELIOSIS HEPATIS

Peliosis hepatis is characterized by the presence in the liver of blood-filled cavities, which may or may not be lined with sinusoidal cells. The individual cysts or cavities usually do not exceed several centimeters in diameter. The lesions may be diffuse or focal. The gross appearance of angiectatic lesions on the cut surface of the liver is distinctive. The lesions are not always limited to the liver and have been found (usually but not invariably in patients with liver lesions) in the spleen, bone marrow, lung, pleura, kidney, and gut.[56,57] There may be slight fibrosis of the walls of the cavities, and hepatocellular necrosis may or may not be associated. The cysts are typically continuous with adjacent, more normal sinusoids and sometimes can be seen in continuity with hepatic venous tributaries. A distinction between phlebectatic and parenchymal types has been made,[58] with attendant pathogenetic implications, but the merit and applicability of this distinction are uncertain. The lesion is usually diagnosed by gross or microscopic examination, but wedged hepatic venography has been reported to reveal quite specific findings.[59] When suspected, it can be diagnosed by percutaneous biopsy.[60-63] Significant bleeding after biopsy seems to be uncommon.[60]

No consistent hepatic functional abnormalities are found in affected patients, but in steroid-associated cases, there may be hepatic failure or rupture and peritoneal hemorrhage.[60]

Associated in the past primarily with wasting diseases such as tuberculosis, malignancy, and chronic suppurative infection, peliosis hepatis is seen most commonly now in association with the administration of anabolic steroids. It is seen also in various clinical disorders[60,61,64] and has been reported in one case of hepatic transplantation.[65] It can occur in human immunodeficiency virus (HIV) infection as an accompaniment of bacterial infection.[66] In the latter setting, it can be treated effectively with antibiotics. Peliosis hepatis occurs in various experimental situations and as a naturally occurring disease in animals.[67]

The pathogenesis of peliosis hepatis is obscure. Among suggested possibilities are necrosis of parenchyma with secondary vascular dilation, congenital weakness of vessel walls, angiitis, vascular (venous) obstruction with secondary dilation, and injury to endothelial cells. Certainly more than one of these factors could operate to give a common morphologic end result. Ultrastructural studies[67,68] and the occurrence of a similar lesion in multiple organs in individual patients suggest that injury to endothelium may be the primary causative basis in many cases. The antibiotic-treatable form in patients with HIV infection suggests the possibility of more than one pathogenesis. Because the lesion usually is found incidentally and may be diffuse, surgical therapy is not considered. Regression of the disease after withdrawal of steroids has been described.[60-62]

HEREDITARY HEPATIC CYSTIC DISEASE

As indicated in Table 49-1, there are a number of hereditary diseases in which hepatic cysts can develop. Renal cysts and a variety of lesions in other viscera also may occur as part of these diseases. Because of advances in molecular biology, the genetic lesion has been defined in a number of them.

In autosomal-dominant polycystic disease two genetic lesions have been identified, and it appears that at least one other remains to be identified. In ADPKD1 the genetic lesion involves a specific locus on chromosome 16. In ADPKD2 the gene lesion involves a specific locus on chromosome 4. The few cases of autosomal-dominant polycystic kidney disease (ADPKD) in which no genetic defect has been found are collectively called ADPKD3. Whether or not there is more than one genetically defined disorder among these latter cases is not known.

In autosomal-recessive polycystic kidney disease (ARPKD), the genetic lesion involves an undetermined locus on chromosome 6. "Isolated" cystic hepatic disease (PLD) has a genetic lesion at 19p13.2-13.1. The genetic lesion in phosphomannoseisomerase deficiency has not been defined.

As suggested throughout this chapter, the genetic lesions in at least some of these disorders may provide an explanation for the cyst formation, as well as possible modes of therapy and/or prevention.

PATHOGENESIS OF HEPATIC CYSTS

Extensive studies of the type done on renal cysts have not been done directly on hepatic cysts per se in any of the heritable hepatic cystic conditions. On the other hand, it is interesting that disturbances of cell-matrix interaction occur in the kidney in ADPKD1 and 2 and that such interaction may be critical for normal development of intrahepatic ducts.[169] This suggests that disturbances in such interactions can contribute to hepatic cyst formation, especially in hepatic cysts associated with DPM. This may be specifically indicated by phosphomannoseisomerase deficiency (see section on this disorder).

POLYCYSTIC LIVER DISEASE

Evidence now clearly suggests that a heritable "isolated" (without renal cysts) polycystic disease exists (i.e., PLD).

A small number of families have been studied in which there is autosomal-dominant inheritance of polycystic liver disease in the absence of cystic liver disease.[70,71]

Affected patients (even those of advanced age) do not have renal cysts demonstrated on tomography. The affected individuals do not have the abnormal genetic findings of either ADPKD1 or ADPKD2. In one such case, however, there was an abnormal locus identified on chromosome 19q13.2-13.1.[70]

The histopathology in these patients has not been determined nor has retrograde cholangiography been performed, so it is not known whether patients have DPM or whether the cysts are communicating.

The pathogenesis of the hepatic cysts is unknown. Because no renal cysts have been detected, there is no basis for thinking that this disease is closely related or identical to ADPKD (so-called ADPKD3), in which neither chromosome lesion ADPKD1 or ADPKD2 is present.

The absence of cholangiographic studies in PLD makes it impossible to comment on its relationship to so-called simple Caroli's disease.

Ductal Plate Malformation

DPM has been shown by Jorgensen[72] to closely resemble the developing, immature portal tract and is apparently an arrest of development. This is significant in hepatic cystic disease because there is a tendency for the ductal structures in these malformed portal tracts to enlarge or become cystic. The ducts communicate with the ductal system.

DPM, a consistent component of ARPKD, is the defining hepatic feature of the clinicopathologic entity of congenital hepatic fibrosis (CHF). It is seen with some frequency in ADPKD, in a variety of congenital anomaly syndromes (see section on Other Malformation Syndromes), and uncommonly in at least one apparently acquired condition, extrahepatic biliary atresia. Desmet describes it as occurring more commonly in the latter and in an even wider variety of conditions[73] than we (or most other pediatric pathologists) have observed.

Phosphomannoseisomerase Deficiency

DPM has been established as an invariable component of phosphomannoseisomerase deficiency.[74-77] This is potentially of great significance because this disorder leads to a defect in glycosylation, thus suggesting a pathway mediating the abnormalities that cause DPM. This may be only one of a number of metabolic abnormalities that lead to this maldevelopment of bile duct. The pathogenesis of DPM has not been established and may be different in different patients (i.e., not all DPM may be the same).

Phosphomannoseisomerase deficiency is especially interesting in the pathogenesis of DPM in light of the work of Terada and colleagues, which shows concomitant changes in epithelium and the matrix elements during the maturation of the portal tracts.[69] One theoretical possibility, therefore, for ductal plate malformation is a disturbance in epithelial-matrix interactions resulting from heritable abnormalities in either or both of these elements. There is no evidence that such disturbances exist in the livers of patients with DPM, but there is interesting evidence that such a disturbance may exist in the kidneys of ADPKD2. However, several types of cystic ducts may occur in ADPKD, and DPM may not occur in all patients. When it does, the distribution of lesions is patchy.

Caroli's Disease

As described in previous editions of this text, Caroli[79] described two entities. In one, there was widespread dilation of the biliary duct system (without choledochal cyst, without significant portal tract or other hepatic pathology, and apparently without other visceral lesions). The other entity, quite clearly, was ARPKD or CHF. Communicating duct cysts occur in both of the "conditions" described by Caroli.

The former is very rare and not known to be heritable; the other is more common and heritable. The former could represent what we have classified as PLD or systemic ductal dilation without choledochal cyst. Radiologists likely will continue to use the term *Caroli's disease* as a description for radiologically demonstrable communicating hepatobiliary duct cysts.

The contention of Desmet[73] that there is a distinct entity with duct dilation limited to a particular level of ducts is interesting but seems to us to lack adequate corroboration. Thus in our opinion, continued use of the terms *Caroli's disease* or *Caroli's syndrome* serves only to complicate the nomenclature (and understanding) of an already rather complex set of heritable disorders.

Non-communicating (Dominant) Polycystic Disease

Reviews of multiple, non-parasitic cysts of the liver represent collections of a number of discrete entities, probably including multiple solitary cysts, choledochal cysts, and both recessively (communicating) and dominantly (non-communicating) inherited cystic diseases of the liver. Such series also include a number of patients with non-communicating multiple cysts and no apparent renal disease. The latter group of patients may have had multiple solitary cysts, or renal disease in these patients may have been overlooked. Alternatively, these patients may have had a purely hepatic type of polycystic disease—that is, multiple heritable, non-communicating cysts of bile ducts. This latter entity has been postulated on the basis of a large series of autopsies[80] and, on occasion, has apparently been observed in families.[81] Nevertheless, it is uncertain that such patients represent a discrete entity or patients with ADPKD, in whom renal cysts were overlooked or were inconspicuous.[82] Because of this uncertainty and because affected families are reported so rarely, this entity is not discussed further in this chapter. The focus instead is on the well-known non-communicating (predominantly) and dominantly inherited polycystic disease commonly called ADPKD.

ADPKD is the most common heritable disorder of the kidneys. Its frequency is estimated to be from 1:1500 to 1:5000 in the general population. It affects approximately 500,000 people in the United States.[83] The disease is inherited in an autosomal-dominant manner with high penetrance. Although somewhat beyond the scope of this chapter, it is worth mentioning recent important molecular genetic findings in this disorder. The findings in the genetics of human and animal polycystic diseases[84] hold great promise in two areas: early diagnosis (including intrauterine)[85] and insight into the pathogenesis of the renal (and presumably the liver) lesions.[86]

Approximately 95 percent of patients with ADPKD have an abnormal locus on chromosome 16 (ADPKD1). A small number of patients have a different locus of abnormality, involving chromosome 4 (ADPKD2), and there is a possibility that at least one additional gene locus may be present in others.[87-89] The presence of the gene for ADPKD1 is said to adversely affect the rate of progression of renal disease.[90,91]

Renal complications of cysts include, in addition to renal failure and hypertension,[92] infection and (uncommonly) perinephric hemorrhage.

The peak incidence for clinical presentation of ADPKD is in adult life (older than 40 years of age), but the disease is also recognized in children, usually in infancy.[93,94] In studying a population of patients with ADPKD using sophisticated imaging techniques, Multinovic and co-workers found recognizable hepatic cysts in 29 percent of 158 patients.[95] A few relatives of such patients may have had hepatic cysts only, demonstrable by imaging techniques[96] (see the earlier discussion of polycystic disease limited to the liver). In an autopsy series of patients with ADPKD, hepatic cysts were found in 17 of 19 patients.[97]

There is considerable variation in the size of the liver in patients with ADPKD; often it is of normal size for many years and then becomes enlarged. This enlargement seems generally to correlate with an increase in the number and size of cysts.[95,98] Thus infants with ADPKD rarely have recognizable cysts of the liver, and the diagnosis of cysts in the liver increases with age. Hepatic cysts also increase in frequency with gender, parity, and severity of renal disease.[99] It has been suggested that the cysts, which are predominantly non-communicating, arise from the von Meyenburg complexes that are typically present (discussed in the following section). This idea has not been proved. The von Meyenburg complexes have been said by different authorities to decrease or increase with age.

The hepatic cysts are lined by biliary epithelium. They usually are diffuse, but they may be localized.[97] The predominant (non-communicating) cysts usually do not communicate with the biliary system and do not contain bile. Occasionally, however, they may rupture into adjacent bile ducts.[97] In uncomplicated cases results of tests of liver function usually are normal or minimally abnormal, even with increasing liver size. Rarely, large cysts cause mechanical obstruction of the biliary system.

In addition to cysts a number of other lesions occur in the liver in patients with ADPKD. These include cystic dilation of the ductal system,[100] dilation of the glands of the intrahepatic ducts,[101] von Meyenburg complexes,[101,102] and DPM.[97,103] The latter was found by Grunfeld and colleagues in 60 percent of patients.[97] Previously, DPM had been reported only rarely in ADPKD.[104] The common presence of both communicating (DPM) and non-communicating lesions of the bile ducts in patients with autosomal-dominant renal disease is surprising and interesting. The precise significance of the observation for understanding the pathogenesis and classification of the polycystic disease is unclear. It could indicate a pathogenetic continuum among the various disorders, although the disorders are not believed to be allelic.

Despite the apparent histologic overlap, it still seems valid to distinguish ADPKD from the recessively inherited, communicating types of polycystic diseases because of (1) the predominance of one type of lesion of the bile ducts (i.e., communicating or non-communicating) over the other in the different diseases, (2) the differing pattern of inheritance (dominant versus recessive), (3) the frequently different symptoms and complications of the hepatic component of each disorder, and (4) different extrahepatic lesions.

A variety of other apparently intrinsic abnormalities, many involving the cardiovascular system, are also found in ADPKD.[105] These appear to be separable from the hypertension, which is common when advanced kidney disease develops.[106,107] It has been speculated, therefore, that the disease involves a generalized defect in connective tissue. Clinically, the most significant of the cardiovascular lesions are intracranial aneurysms. Most of the latter can be detected by non-invasive means.[108] Some evidence shows that certain vascular lesions may tend to occur in families.[109] Additional abnormalities observed include diverticulosis and cysts in multiple organs, including the pancreas, spleen, uterus, and seminal vesicles.

The hepatic lesions in ADPKD have been thought to be insignificant clinically. Some of the small number of symptomatic patients reported previously may have been afflicted with CHF rather than ADPKD (or combinations of the two). Nevertheless, as more patients with ADPKD have survived for longer periods, it has become clear that a significant incidence of liver disease is associated with ADPKD. In the most thorough analysis of this issue, 10.5 percent of the deaths in patients with ADPKD resulted from hepatic complications. In addition, a number of surviving patients had significant liver disease.[97] Hepatic complications included infection of the cysts, cholangiocarcinoma, portal hypertension, and pressure effects due to the cyst. As noted, liver function tests usually are altered minimally in ADPKD; a change in these tests should alert the physician to the development of complications, especially infection. Diagnosis of the latter is facilitated by imaging studies.[110,111] Treatment with antibiotics alone may not suffice; drainage of infected cysts is often required.[110] Analysis of the portal hypertension is obscured by the occurrence of posthepatitic cirrhosis and chronic hepatitis in these patients and by the possible confusion of some patients with CHF or long-surviving patients with ARPKD or both. (This distinction is potentially difficult in light of the occurrence of DPM in ADPKD.) Cholangiocarcinoma may develop from the epithelium of the cystic ducts.[112] Some long-surviving patients may show calcification of both renal and hepatic cysts.[113]

Pressure symptoms from cysts include obstructive jaundice or severe pain,[114] which may be relieved by unroofing as many cysts as possible and draining them into the peritoneal cavity.[114] Some patients with portal hypertension may benefit from portacaval shunting. In the future combined renal and hepatic transplantation may be the treatment of choice in patients with advanced renal and hepatic disease.[115]

RENAL CYST PATHOGENESIS

Although this chapter is devoted to hepatic cysts, there has been much more information developed in recent years pertinent to the pathogenesis of renal cysts, especially in ADPKD. Comparable information (or studies) has not been developed in relation to the hepatic cysts, and, of course, several types of cysts occur in ADPKD, some related to the presence of DPM and some not.

ADPKD is known to be associated with mutations in one of two genes—PKD1 now known to be present on chromosome 16 in a specific locus[17] or in a specific locus on chromosome 4 (PKD2).[117] The former occurs in approximately 85 percent of cases of ADPKD, and the latter in the majority of the remaining cases. In a few cases gene lesions are not found in either site (so-called ADPKD3).

The two known genes seem to act in the same molecular pathway, and it is felt that a loss of function in one or the other is the most likely pathogenetic mechanism in ADPKD. It appears that a somatic "second hit" is also necessary to create the disease.

The gene products polycystin 1 and polycystin 2 are necessary for normal renal tubular maturation, and deficits in their function result in abnormal proliferation, secretion, and matrix.[118-120] The precise role of each of these in creating the cystic tubules is not yet delineated. These findings suggest possible avenues of therapy or prevention of cyst formation.[118]

In terms of ARPKD, the involved chromosome is 6p,[121,122] although the precise gene and its locus have not been identified. In terms of the renal cysts, it has been shown in both human and murine recessive polycystic disease[118] that there is an abnormal localization of epidermal growth factor in cystic renal tubules, implying a role in proliferation and cystogenesis.

PATHOPHYSIOLOGIC CORRELATES OF DUCTAL PLATE MALFORMATION

In addition to its significance as an aid in morphologic diagnosis, DPM is important because it is frequently associated with portal hypertension. This association is most prominent in patients diagnosed clinically as having CHF. Portal hypertension also occurs, however, in other, possibly different, polycystic conditions such as ARPKD. The basis for the association of the lesion of the portal tract with portal hypertension is not clear. Possibilities include an alteration of venous resistance resulting from the fibrosis of the portal tracts, a primary abnormality of the intrahepatic portal veins, and fibrosis around the central veins, particularly in patients with dysplastic kidneys.[123] The early observation of a reduced number of branches of the intrahepatic portal veins in CHF[124] has not been corroborated. Clinically, portal hypertension develops over time, suggesting that it is associated with a change in either the amount or character of the portal fibrosis or with a change in some other element of DPM (e.g., vascular). Interestingly, there is a duplication of intrahepatic radicles of the portal vein in a high percentage of the small number of patients in whom this abnormality was sought.[125,126] There appears to be a strong but not invariable association of portal hypertension with the presence of these radicles.[125]

The Disease of Congenital Hepatic Fibrosis

In 1961 Kerr and colleagues described a group of their own patients and others from the literature with a common disorder, which they called CHF.[124] Their patients had portal hypertension without hepatic parenchymal disease or obstruction of the main portal vein. These patients had a lesion of the portal tract consisting of increased numbers of bile ducts of unusual profiles with a bland fibrosis (i.e., DPM). There also was a paucity of portal vein radicles in the portal tracts, and cystic disease of the kidney was common. The condition appeared to be inherited as an autosomal-recessive trait. Subsequent studies of these patients confirmed the basic pathology except for the finding of a paucity of portal veins at the level of the portal tracts. The passage of time has given rise to the question of whether or not CHF is distinct from ARPKD. Genetic findings in ARPKD seem to suggest that the two are separate entities.

A considerable range of clinical presentations is observed in patients with CHF. Most patients come to a physician's attention because of portal hypertension in the first several decades of life. As might be anticipated from the pathology, ascites is rare in these patients. Some patients present with cholangitis but rarely with hepatic encephalopathy.[118] Still other patients with CHF are discovered only incidentally at autopsy (i.e., latent CHF).[128]

Visceral abnormalities, in addition to those in liver and kidney, found in single patients or small groups of patients with CHF include emphysema, cerebellar hemangioma, enlargement and deformity of the gallbladder, berry aneurysms, congenital heart disease, and intestinal lymphangiectasia or protein-losing enteropathy or both.[128-132] Which of these conditions are coincidental and which intrinsic to the basic disease is not clear.

The renal lesions may be so minimal that they are discernible only at autopsy, but in some patients, the kidney lesions become sufficiently severe to cause hypertension and azotemia and, occasionally, frank renal failure.[125,133] Anatomically the lesions are initially and primarily medullary, with dilation of collecting ducts and distal tubules.[134,135] Later, cortical cysts develop. According to Landing and colleagues, both the extent of initial medullary involvement and the time-dependent variation in the ratio of cystic changes in cortical to medullary areas differ in CHF and ARPKD.[134]

DPM is a characteristic of CHF, but on occasion it is confined to one lobe or a segment of one lobe.[135-137] The lesion is not always equally prominent in all involved portal tracts; therefore, needle biopsy may be unreliable for making the diagnosis. Furthermore, in a few patients the extent of changes in bile ducts has been minimal,[138] and in some patients, profiles of the bile ducts are normal. In terms of hepatic cysts, Jorgensen found an increase in the average diameter of bile ducts in patients with CHF as compared with controls.[139] The incidence of gross cysts, however, is not established, nor is it clear whether or not the incidence of such cysts increases with age. Bouquien and co-workers found formation of cysts in each of five patients studied by cholangiography or injection studies at operation or necropsy.[140] Alvarez and colleagues found cysts in 12 of 17 children.[125] Dilation of the common duct may be present and may exist with or be independent of dilation of intrahepatic ducts. We have seen it so marked that it caused confusion with a sporadic or isolated choledochal cyst, from which it can be differentiated by examination of a liver biopsy specimen. Thus DPM is present in CHF but not in isolated or sporadic instances of choledochal cysts. The distinction is important because CHF is heritable whereas classic sporadic choledochal cysts are not.

Dilation of bile ducts becomes clinically significant when it is associated with either cholangitis or malignant transformation. Although the intrahepatic dilation, when present, tends to be diffuse, occasionally only a single lobe may be involved.[141] In one case a blind but bile-containing dilated duct was observed.[124]

Cholangitis is an uncommon but significant complication of CHF. As noted it may be the presenting symptom of the disorder.[142,143] When it occurs, dilation of the intrahepatic ducts is typically present. Most but not all patients have associated portal hypertension and a considerable number have renal cysts, as seen on biopsy or x-ray films. A number also have cystic dilation of the common duct or gallbladder or both. The ages of affected patients ranged from 1 month to 36 years. Calculi may form in the dilated ducts and may complicate the treatment of patients with preexisting cholangitis or may initiate cholangitis and mandate surgery. The genesis of the cholangitis in patients without calculi is not clear. Operative cholangiography or biliary tract surgery initiates the process in some patients. Perhaps it tends to occur in patients with the most marked dilation of intrahepatic ducts and bile stasis, with or without calculi. In general when cholangitis develops, it is difficult to treat successfully.[143] Biliary tract surgery or operative cholangiography or both may contribute to the poor prognosis.[143] Because of the potentially deleterious effects of operative cholangiography and surgery on the biliary tract, it is suggested that conservative treatment be used as long as possible for all patients with CHF, including those with fever. Chenodeoxycholic acid should be used to prevent formation of calculi.[144] However, the potential for the development of malignancy, together with the possibility of resecting localized ductal dilations as prophylaxis against development of stones and cholecystitis, may constitute reasons for an aggressive approach to the treatment of selected patients with CHF.

When patients have no cholangitis or malignancy, the major problem in treating those with CHF is bleeding esophageal varices. Considerable initial success has been achieved in relieving portal hypertension in both children and adults by portal-systemic shunting. However, the long-term results need evaluation.[145]

An uncommon although significant complication in CHF is the development of malignancy. Cholangiocarcinoma has been the most common tumor observed,[146] and premalignant changes can be found in the epithelium of some resected duct cysts. Ages at tumor development are variable. The tumor is also found in association with choledochal cysts or with cystic dilation of intrahepatic biliary ducts when DPM is not present. It is not clear whether dilation of ducts is a prerequisite for the development of malignancy.

Autosomal-recessive Polycystic Kidney Disease

ARPKD (Potter's type I cystic renal disease) is an autosomal-recessive disorder characterized by a combination of hepatic and renal diseases. The lesion in the liver is DPM. The lesion in the kidney consists of cysts of the collecting ducts.[147]

The cysts in ARPKD are invariably associated with DPM. In terms of molecular biologic findings, an abnormal gene on chromosome 13 has been identified in a mouse model that bears considerable resemblance to ARPKD.[148] In human ARPKD a lesion involving 6p21-cen has been identified.[149] The disease can be recognized in utero by ultrasonography, usually after the second trimester, but can be confused with other conditions. Because no genetic marker is yet available, prenatal counseling and diagnosis should be given with caution.[150]

In the typical postnatal case, the affected infant has bilateral masses in the flanks at birth and survives only a few days, weeks, or months. A few patients, apparently those with less extensive renal disease, survive for prolonged periods.[151,152] Landing and co-workers concluded that the multiple subdivisions of ARPKD proposed by Blyth and Ockenden[151] are not meaningful, a conclusion that was also reached by Gang and Herrin.[152] These conclusions refute the notion that all cases in a single family follow a similar course. This must be taken into account in genetic counseling.

The kidneys in a typical patient present a distinct gross appearance of massive enlargement and radially oriented, minute cysts. This appearance correlates well with the microscopic features (Figure 49-4). Dilation of the collecting ducts is observed.[152] Intervening nephrons are normal and no dysplasia is noted. Renal fibrosis is scant or lacking, but fibrosis may increase with increasing age of surviving patients. With advancing age, there is also a tendency for the cysts to decrease in number, to lose their obvious radial orientation, and to become rounded.[133] It may be difficult to make the diagnosis in such instances without knowing the morphologic appearance of the liver and the family history. Landing and co-workers have emphasized the morphometric differences between the renal lesions of ARPKD and those of CHF.[134,154]

The hepatic lesion is relatively uniform in appearance. Grossly recognizable cysts are present only rarely in a newborn[155]; gross cysts are uncommon even in older patients. The hepatic lesion is DPM (Figure 49-5). The biliary tract is unobstructed, and no parenchymal disease is found. An occasional patient may have only an inconspicuous increase in the number of bile ducts.[133] Reconstruction (stereologic) studies suggest that the ducts communicate both proximally and distally with the remainder of the biliary system. The precise incidence of portal hypertension in ARPKD is unclear. It appears, however, to be less than that in CHF. At least some of the apparent difference in the frequencies of portal hypertension reflects that children with ARPKD often die in infancy. The incidence of portal hypertension in ARPKD may prove to be substantial in children with long survival times. A substantial correlation between the presence of portal hypertension and the presence of duplicated intrahepatic portal vein radicles has been observed in patients with ARPKD-CHF.[126] Some evolution of the hepatic lesion may occur with age, as indicated by the description of Blyth and Ockenden,[151] which suggests that grossly recognizable hepatic cysts may become more frequent with age.

Deaths of patients with ARPKD are often assumed to result from renal failure. Moreover, mortality seems to correlate with the extent of renal abnormality. It has been suggested, however, that the immediate cause of neonatal death usually is pulmonary disease.[133] In patients who survive the neonatal period, hypertension currently seems to be the principal factor determining survival.[133] Renal function abnormalities are non-specific and include a decreased glomerular filtration rate, a decreased ability to concentrate urine, and defective acidification.[152] Portacaval shunting in patients with clinically

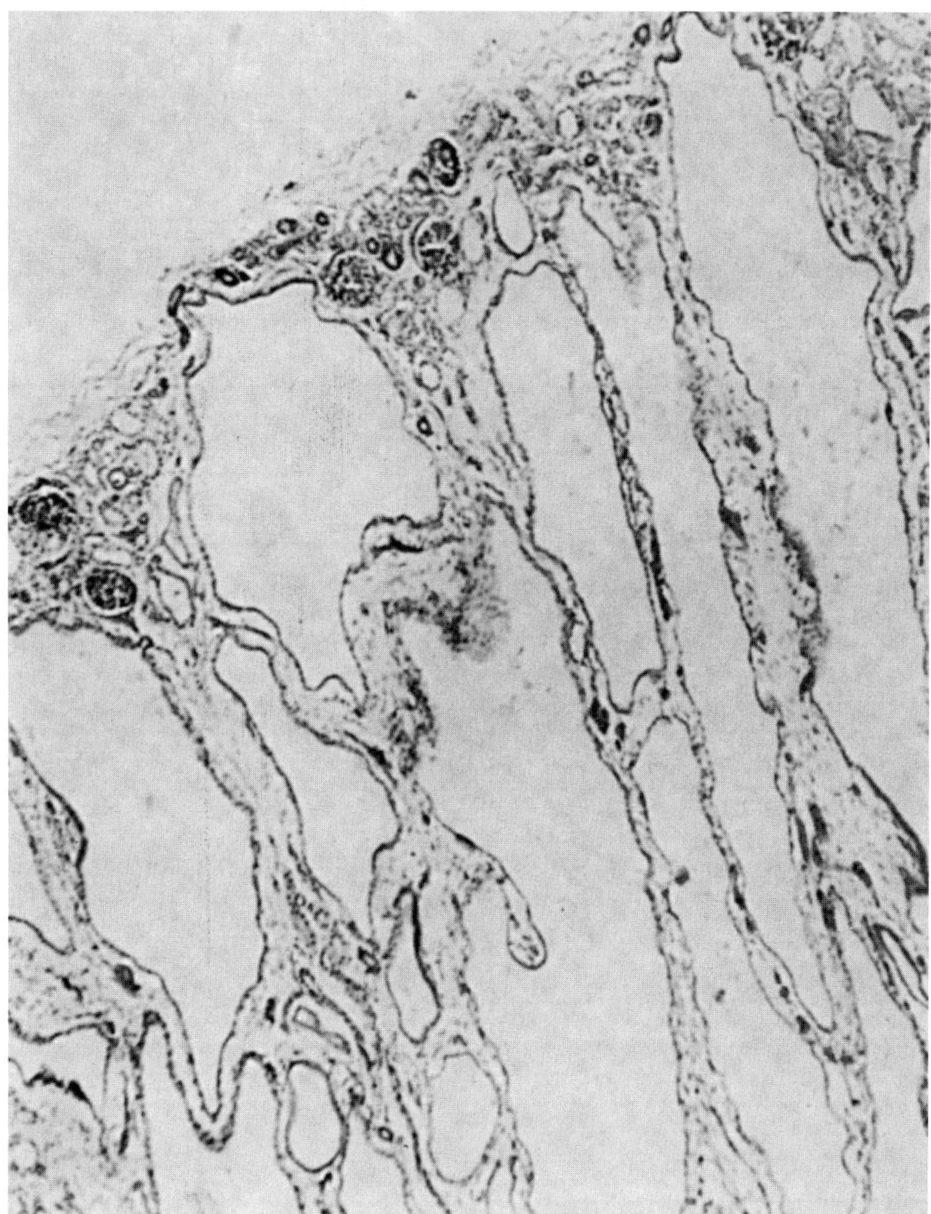

Figure 49-4 Photomicrograph of a kidney from a newborn with infantile polycystic disease, illustrating the typical radially oriented cysts. The cortical surface is at the top of the field (hematoxylin and eosin, ×4).

important portal hypertension results in significant improvement, at least in the short term.[133] Renal transplantation may be indicated. Occasional patients with ARPKD have pancreatic fibrosis with duct dilation or proliferation or both.[133] A few patients with ARPKD-CHF have had intractable diarrhea.[131,132]

Congenital Hepatic Fibrosis-Nephronophthisis

In a small number of patients, severe progressive renal disease has been accompanied by a hepatic lesion bearing a resemblance to DPM.[156,157] The condition is included in this chapter because of the combination of heritability and the simultaneous presence of renal disease and a DPM-like lesion, but hepatic cysts are not a feature in these patients. Several of the patients have had retinal degeneration and cerebellar hypoplasia. The condition bears some similarities to retinal-renal dystrophy, except that there is no associated liver lesion in the latter disease. In all patients reported with the combination of a DPM-like lesion and severe progressive renal disease, the disease has been detected before the patient reached 20 years of age. Most of the patients were frankly uremic by this age. The first observed abnormality of renal function is a concentrating defect. The condition is familial.

The pathologic features of the renal disease are different from those in typical ARPKD and CHF. The renal histopathologic features include interstitial fibrosis and inflammation, tubular atrophy and cyst formation, and

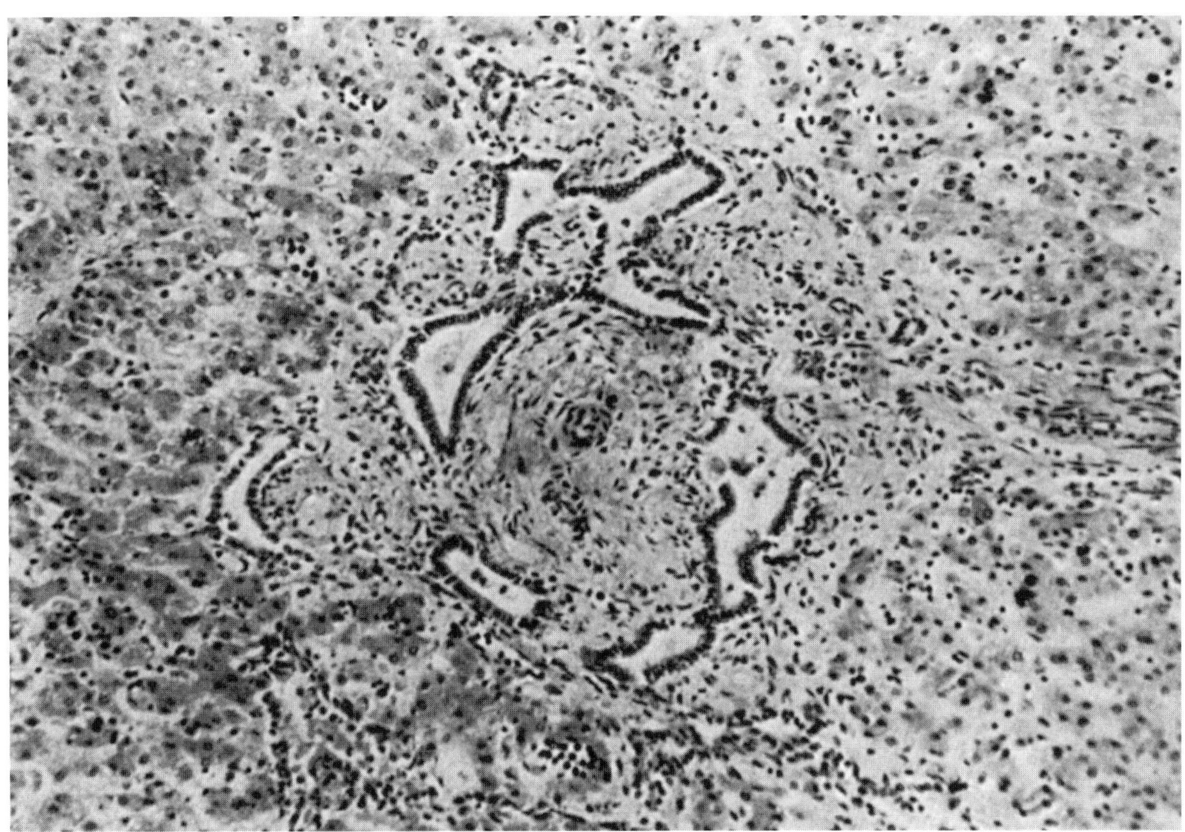

Figure 49-5 Photomicrograph of the portal tract from a newborn with infantile polycystic disease, illustrating congenital hepatic fibrosis lesion. Fibrous tissue and bile ducts are increased. The ducts are slightly dilated and of unusual shapes (hematoxylin and eosin, ×10).

glomerular sclerosis. This histologic picture most closely resembles so-called nephronophthisis, but this is a descriptive impression only. The renal disease may not be similar pathogenetically to the more common juvenile nephronophthisis of Fanconi. The hepatic lesion, although generically consistent with DPM, is nevertheless somewhat atypical. The bile ducts rarely show unusual profiles, and inflammation has been present in a few instances. In one case the portal lesion showed a quite marked change with time. Morphometric studies by Landing and co-workers show that the lesion of the portal tracts in these patients is different from ARPKD and CHF.[67] Hepatomegaly is the most common initial sign of the disease, yet abnormalities of liver function are scant. Splenomegaly is common, but complications of portal hypertension have not been reported.

CHOLEDOCHAL CYST (CONGENITAL CYSTIC DILATION OF THE COMMON BILE DUCT)

Choledochal cysts are associated commonly with dilation of the intrahepatic bile ducts, so it is appropriate to discuss them in this chapter. The combination of intra- and extrahepatic cysts is similar to that in at least one of the polycystic diseases—namely CHF—but choledochal cysts differ significantly from the polycystic diseases because they are not heritable, are not associated with DPM (although hepatic fibrosis as a consequence of obstruction or cholangitis may be present), and are not ordinarily associated with lesions in other organs.

Choledochal cysts are more common in Japan than in Western countries,[158] and Japanese workers deserve the credit for emphasizing that choledochal cysts are frequently associated with dilation of intrahepatic ducts as shared elements of a systemic dilatory change.[159,160] Further, a classification of choledochal cysts has been proposed by Todani and colleagues (Figure 49-6). As noted previously, intrahepatic ductal dilation does not connote the presence of polycystic disease as defined here, and in fact, CHF may be unusual in Japan.[161]

Choledochal cysts, with the exception of one variety, are more common in females. They may present at any age. They have been demonstrated in utero and have been observed to develop in adult life.[162] Approximately 60 percent of patients present before the age of 10 years. Although these cysts are often said to be congenital lesions, it is probably more precise to say that affected patients have a congenital propensity for the development of cysts. Todani and co-workers have defined a subgroup of patients in whom the cysts are cylindric or diffuse.[163,164] Such cases lack a female predominance and differ from other cases of choledochal cysts in a number of respects.[163,164] Other workers have suggested that patients in the pediatric age group can be divided into several different groups.[165] It is important, therefore, to keep in mind that several conditions, differing in origin and

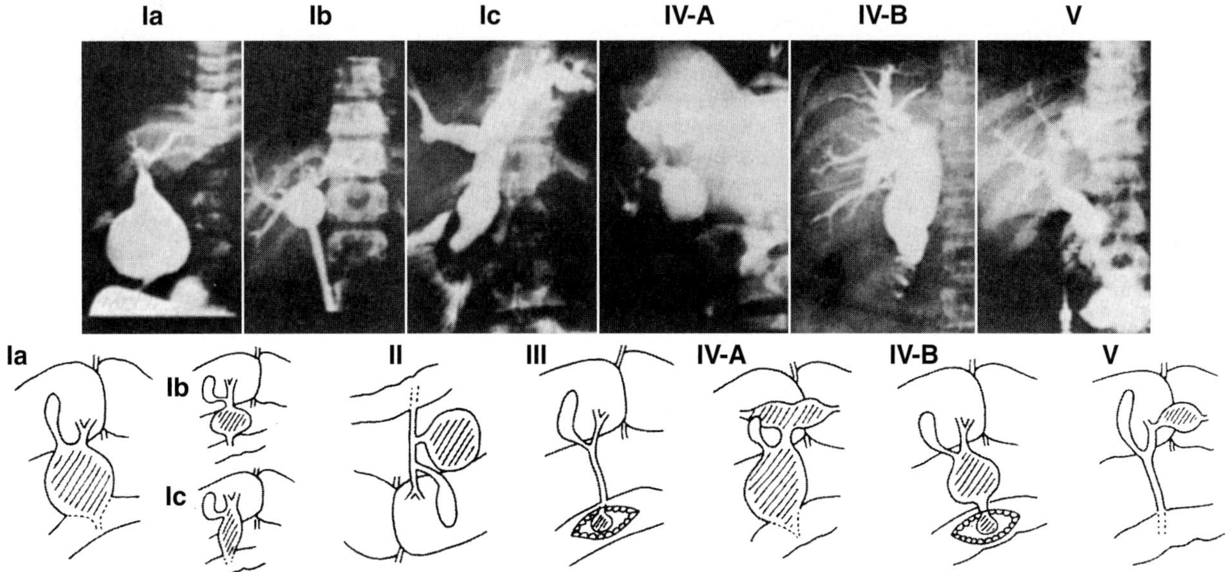

Figure 49-6 *Top,* Operative cholangiograms of congenital biliary duct cysts as classified by Todani and co-workers. *Bottom,* Diagrams of the various types of communicating cysts. *(Left to right), Ia,* common type; *Ib,* segmental dilation; *Ic,* diffuse dilation; *II,* diverticulum; *III,* choledochocele; *IV-A,* multiple cyst (intrahepatic and extrahepatic); *IV-B,* multiple cyst (extrahepatic); *V,* intrahepatic. This classification emphasizes the frequent co-existence of intrahepatic and extrahepatic duct dilation. (From Todani T, et al: Am J Surg 134:263, 1977.)

possibly in other aspects as well, may be included in the broad classification of choledochal cysts without DPM.

The clinical manifestations of choledochal cysts are quite variable.[166,167] Epigastric pain is the most common symptom. Fever and jaundice are the next most common findings in patients with choledochal cysts and intrahepatic duct dilation. In the latter group, abdominal masses are relatively uncommon when compared with patients with only choledochal dilation.[166] The classic triad of pain, jaundice, and an abdominal mass is present in no more than one quarter of patients.[168] Symptoms may develop, regress, and recur in a repetitive fashion.[165]

Although ultrasonography is the initial study of choice[169,170] and may be adequate in pediatric cases, a growing belief is that adult cases benefit from endoscopic retrograde cholangiopancreatography or percutaneous transhepatic cholangiography or both.[170,171] The latter are useful in defining the anatomy precisely, including the presence of intrahepatic ductal cysts, malignancy, and aberrant pancreatic ducts.[170,172]

The pathogenesis of choledochal cyst is a matter of debate and speculation. Suggested possibilities include congenital weakness of the wall, a primary abnormality of the mucosa, and congenital obstruction.[172] As already noted it is by no means clear that all cases have the same pathogenesis. The possible role of pancreatic reflux, associated with an abnormal choledochopancreaticoductal junction, has been emphasized.[173] There are at least two forms of this, depending on which duct joins the other and which is the major duct; the type of choledochal cyst is said to be related to the type of abnormal junction.[174] There is a high incidence but not an invariable occurrence of an abnormal junction. There is also a high incidence of stenosis of the bile duct of variable severity.[164,173] Dysfunction of postganglionic enervation of the common duct has also been suggested,[161] as has defective sphincteric function.[174]

Histologically the cysts have a fibrous wall, typically with absent or mild inflammation (the inflammation is chronic). Most often, the epithelial lining is absent. When this lining is present, its appearance varies from flattened to typically biliary.

As mentioned, intrahepatic dilation of bile ducts often has been demonstrated in association with choledochal cysts. The reported incidence varies widely from country to country. As an example of the problems discussed regarding the indiscriminate use of the term *Caroli's disease*, such cases are referred to in the surgical literature as examples of Caroli's disease despite the obvious differences between them and those described by Caroli (see earlier discussion). Todani and associates found intrahepatic dilation in somewhat less than 30 percent of their patients.[166] It is present less commonly in young children than in older patients.[166] It is sufficiently common that it always should be sought in patients with choledochal cyst. It is diffuse in two thirds of affected patients but may involve only the left lobe of the liver. It is rare that it involves only the right lobe.[163,146] The intrahepatic dilation of bile ducts, at least when associated with the cylindric type of choledochal cyst, tends to regress after excision of the choledochal cyst.[163,164] Dilation of the pancreatic duct is noted with some frequency in patients with choledochal cyst.[176,177]

Complications other than obstruction include stone formation (which occurs in approximately 8 percent of patients),[168] cholangitis, carcinoma, and, rarely, perforation. Perforation is particularly likely to occur when the junction of the bile duct and the pancreatic duct allows free egress of pancreatic secretions into the common duct.[164] Carcinoma is said to develop in 2 to 8 percent of cases.[168,178,179] These figures were derived in large part before the widespread use of excisional therapy, which may substantially reduce the incidence of malignancy. It is unlikely to eliminate it entirely, however, because carcinoma has developed after excision of cysts.[170,180] It is interesting that carcinoma was found in one patient with an abnormal pancreaticobiliary duct system without duct dilation.[181] The incidence of carcinoma increases with age.[178] Tumors may arise in various parts of the pancreaticobiliary system, including the liver, gallbladder, intrahepatic ducts, pancreatic ducts, and pancreas. The usual type is adenocarcinoma, but squamous carcinoma, adenoacanthoma, and undifferentiated carcinoma have been found.[178] The outcome in patients in whom malignancy develops is very poor.

It is now generally agreed that choledochal cysts require surgical treatment. The procedure of choice is excision of the cyst.[159,170,182] This procedure minimizes but does not completely eliminate cholangitis and presumably reduces the incidence of subsequent carcinoma. Todani and colleagues suggested that patients with normal junctions between the bile duct and pancreatic duct may require only an adequate transduodenal sphincteroplasty.[164] Cholecystectomy is usually performed at the same time. Most American surgeons seem to favor Roux-en-Y choledochojejunostomy for restoring biliary-enteric continuity. Todani and colleagues also used hepaticoduodenostomy.[163] Other techniques have also been suggested.[183] A wide anastomosis is important for minimizing cholangitis in situations in which excision of the cyst is not feasible because of the local anatomy or the age and medical status of the patient. A wide anastomosis may reduce the incidence of intrahepatic carcinoma.[184] Roux-en-Y jejunal loop drainage with a large anastomosis may be the operation of choice. In patients with associated dilation of intrahepatic ducts, partial hepatic resection may be appropriate, but only if the dilated ducts are localized to a single lobe.[163,185]

MALFORMATION SYNDROMES

The DPM (with the potential for forming ductal cysts) accompanies a considerable number of malformation syndromes, usually in combination with cystic, dysplastic kidneys.[123] It is likely that the cysts formed are communicating, but reconstruction studies in these cases are rare, as is cholangiography. Nevertheless, because of the character of the portal tract lesion, it seems reasonable to classify these cysts presumptively as communicating.

Meckel-Gruber Syndrome (Dysencephalia Splanchnocystica)

Meckel-Gruber syndrome is inherited as a recessive trait. It is characterized by the presence of many malformations, and death usually occurs perinatally or in early infancy.[186-189] The classic triad of findings in the syndrome—postaxial polydactyly, occipital encephalocele, and cystic kidneys—is not always present. The renal lesion appears to be cystic dysplasia and is quite characteristic. Various central nervous system lesions may be present.[190]

The range of abnormalities that may be present makes diagnosis difficult or uncertain, and a number of different criteria have been proposed for diagnosis.[190] The range of abnormalities raises the possibility that certain other reported malformation constellations,[191] which include DPM, central nervous system lesions, and renal abnormalities, but are not typically included as examples of the Meckel-Gruber syndrome, may be variants. Studies indicate that DPM is nearly always present.[192,194] In some patients dilation of intrahepatic bile ducts results in gross cysts.[187] Some reconstruction studies and occasional reports have suggested that the morphologic features in these patients were similar to ARPKD.[195,196] Other reconstruction studies suggest that the lesions differ in the two conditions.[197] Landing and co-workers determined by morphometric analysis that the lesion of the portal tracts in the Meckel-Gruber syndrome was more fibrotic than that in either CHF or ARPKD.[154] These investigators emphasized a fibrous sheath around canals of Hering. Rarely, pancreatic cysts may be present.[186]

A gene responsible for Meckel-Gruber syndrome in Finland has been mapped to chromosome 17q21-q24.[198] However, this linkage could not be confirmed in most of the non-Finnish families studied. An additional gene for Meckel-Gruber syndrome has been mapped to chromosome 11q13 in families of North African and Middle Eastern ancestry.[199] This genetic heterogeneity could account for the highly variable clinical phenotype.

Jeune's Syndrome (Thoracic Asphyxiating Dystrophy)

Jeune's syndrome is an autosomal-recessive form of dwarfism characterized by an extremely constricted thorax, shortened limbs, abnormalities of the pelvis, and cystic disease of the kidneys. Also apparently associated is a relatively high incidence of hepatic lesions, characterized by portal fibrosis and large numbers of bile ducts.[200-202] Gross cysts have not, to our knowledge, been described. Histologically the hepatic lesions are at least compatible with DPM. Landing and colleagues observed that the morphometric features are generally similar to those in CHF but that the portal tracts are smaller.[154] Bernstein observed microcysts of the pancreas in several cases.[155] The kidney disease is characterized by the development of progressive renal insufficiency. The pathophysiologic features of the liver disease have not been defined.

Ivemark's Syndrome (Renal-Hepatic-Pancreatic Dysplasia)

One of the two syndromes known as Ivemark's syndrome was described by him as a familial dysplasia of the kidneys, liver, and pancreas.[203] The liver lesions appear to be consistent with DPM. Only rare instances of the complete syndrome have been reported.[204] Apparent formes frustes without liver disease are encountered somewhat more frequently.[205] In one case an early biopsy specimen revealed paucity of bile ducts, and a later biopsy sample revealed apparent DPM.[206] A case with pancreatic, hepatic, and renal lesions was reported with trisomy C.[207] The specific diagnosis of renal-hepatic-pancreatic dysplasia can be made only after a number of other malformation syndromes that have comparable findings are precluded.[206]

Other Malformation Conditions

Potter, in her discussion of renal cysts,[208] noted that some patients with what she called type III cystic kidneys have associated liver lesions, and a few of these patients may have pancreatic cysts and fibrosis as well. No familial occurrence was described. In an illustrated case the picture and accompanying description indicate that the hepatic lesions consisted of minimal proliferation of connective tissue and a very slight increase in biliary ducts.[208] Such lesions, as we have indicated, might be considered examples of DPM as broadly interpreted, but Potter states that the hepatic lesions seen in association with type III kidneys can "ordinarily be easily distinguished from those found in type I (ARPKD)." Classification of these cases of Potter with combined liver and pancreatic lesions and type III kidneys is further complicated because type III kidneys are not confined to a single genetic entity, and Potter does not use dysplasia as a diagnostic designation. Landing has pointed out that hepatic lesions of a possibly similar nature may occur in the vaginal atresia syndromes and in tuberous sclerosis,[154] but little information is available on this point.

In one case of the trisomy E syndrome, a fibrocystic liver was observed.[209]

In a single case of Ellis-van Creveld syndrome (chondroectodermal dysplasia), portal fibrosis, an increase in the number of bile ducts, and cystic dysplasia of the kidneys were found.[210]

Bile duct dilation has been reported in Laurence-Moon-Biedl-Bardet syndrome.[211,212] It is not clear from the descriptions whether or not DPM was present. It is interesting that both cited cases were reported from Japan, where choledochal cyst (and intrahepatic duct dilatation) is relatively common. A single case of oral-facial-digital syndrome with renal and pancreatic cysts and "cystadenomatous" bile ducts has been reported.[213]

References

1. Henson SW Jr, Gray HK, Dockerty MB: Benign tumors of the liver. III. Solitary cysts. Surg Gynecol Obstet 103:607, 1956.
2. Flagg RS, Robinson DW: Solitary nonparasitic hepatic cysts: report of oldest known cases and review of the literature. Arch Surg 95:964, 1967.
3. Stoesser AV, Wangensteen OH: Solitary nonparasitic cysts of the liver. Am J Dis Child 38:241, 1929.
4. Caplan LH, Simon M: Nonparasitic cysts of the liver. Am J Roentgenol 96:421, 1966.
5. Desser P, Smith S: Nonparasitic liver cysts in children. J Pediatr 49:297, 1956.
6. Rosch J, Mayer BS, Campbell JR, et al: "Vascular" benign liver cyst in children: report of two cases. Radiology 126:747, 1978.
7. Roemer C, Ferrucci J, Mueller P, et al: Hepatic cysts: diagnosis and therapy by sonographic needle aspiration. Am J Radiol 136:1065, 1981.
8. Bloustein PA: Association of carcinoma with congenital cystic conditions of the liver and bile ducts. Am J Gastroenterol 67:40, 1977.
9. Saini S, Ferrucci J, Mueller PR, et al: Percutaneous aspiration of hepatic cysts done to provide definitive therapy. Am J Radiol 141:559, 1983.
10. Litwin DEM, Taylor BR, Langer B, Greig P: Nonparasitic cysts of the liver. The case of conservative surgical management. Ann Surg 205:45, 1987.
11. Sanchez H, Gagner M, Rossi RL, et al: Surgical management of nonparasitic cystic liver disease. Am J Surg 161:113, 1991.
12. Austin E, Mitchell G, Oliphant M, et al: Solitary hepatic duct polyp: a heretofore unheralded association. Surgery 89:359, 1981.
13. Lambruschu PG, Rudolf LE: Massive unifocal cyst of the liver in a drug abuser. Ann Surg 189:39, 1979.
14. Longmire WP Jr, Sergio AM, Gordon HE: Congenital cystic disease of the liver and biliary system. Ann Surg 174:711, 1971.
15. Andersson R, Jeppsson B, Lunderquist A, Bengmark S: Alcohol sclerotherapy of nonparasitic cysts of the liver. Br J Surg 76:254, 1989.
16. Hagiwara H, Kasahara A, Hayashi N, et al: Successful treatment of a hepatic cyst by one-shot instillation of minocycline chloride. Gastroenterology 103:675, 1992.
17. Henson SW Jr, Hallenbeck GA, Gray HK, et al: Benign tumors of the liver. V. Traumatic cysts. Surg Gynecol Obstet 104:302, 1957.
18. Vauthey JN, Madden GJ, Blumgart LH: Adult polycystic disease of the liver 1-2. Br J Surg 78:524, 1991.
19. Doppman JL, Dunnick NR, Girton RT, et al: Bile duct cysts secondary to liver infarcts: report of a case and experimental production of small vessel hepatic artery occlusion. Radiology 130:1, 1979.
20. Imamoglu KH, Walt AJ: Duplication of the duodenum extending into the liver. Am J Surg 133:628, 1977.
21. Wanless IR, Zahradnik J, Heathcote EJ: Hepatic cysts of periductal gland origin presenting as obstructive jaundice. Gastroenterology 93:894, 1987.
22. Nakanuma Y, Kurumaya H, Ohta G: Multiple cysts in the hepatic hilum and their pathogenesis. Virch Arch A Pathol Anat Histopathol 404:341, 1984.
23. Vick DJ, Goodman ZD, Deavers MT, et al: Ciliated hepatic foregut cyst: a study of six cases and review of the literature. Am J Surg Pathol 23:671, 1999.
24. Wheeler DA, Edmondson HA: Ciliated hepatic foregut cyst. Am J Surg Pathol 8:467, 1984.
25. Vick DJ, Goodman ZD, Ishak KG: Squamous cell carcinoma arising in a ciliated hepatic foregut cyst. Arch Pathol Lab Med 123:1115, 1999.
26. Ishak KG, Willis GW, Cummins SD, et al: Biliary cystadenoma and cystadenocarcinoma. Report of 14 cases and review of the literature. Cancer 39:322, 1977.
27. Marsh JL, Dahms B, Longmire WP: Cystadenoma and cystadenocarcinoma of the biliary system. Arch Surg 109:41, 1974.
28. Takayasu K, Muramatsu Y, Moriyama N, et al: Imaging diagnosis of bile duct cystadenocarcinoma. Cancer 61:941, 1988.
29. Inemoto Y, Kondno Y, Fukamachi S: Biliary cystadenocarcinoma with peritoneal carcinomatosis. Cancer 48:1664, 1988.
30. Keech M: Cystadenomas of the pancreas and intrahepatic bile ducts. Gastroenterology 19:568, 1951.
31. Devine P, Ucci A: Biliary cystadenocarcinoma arising in a congenital cyst. Hum Pathol 16:92, 1985.
32. Wheeler D, Edmonson H: Cystadenoma with mesenchymal stroma (CMS) in the liver and bile ducts. Cancer 56:1434, 1985.
33. Unger PD, Thung SN, Kaneko M: Pseudosarcomatous cystadenocarcinoma of the liver. Hum Pathol 18:521, 1987.
34. Duran ME, Roncero V, Gomez L, et al: Experimental induction of biliary cystadenoma in rats: a morphological study. Histol Histopathol 7:555, 1992.
35. Lewis WD, Jenkins RL, Rossi RL, et al: Surgical treatment of biliary cystadenoma. A report of 15 cases. Arch Surg 123:563, 1988.
36. Marcial M, Hauser S, Cibas E, et al: Intrahepatic biliary cystadenoma. Dig Dis Sci 31:884, 1986.
37. Dehner L, Ewing S, Sumner H: Infantile mesenchymal hamartoma of the liver. Histologic and ultrastructural observations. Arch Pathol 99:379, 1975.
38. Ishak R: Primary hepatic tumors in childhood. Prog Liver Dis 5:636, 1976.
39. Stocker T, Ishak K: Mesenchymal hamartoma of the liver: report of 30 cases and review of the literature. Pediatr Pathol 1:245, 1983.
40. Ros P, Goodman A, Ishak K, et al: Mesenchymal hamartoma of the liver: radiologic-pathologic correlation. Radiology 158:629, 1986.

41. Witzleben CL: Unpublished observations.
42. Bove KE, Blough RI, Soukup S: Third report of t(19q)(13.4) in mesenchymal hamartoma of liver with comments on link to embryonal sarcoma. Pediatr Dev Pathol 1:438, 1998.
43. de Chadarevian JP, Pawel BR, Faerber EN, Weintraub WH: Undifferentiated (embryonal) sarcoma arising in conjunction with mesenchymal hamartoma of the liver. Mod Pathol 7:490, 1994.
44. Lauwers GY, Grant LD, Donnelly WH, et al: Hepatic undifferentiated (embryonal) sarcoma arising in a mesenchymal hamartoma. Am J Surg Pathol 21:1248, 1997.
45. Dehner LP: Hepatic tumors in the pediatric age group: a distinctive clinicopathologic spectrum. In Rosenberg HS, Bolande RP, eds: Perspectives in Pediatric Pathology. Chicago, Year Book Medical Publishers, 1978:217.
46. Ishak KG, Rabin L: Benign tumors of the liver. Med Clin North Am 59:995, 1975.
47. Adam YG, Huvos AG, Fortner JG: Giant hemangiomas of the liver. Ann Surg 172:239, 1970.
48. Hirner A, Haring R: Giant cavernous hemangiomas of the liver. Langenbecks Arch Chir 364:25, 1978.
49. Trastek V, van Heerden J, Sheedy P, et al: Cavernous hemangiomas of the liver: resect or observe. Am J Surg 145:49, 1983.
50. Olmsted WW, Stocker JT: RPC from the AFIP. Diag Radiol 117:59, 1975.
51. Watanabe I, Kasai M, Suzuki S: True teratoma of the liver—report of a case and review of the literature. Acta Hepatogastroenterol 25:40, 1978.
52. Witte D, Kissane J, Askin F: Hepatic teratomas in children. Pediatr Pathol 1:81, 1983.
53. Robinson R, Nelson L: Hepatic teratoma in an anencephalic fetus. Arch Pathol Lab Med 110:655, 1986.
54. DeStephano D, Wesley J, Heidelberger K, et al: Primitive cystic hepatic neoplasm of infancy with mesothelial differentiation. Pediatr Pathol 4:291, 1985.
55. Eisenberg D, Hurwitz L, Yu AC: CT and sonography of multiple bile-duct hamartomas simulating malignant liver disease (case report). Am J Radiol 147:279, 1986.
56. Ichijima K, Lobashi Y, Yamabe H, et al: Peliosis hepatis. An unusual case involving multiple organs. Acta Pathol Jpn 30:109, 1980.
57. Warfel K, Ellis G: Peliosis of the spleen. Arch Pathol Lab Med 106:99, 1982.
58. Yanoff M, Rawson A: Peliosis hepatis: an anatomic study with demonstration of two varieties. Arch Pathol 77:159, 1964.
59. Lyon J, Bookstein J, Cartwright CA, et al: Peliosis hepatis: diagnosis by magnification wedged hepatic venography. Radiology 150:647, 1984.
60. Nadell J, Kosek J: Peliosis hepatis: twelve cases associated with oral androgen therapy. Arch Pathol Lab Med 101:405, 1977.
61. Bagheri A, Boyer J: Peliosis hepatis associated with androgenic-anabolic steroid therapy: a severe form of hepatic injury. Ann Intern Med 81:610, 1974.
62. Poulsen H, Winkler K: Liver disease with periportal sinusoidal dilatation. Digestion 8:441, 1973.
63. Ross R, Kovacs K, Horvath E: Ultrastructure of peliosis hepatis in percutaneous biopsy. Pathol Eur 7:273, 1972.
64. Ishak K: Hepatic lesions caused by anabolic and contraceptive steroids. Semin Liver Dis 1:116, 1981.
65. Scheuer PJ, Schachter LA, Mathur S, et al: Peliosis hepatis after liver transplantation. J Clin Pathol 43:1036, 1990.
66. Perkocha LA, Geaghan SM, Benedict Yen TS, et al: Clinical and pathological features of bacillary peliosis hepatis in association with human immunodeficiency virus infection. N Engl J Med 323:1581, 1990.
67. Lee K: Peliosis hepatis-like lesion in aging rats. Vet Pathol 20:410, 1983.
68. Zafrani E, Cazier A, Baudelot A-M, et al: Ultrastructural lesions of the liver in human peliosis. Am J Pathol 114:349, 1984.
69. Terada J, et al: Normal and abnormal development of the human intrahepatic biliary tree: a review. Tohoku J Exp Med 181:19, 1997.
70. Reynolds D, et al: Identification of a locus for autosomal dominant polycystic liver disease, on chromosome 19p13.2-13.1, Amer J Human Genet 67:1598, 2000.
71. Iglesias D, et al: Isolated polycystic liver disease not linked to polycystic kidney disease 1 and 2. Dig Dis Sci 44:385, 1999.
72. Jorgensen M: The ductal plate malformation. Acta Pathol Microbiol Scand Suppl 257:1, 1977.
73. Desmet VJ: Pathogenesis of ductal plate abnormalities. Mayo Clin Proc 73:80, 1998.
74. De Koning TJ, et al: Congenital hepatic fibrosis in 3 siblings with phosphomannose isomerase deficiency. Virchow's Arch 437:101, 2000.
75. De Koning TJ, et al: Phosphomannose isomerase deficiency as a cause of congenital hepatic fibrosis and protein-losing enteropathy. J Hepatol 31:557, 1999.
76. Niehues R, et al: Carbohydrate-deficient glycoprotein syndrome type Ib: phosphomannose isomerase deficiency and mannose therapy. J Clin Invest 101:1414, 1998.
77. De Koning TJ, et al: A novel disorder of N-glycosylation due to phosphomannose isomerase deficiency. Biochem Biophys Res Comm 245:38, 1998.
78. Jacken J, et al: Phosphomannose isomerase deficiency: a carbohydrate-deficient glycoprotein syndrome with hepatic-intestinal presentation. Am J Human Genet 62:1535, 1998.
79. Caroli J: Diseases of the intrahepatic biliary tree. Clin Gastroenterol 2:147, 1973.
80. Karhunen P, Tenhu M: Adult polycystic kidney and liver diseases are separate entities. Clin Genet 30:29, 1986.
81. Berrebi G, Erickson RB, Markes BW: Autosomal dominant polycystic liver disease: a second family. Clin Genet 21:342, 1982.
82. Norio R: Polycystic disease of liver: an entity of its own or not? Clin Genet 23:78, 1983.
83. Grantham JJ: Clinical aspects of adult and infantile polycystic kidney disease 1-1. Contrib Nephrol 48:178, 1985.
84. Reeders ST: Multilocus polycystic disease. Nat Genet 1:235, 1992.
85. Turco A, Peissel B, Gammaro L: Linkage analysis for the diagnosis of autosomal dominant polycystic kidney disease, and for the determination of genetic heterogeneity in Italian families. Clin Genet 40:387, 1991.
86. Grantham JJ: Polycystic kidney disease—an old problem in a new context. N Engl J Med 319:944, 1988.
87. Reeders ST, Breuning H, Davies KE, et al: A highly polymorphic DNA marker linked to adult polycystic disease on chromosome 16. Nature 317:542, 1985.
88. Germino GG, Somlo S, Weinstat-Saslow D, Reeders ST: Positional cloning approach to the dominant polycystic kidney disease gene, PKD1. Kidney Int 43:S20, 1993.
89. Daoust M, Reynolds D, Bichet D, Somlo S: Evidence for a third genetic locus for autosomal dominant polycystic kidney disease. Genomics 25:733, 1995.
90. Gabow PA, Johnson AM, Kaehny WB, et al: Factors affecting the progression of renal disease in autosomal-dominant polycystic kidney disease. Kidney Int 41:1311, 1992.
91. Bear JC, Parfrey PS, Morgan JM, et al: Autosomal dominant polycystic kidney disease: new information for genetic counselling. Am J Med Genet 43:548, 1992.
92. Gabow PA, Chapman AB, Johnson AM, et al: Renal structure and hypertension in autosomal dominant polycystic kidney disease. Kidney Int 38:1177, 1990.
93. Kaplan BS, Rabin I, Drummond KN: Autosomal dominant polycystic renal disease in children. J Pediatr 90:782, 1977.
94. Shokeir MHK: Expression of "adult" polycystic renal disease in the fetus and newborn. Clin Genet 14:61, 1978.
95. Multinovic J, Fialkow PJ, Rudd TG, et al: Liver cysts in patients with autosomal dominant polycystic kidney disease. Am J Med 68:741, 1980.
96. Levine E, Cooke LT, Grantham JJ: Liver cysts in autosomal-dominant polycystic kidney disease: clinical and computed tomographic study. Am J Radiol 145:229, 1985.
97. Grunfeld JP, Albouze G, Jungers P, et al: Liver changes and complications in adult polycystic kidney disease. Adv Nephrol 14:1, 1985.
98. Comfort MW, Gray HK, Dahlin DC, et al: Polycystic disease of the liver: a study of 24 cases. Gastroenterology 20:60, 1952.
99. Gabow PA, Johnson AM, Kaehny WB, et al: Risk factors for the development of hepatic cysts in autosomal dominant polycystic kidney disease. Hepatology 11:1033, 1990.
100. Terada T, Nakanuma: Congenital biliary dilatation in autosomal dominant adult polycystic disease of the liver and kidneys. Arch Pathol Lab Med 112:1113, 1988.
101. Kida T, Nakanuma Y, Terada T: Cystic dilatation of peribiliary glands in livers with adult polycystic disease and livers with solitary nonparasitic cysts. An autopsy study. Hepatology 16:334, 1992.

102. Ramos A, Torres VE, Holley KE, et al: The liver in autosomal dominant polycystic kidney disease. Arch Pathol Lab Med 114:180, 1990.
103. Cobben JM, Breuning MH, Schoots C, et al: Congenital hepatic fibrosis in autosomal-dominant polycystic kidney disease. Kidney Int 38:880, 1990.
104. Manes JC, Kissane JM, Valdes AJ: Congenital hepatic fibrosis, liver cell carcinoma, and adult polycystic kidneys. Cancer 39:2619, 1977.
105. Christ M, Bechtel U, Schnaack S, et al: Aneurysms of coronary arteries in a patient with adult polycystic kidney disease—arteriosclerosis or involvement by the primary disease. Clin Invest 71:2:150, 1993.
106. Hossack KF, Leddy CL, Johnson AM, et al: Echocardiographic findings in autosomal dominant polycystic kidney disease. N Engl J Med 319:907, 1988.
107. Lozano AM, Leblanc R: Cerebral aneurysms and polycystic kidney disease. A critical review. Can J Neurol Sci 19:222, 1992.
108. Wiebers DO, Torres VE: Screening of unruptured intracranial aneurysms in autosomal dominant polycystic kidney disease. N Engl J Med 327:953, 1992.
109. Fehlings MG, Gentili F: The association between polycystic kidney disease and cerebral aneurysms. Le J Can Sci Neurol 18:505, 1991.
110. Telenti A, Torres VE, Gross JB, et al: Hepatic cyst infection in autosomal dominant polycystic kidney disease. Mayo Clin Proc 65:933, 1990.
111. London RD, Malik AA, Train JS: Infection in a patient with polycystic kidney and liver disease: noninvasive localization and treatment. Am J Med 84:1082, 1988.
112. Landais P, Grunfeld JP, Droz D, et al: Cholangiocellular carcinoma in polycystic kidney and liver disease. Arch Intern Med 144:2274, 1984.
113. Coffin B, Hadengue A, Degos F, Benhamou JP: Calcified hepatic and renal cysts in adult dominant polycystic kidney disease. Dig Dis Sci 35:1172, 1990.
114. Lin T-Y, Chen C-C, Wang S-M: Treatment of nonparasitic cystic disease of the liver: a new approach to therapy with polycystic liver. Ann Surg 168:921, 1968.
115. Starzl TE, Reyes J, Tzakis A, et al: Liver transplantation for polycystic liver disease. Arch Surg 125:575, 1990.
116. Reeders S, et al: A highly polymorphic DNA marker linked to adult polycystic kidney disease on chromosome 16. Nature 317:542, 1985.
117. Kimberling W, et al: Autosomal dominant polycystic disease: localization of the second gene to chromosome 4q13-q23. Genomics 18:467, 1993.
118. Avner E: Cellular pathophysiology of cystic kidney disease: insight into future therapies. Int J Develop Biol 43:457, 1999.
119. Persu A, Devuyst O: Transepithelial chloride secretion and cystogenesis in autosomal polycystic kidney disease. Nephrol Dialysis Transplant 15:747, 2000.
120. Wu G, Somlo S: Molecular genetics and mechanism of autosomal dominant polycystic kidney disease. Molec Genet Metab 69:1, 2000.
121. Perez L, et al: Autosomal recessive kidney disease presenting in adulthood. Molecular diagnosis of the family. Nephrol Dialysis Transplant 13:1273, 1998.
122. Zerres K, et al: Prenatal diagnosis of autosomal recessive kidney disease (ARPKD): molecular genetics, clinical experience, and fetal morphology. Am J Med Genet 76:137, 1998.
123. Bernstein J: Hepatic involvement in hereditary renal syndromes. Birth Defects: Original Article Series 23:115, 1987.
124. Kerr DNS, Harrison CV, Sherlock S, et al: Congenital hepatic fibrosis. Q J Med 30:91, 1961.
125. Alvarez E, Bernard O, Brunelle F, et al: Congenital hepatic fibrosis in children. J Pediatr 99:370, 1981.
126. Odievre M, Chaumont P, Montague J, et al: Anomalies of the intrahepatic portal venous system in congenital hepatic fibrosis. Radiology 122:427, 1977.
127. Richard-Molard B, Couzigou P, Julien J, et al: Fibrose hepatique congenitale tardivement revelee par une encephalopathie hepatique. Gastroenterol Clin Biol 9:449, 1985.
128. Fauvert R, Benhamou J: Congenital hepatic fibrosis. In Schaffner F, Sherlock S, Leery C, eds: The Liver and Its Diseases. New York, Intercontinental Medical Book, 1974:283.
129. Williams R, Scheuer PJ, Heard BE: Congenital hepatic fibrosis with an unusual pulmonary lesion. J Clin Pathol 17:135, 1964.
130. Naveh Y, Roguin N, Ludatscher R, et al: Congenital hepatic fibrosis with congenital heart disease. Gut 21:799, 1980.
131. Pelletier V, Galenao N, Brouchu P, et al: Secretory diarrhea with protein-losing enteropathy, enterocolitis cystic superficialis, intestinal lymphangiectasis and congenital hepatic fibrosis: a new syndrome. J Pediatr 108:61, 1986.
132. Pedersen P, Tygstrup I: Congenital hepatic fibrosis combined with protein-losing enteropathy and recurrent thrombosis. Acta Paediatr Scand 69:571, 1980.
133. Lieberman E, Madrigal-Salinas L, Gwin JL, et al: Infantile polycystic disease of the kidneys and liver: clinical, pathological and radiological correlations and comparisons with congenital hepatic fibrosis. Medicine 50:277, 1993.
134. Landing BH: Some problems in the meanings of terms, as exemplified by tubulointerstitial and medullary cystic diseases of the kidneys. Perspect Pediatr Pathol 12:20, 1988.
135. Hauser R, Alexander R: Localized congenital hepatic fibrosis presenting as an abdominal mass. Hum Pathol 5:473, 1978.
136. Faivre J, Richir C, Deraud C: Agenesis of the left hepatic lobe, persistent ascites. Cruveilhier-Baumgarten's disease. Arch Mal Appar Dig 57:359, 1968.
137. Leong A: Segmental biliary ectasia and congenital hepatic fibrosis in a patient with chromosomal abnormality. Pathology 12:275, 1980.
138. Parker RGF: Fibrosis of the liver as a congenital anomaly. J Pathol Bacteriol 71:359, 1956.
139. Jorgensen M: The ductal plate malformation. Acta Pathol Microbiol Immunol Scand A 257(suppl):1, 1977.
140. Bouquien H, Delumeau G, Lenne Y, et al: Cited by Murray-Lyon IM, Shilkin KB, Laws JW, et al: Non-obstructive dilatation of the intrahepatic biliary tree with cholangitis. Q J Med 41:477, 1973.
141. Vic-Dupont, Mignot J, Halle B: Non-obstructive dilatation of the intrahepatic biliary tree with cholangitis. Q J Med 41:477, 1973.
142. Alvarez F, Hadchoel M, Bernard O: Latent chronic cholangitis in congenital hepatic fibrosis. Eur J Pediatr 139:203, 1982.
143. Murray-Lyon IM, Shilkin ST, Laws JW, et al: Non-obstructive dilatation of the intrahepatic biliary tree with cholangitis. Q J Med 41:477, 1973.
144. Howlett SA, Shulman ST, Ayoub EM, et al: Cholangitis complicating congenital hepatic fibrosis. Case report. Dig Dis Sci 20:790, 1975.
145. Kerr DNS, Okonkwo S, Choa RG: Congenital hepatic fibrosis: the long-term prognosis. Gut 19:514, 1961.
146. Daroca PJ, Tuthill R, Reed RJ: Cholangiocarcinoma arising in congenital hepatic fibrosis. Arch Pathol 99:592, 1975.
147. Holthofer H, Kumpulainen T, Rapola J: Polycystic disease of the kidney. Evaluation and classification based on nephron segment and cell-type specific markers. Lab Invest 62:363, 1990.
148. Moyer J, Lee-Tischler M, Kwon H-Y, et al: Candidate gene associated with a mutation causing recessive polycystic kidney disease in mice. Science 264:1329, 1995.
149. Zerres K, Mucher G, Bachner L, et al: Mapping of the gene for autosomal recessive polycystic kidney disease (ARPKD) to chromosome 6p21-cen. Nature Genet 7:429, 1994.
150. Zerres K: Autosomal recessive polycystic kidney disease. Clin Invest 70:794, 1992.
151. Blyth H, Ockenden BG: Polycystic disease of kidneys and liver presenting in childhood. J Med Genet 8:257, 1971.
152. Anand S, Chang J, Lieberman E: Polycystic disease and hepatic fibrosis in children: renal function studies. Am J Dis Child 130:810, 1975.
153. Gang D, Herrin J: Infantile polycystic disease of the liver and kidneys. Clin Nephrol 25:28, 1986.
154. Landing BH, Wells TR, Claireaux AE: Morphometric analysis of liver lesions in cystic diseases of childhood. Hum Pathol 11(suppl): 549, 1980.
155. Bernstein J: Cystic diseases of the liver in infancy. In Javitt N, ed: Neonatal Hepatitis and Biliary Atresia. Bethesda, Md., Public Health Service, DHEW publication NIH #79-1296, 1979.
156. Boichis H, Passwell J, David R, et al: Congenital hepatic fibrosis and nephronophthisis: a family study. Q J Med 42:221, 1973.
157. Witzleben CL, Sharp A. Nephronophthisis—congenital hepatic fibrosis. An additional hepatorenal disorder. Hum Pathol 13:728, 1982.
158. Hays DM, Goodman GN, Snyder WH, et al: Congenital cystic dilatation of the common bile duct. Arch Surg 98:457, 1969.

159. Saito S, Tsuchida Y, Hashizume K, et al: Congenital cystic dilatation of the biliary ducts: surgical procedures and long-term results. Z Kinderchir 19:49, 1976.
160. Todani T, Watanabe Y, Narusue M, et al: Congenital bile duct cysts. Classification, operative procedures, and review of thirty-seven cases including cancer arising from choledochal cyst. Am J Surg 143:263, 1977.
161. Nonomura A, Ohta G, Yoshida K, et al: Congenital hepatic fibrosis. A case report with study of three dimensional reconstruction of serial sections of the liver. Acta Pathol Jpn 38:949, 1978.
162. Wideman MA, Tan A, Martinez CJ: Fetal sonography and neonatal scintigraphy of a choledochal cyst. J Nucl Med 86:893, 1985.
163. Todani T, Watanabe Y, Fujii T, et al: Congenital choledochal cyst with intrahepatic involvement. Arch Surg 119:1038, 1984.
164. Todani T, Watanabe Y, Fujii T, et al: Cylindrical dilatation of the choledochus: a special type of congenital bile duct dilatation. Surgery 98:964, 1985.
165. Barlow B, Tabor E, Blan WA, et al: Choledochal cyst: a review of 19 cases. J Pediatr 89:934, 1976.
166. Todani T, Naruse M, Watanabe Y, et al: Management of congenital choledochal cyst with intrahepatic involvement. Ann Surg 187:272, 1978.
167. Flanigan DP: Biliary cysts. Ann Surg 177:705, 1973.
168. Yamaguchi M: Congenital choledochal cyst. Analysis of 1433 patients in the Japanese literature. Am J Surg 140:653, 1980.
169. Han BK, Babcock D, Gelfand M: Choledochal cyst with bile duct dilatation: sonography and ^{99m}Tc1DA cholescintigraphy. Am J Radiol 136:1075, 1981.
170. Takiff H, Stone M, Fonkalsrud E: Choledochal cysts: results of primary surgery and need for reoperation in young patients. Am J Surg 150:141, 1985.
171. Hagen G, Kolmannskog F: Radiologic approach to bile duct cysts in adults. Acta Radiol 33:240, 1992.
172. Spitz L: Choledochal cyst. Surg Gynecol Obstet 147:444, 1978.
173. Babbitt D, Starsuk R, Clemett A: Choledochal cyst: a concept of etiology. Am J Radiol 119:57, 1973.
174. Iwai N, Yanagihara J, Tokiwa K, et al: Congenital choledochal dilatation with emphasis on pathophysiology of the biliary tract. Ann Surg 215:27, 1992.
175. Kusunoki M, Yamamura T, Takahaski T, et al: Choledochal cyst. Its possible autonomic involvement in the bile duct. Arch Surg 122:997, 1987.
176. Rattner D, Schapiro RH, Warshaw AL: Abnormalities of the pancreatic and biliary ducts in adult patients with choledochal cyst. Arch Surg 118:1068, 1983.
177. Uno J, Sakoda K, Akita M: Surgical aspects of cystic dilatation of the bile duct. Ann Surg 195:203, 1982.
178. Vogles C, Smadja C, Shands W, et al: Carcinoma in choledochal cysts. Age-related incidence. Arch Surg 118:986, 1983.
179. Todani T, Tabuchi K, Watanabe Y, et al: Carcinoma arising in the wall of congenital bile duct cysts. Cancer 44:1134, 1979.
180. Gallagher P, Mills R, Mitchinson M: Congenital dilatation of the intrahepatic ducts with cholangiocarcinoma. J Clin Pathol 25:804, 1972.
181. Tanaka K, Nishimura A, Yamada K, et al: Cancer of the gallbladder associated with anomalous junction of the pancreatobiliary duct system without bile duct dilatation. Br J Surg 80:622, 1993.
182. Deziel D, Rossi R, Munson L, et al: Management of bile duct cyst in adults. Arch Surg 118:986, 1983.
183. Henne-Bruns D, Kremer B, Thonke F, et al: "Endoscopy friendly" resection technique of choledochal cysts. Endoscopy 25:176, 1993.
184. Todani T, Watanabe Y, Toki A, et al: Reoperation for congenital choledochal cyst. Ann Surg 207:142, 1988.
185. Lorenzo Z, Seed R, Beal J: Congenital dilatation of the biliary tract. Am J Surg 121:510, 1971.
186. Opitz JM, Howe JJ: The Meckel syndrome (dysencephalia splanchnocystica, the Gruber syndrome). Birth Defects 5:167, 1969.
187. Fried K, Liban E, Lurie M, et al: Polycystic kidneys associated with malformations of the brain, polydactyly, and other birth defects in newborn sibs. A lethal syndrome showing the autosomal-recessive pattern of inheritance. J Med Genet 8:285, 1971.
188. Meckel S, Passarge E: Encephalocele, polycystic kidneys, and polydactyly as an autosomal recessive trait simulating certain other disorders: the Meckel syndrome. Ann Genet 14:97, 1971.
189. Hsia YE, Bratu M, Herbordt A: Genetics of the Meckel syndrome (dysencephalica splanchnocystica). Pediatrics 48:237, 1971.
190. Herriot R, Hallam LA, Gray ES: Dandy-Walker malformation in the Meckel syndrome. Am J Med Genet 38:207, 1991.
191. Miranda D, Schinella RA, Finegold MJ: Familial renal dysplasia. Microdissection studies with associated central nervous system and hepatic malformations. Arch Pathol 93:483, 1972.
192. Rapola J, Salonen R: Visceral anomalies in the Meckel syndrome. Teratology 31:193, 1985.
193. Salonen R: The Meckel syndrome: clinicopathological findings in 67 patients. Am J Med Genet 18:671, 1984.
194. Blankenberg TA, Ruebner BH, Ellis WG, et al: Pathology of renal and hepatic anomalies in Meckel syndrome. Am J Med Genet 3:395, 1987.
195. Jorgensen M: A case of abnormal intrahepatic bile duct arrangement submitted to three dimensional reconstruction. Acta Pathol Microbiol Immunol Scand [A] 79:303, 1971.
196. Bernstein J, Brough J, McAdams AJ: The renal lesion in syndromes of multiple congenital malformations. Cerebrohepatorenal syndrome: Jeune asphyxiating thoracic dystrophy; tuberous sclerosis; Meckel syndrome. Birth Defects 10:35, 1974.
197. Adams CM, Danks DM, Campbell PE: Comments upon the classification of infantile polycystic diseases of the liver and kidney based upon three-dimensional reconstruction of the liver. J Med Genet 11:234, 1974.
198. Paavola P, Salonen R, Baumer A, et al: Clinical and genetic heterogeneity in Meckel syndrome. Hum Genet 101:88, 1997.
199. Roume J, Genin E, Cormier-Daire V, et al: A gene for Meckel syndrome maps to chromosome 11q13. Am J Hum Genet 63:1095, 1998,
200. Shokeir MHK, Houston CS, Awen CF: Asphyxiating thoracic chondrodystrophy. Association with renal disease and evidence of possible heterozygous expression. J Med Genet 8:107, 1971.
201. Edelson PJ, Spackham TJ, Belliveau RE, et al: A renal lesion in asphyxiating thoracic dysplasia. Birth Defects 10:51, 1971.
202. Cremin BJ: Infantile thoracic dystrophy. Br J Radiol 43:199, 1970.
203. Ivemark BI, Oldfelt V, Zetterstrom R: Familial dysplasia of kidneys, liver and pancreas. A probably genetically determined syndrome. Acta Paediatr 48:1, 1959.
204. Strayer DS, Kissane J: Dysplasia of the kidneys, liver and pancreas: report of a variant of Ivemark's syndrome. Hum Pathol 19:228, 1978.
205. Yeoh G, Bannatyne P, Russel P, et al: Combined renal and pancreatic dysplasia in the newborn. Pathology 17:653, 1985.
206. Bernstein J, Chandra M, Creswell J, et al: Renal-hepatic-pancreatic dysplasia: a syndrome reconsidered. Am J Med Genet 26:391, 1987.
207. Blair JD: Trisomy C and cystic dysplasia of kidneys, liver and pancreas. Birth Defects 12:139, 1976.
208. Potter E: Normal and abnormal development of the kidney. Chicago, Year Book Medical Publishers, 1972.
209. Butler LJ, Snodgrass GJA, France NE, et al: E(16-18) trisomy syndrome: analysis of 13 cases. Arch Dis Child 40:600, 1965.
210. Bohm N, Fukuda M, Staudt R, et al: Chondroectodermal dysplasia (Ellis-Van Creveld syndrome) with dysplasia of renal medulla and bile ducts. Histopathology 2:267, 1978.
211. Tsuchiya R, Nishimura R, Ito T: Congenital cystic dilatation of the bile duct associated with Laurence-Moon-Biedl-Bardet syndrome. Arch Surg 112:82, 1977.
212. Nakamura F, Sasaki H, Kajihara H, Yamanoue M: Case report: Laurence-Moon-Biedl syndrome accompanied by congenital hepatic fibrosis. J Gastroenterol Hepatol 5:206, 1990.
213. Kennedy SM, Hashida Y, Malatack JJ: Polycystic kidneys, pancreatic cysts, and cystadenomatous bile ducts in the oral-facial-digital syndrome type 1. Arch Pathol Lab Med 115:519, 1991.

CHAPTER

50

Cholestatic Syndromes of Infancy and Childhood

Valeer J. Desmet, MD, PhD, and Tania A. Roskams, MD, PhD

ABBREVIATION

EHBDA extrahepatic bile duct atresia

EXTRAHEPATIC CHOLESTASIS

Various diseases of the extrahepatic bile ducts may cause obstruction to bile flow and cholestasis in neonates and children. By far the most frequent condition in this group is extrahepatic bile duct atresia (EHBDA). Because of its relative frequency, its differential diagnostic problems, and the extensive studies devoted to this condition in the last 25 years, EHBDA is the main subject of this chapter.

ATRESIA OF EXTRAHEPATIC BILE DUCTS

Historic Overview

EHBDA is defined as the lack of a lumen in part or all of the extrahepatic biliary tract, causing complete obstruction to bile flow.[1] This definition is biased by the precision (or lack of precision) of the investigative method used; that is, palpation, macroscopic inspection, or both of transected (whether or not obliterated) ducts, inspection of the ducts through surgical microscopes, operative cholangiography, or microscopic examination of specimens. The reliability of these various investigative approaches differs. In the nineteenth century, observations of EHBDA were made by inspecting with the naked eye the bile ducts at autopsy. By definition, this represented investigation in the end stage of the disease. It is extremely important to study the early stages of the disease, which has become feasible only in recent times.

The earliest observations of EHBDA were made around the middle of the nineteenth century.[2-4] Quite early in the course of study, controversy arose about the etiology and pathogenesis of this disease, which was considered to result from either a lack of development (agenesis) or antenatal infection.[5]

Thomson,[6-8] who published one of the first major reviews of EHBDA (49 patients), concluded that it represented a progressive inflammatory lesion of bile ducts, whatever the cause. Other early investigators also adhered to the idea of a descending cholangitis instead of a malformation.[9] Congenital syphilis, fetal peritonitis, and erythroblastosis fetalis were considered to be causes for this acquired condition.[10] By contrast, several authors favored the concept of a developmental anomaly.[11,12] Controversy over whether the etiology and pathogenesis were developmental or caused by an infection still persists, although the classically invoked infectious agents have been replaced by viruses whose causative role remains to be confirmed.[13] Surgical treatment of EHBDA was first discussed by Holmes in 1916[11]; he predicted that a conventional biliary-enteric anastomosis might be feasible in the 16 percent of patients with dilated, bile-containing proximal segments of extrahepatic ducts.This correctable group of patients was separated from the majority, in whom the entire extrahepatic biliary tract was obliterated. Successful surgery was first reported by Ladd in 1928.[14] One of his early patients was reported to be doing well 37 years later.[15] However, few reports of survival were published in the next four decades; Bill counted only 52 reported successes after operations for biliary atresia performed between 1927 and 1970,[16] and most of them had a limited period of follow-up.

In early clinical reports EHBDA frequently was confused with inspissated bile syndrome (see p. 1518),[17] neonatal hepatitis (see p. 1520), and choledochal cyst (see p. 1520).

In the 1940s curative surgery in the newborn was confined almost exclusively to patients with inspissated bile syndrome.[18] Obstruction in these patients was thought to be a consequence of thick, tenacious bile that required operative irrigation of the extrahepatic bile ducts. This indication for surgery disappeared when it was demonstrated that the vast majority of these patients had a primary hepatic parenchymal disorder associated with massive hemolysis resulting from Rh or ABO incompatibility or acute dehydration, Cholestasis resolved in most patients without surgical intervention.[19] In 1953 Gross documented that EHBDA was the most common condition causing obstructive jaundice in the first months of life,[20] and that most patients had the noncorrectable type of lesion. Early death was an inevitable consequence in these patients.

In the 1950s and 1960s the uselessness of surgery in inspissated bile syndrome and the inability of surgery to correct the lesion in the vast majority of patients with true EHBDA led to delayed operations for jaundice in the newborn. Even infants with remediable lesions were operated on so late that irreversible liver damage had already occurred.[18] This tragedy led Clatworthy and McDonald to advocate brief diagnostic laparotomy and operative cholangiography in the first months of life in all infants with inexplicable jaundice.[21]

In the meantime advances had been made in the distinction of several types of non-obstructive forms of neonatal jaundice and cholestasis of the newborn. It appeared that operation could be harmful in infants with neonatal hepatitis.[22-24] Because the diagnosis of biliary atresia versus neonatal hepatitis could not be established in most infants during the early months of life, it was recommended that surgery be postponed until the patient was 4 months old.[23] The price for avoiding operation in patients with neonatal hepatitis would be paid by those infants with remediable causes of obstructive jaundice.[18] The surgeon's case for early surgery was further inhibited by several reports describing spontaneous cure of biliary atresia.[18] Operative cholangiography was not performed in many of these patients, however, casting doubt on the accuracy of the original diagnosis of biliary atresia. The rather mystic belief that a totally fibrotic extrahepatic duct system might subsequently become patent persisted, nevertheless, because of claims that the development of the bile ducts proceeded for some time after birth.[25] The surgical pessimism in that period produced the feeling that EHBDA represented one of the darkest chapters in pediatric surgery.[26]

A new era in the study and therapy of EHBDA was inaugurated by a new surgical management of this disease, which was developed in Japan. In 1957 Dr. Morio Kasai performed exploratory surgery on an infant and found no patent extrahepatic ducts. He made a shallow exploration into the porta hepatis, just anterior to the portal vein, and found a small amount of bile seepage. He then anastomosed a segment of small bowel to the liver capsule around the raw opening into the liver. A good flow of bile developed in this baby, and the patient remained well for more than 17 years.[27] An account of this surgical approach—hepatic portoenterostomy, or the Kasai operation—was published in Japanese in 1959,[28] in German in 1963,[29] and in the English literature in 1968.[30] Although it originally met with skepticism,[31,32] hepatic portoenterostomy and its subsequent modifications have become the treatment of choice for "non-correctable" EHBDA. In the era of liver transplantation it remains the recommended primary treatment. The Kasai operation has made the non-correctable lesions correctable; therefore, confusion may arise about the term *non-correctable*. In the post-Kasai period truly uncorrectable biliary atresia means a patient with late, severe cirrhosis.[33]

The work of Kasai and colleagues introduced two new concepts into the pathologic study of biliary atresia.[34] First, they showed that intrahepatic bile ducts were patent from the interlobular ducts of the liver to the porta hepatis in nearly all patients during the first 2 or 3 months after birth. Interlobular bile ducts appeared to be destroyed rapidly and their number decreased progressively after 2 months of age. This explained why surgery was most effective for patients younger than 10 weeks of age, which made early and rapid investigation mandatory. Second, the radical approach of portoenterostomy with resection of the obliterated extrahepatic ducts provided unique specimens not hitherto available. Histopathologic study of these fibrous remnants (discussed on p. 1484) confirmed the concept that EHBDA represents an ongoing inflammatory process leading to progressive destruction of the extrahepatic bile ducts.[35,36] It soon became apparent that the intrahepatic bile ducts also participated in the dynamic inflammatory process and were subject to progressive destruction.[16,37,38]

Increased experience worldwide with hepatic portoenterostomy has revealed that the intrahepatic component of duct inflammation and destruction is of great importance in determining the prognosis, even in patients with good bile flow soon after surgery (see the section on Liver Alterations after Portoenterostomy). Hepatic portoenterostomy, including all subsequent variations and technical improvements in the operation, is not tantamount to cure.[13,39-41] A significant number of patients still show abnormalities on liver tests, and signs of portal hypertension may develop.[13,39,41]

Results of treatment today are encouraging but not ideal because the cause or causes of EHBDA are unknown, diagnosis is difficult, and only a minority of infants is truly cured by portoenterostomy.[42] It looks as if a completely satisfactory solution will not be reached without an understanding of the fundamental causes of this disorder.[42,43] The suspicion is growing that EHBDA is the phenotype of several underlying disorders.[13]

Incidence of Extrahepatic Bile Duct Atresia

The incidence of EHBDA was reported in 1963 to be 1:25,000[44]; later studies mentioned a frequency of 1:10,000 to 1:13,000 live births,[34,40,45-47] whereas in recent reviews the incidence was reported to be 1:20,000 in metropolitan France,[48] 1:16,700 in England,[49] and 1:3500 live births in French Polynesia.[48] The suggestion that the Chinese population has a significantly higher incidence was not confirmed in the Chinese population of San Francisco.[50,51] EHBDA occurs more frequently in girls than in boys.[13,52-56] Only a few familial cases have been noted.[35,57-60] Because no specific mode of inheritance for repeated occurrences is evident, genetic counseling is of uncertain value, except for families with more than one affected child, in which the future risk of recurrence is not likely to be less than 20 percent.[61,62]

Pathologic Features of Extrahepatic Bile Duct Atresia

Pathologic Features of the Extrahepatic Bile Ducts

Macroscopic Lesions. EHBDA occurs in various anatomic variants. As early as 1916 Holmes described 116 different configurations of the extrahepatic biliary system and, since then an equal number of different types have been reported. The variations range from total absence of the system at one extreme to complete normality at the other, with presence, or absence, or stenosis, or patency of all or any parts in between. Because of this extreme variation, comparison of the effects of the disease in different patients and consideration of its causes solely on the basis of the anatomy of the extrahepatic biliary tree prove to be impossible.[63]

At one time it appeared useful to distinguish between correctable and non-correctable types of EHBDA.[11] Correctable variants correspond to patients in whom only limited segments of the extrahepatic bile ducts have interrupted permeability; the obliterated segment can be resected and the preserved proximal parts of the extrahepatic system can be reimplanted in the duodenum.[40] Kasai proposed a classification of the numerous observed anatomic variants.[64] The main anatomic groups with types I, II, and III according to Kasai are represented in Figure 50-1. Type I corresponds to atresia of the common bile duct, whereas the more proximal extrahepatic bile duct segments are intact. Type IIa represents obliteration of the common hepatic duct with or without atresia of its main branches; the common bile duct, the cystic duct, and the gallbladder are normal. Re-anastomosis in this type of EHBDA is performed through cystically dilated ducts near the porta hepatis. Type IIb also belongs to the correctable category, although all main branches of the extrahepatic system of bile ducts (common duct, hepatic ducts, and cystic ducts) are obliterated or missing. Re-anastomosis with the duodenum is possible through cystically dilated ducts in the hilum, although the value of this type of corrective surgery has

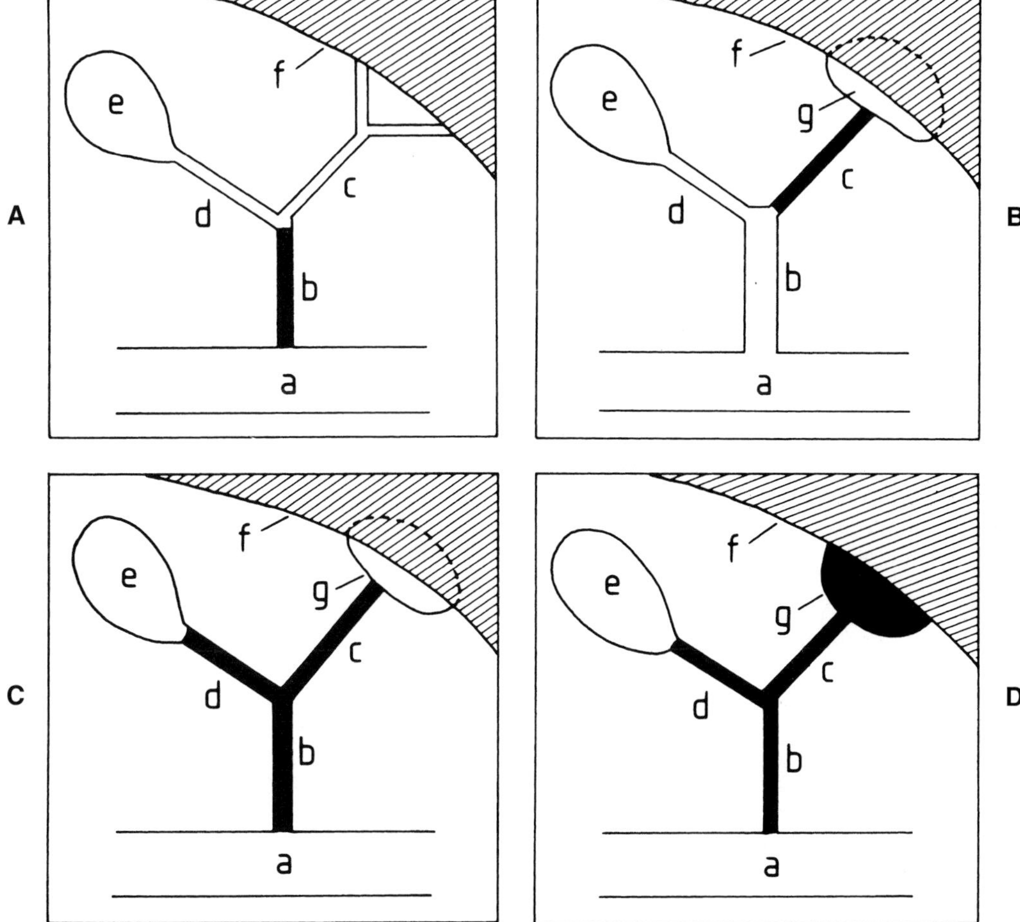

Figure 50-1 Anatomic types of EHBDA according to Kasai. **A,** EHBDA, type I. Correctable form of atresia. The common bile duct is partially or completely occluded or is reduced to a fibrous cord. **B,** EHBDA, type IIa. Correctable form of atresia. Obliteration of common hepatic duct. The common bile duct and cystic duct are patent, and the gallbladder is intact. Presence of cystically dilated bile ducts at the porta hepatis. **C,** EHBDA, type IIb. Correctable form of atresia. Obliteration of common bile duct and hepatic and cystic ducts. Gallbladder is not involved. Presence of cystically dilated bile ducts at the porta hepatis. **D,** EHBDA, type III. Non-correctable form of atresia. Obliteration of common, hepatic, and cystic ducts. No anastomosable ducts at the porta hepatis. Presence of a prehilar fibrous cone. *EHBDA,* Extrahepatic bile duct atresia; *a,* duodenum; *b,* common bile duct; *c,* common hepatic duct; *d,* cystic duct; *e,* gallbladder; *f,* liver; *g,* cystically dilated ducts at the porta hepatis. (Modified from Schweizer P, Müller G: Cholestase-syndrome in Nugeborenen und Saüglingsalter. Stuttgart, Hippokrates Verlag, 1984.)

been questioned.[65] Unfortunately, the correctable types I, IIa, and IIb represent less than 10 percent of all patients with EHBDA.[65] Ninety percent or more of patients cannot be helped by the re-anastomoses mentioned; they belong to Kasai's type III category, which represents non-correctable biliary atresia—that is, the lack of or atresia of common, hepatic, and cystic ducts. There are no cystically dilated hilar ducts that can be used for anastomosis in the type III patients. Often one notes the presence of a peculiar prehilar fibrous cone. The gallbladder is involved in the atretic process in about 80 percent of patients.[66]

Microscopic Lesions. Numerous studies have been performed on the histopathologic characteristics of fibrous remnants of the resected extrahepatic biliary tree.* The authors of these studies have focused their interest on (1) the topography and the nature of the lesions observed in the extrahepatic duct remnants and (2) the correlation between the numbers and sizes of identifiable duct structures at the porta hepatis and the success of increased bile flow after hepatic portoenterostomy.

Topography and Types of Lesions. The histologic procedure usually followed includes serial sectioning of the formalin-fixed extrahepatic fibrous remnant in 2- to 3-mm-thick slices, which are embedded in paraffin for preparation of microscopic slides. A constant finding is complete fibrous obliteration of at least a segment of the extrahepatic biliary tree, confirming the diagnosis of EHBDA at the microscopic level. Usually, however, only a segment is reduced to a fibrous cord, whereas the remaining parts reveal remnants of lumina and inflammatory changes to a variable extent. The variable histologic appearance is categorized usually into three or four types.[71-73,79] One type of histologic picture (type I according to Gautier and co-workers and type III according to Miyano and co-workers and Chandra and Altman)[71,73,79] corresponds to the lack of any lumen lined by biliary epithelium (Figure 50-2). The bile duct segment is replaced by a fibrous cord, often with concentric arrangement of collagen bundles and without inflammatory infiltration.[40,68] A second type of appearance (type II according to Gautier and co-workers and Miyano and co-workers) represents lumina lined by cuboidal epithelia (Figure 50-3).[71,79] The lumina may be distributed randomly or grouped in clusters at the periphery of the section. Some lumina are surrounded by concentric rings of dense connective tissue. Periluminal inflammatory cells are usually found, and signs of necrosis and sloughing of epithelial cells are frequently observed. Bile plugs may be present in the lumina. A third pattern (type III according to Gautier and colleagues) is characterized by a central structure that unquestionably corresponds to an altered bile duct (Figure 50-4).[71] In some specimens the structure contains a loose network of connective tissue without visible epithelium. In a larger proportion of specimens the lumen is filled either with cellular debris and macrophages containing bile or with a biliary concrement. In other instances the lumen appears free but narrowed by surrounding inflammatory tissue; in three quarters of such specimens the epithelial lining is columnar, but it incompletely lines the perimeter of the lumen. Smaller epithelial structures may be seen at the peripheral part of the section and are similar to type II lesions. This type III lesion roughly corresponds to what is termed type I by Miyano and co-workers,[71,79] who further subdivided the specimens into type Ia (luminal diameter more than 300 μm and type Ib (luminal diameter between 100 μm and 300 μm), and to type I by Chandra and Altman (luminal diameter more than 150 μm).[73]

All investigators agree that the variable histologic appearance reflects a dynamic process of progressive in-

*References 36, 37, 40, 43, 64, 67-83.

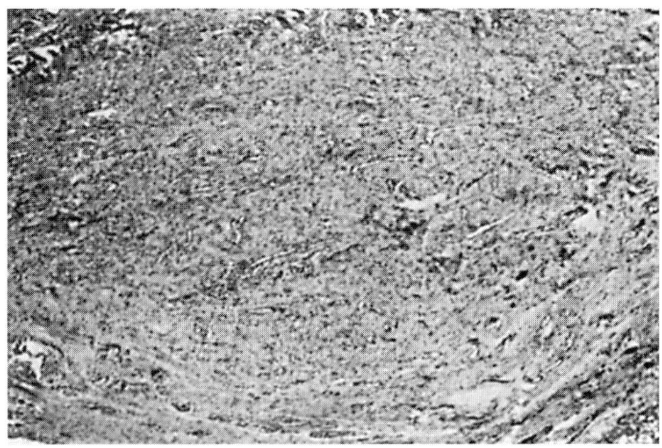

Figure 50-2 EHBDA. Fibrous remnant, Gautier type I. The extrahepatic bile duct has disappeared and is replaced by dense fibrous connective tissue (hematoxylin and eosin, ×64). *EHBDA,* Extrahepatic bile duct atresia.

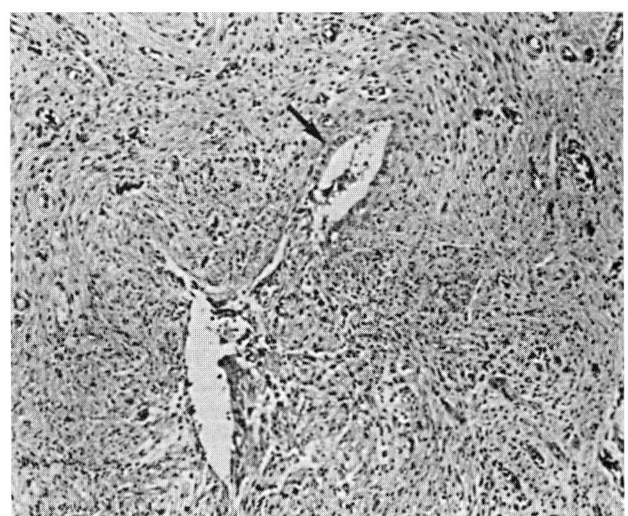

Figure 50-3 EHBDA. Fibrous remnant, Gautier type II. A cluster of small epithelium-lined tubes lies embedded in connective tissue, characterized by inflammatory cell infiltration and beginning fibrosis. Note degenerative changes (e.g., nuclear pyknosis) *(arrow)* in part of the lining epithelial cells (hematoxylin and eosin, ×128). *EHBDA,* Extrahepatic bile duct atresia.

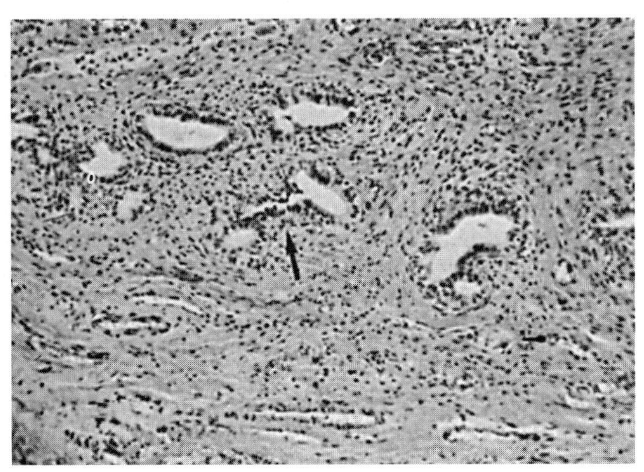

Figure 50-4 EHBDA. Fibrous remnant, Gautier type III. Most of the lining bile duct epithelium is destroyed; some segments remain *(arrow)*. A lumen can still be recognized, surrounded by granulation-like tissue rich in fibroblasts and inflammatory cells (hematoxylin and eosin, ×160). *EHBDA,* Extrahepatic bile duct atresia.

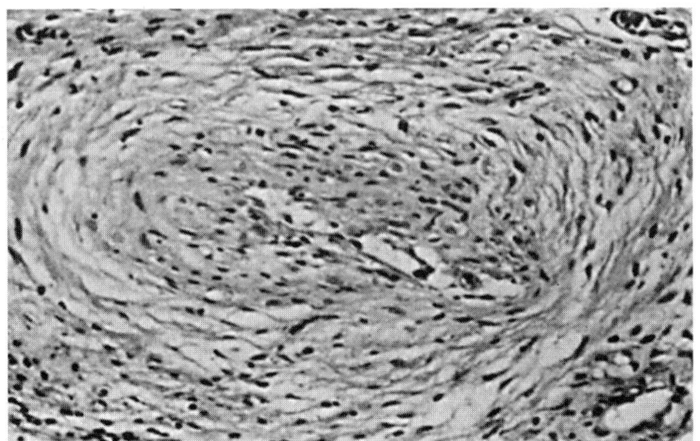

Figure 50-5 EHBDA. Fibrous remnant. Transitional stage between Gautier type III and type I. The epithelial lining of the duct has virtually disappeared. A slit-like lumen is still discernible, surrounded by concentric fibrosis. Collapse of the lumen and further fibrosis would lead to formation of a fibrous cord (hematoxylin and eosin, ×40). *EHBDA,* Extrahepatic bile duct atresia.

flammatory destruction of the extrahepatic bile ducts. The earliest stage corresponds to periductal inflammation with necrosis and sloughing of the epithelial lining, followed by progressive periductal fibrosis and narrowing of the lumen (Figure 50-5). The end stage is a complete fibrous scar of a destroyed epithelium-lined tube that remains identifiable as a fibrous cord in which the collagen texture is more dense than the surrounding connective tissue of the hepatoduodenal ligament and in which the collagen bundles may display a concentric arrangement. The most advanced stage of complete obliteration is frequently seen at the distal end of the common hepatic duct,[70,71,79] whereas the more proximal segments and the prehepatic fibrous cone often show the early stages of inflammatory destruction.[70] This has led to the hypothesis that the lesion represents an ascending progressive inflammatory process.[70] An important observation is that the degree of fibrous obliteration of the extrahepatic ducts increases with the increasing age of the patient, in parallel with increasing fibrosis in the liver.[79] Of equal interest is the finding that epithelial necrobiosis and inflammatory infiltration may be observed distal to regions of complete obstruction, indicating that these changes are not secondary to occlusion of the bile ducts.[37]

Correlation Between Number and Size of Bile Ducts Near the Porta Hepatis and Postoperative Drainage of Bile. The rationale of hepatic portoenterostomy lies in establishing continuity between the bile ducts near the porta hepatis and the intestinal lumen. Theoretically, successful restoration of bile flow is expected in patients with patent biliary structures near the porta hepatis. Postoperative bile flow would be expected to be greatest in patients with biliary structures having the largest diameters or in patients with the greatest numbers of such structures, or both. Investigations by Kasai and co-workers and by Kimura indicated that a satisfactory postoperative flow of bile is obtained only when the diameter of the patent ducts near the porta hepatis is at least 200 μm.[64,75] Suruga and colleagues concluded that duct lumina of 100-μm diameter were sufficient for assuring adequate flow of bile.[84] Some authors recommend intraoperative confirmation by frozen section of the presence of microscopically patent ducts at the level of anastomosis in portoenterostomy.[85-87] However, in the studies mentioned the correlation between the presence of patent ducts and postoperative flow of bile was not 100 percent. Furthermore, other authors reported no correlation between postoperative drainage of bile and the number or size of bile ducts at the porta hepatis.[71,80,88] Gautier and associates found,[71] for example, that 6 of 13 patients with no demonstrable bile ducts at the porta hepatis had an adequate bile flow postoperatively. Later studies have applied a sophisticated computer analysis of the size of bile ducts.[77] From these data no correlation is seen between the degree of postoperative drainage of bile and the number of ducts or the area of the largest bile ducts, but the total area of all bile duct structures (about 100,000 μm^2) was significantly larger in patients with adequate postoperative drainage versus those with poor postoperative drainage (about 30,000 μ^2; $P < 0.05$). More effective bile flow was evident in patients with more than 50,000 μm^2 total area of bile ducts, as compared with those with less than 50,000 μm^2 total area. In four patients, however, there was good postoperative flow of bile despite a small total area for bile ducts at the porta hepatis. Moreover, in all studies bile failed to drain after operation in a significant number of infants with presumably favorable histologic findings. In view of these inconsistencies, further analysis was carried out by Ohi and associates.[82] These authors concluded that distinction should be made among different types of biliary structures at the porta hepatis; that is, among bile ducts, collecting ducts of biliary (periductal) glands, and biliary glands themselves. Only bile ducts, and not collecting ducts and glands, communicate with the intrahepatic biliary system and assure drainage of bile after hepatic portoenterostomy.

Matsukawa concluded from three-dimensional histometry of bile ducts in the porta hepatis that the sites of obstruction may be located very close to the liver tissue and that interruptions of bile duct continuity are found at any level of the fibrous, scarred tissue cone.[78] This finding suggests a preponderant importance of the bile duct configuration high up in the porta hepatis. Although some studies concluded that the size of the bile ducts at the porta hepatis does not have much influence on operative results,[89,90] recent investigations still indicated this an important prognostic parameter.[91-93]

Although refinement in recognition and measurement of bile ducts draining at the porta hepatis might help to assure a better predictive value of operative intervention, the results mentioned previously still do not explain the occurrence of adequate bile flow in patients without recognizable epithelial structures. These puzzling cases raise the question of how bile is drained when there is no duct continuity and point to alternative pathways like lymphatic drainage of bile constituents.[94] The concept of lymphatic drainage forms the basis for some modifications of the Kasai procedure (omentopexy).[40]

Pathologic Features of the Liver and Intrahepatic Bile Ducts in Extrahepatic Bile Duct Atresia

In discussing the changes observed in the liver and intrahepatic bile ducts in EHBDA, it is useful to distinguish between (1) pure EHBDA, (2) EHBDA associated with hypoplasia of intrahepatic bile ducts, and (3) EHBDA associated with hyperplasia of intrahepatic bile ducts.

Pure Extrahepatic Bile Duct Atresia

Interpretation of Histologic Changes

There has been much discussion about the value of liver biopsy in the diagnosis of EHBDA. Although some early studies emphasized the usefulness of liver histopathologic features,[63,95] other authors pointed out the lack of reliability of the histopathologic diagnosis, especially on needle biopsy specimens. From a questionnaire sent to several authorities, Brent obtained divergent opinions about the usefulness of liver biopsy.[35] In 1967 Hays and associates reported the diagnostic accuracy of percutaneous (needle) liver biopsy to be approximately the same as for operative (open) liver biopsy, with a failure rate of 33 percent.[96] Similar figures were given by Landing.[97,98] Alagille and associates found that needle biopsy yielded a firm diagnosis in only one third of cases and a strongly suggestive diagnosis in another third.[99] Surgical liver biopsy was diagnostic in 58 percent of cases and was strongly suggestive in nearly all the remaining cases, with a failure rate of 10 percent. Eliot and associates found that results from needle biopsies correlated fairly well with those from surgical biopsies and concluded that needle biopsy was of great value but could not be used as the sole diagnostic procedure.[100] In more recent years the diagnostic accuracy of liver biopsy is reported to be up to 90 percent and even 95 percent,[40,101-104] at least in biopsies of sufficient size and comprising five to seven portal tracts.[13]

The improvement in accuracy of histopathologic interpretation of liver biopsy specimens in the diagnosis of EHBDA seems to be due to attributing less importance to parenchymal giant cells and more attention to changes in the portal tracts, including interlobular bile duct damage, and, above all, to awareness that the histopathologic changes (including the diagnostic features) are profoundly influenced by the age of the patient. The most important message for the histopathologist is that he or she is studying a snapshot of a dynamic process.

EHBDA is a cause of extrahepatic cholestasis that brings about a series of changes in the liver, the most characteristic of which are those observed in the portal tracts.[83,105] Basically, the neonatal liver reacts to extrahepatic cholestasis in much the same way as does the adult liver. The following description of histologic abnormalities of the liver and intrahepatic bile ducts, observed in preoperative biopsy specimens and in follow-up specimens after hepatic portoenterostomy, is based on reports from the literature and on microscopic study of personally observed specimens partly provided by Prof. Francesco Callea, from patients under the care of Professor Guido Caccia (Brescia, Italy).

The *interpretation* of the histopathologic findings is based on some newer aspects of the histopathologic characteristics of cholestasis in general (e.g., bile acid or cholate stasis without bilirubinostasis), on more recent insights into so-called ductular proliferation, and on renewed interest in the embryologic development of intrahepatic bile ducts (e.g., ductal plates and ductal plate malformation). Hence we place emphasis on features not commonly discussed in the older pertinent literature. Some of these interpretations may be subject to debate, but hopefully they will stimulate further studies into the pathogenesis of EHBDA.

The interpretation of the histopathologic changes relies on the following seven concepts, which were not commonly treated in the pediatric literature until the 1990s: (1) the embryologic development of the intrahepatic bile ducts, (2) the long time it takes for development of the intrahepatic biliary tree throughout fetal life, (3) the apparent fetal type of ductular reaction in early neonatal life in patients with EHBDA, (4) the concept of ductular metaplasia of periportal hepatocytes in longstanding cholestasis, (5) ductular reaction as pacemaker of periportal fibrosis, (6) the diagnostic value of bile acid or cholate stasis without bilirubinostasis, and (7) the diagnostic usefulness of better visualization of ducts and ductules and signs of cholestasis in histologic sections of liver.

Embryologic Development of Intrahepatic Bile Ducts. The intrahepatic bile ducts are derived by transformation from primitive precursors of parenchymal cells. With few exceptions most embryologic studies describe the early formation of intrahepatic ducts by transformation of primitive parenchymal cells (progenitor cells) around the branches of the ingrowing portal vein, which is surrounded by a sheet of mesenchyme.[106] First a layer of primitive hepatoblasts in direct contact with the mesenchymal sheet converts into biliary types of cells (Figure 50-6). This is followed by a similar conversion of a second discontinuous layer of cells, resulting in the formation of a partly double-epithelial cylinder surrounding the portal vein and its accompanying mesenchyme. There is a slit between the two epithelial layers. This primitive bile duct thus assumes the shape of a cylinder, with a cylindric slit-like lumen that is lined on both sides by a biliary type of epithelium. The primitive bile duct with cylindric configuration, located around the primitive portal tract, is termed the *ductal plate.*[107-113] Very soon, and even before completion of the biliary transformation of the outer epithelial layer, some parts of the slit-like lumen dilate (Figure 50-7). Most of the cylindric structure disappears at the same time in relation to ingrowth of mesenchyme. This remodeling of the ductal plate results in an anastomosing system of tube-shaped ducts located within the portal connective tissue.[114] Derangement in, or arrest of, remodeling results in total or partial persistence of the ductal plate; that is, an excess of primitive embryologic structures, appearing as hyperplasia of bile ducts with unusual, curved, and often concentric patterns.[115-117]

Development of Intrahepatic Bile Ducts Throughout Fetal Life. Intrahepatic bile ducts begin their development at the hilum of the liver in the early embryonic stage and proceed toward the periphery throughout fetal life.[63] Distinction should be made between *differentiation* of the intrahepatic bile duct cells from hepatoblasts and *growth* of both hepatocytes and bile duct structures. Differentiation of the bile duct system requires more than differentiation of bile duct cells from hepatoblasts. The primitive cylindric ductal plate is gradually remodeled into an anastomosing system of tubes. The remodeling of ductal plates occurs over a long period, starting with the early ductal plates near the hilum of the liver and continuing until the end of fetal life as more peripheral plates are formed around the terminal ramifications of the portal vein (Figure 50-8).[108-113,115,116,118] Even at the

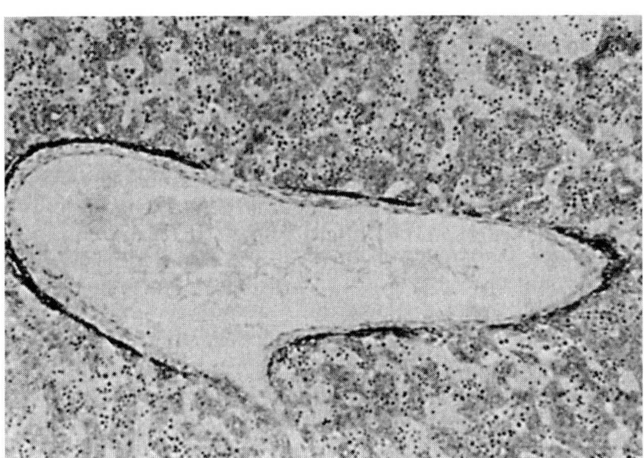

Figure 50-6 Immunoperoxidase stain for cytokeratins 8, 18, and 19 on liver section from an 11-week-old human fetus. This antibody stains cytokeratins in hepatocytes and bile duct structures. A large portal vein is shown, surrounded by a narrow sleeve of mesenchyme. The cell layer in contact with the mesenchyme shows an enhanced expression on cytokeratins, which appear only weakly stained in parenchymal cells. The strongly stained cell layer represents an early ductal plate. (Immunoperoxidase with anti-cytokeratin CAM 5.2 [Becton-Dickinson]. Counterstained with hematoxylin, ×160.)

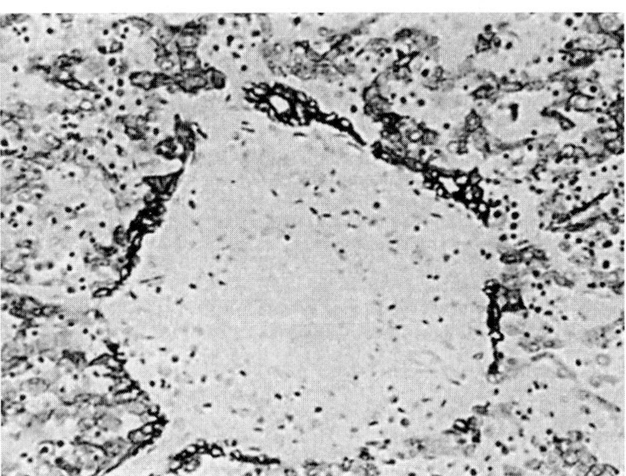

Figure 50-7 Immunoperoxidase stain for cytokeratins 8, 18, and 19 on a liver section from 16-year-old human fetus. This antibody stains cytokeratins in hepatocytes and bile ducts. The picture shows a portal vein with surrounding mesenchyme (portal tract), encircled by a partly double layer of cells with more marked cytokeratin expression (ductal plate). In two places the double epithelial layer molds around a lumen, leading to the primitive form of individualized bile ducts, still located at the periphery of the portal tract. This represents an early stage of remodeling of the ductal plate. (Immunoperoxidase with anti-cytokeratin CAM 5.2 [Becton-Dickinson]. Counterstained with hematoxylin, ×400.)

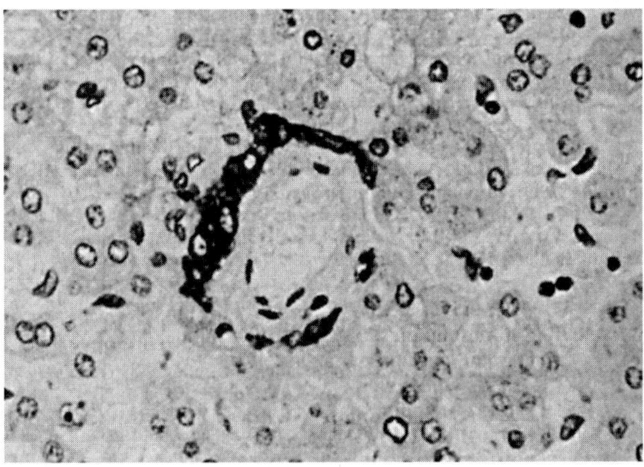

Figure 50-8 Immunoperoxidase stain for epidermal type of keratin on a liver section from a neonate (day 1). Only bile duct epithelium shows positive staining. The parenchymal cells stain negative. At birth, some bile ducts still appear as cylindric structures surrounding smaller (more peripheral) portal tracts. Such ductal plate configuration represents an immature state of bile duct development. (Immunoperoxidase with rabbit polyclonal anti-human cytokeratin [Dako Corporation, Santa Barbara, CA]. Counterstained with hematoxylin, ×640.)

time of birth, the development of the most peripheral branches is not complete, and requires an additional 4 to 6 weeks after birth.[108] Occasional reports in the literature mention the possibility of postnatal maturation of the intrahepatic system of bile ducts in infants initially shown to have a paucity of intrahepatic bile ducts.[119,120]

Postnatal Persistence of the Fetal Type of Duct Formation. The entire complex system for intrahepatic bile duct development—that is, the formation of ductal plates and their remodeling—is potentially susceptible to the action of disturbing factors or influences over a long period. The observation of ductal plates in liver specimens from infants with EHBDA thus suggests an antenatal interference with intrahepatic maturation of bile ducts.

Examination of liver specimens from some infants with EHBDA suggests that formation of ductal plates may continue after birth. This could be due either to retardation in the maturation process of the liver as a whole or to persistence after birth of a fetal type of ductular reaction in response to obstruction in cases of EHBDA. Adequate remodeling of ductal plates appears to be disturbed in EHBDA in view of the frequency with which ductal plates continue to be found after birth.

Ductular Reaction. Any form of extrahepatic cholestasis elicits an intrahepatic "ductular reaction" corresponding to an increase in ductular profiles at the portal tract periphery and indicating an increase in number of the smallest branches of the intrahepatic biliary tree.[105,121] Such ductular increase may be due to multiplication of pre-existing ductules, to a change in phenotype of periportal hepatocytes, or to activation and proliferation of liver progenitor cells.[121,122] Multiplication of pre-existing ductules contributes to ductular reaction mainly in acute biliary obstruction. In chronic, incomplete obstruction the increased number of ductular structures appears to result, at least in part, from ductular metaplasia of periportal hepatocytes.[105,115,123-127] The population of ductular cells derived from cholangiocytic metaplasia of hepatocytes assume the appearance previously described as "atypical ductular proliferation," which also occurs in EHBDA.[128] These newly formed ductules basically retain the labyrinthic anastomosing pattern of the hepatocellular muralia system,[106] as was beautifully illustrated in some three dimensional reconstruction studies.[129] Besides ductular metaplasia of hepatocytes, "atypical ductular reaction" also results from activation and proliferation of liver progenitor cells. Presumed progenitor cells have been demonstrated in EHBDA by immunohistochemistry[130] and electron microscopy.[131]

Ductular Reaction as Pacemaker of Periportal Fibrosis. Ductular reaction is associated with a change in the composition of the surrounding biomatrix and appears to play a pacemaker role in the progression of periductular and periportal fibrosis.[121] In EHBDA the ductular reaction areas are the site of a marked production of matrix components by myofibroblasts, with deposition of collagen types I, III, and IV.[132,133] The profibrogenic cytokine transforming growth factor beta 1 appears to play a key role in periductular fibrogenesis; it is expressed by hepatic stellate cells (Ito cells), ductular epithelial cells, and periseptal hepatocytes.[132-135]

Cholate Stasis and Bilirubinostasis. In conventional terminology histologic cholestasis corresponds to accumulation of bilirubin pigment, most characteristically in the form of intercellular bile plugs.[136] Javitt has insisted that a cholestatic condition is better reflected by a rise in serum bile salt levels than by increased concentrations of conjugated bilirubin in the serum.[137] Thus cholestasis may exist without clinical jaundice and in the presence of normal levels of bilirubin in serum. The same principle applies to the recognition of histologic cholestasis. Especially in cases of low-grade cholestasis (e.g., in patients with long-standing but incomplete obstruction of the biliary passages), the liver parenchyma may show changes reflecting cholestasis without accumulation of bile pigment. Hence it seems useful to distinguish between bilirubinostasis and cholate stasis.[138-140] In several examples of slowly progressive, smoldering cholestasis—for example, in primary biliary cirrhosis or primary sclerosing cholangitis—and in follow-up specimens from patients after successful portoenterostomy for EHBDA-cholate, stasis is a more reliable indicator of a cholestatic state than is bilirubinostasis.[141]

Cholate stasis refers to a microscopic change in periportal hepatocytes. The parenchymal cells appear swollen, with coarsely granular cytoplasm, often associated with intercellular edema, and there is increased fibrosis and infiltration with inflammatory cells, including polymorphs. With time, the cells show gradual accumulation of copper (best demonstrated with the rhodanine stain) and of metallothionein or copper-binding protein (demonstrable with Shikata's orcein stain). In early stages these periportal hepatocytes express the bile duct-type cytokeratin 7. In severe degrees of cholate stasis the altered cells may reflect disturbances in their cytoskeleton by the presence of Mallory bodies.[138,139] Further parenchymal features of cholestasis that are not necessarily accompanied by bilirubinostasis are so-called feathery degeneration and cholestatic liver-cell rosettes.[142] In summary, ductular reaction, cholate stasis, and cholestatic liver-cell rosettes are more reliable histologic markers of a low-grade, smoldering cholestatic state than is the microscopically visible accumulation of bile pigment (bilirubinostasis).

Histologic Visualization of Intrahepatic Bile Ducts. The microscopic identification of intrahepatic bile ducts may be difficult in altered portal tracts with dense inflammatory infiltration. This difficulty is even greater in the case of small ducts, as in liver biopsy specimens from infants and in specimens with damaged, involuted, or disappearing ducts. Histologic analysis of tissue sections from livers with disease of intrahepatic bile ducts is facilitated by staining techniques that help in the visualization of bile duct structures. Several special techniques can be used for this purpose.[106,109] A good and reliable method is the immunohistochemical demonstration, with the use of specific antibodies, of subtypes of intermediate filaments that are specific for bile duct types of cells. Adequate results are obtained with rabbit polyclonal antibodies raised against the epidermal type of keratin and antibodies against cytokeratin 7 (Figure 50-9).[106,109,139,143-145] Immunohistochemical staining for tissue polypeptide antigen (TPA) gives similar results.[146,147] Besides being useful for better visualization of bile ducts, these techniques are useful for revealing mild cholate-static changes in periportal hepatocytes (see Figures 50-11, 50-28, 50-31, 50-33, 50-36, and 50-39).[125,126,139,148-150]

Optimal Time for Diagnostic Liver Biopsy

Even if ductular reaction is accepted as a most reliable but not a pathognomonic criterion in diagnosing extrahepatic obstruction in liver tissue specimens,[46,102] it should be realized that this alteration takes some time to develop. This explains why some authors have recommended postponing liver biopsy until the end of the sixth postnatal week to assure an optimal chance for confident diagnosis of EHBDA.[40] However, our own experience and that of others[92,151] indicates that there is a broad variability in the extent of liver alteration and ductular reaction in patients of the same age, that diagnostic histologic features may be observed in some infants at a younger age than 6 weeks (i.e., 4 weeks), and that in some early severe cases the lesions may be far advanced and close to biliary cirrhosis at the age of 4 to 6 weeks as was observed in 10 patients from a series of 41 cases.[18]

If one accepts that surgical correction should be performed as early as possible, in any case before the liver is severely affected by advanced fibrosis or biliary cirrhosis, it may be unwise to postpone diagnostic liver biopsy until the end of the sixth week of life. Furthermore, it is reasonable to accept that the speed of progress of the disease varies in individual patients, for example, according to the sex of the patient.[56] Moreover, in some patients the pathologic jaundice appears only after the first postnatal month, entailing a similar delay in the development of diagnostic features in the liver. Hence it appears that the optimal time for diagnostic liver biopsy depends to a large extent on clinical judgment and the experience of the pediatrician or pediatric surgeon. A liver biopsy that is obtained too early in the course of the disease may be non-diagnostic, necessitating a second, later biopsy.[152]

Histopathologic Features. It may be of interest to distinguish between classic or typical cases to which most descriptions in published reports correspond and a group of early severe cases, which display somewhat aberrant features in the interlobular bile ducts. The latter group corresponds to what was described as "association between EHBDA and hyperplasia of intrahepatic bile ducts."[40]

Liver specimens with classic features of EHBDA show histologic alterations that change in the course of the disease, allowing some chronologic staging of the lesions in successive periods.[40] As emphasized previously, the timing of the stages is only approximate. The earliest stage (from about 1 to 4 weeks) is characterized by nonspecific features of bilirubinostasis, consisting of granules of bile pigment in hepatocytes and intercellular bile plugs.[40] A few hepatocytes may show degeneration and necrosis. Parenchymal giant cells may be seen, but usually in small numbers and without striking hydropic change. There is no inflammatory infiltration in either the parenchyma or the portal tracts. Branches of the hepatic artery usually appear hyperplastic and hypertrophic.[153] The amount of bilirubin in Kupffer cells increases with the duration of cholestasis. Foci of extramedullary hematopoiesis may persist to a variable extent. The histopathologic features in this early period do not allow for a firm diagnosis.

In the second stage of the disease, from about 4 to 7 weeks,[40] the portal tracts show changes that are characteristic for extrahepatic obstruction of the bile duct. They consist of rounding of the portal tract, edema, dilation of lymph vessels, and ductular proliferation (Figures 50-10, 50-11, 50-12). Some authors also insist on the proliferation of interlobular bile ducts, recognizable by positive

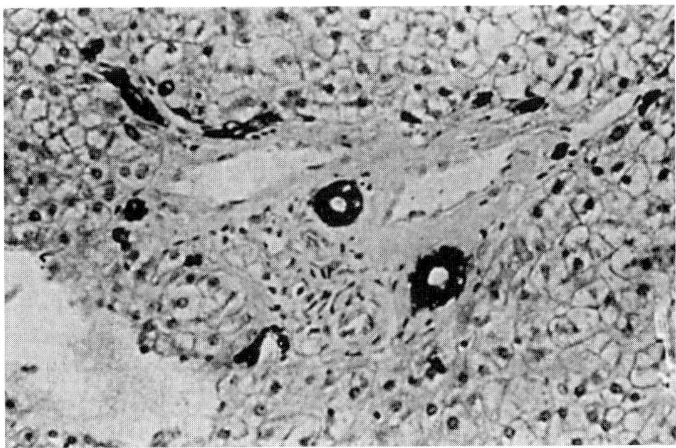

Figure 50-9 Portal tract in normal human adult liver. Immunoperoxidase stain with polyclonal anti-cytokeratin. Only bile ducts in the portal tract and small ductules at the portal-parenchymal interphase show strong positive staining. (Immunoperoxidase stain with polyclonal rabbit anti-keratin, wide-spectrum screening [Dako Corporation, Santa Barbara, CA]. Counterstained with hematoxylin, ×400.)

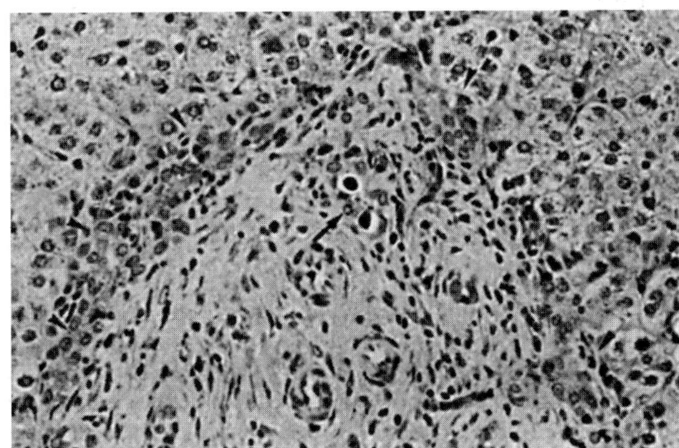

Figure 50-10 EHBDA in infant age 43 days. The portal tract shows mild mononuclear cell infiltration. The bile duct contains bile concrements *(arrow)*. Immediately surrounding the bile duct, an early stage of ductular reaction (mainly ductular metaplasia of hepatocytes) is seen *(arrowheads)* (hematoxylin and eosin, ×400.). *EHBDA,* Extrahepatic bile duct atresia.

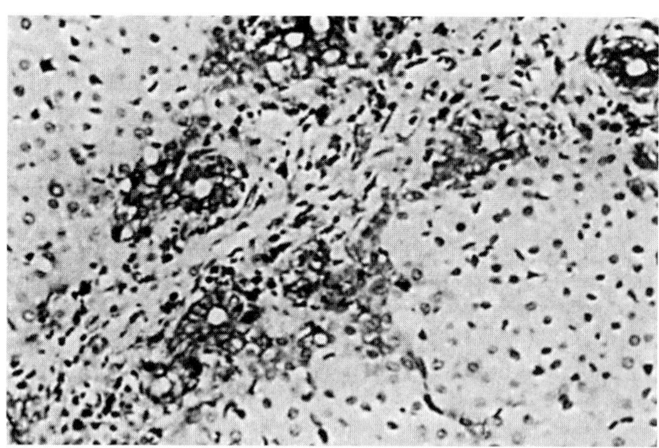

Figure 50-11 EHBDA in infant age 60 days. Immunoperoxidase stain for epidermal type keratin. The figure shows part of a portal tract; it contains several strongly positive staining bile ducts, some of them in close connection with periportal parenchyma. The most peripheral hepatocytes show mild keratin staining, indicating a phenotypic shift toward bile duct type cells (ductular metaplasia of hepatocytes). (Immunoperoxidase with rabbit polyclonal anti-human cytokeratin [Dako Corporation, Santa Barbara, CA]. Counterstained with hematoxylin, ×400.) *EHBDA,* Extrahepatic bile duct atresia.

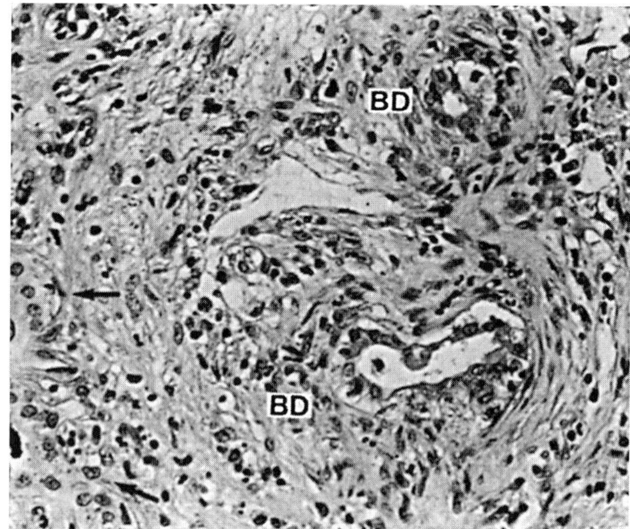

Figure 50-13 EHBDA in infant age 8 weeks. Portal tract with two bile ducts *(BD),* which show swelling, vacuolization, attenuation, and sloughing of their lining epithelial cells. There is mild inflammatory infiltration. Ductular proliferation occurs at the margin of the portal tract *(arrows)* (hematoxylin and eosin, ×400). *EHBDA,* Extrahepatic bile duct atresia.

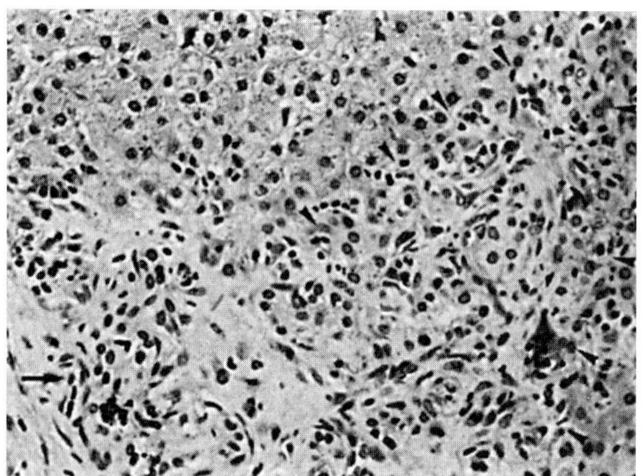

Figure 50-12 EHBDA in infant age 30 days. The figure shows part of a portal tract (lower left). It contains bile ducts, some of them with damaged epithelial lining and bile concrements in the lumen *(arrow).* A wedge-shaped area of ductular proliferation, with admixed inflammatory cells and collagen fibers, extends into the parenchyma *(arrowheads)* (hematoxylin and eosin, ×400). *EHBDA,* Extrahepatic bile duct atresia.

immunostaining for epithelial membrane antigen.[83] The increase in ductules occurs typically at the periphery of the portal tracts, so-called marginal bile duct proliferation.[154] The ductular reaction becomes associated with an inflammatory infiltration, including lymphocytes and polymorphonuclear leukocytes. The density of the inflammatory infiltrate is variable. The ductular reaction in the periphery of the portal tracts creates a diffuse borderline between portal connective tissue and periportal parenchyma, resulting in periportal fibrosis. This stage is considered diagnostic of EHBDA and explains the recommendation by some to postpone diagnostic liver biopsy until the sixth week of life.[40] Most authors agree on the diagnostic usefulness of so-called marginal bile duct proliferation. Also, in older studies ductular proliferation was considered the most reliable histologic change.* It was recognized, however, that ductular proliferation takes some time to reach full development.[99,156-158]

Equally important, from a diagnostic point of view, are the lesions of the portal bile ducts that can be summarized as inflammatory destruction, although this is evaluated by some as an inconsistent finding.[84] The ducts show permeation by inflammatory cells, disruption of their basement membranes, and epithelial abnormalities that include increased acidophilia, vacuolization, flattening, and shedding or necrosis of the epithelium (Figure 50-13; see Figure 50-12). The ductal inflammatory lesions bear striking resemblance to those observed in the extrahepatic bile duct remnants and are responsible for the progressive disappearance of intrahepatic bile duct segments. An occasional portal tract may display bile ducts, usually of small size, in ductal plate configuration.

During a subsequent third stage (from 7 to 8 weeks)[40] portal and periportal fibrosis further develops, associated with extension of the ductular reaction. The density of the inflammatory infiltrate may decrease, and portal edema and lymphangiectasis become less prominent. Bile concrements appear in the lumina of some of the ductular segments, which is typical in EHBDA.[46,66,103] The ductules often show signs of biliary reabsorption as vacuolization, lipofuscin and bilirubin pigment (Figure 50-14),[139,159] and reduplication of the basement membranes on electron micro-

*References 10, 35, 99, 102, 155, 156.

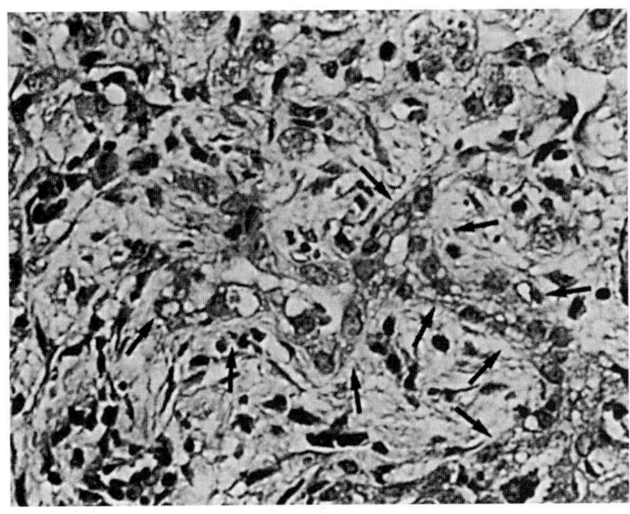

Figure 50-14 EHBDA in infant age 56 days. Edge of an edematous portal tract containing an anastomosing ductular network. The ductular lining cells show striking vacuolation *(arrows)* (hematoxylin and eosin, ×640). *EHBDA,* Extrahepatic bile duct atresia.

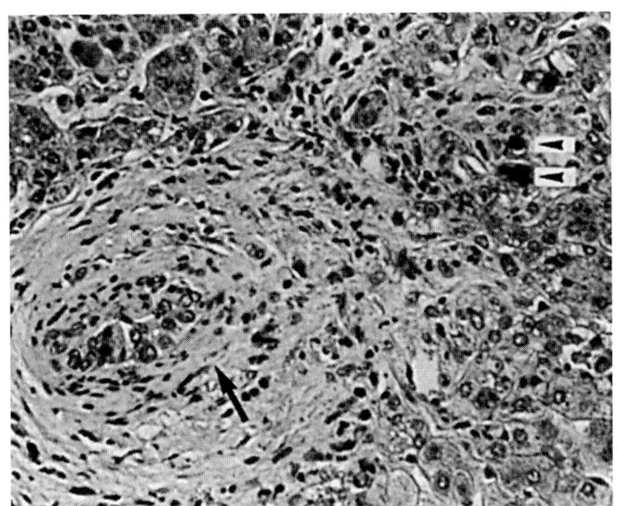

Figure 50-15 EHBDA in infant age 8 weeks. The portal tract contains a bile duct with degenerating epithelial lining, encircled by beginning concentric periductal fibrosis *(arrow)*. Bile plugs are seen in the periportal parenchyma *(arrowheads)* (hematoxylin and eosin, ×400). *EHBDA,* Extrahepatic bile duct atresia.

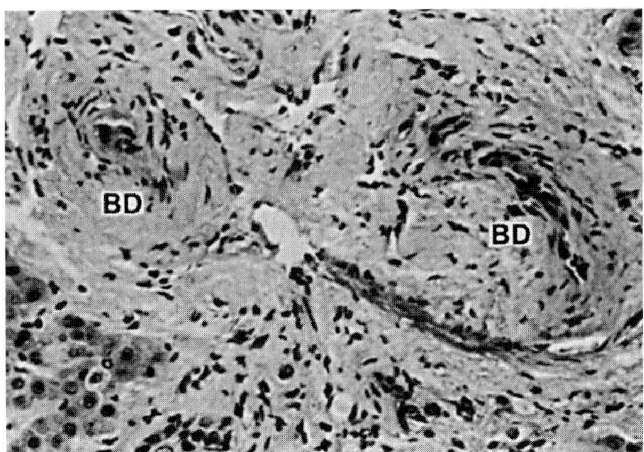

Figure 50-16 EHBDA in infant age 6 months. Portal tract with two bile ducts *(BD)* in advanced stage of destruction: some atrophic lining cells with nuclear pyknosis remain. The ducts are surrounded by broad layers of dense collagen (fibrous obliterating cholangitis) (hematoxylin and eosin, ×400). *EHBDA,* Extrahepatic bile duct atresia.

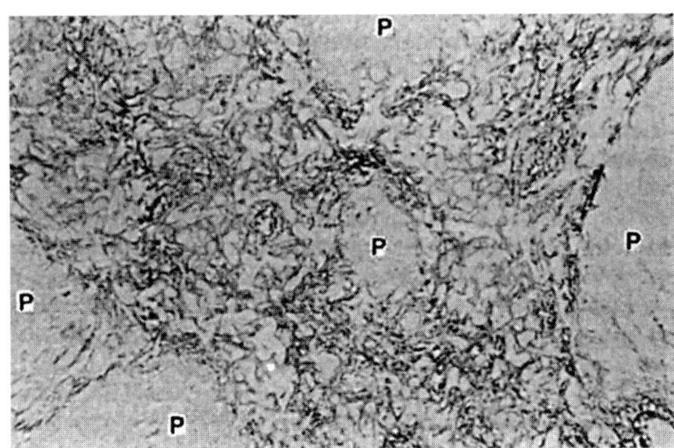

Figure 50-17 EHBDA in infant age 10 months. Stage of biliary cirrhosis. The figure show extensive fibrosis and an increase in ductules between the nodular parenchymal areas *(P)* (Shikata's orcein stain, ×160). *EHBDA,* Extrahepatic bile duct atresia.

scopic examination.[136,160] The parenchymal changes by themselves remain non-diagnostic. The extent and topography of bilirubinostasis are variable; coarse bile plugs are scattered throughout the parenchyma and some hepatocytes show feathery degeneration. Damage to liver cells and necrosis of single cells seem to depend on the degree of bile stasis. There is no appreciable intralobular inflammation. Pigmented macrophages tend to cluster in periportal regions. After about the tenth week of life,[40] the periportal fibrosis extends into the surrounding parenchyma, whereas the density of the inflammatory infiltration tends to decrease. Also, the number of ductular structures seems to decrease and the remaining ductules often show dilation of the lumen and bile concrements. The interlobular bile ducts display fibrous cholangitis, with irregular narrowing of their lumina, thickening of their basement membranes, and development of concentric periductal fibrosis. The strangulated ducts show progressive atrophy of the epithelial lining (Figures 50-15 and 50-16). The progressing periportal fibrosis causes linkage of adjacent portal tracts, reaching the stage of biliary fibrosis but not yet fully developed biliary cirrhosis.[161] The liver lesions at this time are advanced beyond the optimal stage for successful hepatic portoenterostomy, and they indicate a high-risk patient with regard to successful postoperative drainage of bile.

The fifth and final stage (beyond 12 weeks) corresponds to further progression to secondary biliary cirrhosis,[40] characterized by nodular regeneration of the parenchyma and perinodular septal fibrosis (Figure 50-17). Admittedly, the distinction between biliary fibrosis and biliary cirrhosis is not a clear one, especially when judged on needle biopsy specimens. This uncertainty accounts for the controversy concerning the reversibility of biliary cirrhosis.[161] The finding of biliary cirrhosis (the fifth stage of disease) on liver biopsy specimens is a contraindication to corrective surgery.[40]

Several authors have specifically emphasized the alterations that can be observed at the level of the interlobular bile ducts in the central part of the portal tracts.[37,69,162-166] These changes consist of a spectrum of lesions of the bile duct lining cells, including intracellular vacuoles, flattening and condensation of cells with pyknotic nuclei, and necrosis of bile duct cells, and mitosis of these cells. Study of apoptosis and cell proliferation indicates an increased and disorganized bile duct cell turnover.[167] Similar lesions of the lining epithelium of bile ducts were observed in larger intrahepatic ducts at the porta hepatis.[37,43] Based on the distribution of these changes in the original specimens and their persistence after corrective surgery, it was believed that they were not secondary to distal obstruction alone and that they apparently represented an intrahepatic component of the basic disease process affecting the extrahepatic ducts.[37,43] However, there is still some controversy as to the extent to which these lesions might be secondary to obstruction.[83,168,169] Ongoing damage to the bile ducts leads to progressive disappearance of the interlobular ducts,[39,74] also confirmed on hepatectomy specimens at the time of liver transplantation.[170] EHBDA thus represents a "disappearing bile duct disease."[171-173] The lack of interlobular bile ducts in late stages of EHBDA probably results from various causes: damage from distal extrahepatic obstruction,[161] strangulation by progressive fibrosis,[74] ischemia resulting from compression of the peribiliary capillary plexus by portal fibrosis,[142] and, perhaps most importantly, from a relentless progression of the primary process of the sclerosing cholangitis that affects the extra- and intrahepatic ducts.[27,37,170,174-177] This topic is relevant for the discussion of liver lesions in follow-up biopsies after hepatic portoenterostomy.

Lesions of the intrahepatic bile ducts can be recognized by radiographic studies that demonstrate hypoplasia of the intrahepatic biliary tree.[18,65,178-180] Rare lesions that are mentioned in exceptional instances include islands of cartilage near the porta hepatis[83,181] and palisading granulomas around damaged interlobular ducts.[182]

Not only is progression of EHBDA associated with the disappearance of intrahepatic bile ducts, but also the branches of the portal vein often appear strikingly hypoplastic in the sclerosing portal tracts.[183] In later biopsy specimens from patients with EHBDA one may observe fusion between large preterminal portal tracts, which results in enlarged fibrous areas. There is an apparent lack of the finer ramifications of portal tracts. This picture suggests a lack of continued outgrowth of terminal ramifications of the portal tracts and the vessels they contain. Such apparently stunted growth of portal tracts may be part of the previously mentioned retardation in growth and differentiation of intrahepatic bile ducts; it may also be responsible for the hypoplastic pattern of the portal vein.[183]

Studies by Landing and co-workers have disclosed a particular time course for the intrahepatic lesions in untreated or unsuccessfully treated EHBDA.[183] Their data show an early phase of rapid proliferation of bile ductules peaking at 205 days, followed by rapid regression to approximately 400 days. There is a slower progressive loss of intrahepatic ducts thereafter. The connective tissue in the portal tracts increases on a slower course and continues to increase after maximum regression of ducts is reached, indicating a dissociation between the ductular reaction and fibrosis in EHBDA. It was also found that boys with EHBDA show a statistically significant longer survival than girls.[56] Girls show a greater degree of proliferation of intrahepatic ductules in the early phase (less than 200 days) and greater regression of ducts and more rapid development of fibrosis than do boys between 200 and 400 days. The more stormy progression of the disease in girls may be significant from a pathogenetic point of view.

HISTOLOGIC DIFFERENTIAL DIAGNOSIS OF EXTRAHEPATIC BILE DUCT ATRESIA

Histologic Differential Diagnosis Between Extrahepatic Bile Duct Atresia and Neonatal Hepatitis

The histopathologic features of neonatal hepatitis are described on p. 1521. The criteria for differentiating neonatal hepatitis from EHBDA are more pronounced parenchymal changes, focal necrosis, often more numerous parenchymal giant cells with a hydropic change (ballooning) of their cytoplasm, intralobular inflammatory infiltration, and less conspicuous changes in the portal tracts with virtually no ductular proliferation. Immunostaining for pi and alpha isoforms of glutathione-S-transferase may be helpful in differential diagnosis because aberrant expression of pi glutathione-S-transferase can be identified in hepatocytes in most cases of EHBDA and only in a small minority of neonatal hepatitis patients.[184] The histopathologic diagnosis remains in doubt in a small percentage of patients with EHBDA (about 5 percent). The problematic biopsy specimens are those in which ductular proliferation is not prominent and parenchymal damage in the form of giant cell transformation with ballooning and focal necrosis is pronounced. If this histologic appearance is present and other investigations are also inconclusive, it is still advisable to proceed to exploratory laparotomy. This is true despite published warnings that surgery may be harmful to patients with neonatal hepatitis.[23] Several surveys have demonstrated that limited surgery is tolerated well and has no negative effect on prognosis in this condition.[54,64,75,185]

Histologic Differential Diagnosis Between Extrahepatic Bile Duct Atresia and Neonatal Cholestasis

A great number of entities must be considered in the differential diagnosis of neonatal cholestasis (Table 50-1).[186-189] From the point of view of histopathologic differentiation, however, only a few metabolic disorders have to be considered, and they include galactosemia,

TABLE 50-1
Infantile Cholangiopathies

I. Extrahepatic disorders
  A. Biliary atresia
  B. Biliary hypoplasia
  C. Bile duct stenosis
  D. Anomalies of choledochal pancreaticoductal junction
  E. Spontaneous perforation of bile duct
  F. Mass (neoplasia, stone)
  G. Bile/mucous plug
II. Intrahepatic disorders
  A. Idiopathic
    1. Idiopathic neonatal hepatitis
    2. Intrahepatic cholestasis, persistent
      a. Arteriohepatic dysplasia (Alagille's syndrome)[5]
      b. Byler's disease (severe intrahepatic cholestasis with progressive hepatocellular disease)[59]
      c. Inborn errors of bile acid metabolism[59]
        i. Trihydroxycoprostanic acidemia
        ii. Δ^4-3-Oxosteroid-5β-reductase deficiency[60]
        iii. 3β-Hydroxy-Δ^5-steroid dehydrogenase isomerase deficiency[14]
        iv. Zellweger's syndrome (cerebrohepatorenal syndrome) and other peroxisomal disorders
      d. Non-syndromic paucity of intrahepatic ducts (apparent absence of bile ductules)
      e. Microfilament dysfunction[70]
    3. Intrahepatic cholestasis, recurrent (syndromic?)
      a. Familial benign recurrent cholestasis[63]
      b. Hereditary cholestasis with lymphedema (Aagenaes)[1,2]
  B. Anatomic
    1. Congenital hepatic fibrosis/infantile polycystic disease
    2. Caroli's disease (cystic dilation of intrahepatic ducts)
  C. Metabolic disorders
    1. Disorders of amino acid metabolism: tyrosinemia
    2. Disorders of lipid metabolism
      a. Wolman's disease
      b. Niemann-Pick disease
      c. Gaucher's disease
    3. Disorders of carbohydrate metabolism
      a. Galactosemia
      b. Fructosemia
      c. Glycogenosis III/IV

II. Intrahepatic disorders *Continued*
  C. Metabolic disorders *Continued*
    4. Metabolic disease (uncharacterized defect)
      a. α_1-Antitrypsin deficiency
      b. Cystic fibrosis
      c. Idiopathic hypopituitarism
      d. Hypothyroidism
      e. Neonatal iron storage disease (perinatal hemochromatosis)
      f. Infantile copper overload
      g. Multiple acyl-CoA dehydrogenation deficiency (glutaric acid type II)
      h. Familial erythrophagocytic lymphohistiocytosis
  D. Hepatitis
    1. Infectious
      a. Cytomegalovirus
      b. Hepatitis B virus (non-A, non-B virus?)
      c. Rubella virus
      d. Reovirus type 3
      e. Herpes virus
      f. Varicella virus
      g. Coxsackievirus
      h. ECHO virus
      i. Toxoplasmosis
      j. Syphilis
      k. Tuberculosis
      l. Listeriosis
    2. Toxic
      a. Cholestasis associated with parenteral nutrition
      b. Sepsis with possible endotoxemia (urinary tract infection, gastroenteritis)
  E. Genetic/chromosomal
    1. Trisomy E
    2. Down's syndrome
    3. Donahue's syndrome
  F. Miscellaneous
    1. Histiocytosis X
    2. Shock or hypoperfusion
    3. Intestinal obstruction
    4. Polysplenia syndrome
    5. Hemolysis (?)

From Balistreri WF: Interrelationship between the infantile cholangiopathies and paucity of the intrahepatic bile ducts. In Balistreri WF, Stocker JT, eds: Pediatric Hepatology, ed 3. New York, Hemisphere Publishing, 1990:1-3.
CoA, Co-enzyme A; *ECHO,* enteric cythopathic human orphan.

fructose intolerance, and α_1-antitrypsin deficiency (see Chaps. 42 and 48). The other cholestatic syndromes reveal characteristic findings on liver biopsy or can be diagnosed by other means.

Galactosemia and or $_1$-antitrypsin deficiency represent abnormalities that manifest clinically in the same age group as does EHBDA. In both conditions the early stage is characterized by ductular proliferation in the portal tracts, albeit to a lesser extent than in EHBDA. Galactosemia is characterized further by severe histologic cholestasis, with bile plugs in pseudoglandular arrangements of hepatocytes and a constant fatty change.[140,190,191] Fructose intolerance causes a somewhat similar picture, usually with less ductular proliferation and minor cholestasis. Furthermore, most often it causes clinical symptoms at a later age. Beyond the third month of life, α_1-antitrypsin deficiency can be recognized by the characteristic periodic acid–Schiff (PAS)-positive, diastase-resistant globular inclusions in periportal hepatocytes. They can be identified more specifically by means of immunohistochemical methods (immunofluorescence, immunoperoxidase), even on paraffin-embedded tissue.[192-195]

Extrahepatic Bile Duct Atresia Associated with Hypoplasia of Intrahepatic Bile Ducts

Atresia of the intrahepatic bile ducts is usually not complete but consists of a reduced ratio in the number of interlobular bile ducts to the number of portal tracts. This explains why the term *intrahepatic biliary atresia* is replaced by the terms *intrahepatic bile duct hypoplasia* and *paucity of intrahepatic bile ducts.*[120,196,197] Hypoplasia of intrahepatic bile ducts may be an isolated defect or may be associated with other extrahepatic anomalies.[103,198] The latter variety corresponds to arteriohepatic dysplasia or Alagille's syndrome and the cerebrohepatorenal or Zellweger's syndrome (see Chap. 48).[199-204] An isolated or non-syndromic paucity of interlobular bile ducts occurs in patients with congenital rubella, α_1-antitrypsin deficiency, trihydroxy co-prostanic acidemia, Down's syndrome, cystic fibrosis, choledochal cyst, hypopituitarism, Ivemark's syndrome, and lymphedema, and furthermore in patients with no apparent associated disorders (idiopathic forms).[198,205,206]

A sound morphologic diagnosis of hypoplasia of the interlobular bile ducts rests on a sufficient biopsy specimen and morphometric evaluation of bile ducts. Alagille and co-workers recommend a surgical biopsy of the liver.[66,199] Others feel that a simple percutaneous needle biopsy may be adequate.[40,198,207] Between 6 and 20 portal tracts should be present.[40] Clear-cut hypoplasia of intrahepatic bile ducts is diagnosed if the ratio of interlobular bile ducts to the number of portal areas is less than 0.5, whereas in normal children this ratio lies between 0.9 and 1.8.[199,200,208] It may be lower in premature infants.[209] The portal areas without bile ducts usually appear hypoplastic as a whole. Furthermore, it has been shown that the total number of portal tracts per square millimeter of tissue is reduced in patients with hypoplasia in comparison with normal controls.[210] During the last several years, however, this histologic picture of bland, ductless, and somewhat hypoplastic portal areas with a paucity of interlobular bile ducts has been questioned, as will be discussed further in the following paragraph.

Cases of combined EHBDA and hypoplasia of interlobular bile ducts have been described repeatedly.[10,156,190,201,211-213] Schweizer and Muller noted such association in more than 10 percent of their patients with EHBDA (8 of 69 infants).[40] Liver biopsy in such patients reveals the typical portal reaction to EHBDA (edema, ductular proliferation) in those portal areas with an interlobular bile duct, at least when the biopsy is performed during the diagnostic phase of EHBDA. In contrast, the portal areas devoid of an interlobular bile duct show no reaction at all. This histologic picture with both variants of portal tracts is considered diagnostic for combined EHBDA and hypoplasia of interlobular bile ducts.[10,190,211] Because small-needle biopsies may contain only portal tracts lacking an interlobular duct, only paucity of interlobular bile ducts may be diagnosed despite the presence of associated EHBDA. Interestingly, it seems as if the lack of interlobular bile ducts in the portal tracts prevents the development of ductular proliferation in response to extrahepatic obstruction.[120,156,190]

It appears from results of several studies that the interlobular bile ducts are not congenitally lacking in patients with syndromic paucity of intrahepatic bile ducts (Alagille's syndrome). During the first few weeks of life, interlobular bile ducts can be demonstrated in the portal areas of liver biopsy specimens from such patients, but their number gradually diminishes over time.[198,205,207,214-221] The gradual disappearance of portal bile ducts appears to be due to destructive inflammation. There is infiltration with mononuclear leukocytes, and the epithelial lining cells of the bile ducts show desquamation and necrobiosis. Gradually, the lumen is obliterated by connective tissue, with fading of the inflammatory component.[205,215,222-224] The number of interlobular bile ducts decreases with aging of the patient. There is no characteristic age at which bile ducts disappear completely.[215] Some studies document a virtual lack of interlobular ducts during the first 4 weeks of life,[207,225] whereas in another study of five children paucity of interlobular ducts was established after 3 months of age.[205] It would appear therefore that the histopathologic picture, described earlier as typical for combined EHBDA and hypoplasia of intrahepatic bile ducts, applies only to patients in whom destruction of interlobular ducts is far enough advanced to reach the stage of paucity. This age may be around 3 months or even younger.[205,207,225] Hence the histopathologist cannot rely on a lack of portal ducts to diagnose paucity of ducts in earlier stages of Alagille's syndrome.

Whether ductular proliferation in the margin of portal areas carrying a duct remains a valid criterion for diagnosis of EHBDA in association with paucity of intrahepatic ducts appears to be a difficult question. According to some authors[207,218,226-228] there may be ductular proliferation during the phase of inflammatory destruction of ducts in cases of Alagille's syndrome without associated EHBDA. Possibly, all patients with Alagille's syndrome would show an initial proliferation of bile ducts if biopsy was performed early enough.[207] Other authors insist, however, that ductular proliferation is lacking in the destructive phase that leads to a paucity of bile ducts and that the ductular proliferation observed occasionally is secondary to cholangitis.[205,220]

Ductular proliferation must be evaluated carefully in the diagnosis of EHBDA. In 158 cases with adequate clinical follow-up, liver biopsy has been diagnostic in approximately 95 percent. Errors stemmed most often from "over-reading" mild or moderate degrees of bile duct hyperplasia in hepatitis and interpreting the lesion as extrahepatic obstruction.[101,102]

LaBrecque and co-workers state that one should rely on the extrahepatic manifestations (characteristic facies, vertebral abnormalities, heart murmur posterior embryotoxon) for the diagnosis of Alagille's syndrome. It should be realized that not all features are present in every patient.[198,200] In recent years genetic investigation for mutation in the JAG-1 gene may establish the diagnosis.[229] Confirmation of the diagnosis can usually be obtained by a simple percutaneous liver biopsy, which reveals a paucity of intrahepatic ducts. On occasion, the initial biopsy may reveal an increase in ductules, suggesting extrahepatic obstruction and a diagnosis of EHBDA. In such cases exploratory laparotomy may be necessary to confirm patency of the extrahepatic ducts. Patients with extrahepatic biliary atresia have been reported to also have some of the typical features of Alagille's syndrome.[199,201,230] In the non-syndromic type of paucity of intrahepatic bile ducts, biopsy specimens show decreased numbers of interlobular ducts from the first 3 months of life, and evidence is found of inflammatory destruction of remaining ducts. The picture is characterized further by mild periportal fibrosis.[198,206] In one study two patients were mentioned with ductular proliferation in portal tracts. This lesion was found to be due to cholangitis in one patient (age 6 weeks), and EHBDA developed in another infant (age 2 weeks).[206] In the English literature two further patients have been reported with EHBDA in association with paucity of intrahepatic ducts of the non-syndromic type on initial biopsy.[101,206] Repeat biopsy performed 3 weeks later in one of these patients showed development of ductular proliferation,[218] which led to the correct diagnosis of associated EHBDA. Apparently, the first biopsy (at 4 weeks of age) was performed too early for ductular proliferation to have developed; the second biopsy (at 7 weeks of age) was performed in a more diagnostic phase, according to Schweizer and Muller.[40]

The recent reports on paucity of intrahepatic bile ducts, emphasizing that intrahepatic bile ducts may be present but subject to subsequent inflammatory destruction as seen in early liver biopsy specimens from such patients, render the histopathologic diagnosis of associated EHBDA more complicated. Several other observations confuse the issue. EHBDA itself leads to inflammatory destruction of intrahepatic bile ducts, resulting in paucity of bile ducts. Conversely, the disease in Alagille's syndrome need not be limited to the liver and intrahepatic bile ducts but may also affect the major extrahepatic ducts.[201,231,232] A newly described form of sclerosing cholangitis with neonatal onset, leading to disappearance of intrahepatic bile ducts, may result from the same type of bile duct injury as EHBDA, representing a "near-miss" biliary atresia.[233] The main message for the histopathologist from this confusion is that he or she should remain conscious of the evolving nature of the lesions in these obstructive cholangiopathies and realize that histologic recognition of combined intrahepatic paucity and EHBDA in biopsy specimens may be difficult early in life. Interpretation of liver biopsy specimens from such patients requires close collaboration with the clinician.

A further area of controversy with regard to the combination of EHBDA and paucity of intrahepatic bile ducts concerns the nature of the lesion of extrahepatic bile ducts—whether it represents atresia or hypoplasia. Schweizer and Muller mention a 10 percent incidence of associated intrahepatic paucity of ducts (unspecified how many syndromic and non-syndromic types) in patients with verified true EHBDA based on operative cholangiograms and microscopic studies of excised fibrous remnants.[40] The New York group reported five children with Alagille's syndrome.[205,220] Three of these patients had a lesion of the common hepatic duct that was considered hypoplastic, not atretic. Hypoplasia was defined as a narrow but patent lumen on microscopic examination (not complete obliteration). Alagille mentions five patients with extrahepatic manifestations of Alagille's syndrome and intraoperative cholangiograms suggesting atresia of proximal extrahepatic ducts.[234] These patients reportedly had patent but hypoplastic extrahepatic bile ducts on histologic examination of excised tissue. The infant described by Kocoshis and co-workers had clinical stigmata of Alagille's syndrome and apparently diffuse EHBDA.[230] Re-examination of the excised fibrous duct remnants led to the conclusion that this child had severe extrahepatic hypoplasia rather than atresia.[220]

American authors recommend avoiding reconstructive surgery and hepatoportoenterostomy in infants with Alagille's syndrome and associated hypoplasia of the extrahepatic bile ducts to avoid the debilitating effects of cholangitis related to a hepatoportoenterostomy.[207,220] In contrast, German authors recommend hepatoportoenterostomy in patients with combined EHBDA and hypoplasia of intrahepatic bile ducts.[40] This opinion is based on the recognition that the evolution to secondary biliary cirrhosis resulting from EHBDA is slower in patients with both EHBDA and paucity of intrahepatic ducts than in patients with isolated EHBDA. This apparently is so because there is no ductular proliferation in patients with paucity of intrahepatic, interlobular bile ducts. Ductular proliferation may be regarded as the pacemaker for the development of secondary biliary cirrhosis.[161] On reviewing the course of 80 patients with Alagille's syndrome[200] it was noted that the 11 children in whom surgery was performed early because of mistaken diagnosis (EHBDA) or for tentative therapy (cholecystostomy or cholecystojejunostomy) did not have a worse long-term prognosis.

An intriguing finding in patients with Alagille's syndrome and hypoplasia of the common hepatic duct was that changes in bile ducts in the porta hepatis were indistinguishable from those seen in fibrous remnants in EHBDA. Structures of the Gautier types II and III were found.[71,205] The authors' interpretation was that it remained unclear whether these findings reflected hypoplasia of the extrahepatic biliary tree or focal atresia. This finding raises the suspicion, however, that Alagille's syndrome, as with EHBDA, represents a sclerosing cholangitis that may affect the entire biliary tract—extrahepatically as well as intrahepatically.[201] It also raises the intriguing question about a possible common or related pathogenesis in EHBDA and syndromatic paucity of intrahepatic bile ducts.[201,231,232]

Extrahepatic Bile Duct Atresia Associated with Ductal Plate Malformation (Early Severe Forms)

Congenital hyperplasia of the intrahepatic bile ducts is known in the English literature as congenital hepatic fibrosis,[235] in the German literature as cholangiodysplastische Pseudo-Zirrhose and "cholangiodysplasia of the hyperplastic type,"[40,236] and in the French literature as fibroangiodenomatose.[237-239]

The basic lesion of the intrahepatic bile ducts in this entity corresponds to a lack of resorption and remodeling of the excess epithelial structure that is formed in the first embryonic stage of intrahepatic development of bile ducts, that is, the so-called ductal plate.[107] Lack of remodeling into mature bile ducts with persistence of the original embryonic ductal plate structure is termed the *ductal plate malformation.*[240] The bile ducts appear hyperplastic in this condition. The ductal plate malformation constitutes the basic lesion of congenital hepatic fibrosis, infantile polycystic disease, von Meyenburg complexes, Ivemark's syndrome, Meckel's syndrome,[241] Caroli's disease,[115-117,144] and some rare other disorders.[242] However, ductal plate malformation of the intrahepatic bile ducts may also be associated with EHBDA.* In the German literature this was described as "association between EHBDA and cholangiodysplasia of the hyperplastic type" (so-called cholangiodysplastische Pseudo-Zirrhose) in 7 of 69 patients with EHBDA (incidence of 10 percent).[40] The histologic picture seen on preoperative liver biopsy specimens showed a combination of intrahepatic bile duct hyperplasia (ductal plate malformation) and the typical features of EHBDA—edema, inflammatory infiltrate, and marginal ductular proliferation. In two of these patients biopsies were performed 10 and 12 months after successful hepatoportoenterostomy. Interestingly, these biopsy specimens showed regression of the portal alterations caused by EHBDA but persistence of the lesion representing intrahepatic bile duct hyperplasia (or ductal plate malformation) apparently identical to congenital hepatic fibrosis.[40] Similar congenital hepatic fibrosis-like patterns were observed in 5 of 16 "cured" patients followed for 4 to 7 years after successful portoenterostomy and at the time of Kasai's operation in 10 patients of a series of 41 cases.[243,245] The age of these 10 patients at the time of surgical intervention ranged from 30 to 70 days. In all cases, even in the youngest at 4 weeks of age, histologic features revealed already advanced biliary fibrosis, with serpiginous fibrous bands connecting portal tracts (Figure 50-18). These patients thus can be considered early severe cases. The original portal tracts are enlarged and are characterized by excess numbers of branches of the hepatic artery and a relatively small sized portal vein or veins (Figure 50-19). The portal bile ducts display a peculiar pattern, composed of curved segments of variable length surrounding the portal vessels, assuming the basic configuration of an embryonic ductal plate. In several instances the portal vessels are surrounded by two and even three concentric structures, corresponding to interrupted and partially remodeled ductal plates (Figure 50-20). This observation suggests that repetitive formation of ductal plates may occur in successive waves during the first few weeks of life in patients with early severe EHBDA. These ductal plates represent an embryonic type of excess of duct structures, recognized as duct hyperplasia. Several enlarged portal areas seem to correspond to fused clusters of smaller portal tracts because multiple aggregates of complex ductal plates surrounding arterial sprouts may

*References 115, 116, 144, 213, 243, 244.

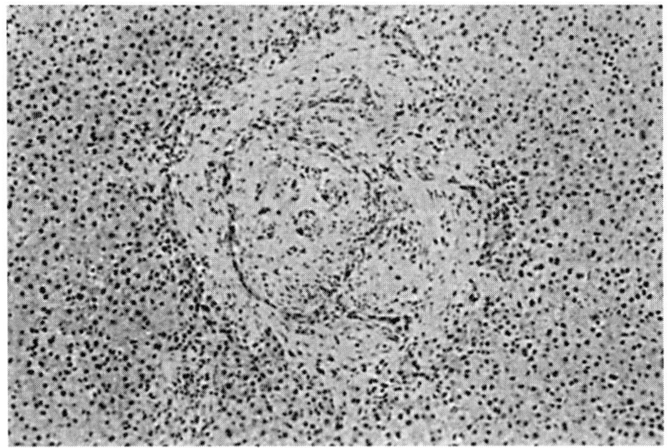

Figure 50-19 EHBDA in infant age 43 days. Portal tract with bile ducts in ductal plate configuration. Some segments of the ductal plate show epithelial irregularities and involution. A mild ductular reaction occurs at the interphase between portal tract and parenchyma. Note prominent arteries and poorly developed portal vein in the portal tract (hematoxylin and eosin, ×160). *EHBDA,* Extrahepatic bile duct atresia.

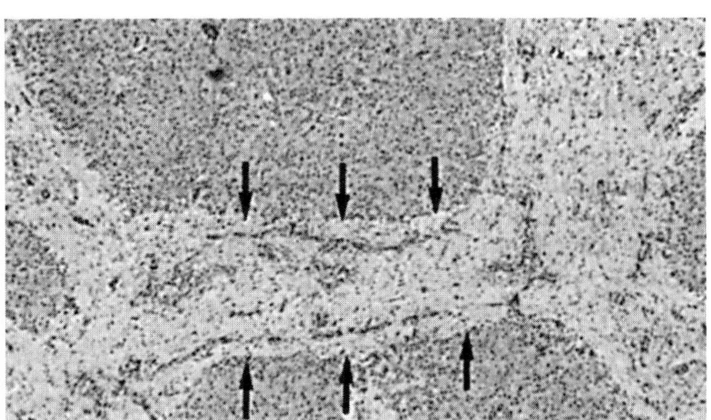

Figure 50-18 EHBDA in infant age 30 days. Disturbed liver architecture by fusion between large portal areas. The latter contain several bile ducts. Some of these appear in ductal plate configuration *(arrows)*. This degree of fibrosis at the age of 30 days represents early, severe EHBDA. Note the resemblance to congenital hepatic fibrosis (hematoxylin and eosin, ×64). *EHBDA,* Extrahepatic bile duct atresia.

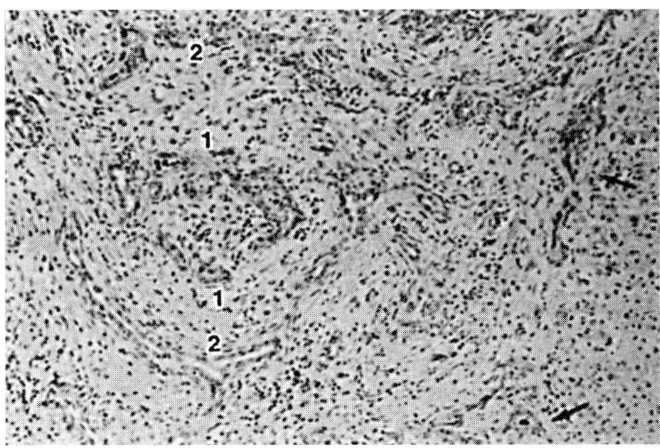

Figure 50-20 EHBDA in infant age 48 days. Enlarged portal tract with moderately dense inflammatory infiltration. Two concentric rings of bile ducts in ductal plate configuration can be recognized *(1, 2)*. Ductular proliferation occurs at the portal-parenchymal interface *(arrows)* (hematoxylin and eosin, ×160). *EHBDA,* Extrahepatic bile duct atresia.

be observed in the same large mesenchymal area (Figures 50-21 and 50-22). Apparently such histologic features result from sectioning through abnormally branching portal tracts: instead of growing by regular tree-like branching, resulting in individualized portal tracts separated by intervening parenchyma, the portal tracts give rise to multiple sprouts of smaller portal twigs that remain in close proximity. Such features may indicate a stunted growth of portal tracts presumably caused by inadequate development (hypoplasia) of the branches of the portal vein.[116,117] This finding would correlate with the observation that portal pressure is often increased at the time of corrective surgery.[246] The immature ducts with ductal plate configuration appear to be subjected to the same fate as their normal or mature counterparts in untreated or progressive EHBDA. They show variable degrees of necrobiosis in their lining cells and become subject to progressive atrophy and fibrous obliteration (Figures 50-23 through 50-26).

In summary, the natural course of EHBDA follows a comparable course in both classic and early severe cases. In both instances progression of the disease is accompanied by variably progressive destruction of intrahepatic segments of bile ducts, either normally shaped, mature ducts in classic cases or immature types of ducts with ductal plate configuration in early severe cases. Reduplication

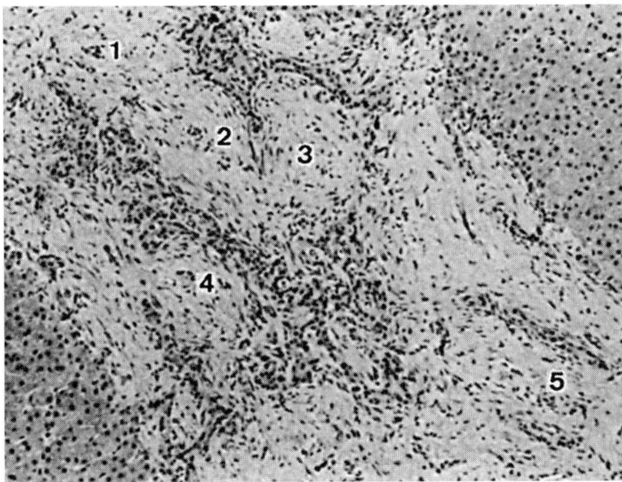

Figure 50-21 EHBDA in infant age 30 days. Large fibrous area containing numerous irregular bile duct segments. This appearance suggests a close approximation of several portal tracts centered by vessels *(1, 2, 3, 4, 5)* with surrounding incomplete ductal plates (hematoxylin and eosin, ×160). *EHBDA,* Extrahepatic bile duct atresia.

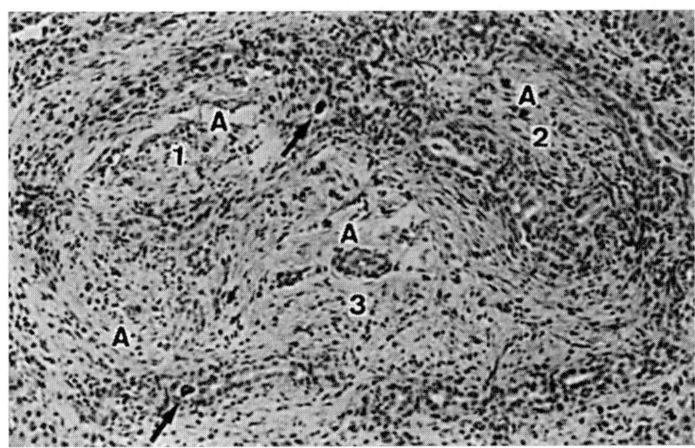

Figure 50-22 EHBDA in infant age 30 days. Large portal tract with numerous abnormal bile duct segments. In analogy with Figure 50-21, this appearance suggests a fusion between adjacent ductal plates (their presumed centers numbered 1, 2, and 3). Note the presence of arterial branches *(A)* but poor development (or lack) of portal vein. Bile concrements are present in some paths of the ductal plates *(arrows)* (hematoxylin and eosin, ×160). *EHBDA,* Extrahepatic bile duct atresia.

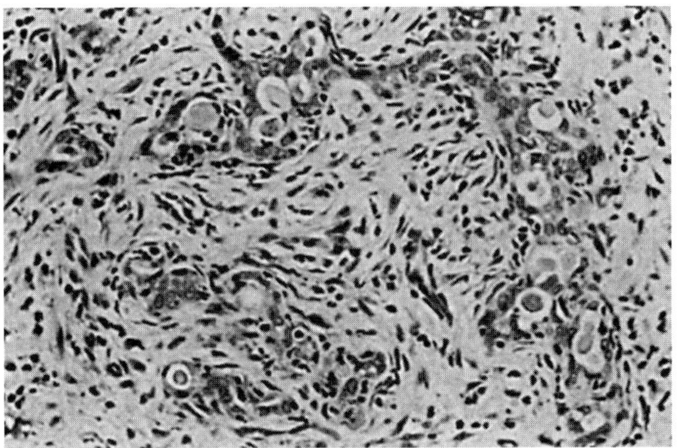

Figure 50-23 EHBDA in infant age 55 days. Detail of portal tract with moderately dense inflammatory infiltration. Bile duct segments (in ductal plate configuration) show irregular dilation of their lumen with bile concrements and interepithelial inflammatory infiltration (hematoxylin and eosin, ×400). *EHBDA,* Extrahepatic bile duct atresia.

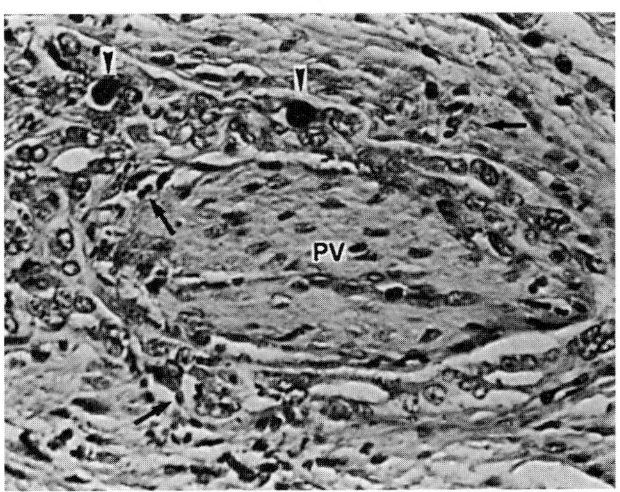

Figure 50-24 EHBDA in infant age 8 weeks. Detail of portal tract with bile duct in ductal plate configuration. Collapsed portal vein *(PV)* in the central connective tissue area. The bile duct epithelium shows degenerative changes like anisocytosis and vacuolization. A few polymorphonuclear leukocytes infiltrate near the bile duct structure *(arrows)*. Occasional bile concrements are found in the lumen of the ductal plate *(arrowheads)* (hematoxylin and eosin, ×640). *EHBDA,* Extrahepatic bile duct atresia.

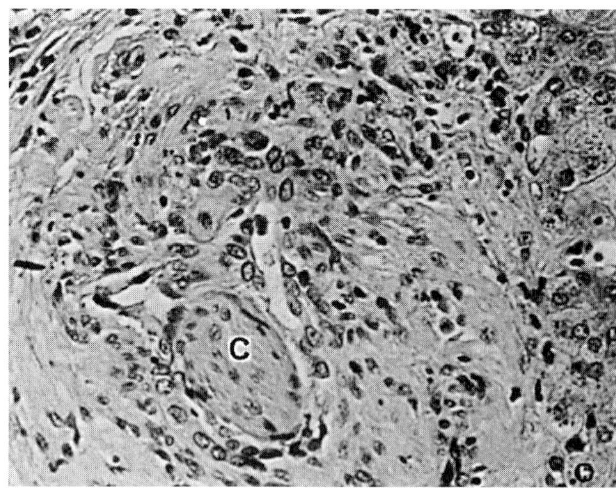

Figure 50-25 EHBDA in infant age 8 weeks. Portal tract containing bile duct in ductal plate configuration with central connective tissue in core *(C)*. The lining epithelial cells display pronounced degenerative changes: anisocytosis, atrophy, vacuolization, and pyknosis of nuclei; the epithelium tends to lift from the mesenchyme (hematoxylin and eosin, ×400). *EHBDA*, Extrahepatic bile duct atresia.

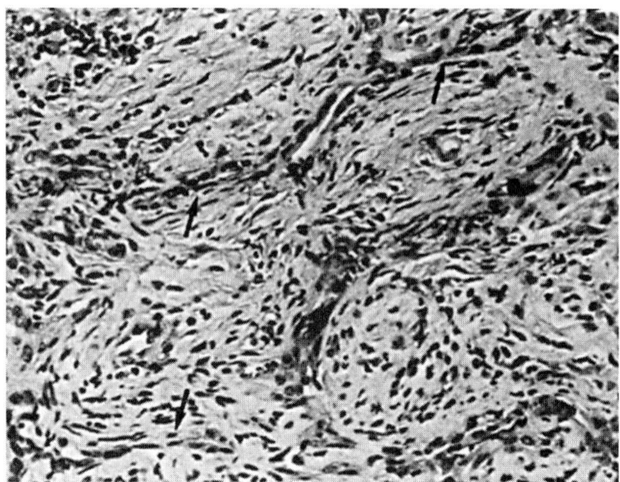

Figure 50-26 EHBDA in infant age 4.5 months. Necroinflammatory ductal plate. Detail from enlarged portal tract containing bile duct structures in ductal plate configuration. The epithelial lining cells show marked degenerative changes: cellular shrinkage and nuclear pyknosis and extreme flattening in some segments *(arrows)*. The surrounding portal connective tissue is highly cellular with moderately dense inflammatory infiltration (hematoxylin and eosin, ×400). *EHBDA*, Extrahepatic bile duct atresia.

of ductal plates followed by variable degrees of destruction of ducts results in a varying degree of duct hyperplasia and resemblance to the pattern of congenital hepatic fibrosis. The hypothesis can be proposed that the duct patterns peculiar to early severe cases are responsible for the later development of a congenital hepatic fibrosis-like pattern—especially when intrahepatic duct destruction is slowed down by relief of the extrahepatic component of obstruction after successful portoenterostomy.[247] The histologic features and clinical course of early severe forms of EHBDA strongly support the concept of an antenatal start of the basic disease process of EHBDA; the latter apparently interferes with the normal maturation and remodeling of the embryonic ductal plates and the normal development of portal vein branches.

Etiology and Pathogenesis of Extrahepatic Bile Duct Atresia

Pathogenesis

EHBDA has been considered a congenital anomaly because of failure of recanalization of the bile duct that was thought to be occluded by proliferated epithelial cells early in fetal life.[12] The other prevailing concept has been that EHBDA represents a progressive destruction of developed extrahepatic and even intrahepatic bile ducts by an inflammatory process of unspecified nature.[6-8] Blanc emphasized that EHBDA was a condition acquired in utero.[35] He based his conviction on the arguments that (1) there was little in traditional embryology to support the hypothesis of the segmental lack of formation of bile ducts; (2) EHBDA is observed rarely in stillborn infants or in autopsies performed on premature infants in the neonatal period; (3) inflammation and progressive obliteration of extrahepatic ducts were observed in surgical specimens from the hilum of the liver taken from areas in which no ducts were grossly visible; (4) when sections of the liver hilum were taken at autopsy, cord-like fibrous remnants of bile ducts were found, indicating that epithelium had been present and then had disappeared possibly as a result of some late fetal or neonatal injury; and (5) the disappearance of the lumen of a duct might result from inflammation. Brent added two further factors to Blanc's ideas: (1) there is inconstant documentation for clay-colored stools early in the disease in patients who eventually had EHBDA, and (2) just as intestinal atresia seldom is reported by experimental teratologists, extrahepatic biliary atresia is also a rarity.[35] A further argument in favor of an acquired disease is the discordance of EHBDA in monozygotic twins.[248,249] Landing proposed the concept of infantile obstructive cholangiopathy based on the histopathologic similarity of the liver lesions in patients with neonatal hepatitis, EHBDA, and choledochal cyst.[97,171] According to this concept, EHBDA is the result of a cholangiopathic process that starts in postnatal life in most cases. The cholangiopathy is due to an inflammatory process, which affects and destroys the liver parenchymal cells and the bile duct epithelium, the latter resulting in obliteration of the bile duct lumina. According to the predominance of parenchymal or duct lesions, the disease corresponds to either neonatal hepatitis or EHBDA. The etiology of the parenchymal and duct inflammatory lesions was presumed to be of viral origin. Parenchymal giant cells were considered the morphologic hallmark of a specific disease process. Although the concept of infantile obstructive cholangiopathy had great impact in the subsequent literature on the subject, it should be realized that it represents a hypothesis. Its main merit is in stimulating thought about EHBDA as an acquired progressive and destructive process. Additional support for this idea was found in resected specimens of remnants of bile ducts, which became available after the introduction of hepatic portoenterostomy as a surgical treatment of EHBDA. At present, some of the facets of the hypothesis of infantile obstructive cholangiopathy are hardly tenable; others remain unconfirmed. The similarity in the histopathologic appearance of the liver in neonatal hepatitis and EHBDA could still be stressed at a time when liver biopsy could not achieve distinction between these two entities in at least 30 percent of cases.[97,171] Currently, however, EHBDA is recognizable by liver histopathologic features in 90 percent to 95 percent of cases,[13,40] and it is difficult to accept a common etiology for diseases with recognizably different histopathologic lesions.[219] One no longer can consider parenchymal giant cells as the morphologic hallmark of a distinct disease process. It is clear that parenchymal giant cell transformation is observed in neonatal liver diseases of diverse causes.[250]

The hypothesis of a viral etiology, more specifically a viral infection with variable impact on parenchymal cells and bile duct cells, remains unrefuted but equally unproved. Somewhat disturbing for the concept of EHBDA as a postnatally acquired disorder is the observation that up to 30 percent of patients have associated malformations.[40,251] Reports on the familial occurrence of EHBDA are also disturbing.[57,59-61] Schweizer and Müller presented a new theory on the pathogenesis of EHBDA,[40] which takes into account most of the observed facts and available information. They propose to distinguish between two types of EHBDA, a fetal-embryonic form and a prenatal, perinatal, or postnatal acquired form of the disease.

It is proposed that the fetal-embryonic form is characterized clinically by the early onset of jaundice. Without a jaundice-free interval, the physiologic jaundice of the newborn turns into a pathologic, conjugated hyperbilirubinuria in the second or third week of life. The level of conjugated bilirubin in serum starts to rise progressively. An analysis of the clinical records from 10 hospitals of 342 children with EHBDA indicates that this type of clinical course is observed in 34 percent of patients.[40] This putative pathogenetic type of EHBDA is characterized morphologically by complete lack of epithelial bile duct remnants in the hepatoduodenal ligament. In their own four patients with this type of disease Schweizer and Muller found associated malformations or malrotation in all four patients and ectopic pancreas in the hepatoduodenal ligament in one patient.[40] This constellation of findings has been taken as evidence that the atresia of bile ducts started in the embryonic or fetal period. The bile duct was missing at the time of birth either because it had not been formed or because it became obliterated completely in the embryonic or fetal period. These patients have a poor prognosis. Postoperative bile flow was not obtained after hepatoportoenterostomy in any of them.

The prenatal, perinatal, or postnatal form of EHBDA is characterized clinically by a longer jaundice-free period after the physiologic jaundice of the newborn. The jaundice-free period often lasts only a few days; in some cases, however, it may be as long as several weeks. As a rule the pathologic jaundice develops after a latent period in the third to fifth weeks of life. From the same study of 342 children with EHBDA observed in 10 different hospitals,[40] it appeared that 66 percent had had a jaundice-free period with a mean duration of 6 days. Bile duct remnants were demonstrated regularly in the hepatoduodenal ligament of these patients in the form of segments with epithelium-lined lumina or epithelial clusters. Associated malformations could not be demonstrated in any of the patients with this form of EHBDA. The constellation of findings in this group suggests that the bile duct was present at birth but that it became obliterated subsequently as the result of an acquired disease. The prognosis in these children is better than in children with the former type of disease. Adequate postoperative flow of bile was achieved in 12 of 16 of these patients.

The ideas of Schweizer and Müller concerning different types of EHBDA are supported by a series of observations. Schweizer and Müller treated a patient with atretic hepatic ducts with hepatoportocholecystostomy because the common bile duct was shown to be patent.[40] Postoperatively, stools became green, and the serum level of conjugated bilirubin dropped from 12.4 mg/dl to 5.2 mg/dl. Three weeks later the patient became more jaundiced and passed acholic stools. At a second operation a complete and microscopically verified occlusion of the cystic and common bile ducts was demonstrated. Thus the obliterative process was progressive and led to complete atresia of the common bile duct over 5 weeks in this patient. A similar observation was reported by Holder.[252]

The development of pathologic jaundice after a jaundice-free period after the physiologic neonatal jaundice indicates that the obliteration of the extrahepatic duct system occurred only after birth. The experimental findings of Holder and Ashcraft support this view.[253] These authors produced bile duct occlusion experimentally in rabbit fetuses and observed that animals born with occluded bile ducts were jaundiced at birth. The presence of normal-colored meconium in the majority of cases of atresia also may be considered an argument in favor of the pre- or perinatally acquired nature of EHBDA and against the dysembryonic hypothesis.[223]

In their microscopic study of resected bile duct remnants Schweizer and Müller often found epithelium-lined luminal segments and epithelial clusters in children operated on in the sixth to eighth weeks of life, whereas no epithelial remnants and only completely obliterated fibrous scars were found in patients operated on later than the twelfth week of life. Furthermore, several investigators have reported that bile duct remnants with microscopic lumina are demonstrable in the connective tissue of the porta hepatis in the early stages of EHBDA.[73,178,254-261] These remnants become obliterated and usually are no longer demonstrable after the twelfth week of life.

At present, the distinction between two clinical forms of EHBDA (an embryonic or fetal type and a perinatal type) is generally accepted,[13] although the incidence of the perinatal type appears to vary from 65 percent[40] to 90 percent.[53]

Etiology

In a disorder manifesting itself in the first weeks of life it is logical to consider genetic factors as causal or contributory. EHBDA is not thought to be inherited in the majority of cases.[13] If genetic factors are a primary cause, they would have to be complex because EHBDA is inconsistently found in families.[35,57-60] For most patients a role for genetic factors is more likely in increasing susceptibility to other insults.[41,262] Human leukocyte antigen (HLA)–identical twins discordant for EHBDA have been described.[248,249,262,263]

Cases in stillbirths or in premature infants are very rare,[264] suggesting a postnatal origin of the inflammatory process.[13,53,97] On the contrary, the less common fetal (embryonic) type of EHBDA apparently begins prenatally, and may have a different etiology than the disorder recognized several weeks after birth. Such considerations support the emerging hypothesis that EHBDA is a common phenotype of several different underlying disorders.[13,265]

The various etiologies that have been considered for EHBDA include disordered morphogenesis, toxic and teratogenic agents, infectious etiology, immune-mediated injury, ischemic damage, reflux of pancreatic juice, and angiofibromatosis.

Defect in Morphogenesis

Observations in favor of a congenital structural anomaly include the cases with ductal plate malformation and the patients with associated anomalies.

The occurrence of ductal plate malformation of the intrahepatic bile ducts has been reported in 20 percent[213] to 25 percent of patients,[245] and even up to more than 80 percent[266] with EHBDA. As mentioned, such "early severe forms" of EHBDA suggest an antenatal start of the basic disease process of EHBDA. Analogous developmental anomalies of the intrahepatic bile ducts in EHBDA include reports on the association with Caroli's disease[267] and the combination of common hepatic duct stricture (possibly a forme fruste of EHBDA) and histologic congenital hepatic fibrosis.[268] Tan and colleagues[269-271] proposed that EHBDA may be caused by failure of remodeling of the ductal plate at the liver hilum, with persistence of fetal bile ducts poorly supported by mesenchyme. Bile leakage from these abnormal ducts may trigger an inflammatory reaction, with subsequent obliteration of the biliary tree. Hepatic innervation is abnormal in EHBDA: neural cell adhesion molecule (NCAM)-positive and S100-positive nerve fibers were found to be increased near branches of the hepatic artery and portal vein, whereas no nerve fibers were observed around bile ducts and periportal ductules that themselves became NCAM-positive.[272,273] The occasionally reported coexistence of EHBDA with other disorders, as with the heterozygous state of galactosemia[274] and α_1-antitrypsin deficiency,[275-277] presumably represents fortuitous associations with different pathogenic processes.

About 20 percent of patients with EHBDA (51 patients from a total of 251 studied) have associated anomalies or malformations.[278] The anomalies segregate into two major groups: one group (29 percent) had various combinations of anomalies within the laterality sequence (polysplenia, cardiovascular defects, asplenia, abdominal situs inversus, intestinal malrotation, and anomalies of the portal vein and hepatic artery); a second major group (59 percent) had single or dual anomalies involving the cardiac, gastrointestinal, and urinary systems that did not follow any recognizable pattern. A third group (12 percent) had intestinal malrotation (some with preduodenal portal vein); these patients show some similarity to the laterality sequence group and may represent a more limited phenotypical result of faulty situs determination.[278] EHBDA within the laterality sequence might prove a suitable candidate for a major gene mutation.[13] Nevertheless, teratogenic, infectious, and polygenic multi-factorial causes may play a more significant role in EHBDA associated with "non-syndromic" organ system anomalies.[13]

Davenport and colleagues[279] specifically studied the splenic malformation syndrome. They analyzed the case records of 308 infants treated between 1975 and 1991 for EHBDA for extrahepatic anomalies. Twenty-three (7.5 percent) infants had polysplenia, four had other splenic malformations (two with double spleen and two with asplenia). The presence of other anomalies such as situs inversus and portal vein anomalies in all the categories of splenic malformation suggested that they formed part of a larger association for which the authors proposed the term *biliary atresia splenic malformation (BASM) syndrome*. The authors concluded that BASM syndrome appears to be a distinct subgroup of patients with EHBDA, which may have a different cause, which tends to have a worse prognosis,[279] and in which special attention to vascular anatomy is required when orthotopic liver transplantation becomes necessary.[280]

Other reported extrahepatic anomalies include intestinal malrotation with partial abdominal heterotaxia and craniofacial anomalies[281]; esophageal, duodenal, and pancreatic atresia[282]; anorectal and esophageal atresia[283]; Kabuki syndrome[284]; and a lethal autosomal recessive syndrome with intrauterine growth retardation and combined esophageal and duodenal atresia.[285]

Toxic and Teratogenic Agents

Some epidemiologic studies on EHBDA have detected a time-space clustering that supports the theory that EHBDA may be caused by environmental exposure (consistent with a viral or a toxic cause) during the perinatal period.[286,287] However, not all studies demonstrate a monthly or seasonal variation in the date of birth or the date of conception of infants with EHBDA.[48,288] Of interest are epidemiologic studies in lambs and calves in New South Wales, Australia, which support a possible environmental cause for EHBDA in these animals.[289] Exposure of pregnant mothers to toxic substances has been considered in discussions on the etiology of EHBDA. An association with amphetamine ingestion by pregnant mothers has been mentioned,[290] but no causative link could be demonstrated with teratogenic drugs or ionizing radiation.[34,35] As a possible endogenous toxic origin, an irritation of the biliary passageways by pathologic bile salts has been proposed.[291] A remarkable case report mentions a neonate with an ectopic liver in the umbilicus in conjunction with EHBDA in the liver proper and an ectopic pancreas in the jejunum; the pathologic features of the ectopic liver and the liver proper were quite similar![292]

Unusual bile acids have been demonstrated in the fetus and newborn infant, and the number of bile acids in fetuses and newborns is closer to 40 compared with the bile acids present in adults.[293,294] Unusual bile acids, including large amounts of 30-hydroxy-cholenoic acid, were detected in the sera of children with Alagille's syndrome,[295] and fetal type bile acids were shown to accumulate in the serum of infants with EHBDA.[296] Biliary injury resembling that observed in EHBDA has been induced by administration of certain bile acids (lithocholic acid, chenodeoxycholic acid) to newborn animals or to their mothers in late pregnancy.[42,297,298] However, no specific abnormality in bile acid metabolism has been described in patients with EHBDA.[47] There is a preponderance of EHBDA in girls.[13,52,53] As mentioned previously, girls show a greater degree of ductular proliferation than do boys in the early phase of EHBDA; they also show a more rapid development of fibrosis.[56] Relevant reported biochemical differences between the sexes that may merit investigation in this regard include the rate of processing of xenobiotics in the hepatocyte's endoplasmic reticulum and differences in the patterns of excretion of bile acids.[299,300]

Infectious Etiology

Since the beginning of this century[9] the hypothesis has been formulated that EHBDA is the result of an infectious hepatitis resulting in destructive cholangitis. Reports were published of families in which one or more of the siblings succumbed to neonatal hepatitis and the others died of EHBDA.[301-303] Some reports mentioned cases of neonatal hepatitis that subsequently evolved to EHBDA.[304,305] A single report of an association with *Listeria monocytogenes* was published.[306] Congenital infections with Epstein-Barr virus and rubella virus have been found occasionally, but the presence of these common agents may be coincidental.[13] Cytomegalovirus infection was considered as a possible cause of EHBDA[307] with subsequent negation[308,309]; repeated reconsideration,[310-312] but overall failure to establish a relationship.[40,41,43,313,314] Of interest is a case report in twins, both of whom had congenital cytomegalovirus infection, one of whom developed EHBDA whereas the other had neonatal hepatitis.[315] A similar lack of relationship was thought to apply to neonatal herpes simplex infection and to viral hepatitis types A, B,[316-319] and C.[320]

Interest arose in infection by reovirus type III because of similarities between the lesions of bile ducts caused by this virus in mice and those of human EHBDA.[321] A higher incidence of reovirus III antibodies was detected in patients with EHBDA than in controls[322-324]; reovirus III immunoreactivity was demonstrated in inflammatory and necrotizing remnants of ducts in a patient with EHBDA,[325-327] and reovirus III antibody titers were found to be elevated in an infant rhesus monkey with EHBDA.[328] Furthermore, the incidence of serum antibodies to reovirus type III in infants with idiopathic neonatal hepatitis was similar to that of patients with EHBDA.[329,330] Other groups could not confirm these results,[331,332] which may result from variation in methods or from different causes of EHBDA in various parts of the world.[333,334] Studies applying newer techniques (polymerase chain reaction) have yielded conflicting results.[335-338]

Rotaviruses of groups A, B, and C are common enteric pathogens in man and have been reported to infect other tissues as well. Group A rotavirus, the most common cause of severe diarrhea in infants, has been shown to cause obstruction (though not atresia) of the biliary tract in mice.[339] Evidence of rotavirus of group C (not A) was found in liver tissue from 10 of 20 infants with EHBDA by reverse transcriptase-polymerase chain reaction in one investigation.[340] However, no evidence of rotavirus of group A, B, or C was found in hepatobiliary specimens from EHBDA patients in a subsequent study.[341] A single case report mentioned isolation of respiratory syncytial virus from liver tissue of a patient with EHBDA.[342] Recent studies have emphasized a high prevalence of human papillomavirus deoxyribonucleic acid in liver tissue from patients with EHBDA.[343]

Immune-mediated Injury

An abnormality in the immune response or the inflammatory reaction in patients with EHBDA has been discussed. An increase in the frequency of the HLA-B12 allele was demonstrated in infants with EHBDA as compared with controls.[344] The increase was most evident (49 percent) in infants with EHBDA who did not have other associated congenital anomalies, favoring an immune mechanism even more strongly. The haplotypes A9-B5 and A28-B35 were also found more frequently.[344] However, the study concerned a small number of patients, and the HLA-B12 allele was also the most common class I major histocompatibility complex in the control population. Further, an increase in frequency of a particular HLA haplotype does not by itself imply an altered immune function.[13] A more recent study found no association of any HLA class I or II haplotypes in Spanish infants with EHBDA.[345] Several other studies have addressed possible immune mechanisms. The immunohistochemically demonstrable expression of HLA antigens and adhesion molecules on the surface of bile duct epithelial cells was investigated. In contrast to normal controls, bile duct epithelial cells in liver specimens from EHBDA patients expressed ICAM-1.[284,346] Co-expression of HLA-DR was observed in some[282,347,348] but not all[284] studies. Expression of HLA-DR on bile duct epithelial cells in cholestatic liver disease may be a secondary epiphenomenon, induced by cholestasis and liver tissue damage per se.[349] Even in this case, however, biliary expression of HLA-DR may play a modulating role in intrahepatic immune reactions associated with bile duct damage.

Ischemic Etiology

An ischemic cause for EHBDA has been suggested repeatedly.[153] It has been proposed that EHBDA could be related to insufficient vascularization of the biliary tree caused by lack of development of some anastomotic loops or their terminal branches in an anatomic region without vessels of its own.[70] Fibrous obliteration of the common duct could be produced experimentally by inducing ischemia of bile ducts.[350] Experimental atresia of bile ducts was induced in fetal rabbits and sheep by ligation of the hepatic artery or its branches.[351,352] Definite proof for an ischemic origin in human EHBDA, however, is lacking.[70]

Reflux of Pancreatic Juice in the Biliary Tree

A further possible cause of EHBDA is reflux of pancreatic juice into the biliary duct system. This could be favored by abnormal anatomic relationships between the common bile duct and the pancreatic duct in the region of the ampulla of Vater. A high incidence of a congenitally abnormal junction of the common bile duct and pancreatic duct—that is, a long common channel and poorly developed musculature of the sphincter of Oddi—was found in autopsies of patients with EHBDA.[353-356] Reflux of pancreatic juice may cause tryptic digestion of the lining of the bile duct, leading to weakening of the wall and eventually choledochal cyst or repetitive cholangitis with progressive stenosing fibrosis.

Angiofibromatosis

Histologic examination of fibrous remnants of extrahepatic bile ducts and fibrous plaques near the porta hepatis often reveals impressive numbers of blood vessels, which may be arranged in nodular areas with concentric fibrosis, giving the impression of an angiofibromatosis.[40,68,72] This hypertrophic arteriopathy has been found to affect the arteries from the trunk of the common hepatic artery up to its peripheral branches supplying the entire biliary tree.[63,153] The suggestion has been made that these vascular anomalies might be causally related to EHBDA.[40]

The conclusion about the etiology of EHBDA is that probably it represents a common phenotype induced by diverse triggering and pathogenetic mechanisms presumably multi-factorial in most instances. Whatever the etiology of this destructive and sclerosing cholangiopathy termed *EHBDA*, the resulting obliteration of variable segments of the biliary tree leads to cholestasis, which involves retention of potentially toxic hydrophobic bile salts and proliferation of reactive ductules producing several cytokines.[13] Retention of chenodeoxycholic acid (or other toxic bile acids) in cholestasis induces hepatocyte apoptosis and necrosis. A key factor appears to be the effect of bile acids on mitochondrial function (altered oxidative metabolism and release of oxygen free radicals). It is proposed that the sequence of mitochondrial injury, oxidant stress, adenosine triphosphate depletion, increased cytosolic free calcium, and activation of degradative hydrolases leads to bile salt–induced hepatocellular injury.[13] The hepatocytes, in turn, release additional factors that stimulate fibrosis.[357] The fibrotic process is enhanced by profibrogenic cytokines released from proliferating ductules.[121] The evolving processes of parenchymal injury and regeneration in a fibrosing environment finally result in secondary biliary cirrhosis.[358]

Experimental Atresia of Extrahepatic Bile Duct Atresia

Several animal models have been attempted for experimental induction of EHBDA; they can be allocated to several categories: ischemic, toxic, viral, genetic, and natural. Ischemic models include the induction of fibrous obliteration of the common bile duct by inducing ischemia,[350] or by ligation of the hepatic artery and its branches in fetal rabbits[253,351] and sheep.[352] In toxic models use has been made of various damaging agents. Intravenous injection of lithocholic acid into preterm rabbits produced obstruction within the biliary tract of newborn rabbits. Obstruction was found in the gallbladder in 2 of 16 rabbits born to mothers given lithocholic acid. No instances of obstruction were observed in 28 controls.[42] Phenylene-1,4-diisothiocyanate is an antihelminthic drug that produces inflammatory changes in the hepatobiliary system of rats.[359] It has been used in experiments set up to simulate EHBDA.[360] Rats given the drug after birth showed dilation of the extrahepatic bile ducts with inflammation. Animals receiving the drug during the fetal period or just after birth showed stenotic or atretic extrahepatic bile ducts caused by thickening and fibrosis of the wall. The results of this experimental model suggest that the differences in the pathologic features in infantile obstructive cholangiopathy (biliary atresia, neonatal hepatitis, and bile duct dilation) may be the result of variation in the developmental stage in which the pathogenic process is acting. When studying clinical cases of EHBDA, these authors came to the conclusion that the correctable type of EHBDA may be due to the impact of the pathogenic process in later developmental stages than is the case in the non-correctable type of EHBDA.[360] Schmeling and colleagues[334,361] infused phorbol myristate acetate into the hamster gallbladder for up to 28 days; the histologic alterations seen in this experimental model were remarkably similar to those observed in patients with EHBDA. Other authors used chemicals that are known to produce intrahepatic ductular proliferation, for example, the aromatic amine p,pl-diaminodiphenylmethane. This toxin was responsible for so-called Epping's jaundice (see Chap. 34).[362] When administered to pregnant rats, this toxin produced ductular proliferation in the mothers but only parenchymal steatosis in the fetal livers.[363]

Viruses used in animals are reovirus type 3 and rhesus rotavirus (RRV) group A. Reovirus type 3 infection damages bile ducts and hepatocytes and causes chronic obstructive jaundice in weanling mice.[321,364] Riepenhoff-Talty and colleagues have reported the development of extrahepatic biliary obstruction in newborn mice orally inoculated with group A rotavirus.[339] Another murine infections model consists I the infection of newborn Balb/c mice with RRV group A.[365] Prophylactic treatment with interferon-alpha prevented the hepatobiliary system from severe damage in this model.[366,367] The morphologic changes of the extrahepatic bile ducts do not follow a particular pattern and mimic most anatomic types of EHBDA in children.[368]

More recent years have seen the development of genetic models. Transgenic mice carrying a recessive insertional mutation in the proximal region of mouse chromosome 4 have anomalies of visceral organ symmetry, including complete abdominal situs inversus, severe jaundice, and death within the first week of life.[369] The mutation, now indicated with the term *inv* mutation, results in a situs abnormality in 100 percent of homozygous mutant mice. The inversin gene, a novel gene with tandem ankyrin-like repeat sequences expressed in liver, kidney, and other tissues early in embryonic life, is partially deleted in the *inv* mouse.[370] A recent study revealed that these transgenic mice with cholestasis and conjugated hyperbilirubinemia and failure to excrete technetium-labeled mebrofenin from the liver into the small intestine suffer from a lack of continuity between the extrahepatic biliary tree and the small intestine, as demonstrated by trypan blue cholangiography.[371] The liver of these animals shows a histologic picture indicative of extrahepatic biliary obstruction with negligible inflammation and necrosis within the hepatic parenchyma.

There is marked increase in intrahepatic bile duct structures that looks identical to the "ductal plate malformation." With a similar spectrum of situs anomalies, a number of characteristics of the *inv* mouse are thus identical to those of human infants with early severe EHBDA and situs inversus. However, there are also several differences between the *inv* mouse and infants with EHBDA, such as cystic kidneys and lack of inflammation, necrosis, or even clear-cut obliteration in the extrahepatic biliary system of the *inv* mouse. It is of interest that infants with EHBDA may have renomegaly (although no cysts) and an increase in plasma levels of hepatocyte growth factor,[372] and that a number of infants with EHBDA also have features of ductal plate malformation such as congenital hepatic fibrosis.[373] On the whole, these results suggest that the inversin gene plays an essential role in the morphogenesis of the hepatobiliary system and raise the possibility that alterations in the human ortholog of inversin could account for some of the cases of EHBDA in which there are also anomalies of situs determination.[371]

A natural animal model of EHBDA is the physiologic involution and atresia of the bile ducts and gallbladder in the lamprey during metamorphosis from the larval (ammocoete) into the adult stage.[374-378] Although it concerns an organism that is far removed from mammals on the taxonomic scale of vertebrates, an interesting aspect concerns the mechanism of bile duct involution and the adaptation of the liver and the organism to survival without a draining biliary system. An analogous problem of ductless livers is encountered in syndromic paucity of intrahepatic bile ducts (Alagille's syndrome) and in some long-term survivors after hepatic portoenterostomy. A first rare case of EHBDA in a dog was recently reported.[379]

Clinical Features—Diagnostic Work-up

The goals of diagnostic investigation in infants with protracted hyperbilirubinemia are to define specific treatable entities and to identify the infant who may benefit from surgical treatment. Prompt identification of cholestasis is imperative because this condition is never benign, in contrast to unconjugated hyperbilirubinuria.[53] The pathophysiologic characteristics and the clinical and biochemical features of cholestasis are considered in Chapters 23 and 39.

Clinical Features

Unfortunately, there is no pathognomonic clinical symptom of extrahepatic biliary atresia because intrahepatic and extrahepatic forms of cholestasis share numerous clinical and biochemical features. Nevertheless, clinical features may aid in the discrimination between EHBDA and the numerous other causes of cholestasis in early childhood mentioned in Table 50-1.

EHBDA occurs more frequently in girls, usually of normal birth weight, whereas neonatal hepatitis appears to be more common in boys (up to 70 percent of cases).[380] Familial cases are rare in EHBDA, whereas a familial incidence is noted in 15 percent to 20 percent of patients with neonatal hepatitis. Associated polysplenia syndrome pleads in favor of EHBDA.[381]

In EHBDA the stools are consistently acholic, whereas incompletely or intermittently decolored stools indicate incomplete cholestasis of the intrahepatic type. However, intrahepatic cholestasis may also be severe and complete, causing a total lack of bile pigment in stools. In neonatal hepatitis the pathologic jaundice follows the physiologic hyperbilirubinemia without interval and is already observed in the second week of life. In EHBDA neonatal physiologic jaundice also persists in about 34 percent of cases; in contrast, in about 66 percent of patients, an intercalated jaundice-free period of about 2 weeks occurs between the physiologic jaundice and the appearance of pathologic icterus.[40] Hepatomegaly is often palpable in the first or second week in neonatal hepatitis, whereas liver enlargement becomes detectable usually in the third or fourth week of life in EHBDA. In view of the importance of an early diagnosis[382] liver disease should be suspected in any infant jaundiced after 14 days of age.[189,383] Simple visual stool inspection remains an important diagnostic screening test.[384] Pathologic jaundice (indicating cholestasis) should be considered present in a patient with hyperbilirubinemia if the conjugated (direct reacting) fraction composes more than approximately 20 percent of the total.[53] In EHBDA, direct-reacting bilirubinemia shows a more progressive rise than in neonatal hepatitis. Serum enzymes are not very helpful in discrimination. In the first 3 months of life neonatal hepatitis may cause higher elevations of aspartate aminotransferase and alanine aminotransferase, whereas γ-glutamyl transpeptidase levels are more abnormal in cases of EHBDA.[385,386]

Different scoring systems based on clinical and laboratory data have been developed in attempts to better differentiate EHBDA from neonatal hepatitis.[387-389] According to Alagille[103] clinical features and laboratory data allow a differentiation between EHBDA and neonatal hepatitis in 83 percent of cases before the age of 3 months. The following features occur significantly more frequently in infants with neonatal hepatitis than in those with EHBDA: male gender (66 percent versus 45 percent), low birth weight (mean 2680 g versus 3230 g), other congenital anomalies (32 percent versus 17 percent), onset of jaundice (mean 23 days versus 11 days of age), onset of acholic stools (mean 30 days versus 16 days), white stools during the first 10 days after admission (26 percent versus 79 percent), and enlarged liver with a firm or hard consistency (53 percent versus 87 percent). Other studies confirm the helpful discriminating value of clinical symptoms.[40]

Further Investigation in the Infant with Protracted Conjugated Hyperbilirubinemia

Further investigations in the diagnostic work-up for differentiating extrahepatic from intrahepatic cholestasis are in two general categories: (1) those that measure hepatobiliary secretion providing information about the patency of the biliary system and (2) those that attempt to establish a definite diagnosis. A series of additional investigations has been introduced for differentiating extrahepatic from intrahepatic cholestasis and hence for checking the patency of extrahepatic bile ducts.[189,390] There is consensus that usually a single diagnostic criterion is insufficient to distinguish the various causes of neonatal jaundice.[189,391]

Alpha Fetoprotein. Zeltzer and co-workers suggested that quantitative estimation of serum alpha fetoprotein (AFP) was of value in distinguishing EHBDA from neonatal hepatitis.[392] The mean serum concentration of AFP in neonatal hepatitis is significantly higher than the mean concentration in infants with EHBDA. Using a sensitive radioimmunoassay method, a peak serum AFP level of greater than 40 ng/ml was diagnostic of neonatal hepatitis.

This conclusion was confirmed in later studies that emphasized the diagnostic value of serum AFP levels during the first 3 months of life.[383] However, in the majority of patients with hepatobiliary disease, there is considerable overlap among the various groups, so discrimination was not possible routinely.

Bile Acids. The serum values of bile acids in infants with biliary atresia or neonatal hepatitis are not increased sufficiently to differentiate these infants from those who are normal (with physiologic cholestasis of the newborn) or to segregate patients according to specific liver disease.[300] Javitt and colleagues proposed that the ratio of chenodeoxycholic acid to cholic acid in serum might help to identify patients with EHBDA, particularly after administration of cholestyramine.[353] Results of other studies failed to substantiate this observation.[393]

Lipoprotein X. Most forms of cholestasis are accompanied by the appearance of an abnormal lipoprotein (lipoprotein X [LPX]) in the serum (see Chap. 54). Cholestyramine-induced stimulation of bile flow decreases the concentration of LPX in serum more in patients with intrahepatic cholestasis than in infants with EHBDA. Poley and co-workers thus recommend the quantitative determination of LPX in serum before and after a 10-day course of cholestyramine as a simple and reproducible screening test for EHBDA.[394] Others use a 3-day course of cholestyramine.[40] EHBDA can be diagnosed only if the value of LPX decreases less than 35 percent. It is agreed that the lack of LPX in the serum excludes EHBDA.[40,394] Combined testing of LPX and γ-glutamyl transpeptidase proposed by some to differentiate between EHBDA and intrahepatic cholestasis[395] remained under debate.[189,396,397]

Vitamin E Absorption Test. Decreased serum levels of vitamin E and an increase in peroxide-induced hemolysis were demonstrated in infants with obstructive jaundice. Although the clinical usefulness of an oral vitamin E tolerance test remains to be clarified, it may be used in conjunction with serum levels of vitamin E to assess the need for parenteral vitamin E supplementation.[398] It is not particularly helpful in the differential diagnosis of cholestasis.[390]

Riboflavin Absorption Test. Children with biliary obstruction have some impairment in the intestinal absorption of the water-soluble vitamin riboflavin, resulting either from alteration in its enterohepatic circulation or from a still unproven role for bile acids in the absorptive process.[399] This test has not gained use in the diagnosis of cholestatic syndromes.

Duodenal Intubation for Bilirubin Content. Greene and co-workers recommended 24-hour collection and visual examination of duodenal fluid as an easy, inexpensive, noninvasive, and rapid method for determining complete cholestasis.[400] They concluded that no laboratory measurements are necessary to detect the typically yellow bilirubin pigment and that quantitation is not necessary to differentiate between the presence or lack of bilirubin pigment. In case of a doubtful result Schweizer and Müller recommend repeating the test after intravenous injection of cholecystokinin.[40] A positive result excludes EHBDA. A negative result allows no discrimination because intrahepatic cholestasis, which also may cause complete lack of bile flow into the intestine.

Other authors find that the bilirubin coloration of intestinal secretions is not reliable because it may be secondary to jaundice, with transmucosal leakage of bilirubin, rather than to true bile flow.[401] The use of qualitative thin-layer chromatography to detect differences in bile acid excretion into the duodenum has been helpful in some cases.[402] However, others found high-performance liquid chromatography of duodenal juice for detection of bile acids to be of limited value.[403]

Endoscopic Retrograde Cholangiopancreatography. Until a few years ago, endoscopic retrograde cholangiopancreatography (ERCP) had been performed successfully and without complication in very few patients with EHBDA.[404,405] Considerable skill and expertise were required on the part of the endoscopist, and even then serious complications such as sepsis, pancreatitis, cholangitis, and rupture of the duodenum occurred.[40,377] Also, the risk of general anesthesia must be calculated. With further technical refinement (i.e., development of instruments designed specifically for pediatric use), this procedure has gained broader applicability in some centers.[406-411]

However, recommendations from a USA National Digestive Diseases Advisory Board Symposium in 1994 are more critical of ERCP[13] and some experienced centers consider that ERCP does not add considerable value to the evaluation of infants with EHBDA.[47] Furthermore, the procedure is costly, requires considerable endoscopic skill, is not widely available for evaluation of infants, and is not without potential complications. Even in the event that ERCP shows findings consistent with EHBDA, a laparotomy is still considered necessary.[47]

Percutaneous Transhepatic Cholangiography. Percutaneous transhepatic cholangiography in infants is a feasible procedure.[412] Demonstration of the intrahepatic bile ducts is possible in 40 percent to 45 percent of cases. Visualization of a patent biliary tract with antegrade flow of contrast medium into the duodenum may negate the need for laparotomy.[390]

Laparoscopy. Application of laparoscopy in neonatal cholestatic jaundice has not found wide acceptance, although diagnoses of EHBDA, choledochal cyst, and neonatal hepatitis have been established by laparoscopy.[413] Laparoscopy has no advantage over a small laparotomy. Both require narcosis and an invasive procedure, but when EHBDA is confirmed at exploratory laparotomy, the surgeon can proceed by enlarging the incision and performing corrective surgery. Laparoscopy also has no role as luminal patency, the key factor in diagnosing EHBDA, is impossible to determine through a laparoscope.[413]

Excretion of Rose Bengal Sodium Iodine-131. Rose bengal sodium iodine-131 (^{131}I) has been used to assess the patency of bile ducts in infants with cholestatic jaundice.[414] After intravenous injection of 0.5 to 1.0 ~μCi of rose bengal sodium ^{131}I, the stools are collected over a 72-hour period and the excreted fraction of ^{131}I is measured. Because rose bengal is excreted with bile, 5 percent to 10 percent, at most, of the injected radioactivity is detected in the stools in patients with extrahepatic biliary obstruction. Isotope in stool in these instances is derived from metabolism of the parent compound. If fecal excretion of isotope is less than 10 percent, one cannot differentiate between EHBDA and intrahepatic cholestasis. In the instance of dubious results the test can be repeated after a 5-day course of cholestyramine or phenobarbital to stimulate bile flow. Biliary excretion of ^{131}I usually increases to greater than 10 percent in patients with intrahepatic cholestasis but remains less than 10 percent in patients with EHBDA.[40] The accuracy of the test was reported to be 91 percent, with a specificity of 88 percent.[415] Other authors consider rose bengal scanning to be of only historic interest,[416] and it is no longer recommended.[13,47]

Hepatobiliary Scintigraphy. Hepatobiliary scintigraphy excludes the diagnosis of EHBDA when biliary excretion of isotope into the intestine is demonstrated.[417-420] The results of hepatobiliary scintigraphy are not specific: patients with cystic fibrosis, severe neonatal hepatitis, and paucity of interlobular bile ducts may fail to excrete isotope into the intestine.[421]

In patients with conjugated hyperbilirubinemia phenobarbital induction may promote excretion of isotope and thus increase the specificity of hepatobiliary scintigraphy. A serious drawback is that phenobarbital induction requires several days.[47] Although biliary scintigraphy is a sensitive diagnostic tool, it cannot identify other structural abnormalities of the biliary tree or vascular abnormalities. Hepatobiliary scintigraphy may be of value in cases where the ultrasonography results are equivocal to confirm that the child does not have EHBDA. For the most part, the usefulness of the diagnostic procedure is limited to most children suspected to have EHBDA.[47] Many centers combine liver biopsy with hepatobiliary scintigraphy, with or without phenobarbital pretreatment.[13] If visualization of both the gallbladder and bowel radioactivity are used as criteria, the specificity of EHBDA on hepatobiliary scintigraphy is said to increase to 86 percent.[422]

Ultrasonography. Abdominal ultrasonography is a useful diagnostic test because it will identify choledocholithiasis, perforation of the bile duct, or other structural abnormalities of the biliary tree such as a choledochal cyst.[417,423-426] Furthermore, in patients with associated malformations abdominal ultrasound will detect polysplenia and vascular malformations.

In EHBDA there is no dilation of the bile ducts, and the gallbladder is either not visualized or appears as a microgallbladder. However, children with intrahepatic cholestasis (idiopathic neonatal hepatitis, cystic fibrosis, or total parenteral nutrition–associated liver disease) may have similar ultrasonographic findings. The sensitivity and specificity of the sonographic investigation may be improved by performing serial ultrasound examination of the abdomen before and after oral feeding because in patients with EHBDA the size of the gallbladder is not affected by oral feeding.[427] However, attention has been drawn to possible pitfalls in biliary ultrasonography.[428] The progressive nature of EHBDA may result in obliteration of biliary passageways that were patent before, thus altering gallbladder behavior over time.[429] One group of investigators has described a specific finding representing the fibrous cone at the porta hepatis; it is described as "triangular cord sign," a triangular or tubular shaped echogenic density just cranial to the portal vein bifurcation on a transverse or longitudinal scan. The "triangular cord sign" is proposed as a simple, time-saving, highly reliable and non-invasive tool in the differentiation of EHBDA from other causes of cholestasis.[430-434] In a small number of patients an antenatal ultrasonographic diagnosis of EHBDA has been reported. Most of them had type I cystic EHBDA and were diagnosed at 19 to 32 weeks of gestation.[435,436]

Magnetic Resonance Cholangiography. Magnetic resonance cholangiography has been used to evaluate its accuracy in visualizing the biliary tree in neonates and infants. The reported preliminary results are not encouraging,[437,438] although T2-weighted, single-shot magnetic resonance cholangiography may reveal a triangular area of high signal intensity in the porta hepatis in some cases, apparently representing cystic dilation of the fetal bile duct.[439]

Liver Histologic Features. Histopathologic examination of a liver biopsy specimen can provide valuable assistance in determining whether exploratory laparotomy is indicated. Several authors consider the liver histopathologic features the most reliable evidence for EHBDA.[13,47,53,101-103,440-444] A liver biopsy specimen can be obtained in most patients by using the Menghini technique of percutaneous aspiration with local anesthesia.[53,442] Because not all portal tracts may show ductular reaction to the same extent, the biopsy specimen should consist of at least five portal tracts.[40] Some authors have recommended postponing liver biopsy until the sixth week of life to give ductular proliferation a chance to develop to a recognizable extent.[40] As discussed previously, it appears that the time of onset or the rate of progression of this lesion, or both, varies in different patients.

Diagnostic Work-up

The first goal in the management of the newborn infant with jaundice is prompt identification of cholestasis and early differentiation from physiologic jaundice or jaundice induced by breast milk. The next goal is early recognition of specific, treatable primary causes of cholestasis.[53] The need for early surgical correction in patients with EHBDA leaves the pediatrician with a short time for diagnostic evaluation. The clinical findings usually allow the experienced pediatrician or surgeon to recognize EHBDA in most patients.[103] A series of additional investigations serves to confirm the diagnosis or to identify other causes of neonatal cholestasis, or both.[189] Table 50-2 represents an example of a recommended staged evaluation of the infant with suspected cholestasis.[186] Similar diagnostic protocols have been published by other authors.[152,445] Whichever plan of investigation is chosen, the emphasis must be on early diagnosis because surgical results are related to the age of the infant at operation.[34]

TABLE 50-2

Staged Evaluation of the Infant with Suspected Cholestasis*

Clinical evaluation (history, physical examination)
Fractionated serum bilirubin or serum bile acid determination
Stool color
Index of hepatic synthetic function (prothrombin time)
Viral and bacterial cultures (blood, urine, spinal fluid)
Viral serology (HBsAg, TORCH) and VDRL titers
α_1-Antitrypsin phenotype
Thyroxine and thyroid-stimulating hormone
Sweat chloride
Metabolic screen (urine or serum amino acids, urine-reducing substances)
Ultrasonography
Hepatobiliary scintigraphy or duodenal intubation for bilirubin content
Liver biopsy

From Balistreri WF: Seminars in Liver Disease, vol 7. New York, Thieme Medical Publications, 1987.
HBsAg, Hepatitis B surface antigen; *TORCH,* toxoplasmosis, other (viruses), rubella, cytomegalovirus, herpes; *VDRL,* Venereal Disease Research Laboratory.

Treatment of Extrahepatic Bile Duct Atresia

The prognosis of untreated EHBDA is very poor. Adelman performed a baseline study for comparison with the results of hepatic portoenterostomy.[446] Follow-up information was obtained for 89 infants who underwent surgical exploration without corrective reconstruction for biliary atresia. The rate of apparent cure was 1.1 percent. The average age at death was 12 months (ranging from 2 months to 4 years); the mean age was 10 months. These findings correlate with other reports,[447,448] which defined the life span of patients with EHBDA who did not undergo corrective surgery at 1 to 2 years.

Hepatic Portoenterostomy

Numerous operative techniques have been applied to reestablish drainage of bile in "uncorrectable" types of EHBDA.[40] Attempts were made to assure drainage through a parenchymal wound by resection of the left lobe of the liver,[449-451] by resection of the quadrate lobe,[452] or by wedge resection of the quadrate lobe.[453] Some surgical techniques included implantation of biliary stents in the liver.[454-456] Other operative procedures attempted to divert bile into hepatic lymph by drainage of the thoracic duct either externally or into the esophagus.[457-460] Alternative methods for lymphatic drainage of bile included connecting lymph nodes of the hepatoduodenal ligament with the intestine.[461] None of these methods was successful because of scarring of parenchymal wounds and obliteration of stents and lymphatic anastomoses.[40] As mentioned in the beginning of this chapter, the hepatic portoenterostomy or Kasai procedure revolutionized the treatment of EHBDA.[30]

Preoperative and Postoperative Prognostic Factors

Preoperative Prognostic Factors. The age at surgery has been identified as a critical determinant of short-term and long-term outcome at multiple centers. The chance for long-term survival decreases with increasing age at surgery.[462] However, even though age is a critical determinant of outcome, a strict upper limit of age for a successful outcome after a portoenterostomy does not exist because the time of onset of disease, its rate of progression, and its severity vary among patients.[47,463] The patterns of obliteration of the distal biliary tree are not indicative of prognosis, but few or absent ductal remnants at the porta hepatitis and absence of portal inflammation ("burnt out" stage) are predictors of poor prognosis,[92] although exceptions do occur.[464] Schweizer and colleagues investigated in a prospective study whether and to what degree the morphology of the porta hepatis has a bearing on the early prognosis. The quantity of bile flow appeared to be a significant function of the total area of the biliary ductules secured in the excised porta hepatis specimen. Only if intact biliary ductules of the two lateral hepatic lobes can be secured (not only the central zone) can a positive prognosis be made.[93] The intraoperative cholangiographic patterns were also mentioned to be of importance for the outcome of surgery.[465] The macroscopic appearance of the degree of hepatobiliary damage assessed by an experienced surgeon at the time of surgery likewise may provide prognostic information. An attempt was made to quantitate the lesions in a "macroscopic appearance at portoenterostomy" score, summated from four features: liver consistency, size of portal remnants, degree of portal hypertension, and associated extrahepatic anomalies.[13]

A further number of investigations or features has been suggested as being of prognostic importance: Doppler sonography of the hepatic blood flow as a noninvasive indicator of disease severity[466]; serum levels of interleukin 18 as marker of progressive inflammation[467]; markers of hepatic fibrosis, including serum hyaluronic acid and type I and type III procollagen propeptides,[468] and serum level of connective tissue growth factor (CTGF)[469]; urinary dosage of D-glucaric acid[470]; determination of biliary bilirubin diconjugate rate[471]; microanalysis by gas chromatography-mass spectrometry of hepatic and serum bile acid composition[472]; and measurement of serum levels of soluble intercellular adhesion molecule-1.[473] Histochemical studies on liver tissue specimens have revealed a prognostic value for the staining patterns of bile canalicular membrane–associated filaments (actin and myosin) in the hepatocytes,[474] and the unfavorable prognosis in case of excessive hepatocellular proliferative response as revealed by proliferating cell nuclear antigen labeling index.[475] An equally dismal sign is marked ductular reaction because it appears to depend on the duration of bile stasis.[476]

A Canadian study attempted to identify preoperative factors that can predict the outcome after a portoenterostomy to spare patients with a poor prognosis needless surgery, to reduce the time to definitive treatment, and to minimize surgical difficulty and morbidity during and after liver transplantation.[477] Histologic criteria predicted outcome in 27 of 31 patients. Fifteen of the 17 clinical successes were correctly predicted, as were 12 of 14 clinical failures (sensitivity, 86 percent; specificity, 88 percent). Individually, the presence of syncytial giant cells, lobular inflammation, focal necrosis, bridging necrosis, and cholangitis was associated with failure of the portoenterostomy. Bile in the lobular periphery was associated with clinical success of the procedure. The study concluded that patients who will not benefit from a Kasai procedure can be identified preoperatively and should be channeled immediately to transplantation.[477]

Follow-up and Postoperative Prognostic Factors. Also for prognostic evaluation and follow-up of patients after portoenterostomy, various types of investigation have been tried with more or less success on larger and smaller series of cases. Serial Doppler ultrasonographic evaluation of the hepatic circulation was reported to provide information about the liver status of children who underwent a Kasai operation.[478] For evaluating the usefulness of magnetic resonance imaging (MRI) in probing liver function, 19 patients with EHBDA after portoenterostomy were subjected to 28 MRI examinations. Results indicated that a normal or high signal area on T1-weighted images represents functional tissue, whereas a high signal area on T2 shows tissue damaged by inflammation and/or fibrosis.[479] Another study attempted to determine the relative value of liver function markers in predicting the magnitude of morbidity and to develop a quantitative estimate of the prognostic risk using a multi-variate regression model. The study sample comprised 37 post-Kasai patients; a computer-based stepwise regression procedure produced the linear predictive models by an equation termed *biliary atresia prognostic index*. The authors claim that these models permit the clinician to evaluate patients for eventual liver transplantation.[480] Fibrosis markers were also studied to monitor the postoperative states of patients with EHBDA. Markers included serum hyaluronic acid[481] and type I and type III procollagen propeptides,[468,482] intrahepatic deposition of collagen type IV and electron microscopical evidence for capillarization of sinusoids,[483] and sandwich enzyme immunoassay for collagen type IV.[484] For evaluation of postoperative liver function, the indocyanine green test was confirmed to be a reliable indicator.[485] It was further found that plasma endothelin levels were significantly increased in EHBDA patients after portoenterostomy, showing higher levels in patients with portal hypertension than in those without.[486] Determination of the chemokine IP-10 (serum interferon-inducible protein-10) by enzyme-linked immunosorbent assay revealed increased serum levels of IP-10 that correlated closely with histologic changes in 30 postoperative EHBDA patients.[487]

Although these investigations have provided interesting results, confirmatory studies on larger series of patients are needed before their broad clinical applicability could be even considered.

More established data are provided by reviews of large numbers of patients over longer periods of time.

Altman and colleagues investigated risk factors for failure after portoenterostomy for EHBDA using univariate and multi-variate methods in a total of 266 patients treated from 1972 to 1996. Age at surgery, surgical decade, and anatomy of atretic bile ducts were identified as independent risk factors.[488] Gauthier and colleagues studied 164 patients treated from 1984 to 1992 by initial Kasai operation and secondary liver transplantation, when necessary. In univariate analysis age younger than 46 days at Kasai operation, favorable extrahepatic biliary lesions pattern (EHBDA with patent gallbladder, cystic dilation of extrahepatic bile duct, or atresia restricted to choledochus), and absence of polysplenia syndrome were significant determinants of a better 10-year outcome regarding actuarial crude survival without or after liver transplantation, actuarial survival with native liver, and jaundice-free actuarial survival with native liver. The biliary lesional pattern was more discriminant than age.[489]

The rationale of hepatic portoenterostomy is the presence of patent ducts at the porta hepatis. The initial goal at operation is to confirm that the diagnosis is EHBDA. The fibrotic biliary remnants should be identified and patency of the distal biliary tract should be assessed by cholangiography. A transection is made in the parenchyma above the fibrous cone of obliterated proximal ducts, and the exposed area of crude liver surface is anastomosed to the intestine (Figure 50-27). Healing of the portoenterostomy is complete in about 6 weeks.[490] Kasai's unorthodox approach was met with skepticism by surgeons and pediatricians in North America,[31,254,491] but nevertheless acquired broad application.[33,178,416] It was recognized at an international meeting in 1977 as the standard procedure for treatment of EHBDA[492] and recommended as primary surgical therapy for EHBDA by the 1983 National Institutes of Health Consensus Conference on Liver Transplantation.[493]

One of the frequent and sometimes fatal complications in patients with successful portoenterostomy and adequate drainage of bile is recurrent cholangitis, especially in the first 2 years after surgery, with a reported incidence of 50 percent to 92 percent.[494] The etiology and pathogenesis of postoperative cholangitis are not entirely clear. It is thought to be due to reflux of intestinal contents from the draining intestinal loop toward the porta hepatis. This has led to several modifications of the original Kasai procedure with construction of external venting conduits. A full discussion of the technical aspects of the various surgical procedures is beyond the scope of this chapter. The most frequently applied techniques (see Figure 50-27) are the Kasai I, Kasai II,[64] Suruga 1,[495] Suruga 11,[496] and the Sawaguchi procedures and the use of a cutaneous double-barreled enterostomy constructed by the Mikulicz technique.[38,497,498] The usefulness of external diversion of bile for preventing the development of cholangitis after portoenterostomy has been a matter of debate. In later studies an external conduit or stoma was not found to be effective.[499,500] The construction of an intussusception-type valve in the Roux-en-Y limb of the portoenterostomy to prevent reflux does not appear to affect the incidence of cholangitis nor the short-term outcome after portoenterostomy.[501,502] Conversely, in believing that postoperative cholangitis is not of ascending origin, some surgeons have recommended lymphatic drainage by omentopexy.[40,251,503]

Specific modifications of the Kasai operation include

- the use of microsurgery,[90]
- extended dissection into the porta hepatis,[504]
- transection of the fibrous cord at the porta hepatis under an appropriate visual field by division of the ligamentum venosum (Arantius' canal),[505]

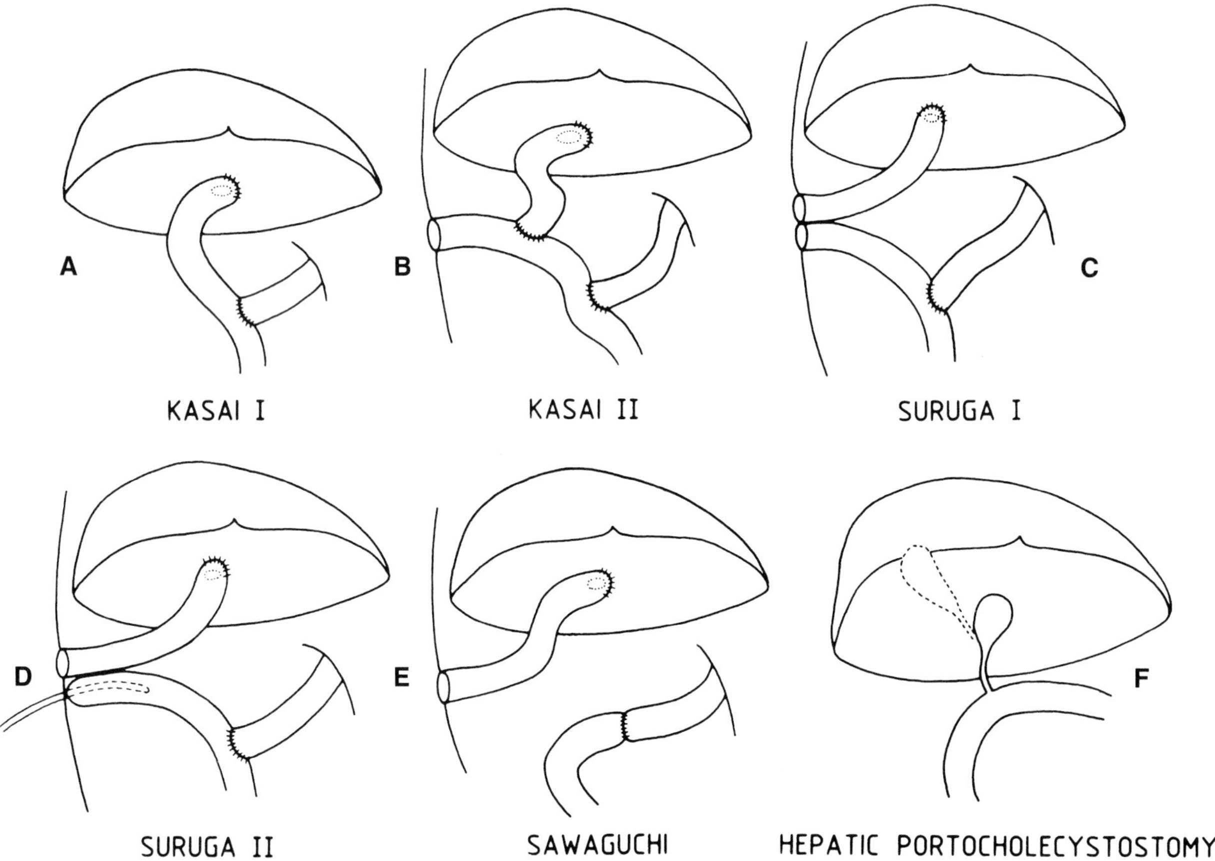

Figure 55-27 The most common surgical procedures for EHBDA. **A,** Kasai I: the original hepatic portoenterostomy. **B,** Kasai II: double Roux-en-Y hepatic portoenterostomy. **C,** Suruga I: double barreled hepatic portoenterostomy. **D,** Suruga II: refinement of Suruga I procedure to include subcutaneous enterostomy for the distal jejunal limb with the insertion of a jejunal tube. **E,** Sawaguchi: hepatic portojejunostomy with external stoma (requires hospitalization until second operation, substitution of fluid and electrolytes, and reinfusion of bile through gastric intubation). **F,** Hepatic portocholecystostomy. *EHBDA,* Extrahepatic bile duct atresia.

- use of a Cavitron ultrasonic suction aspirator for obtaining persistent biliary drainage,[506]
- a procedure designed as invaginating anastomosis, which puts all portal vein branches outside the anastomosis to prevent cicatricial adhesion at the dissected area with the posterior wall of the veins,[507] or
- special techniques for revision of the portoenterostomy in case of inadequate bile flow.[508,509]

In recent years there has been a return to the original Kasai procedure to avoid complicating the technical performance of liver transplantation at a later date in case of failure of the portoenterostomy.[41,47,510]

Hepatic portocholecystostomy or "gallbladder Kasai" (see Figure 50-27) is the method of choice in the approximately 25 percent of patients with obstruction of the common hepatic duct but with a patent distal system: cystic duct, gallbladder, and common bile duct. This type of anastomosis, using biliary conduits for reestablishing continuity, has the advantage of preventing the complications of cholangitis.[47,511]

The important factors contributing to optimal operative results include (1) an early operation, preferably within 60 days after birth; (2) preoperative liver histology and size of ductal remnants; (3) macroscopic appearance of liver and biliary system at surgery; (4) the experience of the surgical team, and (5) the postoperative clearance of jaundice.[47] The earliest reported operation was performed at 76 hours after birth.[512] When the operation is carried out by 60 days of age, excretion of bile is obtained in about 80 percent of the patients. The ability to achieve good postoperative bile flow decreases with the advancing age of the patient.

Over the years the results of portoenterostomy have improved gradually.[513] For about one third of patients, bile flow after portoenterostomy is inadequate; these children develop progressive fibrosis and cirrhosis. Unless they receive a liver transplant, such patients usually die from complications of cirrhosis by the time they are 2 years old.[47]

Cholangitis occurs in up to 50 percent of survivors; the episodes occur on a sporadic to frequent basis, necessitating antibiotic treatment. Histopathologic liver changes of cirrhosis and clinical splenomegaly are present in more than 80 percent of patients. The incidence of complications associated with portal hypertension, in particular esophageal variceal bleeding and, less frequently, hepatopulmonary syndrome, occurs in greater than 60 percent of long-term survivors. Moreover, those patients with cirrhosis and no clinical evidence of portal hypertension may be at risk of developing hepatocellular carcinoma.[47] However, most long-term survivors under adequate supervision and treatment are attending school in an age-appropriate grade, are employed, and achieve normal growth and development.

It is conclusive that, although hepatic portoenterostomy has improved the outcome of patients with EHBDA,[514,515] it has created a population with specific health problems, including recurrent cholangitis, nutritional and growth deficiencies, delayed development, portal hypertension, osteomalacia and osteoporosis, and social and psychiatric difficulties.[516-518] These complications may respond to adequate medical support and therapy, which are detailed in several reviews.[53,189,519,520]

A successful portoenterostomy resulting in adequate bile drainage is not tantamount to cure.[13,47,416] It appears particularly difficult to determine fully and accurately outcome in patients with EHBDA because the short-term or mid-term cure does not clearly reflect the eventual prognosis. A disappointing aspect of hepatic portoenterostomy is the failure of hepatic parenchymal disease to resolve in many patients. It is the exceptional patient who shows histologic improvement after surgery.[40] The histopathologic features of hepatic parenchymal disease after hepatoportoenterostomy are discussed on p. 1511.

After more than three decades of experience with the Kasai procedure (including the pioneer period), multiple reports on long-term results after 10 and 20 years of follow-up have been published.[41,91,521-528] There is no doubt that a small minority of patients with EHBDA can be cured by hepatic portoenterostomy. The overall survival rate without orthotopic liver transplantation 5 years after the initial hepatic portoenterostomy ranges from 40 percent to 60 percent, decreasing to 25 percent to 30 percent at 10 years, and 10 percent to 20 percent by 20 years.[41] The long-term outcome during the 10-year period after the Kasai procedure is that roughly one third of patients with EHBDA will require transplantation in the first 12 to 14 months, another third by their teens, and the rest will live with some degree of liver disease.[13,47] Reports on 20-year follow-up after portoenterostomy reveal that occult progressive liver damage proceeds in long-term survivors,[523,525] that close follow-up is essential even after 20 years or more,[513] especially for patients whose serum total bilirubin exceeds 1.0 mg/dl,[524] and that timing of liver transplantation is a vital management issue.[521]

Liver Transplantation

Human orthotopic liver transplantation was pioneered by Starzl in 1963.[529] Early pediatric cases included patients with EHBDA and concomitant hepatocellular carcinoma.[530] Metabolic liver diseases and EHBDA were the major indications for liver transplantation in the pediatric age group, and results of liver transplantation were better in children than in adults.[531,532]

Since the early days of liver transplantation, continued advances have been made in surgical technique, postoperative care, and immunosuppression. Orthotopic liver transplantation has evolved into an effective and widely accepted therapy for patients with end-stage liver disease, including infants and children. EHBDA remains the most common indication for orthotopic liver transplantation in children, accounting for approximately 50 percent of cases.[131,533] Specific aspects of patient selection, treatment, and complications are discussed in a separate chapter on liver transplantation (see Chap. 55).

Portoenterostomy and Liver Transplantation

Short-term and long-term complications of portoenterostomy on the one hand, and the increasing applicability and success of liver transplantation on the other hand, have created a dilemma about the treatment of choice for the infant with EHBDA. Theoretically, successful liver transplantation represents a more complete treatment of EHBDA because it not only assures re-establishment of bilioenteric continuity but also replaces a diseased organ with a healthy one. However, it should also be stated that in many respects liver transplantation exchanges one disease (EHBDA) for another (the post-transplant immunocompromised state). Over the years there has been a growing consensus that in the present state of affairs a unified approach to the management of EHBDA should be sought. It is recognized that both individual treatment strategies entail imperfect management solutions and that the complementary and sequential utilization of both methods is indicated.[518] This attitude has been advocated in a monograph on EHBDA[508,518] and in several subsequent reports.[41,47,534]

The National Institutes of Health Consensus Conference on Liver Transplantation[493] concluded that (1) hepatic portoenterostomy should be the primary surgical therapy for EHBDA; (2) transplantation is appropriate therapy for patients with EHBDA who fail primary portoenterostomy; (3) liver transplantation should be delayed as long as possible to permit maximum growth; (4) transplantation should be deferred until progressive cholestasis, hepatocellular decompensation, or severe portal hypertension supervenes; and (5) multiple attempts to revise an unsuccessful Kasai procedure are not warranted because they can make liver transplantation more difficult and dangerous.[493] Although these conclusions still form the basis for contemporary management, some debate is still ongoing.

Some authors propose primary transplantation for EHBDA as the procedure of choice for several reasons, including the lack of adhesions when operating on a previously undisturbed abdomen and a decreased need for blood products.[535] The points of concern regarding the concept of primary transplantation for EHBDA center around four issues: (1) shortage of organs for children less than 1 year of age; (2) technical issues in performing transplants on small babies; (3) the success rate of liver transplantation in children younger than 1 year, and, most importantly; (4) the potential long-term palliation or even cure by the Kasai procedure alone.[535] In this debate whether primary portoenterostomy or not, the previous considerations are counterbalanced by the following observations. Organ shortage is progressively compensated by innovative techniques to increase organ availability for young children. These include reduced size and split livers[536] and living related liver transplantation.[536,537] Patients who underwent previous Kasai operations remained on the waiting list significantly longer than those patients who underwent transplantation primarily. The obligatory waiting period to determine whether a Kasai procedure has irretrievably failed may cause a cascade of detrimental effects, including malnutrition.[535] These authors therefore plead that a hepatic portoenterostomy be performed only in those patients in whom it is likely to succeed. They suggest that the histologic criteria of the presence of syncytial giant cells, lobular inflammation, and focal and bridging necrosis in the liver biopsy before a Kasai operation are indicative of poor early outcome and should lead to early referral for transplantation.[477] However, the latter study predicted success with hepatic portoenterostomy correctly in 87 percent of patients. Although encouraging, these data nevertheless indicate that the ability of biopsy results to predict outcome is still imperfect.[534] Prognostic studies of this sort remain in need of validation on larger groups of patients and, in the absence of an accurate predictive scheme, hepatic portoenterostomy should remain the first option,[41,534] except under special circumstances or co-existence of associated anomalies with a more dismal prognosis.[13,538]

Portoenterostomy should preferably be performed before the seventh week of life. Liver transplantation should be considered for the infant who presents beyond this time limit, particularly in the setting of advanced cirrhosis.[47,539,540] The portoenterostomy procedure should be designed to minimize problems with future liver transplantation; a simple retrocolic Roux-en-Y portoenterostomy is most appropriate.[41] Complex variations on the Kasai procedure, the addition of cutaneous venting stomas, and revision portoenterostomies should be avoided because they amplify the complexity and morbidity of the liver transplant procedure. After portoenterostomy, the child should be followed closely. When signs of failure in bile drainage arise, whereas hepatic reserve and nutritional status are still adequate, the child should be referred promptly to a liver transplant center.[541] Late referral of the infant for primary portoenterostomy and death of the child with failed portoenterostomy on a pretransplant waiting list represent missed opportunities.[518] In this comprehensive and sequential approach liver transplantation does not merely represent a therapeutic "safety net" for rescuing the child with a failed portoenterostomy, but instead is considered from the beginning. The Kasai procedure is viewed as a staging operation, which provides a cure for some and a bridge to liver transplantation for the majority.[508] A flow chart for EHBDA management strategy is represented in Table 50-3.

The long-term complications after liver transplantation are mainly the result of immunosuppression and sepsis. Early mortality factors, such as UNOS status, age at transplantation, primary diagnosis, and technical complications, do not predict late deaths.[542] Several recent reports on results of treatment of EHBDA in the transplantation era have appeared.[49,543-548] The reported overall survival in the subgroup of EHBDA patients who underwent a Kasai operation followed by liver transplantation if needed ranges from 66 percent to 100 percent in specialized institutions.[49,548] The French national study[548] is the first study of the overall prognosis of EHBDA that includes all patients with EHBDA from the time of diagnosis. Since both the Kasai operation and liver transplantation became widely available, 5- and 10-year overall survival rates are 70 percent and 68 percent, respectively (Table 50-4). Independent prognostic factors for overall survival were performance of Kasai operation, age at Kasai operation, anatomic pattern of extrahepatic bile ducts, polysplenia syndrome, and experience of the center.[548]

TABLE 50-3

Comprehensive Strategy for the Management of the Infant with Biliary Atresia

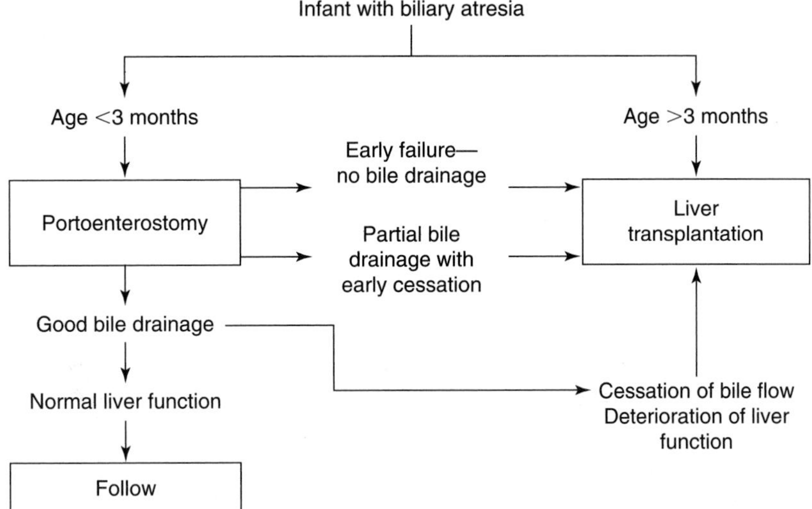

From Hoffman MA: Liver transplantation for biliary atresia. In Hoffman MA, ed: Current controversies in biliary atresia. Austin, Tex, RG Landes, 1992:81.

TABLE 50-4

Survival Rates of Patients with Biliary Atresia

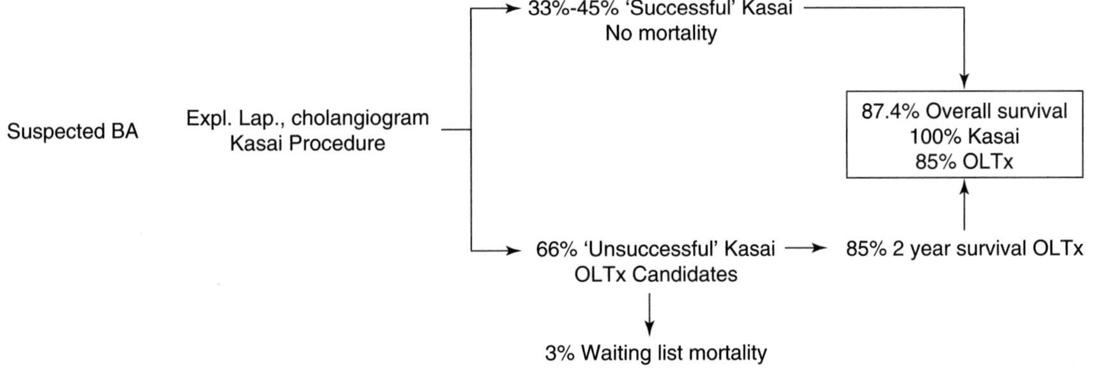

Liver Alterations after Hepatic Portoenterostomy

Most reports on long-term follow-up mention some abnormalities in liver enzymes and serum bile salt levels, as well as hepatomegaly, splenomegaly, and portal hypertension, occasionally with severe bleeding from esophageal varices.[18,39,416,549-557] The time of appearance of such complications as cirrhosis and portal hypertension is variable in different patients. No correlation is found between the development and severity of esophageal varices and the initial lesions at the time of surgery.[558,559] In surgical reports the complication of cirrhosis with portal hypertension is usually ascribed to the occurrence of repetitive episodes of cholangitis. However, there is a probability that the more serious long-term hepatic complications after portoenterostomy reflect the relentless, slow progression of the intrahepatic component of the basic disease process of EHBDA. As formulated by Landing in 1974[97] EHBDA represents a progressive inflammatory destruction of the entire biliary tree—intrahepatic and extrahepatic. The inflammatory destructive process may resolve at any stage and at any level,[97] which probably accounts for some reported instances of spontaneous cure in EHBDA.[18] Hepatic portoenterostomy seems to exert a beneficial effect on the progression of the intrahepatic lesion, not so much by arresting the basic disease process but rather by eliminating the superimposed obstruction caused by progressive obliteration of the extrahepatic bile ducts. This relief of obstruction saves the patient from rapid deterioration to the stage of secondary biliary cirrhosis and is responsible for the increased survival of patients whose prognosis is extremely poor without treatment.[446] However, the basic inflammatory process affecting the intrahepatic branches of the biliary system continues to operate in many patients, albeit at variable speed, similar to destruction of intrahepatic bile ducts in adults with primary biliary cirrhosis or primary sclerosing cholangitis. One report cites a patient who had end-stage cirrhosis at the age of 33 years after a portoenterostomy was performed in infancy.[388] The following section summarizes the major histologic findings in follow-up studies after hepatic portoenterostomy with an attempt at interpretation of the lesions observed.

Description of Histologic Findings

Development of Bile Duct Cysts and Bile Duct Dilation Mostly after Unsuccessful Portoenterostomy

A variety of acquired cystic lesions of the intrahepatic biliary system (biliary cysts or "bile lakes") have been observed in patients with inadequate postoperative flow of bile or attacks of cholangitis after portoenterostomy for EHBDA. In autopsy studies the prevalence of biliary cysts was 24 percent to 36 percent. MRI showed biliary cysts in slightly more than 18 percent of patients. The cysts may be multi-locular in the porta hepatis or unilocular, they may be communicating or not,[560] and they may be associated with a history of clinical cholangitis. The origin of these cysts is not clearly established; they might be due to cholangitis, to therapeutic stimulation of bile flow (choleresis), to obstruction of biliary radicles by surgical portoenterostomy,[561] or to dilation of peribiliary glands.[562] The development of these cysts did not correlate with hepatic function, portoenterostomy surgery, or the extent of morphologic change in the liver.[561] However, biliary cysts have also been found in children with EHBDA who did not have surgery.[258,563] The possibility of associated Caroli's disease has to be considered.[267,424,564]

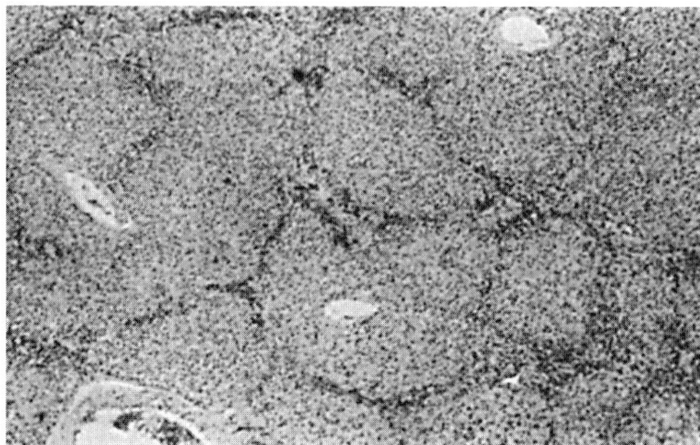

Figure 50-28 EHBDA. Follow-up liver biopsy 4.5 years after successful portoenterostomy (no jaundice). The overall liver architecture is preserved, but the lobules are accentuated by delicate fibrous extensions between adjacent portal tracts, simulating the normal appearance of pig's liver (hematoxylin and eosin, ×64). *EHBDA,* Extrahepatic bile duct atresia.

Improvement in the Histologic Appearance of the Liver after Successful Portoenterostomy

In some histologic studies of liver specimens from patients followed up after hepatic portoenterostomy[553,565,566] an improvement in the hepatic histologic alterations was observed in a few patients. Such improvement included a decrease in parenchymal and ductular cholestasis, in ballooning and damage of liver cells, in the degree of infiltration by inflammatory cells, and in periportal fibrosis.

Progressive Liver Damage Observed in Long-term Follow-up after Successful Portoenterostomy

Successful portoenterostomy in this context implies adequate postoperative flow of bile, disappearance of jaundice, and a patient in generally good condition. These patients may have episodes of cholangitis, especially during the first postoperative year, and portal hypertension develops later in a substantial number of these patients. A variety of histologic abnormalities has been observed in several studies of such patients who were followed for 5 years and longer.[177,245,550,565,567]

Mild Periportal Fibrosis. In some patients only mild periportal fibrosis is observed, with virtual lack of inflammatory infiltration (Figure 50-28). The lobular parenchyma appears normal. This pattern was observed in 4 of a series of 16 cases.[245] In some cases, however, careful analysis often reveals a number of additional abnormalities. Many portal tracts are large and densely collagenized, and a number of smaller terminal portal tracts appear to be missing. An occasional portal tract lacks an identifiable interlobular duct (Figure 50-29). The interlobular ducts may

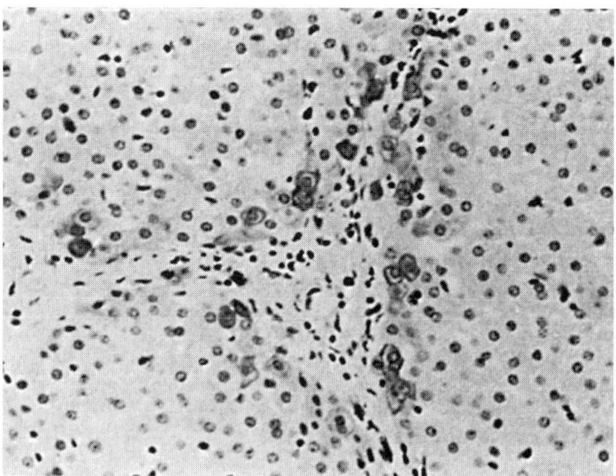

Figure 50-29 EHBDA. Follow-up liver biopsy 4.5 years after successful portoenterostomy (this is the same patient as in Figure 50-28). An occasional portal tract is found in which an interlobular bile duct is missing. The parenchymal cells adjacent to the portal tract show positive staining for bile duct–type cytokeratins, indicating a mild, smoldering cholestasis. (Immunoperoxidase staining with rabbit polyclonal anti-human cytokeratin [Dako Corporation, Santa Barbara, CA]. Counterstained with hematoxylin, ×400.) *EHBDA,* Extrahepatic bile duct atresia.

be ensheathed in a hyaline layer, which is not identical to the laminated concentric periductal fibrosis of classic chronic cholangitis. On PAS-diastase–stained sections the basement membrane of the ducts is more prominent than normal. A few small foci of small ductules usually are found close to or even inside the lobular parenchyma. Almost invariably, one finds some periductular edema and occasional neutrophilic polymorphonuclear leukocytes (PMN), indicating a minimal degree of cholangiolitis. Rhodanine staining for copper usually yields negative results. On immunostains for keratin 7 or TPA, the foci of ductular proliferation are revealed to a better extent. Moreover, the periportal hepatocytes (acinar zone 1) stain positive for keratin or TPA, indicating an early stage of biliary metaplasia and revealing a state of latent cholestasis (see Figure 50-29).[125,139,143,148] Such histologic features are observed in patients who are cured clinically. They have normal levels of bilirubin in sera but often have a mild increase in alkaline phosphatase levels. When the periportal fibrosis is somewhat more pronounced, the lobular pattern of the liver is accentuated, and the histologic appearance at first glance reminds one of the normal histologic appearance of the pig liver.

Congenital Hepatic Fibrosis–like Pattern. In clinically cured cases without jaundice or overt cholestasis the liver histologic appearance may resemble that of so-called congenital hepatic fibrosis (Figure 50-30). This pattern was observed in 5 of a series of 16 cases.[245] The congenital hepatic fibrosis–like histologic appearance is characterized by large portal tracts with dense collagenized stroma and periportal fibrosis. The portal connective tissue areas contain an increased number of bile ducts, occasionally showing curved shapes and even typical circular or nearly circular patterns of ductal plates (Figures 50-31 and 50-32). Several segments of bile ducts show necrobiosis of lining cells, with acidophilic condensation of cytoplasm and pyknosis of nuclei. This lesion may affect a few single cells scattered in the section or the epithelial damage with "melting down" of the bile duct lining may be extensive. Several segments of bile duct are surrounded by thick, hyaline, collagenous sheets (Figure 50-33). Minute foci of intralobular ductules, which are often, but not always, at the periphery of the parenchyma, reveal discrete signs of cholangiolitis. Rhodanine staining for copper yields negative results or minimal positivity. Immunostaining for keratin or TPA emphasizes the duct hyperplasia and shows to better advantage the foci of ductular reaction, but also reveals the keratin positivity of periportal hepatocytes (Figure 50-34). A striking feature often noted in such cases is the hypoplastic size of portal vein branches in the portal tracts. Medial smooth muscle cells develop in the wall of the portal vein branches, correlating with the degree of portal hypertension.[568] A decrease in the caliber of the main portal vein also was observed by abdominal sonography in patients with poor hepatobiliary function.[569] All patients showing a congenital hepatic fibrosis–like picture on follow-up biopsy specimens showed ductal plate malformation of the intrahepatic bile ducts at the time of portoenterostomy.[245]

Secondary Biliary Fibrosis and Cirrhosis. In a proportion of clinically cured cases histologic study of late follow-up biopsy specimens reveals extensive fibrosis with numerous portal-portal connective tissue septa. In some patients the picture is that of secondary biliary cirrhosis. The borderline between biliary fibrosis and biliary cirrhosis is unclear because long-standing cholestasis leads to increasing fibrosis in the periphery of the lobule.[121] Only in later stages does further development of portal-central septa occur (i.e., biliary cirrhosis).[161] Reports in the literature do not always distinguish between advanced biliary fibrosis and secondary biliary cirrhosis.[550,570] For this

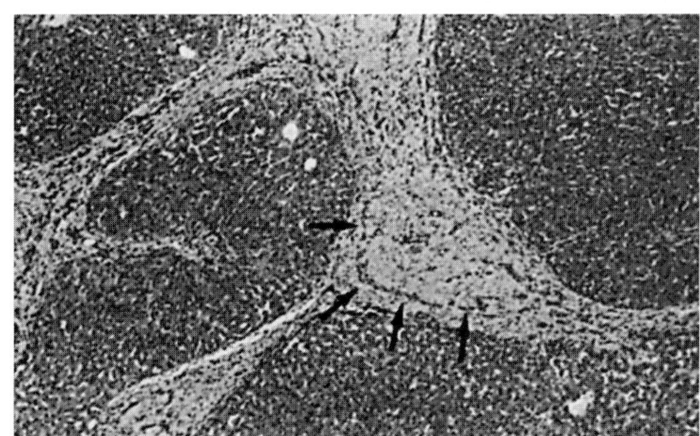

Figure 50-30 EHBDA. Follow-up liver biopsy 4 years after successful portoenterostomy (no jaundice). The overall histologic pattern corresponds to that of congenital hepatic fibrosis. Portal tracts are connected by broad connective tissue bands, containing numerous bile ducts. Some bile ducts appear in ductal plate configuration *(arrows)*. See also Figure 50-31. (Hematoxylin and eosin, ×64.) *EHBDA,* Extrahepatic bile duct atresia.

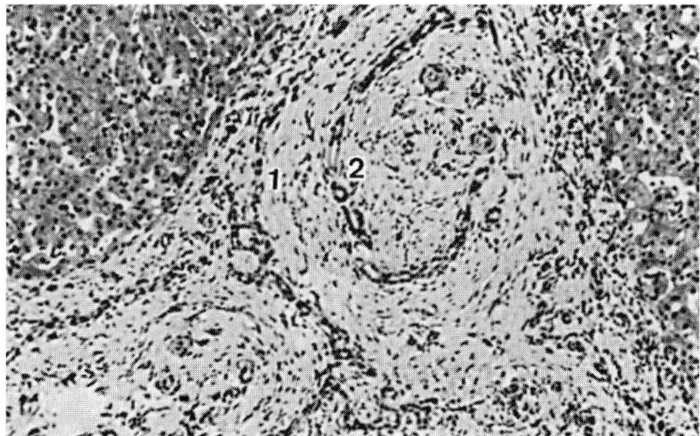

Figure 50-31 EHBDA. Follow-up liver biopsy 4 years after successful portoenterostomy in same patient as in Figure 50-30. Congenital hepatic fibrosis–like appearance. The ducts in the portal tracts and connecting septa often appear in ductal plate configuration. Double concentric ductal plates are often found *(1, 2)*. Compare with ductal plate duplication in early stages (see Figure 50-20) (hematoxylin and eosin, ×160). *EHBDA,* Extrahepatic bile duct atresia.

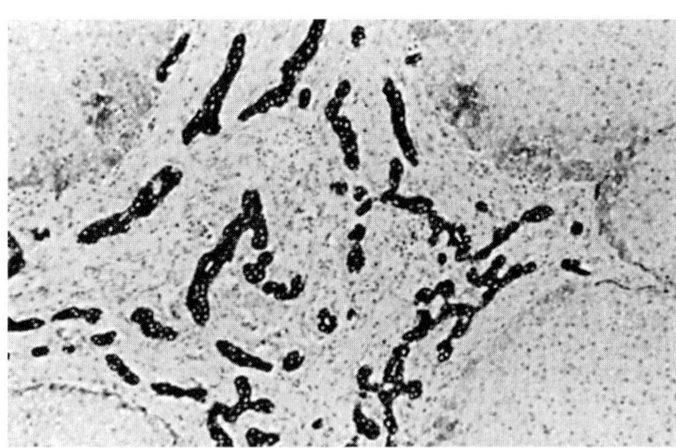

Figure 50-32 EHBDA. Follow-up liver biopsy 4.5 years after successful portoenterostomy (no jaundice). Congenital hepatic fibrosis-like pattern. Immunostaining for bile duct cell markers (TPA) reveals better the numerous bile duct structures, their similarity to ductal plates, and sometimes double concentric layering. Periportal hepatocytes show weakly positive staining, indicating chronic, mild cholestasis. See also Figure 50-34. (Immunoperoxidase staining for TPA. Counterstained with hematoxylin, ×160.) *EHBDA,* Extrahepatic bile duct atresia; *TPA,* tissue polypeptide antigen.

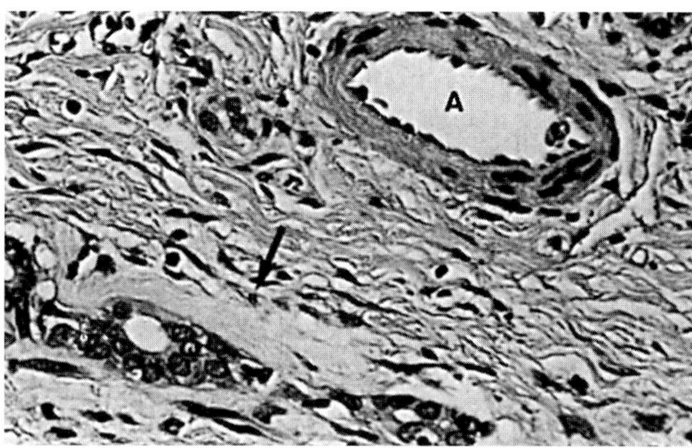

Figure 50-33 EHBDA. Follow-up liver biopsy 4 years after successful portoenterostomy (no jaundice) in same patient as in Figures 50-30 and 50-31. Congenital hepatic fibrosis-like appearance. This higher magnification shows that some of the bile duct segments are encased by broad sheets of fibrillar fibrosis (sclerosing cholangitis) *(arrow). EHBDA,* Extrahepatic bile duct atresia; *A,* hepatic artery. (Hematoxylin and eosin, ×640.)

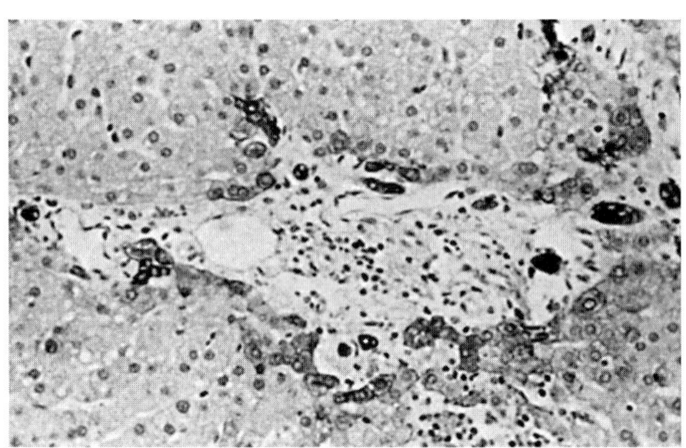

Figure 50-34 EHBDA. Follow-up liver biopsy 4 years after successful portoenterostomy (no jaundice) in same patient as in Figures 50-30 and 50-31. Immunostaining for bile duct cell markers reveals positive reaction in periportal hepatocytes and ductules, suggesting an early stage of ductular metaplasia of zone 1 hepatocytes. This finding indicates mild, smoldering cholestasis. (Immunostaining for TPA. Counterstained with hematoxylin, ×400.) *EHBDA,* Extrahepatic bile duct atresia; *TPA,* tissue polypeptide antigen.

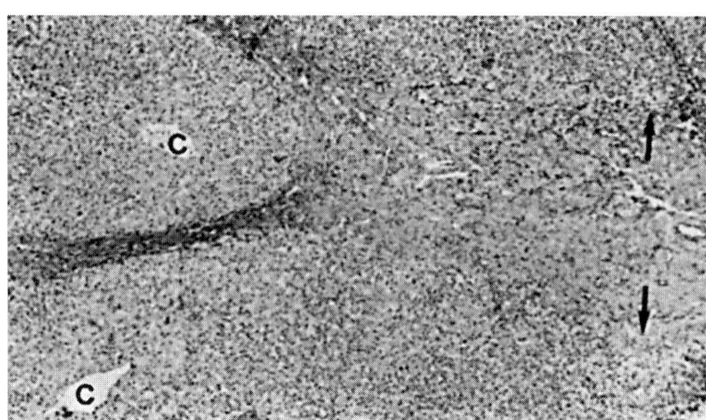

Figure 50-35 EHBDA. Follow-up liver biopsy 4 years after successful portoenterostomy (no jaundice). Acholangic biliary fibrosis. Broad fibrous septa connect adjacent portal tracts. The basic lobular architecture is preserved: parenchymal lobules are centered by draining veins *(C)*. There is total lack of bile ducts inside portal tracts and septa. Occasional foci of ductular proliferation occur at the connective tissue-parenchymal interphase *(arrows),* indicating a very mild cholestatic state. Compare with Figures 50-36 and 50-37 (hematoxylin and eosin, ×64). *EHBDA,* Extrahepatic bile duct atresia.

reason, and because of the admitted difficulty in making this distinction clearly on small specimens of tissue, advanced biliary fibrosis and biliary cirrhosis are treated together. An additional reason for emphasizing this problem is to warn the reader against accepting too easily the concept of reversibility of true biliary cirrhosis, an impression that may arise from occasional reports.[571,572]

In patients with advanced biliary fibrosis the basic pattern of connective tissue is similar to that described in the congenital hepatic fibrosis-like pattern. There is predominance of connective tissue septa from portal area to portal area (Figure 50-35). The parenchyma appears as garland-shaped masses between these septa. The portal vein branches in the portal tracts appear hypoplastic. There may be an increased number of dilated lymphatic channels.[567] They are recognizable by positive staining with Ulex Europeus lectin and by the negativity for factor VIII-related antigen of their lining endothelium.[245] Lymphocytic infiltration may be present, especially in the periphery of the portal tracts; however, usually it does not infiltrate the parenchyma (because of lack of or little interface hepatitis). A striking feature is the lack of interlobular bile ducts (see Figure 50-35). This stage corresponds to acholangic biliary fibrosis, cir-

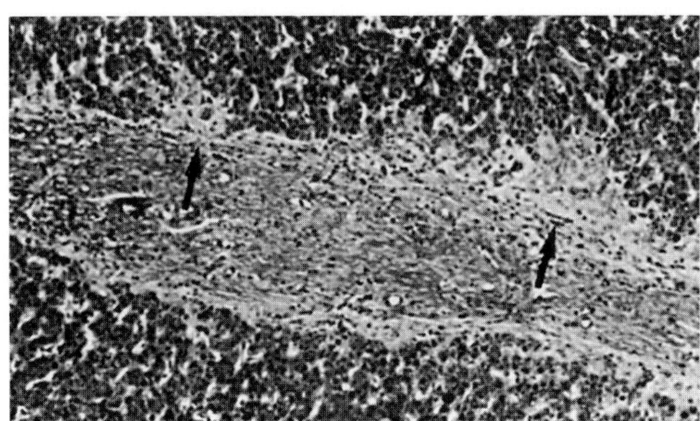

Figure 50-36 EHBDA. Follow-up liver biopsy 4 years after successful portoenterostomy (no jaundice). Acholangic biliary fibrosis. Detail of fibrous septum linking portal tracts. There are no bile ducts inside the portal tract and septum. Higher magnification and use of trichrome stain reveal to a better extent small foci of ductular proliferation at the septal-parenchymal interface *(arrows)*. Compare with Figures 50-35 and 50-37. These alterations indicate a mild, smoldering cholestatic state (Masson's trichrome stain, ×160). *EHBDA,* Extrahepatic bile duct atresia.

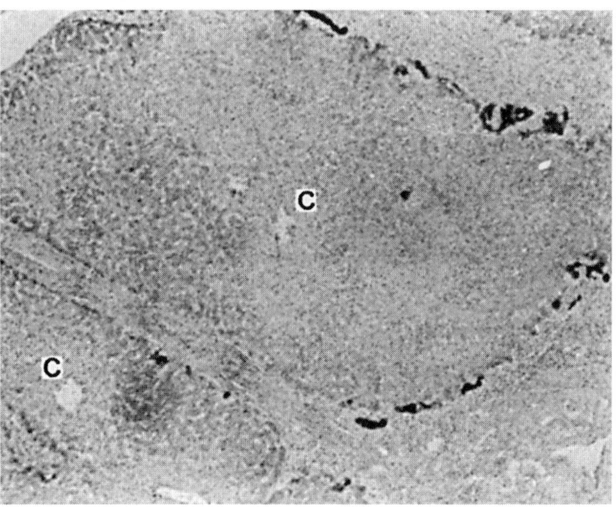

Figure 50-37 EHBDA. Follow-up liver biopsy 4 years after successful portoenterostomy (no jaundice). Acholangic biliary fibrosis. Fibrosis septa connect adjacent portal tracts; parenchymal lobules carry central draining veins *(C)*. There are no interlobular ducts inside portal tracts and septa. Foci of ductular proliferation at the connective tissue–parenchymal interface are better revealed by positive staining for bile duct cell markers. Compare with Figures 50-35 and 50-36. (Immunostaining for TPA. Counterstained with hematoxylin, ×64.) *EHBDA,* Extrahepatic bile duct atresia; *TPA,* tissue polypeptide antigen.

rhosis, or both. This pattern was observed in 2 of a series of 16 patients.[245] Several small foci of cholangiolitis can be found in the form of small clusters of ductules near to or even inside the parenchyma associated with some interstitial edema and a rare neutrophilic PMN (Figure 50-36). In some cases the loss of ducts is not total. An occasional portal tract still contains an interlobular bile duct showing signs of involution and necrobiosis of its lining cells. Such ducts may have normal tubular shape or may exhibit a ductal plate configuration. Occasionally the involuting duct is surrounded by lymphocytes (lymphocytic cholangitis).[573,574] This pattern of paucity of ducts was observed in 5 of a series of 16 patients.[245] The presence of some remaining ducts or ductal plates represents a pattern that is intermediate between the picture described previously as congenital hepatic fibrosis-like and the pattern classified as acholangic biliary fibrosis, cirrhosis, or both. Even in instances of a total lack of interlobular bile ducts, there is no bilirubinostasis either in the parenchyma or in the occasional remaining ducts or ductules.

Rhodanine staining for copper may be negative or may show some accumulation of copper in peripheral hepatocytes, especially in specimens with complete loss of ducts. Immunostaining for the epidermal type of keratin or for TPA emphasizes the decreased number of ducts, emphasizes the foci of ductular proliferation, and shows positive keratin staining of peripheral hepatocytes and of cholestatic liver cell rosettes (Figure 50-37). The latter feature, together with the foci of cholangiolitis, attests to the existence of a mild, smoldering state of cholestasis.

Liver Lesions Observed Near the Time of Clinical Deterioration in Patients with Long-term Clinical Cure. Some patients remain jaundice-free for years after successful portoenterostomy. In some, jaundice reappears after 4 to 7 years. Biopsies performed at this time show active biliary disease. There is seldom periportal fibrosis, more often a congenital hepatic fibrosis–like pattern or a biliary fibrosis–cirrhosis pattern is seen. In a series of 21 patients with long-term follow-up (4 to 7 years) 16 patients were jaundice-free.[245] However, five other patients showed clinical signs of deterioration with appearance of jaundice. The follow-up liver specimens of these children showed lesions of acholangic biliary fibrosis, cirrhosis, or both.[245]

Interface hepatitis also may be present (Figures 50-38 through 50-40).[138,139,575] The peripheral parenchymal cells are separated by interstitial edema and infiltration with inflammatory cells, including mononuclear and polymorphonuclear leukocytes. The dissociated liver cell plates may show features of ductular metaplasia, cholate stasis, or both (Figure 50-41; see Figure 50-40). Bilirubinostasis is found in the parenchyma, usually as intercellular plugs of bile and bilirubin staining of hypertrophic Kupffer cells and macrophages. Some foci of parenchymal cells show features of feathery degeneration.[138] Cholestatic liver cell rosettes are present to a variable extent.[139] The concurrent presence of these features indicates active (instead of slowly smoldering) biliary disease. The portal tracts may still contain an involuting bile duct in tubular or ductal plate configuration, showing atrophy and epi-thelial involution and occasionally lymphocytic infiltration (lymphocytic cholangitis).[573,574] Examples may be found of lymphoid aggregates only, possibly at the site of a preexisting but now vanished duct.

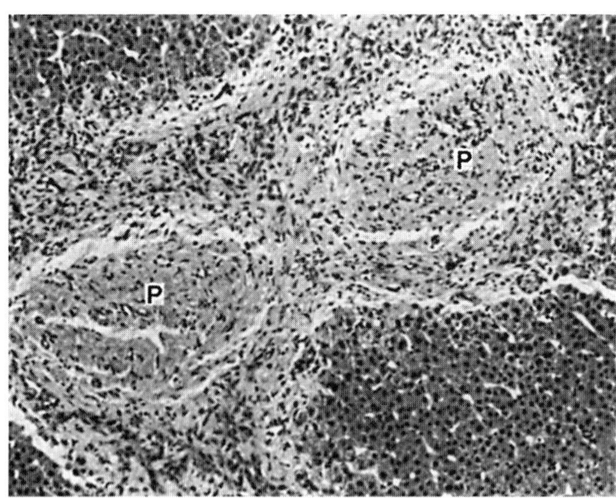

Figure 50-38 EHBDA. Follow-up liver biopsy 5 years after portoenterostomy. The patient was free of jaundice for 5 years but recently a rise of bilirubin in serum developed. The figure shows two interconnected portal tracts *(P)* composed of dense fibrous tissue without interlobular ducts. They are surrounded by a layer of loose connective tissue carrying numerous ductules. The connective tissue–parenchymal interface is irregular because of edema, ductular proliferation, and inflammatory infiltration (so-called biliary piecemeal necrosis). This alteration indicates active biliary disease with progressive cholestatic changes (hematoxylin and eosin, ×160). *EHBDA,* Extrahepatic bile duct atresia.

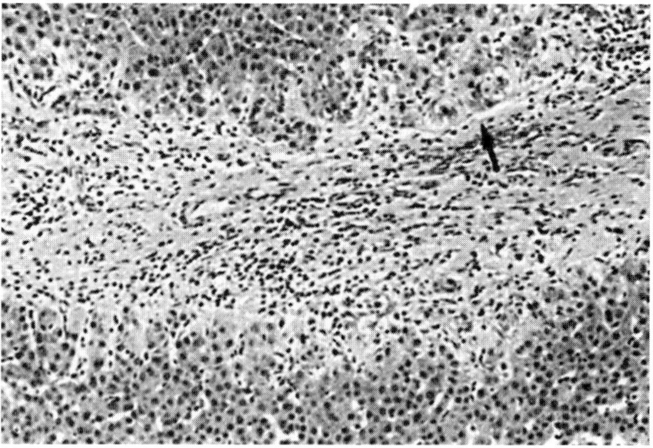

Figure 50-39 EHBDA. Follow-up liver biopsy 5 years after portoenterostomy. The patient was free of jaundice for 5 years, but recently a rise of bilirubin in serum developed. This is the same patient as in Figure 50-38. The figure shows a fibrous septum with moderately dense lymphocytic infiltration. There are no interlobular bile ducts. The septal-parenchymal interface is irregular because of edema, ductular proliferation, and inflammatory infiltration (biliary piecemeal necrosis). Several periseptal hepatocytes appear swollen and coarsely granular (so-called cholate stasis) *(arrow)*. These features indicate active biliary disease with progressive cholestatic changes (hematoxylin and eosin, ×160). *EHBDA,* Extrahepatic bile duct atresia.

Interpretation of Histologic Findings

In patients with an unsuccessful postoperative course the liver lesions correspond to those of the underlying liver disease, possibly aggravated by postoperative complications of ischemia, renewed obstruction, and especially acute cholangitis. In patients with a successful postoperative course the variety of liver lesions observed allows the formulation of the following hypothesis. The core of the hypothesis is not new and refers to EHBDA as a progressive destructive inflammation of intrahepatic and extrahepatic bile ducts.[37,97] The hypothesis further implies that the underlying basic disease process continues at its own pace and during its own and individually determined period of time in spite of successful surgery. The effect of portoenterostomy has been to relieve the patient of extrahepatic obstruction and its own disastrous effects, but it leaves the patient with the intrinsic intrahepatic disease of bile ducts (the basic disease process).[37] Apparently, the basic disease process may resolve spontaneously, resulting in a patient with complete clinical and histologic normalization. There is not much histologic documentation of this course of events. In some patients the intrahepatic disease of bile ducts, with its accompanying inflammation and fibrosis, continues for awhile, resulting in some periportal fibrosis before it finally heals. This course of events would apply to those patients who remain clinically well and biochemically normal but in whom some mild and functionally insignificant periportal fibrosis is found. As described in the section on Pathologic Features of the Liver in Extrahepatic Bile Duct Atresia, several cases are characterized by a particular type of ductular reaction in *the form* of ductal plate formation and even repetitive ductal plate malformation, resulting in often incomplete concentric rings of bile duct structures (early severe EHBDA).

When after successful portoenterostomy the basic disease process causing intrahepatic bile duct destruction stops in an early phase, the liver is left in a state characterized by an excess of immature types of bile duct structures. The bile duct destruction stops, but the remodeling of the ductal plate is deranged. This bile duct hyperplasia, together with the increase in portal and periportal connective tissue accompanying the later waves of ductal plates, creates the histologic appearance described as congenital hepatic fibrosis–like. It is intriguing to speculate whether natural congenital hepatic fibrosis (see Chap. 49) is not brought about by a comparable process of excess stimulation at ductal plate formation with arrest of the normal remodeling process. In this view congenital hepatic fibrosis would represent a fetal type of biliary fibrosis.[247] It is equally intriguing to speculate whether the congenital hepatic fibrosis–like pattern in EHBDA may not be responsible for the development of portal hypertension in the same way that natural congenital hepatic fibrosis is. Development of portal hypertension followed by the complications of esophageal varices and variceal hemorrhage is now recognized universally as a late complication of successful hepatic portoenterostomy,[175,552,559,576-581] although spontaneous alleviation of portal hypertension has been observed in some patients.[554,555,576] It looks as if the arrest in remodeling of the ductal plate may be complete or variably incomplete.

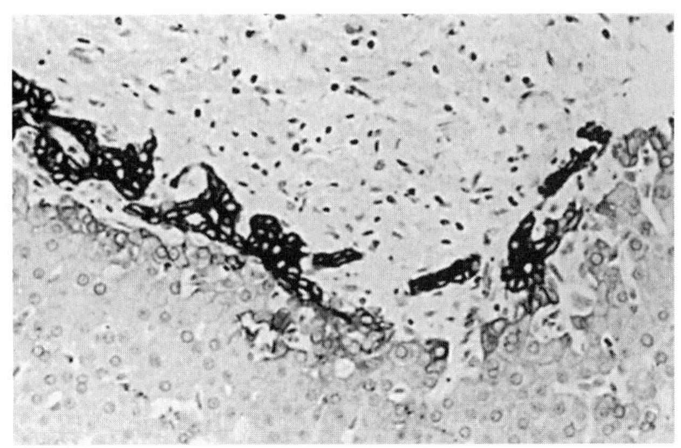

Figure 50-40 EHBDA. Follow-up liver biopsy 5 years after portoenterostomy. The patient was free of jaundice for 5 years, but recently a rise of bilirubin in serum developed. This is the same patient as in Figures 50-38 and 50-39. Detail of septal-parenchymal interface. Immunostaining for bile duct cell markers reveals better the ductular reaction and the moderately positive staining of periseptal hepatocytes. Positive staining is most marked in the periphery of these hepatocytes. (Immunostaining for TPA. Counterstained with hematoxylin, ×400.) *EHBDA,* Extrahepatic bile duct atresia; *TPA,* tissue polypeptide antigen.

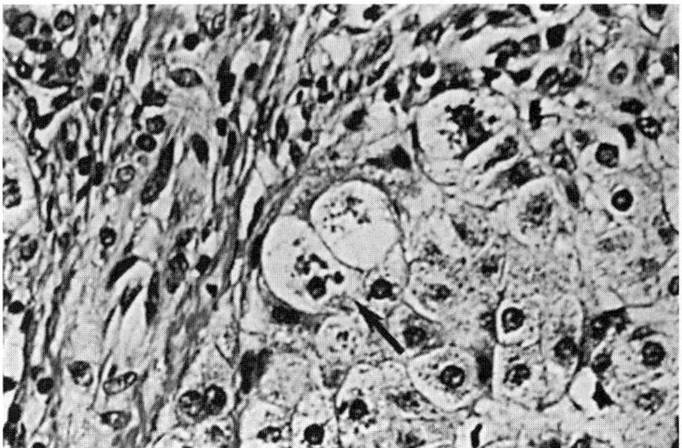

Figure 50-41 EHBDA. Follow-up biopsy 4 years after portoenterostomy. The patient was free of jaundice for nearly 4 years, but recently a rise of bilirubin in serum developed. Detail of septal-parenchymal interphase, with features of cholate stasis in periseptal hepatocytes: they appear swollen and coarsely granular and occasionally contain Mallory bodies *(arrow)* (hematoxylin and eosin, ×640). *EHBDA,* Extrahepatic bile duct atresia.

Complete arrest of remodeling would result in a congenital hepatic fibrosis–like pattern with ductal plate configurations in numerous portal areas. Partial remodeling would result in a congenital hepatic fibrosis-like pattern with ductal plates or ductal plate remnants in some portal tracts and normally shaped (remodeled) ducts in other portal areas. The mechanism of development of portal hypertension in congenital hepatic fibrosis is not established, but presumed mechanisms include the sometimes-documented hypoplasia of interlobular branches of the portal vein and the excess fibrous connective tissue in and around the portal tracts.[183] Whatever the mechanism of development of portal hypertension it may be the only complication in patients who undergo surgery. The liver parenchyma is normal and, because progressive destruction of the intrahepatic bile ducts stops, there is no perpetuation of the state of smoldering cholestasis. Liver test results are normal. The abnormally shaped intrahepatic bile ducts seem to assure adequate drainage of the bile produced by the liver. In several patients however, continued low-grade destruction of intrahepatic bile ducts (in excess numbers and in ductal plate configuration) continues to occur. This is reflected in the histologic picture described: a congenital hepatic fibrosis–like pattern with superimposed signs of smoldering cholestasis. This low-grade destructive cholangitis may lead, over months and years, to progressive disappearance of intrahepatic bile ducts of whatever shape, mature and immature, resulting in ductless portal tracts expanded by increasing amounts of connective tissue and periportal fibrosis. This gradually leads to secondary biliary fibrosis and cirrhosis with virtually complete lack of ducts. The patient may still be free of jaundice. However, the cholestasis will be reflected in raised serum levels of alkaline phosphatase, γ-glutamyl transpeptidase, cholesterol, and bile salts.[400] It is not clear how the liver manages to get rid of bile pigments. The suggestion has been made that drainage occurs through hepatic lymph vessels when no intrahepatic bile ducts are present.[582] The finding of excess numbers of dilated lymphatics is of interest in this respect.[245] This stage may be characterized by portal hypertension.

In some patients a long-term state of clinical cure may deteriorate with reappearance of jaundice. This may be due to clinical episodes of cholangitis, as often is reported in the literature. However, some authors state that there is no correlation between development of biliary cirrhosis in their patients and the presence or lack of repeated episodes of cholangitis.[550] The reason for this deterioration is not clear. It might be late occlusion of the anastomosis at the porta hepatis or late-stage obliteration of the larger intrahepatic draining ducts caused by the basic disease process; a block in lymphatic drainage by slow, progressive fibrosis; or a change in metabolic pathways inside the liver cells. Whatever the mechanism, the clinical deterioration is accompanied, and even preceded by, histologic changes of active biliary disease as described previously. Finally, the non-homogeneous spread of lesions observed in follow-up biopsy specimens from patients after portoenterostomy should be stressed.[567,583] An unequal distribution of the lesions is not surprising in progressive and destructive intrahepatic bile duct disease in view of what is known from experience in adults with primary biliary cirrhosis and sclerosing cholangitis. The lack of homogeneity of lesions throughout the liver, however, causes problems for adequate assessment in liver specimens of restricted size like those obtained by percutaneous needle biopsy. This explains why some authors recommend surgical biopsy to assure a more representative tissue sample.[550] The progressive disappearance of interlobular bile ducts in EHBDA, even after "successful" hepatic portoenterostomy, has been documented in several studies.[168-170,584] As discussed in this chapter we consider this lesion to be a result of the "basic disease process" in EHBDA. Other authors have interpreted the progressive ductopenia as resulting from obstruction of some larger ducts at the porta hepatis, based on the unequal spread of the lesions throughout the liver.[168,169] However, biliary cirrhosis is observed in end-stage liver disease after portoenterostomy in spite of patency of larger ducts at the liver hilum, suggesting an important role for the "basic disease process" of EHBDA in the progressive destruction of interlobular ducts.[170]

For the sake of completeness, it should be mentioned that other mechanisms have been proposed to explain the progression of lesions—for example, immunologic mechanisms and an autonomic fibromatosis of certain fibroblast clones resulting in progressive fibrosis.[585,586] At present, it is not clear whether these mechanisms should be considered alternatives or integral parts of the basic disease process in the hypothesis described earlier.

In conclusion the histologic studies of liver specimens obtained from patients after long-term follow-up for hepatic portoenterostomy allow the conclusion that the basic disease process of the intrahepatic bile ducts continues to run its natural course. This has been proposed on several occasions.[18,34,37,39,170] The advantage of portoenterostomy is in the relief of the extrahepatic bile duct occlusion, which itself is the result of the extrahepatic component of the basic process of sclerosing cholangitis. After reestablishment of bilioenteric continuity, the intrahepatic bile duct disease may heal spontaneously or may progress at variable rates.

The pathologic mechanisms result in progressive obliteration and disappearance of intrahepatic bile ducts accompanied by increasing periportal fibrosis, resulting in the end stage of biliary fibrosis, cirrhosis, or both. The histologic pattern of changes is modulated by the extent to which ductal plate formation and derangements in remodeling of ductal plates have occurred. The persistence of the "basic disease process," even after successful hepatic portoenterostomy, would explain why the majority of patients need subsequent liver transplantation. This emphasizes the need for basic research to solve the mysteries of etiology and pathogenesis of EHBDA.

Bile Duct Hypoplasia

Bile duct hypoplasia is a lesion characterized by an exceptionally small but grossly visible and radiographically patent extrahepatic biliary duct system.[18,36,103] The diagnosis is almost always made at exploratory laparotomy for jaundice in infancy. Bile duct hypoplasia is not a specific disease entity but a manifestation of a variety of hepatobiliary disorders. It may be associated with atresia of extrahepatic ducts and with intrahepatic cholestasis of any cause (see Table 50-1).[103] Bile duct hypoplasia may represent an intermediate stage in the development of EHBDA. Infants have been observed in whom hypoplasia of extrahepatic ducts progressed to total obliteration.[96,252,587] There is also evidence that the obliterating disease that leads to bile duct hypoplasia may stabilize at this stage or may even improve. Resolution of jaundice has occurred spontaneously in patients with hypoplastic extrahepatic bile ducts who underwent operation in infancy,[20,588] but the extent of improvement, if any, of the hypoplastic bile duct system was not substantiated. In patients with persistence of bile duct hypoplasia liver fibrosis is slowly progressive.[589] This slow development of cirrhosis is comparable to the progressive biliary disease that develops in adults with narrowed extrahepatic ducts.[590] A case history has been reported with the documented sequence of choledochal cyst to biliary hypoplasia to biliary atresia.[587] Narrowing and other duct irregularities have been demonstrated by cholangiography in patients suffering from neonatal hepatitis.[96]

Small extrahepatic bile ducts have been demonstrated by operative cholangiography in patients with the homozygous form of α_1-antitrypsin deficiency.[591-593] The hypoplasia of the extrahepatic bile ducts in this setting may represent a form of disuse atrophy caused by decreased bile flow as a result of intrahepatic cholestasis.[96] A similar hypothesis might apply to hypoplasia of the extrahepatic bile duct associated with hypoplasia of intrahepatic ducts as documented in some patients with Alagille's syndrome.[201,205,234,594,595] However, as mentioned previously, histologic study of the extrahepatic bile ducts in some of these patients revealed inflammatory and epithelial degenerative lesions, which were indistinguishable from those observed in fibrous remnants from patients with EHBDA.[205]

Treatment of bile duct hypoplasia depends on the primary hepatobiliary disorder. Bile duct hypoplasia secondary to low flow states (e.g., neonatal hepatitis, α_1-antitrypsin deficiency) cannot be improved by surgery. Patients in whom hypoplastic extrahepatic bile ducts appear to progress to total biliary obstruction should be considered for hepatic portoenterostomy after an observation period of 6 weeks.[18]

Spontaneous Perforation of the Common Bile Duct

Spontaneous perforation of the common bile duct is a highly specific clinical entity in infancy and should always be considered in an infant in whom jaundice develops after an anicteric period of good health.[18,596] It is a rare condition; some 60 cases have been reported since 1932.[597,598] The cause is unknown. In a majority of patients the perforation occurs at the union of the cystic and common ducts. This suggests a developmental weakness at this site,[599] but a viral infection has also been suggested as a cause for this disease.[600] Some cases are associated with distal obstruction resulting from sludge[601] or EHBDA.[602,603] Clinical signs of the disease commonly are noted between 1 week and 2 months after birth, although instances of later onset have been reported.[596] A single case was diagnosed before birth.[604] The clinical presentation may be one of an intra-abdominal catastrophe. Usually, however, fluctuating jaundice, acholic stools, and dark urine slowly develop in these patients. Symptoms may be so mild that the development of an inguinal or umbilical hernia secondary to ascites may be the first sign of illness.[605] In some cases general symptoms of weight loss, irritability, and vomiting may be noted before jaundice.

On clinical examination one notes abdominal distention from bile ascites and sometimes bile staining of the umbilicus or scrotum caused by bile tracking along patent hernial sacs.[596] Signs of peritonitis and pyrexia usually are lacking. Laboratory investigation reveals a moderate rise in serum levels of bilirubin; liver enzyme tests give normal results, a feature that differentiates this condition from EHBDA. Definitive preoperative diagnosis can be made by abdominal paracentesis yielding fluid with a high concentration of bilirubin.[606] Intravenous cholangiography demonstrates a leak in the extrahepatic bile ducts. Scanning with rose bengal sodium ^{131}I or other isotopes indicates free isotope in the peritoneal cavity.[18,596,607] Treatment is surgical. The type of operation performed depends to some extent on the findings in surgery.[18,596,608-610]

Bile Plug Syndrome and Inspissated Bile Syndrome

The terms *bile plug syndrome* and *inspissated bile syndrome* are often used interchangeably,[11,596] although Bernstein and co-workers stated explicitly that obstruction of the common duct by a plug of secretions and bile is to be differentiated from the so-called inspissated bile syndrome.[554] The term *inspissated bile syndrome* was derived in the nineteenth century and used by surgeons to indicate patients with prolonged jaundice in whom the surgeon found normal extrahepatic bile ducts containing inspissated bile at exploration for presumed EHBDA.[17,35] This concept was later extended in pediatric practice to include patients with apparent obstructive jaundice in early infancy in whom jaundice cleared spontaneously after several weeks.[190,611,612] The majority of these infants have massive hemolytic-induced jaundice caused by Rh and ABO blood group incompatibility.[611,612] From a questionnaire sent to 12 leading pediatricians in 1962[35] it appeared that the inspissated bile syndrome in its extended meaning was not considered a disease entity and was felt to represent "a pigment of our imagination." The histologic features of bile plugs in the parenchyma are the result rather than the cause of cholestasis and are caused by bilirubin overload of the liver and by dehydration. Because hemolytic disease of the newborn caused by blood group incompatibility is treated more adequately by exchange transfusion, this form of neonatal cholestasis has become infrequent.[40,211] The bile plug syndrome represents a form of extrahepatic cholestasis in which obstruction is caused by inspissated concrements of secretions and bile in the common bile duct.[613] Usually the syndrome occurs in patients with hemolytic disease.[40] Clinically, bile plug syndrome cannot be differentiated from EHBDA. Ultrasonography may be useful and the diagnosis is usually made at exploratory laparotomy.[614] The inspissated material can be removed by simple irrigation of the biliary tree or use of a mucolytic agent.[615,616] On occasion, inspissation may proceed to the point of production of stones, necessitating manual removal of the calculi, or may resolve spontaneously.[18,96,617] Choledochal cyst formation may also follow inspissated bile syndrome.[618]

Bile Duct Stenosis

A rare cause of extrahepatic obstruction in children beyond the neonatal age is a localized narrowing of the distal part of the common bile duct.[66] Fewer than 15 cases were reported until 2001.[619] In three such cases the proximal segments of the duct were dilated and contained small biliary concrements that had accumulated near the narrowed part of the bile duct. The condition was cured by simple choledochotomy and cleaning of the duct. Mention is made of two cases of post-traumatic stricture of the common bile duct, possibly caused by previous blunt abdominal trauma, and of two patients with partial stenosis of the confluence of the hepatic ducts without evidence of antecedent trauma.[66]

Duplication of the Biliary Tree

Duplication of the biliary tree is a condition of exceptional rarity.[66,620-622] The etiology is probably identical to that of intestinal duplication. Clinical symptoms include abdominal pain and recurring intestinal obstruction. The cholestasis may be anicteric or icteric. A hard mass of variable size is palpated in the right hypochondrium. Usually, the diagnosis is made during surgical intervention for presumed cholangitis or choledochal cyst.

Agenesis of the Extrahepatic Bile Ducts

Schwartz and associates[623] described five neonates with obstructive jaundice in whom exploration revealed absence of the proximal extrahepatic biliary ducts (four cases) or total absence of the extrahepatic ducts and gallbladder (one case). Jaundice was diagnosed from birth to 3 weeks of age. Surgery revealed absence of bile duct remnants, absence of inflammation, and a fibrous mass at the porta hepatis. Liver biopsy specimens showed histologic evidence of cholestasis, minimal bile duct proliferation and fibrosis, and nearly complete absence of inflammation. The authors conclude that this group of patients represents true agenesis of the extrahepatic bile ducts rather than EHBDA and that liver transplantation is the primary mode of treatment in this rare entity.

Gallstones

Cholelithiasis is being reported with increasing frequency in infants and neonates, apparently because of the widespread use of ultrasonography. The pigmentary nature of cholelithiasis has been established in most cases, but the pathogenesis of stone formation remains unclear.[624] Stones in the gallbladder have been described even in the fetus.[625] Gallstone formation can occur in premature infants treated with parenteral nutrition and furosemide.[626-628] Intrahepatic bile stone formation has been ascribed to *Ascaris lumbricoides* infestation.[629] Other possible causes include chronic hemolytic disease (20 percent[630] to 45 percent[631] of cases, but less in infants than in older children), mucoviscidosis, bile duct malformations, and septicemia.[66,628] In contrast with adult gallstone disease, there is no female predominance. Recent reviews of the clinical features, diagnostic procedures, and therapy have been published.[624,630,632]

Bile Duct Tumors

Tumors of the extrahepatic bile ducts are extremely rare in children. The tumors correspond to embryonal rhabdomyosarcoma and exceptionally to liposarcoma.[633-638] The clinical symptoms are those of complete cholestasis with progressive onset; an abdominal mass may be palpable. Operative cholangiography reveals the obstruction, which is often near the ampullary region.[66] Treatment consists of surgical excision. The prognosis is poor.[634,638]

Extramural Compression of the Common Bile Duct

Occasionally, extrahepatic cholestasis in a child is caused by extrinsic compression of the common bile duct. A case has been reported of bile duct obstruction by peritoneal bands, and cure was effected by simple division of the constricting bands.[639] Other causes include malignant tumors of lymph nodes near the porta hepatis (Hodgkin's and non-Hodgkin's lymphomas) and such benign lesions as chronic pancreatitis and post-traumatic cyst of the pancreas.[66] Both benign and malignant tumors of the pancreas or duodenum have been reported as causes of obstructive jaundice in infants (duodenal fibrosarcoma and carcinoma and hemangioendothelioma of the pancreas).[596]

Primary Sclerosing Cholangitis

Primary sclerosing cholangitis (PSC) is characterized by chronic inflammatory constriction of the intra- and extrahepatic biliary tree often associated with ulcerative colitis in adults (see Chap. 40).[144,574] Until recently, the condition was thought to be rare in children. The few cases reported can be separated into several groups:[233] those with sclerosing cholangitis that is somewhat similar to that reported in adults,[640,641] sclerosing cholangitis associated with immunodeficiency syndrome,[642-645] sclerosing cholangitis associated with histiocytosis X,[646-649] and retroperitoneal fibrosis.[66,650,651] A recent study[652] showed that sclerosing cholangitis with diagnostic radiologic features of cholangiopathy can have serologic parameters of autoimmune hepatitis (antinuclear, antismooth muscle or liver-kidney-microsomal type one autoantibodies) and was therefore diagnosed as autoimmune sclerosing cholangitis. This 16-year prospective study showed that autoimmune sclerosing cholangitis was as prevalent (in childhood) as autoimmune hepatitis without radiologic features of cholangiopathy. Probably these two entities lie within the same disease process.

Several studies show that PSC is not rare in children.[653-655] A recent Italian study that compared PSC in children and adults suggests a more severe activity at presentation in children but a better prognosis.[656] An increased awareness of PSC by pediatricians and pathologists, together with the more widespread use of ERCP, should clarify the true incidence of PSC in children.[657] Sokal and associates drew attention to the occurrence of localized forms of PSC.[658] An apparently new subgroup of patients with sclerosing cholangitis of childhood was recently identified.[233] This report described eight children with cholestasis from the first week of life, followed by early cirrhosis and portal hypertension; percutaneous cholecystography (at age 8 months to 9 years) disclosed rarefaction of segmental branches, stenosis, and focal dilation of the intrahepatic bile ducts. The extrahepatic bile ducts were involved in six patients. The authors suggest that this form of PSC with neonatal onset starts before birth and may result from

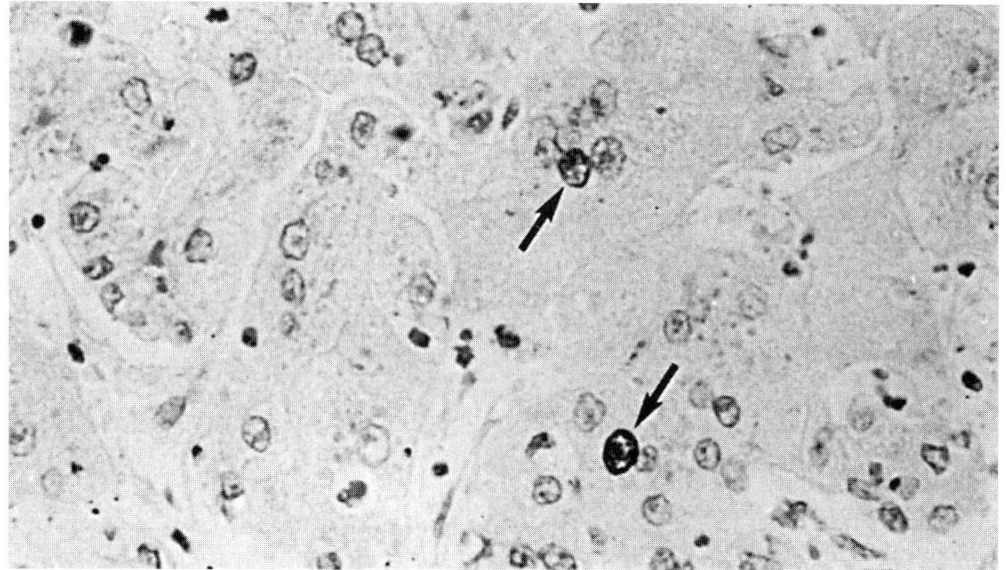

Figure 50-42 Fatal acute viral hepatitis type B in 10-month-old child. Liver biopsy showed multi-lobular bridging hepatic necrosis (not shown). The surviving parenchyma is characterized by parenchymal giant cell transformation. Some of the nuclei in the multi-nucleated giant cells contain hepatitis B core antigen (HBcAg) *(arrows)*. (Immunoperoxidase stain for HBcAg. Counterstained with hematoxylin, ×640.)

the same type of bile duct injury as does EHBDA but without the same extent of damage to the extrahepatic bile ducts, resulting in "near-miss" EHBDA.[233] Treatment with ursodeoxycholic acid has been recently shown to be efficient.[659]

Congenital Dilation of the Intrahepatic Bile Ducts (Caroli's Disease) and Choledochal Cyst

These conditions are described in Chapter 49.

INTRAHEPATIC CHOLESTASIS

Intrahepatic cholestasis comprises all forms of bile secretory failure of the liver in which the pathogenetic mechanisms are operative within the anatomic confines of the organ. This group of diseases can be further divided into two broad categories: (1) those conditions in which the primary lesion is confined to the intrahepatic bile ducts (e.g., paucity of intrahepatic bile ducts) and (2) the diseases that apparently correspond to a primary disturbance of the liver parenchymal cells.[105] In the neonate and young child the latter group of diseases has often been designated with the vague terms *neonatal giant cell hepatitis* or *neonatal hepatitis.* The following discussion is devoted to this apparently multi-factorial category of neonatal hepatitis.

Neonatal Hepatitis

History and Terminology

In 1952 Craig and Landing described a "form of hepatitis in the neonatal period simulating biliary atresia."[660] The disease presented clinically as obstructive jaundice that was indistinguishable from EHBDA and was histologically characterized by parenchymal giant cell transformation. A normal, patent biliary tree was present on abdominal exploration or at postmortem examination. The histopathologic picture was interpreted as "active hepatitis having the characteristics of viral hepatitis." At that time, there were no serologic tests available for viral hepatitis A or B and the viral etiology remained unproved. In the meantime it has become clear that viral hepatitis in the neonate may present a histologic picture with or without parenchymal giant cells (Figure 50-42).[40,211,661-666] In this respect the original authors were right in stating that "perhaps we have overemphasized the diagnostic importance of the multi-nucleate giant cell in this group of cases."[660]

According to the experience of French pediatric hepatologists,[103] neonatal hepatitis or intrahepatic cholestasis was almost as frequent (49.3 percent) as extrahepatic bile duct abnormalities (51.7 percent). The incidence of neonatal hepatitis in southeastern England was found to be 1:2500 live births.[667] Failure to identify a specific viral infection in the majority of cases and the clinical similarity to EHBDA have led to such terms as *neonatal hepatitis syndrome,*[668] *infantile obstructive cholangiopathy,*[97] and *cryptogenic infantile cholestasis type I.*[491] As can be deduced from Table 50-1 the list of specific causes of prolonged, conjugated hyperbilirubinuria in the neonatal age is long and diverse. The early detection of specific infectious diseases, intoxications, and disorders of amino acid, lipid, and carbohydrate metabolism is important because in many instances cholestasis attributable to these factors is treatable and reversible. A similar clinical picture of obstructive jaundice may be seen in homozygous α_1-antitrypsin deficiency and in cystic fibrosis. Endocrine disorders (hypopituitarism and hypothyroidism) may also be associated with cholestasis.[53,188,669] For clinical and therapeutic purposes, then, the terms *neonatal hepatitis syndrome* and *infantile obstructive cholangiopathy* are no longer adequate because they have various connotations and remain too vague.[40,53,66,670]

Distinction between extrahepatic and intrahepatic cholestasis, and then subdivision of the latter into extralobular and intralobular cholestasis, may be more adequate.[105] In the group with intralobular (or parenchymal) cholestasis the disease process is thought to focus on the hepatocyte and not, or only secondarily, on intrahepatic and extrahepatic segments of the biliary tree.[103] Intralobular cholestasis may be due to infectious, metabolic, toxic, and unknown causes.[140,671]

In the infectious category distinction should be made between hepatitis in a neonate and idiopathic neonatal hepatitis.[53] Hepatitis in a neonate refers to infection with a specific, identified virus, such as hepatitis B or cytomegalovirus (see Figure 50-42). These cases represent only a minority (about 10 percent) of cases with neonatal hepatitis syndrome.[491] However, idiopathic neonatal hepatitis remains a form of cholestasis of undetermined cause. This explains why some authors prefer to drop the term *hepatitis* altogether and to use the more objective, non-prejudiced term *cholestasis.*[66] Just as α_1-antitrypsin deficiency, which was formerly included in the idiopathic category, has now become clearly separable as a delineated subcategory, new developments have identified further subcategories as inborn errors of bile acid metabolism.[672-675] some of which are potentially treatable.[676,677] Neonatal hepatitis syndrome thus represents a continuously evolving spectrum of problems.[675]

Because most of the conditions listed in Table 50-1 are treated in other chapters, a detailed discussion of the various causes and diagnostic investigations of neonatal hepatitis syndrome is not given here. Further discussion is limited to the histopathologic features and overall prognosis of idiopathic neonatal hepatitis or idiopathic neonatal cholestasis.

Ever since the recognition of neonatal cholestasis with patent extrahepatic bile ducts, the main challenge for the clinician and the histopathologist has been to differentiate between EHBDA or other anatomic forms of obstruction (e.g., choledochal cyst) on the one hand and neonatal hepatitis without mechanical occlusion of the drainage system on the other. The reasons are the importance of early identification of patients who can be treated by surgery and the concern of avoiding unnecessary and potentially harmful laparotomy in infants with diseased livers.

From a study by Thaler and Gellis[23] it appeared that surgical exploration of the bile ducts had a harmful effect on the prognosis of patients with neonatal hepatitis. In contrast, Lawson and Boggs concluded from their studies that exploratory laparotomy, without biliary duct exploration, need not alter the future course of infants with neonatal hepatitis when they lack a positive family

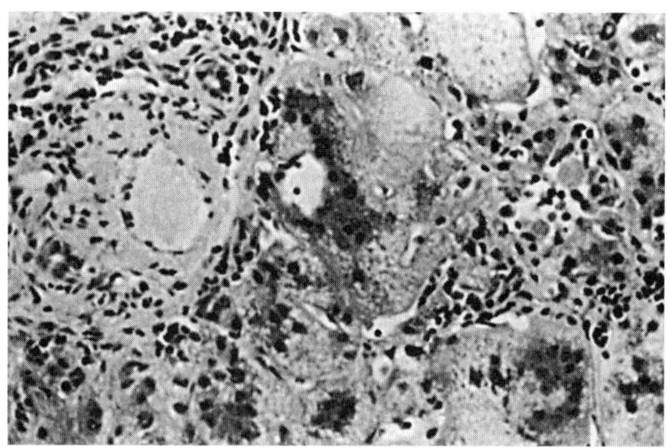

Figure 50-43 Neonatal giant cell hepatitis in infant age 8 weeks. The portal tract (upper left) shows mild mononuclear cell infiltration, the interlobular bile duct appears normal, and there is no ductular proliferation. The lobular parenchyma shows parenchymal giant cell transformation, focal necrosis, and mononuclear cell infiltration (hematoxylin and eosin, ×512).

history.[678] The authors suggested that familial forms of neonatal hepatitis syndrome caused the apparent poor prognosis in their total operative series and that early laparotomy may be safe and useful not only in establishing diagnosis but also in salvaging a number of infants with surgically correctable biliary atresia. In spite of further warning[491] the conclusions from the Lawson and Boggs study were mainly emphasized by pediatric surgeons who insist on early settling of the diagnostic differentiation from EHBDA.[18,679] In a follow-up study from France it was noted that progression to cirrhosis was mainly observed in patients who had undergone surgery,[680] but the authors remarked that the potentially adverse role of laparotomy must be judged with respect to the severity of the liver disease. The majority of their patients who were subjected to surgery had permanently pale stools, hard livers, and histologic features suggesting mechanical bile duct obstruction. Such findings correlate with another study in which poor prognosis was mainly observed in patients with neonatal hepatitis mimicking biliary atresia, that is, severe forms with complete cholestasis.[681] Notwithstanding some controversy about the strategies of diagnostic work-up, no one will doubt the principle that unnecessary surgery should be avoided as much as possible. Clinical features may be helpful in distinguishing neonatal hepatitis from EHBDA, as discussed previously. Liver biopsy may be helpful in discriminating between neonatal hepatitis and EHBDA.

Histopathologic Features

In general the histologic liver alterations in cryptogenic neonatal cholestasis are more prominent in the parenchyma than in the portal tracts (Figure 50-43).[140,157,682] Usually there is more extensive parenchymal giant cell transformation than in patients with EHBDA; giant cells are larger, appear more hydropic or ballooned, and often show degenerative features. Necrosis of parenchymal giant cells may be associated with infiltration by neutrophils[190]; on occasion, this feature has to be differentiated from so-called surgical necrosis in surgically resected wedge biopsy specimens.[683] One study has drawn attention to the occurrence of a peculiar large type of cell with strongly eosinophilic cytoplasm and a bizarrely shaped, homogeneously staining nucleus.[684] It is difficult to differentiate these cells from megakaryocytes, and their nature remains unclear. Foci of extramedullary hematopoiesis are found more often in neonatal hepatitis than in EHBDA, but they do not represent a differentiating feature.[140] Hemosiderin deposition in parenchymal cells and Kupffer cells is more conspicuous in neonatal hepatitis than in EHBDA.[157] Intralobular inflammation and Kupffer cell hyperplasia are usually more striking in neonatal hepatitis, whereas portal and periportal inflammation predominates in EHBDA.[157,682] Bilirubinostasis (histologic cholestasis) is variable but may be marked with pigment granules in parenchymal cells and Kupffer cells and variably sized intercellular plugs of bile. Bile concrements in portal ductules may be seen on occasion but are found more often in EHBDA.[157] Ductular proliferation at the periphery of portal tracts may be observed in some cases, but it never reaches the extent found in EHBDA. However, the finding of mild ductular proliferation may be misleading.[157] The fibrosis is more intralobular in neonatal hepatitis, in contrast to the more periportal predominance of fibrosis in EHBDA.[140,191]

Liver Parenchymal Giant Cells

The multi-nucleated giant cells in neonatal hepatitis are of parenchymal nature, according to their position in liver cell plates and light microscopic and ultrastructural features. The number of nuclei in parenchymal giant cells is variable, as is the location of the nuclei inside the cytoplasmic mass, either central or peripheral. On hematoxylin and eosin–stained sections the cytoplasm is pale staining, possibly because of glycogen or because of a hydropic change in several instances. Giant cells often contain brownish pigment granules, which correspond to bilirubin, lipofuscin, or hemosiderin, or a combination of these pigments. Histochemical characteristics of parenchymal giant cells include intense PAS staining caused by glycogen (diastase-digestible), intense staining for glucose-6-phosphatase, succinic dehydrogenase and nicotinamide adenine dinucleotide and nicotinamide adenine dinucleotide phosphate diaphorases,[685] numerous acid phosphatase positive inclusions, and increased staining for non-specific alkaline phosphatase at the sinusoidal border.[686] Electron microscopic study of parenchymal giant cells reveals well-preserved organelles: normal nuclei, mitochondria, endoplasmic reticulum, and plasma membrane. Apparently, the organelles for energy provision and protein synthesis are normal. An increased number of vacuoles and autophagosomes (cytolysosomes) indicates degenerative changes or increased turnover of organelles, whereas the large number of nuclei can be considered a sign of regeneration.[686] Bile canaliculi can be demonstrated in giant cells[687]; the sinusoidal microvilli are shortened and reduced in number.[686]

Giant cells seem to be deficient in bile secretion, as is seen from the accumulation of bilirubin deposits in their

TABLE 50-5
Conditions Associated with Giant Cell Transformation

Mechanical obstruction	Nonobstructive disease
Extrahepatic biliary atresia	**Diseases of Established Nature**
	Hepatitis B
Choledochal cysts	Rubella
	Cytomegalovirus
Intrahepatic biliary atresia	Herpes simplex
	Coxsackievirus
	Paramyxovirus
	Toxoplasmosis
	Congenital syphilis
	Escherichia coli pyelonephritis
	α_1-Antitrypsin deficiency
	Cystic fibrosis
	Galactosemia
	Inborn errors of bile acid metabolism
	Myeloproliferative disorder
	Niemann-Pick disease
	Gaucher's disease
	Down's syndrome
	17-18 trisomy
	Mucolipidosis
	Turner's syndrome
	Indian childhood cirrhosis
	ABO and Rh incompatibility
	Spherocytosis
	Anomalous pulmonary venous return to portal vein
	Endocardial cushion defect
	Neonatal hepatic necrosis
	Arnold-Chiari malformation
	Disease of Unestablished Nature
	Primary giant cell transformation or neonatal hepatitis

Modified from Ruebner B, Thaler MM: Giant-cell transformation in infantile liver disease. In Javitt NB, ed: Neonatal Hepatitis and Biliary Atresia. US Department of Health, Education and Welfare. DHEW Publication No. (NIH) 79-1296, 1979:2990.

cytoplasm and the delayed excretion of rose bengal sodium ^{131}I.[685] The formation of giant cells has been a matter of debate. Some authors considered parenchymal giant cells to be the result of faulty development of hepatocytes with aplasia of intercellular canaliculi, possibly on a hereditary basis.[688] Others considered the possibility that these multi-nucleated cells arose by nuclear multiplication not followed by cell division, resulting in multi-nucleated plasmodial cells.[689,690] Circumstantial evidence suggests that parenchymal giant cells may represent syncytial masses formed by fusion of several mononuclear hepatocytes. Possibly the cell fusion occurs in liver cell plates with pseudoglandular arrangement.[660,685]

The problem of the spontaneous disappearance of giant cells is similarly unresolved. Serial biopsy specimens from infants with giant cell transformation suggest that giant cells possess a limited life span of only a few months (from 2 or 3 to 6 months).[190,211,685] Their disappearance after several months generally parallels recovery from cholestasis.[685] The biologic significance of parenchymal giant cells remains unsolved. It has been suggested that parenchymal giant cells are not a nonspecific type of reaction to injury but that they represent a morphologic marker of infantile obstructive cholangiopathy.[97] However, parenchymal giant cells may occur in virtually all liver disorders of early infancy.[685] Thus the mere presence or lack of parenchymal giant cells is of relatively limited diagnostic value. A list of neonatal diseases associated with hepatocellular giant cell transformation is given in Table 50-5.[685] It thus may be concluded that parenchymal giant cell transformation (Table 50-5) represents a nonspecific reaction of the infant's hepatocytes to various types of injury.[157,691] Parenchymal giant cell transformation is more age-specific than disease-specific. Even this statement may not be taken too strictly because parenchymal giant cells have also been observed in adult liver disease, as with viral hepatitis and drug-induced liver disease.[692-699] Experimentally, parenchymal giant cell transformation has been induced in the liver by administration of *Escherichia coli* endotoxin to rabbits and rats and aflatoxin B1 to marmosets.[700-703]

Prognosis of Neonatal Hepatitis

A few studies have reported on the follow-up of patients with neonatal hepatitis or cryptogenic neonatal cholestasis. The outcome is highly variable.* In general the outcome is better in sporadic cases without known associated factors, whereas the prognosis is poor in familial cases and in patients with associated conditions such as α_1-antitrypsin deficiency. For example, of the sporadic cases reported by Danks and co-workers,[681] approximately 60 percent of the patients recovered, 10 percent had persisting inflammation or fibrosis, 2 percent had cirrhosis, and 30 percent died. The outcome was worse in familial cases: 30 percent of the patients recovered, chronic liver disease with cirrhosis developed in 10 percent, and 60 percent died. Adverse effects of diagnostic laparotomy are not universally recognized,[23,678,681] but it may be that the patients with the most severe disease causing complete cholestasis and carrying the worst prognosis are the first candidates for diagnostic laparotomy in case of uncertainty after non-invasive investigation.[680]

*References 53, 667, 680, 681, 704, 705.

References

1. Danks DM, Campbell PE, Clarke M, et al: Extrahepatic biliary atresia. The frequency of potentially operable cases. Am J Dis Child 128:684, 1974.
2. Donop CF: De ictero specialisme neonatorum. Inaug Diss, Berlin, 1852. In Schweizer P, Müller G, eds: Gallengangatresie. Cholestase syndrome in Neugeborenen und Säuglingsalter. Stuttgart, Hippokrates Verlag, 1984.
3. Heschl J: Vollständiger Defekt der Gallenwege beobachtet bei einem 7 Monate alt verstorbenen weiblichen Kinde. Wien Med Wochenschr 15:493, 1865.
4. Legg JW: Congenital deficiency of the common bile duct, the custic and hepatic ducts ending in a blind sac; cirrhosis of the liver. Trans Pathol Soc Lond 27:178, 1875-1876.
5. Lomer R: Ueber einen Fall von congenitaler partieller Obliteration der Gallengänge. Arch Pathol Anat Physiol und Klin Medizin 99:130, 1885.
6. Thomson J: On congenital obliteration of the bile ducts. Edinburgh Med J 37:523, 1891.
7. Thomson J: On congenital obliteration of the bile ducts. Edinburgh Med J 37:604, 1892.
8. Thomson J: On congenital obliteration of the bile ducts. Edinburgh Med J 137:724, 1892.
9. Rolleston HD, Hayne LB: A case of congenital hepatic cirrhosis with obliterative cholangtitis (congenital obliteration of the bile ducts). BMJ 1:758, 1901.
10. Moore TC: Congenital atresia of the extrahepatic bile ducts. Surg Gynecol Obstet 96:215, 1953.
11. Holmes JB: Congenital obliteration of the bile ducts. Diagnosis and suggestions for treatment. Am J Dis Child 11:405, 1916.
12. Yippö A: Zwei Fälle von kongenitalem Gallengangverschluss: Fett- und Bilirubin-Stoffwechselversuche bei einem derselbe. Z Kinderheilk 9:319, 1913.
13. Balistreri WF, Grand R, Hoofnagle JH, et al: Biliary atresia: current concepts and research directions. Hepatology 23:1682, 1996.
14. Ladd WE: Congenital atresia and steonosis of the bile ducts. JAMA 91:1082, 1928.
15. Lou MA, Schmutzer KJ, Regan JF: Congenital extrahepatic biliary atresia. Arch Surg 105:771, 1972.
16. Bill AH: World progress in surgery. Biliary atresia—Introduction. World J Surg 2:557, 1978.
17. Ladd WE: Congenital obstruction of bile ducts. Ann Surg 102:742, 1935.
18. Lilly JR, Altman RP: The biliary tree. In Ravitch MM, Welch KJ, Benson CD, et al, eds: Pediatric Surgery, ed 3. Chicago, Year Book Medical Publishers, 1979:827.
19. Dunn PM: Obstructive jaundice and haemolytic disease of the new born. Philadelphia, WB Saunders, 1953.
20. Gross RE: The surgery of infancy and childhood. Philadelphia, WB Saunders, 1953.
21. Clatworthy HWJ, McDonald VGJ: The diagnostic laparotomy in obstructive jaundice in infants. Surg Clin North Am 36:1545, 1956.
22. Thaler MM, Gellis SS: Studies in neonatal hepatitis and biliary atresia. Am J Dis Child 116:257, 1968.
23. Thaler MM, Gellis SS: Studies in neonatal hepatitis and biliary atresia. II. The effect of diagnostic laparotomy on long-term prognosis of neonatal hepatitis. Am J Dis Child 116:262, 1968.
24. Thaler MM, Gellis SS: Studies in neonatal hepatitis and biliary atresia. III. Progression and regression in cirrhosis in biliary atresia. Am J Dis Child 116:271, 1968.
25. Carlson E: Salvage of the "noncorrectable" case of congenital biliary atresia. Arch Surg 81:893, 1960.
26. Herzog B: Zur Gallengangatresie. Helv Chir 35:515, 1968.
27. Bill AH, Brennom WS, Huseby TL: Biliary atresia: new concepts of pathology, diagnosis and management. Arch Surg 109:367, 1974.
28. Kasai M, Suzuki S: A new operation for "non-correctable" biliary atresia: hepatic portoenterostomy. Shujitsu 13:733, 1959.
29. Kasai M, Kimura S, Wagatsuma M, et al: Die chirurgischen Behandlungen der angeborenen Missbildungen des Gallenganges. Therapiewoche 13:710, 1963.
30. Kasai M, Kimura S, Asakura S, et al: Surgical treatment of biliary atresia. J Pediatr Surg 3:665, 1968.
31. Campbell DP:oley JR, Bhatia M, et al: Hepatic portoenterostomy. Is it indicated in the treatment of biliary atresia? J Pediatr Surg 9:329, 1974.
32. Lilly JR: The Japanese operation for biliary atresia: remedy or mischief? Pediatrics 55:12, 1975.
33. Gans SL: Correctable or not correctable: biliary atresia. J Pediatr Surg 18:107, 1983.
34. Howard ER: Extrahepatic biliary atresia. A review of current management. Br J Surg 70:193, 1983.
35. Brent RL: Persistent jaundice in infancy. J Pediatr 61:111, 1962.
36. Witzleben CL: The pathogenesis of biliary atresia. In Javitt NB, ed: Neonatal Hepatitis and Biliary Atresia. US Department of Health, Education and Welfare. DHEW Publication No (NIH) 79-1296, 1979:339.
37. Haas JE: Bile duct and liver pathology in biliary atresia. World J Surg 2:561, 1978.
38. Lilly J, Altman RP, Schroter G, et al: Surgery of biliary atresia. Current status. Am J Dis Child 129:1429, 1975.
39. Alagille D, Valayer J, Odièvre M, et al: Long-term follow-up in children operated on by corrective surgery for extrahepatic biliary atresia. In Kasai M, ed: Biliary Atresia and its Related Disorders. Amsterdam, Excerpta Medica, 1983:233.
40. Schweizer P, Müller G: Gallengangsatresie. Cholestase-Syndrome im Neugeborenen- und Säuglingsalter. ed Stuttgart, Hippokrates Verlag, 1984.
41. Ryckman FC, Alonso MH, Bucuvalas JC, et al: Biliary atresia. Surgical management and treatment options as they relate to outcome. Liver Transpl Surg 4 (suppl 1):S24, 1998.
42. Jenner RE: New perspectives on biliary atresia. Ann R Coll Surg Engl 60:367, 1978.
43. Witzleben CL, Buck BE, Schnaufer L, et al: Studies on the pathogenesis of biliary atresia. Lab Invest 38:525, 1978.
44. Danks D, Bodian M: A genetic study of neonatal obstructive jaundice. Arch Dis Child 38:378, 1963.
45. Tunte W: Zur Häufigkeit der angeborenen Gallengangsatresie. Z Kinderheilk 102:275, 1968.
46. Lefkowitch JH: Biliary atresia. Mayo Clin Proc 73:90, 1998.
47. Bates MD, Bucuvalas JC, Alonso MH, et al: Biliary atresia: pathogenesis and treatment. Semin Liver Dis 18:281, 1998.
48. Chardot C, Carton M, Spire-Bendelac N, et al: Epidemiology of biliary atresia in France: a national study 1986-1996. J Hepatol 31:1006, 1999.
49. McKiernan PJ, Baker AJ, Kelly DA: The frequency and outcome of biliary atresia in the UK and Ireland. Lancet 355:25, 2000.
50. Shim KT, Kasai M, Spence MA: Race and biliary atresia. In Kasai M, Shiraki K, eds: Cholestasis in Infancy. Tokyo, University of Tokyo Press, 1980:5.
51. Thaler MM: Discussion: epidemiological studies in biliary atresia. In Kasai M, Shiraki K, eds: Cholestasis in Infancy. Tokyo, University of Tokyo Press, 1980:24.
52. Lilly JR, Stellin G, Pau CML, et al: Historical background of the biliary atresia registry. In Daum F, ed: Extrahepatic Biliary Atresia. New York, Marcel Dekker, 1983:73.

53. Balistreri WF: Neonatal cholestasis. J Pediatr 106:171, 1985.
54. Balistreri WF, Schubert WK: Liver disease in infancy and childhood. In Schiff L, Schiff ER, eds: Diseases of the Liver, ed 5. Philadelphia, JB Lippincott, 1982:1265.
55. Brough AJ, Bernstein J: Liver biopsy in the diagnosis of infantile obstructive jaundice. Pediatrics 43:519, 1969.
56. Wells TR, Ramicone E, Landing BH, et al: Preferentially longer survival of males than of females with untreated extrahepatic biliary atresia: correlations with time course of intrahepatic lesions and suggestion of possible ethnic influences. Pediatr Pathol 4:321, 1985.
57. Krauss AN: Familial extrahepatic biliary atresia. J Pediatr 65:933, 1964.
58. Lutz-Richner AR, Landolt RF: Familiäre Gallengangsmissbildungen mit tubulärer Niereninsuffizienz. Helv Paediatr Acta 28:1, 1973.
59. Mowat AP:sacharopoulos HT, Williams R: Extrahepatic biliary atresia versus neonatal hepatitis. Review of 137 prospectively investigaed infants. Arch Dis Child 51:763, 1976.
60. Whitten WW, Adie GC: Congenital biliary atresia. J Pediatr 10:539, 1952.
61. Nevin NL, Bell M, Frazer MJL, et al: Congenital extrahepatic biliary atresia in two brothers. J Med Genet 6:379, 1969.
62. Sommer AM, Moody PE, Reiner CB: Familial extrahepatic biliary atresia, report of a case situation. Clin Pediatr 15:267, 1976.
63. Stowens D: Congenital biliary atresia. Ann NY Acad Sci 11:33, 1963.
64. Kasai M: Treatment of biliary atresia with special reference to hepatic porto-enterostomy and its modifications. In Bill AH, Kasai M, eds: Progress of Pediatric Surgery, vol 6. Baltimore, University Park Press, 1974:5.
65. Lilly JR, Hall RJ, Vasquez-Estevez J, et al: The surgery of "correctable" biliary atresia. J Pediatr Surg 22:522, 1987.
66. Alagille D, Odièvre M: Liver and biliary tract disease in children. New York, John Wiley and Sons, 1979.
67. Choulot JJ, Gautier M, Eliot H, et al: Les malformations associées à l'atrésie des voies biliaires extrahépatiques. Arch Fr Pediatr 36:19, 1979.
68. Alagille D, Gautier M: Anatomy II: Anatomic data of the biliary system with respect to extrahepatic biliary atresia. In Bianchi L, Gerok W, Sickinger K, eds: Liver and Bile. Baltimore, University Press, 1977:33.
69. Bill AH, Haas JE, Foster GL: Biliary atresia: histopathologic observations and reflections upon its natural history. J Pediatr Surg 12:977, 1977.
70. Gautier M: L'atrésie des voies biliaires extrahépatiques: hypothèse étiologique basée sur l'étude histologique de 130 reliquats fibreux. Arch Fr Pediatr (suppl) 36:3, 1979.
71. Gautier M, Jehan P, Odièvre M: Histologic study of biliary fibrous remnants in 48 cases of extra-hepatic biliary atresia: correlation with postoperative bile flow restoration. J Pediatr 89:704, 1976.
72. Gautier M, Elliot N: Extrahepatic biliary atresia. Morphological study of 98 biliary remnants. Arch Pathol Lab Med 105:397, 1981.
73. Chandra RS, Altman RP: Ductal remnants in extrahepatic biliary atresia. A histopathological study with clinical correlations. J Pediatr 93:196, 1978.
74. Kasai M: Intra- and extrahepatic bile ducts in biliary atresia. In Javitt NB, ed: Neonatal Hepatitis and Biliary Atresia. US Department of Health, Education and Welfare. DHEW Publication No (NIH) 79-1296, 1979:351.
75. Kimura S: The early diagnosis of biliary atresia. Prog Pediatr Surg 6:91, 1974.
76. Lawrence SP, Sherman KE, Lawson JM, et al: A 39 year old man with chronic hepatitis. Semin Liver Dis 14:97, 1994.
77. Matsuo S, Ikeda K, Yakabe S, et al: Histologic study of the remnant of porta hepatis in patients with extrahepatic biliairy atresia. A computed picture analysis of 30 cases. Z Kinderchir 39:46, 1984.
78. Matsukawa Y: Three-dimensional histometry of bile ducts in the porta hepatis tissue in cases of biliary atresia. Arch Jpn Chir 53:47, 1984.
79. Miyano T, Surugo K, Tsuchiya H: A histopathological study of the remnant of extrahepatic bile duct in so-called uncorrectable biliary atresia. J Pediatr Surg 12:19, 1977.
80. Mustard RJ, Shandling B, Gillam J: The Kasai operation (hepatic portoenterostomy) for biliary atresia—experience with 20 cases. J Pediatr Surg 14:511, 1979.
81. Ohi R, Okamoto A, Kasai M: Morphologic studies of extrahepatic bile ducts in biliary atresia. In Kasai M, Shiraki K, eds: Cholestasis in Infancy. Tokyo, University of Tokyo Press, 1980:157.
82. Ohi R, Shikes RH, Stelling GP, et al: In biliary atresia duct histology correlates with bile flow. J Pediatr Surg 19:467, 1984.
83. Witzleben CL: Pathology of biliary atresia. In Hoffman MA, ed: Current Controversies in Biliary Atresia. Austin, RG Landes Company, 1992.:28.
84. Suruga K, Miyano T, Kimura K, et al: Reoperation in the treatment of biliary atresia. J Pediatr Surg 17:1, 1982.
85. Altman RP: Biliary atresia: a surgical-histopathologic correlation. In Javitt NB, ed: Neonatal Hepatitis and Biliary Atresia. US Department of Health, Education and Welfare. DHEW Publication No (NIH) 79-1296, 1979:391.
86. Altman RP: The portoenterostomy procedure for biliary atresia: a five year experience. Ann Surg 188:357, 1978.
87. Ohya T, Miyano T, Kimura K: Indication for portoenterostomy based on 103 patients with Suruga II modification. J Pediatr Surg 25:801, 1990.
88. Lawrence D, Howard ER, Tsannatos C, et al: Hepatic portoenterostomy for biliary atresia; a comparative study of histology and prognosis after surgery. Arch Dis Child 56:460, 1981.
89. Suruga K, Miyano T, Arai T, et al: A study of patients with long-term bile flow after hepatic portoenterostomy for biliary atresia. J Pediatr Surg 20:252, 1985.
90. Suruga K, Miyano T, Arai T, et al: A study on hepatic portoenterostomy for the treatment of atresia of the biliary tract. Surg Gynecol Obstet 159:53, 1984.
91. Schweizer P, Munzmann K: Extrahepatic bile duct atresia: how efficient is the hepatoporto-enterostomy? Eur J Pediatr Surg 8:150, 1998.
92. Tan CE, Davenport M, Driver M, et al: Does the morphology of the extrahepatic biliary remnants in biliary atresia influence survival? A review of 205 cases. J Pediatr Surg 29:1459, 1994.
93. Schweizer P, Kirschner HJ, Schittenhelm C: Anatomy of the porta hepatis (PH) as rational basis for the hepatoporto-enterostomy (HPE). Eur J Pediatr Surg 9:13, 1999.
94. Schweizer P, Flach A: Lympho-digestive Gallendrainage an der Leberpforte bei extrahepatischer Gallengangsatresie. Tierexperimentelle Studie. Zschr Kinderchir 18:271, 1976.
95. Stowens D: Congenital biliary atresia. Am J Gastroenterol 32:577, 1959.
96. Hays DM, Woolley MM, Snyder WH, et al: Diagnosis of biliary atresia: relative accuracy of percutaneous liver biopsy, open liver biopsy and operative cholangiography. J Pediatr 71:598, 1967.
97. Landing BH: Considerations on the pathogenesis of neonatal hepatitis, biliary atresia and choledochal cyst. The concept of infantile obstructive cholangiopathy. Prog Pediatr Surg 6:113, 1974.
98. Landing BH: Protracted obstructive jaundice in infancy. In Becker FF, ed: The Liver, Normal and Abnormal Functions. Part B. New York, Marcel Dekker, 1975:821.
99. Alagille D, Gautier M, Habib EC, et al: Les données de la biopsie hépatique pré- et peroperatoire au cours des cholestases prolongée du nourrisson. Etude de 128 observations. Arch Fr Pediatr 26:283, 1969.
100. Eliot N, Hadchouel M, Gautier M, et al: Valeur de la biopsie hépatique à l'aiguille et de la biopsie chirurgicale dans le diagnostic des cholestases néonatales. Gastroenterol Clin Biol 2:1025, 1978.
101. Brough HJ, Bernstein J: Conjugated hyperbilirubinemia in early infancy. A reassessment of liver biopsy. Hum Pathol 5:507, 1974.
102. Brough AJ, Bernstein J: Morphologic approach to the evaluation of infantile conjugated hyperbilirubinemia. In Javitt NB, ed: Neonatal Hepatitis and Biliary Atresia. US Department of Health, Education and Welfare. DHEW Publication No (NIH) 79-1296, 1979:381.
103. Alagille D: Cholestasis in the first three months of life. In Popper H, Schaffner F, eds: Progress in Liver Diseases, vol I. New York, Grune and Stratton, 1979:471.
104. Manolaki AG, Larcher VF, Mowat AP, et al: The prelaparotomy diagnosis of extrahepatic biliary atresia. Arch Dis Child 58:591, 1983.
105. Desmet VJ: Cholestasis: extrahepatic obstruction and secondary biliary cirrhosis. In MacSween RNM, Anthony PP, Scheuer PJ, eds: Pathology of the Liver, ed 2. Edinburgh, Churchill Livingstone, 1987:364.
106. Desmet VJ: Modulation of biliary epithelium. In Reutter W, Popper H, Arias IM, et al, eds: Modulation of Liver Cell Expression. Lancaster, MTP Press, 1987:195.
107. Hammar JA: Über die erste Entstehung der nicht kapillaren intrahepatischen Gallengänge beim Menschen. Z Mikrosk Anat Forsch 5:59, 1926.

108. Van Eyken P, Sciot R, Callea F, et al: The development of the intrahepatic bile ducts in man: a keratin-immunohistochemical study. Hepatology 8:1586, 1988.
109. Van Eyken P, Desmet VJ: Bile duct cells. In LeBouton AV, ed: Molecular and Cell Biology of the Liver. Boca Raton, CRC Press, 1993.:475.
110. Shah KD, Gerber MA: Development of intrahepatic bile ducts in humans. Possible role of laminin. Arch Pathol Lab Med 114:597, 1990.
111. Gall JAM, Bathal PS: Liver and biliary: morphological and immunohistochemical assessment of intrahepatic bile duct development in the rat. J Gastroenterol Hepatol 4:241, 1989.
112. Blankenberg TA, Lund JK, Reubner BH: Normal and abnormal development of human intrahepatic bile ducts. An immunohistochemical perspective. In Abramowsky CR, Bernstein J, Rosenberg HS, eds: Perspectives in Pediatric Pathology. Transplantation Pathology—Hepatic Morphogenesis, vol 14. Basel, Karger, 1991:143.
113. Ruebner BH, Blankenberg TA, Burrows DA, et al: Development and transformation of the ductal plate in the developing human liver. Pediatr Pathol 10:55, 1990.
114. Roskams T, Van Eyken P, Desmet V: Human liver growth and development. In Strain A, Diehl AM, eds: Liver Growth and Repair. London, Chapman & Hall, 1998:541.
115. Desmet VJ: Intrahepatic bile ducts under the lens. J Hepatol 1:545, 1985.
116. Desmet VJ: Congenital diseases of intrahepatic bile ducts: variations on the theme "ductal plate malformation." Hepatology 16:1069, 1992.
117. Desmet VJ: Pathogenesis of ductal plate abnormalities. Mayo Clin Proc 73:80, 1998.
118. Van Eyken P, Sciot R, Desmet V: Intrahepatic bile duct development in the rat: a cytokeratin-immunohistochemical study. Lab Invest 59:52, 1988.
119. Lüders D: Hypoplasie der intrahepatischen Gallengänge mit gutartigem Verlauf. Monatsschr Kinderheilkd 121:717, 1973.
120. Gherardi GJ, MacMahon HE: Hypoplasia of terminal bile ducts. Am J Dis Child 120:151, 1970.
121. Desmet VJ, Roskams T, Van Eyken P: Pathology of the biliary tree in cholestasis: ductular reaction. In Manns MP, Boyer JL, Jansen PLM, et al, eds: Cholestatic Liver Diseases. Lancaster, Kluwer Academic Publishers, 1998:143.
122. Desmet V, Roskams T, Van Eyken P: Ductular reaction in the liver. Path Res Pract 191:513, 1995.
123. Nakanuma Y, Ohta G: Immunohistochemical study on bile ductular proliferation in various hepatobiliary diseases. Liver 6:205, 1986.
124. Thung SN: The development of proliferating ductular structures in liver disease. Arch Pathol Lab Med 114:407, 1990.
125. Van Eyken P, Sciot R, Desmet VJ: A cytokeratin immunohistochemical study of cholestatic liver disease: evidence that hepatocytes can express "bile duct-type" cytokeratins. Histopathology 15:125, 1989.
126. Müllhaupt B, Gundat F, Epper R, et al: The common pattern of cytokeratin alteration in alcoholic and cholestatic liver disease is different from that of hepatitic liver damage. A study with the panepithelial monoclonal antibody Lu-5. J Hepatol 19:23, 1993.
127. Van Eyken P, Desmet V: Ductular metaplasia of hepatocytes. In Sirica AE, Longnecker DS, eds: Biliary and Pancreatic Ductal Epithelia. Pathobiology and Pathophysiology. New York, Marcel Dekker Inc, 1997:201.
128. Cocjin J, Rosenthal P, Buslon V, et al: Bile ductule formation in fetal, neonatal, and infant livers compared with extrahepatic biliary atresia. Hepatology 24:568, 1996.
129. Chiba T: Reconstruction of intrahepatic bile ducts in congenital biliary atresia. J Exp Med 115:99, 1975.
130. Crosby HA, Hubscher SG, Joplin RE, et al: Immunolocalization of OV-6, a putative progenitor cell marker in human fetal and diseases pediatric liver. Hepatology 28:980, 1998.
131. Xiao J-C, Ruck P, Kaiserling E: Small epithelial cells in extrahepatic biliary atresia: electron microscopic and immunoelectron microscopic findings suggest a close relationship to liver progenitor cells. Histopathology 35:454, 1999.
132. Lamireau T, Le Bail B, Boussarie L, et al: Expression of collagens type I and IV, osteonectin and transforming growth factor beta-1 (TGFbeta1) in biliary atresia and paucity of intrahepatic bile ducts during infancy. J Hepatol 31:248, 1999.
133. Shirahase I, Ooshima A, Tanaka K, et al: Immunohistochemical demonstration of collagen types III and IV and myofibroblasts in the liver of patients with biliary atresia. J Pediatr Surg 29:639, 1994.
134. Ramm GA, Nair VG, Bridle KR, et al: Contribution of hepatic parenchymal and nonparenchymal cells to hepatic fibrogenesis in biliary atresia. Am J Pathol 153:527, 1998.
135. Rosenweig JN, Omori M, Page K, et al: Transforming growth factor-beta1 in plasma and liver of children with liver disease. Pediatr Res 44:402, 1998.
136. Desmet V: Morphologic and histochemical aspects of cholestasis. In Popper H, Schaffner F, eds: Progress in Liver Diseases, vol 4. New York, Grune and Stratton, 1972:97.
137. Javitt NB: Bile salts and liver disease in childhood. Postgrad Med J 50:354, 1974.
138. Bianchi L: Liver biopsy interpretation in hepatitis. Part I. Presentation of critical morphologic features used in diagnosis (glossary). Pathol Res Pract 178:2, 1983.
139. Desmet VJ: Current problems in diagnosis of biliary disease and cholestasis. Semin Liver Dis 6:233, 1986.
140. Desmet VJ: Pathology of paediatric cholestasis. In Lentze M, Reichen J, eds: Paediatric Cholestasis. Novel Approaches to Treatment. Dordrecht, Kluwer Academic Publishers, 1992:55.
141. Desmet VJ: Histopathology of cholestasis. Verh Dtsh Ges Path 79:233, 1995.
142. International Group: Histopathology of the intrahepatic biliary tree. Liver 3:161, 1983.
143. Butron Vila MM, Haot J, Desmet VJ: Cholestatic features in focal nodular hyperplasia of the liver. Liver 4:387, 1984.
144. Desmet VJ: Cholangiopathies: past, present and future. Semin Liver Dis 7:67, 1987.
145. Van Eyken P, Sciot R, Van Damme B, et al: Keratin-immunohistochemistry in normal human liver. Cytokeratin pattern of hepatocytes, bile ducts and acinar gradient. Virchows Arch [A] 412:63, 1987.
146. Nathrath WBJ, Heidenkummer P, Björklund V, et al: Distribution of tissue polypeptide antigen (TPA) in normal human tissue. Immunological study on unfixed, methanol, ethanol and formalin fixed tissue. J Histochem Cytochem 33:99, 1985.
147. Burt AD, Stewart JA, Aitchison M, et al: Expression of tissue polypeptide antigen (TPA) in fetal and adult liver: changes in liver disease. J Clin Pathol 40:719, 1987.
148. Van Eyken P, Desmet VJ: Cytokeratins and the liver. Liver 13:113, 1993.
149. Treem WR, Krzymowski GA, Cartun RW, et al: Cytokeratin immunohistochemical examination of liver biopsies in infants with Alagille syndrome and biliary atresia. J Pediatr Gastroenterol Nutr 15:73, 1992.
150. Kato T, Yoshino H, Hebiguchi T, et al: Immunohistochemical analysis of portal proliferative bile ductuli in biliary atresia. In Ohi R, ed: Biliary Atresia. Tokyo, ICOM Associates, 1991:47.
151. Bielamowicz A, Weitzman JJ, Alshak NS, et al: Case Report. Successful late Kasai portoenterostomy. J Pediatr Gastroenterol Nutr 14:232, 1992.
152. Ferry GD, Selby ML, Udall J, et al: Guide to early diagnosis of biliary obstruction in infancy. Clin Pediatr 24:305, 1985.
153. Ho CW, Shioda K, Shirasaki K, et al: The pathogenesis of biliary atresia: a morphological study of the hepatobiliary system and the hepatic artery. J Pediatr Gastroenterol Nutr 16:53, 1993.
154. Matzen P, Junge J, Christoffersen P, et al: Reproducibility and accuracy of liver biopsy findings suggestive of an obstructive cause of jaundice. In Brunner H, Thaler H, eds: Hepatology. A Festschrift for Hans Popper. New York, Raven Press, 1985:285.
155. Kasai M, Yakovac W, Koop EC: Liver in congenital biliary atresia and neonatal hepatitis. A histopathologic study. Arch Pathol 74:152, 1962.
156. Gathmann HA, Osswald P, Müller G: Differentialdiagnose und Verlaufsbeobachtungen bei Säuglingen und Kleinkindern mit Längerdauernder Cholestase. Z Kinderheilk 120:259, 1975.
157. Ruebner BH, Miyai K: The pathology of neonatal hepatitis and biliary atresia with particular reference to hemopoiesis and hemosiderin deposition. Ann NY Acad Sci 111:375, 1963.
158. Lorenz G: Histomorphologische Leberveränderungen bei extrahepatischer Gallengangsatresie. Dtsch Z Verdau Stoffwechselkr 39:226, 1979.
159. Hollander M, Schaffner F: Electron microscopic studies in biliary atresia. Am J Dis Child 16:57, 1968.

160. Sasaki H, Schaffner F, Popper H: Bile ductules in cholestasis: morphologic evidence for secretion and absorption in man. Lab Invest 16:84, 1967.
161. Desmet VJ: Cirrhosis: Aetiology and pathogenesis: cholestasis. In Boyer JL, Bianchi L, eds: Liver Cirrhosis. Falk Symposium 44. Lancaster, MTP Press, 1987:101.
162. Ito I, Nagaya M, Niinomi N, et al: Intrahepatic bile ducts in biliary atresia. In Ohi R, ed: Biliary atresia. Tokyo, Professional Postgraduate Services, 1987:62.
163. Suruga K, Tsunoda S, Deguchi E, et al: The future role of hepatic portoenterostomy as treatment of biliary atresia. J Pediatr Surg 27:707, 1992.
164. Arima T, Suita S, Shono T, et al: The progressive degeneration of interlobular bile ducts in biliary atresia: an ultrastructural study. Fukuoka-Igaku-Zasshi 86:58, 1995.
165. Ohya T, Fujimoto T, Shimomura H, et al: Degeneration of intrahepatic bile duct with lymphocyte infiltration into biliary epithelial cells in biliary atresia. J Pediatr Surg 30:515, 1995.
166. Park WH, Kim SP, Park KK, et al: Electron microscopic study of the liver with biliary atresia and neonatal hepatitis. J Pediatr Surg 31:367, 1996.
167. Funaki N, Sasano H, Shizawa S, et al: Apoptosis and cell proliferation in biliary atresia. J Pathol 186:429, 1998.
168. Nietgen GW, Vacanti JP, Perez-Atayde AR: Intrahepatic bile duct loss in biliary atresia despite portoenterostomy: a consequence of ongoing destruction? Gastroenterology 102:2126, 1992.
169. Perez-Atayde AR, Nietgen GW, Vacanti JP: Histological and immunohistochemical study of the liver in early and late extrahepatic biliary atresia. In Ohi R, ed: Biliary Atresia. Tokyo, ICOM Associates, 1991:60.
170. Fabbretti G, Gosseye S, Brisigotti M, et al: Liver transplantation after unsuccessful porto-enterostomy for extra-hepatic biliary atresia (EHBDA): morphologic study of 31 removed livers. In Ohi R, ed: Biliary Atresia. Tokyo, ICOM Associates, 1991:70.
171. Landing BH, Wells TR, Reed GB, et al: Diseases of the bile ducts in children. In Gall EA, Mostofi FK, eds: The Liver by 34 Authors. Baltimore, Williams & Wilkins, 1973:480.
172. Sherlock S: The syndrome of disappearing intrahepatic bile ducts. Lancet 2:493, 1987.
173. Desmet VJ: Vanishing bile duct disorders. In Boyer JL, Ockner RK, eds: Progress in Liver Diseases, vol X. Philadelphia, WB Saunders, 1992:89.
174. Ohi R, Endo N, Kasai M: Histopathological studies of the liver in biliary atresia—further observations. In Kasai M, ed: Biliary Atresia and its Related Disorders, vol 7. Amsterdam, Excerpta Medica, 1983:1.
175. Howard ER, Driver M, McClement J, et al: Prolonged survival after operation for extrahepatic biliary atresia. In Kasai M, ed: Biliary Atresia and its Related Disorders. Amsterdam, Excerpta Medica, 1983:167.
176. Ito T, Horisawa M, Ando H: Intrahepatic bile ducts in biliary atresia—a possible factor determining the prognosis. J Pediatr Surg 18:124, 1983.
177. Altman RP, Chandra R, Lilly J: Ongoing cirrhosis after successful portoenterostomy in infants with biliary atresia. J Pediatr Surg 10:685, 1975.
178. Lilly JR, Altman P: Hepatic portoenterostomy (the Kasai operation) for biliary atresia. Surgery 78:76, 1975.
179. Odièvre M, Valayer J, Razemon-Pinta M, et al: Hepatic portoenterostomy or cholecystostomy in the treatment of extrahepatic biliary atresia. J Pediatr 88:774, 1976.
180. Lilly JR, Karrer FM: Contemporary surgery of biliary atresia. Pediatr Clin North Am 32:1233, 1985.
181. Mirkin LD, Knisely AS: Hyaline cartilage at porta hepatis in extrahepatic biliary atresia. Pediatr Pathol Lab Med 17:587, 1997.
182. Calder CJ, Hubscher SG: Extrahepatic biliary atresia with palisading granulomas. Histopathology 23:585, 1993.
183. Ohuchi N, Ohi R, Takahashi T, et al: Postoperative changes of intrahepatic portal veins in biliary atresia. A 3-D reconstruction study. J Pediatr Surg 21:10, 1986.
184. Mathew J, Cattan AR, Hall AG, et al: Glutathione S-transferases in neonatal liver disease. J Clin Pathol 45:679, 1992.
185. Kasai M, Suzuki H, Ohashi E, et al: Technique and resuls of operative management of biliary atresia. World J Surg 2:571, 1978.
186. Balistreri WF: Foreword. Neonatal cholestasis: lessons from the past, issues for the future. Semin Liver Dis 7:61, 1987.
187. Balistreri WF: Interrelationship between the infantile cholangiopathies and paucity of the intrahepatic bile ducts. In Balistreri WF, Stocker JT, eds: Pediatric Hepatology. New York, Hemisphere Publishing Corporation, 1990:1.
188. Trivedi P, Mieli-Vergani G, Mowat AP: Cholestasis in infancy and childhood: an overview. In Lentze M, Reichen J, eds: Paediatric Cholestasis. Novel approaches to treatment. Dordrecht, Kluwer Academic Publishers, 1992:129.
189. Maller ES, Piccoli DA: Diagnostic evaluation and care of the child with biliary atresia. In Hoffman MA, ed: Current Controversies in Biliary Atresia. Austin, RG Landes Company, 1992:45.
190. Thaler H: Leberkrankheiten. Histopathologie. Pathophysiologie. Klinik. Berlin, Springer, 1982.
191. Scheuer PJ: Liver Biopsy Interpretation, ed 3. London, Bailliere Tindall, 1980.
192. Ray MB, Desmet VJ: Immunofluorescent detection of alpha-1-antitrypsin in paraffin embedded liver tissue. J Clin Pathol 28:717, 1975.
193. Callea F, Fevery J, De Groote J, et al: Detection of PiZ phenotype individuals by alpha-1-antitrypsin (AAT) immunohistochemistry in paraffin-embedded liver tissue specimens. J Hepatol 2:389, 1986.
194. Callea F, Brisigotti M, Faa G, et al: Identification of PiZ gene products in liver tissue by a monoclonal antibody specific for the Z mutant of alpha-1-antitrypsin. J Hepatol 12:372, 1991.
195. Fischer HP, Ortiz-Pallardo ME, Ko Y, et al: Chronic liver disease in heterozygous alpha-1-antitrypsin deficiency PiZ. J Hepatol 33:883, 2000.
196. Ahrens EHJ, Harris RC, MacMahon HE: Atresia of the intrahepatic bile ducts. Pediatrics 8:628, 1951.
197. Sharp HL, Carey JB, White JG, et al: Cholestyramine therapy in patients with a paucity of intrahepatic bile ducts. J Pediatr 71:723, 1967.
198. Kahn E: Paucity of interlobular bile ducts. Arteriohepatic dysplasia and nonsyndromic duct paucity. In Abramowsky CR, Bernstein J, Rosenberg HS, eds: Perspectives in Pediatric Pathology. Transplantation Pathology—Hepatic Morphogenesis, vol 14. Basel, Karger, 1991:168.
199. Alagille D, Odièvre M, Gautier M, et al: Hepatic ductular hypoplasia associated with characteristic facies, vertebral malformations, retarded physical, mental and sexual development and cardiac murmur. J Pediatr 86:63, 1975.
200. Alagille D, Estrade A, Hadchouel M, et al: Syndromic paucity of interlobular bile ducts (Alagille syndrome or arteriohepatic dysplasia): review of 80 cases. J Pediatr 110:195, 1987.
201. Riely CA: Familial intrahepatic cholestatic syndromes. Semin Liver Dis 7:119, 1987.
202. Perrault G: Paucity of interlobular bile ducts: getting to know it better. Dig Dis Sci 26:481, 1981.
203. Kelley RI: Review: the cerebrohepatorenal syndrome of Zellweger: morphologic and metabolic aspects. Am J Med Genet 16:503, 1983.
204. Eyssen H, Eggermont E, Van Eldere J, et al: Bile acid abnormalities and the diagnosis of cerebro-hepato-renal syndrome (Zellweger syndrome). Acta Paediatr Scand 74:539, 1985.
205. Kahn EI, Daum F, Markowitz J, et al: Arteriohepatic dysplasia II. Hepatobiliary morphology. Hepatology 3:77, 1983.
206. Kahn E, Daum F, Markowitz J, et al: Nonsyndromatic paucity of interlobular bile ducts: light and electron microscopic evaluation of sequential liver biopsies in early childhood. Hepatology 6:890, 1986.
207. Labrecque DR, Mitros FA, Nathan RJ, et al: Four generations of arteriohepatic dysplasia. Hepatology 2:467, 1982.
208. Alagille D, Odièvre M, Hadchouel M: Paucity of interlobular bile ducts: recent concepts. In Kasai M, ed: Biliary Atresia and its Related Disorders. Amsterdam, Excerpta Medica, 1983:59.
209. Kahn E, Markowitz J, Aiges H, et al: Human ontogeny of the bile duct to portal space ratio. Hepatology 10:21, 1989.
210. Hadchouel M, Hugon RN, Gautier M: Reduced ratio of portal tracts to paucity of intrahepatic bile ducts. Arch Pathol Lab Med 102:402, 1978.
211. Roschlau G: Leberbiopsie im Kindesalter. VEB Gustav Fischer Verlag, 1978.
212. Alagille D, Le Tan V: L'absence congénitale des voies biliaires intrahépatiques. Rev Medicochir Mal Foie 37:57, 1962.
213. Raweily EA, Gibson AAM, Burt AD: Abnormalities of intrahepatic bile ducts in extrahepatic biliary atresia. Histopathology 17:521, 1990.

214. Schulz R, Schuppan D, Hahn EG: Connective tissue and ductular metaplasia of hepatocytes. In Wolff JR, Sievers J, Berry M, eds: Mesenchymal-epithelial interactions in neural development. Berlin, Springer, 1987:119.
215. Dahms BB, Petrelli M, Wyllie R, et al: Arteriohepatic dysplasia in infancy and childhood: a longitudinal study of six patients. Hepatology 2:350, 1982.
216. Berman MD, Ishak KG, Schaefer EJ, et al: Syndromatic hepatic ductular-hypoplasia (arteriohepatic dysplasia). Dig Dis Sci 26:485, 1981.
217. Heathcote J, Deodhar KP, Scheuer P, et al: Intrahepatic cholestasis in childhood. N Engl J Med 295:801, 1976.
218. Ghishan FK, Labrecque DR, Mitros FA, et al: The evolving nature of infantile obstructive cholangiopathy. J Pediatr 97:27, 1980.
219. Danks DM, Campbell PE, Jack I, et al: Studies on the aetiology of neonatal hepatitis and biliary atresia. Arch Dis Child 52:360, 1977.
220. Markowitz J, Daum F, Kahn EL, et al: Arteriohepatic dysplasia. I. Pitfalls in diagnosis and management. Hepatology 3:74, 1983.
221. Hashida Y, Yunis EJ: Syndromatic paucity of interlobular bile ducts: hepatic histopathology of the early and endstage liver. Pediatr Pathol 8:1, 1988.
222. Pilloud P: Un cas de syndrome de MacMahon-Thannhauser congénital: modalité pathogénique particulière de l'agénésie biliaire intrahépatique. Helv Paediatr Acta 21:327, 1966.
223. Perez-Soler A: The inflammatory and atresia-inducing disease of the liver and bile ducts. In Perez-Soler A, ed: Monographs in Paediatrics, vol 8. Basel, S Karger, 1976.
224. Odawara M, Partin JC, Schubert WK: Intrahepatic biliary atresia: ultrastructural study of three cases. Gastroenterology 60:179, 1971 (abstract).
225. Valencia-Mayoral P, Weber J, Cutz E: Possible defect in the bile secretory apparatus in arteriohepatic dysplasia (Alagille's syndrome). A review with observations on the ultrastructure of the liver. Hepatology 4:691, 1984.
226. Riely CA, La Brecque DR, Ghent C, et al: A father and son with cholestasis and peripheral pulmonic stenosis: a distinct form of intrahepatic cholestasis. J Pediatr 92:406, 1978.
227. Riely CA, Cotlier E, Jensen PS, et al: Arteriohepatic dysplasia: a benign syndrome of intrahepatic cholestasis with multiple organ involvement. Ann Intern Med 91:520, 1979.
228. Novotny NM, Zetterman RK, Antonson DL, et al: Variation in liver histology in Alagille's syndrome. Am J Gastroenterol 75:449, 1981.
229. Birnbaum A, Suchy FJ: The intrahepatic cholangiopathies. Semin Liver Dis 18:263, 1998.
230. Kocoshis SA, Cotrill CM, O'Connor WN, et al: Congenital heart disease, butterfly vertebrae and extrahepatic biliary atresia: a variant of arteriohepatic dysplasia? J Pediatr 99:436, 1981.
231. Yamagiwa I, Obata K, Hatanaka Y, et al: Clinico-pathological studies on a transitional type between extrahepatic biliary atresia and paucity of interlobular bile ducts. Jpn J Surg 23:307, 1993.
232. Maurage C, Brochu P, Garel L, et al: Portoenterostomy in a case of Alagille's syndrome with extrahepatic biliary atresia. J Pediatr Surg 26:111, 1991.
233. Amedee-Manesme O, Bernard O, Brunelle F, et al: Sclerosing cholangitis with neonatal onset. J Pediatr 111:225, 1987.
234. Alagille D: Intrahepatic neonatal cholestasis. In Javitt NB, ed: Neonatal Hepatitis and Biliary Atresia. US Department of Health, Education and Welfare. DHEW Publication No. (NIH) 79-1296, 1979:177.
235. Kerr DNS, Harrison CV, Sherlock S, et al: Congenital hepatic fibrosis. QJM 30:91, 1961.
236. Fink U: Ueber intrahepatische Gallengangshyperplasien und Komplikationen. Zentralbl Allg Pathol 93:497, 1955.
237. Kerneis JP, Ferron ADE, Gordeef A, et al: La fibro-angio-adénomatose du foie avec hypertension portale. II. Anatomie pathologique. Physiopathologie. Nosologie. Presse Med 69:1406, 1961.
238. de Ferron A, Gordeef A, de Ferron C, et al: La fibro-angio-adénomatose du foie avec hypertension portale. I. Clinique. Radiologie. Traitement. Presse Med 69:1147, 1961.
239. Caroli J, Corcos V: Maladies des Voies Biliaires Intrahépatiques Segmentaires. Paris, Masson, 1964.
240. Jørgensen MJ: The ductal plate malformation. A study of the intrahepatic bile duct lesion in infantile polycystic disease and congenital hepatic fibrosis. Acta Pathol Microbiol Scand (Suppl) 257:1, 1977.
241. Sergi C, Kahl P, Otto HF: Contribution of apoptosis and apoptosis-related proteins to the malformation of the primitive intrahepatic biliary system in Meckel syndrome. Am J Pathol 156:1589, 2000.
242. Sergi C, Adam S, Kahl P, et al: Study of the malformation of ductal plate of the liver in Meckel syndrome and review of other syndromes presenting this anomaly. Pediatr Development Pathol 3:568, 2000.
243. Desmet V, Callea F: Ductal plate malformation (DPM) in extrahepatic bile duct atresia (EHBDA). In Ohi R, ed: Biliary Atresia. Tokyo, ICOM Associates Inc, 1991:27.
244. Woolf GM, Vierling JM: Disappearing intrahepatic bile ducts: the syndromes and their mechanisms. Semin Liver Dis 13:261, 1993.
245. Callea F, Facchetti F, Lucini L, et al: Liver morphology in anicteric patients at long-term follow-up after Kasai operation: a study of 16 cases. In Ohi R, ed: Biliary Atresia. Tokyo, Professional Postgraduate Services, 1987:304.
246. Valayer J: Hepatic porto-enterostomy: surgical problems and results. In Berenberg SR, ed: Liver Disease in Infancy and Childhood. The Hague, Martinus Nijhoff Medical Division, 1976.
247. Desmet VJ: What is congenital hepatic fibrosis? Histopathology 20:465, 1992.
248. Hyams JS, Glaser JH, Leichtner AM, et al: Discordance for biliary atresia in two sets of monozygotic twins. J Pediatr 107:420, 1985.
249. Moore TC, Hyman PE: Extrahepatic biliary atresia in one human leucocyte antigen identical twin. Pediatrics 76:604, 1985.
250. Montgomery CK, Ruebner BH: Neonatal hepatocellular giant cell transformation. A review. In Rosenberg HS, Bolande RP, eds: Perspectives in Pediatric Pathology, vol 3. Chicago, Year Book Medical Publishers, 1976:85.
251. Rickham PP, Hirsig J: Biliary atresia: recent advances in aetiology, diagnosis and treatment. Z Kinderchir Grenzgebiete 26:114, 1979.
252. Holder TM: Atresia of the extrahepatic bile duct. Am J Surg 107:458, 1964.
253. Holder TM: The effect of bile duct ligation and inflammation in the fetus. J Pediatr Surg 2:35, 1967.
254. Koop CE: Biliary atresia and the Kasai operation. Pediatrics 55:9, 1975.
255. Koop CE: Progressive extrahepatic biliary obstruction of the newborn. J Pediatr Surg 10:169, 1975.
256. Chiba T: Histopathological studies on the prognosis of biliary atresia. Tohoku J Exp Med 122:249, 1977.
257. Kimura K, Tsugawa C, Kubo M, et al: Technical aspects of hepatic portal dissection in biliary atresia. J Pediatr Surg 14:27, 1979.
258. Fonkalsrud EW, Arima E: Bile lakes in congenital biliary atresia. Surgery 77:384, 1975.
259. Scotto JM, Stralin HG: Congenital extrahepatic biliary atresia. Arch Pathol Lab Med 101:416, 1977.
260. Schweizer P: Die Cholestase im Kindesalter aus chirurgischer Sicht. Monatsschr Kinderheilkd 128:292, 1980.
261. Suruga K, Kono S, Miyano T, et al: Treatment of biliary atresia: microsurgery for hepatic portoenterostomy. Surgery 80:558, 1976.
262. Silveira TR, Salzano FM, Howard ER, et al: Extrahepatic biliary atresia and twinning. Braz J Med Biol Res 24:67, 1991.
263. Werlin S: Extrahepatic biliary atresia in one of twins. Acta Paediatr 70:943, 1981.
264. Dimmick J, Kalousek D: Developmental Pathology of the Embryo and Fetus. Philadelphia, JB Lippincott, 1992:545.
265. Silveira TR, Salzano FM, Howard ER, et al: Congenital structural abnormalities in biliary atresia: evidence for etiopathogenic heterogeneity and therapeutic implications. Acta Paediatr Scand 80:1192, 1991.
266. Terracciano LM, Cathomas G, Vecchione R, et al: Extrahepatic bile duct atresia associated with hyperplasia of the intrahepatic bile ducts ("early severe form"): high incidence in a south-Italian population. Pathol Res Pract 191:192, 1995.
267. Takahashi A, Tsuchida Y, Hatakeyama S, et al: A peculiar form of multiple cystic dilatation of the intrahepatic biliary system found in a patient with biliary atresia. J Pediatr Surg 32:1776, 1997.
268. Brown P, Georgeson K, Mroczek-Musulman E, et al: Common hepatic duct stricture, associated with ductal plate malformation on a 4.5-year-old child. J Pediatr Gastroenterol Nutr 29:221, 1999.
269. Tan CEL, Driver M, Howard ER, et al: Extrahepatic biliary atresia: a first-trimester event? Clues from light microscopy and immunohistochemistry. J Ped Surg 29:808, 1994.
270. Tan CEL, Moscoso GJ: The developing human biliary system at the porta hepatis level between 29 days and 8 weeks of gestation: a way to understanding biliary atresia. Part 1. Pathol Int 44:587, 1994.

271. Tan CEL, Moscoso GJ: The developing human biliary system at the porta hepatis level between 11 and 25 weeks of gestation: a way to understanding biliary atresia. Part 2. Pathol Int 44:600, 1994.
272. Iwami D, Ohi R, Nio M, et al: Abnormal distribution of nerve fibers in the liver of biliary atresia. Tohoku J Exp Med 181:57, 1997.
273. Libbrecht L, Cassiman D, Desmet V, et al: Expression of neural cell adhesion molecule in human liver development and in congenital and acquired liver diseases. Histochem Cell Biol, 116:233-239, 2001.
274. Robertson AF: Case report: the coincidence of biliary atresia and the heterozygous state of galactosemia. Pediatrics 35:1008, 1965.
275. Nord KS, Saad S, Yoshi VV, et al: Concurrence of alpha-1-antitrypsin deficiency and biliary atresia. J Pediatr 111:416, 1987.
276. Fos E, Arcas R, Cabre J, et al: Deficit de alfa-1-antitripsina y atresia de vias biliares. An Esp Pediatr One 25:467, 1986.
277. Christen H, Bau J, Halsband H: Hereditary alpha-1-antitrypsin deficiency associated with congenital extrahepatic bile duct hypoplasia. Klin Wochenschr 53:90, 1975.
278. Carmi R, Magee CA, Neill CA, et al: Extrahepatic biliary atresia and associated anomalies: etiologic heterogeneity suggested by distinctive patterns of associations. Am J Med Genet 45:683, 1993.
279. Davenport M, Savage M, Mowat AP, et al: Biliary atresia splenic malformation syndrome: an etiologic and prognostic subgroup. Surgery 113:662, 1993.
280. Vazquez J, Lopez-Gutierrez JC, Gamez M, et al: Biliary atresia and the polysplenia syndrome: its impact on final outcome. J Pediatr Surg 1995:485, 1995.
281. Erhart NA, Sinatra FR: Biliary atresia, intestinal malrotation, partial abdominal heterotaxia, and craniofacial anomalies in a newborn with intrauterine opiate exposure. J Pediatr Gastroenterol Nutr 18:478, 1994.
282. Nakada M, Nakada K, Kawaguchi F, et al: Immunologic reaction and genetic factors in biliary atresia. Tohoku J Exp Med 181:41, 1997.
283. Dessanti A, Massarelli G, Piga MT, et al: Biliary, anorectal and esophageal atresia: a new entity? Tohoku J Exp Med 181:49, 1997.
284. Dillon PW, Belchis D, Minnick K, et al: Differential expression of the major histocompatibility antigens and ICAM-1 on bile duct epithelial cells in biliary atresia. Tohoku J Exp Med 181:33, 1997.
285. Anneren G, Meurling S, Lilja H, et al: Lethal autosomal recessive syndrome with intrauterine growth retardation, intra- and extrahepatic biliary atresia, and esophageal and duodenal atresia. Am J Med Genet 78:306, 1998.
286. Strickland AD, Shannon K: Studies in the etiology of extrahepatic biliary atresia: time-space clustering. J Pediatr 100:749, 1985
287. Yoon PW, Bresee JS, Olney RS, et al: Epidemiology of biliary atresia: a population-based study. Pediatrics 99:376, 1997.
288. Ayas MF, Hillemeier AC, Olson AD: Lack of evidence for seasonal variation in extrahepatic biliary atresia during infancy. J Clin Gastroenterol 22:292, 1996.
289. Harper PAW, Plant JW, Unger DB: Congenital biliary atresia and jaundice in lambs and calves. Aust Vet J 67:18, 1990.
290. Levin JN: Amphetamine ingestion with biliary atresia. J Pediatr 79:130, 1971.
291. Harris RC, Anderson DH: Intrahepatic bile duct atresia. Am J Dis Child 100:783, 1960.
292. Park WH, Choi SO, Lee SS, et al: Ectopic umbilical liver in conjunction with biliary atresia: uncommon association. J Pediatr Surg 26:219, 1991.
293. Lester R, Pyrek JS, Little JM, et al: Diversity of bile acids in the fetus and newborn infant. J Pediatr Gastroenterol Nutr 2:355, 1983.
294. Colombo C, Zuliani G, Ronchi M, et al: Biliary bile acid composition of the human fetus in early gestation. Pediatr Res 21:197, 1987.
295. Hernanz A, Codoceo R, Jara P, et al: Unusual serum bile acid pattern in children with the syndrome of hepatic ductular hypoplasia. Clin Chim Acta 145:289, 1985.
296. Hata Y, Sasaki F, Takahashi H, et al: Fetal bile acids in congenital biliary atresia. In Ohi R, ed: Biliary Atresia. Tokyo, ICOM Associates, 1991:182.
297. Mcsherry CK, Morrissey KP, Swarm RL, et al: Chenodeoxycholic acid-induced liver injury in pregnant and neonatal baboons. Ann Surg 184:490, 1976.
298. Jenner RE, Howard ER: Unsaturated monhydroxy bile acids as a cause of idiopathic obstructive cholangiopathy. Lancet 2:1073, 1975.
299. Theron CN, Neethling AC, Taljaard JJF: Sex-dependent differences in phenobarbitone-induced oestradiol-2 hydroxylase activity in rat liver. S Afr Med J 60:279, 1981.
300. Javitt NB, Keating JP, Grand RJ, et al: Serum bile acid patterns in neonatal hepatitis and extrahepatic biliary atresia. J Pediatr 90:736, 1977.
301. Scott RB, Wilkins W, Kessler A: Viral hepatitis in early infancy. Report of three fatal cases in siblings simulating biliary atresia. Pediatrics 13:447, 1954.
302. Petermann MG: Neonatal hepatitis in siblings. J Pediatr 50:315, 1957.
303. Suda J, Nakajima S, Okaniwa M, et al: Neonatal hepatitis and extrahepatic biliary atresia in the same sibship. Tohuku J Exp Med 133:445, 1981.
304. Willnow U: Zur Klinik. Morphologie und Pathogenese der mit Riesenzellbildung einhergehenden connatalen Lebererkrankungen. Arch Kinderheilkd 182:153, 1971.
305. McDonald PJ, Stehman FB, Stewart DR: Infantile obstructive cholangiopathy. Am J Dis Child 133:518, 1979.
306. Becroft DM: Biliary atresia associated with prenatal infection by Listeria monocytogenes. Arch Dis Child 47:656, 1972.
307. Oppenheimer EH, Esterly JR: Cytomegalovirus infection: a possible cause of biliary atresia. Am J Pathol 71:2a, 1973.
308. Le Tan Vinh, Tran Van Duc, Thieffry S, et al: Association de malformation congénitale et de cytomégalie: étude de 18 observations anatomo-cliniques. Nouvelle Presse Med 2:1411, 1973.
309. Jevon GP, Dimmick JE: Biliary atresia and cytomegalovirus infection: a DNA study. Pediatr Dev Pathol 2:11, 1999.
310. Lang DJ, Marshall WC, Pincott JR, et al: Cytomegalovirus: association with neonatal hepatitis and biliary atresia. In Javitt NB, ed: Neonatal Hepatitis and Biliary Atresia. US Department of Health, Education and Welfare. DHEW Publication No. (NIH) 79-1296, 1979:33.
311. Finegold MJ, Carpenter RJ: Obliterative cholangitis due to cytomegalovirus: a possible precursor of paucity of intrahepatic bile ducts. Hum Pathol 13:662, 1982.
312. Fischler B, Ehrnst A, Forsgren M, et al: The viral association of neonatal hepatitis in Sweden: a possible link between cytomegalovirus infection and extrahepatic biliary atresia. J Pediatr Gastroenterol Nutr 27:57, 1998.
313. Numazaki Y, Oshima T, Tanaka A, et al: Neonatal liver disease and cytomegalovirus infection. In Kasai M, Shiraki K, eds: Cholestasis in Infancy. Tokyo, University of Tokyo Press, 1980:61.
314. Tarr PI, Haas JE, Christie DL: Biliary atresia, cytomegalovirus, and age at referral. Pediatrics 97:828, 1996.
315. Hart MH, Kaufman SS, Vanderhoof JA, et al: Neonatal hepatitis and extrahepatic biliary atresia associated with cytomegalovirus infections in twins. Am J Dis Child 145:302, 1991.
316. Nahmias AJ, Visintine AM: Liver involvement in neonatal herpes simplex virus infection. In Javitt NB, ed: Neonatal Hepatitis and Biliary Atresia. US Department of Health, Education and Welfare. DHEW Publication No. (NIH) 79-1296, 1979:47.
317. Szmuness W, Stevens CE: Epidemiology of viral hepatitis A and B with particular reference to children. In Javitt NB, ed: Neonatal Hepatitis and Biliary Atresia. US Department of Health, Education and Welfare. DHEW Publication No. (NIH) 79-1296, 1979:59.
318. Shiraki K, Sakurai M, Yoshihara N, et al: Vertical transmission of HB virus and neonatal hepatitis. In Kasai M, Shiraki K, eds: Cholestasis in Infancy. Tokyo, University of Tokyo Press, 1980:67.
319. Balistreri WF, Tabor E, Gerety RJ: Negative serology for hepatitis A and B viruses in 18 cases of neonatal cholestasis. Pediatrics 66:270, 1980.
320. A Kader HH, Nowicki MJ, Kuramoto KI, et al: Evaluation of the role of hepatitis C virus in biliary atresia. Pediatr Infec Dis J 13:657, 1994.
321. Bangaru B, Morecki R, Glaser J, et al: Comparative studies of biliary atresia in the human newborn and reovirus-induced cholangitis in weanling mice. Lab Invest 43:456, 1980.
322. Morecki R, Glaser J, Cho S, et al: Biliary atresia and reovirus type 3 infection. N Engl J Med 307:481, 1982.
323. Glaser JH, Balistreri WF, Morecki R: Role of reovirus type 3 in persistent infantile cholestasis. J Pediatr 105:912, 1984.
324. Richardson SC, Bishop RF, Smith AL: Reovirus serotype 3 infection in infants with extrahepatic biliary atresia or neonatal hepatitis. J Gastroenterol Hepatol 9:264, 1994.
325. Morecki R, Glaser JH, Johnson AB, et al: Detection of reovirus type 3 in the porta hepatis of an infant with extrahepatic biliary atresia: ultrastructural and immunocytochemical study. Hepatology 4:1137, 1984.
326. Morecki R, Glaser JH, Horwitz MS: Etiology of biliary atresia: the role of reo 3 virus. In Daum F, ed: Extrahepatic Biliary Atresia. New York, Marcel Dekker, 1983:1.

327. Glaser JH, Morecki R: Reovirus type 3 and neonatal cholestasis. Semin Liver Dis 7:100, 1987.
328. Cornelius CE, Rosenberg DP: Animal model of human disease. Neonatal biliary atresia. Am J Pathol 118:168, 1985.
329. Morecki R, Glaser J: Pathogenesis of extrahepatic biliary atresia and reovirus type 3 infection. In Kasai M, ed: Biliary Atresia and its Related Disorders. Amsterdam, Excerpta Medica, 1983:20.
330. Glaser J, Morecki R, Balistreri W, et al: Neonatal obstructive cholangiopathy and reovirus type 3 infection. Hepatology 2:719, 1982 (abstract).
331. Dussaix E, Hadchouel M, Tardieu M, et al: Biliary atresia and reovirus type 3 infection. N Engl J Med 310:658, 1984.
332. Brown W, Sokol RJ, Levin M, et al: An immunological search for evidence that infection with reovirus 3 causes extrahepatic biliary atresia or neo-natal hepatitis. Gastroenterology 92:1721, 1987.
333. Morecki R, Glaser JH, Cho S, et al: Biliary atresia and reovirus type 3 infection. N Engl J Med 310:1610, 1984 (letter).
334. Schmeling DJ, Strauch ED, Hoffman MA: Epidemiological and experimental observations of biliary atresia. In Hoffman MA, ed: Current Controversies in Biliary Atresia. Austin, RG Landes Company, 1992:15.
335. Iwami D, Ohi R, Chiba T, et al: Detection of reovirus 3 in patients with biliary atresia by polymerase chain reaction. In Ohi R, ed: Biliary Atresia. Tokyo, ICOM Associates, 1991:7.
336. Sasaki N, Matsui A, Kurihara H, et al: Identification of reovirus type 3 antigens and RNA's in the liver tissues of biliary atresia. In Ohi R, ed: Biliary Atresia. Tokyo, ICOM Associates, 1991:3.
337. Steele MI, Marshall CM, Lloyd RE, et al: Reovirus 3 not detected by reverse transcriptase-mediated polymerase chain reaction analysis of preserved tissue from infants with cholestatic liver disease. Hepatology 21:697, 1995.
338. Tyler KL, Sokol RJ, Oberhaus SM, et al: Detection of reovirus RNA in hepatobiliary tissues from patients with extrahepatic biliary atresia and choledochal cysts. Hepatology 27:1475, 1998.
339. Riepenhoff-Talty M, Schaekel K, Clark F, et al: Group A rotaviruses produce extrahepatic biliary obstruction in orally inoculated newborn mice. Pediatr Res 33:394, 1993.
340. Riepenhoff-Talty M, Gouvea V, Evans MJ, et al: Detection of group C rotavirus in infants with extrahepatic biliary atresia. J Infect Dis 174:8, 1996.
341. Bobo L, Ojeh C, Chiu D, et al: Lack of evidence for rotavirus by polymerase chain reaction/enzyme immunoassay of hepatobiliary samples from children with biliary atresia. Pediatr Res 41:229, 1997.
342. Nadal D, Wunderli W, Meurmann O, et al: Isolation of respiratory syncytial virus from liver tissue and extrahepatic biliary atresia material. Scand J Infect Dis 22:91, 1990.
343. Drut R, Drut RM, Gomez MA, et al: Presence of human papillomavirus in extrahepatic biliary atresia. J Pediatr Gastroenterol Nutr 1998:530, 1998.
344. Silveira TR, Salzano FM, Donaldson PT, et al: Association between HLA and extrahepatic biliary atresia. J Pediatr Gastroenterol Nutr 16:114, 1993.
345. Jurado A, Jara P, Camarena C, et al: Is extrahepatic biliary atresia an HLA-associated disease? J Pediatr Gastroenterol Nutr 25:557, 1997.
346. Dillon P, Belchis D, Tracy T, et al: Increased expression of intercellular adhesion molecules in biliary atresia. Am J Pathol 145:263, 1994.
347. Broome U, Nemeth A, Hultcrantz R, et al: Different expression of HLA-DR and ICAM-1 in livers from patients with biliary atresia and Byler's disease. J Hepatol 26:857, 1997.
348. Kobayashi H, Puri P, O'Brian DS, et al: Hepatic overexpression of MHC class II antigens and macrophage-associated antigens (CD68) in patients with biliary atresia of poor prognosis. J Pediatr Surg 32:590, 1997.
349. Desmet VJ: Expression of MHC molecules during intra- end extrahepatic cholestasis and their pathogenetic implications. In Berg PA, Leuschner U, eds: Bile Acids and Immunology, vol 67-76. Dordrecht, Kluwer Academic Publishers, 1996.
350. Schweizer P: Modell einer extrahepatischen Gallengangsatresie. Z Kinderchir 15:90, 1974.
351. Morgan WW, Rosenkrantz JG, Hill RB: Hepatic arterial interruption in the fetus—an attempt to simulate biliary atresia. J Pediatr Surg 1:342, 1966.
352. Pickett LK, Briggs HC: Biliatry obstruction secondary to hepatic vascular ligation in fetal sheep. J Pediatr 4:95, 1969.
353. Miyano T, Suruga K, Kimura K, et al: A histopathologic study of the region of the ampulla of Vater in congenital biliary atresia. Jpn J Surg 10:34, 1980.
354. Miyano T, Suruga K, Suda K: Abnormal choledocho-pancreatico-ductal junction related to etiology of infantile obstructive jaundice diseases. J Pediatr Surg 14:16, 1979.
355. Suda K, Miyano T, Hashimoto K: The choledocho-pancreatico-ductal junction in obstructive jaundice diseases. Acta Pathol Jpn 30:187, 1980.
356. Chiba T, Ohi R, Mochizuki I: Cholangiographic study of the pancreaticobiliary ductal junction in biliary atresia. J Pediatr Surg 25:609, 1990.
357. Pinzani M, Milani S: Cholestasis and fibrosis. In Manns MP, Boyer JL, Jansen PLM, Reichen J, eds: Cholestatic Liver Diseases. Dordrecht, Kluwer Academic Publishers, 1998:88.
358. Desmet VJ: Modulation of the liver in cholestasis. J Gastroenterol Hepatol 7:313, 1992.
359. Selye H, Szabo S: Experimental production of cholangitis by 1,4-phenylenediisothiocyanate. Arch Pathol 94:486, 1972.
360. Ogawa T, Suruga K, Kojima Y, et al: Experimental study of the pathogenesis of infantile obstructive cholangiopathy and its clinical evaluation. J Pediatr Surg 18:131, 1983.
361. Schmeling DJ, Oldham KT, Guice KS, et al: Experimental obliterative cholangitis. A model for the study of biliary atresia. Ann Surg 213:350, 1991.
362. Kopelman H, Robertson MH, Saunders PG: The Epping jaundice. BMJ 1:514, 1966.
363. Bourdelat D, Moulinoux JP, Chambon Y, et al: Prolifération ductulaire biliaire intrahépatique chez la ratte gestante traitée par le 4,4'diaminodiphenylmethane (4,4 DDPM). Bull Assoc Anat (Nancy) 67:375, 1983.
364. Phillips PA, Keast D, Papadimiriou JM, et al: Chronic obstructive jaundice induced by reovirus type 3 in weanling mice. Pathology 1:193, 1969.
365. Petersen C, Biermanns D, Kuske M, et al: New aspects in a murine model for extrahepatic biliary atresia. J Pediatr Surg 32:1190, 1997.
366. Petersen C, Bruns E, Kuske M, et al: Treatment of extrahepatic biliary atresia with interferon-alpha in a murine infectious model. Pediatr Res 42:623, 1997.
367. Petersen C, Kuske M, Bruns E, et al: Progress in developing animal models for biliary atresia. Eur J Pediatr Surg 8:137, 1998.
368. Petersen C, Grasshoff S, Luciano L: Diverse morphology of biliary atresia in an animal model. J Hepatol 28:603, 1998.
369. Yokoyama T, Copeland NG, Jenkins NA, et al: Reversal of left-right asymmetry: a situs inversus mutation. Science 260:679, 1993.
370. Morgan D, Trurnpenny L, Goodship J, et al: Inversin, a novel gene in the vertebrate left-right axis pathway, is partially deleted in the inv mouse. Nat Genet 20:149, 1998.
371. Mazziotti MV, Willis LK, Heuckeroth RO, et al: Anomalous development of the hepatobiliary system in the Inv mouse. Hepatology 30:372, 1999.
372. Tsau Y-K, Chen C-H, Chang M-H, et al: Nephromegaly and elevated hepatocyte growth factor in children with biliary atresia. Am J Kid Dis 29:188, 1997.
373. Fain JS, Lewin KJ: Intrahepatic biliary cysts in congenital biliary atresia. Arch Pathol Lab Med 113:1383, 1989.
374. De Vos R, De Wolf-Peeters C, Desmet V: A morphologic and histochemical study of biliary atresia in lamprey liver. Z Zellfrosch 136:85, 1973.
375. Sidon EW, Youson JH: Morphological changes in the liver of the sea lamprey, Petromyzon marinus L, during metamorphosis. I. Atresia of the bile ducts. J Morphol 177:109, 1983.
376. Sidon EW, Youson JH: Relocalization of membrane enzymes accompanies biliary atresia in lamprey liver. Cell Tissue Res 236:81, 1984.
377. Youson JH, Sidon EW: Lamprey biliary atresia. First model system for the human condition. Experientia 34:1084, 1978.
378. Youson JH: Biliary atresia in lampreys. Adv Vet Sci Comp Med 37:197, 1993.
379. Schulze C, Rothuizen J, van Sluijs FJ, et al: Extrahepatic biliary atresia in a border collie. J Small Anim Pract 41:27, 2000.
380. Hays DM, Kimura K: Biliary atresia: the Japanese experience. Cambridge, Harvard University Press, 1980.
381. Chandra RS: Biliary atresia and other structural anomalies in congenital polysplenia syndrome. J Pediatr 85:649, 1974.
382. Hussein M, Howard ER, Mieli-Vergani G, et al: Jaundice at 14 days of age: exclude biliary atresia. Arch Dis Child 66:1177, 1991.

383. Andres JM, Lilly JR, Altman RP, et al: Alpha-1-fetoprotein in neonatal hepatobiliary disease. J Pediatr 91:217, 1977.
384. Brown SC, Househam KC: Visual stool examination. A screening test for infants with prolonged neonatal cholestasis. S Afr Med J 77:358, 1990.
385. Maggiore G, Bernard O, Hadchouel M, et al: Diagnostic value of serum gamma-glutamyl transpeptidase activity in liver diseases in children. J Pediatr Gastroenterol Nutr 12:21, 1991.
386. Vajaradul C, Vanprapar N, Chuenmeechow T, et al: Use of serum gamma glutamyl transpeptidase to differentiate between extrahepatic biliary atresia and neonatal hepatitis. J Med Assoc Thai 72:395, 1989.
387. Chiba T, Kasai M: Differentiation of biliary atresia from neonatal hepatitis by routine clinical examinations. Tohoku J Exp Med 115:327, 1975.
388. Shiraki K, Okaniwa M, Landing BH: Cholestatic syndromes of infancy and childhood. In Zakim D, Boyer TD, eds: Hepatology. A Textbook of Liver Disease. Philadelphia, WB Saunders, 1982:1176.
389. Sakurai M, Shiraki K: Quantitative diagnosis of biliary atresia and neonatal hepatitis. In Kasai M, Shiraki K, eds: Cholestasis in Infancy. Tokyo, University of Tokyo Press, 1980:293.
390. Sunaryo FP, Watkins JB: Evaluation of diagnostic techniques for extrahepatic biliary atresia. In Daum F, ed: Extrahepatic Biliary Atresia. New York, Marcel Dekker, 1983:11.
391. Burton EM, Babcock DS, Heubi JE, et al: Neonatal jaundice: clinical and ultrasonographic findings. South Med J 83:294, 1990.
392. Zeltzer PM, Neerhout RC: Differentiation between neonatal hepatitis and biliary atresia by measuring serum alpha-fetoprotein. Lancet 1:373, 1974.
393. Manthorpe D, Mowat AP: Serum bile acids in the neonatal hepatitis syndrome. In Alagille D, ed: Liver Diseases in Children (Hepatologic Infantile). Paris, Editions INSERM, 1976:57.
394. Poley JR, Alaupovic P, Knight-Gibson C, et al: The quantitative determination of serum lipoprotein-X and apolipoproteins in infants with cholestatic liver and biliary tract disease. In Daum F, ed: Extrahepatic Biliary Atresia. New York, Marcel Dekker, 1983:33.
395. Tazawa Y, Yamada M, Nakaawa M, et al: Significance of serum lipoprotein-X and gammaglutamyltranspeptidase in the diagnosis of biliary atresia. A preliminary study in 27 cholestatic young infants. Eur J Pediatr 145:54, 1986.
396. Fung KP: Lipoprotein-X and diagnosis of biliary atresia. Eur J Pediatr 146:312, 1987 (letter).
397. Deutsch J, Kurz R, Mueller WD, et al: Lipoprotein X, gamma-glutamyltranspeptidase and biliary atresia. Eur J Pediatr 146:313, 1987 (letter).
398. Melhorn DK, Gross S, Izant RJ: The red cell hydrogen peroxide hemolysis test and vitamin E absorption in the differential diagnosis of jaundice in infancy. J Pediatr 81:1082, 1972.
399. Jusko WJ, Levy G, Yaffe SJ, et al: Riboflavin absorption in children with biliary obstruction. Am J Dis Child 121:48, 1971.
400. Greene HL, Helinek GL, Moran R, et al: A diagnostic approach to prolonged obstructive jaundice by 24-hour collection of duodenal fluid. J Pediatr 95:412, 1979.
401. Hashimoto S, Tsugawa C, Kimura K, et al: Naso-duodenal tube insertion technique for rapid diagnosis of congenital biliary atresia. J Jpn Soc Pediatr Surg 14:889, 1978.
402. Yamashiro Y, Robinson PG, Lari J, et al: Duodenal bile acids in diagnosis of congenital biliary atresia. J Pediatr Surg 18:278, 1983.
403. Hsu HY, Tang SY, Chang MH: Analysis of duodenal bile acids by high performance liquid chromatography in infants with cholestasis. J Formos Med Assoc 90:487, 1991.
404. Lebwohl O, Waye JD: Endoscopic retrograde cholangio-pancreatography in the diagnosis of extrahepatic biliary atresia. Am J Dis Child 133:647, 1979.
405. Waye JD: Endosopic retrograde cholangiopancreatography in the infant. Am J Gastroenterol 65:461, 1976.
406. Shirai Z, Toriya H, Maeshiro K, et al: The usefulness of endoscopic retrograde cholangiopancreatography in infancts and small children. Am J Gastroenterol 88:536, 1993.
407. Wilkinson ML, Mieli-Vergani G, Ball C, et al: Endoscopic retrograde cholangiopancreatography in infantile cholestasis. Arch Dis Child 66:121, 1991.
408. Derkx HH, Huibregtse K, Taminiau JA: The role of endoscopic retrograde cholangiopancreatography in cholestatic infants. Endoscopy 26:724, 1994.
409. Ohnuma N, Takahashi T, Tanabe M, et al: The role of ERCP in biliary atresia. Gastrointest Endosc 45:365, 1997.
410. Ashida K, Nagita A, Sakaguchi M, et al: Endoscopic retrograde cholangiopancreatography in paediatric patients with biliary disorders. J Gastroenterol Hepatol 13:598, 1998.
411. Iinuma Y, Narisawa R, Iwafuchi M, et al: The role of endoscopic retrograde cholangiopancreatography in infants with cholestasis. J Pediatr Surg 35:545, 2000.
412. Howard ER, Nunnerley HB: Percutaneous cholangiography in prolonged jaundice of childhood. J R Soc Med 72:495, 1979.
413. Leape LL, Ramenofsky ML: Laparoscopy in infants and children. J Pediatr Surg 12:929, 1977.
414. White WE, Welsh JS, Darrow DC, et al: Pediatric application of the radioiodine (I-131) Rose Bengal method in hepatic and biliary system disease. Pediatrics 32:239, 1963.
415. Antico VF, Denhartog P, Ash JM, et al: The I-131 Rose Bengal excretion test is not dead. Clin Nucl Med 10:171, 1985.
416. Ryckman FC, Noseworthy J: Neonatal cholestatic conditions requiring surgical reconstruction. Semin Liver Dis 7:134, 1987.
417. Lai MW, Chang MH, Hsu HC, et al: Differential diagnosis of extrahepatic biliary atresia from neonatal hepatitis: a prospective study. J Pediatr Gastroenterol Nutr 18:121, 1994.
418. Ben-Haim S, Seabold JE, Kao SC, et al: Utility of Tc-99m mebrofenin scintigraphy in the assessment of infantile jaundice. Clin Nucl Med 20:153, 1995.
419. Cox KL, Stadalnik RC, McGahan JP, et al: Hepatobiliary scintigraphy with technetium-99m disofenin in the evaluation of neonatal cholestasis. J Pediatr Gastroenterol Nutr 6:885, 1987.
420. Lin WY, Lin CC, Changlai SP, et al: Comparison of Tc-99m disofenin cholescintigraphy with ultrasonography in the differentiation of biliary atresia from other forms of neonatal jaundice. Pediatr Surg Int 12:30, 1977.
421. Gilmour SM, Hershkop M, Reifen R, et al: Outcome of hepatobiliary scanning in neonatal hepatitis syndrome. J Nucl Med 38:1279, 1997.
422. Lee CH, Wang PW, Lee TT, et al: The significance of functioning gallbladder visualization on hepatobiliary scintigraphy in infants with persistent jaundice. J Nucl Med 41:1209, 2000.
423. Abramson SJ, Berdon WE, Altman RP, et al: Biliary atresia and noncardiac polysplenic syndrome: US and surgical considerations. Radiology 163:377, 1987.
424. Marchal GJ, Desmet VJ, Proesmans WC, et al: Caroli disease: high frequency US and pathologic findings. Radiology 158:507, 1986.
425. Abramson SJ, Treves S, Teele RL: The infant with possible biliary atresia: evaluation by ultrasound and nuclear medicine. Pediatr Radiol 12:1, 1982.
426. Gubernick JA, Rosenberg HK, Ilaslan H, et al: US approach to jaundice in infants and children. Radiographics 20:173, 2000.
427. Ikeda S, Sera Y, Akagi M: Serial ultrasonic examination to differentiate biliary atresia from neonatal hepatitis. Special reference to changes in size of the gallbladder. Eur J Pediatr 148:396, 1989.
428. Rosenthal SJ, Cox GG, Wetzel LH, et al: Pitfalls and differential diagnosis in biliary sonography. Radiographics 10:285, 1990.
429. Ikeda S, Sera Y, Ohshiro H, et al: Gallbladder contraction in biliary atresia: a pitfall of ultrasound diagnosis. Pediatr Radiol 28:451, 1998.
430. Choi SO, Park WH, Lee HJ, et al: "Triangular cord": a sonographic finding applicable in the diagnosis of biliary atresia. J Pediatr Surg 31:636, 1996.
431. Park WH, Choi SO, Lee HJ, et al: A new diagnostic approach to biliary atresia with emphasis on the ultrasonographic triangular cord sign: comparison of ultrasonography, hepatobiliary scintigraphy, and liver needle biopsy in the evaluation of infantile cholestasis. J Pediatr Surg 32:1555, 1997.
432. Choi SO, Park WH, Lee HJ: Ultrasonographic "triangular cord": the most definitive finding for noninvasive diagnosis of extrahepatic biliary atresia. Eur J Pediatr Surg 8:12, 1998.
433. Park WH, Choi SO, Lee HJ: The ultrasonographic "triangular cord" coupled with gallbladder images in the diagnostic prediction of biliary atresia from infantile intrahepatic cholestasis. J Pediatr Surg 34:1706, 1999.
434. Tan-Kendrick AP, Phua KB, Ooi BC, et al: Making the diagnosis of biliary atresia using the triangular cord sign and gallbladder length. Pediatr Radiol 30:69, 2000.
435. Tsuchida Y, Kawarasaki H, Iwanaka T, et al: Antenatal diagnosis of biliary atresia (type I cyst) at 19 weeks' gestation: differential diagnosis and etiologic implications. J Pediatr Surg 30:697, 1995.

436. Redkar R, Davenport M, Howard ER: Antenatal diagnosis of congenital anomalies of the biliary tract. J Pediatr Surg 33:700, 1998.
437. Chan YL, Yeung CK, Lam WW, et al: Magnetic resonance cholangiography, feasibility and application in the paediatric population. Pediatr Radiol 28:307, 1998.
438. Guibaud L, Lachaud A, Touraine R, et al: MR cholangiography in neonates and infants: feasibility and preliminary applications. Am J Roentgenol 170:27, 1998.
439. Kim MJ, Park YN, Han SJ, et al: Biliary atresia in neonates and infants: triangular area of high signal intensity in the porta hepatis at T2-weighted MR cholangiography with US and histopathologic correlation. Radiology 215:395, 2000.
440. Balistreri WF: Neonatal cholestasis. In Lebenthal E, ed: Textbook of Gastroenterology and Nutrition in Infancy, vol 1081. New York, Raven Press, 1981.
441. Mowat AP: Liver Disorders in Children. London, Butterworths, 1979.
442. Mowat AP: Paediatric liver disease: medical aspects. In Wright R, Millward-Sadler GH, Alberti KGMM, Karran S, eds: Liver and Biliary Disease. Pathophysiology, Diagnosis, Management, ed 2. London, Baillière Tindall, WB Saunders, 1985:1201.
443. Ridaura Sanz C, Navarro Castilla E: Role of liver biopsy in the diagnosis of prolonged cholestasis in infants (SPA). Rev Invest Clin 44:193, 1992.
444. Zerbini MCN, Gallucci SDD, Maezono R, et al: Liver biopsy in neonatal cholestasis: a review on statistical grounds. Modern Pathol 10:793, 1997.
445. Altman RP, Levy J: Biliary atresia. Pediatr Ann 14:481, 1985.
446. Adelman S: Prognosis of uncorrected biliary atresia: an update. J Pediatr Surg 13:389, 1978.
447. Hays DM, Snyder WH: Life-span in untreated biliary atresia. Surgery 54:373, 1963.
448. Schweizer M, Schweizer P, Knupfer R, et al: Die extrahepatische Gallengangsatresie. Vergleich zwischen operativer und nichtoperativer Therapie. Monatsschr Kinderheilkd 140:422, 1992.
449. Longmire WPJ, Stanford MC: Intrahepatic-cholangiojejunostomy with partial hepatectomy for biliary atresia. Surgery 24:264, 1948.
450. Krumhaar D, Hecker W, Joppich J, et al: Analyse von 49 Gallenwegserkrankungen im Kindesalter. Arch Kinderheilkd 182:47, 1970.
451. Suruga K, Yamazaki Z, Iwai S, et al: The surgery of infantile obstructive jaundice. Arch Dis Child 40:158, 1965.
452. Hasse W: Studien über die intrahepatische Gefäsztopographie des Frischgeborenen und Säuglings. Erg Chir Orthop 48:1, 1966.
453. Nixon HH: Leberchirurgie im Säuglings-und Kindesalter. Z Kinderchir 1:83, 1964.
454. Sterling JA, Lowenburg AH: Observations of infants with hepatic duct atresia and use of artificial duct prosthesis. Pediatr Clin North Am 9:485, 1962.
455. Aterman K, Lav H, Gillis DA: The response of the liver to implantation of artificial bile ducts. J Pediatr Surg 6:413, 1971.
456. Shimura H, Nakamura Y, Sakai M: Indication of surgical treatment for biliary atresia. Shujitsu 17:872, 1963.
457. Absolon KB, Rikkers H, Aust JB: Thoracic duct lymph drainage in congenital biliary atresia. Surg Gynecol Obstet 120:123, 1965.
458. Hasse W, Waldschmidt J, Grohne H, et al: Experimental studies on thoracic duct anastomosis with the esophagus in dogs. J Pediatr Surg 2:553, 1967.
459. Suruga K, Nagashima N, Hirai Y, et al: A clinical and pathological study of congenital biliary atresia. J Pediatr Surg 2:558, 1967.
460. Williams LF, Dooling JA: Thoracic duct-esophagus anastomosis for relief of congenital biliary atresia. Surg Forum 14:189, 1963.
461. Fonkalsrud EW, Kitawaga S, Longmire WPJ: Hepatic lymphatic drainage to the jejunum for congenital biliary atresia. Am J Surg 112:188, 1966.
462. Mieli-Vergani G, Howard ER, Portmann B, et al: Late referral for biliary atresia—missed opportunities for effective surgery. Lancet I:421, 1989.
463. Toyosaka A, Okamoto E, Kawamura E, et al: Successful Kasai operation for biliary atresia in a 9 month old. J Pediatr Surg 28:1557, 1993.
464. Langenburg SE, Poulik J, Goretsky M, et al: Bile duct size does not predict success of portoenterostomy for biliary atresia. J Pediatr Surg 35:1006, 2000.
465. Deguchi E, Iwai N, Yanagihara J, et al: Relationship between intraoperative cholangiographic patterns and outcomes in biliary atresia. Eur J Pediatr Surg 8:146, 1998.
466. Kardorff R, Klotz M, Melter M, et al: Prediction of survival in extrahepatic biliary atresia by hepatic duplex sonography. J Pediatr Gastroenterol Nutr 28:411, 1999.
467. Urushihara N, Iwagaki H, Yagi T, et al: Elevation of serum interleukin-18 levels and activation of Kupffer cells in biliary atresia. J Pediatr Surg 35:446, 2000.
468. Trivedi P, Dhawan A, Risteli J, et al: Prognostic value of serum hyaluronic acid and type I and III procollagen propeptides in extrahepatic biliary atresia. Pediatr Res 38:568, 1995.
469. Tamatani T, Kobayashi H, Tezkua K, et al: Establishment of the enzyme-linked immunosorbent assay for connective tissue growth factor (CTGF) and its detection in the sera of biliary atresia. Biochem Biophys Res Commun 251:748, 1998.
470. Fujimoto T, Ohya T, Miyano T: A new clinical prognostic predictor for patients with biliary atresia. J Pediatr Surg 29:757, 1994.
471. Ito E, Ando H, Iio K, et al: The prognostic significance of biliary bilirubin conjugates in biliary atresia. Eur J Pediatr Surg 5:271, 1995.
472. Abukawa D, Nakagawa M, Iinuma K, et al: Hepatic and serum bile acid compositions in patients with biliary atresia: a microanalysis using gas chromatography-mass spectrometry with negative ion chemical ionization detection. Tohoku J Exp Med 1998:227, 1998.
473. Minnick KE, Kreisber R, Dillon PW: Soluble ICAM-1 (sICAM-1) in biliary atresia and its relationship to disease activity. J Surg Res 76:53, 1998.
474. Segawa O, Miyano T, Fujimoto T, et al: Actin and myosin deposition around bile canaliculi: a predictor of clinical outcome in biliary atresia. J Pediatr Surg 28:851, 1993.
475. Hossain M, Murahashi O, Ando H, et al: Immunohistochemical study of proliferating cell nuclear antigen in hepatocytes of biliary atresia: a parameter to predict clinical outcome. J Pediatr Surg 30:1297, 1995.
476. Kinugasa Y, Nakashima Y, Matsuo S, et al: Bile ductular proliferation as a prognostic factor in biliary atresia: an immunohistochemical assessment. J Pediatr Surg 34:1715, 1999.
477. Azarow KS, Phillips MJ, Sandler AD, et al: Biliary atresia: should all patients undergo a portoenterostomy? J Pediatr Surg 32:168, 1997.
478. Nakada M, Nakada K, Fujioka T, et al: Doppler ultrasonographic evaluation of hepatic circulation in patients following Kasai's operation for biliary atresia. Surg Today 25:1023, 1995.
479. Takahashi A, Hatakeyama S, Suzuki N, et al: MRI findings in the liver in biliary atresia patients after the Kasai operation. Tohoku J Exp Med 181:193, 1997.
480. Endo M, Masuyama H, Watanabe K, et al: Calculation of biliary atresia prognostic index using a multivariate linear model. J Pediatr Surg 30:1575, 1995.
481. Kobayashi H, Horikoshi K, Yamataka A, et al: Hyaluronic acid: a specific prognostic indicator of hepatic damage in biliary atresia. J Pediatr Surg 34:1791, 1999.
482. Kobayashi H, Miyano T, Horikoshi K, et al: Prognostic value of serum procollagen III peptide and type IV collagen in patients with biliary atresia. J Pediatr Surg 33:112, 1998.
483. Shirahase I, Ooshima A, Tanaka K, et al: Increased deposition and serum level of type IV collagen in patients with extrahepatic biliary atresia. J Pediatr Surg 28:847, 1993.
484. Shirahase I, Ooshima A, Tanaka K, et al: The slow progression of hepatic fibrosis in intrahepatic cholestasis as compared with extrahepatic biliary atresia. Eur J Pediatr Surg 5:77, 1995.
485. Kubota A, Okada A, Fukui Y, et al: Indocyanine green test is a reliable indicator of postoperative liver function in biliary atresia. J Pediatr Gastroenterol Nutr 16:61, 1993.
486. Kobayashi H, Miyano T, Horikoshi K, et al: Clinical significance of plasma endothelin levels in patients with biliary atresia. Pediatr Surg Int 13:491, 1998.
487. Kobayashi H, Narumi S, Tamatani T, et al: Serum IFN-inducible protein-10: a new clinical prognostic predictor of hepatocytes death in biliary atresia. J Pediatr Surg 34:308, 1999.
488. Altman RP, Lilly JR, Greenfeld J, et al: A multivariable risk factor analysis of the portoenterostomy (Kasai) procedure for biliary atresia: twenty-five years of experience from two centers. Ann Surg 226:348, 1997.
489. Gauthier F, Luciani JL, Chardot C, et al: Determinants of life span after Kasai operation at the era of liver transplantation. Tohoku J Exp Med 181:97, 1997.

490. Takemoto H, Tanaka K, Inomata Y, et al: Granulation at the porta hepatis following hepatic portoenterostomy for biliary atresia: the healing of experimental hepatoenterostomy. J Pediatr Surg 24:271, 1989.
491. Thaler MM: Cryptogenic liver disease in young infants. In Popper H, Schaffner F, eds: Progress in Liver Diseases, vol 5. New York, Grune & Stratton, 1976:476.
492. Javitt NB: Neonatal hepatitis and biliary atresia. (An International Workshop, March 1977) US Department of Health, Education and Welfare. DHEW Publications No. (NIH) 79-1296 1978.
493. National Institutes of Health Consensus Development Conference Statement: Liver Transplantation. June 20-23, 1983. Hepatology 4(suppl):107S, 1984.
494. Gottrand F, Bernard O, Hadchouel M, et al: Late cholangitis after successful surgical repair of biliary atresia. Am J Dis Child 145:213, 1991.
495. Suruga K: Congenital biliary atresia. Surgical treatment of congenital biliary atresia. Shujutsu 24:543, 1970.
496. Suruga K, Miyano T, Kitahara T, et al: Treatment of biliary atresia: a study of our operative results. J Pediatr Surg 16:621, 1981.
497. Sawaguchi S, Akiyama Y, Saeki M, et al: The treatment of congenital biliary atresia with special reference to hepatic portoenteroanastomosis. In Fifth Annual Meeting of the Pacific Association of Pediatric Surgeons. Tokyo, 1972.
498. Lilly JR, Hitch DC: Postoperative ascending cholangitis following portoenterostomy for biliary atresia: measures for control. World J Surg 2:581, 1978.
499. Ando H, Ito T, Nagaya M: Use of external conduit impairs liver function in patients with biliary atresia. J Pediatr Surg 31:1509, 1996.
500. Chuang JH, Lee SY, Shieh CS, et al: Reappraisal of the role of the bilioenteric conduit in the pathogenesis of postoperative cholangitis. Pediatr Surg Int 16:29, 2000.
501. Sartorelli KH, Holland RM, Allshouse MJ, et al: The intussusception antireflux valve is ineffective in preventing cholangitis in biliary atresia. J Pediatr Surg 31:403, 1996.
502. Bowles BJ, Abdul-Ghani A, Zhang J, et al: Fifteen years' experience with an antirefluxing biliary drainage valve. J Pediatr Surg 34:1711, 1999.
503. Hirsig J, Rickham PP, Briner J: The importance of hepatic lymph drainage in experimental biliary atresia. Effect of omentopexy on preventation of cholangitis. J Pediatr Surg 14:142, 1979.
504. Toyosaka A, Okamoto E, Okasora T, et al: Extensive dissection at the porta hepatis for biliary atresia. J Pediatr Surg 29:896, 1994.
505. Ando H, Seo T, Ito F, et al: A new hepatic portoenterostomy with division of the ligamentum venosum for treatment of biliary atresia: a preliminary report. J Pediatr Surg 32:1552, 1997.
506. Hashimoto T, Otobe Y, Shimizu Y, et al: A modification of hepatic portoenterostomy (Kasai operation) for biliary atresia. J Am Coll Surg 185:548, 1997.
507. Endo M, Masuyama H, Hirabayashi T, et al: Effects of invaginating anastomosis in Kasai hepatic portoenterostomy on resolution of jaundice, and long-term outcome for patients with biliary atresia. 34:415, 1999.
508. Pearl RH: Surgical management of biliary atresia. In Hoffman MA, ed: Current Controversies in Biliary Atresia. Austin, RG Landes, 1992:62.
509. Hata Y, Uchino J, Kasai Y: Revision of porto-enterostomy in congenital biliary atresia. J Pediatr Surg 20:217, 1985.
510. Shim WKJ, Jin-Zhe Z: Antirefluxing Roux-en-Y biliary drainage valve for hepatic portoenterostomy: animal experiments and clinical experience. J Pediatr Surg 20:689, 1985.
511. Gauthier F, Goulao J, de Dreuzy O, et al: Hepatic portocholecystostomy: 59 cases from a single institution. ed Tokyo, ICOM Associates, 1991:121.
512. Greenholz SK, Lilly JR, Shikes RH, et al: Biliary atresia in the newborn. J Pediatr Surg 21:1147, 1986.
513. Nio M, Ohi R, Shimaoka S, et al: The outcome of surgery for biliary atresia and the current status of long-term survivors. Tohoku J Exp Med 181:235, 1997.
514. Oh M, Hobeldin M, Chen T, et al: The Kasai procedure in the treatment of biliary atresia. J Pediatr Surg 30:1077, 1995.
515. Aronson DC, de Ville de Goyet J, Francois D, et al: Primary management of biliary atresia: don't change the rules. Br J Surg 82:672, 1995.
516. Barkin RM, Lilly JR: Biliary atresia and the Kasai operation: continuing care. J Pediatr 96:1015, 1980.
517. Knisely AS: Biliary atresia and its complications. Ann Clin Lab Sci 20:113, 1990.
518. Hoffman MA: Liver transplantation for biliary atresia. In Hoffman MA, ed: Current Controversies in Biliary Atresia. Austin, RG Landes, 1992:81.
519. Balistreri WF: Clinical aspects. In Ishak KG, ed: Hepatopathology 1985. AASLD Postgraduate Course 1985. American Association for the Study of Liver Diseases. Chicago, 1985:69.
520. Balistreri WF, A-Kader HH, Setchell KDR, et al: Ursodeoxycholic acid therapy in patients with chronic intrahepatic cholestasis and extrahepatic biliary atresia—preliminary results of an open-label, multicenter trial. In Ohi R, ed: Biliary Atresia. Tokyo, ICOM Associates, 1991:167.
521. Okazaki T, Kobayashi H, Yamataka A, et al: Long-term postsurgical outcome of biliary atresia. J Pediatr Surg 34:312, 1999.
522. Ibrahim M, Miyano T, Ohi R, et al: Japanese biliary atresia registry, 1989 to 1994. Tohoku J Exp Med 181:85, 1997.
523. Shimizu Y, Hashimoto T, Otobe Y, et al: Long-term survivors in biliary atresia: findings for a 20-year survival group. Tohoku J Exp Med 181:225, 1997.
524. Matsuo S, Suita S, Kubota M, et al: Long-term results and clnical problems after portoenterostomy in patients with biliary atresia. Eur J Pediatr Surg 8:142, 1998.
525. Nio M, Ohi R, Hayashi Y, et al: Current status of 21 patients who have survived more than 20 years since undergoing surgery for biliary atresia. J Pediatr Surg 31:381, 1996.
526. Karrer FM, Price MR, Bensard DD, et al: Long-term results with the Kasai operation for biliary atresia. Arch Surg 131:493, 1996.
527. Howard ER, Davenport M: The treatment of biliary atresia in Europe 1969-1995. Tohoku J Exp Med 181:75, 1997.
528. Valayer J: Conventional treatment of biliary atresia: long-term results. J Pediatr Surg 31:1546, 1996.
529. Starzl TE, Marchioro TL, von Kaulla KN, et al: Homotransplantation of the liver in humans. Surg Gynecol Obstet 117:659, 1963.
530. Van Wijk J, Halgrimson CG, Giles G, et al: Liver transplantation in biliary atresia with concomitant hepatoma. S Afr Med J 46:885, 1972.
531. Starzl T, Iwatsuki S, Van Thiel D, et al: Evolution of liver transplantation. Hepatology 2:614, 1982.
532. Krom RAF: Liver transplantation (1963-1983): a review of results of the centers Pittsburgh, Cambridge, Hannover, Groningen, Innsbruck and Paris. In Gips CH, Krom RAF, eds: Progress in Liver Transplantation. Dordrecht, Martinus Nijhoff, 1985:3.
533. Balistreri WF: Transplantation for childhood liver disease: an overview. Liver Transpl Surg 4:S18, 1998.
534. Rudolph JA, Balistreri WF: Editorial. Optimal treatment of biliary atresia—"Halfway" there! Hepatology 30:808, 1999.
535. Sandler AD, Azarow KS, Superina RA: The impact of a previous Kasai procedure on liver transplantation for biliary atresia. J Pediatr Surg 32:416, 1997.
536. Otte JB, de Ville de Goyet J, Reding R, et al: Pediatric liver transplantation: from the full-size liver graft to reduced, split, and living related liver transplantation. Pediatr Surg Int 13:308, 1998.
537. Broelsch CE, Stevens LH, Whitington PF: The use of reduced-size liver transplants in children, including split livers and living related liver transplants. Eur J Pediatr Surg 1:166, 1991.
538. Varela-Fascinetto G, Castaldo P, Fox IJ, et al: Biliary atresia-polysplenia syndrome: surgical and clinical relevance in liver transplantation. Ann Surg 227:583, 1998.
539. Kasai M, Mochizuki I, Ohkohchi N, et al: Surgical limitation for biliary atresia: indication for liver transplantation. J Pediatr Surg 24:851, 1989.
540. Lang T, Kappler M, Dietz H, et al: Biliary atresia: which factors predict the success of a Kasai operation? An analysis of 36 patients. Eur J Med Res 27:110, 2000.
541. Ishikawa M, Lynch SV, Balderson GA, et al: Liver transplantation in Japanese and Australian/New Zealand children with biliary atresia: a 10-year comparative study. Eur J Surg 165:454, 1999.
542. Ryckman FC, Alonso MH, Bucuvalas JC, et al: Long-term survival after liver transplantation. J Pediatr Surg 34:845, 1999.
543. Davenport M, Kerkar N, Mieli-Vergani G, et al: Biliary atresia: the King's College Hospital experience (1974-1995). J Pediatr Surg 32:479, 1997.

544. Saing H, Fan ST, Chan KL, et al: Treatment of biliary atresia by portoenterostomy and liver transplantation: the Queen Mary Hospital, Hong Kong experience. Tohoku J Exp Med 181:109, 1997.
545. Lopez-Santamaria M, Gamez M, Murcia J, et al: Long-term follow-up of patients with biliary atresia successfully treated with hepatic portoenterostomy. The importance of sequential treatment. Pediatr Surg Int 13:327, 1998.
546. Ohi R: Surgical treatment of biliary atresia in the liver transplantation era. Surg Today 28:1229, 1998.
547. Goss JA, Shackleton CR, Swenson K, et al: Orthotopic liver transplantation for congenital biliary atresia. An 11 year, single-center experience. Ann Surg 224:276, 1996.
548. Chardot C, Carton M, Spire-Bendelac N, et al: Prognosis of biliary atresia in the era of liver transplantation: French national study from 1986 to 1996. Hepatology 30:606, 1999.
549. Caccia G, Dessanti A, Alberti D: Clinical results in 90 patients with biliary atresia: 2-10 years. In Ohi R, ed: Biliary Atresia. Tokyo, Professional Postgraduate Services, 1987:281.
550. Gautier M, Valayer J, Odièvre M, et al: Histologic liver evaluation 5 years after surgery for extrahepatic biliary atresia: a study of 20 cases. J Pediatr Surg 19:263, 1984.
551. Alagille D: Extrahepatic biliary atresia. Hepatology 4:7S, 1984.
552. Miyata M, Satani M, Uedo T, et al: Long-term results of hepatic portoenterostomy for biliary atresia: special reference to postoperative portal hypertension. Surgery 76:234, 1974.
553. Kasai M, Watanabe I, Ohi R: Follow-up studies of longterm survivors after hepatic portoenterostomy for "non correctable" biliary atresia. J Pediatr Surg 10:173, 1975.
554. Kasai M, Okamoto A, Ohi R, et al: Changes of portal vein pressure and intrahepatic blood vessels after surgery for biliary atresia. J Pediatr Surg 10:152, 1981.
555. Lilly JR, Stellin G: Variceal hemorrhage in biliary atresia. J Pediatr Surg 19:476, 1984.
556. Sondheimer JW, Shandling B, Waber JL, et al: Hepatic function following portoenterostomy for extrahepatic biliary atresia. Can Med Assoc J 118:255, 1978.
557. Howard ER, Mowat AP: Hepatobiliary disorders in infancy: hepatitis, extrahepatic biliary atresia: intrahepatic biliary hypoplasia. In Thomas HC, MacSween RNM, eds: Recent Advances in Hepatology. Edinburgh, Churchill Livingstone, 1983:153.
558. Kang N, Davenport M, Driver M, et al: Hepatic histology and the development of esophageal varices in biliary atresia. J Pediatr Surg 28:63, 1993.
559. Davenport M, Kang N, Driver M, et al: The development of oesophageal varices in extrahepatic biliary atresia. In Ohi R, ed: Biliary Atresia. Tokyo, ICOM Associates, 1991:233.
560. Takahashi A, Tsuchida Y, Suzuki N, et al: Incidence of intrahepatic biliary cysts in biliary atresia after hepatic portoenterostomy and associated histopathologic findings in the liver and porta hepatis at diagnosis. J Pediatr Surg 34:1364, 1999.
561. Betz BW, Bisset GS III, Johnson ND, et al: MR imaging of biliary cysts in children with biliary atresia: clinical associations and pathologic correlation. AJR 162:167, 1994.
562. Kawarasaki H, Itoh M, Mizuta K, et al: Further observations on cystic dilatation of the intrahepatic portoenterostomy: report on 10 cases. Tohoku J Exp Med 181:175, 1997.
563. Danks DM, Campbell PE: Extrahepatic biliary atresia: comments on the frequency of potentially operable cases. J Pediatr 69:21, 1966.
564. Canty TGS: Encouraging results with a modified Sawaguchi hepatoportoenterostomy for biliary atresia. Am J Surg 154:19, 1987.
565. Watanabe I, Ohi R, Okamoto A, et al: Postoperative changes in the histologic picture of the liver in biliary atresia. In Kasai M, Shiraki K, eds: Cholestasis in Infancy. Tokyo, University of Tokyo Press, 1980:381.
566. Dessanti A, Ohi R, Hanamatsu M, et al: Short term histological liver changes in extrahepatic biliary atresia with good postoperative bile drainage. Arch Dis Child 60:739, 1985.
567. Hadchouel M, Gautier M, Valayer J, et al: Histopathology of the liver five years after successful surgery for extrahepatic biliary atresia. In Daum F, ed: Extrahepatic Biliary Atresia. New York, Marcel Dekker, 1983:65.
568. Nio M, Takahashi T, Ohi R: Changes of intrahepatic portal veins in biliary atresia: formation and development of medial smooth muscles correlated with portal hypertension. In Ohi R, ed: Biliary Atresia. Tokyo, Professional Postgraduate Services, 1987:243.
569. Hernandez-Cano AM, Geis JR, Rumack CH, et al: Portal vein dynamics in biliary atresia. J Pediatr Surg 22:519, 1987.
570. Weinbren K, Hadjis NS, Blumgart LH: Structural aspects of the liver in patients with biliary disease and portal hypertension. J Clin Pathol 38:1013, 1985.
571. Bunton GL, Cameron R: Regeneration of liver after biliary cirrhosis. Ann NY Acad Sci 111:412, 1963.
572. Yeong ML, Nicholson GI, Lee SP: Regression of biliary cirrhosis following choledochal cyst drainage. Gastroenterology 82:332, 1985.
573. Ludwig J, Czaja AJ, Dickson R, et al: Manifestations of nonsuppurative cholangitis in chronic hepatobiliary diseases: morphologic spectrum, clinical correlations and terminology. Liver 4:105, 1984.
574. Ludwig J: New concepts in biliary cirrhosis. Semin Liver Dis 7:293, 1987.
575. Popper H: Changing concepts of the evolution of chronic hepatitis and the role of piecemeal necrosis. Hepatology 3:758, 1983.
576. Odièvre M: Long-term results of surgical treatment of biliary atresia. World J Surg 2:589, 1978.
577. Valayer J: Biliary atresia and portal hypertension. In Daum F, ed: Extrahepatic Biliary Atresia. New York, Marcel Dekker, 1983: 105.
578. Akiyama H, Saeki, M, Ogata, T: Portal hypertension after successful surgery for biliary atresia. In Kasai M, ed: Biliary Atresia and its Related Disorders. Amsterdam, Excerpta Medica, 1967:276.
579. Okamoto E, Toyosaka A, Okasora T: Surgical treatment of portal hypertension in biliary atresia. In Kasai M, ed: Biliary Atresia and its Related Disorders. Amsterdam, Excerpta Medica, 1983:283.
580. Grunert D, Stier B, Schoning M: The portal system and the hepatic artery in children with extrahepatic bile duct atresia. 2: Further duplex sonography parameters and flowmetry. Klin Paediatr 202:87, 1990.
581. Dessanti A, Falchetti D, Alberti D, et al: Long term follow-up of portal hypertension in biliary atresia after Kasai operation. In Ohi R, ed: Biliary Atresia. Tokyo, ICOM Associates, 1991:238.
582. Mallet-Guy D, Michoulier J, Beau S: Experimental studies on liver lymph flow: conditions affecting bilio-lymphatic transfer. In Taylor W, ed: The Biliary System. Philadelphia, FA Davis Corporation, 1965:69.
583. Kimura S, Togon H, Sakai K: Histological studies of the liver in long-term survivors. In Ohi R, ed: Biliary Atresia. Tokyo, Professional Postgraduate Services, 1987:299.
584. Nio M, Ohi R, Chiba T, et al: Morphology of intrahepatic bile ducts in jaundice-free patients with biliary atresia. In Ohi R, ed: Biliary Atresia. Tokyo, ICOM Associates, 1991:53.
585. Larcher VF, Vegnente A, Psacharopoulos HT, et al: Immune responses in patients with obstructive jaundice in infancy. Acta Paediatr Scand 72:59, 1983.
586. De Freitas LAR, Chevalier M, Louis D, et al: Human extrahepatic biliary atresia: portal connective tissue activation related to ductular proliferation. Liver 6:253, 1986.
587. Lilly JR: The surgery of biliary hypoplasia. J Pediatr Surg 11:815, 1976.
588. Longmire WP: Congenital biliary hypoplasia. Ann Surg 159:335, 1964.
589. Krant SM, Swenson O: Biliary duct hypoplasia. J Pediatr Surg 8:301, 1973.
590. Afroudakis A, Kaplowitz N: Liver histopathology in chronic common bile duct stenosis due to chronic alcoholic pancreatitis. Hepatology 1:65, 1981.
591. Altman RP, Chandra R: Biliary hypoplasia as a consequnce of alpha-1-antitrypsin deficiency. Surg Forum 27:377, 1976.
592. Odièvre M, Martin JP, Hadchouel M, et al: Alpha-1-antitrypsin deficiency and liver disease in children: phenotypes, manifestations and prognosis. Pediatrics 57:226, 1976.
593. Porter CA, Mowat AP, Cook PJL, et al: Alpha-1-antitrypsin deficiency and neonatal hepatitis. BMJ 3:435, 1972.
594. Gorelick FS, Dobbins JW, Burrell M, et al: Biliary tract abnormalities in patients with arteriohepatic dysplasia. Dig Dis Sci 27:815, 1982.
595. Morelli A, Pelli MA, Vedovelli A, et al: Endoscopic retrograde cholangiopancreatography study in Alagille's syndrome: first report. Am J Gastroenterol 78:241, 1983.
596. Howard ER: Paediatric liver disease: surgical aspects. In Wright R, Millward-Sadler GH, Alberti KGMM, et al., eds: Liver and Biliary Disease, ed 2. London, Baillière Tindall, WB Saunders, 1985:1219.

597. Dijkstra CH: Galuitstorting in de buikholte bij een zuigeling. Maandschr Kindergeneesk 1:409, 1932.
598. Smethurst FA, Carty H: Case report: spontaneous perforation of the common bile duct in infancy. Br J Radiol 66:556, 1993.
599. Johnston JH: Spontaneous perforation of the common bile ducts in infancy. Br J Surg 48:532, 1961.
600. Moore TC: Massive bile peritonitis in infancy due to spontaneous bile duct perforation with portal vein occlusion. J Pediatr Surg 10:537, 1975.
601. Megison SM, Votteler TP: Management of common bile duct obstruction associated with spontaneous perforation of the biliary tree. Surgery 111:237, 1992.
602. Saltzman DA, Snyder CL, Leonard A: Spontaneous perforation of the extrahepatic biliary tree in infancy. A case report. Clin Pediatr (Phila) 29:322, 1990.
603. Davenport M, Heaton ND, Howard ER: Spontaneous perforation of the bile duct in infants. Br J Surg 78:1068, 1991.
604. Chilukuri S, Bonet V, Cobb M: Antenatal spontaneous perforation of the extrahepatic biliary tree. Am J Obstet Gynecol 163:1201, 1990.
605. Caulfield E: Bile peritonitis in infancy. Am J Dis Child 52:1348, 1936.
606. Prevot J, Babut JM: Spontaneous perforations of the biliary tract in infancy. Prog Pediatr Surg 3:187, 1971.
607. Haller JO, Condon VR, Berdon WE, et al: Spontaneous perforation of the common bile duct in children. Radiology 172:621, 1989.
608. Howard ER, Johnston DI, Mowat AP: Spontaneous perforation of common bile duct in infants. Arch Dis Child 51:883, 1976.
609. Lilly JR, Weintraub WH, Altman RP: Spontaneous perforation of the extrahepatic bile ducts and bile peritonitis in infancy. Surgery 75:664, 1974.
610. Dunn DC, Lees VC: Spontaneous perforation of the common bile duct in infancy. Br J Surg 73:929, 1986.
611. Dunn PM: Obstructive jaundice and haemolytic disease of the newborn. Arch Dis Child 38:54, 1963.
612. Hsia DYY, Patterson P, Allen FH, et al: Prolonged obstructive jaundice in infancy. Pediatrics 10:243, 1952.
613. Bernstein J, Braylan R, Brough AJ: Bile plug syndrome: a correctable cause of obstructive jaundice in infants. Pediatrics 43:273, 1969.
614. Heaton ND, Davenport M, Howard ER: Intraluminal biliary obstruction. Arch Dis Child 66:1395, 1991.
615. Rickham PP, Lee EYC: Neonatal jaundice: surgical aspects. Clin Pediatr 3:197, 1964.
616. Brown DM: Bile plug syndrome: successful management with a mucolytic agent. J Pediatr Surg 25:351, 1990.
617. Lang EV, Pickney LE: Spontaneous resolution of bile-plug syndrome. Am J Roentgenol 156:1225, 1991.
618. Lai HS, Duh YC, Chen WJ: Inspissated bile syndrome followed by choledochal cyst formation. Surgery 123:706, 1998.
619. Vazquez Rueda F, Paredes Esteban RM, Escassi Gil A, et al: Isolated congenital stenoses of the extrahepatic bile ducts (SPA). Cir Pediatr 6:40, 1993.
620. Akers DR, Favara BE, Franciosi RA, et al: Duplications of the alimentary tract: report of three unusual cases associated with bile and pancreatic ducts. Surgery 71:817, 1972.
621. Wrenn ElJ, Favara BE: Duodenal duplication (or pancreatic bladder) presenting as double gallbladder. Surgery 69:858, 1971.
622. Kodama T, Iseki J, Murata N, et al: Duplication of common bile duct. A case report. Jpn J Surg 10:67, 1980.
623. Schwartz MZ, Hall RJ, Reubner B, et al: Agenesis of the extrahepatic bile ducts: report of five cases. J Pediatr Surg 25:805, 1990.
624. Debray D, Pariente D, Gauthier F, et al: Cholelithiasis in infancy: a study of 40 cases. J Pediatr 122:385, 1993.
625. Devonald KJ, Ellwood DA, Colditz PB: The variable appearances of fetal gallstones. J Ultrasound Med 11:579, 1992.
626. Whittington PF, Black DD: Cholelithiasis in premature infants treated with parenteral nutrition and furosemide. J Pediatr 97:647, 1980.
627. Randall LH, Shaddy RE, Sturtevant JE, et al: Cholelithiasis in infants receiving furosemide: a prospective study of the incidence and one-year follow-up. J Perinatol 12:107, 1992.
628. Wilcox DT, Casson D, Bowen J, et al: Cholelithiasis in early infancy. Pediatr Surg Int 12:198, 1997.
629. Schulman A: Intrahepatic biliary stones: imaging features and a possible relationship with Ascaris lumbricoides. Clin Radiol 47:325, 1993.
630. Holcomb GWJ, Holcomb GW: Cholelithiasis in infants, children, and adolescents. Pediatr Rev 11:268, 1990.
631. Friesen CA, Roberts CC: Cholelithiasis. Clinical characteristics in children. Case analysis and literature review. Clin Pediatr (Phila) 28:294, 1989.
632. Enriquez G, Lucaya J, Allende E, et al: Intrahepatic biliary stones in children. Pediatr Radiol 22:283, 1992.
633. Taira Y, Nakayama I, Moriuchi A, et al: Sarcoma botryoides arising from the biliary tract of children—a case report with review of the literature. Acta Pathol Jpn 26:709, 1976.
634. Akers DR, Needham ME: Sarcoma botryoides (Rhabdomyosarcoma) of the bile ducts with survival. J Pediatr Surg 6:474, 1971.
635. von der Oelsnitz G, Spaar HJ, Lieber T, et al: Embryonal rhabdomyosarcoma of the common bile duct. Eur J Pediatr Surg 1:161, 1991.
636. Soares FA, Landell GA, Peres LC, et al: Liposarcoma of hepatic hilum in childhood: report of a case and review of the literature. Med Pediatr Oncol 17:239, 1989.
637. Verstandig A, Bar-Ziv J, Abu-Dalu KI, et al: Sarcoma botryoides of the common bile duct: preoperative diagnosis by coronal CT and PTC. Pediatr Radiol 21:152, 1991.
638. Stocker JT: Hepatic tumors. In Balistreri WF, Stocker TJ, eds: Pediatric Hepatology. New York, Hemisphere Publishing Corporation, 1990:399.
639. Nixon HH: Paediatric liver disease: surgical aspects. In Wright R, Alberti KGMM, Karran S, et al., eds: Liver and Biliary Disease, ed 1. London, WB Saunders, 1979:962.
640. Werlin SL, Glicklich M, Jona J, et al: Sclerosing cholangitis in childhood. J Pediatr 96:433, 1980.
641. Spivak W, Grand RJ, Eraklis A: A case of primary sclerosing cholangitis in childhood. Gastroenterology 82:129, 1982.
642. Naveh Y, Mendelsohn M, Spira G, et al: Primary sclerosing cholangitis associated with immunodeficiency. Am J Dis Child 137:114, 1983.
643. Descos B, Brunelle F, Fischer A, et al: Sclerosing cholangitis in children with immunodeficiency. Pediatr Res 18:1059, 1984 (abstract).
644. Record CO, Shilkin KB, Eddleston ALWF, et al: Intrahepatic sclerosing cholangitis associated with a familial immunodeficiency syndrome. Lancet 2:18, 1973.
645. Gremse DA, Bucuvalas JC, Bongiovanni GL: Papillary stenosis and sclerosing cholangitis in an immunodeficient child. Gastroenterology 96:1600, 1989.
646. Leblanc A, Hadchouel M, Jehan P, et al: Obstructive jaundice in children with histiocytosis X. Gastroenterology 80:134, 1981.
647. Concepcion W, Esquivel CO, Terry A, et al: Liver transplantation in Langerhans' cell histiocytosis (histiocytosis X). Semin Oncol 18:24, 1991.
648. Neveu I, Labrune P, Huguet P, et al: Sclerosing cholangitis revealing histiocytosis X. Arch Fr Pediatr 47:197, 1990.
649. Rand EB, Whitington PF: Successful orthotopic liver transplantation in two patients with liver failure due to sclerosing cholangitis with Langerhans cell histiocytosis. J Pediatr Gastroenterol Nutr 15:202, 1992.
650. Hellstrom HR, Perez-Stable EC: Retroperitoneal fibrosis with disseminated vasculitis and intrahepatic sclerosing cholangitis. Am J Med 40:184, 1986.
651. Alpert LI, Jindrak K: Idiopathic retroperitoneal fibrosis and sclerosing cholangitis associated with a reticulum cell sarcoma. Gastroenterology 62:111, 1972.
652. Gregorio GV, Portmann B, Karani J, et al: Autoimmune hepatitis/sclerosing cholangitis overlap syndrome in childhood: a 16-year pospective study. Hepatology 33:544, 2001.
653. El-Shabrawi M, Wilkinson ML, Portmann B, et al: Primary sclerosing cholangitis in childhood. Gastroenterology 92:1226, 1987.
654. Classen M, Götze H, Richter HJ, et al: Primary sclerosing cholangitis in children. J Pediatr Gastroenterol Nutr 6:197, 1987.
655. Roberts EA: Primary sclerosing cholangitis in children. J Gastroenterol Heptol 14:588, 1999.
656. Floreani A, Zancan L, Melis A, et al: Primary sclerosing cholangitis (PSC): clinical, laboratory and survival analysis in children and adults. Liver 19:228, 1999.
657. Nemeth A, Ejderhamn J, Glaumann H, et al: Liver damage in juvenile inflammatory bowel disease. Liver 10:239, 1990.
658. Sokal EM, de Ville de Goyet J, Buts JP, et al: Unifocal stricture of the common bile duct in two children: a localized form of primary sclerosing cholangitis. J Pediatr Gastroenterol Nutr 11:268, 1990.

659. Gilger MA, Gann ME, Opekun AR, et al: Efficacy of ursodeoxycholic acid in the treatment of primary sclerosing cholangitis in children. J Pediatr Gastroenterol Nutr 31:136, 2000.
660. Craig JM, Landing BH: Form of hepatitis in neonatal period simulating biliary atresia. Arch Pathol 54:321, 1952.
661. Thaler MM, Hu F, Heyman MB: Giant cell hepatitis due to hepatitis C virus infection. Hepatology 16:74A, 1992.
662. Chang MH, Huang HH, Huang ES, et al: Polymerase chain reaction to detect human cytomegalovirus in livers of infants with neonatal hepatitis [see comments]. Gastroenterology 103:1022, 1992.
663. Lai MW, Chang MH, Lee CY, et al: Cytomegalovirus-associated neonatal hepatitis. Acta Paediatr Sin 33:264, 1992.
664. Tajiri H, Nose O, Baba K, et al: Human herpesvirus-6 infection with liver injury in neonatal hepatitis. Lancet 335:863, 1990 (letter).
665. Aterman K: Neonatal hepatitis. A viral disease? [classic article]. Pediatr Pathol 9:243, 1989.
666. Phillips MJ, Blendis LM, Poucell S, et al: Syncytial giant cell hepatitis: sporadic hepatitis with distinctive pathology, severe clinical course and paramyxoviral features. N Engl J Med 324:455, 1991.
667. Dick MC, Mowat AP: Hepatitis syndrome in infancy—an epidemiological survey with 10 year follow up. Arch Dis Child 60:512, 1985.
668. Chandra RK: The neonatal hepatitis syndrome. Trop Gastroenterol 2:94, 1981.
669. Felber S, Sinatra F: Systemic disorders associated with neonatal cholestasis. Semin Liver Dis 7:108, 1987.
670. Alagille D: Closing remarks. In Kasai M, ed: Biliary Atresia and its Related Disorders. Amsterdam, Excerpta Medica, 1983:301.
671. Bujanover Y: Prognosis of neonatal cholestatic jaundice. J Pediatr Gastroenterol Nutr 6:163, 1987.
672. Setchell KDR, Piccoli D, Heubi J, et al: Inborn errors of bile acid metabolism. In Lentze M, Reichen J, eds: Paediatric Cholestasis. Novel approaches to treatment. Dordrecht, Kluwer Academic Publishers, 1992:153.
673. Setchell KDR, Street JM: Inborn errors of bile acid metabolism. Semin Liver Dis 7:85, 1987.
674. Witzleben CL, Piccoli DA, Setchell K: A new category of causes of intrahepatic cholestasis. J Pediatr Pathol 12:269, 1992.
675. Watkins JB: Neonatal cholestasis: developmental aspects and current concepts. Semin Liver Dis 13:276, 1993.
676. Daugherty CC, Setchell KDR, Heubi JE, et al: Resolution of liver biopsy alterations in three siblings with bile acid treatment of an inborn error of bile acid metabolism (d4-3-oxosteroid 5b-reductase deficiency). Hepatology 18:1096, 1993.
677. Suchy FJ: Bile acids for babies? Diagnosis and treatment of a new category of metabolic liver disease. Hepatology 18:1274, 1993.
678. Lawson EE, Boggs JD: Long-term follow-up of neonatal hepatitis: safety and value of surgical exploration. Pediatrics 53:650, 1974.
679. Kasai M: Hepatic portoenterostomy for the so-called "noncorrectable" type of biliary atresia. In Daum F, ed: Extrahepatic Biliary Atresia. New York, Marcel Dekker, 1983:79.
680. Odiévre M, Hadchouel M, Landrieu P, et al: Long-term prognosis for infants with intrahepatic cholestasis and patent extrahepatic biliary tract. Arch Dis Child 56:373, 1981.
681. Danks DM, Campbell PE, Smith AL, et al: Prognosis of babies with neonatal hepatitis. Arch Dis Child 52:368, 1977.
682. Ruebner B: The pathology of neonatal hepatitis. Am J Pathol 36:151, 1960.
683. Christoffersen P, Poulsen H, Skeie E: Focal liver cell necrosis accompanied by infiltration of granulocytes arising during operation. Acta Hepatosplenol 17:240, 1970.
684. Kadas I: Neonatal hepatitis: histological and differential diagnostic aspects. Acta Morphol Acad Sci Hung 24:223, 1976.
685. Ruebner B, Thaler MM: Giant-cell transformation in infantile liver disease. In Javitt NB, ed: Neonatal Hepatitis and Biliary Atresia. US Department of Health, Education and Welfare. DHEW Publication No. (NIH) 79-1296, 1979:299.
686. Schaffner F, Popper H: Morphologic studies in neonatal hepatitis with emphasis on giant cells. Ann NY Acad Sci 111:358, 1963.
687. Czenkar B: Pathologie der Riesenzellenhepatitis von Neugeborenen und Säuglingen. Arch Pathol Anat 331:696, 1958.
688. Smetana HF, Edlow JB, Glunz PR: Neonatal jaundice. A critical review of persistent obstructive jaundice in infancy. Arch Pathol 80:553, 1965.
689. Dible JH, Hunt WE, Pugh VW, et al: Foetal and neonatal hepatitis and its sequelae. J Pathol Bacteriol 67:195, 1954.
690. Oledzka-Slotwinska H, Desmet V: Morphologic and cytochemical study on neonatal liver "giant" cell transformation. Exp Mol Pathol 10:162, 1969.
691. Hicks J, Barrish J, Zhu SH: Neonatal syncytial giant cell hepatitis with paramyxoviral-like inclusions. Ultrastruct Pathol 25:65, 2001.
692. Schmid M, Pirovino M, Altorfer J, et al: Acute hepatitis non-A, non-B; are there any specific light microscopic features? Liver 2:61, 1982.
693. Thaler H: Post-infantile giant cell hepatitis. Liver 2:393, 1982.
694. Devaney K, Goodman ZD, Ishak KG: Postinfantile giant-cell transformation in hepatitis. Hepatology 16:327, 1992.
695. Lau JY, Koukoulis G, Mieli-Vergani G, et al: Syncytial giant-cell hepatitis. A specific disease entity? J Hepatol 15:216, 1992.
696. Kumar A, Minuk GY: Postinfantile giant cell hepatitis in association with hypereosinophilia. Gastroenterology 101:1417, 1991.
697. Pessayre D, Degos F, Feldmann G, et al: Chronic active hepatitis and giant multinucleated hepatocytes in adults treated with clometacin. Digestion 22:66, 1981.
698. Altman C, Bedossa P, Dussaix E, et al: Giant cell hepatitis of benign evolution in adults. Gastroenterol Clin Biol 18:389, 1994 (letter).
699. Bianchi L, Terracciano LM: Giant cell hepatitis in adults. Schweiz Rundsch Med Prax 83:1237, 1994.
700. Campbell LVJ: Experimental giant-cell transformation in the liver induced by E. coli endotoxin. Am J Pathol 51:855, 1967.
701. Andres JM, Walker WA: Effect of Escherichia coli endotoxin on the developing rat liver. I. Giant cell induction and disruption in protein metabolism. Pediatr Res 13:1290, 1979.
702. Andres JM, Darby BR, Walker WA: The effect of E. coli endotoxin on the developing rat liver. II. Immunohistochemical localization of alpha-fetoprotein in rat liver multinucleated giant cells. Pediatr Res 17:1017, 1983.
703. Svoboda DJ, Reddy JK, Liu C: Multinucleate giant cells in livers of marmosets given aflatoxin B1. Arch Pathol 91:452, 1971.
704. Deutsch J, Smith AL, Danks DM, et al: Long-term prognosis for babies with neonatal liver disease. Arch Dis Child 60:447, 1985.
705. Suita S, Arima T, Ishii K, et al: Fate of infants with neonatal hepatitis: pediatric surgeons' dilemma. J Pediatr Surg 27:696, 1992.

SECTION

IV F

Special Topics

CHAPTER

51

HIV-Associated Hepatobiliary Disease

C. Mel Wilcox, MD, and Miguel R. Arguedas, MD, MPH

INTRODUCTION

Remarkable progress has been made in our understanding of the human immunodeficiency virus (HIV) and the management of complications related to acquired immunodeficiency syndrome (AIDS). Although the number of newly infected patients and AIDS-related mortality have fallen during the last decade in developed countries,[1] the disease remains devastating worldwide, particularly in Africa, and epidemics are now developing in eastern Europe and Asia.[2,3] After the initial descriptions of AIDS in 1982 the first decade of disease was devoted to characterizing the spectrum of complications and developing an approach to management. When routine prophylaxis against *Pneumocystis carinii* pneumonia (PCP), the most common opportunistic infection in AIDS, was adopted in the late 1980s, the incidence of this infection decreased. The frequency of other opportunistic infections including gastrointestinal and hepatobiliary disorders consequently rose.[4-7] In 1996 protease inhibitors became widely available. These drugs, when combined with other anti-retroviral agents termed *highly active anti-retroviral therapy* (HAART), have had a profound effect on HIV disease. In many patients, particularly those who are naïve to these medications, immunodeficiency can be substantially reversed, resulting in a marked reduction in the incidence of opportunistic infections and improvement in survival.[1,8,9]

Our understanding of the causes, presentations, and diagnostic approaches to liver diseases in HIV-infected patients has continued to evolve. For example, early in the AIDS epidemic some histologic abnormalities of the liver were considered non-specific but are now recognized as an infectious disease (e.g., peliosis hepatis). Likewise, in the 1980s liver biopsies were frequently performed to evaluate abnormal liver tests. We now appreciate that a strategy of routine liver biopsy for abnormal liver tests rarely alters management.[10] Also, the widespread use of HAART has decreased the prevalence of opportunistic disorders.[11] The emergence of drug-induced liver disease has both altered the prevalence of causes and changed our approach to management. Although opportunistic infections and neoplasms are usually first considered when evaluating the HIV-infected patient with liver disease, it is important to recognize that liver disease may be unrelated to HIV infection. In addition, the manifestations of these non-opportunistic disorders may differ from their immunocompetent counterparts.

A thorough understanding of the causes and management of hepatobiliary disease in HIV infection and AIDS is important because of the number of infected patients throughout the world and because of the potential morbidity and mortality that liver and biliary diseases may incur. A decade ago liver disease was infrequently the primary cause of death in HIV-infected patients[12]; more recently, liver-related mortality has risen.[13,14] For example, liver failure was found in one study[14] to be the cause of in-hospital mortality in 12 percent of HIV-infected patients. As the prognosis of HIV infection further improves with advancement in pharmacotherapy, liver disease may become even more important to outcome. To review hepatobiliary disease associated with HIV infection, this chapter addresses the causes of liver disease, the appropriate evaluation and treatment for these disorders, and outlines a diagnostic strategy to evaluate suspected hepatobiliary disease.

CAUSES OF LIVER DISEASE

A number of descriptive studies performed early in the AIDS epidemic characterized the spectrum of hepatobiliary diseases associated with HIV infection.[15-26] More recent studies from throughout the world substantiate and further expand these findings.[27-34] Several trends are evident from these reports. First, the most common opportunistic cause of parenchymal liver disease in AIDS is *Mycobacterium avium* complex (MAC). Second, the identified causes of disease vary between studies because of differences in patient populations—including geographic setting and risk factors for HIV infection, severity of immunodeficiency, and indications for liver biopsy. Studies of intravenous drug users (IVDU) show a high prevalence of viral hepatitis and tuberculosis.[23] Reports from underdeveloped countries uniformly report higher prevalence rates of tuberculosis.[24,31-34] In many earlier studies patients were not stratified by the CD4 lymphocyte count. It is now well established that the likelihood of an opportunistic infection or neoplasm can be based accurately on the absolute CD4 count.[35,36] Thus patients with only modest immunodeficiency (CD4 lymphocyte counts of 200-500/mm^3) are not expected to have MAC or cytomegalovirus (CMV) disease. The method by which liver tissue is acquired will also dictate the spectrum of causes identified. Patients undergoing percutaneous liver biopsy are more likely to have an acute presentation and a specific diagnosis established,[17,23,24] whereas autopsy studies identify disorders that often were clinically silent.[15,20,37,38] Last, although drug-induced liver disease has increased in prevalence coincident with HAART, use of liver biopsy has fallen substantially; therefore, in many patients, the diagnosis of hepatic disease is made by inference.

As shown in Table 51-1, a variety of opportunistic infections and neoplasms are reported to involve the liver in these patients. MAC is the most frequently identified opportunistic cause of liver disease, found in from 4 percent[25] to 50 percent,[17] followed by CMV with a prevalence of 0 percent to 9 percent[10]; autopsy studies often have higher frequencies of identification of CMV. *Mycobacterium tuberculosis* (MTB) is an infrequent cause of liver disease, although in one study,[23] tuberculosis was identified in 25 percent of patients and was more common than MAC. However, this study evaluated an inner-city population consisting primarily of IVDU; these are epidemiologic features associated with a higher prevalence of tuberculosis.[39,40] Studies from Africa and Thailand have also commonly found MTB on liver biopsy and at autopsy.[34] Fungi are uncommon hepatic pathogens in AIDS. Although non-Hodgkin's lymphoma (NHL) is the most frequent symptomatic hepatic neoplasm, Kaposi's sarcoma (KS) is the most common hepatic neoplasm found at autopsy.[10,15,37]

TABLE 51-1

Reported Causes of Hepatic Disease in Patients with HIV Infection

Viral
Hepatitis A, B, C, D, E, and G
Cytomegalovirus
Epstein-Barr syndrome
Herpes simplex type 2
Protozoal
Cryptosporidia
Microsporidia
Isospora organisms
Toxoplasma organisms
Sporothrix organisms
Malaria
Neoplastic
Lymphoma
Kaposi's sarcoma
Hepatoma
Metastatic tumors
Mycobacteria
Mycobacterium avium complex
Mycobacterium tuberculosis
Other mycobacteria
Bacterial
Bartonella henselae
Pneumocystis carinii
Drug-induced
Sulfa
Anti-retrovirals
Anti-fungals
Others
Fungal
Cryptococcus organisms
Histoplasma organisms
Coccidioides organisms
Candida organisms

HIV, Human immunodeficiency virus.

Pathologic Findings

Autopsy and liver biopsy studies have shown that liver histopathology is rarely normal in HIV-infected patients. The most common finding is steatosis, which is usually macrovesicular and clinically unimportant except as a cause of hepatomegaly and abnormal liver tests. It is believed that steatosis is related to malnutrition in most cases. Other potential causes of steatosis include alcohol abuse and total parenteral nutrition (see Chap. 57). A syndrome of severe microvascular steatosis associated with lactic acidosis, hepatic failure, and potential death caused by drug toxicity from anti-retroviral agents has been increasingly recognized (see the following section).[41-44]

Granulomas are the next most common histopathologic abnormality and are seen in 15 percent to 100 percent of patients.[17,35] These granulomas rarely have the typical appearance of epithelioid granulomas with histiocytes and giant cells; rather, they are often poorly formed (Plate 51-1). Foamy blue histiocytes are common in granulomas associated with MAC (Figure 51-1),[19] whereas caseating granulomas are typical for MTB. Approximately 56 percent to 80 percent of granulomas in HIV-infected patients have an infectious etiology, usually MAC, MTB, or fungi,[10,17,18,23-25] although they can be observed in a num-

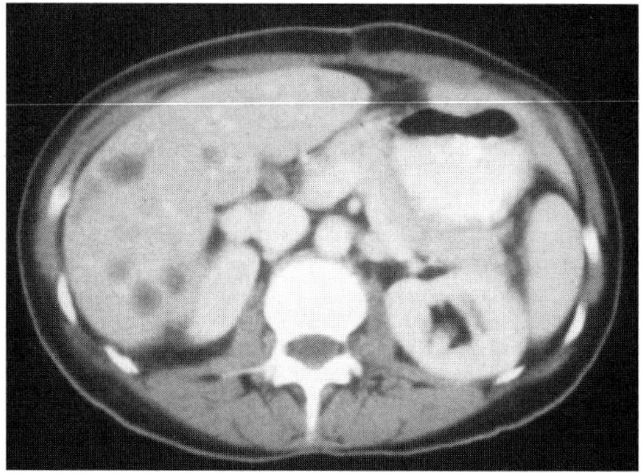

Figure 51-1 Hepatic non-Hodgkin's lymphoma. Multiple filling defects of variable size. Ultrasound-guided biopsy demonstrated high-grade lymphoma.

ber of other conditions (Table 51-2).[16,18,24] Therefore a substantial number of cases (up to 50 percent in some series) remain with no specific identifiable cause for the granulomas.

Histopathologic changes of viral hepatitis are common in HIV-infected patients but are highly dependent on the risk group studied. Reports from early in the AIDS epidemic noted a paucity of severe hepatitis and cirrhosis in patients with chronic hepatitis B virus (HBV) infection,[15,19,22,37,38] with more severe changes appreciated in HIV-infected patients without AIDS. As discussed in the following section, alterations in immune response in AIDS may be the mechanism for reduced liver injury caused by HBV. Cirrhosis has been identified in 10 to 23 percent of patients in some series[10,22] and is usually caused by chronic viral hepatitis or alcohol. Despite marked immunodeficiency, acute alcoholic hepatitis also has been observed.[27]

Non-specific changes including Kupffer cell hyperplasia, mild portal inflammation, bile staining, hemosiderosis,[45] and lymphocyte depletion are of no clinical significance. Peliosis hepatis, previously considered a non-specific finding, has an infectious etiology in some patients (see the following section).

Specific Causes of Liver Disease

Drug-induced Causes

Drugs are probably the most common cause of acute liver injury and should be considered in every patient with suspected liver disease. However, the true prevalence of drug-induced liver disease is difficult to determine. Thus (1) potentially hepatotoxic medications are often discontinued without further investigation when elevated liver enzymes are detected, (2) liver biopsy is rarely performed to evaluate drug-induced hepatic injury, and (3) the histopathologic findings of drug-induced liver disease are often non-specific. It is not surprising that acute, drug-induced liver injury is common in HIV-infected patients given the plethora of medications they receive, many of which have well-established hepatotoxicity. Some medications such as trimethoprim-sulfamethoxazole have an increased risk of toxicity in these patients.[46] The mechanisms of injury can be multifactorial and include drug interactions, the concomitant use of alcohol, or the presence of underlying chronic liver disease. With the advent of HAART it is now recognized that improvement in immune function can exacerbate viral hepatitis, particularly HBV. Although a variety of medications have been linked to hepatotoxicity in HIV-infected patients, we focus on clinical features and toxicity associated with some of the most common offenders.

TABLE 51-2

Causes of Hepatic Granulomas in Patients with HIV

Common*	Uncommon
Mycobacterium avium complex	Cytomegalovirus
Idiopathic	Candida
Other mycobacteria	Microsporidia
Mycobacterium tuberculosis	Schistosoma
Cryptococcus organisms	
Histoplasma organisms	
Medications (trimethoprim-sulfamethoxazole)	

HIV, Human immunodeficiency virus.
*In approximate order of prevalence.

Anti-retroviral Agents

An increasing number of anti-retroviral agents are available for the treatment of HIV infection. Drug-related hepatotoxicity from zidovudine (AZT) is recognized but uncommon.[47] Other agents such as didanosine and zalcitabine have been associated with mild liver hepatocellular injury, although less frequently than has AZT.[43] Lamivudine has little hepatotoxicity and has shown efficacy against other viral pathogens such as HBV.[48]

The most feared liver injury associated with anti-retroviral drugs (nucleoside analogs) is mitochondrial damage.[49] A characteristic multi-system disease has been observed that includes liver injury (jaundice), lactic acidosis, and, frequently, death.[41-44,50] Pancreatitis and myopathy are also frequent. Patients typically present with abdominal pain but may be asymptomatic, the liver tests are usually only slightly increased, and hepatomegaly is typically present. Fortunately, this disorder appears to be rare.[50] Hepatotoxicity caused by the new protease inhibitors is not uncommon. Saquinavir has been implicated most frequently.[51-54] Indinavir has been associated with mild, indirect hyperbilirubinemia and, rarely, acute hepatitis.[55]

Trimethoprim-sulfamethoxazole

The high frequency of side effects, including hepatotoxicity, of trimethoprim-sulfamethoxazole in patients with AIDS became apparent early in the epidemic because of the widespread use of this agent for the treatment of PCP.[46] Trials of trimethoprim-sulfamethoxazole for PCP found drug intolerance in up to 57 percent of patients, with drug-induced hepatitis observed in up to 20 percent.[56] Studies of PCP prophylaxis with lower doses of this agent have also identified drug intolerance and occasional hepatotoxicity.[57] As with most drug-induced liver injuries, hepatitis occurs relatively soon after drug initiation. In keeping with its pathogenesis, features of an allergic reaction including rash, fever, and eosinophilia are frequent.[58] The most common liver test findings are a raised bilirubin associated with mild to marked increases in serum aminotransferases (AST, ALT). Histologically, granulomas may be observed along with bile stasis and hepatocyte necrosis.

Anti-mycobacterial Therapy. Anti-tuberculous agents such as isoniazid and rifampin are common causes of liver injury. Drug-induced hepatotoxicity may be more frequent in HIV-infected patients because of the frequent coexistence of alcoholism and the concomitant use of other drugs.[59,60] In one study of 70 patients from an inner-city hospital treated with isoniazid and rifampin, hepatocellular toxicity was documented in 8 (11.4 percent)[59]; in this study, the risk factors identified for hepatotoxicity were alcoholism and AIDS. In fact, 6 of 22 patients (27 percent) with AIDS developed hepatotoxicity. Isoniazid and rifampin-induced liver injury usually occur within the first several months of drug ingestion but can occur at any time. Clinical features of hepatitis and jaundice are common. Prompt discontinuation of these medications usually results in complete resolution of symptoms. Failure to recognize isoniazid hepatotoxicity with continued drug administration may be fatal, however.

Initial multi-drug regimens for the therapy of MAC, some of which included isoniazid or rifampin, were frequently associated with drug intolerance and liver function abnormalities. Although drug intolerance was high with these older regimens, hepatotoxicity was infrequent. Newer regimens for MAC, which include clarithromycin, azithromycin, ciprofloxacin, and ethambutol, have shown improved efficacy and reduced side effects.[61,62]

Other Agents

Anti-fungal agents are commonly used in AIDS patients because oropharyngeal and esophageal candidiasis and cryptococcal meningitis are common. Mild biochemical abnormalities of liver have been found in 3 percent to 10 percent of patients receiving ketoconazole. More serious liver injury occurs in approximately 1 in 15,000 patients.[63] However, these reports include non–HIV-infected patients. Whether the incidence is higher in HIV patients is unknown, but clinical experience suggests that these drugs are well tolerated and that liver toxicity is rare. The injury caused by anti-fungals is usually of the hepatocellular type, although a mixed hepatocellular-cholestatic picture or cholestasis alone has been described.[63] Fluconazole and itraconazole have been observed to cause abnormalities of liver function tests, but fulminant hepatic failure has not been reported.

Viral Diseases

Viruses are collectively the most important hepatic pathogens in HIV-infected patients. The high prevalence of infection with hepatotropic viruses is not surprising because the risk factors are similar for HIV and hepatotropic viruses. There are a number of important differences in natural history of disease in viral hepatitis patients with AIDS as compared with immunocompetent hosts. Viral hepatitis presents unique diagnostic and management problems in HIV-infected patients.

Hepatitis A Virus

The prevalence, incidence, and outcome of hepatitis A virus (HAV) infection in HIV-infected patients have been little studied. Identified risk factors for the development of HAV infection in homosexual men include the number of sexual partners and oral-anal and digital-rectal intercourse.[64] These identified risk factors have important implications for the prevention of HAV infection. There has been no evidence to suggest a more severe disease or worse outcome as compared to non–HIV-infected patients. A recent report[65] described a transient increase in HIV viral load in two patients acutely infected with HAV. This increase could be the result of HAV-related immune activation.

Hepatitis B Virus

Prevalence. Prior exposure to HBV is common in HIV-infected patients. Serologic studies have shown that 65 percent to 96 percent of patients have had prior exposure as defined by positivity for hepatitis B surface antibody (anti-HBs) or hepatitis B core antibody (anti-HBc).[66,67] However, HBV seropositivity depends on the risk group studied; homosexual men and IVDU have the highest seroprevalence. Risk factors for HBV exposure in homosexual men include anal receptive intercourse, duration of homosexuality, anilingus, and a history of sexually transmitted diseases.[68] Rodriguez-Mendez and coworkers[69] evaluated the prevalence of serologic markers of prior HBV exposure in 585 IVDU. Evidence of prior infection was found in 90 percent of HIV-positive patients compared with 62 percent of HIV-negative patients.

Incidence. Incidence studies of HBV infection in HIV-infected patients are limited. In one study of 57 patients,[70] 6 (10 percent) acquired HBV over a median follow-up of 18 months. Whether the incidence of HBV infection is decreasing among homosexual men as a result of changes in sexual practices is unknown. In a recent study from Switzerland[71] a decreasing incidence rate of HIV and HBV was observed among drug users presenting to a methadone maintenance treatment program, suggesting that public health efforts have modified the risk-taking behavior of these patients.

Natural History

Influence of HIV Infection on HBV Disease. The outcome of HBV infection is altered markedly by co-existent HIV infection. HIV-infected patients who develop acute HBV infection have a high incidence of chronic infection. In a study of HIV-infected homosexual men Hadler and colleagues[72] found that 21 percent of acutely infected men developed a chronic carrier state as compared to 7 percent of homosexual HIV-seronegative controls. No differences in the clinical presentation of acute hepatitis B were observed between the two groups. Others have reported similar findings of a high rate of chronicity after acute HBV.[70] A longitudinal study of 152 patients with HIV/HBV co-infection documented higher levels of HBV deoxyribonucleic acid (DNA) polymerase activity, lower transaminase levels. and lower rate of hepatitis B e antigen (HBeAg) loss compared to HBV+/HIV− controls.[87] HBeAg and HBV DNA are detected more frequently[73] and are of higher levels[74] in HIV-infected as compared with uninfected homosexuals. Spontaneous clearance of HBV DNA is also less likely.[70] The duration of chronic HBV infection has been suggested to play a role in the level of replication.[75]

Studies examining the degree of HBV-related liver injury as assessed by transaminase levels and hepatic histology have yielded conflicting results. Most[70,73,74,76,78] but not all[79,80] studies have found lower ALT levels and less severe histopathologic injury in HIV-infected patients as compared to controls. One study found no differences in ALT levels or histology between HIV-infected and HIV-uninfected patients, although hepatitis C virus (HCV) infection was not excluded in this cohort of primarily IVDU.[81] Using immunoperoxidase stains, hepatocyte staining for hepatitis B surface antigen (HBsAg), hepatitis B core antigen (HBcAg), and HBeAg may be striking in chronically infected patients despite minimal histologic changes.[82]

When stratified by absolute CD4 lymphocyte count, particularly in HBeAg-positive patients, there appears to be a positive correlation of hepatic injury with CD4 count.[73] Bodsworth and colleagues[73] evaluated the course of HBV infection in a large cohort of HIV-seropositive and HIV-seronegative patients. This study found that HIV-infected patients had much higher levels of HBV DNA but lower ALT levels. There was a correlation between the degree of hepatic injury and level of immune dysfunction; CD4 counts were higher in patients with higher ALT levels. Two studies using transaminase levels[79] and liver histology[80] found no differences, however, in ALT levels, HBV DNA levels, or prevalence of reactivation between HIV-infected patients with or without AIDS as compared to controls; HCV infection was not excluded. These conflicting results may be related to levels of CD8 cells. CD8 cells appear to be a major factor for cell-mediated immunity against HBV, and in patients with AIDS, CD8 cells remain relatively normal until very late in the course of the disease.[80] The duration of HBV infection before HIV infection or co-existence of hepatitis C also may be important.

Studies have shown that HIV-infected patients are more likely to lose antibodies to HBV as compared to seronegative controls[70] and to have lower antibody titers.[83] Some patients, who clear HbeAg and become positive for hepatitis B e antibody (anti-HBe), may have return of HBV DNA if they become infected with HIV.[78] Reactivation of disease[67,78] and even reinfection have been described; many of these patients were anti-HBs positive before reactivation. Bonacini and colleagues[80] found 16 percent of patients had reactivation during follow-up and that reactivation was associated with fulminant liver disease. In addition, a recent study found an increased frequency of positive, isolated anti-HBc (with undetectable anti-HBs) in HIV-infected individuals, which likely resulted from failure to develop anti-HBs in the context of immunodeficiency.[69] In this same study[69] 3 percent of HIV-positive and an equal percentage of HIV-negative individuals lost anti-HBs after a median follow-up of approximately 2 years. During follow-up only one HIV-positive patient with evidence of prior exposure to HBV developed elevated serum transaminase levels in association with a detectable HBsAg, HbeAg, and hepatitis delta antigen, suggesting reactivation or possibly reinfection.

Influence of HBV Infection on HIV Disease. Preliminary observations suggested that HBV infection altered the natural history of concomitant HIV infection and was a co-factor for disease progression.[84,85] However, a well-controlled study found that HBV infection had no effect on progression of HIV infection to AIDS.[86] Another recent study[87] also showed no difference in the rates of progression to AIDS or CD4 cell counts in untreated HIV/HBV co-infected patients compared to untreated HIV+/HBV− controls.

Therapy. Interferon-α therapy in HIV-infected patients has been associated with a poor response, which may be related to the overall immunosuppression associated with HIV, presence of inhibitory cytokines, or abnormalities of the interferon-α receptor.[88] Initial trials of interferon for patients with chronic HBV infection yielded a poor response in immunocompromised patients, including those co-infected with HIV.[89,90] Wong and colleagues[91] reported that a response to interferon in patients with HBV infection was likely to occur in only 20 percent of those co-infected with HIV compared to those who were HIV seronegative. The addition of single agent anti-retroviral therapy such as AZT does not appear to improve the efficacy of interferon in these patients.[92]

Lamivudine is a nucleoside analog that is effective in the treatment of chronic HBV infection in non–HIV-infected patients, leading to HBeAg seroconversion in approximately 17 percent at 12 months.[93] Although large controlled studies addressing the loss of HBeAg/HBsAg in HIV-infected individuals are lacking, lamivudine therapy has been associated with a decrease in HBV DNA in patients with co-infection.[94] Resistance of HBV to lamivudine has not been extensively documented in HIV-infected patients. Benhamou and colleagues[95] studied the long-term incidence of HBV resistance to lamivudine in HIV-positive patients. Sixty-six HIV/HBV co-infected patients were studied while they were receiving lamivudine as a part of anti-retroviral therapy. All these patients had a detectable serum HBV DNA at the beginning of therapy. After 2 months of lamivudine, HBV DNA became undetectable in 57 patients (86 percent), and 47 percent had sustained HBV DNA suppression after 2 years of lamivudine. HBV resistance developed because of a mutation at position 550 in the YMDD motif of the DNA polymerase. Patient age, associated protease inhibitor therapy, duration and stage of HIV disease, baseline serum HBV DNA levels, CD4 cell count, and serum ALT at baseline did not predict emergence of resistance to lamivudine. A small study[96] evaluated the effectiveness of combination interferon-α and lamivudine therapy at the time of initiation of anti-retroviral therapy in five co-infected patients. The investigators found that after 6 months of interferon and lamivudine, HBV DNA was undetectable, which was maintained in four patients at 12 months. One patient seroconverted and developed anti-HBs at 12 months. Conversely, severe flares of hepatitis B have been observed with the emergence of HBV mutants after discontinuation of lamivudine.[97,98]

Immune restoration with anti-retroviral therapy has been associated with an acute elevation of serum transaminases (flare) followed by HBV seroconversion, but this phenomenon appears to be relatively infrequent.[99,100]

Prevention. Given the increased prevalence of serologic markers of prior HBV exposure and the high incidence of

HBV infection, particularly among homosexual men and IVDU, vaccination has been recommended.[101] However, as with other immunosuppressed hosts, vaccination is often ineffective,[102,103] especially in those with a lower CD4 count.[103] Vaccination is associated with a reduced HBV antibody titer in homosexual men. Furthermore, Hadler and colleagues[72] found that HIV-infected homosexual men undergoing HBV vaccination, in whom co-incidental acute HBV infection occurred, had a chronicity rate of 56 percent to 80 percent depending on the number of doses of vaccine received. A recent study documented an improvement in response rate to HBV vaccination from 55 percent to 90 percent in HIV-infected individuals when initial nonresponders underwent a second course of monthly hepatitis B vaccine.[104] The reason for this poor response to vaccination in this group of patients is unknown but is perhaps related to immunosuppression and decreased CD4 cell counts. Conversely, the role of immune reconstitution with HAART before vaccination in the hopes of improving the response rate remains to be explored.

Hepatitis Delta Virus

Hepatitis delta virus (HDV) infection is uncommon in the United States as compared to other areas in the world, where prevalence rates of 45 percent (Italy) and 65 percent (Spain) are reported.[105,106] Positivity rates of 15 percent among homosexuals in Los Angeles have been found. Other areas of the United States have very low prevalence rates.[107] The primary risk factor for HDV infection is IVDU,[105] but the number of sexual partners may also play a role.[105,107] HIV infection abrogates the suppressive effects of HDV on HBV replication,[108,109] and HDV antigen clearance may be impaired in HIV-infected patients. Novick and colleagues[110] compared patients with HIV, HBV, and HDV co-infection to patients who had HBV and HDV alone or HIV and HBV alone. They found higher ALT levels in those with concurrent infections. Acute fulminant HBV/HDV co-infection has been reported in a patient with AIDS.[72,111] Given the high levels of HBV DNA associated with HBsAg in some AIDS patients, the data suggest that HDV-infected patients may be at higher risk for significant hepatic injury. However, these studies have not routinely excluded concurrent HCV infection. There is no evidence that HDV infection alters the natural history of HIV infection.[106]

Hepatitis C Virus

Epidemiology. The prevalence of HCV infection among HIV-infected patients is much more variable than HBV. The major risk factors for HCV infection are IVDU and transfusion of blood products.[66] The prevalence of HCV infection is highly dependent on the group studied; among homosexual or bisexual men prevalence rates vary from 1.6 percent to 11.7 percent[112,113] and among IVDU vary from 13 percent[112] to 40 percent.[113] HCV positivity is common in hemophiliacs, approaching 90 percent to 100 percent.[114] A prevalence study from New York[115] showed that a history of IVDU and hemophilia were associated with an increased risk of HCV in HIV/HCV co-infected patients, whereas isolated heterosexual contact was not. These data suggest that HCV infection is uncommon in homosexual men and confirm previous studies of the low transmission rate of HCV through sexual contact.[116] Initial studies documenting prevalence rates of HCV infection by enzyme-linked immunoassay in HIV-infected patients of 14 percent to 50 percent[117-119] may have been an overestimation because hypergammaglobulinemia causes a false positive reaction.[119] Indeed, using second- and third-generation assays with confirmation by recombinant immunoblot assay (RIBA) or HCV ribonucleic acid (RNA), seropositivity rates have approximated 10 percent in homosexual men. Conversely, some patients with HCV infection and co-existent HIV may lose HCV antibody over time,[120] thus potentially underestimating the true prevalence of HCV infection. An indeterminate RIBA is more common in HIV-infected than in uninfected patients and is associated with more frequent viremia (89 percent versus 50 percent).[122]

HCV infection has important implications for both HCV and HIV transmission. HIV infection increases the risk of sexual and parenteral transmission of HCV to HIV-seronegative female sex partners[121] and to newborns of HIV-infected mothers.[123,124] This increased transmission rate may reflect higher levels of HCV viremia in HIV-infected patients. This latter observation has been found to be associated with an increased risk of vertical transmission of HIV in newborns. A study was undertaken to investigate whether co-infection facilitates the heterosexual transmission of HCV. The investigators found that co-infected patients had higher levels of HCV RNA compared to HCV+/HIV− controls and that higher loads were associated with a higher risk of transmission, although statistical significance was not achieved.[125]

Natural History

Influence of HIV Infection on HCV Disease. The outcome of acute HCV infection in HIV-infected patients has only recently undergone investigation. There are no studies comparing the clinical presentation of acute HCV infection in HIV-infected versus HIV-uninfected patients. HCV infection acquired by blood transfusion in patients with AIDS has been associated with fulminant disease shortly after exposure.[126] On the other hand, HIV infection is an important co-factor in progression of chronic HCV disease. HCV RNA is more commonly detected and at higher levels in HIV-infected patients compared with HIV-negative controls,[118,120,121] which suggests an increased rate of viral replication or decreased clearance by the host, perhaps as a result of underlying immunosuppression. Nevertheless, ALT levels are not consistently higher in patients with higher RNA levels. Indeed, several studies have found no difference in ALT levels between HCV+/HIV+ as compared with HCV+/HIV− controls.[120] Nevertheless, histopathologic studies of liver biopsies demonstrate a higher degree of necroinflammatory activity and fibrosis in patients with HIV infection, especially in those with lower CD4 cell counts and HCV genotype 1b.[127,128]

A higher incidence and a more rapid progression to cirrhosis in HCV/HIV individuals have been suggested. Benhamou and colleagues[129] have shown that alcohol use and HIV seropositivity are independent risk factors for the development of cirrhosis in HCV infection. In another study[130] 25 percent of co-infected patients developed cirrhosis at 15 years compared with only 6 percent of HIV-negative patients. It was observed, however, that the incidence of cirrhosis in these groups was no different at 5 and 10 years.[130]

In a cohort study of 183 hemophiliacs in whom the first exposure to donor pool factor concentrates could be determined, follow-up demonstrated hepatic decompensation in 11 (10.8 percent) by 20 years; 10 of these patients were HIV-positive.[131] The median time from concentrate exposure to hepatic decompensation was 16.5 years (range, 7.7-22.9 years), yielding a risk for decompensation of 1.7 percent at 10 years and 10.8 percent at 20 years. For HIV-infected patients the risk of developing liver failure was 21.4 percent.The risk appeared to increase significantly after becoming P24 antigen-positive and was inversely associated with CD4 count. These results are similar to those of Eyster and colleagues.[132] In her cohort of 223 hemophiliacs in whom the date of HIV and HCV seroconversion could be determined, liver failure developed in 8 of 91 (8.8 percent) co-infected with HCV and HIV as compared with none of 58 patients infected with HCV alone.[132] Among the co-infected patients the cumulative incidence of liver failure was 27 percent 40 years after the first blood transfusion. In the 97 patients who were both HCV- and HIV-infected, the cumulative incidence of liver failure was 17 percent 10 years after acquiring HIV infection, and patients developing liver failure had lower median CD4 counts. In another cohort of patients with hemophilia[133] the cumulative risk of death from liver disease and hepatocellular carcinoma was 6.5 percent in co-infected patients at all ages 25 years after the first exposure to potentially infected blood products compared to 1.4 percent in HCV+/HIV− patients. A more recent study[134] of 310 hemophiliacs from England showed that progression rates to death 25 years after exposure to HCV were 57 percent for any cause mortality and 21 percent for liver disease-related mortality in HIV/HCV co-infected patients compared with rates of 8 percent and 3 percent, respectively, in HIV-negative patients. In addition to HIV co-infection, other factors associated with a higher risk of death in this cohort included HCV genotype 1 and increased age at HCV infection.

Eyster and colleagues[135] showed that the level of HCV RNA increased in the first 2 years after HIV infection and overall increased threefold during the study period. There was a significant correlation between HCV RNA levels, low CD4 counts, and AST levels. Using a branched chain DNA assay Cribier and colleagues[120] and Sherman and colleagues[136] also found higher levels of HCV RNA in HIV-infected as compared to HIV-seronegative HCV-positive patients. There was no correlation of the level of HCV with branched chain DNA assays for HIV, and the CD4 count did not correlate with the level of viremia.[120,136] In addition, they found the antibody response to HCV was decreased, probably accounting for some cases of false negative results of the RIBA assay.[120] This study,[120] however, evaluated HCV-infected patients who were primarily IVDU rather than hemophiliacs.

In summary, the preponderance of data show that co-infected patients, especially hemophiliacs, have a greater incidence of progression to cirrhosis and liver-related complications. The mechanisms by which HIV potentiates liver injury from HCV in these latter patients are unknown but may result from a longer period of HCV infection, HCV genotype, or possibly greater levels of viremia. Thus the findings of Wright and colleagues[113] of no increase in mortality in co-infected patients may point to the short duration of HCV infection. The impact of HCV in other immunosuppressive states is illustrated in liver transplant patients with HCV. HCV RNA levels increase with immunosuppressive therapy in these patients, and cirrhosis may occur in up to 8 percent of transplant recipients at 5 years.[137]

Influence of HCV Infection on HIV Disease. The influence of chronic HCV infection on the natural history of HIV and AIDS is less certain. Some studies find no relationship between HCV infection and progression of HIV disease. In a long-term study of 416 HIV-infected non-AIDS patients there was no increased risk for progression to AIDS or CD4 count less than 100/mm^3 for those co-infected with HCV.[138] In a retrospective analysis[139] comparing clinical outcomes in co-infected veterans versus HIV+/HCV− veterans, there was no difference between the cohorts in the time to progression from the diagnosis of HIV to the diagnosis of AIDS and time from the diagnosis of HIV or AIDS to death. One long-term study[113] of HIV+/HCV+ patients found no difference in mortality compared to HIV+/HCV− controls at a median follow-up of 60 months, suggesting that HCV had no independent effect on outcome in AIDS patients. The Italian Seroconversion Study[140] prospectively followed 416 acute HIV seroconverters. Although co-infection with HCV was present in 51.4 percent of participants, these patients also did not experience increased rates of clinical or immunologic progression. In contrast, Sabin and colleagues[141] found that co-infected patients with HCV genotype 1 experienced a more rapid progression to AIDS and death, which was independent of the age at HIV seroconversion, presence of hemophilia, or changes in CD4 cell counts. The authors explain their findings on the basis of increased HIV replication resulting from HCV-triggered CD4 cell proliferation in the liver. Another study[142] did not find significant immunologic progression of HIV disease in co-infected patients versus HIV+/HCV− controls. The authors did identify an increased rate of progression of clinical disease (30 percent or more decrease in Karnofsky's index, 20 percent loss of body weight, AIDS-defining illness or death) in co-infected patients, especially those with an initial CD4 cell count above 600 cells per mm^3. These authors subsequently explored the role of HCV genotype in the clinical and immunologic progression and concluded that HCV genotype was not an important determinant.[143]

A recent prospective study[144] showed that the probability of death or an AIDS-defining illness was increased in HIV-positive individuals with HCV seropositivity. In addition, the degree of CD4 cell recovery after institution of highly active anti-retroviral therapy was smaller. The mechanisms by which HCV infection may interfere with

CD4 cell recovery in patients receiving HAART are unknown, but explanations include HCV-related alteration in the production of CD4 cells or increased apoptosis of CD4 cells.[145]

In summary, the influence of chronic HCV infection on the natural history of HIV and AIDS is controversial. Further studies are recommended to better define the role of HCV in HIV, especially in the setting of HAART.

Influence of HAART. Some studies have shown that the incidence of anti-retroviral-associated liver enzyme elevations and hepatic dysfunction is increased in co-infected patients.[146] Anti-retrovirals such as zidovudine and protease inhibitors such as indinavir have been associated with hepatotoxicity, which ranges from mild hyperbilirubinemia and transaminase elevations to overt liver failure. Some studies have suggested that co-infected patients are also at increased risk of drug hepatotoxicity compared with HCV patients, but, overall, clinically important toxicity appears to be relatively infrequent.[147,148] A recent preliminary observation reported that the incidence of severe hepatotoxicity associated with the use of non-nucleoside reverse transcriptase inhibitors in co-infected patients was similar to the rates observed in HIV+/HCV− patients, but the occurrence of minor elevations in transaminase levels was more common in co-infected patients.[149] The mechanisms of increased hepatotoxicity are unknown. Possible explanations include viral interference (HCV replication facilitated by HIV inhibition), decreased endogenous interferon levels, and immune reconstitution.[150] A study[151] showed that patients with persistently undetectable HIV viral load after institution of HAART frequently developed an increase in ALT that correlated with an increased number of CD8 cells, suggesting T-cell–mediated cytotoxicity. Immune restoration after HAART has been associated with an increase in HCV RNA replication, worsening liver inflammation, and histology and development of hepatic decompensation.[152] Other studies,[153] however, have failed to show an increase in transaminase levels or any changes in HCV RNA associated with HAART.

In summary, anti-retrovirals can be administered safely to co-infected patients with special attention to close monitoring of liver function. Further research into the mechanisms of drug hepatotoxicity and the effects of immune reconstitution is needed.

Therapy. Since the advent of HAART therapy, survival for HIV-infected patients has improved substantially. Given the apparent aggressive course of HCV infection and the potential for increased end-stage liver disease–related mortality in these patients, consideration for anti-HCV therapy is warranted. Indications and contraindications for treating HCV in this population are similar to those that apply to HIV-negative patients.

Several small trials have evaluated the efficacy of interferon-α monotherapy in co-infected patients. The observed end-of-treatment response rates vary between 22 percent and 55 percent with sustained response rates of 0 percent to 44 percent. Unfortunately, dissimilarities between interferon dosing schedules, length of therapy, and definition of response (biochemical versus virologic) exist between these studies. In the largest study,[154] a sustained virologic response was observed in 20 percent of patients treated with interferon for 12 months and was associated with CD4 cell counts of more than 500 cells/mm^3. The role of combination therapy with interferon-α and ribavirin in co-infected patients is currently under investigation.[155-158] Landau and colleagues[158] treated 20 co-infected patients with combination therapy for 6 months; 10 exhibited a virologic end-of-treatment response. However, the sustained response rate was not reported, the study population was heterogeneous (i.e., prior non-responders, cirrhotics), and patients infected with HCV genotype 1 were only treated for 6 months instead of the customary 12 months.[157] Another study[156] evaluated the efficacy of combination therapy administered for 6 months in 21 co-infected individuals who had either failed to achieve a response (20 patients) or had relapsed (1 patient) after initial interferon monotherapy. End-of-treatment and sustained response was achieved in 6 (28.6 percent) and 3 patients (14.3 percent), respectively. Interestingly, HIV viral load and CD4 counts did not significantly change after 6 months of combination therapy when compared with pretreatment values.

There is concern about an increased incidence of side effects related to treating HCV in co-infected patients, particularly the development of anemia in patients receiving ribavirin. Also, interaction of this latter drug with zidovudine, zalcitabine, stavudine, and didanosine may decrease anti-HIV activity or increase concentrations of anti-retrovirals and potential for toxicity. A recent study[155] evaluated the effects of ribavirin in a cohort of co-infected patients receiving anti-HCV combination therapy on stable doses of anti-retrovirals. After 6 months of combination therapy, HIV viral load remained stable and 50 percent of patients experienced a 10 percent to 25 percent decline in the absolute number of CD4 cells. This study and others[158] suggest that although ribavirin may inhibit the phosphorylation of reverse transcriptase inhibitors in vitro and in vivo, ribavirin does not appear to detrimentally affect their anti-retroviral efficacy. No important drug interactions between ribavirin and nucleoside analogs have been noted.[159]

Hepatitis E

Hepatitis E virus (HEV) has been described, primarily in epidemics in immunocompetent patients. One report documented an increased seroprevalence of HEV antibodies (anti-HEV) in HIV-infected as compared to seronegative homosexual men and IVDU.[160] Nevertheless, only 2 of 66 patients were antibody-positive. The high seroprevalence in this one study may be the result of non-specific anti-HIV reactivity when compared to other confirmatory tests. In another study from Russia[161] anti-HEV was found in 11.1 percent of HIV-infected individuals compared to only 1.7 percent of the general population and in 8 percent of non–HIV-infected prisoners. This study also found that the prevalence of anti-HEV increased through successive stages of HIV progression;

43.3 percent of patients with AIDS tested positive. Other studies have failed to show an increased prevalence of anti-HEV in HIV-infected patients.[162] Further studies will be necessary to better characterize the clinical epidemiology, presentation, natural history, and outcome of HEV infection in patients with HIV and AIDS.

Hepatitis G

Hepatitis G virus (HGV) is a recently recognized flavivirus. Infection with HGV is prevalent but is not known to be associated with any chronic disease in healthy individuals. In a study from Spain HGV RNA was been found in 14 percent of individuals infected with HIV compared with only 3 percent of healthy blood donors.[163] A study from the United States[164] found HGV RNA in 23 percent of frozen plasma samples from 192 HIV-infected patients and no difference in the frequency of liver enzyme abnormalities, CD4 counts, or HIV viral load between HGV RNA-positive patients and HGV RNA-negative patients. One study[165] found that HIV-infected hemophiliacs infected with HGV had higher CD4+ lymphocyte counts and 12-year AIDS-free survival rates compared with HGV-negative patients; the significance of these findings is unknown. Therefore although the clinical role of HGV in HIV-infected individuals is understudied and unclear, available data suggest that adverse outcomes from liver disease are unlikely.

HIV

HIV has been identified in liver tissue. In vitro studies show that human Kupffer cells and sinusoidal endothelial cells may be infected in culture, probably via CD4 cell receptors.[166,167] Immunohistochemical studies of liver tissue have demonstrated HIV within Kupffer cells, although rarely within hepatocytes.[168] However, using polymerase chain reaction (PCR), HIV RNA has not been demonstrated consistently in all patients, and no correlations between hepatic histology and concentrations of HIV RNA have been shown.[169,170] Given these findings, it is unclear whether HIV infection of the liver causes non-specific histopathologic abnormalities, dysfunction of Kupffer cells, or serves as a reservoir of viral production.

Cytomegalovirus

Despite being the most common opportunistic infection in AIDS, clinically apparent liver disease caused by CMV is rare. CMV has been demonstrated in liver tissue in up to 9 percent in some series.[10] Although most studies report prevalence rates of less than 5 percent, autopsy studies tend to have higher rates of identification.[171] Histologically, CMV is usually observed in sinusoidal endothelial cells, often with a minimal inflammatory response. It is unclear what role CMV has in causing liver test abnormalities or clinical symptoms. Rarely, CMV may present as acute hepatitis; in these circumstances, anti-viral therapy for CMV results in clinical cure.[27]

Miscellaneous Viral Diseases

Varicella zoster has been reported in a patient with AIDS who developed a clinical picture of hepatitis.[172] Despite prophylaxis with acyclovir, this patient developed chicken pox with severe visceral involvement including acute hepatitis, progressive liver failure, and death. Epstein-Barr virus also may produce acute hepatitis. A single report of hemophagocytic syndrome was described in an HIV-infected patient who presented with fever, abnormal liver tests, and pancytopenia.[173]

Mycobacterial Infections

Mycobacterium Avium *Complex*

Organisms of MAC, *M. avium* and *M. intracellulare,* are among the most common opportunistic infections in patients with AIDS, occurring in up to 43 percent of these patients before the era of HAART.[174-176] The organism is ubiquitous in the environment, and disseminated infection appears to result from recent infection rather than reactivation of previous infection.[177] The gastrointestinal tract and lung are important portals of entry from which the organism may disseminate; culture positivity for MAC in sputum or stool is highly predictive of subsequent dissemination.[178] The major risk factor for infection is the level of immune dysfunction; the mean CD4 count in infected patients is 60/mm^3, with infection rare above 100/mm.[4,35,179] The use of PCP prophylaxis appears to be a significant risk factor for the development of MAC, increasing the prevalence of MAC as the index AIDS illness from 2 percent to 12 percent.[5]

Clinical features that are highly suggestive of disseminated MAC include high fever, anemia, night sweats, diarrhea, and weight loss greater than 10 percent.[179] Abdominal pain, hepatomegaly, and increased alkaline phosphatase are frequently present. Studies evaluating clinical features and diagnostic methods have identified severe anemia (in fewer than 30 percent) and elevated alkaline phosphatase to be predictive of disseminated disease.[179] Another study found that a CD4 count lower than 50/mm^3, fever for more than 30 days, anemia (in fewer than 30 percent), and a serum albumin concentration of less than 3 g/dl to be most predictive, with a 92 percent specificity.[180]

Although the spleen is the most common site of dissemination, the liver is frequently involved as well (Plate 51-1).[181,182] Lymph nodes and bone marrow are also common sites of involvement and play an important role in the clinical expression of disseminated disease. Interestingly, up to 30 percent of patients with MAC bacteremia will have no evidence of MAC at postmortem examination.[183,184]

As previously mentioned, series evaluating liver disease in AIDS have found MAC in from 1 percent to 30 percent of patients.[10,25] Histologically, granulomas often are present but are usually poorly formed (see Plate 51-1).[181,183] Foamy blue histiocytes are the histologic hallmark of MAC infection.[181,183] Mycobacterial staining of biopsy tissue often demonstrates striking numbers of mycobacteria and may be positive in the absence of granulomas. Culture of liver tissue appears to be more sensitive than histology and may be positive in the absence of organisms by special stains.

Because positivity by blood culture may take several weeks, a search for more rapid diagnostic methods has been undertaken. In one study liver biopsy appeared to be more sensitive than bone marrow examination; the diagnosis was established histologically in 75 percent of liver biopsies as compared to 25 percent from bone marrow in patients with documented MAC. Both techniques yielded similar results by culture.[185]

Abdominal imaging may be helpful in suggesting disseminated MAC. Liver and splenic involvement is usually diffuse, causing hepatosplenomegaly; focal abnormalities are rarely identified. Lymphadenopathy is prominent. In contrast to tuberculosis (TB), the involved nodes infrequently have central necrosis.[186]

Before HAART the long-term survival after the diagnosis of disseminated MAC was poor, with a median survival of 3 to 6 months.[179] As with most opportunistic infections, survival has been substantially improved with HAART, and some patients may discontinue long-term anti-mycobacterial therapy.[187,188]

Mycobacterium Tuberculosis

The advent of the AIDS epidemic has been associated with a dramatic resurgence in the prevalence of MTB. Unlike MAC, MTB may occur in earlier stages of immunodeficiency, often with CD4 counts higher than 200/mm^3. Epidemiologically, TB is more common in IVDU and nonwhites than in other risk groups.[189] MTB is also found more frequently in liver tissue from patients residing in developing countries.[190-192] In most patients, disease results from reactivation, not from primary infection. Regardless of the stage of immunodeficiency, pulmonary disease is the most common presentation. With progressive immunodeficiency, however, extrapulmonary manifestations become more frequent[192] and may include involvement of almost any organ. As with MAC, hepatic involvement occurs almost exclusively in the setting of disseminated disease. Liver involvement may be suspected by liver test abnormalities (raised alkaline phosphatase) in the setting of disseminated TB. Similar to MAC, clinical expression of liver disease is rare. Focal liver disease may present with right upper quadrant abdominal pain and fever.[193,194]

Computed tomography (CT) findings of disseminated MTB include lymphadenopathy with central necrosis.[186] In contrast to MAC,[195] focal lesions often occur in other organs and may be necrotic. Hepatic MTB should be suspected when liver lesions are necrotic and when there is associated intra-abdominal adenopathy. Pulmonary disease may be absent.[196] The diagnosis may be established by fine needle aspiration of liver lesions with appropriate staining. Blood cultures are often positive.

Unlike the therapy for MAC, multi-drug regimens for TB yield a clinical and microbiologic cure. Relapse of infection is infrequent. Monitoring of the liver tests in select patients is important so that hepatotoxicity can be detected early. In the HIV-infected patient with a positive PPD, prophylactic therapy with isoniazid has been recommended.[197,198] Although decreasing the incidence of both pulmonary and disseminated tuberculosis, liver toxicity occurs in $\approx$ 10 percent of patients.[199,200]

Fungal Diseases

Despite the prevalence of fungal diseases of other organ systems in AIDS, involvement of the liver is uncommon clinically. Fungal diseases have important differences in prevalence based on the epidemiologic and geographic setting. For example, disseminated histoplasmosis is much more common in the central United States, whereas coccidioidomycosis is a common opportunistic pathogen in the Southwest.

Cryptococcal meningitis is a frequent AIDS-defining illness and is the most common fungus reported to involve the liver.[25] Disseminated disease involving the lung, liver, or bone marrow is uncommon. Amphotericin B is effective for acute disease, whereas fluconazole is administered chronically to maintain a remission.

Disseminated histoplasmosis may involve a variety of organ systems at the time of presentation. In immunocompetent hosts, pulmonary involvement is the most common manifestation; pulmonary involvement is observed in approximately 60 percent of AIDS patients with disseminated histoplasmosis.[201] The most common clinical presentation is recurrent high fever. In some patients there is a clinical picture consistent with disseminated intravascular coagulation.[201,202] Liver involvement is suggested by the presence of abnormal liver function tests, but a clinical presentation of isolated liver disease alone has not been reported. The diagnosis can be established by staining of peripheral blood smears in which the organism may be observed in polymorphonuclear leukocytes, bone marrow biopsy, and occasionally liver biopsy. Bone marrow biopsy with culture may be diagnostic for disseminated histoplasmosis in 60 percent to 90 percent.[201-203] There are no studies comparing the sensitivity of bone marrow biopsy to liver biopsy for the detection of disseminated disease. Blood cultures are usually positive with disseminated disease. Amphotericin B and itraconazole are effective for acute treatment and chronic prophylaxis, respectively. Without immune reconstitution with HAART, as with other opportunistic infections, long-term maintenance anti-fungal therapy is required to maintain a remission.

Hepatic blastomycosis and coccidioidomycosis are rare.[204-205] Because liver disease occurs during widespread dissemination, examination of tissues other than the liver such as bone marrow, lung, or skin or blood cultures usually establishes the diagnosis. In contrast to other immunocompromised hosts, candidal involvement of the liver is very rare.[206]

Bacterial Infections

Bacterial infections of the liver are rare. An unusual bacterial cause of liver disease in patients with bacterial infection is peliosis hepatis. Early in the AIDS epidemic, dilated vascular lakes on liver biopsy, termed *peliosis,* were considered non-specific. In 1989 Perkocha and coworkers[207] identified a bacterium (*Bartonella henselae*) by PCR that is now considered responsible for this disorder. Patients with marked immunodeficiency are at greatest risk and present with disseminated disease involving the skin, bones, and liver similar to cat scratch fever.[208-210] Fever, abdominal pain, and hepatosplenomegaly are common with hepatic involvement.[211] The serum alkaline phosphatase is usually markedly elevated. Abdominal CT scan may demonstrate hepatomegaly with low-density lesions representing these vascular lakes. Biopsy of these lesions reveals vascular channels, and specific stains (Warthin-Starry) aid in identifying the bacteria. Culture of liver tissue also may be positive. Antibiotic therapy with doxycycline or erythromycin is usually effective; relapse may occur.

Protozoal Infections

Protozoa are distinctly uncommon hepatic pathogens. Although rare cases of microsporidial or cryptosporidial hepatitis have been described,[212,213] cryptosporidia and microsporidia typically involve the biliary tree rather than hepatic parenchyma (see the following section).[214] Disseminated *P. carinii* may involve the liver,[215,216] usually in patients using inhaled pentamidine to prevent PCP. Rarely, disseminated disease has been reported in patients taking low-dose trimethoprim-sulfamethoxazole for PCP prophylaxis. Liver involvement is diffuse and thus hepatic mass lesions by CT are uncommon. However, a peculiar radiographic appearance of punctate calcifications of the spleen on ultrasound (US) or CT has been noted,[217] as have focal splenic lesions resembling neoplasms.[216] *Isospora belli* has been reported to cause hepatitis, although it is linked more frequently to biliary disease and cholecystitis (see the following section). Unusual protozoal causes of liver disease include *Leishmania*,[218] *Toxoplasma*,[219] and *Schistosoma* organisms.

Neoplasms

Neoplasms are an important cause of liver disease. Their importance stems from the fact that neoplasms may be the initial manifestation of AIDS and can present with isolated liver involvement. NHL occurs in up to 2.3 percent of HIV-infected patients[220]; this rate has not fallen in the HAART era.[221-224] In contrast to immunocompetent hosts, lymphomas commonly present in extranodal sites in HIV-infected patients. Large studies of patients with HIV-associated lymphoma have found a primary presentation in the liver in 9 percent to 16 percent of patients.[225] In addition, autopsy studies have frequently found hepatic lymphoma, which was unsuspected antemortem.[37,38,226] These tumors occasionally may be observed at an earlier stage of immunodeficiency with CD4 counts of more than 200/mm^3. Hepatic lymphoma is usually manifested by abnormal liver tests, often with striking elevations of the alkaline phosphatase or LDH; jaundice is common.[10,227] Hepatomegaly with or without abdominal pain is frequent, although fever is inconsistent. Peripheral lymphadenopathy is uncommon.

Abdominal US is frequently diagnostic, but abdominal CT is the diagnostic modality of choice for neoplasms.[228,229] Liver involvement appears as one or more focal lesions of variable size (see Figure 51-1). Abdominal lymphadenopathy and splenic involvement are common, whereas mediastinal adenopathy is rare. Magnetic resonance imaging also may be diagnostic. Percutaneous, radiographically directed biopsy of mass lesions safely and reliably establishes the diagnosis. The success rate of chemotherapeutic regimens for NHL is variable, with response rates of more than 50 percent. Complications from chemotherapy are frequent given the underlying immunodeficiency. The long-term prognosis depends on the stage of immunodeficiency rather than the lymphoma itself.

Early in the AIDS epidemic KS was recognized as a common initial manifestation of HIV infection. Similar to NHL, cutaneous KS may appear when the CD4 count is higher than 200/mm^3. Recent evidence strongly supports an infectious etiology resulting from human herpesvirus 8 (HHV-8).[230,231] This virus has also been found in non–HIV-related KS tissue, and its presence in saliva, semen, and prostate tissue suggests the infection may be transmitted sexually.[231,232] Epidemiologically, this tumor is confined primarily to homosexual men. KS is decreasing in incidence, likely because of changes in sexual practices among high-risk patients.[5,233,234] Cutaneous involvement is the most common presentation; rarely, visceral involvement occurs without cutaneous disease. Luminal gastrointestinal disease is common and usually asymptomatic. Hepatic KS is most often clinically silent; autopsy series have identified KS with prevalence rates of up to 22 percent.[10,15] Chemotherapy is relatively effective in controlling disease.[233] Tumor regression has been observed with HAART therapy alone.[233]

Several other tumors involving the liver have been reported in HIV-infected patients, including metastatic adenocarcinoma, melanoma, and hepatoma. Whether the last tumor is related to HIV infection or a complication of other diseases (e.g., HCV) is unknown.

Miscellaneous

Several uncommon liver disorders have been described in HIV-infected patients. It is unclear whether these disorders were specifically related to HIV infection, epidemiologic factors such as risk group, or just an incidental finding. Amyloidosis was found in 5 of 12 patients with AIDS and a history of injection drug use.[235] Clinically these patients presented with hepatomegaly. Underlying myeloma or plasma cell dyscrasia was not identified in any patient. Iron overload has been identified in HIV-infected patients, many of whom received multiple blood transfusions.[236]

Causes of Ascites

Ascites is an uncommon problem in HIV-infected patients. The most common cause of ascites in these patients is cirrhosis and portal hypertension secondary to chronic viral hepatitis.[237] However, opportunistic infections and neoplasms, usually from disseminated disease with peritoneal involvement, account for 25 percent of ascites in patients with HIV.

A syndrome of non-specific peritonitis has been described.[238] Affected patients present with abdominal pain and overt ascites. Ascitic fluid analysis demonstrates high protein concentrations and leukocytosis but no identifiable pathogens. Laparoscopy and laparotomy also fail to disclose a specific etiology. In some patients adhesions and peritonitis were found. The cause of peritoneal disease in these patients is unknown.

Differences in the clinical presentation or ascitic fluid findings between HIV-infected and non-infected patients have been observed.[237] Paracentesis is the most important initial test for evaluating infection and measuring protein concentration. In addition, patients with high-protein ascites should have bacterial, fungal, and mycobacterial cultures performed on the ascitic fluid. Gram staining may be useful to identify bacterial or parasitic disorders.[239] Patients with high-protein ascites also should have a sample submitted for cytologic analysis to exclude NHL.[238] The presence of chylous ascites suggests underlying disruption of the lymphatic system caused by KS[240] or TB.[241] For those patients with high-protein ascites, particularly when it is associated with leukocytosis and absence of pathogens, CT may be useful for identifying peritoneal mass lesions (e.g., NHL) or other intra-abdominal processes. Mass lesions may then be biopsied percutaneously under CT guidance. Laparoscopy with inspection of the liver and peritoneum may be useful when other tests are non-diagnostic.[242]

Biliary Tract Abnormalities

Disorders of the biliary tree in AIDS patients were first reported in 1986.[243] Subsequently, Schneiderman and coworkers reported similar features in eight patients.[244] In both series the clinical presentation consisted of fever, right upper quadrant pain, and striking elevations of the serum alkaline phosphatase; endoscopic retrograde cholangiopancreatography (ERCP) demonstrated intrahepatic or extrahepatic changes characteristic of sclerosing cholangitis or papillary stenosis. Since these seminal observations, a number of studies[245-251] from around the world have documented this disorder, now termed *AIDS cholangiopathy*.

Etiology

The cause of ductal disease in most patients is an infection. Liver biopsies, including biliary ductal epithelium, biopsies of the common bile duct or papilla after endoscopic sphincterotomy, biliary brushings and cytology, and periampullary small bowel biopsies have all identified an infectious cause. The most frequent identifiable pathogens are *Cryptosporidium* organisms[245,248,251-253]; other infectious causes include microsporidia (i.e., *Enterocytozoon bieneusi, Septata intestinalis*),[254-256] *Cyclospora* organisms,[257] CMV, and MAC. Based on autopsy studies and bile duct biopsies at the time of ERCP, these infections cause severe inflammatory changes that result secondarily in the observed cholangiographic abnormalities.[243,253,258] However, in a substantial number of patients, no cause can be found. Non-infectious causes of biliary disease, both benign and malignant, include stones and strictures.

Cholangiographic Patterns

The typical cholangiographic finding is papillary stenosis in association with intrahepatic sclerosing cholangitis occurring in approximately 50 percent of patients with AIDS cholangiopathy syndrome (Table 51-3, Figure 51-2). The next most frequent pattern is intrahepatic and extrahepatic sclerosing cholangitis without papillary stenosis, followed by papillary stenosis alone, or intrahepatic sclerosing cholangitis alone. Isolated strictures of the common bile duct may result from primary common bile duct lymphoma[257] or pancreatic disease caused by chronic pancreatitis, infections, or neoplasms.

Clinical Presentations

The most common presentation of AIDS cholangiopathy is right upper quadrant pain; papillary stenosis is usually present in patients with severe pain and clinical cholangitis. Intrahepatic cholangitis without papillary stenosis typically results in milder pain or may be asymptomatic. Because of the small bowel involvement, patients with cryptosporidia or microsporidia frequently complain of diarrhea. Asymptomatic elevation of liver tests may be the first clue to the diagnosis. Serum alkaline phosphatase is usually elevated, with mean values in most series of 700 to 800 IU/L. Mild increases in ALT are common, although jaundice is rare. In one series[260] liver tests were normal in 20 percent of patients with documented disease by cholangiography.[249]

TABLE 51-3
Cholangiographic Patterns Described in AIDS Cholangiopathy

Reference no.	N	SC/PS	SC	PS	Other
247	4	4	—	—	—
252	20	10	4	3	3
245	15	8	5	1	—
250	8	1	7	—	—
248	26	19	7	—	—
251	45	23	12	4	6

AIDS, Acquired immunodeficiency syndrome; *N*, number of patients in the study; *SC*, sclerosing cholangitis; *PS*, papillary stenosis.

Diagnosis

When using ERCP as the gold standard, US has a sensitivity of approximately 75 percent to 87 percent[245,252] and may demonstrate striking ductal thickening in some patients.[178] HIDA scanning may suggest biliary obstruction when there is delayed excretion of the tracer.[261,262] In the symptomatic patient without jaundice US should be the initial study, with CT reserved for the jaundiced patient in whom intrahepatic masses, abdominal adenopathy, or biliary dilation might be identified.[27] When US or CT are negative, ERCP may be required to confirm the diagnosis and for endoscopic therapy (e.g., sphincterotomy) or biopsy.

Treatment

Treatment of AIDS cholangiopathy is primarily endoscopic. For those patients with abdominal pain or cholangitis associated with papillary stenosis, endoscopic sphincterotomy generally provides symptomatic benefit. Three reports[245,248,252] described long-term relief of symptoms in 70 percent to 100 percent of patients after sphincterotomy for papillary stenosis. In another study, however, a symptomatic response was noted in only 32 percent of patients.[251] Co-existent pancreatic disease may be responsible for incomplete pain relief in some patients.[264] Despite successful sphincterotomy, the serum alkaline phosphatase may continue to rise during long-term follow-up because of progression of associated intrahepatic sclerosing cholangitis.[265] Complications of sphincterotomy in AIDS patients with papillary stenosis and a dilated common bile duct do not appear to be higher than in other groups. There is no evidence that sphincterotomy is beneficial for sclerosing cholangitis in the absence of papillary stenosis and common bile duct dilation. It may be associated with a higher complication rate. For those with a dominant common bile duct stricture, endoscopic stenting or balloon dilation is appropriate.

Patients with diffuse intrahepatic and extrahepatic sclerosing cholangitis alone have no specific treatment options. Although this disorder is usually infectious, medical therapy for cryptosporidia or microsporidia has failed to improve biliary symptoms or cholangiographic abnormalities, probably because the drugs lack efficacy. A profile patient with cryptosporidial cholangitis had clinical, laboratory, and cholangiographic improvement with paromomycin and letrazuril.[266] Despite the efficacy of ganciclovir, CMV-induced biliary disease has not responded to this agent. Trimethoprim-sulfamethoxazole has been curative for cholangitis caused by *Cyclospora* organisms.[257] Although experimental, some have used ursodeoxycholic acid with improvement in liver tests and diminution of pain. The effects of HAART on the natural history of this disorder have not been well described. However, as with other opportunistic processes in AIDS, the frequency of this entity has fallen coincident with the introduction of HAART.

Gallbladder Disease

As with AIDS-associated sclerosing cholangitis, disorders of the gallbladder are caused primarily by infections; *I. belli,* CMV, cryptosporidia, microsporidia, and *Candida albicans* are reported etiologies.[267-271] The most common manifestation of gallbladder disease is acalculous cholecystitis, although symptomatic cholelithiasis may also be seen.[272] The clinical presentation of acalculous cholecystitis includes right upper quadrant pain and fever; abnormal liver tests suggest concomitant sclerosing cholangitis. US may demonstrate a thickened gallbladder wall, pericholecystic fluid, stones, or ductular abnormalities.[262] Isotopic imaging study (HIDA scan) is often diagnostic, demonstrating absence of uptake into the gallbladder

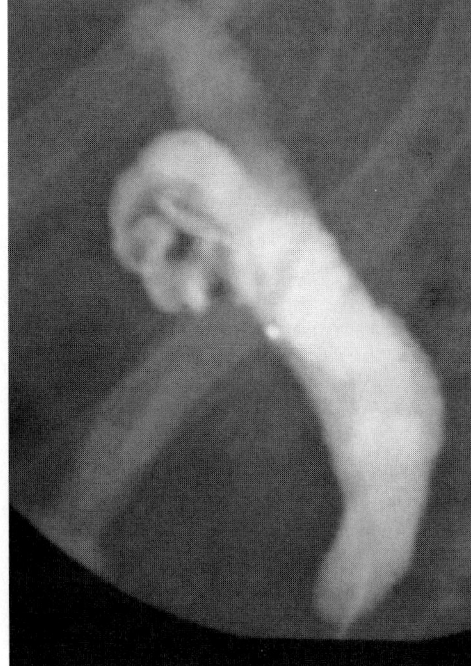

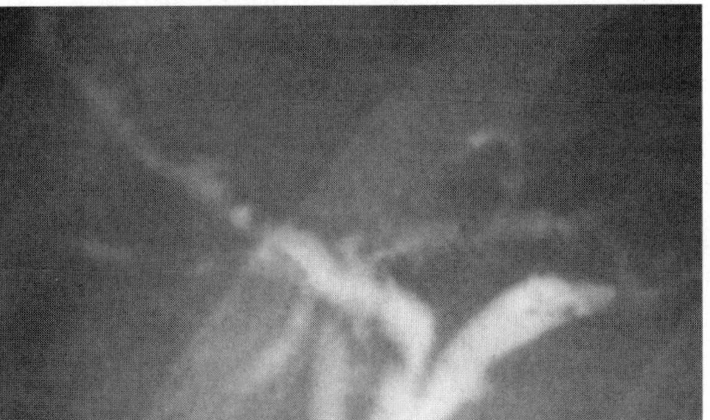

Figure 51-2 AIDS cholangiopathy. **A,** The common bile duct and cystic duct are markedly dilated to the level of the ampulla. There is also nodularity of the duct. **B,** The intrahepatic ducts have areas of stricture and dilation typical for sclerosing cholangitis. A biliary sphincterotomy was performed. *AIDS,* Acquired immunodeficiency syndrome.

despite imaging of the common bile duct.[273] Laparoscopic cholecystectomy is curative and may be associated with less postoperative morbidity than is open cholecystectomy, particularly in malnourished patients.[274,275]

Approach to the Diagnosis of Hepatobiliary Disease

The evaluation of hepatobiliary disease in HIV-infected patients should be tailored to the presenting symptoms and signs, pattern of liver test abnormalities, and severity of immunodeficiency as indicated by the CD4 lymphocyte count. Patients with a CD4 lymphocyte count higher than 200/mm^3 are unlikely to have an opportunistic infection, although some infections (e.g., MTB) and neoplasms including NHL and KS may occur at only modest levels of immunodeficiency. Striking ALT elevations suggest hepatitis possibly due to drugs or viral disease depending on the clinical setting. Alcoholic liver disease generally can be suspected by the history, physical examination, and pattern of liver test abnormalities. Disproportionate elevations of alkaline phosphatase suggest infiltrative disorders or biliary tract disease. Marked elevations of serum alkaline phosphatase are common, having been reported in 17 percent of 90 consecutive AIDS patients in one series.[276] The majority of these patients had no obvious identifiable biliary or hepatocellular disease, although liver biopsy and ERCP were not performed in all patients. Jaundice results most commonly from drug-induced hepatitis, high-grade biliary obstruction, or NHL[20]; jaundice occurs in fewer than 10 percent of patients with AIDS cholangiopathy.

Abdominal imaging studies provide valuable diagnostic information. Patients with marked ALT elevations, however, benefit little from these studies, given the likelihood of hepatitis. In unselected patients undergoing US, most of whom had abnormal liver tests, the studies were abnormal in many patients.[278] Identified abnormalities included both gallbladder and biliary disease and hepatosplenomegaly and hepatomegaly alone. CT is most useful to evaluate possible mass lesions, adenopathy, peliosis, and peritoneal diseases. Infections resulting in diffuse parenchymal liver disease such as TB, MAC, and parasitic diseases rarely show focal abnormalities in these studies. The utility of US as compared to CT in various clinical settings has not been well studied. We employ US in the anicteric patient in whom AIDS cholangiopathy is suspected. We reserve CT for patients with marked hepatomegaly, jaundice, suspected mass lesions, or intra-abdominal processes.

ERCP is most helpful in the patient with biliary ductal dilation when endoscopic therapy is likely. ERCP is also useful in the patient with abdominal or right upper quadrant pain accompanied by marked abnormalities of alkaline phosphatase in whom the US or CT is normal. However, ERCP should be reserved for the symptomatic patient in whom endoscopic therapy is likely. ERCP is also appropriate when bile duct stones are considered.

The role of percutaneous liver biopsy in HIV-infected patients with abnormal liver tests continues to evolve. Studies employing liver biopsy early in the AIDS epidemic revealed a variety of hepatic pathologies; nevertheless, few studies evaluated the effect of the liver biopsy findings on outcome. In one study[10] liver biopsy rarely uncovered disorders not identified in other tissues. As mentioned previously, the majority of opportunistic infections involve the liver secondarily; therefore evaluation of other organ systems may yield a presumptive diagnosis. Because blood cultures may take at least 2 weeks to become positive, liver or bone marrow biopsy may expedite the diagnosis. Bone marrow biopsy has been useful in patients with unexplained fever and severe immunodeficiency.[279] Several studies document the high yield of liver biopsy in HIV-infected patients with fever and abnormal liver tests.[31,34,280,281] Many of these studies are from developing countries where MTB is a common histologic finding. In a prospective study of liver biopsy in 24 patients with unexplained fever and increased alkaline phosphatase or gamma-glutamyl transferase, a microbiologic diagnosis was made in 13 (54 per-

TABLE 51-4

Overview of the Evaluation of Hepatobiliary Disease in Patients with HIV Infection

1. The extent and rapidity of the evaluation should be tailored to the clinical presentation and pattern of liver tests.
2. The CD4 lymphocyte count is essential in formulating the differential diagnosis. Opportunistic infections and neoplasms are most prevalent when the count is $<100/\text{mm}^3$.
3. The liver is an innocent bystander during lympho-hematogenous dissemination of opportunistic infections and neoplasms. Thus evaluation of other organs, such as blood or bone marrow, rather than liver biopsy may establish the diagnosis.
4. Carefully reviewing all medications, both prescription and over-the-counter, and obtaining viral hepatitis serologies should be performed in the patient with marked elevations of the transaminases. Hepatic imaging studies and liver biopsy rarely alter management in this setting.
5. Ultrasound or CT should be performed in the patient with marked elevation of the alkaline phosphatase to exclude mass lesions, infiltrative disorders, or biliary disease. ERCP may be necessary if bile duct dilation is found, especially if the patient has right upper quadrant pain. Liver biopsy may be considered if all studies are negative depending on the clinical setting.
6. In the jaundiced patient CT is the test of choice and will exclude hepatic mass lesions and biliary dilation; ERCP may be necessary for diagnosis and possibly endoscopic therapy if bile duct dilation is found.
7. Mild hepatomegaly is common in AIDS and usually requires no specific evaluation. Marked hepatomegaly is best evaluated with CT; liver biopsy may be useful depending on the clinical presentation and pattern of liver tests.

HIV, Human immunodeficiency virus; *CT*, computed tomography; *ERCP*, endoscopic retrograde cholangiopancreatography; *AIDS*, acquired immunodeficiency syndrome.

cent), in 9 of whom MAC was found.[280] Thus when MAC is suspected and blood and bone marrow cultures are negative, liver biopsy may establish the diagnosis. Given the efficacy and tolerability of newer regimens for MAC, empiric therapy is administered in many centers, in the absence of liver biopsy, pending results of cultures. The use of diagnostic liver biopsy has also decreased over the last decade with improvements in abdominal imaging studies. In addition, US- or CT-guided biopsy has a greater yield for focal abnormalities than does blind percutaneous biopsy. The role of liver biopsy for patients in whom interferon therapy is planned is unknown.

There has been concern regarding the safety of liver biopsy in these patients. Several reports suggested an increased risk of complications from liver biopsies in patients with AIDS.[282,283] However, no comprehensive evidence to date has documented an increased risk of complications—provided coagulation studies are normal. Nevertheless, hemorrhage from vascular lesions such as KS[283] and peliosis hepatis has been noted. A summary of factors guiding the approach to the evaluation of hepatobiliary disease in a patient with HIV infection is provided in Table 51-4.

References

1. Palella FJ, Delaney KM, Moorman AC, et al: Declining morbidity and mortality among patients with advanced human immunodeficiency virus infection. N Engl J Med 338:853-860, 1998.
2. Dehne KL, Pokrovskiy V, Kobyshcha Y, Schwartlander B: Update on the epidemic of HIV and other sexually transmitted infections in the newly independent states of the former Soviet Union. AIDS 14:S75-S84, 2000.
3. Sewankambo NK, Gray RH, Ahmad S, et al: Mortality associated with HIV infection in rural Rakai District, Uganda. AIDS 14:2391-2400, 2000.
4. Bacellar H, Munoz A, Hoover DR, et al for the Multicenter AIDS cohort study: Incidence of clinical AIDS conditions in a cohort of homosexual men with CD4+ cell counts < 100/mm³. J Infect Dis 170:1284-1287, 1994.
5. Selik RM, Chu SY, Ward JW: Trends in infectious diseases and cancers among persons dying of HIV infection in the United States from 1987 to 1992. Ann Intern Med 123: 933-936, 1995.
6. Mocroft A, Sabin CA, Youle M, et al: Changes in AIDS-defining illnesses in a London Clinic, 1987-1998. J Acquir Immune Defic Syndr 21:401-407, 1999.
7. Masliah E, DeTeresa RM, Mallory ME, Hansen LA: Changes in pathological findings at autopsy in AIDS cases for the last 15 years. AIDS 14:69-74, 2000.
8. Rizzardi GP, Tambussi G, Bart PA, et al: Virological and immunological responses to HAART in asymptomatic therapy-naïve HIV-1 infected subjects according to CD4 cell count. AIDS 14:2257-2263, 2000.
9. Kirk O, Gatell JM, Mocroft A, et al: Infections with *Mycobacterium tuberculosis* and *Mycobacterium avium* among HIV-infected patients after the introduction of highly active antiretroviral therapy. Am J Res Crit Care Med 162:865-872, 2000.
10. Schneiderman DJ, Arenson DM, Cello JP, et al: Hepatic disease in patients with the acquired immune deficiency syndrome (AIDS). Hepatology 7:925-930, 1987.
11. Monkemuller KE, Call SA, Lazenby AJ, Wilcox CM: Declining prevalence of opportunistic gastrointestinal disease in the era of combination antiretroviral therapy. Am J Gastroenterol 95:457-468, 2000.
12. Chu SY, Buehler JW, Lieb L, et al: Causes of death among persons reported with AIDS. Am J Public Health 83:1429-1432, 1993.
13. Soriano V, Garcia-Samaniego J, Valencia E, et al: Impact of chronic liver disease due to hepatitis viruses as cause of hospital admission and death in HIV-infected drug users. Eur J Epid 15:1-4, 1999.
14. Puoti M, Spinetti A, Ghezzi A, et al: Mortality of liver disease in patients with HIV infection: A cohort study. J Acquir Immune Defic Syndr 24:211-217, 2000.
15. Glasgow BJ, Anders K, Layfield LJ, et al: Clinical and pathologic findings of the liver in the acquired immune deficiency syndrome (AIDS). Am J Clin Pathol 83:582-588, 1985.
16. Lebovics E, Thung SN, Schaffner F, Radensky PW: The liver in the acquired immunodeficiency syndrome: a clinical and histologic study. Hepatology 5:293-298, 1985.
17. Orenstein MS, Tavitian A, Yonk B, et al: Granulomatous involvement of the liver in patients with AIDS. Gut 26:1220-1225, 1985.
18. Kahn E, Greco A, Daum F, et al: Hepatic pathology in pediatric acquired immunodeficiency syndrome. Hum Pathol 22:1111-1119, 1991.
19. Gordon SC, Reddy KR, Gould EE, et al: The spectrum of liver disease in the acquired immunodeficiency syndrome. J Hepatol 2: 475-484, 1986.
20. Nakanuma Y, Liew CT, Peters RL, et al: Pathologic features of the liver in acquired immune deficiency syndrome (AIDS). Liver 6:158-166, 1986.
21. Kahn SA, Saltzman BR, Klein RS, et al: Hepatic disorders in the acquired immune deficiency syndrome: a clinical and pathological study. Am J Gastroenterol 81:1145-1148, 1986.
22. Dworkin BM, Stahl RE, Giardina MA, et al: The liver in acquired immune deficiency syndrome: emphasis on patients with intravenous drug abuse. Am J Gastroenterol 82:231-236, 1987.
23. Comer GM, Mukherjee S, Scholes JV, et al: Liver biopsies in the acquired immune deficiency syndrome: influence of endemic disease and drug abuse. Am J Gastroenterol 84:1525-1531, 1989.
24. Cappell MS, Schwartz MS, Biempica L: Clinical utility of liver biopsy in patients with serum antibodies to the human immunodeficiency virus. Am J Med 88:123-30, 1990.
25. Wilkins MJ, Lindley R, Dourakis SP, Goldin RD: Surgical pathology of the liver in HIV infection. Histopathology 18:459-464, 1991.
26. Prüfer-Krämer L, Krämer A, Weigel R, et al: Hepatic involvement in patients with human immunodeficiency virus infection: discrepancies between AIDS patients and those with earlier stages of infection. J Infect Dis 163:866-869, 1991.
27. Chalasani N, Wilcox CM: Etiology, evaluation, and outcome of jaundice in patients with acquired immunodeficiency syndrome. Hepatology 23:728-733, 1996.
28. Poles MA, Dieterich DT, Schwartz ED, et al: Liver biopsy findings in 501 patients infected with human immunodeficiency virus (HIV). J Acquir Immune Defic Syndr Hum Retrovirol 11:170-177, 1996.
29. Rathi PM, Amarapurkar DN, Borges NE, et al: Spectrum of liver diseases in HIV infection. Indian J Gastroenterol 16:94-95, 1997.
30. Kennedy M, O-Reilly M, Bergin CJ, McDonald GS: Liver biopsy pathology in human immunodeficiency virus infection. Eur J Gastro Hepatol 10:255-258, 1998.
31. Garcia-Ordonez MA, Colmenero JD, Jimenez-Onate F, et al: Diagnostic usefulness of percutaneous liver biopsy in HIV-infected patients with fever of unknown origin. J Infect 38:94-98, 1999.
32. Lacialle F, Fournet JC, Blanche S: Clinical utility of liver biopsy in children with acquired immunodeficiency syndrome. Ped Infect Dis J 18:143-147, 1999.
33. Chang YG, Chen PJ, Hung CC, Chen MY, et al: Opportunistic hepatic infections in AIDS patients with fever of unknown origin. J Formos Med Assoc 98:5-10, 1999.
34. Piratvisuth T, Siripaitoon P, Sriplug H, Ovartlarnporn B: Findings and benefit of liver biopsies in 46 patients infected with human immunodeficiency virus. J Gastroenterol Hepatol 14:146-149, 1999.
35. Hanson DL, Chu SY, Farizo KM, Ward JW: Distribution of CD4+ T lymphocytes at diagnosis of acquired immunodeficiency syndrome-defining and other human immunodeficiency virus-related illnesses. Arch Intern Med 155:1537-1542, 1995.
36. Mocroft A, Katalama C, Johnson AM, et al: AIDS across Europe, 1994-1998: the EuroSIDA study. Lancet 356:291-296, 2000.
37. Reichert CM, O'Leary TJ, Levens DL, et al: Autopsy pathology in the acquired immune deficiency syndrome. Am J Pathol 112:357-382, 1983.
38. Welch K, Finkbeiner W, Alpers CE, et al: Autopsy findings in the acquired immunodeficiency syndrome. JAMA 252:1152-1159, 1984.
39. Graham NMH, Nelson KE, Soloman L, et al: Prevalence of tuberculin positivity and skin test anergy in HIV-1 seropositive and seronegative drug users. JAMA 267:369-372, 1992.

40. Centers for Disease Control and Prevention: Expanded tuberculosis surveillance and tuberculosis morbidity—United States, 1993. MMWR Morb Mortal Wkly Rep 43:361-366, 1994.
41. Freiman JP, Helfert KE, Hamrell MR, Stein DS: Hepatomegaly with severe steatosis in HIV-seropositive patients. AIDS 7:379-385, 1993.
42. Bissuel F, Bruneel F, Habersetzer F, et al: Fulminant hepatitis with severe lactate acidosis in HIV-infected patients on didanosine therapy. J Intern Med 235:367-371, 1994.
43. Olano JP, Borucki MJK, Wen JW, Haque AK: Massive hepatic steatosis and lactic acidosis in a patient with AIDS who was receiving zidovudine. Clin Infect Dis 21:973-976, 1995.
44. Miller KD, Cameron M, Wood LV, et al: Lactic acidosis and hepatic steatosis associated with use of stavudine: report of four cases. Ann Intern Med 133:192-196, 2000.
45. Al-Khafaji B, Kralovic S, Smith RD: Increased hepatic iron in the acquired immunodeficiency syndrome: an autopsy study. Mod Pathol 10:474-480, 1997.
46. Gordin FM, Simon GL, Wofsy CB, Mills J: Adverse reactions to trimethoprim-sulfamethoxazole in patients with the acquired immunodeficiency syndrome. Ann Intern Med 100:495-499, 1984.
47. Reichman DD, Fischl MA, Grieco MH, et al: The toxicity of azidothymidine (AZT) in the treatment of patients with AIDS and AIDS-related complex. N Engl J Med 317:192-197, 1987.
48. Dienstag JL, Perrillo RP, Schiff ER, et al: A preliminary trial of lamivudine for chronic hepatitis B infection. N Engl J Med 333:1657-1661, 1995.
49. McKenzie R, Fried MW, Sallie R, et al: Hepatic failure and lactic acidosis due to fialuridine (FIAU), an investigational nucleoside analogue for chronic hepatitis B. N Engl J Med 333:1099-1105, 1995.
50. Fortgang IS, Belitsos PC, Chaisson RE, Moore RD: Hepatomegaly and steatosis in HIV-infected patients receiving nucleoside analog antiretroviral therapy. Am J Gastroenterol 90:1433-1436, 1995.
51. Bonfanti P, Valsecchi L, Parazzini F, et al: Incidence of adverse reactions in HIV patient treated with protease inhibitors: a cohort study. J Acquir Immune Defic Syndr 23:236-245, 2000.
52. Saves M, Vandentorren S, Daucourt V, et al: Severe hepatic cytolysis: incidence and risk factors in patients treated by antiretroviral combinations. Aquitaine Cohort, France, 1996-1998. AIDS 13:F115-F121, 1999.
53. Sukowski MS, Thomas DL, Chaisson RE, Moore RD: Hepatotoxicity associated with antiretroviral therapy in adults infected with human immunodeficiency virus and the role of hepatitis C or B virus infection. JAMA 283:74-80, 2000.
54. Gisolf EH, Dreezen C, Danner SA, et al: Risk factors for hepatotoxicity in HIV-1-infected patients receiving ritonavir and saquinavir with or without stavudine. Clin Infect Dis 31:1234-1239, 2000.
55. Brau N, Leaf HL, Wisczorek RL, Margolis DM: Severe hepatitis in three AIDS patients treated with indinavir. Lancet 349:924-925, 1997.
56. Medina I, Mills J, Leoung G, et al: Oral therapy for *Pneumocystis carinii* pneumonia in the acquired immunodeficiency syndrome. N Engl J Med 323:776-782, 1990.
57. Podzamczer D, Salazar A, Jimenez J, et al: Intermittent trimethoprim-sulfamethoxazole compared with dapsone-pyrimethamine for the simultaneous primary prophylaxis of *Pneumocystis* pneumonia and toxoplasmosis in patients infected in HIV. Ann Intern Med 122:755-761, 1995.
58. Lee WM: Drug-induced hepatotoxicity. N Engl J Med 333:1118-1127, 1995.
59. Ozick LA, Jacob L, Comer GM, et al: Hepatotoxicity from isoniazid and rifampin in inner-city AIDS patients. Am J Gastroenterol 90:1978-1980, 1995.
60. Nolan CM, Goldberg DV, Bushkin SE: Hepatotoxicity associated with isoniazid preventive therapy: a 7-year survey from a public health tuberculosis clinic. JAMA 281:1014-1018, 1999.
61. Jacobson MA, Yajko D, Northfelt D, et al: Randomized, placebo-controlled trial of rifampin, ethambutol, and ciprofloxacin for AIDS patients with disseminated *Mycobacterium avium* complex infection. J Infect Dis 168:112-119, 1993.
62. Chaisson RE, Benson CA, Dube MP, et al: Clarithromycin therapy for bacteremic *Mycobacterium avium* complex disease: a randomized, double-blind, dose-ranging study in patients with AIDS. Ann Intern Med 121:905-911, 1994.
63. Lewis JH, Zimmerman J, Benson GD, et al: Hepatic injury associated with ketoconazole therapy. Gastroenterology 86:503-513, 1984.
64. Henning KJ, Bell E, Braun J, Barker ND: A community-wide outbreak of hepatitis A: risk factors for infection among homosexual and bisexual men. Am J Med 99:132-136, 1995.
65. Ridolfo AL, Rusconi S, Antinori S, et al: Persisting HIV-1 replication triggered by acute hepatitis A virus infection. Antivir Ther 5:15-17, 2000.
66. Osmond DH, Charlebois E, Sheppard HW, et al: Comparison of risk factors for hepatitis C and hepatitis B virus infection in homosexual men. J Infect Dis 167:66-71, 1993.
67. Lazizi Y, Grangeot-Keros L, Delfraissy JF, et al: Reappearance of hepatitis B virus in immune patients infected with the human immunodeficiency virus type 1. J Infect Dis 158:666-667, 1988 (letter).
68. Osella AR, Massa MA, Joekes S, et al: Hepatitis B and C virus sexual transmission among homosexual men. Am J Gastroenterol 93:49-52, 1997.
69. Rodriguez-Mendez ML, Gonzalez-Quintela MD, Aguilera A: Prevalence, patterns, and course of past hepatitis B virus infection in intravenous drug users with HIV-1 infection. Am J Gastroenterol 95:1316-1322, 2000.
70. Homann C, Krogsgaard K, Pedersen C, et al: High incidence of hepatitis B infection and evolution of chronic hepatitis B infection in patients with advanced HIV infection. J Acquir Immune Defic Syndr 4:416-420, 1991.
71. Broers B, Junet C, Bourquin M, et al: Prevalence and incidence rate of HIV, hepatitis B and C among drug users on methadone maintenance treatment in Geneva between 1988 and 1995. AIDS 12:2059-2066, 1998.
72. Hadler SC, Judson FN, O'Malley PM, et al: Outcome of hepatitis B virus infection in homosexual men and its relation to prior human immunodeficiency virus infection. J Infect Dis 163:454-459, 1991.
73. Bodsworth N, Donovan B, Nightingale BN: The effect of concurrent human immunodeficiency virus infection on chronic hepatitis B: a study of 150 homosexual men. J Infect Dis 160:577-582, 1989.
74. Mills CT, Lee E, Perrillo R: Relationship between histology, aminotransferase levels, and viral replication in chronic hepatitis B. Gastroenterology 99:519-524, 1990.
75. Koblin BA, Taylor PE, Rubinstein P, Stevens CE: Effect of duration of hepatitis B virus infection on the association between human immunodeficiency virus type-1 and hepatitis B viral replication. Hepatology 15:590-592, 1992.
76. Perrillo RP, Regenstein FG, Roodman ST: Chronic hepatitis B in asymptomatic homosexual men with antibody to the human immunodeficiency virus. Ann Intern Med 105:382-383, 1986.
77. Rustgi VK, Hoofnagle JH, Gerin JL, et al: Hepatitis B virus infection in the acquired immunodeficiency syndrome. Ann Intern Med 101:795-797, 1984.
78. Krogsgaard K, Lindhardt BO, Nielson JO, et al: The influence of HTLV-III infection on the natural history of hepatitis B virus infection in male homosexual HBsAg carriers. Hepatology 7:37-41, 1987.
79. Rector WG, Govindarajan S, Horsburgh CR, et al: Hepatic inflammation, hepatitis B replication, and cellular immune function in homosexual males with chronic hepatitis B and antibody to human immunodeficiency virus. Am J Gastroenterol 83:262-266, 1988.
80. Bonacini M, Govindarajan S, Redeker AG: Human immunodeficiency virus infection does not alter serum transaminases and hepatitis B virus (HBV) DNA in homosexual patients with chronic HBV infection. Am J Gastroenterol 86:570-573, 1991.
81. Housset C, Pol S, Carnot F, et al: Interactions between human immunodeficiency virus-1, hepatitis delta virus and hepatitis B virus infections in 260 chronic carriers of hepatitis B virus. Hepatology 15:578-583, 1992.
82. McDonald JA, Harris S, Waters JA, Thomas HC: Effect of human immunodeficiency virus (HIV) infection on chronic hepatitis B hepatic viral antigen display. J Hepatol 4: 337-342, 1987.
83. Kashala O, Mubikayi L, Kayembe K, et al: Hepatitis B virus activation among central Africans infected with human immunodeficiency virus (HIV) type 1: pre-s2 antigen is predominantly expressed in HIV infection. J Infect Dis 169:628-632, 1994.
84. Eskild A, Magnus P, Petersen G, et al: Hepatitis B antibodies in HIV-infected homosexual men are associated with more rapid progression to AIDS. AIDS 6:571-574, 1992.
85. Jer Twu S, Detels R, Nelson K, et al: Relationship of hepatitis B virus infection to human immunodeficiency virus type I infection. J Infect Dis 167:299-304, 1993.

86. Scharschmidt BF, Held MJ, Hollander HH, et al: Hepatitis B in patients with HIV infection: relationship to AIDS and patient survival. Ann Intern Med 117:837-838, 1992.
87. Gilson RJC, Hawkins AE, Beecham MR, et al: Interactions between HIV and hepatitis B virus in homosexual men: effects on the natural history of infection. AIDS 11:597-606, 1997.
88. McNair ANB, Main J, Thomas HC: Interactions of the human immunodeficiency virus and the hepatotropic viruses. Semin Liver Dis 12:188-196, 1992.
89. Marcellin P, Boyer N, Giostra E, et al: Recombinant human alpha-interferon in patients with chronic non-A, non-B hepatitis: a multicenter randomized controlled trial from France. Hepatology 13:393-397, 1991.
90. McDonald JA, Caruso L, Karayiannis P, et al: Diminished responsiveness of male homosexual chronic hepatitis B virus carriers with HTLV-III antibodies to combinant α-interferon. Hepatology 7:719-723, 1987.
91. Wong DKH, Yim C, Naylor CD, et al: Interferon alfa treatment of chronic hepatitis B: randomized trial in a predominantly homosexual male population. Gastroenterology 108:165-171, 1995.
92. Hess G, Rossol S, Voth R, et al: Treatment of patients with chronic type B hepatitis and concurrent human immunodeficiency virus infection with a combination of interferon alpha and azidothymidine: a pilot study. Digestion 43:56-59, 1989.
93. Dienstag JL, Schiff ER, Wright TC, et al: Lamivudine as initial treatment for chronic hepatitis B in the United States. N Engl J Med 341:156-163, 1999.
94. Nagai K, Hosaka H, Kubo S, et al: Highly active antiretroviral therapy used to treat concurrent hepatitis B and human immunodeficiency virus infections. J Gastroenterol 34:275-281, 1999.
95. Benhamou Y, Bochet M, Thibault V, et al: Long-term incidence of hepatitis B virus resistance to lamivudine in human immunodeficiency virus-infected patients. Hepatology 30:1302-1306, 1999.
96. Nasti G, di Gennaro G, Donada C, et al: Combination therapy with alpha interferon and lamivudine in patients with chronic hepatitis B and HIV infection. AIDS 13:2176-2178, 1999.
97. Altfeld M, Rockstroh JK, Addo M, et al: Reactivation of hepatitis B in a long-term anti-HBs-positive patient with AIDS following lamivudine withdrawal. J Hepatol 29:306-309, 1998.
98. Bessesen M, Ives D, Condreay L, et al: Chronic active hepatitis B exacerbations in human immunodeficiency virus-infected patients following development of resistance to or withdrawal of lamivudine. Clin Infect Dis 28:1032-1035, 1999.
99. Piroth L, Grappin M, Buisson M, et al: Hepatitis B virus seroconversion in HIV/HBV coinfected patients treated with highly active antiretroviral therapy. J Acquir Immune Defic Syndr 23:356-357, 2000.
100. Velasco M, Moran A, Tellez M: Resolution of chronic hepatitis B after ritonavir treatment in an HIV-infected patient. N Engl J Med 340:1765-1766, 1999.
101. Rabeneck L, Risser JMH, Murray NGB, et al: Failure of providers to vaccinate HIV-infected men against hepatitis B: a missed opportunity. Am J Gastroenterol 88:2015-2019, 1993.
102. Collier AC, Corey L, Murphy VL, Handsfield HH: Antibody to human immunodeficiency virus (HIV) and suboptimal response to hepatitis B vaccination. Ann Intern Med 109:101-105, 1988.
103. Keet IPM, van Doornum G, Safary A, Coutinho RA: Insufficient response to hepatitis B vaccination in HIV-positive homosexual men. AIDS 6:509-522, 1992.
104. Rey D, Krantz V, Partisani M, et al. Increasing the number of hepatitis B vaccine injections augments anti-HBs response rate in HIV-infected patients. Effects on HIV viral load. Vaccine 18:1161-1165, 2000.
105. Antinori S, Ridolfo A, Caredda F, et al: Prevalence of delta hepatitis markers among parenteral drug abusers and homosexual men with and without AIDS. J Hepatol 13:380-381, 1991.
106. de Miguel J, Collazos J, Mayo J, et al: Hepatitis D virus infection in drug addicts infected with the human immunodeficiency virus. Clin Infect Dis 19:363-364, 1994.
107. Solomon RE, Kaslow RA, Phair JP, et al: Human immunodeficiency virus and hepatitis delta virus in homosexual men. Ann Intern Med 108:51-54, 1988.
108. Buti M, Esteban R, Espanol MT, et al: Influence of human immunodeficiency virus infection on cell-mediated immunity in chronic D hepatitis. J Infect Dis 163:1351-1353, 1991.
109. Farci P, Orgiana G, Coiana A, et al: The influence of human immunodeficiency virus (HIV) on the course of chronic D hepatitis. J Hepatol 9:S28, 1989.
110. Novick DM, Farci P, Croxson TS, et al: Hepatitis D virus and human immunodeficiency virus antibodies in parenteral drug abusers who are hepatitis B surface antigen positive. J Infect Dis 158:795-803, 1988.
111. Lichtenstein DR, Makadon HJ, Chopra S: Fulminant hepatitis B and delta virus coinfection in AIDS. Am J Gastroenterol 87:1643-1647, 1992.
112. Botti P, Pistelli A, Gambassi A, et al: HBV and HCV infection in I.V. drug addicts; coinfection with HIV. Arch Virol 4:329-332, 1992.
113. Wright TL, Hollander H, Pu X, et al: Hepatitis C in HIV-infected patients with and without AIDS: prevalence and relationship to patient survival. Hepatology 20:1152-1155, 1994.
114. Kumar A, Kulkarni R, Murray DL, et al: Serologic markers of viral hepatitis A, B, C, and D in patients with hemophilia. J Med Virol 41:205-209, 1993.
115. Weinstock DM, Merrick S, Malak SA, et al: Hepatitis C in an urban population infected with the human immunodeficiency virus. AIDS 13:2593-2595, 1999.
116. Melbye M, Biggar RJ, Wantzin P, et al: Sexual transmission of hepatitis C virus: cohort study 1981-9 among European homosexual men. BMJ 301:210-212, 1990.
117. Hayashi PH, Flynn N, McCurdy SA, et al: Prevalence of hepatitis C virus antibodies among patients infected with human immunodeficiency virus. J Med Virol 33:177-180, 1991.
118. Sherman KE, Freeman S, Harrison S, Andron L: Prevalence of antibody to hepatitis C virus in patients infected with the human immunodeficiency virus. J Infect Dis 163:414, 1991 (letter).
119. McHutchison JG, Polito A, Person JL, et al: Assessment of hepatitis C antibody tests in homosexual men with hyperglobulinemia. J Infect Dis 164: 217-218, 1991 (letter).
120. Cribier B, Rey D, Schmitt C, et al: High hepatitis C viraemia and impaired antibody response in patients coinfected with HIV. AIDS 9:1131-1136, 1995.
121. Marcellin P, Martinot-Peignoux M, Elias A, et al: Hepatitis C virus (HCV) viremia in human immunodeficiency virus-seronegative and -seropositive patients with indeterminate HCV recombinant immunoblot assay. J Infect Dis 70:433-435, 1994.
122. Eyster ME, Alter HJ, Aledort LM, et al: Heterosexual co-transmission of hepatitis C virus (HCV) and human immunodeficiency virus (HIV). Ann Intern Med 115:764-768, 1991.
123. Manzini P, Saracco G, Cerchier A, et al: Human immunodeficiency virus infection as risk factor for mother-to-child hepatitis C virus transmission; persistence of anti-hepatitis C virus in children is associated with the mother's anti-hepatitis C virus immunoblotting pattern. Hepatology 21:328-332, 1995.
124. Hershow RC, Riester KA, Lew J, et al: Increased vertical transmission of human immunodeficiency virus from hepatitis C virus-coinfected mothers. J Infect Dis 176:414-420, 1997.
125. Hisada M, O'Brien TR, Rosenberg PS, et al: Virus load and risk of heterosexual transmission of human immunodeficiency virus and hepatitis C virus by men with hemophilia. J Infect Dis 181:1475-1478, 2000.
126. Martin P, Di Bisceglie AM, Kassianides C, et al: Rapidly progressive non-A, non-B hepatitis in patients with human immunodeficiency virus infection. Gastroenterology 97:1559-1561, 1989.
127. Garcia-Samaniego J, Soriano V, Castilla J, et al: Influence of hepatitis C genotypes and HIV on histological severity of chronic hepatitis C. Am J Gastroenterol 92:1130-1134, 1997.
128. Guido M, Rugge M, Fattovich G, et al: Human immunodeficiency virus infection and hepatitis C pathology. Liver 14:314-319, 1994.
129. Benhamou Y, Bochet M, Di Martino V, et al: Liver fibrosis progression in human immunodeficiency virus and hepatitis C virus coinfected patients. Hepatology 30:1054-1058, 1999.
130. Sanchez-Quijano A, Andreu J, Gavilan F, et al: Influence of human immunodeficiency virus type 1 infection on the natural course of parentally acquired hepatitis C. Eur Clin Microbiol Infect Dis 14:949-953, 1995.
131. Telfer P, Sabin C, Devereux H, et al: The progression of HCV-associated liver disease in a cohort of haemophilic patients. Br J Haematol 87:555-561, 1994.
132. Eyster ME, Diamondstone LS, Lien JM, et al: Natural history of hepatitis C virus infection in multitransfused hemophiliacs: effect of

coinfection with human immunodeficiency virus. The Multicenter Hemophilia Cohort Study. J Acquir Immune Defic Syndr 6:602-610, 1993.

133. Darby SC, Ewart DW, Giangrande PLF, et al: Mortality from liver cancer and liver disease in haemophilic men and boys in UK given blood products contaminated with hepatitis C. Lancet 350:1425-1431, 1997.
134. Yee TT, Griffioen A, Sabin CA, et al: The natural history of HCV in a cohort of haemophilic patients infected between 1961 and 1985. Gut 47:845-851, 2000.
135. Eyster ME, Fried MW, Di Bisceglie AM, Goedert JJ: Increasing hepatitis C virus RNA levels in hemophiliacs: relationship to human immunodeficiency virus infection and liver disease. Multicenter Hemophilia Cohort Study. Blood 84:1020-1023, 1994.
136. Sherman KE, O'Brien J, Gutierrez AG, et al: Quantitative evaluation of hepatitis C virus RNA in patients with concurrent human immunodeficiency virus infections. J Clin Microbiol 31:2679-2682, 1993.
137. Vierling JM, Villamil FG, Rojter SE, et al: Morbidity and mortality of recurrent hepatitis C infection after orthotopic liver transplantation. J Viral Hepat 4(suppl 1):117-124, 1997.
138. Dorrucci M, Pezzotti P, Phillips AN, Lepri AC, Rezza F for the Italian Seroconversion Study: Coinfection of hepatitis C virus with human immunodeficiency virus and progression to AIDS. J Infect Dis 172:1503-1508, 1995.
139. Staples CT, Rimland D, Dudas D: Hepatitis C in the HIV Atlanta V.A. Cohort Study (HAVACS): The effect of coinfection on survival. Clin Infect Dis 29:150-154, 1999.
140. Dorucci M, Pezzotti P, Phillips AN, et al: Coinfection of hepatitis C virus with human immunodeficiency virus and progression to AIDS. Italian Seroconversion Study. J Infect Dis 172:1503-1508, 1995.
141. Sabin CA, Telfer P, Phillips AN, et al: The association between hepatitis C virus genotype and human immunodeficiency virus disease progression in a cohort of hemophilic men. J Infect Dis 175:164-168, 1997.
142. Piroth L, Duong M, Quantin C, et al: Does hepatitis C virus coinfection accelerate clinical and immunologic evolution in HIV-infected patients? AIDS 12:381-388, 1998.
143. Piroth L, Bourgeois C, Dantin S, et al: Hepatitis C virus genotype does not appear to be a significant prognostic factor in HIV-HCV coinfected patients. AIDS 13:523-537, 1999.
144. Greub G, Ledergerber B, Battegay M, et al: Clinical progression, survival and immune recovery during antiretroviral therapy in patients with HIV-1 and hepatitis C virus coinfection: the Swiss HIV cohort study. Lancet 356:1800-1805, 2000.
145. Graham CS, Koziel MJ: Why should hepatitis C affect immune reconstitution in HIV-1-infected patients? Lancet 356:1865-1866, 2000.
146. Dieterich DT: Hepatitis C virus and human immunodeficiency virus: clinical issues in coinfection. Am J Med 107(suppl):79-84, 1999.
147. Brau N, Leaf H, Wieczorek R, et al: Severe hepatitis in three AIDS patients treated with indinavir. Lancet 349:924-925, 1997 (letter).
148. Rodriguez-Rosado R, Garcia-Samaniego J, Soriano V: Hepatotoxicity after introduction of highly active antiretroviral therapy. AIDS 12:1256, 1998.
149. Palmon R, Tirelli R, Braun JF, et al: Hepatotoxicity associated with non-nucleoside reverse transcriptase inhibitors for the treatment of human immunodeficiency virus and the effect of hepatitis B or C virus infection. Hepatology 32:312A, 2000.
150. Puoti M, Gargiulo F, Quiros-Roldan E, et al: Liver damage and kinetics of hepatitis C virus and human immunodeficiency virus replication during the early phases of combination antiretroviral therapy. J Infect Dis 181:2033-2360, 2000.
151. Gavazzi G, Bouchard O, Leclercq P, et al: Change in transaminases in hepatitis C virus and HIV-coinfected patients after highly active antiretroviral therapy: differences between complete and partial virologic responders. AIDS Res Hum Retroviruses 16:1021-1023, 2000.
152. Vento S, Garofano T, Renzini C: Enhancement of hepatitis C virus replication and liver damage in HIV-coinfected patients on antiretroviral combination therapy. AIDS 12:116-167, 1998.
153. Zylberberg H, Chaix ML, Rabain C, et al: Tritherapy for human immunodeficiency virus infection does not modify replication of hepatitis c virus in coinfected patients. Clin Infect Dis 26:1104-1106, 1997.
154. Soriano V, Garcia-Sambaing J, Bravo R, et al: Interferon-a for the treatment of chronic hepatitis C in patients infected with human immunodeficiency virus. Clin Infect Dis 23:585-591, 1996.
155. Morsica G, De Bona A, Foppa CU, et al: Ribavirin therapy for chronic hepatitis C does not modify HIV viral load in HIV-1 positive patients under antiretroviral treatment. AIDS 14:1656-1658, 2000.
156. Zylberberg H, Benhamou Y, Lagneaux JL, et al: Safety and efficacy of interferon ribavirin combination therapy in HCV-HIV coinfected subjects: an early report. Gut 47:694-697, 2000.
157. Soriano V, Rodriguez-Rosado R, Perez-Olmeda M, et al: Interferon plus ribavirin for chronic hepatitis C in HIV-infected patients. AIDS 14:2409-2410, 2000.
158. Landau A, Batisse D, Van Huyen JP, et al: Efficacy and safety of combination therapy with interferon-alpha2b and ribavirin for chronic hepatitis C in HIV-infected patients. AIDS 14:839-844, 2000.
159. Landau A, Batisse D, Piketty C, et al: Lack of interference between ribavirin and nucleosidic analogues in HVA/HCV co-infected individuals undergoing concomitant antiretroviral and anti-HCV combination therapy. AIDS 14:1857-1858, 2000.
160. Medrano FJ, Sanchez-Quijano A, Torronteras R, et al: Hepatitis E virus and HIV infection in homosexual men. Lancet 345:127, 1995 (letter).
161. Balayan MS, Fedorova OE, Mikhailov MI, et al: Antibody to hepatitis E virus in HIV-infected individuals and AIDS patients. J Viral Hepat 4:279-283, 1997.
162. Psichogiou M, Tzala E, Boletis J, et al: Hepatitis E virus infection in individuals at high risk of transmission of non-A, non-B hepatitis and sexually transmitted diseases. Scand J Infect Dis 28:443-445, 1996.
163. Puig-Basagoiti F, Cabana M, Guilera M, et al: Prevalence and route of transmission with a novel DNA virus (TTV), hepatitis C virus, and hepatitis G virus in patients infected with HIV. J Acquir Immune Defic Syndr 23:89-94, 2000.
164. Woolley I, Valdez H, Walker C, et al: Hepatitis G virus RNA is common in AIDS patients' plasma but is not associated with abnormal liver function tests or other clinical syndromes. J Acquir Immune Defic Syndr 19:408-412, 1998.
165. Yeo AE, Matsumoto A, Hisada M, et al: Effect of hepatitis G virus infection on progression of HIV infection in patients with hemophilia. Multicenter Hemophilia Cohort Study. Ann Intern Med 132:959-963, 2000.
166. Gendrault JL, Steffan AM, Schmitt MP, et al: Interaction of cultured human Kupffer cells with HIV-infected CEM cells: an electron microscopic study. Pathobiology 59:223-226, 1991.
167. Scoazec JY, Feldmann G: Both macrophages and endothelial cells of the human hepatic sinusoid express the CD4 molecule, a receptor for the human immunodeficiency virus. Hepatology 12:505-510, 1990.
168. Housset C, Lamas E, Courgnaud V, et al: Presence of HIV-1 in human parenchymal and non-parenchymal liver cells in vivo. J Hepatol 19:252-258, 1993.
169. Hoda SA, White JE, Gerber MA: Immunohistochemical studies of human immunodeficiency virus-1 in liver tissues of patients with AIDS. Mod Pathol 4:578-581, 1991.
170. Cao YZ, Dieterich D, Thomas PA, et al: Identification and quantitation of HIV-1 in the liver of patients with AIDS. AIDS 6:65-70, 1992.
171. Hofman P, Saint-Paul MC, Battaglione V, et al: Autopsy findings in acquired immunodeficiency syndrome (AIDS). A report of 395 cases from the south of France. Pathol Res Pract 195:209-217, 1999.
172. Soriani V, Bru F, Gonzalez-Lahoz J: Fatal varicella hepatitis in a patient with AIDS. J Infect 25:107, 1992 (letter).
173. Albrecht H, Schafer H, Stellbrink HJ: Epstein-Barr virus associated hemophagocytic syndrome: a cause of fever of unknown origin in human immunodeficiency syndrome. Arch Pathol Lab Med 121:853-858, 1997.
174. Horsburgh CR, Metchock B, Gordon SM, et al: Predictors of survival in patients with AIDS and disseminated *Mycobacterium avium* complex disease. J Infect Dis 170:573-577, 1994.
175. Nightengale SD, Byrd LT, Southern PM, et al: Incidence of *Mycobacterium avium*-intracellulare complex bacteremia in human immunodeficiency virus-positive patients. J Infect Dis 165:1082-1085, 1992.

176. Chaisson RE, Moore RD, Richman DD, et al: Incidence and natural history of *Mycobacterium avium*-complex infections in patients with advanced human immunodeficiency virus disease treated with zidovudine. Am Rev Respir Dis 146:285-289, 1992.
177. Greene JB, Sidhu GS, Lewin S, et al: *Mycobacterium avium*-intracellulare: a cause of disseminated life-threatening infection in homosexuals and drug users. Ann Intern Med 97:539-546, 1982.
178. Chin DP, Hopewell PC, Yajko DM, et al: *Mycobacterium avium* complex in the respiratory or gastrointestinal tract and the risk of *M. avium* complex bacteremia in patients with human immunodeficiency virus infection. J Infect Dis 169:289-295, 1994.
179. Havlik JA, Horsburgh CR, Metchock B, et al: Disseminated *Mycobacterium avium* complex infection: clinical identification and epidemiologic trends. J Infect Dis 165:577-580, 1992.
180. Chin DP, Reingold AL, Horsburgh CR, et al: Predicting *Mycobacterium avium* complex bacteremia in patients infected with human immunodeficiency virus: a prospectively validated model. Clin Infect Dis 19:668-674, 1994.
181. Wallace JM, Hannah JB: *Mycobacterium avium* complex infection in patients with the acquired immunodeficiency syndrome. Chest 93: 926-932, 1988.
182. Torriani FJ, McCutchan JA, Bozzette SA, et al: Autopsy findings in AIDS patients with *Mycobacterium avium* complex bacteremia. J Infect Dis 170:1601-1605, 1994.
183. Klatt EC, Jensen DF, Meyer PR: Pathology of *Mycobacterium avium*-intracellulare infection in acquired immunodeficiency syndrome. Hum Pathol 18:709-714, 1987.
184. Monforte A, Gori A, Vago L, et al: Atypical mycobacterial disease findings at autopsy in a cohort of 350 AIDS patients in Milan, Italy. J Infect Dis 172:901, 1995 (letter).
185. Prego V, Glatt AE, Roy V, et al: Comparative yield of blood culture for fungi and mycobacteria, liver biopsy, and bone marrow biopsy in the diagnosis of fever of undetermined origin in human immunodeficiency virus-infected patients. Arch Intern Med 150:333-336, 1990.
186. Radin DR: Intraabdominal *Mycobacterium tuberculosis* vs *Mycobacterium avium*-intracellulare infections in patients with AIDS: distinction based on CT findings. AJR 156:487-491, 1991.
187. Baril L, Jouan M, Agher R, et al: Impact of highly active antiretroviral therapy on onset of *Mycobacterium avium* complex infection and cytomegalovirus disease in patients with AIDS. AIDS 14:2593-2596, 2000.
188. Currier JS, Williams PL, Koletar SL, et al: Discontinuation of *Mycobacterium avium* complex prophylaxis in patients with antiretroviral therapy-induces increases in CD4 cell count. Ann Intern Med 133:493-503, 2000.
189. Chaisson RE, Schecter GF, Theuer CP, et al: Tuberculosis in patients with the acquired immunodeficiency syndrome. Am Rev Respir Dis 136:570-574, 1987.
190. Rana FS, Hawken MP, Mwachari C, et al: Autopsy study of HIV-1-positive and HIV-1 negative adult medical patients in Nairobi, Kenya. J Acquir Immune Defic Syndr 24:23-29, 2000.
191. Hsiao CH, Huang SH, Huang SF, et al: Autopsy findings on patients with AIDS in Taiwan. J Micro Imm Infect 30:145-159, 1997.
192. Sunderam G, McDonald RJ, Maniatis T, et al: Tuberculosis as a manifestation of the acquired immunodeficiency syndrome (AIDS). JAMA 256:362-366, 1986.
193. Pottipati AR, Dave PB, Gumaste V, Vieux U: Tuberculosis abscess of the liver in acquired immunodeficiency syndrome. J Clin Gastroenterol 13:549-553, 1991.
194. Kielhofner MA, Hamill RJ: Focal hepatic tuberculosis in a patient with acquired immunodeficiency syndrome. South Med J 84:401-404, 1991.
195. Nyberg DA, Federle MP, Jeffrey RB, et al: Abdominal CT findings of disseminated *Mycobacterium avium*-intracellulare in AIDS. AJR 145:297-299, 1985.
196. Pedro-Botet, Gutierrez J, Miralles R, et al: Pulmonary tuberculosis in HIV-infected patients with normal chest radiographs. AIDS 6:91-93, 1992.
197. Centers for Disease Control and Prevention: Prevention and treatment of tuberculosis among patients with human immunodeficiency virus: principles of therapy and revised recommendations. MMWR Morb Mortal Wkly Rep 47RR-20:1-58, 1998.
198. Whalen CC, Johnson JL, Okwera A: A trial of three regimens to prevent tuberculosis in Ugandan adults infected with the human immunodeficiency virus. N Engl J Med 337:801-808, 1997.
199. Gordin F, Chaisson RE, Matts JP: Rifampin and pyrazinamide vs. isoniazid for prevention of tuberculosis in HIV-infected persons. An international randomized trial. JAMA 283:1445-1450, 2000.
200. Ungo JR, Jones D, Ashkin D, et al: Antituberculosis drug-induced hepatotoxicity. The role of hepatitis C virus and the human immunodeficiency virus. Am J Respir Crit Care Med 157:1871-1876, 1998.
201. Wheat LJ, Connolly-Stringfield PA, Baker RL, et al: Disseminated histoplasmosis in the acquired immune deficiency syndrome: clinical findings, diagnosis and treatment, and review of the literature. Medicine (Baltimore) 69:361-374, 1990.
202. Kurtin PJ, McKinsey DS, Gupta MR, Driks M: Histoplasmosis in patients with acquired immunodeficiency syndrome. Hematologic and bone marrow examination. Am J Clin Pathol 93:367-372, 1990.
203. Lamps LW, Molina CP, West AB, et al: The pathologic spectrum of gastrointestinal and hepatic histoplasmosis. Am J Clin Pathol 113:64-72, 2000.
204. Bronnimann DA, Adam RD, Galgiani JN, et al: Coccidioidomycosis in the acquired immunodeficiency syndrome. Ann Intern Med 106:372-379, 1987.
205. Pappas PG, Pottage JC, Powderly WG, et al: Blastomycosis in patients with the acquired immunodeficiency syndrome. Ann Intern Med 116:847-853, 1992.
206. Girishkumar H, Yousuf AM, Chivate J, Geisler E: Experience with invasive *Candida* infections. Postgrad Med J 75:151-153, 1999.
207. Perkocha LA, Geaghan SM, Yen TS, et al: Clinical and pathological features of bacillary peliosis hepatis in association with human immunodeficiency virus infection. N Engl J Med 323:1581-1586, 1990.
208. Koehler JE, Tappero JW: Bacillary angiomatosis and bacillary peliosis in patients infected with human immunodeficiency virus. Clin Infect Dis 17:612-624, 1993.
209. Slater LN, Welch DF, Min KW: *Rochalimaea henselae* causes bacillary angiomatosis and peliosis hepatis. Arch Intern Med 152:602-606, 1992.
210. Gasquet S, Maurin M, Brouqui P, et al: Bacillary angiomatosis in immunocompromised patients. AIDS 12:1793-1803, 1998.
211. Mohle-Boetani JC, Koehler JE, Berger TG, et al: Bacillary angiomatosis and bacillary peliosis in patients infected with human immunodeficiency virus: clinical characteristics in a case-controlled study. Clin Infect Dis 22:794-800, 1996.
212. Hasan FA, Jeffers LJ, Dickinson G, et al: Hepatobiliary cryptosporidiosis and cytomegalovirus infection mimicking metastatic cancer to the liver. Gastroenterology 100:1743-1748, 1991.
213. Terada S, Reddy KR, Jeffers LJ, et al: Microsporidian hepatitis in the acquired immunodeficiency syndrome. Ann Intern Med 107:61-62, 1987.
214. Kotler DP, Orenstein JM: Clinical syndromes associated with microsporidiosis. Adv Parasitol 40:321-349, 1998.
215. Poblete RB, Rodrigues K, Foust RT, et al: *Pneumocystis carinii* hepatitis in the acquired immunodeficiency syndrome (AIDS). Ann Intern Med 110:737-738, 1989.
216. Rockley PF, Wilcox CM, Moynihan M, et al: Splenic infection simulating lymphoma: an unusual presentation of disseminated *Pneumocystis carinii* infection. South Med J 87:530-536, 1994.
217. Lubat E, Megibow AJ, Balthazar EJ, et al: Extrapulmonary *Pneumocystis carinii* infection in AIDS. CT findings. Radiology 174:157-160, 1990.
218. Angarano G, Maggi P, Rollo MA, et al: Diffuse necrotic hepatic lesions due to visceral leishmaniasis in AIDS. J Infect 36:167-169, 1998.
219. Brion J, Pelloux H, Le Marc'hadour F, et al: Acute toxoplasmic hepatitis in a patient with AIDS. Clin Infect Dis 15:183-184, 1992.
220. Moore RD, Kessler H, Richman DD, et al: Non-Hodgkin's lymphoma in patients with advanced HIV infection treated with zidovudine. JAMA 265:2208-2211, 1991.
221. Tirelli U, Spina M, Gaidano G, et al: Epidemiological, biological and clinical features of HIV-related lymphomas in the era of highly active antiretroviral therapy. AIDS 14:1675-1688, 2000.
222. Masliah E, DeTeresa RM, Mallory ME, Hansen LA: Changes in pathological findings at autopsy in AIDS cases for the last 15 years. AIDS 14:69-74, 2000.
223. Trojan A, Kreuzer KA, Flury R, et al: Liver changes in AIDS. Retrospective analysis of 227 autopsies of HIV-positive patients. Pathologe 19:194-200, 1998.

224. Levine AM: Acquired immunodeficiency syndrome-related lymphoma: clinical aspects. Semin Oncol 27:442-453, 2000.
225. Ziegler JL, Beckstead JA, Volberding PA, et al: Non-Hodgkin's lymphoma in 90 homosexual men. Relation to generalized lymphadenopathy and the acquired immunodeficiency syndrome. N Engl J Med 311:565-570, 1984.
226. Spinello A, Ridolfo AL, Esposito R, et al: Liver involvement in AIDS-associated malignancies. J Hepatol 21:1145-1146, 1994.
227. Scerpella EG, Villareal AA, Casanova PF, Moreno JN: Primary lymphoma of the liver in AIDS. J Clin Gastroenterol 22:51-53, 1996.
228. Townsend RR, Laing FC, Jeffrey RB, Bottles K: Abdominal lymphoma in AIDS: evaluation with US. Radiology 171:719-724, 1989.
229. Radin DR, Esplin JA, Levine AM, Ralls PW: AIDS-related non-Hodgkin's lymphoma: abdominal CT findings in 112 patients. AJR Am J Roentgenol 160:1133-1139, 1993.
230. Chang Y, Cesarman E, Pessin MS, et al: Identification of herpesvirus-like DNA sequences in AIDS-associated Kaposi's sarcoma. Science 266:1865-1869, 1994.
231. Monini P, De Lellis L, Fabris M, et al: Kaposi's sarcoma-associated herpesvirus DNA sequences in prostate tissue and human semen. N Engl J Med 334:1168-1172, 1996.
232. Gnann JW, Pellett PE, Jaffe HW: Human herpes virus 8 and Kaposi's sarcoma in persons infected with human immunodeficiency virus. Clin Infect Dis 30:S72-S76, 2000.
233. Dezube BJ: Acquired immunodeficiency syndrome-related Kaposi's sarcoma: clinical features, staging, and treatment. Semin Oncol 27:424-430, 2000.
234. Jones JL, Hanson DL, Dworkin MS, Jaffe HW: Incidence and trends in Kaposi's sarcoma in the era of effective antiretroviral therapy. J Acquir Immune Defic Syndr 24:270-274, 2000.
235. Osick LA, Lee TP, Pedemonte MB, et al: Hepatic amyloidosis in intravenous drug abusers and AIDS patients. J Hepatol 19:79-84, 1993.
236. Goldin RD, Wilkins M, Dourakis S, et al: Iron overload in multiply transfused patients who are HIV seropositive. J Clin Pathol 46:1036-1038, 1993.
237. Cappell MS, Shetty V: A multicenter, case-controlled study of the clinical presentation and etiology of ascites and of the safety and clinical efficacy of diagnostic abdominal and paracentesis in HIV seropositive patients. Am J Gastroenterol 89:2172-2177, 1994.
238. Wilcox CM, Forsmark CE, Darragh T, et al: High-protein ascites in patients with the acquired immunodeficiency syndrome. Gastroenterology 100:745-748, 1991.
239. Israelski DM, Skowron G, Leventhal JP, et al: Toxoplasma peritonitis in a patient with acquired immunodeficiency syndrome. Arch Intern Med 148:1655-1657, 1988.
240. Lin O, Scholes JV, Lustbader IJ: Chylous ascites resulting from Kaposi's sarcoma in an AIDS patients. Am J Gastroenterol 89:2252-2253, 1994.
241. Arsura EL, Ismail Y, Civrna-Karalian J, Johnson RH: Chylous ascites associated with tuberculosis in a patient with AIDS. Clin Infect Dis 19:973, 1994.
242. Jeffers LJ, Alzate I, Aguilar H, et al: Laparoscopic and histologic findings in patients with the human immunodeficiency virus. Gastrointest Endosc 40:160-164, 1994.
243. Margulis SJ, Honig CL, Soave R, et al: Biliary tract obstruction in the acquired immunodeficiency syndrome [published erratum appears in Ann Intern Med Oct; 105(4:634), 1986]. Ann Intern Med 105:207-210, 1986.
244. Schneiderman DJ, Cello JP, Laing FC: Papillary stenosis and sclerosing cholangitis in the acquired immunodeficiency syndrome. Ann Intern Med 106:546-549, 1987.
245. Bouche H, Housset C, Dumont JL, et al: AIDS-related cholangitis: diagnostic features and course in 15 patients. J Hepatol 17:34-39, 1993.
246. Roulot D, Valla D, Brun-Vezinet F, et al: Cholangitis in the acquired immunodeficiency syndrome: report of two cases and review of the literature. Gut 28:1653-1660, 1987.
247. Dowsett JF, Miller R, Davidson R, et al: Sclerosing cholangitis in acquired immunodeficiency syndrome. Scand J Gastroenterol 23:1267-1274, 1988.
248. Benhamou Y, Caumes E, Gerosa Y, et al: AIDS-related cholangiopathy. Critical analysis of a prospective series of 26 patients. Dig Dis Sci 38:1113-1118, 1993.
249. Forbes A, Blanshard C, Gazzard B: Natural history of AIDS-related sclerosing cholangitis: a study of 20 patients. Gut 34:116-121, 1993.
250. Pol S, Romana CA, Richard S, et al: Microsporidia infection in patients with the human immunodeficiency virus and unexplained cholangitis. N Engl J Med 328:95-99, 1993.
251. Ducreux M, Buffet C, Lamy P, et al: Diagnosis and prognosis of AIDS-related cholangitis. AIDS 9:875-880, 1995.
252. Knapp PE, Saltzman JR, Fairchild P: Acalculous cholecystitis associated with microsporidial infection in a patient with AIDS. Clin Infect Dis 22:195-196, 1996.
252. Cello JP: Acquired immunodeficiency syndrome cholangiopathy: spectrum of disease. Am J Med 86:539-546, 1989.
253. Texidor HS, Godwin TA, Ramirez EA: Cryptosporidiosis of the biliary tract in AIDS. Radiology 180:51-56, 1991.
254. Beaugerie L, Teilhac MF, Deluol AM, et al: Cholangiopathy associated with microsporidia infection of the common bile duct mucosa in a patient with HIV infection. Ann Intern Med 117:401-402, 1992.
255. Pol S, Romana C, Richard S, et al: *Enterocytozoon bieneusi* infection in acquired immunodeficiency syndrome-related sclerosing cholangitis. Gastroenterology 102:1778-1781, 1992.
256. Willson R, Harrington R, Stewart B, Fritsche T: Human immunodeficiency virus 1-associated necrotizing cholangitis caused by infection with *Septata intestinalis.* Gastroenterology 108:247-251, 1995.
257. Teran G, Ruiz-Palacios GM: *Cyclospora cayetanensis* infection in patients with and without AIDS: biliary disease as another clinical manifestation. Clin Infect Dis 21:1092-1097, 1995.
258. Davis JJ, Heyman MB, Ferrell L, et al: Sclerosing cholangitis associated with chronic cryptosporidiosis in a child with a congenital immunodeficiency disorder. Am J Gastroenterol 82:1196-1202, 1987.
259. Kaplan LD, Kahn J, Jacobson M, et al: Primary bile duct lymphoma in the acquired immunodeficiency syndrome (AIDS). Ann Intern Med 110:161-162, 1989.
260. Vakil NB, Schwartz SM, Buggy BP, et al: Biliary cryptosporidiosis in HIV-infected people after the waterborne outbreak of cryptosporidiosis in Milwaukee. N Engl J Med 334:19-23, 1996.
261. Defalque D, Menu Y, Girard PM, Coulaud JP: Sonographic diagnosis of cholangitis in AIDS patients. Gastrointest Radiol 14:143-147, 1989.
262. Romano AJ, VanSonnenberg E, Casola G, et al: Gallbladder and bile duct abnormalities in AIDS: sonographic findings in eight patients. AJR Am J Roentgenol 150:123-127, 1988.
263. Quinn D, Pocock N, Freund J, et al: Radionuclide hepatobiliary scanning in patients with AIDS-related sclerosing cholangitis. Clin Nucl Med 18:417-422, 1993.
264. Teare JP, Daly CA, Rodgers C, et al: Pancreatic abnormalities and AIDS related sclerosing cholangitis. Genitourin Med 73:271-273, 1997.
265. Cello JP, Chan MF: Long-term follow-up of endoscopic retrograde cholangiopancreatography sphincterotomy for patients with acquired immune deficiency syndrome papillary stenosis. Am J Med 99:600-603, 1995.
266. Hamour AA, Bonnington A, Hawthorne B, Wilkins EGL: Successful treatment of AIDS-related cryptosporidial sclerosing cholangitis. AIDS 7:1449-1451, 1993.
267. Wilcox CM, Monkemuller KE: Hepatobiliary disease in patients with AIDS: focus on AIDS cholangiopathy. Dig Dis 16:205-213, 1998.
268. Benator DA, French AL, Beaudet LM, et al: *Isospora belli* infection associated with acalculous cholecystitis in a patient with AIDS. Ann Intern Med 121:663-664, 1994.
269. French AL, Beaudet LM, Benator DA, et al: Cholecystectomy in patients with AIDS: clinicopathologic correlations in 107 cases. Clin Infect Dis 21:852-858, 1995.
270. Adolph MD, Bass SN, Lee SK, et al: Cytomegaloviral acalculous cholecystitis in acquired immunodeficiency syndrome patients. Am Surg 59:679-684, 1993.
271. Brown H, Talamini M, Westra WH: Xanthogranulomatous cholecystitis due to invasive *Candida albicans* in a patient with AIDS. Clin Infect Dis 22:186-187, 1996.
272. Wind P, Chevallier JM, Jones D, et al: Cholecystectomy for cholecystitis in patients with acquired immune deficiency syndrome. Am J Surg 168:244-246, 1994.
273. Cacciarelli AG, Naddaf SY, el-Zeftawy HA, et al: Acute cholecystitis in AIDS patients: correlation of Tc-99m hepatobiliary scintigraphy

with histopathologic laboratory findings and CD4 counts. Clin Nucl Med 23:226-228, 1998.

274. Tanner AG, Hartley JE, Darzi A, et al: Laparoscopic surgery in patients with human immunodeficiency virus. Br J Surg 81:1647-1648, 1994.

275. Leiva JI, Etter EL, Gathe J Jr., et al: Surgical therapy for 101 patients with acquired immunodeficiency syndrome and symptomatic cholecystitis. Am J Surg 174:414-416, 1997.

276. Payne TH, Cohn DL, Davidson AJ, et al: Marked elevations of serum alkaline phosphatase in patients with AIDS. J Acquir Immune Defic Syndr 4:238-243, 1991.

277. Maldonado O, Demasi R, Maldonado Y, et al: Extremely high levels of alkaline phosphatase in hospitalized patients. J Clin Gastroenterol 27:342-345, 1998.

278. Smith FJ, Mathieson JR, Cooperberg PL: Abdominal abnormalities in AIDS: detection at US in a large population. Radiology 192:691-695, 1994.

279. Kilby JM, Marques MB, Jaye DL, et al: The yield of bone marrow biopsy and culture compared with blood cultures in the evaluation of HIV-infected patients for mycobacterial and fungal infections. Am J Med 104:123-128, 1998.

280. Cavicchi M, Pialoux G, Carnot F, et al: Value of liver biopsy for the rapid diagnosis of infection in human immunodeficiency virus-infected patients who have unexplained fever and elevated serum levels of alkaline phosphatase or gamma glutamyl transferase. Clin Infect Dis 20:606-610, 1995.

281. Ruijter TEG, Schattenkerk JKME, VanLeeuwen DJ, Bosma A: Diagnostic value of liver biopsy in symptomatic HIV-1-infected patients. Eur J Gastroenterol Hepatol 5:641-645, 1993.

282. Gordon SC, Veneri RS, McFadden RF, et al: Major hemorrhage after percutaneous liver biopsy in patients with AIDS. Gastroenterology 100:1787, 1991 (letter).

283. Gottesman D, Dyrszka H, Albarran J, Hilfer J: AIDS-related hepatic Kaposi's sarcoma: massive bleeding following liver biopsy. Am J Gastroenterol 88:762-764, 1993.

C H A P T E R

52

The Liver in Systemic Illness

Naga Chalasani, MD, and Oscar W. Cummings, MD

When patients with abnormal liver enzymes or liver function are encountered, it is often assumed that the liver is the primary culprit in the disease process. However, numerous systemic illnesses and diseases of other organs can produce signs and symptoms that are indistinguishable from primary liver diseases. The hepatic manifestations in these disorders may range from mild enzyme abnormalities to significant liver injury and liver failure. In this chapter we will review liver involvement in selected systemic disorders such as heart disease, pulmonary disease, amyloidosis, connective tissue disorders, Reye's syndrome, jejunoileal bypass, and hematologic disorders. Other systemic disorders with hepatic involvement such as sarcoidosis, cystic fibrosis, and sepsis are covered elsewhere in this textbook.

HEART DISEASE

Liver involvement occurs in patients with both acute and chronic heart disease and its spectrum ranges from asymptomatic increases in liver biochemistries to fulminant liver failure. The liver receives a significant portion of the cardiac output. Any condition that decreases cardiac output will lead to a fall in hepatic perfusion. The liver is able to compensate for changes in hepatic blood flow via vasoactive mechanisms and by increasing oxygen extraction during periods of hepatic hypoperfusion.[1] However, when critical levels of left or right heart failure are reached, hepatic injury may occur. It has been suggested that right-sided heart failure is caused by elevation in right atrial pressure, leading to elevation in hepatic venous pressure that causes distention of hepatic sinusoids and liver cell hypoxia. In left-sided heart failure decreased cardiac output results in diminished hepatic perfusion, which leads to hepatic hypoxia. The final common pathway for liver damage appears to be centrolobular hepatocellular necrosis (zone III). This portion of the liver lobule is the most vulnerable to hypoxic injury because of the organization of hepatic blood flow. Highly oxygenated blood enters the hepatic lobule via branches of the hepatic artery and portal vein in the periportal region. As it passes through the hepatic sinusoids toward the terminal hepatic venule, oxygen is extracted and hepatocytes in the centrolobular area are perfused by blood that is the least well oxygenated.[1] In general terms liver involvement in right heart failure is referred to as *congestive hepatopathy,* whereas liver injury resulting from left heart failure is known as *ischemic hepatitis.* However, these two phenomena often co-exist and may be indistinguishable in clinical practice.

Liver in Right Heart Failure (Congestive Hepatopathy)

Liver abnormalities in patients with right heart failure are common. Right heart failure can be isolated (as a result of cor pulmonale or primary pulmonary hypertension) or more likely a consequence of left ventricular failure. In a large study of 175 patients with both acute and chronic right heart failure[2] hepatomegaly was present by physical examination in more than 90 percent and splenomegaly in 20 percent of these patients.[2] Other findings of right heart failure, such as peripheral edema, pleural effusion, and ascites, were also frequently present (Table 52-1). Ascites is more prominent in patients with chronic right heart failure than in acute right heart failure.[2]

Characteristic changes in histology are seen in the liver of patients with congestive heart failure. On gross inspection the congested liver appears enlarged and purple with blunt edges.[3] The classically described "nutmeg" appearance is caused by alternative areas of pale, more

TABLE 52-1
Symptoms and Signs of Congested Livers in 175 Patents with Right-sided Heart Failure

Symptom/sign	Acute heart failure (%)	Chronic heart failure (%)
Hepatomegaly	99	95
Peripheral edema	77	71
Pleural effusion	25	17
Splenomegaly	20	22
Ascites	7	20

Adapted from Richman SM, et al: Am J Med 30:211, 1961.

normal-appearing parenchyma contrasting with congested, hemorrhagic areas that correspond to the centrolobular regions of the liver (Plate 52-1). Microscopically, central veins and sinusoids in the centrolobular region become dilated and engorged with erythrocytes. Inflammation is noticeably absent (Figure 52-1). Adjacent hepatocytes may become compressed and atrophied. With long-standing hepatic congestion, fibrosis and cirrhosis may develop (cardiac cirrhosis) (Figure 52-2).

Hepatic congestion resulting from right heart failure results in numerous biochemical abnormalities (Table 52-2). In chronic congestive heart failure hyperbilirubinemia occurs in more than 20 percent of patients.[2] It is generally mild, less than 3 mg/dl, and composed predominantly of unconjugated bilirubin. Serum aminotransferase levels are usually normal or minimally elevated in compensated, chronic congestive heart failure but may become elevated during exacerbations of heart failure. Prothrombin time is prolonged in the majority of patients with hepatic congestion from right heart failure. Patients anti-coagulated with warfarin sodium (Coumadin) for dilated cardiomyopathy may have decreased Coumadin requirements during exacerbations of congestive heart failure and this effect, if not appreciated, could result in dangerously prolonged prothrombin times. Hepatic biochemical abnormalities generally improve with improvement in cardiac function.

Several signs and symptoms of congestive heart failure (e.g., ascites, pedal edema, mild hyperbilirubinemia) are also seen in patients with decompensated hepatic cirrhosis; distinguishing these two entities may be difficult. In some patients it is particularly difficult to clinically distinguish cardiac ascites from cirrhotic ascites. In such cases characterization of ascitic fluid or measurement of hepatic venous pressure gradient may be of assistance. In a prospective study of 13 patients with cardiac ascites the serum-ascites albumin concentration gradient was equal to or greater than 1.1 g/dl and the to-

TABLE 52-2
Liver Tests of 175 Patients with Right-sided Heart Failure

	Acute heart failure		Chronic heart failure	
Liver tests	**n**	**Abnormal (%)**	**n**	**Abnormal (%)**
Bilirubin	86	37	57	21
BSP retention	71	87	55	71
Alkaline phosphatase	80	10	55	9
Aspartate aminotransferase	67	48	37	5
Alanine aminotransferase	53	15	29	3
Globulins	100	60	67	37
Prothrombin time	68	84	43	74
Albumin	100	32	67	27
Cholesterol	87	49	60	42

Adapted from Richman SM: Am J Med 30:211, 1961.
BSP, Bromsulphalein.

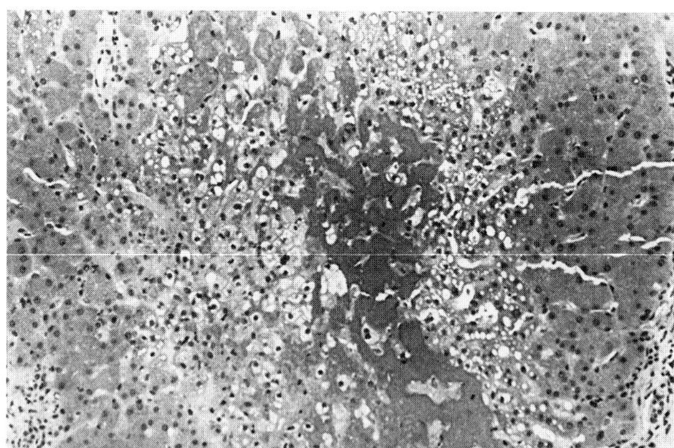

Figure 52-1 Liver congestion. The sinuses around the central vein are distended by normal red cells in congestion. The adjacent hepatocytes are mildly atrophic. There are unremarkable portal tracts at each edge of the photograph. (Hematoxylin and eosin.)

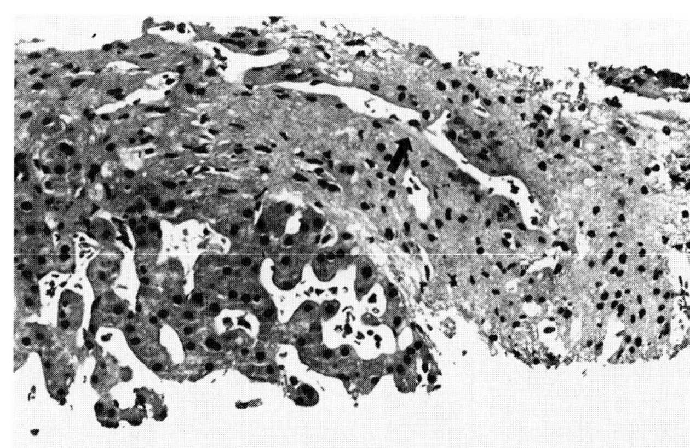

Figure 52-2 Cardiac cirrhosis, with chronic passive congestion secondary to mitral regurgitation. A dense fibrous band adjacent to regenerative hepatocytes surrounds the central vein (arrow). As the fibrosis progresses it tends to form central-central bridges, trapping portal tracts in the center of regenerative nodules. (Hematoxylin and eosin.)

tal protein was 2.5 g/dl.[3] Additionally, cardiac ascites had significantly higher ascitic fluid red cell counts and levels of lactate dehydrogenase as compared to cirrhotic ascites.[3]

Left Heart Failure and Ischemic Hepatitis

Ischemic hepatitis can be defined as hepatocellular necrosis associated with a decrease in hepatic perfusion.[4-6] It is relatively infrequent with a reported incidence of 0.16 percent to 1.5 percent of hospitalized patients. It can affect any age group although it is most frequently reported in older population. This undoubtedly reflects the increased risk of underlying cardiovascular disease in older people. When seen in children, ischemic hepatitis is often seen in association with congenital heart disease or overwhelming sepsis.[7] The term *ischemic hepatitis* is a misnomer because ischemic liver injury is characterized by centrolobular necrosis in the absence of inflammation. The diagnosis of ischemic hepatitis should be considered in any patient with elevations of liver enzymes (i.e., aspartate aminotransferase [AST], alanine aminotransferase [ALT], and lactate dehydrogenase [LDH]) in the setting of documented or suspected systemic hypotension.

Causes and Pathogenesis

Liver is a highly vascular organ, receiving approximately 25 percent of cardiac output. Seventy percent of the hepatic blood flow is derived from the portal system. The other 30 percent is delivered by the hepatic artery, and there is a linear relation between blood pressure and hepatic blood flow.[8] The liver can maintain normal oxygen uptake by increasing oxygen extraction, with as much as 95 percent of the oxygen from the blood being extracted in a single pass through the liver.[6] This remarkable compensatory mechanism most likely accounts for the low incidence of liver damage in shock (resistance to ischemia). Nevertheless, these compensatory mechanisms are overwhelmed in some patients with severely diminished hepatic perfusion leading to ischemic liver injury.

Cardiogenic shock from any cause (e.g., myocardial infarction, tamponade) is the most commonly reported risk factor for the development of ischemic hepatitis. Transiently decreased cardiac output seen in patients with arrhythmia or valvular heart disease may also result in hepatic injury even in the absence of bona fide hypotension (relative hypotension).[9] Episodes of hypotension resulting in ischemic hepatitis may be very brief and sometimes there may not be any documented episodes of hypotension. Although diminished hepatic perfusion from systemic hypotension (either absolute or relative) is essential, a recent study suggests that systemic hypotension or shock alone is insufficient to cause ischemic hepatitis.[10] In this study 31 patients with ischemic hepatitis were compared to a control group consisting of 31 previously healthy subjects with major non-hepatic trauma and marked hypotension (mean systolic pressure of 54 ± 22 mm Hg lasting for a mean of 19 ± 14 minutes). All 31 patients with ischemic hepatitis had organic heart disease and more than 90 percent had demonstrable right heart failure. None of the subjects in the control group developed ischemic hepatitis despite profound hypotension. These findings suggest that right heart failure with passive hepatic congestion is an essential background without which profound but transient systemic hypotension would not cause ischemic hepatitis.[10] Non-cardiogenic causes of ischemic hepatitis include hypovolemic shock from hemorrhage or dehydration, heat stroke, and septic shock.[11-13] Rare episodes of ischemic hepatitis have been reported in patients who ingest vasoactive medication (ergotamine overdose) and after protracted seizures in children.[14,15]

Clinical Syndrome

The clinical picture is usually dominated by the cardiovascular, septic, or hemorrhagic illness that precipitated the hepatic hypoperfusion. A distinctive biochemical pattern is characteristic of this disorder.[16,17] Serum aminotransferase levels rise rapidly after an ischemic episode and peak within 1 to 3 days (Figure 52-3). With treatment of the underlying illness serum aminotransferases return to near normal usually within 7 to 10 days of the initial insult. Persistent elevation of serum aminotransferase levels beyond this period implies a poor prognosis resulting from continued hepatic hypoperfusion.

Serum ALT and AST activity is strikingly elevated and may exceed 200 times the upper limits of normal (see Figure 52-3). Less marked elevations (<500 U/L) have also been reported in biopsy-proven ischemic hepatitis. Serum LDH activity is also markedly elevated in patients with ischemic hepatitis. When fractionated, serum LDH activity is mostly of hepatic origin.[16] The level of LDH may rise to 30 times the upper limits of normal and parallel the pattern of aminotransferase activity with a brisk rise and rapid resolution. Of note, the serum LDH is usually only slightly elevated in patients with acute viral hepatitis. Marked elevations of alkaline phosphatase or serum bilirubin are unusual in ischemic hepatitis, and cholestasis has not been demonstrated on liver biopsies of those patients. Mild elevations of serum bilirubin may be seen but rarely exceed four times the upper limit of normal.[16]

In one series of patients with ischemic hepatitis additional biochemical features were noted that might be helpful in diagnosis.[7] All patients in this series had transient abnormalities of serum creatinine and blood urea nitrogen. These changes were sometimes marked, consistent with acute renal failure, but resolved over 7 to 10 days. They speculated that the same hypotensive insult to the liver had similar adverse effects on the kidney. Both hyperglycemia and hypoglycemia can be seen.[5,16,17] In one series two thirds of patients with ischemic hepatitis had new onset hyperglycemia that occurred within 48 hours of their illness.[17] In another report hypoglycemia was seen in 33 percent of the patients with ischemic hepatitis.[5]

Histologic studies of ischemic hepatitis are limited. Patients in whom a diagnosis of ischemic hepatitis is being considered are usually critically ill, often with multi-organ failure, making a liver biopsy impractical. Nevertheless, the hallmark of ischemic hepatitis is centrolobular necrosis in the absence of an inflammatory

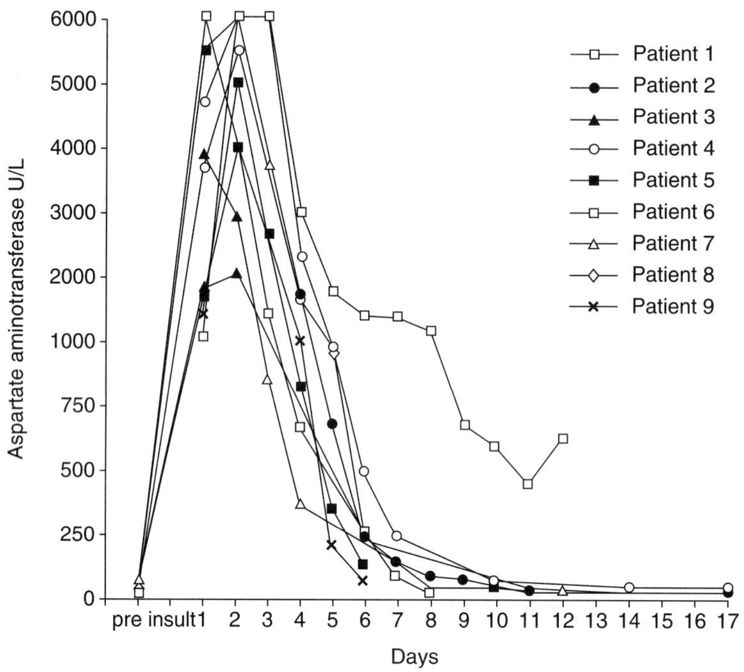

Figure 52-3 Ischemic hepatitis. Serial ALT levels in patients with ischemic hepatitis. *ALT,* Alanine aminotransferase. (Adapted from Gitlin N, Serio KM: Ischemic hepatitis: widening horizons. Am J Gastroenterol 87:831, 1992.)

infiltrate.[18] Gibson and Dudley studied 17 patients with these characteristic histologic findings and concluded that a diagnosis of ischemic hepatitis could be made without a liver biopsy in the appropriate clinical setting (patients who had a potential cause for a fall in cardiac output and a rapid rise in levels of serum aminotransferases and LDH).[16]

Differential Diagnosis

Few primary liver diseases will give such marked elevations of serum aminotransferases followed by rapid resolution. The diagnosis of ischemic hepatitis can be made readily in a patient in the intensive care unit with a rapid and striking increase of serum aminotransferase and LDH activities who has recently suffered a documented, acute hypotensive episode that required pressor support.

Acute viral hepatitis may mimic the clinical picture seen with ischemic hepatitis. Viral hepatitis will usually be accompanied by a symptomatic prodrome or a history of exposure that can be ascertained in the medical history; serologies will help to exclude a viral etiology. Serum LDH activity is only mildly elevated in patients with hepatitis. In patients who have only modest elevations in serum aminotransferases, chronic hepatitis B and hepatitis C should be excluded by history and appropriate serologic tests. Examination of previous liver enzyme results before the current illness may be invaluable in distinguishing the acute illness from chronic viral hepatitis.

Special care should be taken to identify all medications taken by the patient before admission and those started since hospitalization. Drug hepatoxicity can be associated with striking elevations of serum aminotransferase and LDH activities. Acetaminophen toxicity should always be considered in patients with marked elevations of serum aminotransferase levels and renal insufficiency. Amiodarone is an anti-arrhythmic agent that is being increasingly used in the management of unstable tachyarrhythmias. Its toxicity should also be considered in the differential diagnosis because several cases of acute hepatitis and fulminant liver failure have been reported with intravenous loading doses of amiodarone.[18-20]

Other causes of marked, acute elevations of serum AST activity include rhabdomyolysis, acute myocardial infarction, acute cholangitis, hepatic trauma, and hepatic infarction, all of which should be distinguishable from ischemic hepatitis by history and additional laboratory investigation.

Treatment and Prognosis

The treatment of ischemic hepatitis is directed at the underlying illness. Therapy to improve cardiac output with inotropes and pressors will improve hepatic perfusion and result in resolution of the ischemic hepatitis. Similarly, volume resuscitation for patients with hemorrhagic shock and appropriate treatment for septic shock will indirectly improve cardiac output and hepatic perfusion.

Special consideration should be given to prescribing medications in patients with circulatory failure and ischemic hepatitis. The clearance of certain medications (e.g., lidocaine, calcium channel blockers) is dependent on hepatic blood flow and their clearance can be greatly diminished in this setting. Indeed, an association has been reported between the use of calcium channel blockers and anti-arrhythmic agents in patients with ischemic hepatitis and an increase in mortality, although it was not clear from that study if the worse prognosis was merely related to the presence of more severe cardiac disease.[21] Opiates and analgesics that are often prescribed for these critically ill patients also have the potential to accumulate and cause neurologic and respiratory depression. It has been suggested that the risk of acetaminophen toxicity is increased in patients with underlying cardiomyopathy, even at low doses in the absence of alcohol ingestion.[22]

The prognosis of ischemic hepatitis is largely dependent upon the prognosis of the underlying illness. Mortality has been reported to be as high as 50 percent in patients with ischemic hepatitis. However, despite the massive hepatitic necrosis that may occur, deaths due to hepatic failure are extremely rare; the cause of death is usually a result of poor cardiac reserve.[4] The aminotransferase levels do not seem to have any prognostic significance. When stratified according to peak AST activity, the survival for patients with AST levels lower than 2000 was 43 percent compared to 41 percent for patients with a peak AST activity above this value. The pattern of AST activity, however, does seem to have some prognostic value. In patients with ischemic hepatitis who died, the level of serum AST did not drop appreciably from peak values whereas in those who survived, AST levels rapidly returned towards normal.[4]

Liver in Constrictive Pericarditis

Constrictive pericarditis may masquerade as a primary liver disease.[23-25] Pulsatile hepatomegaly, splenomegaly, and ascites are often present in patients with constrictive pericarditis.[26] Other important physical findings include elevated jugular venous pressure, pulsus paradoxus, and pericardial knock. It has been noted that ascites is more prominent than pedal edema.[27] Histologic features are usually non-specific; diffuse centrolobular congestion, necrosis, and fibrosis are the most common, but there may be mild abnormalities such as patchy fibrosis without congestion. Occasionally, there can be prominent sinusoidal dilation and hemorrhagic necrosis with hepatic vein thrombosis leading to a misdiagnosis of Budd-Chiari syndrome.[28,29] Tuberculosis remains an important cause of constrictive pericarditis, but other etiologies such as cardiac surgery, connective tissue disorders, subclinical viral pericarditis, and malignancy are becoming increasingly frequent in recent years. Pericardial calcification on chest radiography and low voltage on electrocardiography, when present, are very suggestive of constrictive pericarditis.

Liver Injury Resulting from Arterial Hypoxemia

Hepatic hypoxia is an important determinant of liver injury and can result from multiple etiologies. Most cases of hepatic hypoxia are related to altered hepatic perfusion (e.g., congestive heart failure); however, severe arterial hypoxemia resulting from respiratory diseases can also lead to hepatic injury independent of hepatic perfusion abnormalities (hypoxic hepatitis).[30-33] A recent study investigated the details of hemodynamic and oxygen transportation abnormalities in 17 consecutive patients with hypoxic hepatitis caused by acute exacerbation of chronic respiratory failure without left heart failure.[33] These patients had marked arterial hypoxemia (arterial oxygen pressure of 34 mm Hg) with elevated central venous pressure but an elevated cardiac index and low systemic vascular resistance. Oxygen delivery was significantly decreased in these patients despite a maintained hepatic blood flow as measured by the low dose galactose clearance test. The authors suggested that hypoxic hepatitis induced by acute exacerbation of chronic respiratory failure is due to severe arterial hypoxemia in the background of elevated central venous pressure and passive hepatic congestion.[33] Most patients with hypoxic hepatitis caused by respiratory diseases have accompanying cardiac dysfunction; however, there are reports of severe obstructive sleep apnea leading to hypoxic hepatitis in the absence of any cardiac dysfunction.[31]

JEJUNOILEAL BYPASS

Jejunoileal bypass surgery was introduced in the 1960s as a surgical treatment for morbid obesity.[34] Initial enthusiasm for this radical weight loss procedure was tempered by the recognition of a myriad of associated complications, including electrolyte abnormalities, kidney problems, gallstones, severe malnutrition, and liver disease.[34-38] The hepatic effects of jejunoileal bypass include fatty infiltration, cirrhosis, and progressive liver failure. This procedure is rarely, if ever, performed today; therefore, new diagnoses of liver disease related to jejunoileal bypass are unusual. However, patients who have had surgery decades ago may present with end-stage liver disease, on occasion being referred to centers for consideration of liver transplantation. Rarely, non-alcoholic steatohepatitis has been reported after gastric partitioning surgery.[39]

Mechanism of Hepatic Injury

Numerous theories have been proposed to explain the liver injury associated with jejunoileal bypass. The bypass procedure results in malabsorption of a number of nutrients, which accounts for some of its weight-loss effects and many of the associated complications. Early researchers noted the similarities of fatty infiltration seen in patients with protein malnutrition and in patients after jejunoileal bypass.[40] Serum levels of essential amino acids were decreased when measured during the period of rapid weight loss and there was a concurrent increase in fatty infiltration of the liver. In a control group of patients who had stable weights after jejunoileal bypass, serum amino acid levels were higher and there was less hepatic steatosis. Nutritional supplements were reported to decrease the extent of hepatic injury in some patients, although others experienced continued deterioration.

Animal models and studies in patients after jejunoileal bypass implicated bacterial overgrowth as a possible etiologic factor in the development of hepatic steatosis. In a dog model of jejunoileal bypass Vibramycin treatment prevented the appearance of fatty liver and death from liver failure.[41] In rats metronidazole therapy also seemed to ameliorate the postoperative changes to the liver, but to a lesser degree than did protein supplementation.[42]

Genetically obese ob/ob mice with hepatic steatosis were shown to have age-related increases in the production of endogenous ethanol resulting from intestinal microflora.[43] Drenick and associates[44] treated patients with metronidazole administered at random time intervals after jejunoileal bypass. In untreated patients hepatic lipid content as measured by morphologic assessment was elevated and remained abnormal over a 12-month period in most patients. In patients treated with metronidazole hepatic fat content that was initially elevated after the bypass surgery decreased after the drug was started. In another group, in whom metronidazole was administered intermittently, levels of hepatic fat increased and then decreased in concert with antibiotic therapy. Moreover, in this study there was no correlation between hepatic steatosis and protein malnutrition. The agent resulting from bacterial overgrowth that may act as the direct hepatoxin is not known.

Pathology of Liver Disease

The hepatic histology found in patients who have undergone jejunoileal bypass often resembles the changes seen in alcoholic liver disease. The most common findings include macrovesicular steatosis, Mallory's hyaline, sinusoidal fibrosis, and infiltrates of polymorphonuclear leukocytes.[45,46] The histologic changes of hepatic steatosis are often at their worst in the first year after surgery and then may improve in some patients, whereas others show continued progression to cirrhosis and liver failure.

Vyberg and co-workers[47] performed serial liver biopsies on 34 morbidly obese patients undergoing jejunoileal bypass. Postoperatively, 44 percent of patients had no or minimal histologic changes, whereas the remainder had varying degrees of steatosis, steatohepatitis, and perivenular fibrosis. From 5 to 9 months postoperatively, liver biopsies revealed progression of the hepatic injury in almost all patients. In the group of patients with minimal preoperative changes 85 percent had developed moderate to marked steatosis. Those patients with more severe changes preoperatively showed increased steatohepatitis and fibrosis; 18 percent developed bridging fibrosis and 9 percent had changes of cirrhosis. Mallory's hyaline was seen in almost one third of patients.

Nasrallah and colleagues[48] attempted to identify pre- and postoperative variables that may predict histologic liver injury after jejunoileal bypass. Preoperatively, 59 percent of morbidly obese patients had normal liver histology. There was no correlation between preoperative histology, serum biochemical parameters, use of small amounts of alcohol, or the amount of weight loss and the postoperative histologic changes.

Clinical Manifestations

Liver injury after jejunoileal bypass may range from asymptomatic elevations of serum hepatic enzymes to cirrhosis with liver failure. It has been estimated that up to 2 percent of patients died of liver failure after this procedure.[35,49] Liver injury may become clinically apparent within months of surgery or progress insidiously for more than 10 years before presenting with signs and symptoms of cirrhosis. Requarth and co-workers[50] reported on long-term morbidity after jejunoileal bypass in 453 patients. During the follow-up 24 patients developed acute liver failure (7 percent), and the actuarial 15-year probability of cirrhosis was 8.1 percent. In the early stages of hepatic injury associated with jejunoileal bypass, liver enzyme abnormalities do not correlate with histologic findings and are therefore of limited value in identifying patients at risk for liver failure.[48,49,51] Mild elevations of serum aminotransferases and alkaline phosphatase levels may occur, but many patients with significant histologic changes have no biochemical abnormalities. Serial liver biopsies may be helpful to follow the progression of liver disease. After overt liver failure develops, elevation of serum bilirubin, a further fall in serum albumin, and prolongation of prothrombin time will be evident. In these patients a trial of parenteral vitamin K administration is worthwhile to exclude malabsorption as a contributing cause to the coagulopathy.

Patients who are discovered to have progressive liver injury may benefit from reversal of the bypass operation.[38,52] In one series nine patients with cirrhosis had reversal of the bypass to re-establish continuity of the small intestine. Seven patients survived for at least 3 years after the surgery. Follow-up liver biopsies showed histologic improvement in four patients with decreased steatosis and inflammation, whereas three had no obvious changes on liver histology. Two patients died of liver failure shortly after the reversal procedure; both of these patients had preoperative ascites, indicating that after decompensation has occurred the prognosis is very poor.

For patients who have already developed decompensated cirrhosis, liver transplantation may be the only therapeutic option available to improve quality of life and prolong survival.[53-56] In general, it is believed that jejunoileal bypass should be reversed either during or immediately after the liver transplantation.[54,55] One should avoid the takedown of jejunoileal bypass in patients with advanced liver disease before transplantation because such surgical interventions are poorly tolerated. If the jejunoileal bypass is not reversed, there is a substantial risk of recurrent steatosis and progressive liver damage in the allografts.[56] In such patients liver biopsies should be performed on a regular basis during the post-transplant period to detect progressive liver damage. Morbid obesity is common in the post-transplant period when jejunoileal bypass is reversed, but allograft abnormalities are uncommon in relation to such weight gain.[54-56]

CONNECTIVE TISSUE DISEASES

Patients with connective tissue disorders such as systemic lupus erythematosus (SLE), rheumatoid arthritis, Sjögren's syndrome, and scleroderma may have clinical and biochemical evidence of associated liver disease. The severity of liver involvement can range from asymptomatic elevations of serum aminotransferases to cirrhosis and liver failure. Unusual liver lesions such as nodular regenerative hyperplasia have been reported with increasing frequency in patients with connective tissue disorders. Over the last decade, there have been numerous reports associating chronic hepatitis C infection with Sjögren's syndrome.

Systemic Lupus Erythematosus

SLE is an autoimmune disorder involving the skin, kidneys, cardiovascular system, and central nervous system. Strict criteria reflecting multi-organ involvement have been established by the American College of Rheumatology to uniformly diagnose SLE and distinguish it from other connective tissue disorders; patients are required to have 4 of 11 criteria before a diagnosis of SLE is established.[57] All criteria need not be present at one time, but may develop sequentially over many years. Abnormalities of liver function are not part of these diagnostic criteria and the liver is generally not a major target for end-organ damage in patients with SLE. Nevertheless, many patients with SLE may have clinically significant liver disease.

Runyon and associates[58] reviewed more than 200 patients who met the criteria for SLE. Twenty-one percent of patients had abnormal liver enzymes at some point during their illness, and these elevations usually could not be attributed to other non-hepatic etiologies or co-morbid conditions. In 20 percent of patients the first liver enzyme elevations were noted during an exacerbation of SLE. Elevations of aminotransferase and alkaline phosphatase levels were usually mild, less than fourfold the upper limits of normal. However, more severe liver disease occurred, and approximately 25 percent of the patients with abnormal liver enzymes were jaundiced. Three patients died of liver failure. Liver biopsy specimens were available from 33 patients and revealed a variety of hepatic lesions, including non-specific portal inflammation, chronic hepatitis, and established cirrhosis. The most common finding was hepatic steatosis that was seen in more than one third of patients.

In an autopsy study published in 1992 Matsumoto and associates[59] studied liver specimens and clinical data from 52 patients with SLE. None of these patients died as a result of liver failure. One third of these patients had abnormalities of at least two different liver enzymes. The most common finding was hepatic congestion, although the authors felt that this lesion was most likely a result of the terminal event. As in the previous study hepatic steatosis was very common and was found in 73 percent of patients. Twelve percent of patients had chronic hepatitis. Of interest, 21 percent of patients had histologic evidence of arteritis, a finding previously considered rare in patients with SLE. Hepatic infarction occurred in one patient. Nodular regenerative hyperplasia, a lesion characterized by diffuse nodularity in the absence of associated fibrosis, was seen in three patients.

The interpretation of any studies of liver disease in patients with SLE is complicated by co-morbid conditions and the potential for drug toxicities that may mimic chronic liver disease. All of the previously mentioned studies were performed before the availability of hepatitis C (HCV) testing. Thus HCV cannot be excluded as a cause for some of the liver enzyme elevation or abnormal hepatic histology. This is particularly important because a substantial number of patients with SLE received blood transfusions before 1991. In addition, most patients in these studies received varying doses of prednisone; this certainly could explain the frequent finding of hepatic steatosis in these patients.

Hepatic injury from salicylates may also be a factor in producing some of the liver dysfunction associated with SLE and other connective tissue disorders.[60] Salicylate-induced hepatotoxicity appears to be dose-dependent. Hepatic injury is not evident in doses less than 2.5 g/day or with a blood salicylate level less than 25 mg/dl. Furthermore, there is a correlation between blood salicylate levels and the serum ALT activity.[61] Features of a hypersensitivity reaction, such as fever or rash, are usually not present. The elevation in the liver enzymes reflects hepatocellular injury with elevations of serum aminotransferases sometimes exceeding 1000 U/L. Discontinuation of aspirin results in prompt improvement of liver enzymes with no chronic sequelae.

Ascites has been reported in several patients with SLE in the absence of liver disease or other secondary conditions.[62] The pathogenesis of ascites in these patients is due to serositis with associated weeping of lymphatics. Ascites may be present even when SLE is relatively quiescent and other symptoms or signs of the disease are inactive. Increased immunosuppression with prednisone may be beneficial in reducing SLE-related ascites after other etiologies have been carefully excluded.

Rheumatoid Arthritis

Elevations of alkaline phosphatase are the most frequently reported liver test abnormalities associated with rheumatoid arthritis, and may be seen in as many as 50 percent of patients, whereas serum aminotransferase levels are usually normal.[63] The source of alkaline phosphatase, bone versus liver, is somewhat controversial. In studies of alkaline phosphatase fractions almost one third of patients with rheumatoid arthritis had elevated levels of hepatobiliary alkaline phosphatase, suggesting liver involvement. However, other serum enzymes, such as 5′-nucleotidase and gamma glutamyl transpeptidase, which are often used as supplementary assays to support the hepatic origin of alkaline phosphatase, are frequently normal in patients with rheumatoid arthritis.[63,64] Furthermore, alkaline phosphatases have been shown to have higher levels in the joint space than in serum, implying that they may originate from inflamed joints. Other investigators have demonstrated that the degree of total alkaline phosphatase elevation varies with the number of joints involved.[65] Finally, the pattern of predominant alkaline phosphatase fractions in patients may vary over time.[66] Thus abnormal serum liver-associated enzymes in patients with rheumatoid arthritis must be interpreted with caution.

Several liver diseases have been reported in patients with adult and juvenile rheumatoid arthritis (Table 52-3). In 1997 Ruderman and associates[67] published an autopsy study that discussed the hepatic histology in 182 patients with rheumatoid arthritis. The most common finding was hepatic congestion, although it is likely that this lesion was mostly a result of the terminal event. As in SLE, hepatic steatosis was common and was found in 23

TABLE 52-3
Liver Disease Associated with Adult and Juvenile Rheumatoid Arthritis

Adult rheumatoid arthritis	Juvenile rheumatoid arthritis
Hepatic steatosis	Acute hepatitis
Primary biliary cirrhosis	Chronic non-specific hepatitis
Autoimmune hepatitis	Massive liver enlargement
Nodular regenerative hyperplasia	Drug toxicity
Amyloidosis	
Salicylate or methotrexate hepatotoxicity	

TABLE 52-4
Liver Complications in Coagulopathy

1. Budd-Chiari syndrome
2. Hepatic veno-occlusive disease
3. Nodular regenerative hyperplasia
4. Transient elevation of hepatic enzymes resulting from multiple fibrin thrombi
5. Infarction of liver
6. Autoimmune hepatitis

percent of the patients. Of these, 11 percent of patients had fibrosis, 2.7 percent had established cirrhosis, and 5 percent had evidence of amyloidosis. Other disorders that are described in association with rheumatoid arthritis, such as primary biliary cirrhosis (PBC) and nodular regenerative hyperplasia, were not seen in this series.

Nodular regenerative hyperplasia has been reported in association with rheumatoid arthritis, often with Felty's syndrome and active joint disease.[68] Features of portal hypertension, such as varices and ascites, are common in this latter group of patients.[59] The pathogenesis of nodular regenerative hyperplasia is not known, although some authors have suggested that it is related to drug toxicity or underlying portal venous thromboses.[59,68] The latter hypothesis is intriguing given the frequency of anti-phospholipid syndrome in patients with connective tissue diseases, the same population with an increased incidence of nodular regenerative hyperplasia.

As with SLE, drug toxicities—particularly aspirin and other salicylates—may play a role in the liver abnormalities associated with rheumatoid arthritis. Gold therapy may cause intrahepatic cholestasis with features of a hypersensitivity reaction, including a skin rash and eosinophilia.[69-71] Prolonged, high-dose gold salt therapy has also been reported to produce a dose-related form of toxicity characterized by jaundice and severe hepatocellular necrosis in one patient. Liver biopsy revealed submassive hepatic necrosis with lobular and portal inflammation. Brown-black pigment, identified as gold granules, was seen in macrophages, and electron microscopy demonstrated gold particles in lysosomes. It was believed that hepatic injury occurred after the concentration of gold exceeded the lysosomal storage capacity.[72]

Perhaps the most controversial issue in drug therapy and hepatotoxicity involves using methotrexate for the treatment of rheumatoid arthritis. This topic is reviewed elsewhere (see Chap. 27).

Anti-phospholipid Syndrome

Anti-phospholipid syndrome (APS) is characterized by the presence of anti-phospholipid antibodies (anti-cardiolipin antibodies or lupus anticoagulant) in association with venous and arterial thromboses, recurrent fetal loss, and thrombocytopenia. Although APS can be a primary disorder, it is frequently seen in patients with SLE and other connective tissue disorders. The most commonly described hepatic manifestation of APS is Budd-Chiari syndrome.[73,74] Pelletier and colleagues[75] reported that of their 22 patients with Budd-Chiari syndrome, 4 had anti-phospholipid antibodies with no other cause of hepatic vein thrombosis (see Chaps. 21 and 53). Several other liver disorders have been reported in patients with APS and are summarized in Table 52-4.[73-75]

Sjögren's Syndrome

Sjögren's syndrome is an autoimmune disorder that mainly affects exocrine glands and usually presents as a persistent dryness of the mouth and eyes resulting from functional impairment of the salivary and lacrimal glands. PBC is common in both primary and secondary forms of Sjögren's syndrome. In a study of 300 patients with primary Sjögren's syndrome 7 percent of the patients had elevated anti-mitochondrial antibody (AMA) titers.[76] Of these, 60 percent had elevations of alkaline phosphatase. Liver biopsies revealed changes of early PBC, even in many patients with normal liver enzymes.[76]

Over the last decade there have been numerous investigations exploring the relationship between HCV and Sjögren's syndrome. In 1992 Haddad and colleagues[77] postulated a causal relationship between Sjögren's syndrome and HCV. An excellent review of current understanding of the relationship between Sjögren's syndrome and HCV has been recently published.[78] The reported prevalence of HCV in patients with Sjögren's syndrome depends on the methods of detection, the population studied, and the criteria for diagnosing primary Sjögren's syndrome. In European patients the prevalence ranges between 14 percent and 19 percent by third-generation enzyme-linked immunoassay and 5 percent to 19 percent by the recombinant immunoblot assay (RIBA)-2 method, whereas its prevalence by RIBA-2 was only 0 percent to 1 percent in American patients.[78] The prevalence of Sjögren's syndrome is much lower when the polymerase chain reaction method was used to detect HCV or when more objective criteria are applied to define primary Sjögren's syndrome.[78] Based on the current evidence HCV seems to be a rare cause of primary Sjögren's syndrome except in patients with cryoglobulinemia.[78] Furthermore, HCV is a sialotropic virus, and morphologic evidence of sialadenitis is found in up to 50 percent of the patients with chronic HCV infection.[78-81] In HCV-related sialadenitis the lymphocytic infiltrate is predominantly pericapillary (unlike periductal in primary Sjögren's syndrome), and clinical symptoms of dryness are infrequent.

Scleroderma

Reynolds and colleagues[82] described six patients with typical primary biliary cirrhosis and varying features of scleroderma and CREST (calcinosis, Raynaud's phenomenon, esophageal dysmotility, sclerodactyly, and telangiectasia) syndrome. Since then, the association between these two autoimmune disorders has been well established. The close immunologic association between PBC and scleroderma is supported by the finding of a positive AMA in more than one quarter of patients with scleroderma and anti-centromere antibody in one quarter of patients with PBC. In a recent study of 40 patients with systemic and localized scleroderma, liver biopsy-confirmed PBC was seen in 5 patients (12.5 percent).[83] Sometimes, patients with PBC develop symptomatology consistent with scleroderma. In a review of 558 patients with PBC 4 percent were found to have symptoms of CREST syndrome.[84] Clinical manifestations of CREST syndrome often antedate the development of PBC by as long as 28 years.

REYE'S SYNDROME

Reye's syndrome is an acute illness characterized by encephalopathy and fatty infiltration of the liver. It was first reported in 1963 by Reye and colleagues, who described 21 Australian children who developed loss of consciousness, vomiting, fever, and hypoglycemia shortly after a viral prodrome.[85] More than 80 percent of patients in this series died. At autopsy, extensive fatty infiltration was noted in the liver and kidney, and to a lesser extent in the myocardium and pancreas.

Epidemiology

The Centers for Disease Control and Prevention (CDC) defines a case of Reye's syndrome as one in which there is (1) acute, non-inflammatory encephalopathy manifested clinically by alterations in the level of consciousness and documented—when such results are available—by the measurement of 8 or fewer leukocytes per cubic millimeter of cerebrospinal fluid or by the presence of cerebral edema without perivascular or meningeal inflammation in the histologic section of the brain; (2) hepatopathy documented by liver biopsy or autopsy or a threefold or greater rise of AST, ALT, or serum ammonia; and (3) no other, more reasonable, explanation for the cerebral or hepatic abnormalities.[86,87] Reye's syndrome predominantly affects children in the first decade of life, but up to 20 percent of patients may be older than age 15 years and thus may be seen by adult gastroenterologists and hepatologists.[87-89] A recent study demonstrated decreasing incidence of Reye's syndrome based on the epidemiologic characteristics of 1207 cases reported to the National Reye Syndrome Surveillance System (NRSSS) from December 1, 1980, through November 30, 1997.[87] A peak of 555 cases was reported in surveillance year 1980. From 1987 through 1993 no more than 36 cases were reported each year; from 1994 through 1997 no more than 2 cases were reported each year (Figure 52-4).[87] A similar decline in the incidence of Reye's syndrome has been noted in Great Britain and elsewhere (Figure 52-5).[89]

Since the original description of Reye's syndrome, epidemiologic studies have suggested an association between Reye's syndrome and the use of aspirin during influenza or varicella infections.[87,89-92] Before 1990 the incidence of Reye's syndrome was higher in years with

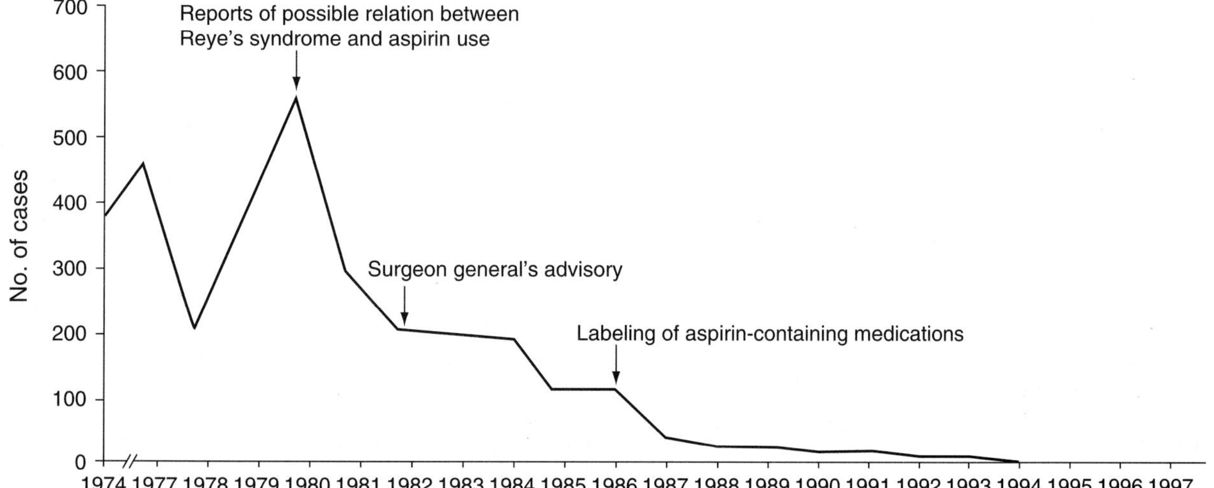

Figure 52-4 Number of reported cases of Reye's syndrome in relation to the public announcement of the epidemiologic association of Reye's syndrome with aspirin ingestion and the labeling of aspirin-containing medications. (Redrawn from Belay ED, et al: Reye's syndrome in the United States from 1981 through 1997. N Engl J Med 340:1377, 1999.)

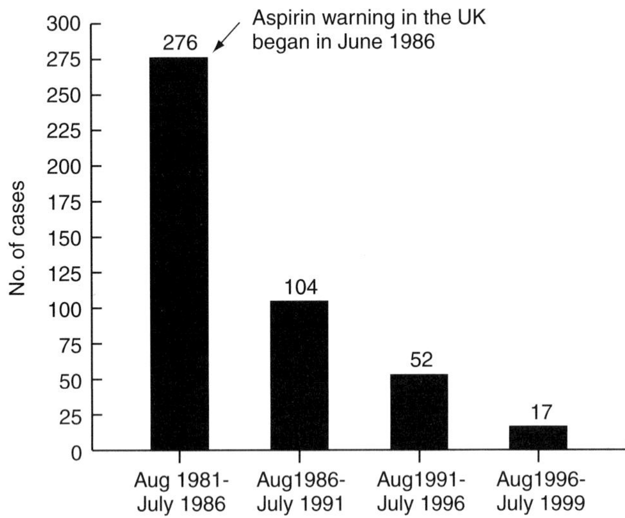

Figure 52-5 Number of cases of Reye's syndrome reported to the British Paediatric Surveillance Unit. (Adapted from Hall SM, Lynn R: Reye's syndrome. N Engl J Med 341:845, 1999.)

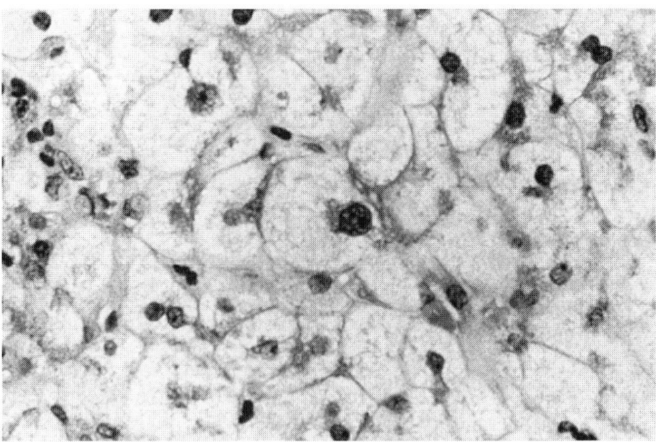

Figure 52-6 Liver in Reye's syndrome. In Reye's syndrome the hepatic architecture is preserved and the portal tracts are unremarkable. The hepatocyte cytoplasm is finely vacuolated because of accumulated lipid. Note that the nuclei remain in the center of the cell, a feature of microvesicular steatosis. (Hematoxylin and eosin.)

epidemics of influenza B than in years with epidemics of influenza A (H3N2 or H1N1), but this association was not found subsequently.[87] Patients who developed Reye's syndrome were much more likely to have received salicylates during a prodromal illness than were those who did not develop the syndrome.[91,92] In a previous study from the CDC the odds ratio of developing Reye's syndrome in association with a viral illness treated with aspirin was 16.1.[92] Children chronically treated with salicylates for illnesses such as juvenile rheumatoid arthritis and Kawasaki's disease are also at increased risk for Reye's syndrome.[87,93] Based upon these observations, in 1986 aspirin and aspirin-containing medications were required to be labeled with an advisory not to administer to children with flulike illnesses. The declining incidence of Reye's syndrome in the United States and United Kingdom is temporally associated with public health warnings about the risk of Reye's syndrome after the use of aspirin in children with varicella and influenza-like illnesses.[87,89] In countries where aspirin is inadvertently used in children with viral illnesses Reye's syndrome continues to be a significant problem.[94] Erroneous diagnosis of Reye's syndrome was not uncommon when presumptive criteria were used to establish the diagnosis. Several inherited metabolic disorders present with signs and symptoms that are indistinguishable from Reye's syndrome (see the following section). When the charts of 49 patients who were originally diagnosed with Reye's syndrome were blindly reviewed, only one case was felt to be truly the result of Reye's syndrome.[95] In the United Kingdom 12.7 percent of patients who were originally reported with Reye's syndrome between 1981 and 1998 were subsequently diagnosed with an inherited metabolic disorder.[89] Because Reye's syndrome is now very rare, it has been suggested that any infant or child suspected of having this disorder should undergo investigation to exclude the presence of inborn metabolic disorders that can mimic Reye's syndrome.[87]

Histopathology and Pathogenesis

Liver specimens in patients with Reye's syndrome exhibit several characteristic histologic abnormalities (Figure 52-6). Microvesicular steatosis and decreased or absent glycogen stores are common and appear to correlate with severity of illness and survival.[96] There is minimal hepatocellular necrosis associated with these lesions. Hepatic glycogen content in biopsies taken within 24 to 48 hours of the onset of encephalopathy was significantly lower in patients who died. These lesions also appear to evolve over time so that in serial biopsy specimens glycogen stains and microvesicular steatosis may initially worsen and then improve within 1 to 2 weeks of the onset of encephalopathy. In survivors liver biopsies performed 1 to 13 months after clinical improvement showed essentially normal histology, indicating that the hepatic lesions of Reye's syndrome are completely reversible.

Electron microscopic studies of the liver in Reye's syndrome have also demonstrated characteristic findings that are consistent with the presumed pathogenesis of the disease. Ultrastructural study has shown that mitochondria within the hepatocytes of children with Reye's syndrome are swollen and irregularly shaped with expansion of the matrix space.[97] These changes also regress in parallel with clinical improvement. An excellent review of metabolic abnormalities seen in Reye's syndrome and other inherited disorders was published in 1994.[98] Hyperammonemia may result from a decrease in the activity of enzymes involved in the urea cycle—carbamyl phosphate synthetase and ornithine transcarbamylase (OTC). Both of these enzymes are normally found predominantly within the mitochondria; however, in patients with Reye's syndrome, OTC activity is shifted to the cytosol, presumably because of damage to the mitochondrial membrane.[99] The decreased levels of enzyme activity are transient and correlate with the clinical status of the patient.[100] Increase in nitrogen load result-

TABLE 52-5
Outcome of Reye's Syndrome According to the Level of Consciousness

		OUTCOME			
			CNS SEQUELAE		
Stage	Total	Complete Recovery	Mild	Severe	Death
0-1	505	391 (77%)	16 (3%)	4 (0.8%)	94 (19%)
2-3	473	289 (61%)	32 (6.7%)	10 (2.1%)	142 (30%)
4-5	128	15 (12%)	5 (4%)	8 (6.2%)	100 (78%)

Redrawn from Belay ED: Reye's syndrome in the United States from 1981 through 1997. N Engl J Med 340:1377, 1999.
CNS, Central nervous system.

ing from muscle breakdown has also been reported in patients with Reye's syndrome and contributes to the profound hyperammonemia that may be seen.[98]

The metabolism of fatty acids is also impaired in patients with Reye's syndrome. Numerous intermediate metabolites are abnormally elevated in the liver, plasma, or urine of these patients, and high levels of these compounds are believed to further inhibit mitochondrial enzymes involved in ureagenesis, gluconeogenesis, and fatty acid oxidation.[98] Salicylates may inhibit mitochondrial enzymes involved in fatty acid oxidation, which may explain the association between these drugs and the development of Reye's syndrome.[98] Furthermore, in mice, infection with influenza virus potentiated the inhibitory effects of salicylates on mitochondrial fatty acid oxidation.[101] Some of the deleterious effects of salicylates on mitochondrial structure and function may be cytokine-mediated; pretreatment with α-interferon ameliorated salicylate-induced damage to isolated rat liver mitochondria.[102]

Clinical Features, Differential Diagnosis, and Treatment

Reye's syndrome is seen predominantly in young children and adolescents but has been reported to occur infrequently in adults.[103-105] Belay and colleagues found that 8 percent of the cases in the United States involved patients who were 15 years of age or older.[87] Other illnesses such as Jamaican vomiting sickness and drug toxicity from valproic acid or fialuridine may present with similar changes of microvesicular steatosis. Several inborn metabolic disorders often present with signs and symptoms that are indistinguishable from Reye's syndrome.[106-108] The most common metabolic disorder mimicking Reye's syndrome is medium-chain acyl-coenzyme-A dehydrogenase deficiency.[108] Most of these inherited disorders are specific enzymatic defects that usually become evident before the age of 3 years. These disorders are characterized by recurrent episodes, the presence of a similar disorder in siblings, frequent hypoglycemia, cardiac enlargement, and muscle weakness. The most consistent distinguishing features of Reye's syndrome on electron microscopy are ultrastructural changes in liver tissue, specifically the proliferation of smooth endoplasmic reticulum and peroxisomes and the presence of enlarged and pleomorphic mitochondria with loss of dense granules.[107,109] In enzymatic defects with Reye's manifestations the mitochondria are normal in size and appearance.

The illness begins with a viral prodrome that may begin to resolve. Within several days patients present with intractable vomiting and mental status changes, ranging from irritability to mild encephalopathy with confusion and disorientation that may progress to deep coma. Serum aminotransferase levels are elevated as much as 50 times the upper limits of normal. Prothrombin time is usually prolonged and serum ammonia is elevated. Serum bilirubin levels are almost invariably normal or just slightly elevated so that jaundice is conspicuously absent in Reye's syndrome.[103]

Treatment of Reye's syndrome is generally supportive with careful attention to hypoglycemia and electrolyte disturbances. High-concentration glucose solutions are required to maintain adequate serum glucose levels. With neurologic deterioration consideration should be given to intracranial pressure monitoring to guide the effects of various interventions, such as hyperventilation and mannitol infusions, which may be used to decrease intracranial pressure. In the CDC report that described the outcomes of 1207 Reye's syndrome cases reported to NRSSS, the overall case fatality rate was 31.3 percent.[87] The level of consciousness at admission was a strong predictor of death; the mortality rate increased from 17.8 percent in stage 0 (alert and wakeful) to 89.6 percent in stage 5 patients (unarousable, areflexia, and fixed pupils) (Table 52-5). Additionally, age younger than 5 years and serum ammonia concentration above 45 μg/dl were independent predictors of mortality. Residual neurologic deficits were reported in 9.8 percent of patients; the deficits were mild in 6.9 percent and severe in 2.8 percent.[87] Patients with serum ammonia above 45 μg/dl had significantly higher risk of neurologic complications (relative risk, 4.1; 95 percent confidence interval, 1.2-14.0).[87]

STAUFFER'S SYNDROME

Stauffer's syndrome (nephrogenic hepatic dysfunction) is a paraneoplastic syndrome of liver test abnormalities in patients with renal cell carcinoma. This was first reported in 1961 by Stauffer, who described five patients with renal cell carcinoma and associated abnormalities of liver function in the absence of hepatic metastases.[110] In the early literature Stauffer's syndrome incidence ranged from 4 percent to 40 percent.[111-113] Its true incidence is difficult to ascertain from these early reports because of the limitations in their ability to adequately exclude hepatic metastases as a cause for liver abnormalities. In a recent study that reviewed the records of 365 patients with renal cell carcinoma 21 percent had paraneoplastic elevation of alkaline phosphatase. In this study hepatic and bone metastases were excluded by computed tomography scans and bone scans.[114]

Recent evidence suggests that interleukin (IL)-6 is responsible for causing various paraneoplastic syndromes seen in renal cell carcinoma.The following evidence supports IL-6 as the cytokine involved: (1) when given systemically IL-6 induces findings similar to paraneoplastic syndromes associated with renal cell carcinoma (fever, elevated alkaline phosphatase)[115,116]; (2) IL-6 is expressed by most of the renal cell cancer cell lines, and strong correlation exists between serum IL-6 and paraneoplastic elevation of alkaline phosphatase[117,118]; and (3) administration of anti–IL-6 monoclonal antibodies normalized the alkaline phosphatase levels in patients with Stauffer's syndrome.[119]

Strickland and Schenker reviewed 29 published cases of nephrogenic hepatic dysfunction in which sufficient data were available to apply strict criteria for the diagnosis.[120] Fever and weight loss were the most common symptoms. Hepatomegaly was present in two thirds of patients. Elevation of alkaline phosphatase was the most common biochemical abnormality, occurring in 90 percent of reported cases, whereas abnormalities of serum aminotransferases and serum bilirubin were much less common. Histologic examination of the liver in patients with nephrogenic hepatic dysfunction has shown only non-specific changes. Steatosis, mild focal hepatocyte necrosis, portal lymphocytic infiltration, and Kupffer cell hyperplasia have all been reported.[111,120,121] Although elevations in alkaline phosphatase are frequent, jaundice and pruritus from cholestasis are very infrequent.

The importance of recognizing this syndrome lies in the decision concerning resection of the tumor and differentiating these benign liver enzyme abnormalities from metastatic disease. Abnormalities of hepatic function usually resolve 1 to 2 months after the primary tumor has been resected; indeed, this is an important feature in the diagnosis of this syndrome.[110-113,120,121] With recurrence of renal cell carcinoma clinical and biochemical characteristics of nephrogenic hepatic dysfunction may again become evident.[121]

AMYLOIDOSIS

Hepatic involvement is common in patients with systemic amyloidosis. It is a disorder of abnormal protein deposition in various organs. On histologic examination all amyloid proteins show extracellular, amorphous, eosinophilic hyaline-like material. This material stains with Congo red dye and shows apple-green birefringence when examined under polarized light. The precursor proteins, although vastly different chemically, share the conformational property of forming beta-pleated sheets as they precipitate. It is the beta-pleated sheet arrangement that leads to the characteristic histochemical findings.

Primary and Secondary Amyloidosis

Amyloid is currently classified by placing an A in front of the abbreviation for the precursor protein (Table 52-6). There are at least 16 different variants. Many of these occur only focally in aged or tumorous organs and do not directly involve the liver.

Primary, or AL amyloidosis, is related to the deposition of immunoglobulin light or heavy chain protein.[122,122a] This is probably the most common form of systemic amyloidosis in the United States. Immunoglobulin is a normal component of the humoral immune system and can be found normally in the serum in a 2:1 ratio, kappa to lambda. In lymphoplasmacytic disorders such as multiple myeloma or Waldenström's macroglobulinemia, there is an overproduction of portions of the immunoglobulin molecule, generally the light chain. The light chain protein itself or its breakdown products then precipitate out of the serum to form amyloid. Most patients with amyloidosis have precipitated lambda light chains, suggesting that this form is more likely to produce the beta-pleated sheet arrangement.

AA, or secondary, amyloid is associated with chronic infections such as osteomyelitis or tuberculosis. Cytokines associated with the inflammation, such as IL-1, IL-6, and tumor necrosis factor, stimulate the liver to produce serum amyloid A.[123,123a] This protein is an injury-specific component of high-density lipoprotein. This protein is continuously produced during chronic infections.[124] People vary greatly in their ability to clear this protein. Although most individuals cleave this protein into small peptides, some patients can only cleave it into larger sizes consistent with the amyloid subunit. The normal human AA protein exists as three isoforms and is coded by three genes on the short arm of chromosome 11.

Familial Mediterranean fever (FMF) is an autosomal-recessive disorder associated with recurrent episodes of fever, arthritis, serositis, and skin rash. It is predominantly seen in non-Ashkenazi Jews and Turkish people. These patients develop renal disease and ultimately renal failure, which can be generally controlled with colchicine administration. Recently a genetic defect has been located on the short arm of chromosome 16 in patients with FMF.[125,126] The defect occurs in a gene coding for a protein known as pyrin/marenostrin. It is unclear how this gene product interacts with the serum A protein to produce amyloidosis.

Mutations in the transthyretin gene are associated with familial amyloidotic polyneuropathy (FAP).[127] This is the most common type of heritable amyloidosis. The transthyretin gene product is a normal serum protein largely produced by the liver; it carries serum thyroxin and retinal-binding protein. The protein is a tetramer of identical subunits that is encoded by a single gene on chromosome 18. At least 78 different amino acid substitutions occurring at least 51 different sites in the transthyretin gene have been reported.[127] Most of these mutations are amyloidogenic. Although inherited as an

TABLE 52-6
Different Types of Amyloidosis

Variant	Precursor protein	Sites involved	Disease	Mutation
AL	Immunoglobulin light chain	Systemic	Myeloma	
ATTR	Transthyretin	Systemic	Hereditary	Chromosome 18;Val30Met most common
AA	(Apo)serum AA	Systemic	Chronic infection	AA gene on 11p; FMF 16p
Aβ_2M	β_2-Microglobulin	Systemic	Chronic hemodialysis	
AapoAI	Apoprotein AI	Nerves, kidney, liver	Hereditary	Chromosome 11; Gly26Arg most common
Alys	Lysozyme variants	Kidney	Hereditary	
Agel	Gelsolin	Cornea, nerves, skin	Hereditary	
Afib	Fibrinogen a-chain	Kidney	Hereditary	
Acys	Cystatin C	Cerebral blood vessels	Hereditary	
Aβ	Aβ-protein precursor	Brain	Alzheimer's disease	Chromosome 21
AprPsc	Prion protein	Nervous system	Spongiform encephalopathy	PRNP gene Chromosome 20
Acal	(Pro)calcitonin	Thyroid	Medullary carcinoma	
AIAPP	Islet amyloid protein	Islet of Langerhans		
AANF	Atrial natriuretic factor	Heart		
Apro	Prolactin	Aging pituitary	Prolactinoma	

FSM, Familial Mediterranean fever.

autosomal-dominant disorder, symptoms generally do not arise until the third to fourth decade. The disorder has been seen in Portugal, Sweden, Japan, and the United States. The U.S. kindreds usually exhibit the defects associated with their country of origin. The clinical onset can be quite variable among these ethnic groups, even in those patients with the same mutation. The patients usually present with a lower limb nephropathy, which progresses to the upper limbs. Autonomic nervous system involvement also is usually extensive, often resulting in diarrhea. Changes in the joints, skin, and cornea are also present. Rarely, other organs can be involved.

Patients undergoing chronic hemodialysis develop amyloid secondary to precipitation of the β_2-microglobulin protein.[128] β_2-Microglobulin is a normal serum protein. The hemodialysis itself is thought to produce localized excess concentration of this protein, resulting in the deposition of amyloid. Generally, the musculoskeletal system and the kidneys are involved.

Although amyloid is relatively homogeneous in its appearance, it is clear that its etiology can be quite variable. The mechanism of amyloid formation is likewise complex; most likely, various mechanisms are at work depending on different forms of the disease. For instance, in the FAP disorders it is thought that the inheritable mutation causes beta-pleated sheet-type fibrils to form on normal proteolysis. This is contrasted to secondary amyloidosis, in which not only overexpression of the AA protein but perhaps also abnormal proteolysis result in the deposition of fibrils.

Clinical Features, Diagnosis, and Treatment

Amyloidosis can present as renal dysfunction and renal failure, heart failure and cardiomyopathy, peripheral neuropathy, skin rash, and blood dyscrasias.[129] The most common finding related to the liver is hepatomegaly.[129a] Several other forms of presentation of hepatic amyloidosis are summarized in Table 52-7. Jaundice and cholestasis can be one of the initial manifestations of hepatic amyloidosis.[130-136] When present, it is an ominous finding and suggests a short survival time. Amyloid can also present catastrophically as liver failure or hepatic rupture.[137] Ascites resulting from sinusoidal occlusion can also be a presenting symptom.[138] Generally, the transaminases are minimally elevated, although they can be quite high in the rare cases of fulminant failure. Jaundice is also infrequent except for the rare cholestatic cases. Imaging studies may show an infiltrative process but are generally not helpful in gauging the extent of disease.

TABLE 52-7
Manifestations of Hepatic Amyloidosis

Hepatosplenomegaly
Splenomegaly
Ascites
Prolongation of prothrombin time resulting from acquired factor X deficiency
Cholestasis
Jaundice
Acute liver failure
Spontaneous rupture

Demonstration of amyloid deposition is generally required to support the diagnosis. Fat-pad aspirations are the easiest and most common approach to diagnose amyloidosis. If that is negative, rectal or skin biopsies are obtained, with biopsies of affected organs if needed. Amyloid deposition in the liver occurs in three basic patterns. The most common pattern is protein deposition in the spaces of Disse (Figure 52-7). As the material accumulates it encroaches on the hepatocytes, causing extensive atrophy. It clearly increases the mass of the liver, producing hepatomegaly, but only rarely compromises sinusoidal blood flow leading to portal hypertension. Another pattern is deposition of amyloid only in the walls of hepatic arterioles; the third pattern is globular clusters of amyloid, again in the space of Disse. The latter pattern appears to be most uncommon. The Congo red stain is the mainstay of diagnosis.[127,139] Although commonly used as a diagnostic test, the Congo red stain can be difficult to perform correctly. The characteristic staining is highly dependent on the pH, salt concentration, and thickness of the material stained. Any variation in these parameters can greatly affect the quality of staining. The Congo red staining is relatively specific for amyloid when properly performed; however, under some conditions, one can also see staining of fibrin, elastin, and collagen. However, these are usually not birefringent under polarized light. The staining properties with Congo red are related to the beta-pleated sheet arrangement of the proteins. Generally, all types of amyloid stain with the Congo red dye. However, in some patients with AL amyloid, it may be very difficult to obtain a satisfactory staining reaction. In these cases it may be useful to attempt other stains such as Thioflavin T and S, crystal violet, or methyl violet. Electron microscopy has been a gold standard for detection of amyloidosis. Ultrastructural examination shows nonbranching fibrillar structures of indefinite length with a width of approximately 9.5 nm.

Therapy is generally directed at treating the underlying condition.[140,141] In the case of primary amyloid, therapy directed against the underlying lymphoplasmacytic neoplasm can sometimes improve survival.[142,143] Liver transplantation has been performed in this disorder and short-term survivors have been noted.[144] However, generally the disease progresses and fatal complications from cardiac or renal failure eventually ensue. Stem cell transplantation therapy has also been employed with mixed results.[145,146] In the case of amyloidosis resulting from chronic infections eradication of underlying infection should be attempted. Colchicine is the treatment of choice in patients with FMF. Orthotopic liver transplantation has been very successful in patients with FAP.[147-154] Most centers recommend transplantation for FAP as soon as symptoms occur because liver transplantation has been shown to diminish the disease progression. In general, there is little improvement in the autonomic dysfunction that is already established.[153,154] Patients with advanced FAP, including both upper and lower motor neuron symptoms, generally do poorly.[153,154]

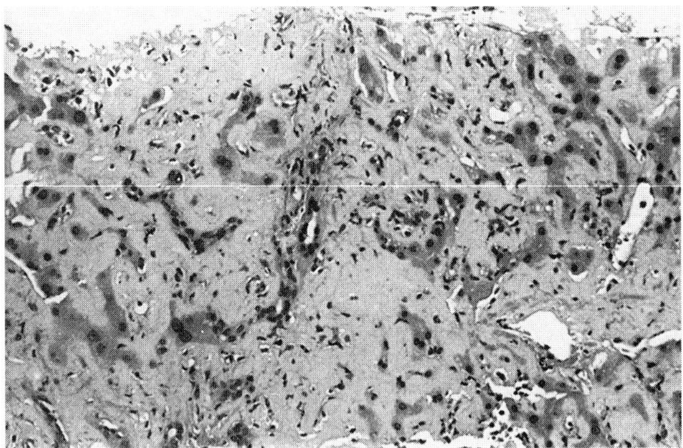

Figure 52-7 Liver in amyloidosis. Amyloid deposited in the space of Disse expands such that the hepatocytes become sunken ribbons. A portal tract is present near the center of the photograph.

LIVER IN HEMATOLOGIC DISEASES

Sickle Cell Anemia

Patients with sickle cell anemia may have a variety of hepatic abnormalities involving both the hepatic parenchyma and the biliary tract. These abnormalities may be present during the asymptomatic phase of sickle cell disease and during the episodes of sickle crisis. The incidence of hepatic involvement is difficult to estimate because the confounding effects of chronic hemolysis may elevate serum bilirubin levels and aminotransferase activity. Of 100 consecutive patients seen as outpatients or inpatients at a university hospital, 24 percent had one or more chronic abnormalities of liver enzymes.[155] The vast majority of the abnormalities were due to concurrent illnesses ranging from chronic viral hepatitis to congestive heart failure.[155] Similarly, in another series serum alkaline phosphatase was abnormal in 64 percent of patients with sickle cell disease, although it appears that the alkaline phosphatase was mostly of bone origin.[156] Thus the true incidence of hepatic involvement is greatly dependent upon the criteria used to define liver disease in this population.

Hepatic Crisis

Hepatic crisis in sickle cell disease is characterized by right upper quadrant abdominal pain, jaundice, hepatomegaly, and fever. This constellation of findings is also suggestive of acute cholecystitis or cholangitis—and differentiating these entities may be difficult. It has been estimated that 7 percent to 10 percent of hospitalizations for sickle cell anemia were complicated by hepatic crises.[157,158] The most marked serum biochemical abnormality during hepatic crisis is elevation in serum bilirubin. Total bilirubin is usually less than 15 mg/dl although extreme levels of hyperbilirubinemia, greater than 50 mg/dl, may occur. This marked hyperbilirubinemia may not necessarily be associated with a worse prognosis.[159-161] A large component of this bilirubin is the direct fraction, which may be as much as 50 percent of the total bilirubin in many cases. Serum aminotransferases are abnormal, with levels usually less than 10 times the upper limits of normal. Elevation of serum LDH activity, disproportionate to the increase of serum aminotransferases, is also common and reflects the ongoing hemolysis associated with sickle crisis.[132,156] Evidence of extrahepatic sickle crisis, such as joint and flank pain, is usually but not invariably, present.

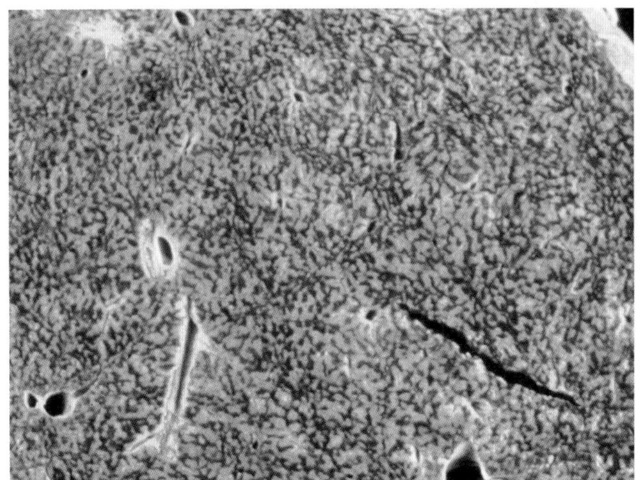

Plate 52-1 Nutmeg liver. In chronic passive congestion of the liver, red cells pool and distend the sinuses around the central vein. These regions develop a darker red-violet color in contrast to the surrounding tan liver parenchyma. This color stippling is reminiscent of the cut surface of a nutmeg.

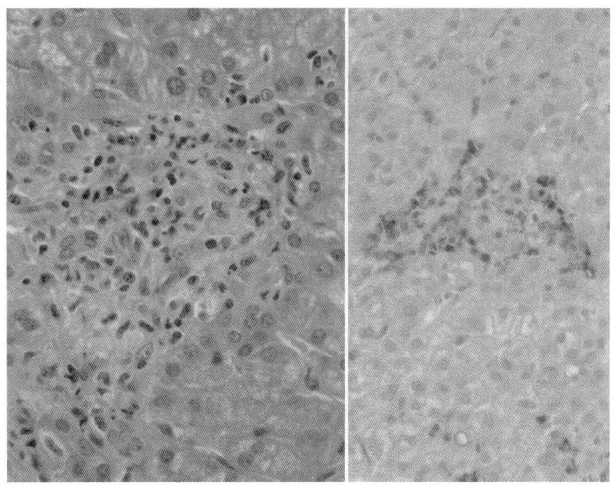

Plate 52-2 *Left,* Hepatic mastocytosis may involve the portal tracts, lobule, or both. (Hematoxylin and eosin.) The lesion is a stellate region of fibrosis occupied by lymphocytes, eosinophils, and cells with larger pale nuclei—mast cells. ***Right,*** Hepatic mastocytosis (Leder). In this section of the liver the numerous mast cells of systemic mastocytosis stand out against the background counterstain. (Chloroacetate esterase [Leder] stain.)

A 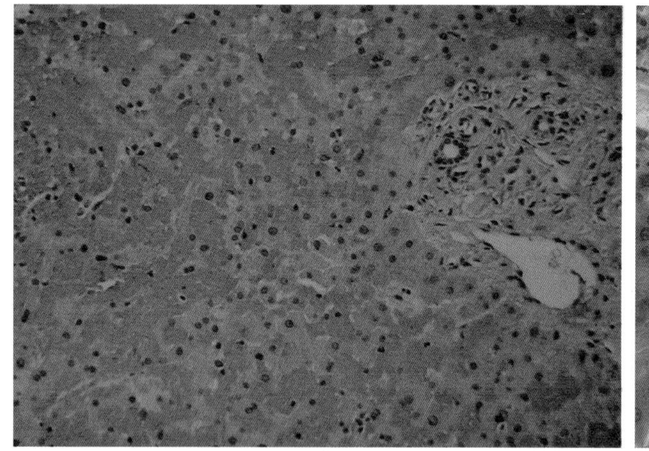

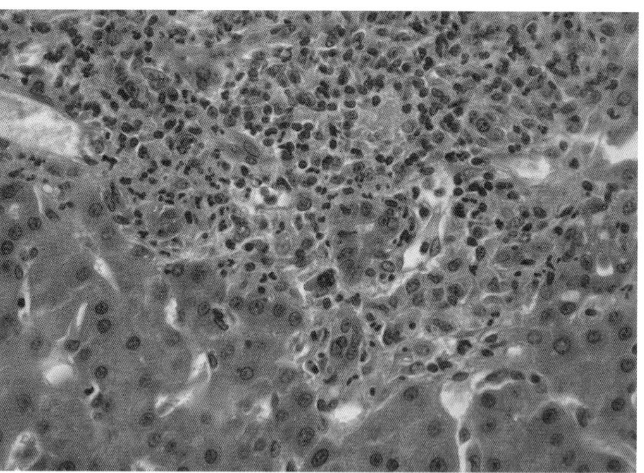 B

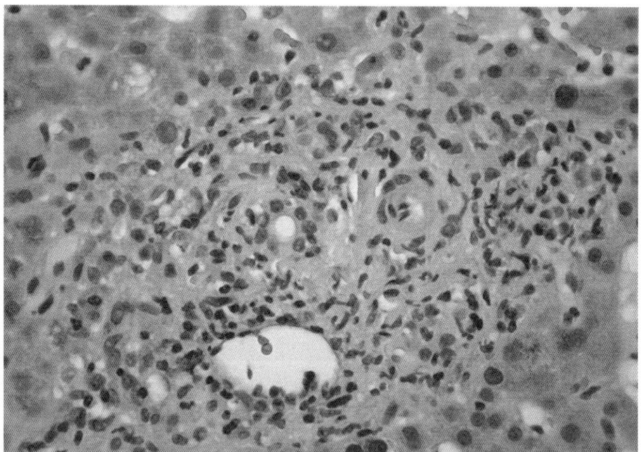 C

Plate 58-1 **A,** In this biopsy specimen, recent onset of veno-occlusive disease is marked by prominent centrizonal hemorrhagic necrosis in which central veins have been obliterated *(left).* Hemorrhage has swollen the adjacent sinusoids and resulted in accumulation of occasional hemosiderin laden macrophages and Kupfer cells. By contrast, the portal triads remain intact *(right).* The lack of significant fibrosis is suggestive of a recent onset of disease. **B,** Graft-versus-host disease in the liver is characterized by injury to interlobular bile ducts. The bile duct, located centrally, displays apoptotic cells and nuclear pleomorphism. A few lymphocytes are seen within the epithelial layer. In addition, the surrounding portal tract shows a predominantly mononuclear infiltrate, though occasional neutrophils, eosinophils, and macrophages are present. Hepatocellular damage is negligible. **C,** Endothelialitis represents the most diagnostic feature of graft-versus-host disease in the liver. Mild endothelialitis, characterized by a small lymphocytic infiltrate within the endothelium, is shown in the portal vein in the lower center within this portal tract. Mild damage to the bile duct in the center is also displayed.

With general supportive care clinical improvement is seen within several days, although hyperbilirubinemia may persist for several weeks. Deaths related to fulminant hepatic failure in the absence of other identifiable etiologies have been reported.[156]

Biliary Tract Disease

Pigment gallstones are frequently found in patients with sickle cell anemia, with estimates of the prevalence ranging between 40 percent and 80 percent.[156,162-164] The incidence varies directly with the age of the patient.[156] Choledocholithiasis was found in 18 percent of 65 patients undergoing cholecystectomy.[156]

Hepatic crisis will resolve quickly with supportive care, whereas cholecystitis and cholangitis will ultimately require endoscopic or surgical intervention. Therefore establishing the correct diagnosis is especially important because of the implications of hepatobiliary surgery in these patients. There is a suggestion that the operative complications of cholecystectomy in patients with sickle cell anemia are greater than in the general population.[165] Schubert reviewed published reports on 97 patients who underwent cholecystectomy and found 15 percent of patients had complications that were deemed serious, including pneumonia, seizures, and sickle crisis.[156,165] Thus cholecystectomy should be reserved for those patients with documented gallstones whose symptoms are clearly of biliary tract origin or for those in whom hepatic crisis and biliary tract disease cannot be adequately differentiated.[156,165] Careful preoperative management with special attention to transfusion requirements and volume status is important.

Viral Hepatitis

As expected from the large numbers of transfusions required by many patients with sickle cell anemia, viral hepatitis has been reported to occur, although from published reports, the incidence is difficult to determine. In patients with liver test abnormalities, the incidence of hepatitis B virus or histologic changes of chronic hepatitis has ranged from 5 percent to 47 percent.[155,162,166,167] The reported prevalence of hepatitis C in patients with sickle cell anemia is 10 percent to 20 percent.[168,169] Not surprisingly, the risk of hepatitis C was directly related to the number of transfusions received. The impact of hepatitis C infection on the natural history of patients with sickle cell anemia is currently unknown.

Hepatic Histology

Several studies have evaluated the histopathologic changes in the livers of patients with sickle cell disease.[159,167,170,171] These studies included biopsies from patients during hepatic crisis and biopsies during quiescent periods. Hepatic sinusoidal distention, erythrocyte sickling, and erythrophagocytosis were found in almost all patients (Figure 52-8).[167] In a study of pregnant women given prophylactic red cell transfusions, erythrocyte sickling and erythrophagocytosis were present in all patients in the absence of hepatic crisis.[170] Thus these changes appear to be characteristic of sickle cell anemia and do not correlate with aminotransferase levels or activity of the liver disease.

The presence of other histologic lesions may also be detected in the livers of patients with sickle cell anemia; these findings further confuse the clinical picture. Massive iron deposition is frequently identified by routine iron stains in the majority of patients.[151,166,167,170] Also, of 19 patients with sickle cell anemia on whom biopsies were performed because of abnormal liver tests, 9 (47 percent) had changes consistent with acute or chronic viral hepatitis.[167] Cirrhosis has been reported to occur in 15 percent to 20 percent of patients with sickle cell anemia and may be due to hypoxic injury from sickling and intrasinusoidal sludging of erythrocytes, chronic viral hepatitis, or hepatic hemosiderosis.[156,167,172]

Hodgkin's Lymphoma

Hepatic involvement in Hodgkin's lymphoma has been reported to occur in 5 percent of patients at the time of diagnosis, 30 percent during the course of the disease, and up to 50 percent at the time of autopsy.[173]

The histology of liver involvement in malignant lymphomas has been reviewed.[174] The extent of tissue sampling correlates with the ability to accurately stage hepatic involvement in Hodgkin's disease; percutaneous liver biopsy has the lowest yield, whereas laparoscopy and laparotomy compare favorably. A diagnosis of hepatic involvement in Hodgkin's disease requires the finding of the Reed-Sternberg cell (Figure 52-9). Non-specific inflammatory infiltrates are seen in 50 percent of liver biopsies in patients with Hodgkin's disease and, alone, do not constitute grounds for diagnosing hepatic involvement. Non-caseating epithelioid granulomas may be seen in 25 percent of patients with Hodgkin's disease.[174,175] Granulomas may be seen in the portal tract and the hepatic lobules and do not necessarily indicate hepatic involvement by Hodgkin's disease.

Elevation of serum alkaline phosphatase levels is the most frequently abnormal liver test found in patients with Hodgkin's disease. In a review of 111 inpatients with

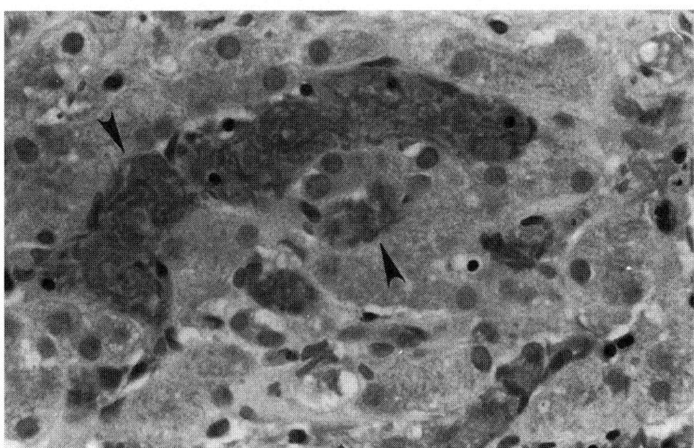

Figure 52-8 Liver in sickle cell anemia. Numerous sickled red blood cells distend the sinuses of the liver *(arrow)*. (Hematoxylin and eosin.)

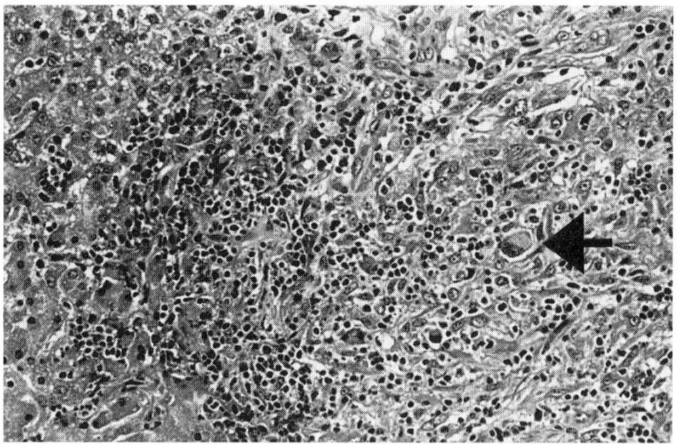

Figure 52-9 Liver in Hodgkin's lymphoma. Classic Reed-Sternberg cell *(arrow)* is seen in a polymorphous background of lymphocytes, plasma cells, and eosinophils, which greatly expands a portal tract. (Hematoxylin and eosin.)

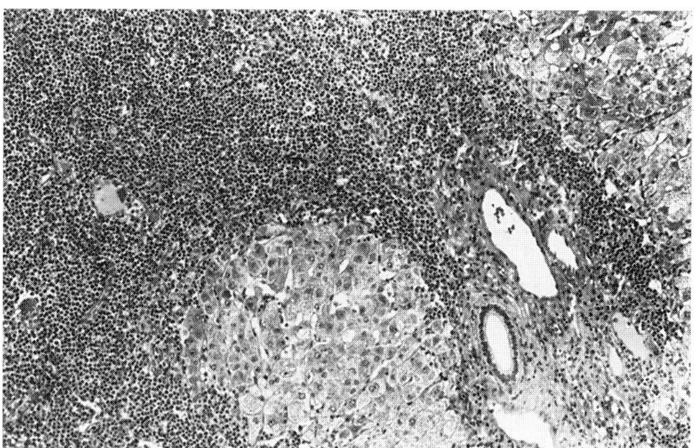

Figure 52-10 Hepatic B-cell lymphoma. Sheets of small lymphocytes surround a regenerative liver nodule. The portal tract also appears to be involved. The B-cell nature of the infiltrate can be confirmed by immunohistochemistry or flow cytometry. (Hematoxylin and eosin.)

Hodgkin's disease 41 percent had abnormal serum alkaline phosphatase levels.[176] Patients with more advanced stages of Hodgkin's disease were more likely to have elevations of this enzyme; 14 percent of patients with stage I or II disease and 65 percent and 81 percent of patients with stage III or stage IV disease, respectively, had abnormal serum alkaline phosphatase levels. The elevations were generally mild, 1.5 to 2 times the upper limits of normal, although more marked increases were noted in patients with stage IV disease. The liver was felt to be the source of the alkaline phosphatase in the majority of patients, although several patients, adolescents with potential for bone growth, had elevation of the bone fraction.[176] Abnormalities in alkaline phosphatase were seen in several patients in the absence of hepatic involvement, more commonly in patients with fever as a systemic manifestation of Hodgkin's disease. Thus in some patients abnormal serum alkaline phosphatase could represent the equivalent of an acute phase reaction.[148]

Jaundice occurs infrequently in Hodgkin's lymphoma except in the late stages of the illness. The most frequent cause of jaundice is direct intrahepatic infiltration, which was seen in 45 percent of jaundiced patients at the time of autopsy.[173,177,178] Extrahepatic biliary tract obstruction occurs much less frequently and accounts for only 5 percent to 10 percent of jaundiced patients.[177-179] A small number of patients with Hodgkin's lymphoma have been described who have evidence of severe intrahepatic cholestasis with dramatic elevations in serum bilirubin and alkaline phosphatase levels in the absence of tumor infiltration or bile duct obstruction.[173,179] The etiology of this syndrome is not known, but one report suggested that it could be related to vanishing bile duct syndrome.[180,181] An association between primary sclerosing cholangitis and Hodgkin's lymphoma has also been suggested.[182] Acute liver failure with encephalopathy, jaundice, and coagulopathy has also been reported in patients with Hodgkin's and non-Hodgkin's lymphoma either resulting from direct lymphomatous involvement of the liver[183,184] or as a paraneoplastic syndrome.[185]

Non-Hodgkin's Lymphoma

Hepatic involvement in non-Hodgkin's lymphomas occurs very frequently, with estimates ranging between 24 percent and 43 percent.[186,187] The hepatic infiltrate usually involves the portal triads and has a nodular appearance (Figure 52-10).[174] Epithelioid granulomas may also be seen in the liver of these patients. Immunophenotyping using monoclonal antibodies may be performed on snap-frozen liver biopsy tissues to characterize the infiltrates.[188] Rarely, primary hepatic lymphoma in the absence of systemic lymphoma has been reported.[189-190]

The clinical manifestations of hepatic infiltration with non-Hodgkin's lymphoma are similar to those seen with Hodgkin's disease. Patients may remain asymptomatic despite extensive hepatic infiltration. Mild to moderate elevations in serum alkaline phosphatase and moderate to marked elevations of LDH activities may be present. In contrast to Hodgkin's disease, non-Hodgkin's lymphomas are more likely to produce jaundice as a result of extrahepatic obstruction, usually at the porta hepatis, rather than by direct hepatic infiltration.[173] Reactivation of chronic hepatitis B in patients receiving cytotoxic therapy is well documented.[191,192] Recent data suggest that lamivudine can prevent such reactivation of hepatitis B in patients receiving chemotherapy.[193] Although some reports have suggested that hepatitis C virus may have a role in the development of non-Hodgkin's lymphoma,[194,195] other reports have failed to confirm such an association.[196,197]

Multiple Myeloma

Liver may be directly involved by plasma cell infiltrate in up to 30 percent of patients with multiple myeloma. The patients generally present with hepatomegaly or ascites.[198] It is important to distinguish myeloma involvement of the liver from autoimmune hepatitis. In myeloma, the plasma cell infiltrate predominantly involves the sinusoids with relative sparing of the portal tracts. This is distinct from autoimmune hepatitis in which the infiltrate is predominantly in the portal area. Another pattern of liver injury in myeloma patients is nodular regenerative hyperplasia.[199]

Waldenström's macroglobulinemia is a neoplastic disorder of B lymphocytes and plasma cells that has been alluded to previously.[200] The neoplastic cells secrete immunoglobulin heavy chain, which rarely has been associated with the development of amyloidosis. The lymphoplasmacytic tumor can directly involve the liver. Clinical liver disease in these patients is often mild, with minimal elevation of transaminases and alkaline phosphatase. Their symptoms are usually due to the extrahepatic problems associated with the disease. Histologically, the infiltrate shows expanded portal tracts with lymphocytes and plasma cells and larger atypical cells with occasional mitotic figures.

Mastocytosis

Mastocytosis is commonly seen in children as a skin rash called urticaria pigmentosa. However, the disease can become systemic and involve the liver, especially in adult patients.[201] When seen in adults, it is often presents with fever, hepatosplenomegaly, steatorrhea or diarrhea, and weight loss. The liver chemistries are usually minimally abnormal; radiologic studies are often not contributory. A liver biopsy demonstrates the characteristic lesions that are similar to those seen in other organs, including spleen and lymph nodes. This is characterized by irregular areas of fibrosis containing numerous eosinophils and a background of lymphocytes and other mononuclear cells (Plate 52-2).[202] These mononuclear cells are mast cells that may be recognized by a number of methods. Because the cells are often degranulated, toluidine blue staining may not be helpful. Chloroacetate esterase staining, however, is usually diagnostic; the cells also exhibit c-kit (CD-117). These fibrotic clusters may be located either in the portal tracts or in the parenchyma. When the lesions abut the central veins they may be responsible for the rare cases of portal hypertension associated with the disease.[203,204]

References

1. Lautt WW, Greenway CV: Conceptual review of the hepatic vascular bed. Hepatology 7:952, 1987.
2. Richman SM, Delman AJ, Grob D: Alterations in indices of liver function in congestive heart failure with particular reference to serum enzymes. Am J Med 30:211, 1961.
3. Runyon BA: Cardiac ascites: a characterization. J Clin Gastroenterol 10:410, 1988.
4. Hickman PE, Potter JM: Mortality associated with ischemic hepatitis. Aust NZ J Med 20:32, 1990.
5. Fuchs S, Bogomolski-Yahalom V, Paltiel O, et al: Ischemic hepatitis. Clinical and laboratory observations of 34 patients. J Clin Gastroenterol 26:183, 1998.
6. Bacon BR, Joshi SN, Granger DN: Ischemia, congestive heart failure, Budd-Chiari syndrome, and veno-occlusive disease. In Kaplowitz N, ed: Liver and Biliary Diseases, ed 2. Philadelphia, Williams and Wilkins, 1996:421.
7. Garland JS, Werlin SL, Rice TB: Ischemic hepatitis in children, diagnosis and clinical course. Crit Care Med 16:1209, 1988.
8. Naschitz JE, Slobodin G, Lewis RJ, et al: Heart diseases affecting the liver and liver diseases affecting the heart. Am Heart J 140:111, 2000.
9. Naschitz JE, Yeshurun D, Shahar J: Cardiogenic hepatorenal syndrome. Angiology 41:893, 1990.
10. Seeto R, Fenn B, Rockey DC: Ischemic hepatitis: clinical presentation and pathogenesis. Am J Med 109:109, 2000.
11. Kew M, Bersohn I, Seftel H, et al: Liver damage in heat stroke. Am J Med 49:192, 1970.
12. Hassanein T, Razack A, Gavaler J, et al: Heat stroke: its clinical and pathological presentation, with particular attention to the liver. Am J Gastroenterol 87:1382, 1992.
13. Rubel LR, Ishak KG: The liver in fatal exertional heat stroke. Liver 3:249, 1983.
14. Deviere J, Reuse C, Askenasi R: Ischemic pancreatitis and hepatitis secondary to ergotamine poisoning. J Clin Gastroenterol 9:350, 1987.
15. Ussery XT, Henar EL, Black DD, et al: Acute liver injury after protracted seizures in children. J Pediatr Gastroenterol Nutr 9:421, 1989.
16. Gibson PR, Dudley FJ: Ischemic hepatitis: clinical features, diagnosis, and prognosis. Aust NZ J Med 14:822, 1984.
17. Gitlin N, Serio KM: Ischemic hepatitis: widening horizons. Am J Gastroenterol 87:831, 1992.
18. Bynum TE, Boitnott JK, Maddrey WC: Ischemic hepatitis. Dig Dis Sci 24:129, 1979.
19. Rhodes A, Eastwood JB, Smith SA: Early acute hepatitis with parenteral amiodarone: a toxic effect of the vehicle? Gut 34:565, 1993.
20. Tosetti C, Ongari M, Evangelisti A, et al: Acute hepatotoxicity from amiodarone. Minerva Med 86:387, 1995.
21. Potter JM, Hickman PE: Cardiodepressant drugs and the high mortality rate associated with ischemic hepatitis. Crit Care Med 20:474, 1992.
22. Bonkovsky HL, Kane RE, Jones DP, et al: Acute hepatic and renal toxicity from low doses of acetaminophen in the absence of alcohol abuse or malnutrition: evidence for increased susceptibility to drug toxicity due to cardiopulmonary and renal insufficiency. Hepatology 19:1141, 1994.
23. Lowe MD, Harcombe AA, Grace AA, et al: Restrictive-constrictive heart failure masquerading as liver disease. BMJ 318:585, 1999.
24. Van der Merwe S, Dens J, Daenen W, et al: Pericardial disease is often not recognized as a cause of chronic severe ascites. J Hepatol 32:164, 2000.
25. Arora A, Seth S, Acharya SK, et al: Hepatic coma as a presenting feature of constrictive pericarditis. Am J Gastroenterol 88:430, 1993.
26. Manga P, Vythilingum S, Mitha AS: Pulsatile hepatomegaly in constrictive pericarditis. Br Heart J 52:465, 1984.
27. Braunwald E: Pericardial disease. In Fauci AS, Braunwald E, Isselbacher KJ, et al, eds: Harrison's Principles of Internal Medicine, ed 14. Philadelphia, McGraw-Hill, 1998:1334-1341.
28. Solano FX, Young E, Talamo TS, et al: Constrictive pericarditis mimicking Budd-Chiari syndrome. Am J Med 80:113, 1986.
29. Arora A, Tandon N, Sharma MP, et al: Constrictive pericarditis masquerading as Budd-Chiari syndrome. J Clin Gastroenterol 13:178, 1991.
30. Whelan G, Pierce AK, Schenker S, et al: Hepatic function in patients with hypoxaemia due to chronic pulmonary disease. Aust Ann Med 18:243, 1969.
31. Mathurin P, Durand F, Ganne N, et al: Ischemic hepatitis due to obstructive sleep apnea. Gastroenterology 109:1682, 1995.
32. Henrion J, Colin L, Schapira M, et al: Hypoxic hepatitis caused by severe hypoxemia from obstructive sleep apnea. J Clin Gastroenterol 24:245, 1997.
33. Henrion J, Minette P, Colin L, et al: Hypoxic hepatitis caused by acute exacerbation of chronic respiratory failure: a case-controlled, hemodynamic study of 17 consecutive cases. Hepatology 29:427, 1999.
34. Scott HW, Law DH, Sandstead HH, et al: Jejunoileal shunt in surgical treatment of morbid obesity. Ann Surg 171:770, 1970.
35. Bo-Linn G: Obesity, anorexia nervosa, bulimia, and other eating disorders. In Sleisinger MH, Fordtran JS, eds: Gastrointestinal Disease, ed 4. Philadelphia, WB Saunders Co., 1989.
36. Jewell WR, Hermreck AS, Hardin CA: Complications of jejunoileal bypass for morbid obesity. Arch Surg 110:1039, 1975.
37. Kirkpatrick JR: Jejunoileal bypass: a legacy of late complications. Arch Surg 122:610, 1987.

38. Dean P, Joshi S, Kaminski D: Long-term outcome of reversal of small intestinal bypass operations. Am J Surg 159:118, 1990.
39. Hamilton DL, Vest TK, Brown BS, et al: Liver injury with alcoholic like hyaline after gastroplasty for morbid obesity. Gastroenterology 85:722, 1983.
40. Moxley RT, Pozefsky T, Lockwood DH: Protein nutrition and liver disease after jejunoileal bypass for morbid obesity. N Engl J Med 290:921, 1974.
41. Hollenbeck JI, O'Leary JP, Maher JW, Woodward ER: An etiologic basis for fatty liver after jejunoileal bypass. J Surg Res 18:83, 1975.
42. Lewin MR, Aranjo JG, Sarmiento JL, et al: Bypass induced liver disease: an experimental study of post-operative protein supplementation and metronidazole therapy in an animal model. Br J Exp Pathol 68:15, 1987.
43. Cope K, Risby T, Diehl AM: Increased gastrointestinal ethanol production in obese mice: implications for fatty liver disease pathogenesis. Gastroenterology 119:1340, 2000.
44. Drenick EJ, Fisler J, Johnson D: Hepatic steatosis after intestinal bypass—prevention and reversal by metronidazole, irrespective of protein calorie malnutrition. Gastroenterology 82:535, 1982.
45. Peters RL, Gay T, Reynolds TB: Post-jejunoileal bypass hepatic disease. Am J Clin Pathol 63:318, 1975.
46. Snover DC: Biopsy Diagnosis of Liver Disease. Baltimore, Williams and Wilkins, 1992:183.
47. Vyberg M, Ravn V, Anderson B: Pattern of progression of liver injury following jejunoileal bypass for morbid obesity. Liver 7:271, 1987.
48. Nasrallah SM, Wills CE, Galambos JT: Liver injury following jejunoileal bypass: are there markers? Ann Surg 192:726, 1980.
49. Weismann RE, Johnson RE: Fatal hepatic failure after jejunoileal bypass. Am J Surg 134:253, 1977.
50. Requarth JA, Burchard KW, Colacchio TA, et al: Long-term morbidity following jejunoileal bypass. The continuing potential need for surgical reversal. Arch Surg 130:318, 1995.
51. Brown RG, O'Leary JP, Woodward ER: Hepatic effects of jejunoileal bypass for morbid obesity. Am J Surg 127:53, 1974.
52. Soyer MT, Ceballos R, Aldrete JS: Reversibility of severe hepatic damage caused by jejunoileal bypass after re-establishment of normal intestinal continuity. Surgery 79:601, 1976.
53. Burke GW, Cirocco R, Hensley G, et al: Liver transplantation for cirrhosis following jejuno-ileal bypass—regional cytokine differences associated with pathological changes in the transplant liver. Transplantation 54:374, 1992.
54. Markowitz JS, Seu P, Goss JA, et al: Liver transplantation for decompensated cirrhosis after jejunoileal bypass: a strategy for management. Transplantation 65:570, 1998.
55. Lowell JA, Shenoy S, Ghalib R, et al: Liver transplantation after jejunoileal bypass for morbid obesity. J Am Coll Surg 185:123, 1997.
56. D'Souza-Gburek SM, Batts KP, Nikias GA, et al: Liver transplantation for jejunoileal bypass-associated cirrhosis: allograft histology in the setting of an intact bypassed limb. Liver Trans Surg 3:23, 1997.
57. Schur PH: Clinical features of SLE. In Kelley WN, Harris ED, Ruddy S, Sledge CB, eds: Textbook of Rheumatology. Philadelphia, WB Saunders Co., 1993:1017.
58. Runyon BA, LaBrecque DR, Anuras S: The spectrum of liver disease in systemic lupus erythematosus. Am J Med 69:187, 1980.
59. Matsumoto T, Yoshimine T, Shimouchi K, et al: The liver in systemic lupus erythematosus: pathologic analysis of 52 cases and review of Japanese autopsy registry data. Hum Pathol 23:1151, 1992.
60. Seaman WE, Ishak KG, Plotz PH: Aspirin induced hepatotoxicity in patients with systemic lupus erythematosus. Ann Intern Med 80:1, 1974.
61. Farrell GC: Drug-Induced Liver Disease. London, Churchill Livingstone, 1994:372-376.
62. Schousboe JT, Koch AE, Chang RW: Chronic lupus peritonitis with ascites: review of the literature with a case report. Semin Arthritis Rheum 18:121, 1988.
63. Thompson PE, Houghton BJ, Clifford C, et al: The source and significance of raised serum enzymes in rheumatoid arthritis. Q J Med 280:869, 1990.
64. Rau R, Pfenninger K, Boni A: Proceedings: liver function tests and liver biopsies in patients with rheumatoid arthritis. Ann Rheum Dis 34:198, 1975.
65. Cimmino MA, Buffrini L, Barisone G, et al: Alkaline phosphatase activity in the serum of patients with rheumatoid arthritis. Z Rheumatol 49:143, 1990.
66. Cimmino MA, Accardo S: Changes in the isoenzyme pattern of alkaline phosphatase in patients with rheumatoid arthritis. Clin Chem 36:1376, 1990.
67. Ruderman EM, Crawford JM, Maier A, et al: Histologic liver abnormalities in an autopsy series of patients with rheumatoid arthritis. Br J Rheum 36:210, 1997.
68. Wanless IR, Godwin TA, Allen F, Feder A: Nodular regenerative hyperplasia of the liver in hematologic disorders: a possible response to obliterative portal venopathy. Medicine 59:367, 1980.
69. Favreau M, Tannenbasum H, Lough J: Hepatic toxicity associated with gold therapy. Ann Intern Med 87:717, 1977.
70. Hanissian AS, Rothschild BM, Kaplan S: Gold: hepatotoxic and cholestatic reactions. Clin Rheumatol 4:183, 1985.
71. Farrell GC: Drug-Induced Liver Disease. London, Churchill Livingstone, 1994:388.
72. Fleischner GM, Morecki R, Hanaichi T, et al: Light and electron microscopical studies of a case of gold salt-induced hepatotoxicity. Hepatology 14:422, 1991.
73. Tsutsumi A, Koike T: Hepatic manifestations of the antiphospholipid syndrome. Intern Med 39:6, 2000.
74. Asherson RA, Khamashta MA, Hughes GR: The hepatic complications of the antiphospholipid antibodies. Clin Exp Rheumatol 9:341, 1991.
75. Pelletier S, Landi B, Piette C, et al: Antiphospholipid syndrome as the second cause of non-tumorous Budd-Chiari syndrome. J Hepatol 21:76, 1994.
76. Skopouli FN, Barbatis C, Moutsopoulos HM: Liver involvement in primary Sjögren's syndrome. Br J Rheumatol 33:745, 1994.
77. Haddad J, Deny P, Munz-Gotheil C, et al: Lymphocytic sialadenitis of Sjögren's syndrome associated with chronic hepatitis C virus liver disease. Lancet 339:321, 1992.
78. Ramos-Casals M, Garcia-Carrasco M, Cervera R, et al: Sjögren's syndrome and hepatitis C virus. Clin Rheumatol 18:93, 1999.
79. Poet JL, Tonelli-Serabian Y, Garnier PP: Chronic hepatitis C and Sjögren's syndrome. J Rheumatol 21:1376, 1994.
80. Pirisi M, Scott C, Fabris C, et al: Mild sialoadenitis: a common finding in patients with hepatitis C virus infection. Scand J Gastroenterol 29:940, 1994.
81. Pawlotsky JM, Roudot-Thoraval F, Simmonds P, et al: Extrahepatic immunologic manifestations in chronic hepatitis C virus serotypes. Ann Intern Med 122:169, 1995.
82. Reynolds TB, Denison EK, Frankl HD, et al: Primary biliary cirrhosis with scleroderma, Raynaud's phenomenon, and telangiectasia. Am J Med 50:302, 1970.
83. Goring HD, Panzer M, Lakotta W, et al: Coincidence of scleroderma and primary biliary cirrhosis: results of a systematic study of a dermatologic patient sample. Hautarzt 49:361, 1998.
84. Powell FC, Schroter AL, Dickinson ER: Primary biliary cirrhosis and the CREST syndrome: a report of 22 cases. Q J Med 62:75, 1987.
85. Reye RDK, Morgan G, Baral J: Encephalopathy and fatty degeneration of the viscera: a disease entity in childhood. Lancet 2:749, 1963.
86. Hurwitz ES, Nelson DB, Davis C, et al: National surveillance for Reye's syndrome: a five year review. Pediatrics 70:895, 1982.
87. Belay ED, Bresee JS, Holman RC, et al: Reye's syndrome in the United States from 1981 through 1997. N Engl J Med 340:1377, 1999.
88. Anonymous: Reye syndrome surveillance—US, 1986. MMWR 36:689, 1987.
89. Hall SM, Lynn R: Reye's syndrome. N Engl J Med 341:845, 1999.
90. Starko KM, Ray CG, Dominguez LB, et al: Reye's syndrome and salicylate use. Pediatrics 6:859, 1980.
91. Walkmann RJ, Hall WN, McGee H, Van Amburg G: Aspirin as a risk factor in Reye's syndrome. JAMA 247:3089, 1982.
92. Hurwitz ES, Barrett MJ, Bregman D, et al: Public health service study of Reye's syndrome and medications: report of a pilot phase. N Engl J Med 313:849, 1985.
93. Remington PL, Shabino CL, McGee H, et al: Reye syndrome and juvenile rheumatoid arthritis in Michigan. Am J Dis Child 139:870, 1985.
94. Ghosh D, Dhadwal D, Aggarwal A, et al: investigation of an epidemic of Reye's syndrome in northern region of India. Indian Pediatr 36:1097, 1999.
95. Gauthier M, Guay J, LaCroix J, Lortie A: Reye's syndrome: a reappraisal of diagnosis in 49 presumptive cases. Am J Dis Child 143:1181, 1989.

96. Bove KE, McAdams AJ, Partin JC, et al: The hepatic lesion in Reye's syndrome. Gastroenterology 69:685, 1975.
97. Partin JC, Schubert WK, Partin JS: Mitochondrial ultrastructure in Reye's syndrome (encephalopathy and fatty degeneration of the viscera). N Engl J Med 285:1339, 1971.
98. Teem WR: Inherited and acquired syndromes of hyperammonemia and encephalopathy in children. Semin Liver Dis 14:236, 1994.
99. Teem WR: Inherited and acquired syndromes of hyperammonemia and encephalopathy in children. Semin Liver Dis 14:236, 1994.
100. Woodfin BM, Davis LE: Displacement of hepatic carbamoyl transferase activity from mitochondria to cytosol in Reye's syndrome. Biochem Med Metab Biol 46:255, 1991.
101. Trauner DA, Horvath E, David LE: Inhibition of fatty acid β-oxidation by influenza B virus and salicylic acid in mice: implications for Reye's syndrome. Neurology 38:239, 1988.
102. Tomoda T, Taked K, Jurashige T, et al: Experimental study on Reye's syndrome: inhibitory effect of interferon alfa on acetylsalicylate-induced injury to rat liver mitochondria. Metabolism 41:887, 1992.
103. Meythaler JM, Varma RR: Reye's syndrome in adults. Arch Intern Med 147:61, 1987.
104. Peters J, Wiener GJ, Gilliam J, et al: Reye's syndrome in adults: a case report and review of the literature. Arch Intern Med 146:2401, 1986.
105. Kirkpatrick DB, Ottoson C, Bateman LL: Reye's syndrome in an adult patient. West J Med 144:223, 1986.
106. Chang PF, Huang SF, Hwu WL, et al: Metabolic disorders mimicking Reye's syndrome. J Formos Med Assoc 99,295, 2000.
107. Green A, Hall SM: Investigations of metabolic disorders resembling Reye's syndrome. Arch Dis Child 145:964, 1995.
108. Clayton PT, Doig M, Ghafari S, et al: Screening for medium chain acyl-CoA dehydrogenase deficiency using electrospray ionization tandem mass spectrometry. Arch Dis Child 79:109, 1998.
109. Partin JS, Daugherty CC, McAdams AJ, et al: A comparison of liver ultrastructure in salicylate intoxication and Reye's syndrome. Hepatology 4:687, 1984.
110. Stauffer MH: Nephrogenic hepatosplenomegaly. Gastroenterology 40:694, 1961 (abstract).
111. Utz DC, Warren MM, Gregg JA, Ludwig J: Reversible hepatic dysfunction associated with hypernephroma. Mayo Clin Proc 45:161, 1970.
112. Ramos CV, Taylor HB: Hepatic dysfunction associated with renal cell carcinoma. Cancer 29:1287, 1972.
113. Walsh PN, Kissane JM: Nonmetastatic hypernephroma with reversible hepatic dysfunction. Arch Intern Med 122:214, 1968.
114. Chuang YC, Lin ATL, Chen KK, et al: Paraneoplastic elevation of serum alkaline phosphatase in renal cell carcinoma: incidence and implication on prognosis. J Urol 158:1684, 1997.
115. Weber J, Gunn H, Yang J, et al: A phase I trial of intravenous interleukin-6 in patients with advanced cancer. J Immunother Emph Tumor Immunol 15:292, 1994.
116. Nieken J, Mulder NH, Buter J, et al: Recombinant human interleukin-6 induces a rapid and reversible anemia in cancer patients. Blood 86:900, 1995.
117. Walther MM, Johnson B, Culley D, et al: Serum interleukin-6 levels in metastatic renal cell carcinoma before treatment with interleukin-6 correlates with paraneoplastic syndromes but not patient survival. J Urol 159:718, 1998.
118. Tsukamoto T, Kumamoto Y, Miyao N, et al: Interleukin-6 in renal carcinoma. J Urol 148:1778, 1992.
119. Blay JY, Rossi JF, Wijdenes J, et al: Role of interleukin-6 in the paraneoplastic inflammatory syndrome associated with renal-cell carcinoma. Int J Cancer 72:424, 1997.
120. Strickland RC, Schenker S: The nephrogenic hepatic dysfunction syndrome: a review. Dig Dis 22:49, 1977.
121. Jacobi GH, Philipp T: Stauffer's syndrome: diagnostic help in hypernephroma. Clin Nephrol 4:113, 1975.
122. Gertz MA, Lacy MQ, Dispenzieri A: Amyloidosis. Hematol Oncol Clin North Am 13:1211, 1999.
122a. Gillmore JD, Lovat LB, Hawkins PN: Amyloidosis and the liver. J Hepatol 30:117, 1999.
123. Rienhoff HY Jr, Huang JH, Li XX, Liao WS: Molecular and cellular biology of serum amyloid A. Mol Biol Med 7: 282, 1990.
123a. Pepys MB, Baltz ML: Acute phase proteins with special reference to C-reactive protein and related proteins (pentaxins) and serum amyloid A protein. Adv Immunol 34:141, 1983.
124. Urieli-Shoval S, Linke RP, Matzner Y: Expression and function of serum amyloid A, a major acute-phase protein, in normal and disease states. Curr Opin Hematol 7:64, 2000.
125. Aksentijevich I, Torosyan Y, Samules J, et al: Mutation and haplotype studies of familial Mediterranean fever reveal new ancestral relationships and evidence for a high carrier frequency with reduced penetrance in the Ashkenazi Jewish population. Am J Hum Genet 64:939, 1999
126. Mulley JC: The genetic basis for periodic fever. Am J Hum Genet 64:939, 1999.
127. Murakami T, Uchino M, Ando M: Genetic abnormalities and pathogenesis of familial amyloidotic polyneuropathy. Pathol Int 45:1, 1995.
128. Drueke TB: Beta2-microglobulin and amyloidosis. Nephrol Dial Transplant 15:17, 2000.
129. Gertz MA, Kyle RA: Hepatic amyloidosis: clinical appraisal in 77 patients. Hepatology 25:118, 1997.
129a. Gillmore JD, Lovat LB, Hawkins PN: Amyloidosis and the liver. J Hepatol 30:117, 1999.
130. Faa G, Van Eyken P, De Vos R, et al: Light chain deposition disease of the liver associated with AL-type amyloidosis and severe cholestasis. J Hepatol 12:75, 1991.
131. Girelli CM, Lodi G, Rocca F: Kappa light chain deposition disease of the liver. Eur J Gastroenterol Hepatol 10:429, 1998.
132. Hoffman MS, Stein BE, Davidian MM, et al: Hepatic amyloidosis presenting as severe intrahepatic cholestasis: a case report and review of the literature. Am J Gastroenterol 83:783, 1988.
133. Iwai M, Ishii Y, Mori T, et al: Cholestatic jaundice in two patients with primary amyloidosis: ultrastructural findings of the liver. J Clin Gastroenterol 28:162, 1999.
134. Mohr A, Miehlke S, Klauck S, et al: Hepatomegaly and cholestasis as primary clinical manifestations of an AL-kappa amyloidosis. Eur J Gastroenterol Hepatol 11:921, 1999.
135. Peters RA, Koukoulis G, Gimson A, et al: Primary amyloidosis and severe intrahepatic cholestatic jaundice. Gut 35:1322, 1994.
136. Qureshi WA: Intrahepatic cholestatic syndromes: pathogenesis, clinical features and management. Dig Dis 17:49, 1999.
137. Bujanda L, Beguiristain A, Alberdi F, et al: Spontaneous rupture of the liver in amyloidosis. Am J Gastroenterol 92:1385, 1997.
138. Bion E, Brenard R, Pariente EA, et al: Sinusoidal portal hypertension in hepatic amyloidosis. Gut 32:227, 1991.
139. Elghetany MT, Saleem A: Methods for staining amyloid in tissues: a review. Stain Technol 63:201, 1988.
140. Gertz MA, Kyle RA: Amyloidosis: prognosis and treatment. Semin Arthritis Rheum 24:124, 1994.
141. Tan SY, Pepys MB, Hawkins PN: Treatment of amyloidosis. Am J Kid Dis 26:267, 1995.
142. Comenzo RL, Vosburgh E, Falk RH, et al: Dose-intensive melphalan with blood stem-cell support for the treatment of AL (amyloid light-chain) amyloidosis: survival and responses in 25 patients. Blood 91:3662, 1998.
143. Dhodapkar MV, Jagannath S, Vesole D, et al: Treatment of AL-amyloidosis with dexamethasone plus alpha interferon. Leuk Lymph 27:351, 1997.
144. Nowak G, Westermark P, Wernerson A, et al: Liver transplantation as rescue treatment in a patient with primary AL kappa amyloidosis. Transplant Int 13:92, 2000.
145. Comenzo RL: Hematopoietic cell transplantation for primary systemic amyloidosis: what have we learned. Leuk Lymph 37:245, 2000.
146. Patriarca F, Geromin A, Fanin R, et al: Improvement of amyloid-related symptoms after autologous stem cell transplantation in a patient with hepatomegaly, macroglossia and purpura. Bone Marrow Transplant 24:433, 1999.
147. Ericzon BG, Holmgren G, Lundgren E, et al: New structural information and update on liver transplantation in transthyretin-associated amyloidosis. Report from the 4th International Symposium on Familial Amyloidotic Polyneuropathy and Other Transthyretin Related Disorders & the 3rd International Workshop on Liver Transplantation in Familial Amyloid Polyneuropathy, Umea, Sweden, June 1999. Amyloid 7:145, 2000.
148. Fournier B, Giostra E, Mentha G, et al: Three cases of liver transplantation for type I familial amyloid polyneuropathy. Transplant Proc 29:2416, 1997.
149. Garcia-Herola A, Prieto M, Pascual S, et al: Progression of cardiomyopathy and neuropathy after liver transplantation in a

patient with familial amyloidotic polyneuropathy caused by tyrosine-77 transthyretin variant. Liver Transplant Surg 5:246, 1999.
150. Hemming AW, Cattral MS, Chari RS, et al: Domino liver transplantation for familial amyloid polyneuropathy. Liver Transplant Surg 4:236, 1998.
151. Monteiro E, Perdigoto R, Furtado AL: Liver transplantation for familial amyloid polyneuropathy. Hepatogastroenterology 45:1375, 1998.
152. Shaz BH, Gordon F, Lewis WD, et al: Orthotopic liver transplantation for familial amyloidotic polyneuropathy: a pathological study. Human Pathol 31:40, 2000.
153. Suhr OB, Herlenius G, Friman S, et al: Liver transplantation for hereditary transthyretin amyloidosis. Liver Transplant 6:263, 2000.
154. Tashima K, Ando Y, Terazaki H, et al: Outcome of liver transplantation for transthyretin amyloidosis: follow-up of Japanese familial amyloidotic polyneuropathy patients. J Neuro Sci 17:119, 1999.
155. Johnson CS, Omata M, Tong MJ, et al: Liver involvement in sickle cell disease. Medicine 64:349, 1985.
156. Schubert T: Hepatobiliary system in sickle cell disease. Gastroenterology 90:2013, 1986.
157. Diggs LW: Sickle cell crisis. Am J Clin Pathol 44:1, 1965.
158. Sheehy TW: Sickle cell hepatopathy. South Med J 70:533, 1977.
159. Rosenblate HJ: Eisenstein R, Holmes AW: The liver in sickle cell anemia. Arch Pathol 90:235, 1970.
160. Sheehy TW: Sickle cell hepatopathy. South Med J 70:533, 1977.
161. Buchanan GR, Blader BE: Benign course of extreme hyperbilirubinemia in sickle cell disease: analysis of six cases. J Pediatr 91:21, 1977.
162. Ballas SK, Lewis CN, Noone AM, et al: Clinical, hematological, and biochemical features of HbSC disease. Am J Hematol 13:37, 1982.
163. Phillips JC, Gerald BE: The incidence of cholethiasis in sickle cell disease. AJR Am J Roentgenol 113:27, 1971.
164. Sarnaik S, Slovis TL, Corbett DP, et al: Incidence of cholelithiasis in sickle cell anemia using the ultrasonic gray-scale technique. J Pediatr 96:1005, 1980.
165. Flye MW, Silver D: Biliary tract disorders and sickle cell disease. Surgery 72:361, 1972.
166. Comer GM, Ozick LA, Sachdev RK, et al: Transfusion related chronic liver disease in sickle cell anemia. Am J Gastroenterol 86:1232, 1991.
167. Omata M, Johnson CS, Tong M, Tatter D: Pathological spectrum of liver disease in sickle cell disease. Dig Dis Sci 31:247, 1986.
168. De Vault KR, Friedman LS, Westerberg S, et al: Hepatitis C in sickle cell anemia. Am J Gastroenterol 18:206, 1994.
169. Hasan MF, March F, Posner G, et al: Chronic hepatitis C in patients with sickle cell disease. Am J Gastroenterol 91:1204, 1996.
170. Yeomans E, Lowe TW, Eigenbrodt EH, Cunningham FG: Liver histopathologic findings in women given prophylactic transfusion during pregnancy. Am J Obstet Gynecol 163:958, 1990.
171. Mills LR, Mwakyusa D, Milner PF: Histopathologic features of liver biopsy specimens in sickle cell disease. Arch Pathol Lab Med 112:290, 1988.
172. Bauer TW, Moore GW, Hutchins GM: The liver in sickle cell disease: a clinicopathologic study of 70 patients. Am J Med 69:833, 1980.
173. Birrer MJ, Young RC: Differential diagnosis of jaundice in lymphoma patients. Semin Liver Dis 7:269, 1987.
174. Jaffe ES: Malignant lymphomas: pathology of hepatic involvement. Semin Liver Dis 7:257, 1987.
175. Kadin ME, Donaldson SS, Dorfman RF: Isolated granulomas in Hodgkin's disease. N Engl J Med 283:859, 1970.
176. Aisenberg AC, Kaplan MM, Rieder SV, Goldman JM: Serum alkaline phosphatase at the onset of Hodgkin's disease. Cancer 26:318, 1970.
177. Bouroncle BA, Old JW, Vazques AG: Pathogenesis of jaundice in Hodgkin's disease. Arch Intern Med 110:872, 1962.
178. Levitan R, Diamond HD, Craver LF: Jaundice in Hodgkin's disease. Am J Med 30:99, 1961.
179. Perera DR, Greene ML, Fenster F: Cholestasis associated with extrabiliary Hodgkin's disease. Gastroenterology 67:680, 1974.
180. Hubscher SG, Lumley MA, Elias E: Vanishing bile duct syndrome: a possible mechanism for intrahepatic cholestasis in Hodgkin's lymphoma. Hepatology 17:70, 1993.
181. Crosbie OM, Crown JP, Nolan NP, et al: Resolution of paraneoplastic bile duct paucity following successful treatment of Hodgkin's disease. Hepatology 26:5, 1997
182. Man KM, Drejet A, Keeffe EB, et al: Primary sclerosing cholangitis and Hodgkin's disease. Hepatology 18:1127, 1993.
183. Woolf GM, Petrovic LM, Rojter SE, et al: Acute liver failure due to lymphoma: a diagnostic concern when considering liver transplantation. Dig Dis Sci 39:1351, 1994.
184. Rowbotham D, Wendon J, Williams R: Acute liver failure secondary to hepatic infiltration: a single center experience of 18 cases. Gut 42:576, 1998.
185. Dourakis SP, Tzemanakis E, Deutsch M, et al: Fulminant hepatic failure as a presenting paraneoplastic manifestation of Hodgkin's disease. Eur J Gastroenterol Hepatol 11:1055, 1999.
186. Memeo L, Pecorello I, Ciardi A, et al: Primary non-Hodgkin's lymphoma of the liver. Acta Oncol 38:655, 1999.
187. Lei KI: Primary non-Hodgkin's lymphoma of the liver. Leuk Lymph 29:293, 1998.
188. Verdi CJ, Grogan TM, Protell R, et al: Liver biopsy immunotyping to characterize lymphoid malignancies. Hepatology 6:6, 1986.
189. Ryoo JW, Manaligod JR, Walker MJ: Primary lymphoma of the liver. J Clin Gastroenterol 8:308, 1986.
190. Osborne BM, Butler JJ, Guarda LA: Primary lymphoma of the liver. Cancer 56:2902, 1985.
191. Pinto PC, Hu E, Bernstein-Singer M, et al: Acute hepatic injury after withdrawal of immunosuppressive chemotherapy in patients with hepatitis B. Cancer 65:878, 1990.
192. Markovic S, Drozina G, Vovk M, et al: Reactivation of hepatitis B but not hepatitis C in patients with malignant lymphoma and immunosuppressive therapy. A prospective study of 305 patients. Hepatogastroenterology 46:2925, 1999.
193. Al-Taie OH, Mork H, Gassel AM, et al: Prevention of hepatitis B flare-up during chemotherapy using lamivudine: case report and review of the literature. Ann Hematol 78:247, 1999.
194. Ferri C, Caracciolo F, Zignego AL, et al: Hepatitis C virus infection in patients with non-Hodgkin's lymphoma. Br J Hematol 88:392, 1994.
195. Ferri C, La Civita L, Monti M, et al: Chronic hepatitis C and B-cell non-Hodgkin's lymphoma. QJM 89:117, 1996.
196. Collier JD, Zanke B, Moore M, et al: No association between hepatitis C and B-cell lymphoma. Hepatology 29:1259, 1999.
197. Pioltelli P, Gargantini L, Cssi E, et al: Hepatitis C virus in non-Hodgkin's lymphoma. A reappraisal after a prospective case-control study of 300 patients. Am J Hematol 64:95, 2000.
198. Karp SJ, Shareef D: Ascites as a presenting feature multiple myeloma. J Royal Soc Med 80:182, 1987.
199. Kitazono M, Saito Y, Kinoshita M, et al: Nodular regenerative hyperplasia of the liver in a patient with multiple myeloma and systemic amyloidosis. Acta Pathol Jpn 35:961, 1985.
200. Dimopoulos MA, Galani E, Matsouka C: Waldenström's macroglobulinemia. Hematol Oncol Clin North Am 13:1351, 1999.
201. Pauls JD, Brems J, Pockros PJ, et al: Mastocytosis: diverse presentations and outcomes. Arch Intern Med 15:9401, 1999.
202. Horny H-P, Ruck P, Krober S, et al: Systemic mast cell disease (mastocytosis). General aspects and histopathological diagnosis. Histo Histopathol 12:1081, 1997.
203. Ghandur-Mnaymneh L, Gould E: Systemic mastocytosis with portal hypertension; autopsy findings and ultrastructural study of the liver. Arch Pathol Lab Med 10:976, 1985.
204. Kyriakou D, Kouroumalis E, Konsolas J, et al: Systemic mastocytosis: a rare cause of non-cirrhotic portal hypertension simulating autoimmune cholangitis—report of four cases. Am J Gastroenterol 93:106, 1998.

CHAPTER

53

Budd-Chiari Syndrome

J. Michael Henderson, MD, and Thomas D. Boyer, MD

Budd-Chiari syndrome (BCS) encompasses all of the disorders arising from obstruction of hepatic venous outflow. There are two types of obstruction of hepatic venous outflow: (1) obstruction of the main hepatic veins or the suprahepatic vena cava or (2) diffuse obstruction of the hepatic venules without involvement of the main hepatic veins.

Although the eponym, as originally described by Budd in 1846[1] and Chiari in 1899,[2] describes obstruction of the major veins, the pathophysiology and principles of management of all types of hepatic venous outflow obstruction are the same. The evaluation and management of patients focus on the following factors:

- Is there a mechanical outflow obstruction?
- Is there ongoing acute liver damage?
- What is the extent of chronic liver injury?
- What is the underlying etiology of the syndrome?
- What are the treatment options?

The investigation and management of this group of disorders require a multi-disciplinary approach. Input from hepatology, hematology, radiology, and surgery is essential. The rarity of these syndromes often leads to a delay in diagnosis, but suspicion of hepatic venous outflow obstruction mandates a careful workup with priorities as outlined previously.

PATHOPHYSIOLOGY

The clinical and histologic changes in BCS result from hepatic venous outflow obstruction although there is continued inflow of blood to the liver.[3-10] There must be a significant degree of obstruction of outflow for clinical manifestations to occur. A single hepatic vein obstruction is usually clinically silent, results in histologic changes to the affected lobe only, and may only be detected at autopsy if the other veins are spared. Clinical signs sometimes develop when two, or if all, hepatic veins are occluded. The normal hepatic venous outflow from the liver is by the right, middle, and left hepatic veins, which enter the inferior vena cava (IVC) just below the diaphragm and drain their respective segments of the liver. In addition, there are several smaller hepatic veins passing directly from the right lobe and the caudate lobe of the liver to the intrahepatic IVC. Outflow obstruction may not affect all of these veins, so in evaluating patients in whom this syndrome is suspected it is important to assess the different parts of the liver. A total obstruction leads to severe congestion of the entire liver, causing significant hepatomegaly, stretching of Glisson's capsule, and pain. The increased sinusoidal pressure leads to early development of ascites. However, if only one or two of the hepatic veins are involved and there is still adequate outflow through a third vein and the accessory veins, the clinical syndrome may not be significant. This may lead to silent "damage" to the obstructed segments of the liver with significant architectural distortion and later sequelae.

The pathophysiologic consequences of outflow obstruction that are seen histologically are initial sinusoidal dilation and congestion, predominantly in the central area of the hepatic lobules.[3,10-12] If the outflow obstruction is severe, sinusoidal pressure rises significantly and can lead to centrolobular hepatocyte necrosis. This is the active hepatocyte injury of BCS. This high sinusoidal pressure is also the driving force behind the formation of ascites. Within a few weeks of obstruction, particularly when there has been ongoing hepatocyte necrosis, the next phase of the pathophysiology is development of a centrolobular fibrosis. Associated with this there may be lobular collapse and nodular regeneration, which can occur in differing patterns depending on the extent of injury but effectively leads to cirrhosis.

Veno-occlusive disease (see Chap. 58) presents with different pathophysiology but a similar outcome. In this condition there is a non-thrombotic occlusion of the small sublobular branches of the hepatic veins that effectively lead to a sinusoidal outflow obstruction identical to large vein occlusion and BCS. The primary pathology in veno-occlusive disease is subendothelial sclerosis with secondary thrombosis and occlusion of these hepatic venules. This has been seen with exposure to pyrrolizidine toxins[13] and in patients receiving chemotherapy, hepatic irradiation, or bone marrow transplantation.[14,15]

ETIOLOGY

The etiologies of BCS are listed in Table 53-1. The main mechanical causes of this syndrome are:[10,16-19]

TABLE 53-1
Etiologies of Budd-Chiari Syndrome

Myeloproliferative disorders
Hypercoagulable status
Pregnancy and oral contraceptives
Mechanical obstructions
Paroxysmal nocturnal hemoglobin
Anti-phospholipid autoantibodies

TABLE 53-2
Prevalence of Different Factors Associated with Budd-Chiari Syndrome

Factor	% with disorder
Prothrombotic disorder	87
1° myeloproliferative	31
Coagulation disorder	33
1° myeloproliferative + coagulation disorder	22
Type coagulation disorder	
Anti-phospholipid antibodies	19
G1691A factor V mutation (Leiden)	22
G20210A factor II mutation	6
C677T MTHFR mutation	13
Protein S deficiency	0
Protein C deficiency	20
Antithrombin deficiency	0

Data from Denninger M-H, Chait Y, Casadevall N, et al: Cause of portal or hepatic venous thrombosis in adults: the role of multiple concurrent factors. Hepatology 31:587, 2000.
MTHFR, Methylene-tetrahydrofolate-reductase.
The study was of 32 patients with hepatic vein thrombosis. Some of the patients had more than one coagulation disorder.

- Membranous obstruction of IVC
- Tumor obstruction
- Extrinsic compression by space-occupying lesions
- Kinking of hepatic venous outflow post-liver transplant

Membranous webs occur at the diaphragmatic suprahepatic IVC. As an etiology for BCS these webs are common in South Africa, Japan, and to a lesser extent India. The main portion of the IVC is usually not obstructed, and significant collaterals will develop from the infrahepatic IVC through the azygous system to return blood to the right atrium. However, build-up of pressure leading to a full-blown BCS can develop and may be associated with other thrombotic events as outlined in the following section.

Tumors that cause BCS range from intrahepatic hepatomas directly invading hepatic venous outflow, to a non-liver tumor ingrowth of the IVC leading to obstruction. The classic tumor in this latter group is renal cell carcinoma, which can grow along the renal veins and up the IVC. However, other rare tumors such as adrenocortin carcinomas, leiomyosarcomas of the IVC, myxomas of the right atrium, and Wilms' tumors can cause hepatic vein outflow obstruction through vascular endoluminal invasion.

Extrinsic compression of hepatic venous outflow has been reported after trauma, with aortic aneurysms and with infectious space-occupying diseases such as amebic abscesses.

Several reports have now appeared in the literature about hepatic venous outflow obstruction after liver transplantation, particularly when the piggyback technique is used.[20,21] This obstruction can occur if there is a redundant length of hepatic vein or IVC used at the suprahepatic anastomosis. It is important that this obstruction is identified at the time of surgery because the newly transplanted liver has no opportunity to develop decompressing collaterals to decompress the obstructed sinusoids. Undetected, this can be a cause of graft loss.

Thrombotic Causes

Thrombotic causes of BCS continue to be recognized and their mechanisms clarified (Table 53-2). The largest group of these are the myeloproliferative disorders.[10,22-24] The most common cause is polycythemia rubra vera, but other disorders such as myelofibrosis, essential thrombocythemia, and chronic lymphocytic leukemia may cause hepatic venous thrombosis. These disorders are characterized by a common origin of malignant stem cell change with subsequent proliferation. Increased viscosity, low-grade disseminated intravascular coagulation, and active fibrinolysis appear to contribute to the overall thrombosis. Because the liver is the main site of clearance of plasminogen activator, a deficiency of hepatic anti-plasmin may contribute to localization of the thrombosis in the hepatic veins. Detection of these hematologic disorders may be more difficult in patients with BCS compared to their usual occurrence because of the associated portal hypertension. Increased plasma volume and splenomegaly may mask the increased red blood cell mass of polycythemia rubra vera and the changes of thrombocythemia. Recognition of "occult" myeloproliferative disorders has led to the demonstration of spontaneous formation of erythroid colonies as the marker for this diagnosis.[22]

Pregnancy and Oral Contraceptives

BCS has been reported during and after pregnancy, usually in the first 2 months of pregnancy.[25,26] It has been postulated that this increased risk of thrombosis may be related to elevated factors VII, VIII, and fibrinogen. The reported increased risk of patients on the oral contraceptive pill for developing hepatic vein thrombosis is 2.4-fold greater than age-matched controls.[28] However, other etiologic factors should also be sought in these patients because there may also be an underlying hematologic disorder.

Paroxysmal Nocturnal Hemoglobinuria

This devastating syndrome is seen in patients who usually have other hematologic disorders such as aplastic anemia and acute leukemias. Complement-induced platelet activation contributes to the increased risk of thrombosis. Hepatic vein occlusion in this setting is often associated with a fulminant course.[29,30]

Anti-phospholipid Autoantibodies

The presence of various anti-phospholipid autoantibodies, such as described in systemic lupus erythematosus and other connective tissue disorders, has increasingly been recognized as an etiology of hepatic vein thrombosis.[31-33] Patients are at increased risk of arterial and venous thrombosis with these autoantibodies and are particularly prone to hepatic venous thrombosis if anticoagulant therapy is discontinued.

Hypercoagulable States

The classic deficiencies of anti-thrombin III, protein C, or protein S are common causes of hepatic vein thrombosis.[34] However, the resistance to activated protein C with factor V Leiden has been recognized in the last several years to be a significant factor in the development of hepatic vein thrombosis.[35,36] Factor V Leiden is a common mutation, which appears to precipitate thrombosis when combined with another hematologic risk factor.[37,38] Mutations in the genes for factor II and methylene-tetrahydrofolate-reductase are also associated with a prothrombotic state and increased risk of hepatic venous thrombosis.[33]

CLINICAL PRESENTATION

BCS may present as an acute, subacute, or chronic illness.[39,40] The acute fulminant presentation is uncommon and requires total obstruction of all venous outflow with severe ongoing necrosis of hepatic parenchyma secondary to the congestion.[40,41] Most commonly patients present with a vague illness of less than 6 months' duration with ascites.[40,42]

The triad of ascites, hepatomegaly, and right upper quadrant abdominal pain may be present. Ascites is usually manageable with diuretics, but occasionally may be intractable. The failure to have an obvious clinical explanation for ascites, such as known cirrhosis, right heart failure, or an intra-abdominal malignancy, should always raise the question of a hepatic venous outflow obstruction. Frequently patients will have been seen by many other physicians and diagnoses such as gynecologic or gastrointestinal malignancies or inflammatory processes entertained. BCS is rare, and unless the diagnosis is considered it is often missed. Other clinical stigmata of severe liver damage are usually absent. Jaundice is unusual, and when present is slight. Other signs of chronic liver disease such as spider angioma and muscle wasting are usually absent. The patient should be examined for jugular venous distention because failure to demonstrate this or failure to show hepatojugular reflux on abdominal pressure is helpful in excluding a central cardiac cause for hepatic congestion. Occasionally, pedal edema may be a feature if there is associated obstruction of the IVC.

LABORATORY STUDIES

The degree of liver test abnormalities is unusually minimal.[4,7,40,42] This is somewhat surprising when one subsequently views the pathologic changes. In general the aminotransferases and bilirubin levels are slightly elevated, serum albumin level slightly decreased, and prothrombin time marginally prolonged. Significant changes in hepatocellular enzymes usually indicate severe hepatocyte damage requiring emergency decompression of the congested liver.

The protein content of BCS' ascites is variable and can be high (more than 3 g/dl) or low.[4,5] The ascites cell count is variable, with most patients having fewer than 100 white blood cells per cubic millimeter. Spontaneous bacterial peritonitis does not occur in these patients.

DIAGNOSIS

The diagnosis of BCS depends on appropriate radiologic imaging and liver biopsy. Because this is a rare entity, a high index of suspicion is required to conduct the appropriate studies.

Radiologic investigations should follow an appropriate management algorithm. If there is a suspicion of BCS, hepatic ultrasound concentrating on the hepatic veins and combined with Doppler flow studies should be the initial non-invasive screening test.[43,44] The typical appearance and phasic flow pattern in a normal hepatic vein is shown in Figure 53-1. In a normal subject, the three major hepatic veins can be readily visualized and phasic flow recorded. The inability to demonstrate these veins, or the findings small and stenotic vessels in which phasic flow cannot be demonstrated, should raise suspicion for hepatic vein occlusion. At the same time the portal vein should be visualized to document its patency and the presence of flow within it because this may become important in further management. Retrograde flow in the portal vein is observed frequently.

Hepatic scintigraphy,[45] computed tomography scanning,[46] and magnetic resonance imaging[47] have all been used and can contribute to the diagnosis of BCS. Although each of these may provide supportive evidence either by patterns of uptake or by morphologic change in either the parenchyma or the vessels, they are not specifically diagnostic of BCS.

Although angiography with hepatic venography and celiac and superior mesenteric arteriography was formerly indicated for most patients with a suspicion of BCS,[40,42,48] this is no longer true. The indication for hepatic venography is now restricted to patients in whom the diagnosis cannot be made with ultrasound or when a biopsy is going to be most safely achieved through a transjugular route. In these patients in whom the diagnosis remains in doubt, an attempt should be made to directly cannulate and image each of the major hepatic veins for study. This allows definition of differential disease with varying degrees of outflow block. The typical appearance of the hepatic veins with the spider's web is shown in Figure 53-2. These collaterals are attempting to decompress the hepatic sinusoids and no normal hepatic vein is identified. Venography also plays a role when surgical decompression is being considered with measurement of pressures in the right atrium and in the intrahepatic and infrahepatic IVC (Figure 53-3). Understanding what the pressure gradient is across the liver is important in determining the type of decompressive shunt to be used when indicated. The only indication for a superior mesenteric arteriography is in the patient in

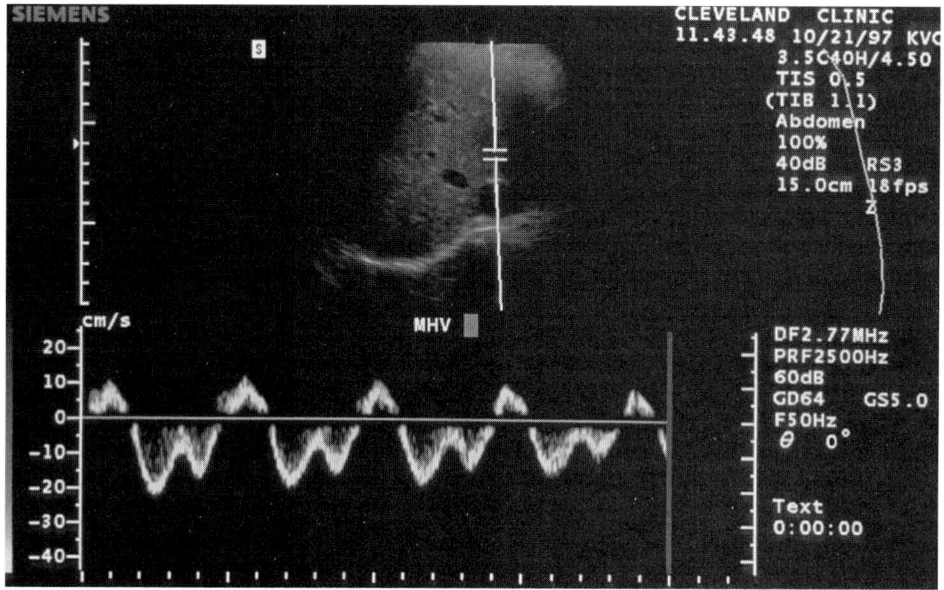

Figure 53-1 Ultrasound evaluation of normal MHV, with Doppler demonstration of phasic flow. The veins may not be visualized or phasic flow is lost in BCS. *MHV,* Middle hepatic vein; *BCS,* Budd-Chiari syndrome.

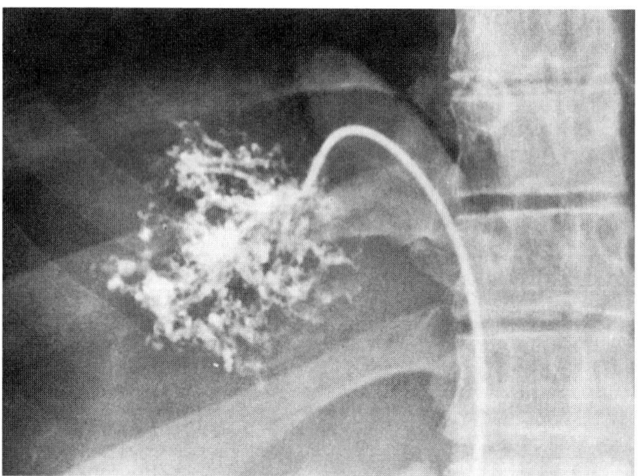

Figure 53-2 Hepatic vein contrast study showing the "spider's web" of Budd-Chiari syndrome. The sinusoids are attempting to drain through capsular collaterals.

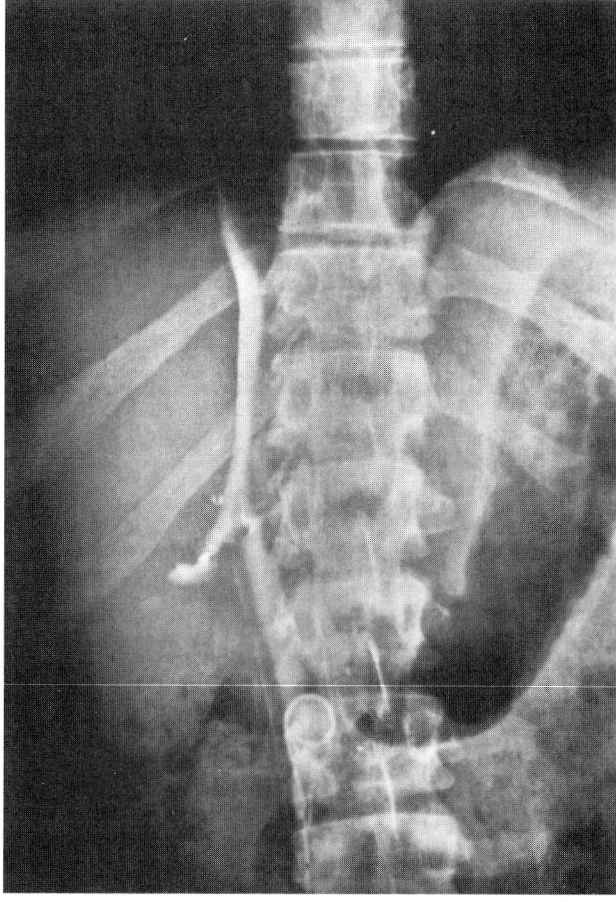

Figure 53-3 An inferior vena cava contrast study. The swollen liver of Budd-Chiari syndrome is compressing the cava, but this has not led to thrombosis for this patient. Measurements of the right atrial to infrahepatic pressure gradient will determine the type of shunt that should be used.

A

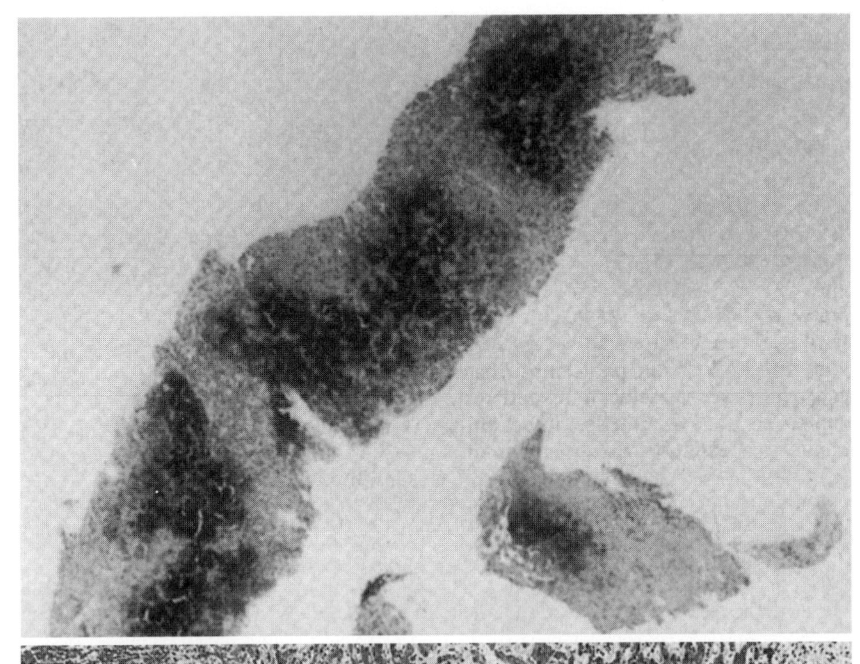

B

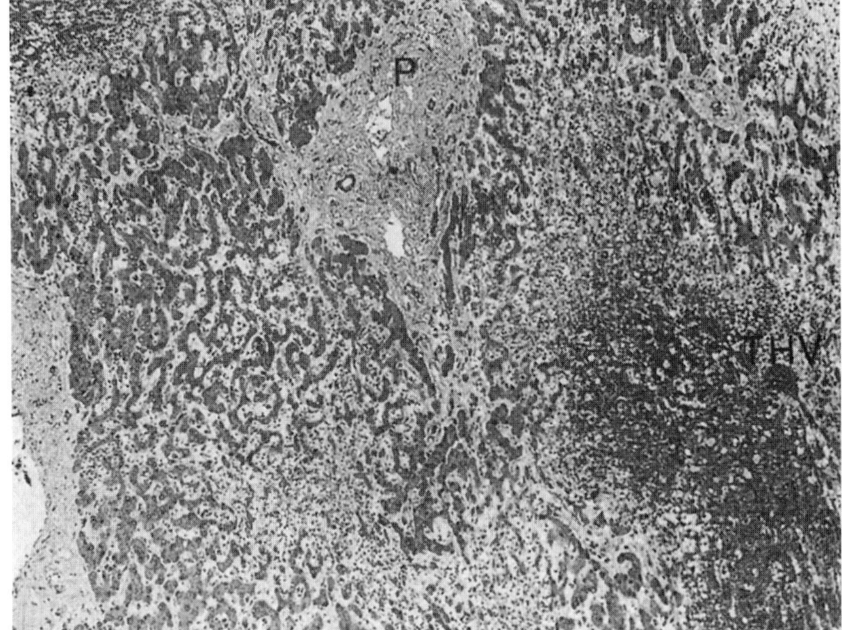

Figure 53-4 **A,** Low-power (× 10) photomicrograph of a needle liver biopsy from a patient with hepatic vein thrombosis. Notice the intense congestion (dark areas) near the terminal hepatic vein. **B,** Medium-power photomicrograph of a liver biopsy from a patient with hepatic vein thrombosis. There is vascular congestion near the terminal hepatic vein (THV) with loss of hepatocytes. In the midzonal region, the hepatocytes are atrophic, whereas they are preserved near the portal areas (p). (Courtesy of R Peters.)

whom the portal vein cannot be identified on ultrasound study. In this situation, proof that there is thrombosis of the portal vein is important because it dictates further management. An arteriogram is the final step in that proof.

Liver biopsy is an important diagnostic step to confirm histologic diagnosis and also assesses the degree of hepatocellular damage. Biopsy helps in planning appropriate therapy for patients with BCS.[7,29,42,48] Massive ascites and severe coagulopathy are unusual in BCS but indicate an even more urgent need for biopsy. The choice of the route for biopsy depends on the patient's overall condition. Although percutaneous bilobar biopsy can be performed if there is minimal ascites, it may be preferable to biopsy the liver through a transjugular route when there is significant ascites. Even through the transjugular route attempts can be made to get differential biopsies of the right and left lobes, even if this means an approach from the IVC or a hepatic vein stump. Occasionally a laparoscopy may be indicated to allow visualization of the liver and differential lobar biopsies.

The essential features to be identified on the histology are central vein thrombosis, the centrizonal congestion, and the degrees of hepatocellular necrosis, lobular collapse, and finally fibrosis and cirrhosis (Figures 53-4 and 53-5). Careful grading of biopsy specimens from both sides of the liver will document the extent of the disease and determine the course of management. When there is congestion but no histologic evidence of ongoing necrosis, expectant management with repeat biopsy in 3 to 6 months may be indicated. Patients with severe congestion

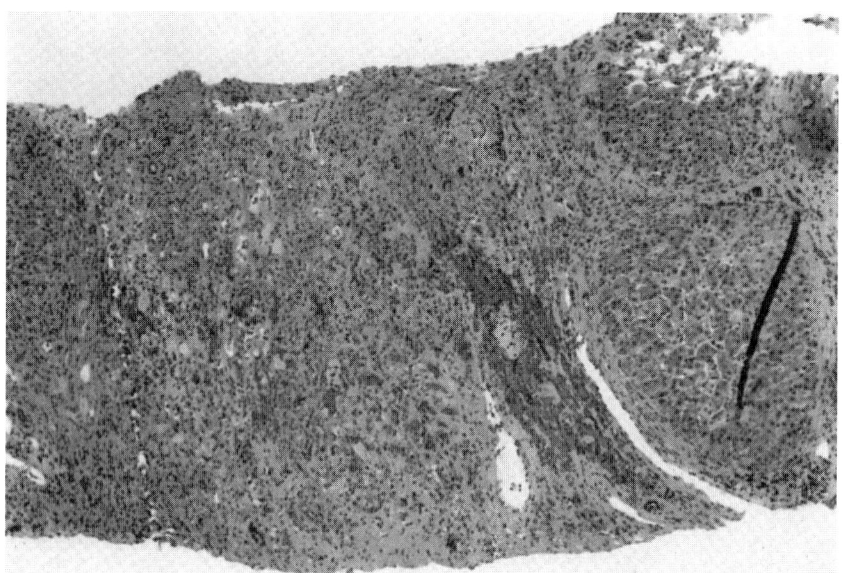

Figure 53-5 A low-power photomicrograph of a liver biopsy from a patient with chronic Budd-Chiari syndrome. The extensive fibrosis is indicative of irreversible damage, with only small islands of regenerative hepatocytes visible.

TABLE 53-3

Hematologic Evaluation of Patients with Budd-Chiari Syndrome

Routine hematology with blood smear
Bone marrow, to include reticulin stain and cytogenetics
Leukocyte alkaline phosphatase
Platelet aggregometry
Red blood cell mass
Sucrose hemolysis
Protein C, protein S, antithrombin III
Factor V Leiden
Anti-phospholipid autoantibodies

and ongoing hepatocyte necrosis but a maintained lobular pattern can be managed by a decompressive procedure. In contrast, patients with severe fibrosis and cirrhosis have progressed to a stage that will probably require liver transplantation.

Hematologic evaluation should be conducted as soon as a radiologic and biopsy diagnosis of BCS is made. This is summarized in Table 53-3 and requires the input of an experienced hematologist.[22,24]

MANAGEMENT

A management algorithm for BCS is given in Figure 53-6. When BCS is untreated the mortality rate for patients is high. In one series, 17 of 19 patients died within 3.5 years of diagnosis,[7] although not all series have such dismal results. Long-term survival of untreated patients is reported and appears to depend on a chronic course and sufficient time for the liver to develop adequate decompressive collaterals from the sinusoids to the diaphragm.[4]

Management is dictated by the combination of imaging studies and liver biopsy. When there is documented hepatic vein thrombosis, the biopsy is used to define the current status of the hepatocytes. Standard liver tests are not sufficient in BCS to define the status of the liver. If there is only a mild degree of outflow obstruction or if adequate collaterals have developed, there may be no ongoing hepatocyte necrosis. When there is significant obstruction, the biopsy may show severe congestion and a variable degree of continuing hepatocyte necrosis. When the obstruction is long-standing, and there has been failure to develop adequate collateral outflow from the liver, there may have been a progression to lobular collapse, severe fibrosis, and even regeneration and cirrhosis.

Non-surgical management may be indicated in some patients in whom the biopsy shows no evidence of hepatocyte necrosis. However, such a "watch and wait" strategy must be accompanied by careful follow-up and repeat biopsies in 3 to 6 months. If such a patient has ascites, it is appropriate to manage the ascites with salt restriction and diuretics. A peritoneovenous shunt is not appropriate therapy for the management of ascites of BCS. The ascites is a symptom of the hepatic vein outflow obstruction; removal of the ascites will not reverse that process. Thrombolytic therapy with streptokinase or urokinase has been reported to relieve symptoms in some patients.[4,49] Thrombolytic therapy may be indicated in the patient with an acute onset in whom there is not severe ongoing necrosis and for whom time allows for a trial of this therapy. Long-term successful therapy with anticoagulants has also been reported.[50] However, the medical approach must be accompanied with full liver evaluation and careful follow-up to prevent progressive silent liver injury.

Invasive radiologic procedures have been used as a non-operative method to relieve obstruction.[51,52] This is

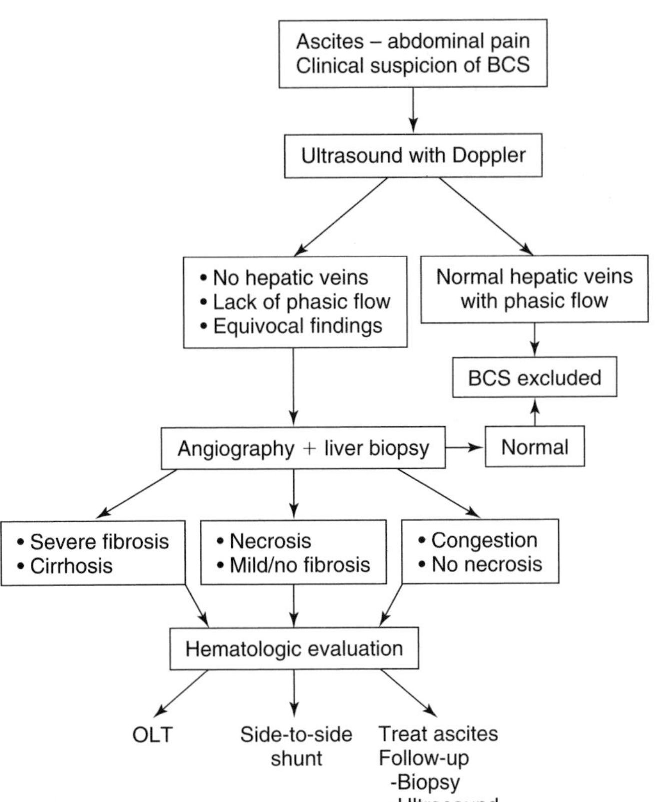

Figure 53-6 Algorithm for the diagnosis and management of BCS. *OLT,* Orthotopic liver transplantation; *BCS,* Budd-Chiari syndrome.

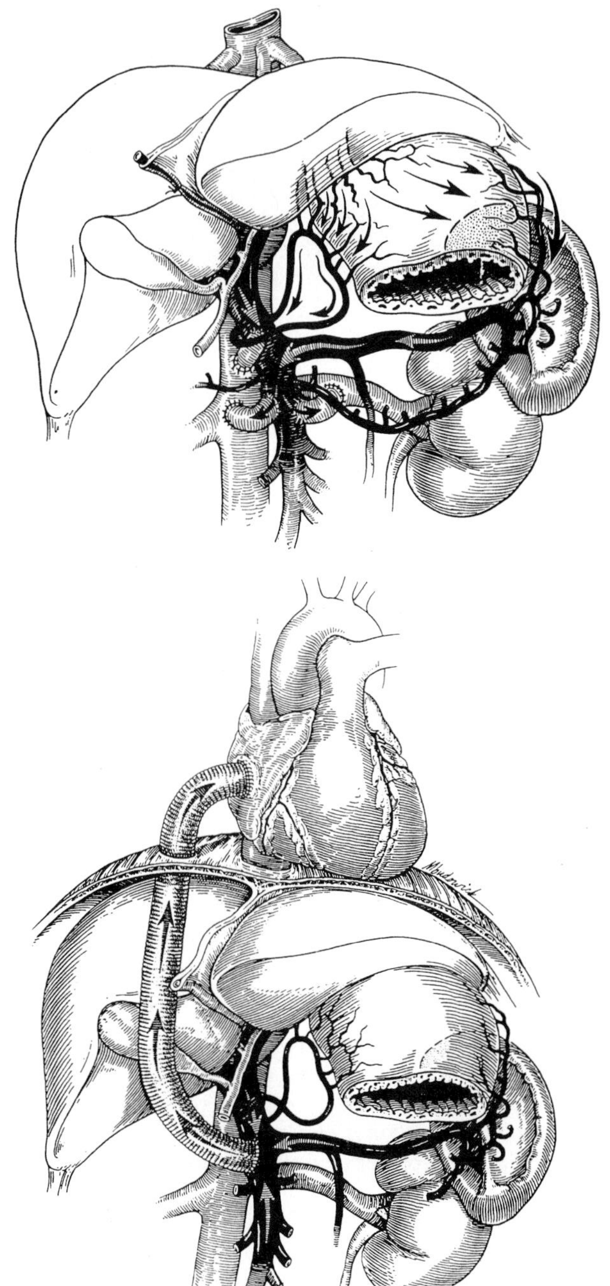

Figure 53-7 **A,** Side-to-side interposition total portal-systemic shunts. The portal vein serves as an outflow from the obstructed sinusoids. **B,** Mesoatrial shunt applies the same principle as in *A* for decompression of the sinusoids. However, inferior vena caval obstruction requires the long shunt to bypass the intrahepatic, occluded cava. (**A** and **B** from Henderson JM, Warren WD: Portal hypertension. In Current Problems in Surgery 25:149, 1988.)

particularly applicable in patients with webs or a limited stenosis of the hepatic veins. Percutaneous transluminal angioplasty has been used to dilate such strictures or webs and with the current technology may be combined with a stent.[53] The further extension of such therapy is the radiologic placement of an intrahepatic shunt from a hepatic vein stump through the liver to the portal vein with a stent deployed in a balloon-dilated track. Experience with this transjugular intrahepatic portosystemic shunt (TIPS) is growing as discussed later.

Surgical management has been used extensively in BCS.[42] In the 1990s this was simplified to side-to-side portosystemic shunts to decompress acutely congested livers and orthotopic liver transplantation to replace irrevocably damaged livers. The use of peritoneovenous shunting in BCS is not indicated, and the direct excisional approach to hepatic vein obstruction advocated by Senning has not been used by other groups.[54] The choice between a decompressive shunt and transplant is based on careful evaluation. The liver biopsy plays a key role in this choice, with the features of congestion, necrosis, and fibrosis being paramount. Equally, an assessment of hepatic function will help determine the wisdom of saving the patient's own liver.

Decompressive shunts aim to relieve sinusoidal congestion by using the portal vein as an outflow.[24,42,55-61] Thus the classic side-to-side portacaval shunt, or an interposition shunt between the portal vein, the superior mesenteric vein or splenic vein, and the vena cava will work equally well. By using the portal vein as an outflow tract from the obstructed sinusoids, the ongoing necrosis is halted, allowing hepatocyte regeneration on an intact lobular reticular framework. If the decision is made to use a decompressive shunt, the surgeon must decide on the choice between an infrahepatic and a suprahepatic shunt (Figure 53-7). This choice is based on the status of

TABLE 53-4

Experience and Outcome of Side-to-Side Portal-systemic Shunt for Acute Budd-Chiari Syndrome

Center, reference no.	Publication year	No. patients	Intrahepatic	Suprahepatic	Survival
Hopkins (56)	2001	43	24	19	75% (5 yr)
Emory (24)	1990	24	10	11	86% (3 yr)
San Diego (57)	2000	50	32	18	86% (10 yr)
Mayo (58)	1985	10	9	1	90% (5 yr)
Baylor (59)	1992	10	3	7	70% (3 yr)
Paul Brousse (60)	1990	21	20	1	96% (5 yr)
Milan (61)	1984	6	6	—	67% (2 yr)

TABLE 53-5

Experience and Outcome of Orthotopic Liver Transplantation for Budd-Chiari Syndrome

Center, reference no.	Publication year	No. patients	Hospital mortality (%)	Survival
Pittsburgh (65)	1989	23	30	58% (5 yr)
Cambridge (66)	1988	17	12	71% (2 yr)
Baylor (59)	1992	14	14	76% (3 yr)

the intrahepatic IVC. When this is thrombosed or severely compromised by liver swelling and the pressure gradient from the atrium to the infrahepatic IVC exceeds portal pressure, an infrahepatic shunt will not work. In this situation a mesoatrial shunt is required. Reported experience with decompressive shunts for acute BCS is summarized in Table 53-4. These series report remarkably similar results, with survival in appropriately selected patients with the acute syndrome and good hepatocellular function ranging from 65 to more than 90 percent at 3 to 5 years. Such results are only achieved when there is early referral of patients and when decompression can be provided before there is irrevocable hepatocellular damage.

TIPS has been increasingly used for decompression of BCS patients in the past decade.[62-64] This shunt obeys basic physiologic principles of a side-to-side portacaval shunt using the portal vein as an outflow from the obstructed sinusoid. Thus when there is a sufficient hepatic vein orifice to allow insertion of a TIPS, this is a reasonable approach. Equally, TIPS has been used in patients with veno-occlusive disease with ongoing severe liver damage with reported mixed results. The theoretic disadvantage of TIPS is the increased risk of stenosis and thrombosis in patients who already have a thrombotic disorder. However, if the hematologic process is being appropriately and aggressively treated, this theoretic disadvantage may be negated. Long-term follow-up of patients with BCS receiving TIPS is still awaited.[62-64]

Liver transplantation is indicated for patients with advanced disease.[24,42,59,65,66] Significant fibrosis and cirrhosis on the liver biopsy, usually combined with poor hepatocellular reserve, can only be treated with transplantation. It should be noted that technically these are some of the more difficult transplants to perform because of the severe distortion of the liver parenchyma and the inexorable attempt of the liver to drain itself through collaterals to the diaphragm. This makes the recipient hepatectomy exceedingly hazardous. The reported experience of patients with BCS managed by liver transplantation is summarized in Table 53-5. In these series, which include some early experience, the outcome appears to be similar to liver transplantation for other diseases. Three- to 5-year survival ranging from 58 to 76 percent has been achieved (see Chap. 55).

Hematologic management issues must be addressed along with the surgical approach. An early and aggressive work-up for hematologic problems must accompany the choice of therapy. A myeloproliferative disorder should be treated preoperatively and with continuing therapy in the perioperative period. If the underlying hematologic disorder is not recognized and appropriately managed, the risk of shunt thrombosis, or thrombosis in the transplanted liver, is high. The specifics of hematologic therapy are beyond the scope of this chapter, but usually require specific therapy for any underlying myeloproliferative disorder and anticoagulation.

SUMMARY

BCS is uncommon but it must be entertained as a possible diagnosis in patients with unexplained ascites. An etiology, usually a hematologic disorder, can be defined in most patients. Evaluation is based on radiologic imaging and liver biopsy. Therapy aims at halting progressive liver damage, but must be combined with management of the etiologic disorder. When irrevocable liver damage has occurred, liver transplantation is the treatment of choice.

References

1. Budd G: On Diseases of the Liver. London, John Churchill, 1846.
2. Chiari H: Ueber die selbstandige phlebitis oliterans der haupstamme der venae hepaticae als todesurache. Beitr Z Pathol Anat 26:1, 1845.
3. Parker R: Occlusion of hepatic veins in man. Medicine 38:369, 1959.
4. Mitchell MC, Boitnott JK, Kaufman S, et al: Budd-Chiari syndrome: etiology, diagnosis and management. Medicine 61(4):199, 1982.
5. Gupta S, Blumgart LH, Hodgson HJ: Budd-Chiari syndrome: long-term survival and factors affecting mortality. Q J Med 60(232):781, 1986.
6. Cameron JL, Herlong F, Safey H, et al: The Budd-Chiari syndrome. Treatment by mesenteric-systemic venous shunts. Ann Surg 198:335, 1983.
7. Tavill AS, Wood EJ, Kreel L, et al: The Budd-Chiari syndrome: correlation between hepatic scintigraphy and the clinical, radiological, and pathological findings in nineteen cases of hepatic venous outflow obstruction. Gastroenterology 68(3):509, 1975.
8. Zeitoun G, Escolano S, Hadengue A, et al: Outcome of Budd-Chiari syndrome: a multivariate analysis of factors related to survival including surgical portosystemic shunting. Hepatology 30(1):84, 1999.
9. Denninger MH, Chait Y, Casadevall N, et al: Cause of portal or hepatic venous thrombosis in adults: the role of multiple concurrent factors. Hepatology 31(3):587, 2000.
10. Valla D, Benhamon J-P: Obstruction of the hepatic venous system. In Bircher J, Benhamon J-P, Mintyre N, et al, eds: Oxford Textbook of Clinical Hepatology, ed 2. Oxford, Oxford Medical Publications, 1999:1469-1478.
11. Wanless IR, Godwin TA, Allen F, Feder A: Nodular regenerative hyperplasia of the liver in hematologic disorders: a possible response to obliterative portal venopathy. A morphometric study of nine cases with an hypothesis on the pathogenesis. Medicine 59(5):367, 1980.
12. Tanaka M, Wanless IR: Pathology of the liver in Budd-Chiari syndrome: portal vein thrombosis and the histogenesis of veno-centric cirrhosis, and large regenerative nodules. Hepatology 27(2):488, 1998.
13. Bras G, Jelliffe D, Stuart K: Veno-occlusive disease of liver with nonportal type of cirrhosis, occurring in Jamaica. Arch Pathol 57:285, 1954.
14. Berk PD, Popper H, Krueger GR, et al: Veno-occlusive disease of the liver after allogeneic bone marrow transplantation: possible association with graft-versus-host disease. Ann Intern Med 90(2):158, 1979.
15. McDonald GB, Hinds MS, Fisher LD, et al: Veno-occlusive disease of the liver and multiorgan failure after bone marrow transplantation: a cohort study of 355 patients. Ann Intern Med 118:255, 1993.
16. Simson IW: Membranous obstruction of the inferior vena cava and hepatocellular carcinoma in South Africa. Gastroenterology 82(2):171, 1982.
17. Dilawari JB, Bambery P, Chawla Y, et al: Hepatic outflow obstruction (Budd-Chiari syndrome). Experience with 177 patients and review of the literature. Medicine 73:21, 1994.
18. Hirooka M, Kimura C: Membranous obstruction of the hepatic portion of the inferior vena cava. Surgical correction and etiology study. Arch Surg 100:656, 1970.
19. Okuda K, Ostrow D: Clinical conference: membranous type of Budd-Chiari syndrome. J Clin Gastroenterol 6(1):81, 1984.
20. Stieber AC, Gordon RD, Bassi N: A simple solution to a technical complication in "piggyback" liver transplantation. Transplantation 64(4):654, 1997.
21. Boggi U, Filipponi R, Mosca F: Water-glove balloon system: a useful option to salvage liver grafts with postreperfusion outflow obstruction. Transplantation 66(10):1317, 1998.
22. Valla D, Casadevall N, Lacombe C, et al: Primary myeloproliferative disorder and hepatic vein thrombosis. A prospective study of erythroid colony formation in vitro in 20 patients with Budd-Chiari syndrome. Ann Intern Med 103(3):329, 1985.
23. Klein AS, Cameron JL: Diagnosis and management of the Budd-Chiari syndrome [see comments]. Am J Surg 160(1):128, 1990.
24. Henderson JM, Warren WD, Millikan WJ Jr, et al: Surgical options, hematologic evaluation, and pathologic changes in Budd-Chiari syndrome. Am J Surg 159(1):41, discussion 48, 1990.
25. Ilan Y, Oren R, Shouval D: Postpartum Budd-Chiari syndrome with prolonged hypercoagulability state. Am J Obstet Gynecol 162(5): 1164, 1990.
26. Khuroo MS, Datta DV: Budd-Chiari syndrome following pregnancy. Report of 16 cases, with roentgenologic, hemodynamic and histologic studies of the hepatic outflow tract. Am J Med 68(1):113, 1980.
27. Hoyumpa AM Jr, Schiff L, Helfman EL: Budd-Chiari syndrome in women taking oral contraceptives. Amer J Med 50(1):137, 1971.
28. Valla D, Le MG, Poynard T, et al: Risk of hepatic vein thrombosis in relation to recent use of oral contraceptives. A case-control study. Gastroenterology 90(4):807, 1986.
29. Valla D, Dhumeaux D, Babany G, et al: Hepatic vein thrombosis in paroxysmal nocturnal hemoglobinuria. A spectrum from asymptomatic occlusion of hepatic venules to fatal Budd-Chiari syndrome. Gastroenterology 93(3):569, 1987.
30. Hartmann RC, Luther AB, Jenkins DE Jr, et al: Fulminant hepatic venous thrombosis (Budd-Chiari syndrome) in paroxysmal nocturnal hemoglobinuria: definition of a medical emergency. Johns Hopkins Med J 146(6):247, 1980.
31. Bisbocci D, De Micheli AG, Tamanti P, et al: Association of the Budd-Chiari syndrome with lupus anticoagulant. Case report and critical review. Ann Ital Med Interna 6(2):251, 1991.
32. Pelletier S, Landi B, Peitte JC, et al: Antiphospholipid syndrome as the second cause of non-tumorous Budd-Chiari syndrome. J Hepatol 21(1):76, 1994.
33. Denninger M-H, Chait Y, Casadevall N, et al: Cause of portal or hepatic venous thrombosis in adults: the role of multiple concurrent factors. Hepatology 31:587, 2000.
34. Bourliere M, Le Treut YP, Arnoux D, et al: Acute Budd-Chiari syndrome with hepatic failure and obstruction of the inferior vena cava as presenting manifestations of hereditary protein C deficiency. Gut 31:949, 1990.
35. Denninger MH, Beldjord K, Durand F, et al: Budd-Chiari syndrome and factor V Leiden mutation. Lancet 345(8948):525, 1995.
36. Mahmoud AE, Elias E, Beauchamp N, Wilde JT: Prevalence of the factor V Leiden mutation in hepatic and portal vein thrombosis. Gut 40(6):798, 1997.
37. Janssen HL, Meinardi JR, Vleggaar FP, et al: Factor V Leiden mutation, prothrombin gene mutation, and deficiencies in coagulation inhibitors associated with Budd-Chiari syndrome and portal vein thrombosis: results of a case-control study. Blood 96(7):2364, 2000.
38. Deltenre P, Denninger MH, Hillaire S, et al: Factor V Leiden related Budd-Chiari syndrome. Gut 48:264, 2001.
39. Clain D, Freston J, Kreel L, Sherlock S: Clinical diagnosis of the Budd-Chiari syndrome. A report of six cases. Am J Med 43(4):544, 1967.
40. Millikan WJ Jr, Henderson JM, Sewell CW, et al: Approach to the spectrum of Budd-Chiari syndrome: which patients require portal decompression? Am J Surg 149(1):167, 1985.
41. Powell-Jackson PR, Ede RJ, Williams R: Budd-Chiari syndrome presenting as fulminant hepatic failure. Gut 27(9):1101, 1986.
42. Klein AS, Stizmann JV, Coleman J, et al: Current management of Budd-Chiari syndrome. Ann Surg 212:144, 1990.
43. Bolondi L, Gaiani S, Li Bassi S, et al: Diagnosis of Budd-Chiari syndrome by pulsed Doppler ultrasound. Gastroenterology 100:1324, 1991.
44. Ralls PW, Johnson MB, Radin DR, et al: Budd-Chiari syndrome: detection with color Doppler sonography. Am J Roentgenol 159(1):113, 1992.
45. Powell-Jackson PR, Karani J, Ede RJ, et al: Ultrasound scanning and 99mTc sulphur colloid scintigraphy in diagnosis of Budd-Chiari syndrome. Gut 27(12):1502, 1986.
46. Vogelzang RL, Anschuetz SL, Gore RM: Budd-Chiari syndrome: CT observations. Radiology 163(2):329, 1987.
47. Friedman AC, Ramchandani P, Black M, et al: Magnetic resonance imaging diagnosis of Budd-Chiari syndrome. Gastroenterology 91(5):1289, 1986.
48. Shill M, Henderson JM, Tavill AS: The Budd-Chiari syndrome revisited. Gastroenterologist 2:27, 1994.
49. Sholar PW, Bell WR: Thrombolytic therapy for inferior vena cava thrombosis in paroxysmal nocturnal hemoglobinuria. Ann Intern Med 103(4):539, 1985.
50. Min AD, Atillasoy EO, Schwartz ME, et al: Reassessing the role of medical therapy in the management of hepatic vein thrombosis. Liver Transplant Surg 3:423, 1997.

51. Sparano J, Chang J, Trasi S, Bonanno C: Treatment of the Budd-Chiari syndrome with percutaneous transluminal angioplasty. Case report and review of the literature. Am J Med 82(4):821, 1987.
52. Martin LG, Henderson JM, Millikan WJ Jr, et al: Angioplasty for long-term treatment of patients with Budd-Chiari syndrome. Am J Radiol 154(5):100, 1990.
53. Lopez RR Jr, Benner KG, Hall L, et al: Expandable venous stents for treatment of the Budd-Chiari syndrome. Gastroenterology 100(5):1435, 1991.
54. Senning A: Transcaval posterocranial resection of the liver as treatment of the Budd-Chiari syndrome. World J Surg 7:632, 1983.
55. McDermott WV, Stone MD, Bothe A Jr, Trey C: Budd-Chiari syndrome. Historical and clinical review with an analysis of surgical corrective procedures. Am J Surg 147(4):463, 1984.
56. Slakey DP, Klein AS, Venbrux AC, Cameron JL: Budd-Chiari syndrome: current management options. Ann Surg 233(4):522, 2001.
57. Orloff JM, Daily PO, Orloff SL, et al: A 27-year experience with surgical treatment of Budd-Chiari syndrome. Ann Surg 232(3):340, 2000.
58. McCarthy PM, van Heerden JA, Adson MA, et al: The Budd-Chiari syndrome. Medical and surgical management of 30 patients. Arch Surg 120(6):657, 1985.
59. Shaked A, Goldstein RM, Klintmalm GB, et al: Portosystemic shunt versus orthotopic liver transplantation for the Budd-Chiari syndrome. Surg Gynecol Obstet 174(6):453, 1992.
60. Bismuth H, Sherlock DJ: Portasystemic shunting versus liver transplantation for the Budd-Chiari syndrome. Ann Surg 214(5):581, 1991.
61. Pezzuoli G, Spina GP, Opocher E, et al: Portacaval shunt in the treatment of primary Budd-Chiari syndrome. Surgery 98(2):319, 1985.
62. Ochs A, Sellinger M, Haag K, et al: Transjugular intrahepatic portosystemic stent-shunt (TIPS) in the treatment of Budd-Chiari syndrome. J Hepatol 18:217, 1993.
63. Blum U, Rossle M, Haag K, et al: Budd-Chiari syndrome: technical, hemodynamic, and clinical results of treatment with transjugular intrahepatic portosystemic shunt. Radiology 197(3):805, 1995.
64. Ganger DR, Klapman JB, McDonald V, et al: Transjugular intrahepatic portosystemic shunt (TIPS) for Budd-Chiari syndrome or portal vein thrombosis: review of indications and problems. Am J Gastroenterol 94(3):603, 1999.
65. Halff G, Todo S, Tzakis AG, et al: Liver transplantation for the Budd-Chiari syndrome. Ann Surg 211(1):43, 1990.
66. Campbell DA Jr, Rolles K, Jamieson N, et al: Hepatic transplantation with perioperative and long term anticoagulation as treatment for Budd-Chiari syndrome. Surg Gynecol Obstet 166(6):51, 1988.

CHAPTER

54

The Liver in Pregnancy

Rebecca W. Van Dyke, MD

The pregnant state is associated with physiologic changes in hepatic function that may cause uncertainty about the presence or absence of liver disease. In addition, common disorders of the liver may present with unusual features during pregnancy. Finally, several types of liver disease are unique to pregnancy. The aspects of liver function and liver disease during pregnancy discussed in this chapter include (1) normal changes in hepatic function during pregnancy, (2) unusual aspects of common liver disorders, (3) liver disorders related to pregnancy, and (4) liver disorders unique to pregnancy.

CHANGES IN LIVER ANATOMY AND FUNCTION DURING PREGNANCY

Liver Anatomy and Histology

Liver size and gross appearance do not change during normal pregnancy.[1,2] Subtle changes in histologic appearance may be seen but are non-specific in nature. These changes include (1) increased variability in hepatocyte size and shape,[3,4] (2) granularity of hepatocyte cytoplasm,[3] (3) more frequent cytoplasmic fat vacuoles in centrolobular hepatocytes,[4] and (4) hypertrophied Kupffer cells.[5] Hepatocytes in women during normal pregnancy also exhibit proliferation of the smooth and rough endoplasmic reticulum; enlarged, rod-shaped, and giant mitochondria with paracrystalline inclusions; and increased numbers of peroxisomes.[6,7] Many of these changes are seen in women taking oral contraceptives.[8-10]

Liver Blood Flow

Blood volume increases 40 percent to 50 percent[11-13] accompanied by an increase in cardiac stroke volume and output and a decrease in peripheral resistance.[11] Hepatic blood flow, measured as clearance of sulfobromophthalein (BSP) or iodine-125-denatured albumin, is unaltered during pregnancy.[14,15] Therefore hepatic blood flow in late pregnancy amounts to a smaller fraction of cardiac output.[14]

Changes in Liver Function

Plasma Proteins

Serum albumin concentrations in pregnancy and during use of oral contraceptives are 10 percent to 60 percent below those in control women, reflecting the increase in plasma volume in pregnancy and a decrease in albumin synthesis.[16-21] Similarly, plasma levels of anti-thrombin III and haptoglobin fall during pregnancy or use of oral contraceptives and are attributed to decreased hepatic synthesis.[20,22] Plasma concentrations of other serum proteins (e.g., ceruloplasmin, fibrinogen, thyroxine-binding globulin, corticosteroid-binding globulin, transferrin, other $\alpha1$, $\alpha2$, and β globulins) are increased in pregnant women[17,20,23] and in women receiving oral contraceptives.[17,22] Prothrombin times remain normal during pregnancy.[24]

Plasma Lipids

There is increased peripheral lipolysis of triglycerides, increased flux of free fatty acids through the liver, increased hepatic synthesis of triglycerides, and increased hepatic synthesis and secretion of very low-density lipoprotein, high-density lipoprotein, and low-density lipoprotein during pregnancy.[17,25-27] These changes are reflected in a progressive increase in plasma triglycerides (up to 300 percent), cholesterol (25 percent-60 percent), and phospholipids during pregnancy.[19,25,26] The increased hepatic fat in biopsies of some pregnant women may be due to these changes in triglyceride and lipoprotein metabolism.

Drug Metabolism

17-Ethynyl estrogens decrease cytochrome P450 activity, probably via suicide inactivation of the enzyme.[28] Pharmacokinetic studies suggest impaired metabolism of promazine, pethidine, and cortisol[29,30] and increased clearance of phenytoin, carbamazepine, metoprolol, and cyclosporine[31-34] in pregnant women and depressed antipyrine metabolism in women receiving oral contraceptives.[35-37] Estrogens and pregnancy have been shown to impair hepatic activity of glucuronosyltransferase activity, whereas progestational agents induce hepatic mixed-function oxidase activity in animals[38,39] and oral contraceptives increase morphine clearance in humans.[40] Thus pregnancy and oral contraceptives appear to alter drug metabolism but the effects on any one drug are not readily predictable. The clinical significance of these changes in humans remains unclear.

Bile Formation

Organic anion transport, including bilirubin[41-43] and BSP,[2,44-46] is impaired during pregnancy or during use of estrogens or oral contraceptives. These changes are likely primarily the result of estrogen- or pregnancy-induced decreases in the canalicular organic anion-transporting pump multidrug resistance-associated protein 2 (MRP2).[47]

Concentrations of bile salts in blood are within the normal range in most pregnant women, but levels of glycocholate, taurocholate, and chenodeoxycholate may rise progressively until term and exceed levels measured early in pregnancy by twofold to threefold.[48-51] Pregnancy- or estrogen-induced decreases in bile salt transport (and bile formation) are likely the result of decreases in sinusoidal and, more importantly, canalicular bile salt transporters (see Chap. 10).[47,52,53]

Liver Tests

During normal pregnancy alkaline phosphatase activity rises progressively, particularly during the last 4 months (Figure 54-1, Table 54-1). At term, 42 percent to 77 percent of women exhibit alkaline phosphatase activities above the upper limit of normal,[19,21,44,54,55] although values rarely exceed two times the upper limit of normal.[19,24,26,54] The origin of the elevated plasma alkaline phosphatase activity during pregnancy is the placenta, not the liver.[56-59] Plasma leucine aminopeptidase activity also rises during pregnancy[60] (Figure 54-1) because of the release of a placental enzyme. 5-Nucleotidase is reported either to increase during pregnancy or not to change.[60,61]

Plasma levels of gamma glutamyl transferase activity (GGTP) may fall slightly during pregnancy (see Figure 54-1).[21,60,62] Levels of GGTP in women who have viral hepatitis and who also are either late in pregnancy or taking oral contraceptives are inappropriately low.[63] Serum aminotransferase activities (aspartate aminotransferase [AST] and alanine aminotransferase [ALT]) remain within the normal range during pregnancy,[21,24,26,44] making them useful tests for identifying hepatocellular injury in the pregnant patient. Because of hemodilution and decreased serum albumin concentrations serum bilirubin levels tend to be lower during pregnancy.[21]

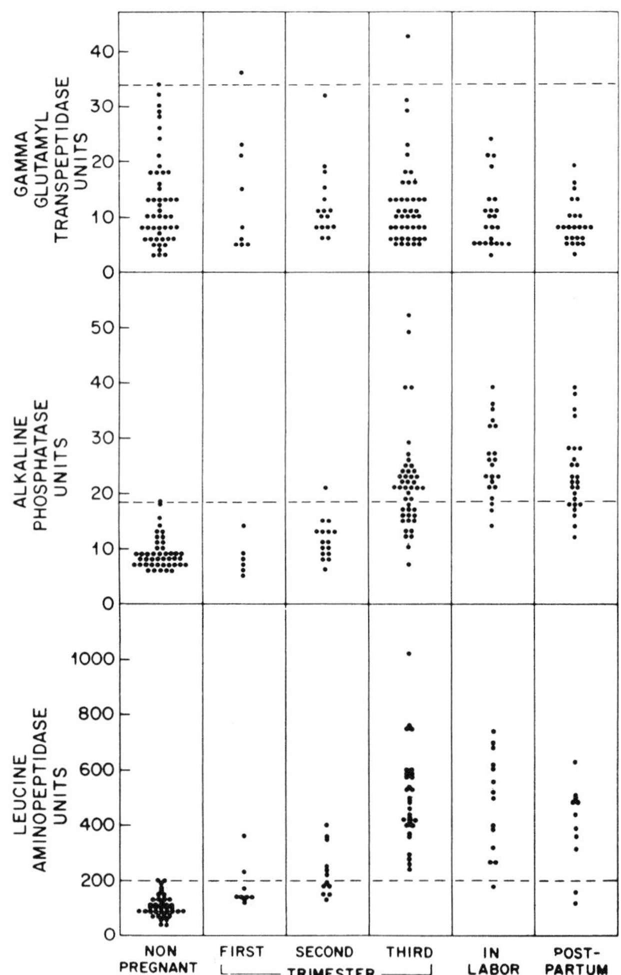

Figure 54-1 Serum activities of three enzymes in normal non-pregnant women and in various stages of pregnancy. The broken lines indicate the highest value obtained for each enzyme in non-pregnant women. (From Walker FB, Hoblit DL, Cunningham FG, et al: Gamma glutamyl transpeptidase in normal pregnancy. Obstet Gynecol 43:745, 1974.)

Skin Manifestations of Liver Disease

Several cutaneous vascular changes, usually associated with chronic liver disease, often appear during pregnancy. Vascular spiders in pregnancy were first reported in 1914.[64] They generally begin as a pale area of skin. A small, central red spot develops and is followed by branching radicles and surrounding erythema.[65] The spiders are distributed on the face, neck, anterior chest, lower arms, and dorsum of the hand. Bean and colleagues[65] observed vascular spiders in 67 percent of 484 white women and 14 percent of 749 black women at term. In contrast, spiders were seen in only 12 percent of non-pregnant white women. Spiders appeared from the second month of pregnancy, with the peak incidence at term. The spiders had disappeared in 75 percent of affected women by 7 weeks postpartum. A few women, particularly those with frequent pregnancies, continued to exhibit vascular spiders indefinitely.

Palmar erythema is observed during pregnancy in 63 percent of white women and 39 percent of black women[65] beginning in the second month of pregnancy and increasing in incidence to a peak at term. By 7 weeks postpartum only 9 percent of white women and 4 percent of black women continued to exhibit palmer erythema.

TABLE 54-1
Liver Tests During Pregnancy

Test	Change during pregnancy	Physiology
Serum bilirubin	None to slight increase	Mild impairment of bilirubin transport with decreased hepatic clearance
Serum bile acids	Progressive increase in serum levels during pregnancy to 200%-300% of non-pregnant values	Impaired hepatic transport and biliary secretion
Sulfobromophthalein	Progressive increase in plasma retention 45 min after administration and decrease in plasma clearance	Slightly increased storage capacity(s) to 122% of non-pregnant values Decrease in biliary transport maximum to 27%-70% of non-pregnant values
Alkaline phosphatase	Progressive increase in serum activity to 1.5-2× non-pregnant values	Release of placental alkaline phosphatase
Leucine aminopeptidase	Progressive increase in serum activity	Release of placenta enzyme
Gamma glutamyl transpeptidase	Serum activity normal or low	Impaired release, particularly in disease states
Aminotransferases	No change	
Serum albumin	Decreased levels	Hemodilution; decrease in synthesis
Prothrombin time	No change	

TABLE 54-2
Acute Viral Hepatitis in Pregnancy*

Features	Observations
Incidence	0.026%-1.2% of gestations
Time of onset (trimester)	
I	13.9%
II	33.5%
III	52.6%
Etiology	4 series: epidemics of NANB hepatitis 1 series: epidemic of hepatitis A 5 series: 11%-78% hepatitis B
Fulminant hepatic failure	31.4% (range 0%-60%)
Maternal mortality	21.4% (range 0%-54%) 1.2% in the United States, Australia, Israel; 27.0% in India, Middle East
Premature birth	24.6% (range 8.3%-54%)
Fetal/neonatal death	29.4% (range 4%-89%) 8.1% in the United States, Australia, Israel; 48.8% in India, Middle East

NANB, Non-A, non-B.
*Data derived from 1346 cases in references 68-85.

COINCIDENT OCCURRENCE OF LIVER DISEASE AND PREGNANCY

This section comprises a brief review of the manifestations of fairly common liver diseases in the pregnant woman. The reader is referred to other chapters for complete discussions of these disorders.

Acute Viral Hepatitis

In 17 reviews of jaundice during pregnancy, hepatitis, presumably viral in etiology, accounted for 40 percent of 654 cases of clinical jaundice.[24,54,66] The true incidence of clinical and subclinical viral hepatitis in pregnancy is not known, but from 1970 to 1974 at Parkland Hospital in Dallas, an incidence of 1 in 700 deliveries was noted.[67] The data in Table 54-2 (collected from refs. 68 through 85) indicate the important features of the disease for mother and fetus.

Maternal Features

The clinical manifestations of acute viral hepatitis in pregnant women do not differ from those noted in non-pregnant women or in men. Similarly, laboratory data, when reported, are similar to values in non-pregnant individuals. In developed countries maternal mortality from fulminant viral hepatitis and liver failure is low. In contrast, in India and the Middle East pregnant women, predominantly with hepatitis E, appear to manifest more severe disease (see Table 54-2).[80,81,86,87] Acute viral hepatitis of any cause is associated with a greater, albeit still small, rate of fetal loss or premature birth even in well-nourished mothers.

Vertical Transmission

Vertical transmission of hepatitis viruses from acutely infected mothers to infants has been reported when mothers are viremic at the time of birth but is generally rare.[85,88-92] Infants exposed to hepatitis A may be given immune serum globulin and the first dose of hepatitis A vaccine immediately after delivery.[88,89] Infants exposed to hepatitis B should receive hepatitis B immunoglobulin and hepatitis B vaccine as recommended for infants of chronically infected mothers.[93] There is no known prophylaxis against vertical transmission of hepatitis C, E, or non-A, non-B, non-C viruses, but hepatitis E may cause severe disease in infected infants.[94]

Alcohol and Pregnancy

The unique aspect of alcohol ingestion during pregnancy is fetal involvement and the fetal alcohol syndrome. This syndrome generally includes facial abnormalities, congenital malformations, growth retardation, and central nervous system dysfunction. Liver dysfunction also has been found in some affected infants.[95-97] In five infants hepatomegaly and elevated serum levels of transaminases and alkaline phosphatase were noted. Liver histology was abnormal in all cases, with varying degrees of fatty infiltration, centrizonal hepatocyte degeneration, perivenular sclerosis, portal and perisinusoidal fibrosis, and proliferation of bile ducts. One affected child exhibited cirrhosis and esophageal varices by age 8 years.[97] These reports suggest that maternal ethanol intake can cause chronic liver disease in offspring. Analysis of additional cases will be needed to define the spectrum of liver pathology.

Chronic Liver Disease

Impact of Chronic Liver Disease on Pregnancy

Women with well-controlled, mild, chronic hepatitis and normal liver function appear to have normal fertility and to tolerate pregnancy well without adverse fetal or maternal outcomes.[98] However, women with active liver disease, significant liver dysfunction, or cirrhosis exhibit decreased fertility,[99-101] may experience liver deterioration during pregnancy, and have higher rates of spontaneous abortion, premature birth, and perinatal death. Indeed, women with alcoholic liver disease often exhibit severe and irreversible gonadal failure, amenorrhea, and infertility, and rarely become pregnant (see Chap. 30). Infants born alive, however, are generally normal and do well, although mothers with clinically significant liver disease are more likely to die before their children reach adulthood. Contraceptive options for women with chronic liver disease include sterilization, barrier methods, and progestin-containing contraceptives.[102] Pregnancy-related issues for specific liver diseases are outlined in the following section.

Autoimmune Hepatitis

Women with autoimmune hepatitis (see Chap. 38) treated with immunosuppressive drugs are surviving for longer periods and when undergoing therapy many regain fertility and some become pregnant. In general, women with well-controlled autoimmune hepatitis receiving immunosuppressive therapy appear to tolerate pregnancy fairly well.[99,103-109] Modest deteriorations in liver tests, particularly the serum bilirubin and alkaline phosphatase, occur. These changes usually return to the patient's previous baseline values after delivery and most likely represent the imposed cholestatic effects of pregnancy. Reports of severe flares, liver failure, and even death in women who stopped immunosuppressive therapy during pregnancy or who were not on therapy during pregnancy indicate that successful therapy should not be stopped and that patients need continued monitoring.[99,107,109] Whether these flares are due to pregnancy per se is not known; remission during pregnancy has also been reported.[108] Autoimmune hepatitis is associated with increased fetal morbidity and mortality, with 7 spontaneous abortions and 9 perinatal deaths reported in 75 pregnancies.[99,103-107] The infants born alive were healthy and did well. With use of immunosuppressive therapy, it appears that women with autoimmune hepatitis can conceive and deliver healthy children with relative safety.

Wilson's Disease

Chelation therapy has allowed patients with Wilson's disease to survive in good health into and through the reproductive years. Many such patients become pregnant and bear children (see Chap. 41). Amenorrhea, infertility, and spontaneous abortions are common in symptomatic untreated women (resulting in part from high tissue copper levels and from the effects of liver dysfunction), but therapy restores fertility and allows a normal reproductive life.[110-115] Some women with Wilson's disease, although satisfactorily treated with chelators, have liver disease, including cirrhosis, that antedates initiation of therapy. These women have increased fetal and maternal morbidity and mortality.

In both normal women and women with Wilson's disease concentrations of copper and ceruloplasmin in serum and urine increase during pregnancy or use of estrogens.[23,111,112,116] In women with Wilson's disease ceruloplasmin and copper concentrations in sera may double by the third trimester of pregnancy. The former may increase into the low-normal range.

Currently patients are treated lifelong with D-penicillamine, trientine (triethylene tetramine dihydrochloride), or zinc.[112,115,117,118] Discontinuing therapy with D-penicillamine during pregnancy has been associated with symptomatic, and occasionally fatal, flare-ups of disease activity.[110,119-121] Although D-penicillamine is potentially teratogenic, in 153 babies born to 111 mothers receiving the drug for Wilson's disease, there were only 2 miscarriages, 3 premature births, 1 baby with a chromosomal defect, and 1 with cleft palate.[115] Trientine and zinc appear to be similarly well tolerated during pregnancy.[112,115,117] It is recommended that treatment with D-penicillamine or trientine (0.75-1.0 g/day during the first two trimesters and 0.5 g/day during the third trimester) or zinc be continued throughout pregnancy.* Also, because of the anti-pyridoxine effects of D-penicillamine, oral supplementation with pyridoxine is recommended.

Cirrhosis

Women with cirrhosis can and do become pregnant, although pregnancy in these women is uncommon.[100,101] Reports of at least 156 pregnancies in 125 women with cirrhosis of varying etiology have been published.[103,123-139] Evaluating the actual risk of hepatic complications during pregnancy is difficult, however, as only one study[124] identified a potential control group of non-pregnant, cirrhotic women. Similarly, few authors have compared rates of obstetric complications in women with cirrhosis to rates in women without liver disease.

During the course of pregnancy, liver tests (most commonly serum bilirubin and alkaline phosphatase activity) were reported to deteriorate in 30 percent to 40 percent of cirrhotic women,[103,125-127] but in two thirds of these cases, postpartum tests returned to baseline values. Much of this apparent deterioration may, in fact, reflect the cholestatic effect of pregnancy.

Maternal morbidity and mortality are high during pregnancy (10.5 percent mortality in the 115 reported cases). Development of jaundice, ascites, hepatic encephalopathy, and postpartum hemorrhage is also common (Table 54-3). Maternal deaths are primarily the result of gastrointestinal hemorrhage from varices with liver failure, accounting for many of the remaining deaths (see Table 54-3). This degree of morbidity and mortality may not differ greatly from the natural history of cirrhosis in these women. Borhanmanesh and Hagighi[124] noted, over a 40-month period, 2 deaths among 9 pregnant cirrhotic women and 3 deaths among 12 age-matched, non-pregnant, cirrhotic women.

Bleeding from esophageal varices occurs in 18 percent to 32 percent of pregnant women with cirrhosis, but in up to 50 percent of women known to have portal hypertension.[127,140] Patients with a history of variceal bleeding may or may not bleed again during pregnancy.[127,131-133] There are no data to indicate whether prophylactic treatment of varices with propranolol, sclerotherapy, or banding reduces bleeding and mortality during pregnancy. Variceal bleeding can be treated with sclerotherapy, banding, placement of a transjugular intrahepatic portal-systemic shunt, or by surgical portal-systemic shunting.† Octreotide infusions and balloon tamponade may also be used. Finally, although elective delivery by cesarean section has been recommended to avoid the strain of labor and risk of precipitating variceal hemorrhage, there is no evidence that vaginal deliveries precipitate hemorrhage and intraabdominal collaterals may complicate surgery.[127,139]

*References 110, 112, 115, 117, 119, 122.

†References 125, 127, 131-134, 137, 138, 140.

As outlined in Table 54-3 the rates of spontaneous abortion, premature birth, and perinatal death are all greater than expected in women with cirrhosis. Infants born alive, however, generally are normal and do well. Fetal distress and perinatal mortality may be due, in part, to maternal hepatic decompensation and its attendant metabolic abnormalities. For example, two well-documented cases of severe maternal hyperbilirubinemia (16 and 33 mg/dl) have been reported[141,142] in which the infants were born severely jaundiced because of maternal-to-infant placental transfer of unconjugated bilirubin. Both infants exhibited fetal distress in utero, required multiple exchange transfusions after birth, and experienced many complications during the first few days of life. One infant exhibited neurologic signs of kernicterus.[141] With therapy both infants improved and on follow-up appeared to be normal neurologically. It would seem prudent to monitor closely the fetuses of cirrhotic women and to consider early delivery when fetal distress or severe maternal hyperbilirubinemia is detected.

Viral Hepatitis B

Chronic hepatitis B infection (see Chap. 32) per se does not appear to alter fertility, conception, or pregnancy beyond the effects of liver dysfunction or cirrhosis itself.[123,143] Vertical transmission of hepatitis B virus (HBV) from chronically infected mothers to offspring occurs during pregnancy or at delivery (see Chap. 32). Prevention of vertical transmission of HBV is an important clinical issue because more than 90 percent of infected infants become chronically infected.[85,144,145] The risk of vertical transmission is related to the HBV viral load and replication rate, and is up to 90 percent in infants of women who have detectable serum hepatitis B e antigen or HBV deoxyribonucleic acid.[85,144,145] Therefore the American College of Obstetrics and Gynecology and the Centers for Disease Control and Prevention recommend

TABLE 54-3
Pregnancy and Cirrhosis*

Features	Shunted (29 women) (%)	Unshunted (83 women) (%)
Variceal hemorrhage	0	18-32
Maternal death	3.5	13.1
Gastrointestinal hemorrhage	0	40-70
Liver failure	100	20-25
Other	0	10-35
Complications		
Jaundice	NA	26.5
Ascites	NA	16.2
Hepatic encephalopathy	NA	4.4
Spontaneous abortions	2.8	17.2
Premature births	NA	20.7
Prenatal deaths	16.7	20.3
Postpartum hemorrhage	24.1	5.9

NA, Data not available.
*Data compiled from references 103, 124-126, and 130-134.

universal screening for hepatitis B surface antigen (HBsAg) of all pregnant women during the third trimester.[93] Infants of HBsAg-positive women should be treated immediately after birth (within 24 hours) with a single intramuscular injection of hepatitis B immunoglobulin and one injection of hepatitis B vaccine.[93] Further doses of vaccine should be given at 1 and 6 months of age. This immunoprophylaxis is highly effective in preventing more than 80 percent of vertically transmitted HBV infection and provides future protection against horizontal transmission of both HBV and hepatitis D.[146-149]

Viral Hepatitis C

Most women with chronic hepatitis C (see Chap. 33) have mild disease and normal liver function and experience uncomplicated pregnancies. However, during pregnancy many women exhibit normalization of serum transaminase levels (AST, ALT), often associated with an increase in the hepatitis C virus (HCV) viral load, that reverses after delivery.[150,151] These changes may be related to subtle immunologic shifts during pregnancy. The long-term consequences, if any, are not known, but a preliminary report[152] suggests that after pregnancy HCV-infected women may experience worsening of necroinflammatory activity and fibrosis changes on liver biopsy. Finally, an epidemiologic study of more than 16,000 pregnant women identified a greater rate of cholestasis of pregnancy in HCV-positive women (15.9 percent) compared to HCV-negative women (0.8 percent), although the mechanism for this association is unclear.[153]

Hepatitis C is transmitted vertically from HCV ribonucleic acid (RNA)–positive mothers to about 5 percent of their offspring.[150,154-156] Although breast milk may contain HCV,[156,157] neither breast-feeding nor cesarean section seem to be risk factors for transmission.[150,154,155] Vertical transmission is more common (up to 20 percent-30 percent) from mothers also infected with human immunodeficiency virus, although adequate anti-retroviral therapy may decrease this risk considerably.[150,154,155] Transient HCV viremia may be seen in another 5 percent of offspring of infected mothers, and some infants will not develop detectable viremia for 3 to 6 months or more after birth.[150,155] Further, maternal anti-HCV antibodies can persist in uninfected infants for up to 18 months.[150,155] Therefore to accurately assess persistent infection, tests for HCV RNA should be run several times between 3 and 12 months of life. Because HCV-positive women cannot be reliably identified by history or examination, broad-based prenatal screening for HCV RNA is being considered to counsel infected women and provide for long-term follow-up and eventual treatment of these women and any infected offspring.[158,159]

The safety and efficacy of treating pregnant HCV-positive women with interferon-based regimens are not known. A few case reports suggest safety; however, interferon is an abortifacient in some animals. The long-term outcomes of infants infected with HCV at birth are also not known, although a 20-year follow-up of children infected with HCV through blood transfusions for cardiac surgery found only one patient with cirrhosis (2.7 percent); all other patients had normal liver tests.[160] The safety, efficacy, and outcome of treating those infants who do become infected also are not known.

Primary Biliary Cirrhosis and Primary Sclerosing Cholangitis

Cholestasis and pruritus in these disorders may be exacerbated or spontaneously improve during pregnancy and may respond to ursodeoxycholic acid therapy (see Chaps. 39, 40).[161-164] Pregnancy outcome is more dependent on liver function and portal hypertension than on the disease per se.

Liver Masses

A variety of liver masses may be identified coincidentally during pregnancy, including intrahepatic pregnancy, hepatic hemangioma, and hepatocellular carcinoma (see Chap. 45).[165-170] Evaluation and management need to be individualized.

Dubin-Johnson Syndrome

Pregnancy or use of oral contraceptives in women with Dubin-Johnson syndrome causes a reversible 2-fold to 2.5-fold increase in plasma concentrations of bilirubin (see Chap. 9).[171-173] Plasma concentrations of bile acids remain normal.[171] Affected women may be deeply jaundiced during pregnancy, but pruritus and other signs of generalized cholestasis are not seen. This transient exacerbation of Dubin-Johnson syndrome is related, presumably, to the cholestatic effects of estrogens superimposed upon a liver with markedly impaired capacity for canalicular excretion of conjugated bilirubin.

Pregnancy After Liver Transplantation

Although women with cirrhosis and severe liver dysfunction are usually amenorrheic and infertile,[100,101] premenopausal women usually regain menstrual function and fertility after successful liver transplantation (see Chap. 55),[100,101,174] most by 7 months after surgery. Pregnancy has been reported as early as 3 weeks post-transplantation[101]; therefore, contraceptive methods should be discussed soon after transplantation.[100-102]

Immunosuppressive drugs must be continued throughout pregnancy and blood levels monitored because changes in drug metabolism, especially of cyclosporine, may occur.[101] Although azathioprine is teratogenic in animals and immunosuppressive drugs other than corticosteroids have not been adequately tested for safety in pregnancy,[100,175] to date there is no evidence of increased fetal malformations in offspring of mothers with liver or kidney transplants.[101,175,176]

Pregnancy after liver transplantation is high risk with approximately 18 percent spontaneous abortions, 2 percent stillbirths, 36 percent premature births, 31 percent low birth weights, and 25 percent neonatal complications in 136 pregnancies in 130 women.[175] Only 70 percent of pregnancies resulted in a live birth; however, these babies all did well. Mothers experience a variety of medical problems, including hypertension (40 percent), pre-eclampsia (25 percent), infections (30 percent, including cytomegalovirus infections that may adversely affect the fetus), and acute rejection (10 percent).[175] Complications of pregnancy may be increased in women with pre-existing decreased renal function. Maternal mortality is low and related to recurrent liver disease and renal failure rather than to pregnancy per se. Liver transplantation has been performed during pregnancy, usually but not always resulting in fetal loss.

LIVER DISORDERS PROBABLY RELATED TO PREGNANCY

Biliary Tract Disease

Gallstone Formation

Women develop cholesterol gallstones (see Chap. 59) and clinical symptoms related to gallstones more frequently than do men (see Chap. 59).[177,178] The increased incidence of gallstone formation begins at puberty, is related to the number of pregnancies, and tapers off after menopause, suggesting that sex hormones may be important etiologic factors.[179] Compared with men, women exhibit increased saturation of bile with cholesterol and have a smaller pool of bile acids (see Chaps. 5 and 59).[177] Use of oral contraceptives[22,177,180-183] or pregnancy[183,184] increases the concentration of cholesterol and its total output in hepatic and gallbladder bile. The pool of bile acids is also increased but more of the bile acid pool is sequestered in the gallbladder and intestine because of decreased motility.[184] As a result, there is little change or even a decrease in bile acids secreted into bile, and the enterohepatic cycling of bile acids is decreased in pregnancy, as is the proportion of chenodeoxycholic acid relative to cholic acid. All of these changes predispose to precipitation of cholesterol. Further, development of gallstones is promoted by pregnancy and oral contraceptive-induced decreases in gallbladder contractility.[182-187]

During pregnancy biliary sludge develops in about one third of women and by the time of delivery 10 percent to 12 percent of women exhibit gallstones on ultrasonographic examination.[188-191] During pregnancy biliary colic occurs in approximately one third of those with existing stones, but not in those with sludge or a normal gallbladder.[188,189] Biliary pain in most women responds to conservative medical management. Postpartum, biliary sludge disappears in virtually all women, but only about one third of small stones disappear.

Epidemiologic studies from pregnant women, women taking oral contraceptives, postmenopausal women receiving estrogens, men treated with diethylstilbestrol, and young women undergoing cholecystectomy suggest that estrogen exposure may accelerate the development of symptoms in patients with pre-existing gallstones.[192-196] Thus pregnancy may predispose not only to formation of gallstones but also to presentation with clinical symptoms.

Biliary Tract Disease During Pregnancy

Acute cholecystitis is second to appendicitis as the most common cause of non-obstetric surgery during pregnancy, accounting for 1 to 8 cases per 10,000 pregnancies.[197-199] Furthermore, common duct stones are a common cause of jaundice during pregnancy.[24] Diagnosis of biliary tract disease, with modern ultrasound, is straightforward.[199-202] Technetium-99 hepatoiminodiacetic acid and other nuclear medicine scans are probably best avoided during pregnancy.

Therapy for symptomatic disease during pregnancy is often conservative (see Chaps. 60 and 61). About 55 percent to 85 percent of pregnant women with biliary colic, acute cholecystitis, or gallstone pancreatitis respond to general medical management, and surgery may be postponed until after delivery.[199,203-205] Patients with recurrent or worsening symptoms or common bile duct obstruction may require treatment during pregnancy. This can be accomplished with relatively little maternal or fetal mortality even with open cholecystectomy.[197-199,203-207] Laparoscopic cholecystectomy may be even safer during pregnancy because more than 180 such operations have been performed with no maternal mortality, 1.7 percent spontaneous abortions, and 3.9 percent premature deliveries.[208-211] Endoscopic management of gallstone pancreatitis or biliary obstruction during pregnancy also appears to be safe and effective in the few cases reported.[212,213]

Herpes Simplex Virus Hepatitis

Although herpes simplex virus hepatitis (types I or II) (see Chap. 34) is rare in previously healthy adults, about half the cases reported have occurred in association with pregnancy and the mortality rate is about 40 percent.[214-218] Patients generally present with a 4- to 14-day history of fever, systemic viral-type symptoms, and abdominal or right upper quadrant pain. Hepatitis is characterized by very high aminotransferase levels (more than 1000 units), an increased prothrombin time, and a low bilirubin level of typically less than 3 mg/dl. Liver biopsy may be diagnostic, showing areas of focal or confluent hemorrhagic and coagulative necrosis, relatively little inflammatory infiltrate, and ground-glass nuclear inclusions or Cowdry type A inclusions at the periphery of areas of necrosis that are positive on immunohistochemical stain.[216] Liver, vaginal, cervical, or throat cultures are often positive. Because therapy with agents such as acyclovir has been successful in salvaging both mothers and infants,[214,215,218] aggressive evaluation of pregnant women who exhibit fever, a viral syndrome, and elevated transaminase values with a modestly elevated or low serum bilirubin should be initiated followed by immediate institution of anti-viral therapy. Although vertical transmission of herpes simplex to infants, either in utero or at the time of delivery, is not inevitable, infants born to these women should be closely observed and treated as appropriate.

Estrogen-responsive Hepatic Neoplasms and Pregnancy

The liver is an estrogen-responsive organ.[219] Estrogens, either endogenous or exogenous, are thought to be responsible for several hepatic vascular and neoplastic processes. These include hepatic sinusoidal dilation, focal nodular hyperplasia, hepatocellular adenoma, and possibly, some cases of hepatocellular carcinoma (see Chap. 45).[220,221] Strong but circumstantial epidemiologic evidence links these processes to use of oral contraceptives; the association between pregnancy and these abnormalities is based on case reports and by analogy to the effects of oral contraceptive use. With the widespread availability of high-quality ultrasonography and magnetic resonance imaging (MRI), hepatic mass lesions may be safely identified and monitored throughout pregnancy.[165]

Hepatic sinusoidal dilation with associated hepatomegaly and abdominal pain has been reported in a few women receiving oral contraceptives. The lesion has been noted in livers that contained oral contraceptive–associated adenomas.[220,222-224] Improvement occurs after oral contraceptives are discontinued. The prognosis is benign.[222-224]

Focal nodular hyperplasia is a benign lesion consisting of normal liver elements disposed around a central stellate scar and is often found incidentally. The lesion occurs almost exclusively in women (see Chap. 45).[225] An association with oral contraceptive use has been suggested.[225-227] Because lesions may increase in size during pregnancy, surgery should be considered prophylactically in those women with estrogen-responsive lesions who desire to bear children,[227] although 10 women with focal nodular hyperplasia lesions of 4 to 13 cm tolerated 13 pregnancies without complications or an increase in tumor size.[228]

Hepatocellular adenomas are benign hepatocellular tumors linked causally to estrogens and use of oral contraceptives (see Chap. 45).[225,226,229,230] It is not clear whether estrogens actually initiate the adenomas, but they do promote growth[231] and the development of clinical symptoms such as a mass lesion, abdominal pain, acute hemorrhage, necrosis, or rupture.[232] Conversely, many adenomas regress after removal of estrogens.[233] Pregnancy has not been associated with an increased incidence of hepatocellular adenomas, but pregnancy is associated with growth of adenomas, development of symptoms (nausea, vomiting, right upper-quadrant pain), and a propensity to rupture.[228,229,234,235] Surgical excision, which is usually well tolerated, should be considered for large, symptomatic tumors, for tumors that do not shrink after stopping oral contraceptives, and for tumors larger than 5 cm in women who desire to bear children.[165,236] Surgical resection of large adenomas has been successfully carried out during pregnancy.[237,238]

Budd-Chiari Syndrome

Budd-Chiari syndrome associated with use of oral contraceptives was noted as early as 1966, and the association has been well documented (see Chap. 53).[239-245] Development of hepatic vein thrombosis is attributed to an oral contraceptive–induced increase in clotting factors plus a generalized propensity to venous thrombosis.[239,246,247] Budd-Chiari syndrome associated with pregnancy is much less common. Thirty cases have been reported.[245-254] The predisposing factors for hepatic vein occlusion are thought to be the estrogen-related increases in clotting factors associated with a decrease in the activity of plasma anti-thrombin III and, in one patient, factor V Leiden mutation.[254] In some women hepatic vein occlusion is associated with widespread venous thrombosis and may represent local propagation of clot originating in the iliac veins and inferior vena cava. Clinical symptoms of Budd-Chiari syndrome frequently begin postpartum or immediately after an abortion rather than during the pregnancy itself. Another syndrome that clinically resembles Budd-Chiari syndrome, hepatic veno-occlusive disease, has been reported in three women postpartum[255] and in one woman receiving an oral progestational agent for contraceptive purposes.[256]

LIVER DISORDERS UNIQUE TO PREGNANCY

Four unique syndromes of liver dysfunction have been identified during pregnancy: hepatic involvement in hyperemesis gravidarum, intrahepatic cholestasis of pregnancy, acute fatty liver of pregnancy, and pre-eclampsia and eclampsia-related liver disease.

Hepatic Involvement in Hyperemesis Gravidarum

Hyperemesis gravidarum is not a liver disease but liver dysfunction occurs in severe cases. For example, among women affected severely enough to require hospitalization for dehydration and weight loss, liver dysfunction and jaundice were noted in 13 percent to 33 percent and 10 percent to 13 percent, respectively.[24,257-259]

Liver dysfunction usually presents in the first trimester within 1 to 3 weeks after the onset of severe vomiting. Jaundice, dark urine, and occasionally pruritus are the major hepatic manifestations.[24,54,257-262] Mild hyperbilirubinemia is the most frequently noted laboratory abnormality (mean value 1-7 mg/dl). Moderate increases in serum transaminase activities (two to three times normal) occur in slightly more than half the patients and rarely values up to 800 IU/L have been noted.[258] Alkaline phosphatase activities are elevated in a minority of patients. BSP excretion, which is a sensitive indicator of hepatic capacity for organic anion transport, is markedly impaired in women with liver dysfunction and hyperemesis compared with control pregnant women.[260] Autopsy specimens from 19 women who died of hyperemesis (6 of whom were jaundiced) exhibited excess pigment in centrolobular areas but no necrosis. Moderate deposits of fat in large vacuoles, usually in centrolobular hepatocytes, were seen in 12 patients.[263] Cholestasis has been seen in liver biopsies from some affected women,[261] but most biopsies are normal.[257] The etiology of hepatic dysfunction is unknown, but may be related to dehydration and malnutrition.[264,265] Hepatic dysfunction in hyperemesis gravidarum is a relatively benign process with little clinical consequence. Women who have died of hyperemesis did so from starvation and dehydration, not from liver failure. If vomiting is controlled the hepatic dysfunction rapidly resolves, usually within a few days, although it may recur in subsequent pregnancies.[24,54,257,261,262]

Intrahepatic Cholestasis of Pregnancy

Intrahepatic cholestasis of pregnancy (IHCP) is a relatively benign cholestatic disorder that generally commences late in pregnancy, disappears abruptly after delivery, and frequently recurs with subsequent pregnancies. The main clinical manifestations are pruritus and jaundice. The term *pruritus gravidarum* is frequently applied to women with pruritus and biochemical cholestasis, whereas the term *cholestatic jaundice of pregnancy* or *cholestasis of pregnancy* is often applied to those women who also develop clinically apparent jaundice.

Incidence

IHCP is identified in less than 2 percent of pregnancies in the United States and Europe (Table 54-4). The disorder appears to be more frequent in Scandinavia and in Chile, being reported in 1 percent to 6 percent of all pregnancies in those countries.* It accounts for 20 percent to 50 percent of all causes of jaundice in pregnancy in a series reported from Scandinavia[24,54,266]; however, the overall incidence appears to exhibit seasonal fluctuations and to have decreased in the past two decades.[277,281,293,294] In an Italian population IHCP was diagnosed more commonly (16 percent) in women who also had hepatitis C than in those who did not (0.8 percent) although the basis for this association is not known.[153]

Etiology

The etiology and pathogenesis of IHCP remain poorly defined but both genetic and hormonal factors appear to be important. The best hypothesis is that IHCP reflects a genetic sensitivity to the cholestatic effects of estrogens, although IHCP also has been associated with altered plasma levels of selenium, zinc, and copper and changes in biliary secretion of sulfated progesterones.[295-297]

*References 266, 268, 269, 273, 274, 278-280.

TABLE 54-4

Intrahepatic Cholestasis of Pregnancy*: Clinical Features

Incidence in pregnancy	United States and Europe: 0.1%-1.7% India: 0.8%-1.4% Scandinavia: 1%-3% Chile: 4.7%-6.5%
Onset	70% third trimester 30% before third trimester
Onset of pruritus	Average: 28-30 weeks; range: 7-40 weeks
Onset of jaundice	1-4 weeks later
Recurrence in subsequent pregnancies	21%-70%
Pruritus	100%
Jaundice	10%-25%
Nausea, vomiting	5%-75%
Abdominal pain	9%-24%
Skin excoriations	Common

*Data derived from references 266-290.

At high doses in experimental studies estrogens, especially ethinyl estradiol and its 17-β-glucuronide metabolite, reproducibly cause mild cholestasis in both humans and experimental animals, likely through inhibition of the hepatocyte canalicular bile salt efflux pump (BSEP) (see Chap. 10).[47,53,298] After the clinical introduction of oral contraceptives (containing high doses of estrogen) a number of women developed cholestasis that resembled IHCP.[299-301] Further, as much as 50 percent of women who experienced IHCP were observed to develop pruritus and cholestasis when given these same oral contraceptives.[270,302,303]

Heritable factors are likely because IHCP frequently affects female relatives of index cases,[269,275,277,282] including up to three generations of women in some families.[278,304,305] IHCP and familial benign recurrent intrahepatic cholestasis have been observed in the same family.[306] IHCP or estrogen-related cholestasis is frequent in both mothers (14 percent) and sisters (15 percent) of women who developed cholestasis while receiving oral contraceptives.[307] Further, ethinyl estradiol administration impairs biliary excretion of the organic anion BSP (a substrate for the canalicular bilirubin transporter MRP2) in both men and women, and the effect is much more marked both in women with a history of IHCP and in women and men with a family history of IHCP.[308]

Mutations in MD3R, the canalicular phospholipid pump,[309,310] have been reported in women from two families who developed IHCP while carrying homozygously affected fetuses.[311,312] Therefore IHCP may occur when women with genetic mutations (polymorphisms) that alter either the production of cholestatic estrogen or progesterone metabolites or the transport capacity of the BSEP and/or the phospholipid transporter are exposed to increased sex steroid hormones, such as during pregnancy. Prolonged IHCP resulting in chronic liver disease has been reported in one family, presumably related to additional genetic or environmental factors.[313]

Clinical Features

The clinical and laboratory features of IHCP[284,293,314] are summarized in Tables 54-4 and 54-5 and Figure 54-2. In addition, lipoprotein X may be identified in plasma,[282] and gallbladder size and residual volume are often increased in IHCP.[315] Serum transaminase activities in a few patients with IHCP are high enough to overlap with those typical of hepatocellular disorders, such as acute viral hepatitis. Serologic tests for hepatitis viruses A and B, and the clinical course of the disease, particularly after delivery, may be helpful in the differential diagnosis. Liver biopsy is generally unnecessary for diagnosis. Liver failure and hepatic encephalopathy are not reported in IHCP and their appearance indicates another etiology for the liver disease.

The pruritus can be disabling, and in exceptional cases, can be so severe as to mandate termination of

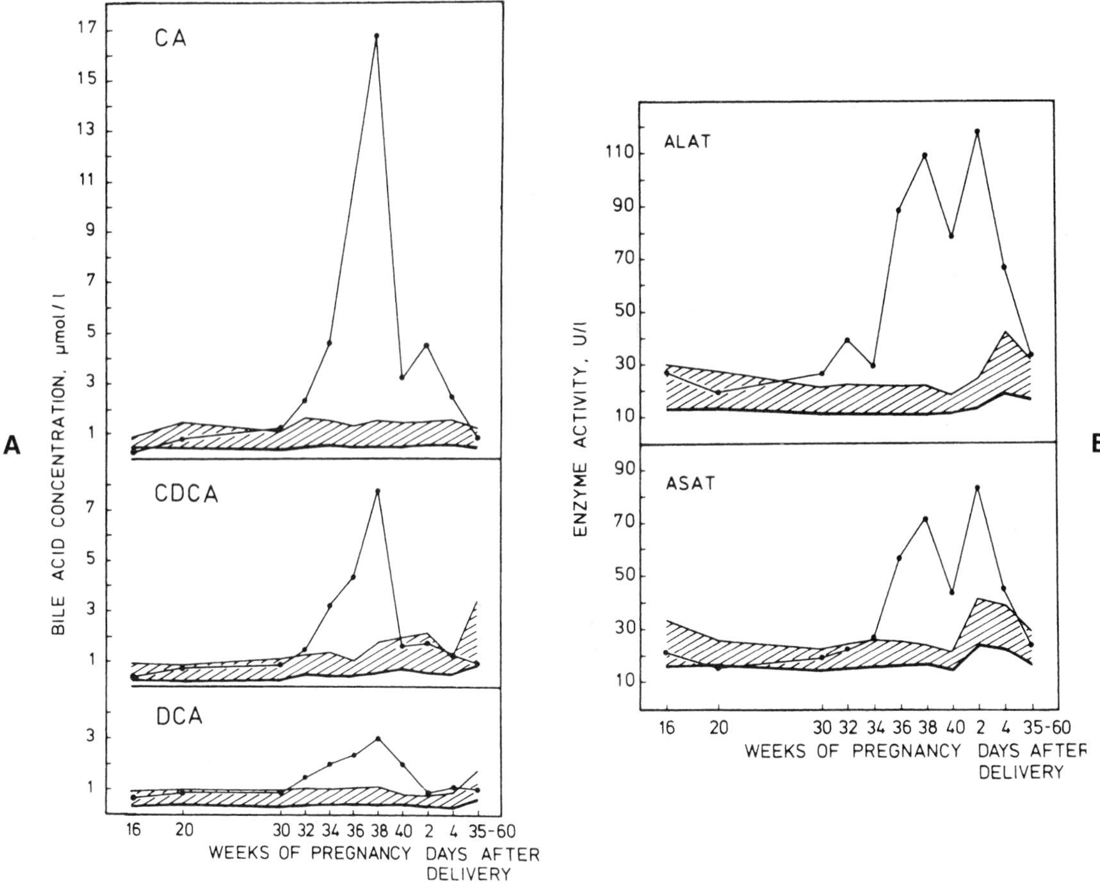

Figure 54-2 Serum bile acid concentrations **(A)** and liver tests **(B)**, during pregnancy in control women (shaded areas; mean ± 2 standard deviations) and in eight women who developed intrahepatic cholestasis of pregnancy (line; mean values). *CA,* Cholic acid; *CDCA,* chenodeoxycholic acid; *DCA,* deoxycholic acid; *ALAT,* alanine aminotransferase; *ASAT,* aspartate aminotransferase. (From Heikkinen J: Serum bile acids in the early diagnosis of intrahepatic cholestasis of pregnancy. Obstet Gynecol Scand 54:437, 1975.)

TABLE 54-5
Intrahepatic Cholestasis of Pregnancy: Laboratory Findings*

Test	Patients (n)	Women with abnormal value (%)	Average reported value	Range of reported values	Normal values†
Bilirubin	736	27	1.0 (all patients) 2.9 (jaundiced patients)	0.4-8.4	≤1.1 mg/dl
Alkaline phosphatase	753	73 (at least 2.4-fold upper limit of normal)	146 ± 66 (up to 12.5-fold upper limit of normal)	nl-750	≤60 IU/L
AST	587	64	125	nl-736	≤40 IU/L
ALT	499	62	155	nl-1030	≤40 IU/L
Serum bile salts	277	96	48 µM	nl-430 µM	≤6.5 µM
Serum cholic acid	91	79	24 µM	nl-148 µM	≤5 µM
BSP retention at 45 min	77	97-100	23%	10%-33%	≤12%
Prothrombin time	177	14‡	—	—	—
Fecal fat					
Patients with jaundice	12	—	14.0	2-31	≤7 g/24 hr
Patients with pruritus	11	—	4.0	1-10	≤7 g/24 hr

nl, Normal; *AST,* aspartate aminotransferase; *ALT,* alanine aminotransferase; *BSP,* bromosulfophthalein.
*Data derived from references 50, 266-282, 284, and 288-292.
†For non-pregnant individuals.
‡All corrected with vitamin K.

pregnancy. Fat malabsorption and vitamin K deficiency[273] may develop in severe cases and may be responsible for some instances of maternal postpartum hemorrhage.[314]

Pathology

The histopathology of IHCP is that of intrahepatic cholestasis (Figure 54-3). Typical findings include centrolobular cholestasis, canaliculi containing bile plugs, and bile pigment in hepatocytes.[24,316] Cholestasis may be patchy and subtle. Inflammation and hepatocellular necrosis usually are absent. Portal tracts and interlobular bile ducts are normal. Electron microscopic examination shows dilated bile canaliculi with loss of microvilli and occasional abnormal mitochondria.[316,317] All histologic changes disappear after delivery and after resolution of clinical symptoms.[24,316]

Natural History and Prognosis

The cholestasis of IHCP generally progresses until the time of delivery or termination of pregnancy.[284,293,314] The severity of cholestasis and of laboratory abnormalities can be quite variable, however, both during one pregnancy and between different pregnancies, with recurrence rates of 21 percent to 70 percent.[274,284,288,293] For example, serum transaminase activities and even bilirubin concentrations may fluctuate and even temporarily normalize as pregnancy progresses.[274,284,290,318] Pruritus, however, rarely improves before delivery. After delivery pruritus quickly disappears, usually within 24 to 48 hours. Biochemical abnormalities and histologic findings resolve over the following weeks to months.[44] Rarely, symptoms may persist for several weeks postpartum and respond to a short course of prednisone.[319] Cholestasis may recur during treatment with oral contraceptives, although this appears to be uncommon with low-dose estrogen contraceptives.[284] During long-term (up to 15 years) follow-up, prognosis for women who have had IHCP is excellent, aside from a higher incidence (1.4-fold to 2.3-fold) of cholelithiasis and gallbladder disease.[54,268,282,320]

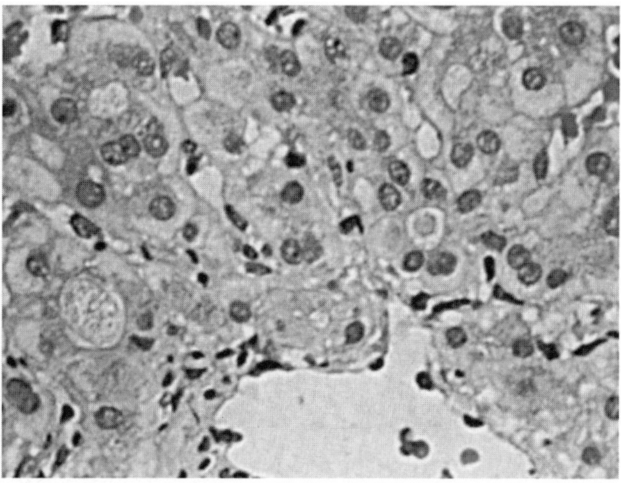

Figure 54-3 Intrahepatic cholestasis of pregnancy showing canalicular bile plugs, well-preserved hepatocytes, and a terminal hepatic venule at the bottom of the field. (Hematoxylin and eosin; ×630.) (From Rolfes DB, Ishak KG: Liver disease in pregnancy. In Histopathology 10:555, 1986.)

The prognosis for the fetus is not as benign as for the mother. Earlier series document high rates of premature labor and neonatal death (11 percent).[50,266-283,321-323] Fetal monitoring has documented high rates of premature labor and delivery,[288] fetal distress during labor (19 percent-60 percent), and meconium staining (35 percent-45 percent).* The true incidence of fetal death resulting from IHCP is not known; however, when several large series are combined, there is a trend toward increased fetal complications and death related to IHCP (1.75 percent mortality in 679 infants born to women with IHCP compared to 1.01 percent mortality in 710 infants born to unaffected women).† The mechanism(s) of premature labor, fetal death, and meconium staining are not known but these events are attributed to elevated bile acids leading to increased uterine and fetal colonic muscle contractions and acute fetal anoxia.[289,314]

These findings have prompted experienced physicians to recommend aggressive obstetric management. It is recommended that all women with IHCP be closely followed during the third trimester, possibly including weekly fetal non-stress tests, especially if onset of IHCP is before 32 weeks, if there is a twin pregnancy, if jaundice occurs, or if there is a history of a fetal death. Babies should be delivered promptly if any signs of fetal distress are found but even in the absence of fetal distress, labor should be induced, after fetal lung maturity has been documented, at 38 weeks for mild IHCP and at 36 weeks for women who are jaundiced.‡ Some have advocated even more aggressive care, including hospitalization and fetal non-stress tests at least once per day.[289,327,328] Although this more aggressive management appears to be associated with fewer sudden fetal deaths, fetuses still die in utero within hours or days of normal tests.[288,289,325,328]

Therapy

In the past women were treated symptomatically for pruritus with cholestyramine,[314,329] phenobarbital,[329] or hypnotics. Success was variable and these agents did not improve fetal outcome. Fetal hemorrhage has been reported resulting from vitamin K deficiency from IHCP and treatment with cholestyramine[314,330] and thus vitamin K supplementation should be given near term to all women with jaundice or prolonged cholestasis.

Ursodeoxycholic acid (UCDA)—a hydrophilic bile acid that improves other cholestatic liver diseases, possibly by stimulating biliary excretion of other, potentially toxic, bile acids or sulfated progesterones—is the most promising treatment for IHCP (see Chap. 39).[293,297,331] UDCA appears to be safe because no adverse outcomes have been reported in more than 104 pregnancies.[290-292,318,323,332-335a] During both open-label and placebo-controlled treatment trials (especially when doses of more than 1 g, or 15 mg/kg, per day were used) most women receiving UDCA exhibit substantial

*References 280, 288, 289, 321, 324, 325.

†References 44, 59, 268, 269, 288, 326.

‡References 269, 273, 275, 278, 288, 293, 294, 314, 325.

improvement in pruritus, liver tests, and serum bile acid levels[290-292,318,332-336] and better placental bile acid transport[292] and delivery later in pregnancy.[318,332,334,335a] It is not clear whether UDCA actually improves fetal outcome when pregnancies also are aggressively managed, although anecdotal reports suggest this may be the case.[323,333]

Other, less well-studied therapeutic options include S-adenosyl-L-methionine (SAME), which methylates phospholipids and improves experimental cholestasis,[337,338] and dexamethasone.[339] SAME, which must be given parenterally and is not widely available, has been tested in four trials[290,335,340,341] with either no[335,340] or slight[290,341] benefits for the mother. Overall, UDCA would appear to be the treatment of first choice.

Acute Fatty Liver of Pregnancy

Acute fatty liver of pregnancy (AFLP) is a rare and potentially fatal idiopathic disorder that appears during the third trimester of pregnancy.[342-344] Its principal and distinctive histologic feature is infiltration of hepatocytes with microvesicular fat, histology strikingly similar to that in Reye's syndrome, Jamaican vomiting sickness, valproic acid hepatotoxicity, tetracycline hepatotoxicity, and medium- and long-chain acyl-co-enzyme A (CoA) dehydrogenase deficiency.[343,345-349] This group of disorders collectively has been termed the hepatic microvesicular steatoses and they share many clinical and laboratory features as well, suggesting a common abnormality in lipid metabolism and, perhaps, related etiology.

Incidence

The frequency of AFLP is between 1 in 7000 to 16,000 pregnancies[344,350,351] but instances of mild disease are now being identified more frequently. AFLP accounts for 16 percent to 70 percent of cases of severe liver disease during pregnancy and, consequently, a significant number of maternal and fetal deaths.[352-354] AFLP is more common in primigravidas, twin pregnancies, and pregnancies with a male fetus (Table 54-6), although it can occur with any pregnancy.

TABLE 54-6

Acute Fatty Liver of Pregnancy: Features and Presentation in 202 Cases*

Feature	Frequency
Incidence	1/7000-1/16,000 deliveries
Age	28 years (range, 16-40)
Primigravidas	46%
Twin gestations	10%
Male fetus	71%
Recurrences	3/22
Onset	35.5 weeks (range, 26-40)
Pre-eclampsia	28%

*Data derived from references 344, 350-352, and 354-386.

Etiology

AFLP, as with other microvesicular steatoses, may be due to a combination of increased flux of triglycerides and fatty acids from adipose tissue to the liver and defects in mitochondrial β-oxidation of fatty acids.[349,355-357,387-389] During late pregnancy increased plasma levels of triglycerides and fatty acids and mildly impaired β-oxidation have been documented in experimental animals and humans, possibly resulting from the effects of estrogens, progesterones, and fetal metabolic demands.[349,388,390] In women who develop AFLP it is thought that additional factors further impair β-oxidation and lead to steatosis, decreased adenosine triphosphate (ATP) generation, lipid peroxidation, toxic effects of elevated free fatty acids, inhibition of gluconeogenesis and, ultimately, liver failure.[349] Potential triggering factors may include drugs, such as aspirin or non-steroidal anti-inflammatory drugs that are known to impair β-oxidation,[389,391] inflammatory cytokines,[349] or pre-eclampsia, which is also associated with increased fatty acid fluxes.[388]

Although most cases of AFLP appear to be sporadic, some cases, perhaps from 10 percent to 20 percent,[349,392] are likely the result of a specific mutation in the gene for long-chain 3-hydroxyacyl-CoA dehydrogenase (LCHAD), which catalyzes an essential step in mitochondrial β-oxidation.[349,385,387,393-396] Children homozygous for LCHAD mutations usually present early in life with rapidly fatal hypoketotic hypoglycemia, fatty liver, a Reye syndrome–like condition, and skeletal or cardiac myopathies. The mothers of these children appear to be at high risk for AFLP. Indeed, during 68 pregnancies in which 52 mothers heterozygous for LCHAD mutations carried homozygous affected fetuses, AFLP occurred in 44 percent and pre-eclampsia occurred in 29 percent.[385,387,393-396] These same women had 60 pregnancies with normal or heterozygous fetuses, and AFLP (3.3 percent) and pre-eclampsia (1.7 percent) were virtually absent. Therefore in women heterozygous for LCHAD deficiency AFLP likely develops because of the combination of maternal genetic and pregnancy-related defects in mitochondrial β-oxidation of fatty acids exacerbated by unknown toxic factors generated by a homozygous affected fetus and, possibly, pre-eclampsia.[349,388]

Although homozygous LCHAD deficiency is very rare (only about 100 reported cases), heterozygosity occurs in European-derived populations at rates of 1 in 150 to 1 in 680[349,385]; some other genetic defects in fatty acid oxidation may also play a role in AFLP.[387,397] It is possible, therefore, that more subtle defects in maternal or fetal β-oxidation may be important co-factors in precipitating "spontaneous" AFLP.

Based on these findings it is recommended that in all cases of AFLP, both baby and mother be tested for at least the most common LCHAD mutation (Glu474Gln), that babies be screened for abnormal organic acids, acyl CoAs and acyl carnitines, and that babies be kept on a high-carbohydrate diet with frequent feedings until metabolic abnormalities have been excluded.[349,395-397] Testing for the common LCHAD mutation is available on a fee-for-service basis through several institutions, including the Washington University Molecular Diagnostic Laboratory.[397a] Determination of other mutations would likely require analysis by research laboratories.

Clinical Features

The clinical and laboratory features of AFLP are summarized in Tables 54-6 through 54-9. Illness usually begins in the third trimester, around 35 weeks of gestation. Onset of illness as early as 26 weeks and as late as the immediate postpartum period has been reported. The early manifestations are non-specific. Nausea, fatigue, malaise, vomiting, and abdominal distress (right upper quadrant or epigastric pain) are the most common symptoms. Fever, headache, diarrhea, back pain suggestive of pancreatitis, and myalgias are reported in some patients. Clinical signs of liver dysfunction and even frank liver failure, such as jaundice, hepatic encephalopathy, or bleeding, ensue 1 to 2 weeks later.

Physical findings often are minimal. Early on, right upper quadrant tenderness may be the only abnormality found. The liver is generally small and not palpable. As the disease progresses jaundice, changes in mental status, edema, and ascites may appear. Pre-eclampsia and its hepatic complications are seen in 28 percent or more of patients.[344,354,382,395,398] This is a much greater incidence than in normal pregnancies and may reflect roles for abnormalities in triglyceride and fatty acid metabolism in both AFLP and pre-eclampsia.[349,388]

AFLP is associated with a number of abnormal laboratory findings (see Table 54-8). The blood smear frequently contains nucleated red blood cells and, in those patients with disseminated intravascular coagulopathy (DIC), fragmented erythrocytes and Burr cells. Leukocytosis is frequent, even in women with no evidence of infection. Coagulation disorders are common, occasionally progressing to frank DIC. The abnormalities in clotting factors probably represent impaired hepatic synthesis and accelerated consumption. Indeed, a profound decrease in plasma anti-thrombin III activity has been found in all tested patients, even before the onset of AFLP.[379,386,399,400]

Liver test abnormalities include hyperbilirubinemia, increases in alkaline phosphatase activity, and modest elevations of serum transaminase activities (usually ≤ 350 IU/L). A few patients, with otherwise typical AFLP however, do exhibit markedly elevated serum transaminase values. The generally modest abnormalities of liver tests can be misleading because they do not reflect accurately the severe degree of liver dysfunction in these patients. For example, many patients may have evidence of fulminant hepatic failure, such as hypoglycemia, impaired synthesis of clotting factors, and hepatic encephalopathy. Hypoglycemia, often requiring administration of concen-

TABLE 54-7
Acute Fatty Liver of Pregnancy: Signs and Symptoms*

Feature	No. of patients for which data are available	Frequency (%)
Nausea, vomiting	198	77
Abdominal pain; epigastric distress	202	54
Encephalopathy	195	56
Jaundice	202	86
Hypoglycemia	199	44
Ascites	88	32
Extrahepatic Manifestations		
Gastrointestinal hemorrhage	132	32
Renal impairment	158	84
Pancreatitis	77	13

*Data derived from references 344, 350-352, and 354-385.

TABLE 54-8
Acute Fatty Liver of Pregnancy: Laboratory Abnormalities*

	No. of patients	Frequency of abnormal results (%)	ABNORMAL VALUES	
			Average	Range
RBC smear	38	50†		
White blood count	142	93	—	12,000-46,000
Platelet count	167	73	—	5000-121,000
Prothrombin time	182	92	22 sec prolonged	nl to 78 sec
Anti-thrombin III level	30	100	11% of normal	—
Bilirubin	202	95	12.2 mg%	1.8-36 mg%
Alkaline phosphatase	141	90	4.4-fold upper limit of normal	nl to tenfold upper limit of normal
AST (nl ≤ 40)	100	99	218 IU/L	nl-1300
ALT (nl ≤ 40)	108	95	366 IU/L	nl-3670
Serum uric acid	76	89	—	Up to 18.5 mg%
Serum creatinine	144	87	3.0 mg/dl	Up to 6.6 mg/dl

RBC, Red blood cell; *nl,* normal; *AST,* aspartate aminotransferase; *ALT,* alanine aminotransferase; *DIC,* disseminated intravascular coagulopathy.
*Data derived from references 344, 350-352, and 354-386.
†Nucleated RBCs seen frequently; RBC fragments in those with DIC.

TABLE 54-9
Acute Fatty Liver of Pregnancy: Outcome

Maternal Mortality	
All reports*	27% (59/219 reported cases)
Reports from 1991-1999 in which delivery was initiated promptly†	5% (5/96 cases)
Infant Mortality	
All reports*	32% (78/244 cases)
Reports from 1991-1999 in which delivery was initiated promptly†	8% (8/103 cases)

*Data derived from references 344, 350, 351, 354, 378-385, and 387.
†Data derived from references 344, 354, 382-385, and 387.

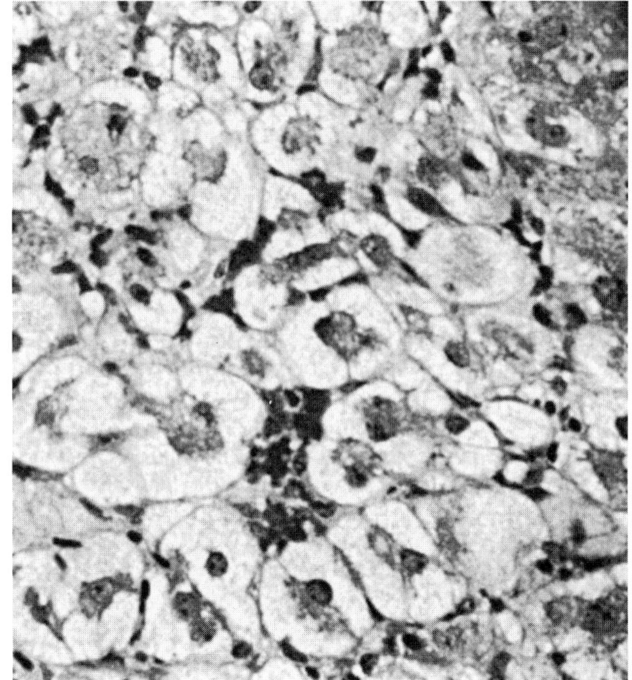

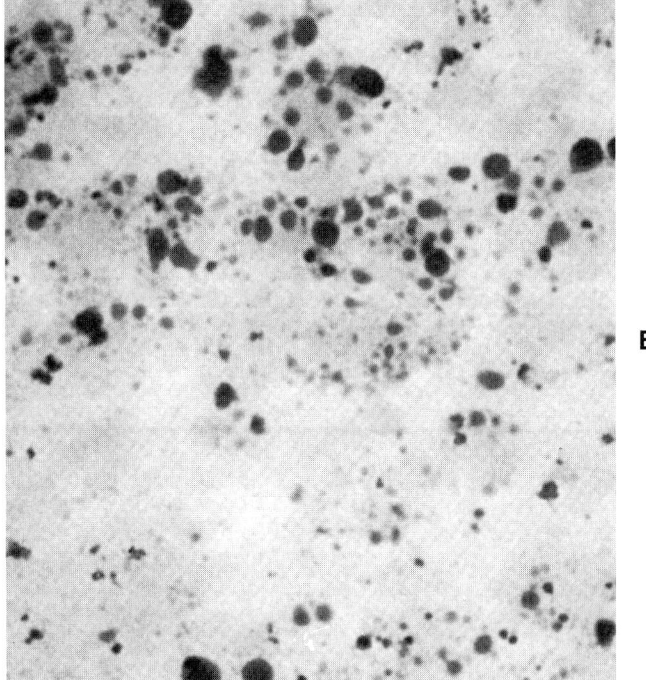

Figure 54-4 Acute fatty liver of pregnancy showing microvesicular fatty infiltration. **A,** Hematoxylin and eosin. **B,** Oil red O stain.

trated glucose, occurs in as many as 44 percent of patients and blood glucose levels should be monitored frequently until AFLP resolves.

Modest renal dysfunction with elevation of blood urea nitrogen, creatinine, and uric acid values occurs in most patients with AFLP. Frank renal failure may occur in severe cases and require interim dialysis. The cause of renal failure is not known, although renal steatosis could be responsible. The characteristic increase in plasma uric acid often occurs before the onset of renal insufficiency, suggesting an early defect in renal tubular function.

Imaging studies of the liver using ultrasound, computed tomography (CT), or MRI may suggest the presence of a fatty liver; however, sensitivity and specificity of these findings are poor, and a normal study does not rule out the diagnosis of AFLP.[344,382,401,402]

Pathology

The histologic appearance of AFLP is well described.* At the light microscopic level lobular architecture is intact, but the lobules are swollen. Infiltration of hepatocytes with microvesicular fat is the key feature of AFLP (Figure 54-4), although diffuse cytoplasmic ballooning or large fat vacuoles may be seen.[377] Fat deposits are predominantly centrolobular (zone 3) with a more variable involvement of zones 1 and 2. The fat is readily appreciated when fat stains are used on frozen sections of tissue. The lesion is missed frequently when fixed tissue is examined because the fat is removed during the fixation process. In addition to fatty metamorphosis centrolobular cholestasis, as indicated by bile canalicular plugs and bile-stained hepatocytes, frequently is seen.

Although widespread hepatic necrosis is virtually never seen, subtle signs of hepatocyte necrosis and hepatocytolysis are evident. Other clues suggesting that substantial loss of hepatocytes has in fact occurred include the small size of livers at autopsy,[342,377] close apposition of portal tracts and central veins, prominent lipid- and lipofuscin-laden Kupffer cells, occasional acidophilic bodies, and numerous mitotic figures.[377] Confluent centrizonal coagulative necrosis is seen in occasional patients who experience preterminal shock and is most likely a superimposed lesion of hepatic ischemia.[377]

Inflammation commonly is subtle and may be absent, although up to 25 percent of biopsies may exhibit substantial infiltration by lymphocytes and plasma cells in

*References 342, 350, 357, 359, 360, 377, 378.

the lobule or portal tracts. In addition, in these patients the histologic picture can resemble that of acute viral hepatitis, particularly if fat stains are not performed on frozen tissue.

At the electron microscopic level the swollen hepatocytes contain numerous small, non-membrane-bound cytoplasmic lipid droplets.[359,370,377,403] Fat has also been reported in lysosomes,[404] in endoplasmic reticulum, and in the Golgi apparatus.[405] Mitochondria are large, pleomorphic, and ameboid-shaped and contain lamellar crystalline inclusions. Bile canaliculi are dilated with loss of microvilli. Precipitated material is seen in canalicular lumens and in intracellular pericanalicular vesicles.

Other organs also may be involved in this disease, and fatty metamorphosis of pancreatic acinar cells and renal tubular epithelia is well described.[357,378,380]

Natural History and Prognosis

All the complications of fulminant hepatic failure (see Chap. 16) can occur in AFLP, including cerebral edema, gastrointestinal hemorrhage, renal failure, and infection. After severe liver dysfunction has become evident, spontaneous labor or fetal death in utero commonly ensues, and delivery is often complicated by postpartum hemorrhage. After delivery liver function rapidly improves, although some women experience transient worsening during the first few days postpartum. Signs, symptoms, liver function, and liver histology resolve over several weeks after delivery and there is no evidence of chronic liver disease.[361,363]

Overall outcome is summarized in Table 54-9. Both maternal and fetal mortality used to be high but have improved in recent series in which prompt delivery was undertaken along with improved medical treatment for fulminant liver failure and for premature infants. Improved outcome likely also reflects increased detection of milder cases that resolve quickly after delivery. Maternal morbidity, however, remains high with—even in recent series—average hospital stays of 11 to 16 days. Fetal mortality is related to rapid maternal decompensation, premature delivery, and maternal DIC with fibrin deposition in the placenta leading to placental infarcts and insufficiency and fetal asphyxia.[406]

AFLP seems to be sporadic disease except in families with genetic mutations in fatty acid oxidation. At least 22 women without known genetic mutations who survived the disorder have become pregnant again (10 months to 7 years later), 4 of them twice. AFLP recurred in only three cases.*

Therapy

There is no specific therapy for AFLP. Based on the observations that the disease occurs only in pregnancy, usually progresses relentlessly and rapidly during pregnancy, improves only after delivery, and has a potentially high fatality rate, prompt termination of pregnancy as soon as the diagnosis is suspected or made seems appropriate.[344,382] Because AFLP usually presents late in pregnancy and affected infants often die in utero with little warning, immediate delivery would be expected to improve fetal survival as well. Mothers with liver failure should be transferred to centers experienced in the care of acute liver failure. Liver transplantation has been used successfully in at least two patients with fulminant hepatic failure and AFLP.[410,411] The decision to proceed with transplantation should be made only after careful consideration because AFLP usually resolves rapidly after delivery.

Liver Disease Related to Pregnancy-induced Hypertension

Pre-eclampsia is a hypertensive disorder of pregnancy characterized by the trilogy of hypertension, proteinuria, and edema, whereas progression to seizures defines eclampsia. Although pre-eclampsia and eclampsia are not primarily liver diseases any organ system can be involved in the disease process, and a substantial fraction of affected women manifest some degree of liver damage, ranging from mild hepatocellular necrosis to hepatic rupture.

Incidence of Pregnancy-induced Hypertension

Pre-eclampsia develops in 5 percent to 10 percent of all pregnancies, more frequently in younger primigravidas, and at an extraordinarily high rate in women with the lupus anti-coagulant. The disorder can be mild or can progress rapidly to multi-organ damage.

Pathophysiology

The pathophysiology underlying pregnancy-induced hypertension, pre-eclampsia, and eclampsia is not well understood; however, defective placental invasion of the maternal circulation and poor placental perfusion are thought to lead to maternal endothelial activation, increased vascular tone, hypertension, and activation of platelets and fibrinogen.[412-415] Platelet aggregation and development of fibrin thrombi lead to thrombocytopenia, microangiopathic hemolytic anemia, and ischemic injury of a variety of organs, including the liver.

Abnormal lipid metabolism may also play a role in pre-eclampsia because plasma free fatty acids and triglycerides are increased in women with the disease[349,388,414] and animal data suggest that increased hepatic flux of fatty acids may trigger hypertension.[416] However, documented genetic mutations in fatty acid metabolism have been identified in only 1 of 180 women with pre-eclampsia-related liver disease.[392,417]

Liver Involvement

Although most women with pre-eclampsia exhibit no clinical or laboratory evidence of liver disease,[44] the liver is involved in at least 10 percent to 20 percent of women with pre-eclampsia.[24,418-421] Pre-eclampsia-related liver disease occurs in 0.1 percent to 1 percent of all deliveries[286,422,423] and accounts for about 5 percent of cases of

*References 350-352, 366, 375, 381, 382, 384, 407-409.

jaundice in pregnancy. Liver involvement is more common, up to 70 percent, in severe pre-eclampsia[423] or eclampsia,[424] constituting the primary cause of death in 15 percent to 21 percent of fatal cases of eclampsia.[424,425] Two distinct syndromes of liver disease in pre-eclampsia have been described. One is a moderate to severe disorder of patchy hepatocyte necrosis associated with thrombocytopenia, termed *HELLP* (hemolysis, elevated liver enzymes, and low platelet) *syndrome*. The second is acute liver hemorrhage and rupture, a rare but often fatal event.

Hepatic Pathology

Although liver biopsies in most women with pre-eclampsia are normal[4,5,426,427] 17 percent or more of women with pre-eclampsia and 70 percent of women dying with eclampsia exhibit histologic liver injury.[4,5,426-430] The characteristic hepatic lesions of pre-eclampsia consist of three features. First is diffuse deposition of fibrin along the sinusoids and, occasionally, in portal tract capillaries, hepatic arterioles, and portal veins.[426,431] Second is ischemic necrosis of hepatocytes, usually focal but occasionally confluent (Figure 54-5).[4,5,424,426-428,431] Third is periportal and portal tract hemorrhage.[4,5,428,431] In cases with severe liver necrosis diffuse patchy areas of hemorrhage and necrosis are visible grossly both within the parenchyma of the liver and in subcapsular locations. Large hematomas may form beneath the capsule and rupture, resulting in exsanguination.

HELLP Syndrome

HELLP syndrome was defined in 1982[432] and occurs in about 10 percent of all women with pre-eclampsia.[419,421,433,434] Patients with the HELLP syndrome probably represent the middle of the spectrum of liver involvement in pre-eclampsia. Accepted criteria for diagnosis usually include abnormal red blood cell morphology or increased lactic dehydrogenase, increased AST (or ALT), and a platelet count of less than 100,000 or 150,000.[413] Although liver damage is considered part of the HELLP syndrome AST levels may reflect injury to organs other than the liver; a few patients who fit these criteria actually may have little or no histologic liver injury.[4,5,426,427]

Clinical features are summarized in Table 54-10. Approximately 30 percent of cases present postpartum.[422,423,447] The relationship between HELLP syndrome and clinically evident pre-eclampsia is variable because hypertension is mild in 25 percent of patients with HELLP syndrome and is absent in 10 percent of cases,[413,422,423] although the other clinical features and characteristic liver histologic changes are present.[435] Some women exhibit considerable hepatic tenderness, whereas large-volume transudative ascites occurs in 8 percent to 10 percent of cases.[422,449,450]

Characteristic laboratory abnormalities are summarized in Table 54-11.

Evidence of true disseminated intravascular coagulopathy is found in 8 percent to 21 percent of patients.[422,447,451] The degree to which overall liver function is impaired may be difficult to assess. For example, hyperbilirubinemia, present in up to 42 percent of reported cases, is likely the result of a combination of hemolysis and liver dysfunction, whereas elevated values for the prothrombin time probably reflect a combination of decreased synthesis and increased consumption. Mild renal dysfunction is virtually universal.

Maternal morbidity from HELLP syndrome is high, especially in severe cases identified by a platelet count of less than 50,000.[415,423] Approximately 50 percent of such women develop cardiopulmonary, renal, hepatic, central nervous system, or bleeding complications with a mean

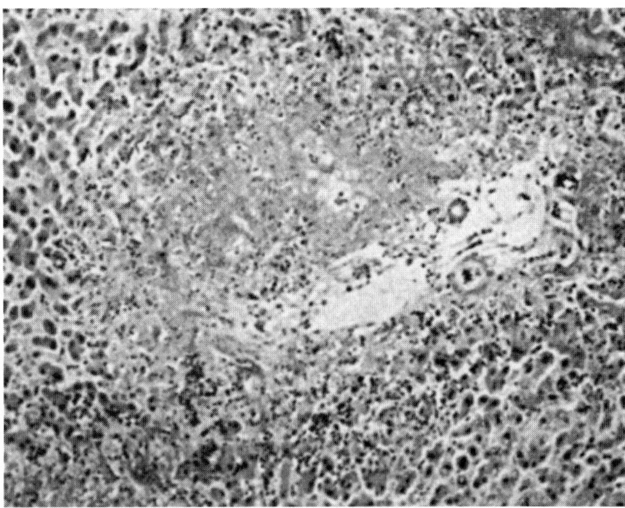

Figure 54-5 Liver in eclampsia showing periportal hemorrhage and patchy necrosis. Hematoxylin and eosin. (Courtesy of Dr. L. Ferrell.)

TABLE 54-10
HELLP Syndrome: Clinical Features*

Feature	Average value
Age	24 years (range, 13-40)
Gestational duration	32.3 weeks (range, 23-40)
Postpartum onset	28%
Primiparas	53%
Frequency among all women with pre-eclampsia	10%
Hypertension†	89%
Proteinuria†	80%
Nausea, vomiting	31%
Epigastric/right upper quadrant pain†	52%
Headache†	48%
Edema†	54%

HELLP, Hemolysis, elevated liver enzymes, and low platelet.
*Data compiled from 1695 patients from references 419-423, 432, and 435-447. Not all data are available for all patients.
†Signs and symptoms also commonly seen in women with pre-eclampsia who do not manifest the characteristic laboratory abnormalities of HELLP syndrome.

TABLE 54-11
HELLP Syndrome: Laboratory Abnormalities*

Test	Percentage with abnormal values	Average value	Range of values
Abnormal RBC morphology	89.5†	—	—
Lactic dehydrogenase	98	—	nl-5000
Thrombocytopenia	95	—	12,000-100,000
Fibrinogen	8-16	Decreased	—
Fibrin degradation products	8-42	Increased	—
Prothrombin time	13	Increased	—
Partial thromboplastin time	13	Increased	—
Serum bilirubin	5-42	—	nl-26 mg/dl
AST (nl ≤ 40)	89	293 IU/L	nl-6200 IU/L
ALT (nl ≤ 40)	67	173 IU/L	nl-702 IU/L
BUN, Cr	50-100	Increased	Usually mild

HELLP, Hemolysis, elevated liver enzymes, and low platelet; *RBC,* red blood cell; *nl,* normal; *AST,* aspartate aminotransferase; *ALT,* alanine aminotransferase; *BUN,* blood urea nitrogen; *Cr,* creatinine.
*Data compiled from 1512 cases from references 419-423, 432, 435-446, and 448. Not all data are available on all patients.
†RBC fragments, schistocytes, spherocytes; signs of microangiopathic hemolytic anemia.

hospital stay of 6 days.[423] Maternal mortality ranges from 0 percent to 3.5 percent in experienced centers.[413,414,423,447,452] Because maternal (and fetal) outcomes are worse when pre-eclampsia is complicated by HELLP syndrome,[423] some have recommended laboratory screening of all women with pre-eclampsia[453] although it is not known if early identification alters treatment decisions or outcome.

HELLP syndrome rapidly resolves after delivery although laboratory abnormalities, including liver tests, may not peak until 24 to 48 hours postpartum.[454] Long-term outcome is excellent because the liver lesions heal completely, although one series identified a higher than expected incidence of Gilbert's syndrome.[455] Pre-eclampsia (and HELLP syndrome) may develop in subsequent pregnancies, with rates of 3 percent to 27 percent being reported.[456,457]

Pre-eclampsia and HELLP are far more dangerous to the fetus than to the mother, with high rates of intrauterine growth retardation and premature delivery and fetal and neonatal death rates of 6 percent to 37 percent.* Fetal deaths are likely the result of placental insufficiency and hypoxia.[433]

Therapy is directed primarily at urgent delivery because progressive damage to the liver and other organs and fetal death can take place quickly, yet the disease resolves rapidly after delivery. Babies with adequate lung maturity are usually delivered within 24 hours, whereas less mature babies often are delivered after a few days of steroid treatment.[413-415] High-dose steroid therapy or plasmapheresis has been used, with apparent success in preliminary studies, to improve pre-eclampsia and HELLP syndrome in severely affected women before delivery or for those women whose disease worsens postpartum.[413-415,454,459,460]

*References 413, 414, 423, 447, 452, 458.

Overlap Between AFLP and Pre-eclampsia/HELLP Syndrome

The very rare AFLP and the more common pre-eclampsia/HELLP syndrome appear to co-exist much more frequently than would be expected by chance alone—28 percent or more of women with AFLP also manifest pre-eclampsia and HELLP syndrome.[344,354,382,395,398] Conversely, liver biopsies from 51 women with pre-eclampsia all showed microvesicular steatosis characteristic of AFLP.[429,430] A common factor may be the abnormal lipid metabolism characteristic of both disorders.[349,388,414] Indeed, women heterozygous for LCHAD deficiency have a 30 percent incidence of pre-eclampsia and HELLP syndrome whether they carry normal or affected fetuses.[385,387,395] However, additional genetic, fetal, or environmental factors may determine whether a pregnant woman develops one or both of these disorders or neither.

Hepatic Hemorrhage and Rupture

Hepatic rupture in pregnancy was first described by Abercrombie in 1844.[461] More than 300 cases have been reported.[418,424,461-464] Hepatic hemorrhage or rupture is probably the result of confluent hepatic necrosis from pre-eclampsia and is reported to occur in between 1 in 15,000 and 1 in 45,000 deliveries and in 1 percent to 2 percent of women with pre-eclampsia.[418,422-424,461,462] The highest figures are derived from a study in which abdominal CT scans were used to identify contained hepatic hematomas in women with few symptoms other than right upper quadrant abdominal pain.[418]

Hemorrhage occurs late in pregnancy or up to 48 hours postpartum. Clinical or histologic features of pre-eclampsia are found in 80 percent to 90 percent of cases,[461] and many patients would satisfy the criteria for HELLP syndrome. Hepatic hemorrhage and rupture are heralded by the sudden onset of right upper quadrant pain, which may, rarely, recur over several days.[465]

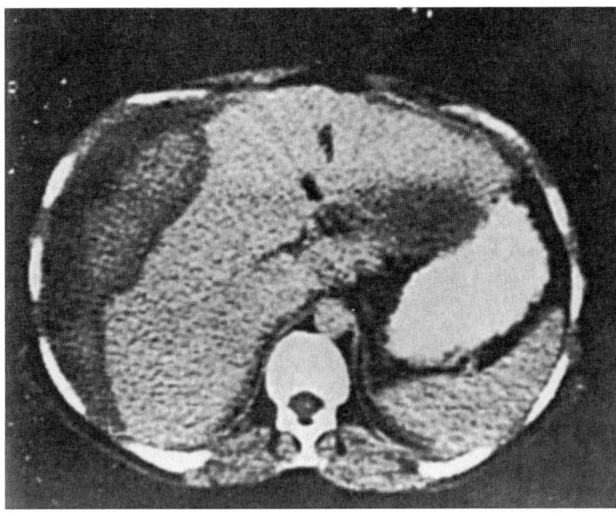

Figure 54-6 Abdominal computed tomography scan showing a subcapsular hematoma *(arrow)* along the right margin of the liver. (From Manas KJ, Welsh JD, Rankin RA, et al: Hepatic hemorrhage without rupture in preeclampsia. N Engl J Med 312:424, 1985.)

Hepatic tenderness, diffuse abdominal pain, peritoneal findings, chest pain, or shoulder pain are noted in some patients. Shock ensues in more than half of patients within a few hours of the onset of pain or after up to 48 hours in women with contained hematomas. Anemia or a rapid drop in hematocrit is noted in many patients. These signs and symptoms are not diagnostic and are similar to those seen in a variety of intra-abdominal catastrophes, including rupture of a hepatic adenoma, abruptio placentae, perforated viscus, or intestinal infarction.

Diagnosis is based on clinical suspicion and visualization of the liver, either radiologically or at laparotomy. Abdominal CT scans (Figure 54-6) may be the most sensitive and specific way to detect hepatic hemorrhage or rupture.[418,461,466] Liver and spleen scans, ultrasound, and angiograms may also be useful. Paracentesis can confirm intra-abdominal hemorrhage but does not clarify the site of bleeding and will be negative in patients with contained hematomas. MRI scans display chronic hematomas well but are less accurate than CT scans in detecting acute hemorrhage.

Survival of an untreated liver rupture has never been reported. In contrast, hemorrhage into a contained hematoma may resolve with medical support.[418,461,463] Treatment of hepatic rupture requires rapid diagnosis and intensive therapy by a multi-disciplinary team. The most important factors in ensuring maternal survival are identification of the disorder before irreversible shock has occurred, rigorous hemodynamic support with large-volume transfusions of blood and platelets, and control of bleeding by surgical or angiographic means.[461]

At surgery hematomas are drained and hemostasis attempted with packing, sutures, or lobectomy. Outcome may be better with packing and drainage than with lobectomy.[464] Surgical or angiographic hepatic artery interruption has been successful as well.[461-464] Liver transplantation was successful in salvaging one woman with uncontrollable hemorrhage.[467]

Women with contained hepatic hematomas may do well without surgery if they receive adequate hemodynamic support and are followed closely.[418,461,463] Exploratory laparotomy should be undertaken, however, if there is any suspicion of free rupture into the peritoneum.

Overall maternal and fetal mortality is high, approximately 50 percent and 60 percent to 70 percent, respectively. Mortality is lower in those with contained hematomas and in those in whom the diagnosis of liver rupture is made at or shortly after delivery.[462] In those who survive, hematomas slowly resolve[418,468] and subsequent successful pregnancy has been reported. Recurrence in a subsequent pregnancy has been reported once.[461]

Differential Diagnosis of Severe Liver Disease in Pregnancy

The principal liver diseases that cause severe disease during pregnancy are acute viral hepatitis, AFLP, pre-eclampsia–related liver disease, and, in the past, tetracycline-induced fatty liver.[469] The clinical presentations of all four diseases can be similar, but laboratory tests are helpful in distinguishing them. Diagnosis of AFLP is based on compatible clinical and laboratory abnormalities in a women in the third trimester of pregnancy in conjunction with a liver biopsy (including fat stains on frozen tissue) showing microvesicular fat. In contrast to AFLP, acute viral hepatitis may present at any time during pregnancy. A history of exposure to an individual with hepatitis is often obtained, serologic tests for hepatitis viruses A or B may be positive, coagulopathy or DIC are uncommon, and serum transaminase values tend to be much higher than is seen in AFLP. Pre-eclampsia–related liver disease is associated with hypertension and proteinuria, whereas pre-eclampsia is often absent in AFLP. Pre-eclampsia–related liver disease exhibits a greater degree of hematologic abnormalities and of hepatocellular necrosis than does AFLP. Indeed, in severe cases liver infarction and hemorrhage are frequently seen. However, some women exhibit both AFLP and pre-eclampsia–related liver disease. In the past tetracycline, particularly when administered in high doses or to patients with impaired renal function, caused a syndrome that was virtually identical to AFLP.[348,358,469] Although tetracycline-induced fatty liver has virtually disappeared, at least one case is related to use of tetracycline for treatment of acne.[470]

It is important to distinguish AFLP and pre-eclampsia from other causes of liver disease in pregnancy because treatment for these two disorders, early delivery, and supportive care are critical to the outcome of both mother and child.

References

1. Sheehan HL: Jaundice in pregnancy. Am J Obstet Gynecol 181:427, 1961.
2. Combes B, Shibata H, Adams R, et al: Alterations in sulfobromophthalein sodium-removal mechanisms from blood during normal pregnancy. J Clin Invest 42:1431, 1963.

3. Nixon WCW, Egeli ES, Laquer W, et al: Icterus in pregnancy. J Obstet Gynecol Brit Emp 54:642, 1947.
4. Ingerslev M, Teilum G: Biopsy studies on the liver in pregnancy I, II, III. Acta Obstet Gynecol Scand 25:339, 1945/46.
5. Anita FP, Bharadwaj TP, Watsa MC, et al: Liver in normal pregnancy, pre-eclampsia, and eclampsia. Lancet 2:776, 1958.
6. Gonzales-Angulo A, Anzar-Ramos R, Marquez-Monter H, et al: Ultrastructure of liver cells in women under steroid therapy. I. Normal pregnancy and trophoblastic growths. Acta Endocrinol 65:193, 1970.
7. Perez V, Gorodisch S, Casavilla F, et al: Ultrastructure of human liver at the end of normal pregnancy. Am J Obstet Gynecol 110:428, 1971.
8. Larsson-Chon U, Stenram U: Liver ultrastructure and function in icteric and non-icteric women using oral contraceptive agents. Acta Med Scand 181:257, 1967.
9. Martinez-Manautou J, Aznar-Ramos R, Bautista-O'Farrill J, et al: The ultrastructure of liver cells in women under steroid therapy. II. Contraceptive therapy. Acta Endocrinol 65:7, 1970.
10. Perez V, Gorodisch S, de Martire J, et al: Oral contraceptives: long-term use produces fine structural changes in liver mitochondria. Science 165:805, 1969.
11. Rovinsky JJ, Jaffin H: Cardiovascular hemodynamics in pregnancy. Am J Obstet Gynecol 95:787, 1966.
12. Pritchard JA: Changes in the blood volume during pregnancy and delivery. Anesthesiology 26:393, 1965.
13. Lund CJ, Donovan JC: Blood volume during pregnancy. Am J Obstet Gynecol 98:393, 1967.
14. Munnell EW, Taylor HC Jr: Liver blood flow in pregnancy—hepatic vein catheterization. J Clin Invest 26:952, 1947.
15. Laakso L, Ruotsalainen P, Punnonen R, et al: Hepatic blood flow during late pregnancy. Acta Obstet Gynecol Scand 50:175, 1971.
16. Iber FL: Jaundice in pregnancy—a review. Am J Obstet Gynecol 91:721, 1965.
17. Song CS, Rifkind AB, Gillette PN, et al: Hormones and the liver. The effects of estrogens, progestins, and pregnancy on hepatic function. Am J Obstet Gynecol 105:813, 1969.
18. Adlercreutz H, Tenhunen R: Some aspects of the interaction between natural and synthetic female sex hormones and the liver. Am J Med 49:630, 1970.
19. McNair RD, Jaynes RV: Alterations in liver function during normal pregnancy. Am J Obstet Gynecol 80:500, 1960.
20. Ramcharan S, Sponzilli EE, Wingerd JC: Serum protein fractions. Effects of oral contraceptives and pregnancy. Obstet Gynecol 48:211, 1976.
21. Bacq Y, Zarka O, Brechot J-F, et al: Liver function tests in normal pregnancy: a prospective study of 103 pregnant women and 103 matched controls. Hepatology 23:1030, 1996.
22. Shaaban MM, Hammad WA, Fathalla MF, et al: Effects of oral contraception on liver function tests and serum proteins in women with past viral hepatitis. Contraception 26:65, 1982.
23. Burrows S, Pekala B: Serum copper and ceruloplasmin in pregnancy. Am J Obstet Gynecol 109:907, 1971.
24. Haemmerli P: Jaundice during pregnancy with special emphasis on recurrent jaundice during pregnancy and its differential diagnosis. Acta Med Scand 179(suppl 444):1, 1966.
25. Svanborg A, Vikrot O: Plasma lipid fractions, including individual phospholipids, at various stages of pregnancy. Acta Med Scand 178:615, 1965.
26. Knopp RH, Warth MR, Carrol CJ: Lipid metabolism in pregnancy. I. Changes in lipoprotein triglyceride and cholesterol in normal pregnancy and the effects of diabetes mellitus. J Reprod Med 10:95, 1973.
27. Novikoff PM: Intracellular organelles and lipoprotein metabolism in normal and fatty livers. In Arias IM, Popper H, Schachter D, et al, eds: The Liver: Biology and Pathobiology. New York, Raven Press, 1982:143.
28. Schmid SE, Au WYW, Hill DE, et al: Cytochrome P-450-dependent oxidation of the 17a-ethinyl group of synthetic steroids. D-homoannulation or enzyme inactivation. Drug Met Disp 11:531, 1983.
29. Crawford JS, Rudofsky S: Some alterations in the pattern of drug metabolism associated with pregnancy, oral contraceptives, and the newly-born. Br J Anaesth 38:446, 1966.
30. Vore M, Bauer J, Pascucci V: The effect of pregnancy on the metabolism of [^{14}C] phenytoin in the isolated perfused rat liver. J Pharmacol Exp Ther 206:439, 1978.
31. Landon MJ, Kirkley M: Metabolism of diphenylhydantoin (phenytoin) during pregnancy. Br J Obstet Gynaecol 86:125, 1979.
32. Dam M, Christiansen J, Munck O, et al: Antiepileptic drugs: metabolism in pregnancy. Clin Pharmacokinet 4:53, 1979.
33. Hogstedt S, Lindberg B, Peng DR, et al: Pregnancy-induced increase in metoprolol metabolism. Clin Pharmacol Ther 37:688, 1985.
34. Casele HL, Laifer SA: Pregnancy after liver transplantation. Semin Perinatol 22:149, 1998.
35. Homeida M, Halliwell M, Branch RA: Effects of an oral contraceptive on hepatic size and antipyrine metabolism in premenopausal women. Clin Pharm Ther 24:228, 1978.
36. Carter DE, Goldman JM, Bressler R, et al: Effect of oral contraceptives on drug metabolism. Clin Pharmacol Ther 15:22, 1973.
37. O'Malley K, Stevenson IH, Crooks J: Impairment of human drug metabolism by oral contraceptive steroids. Clin Pharm Ther 13:552, 1972.
38. Brock WJ, Vore M: Hepatic morphine and estrone glucuronyltransferase activity and morphine biliary excretion in the isolated perfused rat liver. Drug Met Disp 10:336, 1982.
39. Vore M, Montgomery C: The effect of estradiol-17b treatment on the metabolism and biliary excretion of phenytoin in the isolated perfused rat liver and in vivo. J Pharmacol Exp Ther 215:71, 1980.
40. Watson KJR, Ghabrial H, Mashford ML, et al: The oral contraceptive pill increases morphine clearance but does not increase hepatic blood flow. Gastroenterology 90:1779, 1986 (abstract).
41. Schreiber AJ, Simon FR: Estrogen-induced cholestasis: clues to pathogenesis and treatment. Hepatology 3:607, 1983.
42. Soffer LJ: Bilirubin excretion as a test for liver function during normal pregnancy. Bull Johns Hopkins Hosp 52:365, 1933.
43. Sullivan CF, Tew WP, Watson EM: The bilirubin excretion test of liver function in pregnancy. J Obstet Gynecol Brit Emp 41:347, 1934.
44. Ylostalo P: Liver function in hepatosis of pregnancy and pre-eclampsia with special reference to modified bromsulphthalein tests. Acta Obstet Gynecol Scand 49(suppl 4):4, 1970.
45. Mueller MN, Kappas A: Estrogen pharmacology. I. The influence of estradiol and estriol on hepatic disposal of sulfobromophthalein (BSP) in man. J Clin Invest 43:1905, 1964.
46. Kleiner GJ, Kresh L, Arias IM: Studies of hepatic excretory function. II. The effect of norethynodrel and mestranol on bromsulphalein sodium metabolism in women of childbearing age. N Engl J Med 273:420, 1965.
47. Cao J, Huang L, Liu Y, et al: Differential regulation of hepatic bile salt and organic anion transporters in pregnant and postpartum rats and the role of prolactin. Hepatology 33:140, 2001.
48. Jarnfelt-Samsioe A, Eriksson B, Waldenstrom J, et al: Serum bile acids, gamma-glutamyltransferase and routine liver function tests in emetic and nonemetic pregnancies. Gynecol Obstet Invest 21:169, 1986.
49. Fulton HC, Douglas JG, Hutchon DJR, et al: Is normal pregnancy cholestatic? Clin Chim Acta 130:171, 1983.
50. Heikkinen J: Serum bile acids in the early diagnosis of intrahepatic cholestasis of pregnancy. Obstet Gynecol Scand 54:437, 1975.
51. Lunzer M, Barnes P, Byth K, et al: Serum bile acid concentrations during pregnancy and their relationship to obstetric cholestasis. Gastroenterology 91: 825, 1986.
52. Trauner M, Arrese M, Soroka DJ, et al: The rat canalicular conjugate export pump (Mrp2) is down-regulated in intrahepatic and obstructive cholestasis. Gastroenterology 113:255, 1997.
53. Lee J, Boyer JL: Molecular alterations in hepatocyte transport mechanisms in acquired cholestatic liver disorders. Semin Liver Dis 20:373, 2000.
54. Thorling L: Jaundice in pregnancy. A clinical study. Acta Med Scand 151(suppl 302):1, 1955.
55. Kessler WB, Andros GJ: Hepatic function during pregnancy and puerperium. Obstet Gynecol 23:372, 1964.
56. Romslo I, Sagen N, Haram K: Serum alkaline phosphatase in pregnancy. Acta Obstet Gynecol Scand 54:437, 1975.
57. Sammour MB, Ramadan MA, Khalil FK, et al: Serum and placental lactic dehydrogenase and alkaline phosphatase isoenzymes in normal pregnancy and in pre-eclampsia. Acta Obstet Gynecol Scand 54:393, 1975.
58. Sussman HH, Bowman M, Lewis JL: Placental alkaline phosphatase in maternal serum during normal and abnormal pregnancy. Nature 218:359, 1968.

59. Birkett DJ, Done J, Neale FC, et al: Serum alkaline phosphatase in pregnancy: an immunological study. BMJ 1:1210, 1966.
60. Walker FB, Hoblit DL, Cunningham FG, et al: Gamma glutamyl transpeptidase in normal pregnancy. Obstet Gynecol 43:745, 1974.
61. Seitanidis B, Moss DW: Serum alkaline phosphatase and 5'-nucleotidase levels during normal pregnancy. Clin Chim Acta 25:183, 1969.
62. Rosalski SB, Rau D, Lehmann D, et al: Determination of serum g-glutamyl transpeptidase activity and its clinical applications. Ann Clin Biochem 7:143, 1970.
63. Combes B, Shore GM, Cunningham FG, et al: Serum g-glutamyl transpeptidase activity and in viral hepatitis: suppression in pregnancy and by birth control pills. Gastroenterology 72:271, 1977.
64. Bean WB: The cutaneous arterial spider: a survey. Medicine 24:243, 1945;
65. Bean WB, Cogswell R, Dexter M: Vascular changes of the skin in pregnancy. Surg Obstet Gynecol 88:739, 1949.
66. Friedlander P, Osler M: Icterus and pregnancy. Am J Obstet Gynecol 97:894, 1967.
67. Hieber JP, Dalton D, Shorey J, et al: Hepatitis and pregnancy. J Pediatr 91:545, 1977.
68. Cahill KM: Hepatitis in pregnancy. Surg Gynecol Obstet 114:545, 1962.
69. Adams RH, Combes B: Viral hepatitis during pregnancy. JAMA 192:195, 1965.
70. Parker MLM: Infectious hepatitis in pregnancy. Med J Aust 2:967, 1965.
71. Bennett NM, Forbes JA, Lucas CR, et al: Infective hepatitis and pregnancy: analysis of liver function test results. Med J Aust 2:974, 1967.
72. Rao AVN, Devi CS, Savithri P, et al: Infectious hepatitis in pregnancy and puerperium—a study of 60 cases. Indian J Med Sci 23:471, 1969.
73. D'Cruz IA, Balani SG, Iyer LS: Infectious hepatitis and pregnancy. J Am Coll Obstet Gynecol 31:449, 1968.
74. Gelpi AP: Fatal hepatitis in Saudi Arabian women. Am J Gastroenterol 53:41, 1970.
75. Borhanmanesh F, Haghighi P, Hekmat K, et al: Viral hepatitis during pregnancy. Severity and effect on gestation. Gastroenterology 64:304, 1973.
76. Christie AB, Allam AA, Aref MKJ, et al: Pregnancy hepatitis in Libya. Lancet 2:827, 1976.
77. Adams WH, Shrestha SM, Adams DG: Coagulation studies of viral hepatitis occurring during pregnancy. Am J Med Sci 272:139, 1976.
78. Gelpi AP: Viral hepatitis complicating pregnancy: mortality trends in Saudi Arabia. Int J Gynecol Obstet 17:73, 1979.
79. Singh DS, Balasubramaniam M, Krishnaswami S, et al: Viral hepatitis during pregnancy. J Indian Med Assoc 73:90, 1979.
80. Khuroo MS, Teli MR, Skidmore S: Incidence and severity of viral hepatitis in pregnancy. Am J Med 70:252, 1981.
81. Mallia CP, Nancekivell AF: Fulminant virus hepatitis in late pregnancy. Ann Trop Med Parasitol 76:143, 1982.
82. Mandal D, Chowdhury NNR: Viral hepatitis in pregnancy. J Indian Med Assoc 79:96, 1982.
83. Shalev I, Bassan HM: Viral hepatitis in pregnancy in Israel. Br J Gynaecol Obstet 20:73, 1982.
84. Pain GC, Chakraborty AK, Choudhury NR: Outbreak of non-A non-B type viral hepatitis in a Calcutta slum. J Indian Med Assoc 80:125, 1983.
85. Tong MJ, Thursby M, Rakela J, et al: Studies on the maternal-infant transmission of the viruses which cause acute hepatitis. Gastroenterology 80:999, 1981.
86. Harrison TJ: Hepatitis E virus—an update. Liver 19:171, 1999.
87. Hamid SS, Jafri SMW, Khan H, et al: Fulminant hepatic failure in pregnant women: acute fatty liver or acute viral hepatitis? J Hepatol 25:20, 1996.
88. Michielsen PP, Van Damme P: Viral hepatitis and pregnancy. Acta Gastroenterol Belg 62:21, 1999.
89. Duff P: Hepatitis in pregnancy. Semin Perinatol 22:277, 1998.
90. Dinsmoor MJ: Hepatitis in the obstetric patient. Infect Dis Clin North Am 11:78, 1997.
91. Watson JC, Fleming DW, Borella AJ, et al: Vertical transmission of hepatitis A resulting in an outbreak in a neonatal intensive care unit. J Infect Dis 167:567, 1993.
92. Wejstal R, Norkrans G: Chronic non-A, non-B hepatitis in pregnancy: outcome and possible transmission to the offspring. Scand J Infect Dis 21:485, 1989.
93. ACOG Committee Opinion: Committee on Obstetrics: Maternal and Fetal Medicine. Guidelines for hepatitis B virus screening and vaccination during pregnancy. Int J Gynecol Obstet 40:172, 1993.
94. Khuroo MS, Saleem K, Shahid J: Vertical transmission of hepatitis E virus. Lancet 345:1025, 1995.
95. Lefkowitch JH, Rushton AR, Feng-Chen K-C: Hepatic fibrosis in fetal alcohol syndrome. Gastroenterology 85:951, 1983.
96. Moller J, Brandt NJ, Tygstrup I: Hepatic dysfunction in patient with fetal alcohol syndrome. Lancet i:605, 1979.
97. Habbick BF, Casey R, Zaleski WA, et al: Liver abnormalities in three patients with fetal alcohol syndrome. Lancet i:580, 1979.
98. Infeld DS, Borkowf HI, Varma RR: Chronic-persistent hepatitis and pregnancy. Gastroenterology 77:524, 1979.
99. Steven MM, Buckley JD, Mackay IR: Pregnancy in chronic active hepatitis. QJM 48:519, 1979.
100. Armenti VT, Herrine SK, Moritz MJ: Reproductive function after liver transplantation. Clin Liver Dis 1:471, 1997.
101. Laifer SA, Guido RS: Reproductive function and outcome of pregnancy after liver transplantation in women. Mayo Clin Proc 70:388, 1995.
102. Connolly TJ, Zuckerman AL: Contraception in the patient with liver disease. Semin Perinatol 22:178, 1998.
103. Whelton MJ, Sherlock S: Pregnancy in patients with hepatic cirrhosis. Lancet ii:995, 1968.
104. Joske RA, Pawsey HK, Martin JD: Chronic active liver disease and successful pregnancy. Lancet ii:712, 1963.
105. Choudhury KL, Chogtu L: Chronic active hepatitis and pregnancy. J Indian Med Assoc 63:196, 1974.
106. Powell D: Pregnancy in active chronic hepatitis on immunosuppressive therapy. Postgrad Med J 45:292, 1969.
107. Heneghan MA, Norris SM, O'Grady JG, et al: Management and outcome of pregnancy in autoimmune hepatitis. Gut 48:97, 2001.
108. Colle I, Hautekeete M: Remission of autoimmune hepatitis during pregnancy: a report of two cases. Liver 19:55, 1999.
109. Levine AB: Autoimmune hepatitis in pregnancy. Obstet Gynecol 95:1033, 2000.
110. Scheinberg IH, Sternlieb I: Pregnancy in penicillamine-treated patients with Wilson's disease. N Engl J Med 293:1300, 1975.
111. Toaff R, Toaff ME, Peyser MR, et al: Hepatolenticular degeneration (Wilson's disease) and pregnancy. Obstet Gynecol Survey 32:497, 1977.
112. Walshe JM: The management of pregnancy in Wilson's disease treated with trientine. QJM 58:81, 1986.
113. Schagen van Leeuwen JH, Christiaens GCML, Hoogenraad TU: Recurrent abortion and the diagnosis of Wilson disease. Obstet Gynecol 78:547, 1991.
114. Mustafa MS, Shamina AH: Five successful deliveries following 9 consecutive spontaneous abortions in a patient with Wilson disease. Aust N Z J Obstet Gynaecol 38:312, 1998.
115. Sternlieb I: Wilson's disease and pregnancy. Hepatology 31:531, 2000.
116. German JL III, Bearn AG: Effect of estrogens on copper metabolism in Wilson's disease. J Clin Invest 40:445, 1961.
117. Brewer GJ, Johnson VD, Dick RD, et al: Treatment of Wilson's disease with zinc. XVII: treatment during pregnancy. Hepatology 31:364, 2000.
118. Walshe JM: Treatment of Wilson's disease with trientine (triethylene tetramine) dihydrochloride. Lancet i:643, 1982.
119. Marecek Z, Graf M: Pregnancy in penicillamine-treated patients with Wilson's disease. N Engl J Med 295:841, 1976.
120. Shimono N, Ishibashi H, Ikematsu H, et al: Fulminant hepatic failure during perinatal period in a pregnant woman with Wilson's disease. Gastroenterol Jpn 26:69, 1991.
121. Nunns D, Hawthorne B, Goulding P, et al: Wilson's disease in pregnancy. Eur J Obstet Gynecol Reprod Biol 62:141, 1995.
122. Walshe JM: Pregnancy in Wilson's disease. QJM 46:73, 1977.
123. Schweitzer IL, Peters RL: Pregnancy in hepatitis B antigen positive cirrhosis. Obstet Gynecol 48(suppl 1):53S, 1976.
124. Borhanmanesh F, Haghighi P: Pregnancy in patients with cirrhosis of the liver. Obstet Gynecol 36:315, 1970.
125. Schreyer P, Caspi E, El-Hindi JM, et al: Cirrhosis—pregnancy and delivery: a review. Obstet Gynecol Survey 37:304, 1982.

126. Cheng Y-S: Pregnancy in liver cirrhosis and/or portal hypertension. Am J Obstet Gynecol 128:812, 1977.
127. Britton RC: Pregnancy and esophageal varices. Am J Surg 143:421, 1982.
128. Moore RM, Hughes PK: Cirrhosis of the liver in pregnancy. Obstet Gynecol 15:753, 1960.
129. Varma RR, Michelsohn NH, Borkowf HI, et al: Pregnancy in cirrhotic and noncirrhotic portal hypertension. Obstet Gynecol 50:217, 1977.
130. Niven P, Williams D, Zeegen R: Pregnancy following the surgical treatment of portal hypertension. Am J Obstet Gynecol 110:1100, 1971.
131. Salam AA, Warren WD: Distal splenorenal shunt for the surgical treatment of variceal bleeding during pregnancy. Arch Surg 105:643, 1972.
132. Chattopadhyay TK, Kapoor VK, Iyer KS, et al: Successful splenorenal shunt performed during pregnancy. Jpn J Surg 14:405, 1984.
133. Brown HJ: Splenorenal shunt during pregnancy. Am Surg 37:441, 1971.
134. Krol-Van Straaten J, De Maat CEM: Successful pregnancies in cirrhosis of the liver before and after portacaval anastomosis. Neth J Med 27:14, 1984.
135. Cerqui AJ, Haran M, Brodribb R: Implications of liver cirrhosis in pregnancy. Aust N Z J Obstet Gynaecol 38:93, 1998.
136. Aggarwal N, Sawnhey H, Suril V, et al: Pregnancy and cirrhosis of the liver. Aust N Z J Obstet Gynaecol 39:503, 1999.
137. Starkel P, Horsmans Y, Geubel A: Endoscopic band ligation: a safe technique to control bleeding esophageal varices in pregnancy. Gastrointest Endosc 48:212, 1998.
138. Zeeman GG, Moise KJ: Prophylactic banding of severe esophageal varices associated with liver cirrhosis in pregnancy. Obstet Gynecol 94:842, 1999.
139. Russell MA, Craigo SD: Cirrhosis and portal hypertension in pregnancy. Semin Perinatol 22:156, 1998.
140. Pajor A, Lehoczky D: Pregnancy and extrahepatic portal hypertension. Gynecol Obstet Invest 30:193, 1990.
141. Waffarn F, Carlisle S, Pena I, et al: Fetal exposure to maternal hyperbilirubinemia. Am J Dis Child 136:416, 1982.
142. Cotton DB, Brock BJ, Schifin BS: Cirrhosis and fetal hyperbilirubinemia. Obstet Gynecol 57(suppl):25S, 1981.
143. Wong S-J, Chan LY-S, Yu V, et al: Hepatitis B carrier and perinatal outcome in singleton pregnancy. Am J Perinatol 16:485, 1999.
144. Zanetti AR, Ferroni P, Magliano EM, et al: Perinatal transmission of the hepatitis B virus and of the HBV-associated delta agent from mothers to offspring in Northern Italy. J Med Virol 9:139, 1982.
145. Stevens CE, Neurath RA, Beasley RP, et al: HBeAg and anti-HBe detection by radioimmunoassay: correlation with vertical transmission of hepatitis B virus in Taiwan. J Med Virol 3:237, 1979.
146. Beasley RP, Hwang L-Y, Lee G C-Y, et al: Prevention of perinatally transmitted hepatitis B virus infections with hepatitis B immune globulin and hepatitis B vaccine. Lancet 2:1099, 1983.
147. Stevens CE, Toy PT, Tong MJ, et al: Perinatal hepatitis B virus transmission in the United States. Prevention by passive-active immunization. JAMA 253:1740, 1985.
148. Huang K-Y, Lin S-R: Nationwide vaccination: a success story in Taiwan. Vaccine 18:S35, 2000.
149. Roome A, Rak M, Hadler J: Follow-up of infants of hepatitis B-infected women after hepatitis B vaccination, Connecticut, 1994 to 1997. Pediatr Infect Dis J 19:573, 2000.
150. Conte D, Fraquelli M, Prati D, et al: Prevalence and clinical course of chronic hepatitis C virus (HCV) infection and rate of HCV vertical transmission in a cohort of 15,250 pregnant women. Hepatology 31:751, 2000.
151. Gervais A, Bacq Y, Bernuau J, et al: Decrease in serum ALT and increase in serum HCV RNA during pregnancy in women with chronic hepatitis C. J Hepatol 32:293, 2000.
152. Fontaine H, Nalpas B, Gillet A: Worsening of HCV-related hepatitis after pregnancy. Hepatology 32:278A, 2000.
153. Locatelli A, Roncaglia N, Arreghini A, et al: Hepatitis C virus infection is associated with a higher incidence of cholestasis of pregnancy. Br J Obstet Gynaecol 106:498, 1999.
154. Eriksen NL: Perinatal consequences of hepatitis C. Clin Obstet Gynecol 42:121, 1999.
155. Zanetti AR, Tanzi E, Newell ML: Mother-to-infant transmission of hepatitis C virus. J Hepatol 31(suppl 1):96, 1999.
156. Ruiz-Extremera A, Salmeron J, Torres C, et al: Follow-up of transmission of hepatitis C to babies of human immunodeficiency virus-negative women: the role of breast-feeding in transmission. Pediatr Infect Dis J 19:511, 2000.
157. Polywka S, Schroter M, Feucht H-H, et al: Low risk of vertical transmission of hepatitis C virus by breast milk. Clin Infect Dis 29:1327, 1999.
158. Burns DN, Minkoff H: Hepatitis C: screening in pregnancy. Obstet Gynecol 94:1044, 1999.
159. Ward C, Tudor-Williams G, Cotzias T, et al: Prevalence of hepatitis C among pregnant women attending an inner London obstetric department: uptake and acceptability of named antenatal testing. Gut 47:277, 2000.
160. Vogt M, Lang T, Klingler C, et al: Prevalence and clinical outcome of hepatitis C infection in children who underwent cardiac surgery before the implementation of blood-donor screening. N Engl J Med 341:866, 1999.
161. Olsson R, Loof L, Wallerstedt S: Pregnancy in patients with primary biliary cirrhosis—a case for dissuasion? Liver 13:316, 1993.
162. Nir A, Sorokin Y, Abramovici H, et al: Pregnancy and primary biliary cirrhosis. Int J Gynaecol Obstet 28:279, 1989.
163. Chazouilleres O, Poupon R, Bonnand AM, et al: Pregnancy and ursodeoxycholic acid (UDCA) treatment induce remission of primary biliary cirrhosis (PBC). Hepatology 28:545A, 1998.
164. Janczewska I, Olsson R, Hultcrantz R, et al: Pregnancy in patients with primary sclerosing cholangitis. Liver 16:326, 1996.
165. Athanassiou AM, Craigo SD: Liver masses in pregnancy. Semin Perinatol 22:166, 1998.
166. Delabrousse E, Site O, Le Mouel A, et al: Intrahepatic pregnancy: sonography and CT findings. Am J Roentgenol 173:1377, 1999.
167. Marques R, Taborda F, Jorge CS, et al: Successful outcome in a pregnancy complicated by large hepatic hemangioma. Acta Obstet Gynecol Scand 76:606, 1997.
168. Entezami M, Becker R, Ebert A, et al: Hepatocellular carcinoma as a rare cause of excessive rise in alpha-fetoprotein in pregnancy. Gynecol Oncol 62:405, 1996.
169. Jeng LBB, Lee W-C, Wang CC, et al: Hepatocellular carcinoma in a pregnant woman detected by routine screening of maternal alpha-fetoprotein. Am J Obstet Gynecol 172:219, 1995.
170. Gisi P, Floyd R: Hepatocellular carcinoma in pregnancy. A case report. J Reprod Med 44:65, 1999.
171. Cohen L, Lewis C, Arias IM: Pregnancy, oral contraceptives, and chronic familial jaundice with predominantly conjugated hyperbilirubinemia (Dubin-Johnson syndrome). Gastroenterology 62:1182, 1972.
172. Di Zoglio JD, Cardillo E: The Dubin-Johnson syndrome and pregnancy. Obstet Gynecol 42:560, 1973.
173. Shani M, Seligsohn U, Gilon E, et al: Dubin-Johnson syndrome in Israel. QJM 39:549, 1970.
174. Cundy TF, O'Grady JG, Williams R: Recovery of menstruation and pregnancy after liver transplantation. Gut 31:337, 1990.
175. Armenti VT, Herrine SK, Radomski JS, et al: Pregnancy after liver transplantation. Liver Transpl 6:671, 2000.
176. Wu A, Nashan B, Messner U, et al: Outcome of 22 successful pregnancies after liver transplantation. Clin Transplant 12:454, 1998.
177. Bennion LJ, Grundy SM: Risk factors for the development of cholelithiasis in man. N Engl J Med 299:1221, 1978.
178. Thistle JL: Gallstones in women. Med Clin North Am 58:811, 1974.
179. Glasnovic JC, Mege RM, Mannovic I, et al: Cholelithiasis in young women. Gastroenterology 104:A76, 1993 (abstract).
180. Pertsemlidis D, Panveliwalla D, Ahrens EH: Effects of clofibrate and of an estrogen-progestin combination on fasting biliary lipids and cholic acid kinetics in man. Gastroenterology 66:565, 1974.
181. Bennion JL, Mott DM, Howard BV: Oral contraceptives raise the cholesterol saturation of bile by increasing biliary cholesterol secretion. Metabolism 29:18, 1980.
182. Kern F, Everson GT, DeMark B: Biliary lipids, bile acids, and gallbladder function in the human female: effects of contraceptive steroids. J Lab Clin Med 99:798, 1982.
183. Kern F, Everson GT, DeMark B, et al: Biliary lipids, bile acids, and gallbladder function in the human female. Effects of pregnancy and the ovulatory cycle. J Clin Invest 68:1229, 1981.
184. Everson GT: Pregnancy and gallstones. Hepatology 17:159, 1993.

185. Braverman DZ, Johnson ML, Kern F Jr: Effects of pregnancy and contraceptive steroids on gallbladder function. N Engl J Med 302:362, 1980.
186. Everson RB, Byar DP, Bischoff AJ: Estrogen predisposes to cholecystectomy but not to stones. Gastroenterology 82:4, 1982.
187. Braverman DZ, Herbet D, Goldstein R, et al: Postpartum restoration of pregnancy-induced cholecystoparesis and prolonged intestinal transit time. J Clin Gastroenterol 10:642, 1988.
188. Maringhini A, Ciambra M, Baccelliere P, et al: Biliary sludge and gallstones in pregnancy. Ann Intern Med 119:116, 1993.
189. Valdivieso V, Covarrubias C, Siegel F, et al: Pregnancy and cholelithiasis. Hepatology 17:1, 1993.
190. Van Bodegraven AA, Bohmer CJM, Manoliu RA, et al: Gallbladder contents and fasting gallbladder volumes during and after pregnancy. Scand J Gastroenterol 33:993, 1998.
191. Ko CW, Sekijima JH, Lee SP: Biliary sludge. Ann Intern Med 130:301, 1999.
192. Wingrave SJ, Kay CR: Oral contraceptives and gallbladder disease. Royal College of General Practitioners oral contraception study. Lancet ii:957, 1982.
193. Oral contraceptives and venous thromboembolic disease, surgically confirmed gallbladder disease, and breast tumors. Report from the Boston Collaborative Drug Surveillance Programme. Lancet i:7817, 1973.
194. Surgically confirmed gallbladder disease, venous thromboembolism, and breast tumors in relation to postmenopausal estrogen therapy. Report from the Boston Collaborative Drug Surveillance Program. N Engl J Med 290:15, 1974.
195. Everson GT, McKinley C, Lawson M: Gallbladder function in the human female: effect of the ovulatory cycle, pregnancy, and contraceptive steroids. Gastroenterology 82:711, 1982.
196. Glenn F, McSherry CK: Gallstones and pregnancy among 300 young women treated by cholecystectomy. Surg Gynecol Obstet 127:1067, 1968.
197. Friley MD, Douglas G: Acute cholecystitis in pregnancy and the puerperium. Am Surg 38:314, 1972.
198. Hill LM, Johnson CE, Lee RA, et al: Cholecystectomy in pregnancy. Obstet Gynecol 46:291, 1975.
199. Landers D, Carmona R, Crombleholme W, et al: Acute cholecystitis in pregnancy. Obstet Gynecol 69:131, 1987.
200. Bartoli E, Calonaci N, Nenci R: Ultrasonography of the gallbladder in pregnancy. Gastrointest Radiol 9:35, 1984.
201. Williamson SL, Williamson MR: Cholecystosonography in pregnancy. J Ultrasound Med 3:329, 1984.
202. Mintz MC, Grumbach K, Arger PH, et al: Sonographic evaluation of bile duct size during pregnancy. Am J Radiol 145:575, 1985.
203. Davis A, Katz VL, Cox R: Gallbladder disease in pregnancy. J Reprod Med 40:759, 1995.
204. Ghumman E, Barry M, Grace PA: Management of gallstones in pregnancy. Br J Surg 84:1646, 1997.
205. Glasgow RE, Visser BC, Harris HW, et al: Changing management of gallstone disease during pregnancy. Surg Endosc 12:241, 1998.
206. Hiatt JR, Hiatt JCG, Williams RA: Biliary disease in pregnancy: strategy for surgical management. Am J Surg 151:263, 1986.
207. McKellar DP, Anderson CT, Boynton CJ, et al: Cholecystectomy during pregnancy without fetal loss. Surg Gynecol Obstet 174:465, 1992.
208. Graham G, Baxi L, Tharakan T: Laparoscopic cholecystectomy during pregnancy: a case series and review of the literature. Obstet Gynecol Surv 53:566, 1998.
209. Sungler P, Heinerman PM, Steiner H, et al: Laparoscopic cholecystectomy and interventional endoscopy for gallstone complications during pregnancy. Surg Endosc 14:267, 2000.
210. Affleck DG, Handrahan DL, Egger MJ, et al: The laparoscopic management of appendicitis and cholelithiasis during pregnancy. Am J Surg 178:523, 1999.
211. Cosenza CA, Saffari B, Jabbour N, et al: Surgical management of biliary gallstone disease during pregnancy. Am J Surg 178:545, 1999.
212. Nesbitt TH, Kay HH, McCoy MC, et al: Endoscopic management of biliary disease during pregnancy. Obstet Gynecol 87:806, 1996.
213. Barthel JS, Chowdhury T, Miedema BW: Endoscopic sphincterotomy for the treatment of gallstone pancreatitis during pregnancy. Surg Endosc 12:394, 1998.
214. Kang AH, Graves CR: Herpes simplex hepatitis in pregnancy: a case report and review of the literature. Obstet Gynecol Surv 54:463, 1999.
215. Glorioso DV, Molloy PJ, Van Thiel DH, et al: Successful empiric treatment of HSV hepatitis in pregnancy. Dig Dis Sci 41:1273, 1996.
216. Jacques SM, Qureshi F: Herpes simplex virus hepatitis in pregnancy. Hum Pathol 23:183, 1992.
217. Goyert GL, Bottoms SF, Sokol RJ: Anicteric presentation of fatal herpetic hepatitis in pregnancy. Obstet Gynecol 65:585, 1985.
218. Klein NA, Mabie WC, Shaver DC, et al: Herpes simplex virus hepatitis in pregnancy. Gastroenterology 100:239, 1991.
219. Porter LE, Elm MS, Van Thiel DH, et al: Characterization and quantitation of human hepatic estrogen receptor. Gastroenterology 84:704, 1983.
220. Ishak KG: Hepatic lesions caused by anabolic and contraceptive steroids. Semin Liver Dis 1:116, 1981.
221. Christopherson WM, Mays ET, Barrows GHA: Liver oncogenesis and steroids. In Ariel IM, ed: Progress in Clinical Cancer, vol. III. New York, Grune and Stratton, 1978:153.
222. Winkler K, Poulsen H: Liver disease with perioportal sinusoidal dilatation. A possible complication to contraceptive steroids. Scand J Gastroenterol 10:699, 1975.
223. Spellberg MA, Mirro J, Chowdhury L: Hepatic sinusoidal dilatation related to oral contraceptives. Am J Gastroenterol 72:218, 1979.
224. Thung SN, Gerber MA: Precursor stage of hepatocellular neoplasm following long exposure to orally administered contraceptives. Hum Pathol 12:472, 1981.
225. Kerlin P, Davis GL, McGill DB, et al: Hepatic adenoma and focal nodular hyperplasia: clinical, pathologic, and radiologic features. Gastroenterology 84:994, 1983.
226. Klatskin G: Hepatic tumors. Possible relationship to use of oral contraceptives. Gastroenterology 73:386, 1977.
227. Scott LD, Katz AR, Duke JH, et al: Oral contraceptives, pregnancy, and focal nodular hyperplasia of the liver. JAMA 251:1461, 1984.
228. Weimann A, Mossinger M, Fronhoff K, et al: Pregnancy in women with observed focal nodular hyperplasia of the liver. Lancet 351:1251, 1998.
229. Rooks JB, Ory HW, Ishak KG, et al: Epidemiology of hepatocellular adenoma. JAMA 242:644, 1979.
230. Edmondson HA, Henderson B, Benton B: Liver-cell adenomas associated with use of oral contraceptives. N Engl J Med 294:470, 1976.
231. Wanless IR, Medline A: Role of estrogens as promoters of hepatic neoplasia. Lab Invest 46:313, 1982.
232. Guzman IJ, Gold JH, Rosai J, et al: Benign hepatocellular tumors. Surgery 82:495, 1977.
233. Buhler H, Pirovino M, Akovbiantz A, et al: Regression of liver cell adenoma. Gastroenterology 82:775, 1982.
234. Hayes D, Lamki H, Hunter IWE: Hepatic-cell adenoma presenting with intraperitoneal hemorrhage in the puerperium. BMJ 3:1394, 1977.
235. Kent DR, Nissen ED, Nissen SE, et al: Maternal death resulting from rupture of liver adenoma associated with oral contraceptives. Obstet Gynecol 50(suppl):5S, 1977.
236. Check JH, King LC, Rakoff AE: Uncomplicated pregnancy following oral contraceptive-induced liver hepatoma. Obstet Gynecol 52(suppl):28S, 1978.
237. Terkivatan T, De Wilt JHW, De Man RA, et al: Management of hepatocellular adenoma during pregnancy. Liver 20:186, 2000.
238. Hill MA, Albert T, Zieske A, et al: Successful resection of multifocal hepatic adenoma during pregnancy. South Med J 90:357, 1997.
239. Irey NS, Manion WC, Taylor HB: Vascular lesions in women taking oral contraceptives. Arch Pathol 89:1, 1970.
240. Hoyumpa AM, Schiff L, Helfman EL: Budd-Chiari syndrome in women taking oral contraceptives. Am J Med 50:137, 1971.
241. Alpert LI: Veno-occlusive disease of the liver associated with oral contraceptives: case report and review of the literature. Hum Pathol 7:709, 1976.
242. Wu S-M, Spurny OM, Klotz AP: Budd-Chiari syndrome after taking oral contraceptives. A case report and review of 14 cases. Dig Dis Sci 22:623, 1977.
243. Powell-Jackson PR, Melia W, Canalese J, et al:. Budd-Chiari syndrome: clinical patterns and therapy. QJM 51:79, 1982.
244. Lewis JH, Tice HL, Zimmerman HJ: Budd-Chiari syndrome associated with oral contraceptive steroids. Review of treatment of 47 cases. Dig Dis Sci 28:673, 1983.
245. Singh V, Sinha SK, Nain CK, et al: Budd-Chiari syndrome: our experience of 71 patients. J Gastroenterol Hepatol 15:550, 2000.

246. Van Steenbergen W, Beyls J, Vermylen J, et al: "Lupus" anticoagulant and thrombosis of the hepatic veins (Budd-Chiari syndrome). J Hepatol 3:87, 1986.
247. Mackworth-Young CG, Melia WM, Harris EN, et al: The Budd-Chiari syndrome. Possible pathogenetic role for anti-phospholipid antibodies. J Hepatol 3:83, 1986.
248. Hancock KW. The Budd-Chiari syndrome in pregnancy. J Obstet Gynaecol Br Cwlth 75:746, 1968.
249. Oettinger M, Levy N, Lewy Z, et al: The Budd-Chiari syndrome after pregnancy. J Obstet Gynaecol Br Cwlth 77:174, 1970.
250. Rosenthal T, Shani M, Deutsch V, et al: The Budd-Chiari syndrome after pregnancy. Am J Obstet Gynecol 113:789, 1972.
251. Khuroo MS, Datta DV: Budd-Chiari syndrome following pregnancy. Report of 16 cases, with roentgenologic, hemodynamic and histologic studies of the hepatic outflow tract. Am J Med 68:113, 1980.
252. Artigas JMG, Estabanez, Faure MR: Pregnancy and the Budd-Chiari syndrome. Dig Dis Sci 27:89, 1992.
253. Covillo FV, Nyong AO, Axelrod JL: Budd-Chiari syndrome following pregnancy. Mo Med 81:356, 1984.
254. Fickert P, Ramschak H, Kenner L, et al: Acute Budd Chiari syndrome with fulminant hepatic failure in a pregnant woman with factor V Leiden mutation. Gastroenterology 111:510A, 1996.
255. Hodkinson HJ, McKibbin JK, Tim JO, et al: Postpartum veno-occlusive disease treated with ascitic fluid reinfusion. S Afr Med J 54:366, 1978.
256. Girardin M-FS-M, Zafrani ES, Prigent A, et al: Unilobular small hepatic vein obstruction: possible role of progestogen given as oral contraceptive. Gastroenterology 84:630, 1983.
257. Adams RH, Gordon J, Combes B: Hyperemesis gravidarum. I. Evidence of hepatic dysfunction. Obstet Gynecol 31:659, 1968.
258. Abell TL, Riely CA: Hyperemesis gravidarum. Gastroenterol Clin North Am 21:835, 1992.
259. Morali GA, Braverman DZ: Abnormal liver enzymes and ketonuria in hyperemesis gravidarum. J Clin Gastroenterol 12:303, 1990.
260. Combes B, Adams RH, Gordon J, et al: Hyperemesis gravidarum. II. Alterations in sulfobromophthalein sodium-removal mechanisms from blood. Obstet Gynecol 31:665, 1968.
261. Larrey D, Rueff B, Feldman G, et al: Recurrent jaundice caused by recurrent hyperemesis gravidarum. Gut 25:1414, 1984.
262. Chatwani A, Schwartz R: A severe case of hyperemesis gravidarum. Am J Obstet Gynecol 143:964, 1982.
263. Sheehan HL: The pathology of hyperemesis and vomiting of late pregnancy. J Obstet Gynecol Br Emp 46:685, 1939.
264. Verdy M: BSP retention during total fasting. Metabolism 15:769, 1966.
265. Webber BL, Freiman I: The liver in kwashiorkor. Arch Pathol 98:400, 1974.
266. Haemmerli UP, Wyss HI: Recurrent intrahepatic cholestasis of pregnancy. Report of six cases, and review of the literature. Medicine 46:299, 1967.
267. Rencoret R, Aste H: Jaundice during pregnancy. Med J Aust 1:167, 1973.
268. Johnson P, Samsioe G, Gustafson A: Studies in cholestasis of pregnancy. I. Clinical aspects and liver function tests. Acta Obstet Gynecol Scand 54:77, 1975.
269. Ylostalo P, Ylikorkala O: Hepatosis of pregnancy. A clinical study of 107 patients. Ann Chir Gynaecol Fenniae 64:128, 1975.
270. Medline A, Ptak T, Gryfe A, et al: Pruritus of pregnancy and jaundice induced by oral contraceptives. Am J Gastroenterol 65:156, 1976.
271. Wilson BRI, Haverkamp AD: Cholestatic jaundice of pregnancy: new perspectives. Obstet Gynecol 54:650, 1979.
272. Johnston WG, Baskett TF: Obstetric cholestasis. Am J Obstet Gynecol 133:299, 1979.
273. Reyes H, Radrigan ME, Gonzalez MC, et al: Steatorrhea in patients with intrahepatic cholestasis of pregnancy. Gastroenterology 93:584, 1987.
274. Reyes H, Gonzalez MC, Ribalta J, et al: Colestasia intrahepatica de la embarazada: variabilidad clinica y bioquimica. Rev Med Chile 110:631, 1982.
275. Shaw D, Frohlich J, Witmann BAK, Willms M: A prospective study of 18 patients with cholestasis of pregnancy. Am J Obstet Gynecol 142:621, 1982.
276. Zhong-da Q, Qi-nan W, Yue-han L, et al: Intrahepatic cholestasis of pregnancy. Chin Med J 96:902, 1983.
277. Berg B, Helm G, Petersohn L, et al: Cholestasis of pregnancy. Acta Obstet Gynecol Scand 65:107, 1986.
278. Reyes H: The enigma of intrahepatic cholestasis of pregnancy: lessons from Chile. Hepatology 2:87, 1982.
279. Reyes H, Gonzalez MC, Ribalta J, et al: Prevalence of intrahepatic cholestasis of pregnancy in Chile. Ann Int Med 88:487, 1978.
280. Reyes H, Taboada G, Ribalta J: Prevalence of intrahepatic cholestasis of pregnancy in La Paz, Bolivia. J Chronic Dis 32:499, 1979.
281. Glasinovic JC, Marinovic I, Vela P: The changing scene of cholestasis of pregnancy in Chile. An epidemiological study. Hepatology 6:1161, 1986 (abstract).
282. Furhoff A-K: Itching in pregnancy. Acta Med Scand 196:403, 1974.
283. Misra PS, Evanov FA, Wessely Z, et al: Idiopathic intrahepatic cholestasis of pregnancy. Am J Gastroenterol 73:54, 1980.
284. Bacq Y, Sapey T, Brechot MC, et al: Intrahepatic cholestasis of pregnancy: a French prospective study. Hepatology 26:358, 1997.
285. Shanmugam S, Thappa DM, Habeebullah S: Pruritus gravidarum: a clinical and laboratory study. J Dermatol 25:582, 1998.
286. Ch'ng CL, Kingham JG, Morgan M: Prospective study of liver dysfunction in pregnancy in south Wales, UK. Gastroenterology 118:A1008, 2000.
287. Abedin P, Weaver JB, Egginton E: Intrahepatic cholestasis of pregnancy: prevalence and ethnic distribution. Ethn Health 4:35, 1999.
288. Rioseco AJ, Ivankovic MB, Manzur A, et al: Intrahepatic cholestasis of pregnancy: a retrospective case-control study of perinatal outcome. Am J Obstet Gynecol 170:890, 1994.
289. Gaudet R, Merviel P, Berkane N, et al: Fetal impact of cholestasis of pregnancy: experience at Tenon Hospital and literature review. Fetal Diagn Ther 15:191, 2000.
290. Nicastri PL, Diaferia A, Tartagni M, et al: A randomised placebo-controlled trial of ursodeoxycholic acid and S-adenosylmethionine in the treatment of intrahepatic cholestasis of pregnancy. Br J Obstet Gynaecol 105:1205, 1998.
291. Brites D, Rodrigues CMP, Oliveira N, et al: Correction of maternal serum bile acid profile during ursodeoxycholic acid therapy in cholestasis of pregnancy. J Hepatol 28:91, 1998.
292. Serrano MA, Brites D, Larena MG, et al: Beneficial effect of ursodeoxycholic acid on alterations induced by cholestasis of pregnancy in bile acid transport across the human placenta. J Hepatol 28:829, 1998.
293. Reyes H: Intrahepatic cholestasis. A puzzling disorder of pregnancy. J Gastroenterol Hepatol 12:211, 1997.
294. Heinonen S, Kirkinen P: Pregnancy outcome with intrahepatic cholestasis. Obstet Gynecol 94:189, 1999.
295. Reyes H, Sjovall J: Bile acids and progesterone metabolites in intrahepatic cholestasis of pregnancy. Ann Med 32:94, 2000.
296. Reyes H, Baez ME, Gonzalez MC, et al: Selenium, zinc and copper plasma levels in intrahepatic cholestasis of pregnancy, in normal pregnancies and in healthy individuals, in Chile. J Hepatol 32:542, 2000.
297. Elias E: URSO in obstetric cholestasis: not a bear market. Gut 45:331, 1999.
298. Stieger B, Fattinger K, Madon J, et al: Drug- and estrogen-induced cholestasis through inhibition of the hepatocellular bile salt export pump (Bsep) of rat liver. Gastroenterology 118:422, 2000.
299. Cullberg G, Lundstrom R, Stenram U: Jaundice during treatment with an oral contraceptive, lyndiol. BMJ 1:695, 1965.
300. Eisalo A, Jarvinen PA, Luukkainen T: Hepatic impairment during the intake of contraceptive pills: clinical trial with postmenopausal women. BMJ 2:426, 1964.
301. Thulin KE, Nermark J: Seven cases of jaundice in women taking an oral contraceptive, anovlar. BMJ 1:684, 1966.
302. Kreek MJ, Weser E, Sleisenger MH, et al: Idiopathic cholestasis of pregnancy. N Engl J Med 277:1391, 1967.
303. Kreek MJ, Sleisenger MH, Jeffries GH: Recurrent cholestatic jaundice of pregnancy with demonstrated estrogen sensitivity. Am J Med 43:795, 1967.
304. Reyes H, Ribalta J, Gonzalez-Ceron M: Idiopathic cholestasis of pregnancy in a large kindred. Gut 17:709, 1976.
305. Holzbach RT, Sivak DA, Braun WE: Familial recurrent intrahepatic cholestasis of pregnancy: a genetic study providing evidence for transmission of a sex-limited, dominant trait. Gastroenterology 85:175, 1983.
306. De Pagter AGF, van Berge Henegouwen GP, ten Bokkel Huinink JA, et al: Familial benign recurrent intrahepatic cholestasis. Gastroenterology 71:202, 1976.

307. Dalen E, Westerholm B: Occurrence of hepatic impairment in women jaundiced by oral contraceptives and in their mothers and sisters. Acta Med Scand 195:459, 1974.
308. Reyes H, Ribalta J, Gonzalez C, et al: Sulfobromophthalein clearance tests before and after ethinyl estradiol administration, in women and men with familial history of intrahepatic cholestasis of pregnancy. Gastroenterology 81:226, 1981.
309. Jansen PLM, Muller M: Genetic cholestasis: lessons from the molecular physiology of bile formation. Can J Gastroenterol 14:233, 2000.
310. Thompson R, Jansen PLM: Genetic defects in hepatocanalicular transport. Semin Liver Dis 20:365, 2000.
311. Jacquemin E, Cresteil D, Manouvrier S, et al: Heterozygous nonsense mutation of the MDR3 gene in familial intrahepatic cholestasis of pregnancy. Lancet 353:210, 1999.
312. Dixon PH, Weerasekera N, Linton KJ, et al: Heterozygous MDR3 missense mutation associated with intrahepatic cholestasis of pregnancy: evidence for a defect in protein trafficking. Hum Mol Genet 9:1209, 2000.
313. Leevy CB, Koneru B, Klein KM: Recurrent familial prolonged intrahepatic cholestasis of pregnancy associated with chronic liver disease. Gastroenterology 113:966, 1997.
314. Davidson KM: Intrahepatic cholestasis of pregnancy. Semin Perinatol 22:104, 1998.
315. Kirkinen P, Ylostalo P, Heikkinen J, et al: Gallbladder function and maternal bile acids in intrahepatic cholestasis of pregnancy. Eur J Obstet Gynecol Reprod Biol 18:29, 1984.
316. Adlercreutz H, Svanborg A, Anberg A: Recurrent jaundice in pregnancy. I. A clinical and ultrastructural study. Am J Med 42:335, 1967.
317. Van Haelst U, Bergstein N: Electron microscopic study of the liver in so-called idiopathic jaundice of late pregnancy. Pathol Eur 5:198, 1970.
318. Zapata R, Sandoval L, Palma J, et al: Ursodeoxycholic acid in the treatment of intrahepatic cholestasis of pregnancy. A 10-year experience on its efficacy, safety and the perinatal outcome. Gastroenterology 118:A1008, 2000.
319. Olsson R, Tysk C, Aldenborg F, et al: Prolonged postpartum course of intrahepatic cholestasis of pregnancy. Gastroenterology 105:267, 1993.
320. Furhoff A-K, Hellstrom K: Jaundice in pregnancy. A follow-up study of the series of women originally reported by L. Thorling. II. Present health of the women. Acta Med Scand 196:181, 1974.
321. Laatikainen T, Ikonen E: Fetal prognosis in obstetric hepatosis. Ann Chir Gynaecol Fenniae 64:155, 1975.
322. Reid R, Ivey KJ, Rencoret RH, et al: Fetal complications of obstetric cholestasis. BMJ 1:870, 1976.
323. Davies MH, da Silva RCMA, Elias E, et al: Fetal mortality associated with cholestasis of pregnancy and the potential benefit of therapy with ursodeoxycholic acid. Gut 37:580, 1995.
324. Laatinainen T, Tulenheimo A: Maternal serum bile acid levels and fetal distress in cholestasis of pregnancy., Int J Gynaecol Obstet 22:91, 1984.
325. Alsulyman OM, Ouzounian JG, Ames-Castro M, et al: Intrahepatic cholestasis of pregnancy: perinatal outcome associated with expectant management. Am J Obstet Gynecol 175:957, 1996.
326. Laatikainen T, Ikonen E: Serum bile acids in cholestasis of pregnancy. Obstet Gynecol 50:313, 1977.
327. Savonius H, Riikonen S, Gylling H, et al: Pregnancy outcome with intrahepatic cholestasis. Acta Obstet Gynecol Scand 79:323, 2000.
328. Matos A, Bernardes J, Ayres-de-Campos D, et al: Antepartum fetal cerebral hemorrhage not predicted by current surveillance methods in cholestasis of pregnancy. Obstet Gynecol 89:803, 1997.
329. Heikkinen J, Maentausta O, Ylostalo P, et al: Serum bile acid levels in intrahepatic cholestasis of pregnancy during treatment with phenobarbital or cholestyramine. Eur J Obstet Gynecol Reprod Biol 14:153, 1982.
330. Sadler LC, Lane M, North R: Severe fetal intracranial haemorrhage during treatment with cholestyramine for intrahepatic cholestasis of pregnancy. Br J Obstet Gynaecol 102:169, 1995.
331. Trauner M, Graziadei IW: Mechanisms of action and therapeutic applications of ursodeoxycholic acid in chronic liver diseases. Aliment Pharmacol Ther 13:979, 1999.
332. Palma J, Reyes H, Ribalta J, et al: Effects of ursodeoxycholic acid in patients with intrahepatic cholestasis of pregnancy. Hepatology 15:1043, 1992.
333. Palma J, Reyes H, Ribalta J, et al: Ursodeoxycholic acid in the treatment of cholestasis of pregnancy: a randomized, double-blind study controlled with placebo. J Hepatol 27:1022, 1997.
334. Diaferia A, Nicastri PL, Tartagni M, et al: Ursodeoxycholic acid therapy in pregnant women with cholestasis. Int J Gynaecol Obstet 52:133, 1996.
335. Floreani A, Paternoster D, Melis A, et al: S-adenosylmethionine versus ursodeoxycholic acid in the treatment of intrahepatic cholestasis of pregnancy: preliminary results of a controlled trial. Eur J Obstet Gynecol Reprod Biol 67:109, 1996.
335a. Mazzella G, Nicola R, Francesco A, et al: Ursodeoxycholic acid administration in patients with cholestasis of pregnancy: effects on primary bile acids in babies and mothers. Hepatology 33:504, 2001.
336. Meng L-J, Reyes H, Palma J, et al: Effects of ursodeoxycholic acid on conjugated bile acids and progesterone metabolites in serum and urine of patients with intrahepatic cholestasis of pregnancy. J Hepatol 27:1029, 1997.
337. Di Padova C, Tritapepe R, Cammareri G, et al: S-adenosyl-L-methionine antagonizes ethynylestradiol-induced bile cholesterol supersaturation in humans without modifying the estrogen plasma kinetics. Gastroenterology 82:233, 1982.
338. Stramentinoli G, di Padova C, Gualano M, et al: Ethynylestradiol-induced impairment of bile secretion in the rat: Protective effects of S-adenosyl-L-methionine and its implication in estrogen metabolism. Gastroenterology 80:154, 1981.
339. Hirvioja M-L, Tuimala R, Vuori J: The treatment of intrahepatic cholestasis of pregnancy by dexamethasone. Br J Obstet Gynaecol 99:109, 1992.
340. Ribalta J, Reyes H, Gonzalez M, et al: *S*-Adenosyl-L-methionine in the treatment of patients with intrahepatic cholestasis of pregnancy: A randomized, double-blind, placebo-controlled study with negative results. Hepatology 13:1084, 1991.
341. Frezza M, Centini G, Cammareri G, et al: S-adenosylmethionine for the treatment of intrahepatic cholestasis of pregnancy. Results of a controlled clinical trial. Hepatogastroenterology 37(suppl II):122, 1990.
342. Sheehan HL: The pathology of acute yellow atrophy and delayed chloroform poisoning. J Obstet Gynaecol Brit Emp 47:40, 1940.
343. Sherlock S: Acute fatty liver of pregnancy and the microvesicular fat diseases. Gut 24:265, 1983.
344. Castro MA, Fassett MJ, Reynolds TB, et al: Reversible peripartum liver failure: a new perspective on the diagnosis, treatment, and cause of acute fatty liver of pregnancy, based on 28 consecutive cases. Am J Obstet Gynecol 181:389, 1999.
345. Partin JC, Schubert WK, Partin JS: Mitochondrial ultrastructure in Reye's syndrome (encephalopathy and fatty degeneration of the viscera). N Engl J Med 285:1339, 1971.
346. Bourgeois C, Olson L, Comer D, et al: Encephalopathy and fatty degeneration of the viscera: a clinicopathologic analysis of 40 cases. Am J Clin Pathol 56:558, 1971.
347. Heubi JE, Partin JC, Partin JS, et al: Reye's syndrome: current concepts. Hepatology 7:155, 1987.
348. Combes B, Whalley PJ, Adams RH: Tetracycline and the liver. In Popper H, Schaffner F, eds: Progress in Liver Diseases, vol. IV. New York, Grune and Stratton, 1972:5.
349. Strauss AW, Bennett MJ, Rinaldo P, et al: Inherited long-chain 3-hydroxyacyl-CoA dehydrogenase deficiency and a fetal-maternal interaction cause maternal liver disease and other pregnancy complications. Semin Perinatol 23:100, 1999.
350. Pockros PJ, Peters RL, Reynolds TB: Idiopathic fatty liver of pregnancy: findings in ten cases. Medicine 63:1, 1984.
351. Reyes H, Sandoval L, Wainstein A, et al: Acute fatty liver of pregnancy: a clinical study of 12 episodes in 11 patients. Gut 35:101, 1994.
352. Davies MH, Wilkinson SP, Hanid MA, et al: Acute liver disease with encephalopathy and renal failure in late pregnancy and early puerperium: a study of fourteen patients. Br J Obstet Gynaecol 87:1005, 1980.
353. Sheehan HL: Jaundice in pregnancy. Am J Obstet Gynecol 81:427, 1961.
354. Pereira SP, O'Donohue J, Wendon J, et al: Maternal and perinatal outcome in severe pregnancy-related liver disease. Hepatology 26:1258, 1997.
355. Eisele JW, Barker EA, Smuckler EA: Lipid content in the liver of fatty metamorphosis of pregnancy. Am J Pathol 81:545, 1975.
356. Kahil ME, Fred HL, Brown H, et al: Acute fatty liver of pregnancy. Arch Int Med 113:64, 1964.
357. Ober WB, LeCompte PM: Acute fatty metamorphosis of the liver associated with pregnancy. Am J Med 19:743, 1955.
358. Kunelis CT, Peters JL, Edmondson HA: Fatty liver of pregnancy and its relationship to tetracycline therapy. Am J Med 38:359, 1965.

359. Weber FL Jr, Snodgrass PJ, Powell DE, et al: Abnormalities of hepatic mitochondrial urea-cycle enzyme activities and hepatic ultrastructure in acute fatty liver of pregnancy. J Lab Clin Med 94:27, 1979.
360. Duma J, Dowling EA, Alexander HC, et al: Acute fatty liver of pregnancy. Ann Int Med 63:851, 1965.
361. Joske RA, McCully DJ, Mastaglia FL: Acute fatty liver of pregnancy. Gut 9:489, 1968.
362. Breen KJ, Perkins KW, Mistilis SP, et al: Idiopathic acute fatty liver of pregnancy. Gut 11:822, 1970.
363. Hatfield AK, Stein JH, Greenberger NJ, et al: Idiopathic acute fatty liver of pregnancy. Dig Dis Sci 17:167, 1972.
364. Holzbach RT: Acute fatty liver of pregnancy with disseminated intravascular coagulation. Obstet Gynecol 43:740, 1974.
365. Cano RI, Delman MR, Pitchumoni CS, et al: Acute fatty liver of pregnancy. JAMA 231:159, 1975.
366. MacKenna J, Pupkin M, Crenshaw C Jr, et al: Acute fatty metamorphosis of the liver. Am J Obstet Gynecol 127:400, 1977.
367. Moldin P, Johansson O: Acute fatty liver of pregnancy with disseminated intravascular coagulation. Acta Obstet Gynecol Scand 57:179, 1978.
368. Varner M, Rinderknecht NK: Acute fatty metamorphosis of pregnancy. J Reprod Med 24:177, 1980.
369. Koff RS: Weekly clinicopathological exercises. N Engl J Med 304:216, 1981.
370. Burroughs AK, Seong NH, Dojcinov DM, et al: Idiopathic acute fatty liver of pregnancy in 12 patients. QJM 51:481, 1982.
371. Korula J, Malatjalian DA, Badley BWD: Acute fatty liver of pregnancy. CMAJ 127:575, 1982.
372. Cheng CY: Acute fatty liver of pregnancy—survival despite associated severe preeclampsia, coma and coagulopathy. Aust N Z J Obstet Gynaecol 23:120, 1983.
373. Bernuau J, Degott C, Nouel O, et al: Non-fatal acute fatty liver of pregnancy. Gut 24:340, 1983.
374. Hague WM, Fenton DW, Duncan SLB, et al: Acute fatty liver of pregnancy. J Royal Soc Med 76:652, 1983.
375. Ebert EC, Sun EA, Wright SH, et al: Does early diagnosis and delivery in acute fatty liver of pregnancy lead to improvement in maternal and infant survival? Dig Dis Sci 29:453, 1984.
376. Hou SH, Levin S, Ahola S, et al: Acute fatty liver of pregnancy. Dig Dis Sci 29:449, 1984.
377. Rolfes DB, Ishak KG: Acute fatty liver of pregnancy: a clinicopathologic study of 35 cases. Hepatology 5:1149, 1985.
378. Czernobilsky B, Bergnes MA: Acute fatty metamorphosis of the liver in pregnancy with associated liver cell necrosis. Obstet Gynecol 26:792, 1965.
379. Laursen B, Frost L, Mortensen JZ, et al: Acute fatty liver of pregnancy with complicating disseminated intravascular coagulation. Acta Obstet Gynecol Scand 62:403, 1983.
380. Slater DN, Hague WM: Renal morphological changes in idiopathic acute fatty liver of pregnancy. Histopathology 8:567, 1984.
381. Sakamoto S, Tsuji Y, Koga S, et al: Idiopathic fatty liver of pregnancy with a subsequent uncomplicated pregnancy and a progressive increase in serum cholinesterase activity during the third trimester. A case report. Hepatogastroenterology 33:9, 1986.
382. Usta IM, Barton JR, Amon EA, et al: Acute fatty liver of pregnancy: an experience in the diagnosis and management of fourteen cases. Am J Obstet Gynecol 171:1342, 1994.
383. Schoeman MN, Batey RG, Wilcken B: Recurrent acute fatty liver of pregnancy associated with a fatty-acid oxidation defect in the offspring. Gastroenterology 100:544, 1991.
384. Visconti M, Manes G, Giannattasio F, et al: Recurrence of acute fatty liver of pregnancy. J Clin Gastroenterol 21:243, 1995.
385. Tyni T, Ekholm E, Pihko H: Pregnancy complications are frequent in long-chain 3-hydroxyacyl-coenzyme A dehydrogenase deficiency. Am J Obstet Gynecol 178:603, 1998.
386. Castro MA, Goodwin TM, Shaw KJ, et al: Disseminated intravascular coagulation and antithrombin III depression in acute fatty liver of pregnancy. Am J Obstet Gynecol 174:211, 1996.
387. Ibdah JA, Bennett MJ, Rinaldo P, et al: A fetal fatty-acid oxidation disorder as a cause of liver disease in pregnant women. N Engl J Med 340:1723, 1999.
388. Sattar N, Gaw A, Packard CJ, et al: Potential pathogenic roles of aberrant lipoprotein and fatty acid metabolism in pre-eclampsia. Br J Obstet Gynaecol 103:614, 1996.
389. Fromenty B, Berson A, Pessayre D: Microvesicular steatosis and steatohepatitis: role of mitochondrial dysfunction and lipid peroxidation. J Hepatol 26 (suppl 1):13, 1997.
390. Grimbert S, Fisch C, Deschamps D, et al: Effects of female sex hormones on mitochondria: possible role in acute fatty liver of pregnancy. Am J Physiol 268:G107, 1995.
391. Baldwin GS: Do NSAIDs contribute to acute fatty liver of pregnancy? Med Hypotheses 54:846, 2000.
392. Ibdah JA, Viola J, Zhao Y: Frequency of the association between maternal liver disease and fetal long chain 3-hydroxyl-CoA dehydrogenase deficiency. Gastroenterology 118:A1006, 2000.
393. Wilcken B, Leung K-C, Hammond J, et al: Pregnancy and fetal long-chain 3-hydroxyacyl coenzyme A dehydrogenase deficiency. Lancet 341:407, 1993.
394. Treem WR, Rinaldo P, Hale DE, et al: Acute fatty liver of pregnancy and long-chain 3-hydroxyacyl-coenzyme A dehydrogenase deficiency. Hepatology 19:339, 1994.
395. Treem WR, Shoup ME, Hale DE, et al: Acute fatty liver of pregnancy, hemolysis, elevated liver enzymes, and low platelets syndrome, and long chain 3-hydroxyacyl-coenzyme A dehydrogenase deficiency. Am J Gastroenterol 91:2293, 1996.
396. Isaacs JD, Sims HF, Powell CK, et al: Maternal acute fatty liver of pregnancy associated with fetal trifunctional protein deficiency: molecular characterization of a novel maternal mutant allele. Pediatr Res 40:393, 1996.
397. Tein I: Metabolic disease in the fetus predisposes to maternal hepatic complications of pregnancy. Pediatr Res 47:6, 2000.
397a. Washington University-St. Louis website. http://www.surgery.wustl.edu/bjcmdl/
398. Riely CA, Latham PS, Romero R, et al: Acute fatty liver of pregnancy: a reassessment based on observations in nine patients. Ann Int Med 106:703, 1987.
399. Liebman HA, McGehee WG, Patch MJ, et al: Severe depression of antithrombin III associated with disseminated intravascular coagulation in women with fatty liver of pregnancy. Ann Int Med 98:330, 1983.
400. Mosvold J, Abildgaard U, Henssen H, et al: Low antithrombin III in acute hepatic failure at term. Scand J Haematol 29:48, 1982.
401. Farine D, Newhouse J, Owen J, et al: Magnetic resonance imaging and computed tomography scan for the diagnosis of acute fatty liver of pregnancy. Am J Perinatol 7:316, 1990.
402. Clements D, Young WT, Thornton JG, et al: Imaging in acute fatty liver of pregnancy. Br J Obstet Gynaecol 97:631, 1990.
403. Maier J, Daugherty CC, Hug G, et al: Hepatic mitochondrial enzymes and ultrastructural abnormalities in acute fatty liver of pregnancy (AFLP). Gastroenterology 82:1123, 1982 (abstract).
404. Malatjalian DA, Badley BWD: Acute fatty liver of pregnancy. Light and electron microscopic studies. Gastroenterology 84:1384, 1983 (abstract).
405. Bertram PD, Anderson GD, Kelly S, et al: Ultrastructural alterations in acute fatty liver of pregnancy: similarity to Reye's syndrome. Gastroenterology 74:1008, 1978 (abstract).
406. Moise KJ Jr, Shah DM: Acute fatty liver of pregnancy: etiology of fetal distress and fetal wastage. Obstet Gynecol 69:482, 1987.
407. Breen KJ, Perkins KW, Schenker S, et al: Uncomplicated subsequent pregnancy after idiopathic fatty liver of pregnancy. Obstet Gynecol 40:831, 1972.
408. Barton JR, Sibai BM, Mabie WC, et al: Recurrent acute fatty liver of pregnancy. Am J Obstet Gynecol 163:534, 1990.
409. Purdie JM, Walters BNJ: Acute fatty liver of pregnancy: clinical features and diagnosis. Aust N Z J Obstet Gynaecol 28:62, 1988.
410. Ockner SA, Brunt EM, Cohn SM, et al: Fulminant hepatic failure caused by acute fatty liver of pregnancy treated by orthotopic liver transplantation. Hepatology 11:59, 1990.
411. Amon E, Allen SR, Petrie RH, et al: Acute fatty liver of pregnancy associated with preeclampsia. Am J Perinatol 8:278, 1991.
412. VanWijk MJ, Kublickiene K, Boer K, et al: Vascular function in preeclampsia. Cardiovasc Res 47:38, 2000.
413. Saphier CJ, Repke JT: Hemolysis, elevated liver enzymes, and low platelets (HELLP) syndrome: a review of diagnosis and management. Semin Perinatol 22:118, 1998.
414. Ellison J, Sattar N, Greer I: HELLP syndrome: mechanisms and management. Hosp Med 60:243, 1999.
415. Magann EF, Martin JN: Twelve steps to optimal management of HELLP syndrome. Clin Obstet Gynecol 42:532, 1999.
416. Grekin RJ, Dumont CJ, Vollmer AP, et al: Mechanisms in the pressor effects of hepatic portal venous fatty acid infusion. Am J Phys 273:R324, 1997.
417. den Boer ME, Ijlst L, Wijburg FA, et al: Heterozygosity for the common LCHAD mutation (1528G>C) is not a major cause of HELLP

syndrome and the prevalence of the mutation in the Dutch population is low. Pediatr Res 48:151, 2000.
418. Manas KJ, Welsh JD, Rankin RA, et al: Hepatic hemorrhage without rupture in preeclampsia. N Engl J Med 312:424, 1985.
419. MacKenna J, Dover NL, Brame RG: Preeclampsia associated with hemolysis, elevated liver enzymes, and low platelets—an obstetric emergency? Obstet Gynecol 62:751, 1983.
420. Beller FK, Dame WR, Ebert C: Pregnancy induced hypertension complicated by thrombocytopenia, haemolysis and elevated liver enzymes (HELLP) syndrome. Renal biopsies and outcome. Aust N Z J Obstet Gynecol 25:83, 1985.
421. Sibai BM, Taslimi MM, El-Nazer A, et al: Maternal-perinatal outcome associated with the syndrome of hemolysis, elevated liver enzymes, and low platelets in severe preeclampsia-eclampsia. Am J Obstet Gynecol 155:501, 1986.
422. Sibai BM, Ramadan MK, Usta I, et al: Maternal morbidity and mortality in 442 pregnancies with hemolysis, elevated liver enzymes, and low platelets (HELLP syndrome). Am J Obstet Gynecol 169:1000, 1993.
423. Martin JN, Rinehart BK, May WL, et al: The spectrum of severe preeclampsia: comparative analysis by HELLP (hemolysis, elevated liver enzyme levels, and low platelet count) syndrome classification. Am J Obstet Gynecol 180:1373, 1999.
424. Villegas H, Azuela JC, Maqueo M: Spontaneous rupture of liver in toxemia of pregnancy. Int J Gynecol Obstet 8:836, 1970.
425. Hibbard LT: Maternal mortality due to acute toxemia. Obstet Gynecol 42:263, 1973.
426. Maqueo M, Ayala LC, Cervantes L: Nutritional status and liver function in toxemia of pregnancy. Obstet Gynecol 23:222, 1964.
427. Arias F, Mancilla-Jimenez R: Hepatic fibrinogen deposits in preeclampsia. N Engl J Med 295:578, 1976.
428. Sheehan HL, Lynch JB: Pathology of Toxemia of Pregnancy. Edinburgh, Churchill Livingstone, 1973:328.
429. Minakami H, Oka N, Sato T, et al: Preeclampsia: a microvesicular fat disease of the liver? Am J Obstet Gynecol 159:1043, 1988.
430. Dani R, Mendes GS, Medeiros JDL, et al: Study of the liver changes occurring in preeclampsia and their possible pathogenetic connection with acute fatty liver of pregnancy. Am J Gastroenterol 91:292, 1996.
431. Barton JR, Riely CA, Adamee TA: Hepatic histopathologic condition does not correlate with laboratory abnormalities in HELLP syndrome (hemolysis, elevated liver enzymes, and low platelet count). Am J Obstet Gynecol 167:1538, 1992.
432. Weinstein L: Syndrome of hemolysis, elevated liver enzymes, and low platelet count: A severe consequence of hypertension in pregnancy. Am J Obstet Gynecol 142:159, 1982.
433. Reubinoff BE, Schenker JG: HELLP syndrome—a syndrome of hemolysis, elevated liver enzymes and low platelet count—complicating preeclampsia-eclampsia. Int J Gynecol Obstet 36:95, 1991.
434. Sibai BM: The HELLP syndrome (hemolysis, elevated liver enzymes, and low platelets). Am J Obstet Gynecol 162:311, 1990.
435. Aarnoudse JG, Houthoff HJ, Weits J, et al: A syndrome of liver damage and intravascular coagulation in the last trimester of normotensive pregnancy. A clinical and histopathological study. Br J Obstet Gynaecol 93:145, 1986.
436. Pritchard JA, Weisman R Jr, Ratnoff OD, et al: Intravascular hemolysis, thrombocytopenia and other hematologic abnormalities associated with severe toxemia of pregnancy. N Engl J Med 250:89, 1954.
437. Killam AP, Dillard SH Jr, Patton RC, et al: Pregnancy-induced hypertension complicated by acute liver disease and disseminated intravascular coagulation. Am J Obstet Gynecol 123:823, 1975.
438. Goodlin RC: Severe pre-eclampsia. Another great imitator. Am J Obstet Gynecol 125:747, 1976.
439. Long RG, Scheuer PJ, Sherlock S: Pre-eclampsia presenting with deep jaundice. J Clin Pathol 30:212, 1977.
440. Goodlin RC, Cotton DB, Haesslein HC: Severe enema-proteinuria-hypertension gestosis. Am J Obstet Gynecol 132:595, 1978.
441. Goodlin RC, Holt D: Impending gestosis. Obstet Gynecol 58:743, 1981.
442. Schwartz ML, Brenner WE: Pregnancy-induced hypertension presenting with life-threatening thrombocytopenia. Am J Obstet Gynecol 146:756, 1983.
443. Thiagarajah S, Bourgeois FJ, Harbert GM Jr, et al: Thrombocytopenia in preeclampsia: Associated abnormalities and management principles. Am J Obstet Gynecol 150:1, 1984.
444. Bertakis KD, Hufford DB: Hemolysis, elevated liver enzymes and low platelet count. West J Med 144:81, 1986.
445. Clark SL, Phelan JR, Allen SH, et al: Antepartum reversal of hematologic abnormalities associated with the HELLP syndrome. J Reprod Med 31:70, 1986.
446. Weinstein L: Preeclampsia/eclampsia with hemolysis, elevated liver enzymes, and thrombocytopenia. Obstet Gynecol 66:657, 1985.
447. Haddad B, Barton JR, Livingston JC, et al: Risk factors for adverse maternal outcomes among women with HELLP (hemolysis, elevated liver enzymes, and low platelet count) syndrome. Am J Obstet Gynecol 183:444, 2000.
448. Cunningham FG, Lowe T, Guss S, et al: Erythrocyte morphology in women with severe preeclampsia and eclampsia. Am J Obstet Gynecol 153:358, 1985.
449. Calvin S, Silva M, Weinstein L, et al: Characterization of ascites present at cesarean section. Am J Perinatol 8:99, 1991.
450. Woods JB, Blake PG, Perry KG Jr, et al: Ascites: A portent of cardiopulmonary complications in the preeclamptic patient with the syndrome of hemolysis, elevated liver enzymes, and low platelets. Obstet Gynecol 80:87, 1992.
451. Freund G, Arvan DA: Clinical biochemistry of preeclampsia and related liver diseases of pregnancy. Clin Chim Acta 191:123, 1990.
452. Faridi A, Heyl W, Rath W: Preliminary results of the International HELLP-Multicenter-Study. Int J Gynaecol Obstet 69:279, 2000.
453. Rath W, Loos W, Kuhn W, et al: The importance of early laboratory screening methods for maternal and fetal outcome in cases of HELLP syndrome. Eur J Obstet Gynecol Reprod Biol 36:43, 1990.
454. Martin JN Jr, Blake PG, Perry KG Jr, et al: The natural history of HELLP syndrome. Am J Obstet Gynecol 164:1500, 1991.
455. Knapen MF, van Altena AM, Peters WH, et al: Liver function following pregnancy complicated by the HELLP syndrome. Br J Obstet Gynaecol 105:1208, 1998.
456. Sullivan CA, Magann EF, Perry KG, et al: The recurrence risk of the syndrome of hemolysis, elevated liver enzymes, and low platelets (HELLP) in subsequent gestations. Am J Obstet Gynecol 171:940, 1994.
457. Sibai BM, Ramadan MK, Chari RS, et al: Pregnancies complicated by HELLP syndrome (hemolysis, elevated liver enzymes, and low platelets): subsequent pregnancy outcome and long-term prognosis. Am J Obstet Gynecol 172:125, 1995.
458. Brazy JE, Grimm JK, Little VA: Neonatal manifestations of severe maternal hypertension occurring before the thirty-sixth week of pregnancy. J Pediatr 100:265, 1982.
459. Martin JN, Perry KG, Blake PG, et al: Better maternal outcomes are achieved with dexamethasone therapy for postpartum HELLP (hemolysis, elevated liver enzymes, and thrombocytopenia) syndrome. Am J Obstet Gynecol 177:1011, 1997.
460. Tompkins MJ, Thiagarajah S: HELLP (hemolysis, elevated liver enzymes, and low platelet count) syndrome: the benefit of corticosteroids. Am J Obstet Gynecol 181:304, 1999.
461. Ralston SJ, Schwaitzberg SD: Liver hematoma and rupture in pregnancy. Semin Perinatol 22:141, 1998.
462. Stain SC, Woodburn DA, Stephens AL: Spontaneous hepatic hemorrhage associated with pregnancy treatment by hepatic arterial interruption. Ann Surg 224:73, 1996.
463. Sheikh RA, Yasmeen S, Pauly MP, et al: Spontaneous intrahepatic hemorrhage and hepatic rupture in the HELLP syndrome. J Clin Gastroenterol 28:323, 1999.
464. Smith LG Jr, Moise KJ Jr, Dildy GA III, et al: Spontaneous rupture of liver during pregnancy. Obstet Gynecol 77:171, 1991.
465. Gordon SC, Meyer RA, Rosenberg BF: Laparoscopic diagnosis of subcapsular hepatic hemorrhage in pre-eclamptic liver disease. Gastrointest Endosc 38:718, 1992.
466. Dammann HG, Hagemann J, Runge M, et al: In vivo diagnosis of massive hepatic infarction by computed tomography. Dig Dis Sci 27:73, 1982.
467. Hunter SK, Martin M, Benda JA, et al: Liver transplant after massive spontaneous hepatic rupture in pregnancy complicated by preeclampsia. Obstet Gynecol 85:819, 1995.
468. Lavery JP, Berg J: Subcapsular hematoma of the liver during pregnancy. South Med J 82:1568, 1989.
469. Schiffer MA: Fatty liver associated with administration of tetracycline in pregnant and nonpregnant women. Am J Obstet Gynecol 96:326, 1966.
470. Wenk RE, Gebhardt FC, Bhagavan BS, et al: Tetracycline-associated fatty liver of pregnancy, including possible pregnancy risk after chronic dermatologic use of tetracycline. J Reprod Med 26:135, 1981.

C H A P T E R

55

Liver Transplantation

Andy S. Yu, MD, and Emmet B. Keeffe, MD

Liver transplantation is a major advance in modern medicine. It has been an established therapy for a wide variety of acute and chronic liver diseases since the early 1980s. Liver transplantation has evolved from an experimental procedure with modest success before 1980 to a standard operation with excellent survival rates for patients who previously carried a grim prognosis from advanced and irreversible liver failure.

EARLY DEVELOPMENT OF LIVER TRANSPLANTATION AND IMMUNOSUPPRESSION

Initial Experience with Human Liver Transplantation

Key events in the development of liver transplantation are summarized in Table 55-1.[1,2] The first experimental liver transplantations were attempted by Welch in 1955[3] and Cannon in 1956.[4] It was not until 1963 that Starzl and his colleagues performed the first liver transplantations in humans.[2,5] Three patients underwent attempted transplantation in that year, but all died either on the table or on postoperative days 7 and 22, respectively. The first 1-year survival after liver transplantation was achieved in 1967, when a pediatric patient transplanted for hepatoblastoma survived 18 months before succumbing to metastases. Starzl and his team performed approximately one liver transplant per month at the University of Colorado from 1968 to 1980, with a 1-year mortality of greater than 50 percent but long-term survival rate of only 30 percent.[6] Prednisone, azathioprine, and polyclonal anti-lymphocyte globulin was the usual immunosuppressive regimen in this early experience. With the very narrow efficacy-to-safety margin of these medications, rejection and sepsis were quite common.

TABLE 55-1
Key Events in the Development of Liver Transplantation

Year	Event
1955	First experimental auxiliary liver transplantation (Welch)
1956	First experimental orthotopic liver transplantation (Cannon)
1963	Use of azathioprine and prednisone for immunosuppression
1963	First human liver transplantations (Starzl)
1966	Introduction of anti-lymphocyte globulin
1967	First 1-year survival after human liver transplantation (Starzl)
1980	Introduction of cyclosporine for immunosuppression
1983	NIH Consensus Development Conference on liver transplantation
1987	Use of University of Wisconsin solution for improved organ preservation
1989	Introduction of tacrolimus for immunosuppression

Modified from Keeffe EB: Liver transplantation at the millennium: past, present, and future. Clin Liver Dis 4:241-255, 2000.

Evolution of Immunosuppression

The development of more effective and safer immunosuppressive regimens was the key factor that facilitated expansion of liver and other solid organ transplantation (Table 55-2). The single most important factor responsible for long-term survival after liver transplantation was the development of the calcineurin inhibitor cyclosporine. This drug was used initially as a single agent in renal transplantation and was introduced subsequently to liver transplantation in combination with corticosteroids.[7,8] This combination was associated with an increase in the 1-year survival after liver transplantation from approximately 30 percent to more than 70 percent by the late 1970s and early 1980s.[9-12] These developments led the National Institutes of Health (NIH) Consensus Development Conference to conclude that liver transplantation should be classified as a therapeutic modality that deserved broader application and appropriate funding.[13] This meeting initiated the modern era of liver transplantation, stimulated the provision of financial coverage by the various third-party payers, and led to the development of liver transplantation centers across the United States.

TABLE 55-2
Evolution of Immunosuppressive Drug Regimens

Year	Agent
1962	Azathioprine
1963	Azathioprine plus corticosteroids
1966	Polyclonal antibodies; anti-lymphocyte globulin as an adjunct
1970	Cyclophosphamide substituted for azathioprine
1978	Cyclosporine use in humans
1980	Cyclosporine plus corticosteroids
1981	Development of monoclonal antibodies (e.g., muromonab-CD3)
1989	Tacrolimus plus corticosteroids
1990s	Development of newer agents (e.g., mycophenolate mofetil, sirolimus [rapamycin], anti-interleukin-2 receptor antibodies basiliximab and daclizumab)

Modified from Keeffe EB: Liver transplantation at the millennium: past, present, and future. Clin Liver Dis 4:241-255, 2000.

Further advances in immunosuppressive regimens included the development of tacrolimus and anti-lymphocyte antibody therapy. Tacrolimus is another calcineurin inhibitor that has some improved features over cyclosporine. When compared directly with cyclosporine as the basis of a multiple-drug immunosuppressive regimen, tacrolimus achieved similar recipient and graft survivals, significantly fewer episodes of acute cellular rejection and steroid-resistant rejection, lower cumulative dose of steroid exposure, less use of muromonab-CD3, and a less adverse short-term cardiovascular risk profile.[14-19]

Anti-lymphocyte antibody therapy, including muromonab-CD3, has been used as part of induction regimens to reduce the incidence and severity of acute allograft rejection and, more often, to treat steroid-resistant acute rejection.[20-22] It is occasionally used as induction therapy without calcineurin inhibitors in the setting of renal insufficiency. Muromonab-CD3 initially replaced earlier anti-lymphocyte and anti-thymocyte preparations but in recent years has been superseded by newer agents that lower risks of post-transplant lymphoproliferative disorders (PTLD), earlier and more severe allograft injury from hepatitis C, and infections from cytomegalovirus (CMV) and Epstein-Barr virus (EBV) associated with muromonab-CD3.

Other drugs that are effective in kidney transplantation are being tested in clinical trials to determine their role in liver transplantation. These include mycophenolate mofetil, sirolimus, and two anti-interleukin-2 receptor antibodies, basiliximab and daclizumab.[23,24] Both basiliximab and daclizumab have no major side effects and may be important in the future for immunosuppression in patients at risk of calcineurin-induced side effects.

More Recent Developments in Liver Transplantation

Better immunosuppressive drug regimens, further technical advances, and improved perioperative care have resulted in current 1-year post–liver transplantation survival rates of 85 percent.[25] The diagnosis and treatment of acute cellular rejection and chronic ductopenic rejection have improved.[26] The use of long-term steroid-free and low-dose immunosuppressive regimens is safer and has less toxicity. Better patient selection, refinement and standardization of organ procurement and implantation techniques, perioperative management of hemodynamic and metabolic problems by dedicated liver transplant anesthesiologists, and introduction of venovenous bypass have contributed to the improved outcomes of liver transplantation. The use of primary duct-to-duct anastomosis without T-tubes or stents has reduced the rate of biliary complications from 50 percent to less than 15 percent.[6,27] Radiologic and endoscopic diagnostic and therapeutic procedures have facilitated the management of biliary complications with lower rates of morbidity. Venovenous bypass is seldom used now but was once an effective technique to support a patient's hemodynamics during the anhepatic phase of surgery. Currently, the use of blood during surgery averages less than 10 U, and up to 30 percent of liver transplantations can be performed without transfusion.[28] The prophylaxis and treatment of opportunistic infections in immunocompromised recipients have also improved.[29] Routine prophylactic regimens after liver transplantations for bacterial, fungal, and viral infections, including CMV and *Pneumocystis carinii* infections, have decreased these potentially serious infectious complications of transplantation.

SELECTION OF PATIENTS FOR LIVER TRANSPLANTATION

Indications and Selection Criteria

The goals of liver transplantation are to prolong and improve the quality of life. Published data support that these objectives are achievable. The 1-year recipient survival rates are 85 percent to 90 percent for most liver diseases (Table 55-3).[30] The only exception is hepatic malignancies, which are associated with a 72 percent 1-year survival. Additionally, multiple quality-of-life studies show that liver transplantation significantly improves the physical, cognitive, and psychologic functioning of recipients.[31-34] Recently, the rapidly escalating disparity between the limited supply of cadaver donor organs and the increased need for liver transplantation and the contraction in funding for transplantation have created a mandate to optimize resources and cost-effectiveness and avoid retransplantation.[35-37]

The indications and contraindications for liver transplantation, optimal timing of transplantation, and the most appropriate candidates to receive the scarce organs continue to evolve and be debated.[38,39] The diseases for which liver transplantation has been performed in adults can be divided into the broad categories of cirrhosis with end-stage liver disease, acute liver failure, hepatic malignancies—particularly hepatocellular carcinoma—and metabolic diseases in which the inborn error of metabolism resides in the hepatocytes.

Many miscellaneous metabolic diseases have been treated with liver transplantation.[30] The indications for

TABLE 55-3

Survival after Adult Liver Transplantation by Diagnosis

	SURVIVAL (%)*		
Diagnosis	**1 yr**	**4 yr**	**7 yr**
Primary sclerosing cholangitis	91	84	78
Primary biliary cirrhosis	89	84	79
Autoimmune hepatitis	86	81	78
Chronic hepatitis C	86	75	67
Alcoholic liver disease	85	76	63
Cryptogenic cirrhosis	84	76	67
Chronic hepatitis B	83	71	63
Malignancy	72	43	34

Data from Seaberg EC, Belle SH, Beringer KC, et al: Liver transplantation in the United States from 1987-1998: updated results from the Pitt-UNOS liver transplant registry. In Cecka JM, Terasaki PI, eds: Clinical Transplants 1998. Los Angeles, UCLA Tissue Typing Laboratory, 1999:17-37.
*UNOS database 1987-1998; n = 24,900 patients.

transplantation in patients with various metabolic disorders include liver failure, incipient failure of a second organ, or development of an early hepatocellular carcinoma. The majority of the cases are dominated clinically by obvious parenchyma liver disease, and patients are transplanted for liver failure or early development of a malignant hepatic tumor. Examples of this former category include hemochromatosis, α_1-antitrypsin deficiency, Wilson's disease, tyrosinemia, and glycogen storage disease types I, III, and IV.[40-44] However, patients with histologically normal livers have also undergone liver transplantation to correct the metabolic defect that resides in extrahepatic organs, such as in type I hyperoxaluria, familial homozygous hypercholesterolemia, urea cycle enzyme deficiency, and hemophilia A and B.[44-49]

The most common indications for liver transplantation are chronic hepatitis C and alcoholic liver disease in adults, biliary atresia, and α_1-antitrypsin deficiency in children.[30] Other common indications for adult liver transplantation are primary biliary cirrhosis, primary sclerosing cholangitis, autoimmune hepatitis, chronic hepatitis B, metabolic diseases including hemochromatosis and Wilson's disease, acute liver failure, and hepatocellular carcinoma (Table 55-4).[30]

Tables 55-5 and 55-6 list the general criteria that should be considered in the referral and selection of patients with end-stage liver disease and acute liver failure for liver transplantation.[38,50,51] Besides accepted indications for liver transplantation, other general patient selection criteria, in considering referral for liver transplantation, are the absence of alternative forms of therapy that may reverse liver failure and the absence of any absolute contraindication to transplantation. (Contraindications are discussed in the following section.) Another important criterion, which is often subjective and more difficult to determine, is that the patient should be willing to accept liver transplantation and be able to comply with follow-up care. Finally, patients should be able to meet the huge financial costs of liver transplantation and the pretransplant evaluation and the follow-up medical care, including medications that may be expensive. Insurance coverage for transplantation should be determined before referral by a financial counselor at the transplant center.

The available clinical, laboratory, radiologic, histologic, psychosocial, and financial data of a potential candidate are first reviewed to determine whether these selection criteria are met. The worsening disparity between the paucity of cadaveric donor livers and the increasing number of potential transplant recipients has resulted in increased pretransplant deaths, which currently approximates 20 percent of listed patients, and

TABLE 55-4

Liver Disease of Adult Transplant Recipients in the United States*

Primary liver disease	Number	Percent
Chronic hepatitis C	5155	20.7
Alcoholic liver disease	4258	17.1
Alcoholic liver disease and hepatitis C	1106	4.4
Chronic hepatitis B	1368	5.5
Cryptogenic cirrhosis	2719	10.9
Primary biliary cirrhosis	2317	9.3
Primary sclerosing cholangitis	2178	8.7
Autoimmune hepatitis	1194	4.8
Acute liver failure	1555	6.2
Hepatic malignancy	951	3.8
Metabolic diseases	923	3.7
Other	1050	4.2
Unknown	126	0.5

Adapted from Seaberg EC, Belle SH, Beringer KC, et al: Liver transplantation in the United States from 1987-1998: updated results from the Pitt-UNOS liver transplant registry. In: Cecka JM, Terasaki PI, eds: Clinical Transplants 1998. Los Angeles, UCLA Tissue Typing Laboratory, 1999:17-37.
*UNOS database 1987-1998; n = 24,900.

TABLE 55-5

Patient Selection for Liver Transplantation

Accepted indications for liver transplantation
- Advanced chronic liver failure
- Acute liver failure
- Hepatocellular carcinoma
- Miscellaneous liver diseases

No alternative forms of therapy
No absolute contraindications to liver transplantation
Willingness and ability to accept liver transplantation and comply with follow-up care
Ability to provide for the costs of liver transplantation and post-transplant care

From Keeffe EB: Selection of patients for liver transplantation. In Maddrey WC, Sorrell MF, Schiff ER, eds: Transplantation of the Liver, ed 3. Philadelphia, Lippincott Williams & Wilkins, 2001:5-34.

TABLE 55-6

Criteria for Liver Transplantation in Fulminant Hepatic Failure

Criteria of King's College, London[1]

Acetaminophen patients

pH < 7.3 or prothrombin > 6.5 (INR) and serum creatinine > 3.4 mg/dl

Non-acetaminophen Patients

Prothrombin time > 6.5 (INR) or any three of the following variable:

1. Age < 10 or > 40 years
2. Etiology: non-A, non-B hepatitis; halothane hepatitis; idiosyncratic drug reaction
3. Duration of jaundice before encephalopathy > 7 days
4. Prothrombin time > 3.5 (INR)
5. Serum bilirubin > 17.6 mg/dl

Criteria of Hospital Paul-Brousse, Villejuif, France[2]

Hepatic encephalopathy and

1. Factor V level < 20% in patient younger than 30 years of age or
2. Factor V level < 30% in patient 30 years of age or older

Adapted from O'Grady JG, Alexander GJ, Hayllar KM, Williams R: Early indicators of prognosis in fulminant hepatic failure. Gastroenterology 97(2):439-445, 1989; Bernuau J, Samuel D, Durand F, et al: Criteria for emergency liver transplantation in patients with acute viral hepatitis and factor V below 50% of normal: a prospective study. Hepatology 14:49A, 1991 (abstract); Keeffe EB: Selection of patients for liver transplantation. In Maddrey WC, Sorrell MF, Schiff ER, eds: Transplantation of the Liver, ed 3. Philadelphia, Lippincott Williams & Wilkins, 2001:5-34.
INR, International normalized ratio.

TABLE 55-7

Contraindications to Liver Transplantation*

Compensated cirrhosis without complications (Child-Turcotte-Pugh score 5-6)
Extrahepatic malignancy
Active untreated sepsis
Advanced cardiopulmonary disease
Active alcoholism or substance abuse
Anatomic abnormality precluding liver transplantation

*In most, but not all, centers cholangiocarcinoma and human immunodeficiency virus infection are also considered contraindications to liver transplantation.

TABLE 55-8

Non–disease-specific Minimal Listing Criteria

Immediate need for liver transplantation
Estimated 1-year survival ≤ 90%
CTP class B or C (CTP score ≥ 7)
Portal hypertensive bleeding or a single episode of spontaneous bacterial peritonitis, irrespective of CTP score

Adapted from Lucey MR, Brown KA, Everson GT, et al: Minimal criteria for placement of adults on the liver transplant waiting list: a report of a national conference organized by the American Society of Transplant Physicians and the American Association for the Study of Liver Diseases. Liver Transpl Surg 3(6):628-637, 1997.
CTP, Child-Turcotte-Pugh.

the performance of liver transplantation in sicker patients. In general, patients should be referred when hepatic decompensation first develops. Recipient survival significantly decreases and the costs of transplantation markedly increase by the time multi-organ failure occurs. The greatest likelihood of survival and return to an excellent quality of life occurs in recipients who undergo liver transplantation before repeated hospitalizations are necessary. The contraindications to liver transplantation, which have evolved over the past two decades by broad consensus, are noted in Table 55-7.

Minimal Listing Criteria for Liver Transplantation

Minimal listing criteria for liver transplantation were developed at a consensus conference held at the NIH in 1997 and organized by the American Society of Transplant Physicians and the American Association for the Study of Liver Diseases (Table 55-8).[52] The goal of this conference was to establish rational and uniform listing criteria for placing patients with advanced chronic liver disease on the United Network for Organ Sharing (UNOS) waiting list for liver transplantation. It was hoped that the practice of padding the list with patients with less severe liver disease—for them to achieve longer waiting times and a higher priority for a donor organ—could be avoided.

The natural history of compensated and decompensated cirrhosis was the most important factor used for establishing the so-called minimal listing criteria. The survival of patients with cirrhosis is significantly reduced after the development of decompensation (e.g., ascites, portal hypertensive bleeding, encephalopathy).[53-55] In a natural history study of patients with chronic hepatitis C and compensated cirrhosis, the probabilities of decompensation after the diagnosis of cirrhosis were 18 percent at 5 years and 29 percent at 10 years. The 5-year survival was 91 percent in patients who remained without decompensation versus 50 percent in patients with decompensation.[55] Ascites carries a poor prognosis in part because of the associated risks of spontaneous bacterial peritonitis and hepatorenal syndrome. The University of Barcelona reported 1-year survival rate of 66 percent for patients without versus 38 percent for those with an episode of spontaneous bacterial peritonitis.[56] The development of hepatorenal syndrome confers a very poor prognosis, with a median survival of only 1.7 weeks in one study.[57] Finally, mortality after variceal bleeding is high, despite treatment with endoscopic therapy with band ligation or sclerotherapy, transjugular intrahepatic portosystemic shunt (TIPS), or a surgical shunt.[58,59] The

TABLE 55-9

Child-Turcotte-Pugh Classification*

	1 point	2 points	3 points
Bilirubin (mg/dl)	<2	2-3	>3
PBC and PSC patients	<4	4-10	>10
Albumin (g/dl)	<3.5	2.8-3.5	<2.8
PT: seconds prolonged	1-3	4-6	>6
INR	<1.7	1.7-2.3	>2.3
Ascites	None	Slight, or controlled medically	Moderate or severe
Encephalopathy	None	Stage 1-2	Stage 3-4

From Child CG III, Turcotte JG: Surgery and portal hypertension. In Child CG III, ed: The Liver and Portal Hypertension. Philadelphia, WB Saunders Co., 1964:50-64; Pugh RNH, Murray-Lyon IM, Dawson JJ, et al: Transection of the oesophagus for bleeding oesophageal varices. Br J Surg 60(8):646-649, 1973.

PBC, Primary biliary cirrhosis; *PSC,* primary sclerosing cholangitis; *PT,* prothrombin time; *INR,* international normalized ratio.

*Child-Turcotte-Pugh class and score: A = 5-6 points, B = 7-9 points, C = 10-15 points.

definitive therapy for patients with cirrhosis and variceal bleeding is liver transplantation.

The minimal listing criteria were based on the premise that a suitable candidate for liver transplantation should have an estimated 90 percent or less chance of surviving 1 year with supportive care (i.e., an estimated survival rate based on the natural history of the underlying liver disease is less than that expected with liver transplantation at most centers). The Child-Turcotte-Pugh (CTP) scoring system is now used routinely in the assessment of candidacy for liver transplantation (Table 55-9).[60,61] A patient with CTP score of 5 or 6 (Child's A cirrhosis) without a history of portal hypertensive bleeding or spontaneous bacterial peritonitis is likely to remain stable for a considerable period and not require listing. Criteria for listing should be clinical decompensation of cirrhosis, particularly portal hypertensive bleeding or spontaneous bacterial peritonitis, or combined clinical decompensation and biochemical deterioration of synthetic and excretory functions that yield a CTP score of 7 or greater (Child's class B or C). The minimal listing criteria imply that after a transplant center lists a patient, it is prepared to transplant that patient immediately should the donor liver become available.

Biochemical and Clinical Indications for Liver Transplantation

Advanced chronic end-stage liver disease and acute liver failure are usually associated with a parallel deterioration in the quality of life and worsening of liver biochemistry compatible with impaired synthetic and excretory liver functions. Identification of threshold laboratory indices or specific clinical complications of liver disease should prompt referral and initiation of the process leading to liver transplantation.[38,62-68] Table 55-10 outlines the major clinical and biochemical indications for liver transplantation. Mild hepatic encephalopathy alone is not an indication for liver transplantation because it generally responds well to medical therapy, including lactulose or neomycin, and modest restriction of dietary protein.[69] Encephalopathy of recent onset should prompt search for a precipitant factor. On the other hand, progressive or recurrent hepatic encephalopathy should prompt consideration for liver transplantation.

TABLE 55-10

Biochemical and Clinical Indications for Liver Transplantation in Chronic Liver Disease

I. Cholestatic liver disease
   A. Bilirubin > 10 mg/dl
   B. Intractable pruritus
   C. Progressive cholestatic bone disease
   D. Recurrent bacterial cholangitis
II. Hepatocellular liver disease
   A. Serum albumin < 3.0 g/dl
   B. Prothrombin time > 3 seconds above control
III. Both cholestatic and hepatocellular liver diseases
   A. Recurrent or severe hepatic encephalopathy
   B. Refractory ascites
   C. Spontaneous bacterial peritonitis
   D. Recurrent portal hypertensive bleeding
   E. Severe chronic fatigue and weakness
   F. Progressive malnutrition
   G. Development of hepatorenal syndrome
   H. Detection of small hepatocellular carcinoma

From Keeffe EB: Selection of patients for liver transplantation. In Maddrey WC, Sorrell MF, Schiff ER, eds: Transplantation of the Liver, ed 3. Philadelphia, Lippincott Williams & Wilkins, 2001:5-34.

Ascites becomes refractory when it can no longer be mobilized because of (1) a lack of response to dietary sodium restriction and intensive diuretic treatment or (2) diuretic-induced complications precluding use of an effective diuretic regimen.[70] One-year survival is 25 percent for cirrhotic patients with refractory ascites.[71] TIPS has emerged as the therapy of choice for selected patients with refractory ascites that recurs despite serial large-volume paracenteses but without far-advanced liver failure.[72,73] Improved survival without liver transplantation after placement of TIPS may be due to improved nutritional status and decreased risk of spontaneous bacterial peritonitis with resolution of ascites.[74] In light of the organ shortage, referral for liver transplantation should not be delayed until the onset of ominous clinical features such as refractory ascites or spontaneous bacterial peritonitis.[75]

In the setting of spontaneous bacterial peritonitis most transplant programs will defer transplantation until antibiotic treatment has been commenced for 48 hours and resolution of infection is documented on repeat paracentesis.[38] Ascitic fluid becomes sterile in 86 percent of patients after one dose of cefotaxime, and the corresponding neutrophil count achieves an average of 75 percent reduction at 48 hours of therapy.[76] Moreover, 5 days of cefotaxime is as efficacious as 10 days and is significantly less expensive.[77,78] Use of antibiotic prophylaxis is effective in decreasing recurrent infections but does not improve survival.[79-82] After a patient has had an episode of spontaneous bacterial peritonitis, the outcome after liver transplantation is not as favorable.[83]

A single episode of variceal bleeding meets the minimal listing criteria for liver transplantation.[52] Patients who experienced esophagogastric variceal bleeding have a poor 5-year prognosis irrespective of treatment.[84-87] The likelihood of developing varices in patients with cirrhosis ranges from 35 percent to 80 percent. After esophageal varices develop, bleeding occurs in 25 percent to 30 percent of cases within the first 2 years.[84,86] The success rate of controlling the initial variceal bleeding is 70 percent to 90 percent, and 70 percent of variceal bleeders will rebleed within 1 year after the index event. Each bleeding event carries a mortality rate of 35 percent to 50 percent.

TIPS serves as the most ideal "bridge" to liver transplantation for patients without advanced liver failure and with portal hypertensive bleeding refractory to conventional endoscopic therapy.[88-90] TIPS usually avoids the need for a surgical shunt procedure that carries high morbidity and mortality, alters the extrahepatic anatomy, and renders future hepatobiliary surgery technically difficult.[91] Nevertheless, a poorly positioned TIPS also may complicate subsequent liver transplantation.[92] TIPS carries 23 percent risk of hepatic encephalopathy,[93] may worsen liver function, and may even precipitate liver failure by diverting portal blood.[94] Other complications of TIPS include postprocedural bleed, stent occlusion from early thrombosis or late neointimal hyperplasia, congestive heart failure from volume redistribution, contrast nephropathy, infection and mechanical hemolysis.[95] TIPS does not have a positive impact on the course of liver transplantation surgery (i.e., less operative blood loss) and thus should not be employed solely for preoperative portal decompression in the absence of refractory variceal hemorrhage.[96]

Emergency surgical shunts remain the last therapeutic resort for refractory portal hypertensive bleeding, but mortality is high and subsequent liver transplantation becomes technically more difficult.[97] The distal splenorenal shunt (Warren shunt) and mesocaval shunt avoid the porta hepatis and do not complicate future transplant surgery.[98-100] Either surgical shunt may be offered to patients whose liver disease is otherwise well compensated and whose principal liver complication is variceal bleeding.[101]

Progressive and incapacitating fatigue may occasionally be the predominant manifestation of advanced chronic liver disease and interfere with daily activities. When fatigue is a predominant manifestation of advanced liver disease, all other potentially contributing medical conditions, particularly depression and hypothyroidism, should be excluded. However, fatigue may occasionally be the dominant indication for liver transplantation, especially when found in association with major impairment of hepatic synthetic function.[38]

Malnutrition is frequent in end-stage liver disease.[102] The presence of muscle wasting with reduced strength should be assessed during the history and physical examination and should lead, when present, to prompt referral for liver transplantation. Malnutrition was first recognized by Child and Turcotte in 1964 as a negative prognostic factor for patients with cirrhosis.[60] The severity of malnutrition correlates significantly with mortality and duration of ventilator support, intensive care monitoring, and inpatient hospitalization after liver transplantation.[103-105] On the other hand, malnutrition is potentially reversible because cirrhotic patients provided with a nasogastric enteral diet increase serum albumin and improve in their overall clinical condition expressed as Child's score.[106] Strict low-protein diets should be avoided in cirrhotic patients without hepatic encephalopathy because they may worsen preexisting malnutrition.

Hepatorenal syndrome is a functional renal failure in patients with end-stage liver disease in the absence of data suggesting other causes of renal impairment.[107] The International Ascites Club has proposed new and revised criteria for the diagnosis of hepatorenal syndrome (Table 55-11).[108] The pathogenesis appears to be related to portal hypertension with sequestration of blood in the splanchnic circulation, resulting in decreased effective intravascular volume and alteration of many vascular control systems that lead to diminished renal blood flow and reduced glomerular filtration rate. Patients have usually been approved for liver transplantation before the development of hepatorenal syndrome, which occurs late in the natural history of advanced cirrhosis. A higher priority for transplantation should be assigned at the onset of hepatorenal syndrome in light of the poor prognosis of the condition. If a patient had not been previously considered for liver transplantation, urgent referral and expedited evaluation are required. Supportive therapy such as hemodialysis and continuous arteriovenous hemofiltration have been attempted with limited success.[109-111] Recently, an extracorporeal liver support device using an albumin-containing dialysate appears to be the most promising temporizing measure.[112,113] Liver transplantation remains the definitive therapy and reverses the hepatorenal syndrome in most cases, with 3-year survival after surgery approximating 60 percent.[114-118]

Liver transplantation optimizes the chance for curing small hepatocellular carcinoma in the setting of cirrhosis by removing both the tumor and the preneoplastic condition of a cirrhotic liver.[119] Disease-free survival rate after liver transplantation of more than 80 percent was found in patients with either solitary tumors less than 5 cm or up to three tumors with each less than 3 cm.[120] On the other hand, surgical resection as the alternative therapeutic modality carries poor long-term survival with

TABLE 55-11

Diagnostic Criteria of Hepatorenal Syndrome According to the International Ascites Club

Major Criteria*

1. Low GFR, indicated by serum creatinine > 1.5 mg/dl or 24-hour creatinine clearance < 40 ml/min
2. Absence of shock, ongoing bacterial infection, and fluid losses and current treatment with nephrotoxic drugs
3. No sustained improvement in renal function (decrease in serum creatinine to ≤1.5 mg/dl or increase in creatinine clearance to ≥40 ml/min) after diuretic withdrawal and expansion of plasma volume with 1.5 L of plasma expander
4. Proteinuria < 500 mg/day of protein and no ultrasonographic evidence of obstructive uropathy or parenchymal renal disease

Additional Criteria

1. Urine volume < 500 ml/day
2. Urine sodium < 10 mEq/L
3. Urine osmolality > plasma osmolality
4. Urine red blood cells < 50/high-power field
5. Serum sodium concentration < 130 mEq/L

Adapted from Arroyo V, Ginès P, Gerbes AL, et al: Definition and diagnostic criteria of refractory ascites and hepatorenal syndrome in cirrhosis. International Ascites Club. Hepatology 23(1):164-176, 1996.
*Only major criteria are necessary for the diagnosis of hepatorenal syndrome.

frequent tumor recurrence.[121] The risk of recurrence after transplantation or resection increases with tumor size, tumor number, bilobar involvement, and vascular invasion.[121-123]

A thorough evaluation should be performed on patients with hepatocellular carcinoma referred for liver transplantation. Metastatic disease must be excluded by bone scan, as well as computed tomography (CT) of the chest, abdomen, and pelvis. Because of the long waiting time for a donor organ in many areas of the United States, patients are often enrolled into experimental protocols for neoadjuvant therapy pending transplantation, of which chemo-embolization is used most commonly. Because of the possibility of finding intra-abdominal metastases at the time of abdominal exploration, the patient is often brought to the hospital together with a backup recipient when an organ is offered.

Clinical indications for liver transplantation unique to patients with cholestatic liver diseases consist of progressive osteodystrophy,[124,125] intractable pruritus,[126,127] recurrent bacterial cholangitis in the setting of primary sclerosing cholangitis, or xanthomatous neuropathy, which is a rare but disabling complication of severe cholestasis.[128] The biochemical indications differ between patients with hepatocellular diseases, such as alcoholic liver disease and chronic viral hepatitis, and those with cholestatic liver diseases, such as primary biliary cirrhosis and primary sclerosing cholangitis (see Table 55-10). For example, patients with primary biliary cirrhosis should be considered for liver transplantation when the serum bilirubin rises above 10 mg/dl.[129] Patients with alcoholic cirrhosis warrant transplant evaluation when the serum albumin is less than 3 g/dl or the prothrombin time is more than 3 seconds above control. Hypoalbuminemia resulting from gastrointestinal bleeding or spontaneous bacterial peritonitis may be transient and reversible, but fixed serum albumin levels less than 3 g/dl should prompt referral for liver transplantation.

These biochemical parameters should serve only as guidelines and be considered within the context of clinically decompensated liver disease that is typically but not invariably present with advanced chronic liver disease. However, an occasional patient may have advanced cholestasis or significantly impaired hepatic synthetic function without clinically decompensated liver disease. Biochemical indices indicating a CTP score greater than 7 will serve as the primary stimulus for listing this patient for liver transplantation.[38] By contrast, a patient with good synthetic function may suffer from progressive hepatic encephalopathy resulting from a spontaneous distal splenorenal shunt or retrograde flow though a recanalized umbilical vein. Similarly a patient with early primary biliary cirrhosis and normal synthetic function may develop portal hypertensive bleeding, which meets minimal listing criteria, from presinusoidal obstruction by regenerative hyperplasia or fibrotic portal tracts.[130] Hence the final decision to list a potential candidate rests on the clinical judgment and assessment of the overall patient, not on the static biochemical parameters.[52]

Certain pretransplant patient characteristics may predict the postoperative outcome and be helpful in determining referral and selection of patients for liver transplantation. A retrospective review of more than 200 recipients identified CTP class C, preoperative renal dysfunction, and intensive care unit stay immediately before transplantation as predictors of high mortality from liver transplantation.[131] Earlier studies had also noted a correlation between pretransplant renal failure and posttransplant sepsis and death.[132,133] Another study reported that survival at 6 months post-transplant was inversely correlated with intraoperative blood loss and preoperative level of coma, degree of malnutrition, serum bilirubin level, and prothrombin time.[134] Thus patients should be referred and transplanted, if possible with the scarcity of organs, before the development of parameters that predict a poor outcome after liver transplantation. Although somewhat cumbersome, there may be a role in patient selection for liver transplantation based on the results of quantitative dynamic liver function tests, such as the indocyanine green half-life and the monoethylglycinexylidide lidocaine metabolism test. In addition, combining one of these tests with CTP score may improve the selection and timing of liver transplantation.[135,136]

Final Candidate Selection and Listing for Liver Transplantation

Before final selection and listing for liver transplantation, the prospective candidate undergoes a pretransplant evaluation to define the status of systemic diseases and to determine whether absolute or relative contraindications are present. Routine evaluation includes blood bank and hematologic studies, complete liver and kidney chemistry profiles, viral serologies (hepatitis B virus [HBV], hepatitis C virus [HCV], human immunodeficiency virus [HIV], CMV), chest radiograph, and CT of the abdomen or abdominal ultrasound with Doppler of the hepatic vasculature. Additional routine tests include purified protein derivative (PPD) for tuberculosis, kidney function by creatinine clearance, electrocardiogram, and, in presence of lung disease, a pulmonary function test. Patients at risks for coronary artery disease undergo cardiology consultation and, oftentimes, cardiac stress test or cardiac catheterization. Carotid Doppler ultrasound also may be appropriate. Cancer screening, depending on age and gender, includes Pap smear, mammogram, occult fecal blood testing, and lower gastrointestinal endoscopy. Consultations with a social worker, financial counselor, and psychiatrist are routine in most transplant centers (Table 55-12).

After the pretransplant evaluation is complete, the patient is presented to the liver transplantation selection committee, which is composed of the entire transplant team. Patients are generally assigned to one of four categories: (1) suitable and ready, with listing for a donor organ; (2) suitable but too well, with placement on inactive status and continued follow-up with the referring physician; (3) potentially reversible current contraindication, with treatment and recategorization at a later date; and (4) absolute contraindication, with denial of transplantation. Patients who are approved for liver transplantation by the selection committee are listed for a donor organ with UNOS, and final approval by the insurance carrier or third-party payer is sought.

TABLE 55-12
Pretransplant Evaluation for Liver Transplantation

Standard Blood Tests
Complete blood count, liver chemistry, kidney profile, coagulation profile (PT, PTT)
Iron studies, ceruloplasmin, α_1-antitrypsin phenotype
ANA, smooth muscle antibody, AMA
EBV, CMV, HSV, VZV, HIV, syphilis
HAV, HBV, HCV, and HDV serologies
Alpha-fetoprotein
Other Standard Tests
Abdominal ultrasound with Doppler, electrocardiogram, chest radiograph, pulmonary function tests, endoscopic evaluations
PPD skin tests
Standard Consultations
Dietary
Psychosocial
Women's health (Pap smear, mammogram in women older than age 35 years)
Financial (insurance clearance must be obtained)
Overall assessment of patient (clinical judgment in addition to biochemical parameters)
Other Optional Tests
MRI or CT (to exclude hepatocellular carcinoma)
Angiography (to exclude vascular abnormalities)
Carotid duplex scanning (for older or cardiovascular patients)
Contrast echocardiography (for suspected hepatopulmonary syndrome)
Cardiac catheterization (for suspected CAD)
Colonoscopy (history of IBD, PSC, polyps, family history of colon cancer, hematochezia, guaiac (+) stool)
ERCP (in PSC)
Liver biopsy
Fungal serologies (in areas endemic for dimorphal fungi)
Optional Measures
Pretransplant vaccines, if needed (hepatitis A and B, pneumococcal vaccine, influenza vaccine, tetanus booster)

PT, Prothrombin time; *ANA,* anti-nuclear antibody; *AMA,* anti-mitochondrial antibody; *EBV,* Epstein-Barr virus; *CMV,* cytomegalovirus; *HSV,* herpes simplex virus; *VZV,* varicella-zoster virus; *HIV,* human immunodeficiency virus; *HAV,* hepatitis A virus; *HDV,* hepatitis D virus; *PPD,* purified protein derivative; *CTP,* Child-Turcotte-Pugh; *MRI,* magnetic resonance imaging; *CT,* computed tomography; *CAD,* coronary artery disease; *IBD,* inflammatory bowel disease; *PSC,* primary sclerosing cholangitis; *ERCP,* endoscopic retrograde cholangiopancreatography.

Absolute Contraindications to Liver Transplantation

Compared with the early experience with liver transplantation in the 1980s, the list of contraindications to transplantation is now quite short (see Table 55-7). The absolute contraindications have been established by consensus and are generally agreed upon by all transplant centers.

There are also clinical situations in which the likelihood of a successful outcome with liver transplantation is so remote that the surgery should not be attempted. These so-called relative contraindications are not as well established and are not uniform among transplant centers. They often include subjective factors, such as the presence of co-morbidities, advanced age, or far-advanced liver disease with beginning multi-organ failure. However, they allow the identification and exclusion of high-risk candidates, which limits the economic costs and emotional burden of further evaluating patients unfit for transplantation.

Advanced Cardiac Disease

The decision to exclude a patient from liver transplantation because of significant cardiac disease often rests on the consensus opinion of consulting physicians and members of the transplant team.[38] Pretransplant cardiac evaluation may overestimate cardiac function after liver transplantation because of the lower systemic vascular resistance associated with end-stage liver disease.[137] Cardiac insufficiency may be unmasked after liver transplantation by the loss of cardioprotective effect of low systemic vascular resistance, the volume overload from blood and other intravenous products, and the increased afterload due to various immunosuppressive agents.[130] A classic example was seen in a group of nine patients with hemochromatosis, who had normal pretransplant cardiac evaluations. Seven of these patients developed congestive heart failure or arrhythmias after liver transplantation.[138] Patients are not candidates for liver transplantation if they have poor ventricular function (e.g., cardiomyopathy associated with alcoholic cirrhosis or hemochromatosis) or pulmonary hypertension associated with severe valvular heart disease.[30,62,139] Patients with aortic stenosis must be evaluated carefully because a significant pressure gradient associated with poor ventricular function confers an unfavorable outcome after liver transplantation.

Liver transplantation poses high risks of myocardial ischemia or infarction in patients with coronary artery disease, particularly in those with three-vessel or left main coronary disease.[38] Coronary artery disease, if anatomically reversible by angioplasty or bypass surgery, is not a contraindication to listing, as long as left ventricular function is adequate.[140,141] Angioplasty is the preferred therapeutic modality because it obviates the need for surgery; the latter may precipitate postoperative liver failure, hemorrhage, and renal failure.[141] Combined coronary bypass grafting and liver transplantation has been published as case reports but cannot be recommended because it is usually associated with significant morbidity and high expense.[142-144]

A study from the University of Pittsburgh documented a poor outcome among 32 patients with coronary artery disease who underwent liver transplantation, with an overall 81 percent morbidity and 50 percent mortality.[145] Coronary artery disease was managed medically by angioplasty or surgically before transplantation. The nine patients who were managed medically had 100 percent morbidity and 56 percent mortality. The single patient who underwent angioplasty survived without major cardiac morbidity. In the subgroup of two patients who underwent simultaneous bypass grafting and liver transplantation, one died intraoperatively. The other required pacer insertion and inotropic agents postoperatively. The remaining 20 patients with prior bypass grafting suffered an overall 80 percent morbidity and 50 percent mortality post-transplant. If these poor results are confirmed, issues of cost-effectiveness and the scarcity of donor organs may limit the application of liver transplantation in patients with documented coronary artery disease, whether treated or not.[38]

Advanced Pulmonary Disease

Half of all liver transplant candidates have abnormal arterial oxygenation[146]; however, only patients with advanced chronic obstructive pulmonary diseases or pulmonary fibrosis are precluded from liver transplantation. Reversible conditions such as asthma, respiratory impairment from ascites, and muscle weakness resulting from chronic liver failure should not prohibit referral for transplant evaluation.[65] Even patients who were transplanted for α_1-antitrypsin deficiency may have improvement in pulmonary function postoperatively.[147] Previous tuberculosis is not a contraindication to liver transplantation. Active tuberculosis should be treated for at least 2 to 3 weeks and preferably several months before and up to 1 year after liver transplantation.[130,148] PPD testing is an essential part of the liver transplant evaluation. If the test is positive, prophylaxis with either isoniazid and pyridoxine or ofloxacin should be given for 6 months.

Hepatopulmonary syndrome, as manifested by a triad of chronic liver disease complicated by portal hypertension, intrapulmonary vascular dilation (with right-to-left shunting), and arterial hypoxemia,[149] was previously considered an absolute contraindication to liver transplantation.[150] More recent data indicate that liver transplantation can reverse hepatopulmonary syndrome associated with moderate to even severe hypoxemia, provided the patient can be supported through the postoperative period.[151-160] The presumed vascular remodeling may take up to 15 months post-transplant to normalize oxygenation.[149] The post-transplant mortality correlates with the severity of pretransplant hypoxemia, and increases from 4 percent to 30 percent when pretransplant arterial oxygen pressure drops below 50 mm Hg.[158] Progressive deterioration of hepatopulmonary syndrome may be considered an indication for earlier liver transplantation rather than a contraindication.[161] The main contributors to perioperative mortality include refractory hypoxemia with multi-organ failure, intracerebral hemorrhage, sepsis from bile leak, and portal vein thrombosis.[158-160] A few case reports have shown that TIPS may appreciably improve the hypoxemia associated with severe hepatopulmonary syndrome.[162-165] Nitric oxide may favorably alter the ventilation-perfusion mismatch and improve the hypoxemia in the perioperative period.[153,154]

In contrast to hepatopulmonary syndrome, portopulmonary hypertension is associated with high operative cardiopulmonary mortality and frequently unaltered pulmonary hemodynamics even after liver transplantation.[166-168] It is the most significant type of pulmonary hypertension and may be present in up to 9 percent of all patients with advanced liver disease.[169] Albert Einstein Medical Center identified six predictors for pulmonary hypertension, including systemic arterial hypertension, loud pulmonary component of the second heart sound and right ventricular heave on physical examination, and right ventricular dilation, right ventricular hypertrophy, and an estimated systolic pulmonary artery pressure (PAP) higher than 40 mm Hg on echocardiogram.[170] These predictors have a specificity of more than 90 percent, but a sensitivity of 67 percent for identifying liver transplant candidates with pulmonary hypertension. The Mayo Clinic reported that systolic right ventricular pressure of 50 mm Hg or higher can accurately detect moderate to severe pulmonary hypertension with 97 percent sensitivity and 77 percent specificity, and recommended right heart catheterization as follow-up to characterize pulmonary hemodynamics.[171] Retrospective analysis of published data combined with the Mayo Clinic experience has established recommendations on the advisability of liver transplantation at different levels of portopulmonary hypertension.[172] A patient with mean PAP of 50 mm Hg or higher carries 100 percent cardiopulmonary mortality and is absolutely contraindicated against liver transplantation. On the other hand, a patient with mean PAP of less than 35 mm Hg can safely proceed with surgery without increased risk of mortality. For the remaining patients with mean PAP between 35 mm Hg and 50 mm Hg, a pulmonary vascular resistance of 250 dynes per second/cm^5 or greater predicts 50 percent cardiopulmonary mortality. Chronic epoprostenol infusion may reduce PAP sufficiently to allow eventual liver transplantation or may reverse progressive portopulmonary hypertension after surgery.[173-178] The beneficial effects of nitric oxide on the pulmonary vasculature in patients with portopulmonary hypertension have not been established.[178-181]

HIV Disease

Patients who are HIV positive are generally excluded a priori from liver transplantation. The published literature suggests that progression to full-blown acquired immunodeficiency syndrome (AIDS) in HIV-positive patients is more rapid after liver transplantation than in nontransplanted patients.[182-184] One study of 12 patients who were HIV-negative at the time of liver transplantation but acquired HIV disease from infected donor organs or blood products demonstrated a poor outcome. Three patients developed AIDS, and four patients died after a mean follow-up of 37 months post-transplant.[182] Among 10 additional patients known to be HIV-positive at the time of liver transplantation, 9 subsequently died, with the majority dying AIDS-related deaths. The University of Pittsburgh reported similar data for liver transplantation in HIV-positive patients, with AIDS being the leading cause of death post-transplant.[183,184] Furthermore, transplantation plus immunosuppression seemed to shorten the AIDS-free time in HIV-positive patients as compared to non-transplant controls. Whether or not newer antiretroviral drug regimens will improve the outcome after liver transplantation remains unknown, but enthusiasm to perform liver transplantation in HIV-infected individuals is limited.

Active, Untreated Infection

Active, untreated infection should be controlled before liver transplantation. As noted previously, most transplant programs will defer transplantation in the setting of spontaneous bacterial peritonitis until antibiotic treatment has been under way for 48 hours and resolution of infection is documented on repeat paracentesis.[38] Sepsis and pneumonia remain absolute contraindications to liver transplantation. Serious chronic infections such as osteomyelitis, chronic fungal diseases, and abscesses preclude transplantation unless they can be treated effectively.[130]

Extrahepatic Malignancy

Liver transplantation is not performed in the presence of extrahepatic malignancy. The only potential exception is liver transplantation for patients with liver metastases from slow-growing neuroendocrine tumors,[185] such as gastrinomas, insulinomas, glucagonomas, somatostatinomas, and carcinoid tumors.[186] In the setting of neuroendocrine tumors the best indication for transplantation seems to be patients with metastases restricted to the liver and unresponsive to all other feasible surgical and non-surgical treatment options.[186,187] Liver transplantation remains a high-risk operation in such highly selected patients, but it can yield long-term survival. Transplantation in most cases can achieve sustained relief of clinical symptoms, but cure of tumor is unusual.[187-192] However, the increasing donor shortage and lower patient survival may be arguments against liver transplantation in this population of patients. In a recent review of 103 cases in the literature the 2-year and 5-year survival rates were, respectively, 60 percent and 47 percent but the recurrence-free, 5-year survival did not exceed 24 percent. Multi-variate analysis identified a few adverse prognostic factors, including age greater than 50 years and transplantation combined with upper abdominal exenteration or Whipple's operation.[190]

Cholangiocarcinoma

The results of liver transplantation are so poor with cholangiocarcinoma that most centers consider the pretransplant diagnosis of this tumor an absolute contraindication.[185,193,194] This pessimism reflects that most patients with a tumor of small macroscopic size already have extensive microscopic involvement.[186] Unless the tumor can be excised completely with negative margins and negative nodes, the chance of cure is remote. The University of Pittsburgh reported 5-year post-transplant survival rates of 30 percent for advanced disease, but 70 percent for patients with tumors of stage I and II.[195] The same center subsequently described a series of 11 patients with cholangiocarcinoma who underwent neoadjuvant external-beam radiotherapy, brachytherapy, and chemotherapy with fluorouracil.[196] All patients were alive at the time of report, with a median follow-up of 44 months; only one patient developed tumor recurrence. A unique feature in this series was the rigorous attempt to exclude extrahepatic disease by a pretransplant evaluation that included body CT, bone scan, and exploratory laparotomy. This study highlights the significance of patient selection for liver transplantation, but the contribution of neoadjuvant chemoirradiation to a successful outcome remains to be proven.[197,198] If these clinical results are confirmed by other centers, cholangiocarcinoma may become a relative rather than absolute contraindication to liver transplantation.[197]

Active Alcohol or Substance Abuse

Active alcoholism and substance abuse are absolute contraindications to liver transplantation. Most programs accept patients with alcoholic liver disease as liver transplant candidates only after proven alcohol abstinence for at least 6 months and completion of an inpatient or outpatient rehabilitation program. One study found that the incidence of recidivism is significantly lower in patients who had been sober for at least 6 months compared with those who had quit drinking for a shorter interval.[199] However, few of the other published series have applied the 6-month rule, and little evidence exists in the literature on alcoholism to support the rule's utility as a predictor of future abstinence.[200] Furthermore, in many treatment studies and in longitudinal natural history cohorts, a majority of patients who continue to abuse alcohol had achieved 6 months of abstinence at some time in their past.[201]

Anatomic Abnormalities Precluding Liver Transplantation

The number of anatomic abnormalities that preclude liver transplantation has diminished with refinement of surgical techniques. Isolated portal vein thrombosis, previously considered an absolute contraindication, is now only a relative problem in light of novel reconstructive innovations, including thrombectomy or jump grafts.[202-207] Two recent large clinical series recognized the extent of thrombosis as an adverse prognostic indicator for liver transplantation. A French group identified complete portal vein thrombosis as a significant risk factor for rethrombosis, a condition that may predipose patients to acute graft failure and portal hypertensive complications after liver transplantation. Furthermore, post-transplant mortality increased to 33 percent when the complete portal vein thrombosis extended into the splanchnic circulation.[208] A separate British series noted a similar negative impact on post-transplant survival from portal vein thrombosis that extends into the superior mesenteric vein.[209]

Relative Contraindications to Liver Transplantation

Relative contraindications are clinical conditions that affect survival negatively but do not preclude transplantation. The relative importance of such factors on the decision to proceed with transplantation varies considerably from one transplant center to another. Often, it is a combination of clinical factors, not a single one, that excludes a patient from liver transplantation.

Advanced Age

Advanced age per se is not a contraindication to liver transplantation. Patient selection should be based on an assessment of biologic age rather than arbitrary chronologic age cut-off.[210] Patients older than 60 years of age are undergoing transplantations with increasing frequency and experiencing a favorable outcome in many transplant centers. Data from 1987 through 1998 published by UNOS show a significantly reduced survival after liver transplantation in recipients of ages 50 to 59 (1.5-fold relative risk of death) and even more so in recipients of age 60 or older.[30] However, data published from individual liver transplant centers show no survival difference between older and younger patients.[211-219] Furthermore, more than two thirds of older recipients who survive liver transplantation are fully functional.[213] The diminished immune function of older subjects theoretically may improve the transplant outcome because of a lesser likelihood of allograft rejection,[212,220-221] but may have a negative impact on long-term survival because of an increasing incidence of malignancies.[222]

Older liver recipients nevertheless require more rigorous pretransplant assessment. Appropriate screening tests and consultations should be carried out in light of the increased risk of co-morbid conditions such as cardiopulmonary disease and malignancy. Preoperative hormonal replacement therapy is reasonable for older female patients who are at particular risk for osteoporosis. Data from the University of Nebraska and Baylor University Medical Centers demonstrate that the severity of liver disease has a greater impact on survival in older patients. Patients classified preoperatively as being high risk have a significantly poorer outcome than their low-risk counterparts.[223,224] Older recipients can achieve excellent post-transplant outcome, however, when transplanted in a timely fashion before dwindling into the late stages of liver failure.

Renal Failure

Patients undergoing evaluation for liver transplantation may have miscellaneous types of renal dysfunction, such as hepatorenal syndrome, chronic renal failure, or reversible acute renal failure, that may be related to intercurrent events such as spontaneous bacterial peritonitis, gastrointestinal bleeding, or excessive diuresis.[225,226] Chronic renal failure secondary to intrinsic kidney disease is not a contraindication to liver transplantation but necessitates consideration for dual transplantation of liver and kidney. Transient deterioration in renal function resulting from an acute injury is usually not a problem unless complicated by the development of hepatorenal syndrome.

A unique clinical dilemma in the setting of moderate renal failure is to determine whether renal dysfunction is likely to reverse after liver transplantation or to progress, which would indicate the need for combined liver and kidney transplantation.[38] Analysis of the National Institute of Diabetes and Digestive and Kidney Diseases (NIDDK) Liver Transplantation Database showed that renal insufficiency in fulminant hepatic failure or in the setting of dialysis or combined liver and kidney transplantation predicts lower patient and graft survival rates, longer intensive care monitoring and hospitalization, and higher costs of transplantation.[227] In general, a low, fixed glomerular filtration rate leads to combined liver and kidney transplantation, which typically has a favorable outcome. A well-functioning kidney facilitates postoperative management and avoids severe complications associated with renal failure. In one series of seven patients undergoing combined transplantation all but one were alive with functioning grafts. The rate of acute liver allograft rejection was only 37.5 percent compared with 59.3 percent in patients undergoing liver transplantation alone.[228]

Patients with end-stage liver disease complicated by renal failure should undergo a detailed pretransplant evaluation with the assistance of a transplant nephrologist. A kidney biopsy may be recommended when the renal diagnosis is obscure or when the reversibility of renal failure is uncertain after analyzing the historic information and imaging studies. When coagulopathy contraindicates a percutaneous kidney biopsy, either a transjugular approach or an open kidney biopsy should be considered.[229]

Prior Hepatic Surgery

Prior abdominal surgery can cause extensive adhesions with portal hypertensive collaterals, but meticulous surgical techniques can usually overcome this problem, despite longer operative time and increased intraoperative blood loss.[230,231] These vascular problems may occur from major operations such as the creation of a surgical shunt for refractory variceal bleeding or biliary decompressive procedures in patients with primary sclerosing cholangitis. However, even a previous small operation such as cholecystectomy may have a negative impact on the amount of surgical dissection and blood loss during liver transplantation. Hence for the long-term management of patients with chronic liver disease, alternative non-surgical interventions should be taken (e.g., TIPS for refractory portal hypertensive bleeding, endoscopic or radiologic approaches to dominant biliary strictures in patients with primary sclerosing cholangitis).

Severe Obesity

A favorable outcome of liver transplantation in patients with severe obesity was reported initially in 1994.[232] A previous report had shown a proclivity for excessive weight gain in obese subjects after liver transplantation.[233] However, in the 1994 report, 18 patients with severe or morbid obesity underwent liver transplantation, with a survival rate of 100 percent and stable weight on post-transplant follow-up. Morbidity included the expected wound infections, which occurred in 61 percent of recipients, and some unique complications associated with obesity. A separate study showed significantly increased post-transplant morbidity in the form of respiratory failure or systemic vascular complications in the severely obese.[234] This latter study together with two additional series confirmed that the long-term survival after liver transplantation is not different in these patients.[234-236]

Previous Non-hepatic Malignancies

As the number of older patients referred for liver transplantation increases, it becomes more relevant to examine the impact of specific non-hepatic tumors on post-transplant outcome, and the feasibility and timing of such transplantation. Many of the available data are derived from the literature on renal transplantation. In an experience with 939 preexisting malignancies in renal transplant recipients some general recommendations were established.[237] Low post-transplant recurrence rates of up to 10 percent were noted with incidental renal tumors, lymphomas, and testicular, uterine, cervical, and thyroid carcinomas. Intermediate recurrence rates of 11 percent to 25 percent were associated with carcinomas of the uterine body, Wilms' tumor, and carcinomas of the colon, prostate, and breast. High recurrence rates (more than 25 percent) occurred with carcinomas of the bladder, sarcomas, malignant melanomas, symptomatic renal carcinomas, non-melanomatous skin cancers, and myelomas. The investigators recommended a 2-year waiting period between cancer treatment and liver transplantation for most cancers. However, a waiting period of more than 2 years is necessary for malignant melanomas and breast and colon carcinomas.

The King's College Hospital recently reported the outcome of its liver transplant patients with preexisting malignant conditions, including 12 cases of solid-organ or skin malignancy and 8 cases of myeloproliferative disorders (MPD).[238] Three patients developed malignancies post-transplant: recurrence of non-Hodgkin's lymphoma, de novo post-transplant lymphoproliferative disorder (PTLD), and acute leukemic transformation from MPD. Among the 1079 liver transplantations in patients without preexisting neoplasia, 34 patients (3.1 percent) developed de novo malignancies. The authors concluded that MPD or previous non-hepatic malignancy should not be considered a contraindication to liver transplantation.

Timing of Liver Transplantation

Timely performance of liver transplantation in the early phase of decompensated liver disease is associated with an improved outcome and reduced costs. At one center the 1-year survival rates for patients who were not hospitalized when transplanted compared to those who were in the intensive care unit at the time of transplantation were 86 percent and 70 percent, respectively.[12] On the other hand, the average 15 percent 1-year mortality rate associated with liver transplantation dictates not performing transplantation too early but waiting for the appearance of major clinical decompensation of cirrhosis or biochemical evidence of severe hepatic dysfunction. Patients should be referred and listed for transplantation when an estimated survival of longer than 1 year is unlikely, but before the onset of advanced and refractory complications of chronic liver disease. The biochemical and clinical indications for liver transplantation in Tables 55-5, 55-6, and 55-10 have been established for patients with chronic liver diseases and acute liver failure. In general, patients with primary sclerosing cholangitis should be referred somewhat earlier for liver transplantation because of the risk of cholangiocarcinoma in more advanced disease.

Prognostic survival models to assist in the timing and predict the outcome of liver transplantation have been developed and validated for primary biliary cirrhosis, a disease with a reasonably predictable natural history.[129,239-242] The variables employed most commonly in these models were age, serum bilirubin, serum albumin, and histology, among which serum bilirubin is the most important.[129,241] Primary biliary cirrhosis is characterized by a long stable phase with normal serum bilirubin, followed by an accelerated preterminal phase of hyperbilirubinemia. The mean patient survival decreases to 1.4 years when serum bilirubin exceeds 10 mg/dl.

The Mayo model for primary biliary cirrhosis has demonstrated that liver transplantation favorably interrupts the natural history of the disease and improves survival as compared to conservative medical management.[240,241] The Mayo model includes five independent prognostic variables predictive of survival, including age, serum levels of bilirubin and albumin, prothrombin time, and the presence of peripheral edema. A Mayo risk score of 7.8 correlates with the optimal timing of liver transplantation. The risk of death post-transplant remains low as long as the risk score is below 7.8, but increases progressively when the risk score exceeds 7.8.[243] When measured serially the risk score predicts poor prognosis and indicates proceeding with liver transplantation when it increases abruptly.[244]

The model has been validated using populations within and outside the Mayo Clinic[242,245] and is superior to CTP score in predicting outcome for liver transplantation.[246] It facilitates patient selection and the timing of liver transplantation. Furthermore, the Mayo risk score accurately predicts the level of resource utilization after liver transplantation, including intraoperative blood requirement, and the length of time on the ventilator, in the intensive care unit, and in the hospital.[246] The Mayo model gained popularity over other models for two reasons: the rigorous validation to which the model was subjected and the advantage of not requiring liver histology.[247]

Mayo Clinic investigators recently developed a simplified version of the primary biliary cirrhosis natural history model.[248] Based on the five prognostic variables of the original Mayo model that are incorporated into a tabular method similar to the CTP score, an abbreviated risk score is determined. A risk score of 6 predicts 1-year survival of 90.6 percent, which approximates the current minimal listing criteria for liver transplantation.

Primary sclerosing cholangitis has a less predictable natural history. The disease usually progresses insidiously but may be punctuated by episodes of recurrent bacterial cholangitis or jaundice from dominant strictures.[249-254] Furthermore, cholangiocarcinoma may develop and preclude liver transplantation. In the recently revised Mayo model for primary sclerosing cholangitis several independent prognostic indicators were found, including age, serum bilirubin, histologic stage, and the presence or absence of splenomegaly.[241,249,250] Analysis of the NIDDK Database, however, demonstrated that CTP score was a better overall predictor of both resource utilization and survival for patients who underwent liver transplantation.[255]

The guidelines for referral or performance of liver transplantation in patients with chronic liver diseases, especially hepatocellular diseases, are broad and need better definition. The Model for End-Stage Liver Disease (MELD), previously created to estimate survival of patients undergoing TIPS,[256] is being proposed to replace the CTP score to predict survival of patients with end-stage liver disease and determine priority for allocation of donor livers to patients on the UNOS waiting list.[257] Calculation of the MELD score is based on serum bilirubin, prothrombin time as expressed by international normalized ratio, and serum creatinine. The model was validated in four independent populations. The MELD score, when compared to the CTP score, has the advantages of (1) using objective laboratory parameters only rather than subjective factors such as ascites and encephalopathy and (2) increasing continuously as the three constituent parameters deteriorate. The individual scoring elements in the CTP score range from 5 to 15 and remain fixed after a threshold has been reached.[258]

Disease-specific Indications for Liver Transplantation

As shown in Table 55-4 the most common indications for liver transplantation are cirrhosis of various etiologies, including the chronic cholestatic liver diseases. The various causes of cirrhosis contribute to more than 80 percent of all liver transplantations. What most often troubles transplant physicians is not whether an individual patient should be transplanted but the timing of transplantation and the impact of co-existent systemic diseases.

Chronic Hepatitis C

Chronic hepatitis C is now the most common disease for which liver transplantation is performed. It is also the major cause of post-transplant hepatitis.[259] Liver transplantation is the treatment of choice for decompensated cirrhosis resulting from HCV infection. However, HCV reinfection poses challenging management issues post-transplant.[260,261] Reinfection with HCV occurs in more than 95 percent of recipients, with viremia increasing markedly post-transplant.[259,260] The spectrum of recurrent hepatitis C ranges from asymptomatic mild hepatitis to severe chronic hepatitis and cirrhosis.[259,260,262-264] Histologic recurrence is seen in 40 percent to 60 percent of patients. Cirrhosis develops in 20 percent of patients within 5 years.[265]

Furthermore, 5 percent to 10 percent of patients require retransplantation because of graft failure. Within 2 years post-transplant, 2 percent to 8 percent of patients develop a severe form of cholestatic hepatitis. Graft and patient survival rates for the first 10 years after liver transplantation, however, appear to be unaffected by the HCV serostatus of the recipient.[261] It is possible that longer follow-up may demonstrate reduced survival with recurrent hepatitis C.

The underlying cause for recurrent HCV infection with progressive liver disease is probably multifactorial.[261,267-292] Certain characteristics associated with the virus, the recipient, and the type of immunosuppressive regimen have been identified as possibly affecting the course of post-transplant HCV infection (Table 55-13). HCV genotype 1b has been associated with rapidly progressive liver disease post-transplant in most,[261,276-279] but not all,[293] trials. High levels of serum HCV ribonucleic acid (RNA), either pretransplant[282] or post-transplant,[276,280,289] are associated with more rapid disease progression. Fibrosing cholestatic hepatitis is the most severe form of HCV recurrence and is associated with very high pretransplant HCV RNA levels in the native explant.[275]

Pretransplant quasispecies do not persist postoperatively but may predict HCV-induced hepatitis and fibrosis post-transplant.[282] Co-infection with CMV potentiates the graft injury induced by HCV.[287] The presence of anti-HCV core immunoglobulin (Ig)M post-transplant

TABLE 55-13

Risk Factors for More Severe Recurrence of HCV after Liver Transplantation

Pretransplantation	Reference
HLA matching	281
Age	278
Nonwhites	269, 271
Genotype 1b	261, 276, 277, 278, 279
Pretransplant HCV quasispecies	282
High (>1 × 10^6 Eq/ml) pretransplant HCV RNA levels	269, 271, 274
High pretransplant HCV RNA levels in native explant	275
CMV viral co-infection	287
Absence of pretransplant co-infection with HBV	272, 278, 291
Prolonged rewarming time during allograft implantation	267
Year of transplant (recent year associated with rapid progression rate)	269, 271
Post-transplantation	
Presence of IgM anti-HCV core antibodies after transplantation	273
High serum or liver, early post-transplantation HCV RNA viral load	276, 280, 289
Early post-transplant histologic injury	276, 285, 288
Persistent elevation of serum transaminase levels	283
Post-transplant HCV quasispecies	284, 285
High level of immunosuppression	270, 289
Episodes of rejection	270, 290, 292
Mycophenolate use	270
Muromonab-CD3 use	270, 285, 286, 290
Methylprednisone boluses	270, 271, 285, 290
High cumulative steroid dose	292

HCV, hepatitis C virus; *HLA,* human leukocyte antigen; *RNA,* ribonucleic acid; *CMV,* cytomegalovirus; *HBV,* hepatitis B virus; *IgM,* immunoglobulin M.

correlates with the recurrence and severity of hepatitis C.[273] The measurement of this antibody may help to monitor the treatment of viral recurrence post-transplant.

Additional risk factors for severe hepatitis C recurrence post-transplant include age greater than 49 years,[278] persistently elevated serum aminotransferases post-transplant,[283] prolonged rewarming time,[267] and intense post-transplant immunosuppression such as methylprednisolone boluses, high cumulative steroid dose, muromonab-CD3, and mycophenolate.* The rate at which fibrosis develops not only is accelerated compared with immunocompetent individuals, but is increasing in recent years.[269,271] The estimated chance of severe disease within the first year post-transplant was 19 percent, 40 percent, and 65 percent, respectively, after 30, 60, or 90 minutes of ischemic rewarming.[267] Reduction of rewarming time should be stressed in liver transplantation, especially for patients with liver failure from hepatitis C. Absence of pretransplant co-infection with HBV is associated with more severe recurrent hepatitis C in the allograft. Furthermore, hepatitis D infection is associated with mild histologic inflammation and suppressed HCV replication in transplant recipients who are co-infected with HBV and HCV.[294]

There are numerous emerging anti-viral treatment strategies that have been suggested for recurrence of HCV after liver transplantation (Table 55-14). Interferon-

*References 270, 271, 285, 286, 290, 292.

TABLE 55-14

Management of Recurrent Hepatitis C after Liver Transplantation

Pretransplantation
Preemptive anti-viral therapy
Post-transplantation
Early post-transplant treatment
Treatment of recurrent hepatitis C
Selection of immunosuppressive agents
Retransplantation

based therapy can be used to suppress viral replication in patients with cirrhosis because pretransplant reduction in the level of viremia may have a positive impact on recurrent hepatitis post-transplant. Prophylactic use of interferon post-transplant, either alone or in combination with ribavirin, has failed to alter the natural history of recurrent hepatitis C.[295-297] An additional drawback of this approach is the immunomodulatory effect of interferon that may lead to allograft rejection. Interferon monotherapy rarely achieved sustained virologic response in patients with recurrent hepatitis C post-transplant.[298,299] Ribavirin alone does not clear the virus either.[300-302] Results differ among pilot studies using combination interferon and ribavirin therapy, with sustained virologic responses varying from 8 percent to 48 percent.[303-305]

The choice of immunosuppression can be a critical factor in the outcome of an allograft infected with HCV.[306] No difference was observed in the graft and recipient survival rates with the use of tacrolimus- versus cyclosporine-based induction regimen. Because severe recurrent hepatitis C may occur with muromonab-CD3 and increasing number of methylprednisolone doses,[270,271,285,286,290] less aggressive anti-rejection therapy should be instituted in patients with acute cellular rejection. Furthermore, rejection must be documented histologically before anti-rejection treatment. Hepatitis C and acute rejection may resemble each other histologically,[263] and patients with inconclusive liver biopsies should not be treated empirically with steroids.

The Cedars-Sinai Medical Center retrospectively compared histopathologic features of liver biopsy specimens between recipients with unequivocal recurrent hepatitis C and those with unequivocal acute cellular rejection.[307] The index biopsies from patients between the two groups differed significantly for 11 features. The only statistically significant feature associated with early recurrent HCV was sinusoidal dilation. On the other hand, 10 features were significantly associated with acute cellular rejection: portal inflammatory cells, eosinophils, and histiocytes; bile duct epithelial cell overlap, lymphocytic infiltration, and necrosis; endothelialitis; zone 3 and canalicular cholestasis; and hepatocyte necrosis. Stepwise discriminant analysis showed that bile duct necrosis and portal inflammatory cells and eosinophils were associated independently with acute cellular rejection. However, serial biopsies from patients with recurrent hepatitis C demonstrated statistically significant progression in scores for portal inflammation, portal lymphoid aggregates, and lobular inflammation.

Retransplantation remains the only viable option for patients who suffer allograft failure from recurrent hepatitis C.[308] Prognosis after retransplantation is extremely poor, however, in the setting of recurrent HCV infection. One-year survival is less than 50 percent whether or not there are concurrent causes of graft failure (e.g. hepatic artery thrombosis, biliary complications, chronic ductopenic rejection).[309-313] Multi-variate logistic regression analysis has established hepatitis C as an independent risk factor for mortality after retransplantation.[314] Furthermore, progressive hyperbilirubinemia and renal failure were independent prognostic factors for poor outcome after retransplantation of patients with recurrent hepatitis C.[314] A separate study reported more favorable outcome when retransplantation was performed before development of renal insufficiency or infectious complications.[310] In light of critical organ shortage a controversial issue is whether retransplantation should be offered to a patient with liver failure from recurrent hepatitis C when the anticipated postsurgical outcome is poor.

Alcoholic Liver Disease

Alcoholic liver disease remains the second most common indication for liver transplantation. In addition, some patients have both alcohol- and HCV-induced cirrhosis. Initial concerns regarding transplanting patients with alcoholic liver disease included poor patient survival,[315] post-transplant recidivism,[316] negative impact on surgery from alcohol damage to other organs,[200] and societal disapproval of treating a self-inflicted disease.[317] As a result of subsequent series demonstrating low recidivism rates that averaged 15 percent and resource utilization and long-term survival rates comparable to those of patients transplanted for non-alcoholic liver disease,[318-322] alcoholic cirrhosis became the most common indication for liver transplantation in the United States by 1992,[323] but more recently has been replaced by chronic hepatitis C as the leading indication for replacement of the liver.

The most controversial issue regarding liver transplantation for alcoholic cirrhosis is the specific criteria for selection or exclusion from transplantation.[38] Besides the aforementioned "6-month rule" as advocated by the University of California, San Francisco,[199] the University of Michigan used an "alcoholism prognosis scale" based on factors such as acceptance of the diagnosis of alcoholism by the patient and family; the presence of prognostic indices such as substitute activities, social relationships, and self-esteem; and documentation of indicators of social stability and functioning such as employment, permanent residence, and marriage.[319] The California Pacific Medical Center transplant program ranked their candidates by a multi-disciplinary team approach as low-, moderate-, or high-risk for recidivism or non-compliance.[320,321] Respectively, these risk-stratified patients were approved and listed for transplantation, followed by both the referring physicians and the transplant team to confirm compliance before listing, or denied transplantation. Non-compliance with alcohol post-transplant was documented in 16 percent (all transiently) of the low-risk group and 80 percent to 100 percent of the moderate- to high-risk groups, thus confirming the validity of this multi-disciplinary approach.

Despite earlier data suggesting that alcohol recidivism rarely contributes to post-transplant mortality[318] and that alcohol may protect a recipient from allograft rejection,[324] one recent study demonstrated that return to pathologic drinking after liver transplantation is associated with considerable mortality.[325] The recidivists had a higher rate of medical problems, including pneumonia, cellulitis associated with "skin-popping" cocaine, recurrent alcoholic pancreatitis, non-compliance with immunosuppressant protocol, and, occasionally, graft loss and death. Among the 23 recidivists in a separate series reported by the University of Pittsburgh, all developed Mallory's hyaline on histology and 4 developed allograft cirrhosis.[326] Furthermore, alcohol recidivism was recently shown to have a negative impact on job employment after liver transplantation. A meta-analysis by Stanford University indicates that substantially more recipients transplanted for non-alcoholic liver disease were employed before transplantation and at long-term follow-up when compared to those transplanted for alcoholic liver disease.[327]

Although the specific selection criteria for candidates with alcoholic liver disease have a subjective component and continue to be debated, the performance of liver transplantation in recovered alcoholics is no longer controversial. Nearly all third-party payers, including Medicare and most state Medicaid programs, fund liver transplantation in carefully selected patients who have a documented 6-month period of abstinence and psychosocial predictors for long-term sobriety.

Chronic Hepatitis B

The historically low post-transplant survival of hepatitis B surface antigen (HBsAg)-positive patients had made chronic hepatitis B a controversial indication for liver transplantation.[328] The major contributor to poor outcome was graft reinfection. This may present as an asymptomatic HBsAg carrier state. But more commonly chronic active hepatitis and fibrosing cholestatic hepatitis in the form of a rapidly progressive and usually fatal form of liver disease[328-330] may progress to cirrhosis and liver failure over an accelerated time course. Development of hepatocellular carcinoma has been reported.[331] Fibrosing cholestatic hepatitis is reflective of enhanced viral replication with strong histologic expression of viral proteins such as hepatitis B core antigen (HBcAg) and HBsAg, thus supporting a direct cytopathic role of HBV in the pathogenesis.[332] It has also been reported in association with actively replicating precore mutant virus that produces HBcAg but not hepatitis B e antigen (HBeAg).[333,334]

Recurrence of HBV infection is defined as the reappearance of HBsAg in the serum. In a retrospective analysis of 17 European centers performing 372 consecutive liver transplantations for patients with HBV infection, viral recurrence occurred frequently (67 percent) among the recipients transplanted for HBV cirrhosis and was highest (83 percent) in those who were seropositive for HBV deoxyribonucleic acid (DNA) but lowest (58 percent) in those who were seronegative for both HBV DNA and HBeAg.[335] The lowest risks of recurrence were observed in recipients who were transplanted for fulminant hepatitis B (17 percent) or had co-infection with the hepatitis D virus (32 percent). The 1-year (90 percent versus 73 percent) and 3-year (83 percent versus 54 percent) survival rates of patients who remained HBsAg-negative compared favorably against those who developed recurrent hepatitis B.[335]

A recent series suggested that Asian recipients had worse outcomes than non-Asians when transplanted for chronic hepatitis B, with higher early mortality (31 percent versus 3 percent), more frequent HBV reinfection (72 percent versus 32 percent), and higher mortality resulting from recurrent hepatitis B (87 percent versus 22 percent).[336] Data from Stanford University did not confirm a higher HBV reinfection rate or worse late mortality in Asians, but did confirm a higher early mortality that appeared to be related to late referral and more advanced liver disease at the time of transplantation.[337]

The use of long-term passive immunoprophylaxis with hepatitis B immunoglobulin (HBIg), based on the presumed mechanism of neutralizing circulating HBV,[338] reduces the incidence of viral recurrence to 36 percent, when compared to short-term HBIg of less than 6 months or no HBIg at all.[335] The rate of HBV reinfection despite HBIg prophylaxis was distinctly greater in patients with HBeAg or detectable HBV DNA than in those negative for both markers (greater than 90 percent versus less than 30 percent).[335] HBIg is typically administered, starting at 10,000 IU/L during the anhepatic phase, to maintain an antibody to hepatitis B surface antigen (anti-HBs) level greater than 100 to 200 mIU/ml[339,340] and even 500 mIU/ml in more aggressive protocols.[341] Lifelong therapy and high cost are the two major drawbacks of HBIg prophylaxis.[342] In an effort to contain cost and to reduce HBIg-induced adverse effects such as myalgias, an intramuscular form of the medication with titration to specific anti-HBs levels has been adopted in some transplant centers.[338,342]

More recently the nucleoside analog lamivudine,[343,344] which is the first effective oral treatment for chronic hepatitis B,[345-347] has been employed as prophylaxis against HBV recurrence. It is well tolerated and does not require dose adjustment for patients with impaired liver function.[348,349] Lamivudine, 100 mg daily, may suppress viral replication, stabilize end-stage liver function, and improve pretransplant survival for patients with hepatitis B cirrhosis.[350-354] When used alone as prophylaxis it reduces the incidence of recurrent hepatitis B post-transplant, but lamivudine-resistant mutations within the YMDD locus of the HBV genome develop in more than 20 percent of recipients and lead to progressive liver disease.[348,353-357]

The combination of HBIg and lamivudine is much more efficacious in the prevention of HBV recurrence. The University of California at Los Angeles reported 92 percent 1-year patient survival and no treatment failure among 13 patients using the combination regimen.[358] An updated experience that includes 59 patients and longer follow-up confirms the efficacy of the approach with no viral recurrence.[359] This prophylactic approach is equally effective and less costly when HBIg is administered intramuscularly at lower dosages.[360-362] The University of Pittsburgh advocates an alternative regimen that uses HBIg alone for at least 2 years post-transplant followed by long-term lamivudine. All 16 recipients in this latter series remained HBsAg-negative, with an average follow-up of more than 4 years.[363] In a separate series, combined HBIg and lamivudine prophylaxis prevented graft reinfection in all patients who developed precore mutants before transplant.[364]

Recurrent hepatitis B may lead to rapidly progressive disease.[328] In one study patients with recurrent hepatitis B had much higher mortality after liver retransplantation if graft failure was due to the viral disease rather than other etiologies.[365] Nevertheless, recent evidence suggests that retransplantation in combination with HBIg therapy can be successful.[341] Medical management of recurrent hepatitis B is also challenging. The use of oral lamivudine for 1 year led to the losses of HBV DNA and HBeAg in 60 percent and 30 percent of cases, respectively, in a multi-center trial. Emergence of YMDD mutants occurred in 27 percent of cases.[366] Suppression of viral replication and improvement in liver histology also may be achieved with other nucleoside analogs as salvage therapy, including oral adefovir, oral famciclovir, and intravenous ganciclovir.[367-371] Intravenous and oral prostaglandin E treatment achieved histologic improvement and reduction of viral antigen staining in 8 of 10 patients in one pilot study.[372]

Primary Biliary Cirrhosis

Primary biliary cirrhosis is a relatively common and well-accepted indication for liver transplantation.[373] Prognostic models, despite their great utility in defining the need for transplantation, do not take into account less quantifiable complications such as fatigue, pruritus, and metabolic bone disease.[374,375] Irrespective of the prognostic score, transplantation is indicated when pain from recurrent fractures, particularly vertebral collapse, occurs. Osteopenia and reduced bone mineral density are almost universally present in patients with advanced primary biliary cirrhosis, but are often unrecognized until fractures occur. Hence bone density should be assessed pre-transplant and monitored post-transplant. Metabolic bone disease, further aggravated by immobilization and high-dose steroids after liver transplantation, worsens in the initial 3 to 6 months post-transplant but then improves to baseline by 12 months.[376] The potential pre-transplant or post-transplant role of therapy with calcitonin, biphosphonates, and estrogens is undergoing study.[377]

Patients with primary biliary cirrhosis are generally good candidates for liver transplantation because the majority are middle-aged and do not have major comorbidities.[38,62,64-68] The long-term outcome is good, with 5-year survival ranging from 60 percent to 80 percent.[129,239,242,373] Furthermore, liver transplantation for patients with chronic cholestatic liver disease improves the overall quality of life.[378]

Some, but not all, centers report recurrence of primary biliary cirrhosis after liver transplantation.[379-385] This diagnosis is challenging because histologic appearances of the preexisting disease and chronic allograft rejection are similar, and the anti-mitochondrial antibody persists post-transplant, usually at a lower titer. Among 60 patients who underwent liver transplantation in the Mayo Clinic, 5 developed histologic features of recurrent primary biliary cirrhosis marked by florid duct lesions and portal granulomas. All five patients were asymptomatic and had normal test results.[385] The incidence and clinical impact of recurrence of primary biliary cirrhosis remain uncertain.[386]

Primary Sclerosing Cholangitis

A unique feature of primary sclerosing cholangitis is the risk of superimposed cholangiocarcinoma.[251,387-389] Clinical and laboratory clues to the diagnosis of cholangiocarcinoma include the rapid onset of jaundice, weight loss, and a marked rise in alkaline phosphatase and serum bilirubin. Endoscopic retrograde cholangiography typically reveals segmental dilation of intrahepatic ducts. Repeated brushing for cytology and biopsy for tissue should be attempted to exclude cholangiocarcinoma when a dominant biliary stricture is identified.[390] As mentioned previously, cholangiocarcinoma is considered by most centers an absolute contraindication to liver transplantation because of its poor post-transplant outcome.[185,193,194] Patients who have primary sclerosing cholangitis should proceed to transplantation somewhat earlier in their natural history, and Roux-en-Y loop anastomosis is used during the surgery because of the theoretic risk of cholangiocarcinoma if the recipient bile duct is not removed entirely.

When performed before the development of cholangiocarcinoma or advanced liver failure, liver transplantation for primary sclerosing cholangitis improves patient survival and quality of life.[391] Five-year patient and graft survival rates of approximately 85 percent and 75 percent, respectively, have been achieved.[392-394] Primary sclerosing cholangitis recurs with an incidence of 9 percent to 20 percent after transplantation, but the overall patient and graft survival is unaffected.[393,394] Classic fibro-obliterative lesions and fibrous cholangitis are seen. Although disease recurrence is mild in most cases, severe biliary stricturing with graft failure may occasionally occur.[394,395]

Ulcerative colitis is present in more than two thirds of all patients with primary sclerosing cholangitis. It does not have a negative impact on allograft function post-transplant, and the course of the colitis generally remains unchanged after transplantation.[396] However, one report suggested that patients with both ulcerative colitis and primary sclerosing cholangitis are at increased risk for developing precancerous changes in the colonic mucosa,[397] and the development of colon cancer may be accelerated by liver transplantation and chronic immunosuppression.[398] In a separate series colon cancer represented the most common cause of death post-transplant in patients with primary sclerosing cholangitis.[392] In general, liver transplantation takes precedence over colectomy; the latter can be safely performed post-transplant when normal hepatic function and coagulation parameters are restored.[38,67]

Autoimmune Hepatitis

The term autoimmune hepatitis encompasses at least three types of disease based on differences in autoantibody profiles, age, demographics, immunogenetics, and natural history.[399-401] Patients with autoimmune hepatitis are appropriate candidates for liver transplantation when they present either as decompensated cirrhosis or acute liver failure.[38,65-67] Immunosuppressive therapy prolongs life but does not prevent cirrhosis.[402,403] Only a small number of patients enter a permanent remission; the majority require long-term immunosuppressive drug therapy, with liver failure developing insidiously. Additionally, some patients with autoimmune hepatitis are undiagnosed and untreated until severe liver decompensation occurs, leaving liver transplantation the only alternative. An important consideration in the timing of liver transplantation is the severity of steroid-induced osteoporosis, because most patients require long-term immunosuppressive therapy.[404]

Several factors have been identified that appear to be associated with progression of autoimmune hepatitis and need for liver transplantation.[405-409] These include male gender; anti-nuclear antibody seronegativity in patients with type 1 autoimmune hepatitis; younger patients with type 2 autoimmune hepatitis; acute liver failure; failure to achieve remission within 4 years of immunosuppression; spontaneous development of ascites; certain human leukocyte antigen (HLA) haplotypes (HLA-A1, B8, DR3; DR4-negative and specific alleles such as DRB1*0301 and DRB3*0101); and absence of concurrent immunologic disease. However, no prognostic risk score has yet been developed for autoimmune hepatitis.

Liver transplantation is an established therapy for patients with end-stage autoimmune hepatitis, with 1-year and 7-year survival rates of 86 percent and 78 percent, respectively.[30] Nevertheless, acute cellular and chronic ductopenic rejections have been documented to occur at a higher frequency in patients transplanted for autoimmune hepatitis.[410] Furthermore, approximately 15 percent to 30 percent of recipients develop recurrent disease biochemically, serologically, histologically, or in various combinations.[411-415] Disease recurrence often is related to suboptimal immunosuppression because biochemical and histologic features rapidly resolve after adequate immunosuppression is restored.[411] Nevertheless, recurrent autoimmune hepatitis may behave aggressively and progress to graft failure.[411-414] Disease recurrence has been documented in patients who underwent retransplantation.[414]

Drug-induced Liver Failure

The diagnosis of drug-induced liver failure is one of exclusion of viral, autoimmune, and genetic causes of liver disease in the setting of recent use of a medication and its reported pattern of hepatotoxicity. Drug-induced liver disease is relatively more common in the elderly, who often use a large number of medications. Drug-induced hepatotoxicity may lead to the development of fulminant or, more commonly, subfulminant liver failure. Chronic indolent liver failure may be induced by medications, such as methotrexate or isoniazid.[416,417]

Cryptogenic Cirrhosis and Non-alcoholic Steatohepatitis

Most patients with chronic liver disease will have an etiology determined after thorough clinical evaluation, serologic and virologic testing, tests for autoimmune and metabolic liver diseases, and liver biopsy. However, a subset of patients have true cryptogenic cirrhosis that does not appear to be autoimmune or viral.[418,419] In the UNOS database of types of cirrhosis leading to liver transplantation 10.9 percent of the 58 percent of cases diagnosed as cirrhosis were unspecified in terms of etiology.[30] Patients with cryptogenic chronic liver disease generally represent good candidates for liver transplantation, but the Mayo Clinic series showed shorter 1-year and 5-year patient survival rates compared to patients transplanted for other indications, mostly due to high rates of infectious complications.[420]

A large number of cases previously termed cryptogenic cirrhosis later become labeled as hepatitis C with the development of more sensitive virologic testing.[421] Because of sampling errors of liver biopsy, the diagnostic periodic acid-Schiff positive and diastase-resistant globules of α_1-antitrypsin deficiency may be missed until post-transplant examination of the surgical explant.[422] Patients with advanced cryptogenic cirrhosis are more likely to be obese and diabetic when compared with age- and sex-matched controls, suggesting non-alcoholic steatohepatitis (NASH) as an etiologic factor.[423] In a retrospective analysis of patients with the phenotype of NASH-related cirrhosis, allograft steatosis occurred in all patients by 5 years after liver transplantation, with histologic progression to steatohepatitis in 10 percent of cases.[424] Recurrence of NASH after liver transplantation with progression to fibrosis and cirrhosis has been reported.[425,426]

Hemochromatosis

The cure provided by liver transplantation for patients with metabolic liver diseases is functional and phenotypic but not genetic.[427] Post-transplant metabolic diseases do not recur clinically, except for hereditary hemochromatosis, which is due to a genetic defect expressed in the enterocyte not the hepatocyte.[428] Despite early series from the University of Pittsburgh reporting good outcomes after transplantation for hemochromatosis complicated by liver failure,[429] more recent studies reported 1-year and 5-year survival rates of less than 60 percent and 50 percent, respectively.[138,430-433] The diagnosis of hemochromatosis was often unsuspected preoperatively.[138,433] Furthermore, these patients had a high prevalence of hepatocellular carcinoma, with the majority undetected before transplantation.[433] Iron reaccumulation was noted histologically in the liver allografts. Infections, cardiac complications, and malignancies were the most common causes of death post-transplant.[138,430-432] Dilated cardiomyopathy may continue to progress after liver transplantation.[434] Combined liver and heart transplantation has been reported for end-stage liver disease complicated by class IV congestive heart failure.[435] Anticipation of infectious and cardiac problems, and possibly the initiation of pretransplant phlebotomy to unload myocardial iron, might lead to improved survival post-transplant.[38] One-year patient survival ranged from 75 percent to 83 percent in clinical series in which the majority of patients underwent iron depletion therapy pretransplant in the form of either phlebotomy or desferoxamine.[429,436]

Wilson's Disease

Liver transplantation is indicated in patients with Wilson's disease for severe hepatic insufficiency that is unresponsive to several months of chelation therapy such as D-penicillamine. It is also indicated in the scenario of Wilsonian fulminant liver failure, whether occurring as the initial manifestation of the disease or after discontinuation of medical therapy due to non-compliance. Three series reported good prognosis after liver transplantation, with 1-year survival rates of 72 percent to 90 percent for patients presented with chronic liver failure and 67 percent to 90 percent for those presented with fulminant or subfulminant liver failure.[437-439] Transplant recipients obtained a complete reversal of biochemical abnormalities characteristic of Wilson's disease with no risk of phenotypic recurrence.[440] Furthermore, substantial neuropsychiatric improvement may be achieved post-transplant.[438,439] Several reports described liver transplantation for patients presenting only with severe neurologic manifestations that significantly improved post-transplant.[441-446] However, transplant solely for neurologic indications remains controversial,[447] and is strongly opposed by some investigators.[448]

α_1-Antitrypsin Deficiency

The majority of patients with significant liver disease from α_1-antitrypsin deficiency have the Pi (protease inhibitor) ZZ phenotype,[449] whereas the rest are heterozygotes and carry a single PiZZ allele.[450,451] Many patients with severe liver involvement, and even cirrhosis or portal hypertension, may lead a normal life for extended periods because of a relatively slow rate of disease progression.[452,453] Liver transplantation remains the only proven therapy when patients eventually develop end-stage liver disease, with 1-year and 5-year survival rates for children approaching 90 percent and 80 percent, respectively.[454-459] Replacement of the cirrhotic liver results in acquisition of donor phenotype and rise in serum levels of α_1-antitrypsin,[456-460] but its impact on pulmonary function has not yet been adequately studied.[461] Periodic acid-Schiff positive, diastase-resistant globules that are diagnostic of α_1-antitrypsin deficiency in the explant liver do not recur in the allograft.[459,462] Furthermore, membranoproliferative glomerulonephritis, which is an extrahepatic association with α_1-antitrypsin deficiency, may reverse with liver transplantation alone.[463]

Hepatic Malignancies

One of the most controversial areas in the management of hepatic malignancy is the role of liver transplantation versus resection. A number of studies confirm that liver transplantation has survival and cost-effectiveness advantages over resection in patients with cirrhosis.[122,123,464] Long-term, disease-free, post-transplant survival is greater than 80 percent for patients with solitary tumors smaller than 5 cm or up to three tumors of less than 3 cm each.[120] Using preoperative chemoembolization to retard the rate of disease progression the risk of intraoperative dissemination of tumor, the Mayo Clinic reported 1- and 2-year tumor-free survival rates of 91 percent and 84 percent, respectively, in 27 recipients post-transplant.[465] Hepatocellular carcinoma, when discovered incidentally on explant, is associated with better survival and lower recurrence rate.[123,466]

The fibrolamellar variant of hepatocellular carcinoma is an unusual and less aggressive cancer that tends to occur in younger patients in the absence of preexisting liver disease or elevated alpha fetoprotein.[123,467,468] Compared with hepatocellular carcinoma, the fibrolamellar variant has the same recurrence rate of 39 percent but better survivals at 2 years (60 percent versus 30 percent) and 5 years (55 percent versus 18 percent) after transplantation.[466] Among the uncommon primary hepatic malignancies treated by liver transplantation, the results are reasonably good with epithelioid hemangioendothelioma and hepatoblastoma. Post-transplant survival is poor with hemangiosarcoma and metastatic lesions to the liver other than those that are neuroendocrine tumors.

Uncommon Indications for Liver Transplantation

There is a long list of uncommon but accepted indications for liver transplantation, including a large number of rare metabolic diseases. The published experience with any one of these diseases is often scant. Only a few selected indications for liver transplantation will be reviewed.

Budd-Chiari Syndrome

Budd-Chiari syndrome is associated with thrombotic or non-thrombotic occlusion of the major hepatic veins, inferior vena cava, or both.[469] The liver disease is typically but not invariably progressive with ultimate decompensation caused by outflow congestion with centrolobular necrosis, fibrosis, and ultimately cardiac-type cirrhosis. Liver biopsy is pivotal in deciding between liver transplantation for advanced fibrosis and cirrhosis versus decompressive shunt surgery for earlier disease.[470-472] Good long-term results are reported with liver transplantation.[470-476] Recurrent venous thrombosis is unusual but may prompt the use of long-term anti-coagulation especially in the setting of preexisting coagulopathy.[477,478]

Polycystic Liver Disease

Polycystic liver disease presents almost exclusively in middle-aged women.[479] Its symptoms are due more often to associated polycystic kidney disease.[480] However, multiple liver cysts may be complicated by hemorrhage, infection, abdominal pain, portal hypertension with ascites, biliary obstruction, massive hepatomegaly with cystic enlargement, and rarely malignant transformation into cholangiocarcinoma despite well-preserved liver function.[479] Liver transplantation reverses severe physical and social debilitation but remains controversial because affected patients do not have liver failure.[481] In the University of Birmingham series of 16 adult women with polycystic liver disease, 14 of whom had concomitant polycystic kidney disease, indications for transplantation included massive hepatomegaly causing physical handicaps ($n = 16$), social handicaps ($n = 16$), malnutrition ($n = 4$), and cholestasis or portal hypertension ($n = 5$). Concurrent kidney transplantation was performed in one patient who had severe renal dysfunction. Over a follow-up of 3 months to 9 years post-transplant, survival was 87.5 percent, with resumption of fully active lifestyle in most recipients.[482]

MANAGEMENT AFTER LIVER TRANSPLANTATION

Allograft Dysfunction

Allograft dysfunction is the most important complication after liver transplantation. Different etiologies that lead to allograft dysfunction occur at different times postoperatively (Table 55-15).[483] Liver biopsy is critical in

TABLE 55-15

Differential Diagnosis of Allograft Dysfunction

1-5 Days Post-transplant
Hepatic artery thrombosis
Primary non-function
Hyperacute rejection
5-30 Days Post-transplant
Acute cellular rejection
Bile leaks
Azathioprine toxicity
Preservation injury
More Than 30 Days Post-transplant
Acute cellular rejection
Chronic ductopenic rejection
Biliary strictures
Recurrent diseases, including
Viral hepatitis: hepatitis B or hepatitis C
Autoimmune liver diseases
Non-B, non-C hepatitis: CMV, EBV, HSV, adenovirus
Post-transplant lymphoproliferative disorders

Modified from Lake JR, Gournay J: Liver transplantation. In Feldman M, Scharschmidt BF, Sleisenger MH, eds: Sleisenger & Fordtran's Gastrointestinal and Liver Disease: Pathophysiology/Diagnosis/Management, ed 6. Philadelphia, WB Saunders Co, 1998:1404-1416.
CMV, Cytomegalovirus; *EBV*, Epstein-Barr virus; *HSV*, herpes simplex virus.

differentiating between these because many share similar, non-specific clinical and biochemical presentations. Diagnostic evaluations may also include cholangiogram and duplex ultrasound of the vessels supplying the liver because the allograft and its bile duct epithelium are exquisitely sensitive to diminished blood flow.

Vascular Complications after Liver Transplantation

Hepatic artery thrombosis (HAT) occurs in 7 percent of adults and 10 percent to 40 percent of children who undergo liver transplantation.[484-486] Risk factors for the complication include technical aspects associated with the arterial anastomosis, low donor:recipient age ratio, presence of immunologic factors such as anti-cardiolipin antibodies or clotting abnormalities, tobacco use, and infection with CMV.[487] Early, acute HAT may present as fulminant liver failure during the first 2 weeks post-transplant. Other complications from HAT are bile leak, intrahepatic biloma, biliary strictures, liver abscesses, secondary biliary cirrhosis, or relapsing bacteremia.[488] HAT occurring later than 2 months post-transplant may progress slowly as stenosis or intimal hyperplasia, with eventual rearterialization from collaterals.[489,490] Angiography should be pursued if duplex ultrasonography of the hepatic artery is equivocal. Early HAT should prompt immediate revascularization by thrombectomy or use of a surgical conduit, but often requires urgent retransplantation.[491-493] Percutaneous balloon angioplasty, vascular stenting, or even transcatheter thrombolytic therapy with urokinase may be sufficient for patients with late HAT.[494,495] Hepatic artery stenosis without thrombosis is often associated with multiple ischemic biliary strictures.[499,500] The diagnosis requires duplex ultrasonography followed by angiography. Symptomatic disease during the early post-transplant period necessitates urgent surgical revascularization or percutaneous balloon angioplasty. Liver retransplantation is indicated when diffuse biliary strictures or graft failure develops. The single most important factor in graft outcome is the length of time that the liver lacks hepatic arterial blood supply.[496]

Portal vein thrombosis complicates only 1 percent to 3 percent of liver transplant cases.[203] Early acute portal vein thrombosis leads to fulminant liver failure and requires immediate revascularization or urgent retransplantation. On the other hand, late portal vein thrombosis may be asymptomatic but may manifest as portal hypertension with upper gastrointestinal bleeding, ascites, or hepatic encephalopathy.[497] Diagnosis can be made easily by duplex ultrasonography. Splenorenal or mesocaval shunt can be used in patients with good hepatic reserve. Retransplantation is the only option for those with poor liver reserve or venous anatomy unsuitable for reconstruction.[498]

Hepatic venous or inferior vena caval thrombosis or stenosis may result from malposition of a partial graft. Risk factors for these complications include hypercoagulable states, a pretransplant diagnosis of Budd-Chiari syndrome or hepatocellular carcinoma, or anatomic abnormalities of the outflow tract.[498] Venogram is the gold standard for diagnosis. Treatment depends on the clinical presentation. A partial occlusion of the hepatic vein can be asymptomatic and well tolerated. Development of portal hypertensive complications such as ascites can be treated with a surgical shunt. Complete obstruction of the hepatic vein is catastrophic and requires liver retransplantation.[496]

Massive bleeding may occur in the early post-transplant period and can result from a small anastomotic gap unnoticed at the time of liver transplantation or a ruptured mycotic aneurysm resulting from bacterial seeding of the anastomosis. Hypotension, radiologic detection of arterial bleeding or significant intra-abdominal clot, or transfusion requirement above 5 U of packed red blood cells over a 24 hour period should prompt immediate surgical exploration. Among all patients who undergo liver transplantation, 10 percent to 15 percent require reoperation for intra-abdominal bleeding.[501] Management involves primary repair for small anastomotic leaks. Mycotic aneurysms need to be excised, followed by construction of a surgical conduit.[502-504] Occasionally, mycotic aneurysms may warrant retransplantation after arterial resection and a course of antibiotics.[505]

Ischemic-Preservation-Reperfusion Injury

Primary non-function (PNF), or delayed ischemia-reperfusion injury, is the most common cause of graft loss in the early postoperative period after a technically successful liver transplantation.[506,507] The risks for PNF include donor age of older than 50 years, donor liver fat content of more than 30 percent, and prolonged cold or warm ischemia time.[508-512] Clinical presentation resembles fulminant liver failure and consists of persistent or new hepatic encephalopathy, unresolving coagulopathy, reduced bile production, renal failure, lactic acidosis, hypoglycemia, and elevated serum aminotransferases above 2500 IU/L.[507] Duplex ultrasonography is mandatory to exclude acute thrombosis of the hepatic artery or portal vein. Histology reveals ischemic changes and hepatocyte necrosis. PNF occurs within 3 days post-transplant and often necessitates early retransplantation. Among five recipients with PNF who underwent plasmapheresis at Johns Hopkins University, four achieved restoration of allograft function.[513] Intravenous prostaglandin E_1 improves renal function and shortens intensive care stay when used prophylactically, but does not reverse PNF.[514,515]

Initial poor graft function is characteristic of a marginally functioning graft; however, it typically recovers adequate function after days to weeks post-transplant. Compared to PNF, initial poor graft function has a milder clinical presentation, and the associated serum aminotransferases are usually less than 2500 IU/L. Treatment is largely supportive. Most grafts eventually recover, but some patients may require retransplantation.[498] Risk factors are the same as for PNF.

Recipients with allografts suffering from preservation or reperfusion injury have marked increases in serum aminotransferases during the first 24 to 48 hours postoperatively, possibly followed by a subsequent slow resolution. Graft survival for the first year is significantly impaired in these patients and is particularly susceptible to PNF if the peak serum aspartate aminotransferase (AST) exceeds 5000 IU/L during the first 72 hours post-transplant.[511] Short-term graft survival is proportional to the extent of ischemic injury, but grafts not lost to PNF have equivalent 1- and 2-year survival rates and incidences of biliary complications, acute cellular rejection, and chronic ductopenic rejection independent of initial maximum serum AST.[511,516]

Allograft Rejection

Hyperacute or accelerated rejection is due to preformed anti-donor antibodies against arterial endothelium, with resultant hepatic necrosis and graft failure. The major risk factor is ABO incompatibility. It is extremely rare except for xenotransplantation. Graft rejection occurs within minutes to hours of transplant, with a presentation mimicking HAT or primary graft non-function. Immunoperoxidase staining demonstrates immunoglobulin and complement deposition within the liver microvasculature that is consistent with a humoral immune response. Furthermore, vascular thrombosis and endothelial necrosis with neutrophil margination are seen.[517]

Hyperacute rejection usually requires urgent transplantation.[483] When the recipient has received an ABO-mismatched graft in an urgent situation, such as fulminant hepatic failure, increased immunosuppression and plasmapheresis are required.[518-522]

Acute cellular rejection is the most common form of rejection in liver transplantation, occurring in two thirds of all cases.[523] It occurs between day 5 and the first 3 weeks, with an average of 10 days post-transplant.[483] An acute rejection episode occurring beyond 6 weeks post-transplant should raise suspicion for subtherapeutic immunosuppressive regimen and patient non-compliance. Risks factors for acute cellular rejection include young recipient age, older donor age, dual immunosuppressive regimen (as compared to triple regimen), increased number of HLA-DR donor-recipient mismatches, and certain pretransplant liver conditions such as fulminant hepatic failure and autoimmune liver diseases.[296,523-528] The affected patient is usually asymptomatic and presents with abnormal liver biochemistry. There are simultaneous increases in serum bilirubin, alkaline phosphatase, and γ-glutamyltransferase in the early post-transplant course. The predominant abnormality is in serum aminotransferases when acute rejection occurs several weeks after transplantation.[524] However, recipients can also present with fever, malaise, abdominal pain, or portal hypertensive changes such as ascites. Histologic examination reveals a mixed portal or periportal inflammatory infiltrate (with neutrophils, eosinophils, plasma cells, and lymphocytes) leading to destructive suppurative cholangitis and endothelialitis.[529,530] Liver biopsy should be performed before anti-rejection therapy and repeated when subsequent liver biochemistry does not respond to treatment. Transplant centers performing protocol biopsies may diagnose and treat rejection based solely on histology without requiring an abnormal test result.[498] Treatment consisting of high-dose intravenous methylprednisolone followed by oral prednisone cycle with a quick taper over 7 days can reverse 65 percent to 85 percent of all acute cellular rejection episodes.[531,532] Resolution of liver enzyme abnormalities and clinical defervescence usually occur within 24 to 48 hours after commencement of anti-rejection therapy. Addition of anti-lymphocyte preparations, conversion from cyclosporine to tacrolimus, and, potentially, addition of mycophenolate mofetil are used as rescue therapy if the patient does not respond to high-dose steroids.[533-536] Whether or not adjuvant prophylaxis with ursodeoxycholic acid can decrease the incidence of acute cellular rejection remains controversial.[536-540]

Chronic ductopenic rejection currently approximates 3 percent[541] and has been decreasing in incidence among adult recipients, which is largely the result of earlier diagnosis and better use of immunosuppressants.[14-16,542] It occurs most commonly between 6 weeks and 6 months post-transplant.[541] Predisposing risk factors include young recipient age, dual or insufficient immunosuppressive regimen, HLA donor-recipient matching, positive lymphocytic cross-match, recurrent bouts of acute rejection, chronic ischemia resulting from hepatic artery insufficiency, male donor to female recipient, infection with CMV, previous retransplantation for chronic ductopenic rejection, and autoimmune liver disease as the indication for liver transplantation.[541] Clinical manifestations are insidious in onset, but cholestatic abnormalities (e.g., alkaline phosphatase, γ-glutamyltransferase) relentlessly worsen long before onset of jaundice signals the late stage of chronic ductopenic rejection. Histologic evaluation reveals sparse lymphocytic portal inflammation but progressive loss of interlobular and septal bile ducts in at least half of the portal tracts when more than 20 portal triads are analyzed—a condition known as vanishing bile duct syndrome.[543,544] Earlier diagnosis of chronic ductopenic rejection facilitates medical intervention and can be based on the presence of biliary epithelial atrophy or pyknosis when the majority of the bile ducts are still present.[544] On large, open-wedge biopsies—but less often on percutaneous needle specimens—one may note the pathologic feature of foam cell arteriopathy that is due to progressive intimal expansion and luminal obliteration of medium-sized hepatic arteries by foamy histiocytes. Conversion from cyclosporine to tacrolimus may benefit some early cases especially when serum bilirubin is less than 10 mg/dl and the condition is diagnosed longer than 90 days post-transplant.[545] According to two clinical series in the pre-tacrolimus era, chronic ductopenic rejection may resolve using conventional immunosuppressive therapy in 20 percent to 30 percent of cases.[546,547] Otherwise, progression of vanishing bile duct syndrome to complete absence of interlobular bile ducts leads to graft loss. Approximately 15 percent to 20 percent of retransplantations today are due to chronic ductopenic rejection.[541]

Biliary Complications after Liver Transplantation

Described as the Achilles heel of liver transplantation, the biliary tree has very poor regenerative and reparative capacity when damaged.[548,549] It is the most common site for technical complications post-transplant. Biliary complications occur in 10 percent to 25 percent of all recipients,[483] with more than two thirds of cases diagnosed within 1 month and 80 percent of cases within 6 months post-transplant.[498] Their incidence drops significantly to less than 4 percent annually after the first postoperative year. Causes of biliary complications include technical factors, ischemia such as preservation injury and HAT, immunologic factors, and infection, particularly CMV.[550-552] Bile leaks and strictures are the most common presentations of biliary complications in the first 3 months postoperatively.

Choledochocholedochostomy and choledochojejunostomy are the two methods of primary biliary reconstruction in liver transplantation. Choledochocholedochostomy is performed more commonly because it preserves the sphincter of Oddi and is associated with shorter operating time. This type of anastomosis also maintains endoscopic access to the biliary tree post-transplant. However, it is prone to focal ischemia and stricture. Placement of a T-tube at the time of duct-to-duct anastomosis allows stenting and biliary decompression, monitoring of bile flow and quality to assess allograft function in the early postoperative period, and readily available cholangiographic access. But T-tube drainage interrupts the enterohepatic circulation, thus reducing bile acid supply for micelle formation and adequate enteric absorption of medications such as oral cyclosporine. The University of Northern Carolina team has recently advocated placing a radiopaque Silastic internal biliary stent for decompression.[553] The stent can be passed spontaneously or extracted easily by an endoscope.

Choledochojejunostomy, or Roux-en-Y anastomosis, is used for retransplantation, for transplanting reduced-size liver grafts, for patients with intrinsic disease of the extrahepatic bile ducts or appreciable size disparities between the donor and recipient ducts. The duct-to-duct anastomosis can be converted surgically to a Roux-en-Y anastomosis when necessary. The latter, however, is associated with increased operative time to create a jejunal limb and prevents easy endoscopic access to the biliary tree, thus limiting future biliary imaging to either percutaneous transhepatic cholangiography or hepatobiliary scintigraphy.

Bile leak occurs in up to 25 percent of all recipients. Early bile leaks occur within the first month post-transplant and are due to disruption of the surgical anastomosis. Late bile leaks result from ischemic injury from HAT or removal of T-tube. Less common sites of bile leaks include an incompletely closed cystic duct remnant draining from the liver, a previously unrecognized auxiliary bile duct that is ligated during transplantation, or a cut surface of a split allograft.[554-558] Patients may present with fever, abdominal pain, peritonitis, hypotension, or sepsis with biloma as the source of infection. Liver chemistries may or may not be abnormal. Bile leak can be delineated anatomically by cholangiogram or by biliary scintigraphy if sufficiently large. Duplex ultrasonography is essential to exclude HAT except in cases related directly to removing a T-tube. For patients with a bile leak after T-tube removal, endoscopic placement of a nasobiliary drain or internal plastic stent allows the leakage to heal as the bile flows preferentially through the ampulla.[558-561] Nasobiliary drainage has the additional advantage of easy cholangiographic follow-up. For others with an anastomotic leak post-transplant, surgical creation or revision of a choledochojejunostomy should be attempted only after failure of endoscopic or radiologic interventions.[559-562] Severe bile duct necrosis may require retransplantation.

Anastomotic biliary stricture, which affects 4 percent to 10 percent of all recipients, occurs within the first 6 months post-transplant.[548-550] Clinical presentation is typical of cholangitis but may be asymptomatic with only elevation of cholestatic enzymes (predominantly alkaline phosphatase and γ-glutamyltransferase). Cholangiogram is diagnostic of the condition, but Doppler ultrasound should be performed to rule out HAT. Balloon dilation or endoscopic or radiologic stenting should be attempted before resorting to surgical creation or revision of choledochojejunostomy.[559-561] Retransplantation is considered for poor hepatic function or complete obstruction of the hepatic artery.

Non-anastomotic biliary strictures affect up to 20 percent of all recipients and occur within the first 4 months post-transplant. Possible etiologies include HAT, ABO incompatibility, chronic ductopenic rejection, extended cold preservation of longer than 10 hours, pretransplant diagnosis of primary sclerosing cholangitis, and infections with opportunistic organisms such as cytomegalovirus, *Cryptococcus,* and *Candida.* The hilum and the intrahepatic biliary systems are typically involved. The biliary strictures are usually multiple and may be associated with extrahepatic bile leaks and intrahepatic bile lakes. Duplex ultrasonography should be performed to rule out HAT. Management of these strictures depends on their number, location, severity, and liver function.[559-561,563] Diffuse strictures in the setting of bile leaks and bilomas indicate HAT and the need for retransplantation.[498] Focal intrahepatic strictures may benefit from repeated sessions of balloon dilation and stenting performed endoscopically or radiologically, but the rate of long-term patency is less compared with anastomotic strictures. Intrabiliary casts, which are associated with long graft preservation time, could be very difficult and challenging to manage nonsurgically.[564] Complete surgical extraction is usually not possible, especially when multiple, peripheral biliary branches are involved. Liver retransplantation is usually required.

Ampullary dysfunction resulting from denervation and devascularization of the sphincter of Oddi during the recipient hepatectomy presents as obstruction of bile flow in patients with duct-to-duct anastomosis. Patients present with diffuse dilation of extrahepatic and sometimes intrahepatic bile ducts without cholangiographic evidence of biliary stricture.[565] This can be demonstrated by delayed drainage of contrast after cholangiography, slowed biliary emptying on hepatobiliary scintigraphy, and abnormal sphincter of Oddi manometry. In patients with a T-tube, unclamping the tube improves liver chemistry and decompresses the common duct. The differential diagnosis of ampullary dysfunction includes papillary stenosis, benign common duct stricture, pancreatitis, and pancreatic mass. Transpapillary stenting for 1 to 3 months can be attempted first.[566] Endoscopic sphincterotomy has been successful.[567] Surgical revision to a choledochojejunostomy is the last resort when cholestasis persists or cholangitis recurs.

Azathioprine Toxicity

Azathioprine classically causes cholestatic injury to the liver, but hepatocellular and even mixed damage have been noted.[568-570] This drug may lead to sclerosing hepatitis with prominent chronic cholestasis and marked fibrosis. In combination with steroids azathioprine may lead rarely to sinusoidal dilation, peliosis hepatis, nodular regenerative hyperplasia, hepatoportal sclerosis, and veno-occlusive disease of the liver.[569-572] The prognosis of the hepatic injury varies with the nature of the lesion. Drug withdrawal may lead to resolution of cholestasis, but chronic cholestasis or even cirrhosis may ensue.[573] Veno-occlusive disease of the liver led to death among six of eight renal transplant recipients.[574] It is important to suspect azathioprine as the cause of graft dysfunction before liver injury becomes irreversible.[575]

Non-B, Non-C Hepatitis and Post-transplant Lymphoproliferative Disorders

Infection with CMV is a major cause of morbidity and mortality in the transplant population, occurring in 23 percent to 85 percent of liver recipients in the absence of anti-viral prophylaxis.[576] Infection often occurs within 3 months of transplantation. The peak incidence is in the third or fourth week.[577] Risk factors for infection include CMV-positive donors to CMV-negative recipients, previous anti-lymphocyte therapy for acute cellular rejection, and retransplantation. CMV viral syndrome includes fever, malaise, arthralgia, myalgia, leukopenia, and thrombocytopenia. Patients may present with cholestatic hepatitis[578]; less commonly, patients have gastroenteritis with ulcerations, pneumonia, or chorioretinitis. Cholangitis occurs rarely. Mortality is greater in patients with recurrent versus new CMV infection.[579] CMV also predisposes a transplant recipient to opportunistic infections with bacteria, *P. carinii,* and fungi.[580-583] Furthermore, it increases the severity of recurrent hepatitis C.[330] Kaposi's sarcoma is sometimes associated with CMV infection.[580] CMV potentiates allograft rejection by enhancing the expressions of class I and class II histocompatibility antigens and activating transcription factors for inflammatory responses.[584] Patient and graft survival rates post-transplant are significantly reduced in recipients with CMV infection.[585,586]

The diagnosis of CMV infection can be made by recovering virus from any body tissue or fluid; by serologic conversion in a patient who was previously seronegative; by appearance of anti-CMV IgM antibody; by a fourfold increase in anti-CMV IgG titer; by positive CMV antigenemia assay; and by biopsy of end organs such as liver, esophagus, colon, or lungs.[580] CMV hepatitis is histologically demonstrated by neutrophilic microabscesses and, less often, enlarged hepatocytes with intranuclear inclusion bodies that have a typical "owl's eye" appearance.[577] Intravenous ganciclovir is the mainstay of therapy for CMV infection, despite a recent report of CMV resistance.[587] Neutropenia is the major side effect of ganciclovir and can be exacerbated by concomitant use of trimethoprim-sulfamethoxazole and azathioprine. Alternatively, intravenous foscarnet can be used but its use can be complicated by nephrotoxicity, electrolyte abnormality, gastrointestinal disturbance, and seizures. CMV hyperimmunoglobulin in combination with ganciclovir is used in more serious CMV infections such as pneumonia, disseminated CMV disease, or CMV disease in the setting of invasive fungal infection.[588] Prophylactic ganciclovir followed by oral acyclovir is used in high-risk settings for CMV infections, including the use of tacrolimus or cyclosporine for immunosuppression, CMV-positive donors to CMV-negative recipients, and muromonab-CD3 for either induction therapy or steroid-resistant anti-rejection therapy.[498,589]

Infection with EBV can present as a benign infectious mononucleosis, febrile illness with neutropenia, focal organ involvement such as bowel obstruction or perforation, or post-transplant lymphoproliferative disorders (PTLD). The entity of PTLD, due to unrestricted proliferation of B cells stimulated by EBV, occurs more commonly in primary infection than viral reactivation. It affects 1 percent to 3 percent of adult and 20 percent of pediatric recipients. Most cases occur within the first 2 years post-transplant.[590-592] EBV has an extranodal predilection for the brain, head, neck, gastrointestinal tract, and the liver graft.[593] Three quarters of pediatric recipients with PTLD presented with airway obstruction.[594] Risk factors for PTLD include high-dose immunosuppression particularly with anti-lymphocyte antibody therapy such as muromonab-CD3, lack of previous exposure to EBV, and possibly HCV infection when muromonab-CD3 or anti-thymocyte globulin is used.[591-596] Therapy includes high-dose intravenous acyclovir and ganciclovir plus temporary discontinuation or reduction of immunosuppressants. Localized masses (i.e., lymphoma associated with PTLD) may be treated with chemotherapy or radiation.[597] Disseminated disease and central nervous system lymphomas are usually fatal despite chemoradiation therapy and reduced immunosuppression.

Medical Problems after Liver Transplantation

Infections (see Chap. 58)

Most infections occur within the first 2 months post-transplant when recipients are receiving a high-dose induction immunosuppressive regimen. Bacteria and fungi contribute to more than 90 percent of infections during this period.[580] The risk factors for bacterial infections post-transplant include long operations with high blood loss, retransplantation, and surgical mishaps such as HAT, bile leak, intraperitoneal bleeding, and intestinal perforation.[598] Pneumonia, urinary infection, intra-abdominal and hepatic abscesses, peritonitis, wound infection, and line sepsis are the most common infections.[599] The last decade witnessed a significant increase of infection by multiple-antibiotic-resistant, gram-positive bacteria (e.g., methicillin-resistant *Staphylococcus aureus* and vancomycin-resistant *Enterococcus*).[600] In addition, extended-spectrum beta-lactamase–producing enterobacteria that may not be susceptible to any currently available antibiotics are emerging.[601]

Candida albicans is the most common fungal infection in the immediate post-transplant period. Other frequent fungal diseases include *Aspergillus fumigatus* and non-*albicans candida* species such as *C. tropicalis, C. krusei, C. parapsilosis, and Torulopsis glabrata.* Risk factors for fungal infections include high-dose immunosuppression, prolonged treatment with ciprofloxacin, CMV infection, fulminant hepatic failure, renal insufficiency, prolonged operation, and retransplantation.[602,603] Dissemination of aspergillosis to the central nervous system can lead to fever and acute neurologic decompensation, with mortality approaching 100 percent.[601] Despite its nephrotoxicity, amphotericin B is the treatment of choice for invasive fungal infections. Oral fluconazole, on the other hand, has been established as the standard anti-fungal prophylaxis for the first 6 weeks post-transplant. Amphotericin B lipid complex is recently advocated as a well-tolerated anti-fungal prophylaxis targeted to patients requiring intensive care unit stay for more than 5 days after transplantation.[604]

Evaluation of fever should be guided by symptoms and physical findings. All lines, drains, and tubes should be cultured. Fluid collections should be aspirated and sent for white blood cells, Gram stain, bacterial and fungal cultures, and CMV culture if the patient is more than 3 weeks post-transplant. Further evaluations include CT of the abdomen and cholangiography to look for intra-abdominal abscess and bile duct disease. In patients with focal signs or symptoms suggestive of a neurologic source, head CT or magnetic resonance imaging followed by lumbar puncture should be pursued. Broad-spectrum antibiotics should be initiated without delay after cultures are obtained. Vancomycin is preferable if a wound, vascular source, or catheters are suspected as causes of infections. Aminoglycosides should be avoided because of the additive nephrotoxic effects with tacrolimus and cyclosporine. Macrolides should be used with caution because they inhibit the metabolism of tacrolimus and cyclosporine. Stress-dose steroids are not necessary.

Infection with *P. carinii* presents as fever, cough, and hypoxemia most commonly during the first year post-transplant. The use of trimethoprim-sulfamethoxazole as prophylaxis provides additional coverage against other opportunistic infections, including *Listeria monocytogenes, Toxoplasma gondii,* and *Nocardia asteroides.* Intravenous pentamidine and oral dapsone are alternatives in patients allergic to sulfa. Prophylaxis lasts for 1 year after transplantation but should be extended for an extra year if the patient receives additional high-dose immunosuppressants (e.g., steroid boluses, muromonab-CD3, increased tacrolimus) after the first year post-transplant.

Reactivation of herpes simplex virus as oral and genital lesions may occur within the first month post-transplant. Oral or intravenous acyclovir can be used for treatment. For patients who have recurrent mucocutaneous herpes, a reduced immunosuppressive regimen is indicated. Prophylaxis with oral acyclovir for 3 months post-transplant is advocated even when the recipient does not require CMV prophylaxis. On the other hand, reactivation of varicella-zoster virus (VZV) also occurs in the early post-transplant period. It may present as localized dermatomal vesicles and, in patients who were seronegative for VZV pretransplant, cutaneous and visceral dissemination. Treatment with high-dose acyclovir is effective unless there is simultaneous reactivation of CMV. In this latter scenario intravenous ganciclovir covers both viral infections. VZV vaccine may be administered to transplant candidates who are seronegative. Transplant recipients who are seronegative for VZV should report any exposure to the virus so that varicella-zoster immunoglobulin can be given.

Six months after liver transplantation, recipients with normal allograft function on standard doses of immunosuppressive drugs share the same risks for community-acquired infections as immunocompetent hosts. They are not at increased risk for opportunistic infections. Recipients on increased immunosuppressive drugs as anti-rejection therapy continue to be at high risk for life-threatening, opportunistic infections.[580]

Pulmonary Complications

Pleural effusions are extremely common post-transplant but are usually clinically insignificant. They often resolve within a month of surgery.[605] A paralyzed right hemidiaphragm at surgery also may return to function within a month. Pulmonary infiltrates occur in almost 50 percent of all recipients post-transplant, and at least half of these have an infectious cause.[483] Early infections are predominantly bacterial. Later infections are due to opportunistic microorganisms such as *P. carinii, Cryptococcus neoformans, A. fumigatus,* and *Candida* species. The most common viral pneumonia is due to CMV and can be fatal. Bronchoscopy with bronchoalveolar lavage and, rarely, thoracoscopy or open lung biopsy may be required to make a diagnosis. Broad-spectrum antibiotics should be initiated early after pneumonia is suspected and tailored when sensitivity results are obtained. At least half of the patients are fluid overloaded during the immediate postoperative period because of aggressive intraoperative fluid administration.[606] Renal insufficiency in some patients can further exacerbate the fluid problem, leading to pulmonary edema and congestive heart failure. When aggressive diuresis fails to reverse the congestion, hemofiltration or hemodialysis may be required. The monoclonal antibody muromonab-CD3 can also cause life-threatening non-cardiogenic pulmonary edema.

Renal Failure

Acute renal dysfunction is common after liver transplantation. Predisposing factors include hepatorenal syndrome, baseline chronic liver diseases, acute tubular necrosis from difficult operations, poor allograft function, and drug toxicities of antibiotics and immunosuppressants such as tacrolimus or cyclosporine. For patients with mild to moderate renal insufficiency, dose reduction of nephrotoxic medications usually suffices. However, for those with severe renal dysfunction, temporarily discontinuing tacrolimus or cyclosporine and switching to mycophenolate mofetil are necessary maneuvers. When aggressive diuresis fails, more stable patients can undergo hemodialysis. Hypotensive patients can be treated with continuous venovenous hemofiltration dialysis. A Swan-Ganz catheter can be placed for hemodynamic monitoring and fluid management in the immediate postoperative period.

Gastrointestinal Complications

Postoperative pain is usually not a major complaint, unless the patient had been abusing analgesics on a regular basis before liver transplantation. Abdominal pain should never be attributed immediately to constipation. Other potential causes (e.g., peptic ulcer disease, bile leak, pancreatitis, obstruction, ileus, intestinal perforation) should be explored. Immediate surgical exploration is required for the patient with an acute abdomen.

The evaluation of diarrhea should rule out a bacterial cause. Stool analysis includes white blood cells, culture for pathogens, and assay for *Clostridium difficile* toxin. A limited flexible sigmoidoscopy can be informative if white blood cells are present but *Clostridium* toxin is negative.[483] Differential diagnosis of diarrhea also includes inflammatory bowel disease, side effects of tacrolimus, and graft-versus-host disease (GVHD). GVHD usually occurs within 2 months after liver transplantation and is due to migration of donor lymphocytes from the transplanted organ into the recipient, with a subsequent immune response against the host (see Chap. 58). Clinical presentation includes fever, neutropenia, diarrhea, and skin rash. Diagnosis is based on biopsy of the involved organ, such as the skin or the colon.[607]

Neurologic Disorders

Between 10 percent and 20 percent of recipients develop neurologic complications after liver transplantation.[594] Potential causes of neurologic changes include metabolic encephalopathy, graft dysfunction, electrolyte disturbances, intracranial bleeding, and situational psychosis.[608-610] Infections and medications are the two most common etiologies of neurologic complications once the patient is discharged home.[594] *Streptococcus pneumoniae, Neisseria meningitidis, Haemophilus influenzae,* and *L. monocytogenes* can cause acute meningitis; whereas *C. neoformans, Mycobacterium tuberculosis,* and *Candida immitis* can give a more subacute or chronic presentation. On the other hand, *A. fumigatus, N. asteroides, T. gondii,* and *L. monocytogenes* may cause focal brain lesions.[580] Steroids may induce mental status and personality changes. Cyclosporine and tacrolimus share similar neurotoxicities that include headache, peripheral neuropathy, confusion, seizures, and cortical blindness. Seizures are due most often to electrolyte abnormalities or immunosuppressants, but an intracranial event needs to be excluded. Central pontine myelinolysis is a potentially lethal condition that is preventable by avoiding rapid correction of hyponatremia.[611] Other neurologic complications among transplant recipients include headache, sleep disturbance, psychosis, hemiplegias, spastic quadripareses, cortical blindness, and even coma.[483] Neurologic disorders should prompt a cautious review of the serum electrolyte levels, medication profile, and immunosuppressant levels. Anti-convulsants should be used cautiously because they interfere with hepatic metabolism of cyclosporine and tacrolimus.

Long-term Follow-up of Post-transplant Patients

Long-term management of the liver transplant recipient requires continuing communication and cooperation between the transplant center and the primary care physician. These patients require management of coronary artery disease risk factors, screening for malignancy, and immunization updates and boosters.[612,613]

Hypertension

Hypertension after liver transplantation is related most likely to immunosuppressants such as cyclosporine and tacrolimus. The pathogenesis involves vasoconstriction in the systemic and renal vasculature.[614] Corticosteroids contribute to hypertension through sodium retention, increased plasma volume, and weight gain. Hypertension occurs in 30 percent to 90 percent of recipients.[23] Management of hypertension in liver transplant recipients follows a stepwise approach. Dietary sodium restriction, resumption of physical activity, and weight reduction are the basic steps. Because of the pathophysiology of vasoconstriction in cyclosporine- and tacrolimus-induced hypertension, calcium channel blockers are the drugs of first choice. The preferred calcium channel blockers belong to the dihydropyridine class (e.g., nifedipine, isradipine, amlodipine, felodipine, nitrendipine). Verapamil, diltiazem, and nicardipine are also effective, but increase the drug levels of cyclosporine and tacrolimus. Second-line anti-hypertensive agents are diuretics, beta blockers, and α-adrenergic blockers. Angiotensin-converting enzyme inhibitors should be used with caution. They may aggravate hyperkalemia, and rarely can exacerbate leukopenia, especially when used with mycophenolate mofetil or azathioprine. Hypertension may improve with time as corticosteroids are discontinued and dosages of cyclosporine or tacrolimus are lowered.

Diabetes Mellitus

Diabetes mellitus develops in more than one third of liver recipients post-transplant. The majority of patients are insulin-dependent.[613] The pathogenesis is multifactorial, including genetic predisposition and use of tacrolimus, cyclosporine, and corticosteroids. Hyperglycemia is particularly severe during the immediate post-transplant period and anti-rejection treatment resulting from steroid boluses. Steroid tapering is the key to management of early post-transplant hyperglycemia. The rest of the management is similar to that for the nontransplant population.

Hyperlipidemia

Approximately one quarter of all liver recipients develop hyperlipidemia after transplantation.[483] The pathophysiology is multi-factorial, including genetic predisposition, co-existence of diabetes mellitus, dietary factors, weight gain, and use of corticosteroids. The management of hyperlipidemia includes diabetic control, appropriate dietary restrictions of fat and carbohydrates, weight reduction, regular exercise, and smoking cessation. The preferred medication for patients with resistant hyperlipidemia is 3-hydroxy-3-methylglutaryl co-enzyme A (HMG-CoA) reductase inhibitors. Pravastatin was found to be effective and well tolerated without occurrence of rhabdomyolysis, a complication associated with the use of HMG-CoA reductase inhibitors.[615]

Obesity

At least 40 percent of patients become obese or overweight at 1 year after liver transplantation. Use of corticosteroids, increased caloric intake, reduced physical activity, and co-existence of diabetes mellitus all contribute to weight gain. More recipients developed obesity while on a tacrolimus-based regimen than cyclosporine-based regimen, probably because of the stronger steroid-sparing effect of the former immunosuppressant.[17] Obesity is a major contributing factor to many co-morbid factors post-transplant, including hypertension, diabetes mellitus, hyperlipidemia, coronary artery disease, and osteoporosis. As soon as a patient's weight exceeds 110 percent of ideal body weight, physician counseling and dietary restriction should be initiated. Regular exercise should be reinforced and formal weight reduction programs may be necessary. Pharmacologic therapy for obesity may be available in the future if safety of these medications is proven.

Bone Disease

Bone mineral density decreases further during the first few months post-transplant but eventually regains its preoperative level, with primary biliary cirrhosis being the prototype.[124,263] Fractures most frequently involve trabecular bones such as the vertebrae and ribs. Osteonecrosis or avascular necrosis of the hips and, less often, the knees and humerus bones, may occur. Contributing risk factors to bone disease include preexisting osteopenia, corticosteroids (which inhibit bone formation and activate bone resorption), cyclosporine and tacrolimus (which promote rapid bone turnover), furosemide (which enhances hypercalciuria), original diagnosis of primary biliary cirrhosis or primary sclerosing cholangitis with associated metabolic osteodystrophy, prolonged bedrest, malnutrition, and increased cytokine levels postoperatively. Management includes weight reduction, regular exercise, and pharmacologic therapies such as calcium supplementation, vitamin D derivatives, bisphosphonates, and, for postmenopausal women, estrogen replacement.

Cancer Screening and Prevention of Malignancies

Skin cancer is the most common malignancy occurring in the setting of solid-organ transplantation and immunosuppression. Squamous cell carcinoma is more common than basal cell carcinoma or malignant melanoma in this population. Some transplant recipients may develop hundreds of squamous cell carcinomas that may be life-threatening. Patients should seek medical attention if they have a skin growth that bleeds or crusts, increases in size or thickness, or changes in color or texture.[616] Sunscreen with a sun protection factor of at least 30 is recommended. Patients should undergo at least annual skin examination depending on previous history of skin cancers, with particular attention to sun-exposed areas and the perineum. Prompt referral to a dermatologist expert in the management of these patients is essential to minimize morbidity and mortality.

Colon cancer is a common de novo neoplasia post-transplant. Colon cancer was the most common cause of postoperative death among 37 patients who underwent liver transplantation for primary sclerosing cholangitis at the University of California, San Francisco.[392] Colonoscopic surveillance with multiple biopsies every 6 months for the first 2 years post-transplant followed by annual examination has been recommended for these high-risk patients.[617] Surveillance colonoscopy every 3 years suffices for average-risk recipients.

Immunizations

If not given before liver transplantation, recipients should receive hepatitis A, hepatitis B, and pneumococcal vaccines. Other immunizations include influenza vaccine annually and tetanus toxoid booster every 5 years. Vaccines based on live or attenuated microorganisms should be avoided, including those for measles, mumps, rubella, chickenpox, polio, and bacille Calmette-Guérin (BCG).

Evolving and Novel Approaches to Liver Transplantation

Improved immunosuppressive strategies can potentially increase the success of liver transplantation. There is a movement toward minimal immunosuppression and steroid withdrawal and the development of safer and more effective medications. The growing discrepancy between the available donor organs and the need for transplantation has led to increasing application of novel approaches to liver replacement, including cadaver split liver transplantation, adult living donor liver transplantation and, possibly, in the more distant future, xenotransplantation and transplantation of hepatocytes.

EVOLVING IMMUNOSUPPRESSIVE STRATEGIES

Corticosteroid

Current immunosuppressive strategies are classified as induction regimens, maintenance therapy, and more aggressive therapy to treat rejection. Early in the post-transplant period, when the risk of acute cellular rejection is the highest, induction regimens include high-dose intravenous corticosteroid therapy with rapid tapering to oral doses of 20 mg daily by day 7. The transition from induction to maintenance therapy begins early after transplantation and is gradual over several months. Patients are often tapered off prednisone 3 to 6 months post-transplant. Long-term, low-dose prednisone maintenance, as an exception, may be used to prevent acute cellular rejection and chronic ductopenic rejection in patients transplanted for autoimmune liver diseases.

Calcineurin Inhibitors

The calcineurin inhibitors cyclosporine and tacrolimus are initiated at the time of transplantation and serve as the basis for most maintenance therapy. Both agents have similar toxicity profiles, which include nephrotoxicity, neurotoxicity, gastrointestinal symptoms, and the risk of lymphoproliferative disorders. Hyperglycemia and diarrhea are more common with tacrolimus. Hypertension, hyperkalemia, gingival hyperplasia, and hirsutism are more common with cyclosporine. Azathioprine has often been used as part of a triple-drug regimen, but the greater potency of tacrolimus and the lower incidence of acute cellular rejection have led some transplant centers to adopt the two-drug regimen of prednisone and tacrolimus. Trough tacrolimus levels are maintained at 10 to 15 ng/ml during the early weeks to months post-transplant, but trough levels of 5 to 7 ng/ml are satisfactory for long-term maintenance of immunosuppression even in the absence of prednisone maintenance.

Mycophenolate Mofetil

Mycophenolate mofetil is a new immunosuppressant that exerts its effects by inhibiting de novo purine synthesis and halting T-cell and B-cell proliferation. It may have an advantage over azathioprine because of more specific enzyme inhibition. The usual dosage of mycophenolate mofetil is 2 g daily in divided doses. Its major side effects are leukopenia, gastrointestinal symptoms, and neurologic disturbances. It has been used as part of a multi-drug regimen for steroid-sparing or calcineurin inhibitor–sparing purposes and for anti-rejection therapy.

Sirolimus

Sirolimus, also known as rapamycin, is structurally similar to tacrolimus but acts by a different mechanism. It may play a major role in the immunosuppressive regimens of patients with poor renal function because of its lack of nephrotoxicity. However, it may cause leukopenia, thrombocytopenia, and hyperlipidemia. Early experience is encouraging for combination of sirolimus with cyclosporine or tacrolimus.[618,619]

DONOR ORGAN OPTIONS

Split-liver Transplantation

Split-liver transplantation has been used increasingly over the past 3 to 4 years.[620] This procedure allows two liver transplants from a single cadaver liver. Usually, a right lobe is implanted into an adult recipient and a left lobe or left lateral segment is implanted into a pediatric recipient. This was a logical extension of reduced-sized liver transplantation in children, in which the left lateral segment (segments 2 and 3) or left lobe (segments 2, 3, and 4) was taken from an adult cadaver organ for implantation into a child, whereas the remaining right lobe was discarded.

Two methods are employed for split-liver transplantation: (1) the ex vivo technique (splitting the liver on the bench after its removal from the cadaver) and (2) the in vivo technique (division of the liver in the cadaver before procurement). Early experience with the ex vivo technique had excessive biliary complications and reoperations. Adult and pediatric survival rates were only 67 percent and 20 percent, respectively.[621] The patient and graft survival rates were improved to 90 percent and 80 percent, respectively, in the recent King's College Hospital series.[622] In a series of 102 pediatric and adult patients who received 110 in vivo split grafts at the University of California at Los Angeles overall graft and patient survival rates were not different from rates achieved with standard whole-organ transplantation.[623]

Living Donor Liver Transplantation

Living donor liver transplantation (LDLT) was first reported in children in 1988 and in adults in 1994.[624,625] Adult-to-child LDLT achieved a 1-year survival rate of 82 percent among 149 cases from Kyoto University; these excellent outcomes have been duplicated in many transplant centers.[626] The use of the left lateral segment has become the standard technique for adult-to-child LDLT, with a low risk to the adult donor.

Good results have been achieved in recent years with elective adult-to-adult LDLT using right lobe (segments 5 to 8); left lobe (segments 2 to 4) for small recipients; and right trisegment (segments 4 to 8) for larger recipients to ensure adequate liver volume.[627-629] This operation has also been applied to urgent cases with good outcomes.[630] LDLT allows liver replacement before the development of progressive advanced liver failure that might compromise the operative outcome. Patients with small hepatocellular carcinomas and those with primary sclerosing cholangitis at risk of cholangiocarcinoma are also excellent candidates for an LDLT. Furthermore, a graft obtained from a thoroughly evaluated healthy living donor should be better than a cadaveric liver harvested from a patient who may have suffered ischemic and metabolic insults during a terminal event. Finally, LDLT allows immediate transplantation of the donated liver portion, thus limiting the extracorporeal preservation injury associated with cadaveric organs. Unfortunately, adult-to-adult LDLT is only a partial solution to the donor shortage for adult liver transplantation. After complete evaluation only a relatively small percentage of potential donors are satisfactory candidates. Among 100 potential living donor recipients at the University of Colorado Health Science Center, 51 were rejected based on recipient characteristics. Of the remaining 49 patients, 26 living donors were evaluated but only 15 donor-recipient pairs were satisfactory and led to LDLT.[631]

The evaluation of potential living donors follows a stepwise approach. Stage 1 includes a complete history and physical examination, including screening blood studies such as blood type, complete blood count, liver and kidney chemistry, coagulation profile, and viral serologies. Stage 2 includes a complete psychosocial evaluation, imaging studies such as CT scan of the abdomen, and other studies such as echocardiogram and pulmonary function tests. Many patients are excluded at these stages because of incompatible blood type or detection of previously unrecognized medical or psychosocial problems. Stage 3 encompasses more invasive assessment in some but not all centers, potentially including a liver biopsy to exclude steatosis above 30 percent and celiac and superior mesenteric angiography with portal venous phase to accurately define the vascular anatomy. Often, magnetic resonance cholangiography is performed at stage 4.[632]

The morbidity and mortality to the donor average 10 percent and 0.5 percent, respectively, thus making the donor operation quite formidable and necessitating careful informed consent. Procuring the right lobe from a donor is technically complex, and carries the potential risks of bleeding, bile leak, need for reoperation, and pulmonary embolus and pneumonia. However, living donors are most often highly motivated and willing to accept these risks.

References

1. Starzl TE: History of liver and other splanchnic organ transplantation. In Busuttil RW, Klintmalm GB, eds: Transplantation of the Liver. Philadelphia, WB Saunders, 1996:3.
2. Keeffe EB: Liver transplantation at the millennium: past, present, and future. Clin Liver Dis 4(1):241, 2000.
3. Welch CS: A note on transplantation of the whole liver in dogs. Transplant Bull 2:54, 1955.
4. Cannon JA: Brief report. Transplant Bull 3:7, 1956.
5. Starzl TE, Marchioro TL, Von Kaulla KN, et al: Homotransplantation of the liver in humans. Surg Gynecol Obstet 117:659, 1963.
6. Starzl TE, Iwatsuki S, Van Thiel DH, et al: Evolution of liver transplantation. Hepatology 2(5):614, 1982.
7. Calne RY, White DJ, Thiru S, et al: Cyclosporin A in patients receiving renal allografts from cadaver donors. Lancet 2(8104):1323, 1978.
8. Calne RY, Rolles K, White DJ, et al: Cyclosporin A initially as the only immunosuppressant in 34 recipients of cadaveric organs: 32 kidneys, 2 pancreases, and 2 livers. Lancet 2(8151):1033, 1979.
9. Starzl TE, Klintmalm GB, Porter KA, et al: Liver transplantation with use of cyclosporin A and prednisone. N Engl J Med 305(5):266, 1981.
10. Starzl TE, Demetris AJ, Van Thiel D: Liver transplantation (part I). N Engl J Med 321(15):1014, 1989.
11. Starzl TE, Demetris AJ, Van Thiel D: Liver transplantation (part II). N Engl J Med 321(16):1092, 1989.
12. Iwatsuki S, Starzl TE, Todo S, et al: Experience in 1,000 liver transplants under cyclosporine-steroid therapy: a survival report. Transplant Proc 20(suppl 1):498, 1988.
13. National Institutes of Health Consensus Development Conference Statement: liver transplantation–June 20-23, 1983: Hepatology 4(1 suppl):107S, 1984.
14. The U.S. Multicenter FK506 Liver Study Group: A comparison of tacrolimus (FK506) and cyclosporine for immunosuppression in liver transplantation. N Engl J Med 331(17):1110, 1994.
15. European FK506 Multicentre Liver Study Group: Randomised trial comparing tacrolimus (FK506) and cyclosporin in prevention of liver allograft rejection. Lancet 344(8920):423, 1994.
16. Wiesner RH: A long-term comparison of tacrolimus (FK506) versus cyclosporine in liver transplantation: a report of the United States FK506 Study Group. Transplantation 66(4):493, 1998.
17. Canzanello VJ, Schwartz L, Taler SJ, et al: Evolution of cardiovascular risk after liver transplantation: a comparison of cyclosporine A and tacrolimus (FK506). Liver Transpl Surg 3(1):1, 1997.
18. Canzanello VJ, Textor SC, Taler SJ, et al: Late hypertension after liver transplantation: a comparison of cyclosporine and tacrolimus (FK 506). Liver Transpl Surg 4(4):328, 1998.
19. Manzarbeitia C, Reich DJ, Rothstein KD, et al: Tacrolimus conversion improves hyperlipidemic states in stable liver transplant recipients. Liver Transpl 7(2):93, 2001.
20. Wall WJ, Ghent CN, Roy A, et al: Use of OKT3 monoclonal antibody as induction therapy for control of rejection in liver transplantation. Dig Dis Sci 40(1):52, 1995.
21. Neuhaus P, Bechstein WO, Blumhardt G, et al: Comparison of quadruple immunosuppression after liver transplantation with ATG or IL-2 receptor antibody. Transplantation 55(6):1320, 1993.
22. Reding R, Vraux H, de Ville de Goyet J, et al: Monoclonal antibodies in prophylactic immunosuppression after liver transplantation. A randomized controlled trial comparing OKT3 and anti-IL-2 receptor monoclonal antibody LO-Tact-1. Transplantation 55(3): 534, 1993.
23. Cronin DC, Faust TW, Brady L, et al: Modern immunosuppression. Clin Liver Dis 4(3):619, 2000.
24. Denton MD, Magee CC, Sayegh MH: Immunosuppressive strategies in transplantation. Lancet 53(9158):1083, 1999.
25. Smith CM, Davies DB, McBride MA: Liver transplantation in the United States: a report from the UNOS Liver Transplant Registry. In Cecka JM, Terasaki PI, eds: Clinical Transplants 1999. Los Angeles, UCLA Immunogenetics Center, 2000:23.
26. Snover DC, Freese DK, Sharp HL, et al: Liver allograft rejection. An analysis of the use of biopsy in determining outcome of rejection. Am J Surg Pathol 11(1):1, 1987.
27. Verran DJ, Asfar SK, Ghent CN, et al: Biliary reconstruction without T tubes or stents in liver transplantation: report of 502 consecutive cases. Liver Transpl Surg 3(4):365, 1997.
28. Cacciarelli TV, Keeffe EB, Moore DH, et al: Primary liver transplantation without transfusion of red blood cells. Surgery 120(4):698, 1996.
29. Fishman JA, Rubin RH: Infection in organ-transplant recipients. N Engl J Med 338(24):1741, 1998.
30. Seaberg EC, Belle SH, Beringer KC, et al: Liver transplantation in the United States from 1987-1998: updated results from the Pitt-UNOS Liver Transplant Registry. In Cecka JM, Terasaki PI, eds: Clinical Transplants 1998. Los Angeles, UCLA Tissue Typing Laboratory, 1998:17
31. Bravata DM, Olkin I, Barnato AE, et al: Health-related quality of life after liver transplantation: a meta-analysis. Liver Transpl Surg 5(4):318, 1999.
32. Moore KA, Jones RM, Burrows GD: Quality of life and cognitive function of liver transplant patients: a prospective study. Liver Transpl 6(5):633, 2000.
33. Younossi ZM, McCormick M, Price LL, et al: Impact of liver transplantation on health-related quality of life. Liver Transpl 6(6):779, 2000.

34. Midgley DE, Bradlee TA, Donohoe C, et al: Health-related quality of life in long-term survivors of pediatric liver transplantation. Liver Transpl 6(3):333, 2000.
35. Evans RW, Kitzmann DJ: The "arithmetic" of donor liver allocation. In Cecka JM, Terasaki PI, eds: Clinical Transplants 1996, Los Angeles, UCLA Tissue Typing Laboratory, 1997:338.
36. Showstack J, Katz PP, Lake JR, et al: Resource utilization in liver transplantation: effects of patient characteristics and clinical practice. NIDDK Liver Transplantation Database Group. JAMA 281(15):1381, 1999.
37. Gilbert JR, Pascual M, Schoenfeld DA, et al: Evolving trends in liver transplantation: an outcome and charge analysis. Transplantation 67(2):246, 1999.
38. Keeffe EB: Selection of patients for liver transplantation. In Maddrey WC, Schiff ER, Sorrell MF, eds: Transplantation of the Liver, ed 3. Philadelphia, Lippincott Williams & Wilkins, 2001:5.
39. Carithers RL: Liver transplantation. American Association for the Study of Liver Diseases. Liver Transpl 6(1):122, 2000.
40. Murcia FJ, Vazquez J, Gamez M, et al: Liver transplantation in type I tyrosinemia. Transplant Proc 27(4):2301, 1995.
41. Paradis K: Tyrosinemia: the Quebec experience. Clin Invest Med 19(5):311, 1996.
42. Matern D, Starzl TE, Arnaout W, et al: Liver transplantation for glycogen storage disease types I, III, and IV. Eur J Pediatr 158 (suppl 2):S43, 1999.
43. Faivre L, Houssin D, Valayer J, et al: Long-term outcome of liver transplantation in patients with glycogen storage disease type Ia. J Inherit Metab Dis 22(6):723, 1999.
44. Pratschke J, Steinmuller T, Bechstein WO, et al: Orthotopic liver transplantation for hepatic associated metabolic disorders. Clin Transplant 12(3):228, 1998.
45. Nolkemper D, Kemper MJ, Burdelski M, et al: Long-term results of pre-emptive liver transplantation in primary hyperoxaluria type 1. Pediatr Transplant 4(3):177, 2000.
46. Revell SP, Noble-Jamieson G, Johnston P, et al: Liver transplantation for homozygous familial hypercholesterolaemia. Arch Dis Child 73(5):456, 1995.
47. Todo S, Starzl TE, Tzakis A, et al: Orthotopic liver transplantation for urea cycle enzyme deficiency. Hepatology 15(3):419, 1992.
48. Gibas A, Dienstag JL, Schafer AI, et al: Cure of hemophilia A by orthotopic liver transplantation. Gastroenterology 95(1):192, 1988.
49. Delorme MA, Adams PC, Grant D, et al: Orthotopic liver transplantation in a patient with combined hemophilia A and B. Am J Hematol 33(2):136, 1990.
50. O'Grady JG, Alexander GJ, Hayllar KM, Williams R: Early indicators of prognosis in fulminant hepatic failure. Gastroenterology 97(2):439, 1989.
51. Bernuau J, Samuel D, Durand F, et al: Criteria for emergency liver transplantation in patients with acute viral hepatitis and factor V below 50% of normal: a prospective study. Hepatology 14:49A, 1991 (abstract).
52. Lucey MR, Brown KA, Everson GT, et al: Minimal criteria for placement of adults on the liver transplant waiting list: a report of a national conference organized by the American Society of Transplant Physicians and the American Association for the Study of Liver Diseases. Liver Transpl Surg 3(6):628, 1997.
53. Propst A, Propst T, Zangerl G, et al: Prognosis and life expectancy in chronic liver disease. Dig Dis Sci 40(8):1805, 1995.
54. Gines P, Quintero E, Arroyo V, et al: Compensated cirrhosis: natural history and prognostic factors. Hepatology 7(1):122, 1987.
55. Fattovich G, Giustina G, Degos F, et al: Morbidity and mortality in compensated cirrhosis type C: a retrospective follow-up study of 384 patients. Gastroenterology 112(2):463, 1997.
56. Andreu M, Sola R, Sitges-Serra A, et al: Risk factors for spontaneous bacterial peritonitis in cirrhotic patients with ascites. Gastroenterology 104(4):1133, 1993.
57. Gines A, Escorsell A, Gines P, et al: Incidence, predictive factors, and prognosis of the hepatorenal syndrome in cirrhosis with ascites. Gastroenterology 105(1):229, 1993.
58. Henderson JM, Kutner MH, Millikan WJ, et al: Endoscopic variceal sclerosis compared with distal splenorenal shunt to prevent recurrent variceal bleeding in cirrhosis. A prospective, randomized trial. Ann Intern Med 112(4):262, 1990.
59. Rössle M, Haag K, Ochs A, et al: The transjugular intrahepatic portosystemic stent-shunt procedure for variceal bleeding. N Engl J Med 330(3):165, 1994.
60. Child CG III, Turcotte JG: Surgery in portal hypertension. In Child CG III, ed: The Liver and Portal Hypertension. Philadelphia, WB Saunders Co., 1964:50
61. Pugh RNH, Murray-Lyon IM, Dawson JJ, et al: Transection of the oesophagus for bleeding oesophageal varices. Br J Surg 60(8):646, 1973.
62. Maddrey WC, Friedman LS, Munoz SJ, et al: Selection of the patient for liver transplantation and timing of surgery. In Maddrey WC, ed: Transplantation of the Liver. New York, Elsevier, 1988:23.
63. Keeffe EB, Esquivel CO: Controversies in patient selection for liver transplantation. West J Med 159(5):586, 1993.
64. Yoshida EM, Lake JR: Selection of patients for liver transplantation in 1997 and beyond. Clin Liver Dis 1(2): 247, 1997.
65. Wiesner RH: Current indications, contraindications, and timing for liver transplantation. In Busuttil RW, Klintmalm GB, eds: Transplantation of the Liver. Philadelphia, WB Saunders Co., 1996:71.
66. Rosen HR, Shackleton CR, Martin P: Indications for and timing of liver transplantation. Med Clin North Am 80(5):1069, 1996.
67. Fabry TL, Klion FM: Liver transplantation: selection of patients for referral. In Fabry TL, Klion FM, eds: Guide to Liver Transplantation. New York, Igaku-Shoin, 1992:79.
68. Donovan JP, Zetterman RK, Burnett DA, et al: Preoperative evaluation, preparation, and timing of orthotopic liver transplantation in the adult. Semin Liver Dis 9(3):168, 1989.
69. Mullen KD: Hepatic encephalopathy. In Rector WG Jr, ed: Complications of Chronic Liver Disease. St Louis, Mosby Year Book, 1992:127.
70. Arroyo V, Ginès P, Gerbes AL, et al: Definition and diagnostic criteria of refractory ascites and hepatorenal syndrome in cirrhosis. Hepatology 23(1):164, 1996.
71. Bories P, Garcia-Compean D, Michel H, et al: The treatment of refractory ascites by the LeVeen shunt: a multi-center controlled trials (57 patients). J Hepatol 3(2):212, 1986.
72. Rössle M, Ochs A, Gülberg V, et al: A comparison of paracentesis and transjugular intrahepatic portosystemic shunting in patients with ascites. N Engl J Med 342(23):1701, 2000.
73. Somberg KA, Lake JR, Tomlanovich SJ, et al: Transjugular intrahepatic portosystemic stent shunts for refractory ascites: assessment of clinical and hormonal response and renal function. Hepatology 21(3):1995, 709.
74. Trotter JF, Suhocki PV, Rockey DC, et al: Transjugular intrahepatic portosystemic shunt in patients with refractory ascites: effect on body weight and Child-Pugh Score. Am J Gastroenterol 93(10): 1891, 1998.
75. Yu AS, Hu KQ: Management of ascites. Clin Liver Dis 5(2):541, 2001.
76. Akriviadis EA, Runyon BA: Utility of an algorithm in differentiating spontaneous from secondary bacterial peritonitis. Gastroenterology 98(1):127, 1990.
77. Runyon BA: Four days of antibiotics can be effective therapy of culture-negative neutrocytic ascites or of delayed growth culture-positive spontaneous peritonitis. Hepatology 6(5):1139A, 1986.
78. Runyon BA, McHutchison JG, Antillon MR, et al: Short-course vs long-course antibiotic treatment of spontaneous bacterial peritonitis: a randomized controlled study of 100 patients. Gastroenterology 100(6):1737, 1991.
79. Tító L, Rimola A, Ginés P, et al: Recurrence of spontaneous bacterial peritonitis in cirrhosis: Frequency and predictive factors. Hepatology 8(1):27, 1988.
80. Ginès P, Rimola A, Planas R, et al: Norfloxacin prevents spontaneous bacterial peritonitis recurrence in cirrhosis: results of a double-blind, placebo-controlled trial. Hepatology 12(4):716, 1990.
81. Soriano G, Guarner C, Teixidó M, et al: Selective intestinal decontamination prevents spontaneous bacterial peritonitis. Gastroenterology 100(2):477, 1991.
82. Soriano G, Guarner C, Tomás A, et al: Norfloxacin prevents bacterial infection in cirrhotics with gastrointestinal hemorrhage. Gastroenterology 103(4):1267, 1992.
83. Ukah FO, Merhav H, Kramer D, et al: Early outcome of liver transplantation in patients with a history of spontaneous bacterial peritonitis. Transplant Proc 25:1113, 1993.

84. Graham DY, Smith JL: The course of patients after variceal hemorrhage. Gastroenterology 80(4):800, 1981.
85. Stanley AJ, Hayes PC: Portal hypertension and variceal haemorrhage. Lancet 350(9086):1235, 1997.
86. Lebrec D: Portal hypertension. In Rector WG Jr, ed: Complications of Chronic Liver Disease. St Louis, Mosby Year Book, 1992:24.
87. Roberts LR, Kamath PS: Pathophysiology and treatment of variceal hemorrhage. Mayo Clin Proc 71(10): 973, 1996.
88. Ring EJ, Lake JR, Roberts JP, et al: Using transjugular intrahepatic portosystemic shunts to control variceal bleeding before liver transplantation. Ann Intern Med 116(4):304, 1992.
89. Woodle ES, Darcy M, White HM, et al: Intrahepatic portosystemic vascular stents: a bridge to hepatic transplantation. Surgery 113(3):344, 1993.
90. Jenkins RL: Defining the role of transjugular intrahepatic portosystemic shunts in the management of portal hypertension. Liver Transpl Surg 1(4):225, 1995.
91. Brems JJ, Hiatt JR, Klein AS, et al: Effect of a prior portosystemic shunt on subsequent liver transplantation. Ann Surg 209(1):51, 1989.
92. Millis JM, Martin P, Gomes A, et al: Transjugular intrahepatic portosystemic shunts: impact on liver transplantation. Liver Transpl Surg 1(4):229, 1995.
93. Somberg KA, Riegler JL, LaBerge JM, et al: Hepatic encephalopathy after transjugular intrahepatic portosystemic shunts: Incidence and risk factors. Am J Gastroenterol 90(4):549, 1995.
94. Martinet JP, Fenyves D, Legault L, et al: Treatment of refractory ascites using transjugular intrahepatic portosystemic shunt: a caution. Dig Dis Sci 42(1):161, 1997.
95. Sanyal AJ, Freedman AM, Purdum PP, et al: The hematologic consequences of transjugular intrahepatic portosystemic shunts. Hepatology 23(1):32, 1996.
96. Somberg KA, Lombardero MS, Lawlor SM, et al: A controlled analysis of the transjugular intrahepatic portosystemic shunt in liver transplant recipients. The National Institute of Diabetes and Digestive and Kidney Diseases (NIDDK) Liver Transplantation Database. Transplantation 63(8):1074, 1997.
97. Langnas AN, Marujo WC, Stratta RJ, et al: Influence of a prior portasystemic shunt on outcome after liver transplantation. Am J Gastroenterol 87(6):714, 1992.
98. Esquivel CO, Klintmalm G, Iwatsuki S, et al: Liver transplantation in patients with patent splenorenal shunts. Surgery 101(4):430, 1987.
99. Hillebrand DJ, Kojouri K, Cao S, et al: Small-diameter portacaval H-graft shunt: a paradigm shift back to surgical shunting in the management of variceal bleeding in patients with preserved liver function. Liver Transpl 6(4):459, 2000.
100. Mazzaferro V, Todo S, Tzakis AG, et al: Liver transplantation in patients with previous portasystemic shunt. Am J Surg 160(1):111, 1990.
101. Henderson JM, Nagle A, Curtas S, et al: Surgical shunts and TIPS for variceal decompression in the 1990s. Surgery 128(4):540, 2000.
102. O'Keefe SJ, El-Zayadi AR, Carraher TE, et al: Malnutrition and immuno-incompetence in patients with liver disease. Lancet 2(8195 Pt 1):615, 1980.
103. Pikul J, Sharpe MD, Lowndes R, et al: Degree of preoperative malnutrition is predictive of postoperative morbidity and mortality in liver transplant recipients. Transplantation 57(3):469, 1994.
104. Helton WS: Nutritional issues in hepatobiliary surgery. Semin Liver Dis 14(2):140, 1994.
105. Selberg O, Bottcher J, Tusch G, et al: Identification of high- and low-risk patients before liver transplantation: a prospective cohort study of nutritional and metabolic parameters in 150 patients. Hepatology 25(3):652, 1997.
106. Cabre E, Gonzalez-Huix F, Abad-Lacruz A, et al: Effect of total enteral nutrition on the short-term outcome of severely malnourished cirrhotics. A randomized controlled trial. Gastroenterology 98(3):715, 1990.
107. Ginès A, Escorsell A, Ginès P, et al: Incidence, predictive factors, and prognosis of hepatorenal syndrome in cirrhosis. Gastroenterology 105(1):229, 1993.
108. Arroyo V, Ginès P, Gerbes AL, et al: Definition and diagnostic criteria of refractory ascites and hepatorenal syndrome in cirrhosis. International Ascites Club. Hepatology 23(1):164, 1996.
109. Cárdenas A, Uriz J, Ginès P, et al: Hepatorenal syndrome. Liver Transpl 6(4 suppl 1):S63, 2000.
110. Wilkinson SP, Weston MJ, Parsons V, et al: Dialysis in the treatment of renal failure in patients with liver disease. Clin Nephrol 8(1):287, 1977.
111. Golper TA: Continuous arteriovenous hemofiltration in acute renal failure. Am J Kidney Dis 6(6):373, 1985.
112. Mitzner SR, Stange J, Klammt S, et al: Improvement of hepatorenal syndrome with extracorporeal albumin dialysis MARS: results of a prospective, randomized, controlled clinical trial. Liver Transpl 6(3):277, 2000.
113. Arroyo V: New treatments for hepatorenal syndrome. Liver Transpl 6(3):287, 2000.
114. Iwatsuki S, Popovtzer MM, Corman JL, et al: Recovery from "hepatorenal syndrome" after orthotopic liver transplantation. N Engl J Med 289(22):1155, 1973.
115. Gonwa TA, Morris CA, Goldstein RM, et al: Long-term survival and renal function following liver transplantation in patients with and without hepatorenal syndrome—experience in 300 patients. Transplantation 51(2):428, 1991.
116. Seu P, Wilkinson AH, Shaked A, Busuttil RW: The hepatorenal syndrome in liver transplant recipients. Am Surg 57(12): 806, 1991.
117. Rimola A, Navasa M, Grande L: Liver transplantation in cirrhotic patients with ascites. In Arroyo V, Ginès A, Rodés J, Schrier RW, eds: Ascites and Renal Dysfunction in Liver Disease: Pathogenesis, Diagnosis, and Treatment. Malden, Blackwell Science, 1999:522.
118. Wood RP, Ellis D, Starzl TE: The reversal of the hepatorenal syndrome in four pediatric patients following successful orthotopic liver transplantation. Ann Surg 205(4):415, 1987.
119. Everson GT: Increasing incidence and pretransplantation screening of hepatocellular carcinoma. Liver Transpl 6:S2, 2000.
120. Mazzaferro V, Regalia E, Doci R, et al: Liver transplantation for the treatment of small hepatocellular carcinomas in patients with cirrhosis. N Engl J Med 334(11):693, 1996.
121. Marsh JW, Dvorchik I, Subotin M, et al: The prediction of risk of recurrence and time to recurrence of hepatocellular carcinoma after orthotopic liver transplantation: a pilot study. Hepatology 26(2):444, 1997.
122. Bismuth H, Chiche L, Adam R, et al: Liver resection versus transplantation for hepatocellular carcinoma in cirrhotic patients. Ann Surg 218(2):145, 1993.
123. Iwatsuki S, Starzl TE, Sheahan DG, et al: Hepatic resection versus transplantation for hepatocellular carcinoma. Ann Surg 214(3): 221, 1991.
124. Porayko MK, Wiesner RH, Hay JE, et al: Bone disease in liver transplant recipients: incidence, timing, and risk factors. Transplant Proc 23(1 Pt 2):1462, 1991.
125. Stellon AJ, Webb A, Compston J, et al: Low bone turnover state in primary biliary cirrhosis. Hepatology 7(1):137, 1987.
126. Bergasa NV, Jones EA: The pruritus of cholestasis. Semin Liver Dis 13(4):319, 1993.
127. Poupon RE, Poupon R, Balkau B: Ursodiol for the long-term treatment of primary biliary cirrhosis: the UDCA-PBC Study Group. N Engl J Med 330(19):1342, 1994.
128. Turnberg LA, Mahoney MP, Gleeson MH, et al: Plasmaphoresis and plasma exchange in the treatment of hyperlipidemia and xanthomatous neuropathy in patients with primary biliary cirrhosis. Gut 13(12):976, 1972.
129. Shapiro JM, Smith H, Schaffner F: Serum bilirubin: a prognostic factor in primary biliary cirrhosis. Gut 20(2):137, 1979.
130. Rosen HR, Martin P: Liver transplantation. In Schiff ER, Sorrell MF, Maddrey WC, eds: Schiff's Diseases of the Liver, ed 8. Philadelphia, Lippincott-Raven Publishers, 1999:1589.
131. Baliga P, Merion RM, Turcotte JG, et al: Preoperative risk factor assessment in liver transplantation. Surgery 112(4):704, 1992.
132. Cuervas-Mons V, Millan I, Gavaler JS, et al: Prognostic value of preoperatively obtained clinical and laboratory data in predicting survival following orthotopic liver transplantation. Hepatology 6(5):922, 1986.
133. Danovitch GM, Wilkinson AH, Colonna JO, et al: Determinants of renal failure in patients receiving orthotopic liver transplants. Kidney Int 31:195, 1987 (abstract).
134. Shaw BW, Wood RP, Gordon RD, et al: Influence of selected patient variables and operative blood loss on six-month survival following liver transplantation. Semin Liver Dis 5(4):385, 1985.
135. Oellerich M, Burdelski M, Lautz HU, et al: Assessment of pretransplant prognosis in patients with cirrhosis. Transplantation 51(4):801, 1991.

136. Oellerich M, Burdelski M, Lautz HU, et al: Predictors of one-year pretransplant survival in patients with cirrhosis. Hepatology 14(6):1029, 1991.
137. Seifert RD, Kang YG, Begliomini B, et al: Baseline cardiac index does not predict hemodynamic instability during orthotopic liver transplantation. Transplant Proc 21(3):3523, 1989.
138. Farrell FJ, Nguyen M, Woodley S, et al: Outcome of liver transplantation in patients with hemochromatosis. Hepatology 20(2):404, 1994.
139. Keeffe EB: Comorbidities of alcoholic liver disease that affect outcome of orthotopic liver transplantation. Liver Transpl Surg 3(3):251, 1997.
140. Plotkin JS, Johnson LB, Rustgi V, et al: Coronary artery disease and liver transplantation: the state of the art. Liver Transpl 6(4 suppl 1):S53, 2000.
141. Keeffe BG, Valantine H, Keeffe EB: Detection and treatment of coronary artery disease in liver transplant recipients. Liver Transpl 7(9):755, 2001.
142. Eckhoff DE, Frenette L, Sellers MT, et al: Combined cardiac surgery and liver transplantation. Liver Transpl 7(1):60, 2001.
143. Benedetti E, Massad MG, Chami Y, et al: Is the presence of surgically treatable coronary artery disease a contraindication to liver transplantation? Clin Transplant 13(1 Pt 1):59, 1999.
144. Manas DM, Roberts DR, Heaviside DW, et al: Sequential coronary artery bypass grafting and orthotopic liver transplantation: a case report. Clin Transplant 10(3):320, 1996.
145. Plotkin JS, Scott VL, Pinna A, et al: Morbidity and mortality in patients with coronary artery disease undergoing orthotopic liver transplantation. Liver Transpl Surg 2(6):426, 1996.
146. Battaglia SE, Pretto JJ, Irving LB, et al: Resolution of gas exchange abnormalities and intrapulmonary shunting following liver transplantation. Hepatology 25(5):1228, 1997.
147. Krowka MJ, Cortese DA: Pulmonary aspects of chronic liver disease and liver transplantation. Mayo Clin Proc 60(6):407, 1985.
148. Chaparro SV, Montoya JG, Keeffe EB, et al: Risk of tuberculosis in tuberculin skin test-positive liver transplant patients. Clin Infect Dis 9(1):207, 1999.
149. Krowka MJ: Hepatopulmonary syndrome: recent literature (1997 to 1999) and implications for liver transplantation. Liver Transpl 6(4 suppl 1):S31, 2000.
150. Lange PA, Stoller JK: The hepatopulmonary syndrome. Effect of liver transplantation. Clin Chest Med 17(1):115, 1996.
151. Aboussouan LS, Stoller JK: The hepatopulmonary syndrome. Baillieres Best Pract Res Clin Gastroenterol 14(6):1033, 2000.
152. Scott V, Miro A, Kang Y, et al: Reversibility of the hepatopulmonary syndrome by orthotopic liver transplantation. Transplant Proc 25(2):1787, 1993.
153. Alexander J, Greenough A, Baker A, et al: Nitric oxide treatment of severe hypoxemia after liver transplantation in hepatopulmonary syndrome: case report. Liver Transpl Surg 3(1):54, 1997.
154. Durand P, Baujard C, Grosse AL, et al: Reversal of hypoxemia by inhaled nitric oxide in children with severe hepatopulmonary syndrome, type 1, during and after liver transplantation. Transplantation 65(3):437, 1998.
155. Stoller JK, Moodie D, Schiavone WA, et al: Reduction of intrapulmonary shunt and resolution of digital clubbing associated with primary biliary cirrhosis after liver transplantation. Hepatology 11(1):54, 1990.
156. Stoller JK, Lange PA, Westveer MK, et al: Prevalence and reversibility of the hepatopulmonary syndrome after liver transplantation. The Cleveland Clinic experience. West J Med 163(2):133, 1995.
157. Laberge JM, Brandt ML, Lebecque P, et al: Reversal of cirrhosis-related pulmonary shunting in two children by orthotopic liver transplantation. Transplantation 53(5):1135, 1992.
158. Krowka MJ, Porayko MK, Plevak DJ, et al: Hepatopulmonary syndrome with progressive hypoxemia as an indication for liver transplantation: case reports and literature review. Mayo Clin Proc 72(1):44, 1997.
159. Egawa H, Kasahara M, Inomata Y, et al: Long-term outcome of living related liver transplantation for patients with intrapulmonary shunting and strategy for complications. Transplantation 67(5): 712, 1999.
160. Abrams GA, Rose K, Fallon MB, et al: Hepatopulmonary syndrome and venous emboli causing intracerebral hemorrhages after liver transplantation: a case report. Transplantation 68(11):1809, 1999.
161. Rodriguez-Roisin R, Krowka MJ: Is severe arterial hypoxaemia due to hepatic disease an indication for liver transplantation? A new therapeutic approach. Eur Respir J 7(5):839, 1994.
162. Allgaier HP, Haag K, Ochs A, et al: Hepato-pulmonary syndrome: successful treatment by transjugular intrahepatic portosystemic stent-shunt (TIPS). J Hepatol 23(1):102, 1995.
163. Riegler JL, Lang KA, Johnson SP, et al: Transjugular intrahepatic portosystemic shunt improves oxygenation in hepatopulmonary syndrome. Gastroenterology 109(3):978, 1995.
164. Selim KM, Akriviadis EA, Zuckerman E, et al: Transjugular intrahepatic portosystemic shunt: a successful treatment for hepatopulmonary syndrome. Am J Gastroenterol 93(3):455, 1998.
165. Lasch HM, Fried MW, Zacks SL, et al: Use of transjugular intrahepatic portosystemic shunt as a bridge to liver transplantation in a patient with severe hepatopulmonary syndrome. Liver Transpl 7(2):147, 2001.
166. Krowka MJ: Hepatopulmonary syndrome versus portopulmonary hypertension: distinctions and dilemmas. Hepatology 25(5):1282, 1997.
167. De Wolf AM, Scott VL, Gasior T, et al: Pulmonary hypertension and liver transplantation. Anesthesiology 78(1):213, 1993.
168. Ramsay MA, Simpson BR, Nguyen AT, et al: Severe pulmonary hypertension in liver transplant candidates. Liver Transpl Surg 3(5):494, 1997.
169. Ramsay MA: Perioperative mortality in patients with portopulmonary hypertension undergoing liver transplantation. Liver Transpl 6(4):451, 2000.
170. Pilatis ND, Jacobs LE, Rerkpattanapipat P, et al: Clinical predictors of pulmonary hypertension in patients undergoing liver transplant evaluation. Liver Transpl 6(1):85, 2000.
171. Kim WR, Krowka MJ, Plevak DJ, et al: Accuracy of Doppler echocardiography in the assessment of pulmonary hypertension in liver transplant candidates. Liver Transpl 6(4):453, 2000.
172. Krowka MJ, Plevak DJ, Findlay JY, et al: Pulmonary hemodynamics and perioperative cardiopulmonary-related mortality in patients with portopulmonary hypertension undergoing liver transplantation. Liver Transpl 6(4):443, 2000.
173. Kuo PC, Johnson LB, Plotkin JS, et al: Continuous intravenous infusion of epoprostenol for the treatment of portopulmonary hypertension. Transplantation 63(4):604, 1997.
174. Plotkin JS, Kuo PC, Rubin LJ, et al: Successful use of chronic epoprostenol as a bridge to liver transplantation in severe portopulmonary hypertension. Transplantation 65(4):457, 1998.
175. McLaughlin VV, Genthner DE, Panella MM, et al: Compassionate use of continuous prostacyclin in the management of secondary pulmonary hypertension: a case series. Ann Intern Med 130(9): 740, 1999.
176. Krowka MJ, Frantz RP, McGoon MD, et al: Improvement in pulmonary hemodynamics during intravenous epoprostenol (prostacyclin): a study of 15 patients with moderate to severe portopulmonary hypertension. Hepatology 30(3):641, 1999.
177. Rafanan AL, Maurer J, Mehta AC, Schilz R: Progressive portopulmonary hypertension after liver transplantation treated with epoprostenol. Chest 118(5):1497, 2000.
178. Ramsay MA, Spikes C, East CA, et al: The perioperative management of portopulmonary hypertension with nitric oxide and epoprostenol. Anesthesiology 90(1):299, 1999.
179. Findlay JY, Harrison BA, Plevak DJ, et al: Inhaled nitric oxide reduces pulmonary artery pressures in portopulmonary hypertension. Liver Transpl Surg 5(5):381, 1999.
180. Ramsay MA, Schmidt A, Hein HA, et al: Nitric oxide does not reverse pulmonary hypertension associated with end-stage liver disease: a preliminary report. Hepatology 25(3):524, 1997.
181. Mandell MS: Critical care issues: portopulmonary hypertension. Liver Transpl 6(4 suppl 1):S36, 2000.
182. Erice A, Rhame FS, Heussner RC, et al: Human immunodeficiency virus infection in patients with solid-organ transplants: report of five cases and review. Rev Infect Dis 13(4):537, 1991.
183. Dummer JS, Erb S, Breinig MK, et al: Infection with human immunodeficiency virus in the Pittsburgh transplant population. A study of 583 donors and 1043 recipients, 1981-1986. Transplantation 47(1):134, 1989.
184. Tzakis AG, Cooper MH, Dummer JS, et al: Transplantation in HIV+ patients. Transplantation 49(2):354, 1990.
185. Pichlmayr R, Weimann A, Oldhafer KJ, et al: Role of liver transplantation in the treatment of unresectable liver cancer. World J Surg 19(6):807, 1995.

186. Wall WJ: Liver transplantation for hepatic and biliary malignancy. Semin Liver Dis 20(4):425, 2000.
187. Dousset B, Houssin D, Soubrane O, et al: Metastatic endocrine tumors: is there a place for liver transplantation? Liver Transpl Surg 1(2):111, 1995.
188. Dousset B, Saint-Marc O, Pitre J, et al: Metastatic endocrine tumors: medical treatment, surgical resection, or liver transplantation. World J Surg 20(7):908, 1996.
189. Routley D, Ramage JK, McPeake J, et al: Orthotopic liver transplantation in the treatment of metastatic neuroendocrine tumors of the liver. Liver Transpl Surg 1(2):118, 1995.
190. Lehnert T: Liver transplantation for metastatic neuroendocrine carcinoma: an analysis of 103 patients. Transplantation 66(10): 1307, 1998.
191. Le Treut YP, Delpero JR, Dousset B, et al: Results of liver transplantation in the treatment of metastatic neuroendocrine tumors. A 31-case French multicentric report. Ann Surg 225(4):355, 1997.
192. Alsina AE, Bartus S, Hull D, et al: Liver transplant for metastatic neuroendocrine tumor. J Clin Gastroenterol 12(5):533, 1990.
193. O'Grady JG, Polson RJ, Rolles K, et al: Liver transplantation for malignant disease. Results in 93 consecutive patients. Ann Surg 207(4):373, 1988.
194. Meyer CG, Penn I, James L: Liver transplantation for cholangiocarcinoma: results in 207 patients. Transplantation 69(8):1633, 2000.
195. Iwatsuki S, Todo S, Marsh JW, et al: Treatment of hilar cholangiocarcinoma (Klatskin tumors) with hepatic resection or transplantation. J Am Coll Surg 87(4):358, 1998.
196. De Vreede I, Steers JL, Burch PA, et al: Prolonged disease-free survival after orthotopic liver transplantation plus adjuvant chemoirradiation for cholangiocarcinoma. Liver Transpl 6(3):309, 2000.
197. Bismuth H: Revisiting liver transplantation for patients with hilar cholangiocarcinoma: the Mayo Clinic proposal. Liver Transpl 6(3):317, 2000.
198. Figueras J, Llado L, Valls C, et al: Changing strategies in diagnosis and management of hilar cholangiocarcinoma. Liver Transpl 6(6):786, 2000.
199. Osorio RW, Ascher NL, Avery M, et al: Predicting recidivism after orthotopic liver transplantation for alcoholic liver disease. Hepatology 20(1 Pt 1):105, 1994.
200. Lucey MR: Liver transplantation in the alcoholic patient. In Maddrey WC, Sorrell MF, Schiff ER, eds: Transplantation of the Liver, ed 3. Philadelphia, Lippincott Williams & Wilkins, 2001:319.
201. Vaillant GE: The natural history of alcoholism and its relationship to liver transplantation. Liver Transpl Surg 3(3):304, 1997.
202. Shaw BW Jr, Iwatsuki S, Bron K, et al: Portal vein grafts in hepatic transplantation. Surg Gynecol Obstet 161(1):66, 1985.
203. Lerut J, Tzakis AG, Bron K, et al: Complications of venous reconstruction in human orthotopic liver transplantation. Ann Surg 205(4):404, 1987.
204. Tzakis A, Todo S, Stieber A, et al: Venous jump grafts for liver transplantation in patients with portal vein thrombosis. Transplantation 48(3):530, 1989.
205. Stieber AC, Zetti G, Todo S, et al: The spectrum of portal vein thrombosis in liver transplantation. Ann Surg 213(3):199, 1991.
206. Shaked A, Busuttil RW: Liver transplantation in patients with portal vein thrombosis and central portacaval shunts. Ann Surg 214(6):696, 1991.
207. Moreno Gonzalez E, Garcia Garcia I, Gomez Sanz R, et al: Liver transplantation in patients with thrombosis of the portal, splenic or superior mesenteric vein. Br J Surg 80(1):81, 1993.
208. Manzanet G, Sanjuan F, Orbis P, et al: Liver transplantation in patients with portal vein thrombosis. Liver Transpl 7(2):125, 2001.
209. Yerdel MA, Gunson B, Mirza D, et al: Portal vein thrombosis in adults undergoing liver transplantation: risk factors, screening, management, and outcome. Transplantation 69(9):1873, 2000.
210. Calne R: Contraindications to liver transplantation. Hepatology 20(1 Pt 2):3S, 1994.
211. Zetterman RK, Belle SH, Hoofnagle JH, et al: Age and liver transplantation: a report of the Liver Transplantation Database. Transplantation 66(4):500, 1998.
212. Box TD, Keeffe EB, Esquivel CO: Liver transplantation in elderly patients. Pract Gastroenterol 17:22, 1993.
213. Stieber AC, Gordon RD, Todo S, et al: Liver transplantation in patients over sixty years of age. Transplantation 51(1):271, 1991.
214. Shaw BW Jr: Liver transplantation in patients over 60 years of age. Liver Update: Function and Disease. Cedar Grove, NJ, American Liver Foundation 1992. 5:3.
215. Emre S, Mor E, Schwartz ME, et al: Liver transplantation in patients beyond age 60. Transplant Proc 25(1 Pt 2):1075, 1993.
216. Pirsch JD, Kalayoglu M, D'Alessandro AM, et al: Orthotopic liver transplantation in patients 60 years of age and older. Transplantation 51(2):431, 1991.
217. Bromley PN, Hilmi I, Tan KC, et al: Orthotopic liver transplantation in patients over 60 years old. Transplantation 58(7):800, 1994.
218. De la Pena A, Herrero JI, Snagro B, et al: Liver transplantation in cirrhotic patients over 60 years of age. Rev Esp Enferm Dig 90(1):3, 1998.
219. Annual Report of the U.S. Scientific Registry for Organ Transplantation and the Organ Procurement and Transplantation Network 1990: UNOS, Richmond VA, and the Division of Organ Transplantation, Health Resources and Services Administration, Bethesda, MD.
220. Weigle WO: Effects of aging on the immune system. Hosp Pract 24(12):112, 1989.
221. Ershler WB: Biomarkers of aging: immunological events. Exp Gerontol 23(4-5):387, 1988.
222. Collins BH, Pirsch JD, Becker YT, et al: Long-term results of liver transplantation in older patients 60 years of age and older. Transplantation 70(5):780, 2000.
223. Castaldo P, Langnas AN, Stratta RJ, et al: Liver transplantation in patients over 60 years of age. Gastroenterology 100:A727, 1991 (abstract).
224. Levy MF, Somasundar PS, Jennings LW, et al: The elderly liver transplant recipient: a call for caution. Ann Surg 233(1):107, 2001.
225. McCauley J, Van Thiel DH, Starzl TE, et al: Acute and chronic renal failure in liver transplantation. Nephron 55(2):121, 1990.
226. Arroyo V, Gines P, Navasa M, et al: Renal failure in cirrhosis and liver transplantation. Transplant Proc 25(2):1734, 1993.
227. Brown RS Jr, Lombardero M, Lake JR: Outcome of patients with renal insufficiency undergoing liver or liver-kidney transplantation. Transplantation 62(12):1788, 1996.
228. Gonwa TA, Nery JR, Husberg BS, et al: Simultaneous liver and renal transplantation in man. Transplantation 46(5):690, 1988.
229. Pham PT, Pham PC, Wilkinson AH: The kidney in liver transplantation. Clin Liver Dis 4(3):567, 2000.
230. Shaked A, Colonna JO, Goldstein L, et al: The interrelation between sclerosing cholangitis and ulcerative colitis in patients undergoing liver transplantation. Ann Surg 215(6):598, 1992.
231. Langnas AN, Grazi GL, Stratta RJ, et al: Primary sclerosing cholangitis: the emerging role for liver transplantation. Am J Gastroenterol 85(9):1136, 1990.
232. Keeffe EB, Gettys C, Esquivel CO: Liver transplantation in patients with severe obesity. Transplantation 57(2):309, 1994.
233. Palmer M, Schaffner F, Thung SN: Excessive weight gain after liver transplantation. Transplantation 51(4):797, 1991.
234. Nair S, Cohen DB, Cohen MP, et al: Postoperative morbidity, mortality, costs, and long-term survival in severely obese patients undergoing orthotopic liver transplantation. Am J Gastroenterol 96(3):842, 2001.
235. Braunfeld MY, Chan S, Pregler J, et al: Liver transplantation in the morbidly obese. J Clin Anesth 8(7):585, 1996.
236. Sawyer RG, Pelletier SJ, Pruett TL: Increased early morbidity and mortality with acceptable long-term function in severely obese patients undergoing liver transplantation. Clin Transplant 13(1 Pt 2):126, 1999.
237. Penn I: The effect of immunosuppression on pre-existing cancers. Transplantation 55(4):742, 1993.
238. Saigal S, Norris S, Srinivasan P, et al: Successful outcome of orthotopic liver transplantation in patients with preexisting malignant states. Liver Transpl 7(1):11, 2001.
239. Roll J, Boyer JL, Barry D, et al: The prognostic importance of clinical and histologic features in asymptomatic and symptomatic primary biliary cirrhosis. N Engl J Med 308(1):1, 1983.
240. Markus BH, Dickson ER, Grambsch PM, et al: Efficiency of liver transplantation in patients with primary biliary cirrhosis. N Engl J Med 320(26):1709, 1989.
241. Wiesner RH, Porayko MK, Dickson ER, et al: Selection and timing of liver transplantation in primary biliary cirrhosis and primary sclerosing cholangitis. Hepatology 16(5):1290, 1992.

242. Dickson ER, Grambsch PM, Fleming TR, et al: Prognosis in primary biliary cirrhosis: model for decision making. Hepatology 10(1):1, 1989.
243. Kim WR, Wiesner RH, Therneau TM, et al: Optimal timing of liver transplantation for primary biliary cirrhosis. Hepatology 28(1):33, 1998.
244. Klion FM, Fabry TL, Palmer M, Schaffner F: Prediction of survival of patients with primary biliary cirrhosis. Examination of the Mayo Clinic model on a group of patients with known endpoint. Gastroenterology 102(1):310, 1992.
245. Grambsch PM, Dickson ER, Kaplan M, et al: Extramural cross-validation of the Mayo primary biliary cirrhosis survival model establishes its generalizability. Hepatology 10(5):846, 1989.
246. Gilroy RK, Lynch SV, Strong RW, et al: Confirmation of the role of the Mayo risk score as a predictor of resource utilization after orthotopic liver transplantation for primary biliary cirrhosis. Liver Transpl 6(6):749, 2000.
247. Kim WR, Dickson ER: Timing of liver transplantation. Semin Liver Dis 20(4):451, 2000.
248. Kim WR, Wiesner RH, Poterucha JJ, et al: Adaptation of the Mayo primary biliary cirrhosis natural history model for application in liver transplant candidates. Liver Transpl 6(4):489, 2000.
249. Wiesner RH, Grambsch PM, Dickson ER, et al: Primary sclerosing cholangitis: natural history, prognostic factors and survival analysis. Hepatology 10(4):430, 1989.
250. Dickson ER, Murtaugh PA, Wiesner RH, et al: Primary sclerosing cholangitis: refinement and validation of survival models. Gastroenterology 103(6):1893, 1992.
251. Wee A, Ludwig J, Coffey RJ Jr, et al: Hepatobiliary carcinoma associated with primary sclerosing cholangitis and chronic ulcerative colitis. Hum Pathol 16(7):719, 1985.
252. Farges O, Malassagne B, Sebagh M, et al: Primary sclerosing cholangitis: liver transplantation or biliary surgery. Surgery 117(2):146, 1995.
253. Wiesner RH, LaRusso NF: Clinicopathologic features of the syndrome of primary sclerosing cholangitis. Gastroenterology 79(2):200, 1980.
254. Chapman RW, Arborgh BA, Rhodes JM, et al: Primary sclerosing cholangitis: a review of its clinical features, cholangiography, and hepatic histology. Gut 21(10):870, 1980.
255. Talwalkar JA, Seaberg E, Kim WR, et al: Predicting clinical and economic outcomes after liver transplantation using the Mayo primary sclerosing cholangitis model and Child-Pugh score. Liver Transpl 6(6):753, 2000.
256. Malinchoc M, Kamath PS, Gordon FD, et al: A model to predict poor survival in patients undergoing transjugular intrahepatic portosystemic shunts. Hepatology 31(4):864, 2000.
257. Kamath PS, Wiesner RH, Malinchoc M, et al: A model to predict survival in patients with end-stage liver disease. Hepatology 33(2):464, 2001.
258. Forman LM, Lucey MR: Predicting the prognosis of chronic liver disease: an evolution from Child to MELD. Hepatology 33(3):473, 2001 (editorial).
259. Pessoa MG, Wright TL: Hepatitis C infection in transplantation. Clin Liver Dis 1(3):663, 1997.
260. Ferrell LD, Wright TL, Roberts J, et al: Hepatitis C viral infection in liver transplant recipients. Hepatology 16(4):865, 1992.
261. Gane EJ, Portmann BC, Naoumov NV, et al: Long-term outcome of hepatitis C infection after liver transplantation. N Engl J Med 334(13):815, 1996.
262. Chazouillères O, Kim M, Combs C, et al: Quantitation of hepatitis C virus RNA in liver transplant recipients. Gastroenterology 106(4):994, 1994.
263. Dickson RC, Caldwell SH, Ishitani MB, et al: Clinical and histologic patterns of early graft failure due to recurrent hepatitis C in four patients after liver transplantation. Transplantation 61(5):701, 1996.
264. Fukumoto T, Berg T, Ku Y, et al: Viral dynamics of hepatitis C early after orthotopic liver transplantation: evidence for rapid turnover of serum virions. Hepatology 24(6):1351, 1996.
265. Molmenti EP, Klintmalm GB: Hepatitis C recurrence after liver transplantation. Liver Transpl 6(4):413, 2000.
266. Gordon SC, Bayati N, Silverman AL: Clinical outcome of hepatitis C as a function of mode of transmission. Hepatology 28(2):562, 1998.
267. Baron PW, Sindram D, Higdon D, et al: Prolonged rewarming time during allograft implantation predisposes to recurrent hepatitis C infection after liver transplantation. Liver Transpl 6(4):407, 2000.
268. Berenguer M, Terrault NA, Piatak M, et al: Hepatitis G virus infection in patients with hepatitis C virus infection undergoing liver transplantation. Gastroenterology 111(6):1569, 1996.
269. Berenguer M, Ferrell L, Watson J, et al: Fibrosis progression in recurrent hepatitis C virus (HCV) disease: differences between the U.S. and Europe. Hepatology 28(4 Pt 2):220A, 1998 (abstract).
270. Berenguer M, Prieto M, Cordoba J, et al: Early development of chronic active hepatitis in recurrent hepatitis C virus infection after liver transplantation: association with treatment of rejection. J Hepatol 28(5):756, 1998.
271. Berenguer M, Ferrell L, Watson J, et al: HCV-related fibrosis progression following liver transplantation: increase in recent years. J Hepatol 32(4):673, 2000.
272. Bizollon T, Guichard S, Ahmed SN, et al: Impact of hepatitis G virus co-infection on the course of hepatitis C virus infection before and after liver transplantation. J Hepatol 29(6):893, 1998.
273. Bizollon T, Ahmed SN, Guichard S, et al: Anti-hepatitis C virus core IgM antibodies correlate with hepatitis C recurrence and its severity in liver transplant patients. Gut 47(5):698, 2000.
274. Charlton M, Seaberg E, Wiesner R, et al: Predictors of patient and graft survival following liver transplantation for hepatitis C. Hepatology 28(3):823, 1998.
275. Deshpande V, Burd E, Aardema KL, et al: High levels of hepatitis C virus RNA in native livers correlate with the development of cholestatic hepatitis in liver allografts and a poor outcome. Liver Transpl 7(2):118, 2001.
276. Di Martino V, Saurini F, Samuel D, et al: Long-term longitudinal study of intrahepatic hepatitis C virus replication after liver transplantation. Hepatology 26(5):1343, 1997.
277. Féray C, Gigou M, Samuel D, et al: Influence of the genotypes of hepatitis C virus on the severity of recurrent liver disease after liver transplantation. Gastroenterology 108(4):1088, 1995.
278. Féray C, Caccamo L, Alexander GJ, et al: European collaborative study on factors influencing outcome after liver transplantation for hepatitis C. European Concerted Action on Viral Hepatitis (EUROHEP) Group. Gastroenterology 117(3):619, 1999.
279. Gayowski T, Singh N, Marino IR, et al: Hepatitis C virus genotypes in liver transplant recipients: impact on posttransplant recurrence, infections, response to interferon-alpha therapy and outcome. Transplantation 64(3):422, 1997.
280. Gretch DR, Bacchi CE, Corey L, et al: Persistent hepatitis C virus infection after liver transplantation: clinical and virological features. Hepatology 22(1):1, 1995.
281. Manez R, Mateo R, Tabasco J, et al: The influence of HLA donor-recipient compatibility on the recurrence of HBV and HCV hepatitis after liver transplantation. Transplantation 59(4):640, 1995.
282. Pelletier SJ, Raymond DP, Crabtree TD, et al: Pretransplantation hepatitis C virus quasispecies may be predictive of outcome after liver transplantation. Hepatology 32(2):375, 2000.
283. Pelletier SJ, Iezzoni JC, Crabtree TD, et al: Prediction of liver allograft fibrosis after transplantation for hepatitis C virus: persistent elevation of serum transaminase levels versus necroinflammatory activity. Liver Transpl 6(1):44, 2000.
284. Pessoa MG, Bzowej N, Berenguer M, et al: Evolution of hepatitis C virus quasispecies in patients with severe cholestatic hepatitis after liver transplantation. Hepatology 30(6):1513, 1999.
285. Prieto M, Berenguer M, Rayon JM, et al: High incidence of allograft cirrhosis in hepatitis C virus genotype 1b infection following transplantation: relationship with rejection episodes. Hepatology 29(1):250, 1999.
286. Rosen HR, Shackleton CR, Higa L, et al: Use of OKT3 is associated with early and severe recurrence of hepatitis C after liver transplantation. Am J Gastroenterol 92(9):1453, 1997.
287. Rosen HR, Chou S, Corless CL, et al: Cytomegalovirus viremia: risk factor for allograft cirrhosis after liver transplantation for hepatitis C. Transplantation 64(5):721, 1997.
288. Rosen HR, Gretch DR, Oehlke M, et al: Timing and severity of initial hepatitis C recurrence as predictors of long-term liver allograft injury. Transplantation 65(9):1178, 1998.
289. Schluger LK, Sheiner PA, Thung SN, et al: Severe recurrent cholestatic hepatitis C following orthotopic liver transplantation. Hepatology 23(5):971, 1996.

290. Sheiner PA, Schwartz ME, Mor E, et al: Severe or multiple rejection episodes are associated with early recurrence of hepatitis C after orthotopic liver transplantation. Hepatology 21(1):30, 1995.
291. Taniguchi M, Shakil AO, Vargas HE, et al: Clinical and virologic outcomes of hepatitis B and C viral coinfection after liver transplantation: effect of viral hepatitis D. Liver Transpl 6(1):92, 2000.
292. Testa G, Crippin JS, Netto GJ, et al: Liver transplantation for hepatitis C: recurrence and disease progression in 300 patients. Liver Transpl 6(5):553, 2000.
293. Zhou S, Terrault NA, Ferrell L, et al: Severity of liver disease in liver transplantation recipients with hepatitis C virus infection: relationship to genotype and level of viremia. Hepatology 24(5):1041, 1996.
294. Taniguchi M, Shakil AO, Vargas HE, et al: Clinical and virologic outcomes of hepatitis B and C viral coinfection after liver transplantation: effect of viral hepatitis D. Liver Transpl 6(1):92, 2000.
295. Sheiner PA, Boros P, Klion FM, et al: The efficacy of prophylactic interferon alfa-2b in preventing recurrent hepatitis C after liver transplantation. Hepatology 28(3):831, 1998.
296. Singh N, Gayowski T, Wannstedt CF, et al: Interferon-alpha for prophylaxis of recurrent viral hepatitis C in liver transplant recipients: a prospective, randomized, controlled trial. Transplantation 65(1):82, 1998.
297. Mazzaferro V, Regalia E, Pulvirenti A, et al: Prophylaxis against HCV recurrence after liver transplantation: effect of interferon and ribavirin combination. Transplant Proc 29(1-2):519, 1997.
298. Féray C, Gigou M, Samuel D, et al: The course of hepatitis C virus infection after liver transplantation. Hepatology 20(5):1137, 1994.
299. Wright TL, Combs C, Kim M, et al: Interferon-alpha therapy for hepatitis C virus infection after liver transplantation. Hepatology 20(4 Pt 1):773, 1994.
300. Gane EJ, Tibbs CJ, Ramage JK, et al: Ribavirin therapy for hepatitis C infection following liver transplantation. Transpl Int 8(1):61, 1995.
301. Gane EJ, Lo SK, Riordan SM, et al: A randomized study comparing ribavirin and interferon alfa monotherapy for hepatitis C recurrence after liver transplantation. Hepatology 27(5):1403, 1998.
302. Cattral MS, Hemming AW, Wanless IR, et al: Outcome of long-term ribavirin therapy for recurrent hepatitis C after liver transplantation. Transplantation 67(9):1277, 1999.
303. Bizollon T, Palazzo U, Ducerf C, et al: Pilot study of the combination of interferon alfa and ribavirin as therapy of recurrent hepatitis C after liver transplantation. Hepatology 26(2):500, 1997.
304. Bizollon T, Ducerf C, Chevallier M, et al: Long-term efficacy of ribavirin plus IFN in the treatment of HCV recurrence after liver transplantation. 11th Congress of the European Society for Organ Transplantation. Oslo, 19-24 June 1999 (abstract 20).
305. Gopal DV, Rabkin JM, Berk BS, et al: Treatment of progressive hepatitis C recurrence after liver transplantation with combination interferon plus ribavirin. Liver Transpl 7(3):181, 2001.
306. Charlton M, Seaberg E: Impact of immunosuppression and acute rejection on recurrence of hepatitis C: results of the National Institute of Diabetes and Digestive and Kidney Diseases Liver Transplantation Database. Liver Transpl Surg 5(4 suppl 1):S107, 1999.
307. Petrovic LM, Villamil FG, Vierling JM, et al: Comparison of histopathology in acute allograft rejection and recurrent hepatitis C infection after liver transplantation. Liver Transpl Surg 3(4):398, 1997.
308. Berenguer M, Lopez-Labrador FX, Greenberg HB, et al: Hepatitis C virus and the host: an imbalance induced by immunosuppression? Hepatology 32(2):433, 2000.
309. Rosen HR: Retransplantation for hepatitis C: implications of different policies. Liver Transpl 6(6 suppl 2):S41, 2000.
310. Carithers RL Jr: Recurrent hepatitis C after liver transplantation. Liver Transpl Surg 3(5 Suppl 1):S16, 1997.
311. Sheiner PA, Schluger LK, Emre S, et al: Retransplantation for recurrent hepatitis C. Liver Transpl Surg 3(2):130, 1997.
312. Vierling JM, Villamil FG, Rojter SE, et al: Morbidity and mortality of recurrent hepatitis C infection after orthotopic liver transplantation. J Viral Hepat 4(suppl 1):117, 1997.
313. Casavilla FA, Lee R, Lim J, et al: Outcome of liver retransplantation for recurrent hepatitis C infection. Hepatology 22(4 Pt 2):153A, 1995.
314. Rosen HR, Martin P: Hepatitis C infection in patients undergoing liver retransplantation. Transplantation 66(12):1612, 1998.
315. Scharschmidt BF: Human liver transplantation: analysis of data on 540 patients from four centers. Hepatology 4(1 suppl):95S, 1984.
316. Vaillant GE: What can long-term follow-up teach us about relapse and prevention of relapse in addiction? Br J Addict 83(10):1147, 1988.
317. Neuberger J, Adams D, MacMaster P, et al: Assessing priorities for allocation of donor liver grafts: survey of public and clinicians. BMJ 317(7152):172, 1998.
318. Starzl TE, Van Thiel D, Tzakis AG, et al: Orthotopic liver transplantation for alcoholic cirrhosis. JAMA 260(17):2542, 1988.
319. Lucey MR, Merion RM, Henley KS, et al: Selection for and outcome of liver transplantation in alcoholic liver disease. Gastroenterology 102(5):1736, 1992.
320. Gish RG, Lee AH, Keeffe EB, et al: Liver transplantation for patients with alcoholism and end-stage liver disease. Am J Gastroenterol 88(9):1337, 1993.
321. Keeffe EB: Assessment of the alcoholic patient for liver transplantation: comorbidity, outcome, and recidivism. Liver Transpl Surg 2(5 suppl 1):12, 1996.
322. McCurry KR, Baliga P, Merion RM, et al: Resource utilization and outcome of liver transplantation for alcoholic cirrhosis. A case-control study. Arch Surg 127(7):772, 1992.
323. Belle SH, Kimberly CB, Detre KM: Trends in liver transplantation in the United States. In Terasaki P, Cecka M, eds: Clinical Transplants 1993. Los Angeles, UCLA Tissue Typing Laboratory, 1993:19.
324. Van Thiel DH, Bonet H, Gavaler J, et al: Effect of alcohol use on allograft rejection rates after liver transplantation for alcoholic liver disease. Alcohol Clin Exp Res 19(5):1151, 1995.
325. Lucey MR, Carr K, Beresford TP, et al: Alcohol use after liver transplantation in alcoholics: a clinical cohort follow-up study. Hepatology 25(5):1223, 1997.
326. Baddour N, Demetris AJ, Shah G, et al: The prevalence, rate of onset and spectrum of histologic liver disease in alcohol abusing liver allograft recipients. Gastroenterology 102:A779, 1992 (abstract).
327. Bravata DM, Olkin I, Barnato AE, et al: Employment and alcohol use after liver transplantation for alcoholic and nonalcoholic liver disease: a systematic review. Liver Transpl 7(3):191, 2001.
328. Todo S, Demetris AJ, Van Thiel D, et al: Orthotopic liver transplantation for patients with hepatitis B virus-related liver disease. Hepatology 13(4):619, 1991.
329. Davies SE, Portmann BC, O'Grady JG, et al: Hepatic histological findings after transplantation for chronic hepatitis B virus infection, including a unique pattern of fibrosing cholestatic hepatitis. Hepatology 13(1):150, 1991.
330. Benner KG, Lee RG, Keeffe EB, et al: Fibrosing cytolytic liver failure secondary to recurrent hepatitis B after liver transplantation. Gastroenterology 103(4):1307, 1992.
331. Luketic VA, Shiffman ML, McCall JB, et al: Primary hepatocellular carcinoma after orthotopic liver transplantation for chronic hepatitis B infection. Ann Intern Med 114(3):212, 1991.
332. Mason AL, Wick M, White HM, et al: Increased hepatocyte expression of hepatitis B virus transcription in patients with features of fibrosing cholestatic hepatitis. Gastroenterology 105(1):237, 1993.
333. Fang JW, Tung FY, Davis GL, et al: Fibrosing cholestatic hepatitis in a transplant recipient with hepatitis B virus precore mutant. Gastroenterology 105(3):901, 1993.
334. Angus PW, Locarnini SA, McCaughan GW, et al: Hepatitis B virus precore mutant infection is associated with severe recurrent disease after liver transplantation. Hepatology 21(1):14, 1995.
335. Samuel D, Muller R, Alexander G, et al: Liver transplantation in European patients with the hepatitis B surface antigen. N Engl J Med 329(25):1842, 1993.
336. Jurim O, Martin P, Shaked A, et al: Liver transplantation for chronic hepatitis B in Asians. Transplantation 57(9):1393, 1994.
337. Ho BM, So SK, Esquivel CO, et al: Liver transplantation in Asian patients with chronic hepatitis B. Hepatology 25(1):223, 1997.
338. Terrault NA: Hepatitis B virus and liver transplantation. Clin Liver Dis 3(2):389, 1999.
339. Gish RG, Keeffe EB, Lim J, et al: Survival after liver transplantation for chronic hepatitis B using reduced immunosuppression. J Hepatol 22(3):257, 1995.
340. Terrault NA, Zhou S, Combs C, et al: Prophylaxis in liver transplant recipients using a fixed dosing schedule of hepatitis B immunoglobulin. Hepatology 24(6): 1327, 1996.

341. McGory RW, Ishitani MB, Oliveira WM, et al: Improved outcome of orthotopic liver transplantation for chronic hepatitis B cirrhosis with aggressive passive immunization. Transplantation 61(9): 1358, 1996.
342. Rizzetto M, Marzano A: Posttransplantation prevention and treatment of recurrent hepatitis B. Liver Transpl 6(6 suppl 2):S47, 2000.
343. Chang CN, Skalski V, Zhou JH, et al: Biochemical pharmacology of (+)- and (−)-2′,3′-dideoxy-3′-thiacytidine as anti-hepatitis B virus agents. J Biol Chem 267(31):22414, 1992.
344. Furman PA, Davis M, Liotta DC, et al: The anti-hepatitis B virus activities, cytotoxicities, and anabolic profiles of the (−) and (+) enantiomers of cis-5-fluoro-1-[2-(hydroxymethyl)-1,3-oxathiolan-5-yl]cytosine. Antimicrob Agents Chemother 36(12):2686, 1992.
345. Dienstag JL, Perrillo RP, Schiff ER, et al: A preliminary trial of lamivudine for chronic hepatitis B infection. N Engl J Med 333(25):1657, 1995.
346. Lai CL, Chien RN, Leung NW, et al: A one-year trial of lamivudine for chronic hepatitis B. Asia Hepatitis Lamivudine Study Group. N Engl J Med 339(2):61, 1998.
347. Tassopoulos NC, Volpes R, Pastore G, et al: Efficacy of lamivudine in patients with hepatitis B e antigen-negative/hepatitis B virus DNA-positive (precore mutant) chronic hepatitis B. Lamivudine Precore Mutant Study Group. Hepatology 29(3):889, 1999.
348. Mutimer D, Dusheiko G, Barrett C, et al: Lamivudine without HBIg for prevention of graft reinfection by hepatitis B: long-term follow-up. Transplantation 70(5):809, 2000.
349. Johnson MA, Horak J, Breuel P: The pharmacokinetics of lamivudine in patients with impaired hepatic function. Eur J Clin Pharmacol 54(4):363, 1998.
350. Keeffe EB: End-stage liver disease and liver transplantation: role of lamivudine therapy in patients with chronic hepatitis B. J Med Virol 61:403, 2000.
351. Yao FY, Bass NM: Lamivudine treatment in patients with severely decompensated cirrhosis due to replicating hepatitis B infection. J Hepatol 33(2):301, 2000.
352. Sponseller CA, Bacon BR, Di Bisceglie AM: Clinical improvement in patients with decompensated liver disease caused by hepatitis B after treatment with lamivudine. Liver Transpl 6(6):715, 2000.
353. Van Thiel DH, Friedlander L, Kania RJ, et al: Lamivudine treatment of advanced and decompensated liver disease due to hepatitis B. Hepatogastroenterology 44(15):808, 1997.
354. Perrillo RP, Wright T, Rakela J, et al: A multicenter United States-Canadian trial to assess lamivudine monotherapy before and after liver transplantation for chronic hepatitis B. Hepatology 33(2):424, 2001.
355. Grellier L, Mutimer D, Ahmed M, et al: Lamivudine prophylaxis against reinfection in liver transplantation for hepatitis B cirrhosis. Lancet 348(9036):1212, 1996.
356. Ling R, Mutimer D, Ahmed M, et al: Selection of mutations in the hepatitis B virus polymerase during therapy of transplant recipients with lamivudine. Hepatology 24(3):711, 1996.
357. Ben-Ari Z, Pappo O, Zemel R, et al: Association of lamivudine resistance in recurrent hepatitis B after liver transplantation with advanced hepatic fibrosis. Transplantation 68(2):232, 1999.
358. Markowitz JS, Martin P, Conrad AJ, et al: Prophylaxis against hepatitis B recurrence following liver transplantation using combination lamivudine and hepatitis B immune globulin. Hepatology 28(2):585, 1998.
359. Han SH, Ofman J, Holt C, et al: An efficacy and cost-effectiveness analysis of combination hepatitis B immune globulin and lamivudine to prevent recurrent hepatitis B after orthotopic liver transplantation compared with hepatitis B immune globulin monotherapy. Liver Transpl 6(6):741, 2000.
360. Angus PW, McCaughan GW, Gane EJ, et al: Combination low-dose hepatitis B immune globulin and lamivudine therapy provides effective prophylaxis against posttransplantation hepatitis B. Liver Transpl 6(4):429, 2000.
361. Yao FY, Osorio RW, Roberts JP, et al: Intramuscular hepatitis B immune globulin combined with lamivudine for prophylaxis against hepatitis B recurrence after liver transplantation. Liver Transpl Surg 5(6):491, 1999.
362. Yoshida EM, Erb SR, Partovi N, et al: Liver transplantation for chronic hepatitis B infection with the use of combination lamivudine and low-dose hepatitis B immune globulin. Liver Transpl Surg 5(6):520, 1999.
363. Dodson SF, de Vera ME, Bonham CA, et al: Lamivudine after hepatitis B immune globulin is effective in preventing hepatitis B recurrence after liver transplantation. Liver Transpl 6(4):434, 2000.
364. McCaughan GW, Spencer J, Koorey D, et al: Lamivudine therapy in patients undergoing liver transplantation for hepatitis B virus precore mutant-associated infection: high resistance rates in treatment of recurrence but universal prevention if used as prophylaxis with very low dose hepatitis B immune globulin. Liver Transpl Surg 5(6):512, 1999.
365. Crippin J, Foster B, Carlen S, et al: Retransplantation in hepatitis B—a multicenter experience. Transplantation 57(6):823, 1994.
366. Perrillo R, Rakela J, Dienstag J, et al: Multicenter study of lamivudine therapy for hepatitis B after liver transplantation. Lamivudine Transplant Group. Hepatology 29(5):1581, 1999.
367. Torresi J, Locarnini S: Antiviral chemotherapy for the treatment of hepatitis B virus infections. Gastroenterology 118(2 suppl 1):S83, 2000.
368. Peters MG, Singer G, Howard T, et al: Fulminant hepatic failure resulting from lamivudine-resistant hepatitis B virus in a renal transplant recipient: durable response after orthotopic liver transplantation on adefovir dipivoxil and hepatitis B immune globulin. Transplantation 68(12):1912, 1999.
369. Han SH, Kinkhabwala M, Martin P, et al: Resolution of recurrent hepatitis B in two liver transplant recipients treated with famciclovir. Am J Gastroenterol 93(11):2245, 1998.
370. Gish RG, Lau JY, Brooks L, et al: Ganciclovir treatment of hepatitis B virus infection in liver transplant recipients. Hepatology 23(1):1, 1996.
371. Hadziyannis SJ, Manesis EK, Papakonstantinou A: Oral ganciclovir treatment in chronic hepatitis B virus infection: a pilot study. J Hepatol 31(2):210, 1999.
372. Flowers M, Sherker A, Sinclair SB, et al: Prostaglandin E in the treatment of recurrent hepatitis B infection after orthotopic liver transplantation. Transplantation 58(2):183, 1994.
373. Esquivel CO, Van Thiel DH, Demetris AJ, et al: Transplantation for primary biliary cirrhosis. Gastroenterology 94(5 Pt 1):1207, 1988.
374. Maddrey WC: Bone disease in patients with primary biliary cirrhosis. In Popper H, Schaffner F, eds: Progress in Liver Diseases, vol 9. Philadelphia, WB Saunders Co., 1990:537.
375. Hay JE: Bone disease in liver transplant recipients. Gastroenterol Clin North Am 22:337, 1993.
376. Eastell R, Dickson ER, Hodgson SF, et al: Rates of vertebral bone loss before and after liver transplantation in women with primary biliary cirrhosis. Hepatology 14(2):296, 1991.
377. Heathcote EJ: Management of primary biliary cirrhosis. The American Association for the Study of Liver Diseases practice guidelines. Hepatology 31(4):1005, 2000.
378. Gross CR, Malinchoc M, Kim WR, et al: Quality of life before and after liver transplantation for cholestatic liver disease. Hepatology 29(2):356, 1999.
379. Neuberger J, Portmann B, Macdougall BR, et al: Recurrence of primary biliary cirrhosis after liver transplantation. N Engl J Med 306(1):1, 1982.
380. Polson RJ, Portmann B, Neuberger J, et al: Evidence for disease recurrence after liver transplantation for primary biliary cirrhosis. Clinical and histologic follow-up studies. Gastroenterology 97(3):715, 1989.
381. Wong PY, Portmann B, O'Grady JG, et al: Recurrence of primary biliary cirrhosis after liver transplantation following FK506-based immunosuppression. J Hepatol 17(3):284, 1993.
382. Neuberger J: Recurrence of primary biliary cirrhosis, primary sclerosing cholangitis, and autoimmune hepatitis. Liver Transpl Surg 1(5 suppl 1):109, 1995.
383. Slapak GI, Saxena R, Portmann B, et al: Graft and systemic disease in long-term survivors of liver transplantation. Hepatology 25(1):195, 1997.
384. Neuberger J: Recurrent primary biliary cirrhosis. Baillieres Best Pract Res Clin Gastroenterol 14(4):669, 2000.
385. Balan V, Batts KP, Porayko MK, et al: Histological evidence for recurrence of primary biliary cirrhosis after liver transplantation. Hepatology 18(6):1392, 1993.
386. Gouw AS, Haagsma EB, Manns M, et al: Is there recurrence of primary biliary cirrhosis after liver transplantation? A clinicopathologic study in long-term survivors. J Hepatol 20(4):500, 1994.

387. Rosen CB, Nagorney DM, Wiesner RH, et al: Cholangiocarcinoma complicating primary sclerosing cholangitis. Ann Surg 213(1):21, 1991.
388. Rosen CB, Nagorney DM: Cholangiocarcinoma complicating primary sclerosing cholangitis. Semin Liver Dis 11(1):26, 1991.
389. Miros M, Kerlin P, Walker N, et al: Predicting cholangiocarcinoma in patients with primary sclerosing cholangitis before transplantation. Gut 32(11):1369, 1991.
390. Rabinovitz M, Zajko AB, Hassanein T, et al: Diagnostic value of brush cytology in the diagnosis of bile duct carcinoma: a study in 65 patients with bile duct strictures. Hepatology 12(4 Pt 1):747, 1990.
391. Saldeen K, Friman S, Olausson M, et al: Follow-up after liver transplantation for primary sclerosing cholangitis: effects on survival, quality of life, and colitis. Scand J Gastroenterol 34(5):535, 1999.
392. Narumi S, Roberts JP, Emond JC, et al: Liver transplantation for sclerosing cholangitis. Hepatology 22(2):451, 1995.
393. Goss JA, Shackleton CR, Farmer DG, et al: Orthotopic liver transplantation for primary sclerosing cholangitis. A 12-year single center experience. Ann Surg 225(5):472, 1997.
394. Graziadei IW, Wiesner RH, Marotta PJ, et al: Long-term results of patients undergoing liver transplantation for primary sclerosing cholangitis. Hepatology 30(5):1121, 1999.
395. Rosen HR: Disease recurrence following liver transplantation. Clin Liver Dis 4(3):675, 2000.
396. Shaked A, Colonna JO, Goldstein L, et al: The interrelation between sclerosing cholangitis and ulcerative colitis in patients undergoing liver transplantation. Ann Surg 215(6):598, 1992.
397. Broome U, Lindberg G, Lofberg R: Primary sclerosing cholangitis in ulcerative colitis—a risk factor for the development of dysplasia and DNA aneuploidy? Gastroenterology 102(6):1877, 1992.
398. Higashi H, Yanaga K, Marsh JW, et al: Development of colon cancer after liver transplantation for primary sclerosing cholangitis associated with ulcerative colitis. Hepatology 11(3):477, 1990.
399. Czaja AJ: Diagnosis and therapy of autoimmune liver disease. Med Clin North Am 80(5):973, 1996.
400. Krawitt EL: Autoimmune hepatitis. N Engl J Med 334(14):897, 1996.
401. Johnson PJ, McFarlane IG, Eddleston AL: The natural course and heterogeneity of autoimmune-type chronic active hepatitis. Semin Liver Dis 11(3):187, 1991.
402. Czaja AJ: Natural history of chronic active hepatitis. In Czaja AJ, Dickson ER, eds: Chronic Active Hepatitis: The Mayo Clinic Experience. New York, Marcel Dekker, 1986:9.
403. Maddrey WC, Combes B: Therapeutic concepts for the management of idiopathic autoimmune chronic hepatitis. Semin Liver Dis 11(3):248, 1991.
404. Meyer zum Buschenfelde KH, Lohse AW: Autoimmune hepatitis. N Engl J Med 333(15):1004, 1995.
405. Sanchez-Urdazpal L, Czaja AJ, van Hoek B, et al: Prognostic features and role of liver transplantation in severe corticosteroid-treated autoimmune chronic active hepatitis. Hepatology 15(2):215, 1992.
406. Czaja AJ, Cassani F, Cataleta M, et al: Frequency and significance of antibodies to actin in type 1 autoimmune hepatitis. Hepatology 24(5):1068, 1996.
407. Czaja AJ, Strettell MD, Thomson LJ, et al: Associations between alleles of the major histocompatibility complex and type 1 autoimmune hepatitis. Hepatology 25(2):317, 1997.
408. Czaja AJ, Cassani F, Cataleta M, et al: Antinuclear antibodies and patterns of nuclear immunofluorescence in type 1 autoimmune hepatitis. Dig Dis Sci 42(8):1688, 1997.
409. Milkiewicz P, Ahmed M, Hathaway M, et al: Factors associated with progression of the disease before transplantation in patients with autoimmune hepatitis. Liver 19(1):50, 1999.
410. Hayashi M, Keeffe EB, Krams SM, et al: Allograft rejection after liver transplantation for autoimmune liver diseases. Liver Transpl Surg 4(3):208, 1998.
411. Hubscher SG: Recurrent autoimmune hepatitis after liver transplantation: diagnostic criteria, risk factors, and outcome. Liver Transpl 7(4):285, 2001.
412. Milkiewicz P, Hubscher SG, Skiba G, et al: Recurrence of autoimmune hepatitis after liver transplantation. Transplantation 68(2):253, 1999.
413. Ratziu V, Samuel D, Sebagh M, et al: Long-term follow-up after liver transplantation for autoimmune hepatitis: evidence of recurrence of primary disease. J Hepatol 30(1):131, 1999.
414. Reich DJ, Fiel I, Guarrera JV, et al: Liver transplantation for autoimmune hepatitis. Hepatology 32(4 Pt 1):693, 2000.
415. Gonzalez-Koch A, Czaja AJ, Carpenter HA, et al: Recurrent autoimmune hepatitis after orthotopic liver transplantation. Liver Transpl 7(4):302, 2001.
416. Gilbert SC, Klintmalm G, Menter A, et al: Methotrexate-induced cirrhosis requiring liver transplantation in three patients with psoriasis. A word of caution in light of the expanding use of this "steroid-sparing" agent. Arch Intern Med 150(4):889, 1990.
417. CDC: Severe isoniazid-associated hepatitis—New York, 1991-1993. MMWR Morb Mortal Wkly Rep 42:545, 1993.
418. Greeve M, Ferrell L, Kim M, et al: Cirrhosis of undefined pathogenesis: absence of evidence for unknown viruses or autoimmune processes. Hepatology 17(4):593, 1993.
419. Maor-Kendler Y, Batts KP, Burgart LJ, et al: Comparative allograft histology after liver transplantation for cryptogenic cirrhosis, alcohol, hepatitis C, and cholestatic liver diseases. Transplantation 70(2):292, 2000.
420. Charlton MR, Kondo M, Roberts SK, et al: Liver transplantation for cryptogenic cirrhosis. Liver Transpl Surg 3(4):359, 1997.
421. Brown J, Dourakis S, Karayiannis P, et al: Seroprevalence of hepatitis C virus nucleocapsid antibodies in patients with cryptogenic chronic liver disease. Hepatology 15(2):175, 1992.
422. Vennarecci G, Gunson BK, Ismail T, et al: Transplantation for end stage liver disease related to alpha 1 antitrypsin. Transplantation 61(10):1488, 1996.
423. Poonawala A, Nair SP, Thuluvath PJ: Prevalence of obesity and diabetes in patients with cryptogenic cirrhosis: a case-control study. Hepatology 32(4 Pt 1):689, 2000.
424. Contos MJ, Cales W, Sterling RK, et al: Development of nonalcoholic fatty liver disease after orthotopic liver transplantation for cryptogenic cirrhosis. Liver Transpl (4):363, 2001.
425. Molloy RM, Komorowski R, Varma RR: Recurrent nonalcoholic steatohepatitis and cirrhosis after liver transplantation. Liver Transpl Surg 3(2):177, 1997.
426. Kim WR, Poterucha JJ, Porayko MK, et al: Recurrence of nonalcoholic steatohepatitis following liver transplantation. Transplantation 62(12):1802, 1996.
427. Esquivel CO, Marino IR, Fioravanti V, Van Thiel DH: Liver transplantation for metabolic disease of the liver. Gastroenterol Clin North Am 17(1):167, 1988.
428. Powell LW: Does transplantation of the liver cure genetic hemochromatosis? J Hepatol 16(3):259, 1992.
429. Pillay P, Tzoracoleftherakis E, Tzakis AG, et al: Orthotopic liver transplantation for hemochromatosis. Transplant Proc 23(2):1888, 1991.
430. Kilpe VE, Krakauer H, Wren RE, et al: An analysis of liver transplant experience from 37 transplant centers as reported to Medicare. Transplantation 56(3):554, 1993.
431. Brandhagen DJ, Alvarez W, Therneau TM, et al: Iron overload in cirrhosis—HFE genotypes and outcome after liver transplantation. Hepatology 31(2):456, 2000.
432. Tung BY, Farrell FJ, McCashland TM, et al: Long-term follow-up after liver transplantation in patients with hepatic iron overload. Liver Transpl Surg 5(5):369, 1999.
433. Kowdley KV, Hassanein T, Kaur S, et al: Primary liver cancer and survival in patients undergoing liver transplantation for hemochromatosis. Liver Transpl Surg 1(4):237, 1995.
434. Westra WH, Hruban RH, Baughman KL, et al: Progressive hemochromatotic cardiomyopathy despite reversal of iron deposition after liver transplantation. Am J Clin Pathol 99(1):39, 1993.
435. Surakomol S, Olson LJ, Rastogi A, et al: Combined orthotopic heart and liver transplantation for genetic hemochromatosis. J Heart Lung Transplant 16(5):573, 1997.
436. Poulos JE, Bacon BR: Liver transplantation for hereditary hemochromatosis. Dig Dis 14(5):316, 1996.
437. Bellary S, Hassanein T, Van Thiel DH: Liver transplantation for Wilson's disease. J Hepatol 23(4):373, 1995.
438. Schilsky ML, Scheinberg IH, Sternlieb I: Liver transplantation for Wilson's disease: indications and outcome. Hepatology 19(3):583, 1994.
439. Eghtesad B, Nezakatgoo N, Geraci LC, et al: Liver transplantation for Wilson's disease: a single-center experience. Liver Transpl Surg 5(6):467, 1999.
440. Sternlieb I: Wilson's disease. Clin Liver Dis 4(1):229, 2000.

441. Polson RJ, Rolles K, Calne RY, et al: Reversal of severe neurological manifestations of Wilson's disease following orthotopic liver transplantation. QJM 64(244):685, 1987.
442. Schumacher G, Platz KP, Mueller AR, et al: Liver transplantation: treatment of choice for hepatic and neurological manifestation of Wilson's disease. Clin Transplant 11(3):217, 1997.
443. Chen CL, Chen YS, Lui CC, et al: Neurological improvement of Wilson's disease after liver transplantation. Transplant Proc 29(1-2): 497, 1997.
444. Bax RT, Hassler A, Luck W, et al: Cerebral manifestation of Wilson's disease successfully treated with liver transplantation. Neurology 51(3):863, 1998.
445. Stracciari A, Tempestini A, Borghi A, et al: Effect of liver transplantation on neurological manifestations in Wilson disease. Arch Neurol 57(3):384, 2000.
446. Schumacher G, Platz KP, Mueller AR, et al: Liver transplantation in neurologic Wilson's disease. Transplant Proc 33(1-2):1518, 2001.
447. Eghtesad B, Fung JJ, Rakela J: Response. Liver Transpl 6(5): =663, 2000.
448. Brewer GJ, Askari F: Transplant livers in Wilson's disease for hepatic, not neurologic, indications. Liver Transpl 6(5):662, 2000.
449. Teckman JH, Qu D, Perlmutter DH: Molecular pathogenesis of liver disease in alpha1-antitrypsin deficiency. Hepatology 24(6):1504, 1996.
450. Eigenbrodt ML, McCashland TM, Dy RM, et al: Heterozygous alpha 1-antitrypsin phenotypes in patients with end stage liver disease. Am J Gastroenterol 92(4):602, 1997.
451. Graziadei IW, Joseph JJ, Wiesner RH, et al: Increased risk of chronic liver failure in adults with heterozygous alpha1-antitrypsin deficiency. Hepatology 28(4):1058, 1998.
452. Rakela J, Goldschmiedt M, Ludwig J: Late manifestation of chronic liver disease in adults with alpha-1-antitrypsin deficiency. Dig Dis Sci 32(12):1358, 1987.
453. Qu D, Teckman JH, Perlmutter DH: Review: alpha 1-antitrypsin deficiency associated liver disease. J Gastroenterol Hepatol 12(5): 404, 1997.
454. Esquivel CO, Vicente E, Van Thiel D, et al: Orthotopic liver transplantation for alpha-1-antitrypsin deficiency: an experience in 29 children and ten adults. Transplant Proc 19(5):3798, 1987.
455. Adrian-Casavilla F, Reyes J, Tzakis A, et al: Liver transplantation for neonatal hepatitis as compared to the other two leading indications for liver transplantation in children. J Hepatol 21(6):1035, 1994.
456. Filipponi F, Soubrane O, Labrousse F, et al: Liver transplantation for end-stage liver disease associated with alpha-1-antitrypsin deficiency in children: pretransplant natural history, timing and results of transplantation. J Hepatol 20(1):72, 1994.
457. Vennarecci G, Gunson BK, Ismail T, et al: Transplantation for end stage liver disease related to alpha 1 antitrypsin. Transplantation 61(10):1488, 1996.
458. Hood JM, Koep LJ, Peters RL, et al: Liver transplantation for advanced liver disease with alpha-1-antitrypsin deficiency. N Engl J Med 302(5):272, 1980.
459. Putnam CW, Porter KA, Peters RL, et al: Liver replacement for alpha1-antitrypsin deficiency. Surgery 81(3):258, 1977.
460. Van Furth R, Kramps JA, van der Putten AB, et al: Change in alpha 1-antitrypsin phenotype after orthotopic liver transplant. Clin Exp Immunol 66(3):669, 1986.
461. Goss JA, Stribling R, Martin P: Adult liver transplantation for metabolic liver disease. Clin Liver Dis 2(1):187, 1998.
462. Iezzoni JC, Gaffey MJ, Stacy EK, et al: Hepatocytic globules in end-stage hepatic disease: relationship to alpha1-antitrypsin phenotype. Am J Clin Pathol 107(6):692, 1997.
463. Elzouki AN, Lindgren S, Nilsson S, et al: Severe alpha1-antitrypsin deficiency (PiZ homozygosity) with membranoproliferative glomerulonephritis and nephrotic syndrome, reversible after orthotopic liver transplantation. J Hepatol 26(6):1403, 1997.
464. Sarasin FP, Giostra E, Mentha G, et al: Partial hepatectomy or orthotopic liver transplantation for the treatment of resectable hepatocellular carcinoma? A cost-effectiveness perspective. Hepatology 28(2):436, 1998.
465. Harnois DM, Steers J, Andrews JC, et al: Preoperative hepatic artery chemoembolization followed by orthotopic liver transplantation for hepatocellular carcinoma. Liver Transpl Surg 5(3):192, 1999.
466. Penn I: Hepatic transplantation for primary and metastatic cancers of the liver. Surgery 110(4):726, 1991.
467. Soreide O, Czerniak A, Bradpiece H, et al: Characteristics of fibrolamellar hepatocellular carcinoma. A study of nine cases and a review of the literature. Am J Surg 151(4):518, 1986.
468. Berman MA, Burnham JA, Sheahan DG: Fibrolamellar carcinoma of the liver: an immunohistochemical study of nineteen cases and a review of the literature. Fibrolamellar carcinoma of the liver: an immunohistochemical study of nineteen cases and a review of the literature. Hum Pathol 19(7):784, 1988.
469. Reynolds TB: Budd-Chiari syndrome. In Schiff L, Schiff ER, eds: Diseases of the Liver, ed 6. Philadelphia, JB Lippincott, 1987: 1466.
470. Halff G, Todo S, Tzakis AG, et al: Liver transplantation for the Budd-Chiari syndrome. Ann Surg 211(1):43, 1990.
471. Bismuth H, Sherlock DJ: Portasystemic shunting versus liver transplantation for the Budd-Chiari syndrome. Ann Surg 214(5):581, 1991.
472. Shaked A, Goldstein RM, Klintmalm GB, et al: Portosystemic shunt versus orthotopic liver transplantation for the Budd-Chiari syndrome. Surg Gynecol Obstet 174(6):453, 1992.
473. Campbell DA Jr, Rolles K, Jamieson N, et al: Hepatic transplantation with perioperative and long term anticoagulation as treatment for Budd-Chiari syndrome. Surg Gynecol Obstet 166(6):511, 1988.
474. Orloff MJ, Orloff MS, Daily PO: Long-term results of treatment of Budd-Chiari syndrome with portal decompression. Arch Surg 127(10):1182, 1992.
475. Ringe B, Lang H, Oldhafer KJ, et al: Which is the best surgery for Budd-Chiari syndrome: venous decompression or liver transplantation? A single-center experience with 50 patients. Hepatology 21(5):1337, 1995.
476. Hemming AW, Langer B, Greig P, et al: Treatment of Budd-Chiari syndrome with portosystemic shunt or liver transplantation. Am J Surg 171(1):176, 1996.
477. Seltman HJ, Dekker A, Van Thiel DH, et al: Budd-Chiari syndrome recurring in a transplanted liver. Gastroenterology 84(3):640, 1983.
478. Ruckert JC, Ruckert RI, Rudolph B, et al: Recurrence of the Budd-Chiari syndrome after orthotopic liver transplantation. Hepatogastroenterology 46(26):867, 1999.
479. Sherlock S: Cystic diseases of the liver. In Schiff ER, Sorrell MF, Maddrey WC, eds: Schiff's Diseases of the Liver, ed 8. Philadelphia, Lippincott-Raven Publishers, 1999:1083.
480. Gabow PA: Autosomal dominant polycystic kidney disease. N Engl J Med 329(5):332, 1993.
481. Swenson K, Seu P, Kinkhabwala M, et al: Liver transplantation for adult polycystic liver disease. Hepatology 28(2):412, 1998.
482. Pirenne J, Aerts R, Yoong K, et al: Liver transplantation for polycystic liver disease. Liver Transpl 7(3):238, 2001.
483. Lake JR, Gournay J: Liver transplantation. In Feldman M, Scharschmidt BF, Sleisenger MH, eds: Sleisenger & Fordtran's Gastrointestinal and Liver Disease: Pathophysiology/Diagnosis/Management, ed 6. Philadelphia, WB Saunders Co, 1998:1404.
484. Langnas AN, Marujo W, Stratta RJ, et al: Vascular complications after orthotopic liver transplantation. Am J Surg 161(1):76, 1991.
485. Madalosso C, de Souza NF Jr, Ilstrup DM, et al: Cytomegalovirus and its association with hepatic artery thrombosis after liver transplantation. Transplantation 66(3):294, 1998.
486. Sanchez-Bueno F, Robles R, Acosta F, et al: Hepatic artery complications in a series of 300 orthotopic liver transplants. Transplant Proc 32(8):2669, 2000.
487. Pastacaldi S, Teixeira R, Montalto P, et al: Hepatic artery thrombosis after orthotopic liver transplantation: a review of nonsurgical causes. Liver Transpl 7(2):75, 2001.
488. Valente JF, Alonso MH, Weber FL, Hanto DW: Late hepatic artery thrombosis in liver allograft recipients is associated with intrahepatic biliary necrosis. Transplantation 61(1):61, 1996.
489. Steiber AC, Gordon RD, Galloway JR: Orthotopic liver transplantation. In Zakim D, Boyer TD, eds: Hepatology: A Textbook of Liver Disease, ed 3. Philadelphia, WB Saunders Co, 1996:1759.
490. Rabkin JM, Orloff SL, Corless CL, et al: Hepatic allograft abscess with hepatic arterial thrombosis. Am J Surg 175(5):354, 1998.
491. Yanaga K, Lebeau G, Marsh JW, et al: Hepatic artery reconstruction for hepatic artery thrombosis after orthotopic liver transplantation. Arch Surg 125(5):628, 1990.

492. Pinna AD, Smith CV, Furukawa H, et al: Urgent revascularization of liver allografts after early hepatic artery thrombosis. Transplantation 62(11):1584, 1996.
493. Sheiner PA, Varma CV, Guarrera JV, et al: Selective revascularization of hepatic artery thromboses after liver transplantation improves patient and graft survival. Transplantation 64(9):1295, 1997.
494. Vorwerk D, Gunther RW, Klever P, et al: Angioplasty and stent placement for treatment of hepatic artery thrombosis following liver transplantation. J Vasc Interv Radiol 5(2):309, 1994.
495. Hidalgo EG, Abad J, Cantarero JM, et al: High-dose intra-arterial urokinase for the treatment of hepatic artery thrombosis in liver transplantation. Hepatogastroenterology 36(6):529, 1989.
496. Suhocki P, Chari R, McCann R, et al: Vascular aspects of liver transplantation. In Killenberg PG, Clavien PA, eds: Medical Care of the Liver Transplant Patients. Malden, Blackwell Science, 1997:80.
497. Helling TS: Thrombosis and recanalization of the portal vein in liver transplantation. A case report. Transplantation 40(4):446, 1985.
498. Everson GT, Kam I: Immediate postoperative care. In Maddrey WC, Schiff ER, Sorrell MF, eds: Transplantation of the Liver, ed 3. Philadelphia, Lippincott Williams & Wilkins, 2001:131.
499. Abbasoglu O, Levy MF, Vodapally MS, et al: Hepatic artery stenosis after liver transplantation—incidence, presentation, treatment, and long term outcome. Transplantation 63(2):250, 1997.
500. Orons PD, Zajko AB: Angiography and interventional procedures in liver transplantation. Radiol Clin North Am 33(3):541, 1995.
501. Houssin D, Ortega D, Richardson A, et al: Mycotic aneurysm of the hepatic artery complicating human liver transplantation. Transplantation 46(3):469, 1988.
502. Lebeau G, Yanaga K, Marsh JW, et al: Analysis of surgical complications after 397 hepatic transplantations. Surg Gynecol Obstet 170(4):317, 1990.
503. Fichelle JM, Colacchio G, Castaing D, et al: Infected false hepatic artery aneurysm after orthotopic liver transplantation treated by resection and reno-hepatic vein graft. Ann Vasc Surg 11(3):300, 1997.
504. Goldman DE, Colquhoun SD, Ghobrial RM, et al: Mycotic aneurysm of arterial conduit presenting as massive upper gastrointestinal hemorrhage after liver transplantation. Liver Transpl Surg 4(5):435, 1998.
505. McDonald M, Perkins JD, David R, et al: Postoperative care: Immediate. In Maddrey WC, Sorrell MF, eds: Transplantation of the Liver, ed 3. Norwalk, Appleton & Lange, 1995:171.
506. Quiroga J, Colina I, Demetris AJ, et al: Cause and timing of first allograft failure in orthotopic liver transplantation: a study of 177 consecutive patients. Hepatology 14(6):1054, 1991.
507. Bzeizi KI, Jalan R, Plevris JN, et al: Primary graft dysfunction after liver transplantation: from pathogenesis to prevention. Liver Transpl Surg 3(2):137, 1997.
508. Busuttil RW, Shaked A, Millis JM, et al: One thousand liver transplants. The lessons learned. Ann Surg 219(5):490, 1994.
509. Marsman WA, Wiesner RH, Rodriguez L, et al: Use of fatty donor liver is associated with diminished early patient and graft survival. Transplantation 62(9):1246, 1996.
510. Gayowski T, Marino IR, Singh N, et al: Orthotopic liver transplantation in high-risk patients: risk factors associated with mortality and infectious morbidity. Transplantation 65(4):499, 1998.
511. Rosen HR, Martin P, Goss J, et al: Significance of early aminotransferase elevation after liver transplantation. Transplantation 65(1):68, 1998.
512. Wall WJ: Predicting outcome after liver transplantation. Liver Transpl Surg 5(5):458, 1999.
513. Mandal AK, King KE, Humphreys SL, et al: Plasmapheresis: an effective therapy for primary allograft nonfunction after liver transplantation. Transplantation 70(1):216, 2000.
514. Klein AS, Cofer JB, Pruett TL, et al: Prostaglandin E1 administration following orthotopic liver transplantation: a randomized prospective multicenter trial. Gastroenterology 111(3):710, 1996.
515. Schafer DF, Sorrell MF: Prostaglandins in liver transplantation: a promise unfulfilled. Gastroenterology 111(3):819, 1996.
516. Shackleton CR, Martin P, Melinek J, et al: Lack of correlation between the magnitude of preservation injury and the incidence of acute rejection, need for OKT3, and conversion to FK506 in cyclosporine-treated primary liver allograft recipients. Transplantation 60(6):554, 1995.
517. Terminology of chronic hepatitis, hepatic allograft rejection, and nodular lesions of the liver: summary of recommendations developed by an international working party, supported by the World Congresses of Gastroenterology, Los Angeles, 1994. Am J Gastroenterol 89(8 suppl):S177, 1994.
518. Farges O, Kalil AN, Samuel D, et al: The use of ABO-incompatible grafts in liver transplantation: a life-saving procedure in highly selected patients. Transplantation 59(8):1124, 1995.
519. Mor E, Skerrett D, Manzarbeitia C, et al: Successful use of an enhanced immunosuppressive protocol with plasmapheresis for ABO-incompatible mismatched grafts in liver transplant recipients. Transplantation 59(7):986, 1995.
520. Fang WC, Saltzman J, Rososhansky S, et al: Acceptance of an ABO-incompatible mismatched (AB(−) to O(+)) liver allograft with the use of daclizumab and mycophenolate mofetil. Liver Transpl 6(4):497, 2000.
521. Eid A, Zamir G, Yaron I, Galun E, et al: Liver transplantation across the ABO barrier: the role of plasmapheresis. Transplant Proc 30(3):701, 1998.
522. Lo CM, Shaked A, Busuttil RW: Risk factors for liver transplantation across the ABO barrier. Transplantation 58(5):543, 1994.
523. Wiesner RH, Demetris AJ, Belle SH, et al: Acute hepatic allograft rejection: incidence, risk factors, and impact on outcome. Hepatology 28(3):638, 1998.
524. Harland RC: Rejection of the liver graft. In Killenberg PG, Clavien PA, eds: Medical Care of the Liver Transplant Patients. Malden, Blackwell Science, 1997:147.
525. Mor E, Solomon H, Gibbs JF, et al: Acute cellular rejection following liver transplantation: clinical pathologic features and effect on outcome. Semin Liver Dis 12(1):28, 1992.
526. Bathgate AJ, Hynd P, Sommerville D, et al: The prediction of acute cellular rejection in orthotopic liver transplantation. Liver Transpl Surg 5(6):475, 1999.
527. Seiler CA, Dufour JF, Renner EL, et al: Primary liver disease as a determinant for acute rejection after liver transplantation. Arch Surg 384(3):259, 1999.
528. Neuberger J: Incidence, timing, and risk factors for acute and chronic rejection. Liver Transpl Surg 5(4 zuppl 1):S30, 1999.
529. Demetris A, Adams D, Bellamy C, et al: Update of the International Banff Schema for Liver Allograft Rejection: working recommendations for the histopathologic staging and reporting of chronic rejection. An International Panel. Hepatology 31(3):792, 2000.
530. Ludwig J: Terminology of hepatic allograft rejection (glossary). Semin Liver Dis 12(1):89, 1992.
531. Wiesner RH, Ludwig J, Krom RA, et al: Treatment of early cellular rejection following liver transplantation with intravenous methylprednisolone. The effect of dose on response. Transplantation 58(9):1053, 1994.
532. Wiesner RH, Ludwig J, Krom RA, et al: Hepatic allograft rejection: new developments in terminology, diagnosis, prevention, and treatment. Mayo Clin Proc 68(1):69, 1993.
533. Hebert MF, Ascher NL, Lake JR, et al: Four-year follow-up of mycophenolate mofetil for graft rescue in liver allograft recipients. Transplantation 67(5):707, 1999.
534. Charco R, Murio E, Edo A, et al: Early use of tacrolimus as rescue therapy for refractory liver allograft rejection. Transpl Int 11(suppl 1): S313, 1998.
535. Klein A: Tacrolimus rescue in liver transplant patients with refractory rejection or intolerance or malabsorption of cyclosporine. The US Multicenter FK506 Liver Study Group. Liver Transpl Surg 5(6):502, 1999.
536. Friman S, Persson H, Schersten T, et al: Adjuvant treatment with ursodeoxycholic acid reduces acute rejection after liver transplantation. Transplant Proc 24(1):389, 1992.
537. Barnes D, Talenti D, Cammell G, et al: A randomized clinical trial of ursodeoxycholic acid as adjuvant treatment to prevent liver transplant rejection. Hepatology 26(4):853, 1997.
538. Pageaux GP, Blanc P, Perrigault PF, et al: Failure of ursodeoxycholic acid to prevent acute cellular rejection after liver transplantation. J Hepatol 23(2):119, 1995.
539. Keiding S, Hockerstedt K, Bjoro K, et al: The Nordic multicenter double-blind randomized controlled trial of prophylactic ursodeoxycholic acid in liver transplant patients. Transplantation 63(11):1591, 1997.
540. Fleckenstein JF, Paredes M, Thuluvath PJ: A prospective, randomized, double-blind trial evaluating the efficacy of ursodeoxycholic

acid in prevention of liver transplant rejection. Liver Transpl Surg 4(4):276, 1998.
541. Wiesner RH, Batts KP, Krom RA: Evolving concepts in the diagnosis, pathogenesis, and treatment of chronic hepatic allograft rejection. Liver Transpl Surg 5(5):388, 1999.
542. Gavlik A, Goldberg MG, Tsaroucha A, et al: Mycophenolate mofetil rescue therapy in liver transplant recipients. Transplant Proc 29 (1-2):549, 1997.
543. Wiesner RH, Ludwig J, van Hoek B, et al: Current concepts in cell-mediated hepatic allograft rejection leading to ductopenia and liver failure. Hepatology 14(4 Pt 1):721, 1991.
544. Demetris AJ, Murase N, Lee RG, et al: Chronic rejection. A general overview of histopathology and pathophysiology with emphasis on liver, heart and intestinal allografts. Ann Transplant 2(2):27, 1997.
545. Sher LS, Cosenza CA, Michel J, et al: Efficacy of tacrolimus as rescue therapy for chronic rejection in orthotopic liver transplantation: a report of the U.S. Multicenter Liver Study Group. Transplantation 64(2):258, 1997.
546. Hubscher SG, Buckels JA, Elias E, et al: Vanishing bile-duct syndrome following liver transplantation—is it reversible? Transplantation 51(5):1004, 1991.
547. Noack KB, Wiesner RH, Batts K, et al: Severe ductopenic rejection with features of vanishing bile duct syndrome: clinical, biochemical, and histologic evidence for spontaneous resolution. Transplant Proc 23(1 Pt 2):1448, 1991.
548. Greif F, Bronsther OL, Van Thiel DH, et al: The incidence, timing, and management of biliary tract complications after orthotopic liver transplantation. Ann Surg 219(1):40, 1994.
549. Stratta RJ, Wood RP, Langnas AN, et al: Diagnosis and treatment of biliary tract complications after orthotopic liver transplantation. Surgery 106(4):675, 1989.
550. Porayko MK, Kondo M, Steers JL: Liver transplantation: late complications of the biliary tract and their management. Semin Liver Dis 15(2):139, 1995.
551. Clavien PA, Harvey PR, Strasberg SM: Preservation and reperfusion injuries in liver allografts. An overview and synthesis of current studies. Transplantation 53(5):957, 1992.
552. Sanchez-Urdazpal L, Gores GJ, Ward EM, et al: Diagnostic features and clinical outcome of ischemic-type biliary complications after liver transplantation. Hepatology 17(4):605, 1993.
553. Johnson MW, Thompson P, Meehan A, et al: Internal biliary stenting in orthotopic liver transplantation. Liver Transpl 6(3):356, 2000.
554. Starzl TE, Putnam CW, Hansbrough JF, et al: Biliary complications after liver transplantation: with special reference to the biliary cast syndrome and techniques of secondary duct repair. Surgery 81(2):212, 1977;
555. Lerut J, Gordon RD, Iwatsuki S, et al: Biliary tract complications in human orthotopic liver transplantation. Transplantation 43(1):47, 1987.
556. Klein AS, Savader S, Burdick JF, et al: Reduction of morbidity and mortality from biliary complications after liver transplantation. Hepatology 14(5):818, 1991.
557. Reichert PR, Renz JF, Rosenthal P, et al: Biliary complications of reduced-organ liver transplantation. Liver Transpl Surg 4(5):343, 1998.
558. Saab S, Martin P, Soliman GY, et al: Endoscopic management of biliary leaks after T-tube removal in liver transplant recipients: nasobiliary drainage versus biliary stenting. Liver Transpl 6(5):627, 2000.
559. Osorio RW, Freise CE, Stock PG, et al: Nonoperative management of biliary leaks after orthotopic liver transplantation. Transplantation 55(5):1074, 1993.
560. Rizk RS, McVicar JP, Emond MJ, et al: Endoscopic management of biliary strictures in liver transplant recipients: effect on patient and graft survival. Gastrointest Endosc 47(2):128, 1998.
561. Sawyer RG, Punch JD: Incidence and management of biliary complications after 291 liver transplants following the introduction of transcystic stenting. Transplantation 66(9):1201, 1998.
562. Davidson BR, Rai R, Nandy A, et al: Results of choledochojejunostomy in the treatment of biliary complications after liver transplantation in the era of nonsurgical therapies. Liver Transpl 6(2):201, 2000.
563. Campbell WL, Sheng R, Zajko AB, et al: Intrahepatic biliary strictures after liver transplantation. Radiology 191(3):735, 1994.
564. Chen CL, Wang KL, Chuang JH, et al: Biliary sludge-cast formation following liver transplantation. Hepatogastroenterology 35(1):22, 1988.
565. Branch MS, Clavien PA: Biliary complications following liver transplantation. In Killenberg PG, Clavien PA, eds: Medical Care of the Liver Transplant Patients. Malden, Blackwell Science, 1997:193.
566. Clavien PA, Camargo CA Jr, Baillie J, et al: Sphincter of Oddi dysfunction after liver transplantation. Dig Dis Sci 40(1):73, 1995.
567. Tung BY, Kimmey MB: Biliary complications of orthotopic liver transplantation. Dig Dis 17(3):133, 1999.
568. Sparberg M, Simon N, del Greco F: Intrahepatic cholestasis due to azathioprine. Gastroenterology 57(4):439, 1969.
569. Sterneck M, Wiesner R, Ascher N, et al: Azathioprine hepatotoxicity after liver transplantation. Hepatology 14(5):806, 1991
570. Zimmerman HJ: Drug-induced liver disease. In Zimmerman HJ, ed: Hepatotoxicity: The Adverse Effects of Drugs and Other Chemicals on the Liver. Philadelphia, Lippincott Williams & Wilkins, 1999:427.
571. Mion F, Napoleon B, Berger F, et al: Azathioprine induced liver disease: nodular regenerative hyperplasia of the liver and perivenous fibrosis in a patient treated for multiple sclerosis. Gut 32(6):715, 1991.
572. Gane E, Portmann B, Saxena R, et al: Nodular regenerative hyperplasia of the liver graft after liver transplantation. Hepatology 20 (1 Pt 1):88, 1994.
573. Zarday Z, Veith FJ, Gliedman ML, et al: Irreversible liver damage after azathioprine. JAMA 222(6):690, 1972;
574. Read AE, Wiesner RH, LaBrecque DR, et al: Hepatic veno-occlusive disease associated with renal transplantation and azathioprine therapy. Ann Intern Med 104(5):651, 1986.
575. Washington MK, Howell DN: The role of histopathology in the evaluation of the liver transplant recipient. In Killenberg PG, Clavien PA, eds: Medical Care of the Liver Transplant Patients. Malden, Blackwell Science, 1997:210.
576. Paya CV, Hermans PE, Washington JA, et al: Incidence, distribution, and outcome of episodes of infection in 100 orthotopic liver transplantations. Mayo Clin Proc 64(5):555, 1989.
577. Sampathkumar P, Paya CV: Management of cytomegalovirus infection after liver transplantation. Liver Transpl 6(2):144, 2000.
578. Paya CV, Hermans PE, Wiesner RH, et al: Cytomegalovirus hepatitis in liver transplantation: prospective analysis of 93 consecutive orthotopic liver transplantations. J Infect Dis 160(5):752, 1989.
579. Falagas ME, Snydman DR, Ruthazer R, et al: Cytomegalovirus immune globulin (CMVIG) prophylaxis is associated with increased survival after orthotopic liver transplantation. The Boston Center for Liver Transplantation CMVIG Study Group. Clin Transplant 11(5 Pt 1):432, 1997.
580. Kanj SS: Infection in the liver transplant recipient: approach to the febrile patient. In Killenberg PG, Clavien PA, eds: Medical Care of the Liver Transplant Patients. Malden, Blackwell Science, 199:159.
581. Stratta RJ, Shaeffer MS, Markin RS, et al: Cytomegalovirus infection and disease after liver transplantation. An overview. Dig Dis Sci 37(5):673, 1992.
582. Paya CV, Wiesner RH, Hermans PE, et al: Risk factors for cytomegalovirus and severe bacterial infections following liver transplantation: a prospective multivariate time-dependent analysis. J Hepatol 18(2):185, 1993.
583. George MJ, Snydman DR, Werner BG, et al: The independent role of cytomegalovirus as a risk factor for invasive fungal disease in orthotopic liver transplant recipients. Boston Center for Liver Transplantation CMVIG-Study Group. Cytogam, MedImmune, Inc., Gaithersburg, Maryland. Am J Med 103(2):106, 1997.
584. Kowalik TF, Wing B, Haskill JS, et al: Multiple mechanisms are implicated in the regulation of NF-kappa B activity during human cytomegalovirus infection. Proc Natl Acad Sci U S A 90(3):1107, 1993.
585. Rosen HR, Corless CL, Rabkin J, et al: Association of cytomegalovirus genotype with graft rejection after liver transplantation. Transplantation 66(12):1627, 1998.
586. Falagas ME, Paya C, Ruthazer R, et al: Significance of cytomegalovirus for long-term survival after orthotopic liver transplantation: a prospective derivation and validation cohort analysis. Transplantation 66(8):1020, 1998.
587. Rosen HR, Benner KG, Flora KD, et al: Development of ganciclovir resistance during treatment of primary cytomegalovirus infection after liver transplantation. Transplantation 63(3):476, 1997.

588. Kanj SS, Sharara AI, Clavien PA, et al: Cytomegalovirus infection following liver transplantation: review of the literature. Clin Infect Dis 22(3):537, 1996.
589. Freise CE, Pons V, Lake J, et al: Comparison of three regimens for cytomegalovirus prophylaxis in 147 liver transplant recipients. Transplant Proc 23(1 Pt 2):1498, 1991.
590. McAlister V, Grant D, Roy A, et al: Posttransplant lymphoproliferative disorders in liver recipients treated with OKT3 or ALG induction immunosuppression. Transplant Proc 25(1 Pt 2):1400, 1993.
591. Rustgi VK: Epstein-Barr viral infection and posttransplantation lymphoproliferative disorders. Liver Transpl Surg 1(5 suppl 1):100, 1995.
592. Walker RC, Paya CV, Marshall WF, et al: Pretransplantation seronegative Epstein-Barr virus status is the primary risk factor for posttransplantation lymphoproliferative disorder in adult heart, lung, and other solid organ transplantations. J Heart Lung Transplant 14(2):214, 1995.
593. Penn I: Posttransplantation de novo tumors in liver allograft recipients. Liver Transpl Surg 2(1):52, 1996.
594. Carson KL, Killenberg PG: Medical problems after liver transplantation. In Killenberg PG, Clavien PA, eds: Medical Care of the Liver Transplant Patients. Malden, Blackwell Science, 1997:259.
595. McLaughlin K, Wajstaub S, Marotta P, et al: Increased risk for posttransplant lymphoproliferative disease in recipients of liver transplants with hepatitis C. Liver Transpl 6(5):570, 2000.
596. Hezode C, Duvoux C, Germanidis G, et al: Role of hepatitis C virus in lymphoproliferative disorders after liver transplantation. Hepatology 30(3):775, 1999.
597. Nalesnik MA, Makowka L, Starzl TE: The diagnosis and treatment of posttransplant lymphoproliferative disorders. Curr Probl Surg 25(6):367, 1988.
598. Winston DJ, Emmanouilides C, Busuttil RW: Infections in liver transplant recipients. Clin Infect Dis 21(5):1077, 1995.
599. Kusne S, Dummer JS, Singh N, et al: Infections after liver transplantation. An analysis of 101 consecutive cases. Medicine 67(2):132, 1988.
600. Singh N, Gayowski T, Rihs JD, et al: Evolving trends in multiple-antibiotic-resistant bacteria in liver transplant recipients: a longitudinal study of antimicrobial susceptibility patterns. Liver Transpl 7(1):22, 2001.
601. Singh N: The current management of infectious diseases in the liver transplant recipient. Clin Liver Dis 4(3):657, 2000.
602. Castaldo P, Stratta RJ, Wood RP, et al: Fungal disease in liver transplant recipients: a multivariate analysis of risk factors. Transplant Proc 23(1 Pt 2):1517, 1991.
603. Collins LA, Samore MH, Roberts MS, et al: Risk factors for invasive fungal infections complicating orthotopic liver transplantation. J Infect Dis 170(3):644, 1994.
604. Singhal S, Ellis RW, Jones SG, et al: Targeted prophylaxis with amphotericin B lipid complex in liver transplantation. Liver Transpl 6(5):588, 2000.
605. Krowka MJ, Cortese DA: Pulmonary aspects of liver disease and liver transplantation. Clin Chest Med 10(4):593, 1989.
606. Snowden CP, Hughes T, Rose J, et al: Pulmonary edema in patients after liver transplantation. Liver Transpl 6(4):466, 2000.
607. Sanchez-Izquierdo JA, Lumbreras C, Colina F, et al: Severe graft versus host disease following liver transplantation confirmed by PCR-HLA-B sequencing: report of a case and literature review. Hepatogastroenterology 43(10):1057, 1996.
608. Bronster DJ, Emre S, Boccagni P, et al: Central nervous system complications in liver transplant recipients—incidence, timing, and long-term follow-up. Clin Transplant 14(1):1, 2000.
609. Lee YJ, Lee SG, Kwon TW, et al: Neurologic complications after orthotopic liver transplantation including central pontine myelinolysis. Transplant Proc 28(3):1674, 1996.
610. Sterzi R, Santilli I, Donato MF, et al: Neurologic complications following orthotopic liver transplantation. Transplant Proc 26(6):3679, 1994.
611. Fryer JP, Fortier MV, Metrakos P, et al: Central pontine myelinolysis and cyclosporine neurotoxicity following liver transplantation. Transplantation 61(4):658, 1996.
612. Munoz SJ, Rothstein KD, Reich D, et al: Long-term care of the liver transplant recipient. Clin Liver Dis 4(3):691, 2000.
613. Reich D, Rothstein K, Manzarbeitia C, et al: Common medical diseases after liver transplantation. Semin Gastrointest Dis 9(3):110, 1998.
614. Textor SC, Taler SJ, Canzanello VJ, et al: Posttransplantation hypertension related to calcineurin inhibitors. Liver Transpl 6(5):521, 2000.
615. Imagawa DK, Dawson S 3rd, Holt CD, et al: Hyperlipidemia after liver transplantation: natural history and treatment with the hydroxy-methylglutaryl-coenzyme A reductase inhibitor pravastatin. Transplantation 62(7):934, 1996.
616. Otley CC, Pittelkow MR: Skin cancer in liver transplant recipients. Liver Transpl 6(3):253, 2000.
617. Papatheodoridis GV, Hamilton M, Rolles K, et al: Liver transplantation and inflammatory bowel disease. J Hepatol 28(6):1070, 1998.
618. Watson CJ, Friend PJ, Jamieson NV, et al: Sirolimus: a potent new immunosuppressant for liver transplantation. Transplantation 67(4):505, 1999.
619. McAlister VC, Gao Z, Peltekian K, et al: Sirolimus-tacrolimus combination immunosuppression. Lancet 355(9201):376, 2000.
620. Busuttil RW, Goss JA: Split liver transplantation. Ann Surg 229(3):313, 1999.
621. Broelsch CE, Emond JC, Whitington PF, et al: Application of reduced-size liver transplants as split grafts, auxiliary orthotopic grafts, and living related segmental transplants. Ann Surg 212(3):368, 1990.
622. Rela M, Vougas V, Muiesan P, et al: Split liver transplantation: King's College Hospital experience. Ann Surg 227(2):282, 1998.
623. Ghobrial RM, Yersiz H, Farmer DG, et al: Predictors of survival after in vivo split liver transplantation: analysis of 110 consecutive patients. Ann Surg 232(3):312, 2000.
624. Raia S, Nery JR, Mies S: Liver transplantation from live donors. Lancet 2(8661):497, 1989.
625. Hashikura Y, Makuuchi M, Kawasaki S, et al: Successful living-related partial liver transplantation to an adult patient. Lancet 343(8907):1233, 1994.
626. Inomata Y, Tanaka K, Okajima H, et al: Living related liver transplantation for children younger than one year old. Eur J Pediatr Surg 6(3):148, 1996.
627. Marcos A, Ham JM, Fisher RA, et al: Single-center analysis of the first 40 adult-to-adult living donor liver transplants using the right lobe. Liver Transpl 6(3):296, 2000.
628. Marcos A: Right lobe living donor liver transplantation: a review. Liver Transpl 6(1):3, 2000.
629. Lo CM, Fan ST, Liu CL, et al: Adult-to-adult living donor liver transplantation using extended right lobe grafts. Ann Surg 226(3):261, 1997.
630. Lo CM, Fan ST, Liu CL, et al: Applicability of living donor liver transplantation to high-urgency patients. Transplantation 67(1):73, 1999.
631. Trotter JF, Wachs M, Trouillot T, et al: Evaluation of 100 patients for living donor liver transplantation. Liver Transpl 6(3):290, 2000.
632. Ghobrial RM, Amersi F, Busuttil RW: Surgical advances in liver transplantation. Living related and split donors. Clin Liver Dis 4(3):553, 2000.

CHAPTER

56

Recurrent Disease after Liver Transplantation

Marina Berenguer, MD, and Teresa L. Wright, MD

With significant improvements in immunosuppressive therapy and surgical techniques over the past 2 decades, liver transplantation has become the definitive and effective therapy for patients with end-stage liver disease, with survival rates approaching 90 percent to 95 percent and 65 percent to 80 percent after 1 and 5 years of follow-up, respectively.[1] Among several circumstances that may pose a threat to long-term survival, the one of significant concern is the recurrence of the original liver disease. This situation was first best described for hepatitis B, with more than 80 percent viral recurrence in the era before the introduction of immunoprophylaxis.[2] Although hepatitis B virus (HBV) recurrence has been effectively contained by hepatitis B immunoglobulin (HBIg) with or without lamivudine, there remain other conditions, such as recurrent hepatitis C virus (HCV), that are becoming increasingly challenging problems to the transplant community.[3] In addition, and albeit with less dramatic consequences, recurrence of other diseases that were originally believed not to recur, such as primary sclerosing cholangitis, is now widely accepted. As patients survive longer and enter their second and third decade posttransplantation, it is likely that allograft failure related to primary disease recurrence will become an increasingly serious problem. In this chapter we will summarize the current knowledge of disorders that may recur after liver transplantation, with particular emphasis on the natural history, pathogenesis, and treatment of these conditions.

RECURRENT HEPATITIS B VIRUS INFECTION

In the past few years, there has been a substantial improvement in the management of HBV infection in the liver transplant setting. Historically these patients had done poorly with transplantation. The 5-year survival rate for patients undergoing liver transplantation with HBV infection was reported to be 50 percent compared to survival rates of 70 percent to 85 percent for patients with alcoholic or cholestatic liver diseases.[4] This reduced survival was in large part related to the high rate of HBV recurrence in the absence of specific prophylactic therapies with subsequent graft loss resulting from the development of recurrent liver disease.[2,5] In an early study performed before the introduction of immunoprophylaxis, the reinfection rate was approximately 80 percent, resulting in graft loss in more than 70 percent of patients.[2] Efforts to improve the outcome of these patients were predominantly focused upon strategies to prevent reinfection. In recent years several new therapies have become available[6] that are improving the outcome of this patient group, lending a sense of optimism to clinicians caring for patients with this disease. Currently the debate has shifted from whether liver transplantation is an option for this patient subgroup to selecting the best approaches to prevent reinfection and treat disease before and after transplantation.

Indications for Liver Transplantation

As a result of the initial poor results, the proportion of patients with HBV infection undergoing liver transplantation in the United States declined in the early 1990s from approximately 6 percent in 1990 to 3.5 percent in 1993.[7] With subsequent improvements in patient management, there has been a gradual increase in this indication in most transplant centers. Liver disease secondary to HBV infection, whether acute or chronic, represents 6 percent to 10 percent of the liver transplants performed annually.[1] The indications and contraindications for transplantation in these patients do not differ from those applied to other forms of liver diseases (see Chap. 55) and typically include complications from portal hypertension, liver failure, or the development of hepatocellular carcinoma.

One particular aspect of this infection relates to the virologic status before transplantation. Until the introduction of nucleoside analogs, the presence of HBV replication (HBV deoxyribonucleic acid [DNA]-positive by hybridization methods) was considered by some centers as a contraindication to transplantation because of the high rate of recurrence in these patients compared to those who are HBV DNA-negative and hepatitis B e antigen (HBeAg)-negative before transplantation.[2,5] The availability of new and effective treatments, mainly nucleoside analogs that can reduce the level of viral replication before transplantation, is dramatically changing this approach.[6]

Virus-infected patients are at high risk for developing hepatocellular carcinoma, a circumstance that is not uncommon in the transplant setting. Although the rate of cancer recurrence was very high in early series, more promising results have been recently obtained with an accurate staging of tumors and improved patient selection.[8] Criteria for selecting these patients do not differ from those uninfected with a co-existent hepatocellular carcinoma and include unilobar tumors, less than three in number with no single lesion greater than 3 cm or one lesion less than 5 cm in diameter without macroscopic vascular involvement or extrahepatic spread. Postoperative follow-up should include chest radiographs, abdominal ultrasound, and alpha-fetoprotein levels every 3 to 6 months.

Natural History

HBV infection post-transplantation typically results from the recurrence of an infection present before liver transplantation. The serologic and virologic status before transplantation is the major predictor of post-transplantation reinfection, with lower rates in patients with fulminant hepatitis, hepatitis D virus (HDV) co-infection, and chronic HBV infection without detectable HBeAg or HBV DNA pretransplantation as compared to those with indices of active viral replication.[5] Populations at risk for HBV disease of the allograft are shown in Figure 56-1.

Occasionally HBV infection post-transplantation is a consequence of de novo infection, despite the use of strict screening measures in blood banks with exclusion of hepatitis B surface antigen (HBsAg)-positive donations.[9] The prevalence of de novo HBV ranges from 2 percent to 8 percent, and is generally observed when a liver from an HBsAg-negative anti-hepatitis B core (HBc) positive donor is used. The most significant factor associated with transmission is the serologic status of the recipient, so that the risk is almost zero in patients who are anti-HBs-positive, minor (approximately 10 percent) in those who are anti-HBs-negative but anti-HBc-positive, and high (approximately 50-70 percent) in those without markers of previous exposure to HBV.[9,10] Although there have been reports of severe progression,[11] the natural history of de novo HBV is generally more benign than that described for recurrent HBV.

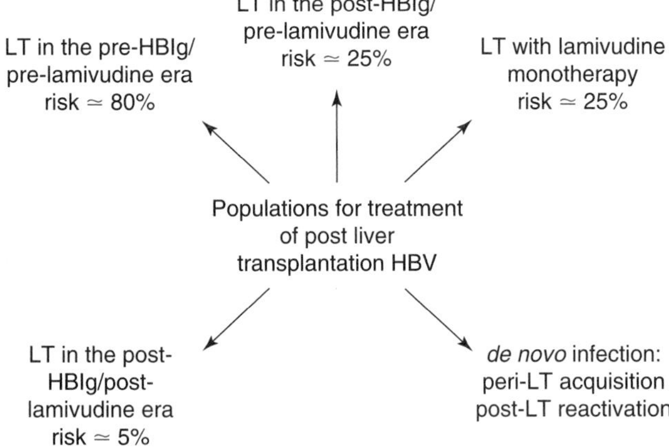

Figure 56-1 Populations for treatment of post-transplantation HBV disease. Recurrent HBV disease is uncommon, but five different groups with HBV disease of the allograft exist. Management of these populations depends on their prior treatment exposure and the presence of treatment-associated HBV variants. *HBV*, Hepatitis B virus.

The natural history of recurrent HBV is more aggressive than that observed in the immunocompetent population. Typically, patients develop acute hepatitis after becoming HBsAg positive in serum, with progression to chronic hepatitis and cirrhosis within 2 years of transplantation.[2] One particular entity initially described in these patients[12] and later among HCV-infected recipients[13] is called fibrosing cholestatic hepatitis. It develops in a small subset of patients and is characterized histologically by the presence of periportal and perisinusoidal fibrosis, ballooned hepatocytes with cell loss, pronounced cholestasis, and a paucity of inflammatory activity.[12] Immunohistochemical stains show high cytoplasmic expression of viral antigens, which in conjunction with the lack of inflammatory infiltrate suggests a direct cytopathic effect of the virus. The clinical course is rapidly progressive with severe cholestasis, hypoprothrombinemia, and liver failure within weeks of onset. High early mortality rate occurs after liver retransplantation; among those surviving the postoperative period, an even more aggressive course of recurrent disease develops.[2,12,14] Recently, the use of specific prophylactic interventions has led to prolonged survival.[15] Patients at risk for this syndrome include those with high levels of viremia pretransplantation[14] and those infected with precore mutants.[16]

The mechanisms by which HBV leads to liver injury after liver transplantation are incompletely understood. Increased levels of HBV replication are typically observed, likely related to the use of immunosuppressive drugs, particularly corticosteroids.[17] This enhanced replication with excess production of viral proteins in conjunction with the altered host immune responsiveness probably contributes to the pathogenesis of liver damage.[18]

Prevention of HBV Graft Reinfection

To prevent reinfection with HBV, lifelong passive immunization with high-dose HBIg is used in most transplant centers and is currently considered the "standard of care" (Figures 56-2 and 56-3).[5,19,20] HBIg consists of polyclonal antibodies directed against the viral envelope and was originally derived from donors positive for antibody to HBV surface antigen (anti-HBsAg). The presumed mechanism of action of this antibody is to neutralize circulating virus by binding to the viral envelope, preventing infection of the transplanted liver.

The administration of HBIg for more than 6 months has been shown to reduce dramatically the rate of HBV recurrence to a median rate of 20 percent after 2 years (Figure 56-3).[5,19,20] In a large European multi-center study recurrence rate was 75 percent in patients receiving no or short-term HBIg versus 33 percent in those receiving long-term HBIg ($p < .001$).[5] Long-term administration of HBIg reduced the rate of recurrence in patients with fulminant HBV to less than 10 percent, in HDV co-infected patients to 10 percent to 15 percent, and in HBV

DNA-negative cirrhotic patients to less than 30 percent. Yet it did not reduce the rate of recurrence in patients with HBV DNA-positive HBV cirrhosis.[5] The adverse prognostic characteristic of active viral replication pre-transplantation may be overcome with more aggressive use of HBIg by maintaining titers higher than 500 IU/L[20,21] or by the use of HBIg in combination with lamivudine post-transplantation.[22]

Various regimens have been described, with most including the administration of 10,000 IU HBIg intravenously during the anhepatic phase and 10,000 IU HBIg daily for the first week post-transplantation. The subsequent dosing is either given on a fixed schedule (generally on a monthly basis) or based on anti-HBs titers (re-administration when anti-HBs is less than 100 IU/L).[5,19-22]

Despite the clear efficacy of prophylactic HBIg, this therapy has limitations. The major disadvantages are high cost and limited availability. Treatment with HBIg in the United States adds $10,000 to $50,000 to the first year's charges for a liver transplantation and $5000 to $20,000

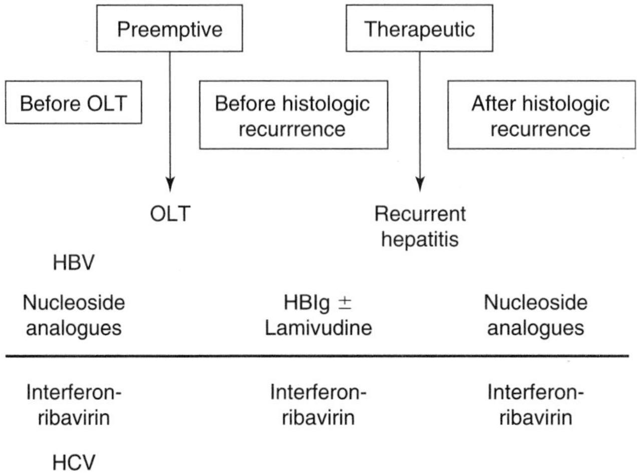

Figure 56-2 Approaches to the prevention and treatment of HBV and HCV infection in the setting of liver transplantation. *HBV,* Hepatitis B virus; *HCV,* hepatitis C virus.

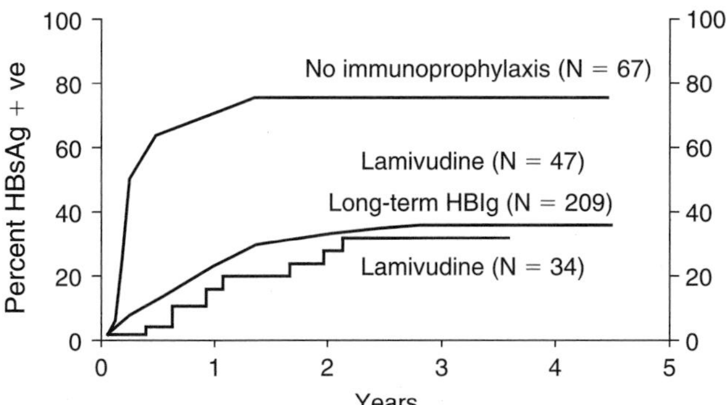

Figure 56-3 Risk of recurrent HBV disease according to pre- and peritransplantation intervention. *HBV,* Hepatitis B virus. (Reproduced with permission of R. Perrillo.)

to each subsequent year. Another important limitation is the lack of efficacy in approximately 20 percent of patients who will become HBsAg-positive despite high doses of HBIg. Graft loss is common in these patients, but treatment with nucleoside analogs has shown promising results with decreases in HBV replication and biochemical and histologic improvement.[23,24]

Causes of breakthrough are probably multi-factorial and include inadequate anti-HBs titers after transplantation, HBV overproduction coming from extrahepatic sites, or mutations in the region of the surface gene of the HBV genome that encodes the "a" determinant region—the putative region for antibody binding—resulting from immune pressure selection. These mutations occur in approximately half of the patients failing HBIg prophylaxis, with the most common mutation being a substitution of glycine for arginine at amino acid position 145.[25-28] Discontinuation of HBIg results in reversion of the mutations to the wild-type virus in the majority of patients (78 percent).

The last limitation of using HBIg is the difficulty of discontinuing this product in the long term. Recurrent infection has been documented in patients stopping prophylaxis with HBIg after 1 year.[19] Furthermore, HBV DNA has been detected by highly sensitive molecular techniques in the serum, liver, and peripheral blood mononuclear cells (PBMC) of HBsAg-negative patients on HBIg prophylaxis,[29] suggesting that indefinite treatment is required.

To overcome the limitations of HBIg, there are several alternatives currently being evaluated (Table 56-1). The first one is the use of anti-viral treatment before transplantation to inhibit viral replication.[30-35] Because of the risk of worsening hepatic decompensation and low tolerability of interferon (IFN) in patients with decompensated liver disease, IFN is not recommended in this situation.[30,31] The introduction of nucleoside analogs has substantially changed the management of patients with HBV infection undergoing liver transplantation. These drugs have a potent anti-viral effect inducing a rapid clearance of HBV DNA from serum. They are very well tolerated, are orally administered, and do not provoke deterioration of the liver function.[32] Recent experience with these drugs in cirrhotic patients awaiting liver transplantation is encouraging.[33] Most of the experience published is with lamivudine.[34-38] With this drug HBV replication is decreased to undetectable levels, allowing liver transplantation to be performed with a low risk of recurrence. The major drawback of this approach is the development of "resistance" to lamivudine with HBV DNA reappearance.[32,33] The risk of a patient awaiting liver transplantation developing lamivudine resistance is dependent on the duration of therapy with lamivudine (in one large series, this risk was 15 percent to 20 percent). Longer periods of therapy will be associated with an increasing risk of lamivudine resistance. Although most patients with resistant mutants continue to have low serum HBV DNA levels because of the decreased replication fitness of the mutants,[39] severe flares have been reported.[40] Against this risk is the potential benefit in improving hepatic synthetic function in those with decompensated liver disease. Although there are no controlled studies, there are reports of improvement in Child's Pugh status and even abrogation of need for liver transplantation. Thus lamivudine appears to be appropriate for patients with decompensated HBV cirrhosis awaiting liver transplantation. Lamivudine also is beneficial in patients with advanced HBV disease who, because of contraindications, are not candidates for liver transplantation.

However, there is some risk in treating the patient who is awaiting liver transplantation with lamivudine monotherapy because the development of active viral replication associated with resistance could alter successful outcomes after transplantation. Because of the overlapping nature of polymerase and surface genes of HBV, there is at least a theoretic risk that lamivudine-associated polymerase mutations could result in alteration of the surface gene such that HBIg would no longer be neutralizing. There are case reports of patients with pretransplantation lamivudine resistance receiving HBIg at the time of transplantation without evidence of post-transplantation recurrence. Moreover, as other HBV therapies are developed, particularly those with demonstrated activity against lamivudine-resistant variants, the risk associated with pretransplantation lamivudine therapy will be greatly outweighed by the potential benefit to the patient in terms of stabilization and even improvement in their decompensated liver disease. There is also consensus that if lamivudine is begun in the decompensated patient awaiting liver transplantation, it should be continued until the patient undergoes liver transplantation. In theory stopping lamivudine therapy in a decompensated patient could result in a "flare" of liver enzymes and worsening of hepatic function.

Famciclovir has also been used as preemptive therapy[41] but given the lower anti-viral effect of this agent when compared to lamivudine, its use as a single agent is unlikely to expand. As with lamivudine, there are concerns regarding the development of famciclovir-resistant mutants, which may in turn demonstrate cross-resistance to lamivudine.[42] There are limited data available on the use of adefovir in this setting. Adefovir may have an advantage over other drugs in the treatment of lamivudine resistance infection because this agent has demonstrated activity in vitro and in vivo against HBV strains with genetic resistance to lamivudine.[43,44]

After liver transplantation is performed, there are several alternatives to long-term HBIg (see Table 56-1), the first of which is to continue the preemptive therapy with lamivudine that was begun before transplantation.[34,35] Although this approach is initially effective and patient management is easy to perform given the good tolerance to this drug, it is limited by the emergence of HBV mutants with prolonged treatment (see the following section).[32,42] Furthermore, because nucleoside analogs have to be administered for long periods to avoid relapse after therapy is stopped, it is likely that monotherapy will be insufficient as prophylaxis of HBV reinfection.[32,42] In an initial report only 1 of 10 patients treated prophylactically with oral lamivudine developed HBV recurrence after 1 year of follow-up.[34] However, with prolonged follow-up, the authors described a higher rate of recurrence (50 percent) as a result of the emergence of escape mutations, mainly in patients with a high level of viral replication before transplantation.[43]

The second alternative is the use of combination therapy with HBIg and nucleoside analogues because treatment failures occur both with HBIg and lamivudine when given as monotherapy. In a preliminary report lamivudine in combination with high doses of HBIg has been shown to be safe and highly effective in preventing HBV recurrence.[22] In this study 13 patients were treated prophylactically with lamivudine (150 mg daily) and

TABLE 56-1

Prevention of Recurrent HBV: Alternatives to High Intravenous Doses of HBV Immunoglobulin

Type and timing of intervention	End point	Available drugs	Potential problems
Pre-transplantation anti-viral therapy	Decrease viral replication	Interferon Nucleoside analogs	Tolerance Development of resistant mutants
Preemptive post-transplantation anti-viral therapy	Prevent HBV recurrent infection	Nucleoside analogs	Development of resistant mutants
Preemptive post-transplantation antiviral therapy in combination with:	Prevent HBV recurrent infection	HBIg in combination with nucleoside analogs	
High doses of HBIg			Cost
Low doses of HBIg			Development of resistant mutants/ lack of efficacy
HBIg in combination with post-transplantation vaccination against HBV	Prevent HBV recurrent infection	Double dose vaccination after discontinuation of HBIg	Failure of vaccination regimen Lack of efficacy

HBV, Hepatitis B virus; *HBIg,* hepatitis B immunoglobulin.

high-dose HBIg starting with 10,000 IU during the anhepatic phase. No treatment failures were observed after 1 year of treatment, and 1-year patient survival reached 92 percent. Whether the frequency of viral resistance will increase with more prolonged follow-up is still unknown. Low doses of intramuscular HBIg and lamivudine have also been shown to be effective (Table 56-2).[46-50] Besides the potential to offer synergy or decrease resistance to HBIg, the economic advantages of this latter approach are apparent.

Several studies are underway to assess the efficacy of nucleoside analogs given either alone or in combination with HBIg as a means of preventing HBV recurrence.

A final alternative recently described is the use of HBIg in combination with post-transplantation vaccination against HBV. In a pilot study HBIg was discontinued in 17 selected liver transplant recipients who had been treated with high intravenous doses during the first month then with low intramuscular doses for a median of 24 months (range 18-67 months) and who had a low spontaneous risk of HBV recurrence.[51] After discontinuation of HBIg, a double dose of recombinant HBV vaccine was administered at 0, 1, and 6 months. Seroconversion to anti-HBs was obtained in 82 percent of cases (in six patients after the first three double doses, and in eight after a second course). These results need to be confirmed in larger series with prolonged follow-up but this approach may potentially become a useful and cost-effective strategy in the prophylaxis of HBV recurrence in selected liver transplant recipients. Evaluation of this approach in high-risk patients should also be investigated.

Treatment of HBV Disease of the Graft

Treatment of HBV-related liver disease in transplant patients is difficult for several reasons, including the high levels of HBV replication and the ongoing immunosuppressive treatment (see Figure 56-3). Interferon has been used in this setting with discouraging results despite a low risk of rejection.[52] New nucleoside analogs are promising because of their potent anti-viral effect and their lack of side effects, particularly regarding the risk of rejection.[32] Resistance, however, is an issue. If this resistance becomes an increasingly important problem, the interest in IFN with or without nucleoside analogs may increase.

Lamivudine is the most widely used nucleoside analog.[23,32,53] In most studies, liver transplant recipients with documented HBV recurrence (elevated serum alanine aminotransferase (ALT) levels, positivity of HBsAg, and detectability of HBV DNA) have been treated with lamivudine, 100 mg daily (adjusted for renal function), with good tolerance and rapid loss of HBV DNA in serum. Good biochemical and virologic responses have been achieved not only in patients with chronic HBV after transplantation,[23,32,53] but also in the setting of acute HBV infection of the graft[54] and in the most severe cases of fibrosing cholestatic hepatitis.[24] Histologic improvements in the inflammatory grade are also achieved with therapy. In a multi-center study based on 52 patients with detectable DNA after liver transplantation, lamivudine given for 1 year resulted in 60 percent loss of HBV DNA in serum and 31 percent HBeAg seroconversion.[53] The downside of this agent is the need for continuous treatment; relapse is the rule after the drug is discontinued.[32] Prolonged therapy is associated with the potential development of breakthrough resulting from the emergence of HBV escape mutants, which has been shown to reach 50 percent.[42]

Famciclovir (500 mg 3 times daily with dosing adjusted to renal function) has also been used to treat liver transplant recipients with HBV recurrence.[55,56] Although

TABLE 56-2

Prevention of Recurrent HBV: Combination with HBV Immunoglobulin and Lamivudine

	Pre-OLT treatment with lamivudine (%)	% DNA + pre-OLT	HBIg regimen	Follow-up (months)	Recurrence rate (%)
Markowitz 1998 (n = 14)	70	7	Standard high IV (10,000 IU day 0 to 7, then weekly during the first month, then monthly)	13	0
Yao 1999 (n = 10)	90	20	10,000 IU IV day 0 (7 days if DNA +), 1111 U IM weekly for 3 weeks, 1111 U IM every 3 weeks	15.6	10
Caughan 1999 (n = 9)	—	—	4000 IU IM (daily for first week, weekly for 3 weeks, then monthly)	15.6	0
Yoshida 1999 (n = 7)	60	0	2170 IU IM 14 days, then twice weekly with progressive reduction until once monthly at 1 year post-OLT	17	0
Angus 2000 (n = 32)	100	50	400-800 IU IM daily the first week and then monthly	18.5 (5-45)	3

OLT, Orthotopic liver transplantation; *DNA,* deoxyribonucleic acid; *HBIg,* hepatitis B immunoglobulin; *IV,* intravenous; *IM,* intramuscular.

initial good results are obtained with this drug in terms of both HBV DNA reduction and transaminase normalization, viral clearance is obtained in a lower percentage of patients than with lamivudine and in the long term, most of the patients treated with this drug relapse.[56]

Emergence of HBV Variants

Monotherapy with both drugs, lamivudine and famciclovir, has resulted in the emergence of HBV mutants that are resistant to these compounds.[32,40,42,57-59] This resistance generally occurs after prolonged therapy (more than 6 months). In both instances the appearance of resistant mutants is associated with a rise in serum HBV DNA and ALT levels, indicating a breakthrough in therapy. Molecular analysis has shown that mutations are located in the viral DNA polymerase gene.[40,57-59]

Resistance to lamivudine is associated with changes in both the B and C domains of the polymerase whereas those associated with famciclovir resistance occur mainly in the B domain. These mutations have been shown to confer reduced sensitivity to lamivudine in vitro and in the duck model.[32,42] When these drugs are stopped, the wild-type variant reemerges as the dominant viral population, but retreatment is again associated with the development of resistant mutants at an accelerated rate.[59] Lamivudine-induced mutations can also occur in the B domain of the polymerase, where changes have also been described with famciclovir.Thus famciclovir-resistant virus may not be sensitive to lamivudine, a situation recently described in several patients. The long-term rate of emergence of drug-resistant mutants and their implications in the natural history of HBV infection are still unknown.Although some cases of histologic and clinical deterioration have been reported when drug-resistant mutants develop, hepatic disease progression[42] frequently is not observed. It is possible that differences in the replicative competence or "fitness" of the mutants may account for these differences in outcome.[60] In vitro studies with adefovir have shown that although cross-resistance occurs between lamivudine and famciclovir, resistant variants to both these drugs remain sensitive to adefovir, suggesting that adefovir may be very important in the treatment of HBV with or without resistance to other oral agents.[43,44]

As has been shown in the management of patients with human immunodeficiency virus, synergistic combination regimens with one or more nucleoside/nucleotide analogs and immune stimulants such as IFN or therapeutic vaccines are likely to be the best strategy in maximizing anti-viral activity and in preventing the development of HBV-resistant variants.

Co-adjuvant Approaches

In non-transplant patients with chronic HBV infection, immunosuppression has been associated with reactivation of quiescent infection and, in some cases, with rapidly progressive disease.[17] Steroids have a deleterious effect, which may be related to the presence of a corticosteroid-responsive promoter region in the HBV genome.The activation of this promoter leads to increased viral replication. Rapid reduction in dose of corticosteroids in liver transplant recipients with HBV infection is common practice in many transplant programs, although the efficacy of this approach is unproven. Neither cyclosporine nor FK 506 given alone has an effect on HBV replication in vitro.[61] These in vitro studies, however, were performed with short-term drug exposure and thus may not correspond to the liver transplant situation in which long-term exposure is typical.

Prevention and Treatment of De Novo HBV Infection

To avoid de novo HBV infection, two complementary approaches may be undertaken. The first is HBV vaccination before liver transplantation of all anti-HBs-negative candidates. An accelerated vaccination regimen with double doses (40 μg) has been adopted at 0, 1, and 2 months with a follow-up vaccine at 6 months. Unfortunately, as with other immunosuppressed populations, the results of vaccination in these cirrhotic patients have been disappointing, with response rates that barely reach 40 percent.[62] A second course of vaccination may slightly increase these results.The second approach is determining the anti-HBc of the donor and the limitation of use of organs from anti-HBc-positive donors to recipients already infected with HBV. To obtain a maximum benefit from these organs while reducing the risk of HBV transmission, these organs may be used in special circumstances in recipients not infected with HBV.The following criteria should then be applied.[9,63] First, because the risk of HBV transmission is almost zero if the recipient is anti-HBs-positive,[9,10] select an anti-HBs-positive recipient. In this group there is no need for additional interventions. Livers from anti-HBc-positive donors can be used in recipients who are anti-HBc-positive and anti-HBs-negative. However, a low risk of HBV transmission appears to exist if no specific HBV prophylactic measures are taken.[9,10] Although initiating prophylaxis all patients will prevent transmission, it has the potential disadvantage of treating a high proportion of recipients who would never have developed an infection.When no individuals with the above criteria exist on the waiting list, anti-HBc-positive donors can be offered to naïve recipients with a critical clinical situation or with hepatocellular carcinoma although, in such cases, prophylaxis of HBV infection with lamivudine is necessary given the high likelihood of HBV transmission.

Treatment of De Novo HBV

Treatment of de novo HBV is similar to that described for recurrent HBV. If started at early points, the results are generally better than those obtained with recurrent HBV. Resistant mutants develop unfortunately at the same rate (see Chap. 32).

Retransplantation

The initial results on retransplantation for patients with graft failure resulting from recurrent HBV were discouraging because of the high rates of HBV reinfection and even more aggressive disease in the second graft.[15,64] Improved outcomes have been achieved with specific interventions, mainly with the use of aggressive immunoprophylaxis to prevent HBV reinfection in combination with lamivudine, which is typically started before retransplantation to inhibit viral replication.[15,64]

Transplantation in Patients Co-infected with HDV

HDV infection is becoming increasingly rare, even in Mediterranean areas where it was originally described. There are convincing data to support the more aggressive natural history of those with HBV/HDV infection versus those with HBV infection alone. Co-infection with HDV is present in a proportion of those with HBV infection undergoing evaluation for liver transplantation, particularly in Europe. In the original descriptions of outcomes after liver transplantation, HDV infection was associated with a lower risk of recurrence as compared to those with HBV alone, presumably reflecting the lower levels of viral replication in the former group.[5] When HDV and HBV infection of the graft occurred, HDV was not injurious to the graft until HBV was also actively replicating.[65] A variety of clinical and histologic outcomes have been described with HDV infection of the graft,[65-68] but currently, with the interventions described previously to prevent HBV recurrence, HDV infection is extremely unusual. HBV immunoglobulin effectively prevents recurrence in the majority of patients.[66] There are limited data on the use of lamivudine in patients with HBV/HDV co-infection, but in the absence of such data in the transplant setting, it appears appropriate to manage patients in the same way as those with HBV infection alone (i.e. with lamivudine before transplantation and then with HBIg in the peri- and postoperative periods in those who undergo liver transplantation).

Conclusions

Although there are limits to all current practices regarding the best approach to preventing HBV recurrence, the management of HBV in the liver transplant setting has improved substantially in recent years, and currently, the likelihood of serious disease resulting from HBV reinfection is unlikely. Treatment with nucleoside analogs before transplantation is limited by the possible development of drug-resistant mutants that, in turn, may impair the ability of HBIg to prevent HBV recurrence. However, the benefit of improving the synthetic function of the liver may outweigh the risks associated with development of resistance in these patients with decompensated liver disease. Prolonged HBIg therapy is limited by the cost and side effects. If lamivudine is to be used in combination with HBIg, the dose and duration of HBIg treatment remain uncertain. With current combination therapy, the risk of post-transplantation disease recurrence is very low so that treatment of HBV disease of the graft will be limited largely to those who have acquired or reactivated HBV infection in the peri- and post-transplantation periods.

RECURRENT HCV INFECTION

HCV-associated end-stage liver disease is a leading diagnosis in patients undergoing liver transplantation.[1] In most centers more than half of transplanted patients are infected with HCV before transplantation. It is likely that that this number will increase in future years, mainly as a consequence of the progressive nature of the disease and the threefold greater prevalence of HCV infection in those who are 30 to 50 years old as compared with younger or older age groups. Viral recurrence defined by the presence of HCV RNA in serum after transplantation occurs almost universally.[69] In spite of viral recurrence early post-transplantation infection generally results in indolent disease with good graft and patient survival. Disease progression is significantly faster, however, than that observed in immunocompetent patients, with a significantly higher rate of cirrhosis occurring within 5 years of infection compared to the non-transplant setting. With longer follow-up the consequences of HCV, recurrence ultimately results in reduced graft and patient survival compared with patients transplanted for non-viral causes. Factors that may influence the outcome include viral factors such as viral load at transplantation and the infecting genotype, host-related factors such as the type of immune response mounted toward the virus and the genetic background (race, HLA), and external factors such as the type and amount of immunosuppression. Other variables include the grade of activity and the stage of fibrosis evidenced early after transplantation and the age of the donor. Preliminary data suggest that the rate of disease progression has increased in recent years. The reasons that explain this worse outcome are under analysis and include the increasing age of the donor population and the use of more potent immunosuppressive drugs with "abrupt reconstitution" of the immune response. The need for an effective treatment derives from the potential seriousness of this disease. Unfortunately, to date, there is no suitable intervention to prevent HCV recurrence, and treatments available are limited to IFN and ribavirin, which are of limited efficacy in the transplant setting.

Indication for Liver Transplantation

Liver transplantation remains the most effective option in patients with decompensated HCV-related cirrhosis. In contrast, traditional medical management is indicated for compensated cirrhosis.[70] As with HBV infection a substantial proportion of HCV-infected candidates have a coincidental hepatocellular carcinoma.[1] The outcome of patients with hepatocellular carcinoma does not differ from that of patients without the tumor if strict selection criteria are followed (see section on hepatitis B virus).[8,71] In one recent multi-center European study the presence of hepatocellular carcinoma was the only variable associated with reduced patient and graft survival.[72] This may be explained by the fact that a substantial percentage of the patients included in this study were recruited from the early years of transplant activity in several centers (late 1980s), at which time strict selection criteria were not generally applied.

Natural History

Histologic evidence of liver injury develops in approximately half of the patients within the first year posttransplantation,[73] during which time severe graft dysfunction is infrequent (Figure 56-4).[74,75] With longer follow-up (5-7 years), the vast majority of patients develop some degree of histologic damage, with a subset, ranging from 8 percent to 30 percent, progressing to HCV-related graft-cirrhosis (Table 56-3).[72,74-78] Furthermore, in a proportion of patients, albeit less than 5 percent, an accelerated course of liver injury leading to rapid development of liver failure has been observed,[79] reminiscent of that previously described in HBV-infected recipients with fibrosing cholestatic hepatitis.[12] In most series published to date, short- and medium-term survivals are unaffected by the HCV status, with survival rates approaching 75 percent to 85 percent at 5 years in both HCV and non-HCV-infected patients.[72,74,75,78,80] It is likely that as we prolong follow-up, there will be differences in outcome. Indeed, based on the histologic evolution of chronic hepatitis in these patients, it has been estimated that the duration of time required to develop graft cirrhosis is approximately 10 to 12 years.[76] From these observations, one can anticipate an increase in HCV-related graft loss in the near future as transplant programs reach their second decade of activity, with a subsequent decrease in both graft and patient survival.[81]

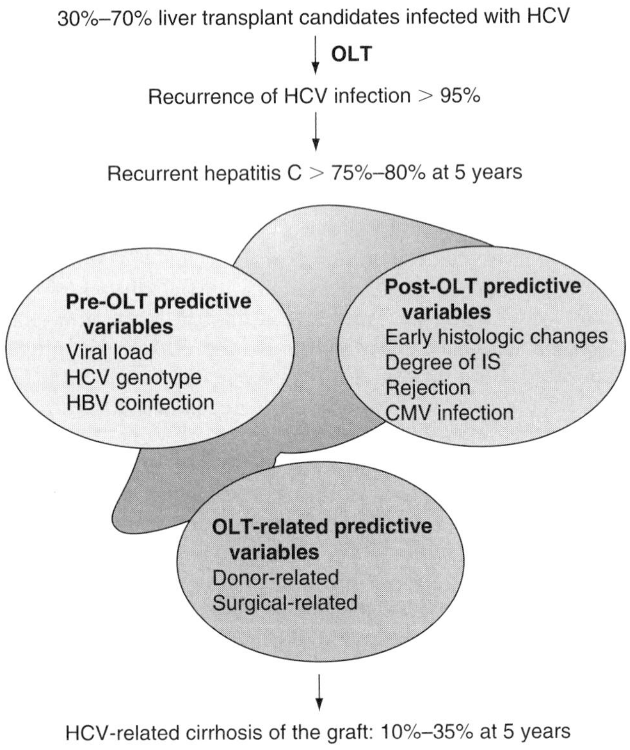

30%–70% liver transplant candidates infected with HCV

↓ OLT

Recurrence of HCV infection > 95%

↓

Recurrent hepatitis C > 75%–80% at 5 years

Pre-OLT predictive variables
Viral load
HCV genotype
HBV coinfection

Post-OLT predictive variables
Early histologic changes
Degree of IS
Rejection
CMV infection

OLT-related predictive variables
Donor-related
Surgical-related

↓

HCV-related cirrhosis of the graft: 10%–35% at 5 years

Figure 56-4 Risk of recurrent HCV infection and variables associated with post-transplantation liver disease progression. Orthotopic pre-transplantation (OLT), transplantation (OLT), and post-transplantation (post-OLT) variables are summarized in distinct circles. *IS*, Immunosuppression.

The natural history of post-transplantation hepatitis C is, however, highly variable, and although some patients develop cirrhosis in less than 1 year because of recurrent infection, others show minimal or no injury in their protocol liver biopsies during years of follow-up, even in the presence of high levels of viremia (see Figure 56-4).[75,82-85] Factors influencing this variability present before or after liver transplantation are poorly understood, and although there are enough data to support the role of some variables such as viral load pretransplantation, the data regarding other variables such as genotype are controversial.

Variables Associated with Disease Severity or Disease Progression

Pretransplant or early post-transplant recognition of patients with a high risk of severe recurrence post-transplantation (Table 56-4) is desirable because these patients can be either targeted for intervention or, in the

TABLE 56-3
Natural History of Recurrent HCV

Author	Incidence of cirrhosis (%)	Median time to cirrhosis	Predictive factors of severe disease or decreased survival
Gane et al, 1996	8	51 months	Genotype 1b
Charlton, 1998	9	NA	Pre-OLT viral load
			Race
			Recipient age
			Child's Pugh score at OLT
Prieto, 1999	15	24 months	Rejection episodes
	28	5-year actuarial rate	Number of MP boluses
			Early histologic changes
Feray, 1999	10	5-year actuarial rate	Absence of HBV co-infection
			Genotype 1b
			Recipient age
Testa, 2000	11	23 months	Early histologic recurrence
Berenguer, 2000	10-31	5-year actuarial rate	Year of transplantation
			Pre-OLT viral load
			Race
			Number of MP boluses

HCV, Hepatitis C virus; *OLT*, orthotopic liver transplantation; *MP*, methylprednisolone; *HBV*, hepatitis B virus.

absence of effective anti-viral therapy, denied transplantation. In contrast to HBV, in which the availability of new therapies has obviated the need for selection of patients based on predictive factors, the elucidation of these predictive factors remains of paramount importance in HCV-infected patients, given the absence of effective prophylactic or therapeutic agents.

Factors influencing the rate of progression relate to either the virus, the host, or environmental or iatrogenic influences on the infected individual (see Tables 56-3 and 56-4, Figure 56-4). The high-risk patient likely derives from the interaction between these factors, particularly between the virus and the immune system.

Host-related Variables

Recent data have strongly implicated the immune system in the pathogenesis of liver injury resulting from HCV.[86] This is further supported by the fact that the course of HCV infection is accelerated in liver transplant recipients when compared to that observed in immunocompetent patients,[76] emphasizing the key role played by the immune system, particularly the deleterious effect of the immunosuppression on progression of HCV-related liver disease.[74-76] Progression is not only faster before the development of cirrhosis but also afterwards, with a shorter natural history of clinically compensated HCV-related graft cirrhosis in transplant patients compared to that observed in the immunocompetent patients.[87] Not only is the immunosuppressed status per se deleterious for the evolution of the hepatitis C, the intensity of the immunosuppression has also been shown to be associated with disease severity, so that patients who are more severely immunosuppressed such as those receiving high doses of steroids or anti-lymphocyte globulin are at higher risk of progressing to cirrhosis than those less immunosuppressed.[75,76,78,88-90] Furthermore, a strong association has been found in one study between the year of transplantation and fibrosis progression, with patients transplanted recently progressing at a faster rate than those transplanted in earlier years.[76] This enhanced aggressivity in the natural history of recurrent HCV may in part be related to the recent introduction of more potent immunosuppressive agents, such as tacrolimus and mycophenolate.[76] Results of the potential association between the type of administered immunosuppression and disease severity are difficult to prove, however, because of the multiplicity of immunosuppressive regimen together with the changes in immunosuppressive drugs in individual patients over time. In that sense the majority of studies have found no differences in patient or graft survival in recipients treated with cyclosporine-based versus those treated with tacrolimus-based induction regimens.[74-78,91,92]

TABLE 53-4

Transplant Recipient at High Risk of Severe HCV-related Liver Disease after Liver Transplantation

Genotype 1b
Viral load pre-transplantation > 1 MEq/ml
Viral load at 4 months post-transplantation > 10 MEq/ml
Donor age > 50 years
Rewarming ischemic time > 60 minutes
Early histologic recurrence (<6 months)
Severe early histologic changes:
Hepatic activity index >3 at 4 months or >8 at 1 year
Fibrosis stage >2 at 1 year
Rejection episodes >2
Treatment with anti-lymphocyte globulin
Rejection treatment with >3 g methylprednisolone

It is likely that the interplay between the immune system and the virus may be modulated by the immunogenetic background, such as the human leukocyte antigen (HLA) system. In that sense specific HLA class II alleles, such as HLA-B14 and HLA-DRB1*04, have emerged as possible modulators of disease severity,[93] and disease severity has been linked to HLA-B sharing between the donor and the recipient in some[94] but not all studies.[74] Last, race has recently been found to influence outcome in patients with recurrent HCV infection, with non-whites doing worse than whites.[76,77] This association deserves further analysis in both immunosuppressed and immunocompetent patients.

Virus-related Variables

Post-transplantation HCV Ribonucleic Acid Levels. Circulating HCV ribonucleic acid (RNA) levels after liver transplantation are typically tenfold to twentyfold higher than levels before transplantation,[82-84] without a clear association between levels of viremia and disease severity. High levels of viremia, however, have been described in the setting of fibrosing cholestatic hepatitis[95] and during the acute phase of recurrent hepatitis C.[83,85] These observations suggest that albeit in most situations, liver damage is immune-mediated, in some instances such as in the setting of this particular syndrome, it may be due to a direct cytopathic effect of HCV.

Altogether, the data on the effects of immunosuppression on HCV RNA levels suggest that in the presence of strong immunosuppression, the inadequate immunologic clearance of HCV virions contributes to high levels of viremia. Because the immune system is "reconstituted," immune-mediated liver damage may occur with progression to severe forms of chronic hepatitis[85,96,97] in a similar way to that described in HCV-infected patients who develop reactivation of chronic HCV and even fulminant liver failure on withdrawal of chemotherapy.[98]

Pretransplantation HCV RNA Levels. Several studies have shown that, as described for HBV, the levels of viremia pretransplantation predict the occurrence and/or severity of recurrent hepatitis C.[76,77,84,96,99]

HCV Genotype. The effect of the infecting genotype on the severity of liver disease post-transplantation is unclear. Some,[72,74,85,100] but not all,[76-78,99,101] studies have implicated genotype 1b in a more severe post-transplantation disease compared to non-1b genotype. Furthermore, a fast HCV-related disease progression has been observed in centers with a high prevalence of genotype 1b,[75,76] thus indirectly implicating this genotype in a more aggressive course of the disease. It may be possible that different strains belonging to genotype 1b may be involved because the majority of positive studies are from Europe whereas those coming from U.S. centers have not found this association.

HCV Diversity. HCV heterogeneity may play a role in the pathogenesis of progressive HCV disease. Results from the few studies published to date are inconclusive and somewhat discrepant, however, and may be related to the small number of patients included, the different methodologies applied to assess HCV heterogeneity, the type of end-point chosen, the region of the genome evaluated, and the definition of disease severity.[102-104]

External Variables

Donor-related Variables. The age of the donor has been found to be independently associated with disease severity, disease progression, and survival.[76,81] The increasing age of the donors may explain the worse outcome seen in recent years.[76,81]

Co-infection with Other Viruses. Patients who develop cytomegalovirus (CMV) viremia may be at increased risk of severe HCV recurrence.[105] The reasons for this association are unknown but likely relate to induction of immune deficiencies, release of tumor necrosis factor by CMV, or the existence of cross-reactive immunologic responses.

Co-infection with other hepatotropic viruses such as HBV may influence histologic disease severity but results are conflicting.[72,106] Although no effect was found in an initial study,[106] co-infected patients appeared to have milder histologic course than patients infected only with HCV.[72] Although viral interactions could explain this phenomenon, the passive transmission of antibodies against HCV in co-infected patients receiving HBIg during the pre-HCV era is a more likely explanation. In contrast, co-infection with other viruses such as HGV[107] does not seem to influence the post-transplantation course of HCV disease.

Other Variables

Histologic Changes. The degree of necroinflammatory activity and fibrosis staging observed on the initial liver biopsy has been used as a variable predictive of subsequent development of severe chronic HCV in some studies.[75,76,85,99,108]

Prolonged rewarming time during allograft implantation has been associated with severe recurrent disease.[109] If these data are confirmed, special care should be taken to minimize rewarming time.

The early detection of anti-HCV core IgM has been correlated with both recurrence of HCV disease in the graft and its severity.[110,111] If these data are confirmed, this marker could be used to select patients early after transplantation for anti-viral therapy.

A lack of association has been found between the rate of fibrosis progression before transplantation and after transplantation, suggesting that variables present at the time of transplantation and those related to post-transplantation management are more important in influencing disease progression than genetic or viral variables unique to the individual.[76]

Year of transplantation was significantly predictive of time to cirrhosis and fibrosis progression in one study, with patients transplanted more recently progressing at a faster rate than patients transplanted in earlier cohorts (Figure 56-5).[76,86] Reasons that explain the worse outcome seen in HCV-infected patients in recent years are not fully understood. Possible factors include: (1) increasing age of the donors, (2) use of stronger induction and initial maintenance immunosuppression, and (3) an earlier and faster reconstitution of the immune system with withdrawal of "secondary immunosuppressive drugs" such as prednisone and azathioprine at earlier times. Because the immune system is "reconstituted," a presumably immune-mediated liver damage may occur with progression to severe forms of chronic hepatitis. The pivotal role of the host immune response in HCV-related disease severity[112] is further supported by the observation of a marked and aberrant intrahepatic expression of molecules involved in antigen recognition together with the evidence of intercellular and vascular adhesion molecules involved in regulating the recruitment and activation of cytotoxic T cells in patients with severe post-transplant HCV.[113]

Prevention of Infection or HCV-related Disease

In contrast to HBV in which HBIg has been shown to be beneficial, there is currently no available intervention to prevent HCV recurrence (see Figure 56-2). In one study, polyclonal immunoglobulins containing anti-HCV were shown to decrease the incidence of recurrent HCV viremia measured 1 year post-transplantation.[114] However, given the humoral immune failure in providing adequate and long-lasting neutralizing immunity against HCV, one would predict that additional approaches will be necessary.

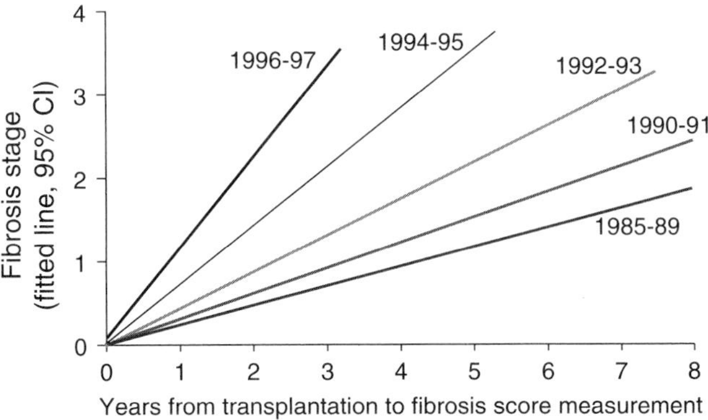

Figure 56-5 Fibrosis progression after liver transplantation. Effect of year of transplantation. (From Berenguer M, Ferrell L, Watson J, et al: HCV-related fibrosis progression following liver transplantation: increase in recent years. J Hepatol 32:673, 2000.)

An alternative to preventing recurrence of HCV infection is post-transplantation preemptive treatment to prevent HCV disease recurrence or diminish the risk of aggressive histologic progression. Interferon alone[115,116] or in combination with ribavirin[117] has been used in this setting with different results. Although treatment with IFN alone does not appear to modify disease progression,[115,116] its combination with ribavirin may produce some benefits.[117] In one study[115] 86 recipients were randomized within 2 weeks of transplantation to receive either IFN alone (n = 38) or placebo (n = 48) for 1 year. Although patient and graft survival at 2 years did not differ between groups and the rate of persistence of HCV was not affected by treatment, histologic disease recurrence was observed less frequently in IFN-treated patients (8 of 30 evaluable at 1 year) than in those who were not treated (22 of 41; $p = .01$). In a second controlled trial,[116] 24 recipients were randomized at 2 weeks posttransplantation to receive IFN or placebo for 6 months. Patient and graft survival and the incidence of histologic recurrence and its severity did not differ between groups. However, IFN treatment delayed the development of HCV hepatitis.

In a case series,[117] 21 recipients were treated with IFN-α2b and ribavirin starting the third week post-transplant. After a median follow-up of 12 months, 4 patients (19 percent) had developed acute recurrent HCV, but only 1 (5 percent) had evolved to chronic active hepatitis, despite presence of viremia in 59 percent of patients. No follow-up data were provided.

Treatment with either drug was well tolerated in these studies, with hemolytic anemia requiring drug reduction or withdrawal in only some cases. Moreover, although there had been concern about using IFN in solid organ transplant recipients for its risk of precipitating allograft rejection, IFN-induced rejection appears to be uncommon in the setting of liver transplantation. Well-designed controlled randomized studies are needed to confirm these encouraging findings.

Treatment of HCV-related Recurrent Disease

As with preemptive therapy, treatment of recurrent HCV disease with IFN or ribavirin as single agents has thus far been disappointing, but initial results from combination therapy with IFN and ribavirin are encouraging (see Figure 56-2).

The experience with IFN alone has been limited and its efficacy appears to be moderate and transient. IFN at doses of 3 million units (MU) 3 times weekly for 6 months has failed to clear serum HCV RNA, despite normalization of ALT values in a subset of patients treated (0 percent-28 percent).[118,119] Relapse after discontinuing treatment is almost the rule, and post-treatment improvement in liver damage is not common.

The experience with ribavirin has also been limited, and results are discouraging when given as a single agent. Its administration induces biochemical improvement in many patients but virologic clearance in none.[120] Furthermore, biochemical relapse is universal after cessation of therapy and no histologic improvement is observed. The main side effect is hemolysis, which usually resolves after the reduction or cessation of therapy. In one randomized trial,[120] 31 liver transplant recipients with chronic HCV in the graft were randomized to receive either IFN or ribavirin for 24 weeks. After 12 months of therapy, ribavirin was superior in achieving normalization of serum aspartate aminotransferase levels (85 percent versus 43 percent, $p < .05$) and in reducing lobular inflammation (64 percent versus 21 percent, $p = .05$), but not in reducing the fibrosis stage or the total histologic activity index. In contrast, patients receiving IFN alone had reduction in HCV RNA but not complete elimination of viremia.

To improve the results obtained with either agent alone, and based on the encouraging results obtained in the immunocompetent population, some authors have attempted combination therapy for patients with recurrent disease. Although initial results with this approach seemed promising,[121,122] more recent data have questioned its efficacy in the transplant setting.[123] In a non-randomized pilot study, 21 patients with early documented recurrent HCV were treated with IFN-α2b (3 MU 3 times per week) and ribavirin (1000 mg/day) for 6 months, and then maintained on ribavirin monotherapy until the end of the study. All patients had normalized ALT, and 50 percent cleared HCV RNA from serum at the end of the treatment period. The remaining patients, although viremic, experienced a 50 percent reduction in viral load. Only one patient had a biochemical relapse during the 6 months on ribavirin alone, despite reappearance of serum HCV RNA in 50 percent who had initially cleared HCV RNA. Most importantly, all but one patient who tolerated the drug showed an improvement in liver histology. Safety and tolerability were satisfactory, with reversible hemolytic anemia being the most common side effect. Off-treatment response rates were not provided in this initial report.

Recent data from a U.S. multi-center study are less enthusiastic for several reasons: (1) tolerability of the treatment with a significant percentage of patients requiring reduction or interruption of ribavirin because of significant side effects and (2) lower virologic response with only 25 percent of patients clearing HCV RNA at the end of the combination treatment phase. The reasons that explain these somewhat discrepant results are unknown but may include differences in timing of intervention, infecting genotype, or in the doses used in the separate studies.

Thus although this use of IFN and ribavirin may be beneficial, results from published studies are controversial and duration of follow-up after therapy is discontinued is still too short to draw valid conclusions.

Alternative Approaches

Because anti-viral therapy is limited in HCV-infected recipients, patient selection and management become important steps in improving the long-term outcome of HCV-infected patients undergoing liver transplantation. Unfortunately, no single variable or combination of variables is capable of predicting accurately which individual will develop serious disease post-transplantation and which individual will not. If anti-viral drugs aimed at reducing viral replication were better tolerated in decompensated cirrhotic patients, HCV RNA levels before transplantation could be used as a screening process. Interferon is, however, poorly tolerated in this setting and may precipitate worsening hepatic function. Modified regimens or combinations with ribavirin are being evaluated in these patients.

Given the deleterious effect of added immunosuppression on the progression of recurrent HCV disease, treatment of rejection episodes should be less aggressive in these patients with use of lower doses of corticosteroids and avoidance of anti-lymphocyte globulin. This is a trend already followed in many transplant centers, but efficacy of this approach has yet to be proven. Additionally, when doubts exist between rejection and hepatitis C as a result of atypical histologic findings (marked ductal injury and venulitis), serial biopsies should be performed to avoid the use of steroids unless absolutely necessary. Features more suggestive of HCV infection include lymphoid aggregates, fatty changes, and sinusoidal dilation[73] whereas those more suggestive of rejection include endotheliitis, bile duct necrosis, and a mixed portal inflammatory infiltrate (eosinophils, neutrophils, and mononuclear cells).

Retransplantation

Retransplantation is the last option for patients with failing grafts resulting from recurrent disease, but the results of retransplantation are inferior to those reported for the initial transplantation.[123] As predicted from natural history studies, the prevalence of HCV infection in patients undergoing retransplantation is progressively increasing in most transplant centers (from 6.5 percent in 1990 to 38.4 percent in 1995).[124] It has thus become imperative to determine whether all patients with graft failure because of recurrent HCV disease are candidates for further transplantation. Some data have suggested that survival after retransplantation is particularly poor in patients with recurrent HCV.[125-128] Other factors such as creatinine, bilirubin, and UNOS status appear, however, to have greater predictive value than HCV status in patients undergoing retransplantation,[127,128] and outcomes are improved if retransplantation is performed before the development of severe hyperbilirubinemia and renal complications.[127,128] Retransplantation is a reasonable option in low-risk patients, independently of HCV status. Whether retransplantation is justifiable in patients with high-risk scores needs to be carefully evaluated. Although not clear to date, the severity of recurrent HCV disease in the first graft does not seem to predict the outcome in the second graft. Larger studies are, however, needed to address this issue.

RECURRENT DISEASE OF PRESUMED AUTOIMMUNE ORIGIN

Although recurrence of viral hepatitis has been clearly demonstrated, recurrence of a number of liver diseases of presumed autoimmune origin such as primary biliary cirrhosis (PBC), primary sclerosing cholangitis (PSC), and autoimmune hepatitis is controversial.[129]

PBC and PSC are chronic cholestatic liver diseases with excellent outcomes after liver transplantation, with survival rates of approximately 80 percent at 5 years.[1] Whether these conditions recur after liver transplantation has been the subject of considerable debate. In both cases there have been reports suggesting recurrence of the original disease in the allograft. However, the diagnosis of recurrent disease has been complicated by the knowledge that there are a variety of potential conditions that may mimic these diseases (Table 56-5), so that their careful exclusion remains of paramount importance before making a diagnosis of recurrent disease. This is of particular relevance because in most instances of suspected recurrence, patients are clinically asymptomatic, liver tests results are non-specific, and markers of autoimmunity frequently recur or persist. Other circumstances such as low number of patients per study, differences in study design and length of follow-up, or differences in immunosuppressive regimen may further explain discrepant results. Finally, HLA disparity between donor and recipient and chronic immunosuppression may modify disease expression within the graft.

In both PBC and PSC, however, liver transplantation continues to be recommended for liver failure, rising hyperbilirubinemia, recurrent cholangitis, uncontrolled pruritus, or severe osteoporosis because both intermediate graft and patient survival are excellent and are not altered by recurrent disease. Long-term studies will be required to address the effect of recurrent disease on long-term graft survival.

TABLE 56-5
Conditions Mimicking Recurrence of the Original Disease

Primary biliary cirrhosis	Primary sclerosing cholangitis	Autoimmune hepatitis
Viral hepatitis	Ischemic strictures (hepatic artery thrombosis, preservation injury)	Viral hepatitis
Biliary obstruction	Strictures secondary to ascending cholangitis after choledochojejunostomy	Acute rejection
Chronic rejection	Chronic rejection	Biliary obstruction
Acute hepatitis	ABO incompatibility	Drug toxicity
Drug toxicity	Viral infections (cytomegalovirus)	
Graft versus host disease		

Primary Biliary Cirrhosis

PBC is a presumed autoimmune disease of the liver that predominantly affects middle-aged women (see Chap. 39). It is caused by granulomatous destruction of the interlobular bile ducts that leads to progressive ductopenia. The major hallmark of PBC is the presence of antimitochondrial antibodies (AMA) that are present in serum in most patients. Specifically, more than 90 percent of patients have antibodies against the E2 subunit of an inner mitochondrial enzyme. Histologically, four stages of the disease have been described, all of which may coincide in a single biopsy specimen. Stage 1 is characterized by a portal hepatitis with granulomatous destruction of bile ducts. Stage 2 is characterized by periportal hepatitis and bile duct proliferation. Stage 3 is identified by septal fibrosis, bile duct loss, and cholestasis. Cirrhosis represents stage 4. Although granulomas are often not seen, granulomatous destruction of bile ducts is considered pathognomonic. Other histologic features, such as portal and periportal inflammatory infiltrates, lymphocytic bile duct loss, and biliary epithelial cell loss, albeit more common, are not diagnostic of PBC.[130]

Several reports have documented recurrent PBC in the allograft (Table 56-6).[131-137] Frequently the diagnosis was suggested by an elevation of bilirubin and alkaline phosphatase, pruritus, reappearance or increase of AMA titers, or development of other conditions believed to be autoimmune in nature such as sicca syndrome or Raynaud's phenomenon. Histologic findings were consistent with recurrent disease, with biopsies revealing both non-specific and specific features of PBC. Other authors however, have been unable to confirm these findings[138-143] (Table 56-6) while emphasizing flaws of previous studies such as the lack of a control group, mismatching of biopsies between groups, inavailability of HCV molecular testing, presence of only non-specific histologic features with absence of florid duct lesions, or lack of exclusion of other conditions mimicking PBC.

Certain aspects add difficulties in making a correct diagnosis of recurrent PBC: (1) antibody titers and IgM fall in the majority of patients after liver transplantation, with no correlation between titers and histologic recurrence[141-143]; (2) histologic findings, considered the gold standard for the diagnosis of recurrent PBC, are often non-specific[144]; (3) a number of conditions that complicate the course of liver transplantation, particularly ductopenic rejection, may mimic recurrent PBC (see Table 56-5); and (4) immunosuppression may delay or even modify the expression of the disease within the graft.

The role of immunosuppression in the natural history of disease recurrence is still a subject of debate. Some authors have suggested that a cyclosporine-based regimen is preferable to tacrolimus.[145,146] Others have suggested that rapid corticosteroid withdrawal may be deleterious in these patients given their presumed genetic predisposition to the development of autoimmune conditions.[138] In that sense there have been recent reports of de novo autoimmune hepatitis developing in patients undergoing liver transplantation for PBC.[147] These cases emphasize the broad-based susceptibility to multiple autoimmune diseases present in some patients, even in the presence of immunosuppression, and raise important questions regarding the method of weaning these patients from immunosuppression.

In conclusion PBC is a common indication for liver transplantation with excellent results, at least for the medium term. Despite initial doubts regarding disease recurrence, it is now widely accepted that PBC may recur in the allograft. Recurrence, however, occurs in the minority, and diagnosis requires careful exclusion of other conditions such as acute or chronic rejection, biliary obstruction, graft versus host disease, or viral/drug hepatitis, all of which may mimic PBC. Liver biopsy remains the gold standard for diagnosis, although the pathognomonic lesion, non-suppurative destructive cholangitis, may not always be found. Therapeutic strategies for the prevention or treatment of recurrent PBC remain to be defined. There are several questions that remain to be answered. What is the actual recurrence rate of PBC with long-term follow-up? Will newer immunosuppressive drugs modify the incidence and natural history of recurrent PBC? Should we increase or change

TABLE 56-6

Recurrence of Primary Biliary Cirrhosis

Author, year	Number of patients/ number of controls	Follow-up (years)	Histologic recurrence rate (%)
Neuberger, 1982	3	3.5-4.5	NA
Demetris, 1988	106/288	>0.5	0
Esquivel, 1988	76	1-6.5	0
Polson, 1989	23/102	>1	90
Hubscher, 1993	83/105	1-8.3	16
Balan, 1993	60/156	>1	8
Gouw, 1994	19/14	1-11	0
Klein, 1994	23	>1	0
Dubel, 1995	16	>4	0
Van De Water, 1996	38/29	>0.3	21
Slapak, 1997	33	>5	24
Sebagh, 1998	69/53	>1	9

immunosuppression in all patients with histologic suspicion of recurrent PBC, regardless of clinical symptoms? Should PBC transplant patients receive ursodeoxycholic acid as preventive therapy? Additional studies will be necessary to answer these questions.

Primary Sclerosing Cholangitis

PSC is a chronic cholestatic liver disease of unknown cause with presumed autoimmune implication. It is characterized by diffuse fibrosing inflammation involving both the intrahepatic and extrahepatic biliary tree (see Chap. 40). The diagnosis is typically made by cholangiography, which shows stricturing, beading, and irregularities of the biliary tree. In the absence of other identifiable causes, liver biopsy may not be necessary. If a biopsy is performed, features compatible with PSC include inflammation and fibrosis of interlobular and septal bile ducts and bile fibrous obliteration with ductopenia or biliary cirrhosis. Liver transplantation remains the only effective therapeutic option for patients with advanced PSC complicated by recurrent cholangitis or intractable pruritus. The outcome after liver transplantation for this disease is excellent, with 5- and 10-year survival rates approaching 85 percent and 70 percent, respectively.[1]

As for PBC, there have been doubts regarding disease recurrence in patients undergoing liver transplantation for PSC.[129] Increasing evidence, however, supports that, albeit at a low incidence, PSC recurs after transplantation.[148-153] An early report demonstrated that PSC patients had a high incidence of histopathologic findings suggestive of recurrent PSC including biliary obstruction, periductal fibrosis, and fibro-obliterative lesions.[149] Subsequent reports either supported this concept[150-154] or refuted it.[155-156] Reasons for these discrepant results likely include differences in length of follow-up, methods of diagnosis (radiologic versus histologic), study design, and lack of a gold standard for the diagnosis. Exclusion of other disorders that produce similar lesions (see Table 56-5) is mandatory before making the diagnosis of recurrent PSC. Indeed, although most studies have demonstrated an increased incidence of biliary strictures after liver transplantation in PSC patients,[148,153,155,156] these can also develop as a consequence of preservation injury, ABO blood type incompatibility, chronic rejection, hepatic arterial thrombosis, or viral infections. Recurrent bacterial cholangitis resulting from reflux from the gastrointestinal tract has been implicated in the development of secondary sclerosing cholangitis in patients with a Roux-en-Y limb biliary reconstruction, a technique frequently performed in PSC patients. Secondary sclerosing cholangitis is cholangiographically and histologically impossible to differentiate from recurrent PSC. The significantly higher incidence of non-anastomotic strictures in patients with PSC compared to non-PSC patients with a Roux-en-Y limb supports the fact that the Roux-en-Y anastomosis is not a risk factor, per se, for the development of biliary strictures post-transplantation.[153]

Using strict inclusion and exclusion criteria, a recent study from the Mayo Clinic provided further evidence of PSC recurrence in recipients.[153] The definition of recurrent PSC was based on either cholangiographic or histologic findings. Patients with any other cause of biliary stricture were excluded, and a control group was used for comparison. Cholangiographic and histologic findings consistent with recurrence were present in 18 percent and 9 percent of patients transplanted for PSC, respectively. The time to cholangiographic and histologic recurrence ranged from 1 to 3.5 years. No specific risk factors were identified that predicted PSC recurrence.

Patients with PSC frequently have concomitant inflammatory bowel disease, mainly ulcerative colitis (see Chap. 40). There are conflicting data as to whether the presence of inflammatory bowel disease has an adverse impact on patient outcome after liver transplantation.[154,157] Overall the data available suggest that post-transplantation survival is similar in PSC patients with or without concomitant inflammatory bowel disease. There are, however, specific differences in patients with PSC and ulcerative colitis who undergo liver transplantation: (1) the incidence of acute and chronic rejection is higher in these patients than in PSC patients without concomitant inflammatory bowel disease[150,153,157] and (2) there is a fourfold increased risk of colon cancer compared to non-transplanted patients with ulcerative colitis.[153,158] Because immunosuppression may enhance the risk of colon cancer, yearly surveillance colonoscopies are recommended in PSC patients, regardless of the presence or absence of ulcerative colitis before transplantation.

In conclusion, in patients with suspected recurrence (elevated alkaline phosphatase levels after the first postoperative year), cholangiography or liver biopsy should be performed. Diagnosis of recurrent PSC requires exclusion of other conditions that may also cause strictures of the biliary tree. Therapeutic options for non-anastomotic strictures include radiologic or surgical therapies or retransplantation. Over the intermediate term, overall patient and graft survival are not affected by recurrence.[150-154] In some instances, however, severe recurrence may evolve into a need for retransplantation. Further follow-up will be necessary to assess the true effect of recurrent PSC on long-term outcome. As with PBC, there is no consensus over the ideal immunosuppressive regimen for these patients. Although some studies have suggested that tacrolimus-based immunosuppression is preferable to cyclosporine,[151] additional studies with a larger number of patients are required to draw definitive conclusions.

Autoimmune Hepatitis

Autoimmune hepatitis is a disease of unknown origin characterized by unexplained periportal hepatitis on histologic examination in association with autoantibodies in serum (see Chap. 38). As with PBC and PSC, altered immunoreactivity to intrinsic or extrinsic antigens appears to be play a role in the pathogenesis of this disease. The majority of patients respond to treatment with prednisone alone or in combination with azathioprine. Deterioration despite therapy occurs in 13 percent of patients. Patients who fail to respond and develop progressive liver disease may eventually require liver transplantation. The 5-year survival after liver transplantation compares favorably to other indications and has been reported to be approximately 95 percent.[1] Given the high survival rates after liver transplantation for these diseases, patients with autoimmune hepatitis are considered excellent candidates for transplantation.

Recurrence of autoimmune hepatitis may, however, become an issue with prolonged follow-up. The first report of autoimmune recurrence was described in a woman who developed histologic and serologic evidence of recurrent autoimmune hepatitis when immunosuppression with corticosteroids was discontinued.[159] Similar reports confirmed this initial report with an incidence ranging from 10 percent to 60 percent.[160-165] In addition to the small number of patients included in each study, differences in length of follow-up, immunosuppressive regimen, or diagnostic criteria used in the different studies may explain the wide range in the incidence rate.

The duration of follow-up appears to be particularly important, with few cases occurring within the first year post-transplantation followed by a progressive increase with longer follow-up.[163,165] In a longitudinal multi-center study from Spain, the risk of recurrence was 8 percent for the first year, 20 percent by the third year, and 68 percent after 5 years of follow-up.[163] The lower incidence rate within the first year compared to that described with prolonged follow-up is likely related to the stronger immunosuppression used during the initial post-transplantation period. Indeed, most studies have emphasized the hazards of discontinuing immunosuppression, particularly corticosteroids, in these patients.[166] The reintroduction of steroids is frequently accompanied by an improvement in liver tests.[162-164] Recurrence has not been linked to a specific immunosuppressive regimen, occurring both in patients using cyclosporine- or tacrolimus-based immunosuppression. Furthermore, triple therapy with cyclosporine, azathioprine, and prednisone does not appear to be always protective.[162,163] A common finding in all series is the steroid dependency, with a majority of patients requiring continuous steroids to keep their disease in remission.[162-165] A slow and careful tapering of immunosuppressive drugs, particularly prednisone, is recommended in these patients. The effect of newer immunosuppressive drugs such as mycophenolate mofetil or rapamycin on the incidence and severity of recurrent autoimmune hepatitis is still unknown.

Initial discrepant results on the existence of recurrent autoimmune hepatitis were also a consequence of a lack of standardized criteria for its diagnosis. A histologic diagnosis of autoimmune hepatitis regardless of other parameters may overdiagnose this entity. Indeed, in some series histologic changes compatible with recurrent autoimmune hepatitis are present in as many as 80 percent of patients, despite the normality of liver tests in a substantial proportion.[161] Furthermore, other disorders such as viral hepatitis or rejection may present with the same histologic features. Thus a more appropriate definition of recurrent autoimmune hepatitis should be based not only on histologic criteria but also on biochemical, serologic, and clinical criteria. Recurrent autoimmune hepatitis should be strongly suspected in recipients with sustained elevation of transaminases, consistent histopathology, and positive autoimmune markers (antinuclear antibody [ANA], antismooth muscle [SMA], anti-liver, kidney, microsomal antibody [anti-LKM]) with or without elevated IgG or gamma-globulin (see Chap. 38). A history of steroid dependency further supports this diagnosis. Other causes of hepatitis such as viral hepatitis, drug toxicity, or alcohol abuse should be excluded.[167] The utility of monitoring autoantibodies after transplantation is controversial. Most studies have described an initial fall or persistence of these markers and a lack of correlation between the titers of autoantibodies and the development or severity of autoimmune hepatitis.[160-162,165] Some, on the contrary, have suggested that a titer exceeding the pretransplantation level indicates recurrence.[165] Additional studies are needed to evaluate this point.

The natural history of recurrent autoimmune hepatitis is just beginning to be delineated. In most instances reintroduction or increase in the immunosuppression is followed by a renormalization of liver tests. This biochemical response is not always associated with histologic resolution or improvement, however, and hepatic inflammation may even worsen with follow-up.[162,165] Regardless of the type of response, patient and graft survival appear to be similar in patients with recurrence compared to those without evidence of recurrence.[163] Longer follow-up will be necessary to assess the consequences of recurrent disease on patient and graft survival. Although at a low rate of approximately 4 percent, severe graft dysfunction with need for retransplantation because of recurrent autoimmune hepatitis occurs.[167] This is particularly true for pediatric patients in whom recurrent severe disease after liver retransplantation has also been reported despite the use of strong immunosuppression.[168]

Although several factors predictive of both recurrence and its severity have been outlined, none consistently predicts this event. Patients who are inadequately immunosuppressed, HLA-DR3-positive recipients who receive HLA-DR3-negative grafts, patients who were diagnosed before transplantation as type I autoimmune hepatitis, and those undergoing liver transplantation for fulminant liver failure appear to be at a higher risk for recurrence.[167] Data regarding these variables are scarce, however, and need confirmation from larger series.

In conclusion, approximately one fourth of the patients undergoing liver transplantation for autoimmune hepatitis develop recurrent disease within the first 5 years after transplantation. It is likely that this incidence rate will increase with more prolonged follow-up. Although a small proportion of these patients develop a serious disease necessitating retransplantation, the majority respond, at least biochemically, to increases in immunosuppression. Graft and patient survival do not appear to be affected, at least in the medium term, by recurrence. Future studies with longer follow-up and use of newer immunosuppressive agents will likely address these issues and improve our understanding of this disease.

References

1. United Network for Organ Sharing: Retrieved January 31, 2000, from the World Wide Web: http://www.unet.org.
2. Todo S, Demetris A, Van Thiel D, et al: Orthotopic liver transplantation for patients with hepatitis B virus-related liver disease. Hepatology 13:619, 1991.

3. Berenguer M, Wright TL: Hepatitis C and liver transplantation. In Liang TJ, Hoofnagle JH, eds: Hepatitis C. Academic Press, 2000:277-294.
4. Detre K: Liver transplantation. Presented at AASLD Single Topic Conference on Viral Hepatitis and Liver Transplantation. Resven, Va, 1995.
5. Samuel D, Muller R, Alexander G, et al: Liver transplantation in European patients with the hepatitis B surface antigen. N Engl J Med 329:1842, 1993.
6. Berenguer M, Wright TL: Antiviral therapy pre and post-transplantation. In Maddrey W, Sorrell M, Schiff E, eds: Transplantation of the Liver. Philadelphia, Lippincott Williams & Wilkins, 2000:343-360.
7. Weisner R, Krom R: Liver transplantation for hepatitis B: the con aspect. Liver Transpl Surg 1:265, 1995.
8. Mazzaferro V, Regalia E, Doci R, et al: Liver transplantation for the treatment of small hepatocellular carcinomas in patients with cirrhosis. N Engl J Med 334:693, 1996.
9. Prieto M, Gómez MD, Berenguer M, et al: De novo hepatitis B after liver transplantation from hepatitis B core antibody-positive donors in an area with high prevalence of anti-HBc positivity in the donor population. Liver Transplant 7:51-58, 2001.
10. Dickson RC, Everhart JE, Lake JR, et al: Transmission of hepatitis B by transplantation of livers from donors positive for antibody to hepatitis B core antigen. The National Institute of Diabetes and Digestive and Kidney Diseases Liver Transplantation Database. Gastroenterology 113:1668, 1997.
11. Crespo J, Fabrega E, Casafont F, et al: Severe clinical course of de novo hepatitis B infection after liver transplantation. Liver Transpl Surg 5:175, 1999.
12. Davies S, Portmann B, O'Grady J, et al: Hepatic histological findings after transplantation for chronic hepatitis B virus infection, including a unique pattern of fibrosing cholestatic hepatitis. Hepatology 13:15, 1991.
13. Schluger L, Sheiner P, Thung S, et al: Severe recurrent cholestatic hepatitis C following orthotopic liver transplantation. Hepatology 23:971, 1996.
14. Benner K, Lee R, Keefe E, et al: Fibrosing cytolytic liver failure secondary to recurrent hepatitis B after liver transplantation. Gastroenterology 103:1307, 1992.
15. Ishitani M, McGory R, Dickson R, et al: Retransplantation of patients with severe posttransplant hepatitis B in the first allograft. Transplantation 64:410, 1997.
16. McMillan J, Bowden D, Angus P, et al: Mutations in the hepatitis B virus precore/core gene and core promoter in patients with severe recurrent disease following liver transplantation. Hepatology 24:1371, 1996.
17. Lok A, Liang R, Chiu E, et al: Reactivation of hepatitis B virus replication in patients receiving cytotoxic therapy. Gastroenterology 100:182, 1991.
18. Missale G, Brems J, Takiff H, et al: Human leukocyte antigen class I-independent pathways may contribute to hepatitis B virus-induced liver disease after liver transplantation. Hepatology 18:491, 1993.
19. Muller R, Samuel D, Fassati L, et al: "EUROHEP" consensus report on the management of liver transplantation for hepatitis B virus infection. J Hepatol 21:1140, 1994.
20. Terrault NA, Zhou S, Combs C, et al: Prophylaxis in liver transplant recipients using a fixed dosing schedule of hepatitis B immunoglobulin. Hepatology 24:1327, 1996.
21. McGory RW, Ishitani MB, Oliveira WM, et al: Improved outcome of orthotopic liver transplantation for chronic hepatitis B cirrhosis with aggressive passive immunization. Transplantation 61:1358, 1996.
22. Markowitz JS, Martin P, Conrad AJ, et al: Prophylaxis against hepatitis B recurrence following liver transplantation using combination lamivudine and hepatitis B immune globulin. Hepatology 28:585, 1998.
23. Nery JR, Weppler D, Rodriguez M, et al: Efficacy of lamivudine in controlling hepatitis B virus recurrence after liver transplantation. Transplantation 65:1615, 1998.
24. Al Faraidy K, Yoshida EM, Davis JE, et al: Alteration of the dismal natural history of fibrosing cholestatic hepatitis secondary to hepatitis B virus with the use of lamivudine. Transplantation 64:926, 1997.
25. Carman WF, Trautwein C, van Deursen FJ, et al: Hepatitis B virus envelope variation after transplantation with and without hepatitis B immune globulin prophylaxis. Hepatology 24:489, 1996.
26. Ghany MG, Ayola B, Villamil FG, et al: Hepatitis B virus S mutants in liver transplant recipients who were reinfected despite hepatitis B immune globulin prophylaxis. Hepatology 27:213, 1998.
27. Protzer-Knolle U, Naumann U, Bartenschlager R, et al: Hepatitis B virus with antigenically altered hepatitis B surface antigen is selected by high-dose hepatitis B immune globulin after liver transplantation. Hepatology 27:254, 1998.
28. Terrault NA, Zhou S, McCory RW, et al: Incidence and clinical consequences of surface and polymerase gene mutations in liver transplant recipients on hepatitis B immunoglobulin. Hepatology 28:555, 1998.
29. Feray C, Zignego A, Samuel D, et al: Persistent hepatitis B virus infection of mononuclear blood cells without concomitant liver infection. Transplantation 49:1155, 1990.
30. Marcellin P, Samuel D, Areias J, et al: Pretransplantation interferon treatment and recurrence of hepatitis B virus infection after liver transplantation for hepatitis B-related end-stage liver disease. Hepatology 19:6, 1994.
31. Perrillo R, Tamburro C, Regenstein F, et al: Low dose, titratable interferon alfa in decompensated liver disease caused by chronic infection with hepatitis B virus. Gastroenterology 109:908, 1995.
32. Berenguer M, Wright TL: Hepatitis B and C viruses: molecular identification and targeted antiviral therapies. Proc Assoc Am Physicians 110:98, 1998.
33. Fontana RJ, Lok ASF. Lamivudine treatment in patients with decompensated cirrhosis: for whom and when? J Hepatol 33:329, 2000.
34. Grellier L, Mutimer D, Ahmed M, et al: Lamivudine prophylaxis against reinfection in liver transplantation for hepatitis B cirrhosis. Lancet 348:1212, 1996.
35. Perrillo R, Rakela J, Martin P, et al: Lamivudine for suppression and/or prevention of hepatitis B when given pre/post transplantation (Abstract). Hepatology 26:260A, 1997.
36. Villeneuve J, Condreay LD, Willems B, et al: Lamivudine treatment for decompensated cirrhosis resulting from chronic hepatitis B. Hepatology 31:207, 2000.
37. Yao FY, Bass NM: Lamivudine treatment in patients with severely decompensated cirrhosis due to replicating hepatitis B infection. J Hepatol 33:301, 2000.
38. Kapoor D, Gutpan RC, Wakil S, et al: Beneficial effects of lamivudine in hepatitis B virus related decompensated cirrhosis. J Hepatol 33:308, 2000.
39. Melegari M, Scaglioni PP, Wands JR: Hepatitis B virus mutants associated with 3TC and famciclovir administration are replication defective. Hepatology 27:628, 1998.
40. Bartholomew MM, Jansen RW, Jeffers LJ, et al: Hepatitis-B-virus resistance to lamivudine given for recurrent infection after orthotopic liver transplantation. Lancet 349:20, 1997.
41. Singh N, Gayowski T, Wannstedt CF, et al: Pretransplant famciclovir as prophylaxis for hepatitis B virus recurrence after liver transplantation. Transplantation 63:1415, 1997.
42. Locarnini S: Hepatitis B virus surface antigen and polymerase gene variants: potential virological and clinical significance. Hepatology 27:294, 1998.
43. Xiong X, Flores C, Yang H, et al: Mutations in hepatitis B DNA polymerase associated with resistance to lamivudine do not confer resistance to adefovir in vitro. Hepatology 28:1669, 1998.
44. Perrillo R, Schiff E, Yoshida E, et al: Adefovir dipivoxil for the treatment of lamivudine-resistant hepatitis B mutants. Hepatology 32:129, 2000.
45. Mutimer D, Pillady D, Dragon E, et al: High pretreatment serum hepatitis B titre predicts failure of lamivudine prophylaxis and graft reinfection after liver transplantation. J Hepatol 30:715, 1999.
46. Naoumov NV, Lopes R, Crepaldi G, et al: Randomized trial of lamivudine (LAM) versus hepatitis B immunoglobulin (HBIG) for prophylaxis of HBV recurrence after liver transplantation (abstract). J Hepatol 30(suppl 1):51, 1999.
47. Yao FY, Osorio RW, Roberts JP, et al: Intramuscular hepatitis B immune globulin combined with lamivudine for prophylaxis against hepatitis B recurrence after liver transplantation. Liver Transpl Surg 5:491, 1999.

48. Yoshida EM, Erb SR, Partovi N, et al: Liver transplantation for chronic hepatitis B infection with the use of combination lamivudine and low-dose hepatitis B immune globulin. Liver Transpl Surg 5:520, 1999.
49. McCaughan GW, Spencer J, Koorey D, et al: Lamivudine therapy in patients undergoing liver transplantation for hepatitis B virus precore mutant-associated infection: high resistance rates in treatment of recurrence but universal prevention if used as prophylaxis with very low dose hepatitis B immune globulin. Liver Transpl Surg 5:512, 1999.
50. Angus P, McCaughan GW, Gane EJ, et al: Combination low dose hepatitis B immune globulin and lamivudine therapy provides effective prophylaxis against posttransplantation hepatitis B. Liver Transpl 6:429, 2000.
51. Sanchez-Fueyo A, Rimola A, Grande L, et al: Hepatitis B immunoglobulin discontinuation followed by hepatitis B virus vaccination: a new strategy in the prophylaxis of hepatitis B virus recurrence after liver transplantation. Hepatology 31:496, 2000.
52. Terrault NA, Holland CC, Ferrell L, et al: Interferon alfa for recurrent hepatitis B infection after liver transplantation. Liver Transpl Surg 2:132, 1996.
53. Perrillo R, Rakela J, Dienstag J, et al: Multicenter study of lamivudine therapy for hepatitis B after liver transplantation. Hepatology 29:1581, 1999.
54. Andreone P, Caraceni P, Grazi GL, et al: Lamivudine treatment for acute hepatitis B after liver transplantation. J Hepatol 29:985, 1998.
55. Kruger M, Tillmann HL, Trautwein C, et al: Famciclovir treatment of hepatitis B virus recurrence after liver transplantation: a pilot study. Liver Transpl Surg 2:253, 1996.
56. Berenguer M, Prieto M, Rayón M, et al: Famciclovir treatment in transplant recipients with HBV-related liver disease: disappointing results. Am J Gastroenterol 96:526-533, 2001.
57. Tipples GA, Ma MM, Fischer KP, et al: Mutation in HBV RNA-dependent DNA polymerase confers resistance to lamivudine in vivo. Hepatology 24:714, 1996.
58. Allen M, Deslauriers M, Andrews C, et al: Identification and characterization of mutations in hepatitis B virus resistant to lamivudine. Hepatology 27:1670, 1998.
59. Chayama K, Suzuki Y, Kobayashi M, et al: Emergence and takeover of YMDD motif mutant hepatitis B virus during long-term lamivudine therapy and re-takeover by wild type after cessation of therapy. Hepatology 27:1711, 1998.
60. Melegari M, Scaglioni PP, Wands JR: Hepatitis B virus mutants associated with 3TC and famciclovir administration are replication defective. Hepatology 27:628, 1998.
61. McMillan JS, Shaw T, Angus PW, Locarnini SA: Effect of immunosuppressive and antiviral agents on hepatitis B virus replication in vitro. Hepatology 22:36, 1995.
62. Chalasani N, Smallwood G, Halcomb J, et al: Is vaccination against hepatitis B infection indicated in patients waiting for or after orthotopic liver transplantation? Liver Transpl Surg 4:128, 1998.
63. Dodson SF, Bonham CA, Geller DA, et al: Prevention of the novo hepatitis B infection in recipients of hepatic allografts from anti-HBc positive donors. Transplantation 68:1058, 1999.
64. Crippin J, Foster B, Carlen S, et al: Retransplantation for hepatitis B—a multicenter experience. Transplantation 57:823, 1994.
65. Ottobrelli A, Marzano A, Smedile A, et al: Patterns of hepatitis delta virus reinfection and disease in liver transplantation. Gastroenterology 101:1649, 1991.
66. Samuel D, Zignego A, Reynes M, et al: Long-term clinical and virological outcome after liver transplantation for cirrhosis caused by chronic delta hepatitis. Hepatology 21:333, 1995.
67. David E, Rahier J, Pucci A, et al: Recurrence of hepatitis D (delta) in liver transplants: histopathological aspects. Gastroenterology 104:1122, 1993.
68. Rosina F, Conoscitore P, Cuppone R, et al: Changing pattern of chronic hepatitis D in Southern Europe. Gastroenterology 117:161, 1999.
69. Wright TL, Donegan E, Hsu H, et al: Recurrent and acquired hepatitis C viral infection in liver transplant recipients. Gastroenterology 103:317, 1992.
70. Fattovitch G, Giustina G, Degos F, et al: Morbidity and mortality in compensated cirrhosis type C: a retrospective follow-up study of 384 patients. Gastroenterology 112:463, 1997.
71. Figueras J, Jaurrieta E, Valls C, et al: Survival after liver transplantation in cirrhotic patients with and without hepatocellular carcinoma: a comparative study. Hepatology 25:1485, 1997.
72. Feray C, Caccamo L, Alexander GJM, et al: European Collaborative Study on factors influencing the outcome after liver transplantation for hepatitis C. Gastroenterology 117:619, 1999.
73. Ferrell L, Wright T, Roberts J, et al: Hepatitis C viral infection in liver transplant recipients. Hepatology 16:865, 1992.
74. Gane E, Portmann B, Naoumov N, et al: Long-term outcome of hepatitis C infection after liver transplantation. N Engl J Med 334:815, 1996.
75. Prieto M, Berenguer M, Rayón M, et al: High incidence of allograft cirrhosis in hepatitis C virus genotype 1b infection following transplantation: Relationship with rejection episodes. Hepatology 29:250, 1999.
76. Berenguer M, Ferrell L, Watson J, et al: HCV-related fibrosis progression following liver transplantation: increase in recent years. J Hepatol 32:673, 2000.
77. Charlton M, Seaberg E, Wiesner R, et al: Predictors of patient and graft survival following liver transplantation for hepatitis C. Hepatology 28:823, 1998.
78. Testa G, Crippin JS, Netto GJ, et al: Liver transplantation for hepatitis C: recurrence and disease progression in 300 patients. Liver Transpl 6:553, 2000.
79. Schluger L, Sheiner P, Thung S, et al: Severe recurrent cholestatic hepatitis C following orthotopic liver transplantation. Hepatology 23:971, 1996.
80. Boker KHW, Dalley G, Bahr MJ, et al: Long-term outcome of hepatitis C virus infection after liver transplantation. Hepatology 25:203, 1997.
81. Berenguer M, Ferrell L, Watson J, et al: HCV-related fibrosis progression following liver transplantation: increase in recent years. J Hepatol 32:673-684, 2000.
82. Chazouilleres O, Kim M, Combs C, et al: Quantitation of hepatitis C virus RNA in liver transplant recipients. Gastroenterology 106:994, 1994.
83. Gretch D, Bacchi C, Corey L, et al: Persistent hepatitis C virus infection after liver transplantation: clinical and virological features. Hepatology 22:1, 1995.
84. Gane E, Naoumov N, Qian K, et al: A longitudinal analysis of hepatitis C virus replication following liver transplantation. Gastroenterology 110:167, 1996.
85. DiMartino V, Saurini F, Samuel D, et al: Long-term longitudinal study of intrahepatic hepatitis C virus replication after liver transplantation. Hepatology 26:1343, 1997.
86. He XS, Rehermann B, López-Labrador FX, et al: Quantitative analysis of hepatitis C virus-specific CD8(+) T cells in peripheral blood and liver using peptide-MHC tetramers. Proc Natl Acad Sci U S A 96:5692, 1999.
87. Berenguer M, Prieto M, Rayon JM, et al: Natural history of clinically compensated HCV-related graft cirrhosis following liver transplantation. Hepatology 32:852, 2000.
88. Sheiner PA, Schwartz ME, Mor E, et al: Severe or multiple rejection episodes are associated with early recurrence of hepatitis C after orthotopic liver transplantation. Hepatology 21:30-34, 1995.
89. Berenguer M, Prieto M, Córdoba J, et al: Early development of chronic active hepatitis in recurrent hepatitis C virus infection after liver transplantation: association with treatment of rejection. J Hepatol 28:756, 1998.
90. Rosen HR, Shackleton CR, Higa L, et al: Use of OKT3 is associated with early and severe recurrence of hepatitis C after liver transplantation. Am J Gastroenterol 92:1453, 1997.
91. Casavilla FA, Rakela J, Kapur S, et al: Clinical outcome of patients infected with hepatitis C virus infection on survival after primary liver transplantation under tacrolimus. Liver Transpl Surg 4:448, 1998.
92. Zervos XA, Weppler D, Fragulidis GP, et al: Comparison of tacrolimus with microemulsion cyclosporine as primary immunosuppression in hepatitis C patients after liver transplantation. Transplantation 65:1044, 1998.
93. Belli S, Zavaglia C, Alberti AB, et al: Influence of immunogenetic background on the outcome of recurrent hepatitis C after liver transplantation. Hepatology 31:1345, 2000.
94. Manez R, Mateo R, Tabasco J, et al: The influence of HLA donor-recipient compatibility on the recurrence of HBV and HCV hepatitis after liver transplantation. Transplantation 59:640, 1994.

95. Doughty AL, Spencer JD, Cossart YE, McCaughan GW: Cholestatic hepatitis after liver transplantation is associated with persistently high serum hepatitis C virus RNA levels. Liver Transpl Surg 4:15, 1998.
96. Pelletier SJ, Raymond DP, Crabtree TD, et al: Hepatitis C-induced hepatic allograft injury is associated with a pre-transplantation elevated viral replication rate. Hepatology 32:418, 2000.
97. Berenguer M, Lopez-Labrador FX, Greenberg HB, Wright TL: Hepatitis C virus and the host: an imbalance induced by immunosuppression. Hepatology 32:433-435, 2000.
98. Vento S, Cainelli F, Mirandola F, Cosco L, et al: Fulminant hepatitis on withdrawal of chemotherapy in carriers of hepatitis C virus. Lancet 347:92, 1996.
99. Sreekumar R, Gonzalez-Koch A, Maor-Kendler Y, et al: Early identification of recipients with progressive histologic recurrence of hepatitis C after liver transplantation. Hepatology 32:1125, 2000.
100. Feray C, Gigou M, Samuel D, et al: Influence of genotypes of hepatitis C virus on the severity of recurrent liver disease after liver transplantation. Gastroenterology 108:1088, 1995.
101. Zhou S, Terrault N, Ferrell L, et al: Severity of liver disease in liver transplantation recipients with hepatitis C virus infection: relationship to genotype and level of viremia. Hepatology 24:1041, 1996.
102. Sullivan DG, Wilson JJ, Carithers RL Jr, et al: Multigene tracking of hepatitis C virus quasispecies after liver transplantation: correlation of genetic diversification in the envelope region with asymptomatic or mild disease patterns. J Virol 72:10036, 1998.
103. Pessoa MG, Bzowej NH, Berenguer M, et al: Evolution of hepatitis C (HCV) quasispecies in patients with severe cholestatic hepatitis following liver transplantation. Hepatology 30:1513, 1999.
104. Pelletier SJ, Raymond DP, Crabtree TD, et al: Pretransplantation hepatitis C virus quasispecies may be predictive of outcome after liver transplantation. Hepatology 32:375, 2000.
105. Rosen H, Chou S, Corless C, et al: Cytomegalovirus viremia. Risk factor for allograft cirrhosis after liver transplantation for hepatitis C. Transplantation 64:721, 1997.
106. Huang E, Wright TL, Lake J, et al: Hepatitis B and C coinfections and persistent hepatitis B infections: clinical outcome and liver pathology after transplantation. Hepatology 23:396, 1996.
107. Berenguer M, Terrault NA, Piatak M, et al: Hepatitis G virus infection in patients with hepatitis C virus infection undergoing liver transplantation. Gastroenterology 111:1569, 1996.
108. Rosen HR, Gretch DR, Oehlke M, et al: Timing and severity of initial hepatitis C recurrence as predictors of long-term liver allograft injury. Transplantation 65:1178, 1998.
109. Baron PW, Sindram D, Higdon D, et al: Prolonged rewarming time during allograft implantation predisposes to recurrent hepatitis C infection after liver transplantation. Liver Transpl 6:407, 2000.
110. Crespo J, Carte B, Lozano JL, et al: Hepatitis C virus recurrence after liver transplantation: relationship to anti-HCV core IgM, genotype and level of viremia. Am J Gastroenterol 92:1458, 1997.
111. Bizollon T, Ahmed SN Si, Guichard S, et al: Anti-hepatitis C virus core IgM antibodies correlate with hepatitis C recurrence and its severity in liver transplant patients. Gut 47:698, 2000.
112. Rosen HR, Hinrichs DJ, Gretch DR, et al: Association of multispecific CD4(+) response to hepatitis C and severity of recurrence after liver transplantation. Gastroenterology 117:926, 1999.
113. Asanza CG, Garcia-Monzon C, Clemente G, et al: Immunohistochemical evidence of immunopathogenetic mechanisms in chronic hepatitis C recurrence after liver transplantation. Hepatology 26:755, 1997.
114. Feray C, Gigou M, Samuel D, et al: Incidence of hepatitis C in patients receiving different preparations of hepatitis B immunoglobulins after liver transplantation. Ann Intern Med 128:810, 1998.
115. Sheiner P, Boros P, Klion FM, et al: The efficacy of prophylactic interferon alfa-2b in preventing recurrent hepatitis C after liver transplantation. Hepatology 28:831, 1998.
116. Singh N, Gayowski T, Wannstedt C, et al: Interferonα for prophylaxis of recurrent viral hepatitis C in liver transplant recipients. Transplantation 65:82, 1998.
117. Mazzaferro V, Regalia E, Pulvirenti A, et al: Prophylaxis against HCV recurrence after liver transplantation. Effect of interferon and ribavirin combination. Transpl Proc 29:519, 1997.
118. Wright TL, Combs C, Kim M, et al: Interferon alpha therapy for hepatitis C virus infection following liver transplantation. Hepatology 20:773, 1994.
119. Feray C, Samuel D, Gigou M, et al: An open trial of interferon alfa recombinant for hepatitis C after liver transplantation: antiviral effects and risk of rejection. Hepatology 22:1084, 1995.
120. Gane EJ, Lo SK, Riordan SM, et al: A randomized study comparing ribavirin and interferon alfa monotherapy for hepatitis C recurrence after liver transplantation. Hepatology 27:1403, 1998.
121. Bizollon T, Palazzo U, Ducerf C, et al: Pilot study of the combination of interferon alfa and ribavirin as therapy of recurrent hepatitis C after liver transplantation. Hepatology 26:500, 1997.
122. Shakil AO, McGuire B, Crippin J, et al: Interferon alfa2b and ribavirin combination therapy in liver transplant recipients with recurrent hepatitis C (abstract). Hepatology 23:216A, 2000.
123. Busuttil RW, Shaked A, Millis JM, et al: One thousand liver transplants. The lessons learned. Ann Surg 219:490, 1994.
124. Rosen HR, Martin P: Hepatitis C infection in patients undergoing liver retransplantation. Transplantation 66:1612, 1998.
125. Sheiner PA, Schluger LK, Emre S, et al: Retransplantation for recurrent hepatitis C. Liver Transpl Surg 3:130, 1997.
126. Rosen H, O'Reilly P, Shackleton C, et al: Graft loss following liver transplantation in patients with chronic hepatitis C. Transplantation 62:1773, 1997.
127. Facciuto M, Heidt D, Guarrera J, et al: Retransplantation for late liver graft failure: predictors of mortality. Liver Transpl 6:174, 2000.
128. Rosen HR, Madden JP, Martin P: A model to predict survival following liver retransplantation. Hepatology 29:365, 1999.
129. Rosen H: Disease recurrence following liver transplantation. Clin Liver Dis 4:675, 2000.
130. Heathcote J: Management of primary biliary cirrhosis. Hepatology 31:1005, 2000.
131. Neuberger J, Portmann B, Macdougall B, et al: Recurrence of primary biliary cirrhosis after liver transplantation. N Engl J Med 306:1, 1982.
132. Polson RJ, Portmann B, Neuberger J, et al: Evidence for disease recurrence after liver transplantation for primary biliary cirrhosis: clinical and histological follow up studies. Gastroenterology 97:715, 1989.
133. Hubscher SG, Elias E, Buckels JAC, et al: Primary biliary cirrhosis: histological evidence of disease recurrence after liver transplantation. J Hepatol 18:173, 1993.
134. Balan V, Batts K, Porayko MK, et al: Histological evidence for recurrence of primary biliary cirrhosis after liver transplantation. Hepatology 18:1392, 1993.
135. Sebagh M, Farges O, Dubel L, et al: Histological features predictive of recurrence of primary biliary cirrhosis after liver transplantation. Transplantation 65:1328, 1998.
136. Van De Water J, Gerson LB, Ferrell LD, et al: Immunohistochemical evidence of disease recurrence after liver transplantation for primary biliary cirrhosis. Hepatology 24:1079, 1996.
137. Slapak GI, Saxena R, Portmann B, et al: Graft and systemic disease in long term survivors of liver transplantation. Hepatology 25: 195, 1997.
138. Demetris AJ, Markus BH, Esquivel C, et al: Pathologic analysis of liver transplantation for primary biliary cirrhosis. Hepatology 8: 939, 1988.
139. Esquivel CO, Van Thiel DH, Demetris AJ, et al: Transplantation for primary biliary cirrhosis. Gastroenterology 94:1207, 1988.
140. Gouw ASH, Haagsma EB, Manns M, et al: Is there recurrence of primary biliary cirrhosis after liver transplantation? A clinicopathologic study in long-term survivors. J Hepatol 20:500, 1994.
141. Klein R, Huizenga JR, Gips CH, Berg PA: Antimitochondrial antibody profiles in patients with primary biliary cirrhosis before orthotopic liver transplantation and titres of antimitochondrial antibody-subtypes after transplantation. J Hepatol 20:181, 1994.
142. Dubel L, Farges O, Bismuth H, et al: Kinetics of anti-M2 antibodies after liver transplantation for primary biliary cirrhosis. J Hepatol 23:674, 1995.
143. Luettig B, Boeker KHW, Schoessler W, et al: The antinuclear antibodies Sp100 and gp210 persist after orthotopic liver transplantation in patients with primary biliary cirrhosis. J Hepatol 28:824, 1998.
144. Ferrell LD, Lee R, Brixko C, et al: Hepatic granulomas following liver transplantation. Transplantation 60:926, 1995.
145. Wong PYN, Portmann B, O'Grady JG, et al: Recurrence of primary biliary cirrhosis after liver transplantation following FK506-based immunosuppression. J Hepatol 17:284, 1993.

146. Dmitrewski J, Hubscher SG, Mayer AD, et al: Recurrence of primary biliary cirrhosis in the liver allograft: the effect of immunosuppression. J Hepatol 24:253, 1996.
147. Jones DE, James OF, Portmann B, et al: Development of autoimmune hepatitis following liver transplantation for primary biliary cirrhosis. Hepatology 30:53, 1999.
148. Sheng R, Zjako AB, Campbell WL, Abu-Elmagd K: Biliary strictures in hepatic transplants: prevalence and types in patients with primary sclerosing cholangitis vs those with other liver diseases. AJR 161:297, 1993.
149. Harrison RF, Davies MH, Neuberger JM, Hubscher SG: Fibrous and obliterative cholangitis in liver allografts: evidence of recurrent primary sclerosing cholangitis? Hepatology 20:356, 1994.
150. Narumi S, Roberts JP, Edmond JC, et al: Liver transplantation for sclerosing cholangitis. Hepatology 22:451, 1995.
151. Yeyarajah DR, Netto GJ, Lee SP, et al: Recurrent primary sclerosing cholangitis after orthotopic liver transplantation: is chronic rejection part of the disease process. Transplantation 66:1300, 1998.
152. Goss JA, Shackleton CR, Farmer DG, et al: Orthotopic liver transplantation for primary sclerosing cholangitis: a 12-year single center experience. Ann Surg 5:472, 1997.
153. Graziadei IW, Wiesner RH, Batts KP, et al: Recurrence of primary sclerosing cholangitis following liver transplantation. Hepatology 29:1050, 1999.
154. Graziadei IW, Wiesner RH, Batts KP, et al: Long-term results of patients undergoing liver transplantation for primary sclerosing cholangitis. Hepatology 30:1121, 1999.
155. Campbell WL, Sheng R, Zajko AB, et al: Intrahepatic biliary strictures after liver transplantation. Radiology 191:735, 1994.
156. Letourneau JG, Day DL, Hunter DW, et al: Biliary complications after liver transplantation in patients with preexisting sclerosing cholangitis. Radiology 167:349, 1988.
157. Miki C, Harrison JD, Gunson BK, et al: Inflammatory bowel disease in primary sclerosing cholangitis: an analysis of patients undergoing liver transplantation. Br J Surg 82:1114, 1995.
158. Bretnall TA, Haggitt RC, Rabinovitch PS, et al: Risk and natural history of colonic neoplasia in patients with primary sclerosing cholangitis and ulcerative colitis. Gastroenterology 110:331, 1996.
159. Neuberger J, Portmann B, Calne R, Williams R: Recurrence of autoimmune chronic active hepatitis following orthotopic liver grafting. Transplantation 37:363, 1984.
160. Wright HL, Bou-Abboud CF, Hassanein T, et al: Disease recurrence and rejection following liver transplantation for autoimmune chronic active liver disease. Transplantation 53:136, 1992.
161. Gotz G, Neuhaus R, Bechstein WO, et al: Recurrence of autoimmune hepatitis after liver transplantation. Transplant Proc 31:430, 1999.
162. Ratziu V, Samuel D, Sebagh M, et al: Long-term follow-up after liver transplantation for autoimmune hepatitis: evidence of recurrence of primary disease. J Hepatol 30:131, 1999.
163. Prados E, Cuervas-Mons V, de la Mata M: Outcome of autoimmune hepatitis after liver transplantation. Transplantation 66:1645, 1998.
164. Milkiewicz P, Hubscher SG, Skiba G, et al: Recurrence of autoimmune hepatitis after liver transplantation. Transplantation 68:253, 1999.
165. Reich DJ, Fiel I, Guarrera JV, et al: Liver transplantation for autoimmune hepatitis. Hepatology 32:693, 2000.
166. Czaja AJ: The immunoreactive propensity of autoimmune hepatitis: is it corticosteroid-dependent after liver transplantation? Liver Transpl Surg 5:460, 1999.
167. Manns MP, Bahr MJ: Recurrent autoimmune hepatitis after liver transplantation: when non-self becomes self? Hepatology 32:868, 2000.
168. Birnbaum AH, Benkov KJ, Pittman NS, et al: Recurrence of autoimmune hepatitis in children after liver transplantation. J Pediatr Gastroenterol Nutr 25:20, 1997.

C H A P T E R

57

Liver Disease and Parenteral Nutrition

Toyomi Fukushima, MD, MPH, and Thomas R. Ziegler, MD

An important landmark in modern medicine occurred in 1968. Wilmore and Dudrick, at the Children's Hospital of Philadelphia, published the first report that year of somatic growth in an infant with extreme short-bowel syndrome treated with long-term total parenteral nutrition (TPN).[1] This was followed in 1969 by a case series of 14 infants treated with TPN at the Children's Hospital in Boston by Filler and colleagues.[2] Home parenteral feeding became a reality with the work of these investigators and that of Shils and colleagues in 1970.[3] Parenteral nutrition (PN) is now a widely available method of nutrition-support in adult and pediatric patients with various ailments.[4-6] The term *TPN* is commonly used for all situations in which PN is administered; however, it is a misnomer in the relatively common situation in which patients consume some enteral diet or receive tube feeds in addition to PN (e.g., short-bowel syndrome). We refer to TPN in this chapter as the specific situation in which minimal or no oral or enteral food is administered. PN is the general use of parenteral feeding.

The most recently available data estimated that approximately 40,000 patients in the United States received PN in 1992.[7-8] With a greater emphasis on shorter hospitalization, use of home PN in the United States doubled between 1989 and 1992, with an average duration of treatment of 60 days. The most prevalent diagnosis for home PN was cancer in more than 40 percent of patients, followed by Crohn's disease and swallowing disorders.[7-8]

Mortality related directly to long-term PN is low.[9] However, morbidity related to PN is common and includes complications related to insertion technique (pneumothorax and hemothorax), use of catheters (infections and occlusions), and metabolic abnormalities (metabolic bone disease, renal and hepatobiliary dysfunction, electrolyte abnormalities, hyperglycemia).[5-6,10] Improved techniques for inserting catheters and better design of catheters have significantly reduced complications related to insertion and indwelling catheters. But PN-associated metabolic complications remain frequent despite improved nutrient formulae and administration.[10]

TPN-associated hepatobiliary complications were first reported in 1971 by Penden and colleagues, who described cholestasis and early cirrhosis on postmortem examination of a premature infant after long-term TPN use.[11] TPN- and PN-associated hepatobiliary abnormalities are now well recognized in both adults and children.[4-5] These range from transient biochemical abnormalities to progressive liver disease leading to cirrhosis and liver failure (Table 57-1).

Two distinct patterns of hepatic complications occur in association with PN, primarily according to the patient's age. Hepatic steatosis predominates in adults.[12-13]

TABLE 57-1
PN-associated Hepatobiliary Complications

Biochemical abnormalities	Hepatic complications	Biliary complications
Hyperbilirubinemia	Steatosis	Acalculous cholecystitis
Cholestasis	Steatohepatitis	Biliary sludge
Transaminitis	Non-specific triaditis	Cholelithiasis
	Intrahepatic cholestasis	Calculous cholecystitis
	Portal and bridging fibrosis	
	Cirrhosis	
	Hepatic failure	
	Hepatoma	

PN, Parenteral nutrition.

Although rare, hepatic steatosis may progress to steatohepatitis and cirrhosis. Occurrence of intrahepatic cholestasis is relatively infrequent among adults, but chronic cholestasis may progress to hepatic fibrosis. Cholestasis, on the other hand, predominates in children and may progress over time to hepatic fibrosis, biliary cirrhosis, portal hypertension, and liver failure, particularly in premature infants treated with TPN.[14-15] Biliary complications of PN include biliary sludge, cholelithiasis, and acalculous and calculous cholecystitis, and are observed equally in both adults and children receiving TPN.[16]

This chapter outlines current understanding of the clinical, biochemical, and histologic features of PN-associated hepatobiliary complications in adults and children. The proposed pathogenesis of these lesions is summarized, as is management. This chapter also reviews currently available data on long-term survival with PN and the risk of end-stage liver disease induced by parenteral feeding.

HEPATIC ABNORMALITIES

Clinical Features Related to TPN-associated Liver Disease

Apart from the presence of preexisting liver disease, the following five clinical features are identified consistently as major risk factors for development of TPN- or PN-associated liver disease: (1) prematurity and low birth weight; (2) longer duration of PN; (3) lack of enteral intake; (4) presence of systemic inflammation or sepsis; and (5) short-bowel syndrome.[10,16,20]

Age (Prematurity and Low Birth Weight)

Age is the most important clinical feature determining the pattern of hepatic injuries. Patients of very young age are at particular risk for developing cholestasis and progressive biliary cirrhosis. Beale and colleagues reviewed liver function data from 62 premature infants receiving TPN.[17] Cholestasis was found in as many as 50 percent of the infants weighing less than 1000 grams and in 18 percent of those weighing 1000 grams to 1500 grams at birth. The lesion occurred in only 7 percent of infants weighing 1500 grams or more.[17] It is suggested that the decreased enterohepatic circulation of premature infants, and their deficiency in hepatic glutathione production, leads to increased production of lithocholic acid, which in turn causes the hepatic injury.[14] Available data suggest that significant liver dysfunction develops in 40 percent to 60 percent of infants requiring long-term TPN for intestinal failure.[18-19]

Duration of PN Administration

Longer duration of PN is strongly associated with increased incidence of liver disease in both adults and children. In a comprehensive recent report from France, Cavicchi and colleagues prospectively followed 90 adults and children with a median age of 45 years (range, 6 to 77 years) who received home PN for permanent intestinal failure.[20] Chronic cholestasis was defined as persistent elevation (more than 1.5 times the upper limit of normal for more than 6 months) in two of three liver tests: gamma glutamyl transpeptidase (GGTP),[51-53] alkaline phosphatase (ALP), and bilirubin. Chronic cholestasis occurred in 58 patients (65 percent) after a median period of PN of 6 months (range, 3 to 132 months). The prevalence of cholestasis increased with time from 55 percent at 2 years (confidence interval [CI], 45 percent to 65 percent), to 64 percent at 4 years (CI, 53 percent to 75 percent), to 72 percent at 6 years (CI, 60 percent to 84 percent). The probability of developing clinical or biologic liver disease also showed an increasing trend with longer duration of PN: 26 percent at 2 years (CI, 17 percent to 35 percent); 39 percent at 4 years (CI, 28 percent to 50 percent); 50 percent at 6 years (CI, 37 percent to 63 percent); and 53 percent at 8 years (CI, 37 percent to 63 percent). A correlation between the development of cholestasis and duration of TPN also was shown by Beale and colleagues.[17] The overall incidence of cholestasis was 23 percent among the 62 premature infants receiving TPN. Infants receiving TPN for more than 60 days had an incidence of 80 percent, which rose to 90 percent in infants treated for more than 3 months.

Lack of Enteral Intake

TPN-associated liver disease is more likely to develop in adults and children who are unable to tolerate any oral or enteral feeding compared with those who feed via the gastrointestinal tract.[21-24] Zamir and colleagues demonstrated that adding some enteral feeding to a TPN regimen significantly reduced the degree of hepatic steatosis when compared with TPN infusion alone.[24] It is noteworthy in this context that prolonged fasting is believed to promote liver injury by uncertain mechanisms and that levels of gut hormones are significantly lower in patients on TPN compared with fed controls.[25-27] Theoretically, as the unfed gut atrophies, intestinal stasis increases. Bacterial overgrowth and translocation of microbes or toxins from the lumen may occur.[28] Bacterial overgrowth may lead to increased local release of endotoxin and increased production of toxic bile acids, both of which can cause cholestasis.[29-33] In humans the metabolic response to endotoxin and cytokines, including tumor necrosis factor alpha (TNFα), is amplified with TPN and bowel rest, further exacerbating liver injuries.[34-35] Prolonged fasting also promotes PN-associated gallbladder disease.[36-38] In one series 33 percent of patients receiving TPN and minimal oral diet developed gallbladder disease within 5 years.[39]

Presence of Systemic Inflammation Manifested as Hypoalbuminemia

In patients receiving adequate protein intake via PN, hypoalbuminemia is often the result of a systemic inflammatory response mediated by the cytokines interleukins 1 and 6 and TNFα.[40] Prospective clinical studies show an increased incidence of PN-associated liver disease in patients with hypoalbuminemia.[41-43] Although the overall rate of PN-associated cholestasis was 50 percent to 60 percent, all patients with albumin levels less than 2 mg/dl had cholestasis. Patients with systemic inflammation or sepsis therefore may be at higher risk of developing PN-associated liver disease.

Short-bowel Syndrome

In the French cohort of 90 patients on long-term TPN reported by Cavicchi and colleagues,[20] a small-bowel remnant less than 50 cm in length was one of two factors strongly associated with the occurrence of liver disease related to home PN (relative risk [RR], 2.1; CI, 1.2-3.7). It is believed that short-bowel syndrome increases the risk for chronic cholestasis[44-46] by interrupting the enterohepatic circulation, which results in abnormal bile acid metabolism.[47-49] In addition, individuals with short-bowel syndrome commonly have bacterial overgrowth and a *theoretical* risk of gut-derived sepsis resulting from bacterial translocation.

Hepatic Biochemical Abnormalities Associated with TPN

Hepatic biochemical abnormalities associated with PN have been observed since the earliest days of PN use.[50] Both reversible and irreversible hepatic injuries are heralded by abnormalities in biochemical liver profiles. Various studies suggest that elevated concentrations of GGTP,[51-53] aspartate aminotransferase (AST),[54-55] alanine aminotransferase (ALT),[56] and ALP[49,57] in blood are sensitive indicators of PN-associated liver abnormalities. Hyperbilirubinemia is commonly noted in children and adults receiving TPN.[16]

Two distinct patterns of PN-associated hepatic biochemical abnormalities exist, primarily according to age.[13,50] Elevated levels of AST and ALT are seen primarily in adults. Elevated levels of bilirubin and ALP (reflecting cholestasis) are seen predominantly in children, particularly premature infants. In adults serum aminotransferase levels usually rise 1 to 2 weeks after initiation of PN, and often resolve without stopping or changing the PN formula.[50] Elevated serum ALP and bilirubin levels occur less frequently in adults, usually after 2 to 3 weeks of PN.[50] In children serum levels of bilirubin may rise as early as 2 weeks after initiation of PN; ALP and aminotransferase levels may rise within 4 to 6 weeks.[14,16]

Various modifications in PN formulae over the past three decades appear to have reduced the frequency of PN-associated liver abnormalities (particularly the avoidance of overfeeding and emphasis on the oral route of feeding). However, the age-specific patterns and the time course of PN-associated hepatic biochemical abnormalities have remained much the same.[13-16,20]

Hepatic Biochemical Abnormalities and High-calorie Dextrose-based TPN

In the era of high-calorie TPN (before 1980) PN consisted primarily of dextrose and amino acid solutions without lipid emulsions (dextrose-based PN). High-volume infusion of dextrose-based PN was typically used to provide 3 to 4 L of solution daily and much higher caloric loads than presently used. Therefore studies before 1980 may not be directly applicable today but provide information regarding effects of overfeeding with PN.[50]

Host and associates first reported hepatic biochemical abnormalities in adult patients receiving dextrose-based TPN in 1972.[58] In that report 6 of 19 patients (32 percent) with normal baselines developed liver enzyme abnormalities after 5 to 10 days of TPN. Serum AST rose threefold in all six patients; ALP rose twofold in four of six; ALT rose twentyfold in two of six. However, these abnormalities were transient and normalized with continued TPN. In 1977 Grant and associates published a review of 100 patients receiving 3 to 4.5 L per day of dextrose-based TPN.[54] The study found elevated serum AST in 93 percent and elevated ALT in 89 percent. AST rose 3 to 5 times' normal and ALT 5 to 10 times normal after 8 to 10 days of TPN. Both AST and ALT normalized while patients continued on TPN during the subsequent 4 to 10 days. The study also described a second peak after 1 month of TPN therapy. Serum bilirubin levels rose twofold in 26 percent of patients after 8 days of TPN; ALP levels rose twofold in 56 percent after 32 days of TPN. A 1982 study by Wagman and associates of 144 cancer patients receiving PN showed similar time lags in the development of biochemical abnormalities.[59] AST and ALT were noted to rise in about 1 week, ALP in about 2 weeks, and bilirubin in about 6 weeks of TPN. Another study by Lindor and associates, in 1979, reported similarly high rates of hepatic biochemical abnormalities associated with TPN.[55] Of 48 patients receiving TPN, elevated AST levels were noted in 68 percent and elevated ALT levels in 54 percent. Peak values occurred after 9 to 12 days of TPN.

In 1979 Lowry and Brennan reported that 83 percent of cancer patients receiving dextrose-based PN had elevated AST, ALT, or ALP after approximately 2 weeks of therapy.[60] A strong correlation between infusion of excess carbohydrate calories as determined by the Harris-Benedict equation[61] and development of hepatic biochemical abnormalities was observed. Among those who developed liver test abnormalities, 97 percent received more than 1.39 times their predicted basal energy expenditure (BEE).[60] Although not confirmed by other investigators[54,59,62] this and other studies suggested a correlation between excess calorie intake and development of hepatic biochemical abnormalities.[63]

Hepatic Biochemical Abnormalities and Lipid-supplemented TPN

In contrast to dextrose-based TPN, PN solutions in the late 1970s routinely replaced a portion of non-protein calories with lipid emulsion, thereby decreasing the amount of dextrose. In 1981 Carpentier and Van Brandt reviewed 36 patients receiving lipid-supplemented TPN in whom the calorie intake was limited to 125 percent of BEE and 50 percent of non-protein calories were supplied by lipids.[64] Increases in ALT and ALP were observed in only 11 percent and 14 percent of the patients, respectively. Because these abnormalities were significantly lower than with dextrose-based TPN,[54-55,58-59] it was suggested that lipid replacement would reduce the risk of hepatic dysfunction. A study published by Tulikoura and Huikuri in 1982 supported this idea.[65] Thirty-seven patients were treated with three types of isocaloric PN solutions: a dextrose group received a dextrose and amino acid mixture with relatively high dextrose content; an amino acid group received a mixture of dextrose and amino acid with higher amino acid content; and a lipid group received a standard lipid emulsion in addition to a carbohydrate and amino acid mixture. No significant hepatic biochemical abnormalities occurred with PN when 56 percent of non-protein calories were lipids.[65] Similarly, a retrospective study suggested that the incidence of hepatic biochemical abnormalities was halved in 25 patients receiving 70 percent of non-protein calories as lipid as compared with 15 patients who received all non-protein calorie as dextrose.[66] In 1984 Meguid and associates published a prospective, randomized study confirming the efficacy of lipid supplementation in PN as a method to reduce hepatic biochemical abnormalities.[67] In this study 88 patients receiving TPN were divided into two groups. In one group, one third of carbohydrate calories were replaced with lipid emulsion. The other study group received isocaloric dextrose solutions (control group). AST levels did not rise in the lipid-supplemented group but increased more than 2.5-fold in the control subjects. ALT values rose 2.5-fold in the lipid-supplemented group over time, but increased more than fivefold in the controls.[67]

Another prospective clinical trial conducted by Buchmiller and associates addressed the significance of the carbohydrate fat ratio in PN.[68] Forty-three patients received either a standard dextrose-based PN formulation (8.5 percent amino acids, 50 percent dextrose, and 7.5 percent of total calories from lipids) or an isocaloric, lipid-based PN solution (8.5 percent amino acids, 30 percent dextrose, and 40 percent of calories from lipids). Those who received lipid-based PN had significantly less abnormalities of AST, ALT, and bilirubin than did patients treated with the standard carbohydrate-based PN. It is now well accepted that PN providing energy as dextrose and lipid emulsion reduces, if not eliminates, the risk of hepatic biochemical abnormalities. The mechanisms for this response remain speculative, but may involve prevention of fatty acid deficiency or decreased metabolic or hormonal effects associated with dextrose provision.

Hepatic Biochemical Abnormalities in Adults Receiving PN

Clarke and colleagues reviewed prospective data for 420 adults who received PN over a 5-year period.[69] Patients with normal liver tests pre-PN (n = 14) developed gradual but progressive increases in serum ALP and AST and small increases in bilirubin. In 56 patients receiving TPN for more than 4 weeks values of serum bilirubin were increased in 31 percent, AST in 27 percent, and ALP in 32 percent. Both AST and ALP values rose progressively in patients on long-term PN throughout the 10-week study duration.[69] Nearly 50 percent of patients experienced a septic episode during PN and were noted to have significantly higher bilirubin levels than those without sepsis. Patients with underlying malignancy were more likely to have aminotransferase abnormalities. These data illustrate that several clinical factors may interact to cause PN-associated liver dysfunction.

Taken together with the data in Cavicchi, this work suggests that 30 percent to 65 percent of adult patients on long-term PN develop chronic abnormal liver tests and are at risk for chronic liver disease.

Hepatic Biochemical Abnormalities in Children Receiving PN

TPN-associated cholestasis is a significant problem for premature infants, many of whom have intestinal failure resulting from congenital abnormalities or necrotizing enterocolitis.[16,70] Postuma and associates described an elevation in bilirubin within 2 weeks of initiating TPN in 34 percent of mostly premature infants.[71] AST and ALP elevations were observed after 4 to 6 weeks in a similar percentage. The most prominent feature on liver biopsy was cholestasis. It is suggested that cholestasis, after it has developed, persists as long as TPN is continued,[17,71-72] but liver tests returned to normal in most infants within 4 weeks of discontinuing TPN.[71]

The reported incidence of TPN-associated hepatic dysfunction in children has varied from 7 percent to 84 percent.[73-74] Greater awareness that TPN-associated cholestasis leads to end-stage liver disease has led to a more prudent use of PN in neonates. There is now increased emphasis on establishing enteral feeds whenever possible. But a recent review reported that 40 percent to 60 percent of children on long-term TPN still develop hepatic biochemical abnormalities.[12]

Hepatic Histopathology Associated with PN

Steatosis and cholestasis are the two most common histologic abnormalities associated with TPN.[63] Although hepatic steatosis is often asymptomatic and reversible, rare cases may progress to steatohepatitis and cirrhosis.[13,75] Non-specific triaditis also has been described in adults receiving TPN for inflammatory bowel disease.[56] It is suggested that non-specific triaditis may be a subtle form of underlying liver disease or an early stage of cholestasis.[63] Intrahepatic cholestasis predominantly found in premature infants has been associated with a high risk for progression to biliary cirrhosis and end-stage liver disease.[14,15,70,76] As mentioned previously, chronic cholestasis in adults receiving long-term home PN is strongly associated with occurrence of end-stage liver disease.[20]

Hepatic Steatosis

Hepatic steatosis is a common complication during short-term administration of PN, primarily in adults.[54-55,57-58] Hepatic steatosis occurred frequently with dextrose-based PN, confirmed by biopsy obtained in the first week or two of treatment. With milder involvement hepatic steatosis was periportal in distribution. With more extensive involvement panlobular or centrolobular distributions were noted, similar to alcoholic or diabetic hepatic steatosis.[63] Host and associates reviewed 30 patients on dextrose-based PN and performed biopsies in six patients who had a threefold increase in AST levels after 10 days of treatment.[58] Three of the six patients also had tenfold increases in ALT. ALP was increased less markedly. Periportal fatty infiltration was found in all six. No abnormalities were found in liver biopsies of two patients with no evidence of biochemical abnormalities. Grant and associates reviewed 100 patients on dextrose-based TPN.[54] As many as 93 percent of the patients (93 of 100) had abnormal AST and ALT levels. Nine patients had liver biopsies. Hepatic steatosis was the predominant finding. In studies by Grant and Host biochemical abnormalities improved despite continued PN. Serial biopsies obtained in a patient on continued TPN for several months showed progressive resolution of extensive hepatitis stenosis without fibrosis after clinical improvement and "cyclic hyperalimentation."[77]

With lipid emulsion–supplemented PN, the occurrence of hepatic steatosis and tender hepatomegaly decreased.[63] Tulikoura and Huikuri obtained liver biopsies before initiation of standard dextrose-based TPN, dextrose with higher amino acid–based TPN, or lipid-supplemented TPN in 28 surgical patients.[65] Repeat liver biopsies were obtained between days 11 and 13. Hepatic steatosis rose from 5 percent to 35 percent ($p < .001$) in the dextrose group and from 7 percent to 23 percent ($p < .01$) in the amino acid group. No patient in the lipid group had progressive steatosis.

Although studies in humans[64,67] and in animals[78,79] show that lipid supplementation of PN can blunt hepatic steatosis, administration of excessive amounts of lipid also can cause hepatic accumulation of fat.[80-81]

Steatohepatitis

For a large majority of adult patients on PN, hepatic steatosis is a transient and generally reversible state. However, rare progression to steatohepatitis and cirrhosis has been reported.[13,75] Craig and associates first reported a case of severe steatohepatitis on TPN in a 63-year-old man who underwent massive small-bowel resection for intestinal ischemia.[75] The patient received daily cyclic infusion of crystalline amino acids and dextrose supplemented weekly with 500 ml of 10 percent lipid emulsion. AST and ALP rose progressively. An initial biopsy obtained 3 months after small-bowel resection showed hepatic steatosis alone. The subsequent three biopsies and a sample obtained at autopsy (death from myocardial infarction) revealed progression from an alcoholic hepatitis-like lesion to micronodular cirrhosis.

Bowyer and associates reported similar features in 9 of 60 patients who received PN for 8 to 95 months because of extensive intestinal disease or small-bowel resection.[13] These patients had progressive increases in AST and ALP. Three had prolonged jaundice; one died from complications of hepatic encephalopathy, a second from prolonged cholestasis, and a third remained ill at the time of report. Liver biopsies were obtained at least once from each of these nine patients, and eight of the nine showed steatohepatitis. The remaining 51 patients had mildly abnormal liver tests at worst and did not undergo liver biopsies.

A review of approximately 70 patients followed for home TPN at the University of Chicago for up to 10 years included three cases of persistently elevated AST levels leading to eventual liver biopsy.[63] Central pericellular fibrosis along with occasional foci of steatohepatitis were noted in all three. These findings were felt to be reminiscent of lesions that may identify risk of steatohepatitis after ileojejunal bypass[82] or precursors of micronodular cirrhosis among alcohol consumers.[83-84]

Non-specific Triaditis

Bengoa and associates from the University of Chicago described non-specific triaditis in association with liver test abnormalities found in patients receiving lipid-supplemented TPN because of inflammatory bowel disease.[56] Five patients with serum ALT values greater than 500 IU/L and moderate increases in ALP and bilirubin while receiving lipid-supplemented TPN underwent liver biopsy. Non-specific triaditis with little evidence of hepatic steatosis or hepatocellular injury was the major histologic feature. Baker and Rosenberg suggested that non-specific triaditis represents an early or mild form of cholestasis.[63] However, the clinical significance of this entity remains speculative at this point.

Intrahepatic Cholestasis

Intrahepatic cholestasis was the first hepatobiliary complication attributed to TPN.[11] Most recent studies indicate that 40 percent to 60 percent of children on long-term TPN will develop intrahepatic cholestasis.[18-19] Besides an increase in conjugated bilirubin, ALP also may increase.[14] It has been suggested that GGTP may be a more sensitive indicator of PN-associated cholestasis.[85] Bile acids also have been used in adults as a sensitive marker.[86] However, in infants up to 6 months of age, bile acid levels are not useful because of a physiologic elevation in cholate and chenodeoxycholate.[87]

TPN-associated cholestasis presents initially with periportal infiltration of lymphocytic and neutrophilic bile plugs. This lesion is followed by non-ductular proliferation and biliary cirrhosis.[88] Dahms and Halpin described the hepatic histopathology of 11 infants with jaundice within 3 weeks of initiating TPN.[72] Biopsies revealed severe cholestasis, associated portal inflammation, and mild portal and periportal fibrosis. No evidence of steatosis was noted, but foci of hepatocyte necrosis and bile duct proliferation were seen. These histologic features were felt to be similar to patients with neonatal hepatitis, extrahepatic biliary obstruction, or biliary atresia. Electron-microscopic features of PN-associated cholestasis included increases in the size of mitochondria, dilated smooth endoplasmic reticulum, collagen fibers in the space of Disse, and proteinaceous material in hepatocyte cytoplasm.[72] All 11 infants in this study recovered. However, it is not uncommon for TPN-associated cholestasis to lead to cirrhosis, hepatic failure, and death.[11,74,89-90]

Cohen and Olsen reviewed the hepatic histology of 31 consecutive autopsies of infants who died while receiving TPN.[74] They found hepatic steatosis in 21 of 29 patients who received TPN for 3 to 90 days. Diffuse steatosis was described in patients treated for the shortest time. In contrast, a centrolobular distribution of fat was noted after at least 10 days of TPN. No inflammatory infiltrate was evident, and severity of liver disease correlated with duration of TPN. Bile duct proliferation was more frequent after 3 weeks of TPN and severe portal fibrosis after more than 90 days of TPN.[74] The only patient with micronodular cirrhosis had received TPN for 217 days. This study clearly demonstrated the progression of PN-associated hepatic steatosis to intrahepatic cholestasis, to bile duct proliferation, to portal fibrosis, and to micronodular cirrhosis. The histologic progression of TPN-associated hepatic diseases is summarized in Figure 57-1.

PN-associated intrahepatic cholestasis also occurs in adults.[20,54,55,57,91] Sheldon and associates documented that hepatic steatosis was the main lesion in their patients who underwent liver biopsies during the first 21 days of TPN, but cholestasis with periportal inflammation was seen in nine biopsies obtained after more than 21 days of TPN.[57] In two of these, portal fibrosis was noted. Table 57-2 shows proposed etiologies for PN-associated cholestasis.[20]

Hepatocellular Carcinoma

A single case of hepatoma was reported in a preterm infant receiving TPN.[92] The infant developed severe cholestasis and periportal fibrosis after 112 days of TPN and hepatocellular carcinoma after 395 days of TPN. Choline deficiency has been associated with hepatocellular carcinoma in rats, and choline supplementation prevents the development of cancer in this setting.[93-94] Additional studies in this area are warranted.

Pathogenesis of Hepatic Steatosis

Various factors contributing to hepatic steatosis have been described in both experimental animals and humans. Proposed etiologies of PN-associated hepatic steatosis are listed in Table 57-3. In the first systemic evaluation of the pathogenesis of hepatic steatosis in parenterally fed rats Hall and associates examined the mechanisms responsible for the rate of entry and the rate of removal of fat from the liver.[95] They found that hepatic triglycerides were produced endogenously in the liver and not derived from circulating fatty acids. This study suggested that TPN-associated hepatic steatosis resulted from enhanced fatty acid synthesis and reduced triglyceride secretion by the liver.[95]

Factors Promoting Hepatic Fatty Acid Synthesis

Among various factors contributing to hepatic steatosis, overfeeding with high carbohydrate loads has been recognized as a potent stimulus for hepatic steatosis in both animals[96] and humans.[57] Burke and associates found the maximal rate of glucose oxidation in man to be 5 to 7 mg/kg per minute.[97] Parenteral infusions of dextrose exceeding this rate result in the hepatic accumulation of acetyl co-enzyme A (CoA) (see Chap. 3), which is the carbon source for synthesis of long-chain fatty acids.[98] Excessive carbohydrate infusion increases acetyl-CoA levels and induces acetyl CoA carboxylase, the rate-limiting enzyme for fatty acid synthesis (see Chap. 3).[96,99]

Meguid and associates proposed that the infusion of hypercaloric TPN promoted hepatic fat deposition by stimulating insulin release.[100] Insulin promotes lipogenesis while inhibiting mitochondrial carnitine acyltransferase, which is rate-limiting for fatty acid oxidation.[100] With a series of experiments in rats using graded variations in carbohydrate, amino acid, and lipid components of TPN, Meguid and associates demonstrated that providing one third of TPN calories as lipid not only reduced hepatic biochemical abnormalities and steatosis, but also aborted the rise of serum insulin by 50 percent compared with dextrose-based TPN.[100-101]

Hepatic lipid metabolism is influenced by the balance between insulin (glycogenic, anti-lipolytic) and glucagon (glycolytic, lipolytic). High-carbohydrate infusions increase the ratio of insulin to glucagon in portal blood.[102] In this regard administration of glucagon via PN prevents[103] or reverses[104] hepatic steatosis. Addition of a lipid emulsion to TPN solutions decreases the ratio of insulin to glucagon in rats, consistent with the observation that lipid-supplemented TPN leads to less hepatic steatosis.[105] The same is likely to occur in humans, but no data are available.

Glutamine supplementation of TPN increases glucagon secretion and lowers the insulin to glucagon ratio in the portal vein of rats.[106] Rats receiving 1 percent to 2 percent glutamine with TPN did not develop hepatic steatosis, whereas steatosis developed in rats receiving standard TPN.[107] Glutamine depletion in critically ill pa-

TABLE 57-2

Proposed Etiologies for PN-associated Cholestasis

PN-dependent etiologies	Patient-dependent etiologies
Excessive amino acid content	Immaturity of hepatobiliary system
Defective amino acid content	Altered biliary secretion
Toxicity from contaminants	Bacterial overgrowth and translocation
Excessive lipid content	Infectious or non-infectious chronic inflammation
Nutrient deficiency (serine, taurine, molybdenum, selenium, vitamin E)	Lack of enteral stimulation
Long duration of TPN	
Continuous infusion	

PN, Parenteral nutrition; *TPN*, total parenteral nutrition.

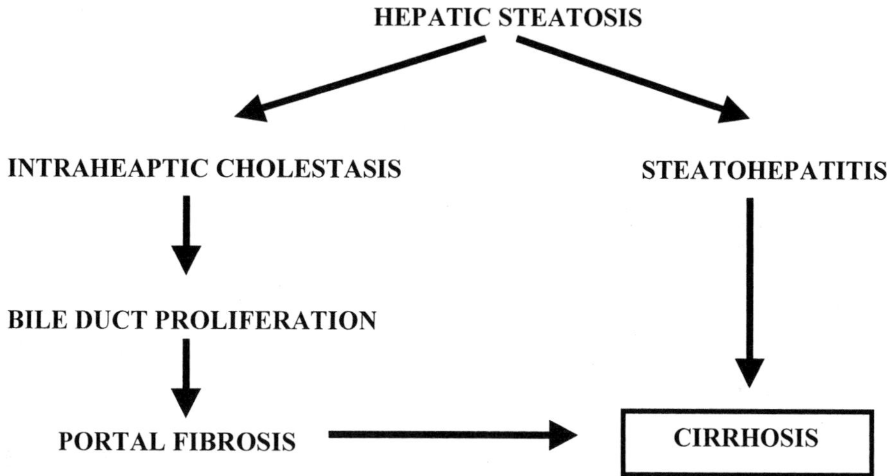

Figure 57-1 Histologic progression of parenteral nutrition–associated liver disease.

tients on TPN has been associated with reduced plasma glutathione (GSH) levels.[108] A decrease in GSH synthesis in liver that may occur because of substrate depletion or increased utilization of GSH can promote liver injury by reducing protection against free radicals.[109]

Factors Suppressing Hepatic Fatty Acid Clearance

Various nutritional deficiencies can suppress hepatic fatty acid clearance and thus lead to hepatic steatosis. Fat-free TPN can result in essential fatty acid deficiency because lack of infused essential fatty acids will eventually deplete essential fatty acids. In turn essential fatty acid deficiency decreases synthesis of hepatic phospholipids. This limits the export of hepatic lipoprotein and leads to hepatic steatosis.[110-112] The condition can be easily corrected in patients receiving PN by providing adequate amounts of essential fatty acids as intravenous fat emulsion, with dietary supplementation as tolerated.[113-114] It is suggested that PN should provide a minimum of 2 percent to 4 percent of total calories as linoleic acid to avoid essential fatty acid deficiency.[105,110-116] Because the fatty acid component of commercial soybean-based lipid emulsions is approximately 50 percent linoleic acid, 4 percent to 8 percent of total calories provided as lipid emulsion should be sufficient to prevent deficiency.

Kwashiorkor (protein malnutrition) is associated with hepatic steatosis.[117] In this condition of extreme malnutrition apoproteins required for production of very low-density lipoprotein (VLDL) are decreased and there is impaired export of triglyceride from the liver. Together with increased circulating free fatty acids, hepatic steatosis is promoted.

Carnitine deficiency may lead to hepatic steatosis because mitochondrial fatty acid oxidation is reduced.[118-119] Although carnitine can be synthesized from the amino acids methionine and lysine and is now available for addition to PN, carnitine is not present in standard PN formulas and may be reduced in patients receiving long-term TPN.[120] It has not been proven that carnitine deficiency causes hepatic steatosis in patients receiving TPN. Bowyer and associates treated four patients on TPN with low carnitine levels and abnormal liver tests.[121-122] However, these studies failed to show that treating carnitine deficiency for several weeks reverses hepatic steatosis. Because infants often develop carnitine deficiency, intravenous, tablet, and oral solutions of carnitine are now available in the United States for pediatric patients (Sigma-Tau Pharmaceuticals, Inc., Gaithersburg, MD).

Phosphatidylcholine is an essential component of VLDL synthesis.[123-124] When choline or methionine becomes deficient, hepatic steatosis develops because hepatic triglyceride cannot be exported through synthesis of VLDL. Hepatocytes isolated from choline-deficient rats cannot export VLDL until choline or methionine is made available.[125] Although some investigators

TABLE 57-3
Proposed Etiologies for PN-associated Hepatic Steatosis

Promoting lipid synthesis	Reducing lipid removal	Others
Hypercaloric infusion	Essential fatty acid deficiency	Bacterial translocation
Hyperinsulinemia	Choline deficiency	Sepsis
Excessive lipid infusion	Carnitine deficiency	Chronic inflammation
Glutamine depletion	Taurine deficiency	Tryptophan metabolites
	Cysteine deficiency	

PN, Parenteral nutrition.

have recently advocated choline as an essential nutrient for humans,[126-127] it is not currently included in conventional PN solutions. But data suggest that choline deficiency exists in up to 90 percent of patients on long-term PN.[127-131] Buchman and associates provided oral lecithin to long-term TPN patients with hepatic steatosis and low free-plasma choline levels. Concentrations of free choline in plasma increased in these patients (although not to normal levels), and hepatic steatosis was significantly decreased.[130] Another study by Demetriau showed that supplementation with oral lecithin raised free choline levels and prevented hepatic steatosis in patients on long-term TPN.[131] TPN-associated hepatic steatosis was completely alleviated by intravenous choline that corrected plasma-free choline to normal levels.[132] Intravenous choline is not yet available commercially in the United States but is being actively investigated in PN-dependent patients.

Other Factors Contributing to PN-associated Hepatic Steatosis

As noted previously, providing a portion of TPN calories as lipid prevents or decreases hepatic steatosis.[78,113] However, infusion of large amounts of lipid may cause fatty infiltration of the liver.[133-134] The infused lipid appears to be taken up directly by hepatocyte lysosomes and Kupffer cells, which is a different mechanism for steatosis within hepatocyte cytoplasm.[135-136] Hepatic phospholipidosis has also been described as a complication of prolonged infusion of lipid emulsion during PN.[137]

There is a well-known association between sepsis and cholestasis. Bacterial overgrowth in animals is associated with the increased production and release of proinflammatory cytokines such as TNFα and endotoxin.[138-141] TNFα released during sepsis has been associated with hepatic steatosis in rats.[142-143] Pappo and associates showed that polymyxin B reduced total cecal flora and, concomitantly, TNFα production and hepatic steatosis during TPN in rats.[142-143] They further demonstrated that TNFα is responsible for hepatic steatosis by showing that anti-TNFα antibodies reduced hepatic steatosis during TPN in rats.[144] Drenick and colleagues reported that hepatic steatosis associated with bacterial overgrowth could be prevented by metronidazole in patients with jejunoileal bypasses.[145] The effectiveness of metronidazole in preventing increased ALP, GGTP, and AST levels during TPN was shown in a prospective clinical study conducted by Lambert and associates.[146]

Bowel rest during TPN has been associated with a significant increase in the number of lactose-positive and lactose-negative aerobes and in anaerobic, gram-negative bacteria in the ceca of rats.[147] A method to prevent or minimize bacterial overgrowth may be avoidance of total bowel rest. In the study by Pappo and colleagues[142] rats infused with saline and free oral feeds had less hepatic steatosis than rats receiving polymyxin B while on TPN.[142]

Taurine and cysteine are metabolites of methionine via the transsulfuration pathway.[70] Taurine and cysteine are now considered "conditionally essential" amino acids in premature infants and are supplemented in commercial pediatric PN and enteral nutrient formulas.[148-149] Thus deficiencies of taurine and cysteine can occur in premature infants, who have immature hepatic enzyme systems. Yan and associates studied the effects of taurine on hepatic lipid metabolism and showed that taurine supplementation reduced hepatic lipid content.[150] The effects of supplementation with taurine on hepatic steatosis during TPN have not been studied. Narkewicz and associates studied weanling rats and found that cysteine replacement was also useful in reducing hepatic steatosis during TPN.[151] This has not been confirmed in man, but some clinicians anecdotally report that parenteral cysteine administration improves liver function tests in occasional patients on chronic PN.

The possibility that toxic contaminants in TPN solutions lead to hepatic steatosis is minimal with present-day nutritional support resources. Periportal hepatic steatosis had been found in rats receiving TPN containing degradation products of tryptophan.[12] Decomposition of tryptophan in TPN solution is not a problem if sodium bisulfite is not used as a preservative and if the solutions are protected from light.[12]

Pathogenesis of PN-associated Intrahepatic Cholestasis

The pathogenesis of PN-associated cholestasis remains uncertain, but is likely multi-factorial in etiology (see Table 57-2). Because PN is often initiated for intestinal failure, it is important to realize that PN-associated cholestasis may be caused not only by administration of components of PN itself, but by conditions existing before administration of PN. PN-dependent mechanisms involved in cholestasis include excessive or defective amino acid content, toxicity from contaminants in PN solutions, excessive lipid content, nutrient deficiency in PN formulation, and long duration or continuous administration of PN.[10,16-18] The patient-dependent mechanisms leading to cholestasis include immaturity of hepatobiliary system, altered biliary secretion, bacterial overgrowth and translocation, and infection or non-infectious conditions of chronic inflammation.[10,16-18] Lack of enteral stimulation, common among most patients receiving PN, seems to underlie or potentiate many of these recipient-related mechanisms. The two mechanistic categories that may lead to PN-associated cholestasis may co-exist and influence one another.

PN-dependent Etiologies of Cholestasis

Both excessive and deficient amino acid intake have been suspected in the pathogenesis of PN-associated cholestasis. Animal studies suggest that amino acids in TPN solutions induce cholestasis.[152-155] Black and associates showed an early, direct, and independent effect of amino acid infusions on the hepatocyte canalicular membrane in the human neonate.[85] Further, Vileisis and associates demonstrated in a prospective study of 82 premature infants that higher daily protein intake (3.6 g/kg/day versus 2.3 g/kg/day) provided in TPN led to a higher total serum bilirubin concentration and a shorter time to onset of cholestasis.[156] Brown and associates proposed that avoidance of amino acid–containing solutions (and substitutions of enterol protein) prevents cholestasis in premature infants.[157] These early studies in children and animals suggest a possible role of excess amino acid in development of PN-associated cholestasis.

Results of early studies on the effect of amino acids in PN solutions possibly were influenced by aluminum contamination from the protein hydrolysate widely used as an amino acid source until early the 1980s.[50] Aluminum toxicity has been associated with hepatic abnormalities in animals.[158-159] Although hepatic aluminum accumulation has been found in children,[160] there is uncertain evidence that aluminum currently contributes to TPN-associated cholestasis.[50] Protein hydrolysates in PN have been replaced with crystalline amino acids, which have significantly decreased aluminum contamination to less than 2 percent of the aluminum content in casein hydrolysate.[161] However, other components of PN solutions may still contain aluminum.[161-162]

The key metabolites of the transsulfuration pathway and their relationship to each other are summarized in Figure 57-2. Recently, Moss and Amli proposed that an excess of methionine included as an essential amino acid in PN may be responsible for PN-associated cholestasis.[70] Methionine is an essential sulfur-containing amino acid, metabolized via the transsulfuration pathway into such important metabolites as S-adenosylmethionine, homocystine, cysteine, taurine, and GSH (see Figure 57-2). Although an essential amino acid, methionine is potentially hepatotoxic.[163-164] Moss and Amli found that PN solutions may be equally hepatotoxic whether given intravenously or enterally in rats.[165] Methionine may be directly toxic to liver and might increase susceptibility to oxidative damage. As methionine is converted to its first metabolite S-adenosylmethionine, an equivalent amount of ATP is consumed. Excessive methionine infusion therefore can deplete hepatic ATP.[164] This might lead to a marked shift in hepatic glutathione from its reduced state (GSH) to glutathione disulfide (GSSG).[166] Because

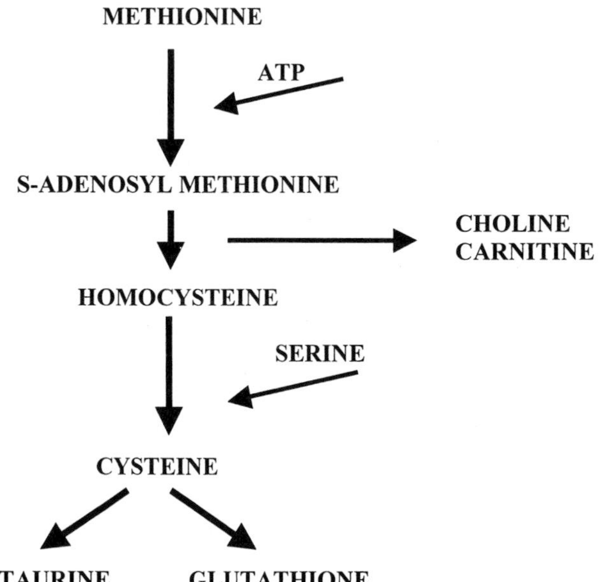

Figure 57-2 Key metabolites of the transsulfuration pathway.

GSH but not GSSG protects against oxidative injury, the liver with excess methionine may be susceptible to oxidative damage. Impairment of the transsulfuration pathway has been demonstrated in cirrhotics and has been shown to lead to methionine excess and a shortage of GSH.[167-168] In premature infants the transsulfuration pathway is also immature and only partially functional, and blockage at the level of cystathionase is common.[149,169] Premature infants thus are thought to be particularly at high risk of developing methionine toxicity and intrahepatic cholestasis.

Deficiencies in specific amino acids could contribute to PN-associated cholestasis. Belli and associates compared two commercial amino acid solutions and found that impaired bile flow occurred only in rats administered amino acid solutions without serine.[48] Cholestasis caused by the serine-free amino acid solution was reversed by addition of serine.

Taurine deficiency apparently can contribute to PN-associated cholestasis in premature infants. As mentioned previously, taurine is probably "conditionally essential" in premature infants, the mechanism being decreased expression of enzymes of the transsulfuration pathway (i.e., cystathionase and cysteine sulfinic acid decarboxylase).[170] Taurine promotes bile secretion as the principal bile acid conjugate in infants[171] and prevents lithocholate toxicity.[172] Relative deficiency of taurine in adults receiving long-term TPN has been demonstrated.[173] Taurine supplementation was indeed shown to promote bile acid secretion in premature infants[174] and in adults with various hepatobiliary disorders.[175] Therefore taurine supplementation in PN solutions has been advocated to prevent cholestasis.[47]

Excessive lipid provided in PN promotes intrahepatic cholestasis. At least 50 percent of patients on long-term PN receiving more than 60 percent of calories as lipid develop hepatic cholestasis.[176-178] Lowering the amount of lipid calories to 1500 kcal/week reverses the biochemical evidence of cholestasis in some patients. Providing only 1 g/kg/day of lipid supplementation prevents the development of biochemical evidence of cholestasis.[176-178] Cavicchi and colleagues also found a higher incidence of chronic cholestasis and severe PN-associated liver diseases in patients receiving more than 1 g/kg/day of parenteral lipid.[20] Thus patients with permanent intestinal failure and long-term PN dependence should receive 20 percent omega-6 rich fat emulsions at quantities of less than 1 g/kg/day.

Deficiencies of specific micronutrients also have been suggested to contribute to development of TPN-associated cholestasis. Molybdenum is a co-factor in the enzyme systems of the transsulfuration pathway. Its deficiency may aggravate methionine toxicity and decrease bile flow.[179] Carnitine deficiency also is believed to cause cholestasis in premature infants receiving TPN.[180] Reversal of hyperbilirubinemia with carnitine supplementation has been reported.[181-182]

TPN-associated cholestasis is often noted in premature infants with immature defense against peroxidative injuries. Selenium and vitamin E are involved in antioxidant defense and are known to be deficient in premature infants.[76] Selenium deficiency has been implicated in intrahepatic cholestasis of pregnancy and may also influence PN-associated cholestasis.[185] Selenium deficiency has been documented in patients receiving short- and long-term TPN.[183-184] Vitamin E deficiency alone does not cause cholestasis, but vitamin E status influences the liver's susceptibility to cholestasis.[186]

Both the composition of PN solutions and how PN is administered may influence development of PN-associated cholestasis. Messing and associates correlated the development of cholestasis with the duration of PN use and continuous (i.e., over 24 hours) versus cyclic infusion (i.e., over 8 to 14 hours).[20,187] One study by Nanji and Anderson suggested, however, that the incidence of PN-associated cholestasis was related more to the underlying disease process than to the duration of PN administration.[91] However, as already noted the most recent data confirm progressive development of chronic cholestasis with longer duration of PN.[20] The prevalence of cholestasis increased from 55 percent at 2 years, to 64 percent at 4 years, to 72 percent after 6 years of chronic PN administration.[20]

Patient-dependent Etiologies of Cholestasis

Prolonged fasting leads to altered biliary secretion, which in turn is thought to contribute to TPN-associated cholestasis.[188] A deficiency of bile acid secretion may occur in all age groups, either from decreased synthesis of bile salts or from a prolonged storage of bile salts in the gallbladder or intestine. In adults and infants, oral feeding releases cholecystokinin, which stimulates the gallbladder to empty 6 to 10 times daily.[189] Bile salts excreted in bile are nearly all reclaimed and re-excreted by the enterohepatic circulation, which helps maintain bile fluidity. With TPN and prolonged fasting, bile stasis and the formation of biliary sludge commonly occur.[190]

Studies showing that cholestasis can be prevented by treatments to maintain biliary secretion provide indirect evidence that PN-associated cholestasis involves altered biliary secretion. Cholecystokinin was effective in preventing TPN-associated cholestasis in high-risk premature infants.[191-193] Simultaneous partial oral feeding also appears to lower the risk of PN-associated cholestasis.[194-195] Whereas cholecystokinin and simultaneous partial feeding primarily promote biliary secretion by enteral stimulation, ursodeoxycholic acid promotes bile acid synthesis and increases the size of the bile acid pool. Lindor and Burnes demonstrated improvement in serum bilirubin levels after ursodeoxycholic acid in a patient with TPN-associated cholestasis.[196] Durkesen and associates successfully prevented TPN-associated cholestasis in piglets using ursodeoxycholic acid.[197] A pilot study conducted by Spagnuolo and associates documented effectiveness of ursodeoxycholic acid in reversing TPN-associated cholestasis in seven children.[198] Further clinical studies are needed to confirm effectiveness and safety of cholecystokinin and ursodeoxycholic acid as methods to treat or prevent PN-associated liver disease.

Bacterial translocation through the gut wall may promote PN-associated cholestasis via ascending cholangitis,[199-200] systemic or portal endotoxemia,[201-202] or abnormal bile acid metabolism, especially overproduction of endogenous lithocholic acid.[49] Consistent with these concepts, use of oral metronidazole or gentamicin to reduce intestinal bacterial overgrowth in TPN-fed patients was effective in preventing PN-associated cholestasis.[203-204]

Although human data are limited, specific nutrients that improve the anatomic and immune barrier functions of the gut may diminish PN-associated liver dysfunction. In animal models TPN administration impairs intestinal mucosal growth and the gut-associated immune system, thus promoting bacterial translocation across the gut wall.[205] In rodents bacterial translocation was increased by both oral and intravenous administration of TPN compared to animals fed an oral diet[206]; this effect was prevented with oral fiber supplementation.[207] Glutamine enrichment of TPN solutions also provided protection against bacterial translocation in rodent models by preventing atrophy of gut mucosa[208] and by preserving intestinal plasma cells that produce immunoglobulin A.[209-211]

Another important role of bacterial overgrowth in development of PN-associated cholestasis is in the formation of lithocholic acid by bacterial hydroxylation of chenodeoxycholic acid.[212] Increased concentrations of lithocholic acid have been associated with intrahepatic cholestasis.[49,212-213] Thus a rationale for treating PN recipients with antibiotics is the associated reduction in intestinal bacterial conversion of chenodeoxy- to lithocholic acid. Inflammatory cytokines can induce cholestasis; therefore, inflammation after infectious and non-infectious etiologies can contribute to PN-associated cholestasis.[214] For example, hematologic malignancy has been shown also to lead to PN-associated cholestasis.[215]

Recently, a role of multi-drug resistance 2 gene (mdr-2 gene) was suggested in development of TPN-associated cholestasis in murine liver.[216] The mdr-2 gene product is involved in biliary secretion of phospholipid.[217] Mdr-2 knockout mice are unable to secrete phospholipids into bile and are used as an animal model of chronic cholestasis.[218] Hepatic cholestasis similar to what occurs in sclerosing cholangitis, primary biliary cirrhosis, and TPN-associated cholestasis develops in these animals.[219] It has been suggested that TPN and endotoxin reduce the level of mdr-2 RNA in mice.[216,220] Therapy with ursodeoxycholic acid in this animal model was effective in reducing histologic cholestasis.[221] Cavicchi and associates suggested that hepatic phospholipidosis and microvacuolar steatosis in hepatocytes and Kupffer cells may be induced by high doses of intravenous fat emulsion PN.[20] Although still speculative, these authors further suggested that hepatic phospholipidosis, together with reduced mdr-2 levels and bacterial translocation, might lead to TPN-associated cholestasis. Gradual development of progressive liver disease may modify the immune system of the liver further and aggravate tendencies for bacterial translocation and endotoxemia.[222-224] In addition, lipid emulsions themselves may contribute directly to the risk of endotoxemia because they reduce clearance of endotoxins and bacteria.[225]

BILIARY TRACT ABNORMALITIES

Acalculous cholecystitis and cholelithiasis with calculous cholecystitis occur with TPN. Acalculous cholecystitis was first recognized as a complication of TPN by Anderson in 1972,[226] 10 years before the association between gallstones and TPN was first appreciated.[187] TPN-associated biliary tract complications tend to be more frequent and severe in pediatric patients.[227-228]

Acalculous Cholecystitis

About 5 percent of acute cholecystitis in adults occurs without gallstones.[50] It appears to be caused by bile stasis and increased bile lithogenicity and often is associated with major trauma, severe systemic illness, and recent major operative procedures.[229-230] Fasting appears to be an important factor for development of biliary sludge and acalculous cholecystitis. Roslyn and associates found the incidence of gallbladder disease (acalculous cholecystitis and cholelithiasis) nearly double in patients with little or no oral intake.[39] Petersen and Sheldon reported eight cases of acute acalculous cholecystitis that were clearly associated with administration of TPN.[231] This problem occurs more frequently in patients receiving prolonged TPN (longer than 3 months).[232] Diagnosis is often more difficult because of the absence of gallstones, and a delayed diagnosis potentially leads to increased morbidity because of perforation of the gallbladder and bile peritonitis.[229,233]

In a prospective study Messing and associates found that gallstones occurred more frequently than acalculous cholecystitis in patients receiving TPN.[234] Of 14 patients who developed gallbladder sludge while receiving TPN, 6 developed gallstones and 1 developed acalculous cholecystitis.[234] This supports the hypothesis that gallbladder stasis leads to sludge formation, which in turn is a precursor to acalculous cholecystitis and gallstones. Gallbladder dilation found in association with acalculous cholecystitis in neonates receiving TPN was shown to resolve after enteral feeding.[235-236]

Biliary Sludge and Cholelithiasis

The prospective analysis by Messing and associates of 23 patients receiving TPN used serial ultrasound to monitor gallbladder status on long-term TPN.[234] No abnormalities were found in the first 12 days of TPN. Sludge developed in 6 percent of patients after 3 weeks, 50 percent in 4 to 6 weeks, and 100 percent after 6 weeks of TPN. Six of 14 sludge-forming patients developed stones, but none without sludge developed stones. Moreover, 1 of 14 with sludge developed acalculous cholecystitis; none without sludge developed acalculous cholecystitis.[234] In eight patients examined after stopping TPN and resuming oral feeding, sludge cleared from all after 4 weeks of oral feeding.

Roslyn and associates reviewed 109 patients receiving long-term TPN who did not have preexisting cholelithiasis.[39] Gallbladder disease developed in 23 percent of patients (19 percent cholelithiasis, 4 percent acalculous cholecystitis). The same group reported an additional 60 patients on long-term TPN without preexisting cholelithiasis.[230] In this analysis gallstones were more prevalent in patients with ileal disorders (39 percent) than in those without (25 percent). Manji and associates also found a significantly increased incidence of TPN-associated cholelithiasis in patients with severe short-bowel syndrome.[237]

Gallstone composition in patients on long-term TPN has characteristics of both black and brown pigment stones.[238] Black stones contain less than 10 percent cholesterol and more than 5 percent calcium salts of fatty acids; brown stones contain 10 to 30 percent cholesterol, less than 1 percent calcium salts of carbonate and phosphate, and moderate amounts of calcium salts of fatty acids.[239] Because PN-associated cholelithiasis appears to follow biliary sludge formation, composition of biliary sludge in patients receiving PN may provide useful information regarding stone composition. Calcium bilirubinate crystals but not cholesterol crystals were found in the bile of nine patients with TPN-associated gallbladder sludge.[240] Although the exact composition of PN-related gallstones may be variable, development of pigment stones appears invariably to be associated with gallbladder stasis.[50] It is also suggested that infectious processes lead to development of pigmented stones.[241-242]

Acute Calculous Cholecystitis

Acute calculous cholecystitis requiring cholecystectomy may occur as an apparent consequence of PN-associated cholelithiasis. In a retrospective analysis Messing and associates found ALP elevation in 14 of 27 patients receiving long-term TPN.[187] Five of these patients required cholecystectomy for stones during their course of TPN. Messing and associates also prospectively followed 23 patients on long-term TPN.[234] In these individuals 6 of 23 developed cholelithiasis; 3 of these patients later developed acute calculous cholecystitis requiring cholecystectomy.

Cholecystectomy is a treatment of choice in acute cholecystitis associated with chronic PN use.[243] However, Roslyn and associates found high complication rates among patients who underwent cholecystectomy for PN-associated cholecystitis. A perioperative morbidity of 54 percent and hospital mortality of 11 percent were observed[244] among 23 adult and 12 pediatric patients who underwent urgent cholecystectomy for PN-associated cholecystitis. These high rates are likely related not only to underlying diseases, but also to delayed diagnosis and adhesions from chronic inflammation. The authors proposed periodic ultrasonographic surveillance and early prophylactic cholecystectomy when cholelithiasis is first demonstrated in patients receiving chronic PN.[244-245]

Pathogenesis

Biliary sludge and cholelithiasis develop at rates proportional to the duration of PN therapy. The risk of cholelithiasis increases with the duration of PN; incidence of cholelithiasis as high as 45 percent had been reported.[232,244,246] Roslyn and associates reviewed 21 children on long-term TPN and found 9 who developed cholelithiasis.[227] Those who developed cholelithiasis were on TPN for an average of 30 months. Pitt and associates reviewed 60 adults on long-term TPN; 21 patients who developed cholelithiasis were on TPN for at least 24 months.[232]

Various proposed causes of PN-associated biliary diseases are listed in Table 57-4. One of the main factors leading to the formation of biliary sludge and subsequent cholelithiasis on PN is reduced gallbladder contractility.[39,234,240,247] Messing and associates demonstrated progressive motor dysfunction of the biliary tract of TPN-treated patients by serial ultrasound.[234,248] Gallbladder stasis and low plasma cholecystokinin levels observed during PN may also contribute to the formation of gallstones.[39,227,239] Fasting and bowel rest during TPN lead to gallbladder stasis, biliary sludge, and cholelithiasis, whereas resumption of oral intake reverses this trend.[227,244,249] With concurrent oral feeding during PN, Roslyn and associates succeeded in reducing the frequency of symptomatic gallbladder disease from 23 percent to 12.5 percent.[39]

Impaired bile flow is another consistent factor related to the formation of biliary sludge and subsequent cholelithiasis with PN.[250-254] Biliary bile acid concentration and bile acid pool were both increased during PN without change in bile acid synthesis in an animal model.[255]

The presence of a relative stagnation of bile acids within the enterohepatic circulation with PN was suggested to explain an apparent lack of choleretic effects during TPN.[254] As noted, ursodeoxycholic acid reversed severe TPN-associated cholestasis.[196] Administration of ursodeoxycholic acid may be helpful in increasing bile flow and choleresis.

Several studies have examined the effects of PN on bile composition.[255-259] Supersaturation of bile with cholesterol usually does not occur during TPN.[243-253,258] However, the concentration of unconjugated bilirubin in gallbladder bile content increases markedly during TPN in animals, predisposing to precipitation of bilirubin.[259] Calcium concentration in bile nearly doubles during TPN, which likely contributes to the formation of calcium bilirubinate crystals.[255,259-262]

Ileal resection or mucosal disease of the ileum predisposes to lithogenic bile, which leads in turn to cholesterol stones.[263-264] TPN-treated patients with ileal disorders appear to develop stones more often than those without ileal disorders.[232,237,245] But the gallstones associated with TPN are usually calcium bilirubinate, not cholesterol.[239,243] It thus is unclear how ileal resection leads to increased formation of these gallstones. Development of pigment stones is thought to often involve an infectious process[241-242]; this may be operative in patients with short-bowel syndrome without an ileum who have frequent catheter- and non-catheter-related infections. Additional studies are needed to address the nature of pigmented gallstone formation and the effects of short-bowel syndrome on gallstone formation in patients receiving long-term PN.

TABLE 57-4

Proposed Etiologies for PN-associated Biliary Disease

Reduced gallbladder contractility from prolonged fasting
Reduced bile flow
Reduced enterohepatic circulation
Ileal resection
Short-bowel syndrome

PN, Parenteral nutrition.

LONG-TERM SURVIVAL AFTER TPN-INDUCED CHRONIC LIVER DISEASE

PN-associated liver abnormalities occur in children and adults at rates ranging from 15 percent to 85 percent.* Kubota and associates reported a 25-year experience with neonates receiving TPN for massive bowel resection or congenital abnormalities.[15] They divided 273 neonates who received TPN for more than 2 weeks into three groups based on treatment periods: 77 patients in group A were treated between 1971 and 1982; 72 patients in group B were treated between 1983 and 1987. and 124 patients in group C were treated between 1992 and 1996. The incidence of TPN-associated cholestasis (defined as serum bilirubin levels greater than 2.0 mg/dl) were 57 percent, 31 percent, and 25 percent ($P < .01$), respectively, in groups A, B, and C. The mortality rate from TPN-associated complications was 13 percent, 3 percent and 3 percent ($P < .05$), respectively. Severe TPN-associated cholestasis developed in only 20 patients in group C, and 4 died from TPN-associated hepatic failure. Thus the incidence of TPN-associated cholestasis in neonates and the mortality resulting from liver complications decreased significantly during 1971 to 1996. However, despite significant improvements in TPN formulae and administration, the mortality rate of 3 percent was the same for the last 11 years of this 25-year series.

The first prospective case study of long-term hepatic complications in adults receiving PN (between 1975 and 1982) included 60 patients with gut failure treated for a total of 2000 patient months. Nine patients had abnormal liver tests that persisted for 8 to 95 months (median, 18 months), prompting one or more liver biopsies per patient. The authors suggested that PN-associated steatohepatitis with or without cholestasis might progress to chronic liver disease.

Messing and associates from two centers in Belgium and seven in France published a comprehensive review of their 10-year experience (1980 through 1989) with adult patients receiving home PN for more than 1 month.[265] Of the 217 patients enrolled 73 died during the survey. The mortality rate from complications of PN was approximately 11 percent. The probabilities of patient survival at 1, 3, and 5 years were 91 percent, 70 percent, and 62 percent, respectively. By multi-variate analysis, patient age younger than 40 years, start of home TPN after 1987, and absence of chronic intestinal obstruction were independent variables associated with decreased risk of death.[265] Two-year survival was 90 percent in patients younger than 60, with very short bowel potentially eligible for small-bowel transplantation. This compares fa-

*References 13, 16, 44, 45, 69, 248.

vorably with survival reported after small-bowel transplantation.[265]

Of 225 patients requiring home PN at the Mayo Clinic between 1975 and 1995, overall 5-year survival was 60 percent (median age, 51 years).[266] The 5-year survival by category of disease was 92 percent for inflammatory bowel disease, 60 percent for ischemic bowel, 54 percent for radiation enteritis, 48 percent for pseudo-obstruction, and 38 percent for cancer. Most deaths during TPN were attributed to the patient's primary disease; 20 deaths were due to PN-related causes. Four of the latter group died from liver failure. Eleven deaths were due to catheter sepsis, two from venous thrombosis, and two from metabolic abnormalities. As expected, underlying disease is the major contributor to PN-associated mortality.

Chan and associates published a retrospective of their 24-year experience with patients receiving home TPN.[267] Six of 42 patients on chronic TPN for more than 1 year developed end-stage liver disease at an average of 10.8 months after the initial elevation of bilirubin. The results in this review suggest that the combination of chronic inflammation and short-bowel syndrome is necessary for developing end-stage liver disease with prolonged TPN.[267]

The data of Cavicchi and colleagues are the most comprehensive prospective study of the prevalence and the natural history of PN-associated chronic liver disease to date in adult patients with permanent intestinal failure.[20] The median duration of PN was 45 months in these patients (range, 6 to 198 months); no patient was lost to follow-up. At the end of the study period 53 patients (59 percent) were still receiving PN, 10 (11 percent) had been weaned, and 27 (30 percent) had died (range, 10 to 140 months on PN). Chronic cholestasis developed after a median of 6 months (range, 3 to 132 months) in 58 patients (65 percent). Thirty-seven of these patients (41.5 percent) developed complicated home PN–related liver disease (bilirubin level greater than 3.5 mg/dl, factor V level less than 50 percent, portal hypertension, encephalopathy, ascites, gastrointestinal bleeding, or histologically proven extensive fibrosis or cirrhosis) after a median of 17 months (range, 2 to 155 months).[20] Seventeen patients in this group had extensive hepatic fibrosis after 26 months (range, 2 to 148 months), and five had cirrhosis after 37 months (range, 26 to 77 months). The prevalence of complicated PN-associated liver disease was 26 percent (CI, 17 percent to 35 percent) at 2 years, 50 percent (CI, 39 percent to 67 percent) at 6 years, and 53 percent (CI, 39 percent to 67 percent) at 8 years.[20] Six patients (22 percent of all deaths) died from PN-associated liver disease, seven (26 percent) from sepsis, and four (15 percent) from primary disease. Variables significantly associated with PN-associated cholestasis by multi-variate analysis in this study are listed in Table 57-5. Chronic cholestasis was significantly associated with a bowel remnant shorter than 50 cm (RR 2.1; CI, 1.2-3.7), known risk of liver disease (e.g., chronic viral hepatitis or portal vein thrombosis [RR 3.1; CI, 1.3-4.1]), and a parenteral lipid intake of 1 g/kg of body weight per day or more (RR 2.3; CI, 1.6-5.9).[20] Furthermore, complicated PN-associated liver disease was significantly associated with chronic cholestasis (RR 4.8; CI, 1.6-13.7) and lipid parenteral intake of 1 g/kg/day or more (RR 3.4; CI, 1.6-6.8).[20]

Taken together, these studies suggest that PN-associated liver disease is a significant source of morbidity and mortality especially among patients with permanent intestinal failure because of short-bowel syndrome. According to the International Registry of Intestinal Transplantation, severe PN-associated liver disease is currently the leading indication for combined liver-intestinal transplantation.[268-270] A total 48 percent of the 260 reported patients underwent combined liver-intestinal transplantation for severe PN-associated liver disease.[268]

RECOMMENDATIONS FOR PREVENTION AND MANAGEMENT OF PN-ASSOCIATED HEPATOBILIARY COMPLICATIONS

Guiding Principles to Prevent PN-associated Hepatobiliary Complications

A few simple principles to reduce the risk of PN-associated hepatobiliary complications are provided in the following sections and summarized in Table 57-6.

TABLE 57-5

Variables Associated with PN-associated Cholestasis

Variables	*P* value or RR (95% CI)
Univariate Analysis	
Small bowel length < 50 cm	.009
Known risk factor for liver disease	.008
Parenteral lipid intake > 1 g/kg/day	.004
Parenteral caloric intake > 80% of basal energy expenditure	.03
Mesenteric infarction	.002
Multi-variate Analysis	
Small bowel length < 50 cm	2.1 (1.2-3.7)
Known risk factor for liver disease	3.1 (1.3-4.1)
Parenteral lipid intake > 1 g/kg/day	2.3 (1.6-5.9)

From Cavicchi M, Beau P, Crenn P, et al: Prevalence of liver disease and contributing factors in patients receiving home parenteral nutrition for permanent intestinal failure. Ann Intern Med 132(7):525-532, 2000.

PN, Parenteral nutrition; *RR,* relative risk; *CI,* confidence interval.

TABLE 57-6

Guiding Principles to Reduce PN-associated Hepatobiliary Complications

Avoid overfeeding
Use intravenous lipid supplementation at a dose < 1 g/kg/day
Use cyclic rather than continuous feeding
Provide oral feeding whenever possible
Monitor liver tests periodically
Diagnose and treat concomitant non-PN causes of hepatobiliary dysfunction

PN, Parenteral nutrition.

Avoid Overfeeding

Excessive quantities of total energy, carbohydrate, fat, and protein should be avoided. The Harris-Benedict equation[61] is useful and practical for predicting basal energy requirements in most patients. Caloric intake by PN of less than 1.2 times the basal energy expenditure as obtained by the Harris-Benedict equation is recommended to reduce hepatic complications.[114] Further, the ratio of non-protein to protein calories should be appropriate for the degree of stress.[271-272] If there is doubt about an individual's caloric requirements, indirect calorimetry can be used to determine resting energy expenditure and respiratory quotient. A respiratory quotient greater than 1.0 indicates that net lipogenesis is occurring and excessive carbohydrate is being administered. However, this result is unusual given that current standards rarely call for long-term administration of PN energy intake at levels more than 1.5 times the estimated basal requirements. Careful clinical assessment, including serial body weights, routine biochemical parameters (e.g., blood glucose, urea nitrogen, electrolytes), and physical examination, is required during long-term PN to assess the adequacy of energy (and protein) administration.

Avoid Excessive Parenteral Lipid Supplementation

Balanced use of lipid supplementation to replace 25 percent to 50 percent of PN carbohydrate intake reduces hepatic steatosis.[67-68] However, when abnormal liver tests develop while the patient is receiving lipid-supplemented TPN, there is little benefit (but potential risk) from increasing the amount of infused lipid.[13,20,273] Infusion of lipid emulsion should not exceed 1 g/kg/day, particularly in patients with permanent intestinal failure.[20] In the presence of lipid intolerance, lipid emulsion should supply a minimum of 4 percent to 8 percent of total calories (2 percent to 4 percent of total calories as linoleic acid) to avoid essential fatty acid deficiency.[105,110-116]

Use Cyclic Rather than Continuous PN Infusion

The incidence of PN-induced cholestasis is reduced with cyclic TPN.[275-276] Cycling PN allows serum glucose concentrations to decrease intermittently, and thereby to prevent prolonged hyperinsulinemia and stimulation of hepatic lipogenesis.[274] Changing patients from continuous to cyclic PN improves abnormal liver enzymes within 2 to 3 weeks.[274-276]

Provide Oral Feeding as Soon as Possible

The safest and surest way to avoid PN-associated hepatic complications is to use the enteral route and minimize PN. Simultaneous enteral feeding with PN reduces hepatic steatosis as compared with TPN alone.[24]

Monitor Liver Tests Periodically

Standard practice of nutritional support includes periodic monitoring of liver-related enzymes in patients on PN. This provides for opportunities to adjust the PN formula and administration with an intention to correct any abnormalities. When abnormalities persist, ultrasonography to monitor hepatic fat content and the biliary system and liver biopsy may be considered. Preexisting liver diseases should be excluded.

Treatment of TPN-associated Hepatobiliary Complications

Various treatments have been proposed to reverse PN-associated hepatobiliary complications (Table 57-7). Many of these were discussed in pathogenesis of various PN-associated hepatobiliary complications, but are briefly summarized in the following section. Most of these treatment options cannot be recommended routinely for lack of data from randomized, blinded clinical trials. However, when the risk of discontinuing PN is greater than continuing it, and the observed abnormalities persist despite following the principles discussed previously, the following therapeutic options may be considered, carefully weighing their potential benefits and risks.

Oral Antibiotics to Diminish Bacterial Overgrowth

Animal studies have shown that antibiotics diminish TPN-associated hepatic steatosis and cholestasis.[142-143,277-278] Metronidazole and gentamicin have been studied in TPN-treated patients to reduce cholestasis,[203-204] but polymyxin B has been studied only in animal models. It is suggested that antibiotics treat bacterial overgrowth within the gut and may diminish circulating levels of endotoxin and TNFα, both of which probably contribute to hepatic steatosis and cholestasis.

TABLE 57-7

Adjunctive Approaches to Prevent or Treat PN-associated Hepatobiliary Complications*

Oral antibiotics to reduce small bowel bacterial overgrowth
Ursodeoxycholic acid (intravenous or oral)
Glutamine supplementation (enteral or parenteral)
Taurine or cysteine supplementation (enteral or parenteral)
Decrease methionine intake
S-adenosyl-L-methionine
Carnitine
Oral lecithin or intravenous choline
Anti-oxidant administration (e.g., vitamin E ± glutamine)
Cholecystokinin
Glucagon
Erythromycin
Cholecystectomy (prophylactic, therapeutic)
Small bowel transplantation
Combined liver–small bowel transplantation

PN, Parenteral nutrition.
*Most of these treatments have not been proven in multi-center, double-blind, randomized controlled trials or are suggested to be beneficial only in anecdotal case reports or animal studies.

Use of Ursodeoxycholic Acid

Ursodeoxycholic acid appears to prevent and even reverse PN-associated cholestasis.[196-198] The efficacy of this drug is probably based on its choleretic and hepatoprotective effects.[279-281] Though promising and safe, larger scale clinical trials will be needed to establish the efficacy of this drug in prevention and treatment of PN-associated cholestasis.

Glutamine Supplementation

Some animal data suggest that supplementation of PN with glutamine will prevent TPN-associated hepatic steatosis.[107] Yeh and associates failed to show any significant benefits of parenteral glutamine supplementation in rats receiving high glucose- or lipid-based TPN.[282-283] On the other hand, Grant and Snyder documented protective effects of parenteral glutamine against TPN-associated hepatic steatosis.[107] No human studies specifically address this, however. A few home infusion agencies in the United States prepare PN solutions with supplemental glutamine. Additional clinical research on the efficacy of this amino acid in PN is needed.

Reduction of Methionine Content

As mentioned previously, infusion of excess methionine can be "toxic" to some patients with hepatic dysfunction.[70] It is suggested, therefore, that the amount of methionine be reduced in PN solutions along with supplementation (enteral or intravenous) of intermediate metabolites (e.g., S-adenosyl-L-methionine, taurine, carnitine) to prevent hepatic cholestasis. These maneuvers are very difficult to achieve in practice given that commercial PN amino acid solutions are available as mixtures. Individualized, custom amino acid components of PN can be prepared, however, by some specialized pharmacies and home infusion networks.

Administration of S-Adenosyl-L-Methionine

Administration of S-adenosyl-L-methionine to animals protects against alcohol,[284] acetaminophen,[285] D-galactosamine,[286] carbon tetrachloride,[287] and ethinyl estradiol toxicity.[288] S-adenosyl-L-methionine given in vivo or in vitro prevents the decrease in bile flow and bile acid secretion and liver damage induced by Cyclosporin A[289] and leukotriene D_4.[290] S-adenosyl-L-methionine treatment preserves membrane adenosinetriphosphatase (ATPase) activities in rats after ligating the common duct and prevents a rise in bilirubin level and transaminases.[291] A preliminary study of S-adenosyl-L-methionine in rats receiving TPN for 5 days showed a preserved bile acid and bile.[292] Further clinical trials are needed to establish the efficacy of this agent in treatment of PN-associated cholestasis.

Supplementation with Carnitine and Taurine

Carnitine deficiency is associated with hepatic steatosis.[119] Taurine deficiency is often found in premature infants and is believed to affect hepatic lipid metabolism.[148-150] Because premature infants tend to be deficient in the enzymes of the transsulfuration pathway, severe deficiency of carnitine or taurine may develop. Taurine and carnitine, therefore, are routinely supplemented in pediatric PN. A carnitine preparation for intravenous administration is available commercially.

Use of Oral Lecithin and Intravenous Choline

Oral lecithin supplementation reverses PN-associated hepatic steatosis in choline-deficient patients.[130-131] Buchman and colleagues showed that intravenous choline administration was effective in reversing hepatic steatosis in patients on chronic PN.[132] Both oral lecithin and intravenous choline supplementation are documented to increase plasma levels of free choline, which may improve hepatic lipid transport and thereby decrease hepatic steatosis.[130-132]

Anti-oxidant Protection with Vitamin E and Other Agents

Potential benefits of anti-oxidant protection via supplementation with vitamin E alone and in combination with other anti-oxidants are based on the idea that tissue injuries are mediated by oxidative stress. No clinical data in PN-associated liver disease are published, although individual anti-oxidants and anti-oxidant "cocktails" are readily available for clinical administration. Further study in this important area is needed.

Use of Cholecystokinin

Use of cholecystokinin to stimulate gallbladder contraction is effective against development of biliary sludge and cholelithiasis in patients on TPN.[293] However, Messing and associates described acute cholecystitis and biliary colic after cholecystokinin infusion in two patients, suggesting that caution is needed regarding use of this agent.[234,248]

Use of Glucagon

TPN infusion increases the ratio of insulin to glucagon in portal blood because of dextrose- and amino acid–induced insulin release, which may promote hepatic steatosis. The simultaneous infusion of glucagon with TPN reversed hepatic steatosis.[103-104] Infusion of glucagon, however, may lead to hyperglycemia by stimulating gluconeogenesis.

Cholecystectomy

Some physicians believe that prophylactic cholecystectomy is indicated if chronic PN is required for patients with preexisting cholelithiasis.[243-245,294] Likewise, prophylactic cholecystectomy may be considered in PN-treated patients who exhibit biliary sludge and cholestasis but not cholelithiasis. These patients have an increased risk of acalculous cholecystitis.[226,294-295]

Small Bowel Transplantation and Combined Liver–Small Bowel Transplantation

Small bowel transplantation is increasing available in academic medical centers and needs to be considered in patients with short-bowel syndrome and PN-associated chronic liver disease.[296] If end-stage liver disease develops while the patient is on PN, combined liver–small bowel transplantation becomes the only treatment option for prolonged survival. Indeed, severe PN-associated liver disease is the leading indication for combined liver-intestinal transplantation.[268-270] Current long-term survival is approximately 50 percent to 75 percent after small bowel transplantation and approximately 40 percent after combined liver–small bowel transplantation.[296-299]

SUMMARY

Hepatobiliary complications of PN are a significant problem in adults and children. Frequently, PN-dependent patients have other acute and chronic risk factors for liver dysfunction, and these likely interact with problems because of PN itself. Major non–PN-related actors that may cause liver dysfunction in parenterally fed patients are shown in Table 57-8.

The risk for liver disease is clearly related to duration of PN therapy and is increased in patients with permanent intestinal failure resulting from short-bowel syndrome. Various hepatobiliary complications of long-term PN have been described, including hepatic steatosis, steatohepatitis, cholestasis, portal fibrosis, cirrhosis, biliary sludge, acalculous cholecystitis, and cholelithiasis. Whereas children manifest primarily cholestatic liver diseases, the adult manifestation is more of steatosis than of cholestasis. It is well recognized that severe PN-associated liver disease of adults and children may lead to hepatic failure. Premature infants on long-term TPN are the most susceptible group.

Although both mortality and morbidity from PN-associated hepatobiliary complications may be decreasing, hepatic failure from severe PN-associated liver disease is the leading indication for combined liver-intestine transplantation.[268]

It is increasingly important to monitor and recognize the earliest signs of PN-associated hepatobiliary complications, especially in those with the highest risk for hepatobiliary complications. No specific pharmacologic or nutritional intervention has been tested rigorously enough to be recommended routinely. However, one or more approaches may be useful in individual patients, as outlined previously. Continued investigations are needed to clarify the efficacy of specific nutritional or pharmacologic interventions and mechanisms for liver disease in patients requiring parenteral feeding.

TABLE 57-8

Common Non-PN–related Causes of Liver Dysfunction and Abnormal Liver Function Tests in Patients Receiving Parenteral Feeding*

Sepsis, infection, or abscess
Dehydration
Positive pressure ventilation
Cholestatic medications
Underlying acute or chronic medical or surgical conditions (e.g., partial biliary obstruction, cholecystitis)

PN, Parenteral nutrition.
*These non-PN-related causes of liver dysfunction are particularly common in hospitalized patients.

References

1. Wilmore DW, Dudrick SJ: Growth and development of an infant receiving all nutrients exclusively by vein. JAMA 203(10):860-864, 1968.
2. Filler RM, Eraklis AJ, Rubin VG, Das JB: Long-term total parenteral nutrition in infants. N Engl J Med 281(11):589-594, 1969.
3. Shils ME, Wright WL, Turnbull A, Brescia F: Long-term parenteral nutrition through an external arteriovenous shunt. N Engl J Med 283(7):341-344, 1970.
4. American Society for Parenteral and Enteral Nutrition: Guidelines for the use of parenteral and enteral nutrition in adults and pediatric patients. J Parenter Enteral Nutr 17(4 suppl):5sa-6sa (III), 1993.
5. Sitzmann J, Pitt H, The Patient Care Committee of the American Gastroenterological Association: Statement on guidelines for total parenteral nutrition. Dig Dis Sci 34(4):489-496, 1989.
6. Howard L, Hassan N: Home parenteral nutrition. 25 years later. Gastroenterol Clin North Am 27(2):481-511, 1998.
7. Howard L, Ament M, Fleming R, et al: Current use and clinical outcome of home parenteral and enteral nutrition therapies in the United States. Gastroenterology 109(2):355-365, 1995.
8. Williams DM: The current state of home nutrition support in the United States. Nutrition 14(4): 416-419, 1998:
9. Howard L, Heaphey L, Flemming CR, et al: Four years of North American registry home parenteral nutrition outcome data and their implications for patient management. J Parenter Enteral Nutr 15(4):384-393, 1991.
10. Buchman AL: Complications of long-term home total parenteral nutrition. Their identification, prevention and treatment. Dig Dis Sci 46(1):1-18, 2001.
11. Peden VH, Witzleben CL, Skelton MA: Total parenteral nutrition. J Pediatr 78(1):180-187, 1971.
12. Bashir RM, Lipman TO: Hepatobiliary toxicity of total parenteral nutrition in adults. Gastroenterol Clin North Am 24(4):1003-1025, 1995.
13. Bowyer BA, Fleming CR, Ludwig J, et al: Does long-term home parenteral nutrition in adult patients cause chronic liver disease? J Parenter Enteral Nutr 9(1):11-17, 1984.
14. Kelly D: Liver complications of pediatric parenteral nutrition—epidemiology. Nutrition 14(1):153-157, 1998.
15. Kubota A, Yonekura T, Hoki M, et al: Total parenteral nutrition-associated intrahepatic cholestasis in infants: 25 years' experience. J Pediatr Surg 35(7):1049-1051, 2000.
16. Quigley EMM, Marsh MN, Shaffer JL, Markin RS: Hepatobiliary complications of total parenteral nutrition. Gastroenterology 104(1):286-301, 1993.
17. Beale EF, Nelson RM, Bucciarelli RL, et al: Intrahepatic cholestasis associated with parenteral nutrition in premature infants. Pediatrics 64:342, 1979.
18. Ricour C, Gorski AM, Goulet O, et al: Home parenteral nutrition in children. 8 years experience with 112 patients. Clin Nutr 9:65, 1990.
19. Suita S: Follow up studies of children treated with long-term intravenous nutrition during the neonatal period. J Pediatr Surg 17:37, 1982.
20. Cavicchi M, Beau P, Crenn P, et al: Prevalence of liver disease and contributing factors in patients receiving home parenteral nutrition for permanent intestinal failure. Ann Intern Med 132(7):525-532, 2000.
21. Benjamin DR: Hepatobiliary dysfunction in infants and children associated with long-term total parenteral nutrition a clinico-pathologic study. Am J Clin Pathol 76:276, 1981.
22. Hodes JE, Grosseld JL, Webert R, et al: Hepatic failure in infants on total parenteral nutrition (TPN): clinical and histologic observations. J Pediatr Surg 17:463, 1982.
23. Colmb BV, Goulet O, Rambau DC, et al: Long-term parenteral nutrition in children; liver and gall bladder disease. Transplant Proc 24:1054, 1992.

24. Zamir O, Nussbaum MS, Bhadra S, et al: Effect of enteral feeding on hepatic steatosis induced by total parenteral nutrition. J Parenter Enteral Nutr 18:20-25, 1994.
25. Ansley-Green A: Plasma hormone concentrations during enteral and parenteral nutrition in the human newborn. J Pediatr Gastroenterol Nutr 2:S108, 1983.
26. Greenberg G, Walman S, Christofides N, et al: Effect of total parenteral nutrition on gut hormone release in humans. Gastroenterology 80:988, 1981.
27. Lucas A, Bloom SR, Aynsley-Green A: Metabolic and endocrine consequences of depriving preterm infants of enteral nutrition. Acta Paediatr Scand 72:245, 1983.
28. Alverdy JC, Oays F, Moss GS: Total parenteral nutrition promotes bacterial translocation from the gut. Surgery 104:185-190, 1988.
29. Rooney JC, Hill DJ, Danks DM: Jaundice associated with bacterial infection in the newborn. Am J Dis Child 122:39, 1971.
30. Noland JP: The role of endotoxin in liver injury. Gastroenterology 69:1346, 1975.
31. Utili R, Abernathy CO, Zimmerman HJ: Cholestatic effects of *Escherichia coli* endotoxin on the isolated perfused rat liver. Gastroenterology 70:248, 1976.
32. Palmer RH, Hruban Z: Production of bile duct hyperplasia and gallstones by lithocholic acid. J Clin Invest 45:1255, 1964.
33. Miyai R, Price VM, Fisher MM: Bile acid metabolism in mammals. Ultra-structural studies on the intrahepatic cholestasis induced by lithocholate and chenodeoxycholic acids in the rat. Lab Invest 24:292, 1971.
34. Fong Y, Marano MA, Barber A, et al: Total parenteral nutrition and bowel rest modify the metabolic responses to endotoxin in humans. Ann Surg 210:449-457, 1989.
35. Saito J, Trocki O, Alexander JW: The effect of route of nutrient administration on the nutritional state, catabolic hormone secretion and gut mucosal integrity after burn injury. J Parenter Enteral Nutr 11:11-24, 1987.
36. Barth RA, Brasch RC, Filly RA: Abdominal pseudotumor in childhood: distended gallbladder with parenteral hyperalimentation. Am J Roentgenol 126:341-343, 1981.
37. Petersen SR, Sheldon GF: Acute acalculous cholecystitis: a complication of hyperalimentation. Am J Surg 138:814-817, 1979.
38. Whitington PF, Black DD: Cholelithiasis in premature infants treated with parenteral nutrition and furosemide. J Pediatr 97:647-649, 1980.
39. Roslyn JJ, Pitt HA, Mann LL, et al: Gallbladder disease in patients on long-term parenteral nutrition. Gastroenterology 84:148-154, 1983.
40. Saad B, Frei K, Scholl FA, et al: Hepatocyte-derived interleukin-6 and tumor-necrosis factor alpha mediate the lipopolysaccharide-induced acute-phase response and nitric oxide release by cultured rat hepatocytes. Eur J Biochem 229:349-355, 1995.
41. Kalfarentzos F, Vagenas K, Spiliotis J, et al: The role of hypoalbuminemia in the development of TPN associated cholestasis. Clin Nutr 5:193, 1986.
42. Nanji A, Anderson F: Relationship between serum albumin and parenteral nutrition associated cholestasis. J Parenter Enteral Nutr 8:438, 1984.
43. Nanji A, Campbell DJ, Pudeck M: Decreased anion gap associated with hypoalbuminemia and polyclonal gammopathy. JAMA 246:859,1981.
44. Stanko RT, Nathan G, Mendelow H, Adibi SA: Development of hepatic cholestasis and fibrosis in patients with massive loss of intestine supported by prolonged parenteral nutrition. Gastroenterology 92:197-202, 1987.
45. Ito Y, Shils ME: Liver dysfunction associated with long-term total parenteral nutrition in patients with massive bowel resection. J Parenter Enteral Nutr 15:271-276, 1991.
46. Messing B, Zarka Y, Lemann M, et al: Chronic cholestasis associated with long-term parenteral nutrition. Transplant Proc 26:1438-1439, 1994 (abstract).
47. Guertin F, Roy CC, Lepage G, et al: Effect of taurine on total parenteral nutrition-associated cholestasis. J Parenter Enteral Nutr 15:247-251, 1991.
48. Belli DC, Fournier LA, Lepage G, et al: Total parenteral nutrition-associated cholestasis in rats: comparison of different amino acid mixtures. J Parenter Enteral Nutr 11:67-73, 1987.
49. Fouin-Fortunet H, Le Quernec L, Erlinger S, et al: Hepatic alterations during total parenteral nutrition in patients with inflammatory bowel disease: a possible consequence of lithocholate toxicity. Gastroenterology 82:932-937, 1982.
50. Klein S, Nealon WH: Hepatobiliary abnormalities associated with total parenteral nutrition. Semin Liver Dis 8(2):237-246, 1988.
51. Nanji AA, Anderson FH: Sensitivity and specificity of liver function tests in the detection of parenteral nutrition-associated cholestasis. J Parenter Enteral Nutr 9:307-308, 1985.
52. Robertson JFR, Garden OJ, Shenkin A: Intravenous nutrition and hepatic dysfunction. J Parenter Enteral Nutr 10:172-176, 1986.
53. Abad-Lacruz A, Gonzalez-Huix F, Esteve M, et al: Liver function test abnormalities in patients with inflammatory bowel disease receiving artificial nutrition: a prospective randomized study of total enteral nutrition vs. total parenteral nutrition. J Parenter Enteral Nutr 14:618-621, 1990.
54. Grant JP, Cox CE, Kleinman LM, et al: Serum hepatic enzyme and bilirubin elevations during parenteral nutrition. Surg Gynecol Obstet 145:573-580, 1977.
55. Lindor KD, Fleming CR, Abrams A, Hirschkorn MA: Liver function values in adults receiving total parenteral nutrition. JAMA 241:2398-2400, 1979.
56. Bengoa JM, Hanauer SB, Sitrin MD, et al: Pattern and prognosis of liver function test abnormalities in patients with inflammatory bowel disease. Hepatology 5(1)79-84, 1985.
57. Sheldon GF, Petersen SR, Sanders R: Hepatic dysfunction during hyperalimentation. Arch Surg 113:504-508, 1978.
58. Host WR, Serlin O, Rush BF: Hyperalimentation in cirrhotic patients. Am J Surg 123:57-62, 1977.
59. Wagman LD, Burt ME, Brennan MF: The impact of total parenteral nutrition on liver function tests in patients with cancer. Cancer 49(6):1249-1257, 1982.
60. Lowry SF, Brennan MF: Abnormal liver function during parenteral nutrition: relation to infusion excess. J Surg Res 26:300-307, 1979.
61. Harris JA, Benedict FG: A Biometric Study of Basal Metabolism in Man. Washington, DC, Carnegie Institute of Washington, 1919.
62. MacFayden BV, Dudrick SJ, Baquero G, et al: Clinical and biochemical changes in liver function during intravenous hyperalimentation. J Parenter Enteral Nutr 3:438-443, 1979.
63. Baker AL, Rosenberg IH: Hepatic complications of total parenteral nutrition. Am J Med 82:489-497, 1987.
64. Carpentier YA, Van Brandt M: Effect of total parenteral nutrition on liver function. Acta Chir Belg 80(2-3):141-144, 1981.
65. Tulikoura I, Huikuri K: Morphological fatty changes and function of the liver, serum free fatty acids, and triglycerides during parenteral nutrition. Scand J Gastroenterol 17(2):177-185, 1982.
66. Wagner WH, Lowry AC, Silberman H: Similar liver function abnormalities occur in patients receiving glucose-based and lipid-based parenteral nutrition. Am J Gastroenterol 78(4):1999-2002, 1983.
67. Meguid MM, Akahoshi MP, Jeffers S, et al: Amelioration of metabolic complications of conventional total parenteral nutrition. A prospective randomized study. Arch Surg 119(11):1294-1298, 1984.
68. Buchmiller CE, Kelinman-Wexler RL, Ephgrave KS, et al: Liver dysfunction and energy source: results of a randomized clinical trial. J Parenter Enteral Nutr 17:301-306, 1993.
69. Clarke PJ, Ball MJ, Kettlewell MG: Liver function tests in patients receiving parenteral nutrition. J Parenter Enteral Nutr 15:54-59, 1991.
70. Moss RL, Amii LA: New approaches to understanding the etiology and treatment of total parenteral nutrition-associated cholestasis. Semin Ped Surg 8(3):140-147, 1999.
71. Postuma R, Trevenen CL: Liver disease in infants receiving total parenteral nutrition. Pediatrics 94:296-298, 1979.
72. Dahms BB, Halpin TC: Serial liver biopsies in parenteral nutrition-associated cholestasis of early infancy. Gastroenterology 81:136-144, 1981.
73. Bell RL, Ferry GD, Smith EO, et al: Parenteral nutrition-related cholestasis in infants. J Parenter Enteral Nutr 10:356-359, 1986.
74. Cohen C, Olsen MM: Pediatric total parenteral nutrition. Liver histopathology. Arch Pathol Lab Med 105:152-156, 1981.
75. Craig RM, Newmann T, Jeejeebhoy KN, Yokoo H: Severe hepatocellular reaction resembling alcoholic hepatitis with cirrhosis after massive small bowel resection and prolonged total parenteral nutrition. Gastroenterology 79:131-137, 1980.

76. Goplerud JM: Hyperalimentation associated hepatotoxicity in the newborn. Ann Clin Lab Sci 22(2):79-84, 1992.
77. Maini B, Blackburn GL, Bistrian BR, et al: Cyclic hyperalimentation: an optimal technique for preservation of visceral protein. J Surg Res 20:515-525, 1976.
78. Buzby GP, Mullen JL, Stein TP, Rosato EF: Manipulation of TPN caloric substrate and fatty infiltration of the liver. J Surg Res 31:46-54, 1981.
79. Stein TP, Buzby GP, Leskiev MJ, et al: Protein and fat metabolism in rats during repletion with total parenteral nutrition. J Nutr 111:154-165, 1981.
80. Boelhouwer RV, King WWK, Kingsnorth AN, et al: Fat-based (Intralipid 20%) versus carbohydrate-based total parenteral nutrition: Effects on hepatic structure and function in rats. J Parenter Enteral Nutr 7:530-533, 1983.
81. Meurling S, Roos KA: Liver changes in rats on continuous and intermittent parenteral nutrition with and without fat (Intralipid 20%). Acta Chir Scand 147:475-480, 1981.
82. Haines NW, Baker AL, Boyer JL, et al: Prognostic indicators of hepatic injury following jejunoileal bypass performed for refractory obesity: a prospective study. Hepatology 1:161-167, 1981.
83. Nasrallah SM, Nassar VH, Galambos JT: Importance of terminal hepatic venule thickening. Arch Pathol Lab Med 104:84-86, 1980.
84. Van Wass L, Lieber CS: Early perivenular sclerosis in alcoholic fatty liver: an index of progressive liver injury. Gastroenterology 73:646-650, 1977.
85. Black DD, Sutle EA, Whitington PF, et al: The effect of short term total parenteral nutrition on hepatic function in the human neonate; a prospective randomized study demonstrating alteration of hepatic canalicular function. J Pediatr 99(3):445-449, 1981.
86. Whitington PF: Cholestasis associated with total parenteral nutrition in infants. Hepatology 84:1055-1058, 1983.
87. Suchy FJ, Balisteri WF, Heubi JE, et al: Physiologic cholestasis: elevation of the primary serum bile acid concentrations in normal infants. Gastroenterology 80:1037-1041, 1981.
88. Angelico M, Guardia PD: Review article: hepatobiliary complications associated with total parenteral nutrition. Aliment Pharmacol Ther 14(2):54-57, 2000.
89. Touloukian RJ, Downing SE: Cholestasis associated with longterm parenteral hyperalimentation. Arch Surg 106(1):58-62, 1973.
90. Brown MR, Putnam TC: Cholestasis associated with central intravenous nutrition in infants. NY State J Med 78(1):27-30, 1978.
91. Nanji AA, Anderson FH: Cholestasis associated with parenteral nutrition develops more commonly with hematologic malignancy than with inflammatory bowel disease. J Parenter Enteral Nutr 8(3):325, 1984.
92. Vileisis RA, Sorensen K, Gonzalez-Crussi F, Hunt CE: Liver malignancy after parenteral nutrition. J Pediatr 100(1):88-90, 1982.
93. Ghoshal AK, Farber E: The induction of liver cancer by dietary deficiency of choline and methionine without added carcinogens. Carcinogenesis 5(10):1367-1370, 1984.
94. Yokoyama S, Sells MA, Reddy TV, Lombardi B: Hepatocarcinogenic and promoting action of a choline-devoid diet in the rat. Cancer Res 45(6):2834-2842, 1985.
95. Hall RI, Grant JP, Ross LH, et al: Pathogenesis of hepatic steatosis in the parenterally fed rat. J Clin Invest 74:1658-1668, 1984.
96. Chang S, Silvis SE: Fatty liver produced by hyperalimentation of rats. Am J Gastroenterol 62:410-418, 1974.
97. Burke JF, Wolfe RR, Mullany CJ, et al: Glucose requirements following burn injury. Parameters of optimal glucose infusion and possible hepatic and respiratory abnormalities following excessive glucose intake. Ann Surg 190(3):274-285, 1990.
98. Spiliotis JD, Kalfarentzos F: Total parenteral nutrition-associated liver dysfunction. Nutrition 10(3):255-260, 1994.
99. Kaminski DL, Adams A, Jellinek M: The effect of hyperalimentation on hepatic lipid content and lipogenic enzyme activity in rats and man. Surgery 88(1):93-100, 1980.
100. Meguid MM, Chen T-Y, Yang Z-J, et al: Effects of continuous graded total parenteral nutrition on feeding indexes and metabolic concomitants in rats. Am J Physol 260:E126-E140, 1991.
101. Campos AC, Oler A, Meguid MM, Chen T-Y: Liver biochemical and histological changes with graded amounts of total parenteral nutrition. Arch Surg 125:447-450, 1990.
102. Li S, Nussbaum MS, Teague D, et al: Increasing dextrose concentrations in total parenteral nutrition (TPN) causes alterations in hepatic morphology and plasma levels of insulin and glucagon in rats. J Surg Res 44:639-648, 1988.
103. Li S, Nussbaum MS, McFadden DW, et al: Addition of glucagon to total parenteral nutrition (TPN) prevents hepatic steatosis in rats by addition of glucagon to total parenteral nutrition (TPN). Surgery 104:350-357, 1988.
104. Li S, Nussbaum MS, McFadden DW, et al: Reversal of hepatic steatosis in rats by addition of glucagon to total parenteral nutrition (TPN). J Surg Res 46:557-566, 1989.
105. Nussbaum MS, Li S, Bower RH, et al: Addition of lipid to total parenteral nutrition prevents hepatic steatosis in rats by lowering the portal venous insulin/glucagon ratio. J Parenter Enteral Nutr 102:1262-1370, 1992.
106. Li S, Nussbaum MS, McFadden DW, et al: Addition of L-glutamine to total parenteral nutrition and its effects on portal insulin and glucagons and the development of hepatic steatosis in rats. J Surg Res 48(5):421-426, 1990.
107. Grant JP, Snyder PJ: Use of L-glutamine in total parenteral nutrition. J Surg Res 44(5):506-513, 1988.
108. Sax HC, Talamini MA, Bracket K, et al: Hepatic steatosis in total parenteral nutrition: Failure of fatty infiltration to correlate with abnormal serum hepatic enzyme levels. Surgery 100:697-703, 1986.
109. Machilin L, Bendich A: Free radical tissue damage: protective role of antioxidant nutrients. FASEB J 1:441-445, 1987.
110. Barr LH, Dunn GD, Brennan MF: Essential fatty acid deficiency during total parenteral nutrition. Ann Surg 193:304-311, 1981
111. Langer B, McHattie JD, Zohrab WJ, Jeejeebhoy KN: Prolonged survival after complete small bowel resection using intravenous alimentation at home. J Surg Res 15:226-233, 1973.
112. Richardson TJ, Sgoutas D: Essential fatty acid deficiency in four adult patients during total parenteral nutrition. Am J Clin Nutr 28:258-263, 1975.
113. McDonald ATJ, Philips MJ, Jeejeebhoy KN: Reversal of fatty liver by Intralipid in patients on total parenteral nutrition. Gastroenterology 64:885, 1973 (abstract).
114. Reif S, Tano M, Oliverio R, et al: Total parenteral nutrition-induced steatosis: reversal by parenteral lipid infusion. J Parenter Enteral Nutr 15(1):102-104, 1991.
115. Faulkner WJ, Flint LM: Essential fatty acid deficiency associated with total parenteral nutrition. Surg Gynecol Obstet 144(5):665-667, 1977.
116. Tashiro T, Ogata H, Yokoyama H, et al: The effect of fat emulsion (Intralipid) on essential fatty acid deficiency in infants receiving intravenous alimentation. J Pediatr Surg 11(4):505-515, 1976.
117. Cook GC, Hutt MSR: The liver after kwashiorkor. BMJ 3:454-457, 1967.
118. Tao RL, Yoshimura NN: Carnitine metabolism and its application in parenteral nutrition. J Parenter Enteral Nutr 4:469-486, 1980.
119. Karpati G, Carpenter S, Engel AG, et al: The syndrome of systemic carnitine deficiency: Clinical, morphologic, biochemical and pathophysiologic features. Neurology (Minneap) 25:16-24, 1975.
120. Bowyer BA, Fleming CR, Ilstrup DM, et al: Plasma and hepatic carnitine levels and patients receiving home parenteral nutrition. Am J Clin Nutr 43:85-91, 1986.
121. Bowyer BA, Miles JM, Haymond MW, et al: L-carnitine therapy in home parenteral nutrition patients with abnormal liver tests and low plasma carnitine concentrations. Gastroenterology 94:434-438, 1988.
122. Bowyer BA, Fleming CR, Haymond MW, Miles JM: L-carnitine: effect of intravenous administration on fuel homeostasis in normal subjects and home-parenteral-nutrition patients with low plasma carnitine concentrations. Am J Clin Nutr 49:618-623, 1989.
123. Yao Z, Vance DE: Head group specificity in the requirement of phosphatidylcholine biosynthesis for very low density lipoprotein secretion from cultured hepatocytes. J Biol Chem 264:11373, 1989.
124. Yao Z, Vance DE: The active synthesis of phosphatidylcholine is required for very low density lipoprotein secretion from rat hepatocytes. J Biol Chem 263:2998, 1988.
125. Lombardi B, Pani P, Schlunk FF: Choline-deficiency fatty liver: impaired release of hepatic triglycerides. J Lipid Res 9(4):437-446, 1968.
126. Zeisel SH: Choline: an essential nutrient for humans. Nutrition 16(7-8):669-671, 2000.
127. Chawla RK, Wolf DC, Kutner MH, et al: Choline may be an essential nutrient in malnourished patients with cirrhosis. Gastroenterology 97(6):1514-1520, 1989.

128. Sheard NF, Tayek JA, Bistrian BR, et al: Plasma choline concentration in humans fed parenterally. Am J Clin Nutr 43(2):219-224, 1986.
129. Burt ME, Hanin I, Brennan MF: Choline deficiency associated with parenteral nutrition. Lancet 2:638-639, 1980.
130. Buchman AL, Dubin M, Jenden D, et al: Lecithin increases plasma free choline and decreases hepatic steatosis in long-term total parenteral nutrition patients. Gastroenterology 102:1363-1370, 1992.
131. Demetriou AA: Lecithin increases plasma free choline and decreases hepatic steatosis in long-term total parenteral nutrition patients. J Parenter Enteral Nutr 16(5):487-488, 1992.
132. Buchman AL, Dubin MD, Moukarzel AA, et al: Choline deficiency: a cause of hepatic steatosis during parenteral nutrition that can be reversed with intravenous choline supplementation. Hepatology 22(5):1399-1403, 1995:
133. Martins FM, Wennberg A, Kihlberg R, et al: Total parenteral nutrition with different ratios of fat/carbohydrate at two entry levels: An animal study. J Parenter Enteral Nutr 9:47-52, 1985.
134. Boelhouwer RV, King WWK, Kingsnorth AN, et al: Fat-based (Intralipid 20%) versus carbohydrate-based total parenteral nutrition: effects on hepatic structure and function in rats. J Parenter Enteral Nutr 7:530-533, 1983.
135. Meurling S, Roos KA: Liver changes in rats on continuous and intermittent parenteral nutrition with and without fat (Intralipid 20%). Acta Chir Scand 147:475-480, 1981.
136. Martins FM, Wennberg A, Meurling S, et al: Serum lipids and fatty acid and composition of tissues in rats on total parenteral nutrition (TPN). Lipids 19:728-737, 1984.
137. Degott C, Messing B, Moreau D, et al: Liver phospholipidosis induced by parenteral nutrition: histologic, histochemical, and ultrastructural investigations. Gastroenterology 95(1):183-191, 1988
138. Deitch EA: The role of intestinal barrier failure and bacterial translocation in the development of systemic infection and multiple organ failure. Arch Surg 125(3):403-404, 1990.
139. Deitch EA, Winterton J, Berg R: Effect of starvation, malnutrition, and trauma on the gastrointestinal tract flora and bacterial translocation. Arch Surg 122:1019-1024, 1987.
140. Deitch EA, Xu D, Berg RD: Bacterial translocation from the gut impairs systemic immunity. Surgery 109(3):69-76, 1991.
141. Freund H: Abnormalities of liver function and hepatic damage associated with total parenteral nutrition. Nutrition 7(1):1-5, 1991.
142. Pappo I, Becovier H, Berry EM, Freund HR; Polymyxin B reduces cecal flora, TNF production and hepatic steatosis during total parenteral nutrition in the rat. J Surg Res 51(2):106-112, 1991.
143. Pappo I, Bercovier H, Berry EM, et al: Polymyxin B reduces total parenteral nutrition-associated hepatic steatosis by its antibacterial activity and by blocking deleterious effects of lipopolysaccharide. J Parenter Enteral Nutr 16(6):529-532, 1992.
144. Pappo I, Bercovier H, Berry E, et al: Antitumor necrosis factor antibodies reduce hepatic steatosis during total parenteral nutrition and bowel rest in the rat. J Parenter Enteral Nutr 19(1):80-82, 1995.
145. Drenick EJ, Fisher J, Johnson D: Hepatic steatosis after intestinal bypass—prevention and reversal by metronidazole, irrespective of protein-calorie malnutrition. Gastroenterology 83:535-548, 1982.
146. Lambert JR, Thomas SM: Metronidazole prevention of serum liver enzyme abnormalities during total parenteral nutrition. J Parenter Enteral Nutr 9(4):501-503, 1985.
147. Freund HR, Muggia-Sullam M, Berry EM, et al: Total parenteral nutrition and bowel rest result in change of cecal flora but not increased bacterial translocation. Surg Res Commun 7:357, 1990.
148. Chesney RW, Helms RA, Christensen M, et al: The role of taurine in infant nutrition. Adv Exp Med Biol 442:453-476, 1998.
149. Vina J, Vento M, Garcia-Sala F. et al. L-cysteine and glutathione metabolism are impaired in premature infants due to cystathionase deficiency. Am J Clin Nutr 61(5):1067-1069, 1995.
150. Yan CC, Bravo E, Cantafora A: Effect of taurine levels on liver lipid metabolism: an in vivo study in the rat. Proc Soc Exp Biol Med 202(1):88-96, 1993.
151. Narkewicz MR, Caldwell S, Jones G: Cysteine supplementation and reduction of total parenteral-nutrition-induced hepatic lipid accumulation in the weanling rat. J Pediatr Gastroenterol Nutr 21(2)18-24, 1995.
152. Lilly JR, Sokol RJ: On the bile sludge syndrome or is total parenteral nutrition cholestasis a surgical disease? Pediatrics 76:992-993, 1985.
153. Presig R, Rennert O: Biliary transport and cholestatic effects of amino acids (abstr). Gastroenterology 73:1240, 1977.
154. King WW, Boelhouwer RU, Kingsnorth AN, et al: Nutritional efficacy and hepatic changes during intragastric, intravenous and pre-hepatic feeding in rats. J Parenter Enteral Nutr 7:443-446, 1983.
155. Merritt RJ, Sinatra FR, Henton DH, Neustein H: Cholestatic effect of intraperitoneal administration of tryptophan to suckling rat pups. Pediatr Res 18:904-907, 1984.
156. Vileisis RA, Inwood RJ, Hunt CE: Prospective controlled study of parenteral nutrition-associated cholestatic jaundice: effect of protein intake. J Pediatr 96:893-897, 1980.
157. Brown MR, Thunberg BJ, Golub JB, et al: Decreased cholestasis with enteral instead of intravenous protein in the very low-birth weight infant. J Pediatr Gastroenterol Nutr 9:21-27, 1989.
158. Klein GL, Sedman AB, Heyman MB, et al: Hepatic abnormalities associated with aluminum loading in piglets. J Parenter Enteral Nutr 11:293-297, 1987.
159. Klein GL, Heyman MB, Lee TC, et al: Aluminum associated hepatobiliary dysfunction in rats: relationships to dosage and duration of exposure. Pediatr Res 23:275-278, 1988.
160. Klein GL, Barquist WE, Ament ME, et al: Hepatic aluminum accumulation in children on total parenteral nutrition. J Pediatr Gastroenterol Nutr 3:740-743, 1984.
161. Klein GL: The aluminum content of parenteral solutions: current status. Nutr Rev 49:74-79, 1991.
162. Klein GL, Alfrey AC, Miller NL, et al: Aluminum loading during total parenteral nutrition. Am J Clin Nutr 35:1425-1429, 1982.
163. Benevenga NJ: Toxicities of methionine and other amino acids. J Agric Food Chem 22:2-9, 1974.
164. Hardwick DF, Applegarth DA, Cockroft DM, et al: Pathogenesis of methionine induced toxicity. Metabolism 19:381-391, 1970.
165. Moss RL, Das JB, Ansari G: Hepatobiliary dysfunction during total parenteral nutrition is caused by infusate, not the route of administration. J Ped Surg 28:391-396, 1993.
166. Corrares F, Ochoa P, Rivas C, et al: Inhibition of glutathione synthesis in the liver leads to S-adenosyl-L-methionine synthetase reduction. Hepatology 14:528-533, 1992.
167. Duce AM, Ortiz P, Cabrero C, et al: S-adenosyl-L-methionine synthetase reduction. Hepatology 8:65-68, 1988.
168. Horowitz JH, Rypins EB, Henderson JM, et al: Evidence for impairment of the trans-sulfuration pathway in cirrhosis. Gastroenterology 81:668-675, 1981.
169. Zlotkin SH, Anderson GH: The development of cystathionase activity during the first year of life. Pediatr Res 16(1):65-68, 1982.
170. Rigo J, Senterre J: Is taurine essential for neonates? Biol Neonate 32:73-76, 1977.
171. Dorvil NP, Yousef IM, Tuchweber B, Roy CC: Taurine prevents cholestasis induced by lithocholate acid sulfate in guinea pigs. Am J Clin Nutr 37:221-232, 1983.
172. Belli DC, Roy CC, Fournier L-A, et al: The effect of taurine on the cholestatic potential of sulfated lithocholate and its conjugates. Liver 11:162-169, 1991.
173. Geggel HS, Ament ME, Heckenlively JR, et al: Nutritional requirement for taurine in patients receiving long-term parenteral nutrition. N Engl J Med 312(3):142-146, 1985.
174. Okamoto E, Rassin DK, Zucker CL, et al: Role of taurine in feeding the low birth-weight infant. J Pediatr 104:936-940, 1984.
175. Wang W-Y, Liaw K-Y: Effect of a taurine-supplemented diet on conjugated bile acids in biliary surgical patients. J Parenter Enteral Nutr 15:294-297, 1991.
176. Allardyce DB, Slavian AJ, Quenville NF: Cholestatic jaundice during total parenteral nutrition. Can J Surg 21:332-339, 1978.
177. Salvian AJ, Allardyce DB: Impaired bilirubin secretion during total parenteral nutrition. J Surg Res 28:547-555, 1978.
178. Allardyce DB: Cholestasis caused by lipid emulsions. Surg Gynecol Obstet 154:641-647, 1982.
179. Klein GL, Rivera D: Adverse metabolic consequences of total parenteral nutrition. Cancer 55(1 suppl):305-308, 1985.
180. Fisher RL: Hepatobiliary abnormalities associated with total parenteral nutrition. Gastroenterol Clin North Am 18(3):645-666, 1989.
181. Palombo JD, Schnure F, Bistrian BR, et al: Improvement of liver function tests by administration of L-carnitine to a carnitine-deficient patient receiving home parenteral nutrition: a case report. J Parenter Enteral Nutr 11(1):88-92, 1987.

182. Worthley LI, Fishlock RC, Snoswell AM: Carnitine deficiency with hyperbilirubinemia, generalized skeletal muscle weakness and reactive hypoglycemia in a patient on long-term total parenteral nutrition: treatment with intravenous L-carnitine. J Parenter Enteral Nutr 7(2):176-180, 1983.
183. Korpela H, Nuutinen LS, Kumpulainen J: Low serum selenium and glutathione peroxidase activity in patients receiving short-term total parenteral nutrition. Int J Vitam Nutr Res. 59(1):80-84, 1989.
184. Cohen HJ, Brown MR, Hamilton D, et al: Glutathione peroxidase and selenium deficiency in patients receiving home parenteral nutrition: time course for development of deficiency and repletion of enzyme activity in plasma and blood cells. Am J Clin Nutr 49(1):132-139, 1989.
185. Kauppila A, Korpela H, Makila UM, Yrjanheikki E: Low serum selenium concentration and glutathione peroxidase activity in intrahepatic cholestasis of pregnancy. BMJ 294(6565):150-152, 1987.
186. Sokol RJ: Fat-soluble vitamins and their importance in patient with cholestatic liver diseases. Gastroenterol Clin North Am 23(4)673-705, 1994.
187. Messing B, De Oliveira FJ, Galian A, Bernier JJ: Cholestase au cours de la nutrition parenterale totale: mise en evidence de facteurs favorisants; association a une lithiase vesiculaire. Gastroenterol Clin Biol 6:740-747, 1982.
188. Hofmann AF: Defective biliary secretion during total parenteral nutrition: probable mechanisms and possible solutions. J Pediatr Gastroenterol Nutr 20(4):376-390, 1995.
189. Briones ER, Iber FL: Liver and biliary tract changes and injury associated with total parenteral nutrition: pathogenesis and prevention. J Am Col Nutr 14(3):219-228, 1995.
190. Carey MC, Cahalane MJ: Wither biliary sludge? Gastroenterology 95:508-523, 1988.
191. Teitelbaum DH, Han-Markey T, Schumacher RE: Treatment of parenteral nutrition-associated cholestasis with cholecystokinin-octapeptide. J Pediatr Surg 30(7):1082-1085, 1995.
192. Rintala RJ, Lindahl H, Pohjavuori M: Total parenteral nutrition-associated cholestasis in surgical neonates may be reversed by intravenous cholecystokinin: a preliminary report. J Pediatr Surg 30(6):827-830, 1995.
193. Teitelbaum DH, Han-Markey T, Drongowski RA, et al: Use of cholecystokinin to prevent the development of parenteral nutrition-associated cholestasis. J Parenter Enteral Nutr 21(2):100-103, 1997.
194. Campos AC, Oler A, Meguid MM, Chen TY: Liver biochemical and histological changes with graded amounts of total parenteral nutrition. Arch Surg 125:447-450, 1990.
195. Whalen GF, Shamberger RC, Perez-Atayde A, Folkman J: A proposed cause for the hepatic dysfunction associated with parenteral nutrition. J Pediatr Surg 25:622-626, 1990.
196. Lindor KD, Burnes J: Ursodeoxycholic acid for the treatment of home parenteral nutrition-associated cholestasis. A case report. Gastroenterology 101:250-253, 1991.
197. Duerksen DR, Van Aerde JE, Gramlich L, et al: Intravenous ursodeoxycholic acid reduces cholestasis in parenterally fed newborn piglets. Gastroenterology 111:1111-1117, 1996.
198. Spagnuolo MI, Iorio R, Vegnente A, Guarino A: Ursodeoxycholic acid for treatment of cholestasis in children on long-term total parenteral nutrition: a pilot study. Gastroenterology 111(3):716-719, 1996.
199. Cooper A, Ross AJ, O'Neill JA, et al: Resolution of intractable cholestasis associated with total parenteral nutrition following biliary irrigation. J Pediatr Surg 20:772-774, 1985.
200. Rintala R, Lindahl H, Pohjavuori M, et al: Surgical treatment of intractable cholestasis associated with total parenteral nutrition in premature infants. J Pediatr Surg 28:716-719, 1993.
201. Keller GA, West MA, Cerra FB, et al: Multiple systems organ failure. Modulation of hepatocyte protein synthesis by endotoxin activated Kupffer cells. Ann Surg 201:87-95, 1985.
202. Nolan JP: Intestinal endotoxins as mediators of hepatic injury—an idea whose time has come again. Hepatology 10:887-891, 1989.
203. Capron JP, Gineston JL, Herve MA, Braillon A: Metronidazole in prevention of cholestasis associated with total parenteral nutrition. Lancet 1(8322):446-447, 1983.
204. Spurr SG, Grylack LJ, Mehta NR: Hyperalimentation-associated neonatal cholestasis: effect of oral gentamicin. J Parenter Enteral Nutr 13(6):633-636, 1989.
205. Alverdy JC, Aoys F, Moss GS: Total parenteral nutrition promotes bacterial translocation from the gut. Surgery 104:185-190, 1988.
206. Spaeth G, Berg RD, Specian RD, Deitch EA: Food without fiber promotes bacterial translocation from the gut. Surgery 108:240-247, 1990.
207. Spaeth G, Specian RD, Berg RD, Deitch EA: Bulk prevents bacterial translocation induced by the oral administration of total parenteral nutrition solution. J Parenter Enteral Nutr 14:442-447, 1990.
208. Souba WW, Klimberg VS, Plumley DA, et al: The role of glutamine in maintaining a healthy gut and supporting the metabolic response to injury and infection. J Surg Res 48:383-391, 1990.
209. Alverdy JA, Aoys E, Weiss-Carrington P, Burke DA: The effect of glutamin-enriched TPN on gut immune cellularity. J Surg Res 52:34-38, 1992.
210. Li J, Kudsk KA, Janu P, Renegar KB: Effect of glutamin-enriched total parenteral nutrition on small intestinal gut-associated lymphoid tissue and upper respiratory tract immunity. Surgery 121(5): 542-549, 1997.
211. Kudsk KA, Wu Y, Fukatsu K, et al: Glutamine-enriched total parenteral nutrition maintains intestinal interleukin-4 and mucosal immunoglobulin A levels. J Parenter Enteral Nutr 24(5):274-275, 2000.
212. Feldhaus S, Gerok W: Influence of hydroxylation and conjugation of bile salts on their membrane damaging properties. Studies on isolated hepatocytes and lipid membrane vesicles. Hepatology 4:661-666, 1984.
213. Mizoguchi Y, Kodama C, Sakagami Y, et al: Effect of bile acids on liver cell injury by cultured supplement of activated liver adherent cells. Gastroenterol Jpn 24:25-30, 1989.
214. Trauner M, Fickert P, Stauber RE: Inflammation-induced cholestasis. J Gastroenterol Hepatol 14(10):946-959, 1999.
215. Nanji AA, Anderson FH: Cholestasis associated with parenteral nutrition develops more commonly with hemorrhagic malignancy than with inflammatory bowel disease. J Parenter Enteral Nutr 8(3):325, 1984.
216. Forbush B, Kiristioglu I, Teitelbaum DH, et al: Multi-drug resistance 2 gene expression in the murine liver: relevance to the development of parenteral nutrition-associated cholestasis. Gastroenterology 114(suppl):124, 1998 (abstract).
217. Lomri N, Fitz JG, Scharschmidt BF: Hepatocellular transport: role of ATP-binding cassette proteins. Semin Liver Dis 16(2):201-210, 1996.
218. Smit JJ, Schinkel AH, Oude Elferink RR, et al: Homozygous disruption of the murine mdr-2 P-glycoprotein gene leads to a complete absence of phospholipid from bile and to liver disease. Cell 75:451-462, 1993.
219. Van den Bosch H, Schutgens RB, Wanders RJ, Tager JM: Biochemistry of peroxisomes. Annu Rev Biochem 61:157-197, 1992.
220. Piquette-Miller M, Pak A, Kim H, Shazamani A: Decreased expression and activity of P-glycoprotein in rat liver during acute inflammation. Pharm Res 15:706-711, 1998.
221. Van Nieuwkerk CM, Elferink RP, Groen AK, et al: Effects of ursodeoxycholate and cholate feeding on liver disease in FVB mice with a disrupted mdr2 P-glycoprotein gene. Gastroenterology 111:165-171, 1996.
222. Scott-Conner CE, Grogan JB: The pathophysiology of biliary obstruction and its effect on phagocytic and immune function. J Surg Res 57:316-336, 1994.
223. Innes GK, Nagafuchi Y, Fuller BJ, Hobbs KE: Increased expression of major histocompatibility antigens in the liver as a result of cholestasis. Transplantation 45:749-752, 1988.
224. Van Devenster SJ, ten Cate JW, Tytgat GN: Intestinal endotoxemia. Clinical significance. Gastroenterology 94:825-831, 1988.
225. Fischer GW, Hunter KW, Wilson SR, Mease AD: Diminished bacterial defenses with Intralipid. Lancet 2:819-820, 1980.
226. Anderson JL: Acalculous cholecystitis. A possible complication of parenteral nutrition. Report of a case. Med Ann DC 41:448-450, 1972.
227. Roslyn JJ, Barquist WE, Pitt HA, et al: Increased risk of gallstones in children receiving total parenteral nutrition. Pediatrics 71:784-789, 1983.
228. Farrell MK, Balistreri WF: Parenteral nutrition and hepatobiliary dysfunction. Clin Perinatol 13:197-212, 1986.
229. Flati G, Flat D, Jonsson PE, et al: Role of cholesterol and calcium bilirubinate crystals in acute postoperative acalculous cholecystitis. Ital J Surg Sci 14:333-336, 1984.
230. Deitch EA, Engel JM: Acute acalculous cholecystitis. Am J Surg 142:290-293, 1981.

231. Petersen SR, Sheldon GF: Acute acalculous cholecystitis: a complication of hyperalimentation. Am J Surg 138:814-815, 1979.
232. Pitt HA, King W, Mann L, et al: Increased risk of cholelithiasis with prolonged total parenteral nutrition. Am J Surg 145:106-112, 1983.
233. Orlando R, Gleason E, Drezner AD: Acute acalculous cholecystitis. Ital J Surg Sci 14:333-334, 1984.
234. Messing B, Bones C, Kunstlinger F, Bernier JJ: Does total parenteral nutrition induce gallbladder sludge formation and lithiasis? Gastroenterology 84:1012-1019, 1983.
235. Liechty EA, Cohen MD, Lemon JA, et al: Normal gallbladder appearing as abdominal mass in neonates. J Dis Child136:468-469, 1982.
236. Saldana RL, Stein CA, Kopelman AE: Gallbladder distention in ill premature infants. Am J Dis Child 137:1179-1180, 1983.
237. Manji N, Bistrian BR, Mascioli EA, et al: Gallstone disease in patients with severe short bowel syndrome dependent on parenteral nutrition. J Parenter Enteral Nutr 13(5):461-464, 1989.
238. O'Brien CB, Berman JM, Fleming CR, et al: Total parenteral nutrition gallstones contain more calcium bilirubinate than sickle cell gallstones. Gastroenterology 90:1752, 1986 (abstract).
239. Soloway RD, Trotman BW, Maddrey WC, Nakayama F: Pigment gallstone composition in patients with hemolysis or infection/stasis. Dig Dis Sci 31:454-460, 1986.
240. Allen B, Bernhoft R, Blanckaert N, et al: Sludge is calcium bilirubinate associated with bile stasis. Am J Surg 141:51-56, 1981.
241. Stewart L, Smith AL, Pellegrini CA, et al: Pigment of gallstones form as a composite of bacterial microcolonies and pigment solids. Ann Surg 206:242-250, 1987.
242. Holzback RT: Gallbladder stasis. Consequence of long-term parenteral hyperalimentation and risk factor for cholelithiasis. Gastroenterology 84:1055-1058, 1983.
243. Bower R, Mrdeza MA, Block GE: Association of cholecystitis and parenteral nutrition. Nutrition 6(2):125-130, 1990.
244. Roslyn JJ, Pitt HA, Mann L, et al: Parenteral nutrition-induced gallbladder disease: a reason for early cholecystectomy. Am J Surg 148(1):58-63, 1984.
245. Roslyn JJ, Pitt HA, Mann LL, et al: Gallbladder disease in patients on long-term parenteral nutrition. Gastroenterology 84(1):140-154, 1983.
246. Pitt HA, Berquist WE, Mann LL, et al: Parenteral nutrition induces calcium bilirubinate gallstones. Gastroenterology 84:1274, 1983.
247. Gafa M, Sarli L, Miselli A, et al: Sludge and microlithiasis of the biliary tract after total gastrectomy and postoperative total parenteral nutrition. Surg Gynecol Obstet 165:413-418, 1987.
248. Messing B, Colanbel JF, Heresbrach D, et al: Chronic cholestasis and macronutrient excess in patients treated with prolonged parenteral nutrition. Nutrition 8:30-36, 1992.
249. Bolondi L, Gaiani S, Testa S, et al: Gallbladder sludge formation during prolonged fasting after gastrointestinal surgery. Gut 26:734-738, 1985.
250. Hamilton RF, Davis WC, Stephenson DV, Magee DF: Effects of parenteral hyperalimentation on upper gastrointestinal tract secretions. Arch Surg 102:348-352, 1971.
251. Van Der Linden W, Nakayama F: Effect of intravenous fat emulsion on hepatic bile: increased lithogenicity and crystal formation. Acta Chir Scand 142:401-406, 1976.
252. Innis SM: Hepatic transport of bile salt and bile composition following total parenteral nutrition with and without lipid emulsion in the rat. Am J Clin Nutr 41:1283-1288, 1985.
253. Lirussi F, Vaja S, Murphy GM, Dowling RH: Cholestasis of total parenteral nutrition: bile acid and bile lipid metabolism in parenterally nourished rats. Gastroenterology 96:493-502, 1989.
254. Das JB, Ghosh S, Cosentino CM, Ansari GG: Hepatic organic anion transport kinetics and bile flow during short-term total parenteral nutrition in the rabbit. Proc Soc Exp Biol Med 195:274-278, 1990.
255. Doty JE, Pitt HA, Porter-Fink V, Den Besten L: The effects of intravenous fat and total parenteral nutrition on biliary physiology. J Parenter Enteral Nutr 8;265-268, 1984.
256. Gimmon Z, Kelly RE, Simko V, Fischer JE: Total parenteral nutrition increases bile lithogenicity in the rat. J Surg Res 32:256-263, 1982.
257. Cano N, Marteau C, DiConstanzo J, et al: Etude de la composition biliare sous nutrition parenterale total chez l'homme. Gasteroenterol Clin Biol 6:673-678, 1982.
258. Innis SM, Boyd MC: Cholesterol and bile acid synthesis during total parenteral nutrition with and without lipid emulsion in the rat. Am J Clin Nutr 38:95-100, 1983.
259. Muller EL, Grace PA, Pitt HA: The effect of parenteral nutrition on biliary calcium and bilirubin. J Surg Res 40:55-62, 1986.
260. Doty JE, Pitt HA, Porter-Fink V, Denbesten L: Cholecystokinin prophylaxis of parentereral nutrition-induced gallbladder disease. Ann Surg 210:76-78, 1985.
261. Messing B, Aprahamian M, Rautureau M, et al: Gallstone formation during total parenteral nutrition: a prospective study in man. Gastroenterology 86:1183, 1984.
262. Roslyn JJ, Denbesten L, Pitt HA, et al: Effects of cholecystokinin on gallbladder stasis and cholesterol gallstone formation. J Surg Res 30:200-204, 1981.
263. Hill GL, Mair WSJ, Goligher JC: Gallstones after ileostomy and ileal resection. Gut 16:932-936, 1975.
264. Dowling RH, Bell GD, White J: Lithogenic bile in patients with ileal dysfunction. Gut 13:415-420, 1971.
265. Messing B, Lemann M, Landais P, et al: Prognosis of patients with nonmalignant chronic intestinal failure receiving long-term home parenteral nutrition. Gastroenterology 108(4):1302-1304, 1995.
266. Scolapio JS, Flemming CR, Kelly DG, et al: Survival of home parenteral nutrition-treated patients: 20 years of experience at the Mayo Clinic. Mayo Clin Proc 74(3):217-222, 1999.
267. Chan S, McCowen KC, Bistrian B, et al: Incidence, prognosis, and etiology of end-stage liver disease in patients receiving home total parenteral nutrition. Surgery 126(1):28-34, 1999.
268. Grant D: Intestinal transplantation: 1997 report of the International Registry Intestinal Transplant Registry. Transplantation 67:1061-1064, 1999.
269. Brousse N, Goulet O: Small bowel transplantation. BMJ 110;312: 261-262, 1996 (editorial).
270. Quigley EM: Small intestinal transplantation: reflections on an evolving approach to intestinal failure. Gastroenterology 110: 2009-2012, 1996.
271. Thorne A, Johansson U, Wahren J, et al: Thermogenic response to intravenous nutrition in patients with cirrhosis. J Hepatol 16:145-152, 1992.
272. Goldstein SA, Elwyn DH: The effect of injury and sepsis on fuel utilization. Annu Rev Nutr 9:445-464, 1989.
273. Williams JW, Sankary HN, Foster PF, et al: Splanchnic transplantation. An approach to the infant dependent on parenteral nutrition who develops irreversible liver disease. JAMA 261:1458-1462, 1989.
274. Fein BI, Holt PR: Hepatobiliary complications of total parenteral nutrition. J Clin Gastroentrol 18:62-66, 1994.
275. Maini B, Blackburn GL, Bistrian BM, et al: Cyclic hyperalimentation: An optimal technique for preservation of visceral protein. J Surg Res 20:515-525, 1976.
276. Ternullo SR, Burkart GJ: Experience with cyclic hyperalimentation in infants. J Parenter Enteral Nutr 3:516, 1979.
277. Keim N: Nutritional effectors of hepatic steatosis induced by parenteral nutrition in the rat. J Parenter Enteral Nutr 11:18-22, 1987.
278. Freund HR, Muggia-Sullam M, LaFrance R, et al: A possible benefit of metronidazole in reducing TPN-associated liver function derangements. J Surg Res 38:356-363, 1985.
279. Beau P, Labat-Labourdette J, Ingrand P, Beuchant M: Is ursodeoxycholic acid an effective therapy for total parenteral nutrition-related liver disease? J Hepatol 20(2):240-244, 1994.
280. Hoffman AF: Defective biliary secretion during total parenteral nutrition: probable mechanisms and possible solutions. J Pediatr Gastroenterol Nutr 20(4):376-390, 1995.
281. Lazardis KN, Gores GJ, Lindor KD: Ursodeoxycholic acid's mechanisms of action and clinical use in hepatobiliary disorders. J Hepatol 35(1):134-146, 2001.
282. Yeh SL, Chen WJ, Huang PC: Effect of L-glutamine on hepatic lipids at different energy levels in rats receiving total parenteral nutrition. J Parenter Enteral Nutr 18(1):40-44, 1994.
283. Yeh SL, Chen WJ, Huang PC: Effects of L-glutamine on induced hepatosteatosis in rats receiving total parenteral nutrition. J Formos Med Assoc 94(10):593-599, 1995.
284. Palmerini CA, Corazzi L, Arienti G: The action of s-adenosyl-L-methionine on the levels of triglyceride and phospholipid precursors in ethanol-intoxicated rat liver. Pharmacol Sci 36:942-946, 1981.
285. Stramentinoli G, Pezzoli C, Galli-Kienle M: Protective role of s-adenosyl-L-methionine against acetaminophen induced mortality and hepatotoxicity in mice. Biochem Pharmacol 28:3567-3571, 1979.

286. Stramentinoli G, Gualano M, Ideo G: Protective role of s-adenosyl-L-methionine on liver injury induced by D-galactosamine in rats. Biochem Pharmacol 27:1431-1433, 1978.
287. Corrales F, Gimenez A, Alvarez L, et al: s-adenosylmethionine treatment prevents carbon tetrachloride-induced s-adenosylmethionine synthetase inactivation and attenuates liver injury. Hepatology 16:1022-1027, 1992.
288. Boelsterli UA, Rakhit G, Balazs T: Modulation by s-adenosyl-L-methionine of hepatic Na+, K+-ATPase, membrane fluidity, and bile flow in rats with ethinyl estradiol-induced cholestasis. Hepatology 3:12-17, 1983.
289. Fernandez E, Galan AI, Moran D, et al: Reversal of cyclosporine A-induced alterations in biliary secretion by s-adenosyl-L-methionine in rats. J Pharmacol Exp Ther 275:442-449, 1995.
290. Cincu RN, Rodriguez-Ortigosa CM, Vesperinas I, et al: S-adenosyl-L-methionine protects the liver against the cholestatic, cytotoxic, and vasoactive effects of leukotriene D4. A study with isolated and perfused rat liver. Hepatology 26:330-335, 1997.
291. Muriel P, Suarez OR, Gonzalez P, et al: Protective effect of s-adenosyl-L-methionine on liver damage induced by biliary obstruction in rats: a histological, ultrastructural and biochemical approach. J Hepatol 21:95-102, 1994.
292. Belli DC, Fournier L-A, Lepage G, et al: S-adenosylmethionine prevents total parenteral nutrition-induced cholestasis in the rat. J Hepatol 21:18-23, 1994.
293. Sitzmann JV, Pitt HA, Steinborn PA, et al: Cholecystokinin prevents parenteral-nutrition induced biliary sludge in humans. Surg Gynecol Obstet 170:25-31, 1990.
294. Sharp KW: Acute cholecystitis. Surg Clin North Am 68:269-279, 1988.
295. Petersen SR, Sheldon GF: Acute acalculous cholecystitis: a complication of hyperalimentation. Am J Surg 138:814-817, 1979.
296. Brook G: Quality of life issues: parenteral nutrition to small bowel transplantation—a review. Nutrition 14(10):813-816, 1988.
297. Kaufman SS, Atkinson JB, Bianchi A, et al: Indications for pediatric intestinal transplantation: a position paper of the American Society of Transplantation. Pediatr Transplant 5(2):80-87, 2001.
298. Thompson JS: Intestinal transplantation. Experience in the United States. Eur J Pediatr Surg 9(4):271-273, 1999.
299. Vanderhoof JA, Langnas AN: Short-bowel syndrome in children and adults. Gastroenterology 113(5):1767-1778, 1997.

CHAPTER

58

The Role of the Liver in Hematopoietic Progenitor Cell Transplantation

Sagar Lonial, MD, David L. Jaye, MD, and Edmund K. Waller, MD, PhD

Hematopoietic progenitor cell (HPC) transplantation involves administration of high doses of chemotherapy or combinations of chemotherapy and total body irradiation (TBI) followed by an intravenous infusion of HPCs that repopulate the marrow and blood cell compartments. The role of high-dose therapy is to eliminate malignant cells that may be resistant to conventional doses of therapy and, in the case of allogeneic transplant, to prevent rejection of the hematopoietic cell graft by host. The patient is protected from fatal marrow aplasia by engraftment of the transplanted hematopoietic repopulating cells with reconstitution of normal blood counts. The patient may serve as the donor and the recipient of the HPCs (autologous transplantation). In autologous transplantation the HPCs are harvested from the patient before the administration of high-dose therapy, cryopreserved, then re-infused after the toxic metabolites of the chemotherapy have cleared from the body. Alternatively, HPC may be harvested from the bone marrow or peripheral blood compartment of a normal donor (allogeneic transplantation). Allogeneic donor lymphocytes administered with the hematopoietic repopulating cells may also exert a powerful graft versus tumor effect.[1] Hematopoietic repopulating cells may be harvested from the bone marrow or from the peripheral blood after administration of myeloid growth factors, granulocyte colony-stimulating factor, or granulocyte-macrophage colony-stimulating factor.[1] For the purposes of simplicity, the term *hematopoietic progenitor cell* transplant is used to include both bone marrow (BM) transplants and peripheral blood stem cell (PBSC) transplants. BM and PBSC differ in the method of collecting the hematopoietic repopulating cells but not with respect to the hepatic complications of the transplant maneuver.

The liver is the target for many of the toxicities of HPC transplantation resulting from (1) the susceptibility of hepatic endothelial cells to injury from chemoradiotherapy, (2) the propensity of allogeneic donor T cells to cause immune injury to the liver, and (3) the development of hepatic infections during periods of impaired immune function. This chapter will review the hepatic disorders that may increase the risk of liver injury during HPC transplantation, the evaluation and management of common hepatic complications of HPC transplantation, and the emerging understanding of the liver as a hematopoietic organ.

EVALUATION OF HEPATIC FUNCTION BEFORE HIGH-DOSE THERAPY AND HEMATOPOIETIC PROGENITOR CELL TRANSPLANTATION

The susceptibility of the liver to injury from the effects of high-dose chemotherapy and radiation administered as part of HPC transplantation makes evaluation of hepatic function of the intended HPC transplant recipient a critically important part of the overall pretransplant evaluation process. Chronic viral hepatitis, cirrhosis, or inherited disorders of hepatocellular function significantly increase the risk of fatal complications after high-dose therapy and HPC transplantation. The usual pretransplant evaluation includes measurement of serum transaminase and bilirubin and serologic tests for the presence of viral hepatitis. Active hepatitis as evidenced by significant transaminase elevation (more than twice the upper limit of normal) warrants a detailed investigation of the cause of hepatocellular injury. Acute viral infection, regardless of the etiologic agent, is a contraindication to proceeding with high-dose treatment and HPC transplantation. Serologic evidence of past infection with hepatitis A is not a contraindication to transplant, so long as the acute infection has resolved (conversion of immunoglobulin [Ig]M antibody response to an IgG antibody response). Evidence of prior hepatitis B infection (presence of IgG surface antibody and IgG core antibody without the presence of hepatitis B antigen in the blood) is not a contraindication to proceeding with high-dose therapy and HPC transplant so long as bilirubin and transaminases are within the normal range. Serologic evidence for past hepatitis B infection without active or chronic hepatitis does not increase the risk of veno-occlusive disease after HPC transplant.[2] The presence of hepatitis B antigenemia is a contraindication to both autologous and allogeneic HPC transplant because the immunosuppression that results from high-dose conditioning therapy results in recrudescence of a virulent active hepatitis in patients with chronic active hepatitis B infection. Evaluation of hepatitis C infection requires tests for serologic evidence of past infection and measurements of viral ribonucleic acid (RNA) in the blood by polymerase chain reaction (PCR). Detection of hepatitis C viral RNA indicates chronic active hepatitis C infection and is a relative contraindication to proceeding with high-dose therapy and HPC transplantation.[3]

TABLE 58-1

Causes of Liver Disease after Hematopoietic Progenitor Cell Transplantation

Veno-occlusive Disease
Graft-versus-host disease
Drug hepatotoxicity
Infections of the liver

Bacterial
Sepsis
Pyogenic liver abscess

Viral
Herpes simplex
Varicella-zoster
Cytomegalovirus
Adenovirus
Hepatitis B
Hepatitis C

Fungal
Candida albicans
Aspergillus species

DIFFERENTIAL DIAGNOSIS OF LIVER INJURY AFTER HEMATOPOIETIC PROGENITOR CELL TRANSPLANTATION

The liver is susceptible to a variety of injuries that may be associated with HPC transplantation, and multiple causes may be simultaneously associated with acute and chronic cholestasis post-transplant (Table 48-1).[4] Injury to the endothelial cells of the venules, and subsequent veno-occlusive disease, may result from the high doses of radiation and chemotherapy administered to patients before hematopoietic cell transplantation. Disruption of the biosynthetic capacities of the liver may lead to accumulation of compounds normally metabolized by the liver. The presence of hematopoietic-derived Kupffer cells in the liver may trigger an immunologic attack by donor T cells infused as part of the allogeneic HPC transplant.

The lengthy differential of hepatic complications of HPC transplantation is divided according to their etiologies and the temporal sequence at which they develop from the time of transplant. Hepatic toxicity that occurs in the first month after HPC transplant is usually related to infections or the toxicity of the conditioning regimen, whereas late hepatic complications (after day 30 post-transplant) are usually immunologic in nature and related to graft-versus-host disease (GVHD). Histologic confirmation of the diagnosis for hepatic injury is often lacking or is obtained late in the natural history of the disease. Because of the morbidity associated with liver biopsy in the context of thrombocytopenia, and the lack of clear pathognomonic histologic findings for many causes of hepatic injury,[4] a clinical diagnosis of the differential diagnosis of the various hepatic complications of HPC transplant is often used as the basis for treatment.

Early Hepatic Complications

Veno-occlusive disease (VOD) of the liver is a known regimen-related complication of high-dose chemotherapy followed by HPC or bone marrow transplantation.[5] Historically the incidence of VOD after autologous or allogeneic transplantation has ranged from as low as 4.1 percent to as high as 50 percent,[6] with most series reporting an incidence of around 20 percent.[7,8] Chemotherapy is thought to play a significant role in the pathogenesis of VOD through sinusoidal endothelial and hepatocyte injury that results in a procoagulant state.[9] The relative risk of VOD is 2.8-fold higher after busulfan-cyclophosphamide conditioning than TBI-based conditioning among allogeneic transplant recipients.[10] Biochemical changes associated with VOD include decreased factor VII and protein C levels,[11,12] increased levels of plasminogen activator inhibitor-1,[13,14] and release of von Willebrand's factor and angiotensin-converting enzyme from injured endothelial cells.[12] It has been demonstrated that the use of pharmacokinetic targeting of busulfan plasma levels has reduced the incidence of toxicity in busulfan-containing regimens.[15,16] However, other commonly used agents such as cyclophosphamide have been linked with glutathione depletion and resultant hepatic toxicity.[17] The incidence of VOD has been correlated with the metabolites of cyclophosphamide,[18] pointing out individual differences in drug metabolism that can alter the toxicity of preparative regimens. The nitrosourea bischloroethylnitrosourea (BCNU)[2] has also been associated with the development of VOD, especially when used in single-fraction, high-dose infusion. Other agents such as melphalan, etoposide, and thiotepa have also been implicated in the development of VOD, especially when used in combination with cyclophosphamide. Patients with pre-existing hepatic dysfunction resulting from disease involvement, acute or subacute viral hepatitis, or cirrhosis also have an increased risk of post-transplant VOD.[2]

The clinical manifestations and features of VOD include painful hepatomegaly, hyperbilirubinemia, and fluid retention. Two systems of diagnostic criteria exist: one developed in Seattle, a second developed in Baltimore. The Seattle criteria require the presence of two of three clinical criteria: (1) jaundice, (2) painful hepatomegaly, and (3) fluid retention before day 20 after transplantation.[6,7] The Baltimore criteria include (1) jaundice and two of the following: (2) hepatomegaly, (3) ascites, or (4) more than 5 percent weight gain.[8] The major difference between the two diagnostic systems is that the Seattle criteria require manifestations of signs and symptoms of VOD within the first 20 days after transplant, thereby excluding approximately one fourth of patients with "late" VOD.[10]

The diagnosis of VOD is based on clinical signs and symptoms of the combination of these criteria: (1) hyperbilirubinemia, (2) unexplained weight gain or ascites, and (3) hepatomegaly or right upper quadrant tenderness. The presence of all three clinical signs has specificity of 92 percent for a histologic diagnosis of VOD. The presence of only two of three clinical criteria has a specificity of only 42 percent for the diagnosis of VOD.[19] Other laboratory studies are not specific to VOD. Elevations of hepatic transferases reflect hepatic necrosis and are prognostic rather than diagnostic, with serum aspartate aminotransferase higher than 750 associated with a poor outcome.[9] The association of decreased factor VII and protein C levels[11,12] and increased levels of plasminogen activator inhibitor-1[13,14] are not sufficiently specific for VOD to be used in place of clinical criteria for diagnosis. Imaging studies can provide objective evidence for the presence of hepatomegaly and ascites. Additionally, the use of ultrasound can sometimes be helpful in determining the portal venous flow, though the sensitivity of this study in early VOD is less than optimal.[20,21] When the clinical diagnosis is unclear a liver biopsy performed by radiologists familiar with transvenous hepatic biopsy may be helpful. The advantage this procedure provides is relative safety for patients with severe thrombocytopenia (refractory thrombocytopenia is often a feature of severe VOD) and the ability to directly measure the hepatic venous pressure gradients.[22] Two separate groups have demonstrated that hepatic venous pressure gradients higher than 10 mm Hg are associated with the diagnosis of VOD and that higher pressures portend poorer outcomes.[23,24]

The histopathologic features associated with early VOD can include edema and obliteration of central hepatic venules, endothelial destruction, enlargement of the sinusoids, and eventual necrosis of zone 3 hepatocytes (Plate 58-1, *A*).[24] Immunohistochemical staining of biopsy specimens demonstrates deposition of factor VIII and other clotting factors at the interface between the hepatic sinusoids and hepatic venules.[25] It has also been demonstrated that a correlation exists between the degree of zone 3 changes and clotting factor deposition and clinical severity of VOD.[26] It is not necessary to see venous obstruction to clearly make the diagnosis of VOD (despite the name) because the intense destruction and fibrosis seen in zone 3 of the liver acinus is more accurately correlated with severity of disease and prognosis. This association suggests that the eventual outcome is determined very early in the course of disease and that interventions must be directed toward early therapy because initial injury predicts the overall severity of VOD.[27]

The contribution of VOD to treatment-related mortality depends upon the definition of VOD used and how the causes of death are defined. Pre-existing hepatitis C infection is a risk factor for severe and fatal VOD post-transplant. Liver biopsies from patients with pre-existing hepatitis C who develop VOD show greater than 100-fold increases in viral ribonucleic acid in liver tissues.[3] Most patients who die after transplantation with concomitant VOD do not die of liver failure but rather of multi-organ dysfunction with prominent manifestations of renal or cardiopulmonary failure. As one would expect, patients with mild VOD have a better overall survival than those with severe VOD (91 percent versus 2 percent)[6]; outcomes can be correlated with the severity of hyperbilirubinemia. To better predict who will require more than supportive care for the management of VOD, a mathematical model was developed by Bearman and colleagues to predict the chance of developing fatal VOD based upon the criteria of weight gain and serum bilirubin at various time points after transplant.[28] This model can be used to determine which patients should receive experimental therapy early in the course of VOD and which patients can be expected to recover with supportive care only (Figure 58-1).

Treatment and prophylaxis strategies for VOD have been directed toward two goals: (1) prophylactic measures to prevent the development of VOD in a high-risk population and (2) to reverse the pathophysiology of VOD early in the course of the disease, before irreversible hepatic injury has occurred. A variety of patients are at increased risk for the development of VOD after HPC transplant, including patients with a history of VOD after previous therapies, those receiving additional high-dose conditioning as part of a planned second HPC transplant, those with active hepatitis and elevated transaminases, and those with pre-existing cirrhosis or fibrosis.[6,29] In high-risk patients the incidence of VOD may be reduced by using lower doses of TBI, administering fractionated doses of BCNU, shielding the liver during TBI, and avoiding the use of cyclophosphamide during conditioning. Because the metabolism of cyclophosphamide is quite variable among different individuals, patients who have received the same relative cyclophosphamide dose (per kilogram or per square meter) may have quite different risks for the development of VOD.

Primary prophylaxis studies have examined the effect of low-dose heparin (100-150 U/kg/day), pentoxifylline, and ursodiol[30] started at the time of conditioning and continued for 2 to 4 weeks post-transplant on incidence of VOD. Two randomized studies of low-dose heparin administered in the peritransplant period showed benefit for prevention of non-fatal VOD but were not powered to show a difference in the incidence of severe VOD.[31,32] In contrast, a third randomized study that examined prophylactic heparin in patients at high risk for VOD found that patients who received heparin had a higher incidence of VOD, with the high-risk group experiencing a 16 percent incidence of VOD.[33] These conflicting results, and the difficulties of using heparin in patients with severe thrombocytopenia, have limited widespread acceptance of the use of heparin for the prophylaxis of VOD.

A randomized study by Gluckman studied the effect of continuous intravenous infusion of prostaglandin $(PG)E_1$ from day -8 to day $+30$ after HPC transplant.[34] PGE_1 is thought to protect the vascular endothelium by causing vasodilation, inhibition of platelet aggregation, and activation of the fibrinolytic pathway. There was a reduction in the incidence of VOD compared to non-treated controls but a subsequent study demonstrated

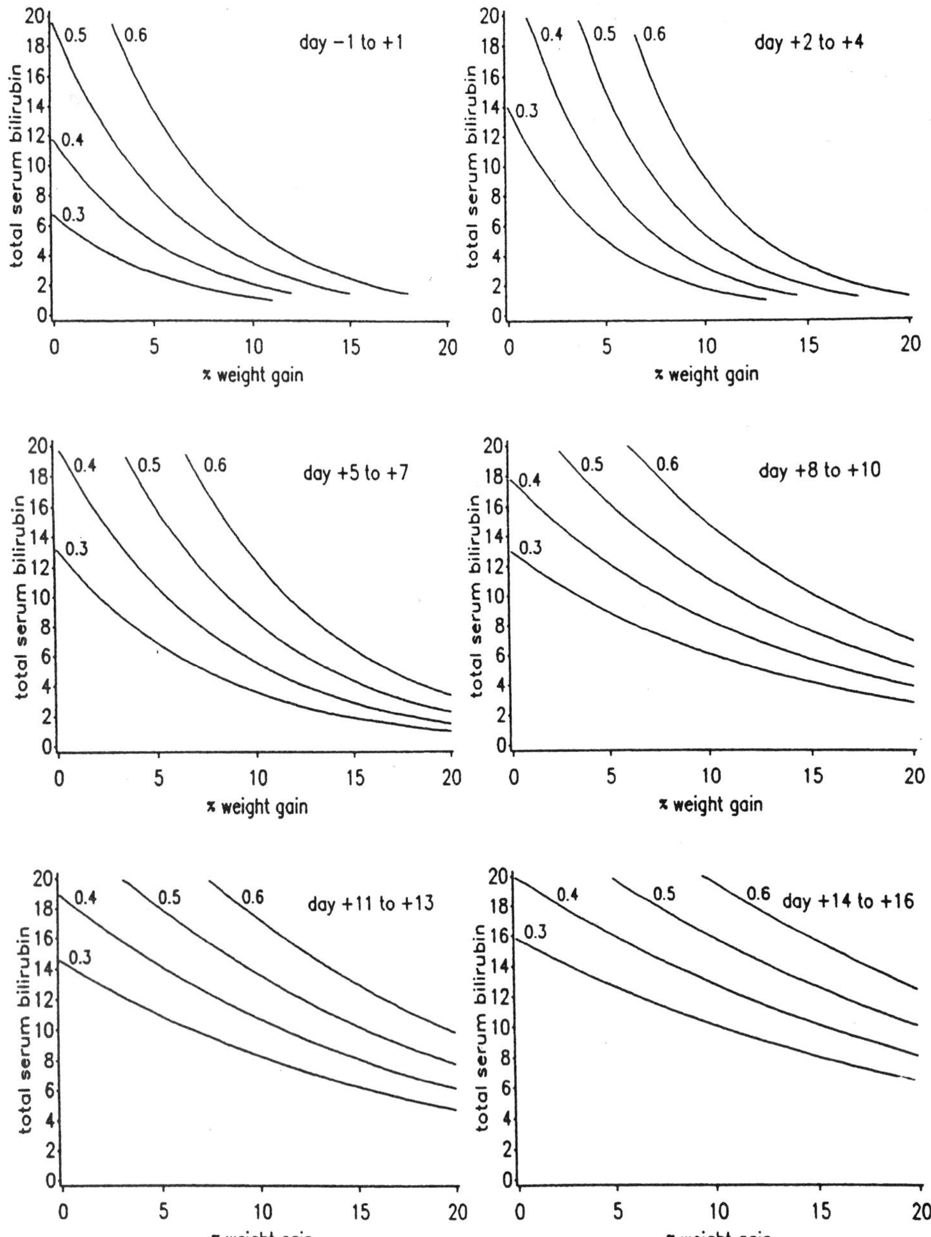

Figure 58-1 Contour lines estimating the probability of developing severe veno-occlusive disease (VOD). The lines refer to the probabilities of at least 30 percent, 40 percent, 50 percent, or 60 percent using total serum bilirubin and percent weight gain above baseline between days +1 and +16 after transplant. If the plotted point is above the probability line, the chance of progressing to severe VOD exceeds the value of that line. This algorithm was based on patients receiving cyclophosphamide-based conditioning regimens. (From Bearman SI, Anderson GL, Mori M, et al: Venoocclusive disease of the liver: development of a model for predicting fatal outcome after marrow transplantation. J Clin Oncol 11:1729-1736, 1993.)

significant toxicity to the PGE_1 infusion[35]; therefore, this approach has been largely abandoned. A large randomized trial addressed the role of pentoxifylline as a prophylactic agent for the prevention of VOD. The mechanism was thought to relate to PGE_2 production and inhibition of macrophage tumor necrosis factor (TNF)α production. Although phase II studies had demonstrated some efficacy of pentoxifylline as prophylaxis for VOD,[36] a prospective, placebo-controlled, double-masked randomized trial of 88 patients undergoing allogeneic BM transplants failed to show any reduction in treatment-related complications among patients who received pentoxifylline.[37]

Ursodiol (ursodeoxycholic acid), a hydrophilic bile acid that is administered orally, is believed to protect the liver from the hepatic injury caused by the enterohepatic recirculation of bile acids. A randomized, placebo-controlled trial of 67 patients who received allogeneic BMT after busulfan and cyclophosphamide conditioning demonstrated a reduced incidence of VOD among recipients of 600 mg of daily ursodiol compared to recipients of placebo.[38]

With prophylaxis studies having shown limited benefit, another approach to the management of VOD is therapeutic intervention early in its course. Most patients with VOD recover with supportive care alone. This usually involves the use of volume expanders to maintain renal function and intravascular volume and the use of diuretics such as spironolactone to reduce extravascular fluid accumulation. Unfortunately, after renal failure or respiratory failure develops there is little evidence that the use of hemodialysis or ventilatory support increases long-term survival.[6,39,40]

Based on the evidence that VOD represents a procoagulant state, a number of studies have examined the role of thrombolytic therapy in the management of patients with severe VOD. A case report of a single patient with severe VOD treated with recombinant tissue plasminogen activator (t-PA) described complete resolution of VOD symptoms.[41] The potential efficacy of t-PA in the management of VOD was supported by additional data that demonstrated safety and efficacy in small series of adult and pediatric patients.[42,43] A large, randomized study did not support an overall clinical benefit among patients treated with t-PA, and additional studies have shown that intracranial bleeding after treatment with t-PA is a significant problem.[44,45] A series of patients with severe VOD who received defibrotide on a compassionate-use basis has also recently been reported.[46] Defibrotide is a large, single-stranded polydeoxyribonucleotide derived from mammalian tissue (porcine mucosa) with anti-thrombotic and thrombolytic activity without significant systemic anti-coagulation. Defibrotide increases levels of endogenous prostaglandins (PGI_2 and PGE_2), reduces levels of leukotriene B4, inhibits monocyte superoxide anion generation, stimulates expression of thrombomodulin in human vascular endothelial cells, modulates platelet activity, and stimulates fibrinolysis by increasing endogenous t-PA function while decreasing activity of type I plasminogen activator inhibitor. Among 19 patients with severe VOD who received defibrotide using a variety of doses and schedules, 8 patients (42 percent) had complete resolution of VOD with minimal side effects and no increased bleeding. Defibrotide therapy is promising, although large randomized studies are needed to confirm its efficacy.[46]

Finally, because deficiencies in the natural anti-coagulants protein C, protein S, and anti-thrombin III (AT-III) have been associated with transplant patients in general—and in patients with VOD[11,47]—a few investigators have used replacement of AT-III as a strategy for the treatment of post-transplant VOD. The clinical data related to AT-III are limited to two small groups of patients with severe VOD. AT-III replacement either alone[48] or in combination with t-PA[49] appeared to have activity in reversing the signs and symptoms of VOD. AT-III therapy has not been tested in large patient populations and warrants further study in a randomized fashion.

TABLE 58-2

Common Drug Reactions After Hematopoietic Progenitor Cell Transplantation

Form of hepatic toxicity	Common drugs
Cholestasis	Fluconazole, rifampin, cyclosporine
	Erythromycin, trimethoprim-sulfamethoxazole, nafcillin
Cholestasis and elevated transaminases	Phenytoin (allergic hepatitis), TPN
Elevated transaminases	Methotrexate
VOD	Busulfan, BCNU, cyclophosphamide

TPN, Total parenteral nutrition; *BCNU,* bischloroethylnitrosourea; *VOD,* veno-occlusive disease.

HEPATIC SIDE EFFECTS OF DRUGS COMMONLY ADMINISTERED DURING HEMATOPOIETIC PROGENITOR CELL TRANSPLANTATION

Several drugs commonly used in the management of patients after HPC transplant are associated with direct hepatotoxicity. In most cases cholestasis or elevations of hepatic transaminases are reversed by stopping the offending agent, and alternative drugs are available to treat most transplant conditions. A list of drugs commonly associated with hepatotoxicity post-transplant is shown in Table 58-2. The management of drug-induced hepatic toxicity is primarily to stop the agents that may be causing hepatic injury.

Graft-versus-Host Disease

GVHD is an immunologically mediated complication of transplantation. The immunologic requirements for the development of GVHD postallogeneic transplantation were defined by Billingham more than 30 years ago.[50] For GVHD to develop there must be (1) immunocompetent cells in the graft, (2) human leukocyte antigen (HLA) disparity between the donor and the recipient, and (3) relative immunoincompetence of the recipient to the extent that the recipient is unable to reject the graft. GVHD is mediated primarily by activated T cells from the donor, which recognize host alloantigen as foreign.[50] After clones of T cells are activated and generate an alloimmune response, they set in motion a large cascade of events that include recruitment of additional immune cells, proliferation of the alloreactive clone, and secretion of cytokines, and result in the manifestations of GVHD.

GVHD has been divided into two clinical phases—acute (usually developing before day +100) and chronic (usually developing after day +100). Acute GVHD is characterized by an inflammatory process with injury to the epithelial cells of the skin, gastrointestinal (GI) tract, and bile ducts. Chronic GVHD is usually defined as GVHD that occurs beyond day +100 post-transplant and resembles autoimmune processes that produce fibrosis and obstruction in the lacrimal and salivary glands, bile ducts, pulmonary bronchioles, and sclerodermatous changes in the skin. There is clearly an overlap between acute and chronic GVHD with respect to the time of presentation. Some patients develop typical signs and symptoms of chronic GVHD before day 100, whereas some patients develop signs and symptoms typical of acute GVHD after day 100, particularly when immunosuppressive medications are tapered. The severity of GVHD and the frequency with which acute GVHD and chronic GVHD develop depend upon the degree of HLA disparity between the donor and the recipient and the numbers of T cells in the graft.[51] Data from a murine BM transplantation model indicate that the presence of host antigen-presenting cells in the liver is necessary for hepatic GVHD to develop.[52] Mortality from acute GVHD varies depending on the severity, with overall survival for patients with grade 4 GVHD being on the order of 10 percent.[53,54]

Acute GVHD occurs in 40 percent to 65 percent of all patients undergoing allogeneic transplant from HLA-matched siblings.[53,55] The clinical manifestations of acute GVHD usually involve the skin, GI tract, and liver. The extent of damage to each organ system by acute GVHD is graded according to its severity, with grade 1 representing mild injury and grade 4 representing life-threatening injury. Skin manifestations begin with mild erythema and can progress to erythroderma and finally bullous skin disease. GI tract involvement may include persistent nausea and vomiting (upper tract disease) or cramping abdominal pain and watery or bloody diarrhea (lower GI tract). Liver involvement by acute GVHD usually manifests as jaundice with elevated alkaline phosphatase. Mild hepatic GVHD (stage 1) is associated with elevation of serum bilirubin of 2 to 3 mg/ml; moderate hepatic GVHD is associated with elevation of serum bilirubin of 3 to 6 mg/ml (stage 2); severe acute GVHD is associated with elevation of serum bilirubin of 6 to 15 mg/ml (stage 3); and more than 15 mg/ml (stage 4).[56] Elevations in the hepatic transaminases up to 5 times the upper limit of normal values may also occur with acute hepatic GVHD.

The overall clinical stage of acute GVHD represents a combination of the different organ-specific stages.[56] Isolated liver involvement with acute GVHD is rare. Acute GVHD most commonly presents with skin and GI tract involvement; liver involvement is usually associated with a higher overall clinical grade of acute GVHD. Histopathologically, acute GVHD of the liver manifests as epithelial degeneration of interlobular bile ducts with cholestasis. Later, the portal tracts may be infiltrated with lymphocytes, and as disease progress, bile duct destruction and obstruction of the lumen result from necrotic material (Plate 58-1, *B* and *C*). Eventually, severe hepatic GVHD results in ballooning degeneration of hepatocytes, Kupffer cell hyperplasia, and bridging and piecemeal necrosis.[57-60] In many cases the presence of hyperbilirubinemia in the first 3 months post-transplant has multiple clinical and pathologic etiologies.[4] GVHD may be present simultaneously with viral hepatitis, particularly hepatitis C, VOD, or drug toxicities,[4] emphasizing the need for careful clinical and histologic evaluation of all potential causes of hyperbilirubinemia in the post-transplant setting.[4]

Chronic GVHD has a pathophysiology similar to an autoimmune collagen vascular disorder and less like an acute inflammatory disorder.[61] The skin manifestations of chronic GVHD result in dermal fibrosis and a scleroderma-like picture. GI tract involvement usually appears as malabsorption and chronic diarrhea. Patients can also develop multi-system disease with pulmonary fibrosis, esophageal stricture and dysphagia, and a sicca-like syndrome with xerostomia and keratoconjunctivitis.[62] Hepatic chronic GVHD presents with a chronic lobular, chronic persistent, or chronic active hepatitis with a lobular, portal, or periportal inflammatory reaction.[58,63] As the disease progresses portal inflammation and fibrosis result in a significant reduction of small interlobular bile ducts and a concentric periductal fibrosis that can appear like primary sclerosing cholangitis.[64]

Treatments for both acute and chronic GVHD of the liver involve using systemic immunosuppression. For the treatment of acute GVHD, steroids remain the mainstay of therapy, to which the calcineurin inhibitors (cyclosporine A or tacrolimus) are added when steroids alone are not sufficient. Historically, treatment for steroid-refractory acute GVHD has been anti-thymocyte globulin. The response rate for steroid-refractory GVHD is usually less than 50 percent, and most patients die of infectious complications related to either mucosal barrier disruption from GVHD or T-cell deficiency.[65,66] Newer drugs such as mycophenolate mofetil and the anti–TNFα agents infliximab (Remicade) and etanercept (Enbrel) are also being used increasingly for the treatment of acute GVHD, especially when the GI tract or liver is the site of disease. The treatment of chronic GVHD is prolonged therapy with combination immunosuppressive drugs that are typically a combination of alternating-day treatment with steroids and a calcineurin inhibitor.[67] Patients with chronic GVHD are at risk for significant infectious problems related to immunosuppressive drug therapy and underlying T-cell– and B-cell–mediated dysfunction related to chronic GVHD.

HEPATIC INFECTIONS COMPLICATING TRANSPLANTATION

Infections form a large part of the complications associated with HPC transplantation. The type of infections that commonly develop post-transplant is most related to the time after transplantation. In the very early post-transplant period before engraftment, bacteria are the most common pathogens and are rarely involved in primary hepatic infections. Hematopoietic engraftment typically occurs within the first 30 days post-transplant; between the time of engraftment and day 100 the incidence of viral infections rises. Although patients may have normal granulocyte counts they have profound cell-mediated immunodeficiency that makes them susceptible to viral infections. Fungal infections from pretransplant "seeding" of the liver may also become manifest during the first 2 months after hematopoietic engraftment. After the first 100 days have passed and if chronic GVHD is established, the development of fungal and viral infections is likely the result of concomitant administration of immunosuppression and the profound immune deficiency associated with chronic GVHD.[60]

Bacterial Infections

Although the incidence of bacteremia is high after HPC transplantation, the incidence of bacterial hepatic abscess is quite low. This may be related in part to early empiric antibiotics for fever of unknown origin and the use of prolonged prophylaxis during periods of neutropenia. The spectrum of bacterial disease has shifted away from gram-negative rods (which were the predominant organisms previously) to gram-positive organisms such as *Staphylococcus* and *Streptococcus* species.[68,69] This has occurred because of the increased use of indwelling catheters for transplant patients and because of routine gram-negative prophylaxis. On rare occasions patients with prolonged immunosuppression may reactivate latent mycobacterial infection within the liver. Diagnosis requires biopsy and pathologic confirmation using special stains and culture.[70]

Viral Infections

Herpes Simplex Virus

The routine use of acyclovir has all but eliminated the occurrence of herpes simplex virus (HSV)-related hepatitis. The typical clinical presentation is that of rapidly rising hepatic aminotransferases with fever, abdominal pain, and often oral or skin herpetic lesions, although skin findings may be absent. Histologic changes within the liver demonstrate necrosis, which may be non-specific, but immunohistochemistry with specific HSV1 and HSV2 antibodies usually aids in the diagnosis[71,72] if characteristic viral inclusions are absent. Computed tomography (CT) scanning may show multiple necrotic abscesses but this too is non-specific and requires biopsy for confirmation.[73] Treatment involves using high-dose acyclovir.

Varicella-Zoster Virus

Varicella-zoster virus (VZV) infections usually occur as a result of reactivation of a latent virus in a seropositive patient. The overall incidence of VZV reactivation varies between 16 percent and 40 percent and usually occurs about 5 months after transplant,[74] with most infections occurring within the first 7 months after transplant.[75,76] Prophylactic acyclovir can reduce the incidence of early reactivation but late reactivation can still occur after acyclovir is discontinued.[77] VZV reactivation can occur as localized dermatomal disease, widespread cutaneous disease, or visceral dissemination. Although local reactivation may be painful or yield scarring, visceral disease carries a mortality of up to 50 percent and may manifest as pneumonitis, hepatitis, or fulminant hepatic failure.[78] Because the disease can progress so rapidly in recipients of HPC grafts, it is recommended that any patient who develops rapidly rising hepatic transaminases receive empiric high-dose acyclovir before diagnostic testing is started. Liver histology again demonstrates hepatocyte necrosis with multi-nuclear giant cells and intranuclear inclusions. Immunohistochemistry and VZV-specific antibodies are needed to clearly relate disease to the histologic findings[79,80] because the findings may be nonspecific.

Cytomegalovirus

Cytomegalovirus (CMV) infection usually occurs as a result of reactivation of latent CMV in an allogeneic HPC transplant recipient. The risk factors associated with increased risk of infection are the use of a seropositive donor, the use of seropositive blood products, and the presence of acute GVHD.[81] With the use of aggressive pre-emptive anti-viral therapy, the incidence of acute CMV infection has been reduced, with CMV infection usually being limited to those patients undergoing unrelated donor or T-cell–depleted allogeneic transplants.[82,83] It is unusual for CMV to affect the liver alone, and the liver is most often a site of involvement when CMV disease has disseminated.[81] The timing of infection usually occurs between days +30 and +100 after transplant. Symptoms may include fever, pneumonitis, hepatitis, enteritis, and graft failure.[60] The symptoms may resemble acute GVHD, and because the therapies are quite divergent it is important to obtain tissue confirmation of either CMV or GVHD. Pathologic situations in which both GVHD and CMV are diagnosed should be extensively reviewed and confirmed because immunosuppression required for the treatment of acute GVHD may hasten the progression of CMV. Pathologic diagnosis of CMV invasive disease is most sensitive when PCR or in situ hybridization is used. Routine histologic findings (intranuclear or intracytoplasmic inclusions), viral culture, or immunohistochemistry is quite insensitive in the setting of hepatic CMV disease.[84] Treatment involves the use of induction doses of ganciclovir followed by maintenance dosing. Patients with evidence of end-organ disease can be considered for concomitant use of intravenous gamma globulin. Patients with PCR evidence of progression despite the use of induction doses of ganciclovir should be considered for therapy with foscarnet for the treatment of ganciclovir-resistant CMV.

Adenovirus

Adenovirus infection in the context of allogeneic hematopoietic progenitor cell transplantation may manifest as enteritis, pneumonitis, myocarditis, hemorrhagic cystitis, nephritis, encephalitis, or fulminant hepatitis.[85-87] Despite the cataclysmic complications of disseminated disease, most patients do not develop disseminated disease. Hepatitis presents with rapidly elevating hepatic transaminases, which can result in coagulopathy and encephalopathy. Antemortem diagnosis requires an urgent liver biopsy, which may demonstrate coagulative necrosis surrounded by rims of hepatocytes that contain intranuclear inclusions. Immunohistochemistry, viral culture, and PCR of involved tissue are also quite helpful, although they may not be available in a manner rapid enough to affect the disease. Treatment involves the use of intravenous ribavirin but it is important to start therapy early because the disease may progress quite rapidly.[88,89] Because the clinical scenario is quite similar to CMV infection, empiric ganciclovir is often started, and has demonstrated in vitro activity against adenovirus.[90]

Hepatitis B Virus

Hepatitis B virus (HBV) infections can affect recipients of allogeneic transplantation in three ways. Patients can have a progression of active viral disease that was present before transplant, activation of latent HBV, or transmission of HBV from an infected donor. Patients who receive immunosuppression may develop high viral levels in the blood without evidence of hepatitis. This can continue until either immune reconstitution or a tapering of immunosuppression occurs. Elevations of transaminases and jaundice can be a result of HBV or GVHD; liver biopsy is an important tool to help distinguish if one or both conditions are involved. A clinical flare of hepatitis at the time of tapering immunosuppression can make a distinction between GVHD and viral hepatitis difficult when patients have previously been diagnosed with GVHD.[91] In patients with GVHD diagnosed by histologic criteria, increasing immunosuppression may reduce the laboratory evidence of hepatitis, but viral replication increases unless additional anti-viral medications are used.[27]

Treatment options for patients who are at risk for developing hepatitis B or who are at risk for the reactivation of latent infections are different from those used for patients not undergoing HPC transplantation. Ganciclovir has been used in patients with concomitant CMV disease, although after the drug is discontinued, rapid return of hepatitis occurs.[92] The anti-viral agents famciclovir and lamivudine also have demonstrated efficacy in preventing post-transplant hepatitis and have fewer side effects than ganciclovir. With the use of these agents, hepatitis may also recur after the drugs are stopped; therefore, long-term therapy is recommended to prevent fulminant hepatic failure or hepatitis in patients known to be hepatitis B surface antigen positive.[93] Cirrhosis resulting from HBV has not emerged as a problem for long-term survivors after transplantation.

Hepatitis C Virus

Hepatitis C virus (HCV) infection after HPC transplant occurs either from a progression of pretransplant disease[3] or from transmission of HCV in either the HPC product or transfused blood products. As is seen in patients with HBV infections chronic hepatitis usually resolves around the time of conditioning because the immune response is blunted. After immune reconstitution begins, asymptomatic elevations in the hepatic transaminases occur, again coincident with tapering of immunosuppression.[94,95] Elevation of liver tests may occur concomitant with tapering of immunosuppression, leading to the clinical question of whether GVHD has developed. Liver biopsy is central to making this distinction. If the disease is related to GVHD, more intense immunosuppression is needed; if HCV infection is the culprit, supportive care is indicated because most HCV flares are self-limited. The development of liver failure as is reported with HBV is less common with HCV.[96]

Treatment of patients with early HCV infections is not indicated, and patients should not receive anti-viral therapy until off immunosuppression and without evidence of GVHD. Patients often return to a previous pattern of chronic hepatitis after the initial flare has resolved.[97] Previous data have demonstrated a low incidence of cirrhosis 10 years after transplantation, but most of these patients did have HCV—and several have required liver transplantation.[27] The reported low incidence may be due to the relatively short follow-up of patients with diagnosed HCV and may increase because testing is now more common. Patients who have been off immunosuppression for longer than 6 months and have no evidence of GVHD or immune dysfunction are candidates for interferon therapy, although the presence of iron overload can reduce the efficacy of anti-viral therapy.[98]

Fungal Infections

Candida albicans has been the most common fungal pathogen seen in patients undergoing HPC transplantation, with an estimated incidence of 10 percent to 20 percent. Hepatic and splenic abscesses were common presentations; the clinical scenario usually involved fever of unknown origin at the time of neutrophil recovery. Hepatic involvement usually occurs in the context of systemic disease, though it is possible to have isolated hepatic involvement.[99] A more recent autopsy survey reported a virtual absence of hepatic *Candida* infections in patients receiving fluconazole prophylaxis (3 percent), compared with a 16 percent incidence in patients not receiving fluconazole.[100] The overall incidence of *Candida* infections in this series was 28 percent without prophylaxis, compared with 7 percent in patients receiving prophylaxis. Clinical experience has demonstrated a marked decrease in the incidence of *C. albicans* infections in the postfluconazole era. Unfortunately, with a decrease in the incidence of *C. albicans* infection has come an increase in the incidence of *Candida krausei* and *Torulopsis glabrata* (previously *Candida glabrata*) infections.[101] These pathogens are known to be resistant to fluconazole therapy since the drug's inception in the 1980s. Radiologic studies are often not helpful except to identify sites for biopsy. Typical bull's-eye lesions may not be seen without neutrophil recovery. As with other unusual pathogens it is important to clearly identify the pathogen—often this requires biopsy and culture confirmation for the presence of yeast. For patients with disseminated disease the prolonged administration of amphotericin B (or liposomal preparations) is often needed.[60]

Aspergillus species infections occurred in 4.5 percent of patients undergoing HPC transplantation between 1980 and 1987 in one series,[102] but more recent series place the incidence between 10 percent and 20 percent, especially among recipients of unrelated donor transplants.[103] Aspergillosis may affect the liver but most commonly involves the lungs initially; liver involvement is usually a sign of disseminated disease. Treatment involves the use of amphotericin B (or liposomal preparations), though newer agents such as the echinocardius are in development for the treatment of *Aspergillus* species infections. Therapy is usually long term and requires frequent CT scan monitoring to assess disease response. The overall prognosis in patients with *Aspergillus* species infections is quite poor unless immunosuppression can be withdrawn and T-cell–mediated immunity can be restored.

THE LIVER IS A SOURCE OF HEMATOPOIETIC STEM CELLS

Orthotopic allogeneic liver transplant has been associated with the development of mixed hematopoietic chimerism with the presence of small numbers of hematopoietic cells of donor origin in the peripheral blood and bone marrow compartments of transplant recipients.[104] The presence of mixed chimerism after allogeneic liver transplant is associated with a reduced risk of graft rejection.[105] The liver is a significant source for hematopoietic stem cells during fetal development,[106,107] and hematopoietic stem cells persist in the adult liver.[108] Recent data on the ontologic potential of stem cell populations have demonstrated that highly purified hematopoietic stem cells have the ability to differentiate into hepatocytes and repopulate the liver after intravenous transplantation.[109] Two new competing paradigms are emerging: (1) that pluripotent progenitor cells with multi-lineage differentiation potential are present at low levels in many, if not all, tissues; and (2) that tissue specific pluripotent progenitor cells retain the ability for "trans-differentiation" when placed in the appropriate microenvironment.[109] The identification of a common source for both hematopoietic and hepatic progenitor cells is blurring the distinction between solid organ and blood progenitor cell transplantation and raises the possibility of treating hepatic disorders by HPC transplantation.

ACKNOWLEDGMENT

The authors would like to thank Sylvia D. Ennis for her editorial assistance.

References

1. Thomas ED, Blume KG: Historical markers in the development of allogeneic hematopoietic cell transplantation. Biol Blood Marrow Transplant 5:341-346, 1999.
2. Ayash LJ, Hunt M, Antman K, et al: Hepatic venoocclusive disease in autologous bone marrow transplantation of solid tumors and lymphomas. J Clin Oncol 8:1699-1706, 1990.
3. Frickhofen N, Wiesneth M, Jainta C, et al: Hepatitis C virus infection is a risk factor for liver failure from veno-occlusive disease after bone marrow transplantation [see comments]. Blood 83:1998-2004, 1994.
4. Bertheau P, Hadengue A, Cazals-Hatem D, et al: Chronic cholestasis in patients after allogeneic bone marrow transplantation: several diseases are often associated. Bone Marrow Transplant 16:261-265, 1995.
5. Bearman SI, Appelbaum FR, Buckner CD, et al: Regimen-related toxicity in patients undergoing bone marrow transplantation. J Clin Oncol 6:1562-1568, 1988.
6. McDonald GB, Hinds MS, Fisher LD, et al: Veno-occlusive disease of the liver and multiorgan failure after bone marrow transplantation: a cohort study of 355 patients. Ann Intern Med 118:255-267, 1993.
7. McDonald GB, Sharma P, Matthews DE, et al: Venocclusive disease of the liver after bone marrow transplantation: diagnosis, incidence, and predisposing factors. Hepatology 4:116-122, 1984.
8. Jones RJ, Zuehlsdorf M, Rowley SD, et al: Variability in 4-hydroperoxycyclophosphamide activity during clinical purging for autologous bone marrow transplantation. Blood 70:1490-1494, 1987.
9. Shulman HM, McDonald GB, Matthews D, et al: An analysis of hepatic venocclusive disease and centrilobular hepatic degeneration following bone marrow transplantation. Gastroenterology 79:1178-1191, 1980.
10. Rozman C, Carreras E, Qian C, et al: Risk factors for hepatic veno-occlusive disease following HLA-identical sibling bone marrow transplants for leukemia. Bone Marrow Transplant 17:75-80, 1996.
11. Faioni EM, Krachmalnicoff A, Bearman SI, et al: Naturally occurring anticoagulants and bone marrow transplantation: plasma protein C predicts the development of venoocclusive disease of the liver. Blood 81:3458-3462, 1993.
12. Scrobohaci ML, Drouet L, Monem-Mansi A, et al: Liver veno-occlusive disease after bone marrow transplantation. Changes in coagulation parameters and endothelial markers. Thromb Res 63:509-519, 1991.
13. Salat C, Holler E, Wolf C, et al: Laboratory markers of veno-occlusive disease in the course of bone marrow and subsequent liver transplantation. Bone Marrow Transplant 19:487-490, 1997.
14. Salat C, Holler E, Kolb HJ, et al: Plasminogen activator inhibitor-1 confirms the diagnosis of hepatic veno-occlusive disease in patients with hyperbilirubinemia after bone marrow transplantation. Blood 89:2184-2188, 1997.
15. Yeager AM, Wagner JE Jr, et al: Optimization of busulfan dosage in children undergoing bone marrow transplantation: a pharmacokinetic study of dose escalation. Blood 80:2425-2428, 1992.
16. Demirer T, Buckner CD, Appelbaum FR, et al: Busulfan, cyclophosphamide and fractionated total body irradiation for autologous or syngeneic marrow transplantation for acute and chronic myelogenous leukemia: phase I dose escalation of busulfan based on targeted plasma levels. Bone Marrow Transplant 17:491-495, 1996.
17. DeLeve LD, Wang X, Kuhlenkamp JF, Kaplowitz N: Toxicity of azathioprine and monocrotaline in murine sinusoidal endothelial cells and hepatocytes: the role of glutathione and relevance to hepatic venoocclusive disease. Hepatology 23:589-599, 1996.
18. Slattery JT, Kalhorn TF, McDonald GB, et al: Conditioning regimen-dependent disposition of cyclophosphamide and hydroxycyclophosphamide in human marrow transplantation patients. J Clin Oncol 14:1484-1494, 1996.
19. Carreras E, Granena A, Navasa M, et al: On the reliability of clinical criteria for the diagnosis of hepatic veno-occlusive disease. Ann Hematol 66:77-80, 1993.
20. Hommeyer SC, Teefey SA, Jacobson AF, et al: Venocclusive disease of the liver: prospective study of US evaluation. Radiology 184:683-686, 1992.
21. Herbetko J, Grigg AP, Buckley AR, Phillips GL: Venoocclusive liver disease after bone marrow transplantation: findings at duplex sonography. AJR Am J Roentgenol 158:1001-1005, 1992.
22. Bearman SI: The syndrome of hepatic veno-occlusive disease after marrow transplantation. Blood 85:3005-3020, 1995.
23. Carreras E, Granena A, Rozman C: Hepatic veno-occlusive disease after bone marrow transplant. Blood Rev 7:43-51, 1993.
24. Shulman HM, Gooley T, Dudley MD, et al: Utility of transvenous liver biopsies and wedged hepatic venous pressure measurements in sixty marrow transplant recipients [see comments]. Transplantation 59:1015-1022, 1995.
25. Shulman HM, Gown AM, Nugent DJ: Hepatic veno-occlusive disease after bone marrow transplantation. Immunohistochemical identification of the material within occluded central venules. Am J Pathol 127:549-558, 1987.
26. Shulman HM, Fisher LB, Schoch HG, et al: Veno-occlusive disease of the liver after marrow transplantation: histological correlates of clinical signs and symptoms. Hepatology 19:1171-1181, 1994.
27. Strasser SI, McDonald G: Gastrointestinal and hepatic complications. In Thomas ED, Blume KG, Forman SJ, eds: Hematopoietic Cell Transplantation, ed 2. Malden, Mass., Blackwell Science Inc, 1999:627-658.
28. Bearman SI, Anderson GL, Mori M, et al: Venoocclusive disease of the liver: development of a model for predicting fatal outcome after marrow transplantation. J Clin Oncol 11:1729-1736, 1993.
29. Radich JP, Sanders JE, Buckner CD, et al: Second allogeneic marrow transplantation for patients with recurrent leukemia after initial transplant with total-body irradiation-containing regimens. J Clin Oncol 11:304-313, 1993.

30. Essell JH, Thompson JM, Harman GS, et al: Pilot trial of prophylactic ursodiol to decrease the incidence of veno-occlusive disease of the liver in allogeneic bone marrow transplant patients. Bone Marrow Transplant 10:367-372, 1992.
31. Attal M, Huguet F, Rubie H, et al: Prevention of hepatic veno-occlusive disease after bone marrow transplantation by continuous infusion of low-dose heparin: a prospective, randomized trial [see comments]. Blood 79:2834-2840, 1992.
32. Bearman SI, Hinds MS, Wolford JL, et al: A pilot study of continuous infusion heparin for the prevention of hepatic veno-occlusive disease after bone marrow transplantation. Bone Marrow Transplant 5:407-411, 1990.
33. Marsa-Vila L, Gorin NC, Laporte JP, et al: Prophylactic heparin does not prevent liver veno-occlusive disease following autologous bone marrow transplantation. Eur J Haematol 47:346-354, 1991.
34. Gluckman E, Jolivet I, Scrobohaci ML, et al: Use of prostaglandin E1 for prevention of liver veno-occlusive disease in leukaemic patients treated by allogeneic bone marrow transplantation [see comments]. Br J Haematol 74:277-281, 1990.
35. Bearman SI, Shen DD, Hinds MS, et al: A phase I/II study of prostaglandin E1 for the prevention of hepatic venocclusive disease after bone marrow transplantation. Br J Haematol 84:724-730, 1993.
36. Bianco JA, Appelbaum FR, Nemunaitis J, et al: Phase I-II trial of pentoxifylline for the prevention of transplant-related toxicities following bone marrow transplantation [published erratum appears in Blood Jun 15;79(12):3397, 1992] [see comments]. Blood 78:1205-1211, 1991.
37. Clift RA, Bianco JA, Appelbaum FR, et al: A randomized controlled trial of pentoxifylline for the prevention of regimen-related toxicities in patients undergoing allogeneic marrow transplantation. Blood 82:2025-2030, 1993.
38. Essell JH, Schroeder MT, Harman GS, et al: Ursodiol prophylaxis against hepatic complications of allogeneic bone marrow transplantation. A randomized, double-blind, placebo-controlled trial. Ann Intern Med 128:975-981, 1998.
39. Zager RA, O'Quigley J, Zager BK, et al: Acute renal failure following bone marrow transplantation: a retrospective study of 272 patients. Am J Kidney Dis 13:210-216, 1989.
40. Rubenfeld GD, Crawford SW: Withdrawing life support from mechanically ventilated recipients of bone marrow transplants: a case for evidence-based guidelines [see comments]. Ann Intern Med 125:625-633, 1996.
41. Baglin TP, Harper P, Marcus RE: Veno-occlusive disease of the liver complicating ABMT successfully treated with recombinant tissue plasminogen activator (rt-PA). Bone Marrow Transplant 5:439-441, 1990.
42. Bearman SI, Shuhart MC, Hinds MS, McDonald GB: Recombinant human tissue plasminogen activator for the treatment of established severe venocclusive disease of the liver after bone marrow transplantation. Blood 80:2458-2462, 1992.
43. Yu LC, Malkani I, Regueira O, et al: Recombinant tissue plasminogen activator (rt-PA) for veno-occlusive liver disease in pediatric autologous bone marrow transplant patients. Am J Hematol 46:194-198, 1994.
44. Terra SG, Spitzer TR, Tsunoda SM: A review of tissue plasminogen activator in the treatment of veno-occlusive liver disease after bone marrow transplantation. Pharmacotherapy 17:929-937, 1997.
45. Hagglund H, Ringden O, Ericzon BG, et al: Treatment of hepatic venoocclusive disease with recombinant human tissue plasminogen activator or orthotopic liver transplantation after allogeneic bone marrow transplantation. Transplantation 62:1076-1080, 1996.
46. Richardson PG, Elias AD, Krishnan A, et al: Treatment of severe veno-occlusive disease with defibrotide: compassionate use results in response without significant toxicity in a high-risk population. Blood 92:737-744, 1998.
47. Gordon B, Haire W, Kessinger A, et al: High frequency of antithrombin 3 and protein C deficiency following autologous bone marrow transplantation for lymphoma. Bone Marrow Transplant 8:497-502, 1991.
48. Morris JD, Harris RE, Hashmi R, et al: Antithrombin-III for the treatment of chemotherapy-induced organ dysfunction following bone marrow transplantation. Bone Marrow Transplant 20:871-878, 1997.
49. Patton DF, Harper JL, Wooldridge TN, et al: Treatment of veno-occlusive disease of the liver with bolus tissue plasminogen activator and continuous infusion antithrombin III concentrate. Bone Marrow Transplant 17:443-447, 1996.
50. Billingham RE: The biology of graft-versus-host reactions. Harvey Lect 62:21-78, 1966.
51. Aversa F, Tabilo A, Velardi A, et al: Treatment of high-risk acute leukemia with T-cell depleted stem cells from related donors with one fully mismatched HLA haplotype. N Engl J Med 339:1186-1193, 1998.
52. Shlomchik WD, Couzens MS, Tang CB, et al: Prevention of graft versus host disease by inactivation of host antigen-presenting cells. Science 285:412-415, 1999.
53. Gratwohl A, Hermans J, Apperley J, et al: Acute graft-versus-host disease: grade and outcome in patients with chronic myelogenous leukemia. Working Party Chronic Leukemia of the European Group for Blood and Marrow Transplantation. Blood 86:813-818, 1995.
54. Rowlings PA, Przepiorka D, Klein JP, et al: IBMTR Severity Index for grading acute graft-versus-host disease: retrospective comparison with Glucksberg grade. Br J Haematol 97:855-864, 1997.
55. Deeg HJ, Storb R: Graft-versus-host disease: pathophysiological and clinical aspects. Annu Rev Med 35:11-24, 1984.
56. Przepiorka D, Weisdorf D, Martin P, et al: 1994 Consensus Conference on Acute GVHD Grading. Bone Marrow Transplant 15:825-828, 1995.
57. Sale GE, Storb R, Kolb H: Histopathology of hepatic acute graft-versus-host disease in the dog. A double blind study confirms the specificity of small bile duct lesions. Transplantation 26:103-106, 1978.
58. Wick MR, Moore SB, Gastineau DA, Hoagland HC: Immunologic, clinical, and pathologic aspects of human graft-versus- host disease. Mayo Clin Proc 58:603-612, 1983.
59. Snover DC, Weisdorf SA, Ramsay NK, et al: Hepatic graft versus host disease: a study of the predictive value of liver biopsy in diagnosis. Hepatology 4:123-130, 1984.
60. Ayash L: Hepatic complications of bone marrow transplantation. In Armitage GO, Antman K, eds: High-Dose Cancer Therapy: Pharmacology, Hematopoietins, Stem Cells, ed 3. Philadelphia, Lippincott Williams & Wilkins, 2000:575-593.
61. Shulman HM, Sullivan KM, Weiden PL, et al: Chronic graft-versus-host syndrome in man. A long-term clinicopathologic study of 20 Seattle patients. Am J Med 69:204-217, 1980.
62. Ferrara JL, Levy R, Chao NJ: Pathophysiologic mechanisms of acute graft-vs.-host disease. Biol Blood Marrow Transplant 5:347-356, 1999.
63. McDonald GB, Shulman HM, Sullivan KM, Spencer GD: Intestinal and hepatic complications of human bone marrow transplantation. Part I. Gastroenterology 90:460-477, 1986.
64. Epstein O, Thomas HC, Sherlock S: Primary biliary cirrhosis is a dry gland syndrome with features of chronic graft-versus-host disease. Lancet 1:1166-1168, 1980.
65. Deeg HJ, Loughran TP Jr, Storb R, et al: Treatment of human acute graft-versus-host disease with antithymocyte globulin and cyclosporine with or without methylprednisolone. Transplantation 40:162-166, 1985.
66. Deeg HJ, Henslee-Downey PJ: Management of acute graft-versus-host disease. Bone Marrow Transplant 6:1-8, 1990.
67. Sullivan KM, Shulman HM, Storb R, et al: Chronic graft-versus-host disease in 52 patients: adverse natural course and successful treatment with combination immunosuppression. Blood 57:267-276, 1981.
68. Chanock SJ, Pizzo PA: Infectious complications of patients undergoing therapy for acute leukemia: current status and future prospects. Semin Oncol 24:132-140, 1997.
69. Hughes WT, Armstrong D, Bodey GP, et al: 1997 guidelines for the use of antimicrobial agents in neutropenic patients with unexplained fever. Infectious Diseases Society of America. Clin Infect Dis 25:551-573, 1997.
70. Navari RM, Sharma P, Deeg HJ, et al: Pneumatosis cystoides intestinalis following allogeneic marrow transplantation. Transplant Proc 15:1720-1724, 1983.
71. Johnson JR, Egaas S, Gleaves CA, et al: Hepatitis due to herpes simplex virus in marrow-transplant recipients. Clin Infect Dis 14:38-45, 1992.

72. Gleaves CA, Rice DH, Bindra R, et al: Evaluation of a HSV specific monoclonal antibody reagent for laboratory diagnosis of herpes simplex virus infection. Diagn Microbiol Infect Dis 12:315-318, 1989.
73. Gruson D, Hilbert G, Le Bail B, et al: Fulminant hepatitis due to herpes simplex virus-type 2 in early phase of bone marrow transplantation. Hematol Cell Ther 40:41-44, 1998.
74. Locksley RM, Flournoy N, Sullivan KM, Meyers JD: Infection with varicella-zoster virus after marrow transplantation. J Infect Dis 152:1172-1181, 1985.
75. Wingard JR: Advances in the management of infectious complications after bone marrow transplantation. Bone Marrow Transplant 6:371-383, 1990.
76. Schuchter LM, Wingard JR, Piantadosi S, et al: Herpes zoster infection after autologous bone marrow transplantation. Blood 74:1424-1427, 1989.
77. Ljungman P, Wilczek H, Gahrton G, et al: Long-term acyclovir prophylaxis in bone marrow transplant recipients and lymphocyte proliferation responses to herpes virus antigens in vitro. Bone Marrow Transplant 1:185-192, 1986.
78. Straus SE, Ostrove JM, Inchauspe G, et al: NIH conference. Varicella-zoster virus infections. Biology, natural history, treatment, and prevention [published erratum appears in Ann Intern Med 109(5):438-439, 1988]. Ann Intern Med 108:221-237, 1988.
79. Nikkels AF, Debrus S, Sadzot-Delvaux C, et al: Immunohistochemical identification of varicella-zoster virus gene 63-encoded protein (IE63) and late (gE) protein on smears and cutaneous biopsies: implications for diagnostic use. J Med Virol 47:342-347, 1995.
80. Nikkels AF, Delvenne P, Sadzot-Delvaux C, et al: Distribution of varicella zoster virus and herpes simplex virus in disseminated fatal infections. J Clin Pathol 49:243-248, 1996.
81. Meyers JD, Flournoy N, Thomas ED: Risk factors for cytomegalovirus infection after human marrow transplantation. J Infect Dis 153:478-488, 1986.
82. Takenaka K, Gondo H, Tanimoto K, et al: Increased incidence of cytomegalovirus (CMV) infection and CMV-associated disease after allogeneic bone marrow transplantation from unrelated donors. The Fukuoka Bone Marrow Transplantation Group [see comments]. Bone Marrow Transplant 19:241-248, 1997.
83. Couriel D, Canosa J, Engler H, et al: Early reactivation of cytomegalovirus and high risk of interstitial pneumonitis following T-depleted BMT for adults with hematological malignancies. Bone Marrow Transplant 18:347-353, 1996.
84. Einsele H, Waller HD, Weber P, et al: Cytomegalovirus in liver biopsies of marrow transplant recipients: detection methods, clinical, histological and immunohistological features. Med Microbiol Immunol (Berl) 183:205-216, 1994.
85. Shields AF, Hackman RC, Fife KH, et al: Adenovirus infections in patients undergoing bone-marrow transplantation. N Engl J Med 312:529-533, 1985.
86. Bertheau P, Parquet N, Ferchal F, et al: Fulminant adenovirus hepatitis after allogeneic bone marrow transplantation. Bone Marrow Transplant 17:295-298, 1996.
87. Somervaille TC, Kirk S, Dogan A, et al: Fulminant hepatic failure caused by adenovirus infection following bone marrow transplantation for Hodgkin's disease. Bone Marrow Transplant 24:99-101, 1999.
88. Liles WC, Cushing H, Holt S, et al: Severe adenoviral nephritis following bone marrow transplantation: successful treatment with intravenous ribavirin [see comments]. Bone Marrow Transplant 12:409-412, 1993.
89. Jurado M, Navarro JM, Hernandez J, et al: Adenovirus-associated haemorrhagic cystitis after bone marrow transplantation successfully treated with intravenous ribavirin. Bone Marrow Transplant 15:651-652, 1995 (letter).
90. Chen FE, Liang RH, Lo JY, et al: Treatment of adenovirus-associated haemorrhagic cystitis with ganciclovir. Bone Marrow Transplant 20:997-999, 1997.
91. Webster A, Brenner MK, Prentice HG, Griffiths PD: Fatal hepatitis B reactivation after autologous bone marrow transplantation. Bone Marrow Transplant 4:207-208, 1989.
92. Mertens T, Kock J, Hampl W, et al: Reactivated fulminant hepatitis B virus replication after bone marrow transplantation: clinical course and possible treatment with ganciclovir. J Hepatol 25:968-971, 1996.
93. Lau GK, Yuen ST, Au WY, et al: Histological changes during clearance of chronic hepatitis B virus infection by adoptive immunity transfer. J Gastroenterol Hepatol 14:262-268, 1999.
94. Shuhart MC, Myerson D, Childs BH, et al: Marrow transplantation from hepatitis C virus seropositive donors: transmission rate and clinical course. Blood 84:3229-3235, 1994.
95. Maruta A, Kanamori H, Fukawa H, et al: Liver function tests of recipients with hepatitis C virus infection after bone marrow transplantation. Bone Marrow Transplant 13:417-422, 1994.
96. Ljungman P, Johansson N, Aschan J, et al: Long-term effects of hepatitis C virus infection in allogeneic bone marrow transplant recipients. Blood 86:1614-1618, 1995.
97. Norol F, Roche B, Girardin MF, et al: Hepatitis C virus infection and allogeneic bone marrow transplantation. Transplantation 57:393-397, 1994.
98. Bonkovsky HL, Banner BF, Rothman AL: Iron and chronic viral hepatitis. Hepatology 25:759-768, 1997.
99. Thaler M, Pastakia B, Shawker TH, et al: Hepatic candidiasis in cancer patients: the evolving picture of the syndrome. Ann Intern Med 108:88-100, 1988.
100. van Burik JH, Leisenring W, Myerson D, et al: The effect of prophylactic fluconazole on the clinical spectrum of fungal diseases in bone marrow transplant recipients with special attention to hepatic candidiasis. An autopsy study of 355 patients. Medicine (Baltimore) 77:246-254, 1998.
101. Wingard JR: Importance of *Candida* species other than *C. albicans* as pathogens in oncology patients. Clin Infect Dis 20:115-125, 1995.
102. Meyers JD: Fungal infections in bone marrow transplant patients. Semin Oncol 17:10-13, 1990.
103. Bowden R: Fungal infections after hematopoietic cell transplantation. In Thomas ED, Blume K, Forman SJ, eds: Hematopoietic Cell Transplantation, ed 2. Malden, Mass., Blackwell Scientific, 1999:550-559.
104. Starzl T, Demetris A, Trucco M, et al: Systemic chimerism in human female recipients of male livers. Lancet 340:876-877, 1992.
105. Starzl TE, Murase N, Thomson A, Demetris A: Liver transplants contribute to their own success. Nat Med 2:198-203, 1996.
106. Lansdorp PM, Dragowska W, Mayani H: Ontogeny related changes in the proliferative potential of human hematopoietic cells. J Exp Med 178:787-791, 1993.
107. Bacchetta R, Vanderkerckhove BAE, Touraine J-L, et al: Chimerism and tolerance to host and donor in severe combined immunodeficiencies transplanted with fetal liver stem cells. J Clin Invest 91:1067, 1993.
108. Taniguchi H, Toyoshima T, Fukao K, Nakauchi H: Presence of hematopoietic stem cells in the adult liver. Nat Med 2:198-203, 1996.
109. Lagasse E, Connors H, Al-Dhalimy M, et al: Purified hematopoietic stem cells can differentiate into hepatocytes in vivo. Nat Med 6:1229-1234, 2000.

SECTION

IV G

Diseases of the Biliary Tract

CHAPTER

59

Pathogenesis of Gallstones

David E. Cohen, MD, PhD

More than 20 million individuals in the United States have gallstones. Prevalences, which vary according to gender and ethnicity, range from 5.3 percent in non-Hispanic black men to 26.7 percent in Mexican-American women.[1] Gallstones ranked as the second most costly digestive disease in 2000, with a cost of $6.5 billion.[2] This chapter focuses on the pathophysiology of gallstone formation. Clinical aspects and management of cholelithiasis are the topic of a separate chapter.[3]

TYPES OF GALLSTONES

Based upon their chemical compositions, gallstones may be categorized into three types: cholesterol stones, black pigment stones, and brown pigment stones. Although their clinical presentations may be quite similar, these different types of gallstones result from distinct pathophysiologic processes. And, as a general rule, gallstones present in a single gallbladder are similar in composition.[4] The co-existence of cholesterol and black pigment stones has been reported as a rare occurrence, however.[5]

Cholesterol Stones

Approximately 75 percent of gallstones in Western populations are cholesterol stones. Although defined as gallstones composed of greater than 50 percent cholesterol, these stones contain more than 80 percent cholesterol in most patients.[6] The remaining components of cholesterol gallstones are calcium bilirubinate, inorganic calcium salts, mucin glycoproteins, and traces of other bile components. The number, size, shape, and appearance of cholesterol gallstones may be quite varied.[6] Most cholesterol stones contain a pigmented center composed of calcium bilirubinate.[7] Commonly, there is cyclical deposition of calcium bilirubinate and variable crystal forms of calcium carbonate,[8] which lead to a ringed appearance of cholesterol gallstones.[9] The majority of cholesterol gallstones form within the gallbladder. But intrahepatic calculi with high cholesterol content are reported in Asia.[10,11]

Black Pigment Stones

Approximately 20 percent to 25 percent of stones are black pigment stones. These stones form in the gallbladder and usually are small, multiple, and spiculated.[6] Black pigment stones are composed principally of calcium bilirubinate. They have varying amounts of calcium phosphate and calcium carbonate.[12] Black pigment stones may contain up to 30 percent cholesterol, but most have cholesterol contents of less than 10 percent.[6] Compared with brown pigment stones, a greater proportion of calcium bilirubinate is polymerized in black stones.[13]

Brown Pigment Stones

Brown pigment stones make up less than 5 percent of gallstones in the West,[14] but are more common in the Far East.[13] Unlike cholesterol and black pigment stones, which are found in sterile biles, brown pigment stones form in the setting of chronic infection.[12,14] These stones occur in extrahepatic and intrahepatic ducts.[13] Their rare presence in the gallbladder represents a consequence of acute cholecytitis.[14] Brown pigment stones are laminated and contain calcium salts of bilirubin, fatty acids and phosphates, and cholesterol.[13]

BILIARY PHYSIOLOGY AND THE ENTEROHEPATIC CIRCULATION

Bile

Bile is an exocrine secretion of the liver, providing a pathway for elimination of cholesterol and other sparingly soluble molecules (e.g., bilirubin and lipophilic drugs) from the body. The components of bile are critically important for digestion and absorption of dietary fats, fat-soluble vitamins, and cholesterol.

Figure 59-1 presents the average solute composition of bile in a healthy human being. Bile salts are the most abundant class of molecules, followed by phospholipids and cholesterol. In contrast to plasma—in which most

---

The terms *bile salt* and *bile acid* are often used interchangeably in the literature. This chapter uses *bile salt* exclusively. As described elsewhere in this chapter (see ref. 36), it is important to consider that the undissociated and ionized forms differ substantially in their physical properties.

Human genes are denoted using all capital letters that are italicized. Protein products of human genes are capitalized but not italicized. Rodent genes are italicized; only the first letter is capitalized. Protein products of rodent genes are not italicized, and generally the first letter is capitalized. To facilitate their recognition, this chapter uses the commonly reported abbreviations for genes and proteins in cases in which these conventions have not been widely adopted.

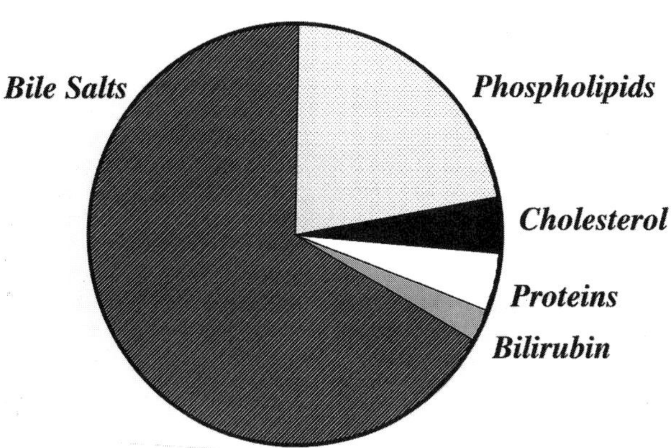

Figure 59-1 Solute composition of gallbladder bile of a healthy human being. (Modified from Carey MC, Duane WC: Enterohepatic circulation. In Arias IM, Boyer JL, Fausto N, et al, eds: The Liver: Biology and Pathobiology. New York, Raven Press, Ltd., 1994:719.)

cholesterol is esterified to fatty acids—all cholesterol in bile is unesterified.[15] Bilirubin conjugates[16] constitute a relatively small fraction of biliary solutes. Proteins in bile originate from serum, liver, and the epithelial lining of the biliary tree.[17,18]

From anatomic and functional perspectives, it is useful to classify bile as "hepatic" or "gallbladder." Hepatic bile is characterized by an average solute concentration of 3 g/dl and pH in the range of 7.3 to 8.3.[19] The average solute concentration of gallbladder bile is 10 g/dl with pH that ranges from 6.2 to 7.4.[20]

The liver produces 500 to 1200 ml of bile daily. Water secretion is passive and occurs in response to active or facilitated transport of a number of solutes within hepatocytes or bile ductular cells. Mechanisms of bile water and solute secretion are the topic of a separate chapter in this book.[21]

Cholesterol Homeostasis

Cholesterol gallstones are a consequence of an imbalance in cholesterol homeostasis. Cholesterol is an insoluble molecule essential for cellular function and for metabolic homeostasis of the organism. In cell membranes cholesterol helps to maintain the structural integrity of the lipid bilayer. Cholesterol in plasma membranes may also promote formation of functional microdomains such as rafts and caveolae that are important in signal transduction.[22,23] Cholesterol is synthesized by most cells in the body and is also obtained in the diet. A 70-kg human synthesizes cholesterol at rates of 600 to 900 mg/day.[24,25] Absorption of cholesterol from the diet is incomplete, with percentages that range from 25 percent to 80 percent[26-28] and average approximately 50 percent. Dietary cholesterol contents vary considerably (200 to 1000 mg)[26,28] so that approximately 100 to 500 mg of cholesterol are assimilated daily. Because excess cholesterol is toxic to cells, an amount equal to endogenous synthesis plus absorbed cholesterol must be eliminated each day.

Few tissues are capable of catabolizing cholesterol. In adrenal glands, testes, and ovaries cholesterol is a substrate for biosynthesis of glucocorticoids, mineralocorticoids, and reproductive hormones. Minor losses of cholesterol are attributable to biosynthesis of steroid hormone (50 mg/day) and to sloughing of skin cells (85 mg/day).[29] The liver eliminates virtually all excess cholesterol from the body (400 to 1350 mg/day).

Reverse cholesterol transport is the process by which excess cholesterol is routed from peripheral tissues to the liver.[30] This is achieved when high-density lipoproteins (HDL) in plasma accept excess cholesterol from cells in the periphery. Transfer of cellular cholesterol occurs principally by diffusion of free (i.e., unesterified) cholesterol from plasma membranes of cells to nearby HDL particles.[31] In plasma, cholesterol is esterified by the circulating enzyme lecithin:cholesterol acyl transferase to form cholesteryl esters.[30] Cholesteryl ester molecules that have accumulated in HDL are then returned to the liver, where they are taken up via an HDL receptor known as scavenger receptor class B type I (SR-BI). A fraction of the cholesteryl esters in HDL take an alternate route to the liver. These are transferred by a circulating protein known as cholesteryl ester transfer protein to triglyceride-rich lipoproteins (i.e., remnants of chylomicrons and very low-density lipoproteins [VLDL]), which are removed from the circulation by specific receptors in the liver.[32]

While processing cholesterol delivered from extrahepatic sources, the liver must also maintain a steady state content of free cholesterol that is suitable for hepatocellular function. Figure 59-2 illustrates schematically the general metabolic pathways by which this balance is achieved. Hepatic cholesterol is derived from lipoproteins, from de novo synthesis that is rate-limited by the microsomal enzyme 3-hydroxy-3-methylglutaryl coenzyme A (HMG-CoA) reductase[33] and from hydrolysis of stored cholesteryl esters by the action of a cholesteryl ester hydrolase.[34] Excess cholesterol may be exported into plasma by incorporation into HDL or VLDL particles. The liver also can store cholesterol by synthesizing cholesterol esters in a transacylation reaction catalyzed by acyl-CoA:cholesterol acyltransferase enzymes.[35] Finally, cholesterol may be eliminated from the body via bile. This is achieved by conversion of cholesterol to bile salts (see the following section) at rates of 200 to 600 mg/day[36] and by secretion of unmodified cholesterol into bile at rates of 400 to 1500 mg/day.[37-40] Fecal losses of bile salts balance synthetic rates for bile salts, accounting for 200 to 600 mg/day of cholesterol losses.[36] Approximately 50 percent of biliary cholesterol is reabsorbed in the intestine,[41] resulting in net cholesterol losses of 200 to 750 mg/day.

Enterohepatic Circulation of Bile Salts

Bile formation and fat digestion necessitate the biliary secretion of an average of 1 g/hr of bile salts.[36] Efficient mechanisms have evolved to recycle bile salts from the intestine to liver in an enterohepatic circulation (Figure 59-3). The bile salt pool is the total mass of bile salts within the enterohepatic circulation and amounts to approximately 3 g in humans. Each molecule in the bile salt pool completes 4 to 12 cycles between the liver and intestine per day. When enterohepatic circulation is intact

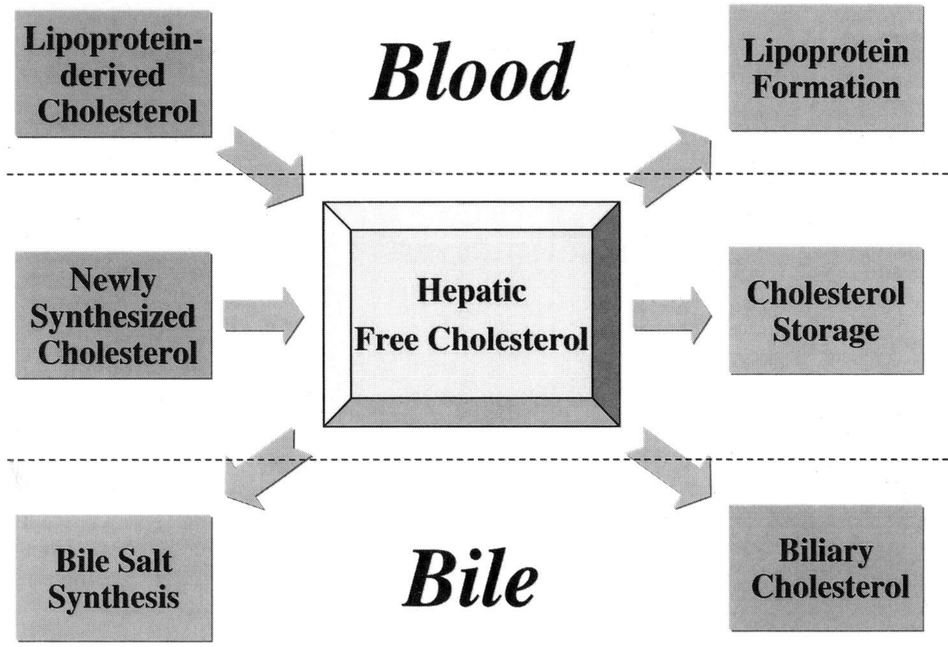

Figure 59-2 Schematic diagram of hepatic cholesterol balance.

the liver synthesizes only 200 to 600 mg/day to compensate for losses in feces. This implies a greater than 95 percent efficiency of the intestine for reclaiming bile salts.

Bile Salt Synthesis

Bile salt molecules synthesized by catabolism of cholesterol within the liver are referred to as primary bile salts. Cholesterol used for synthesis of bile salts derives principally from apolipoprotein B–containing lipoproteins (e.g., low-density lipoproteins).[42,43]

In humans there are two molecular species of primary bile salts: 3α,7α,12α-trihydroxy-5β-cholanoate (cholate) and 3α,7α-dihydroxy-5β-cholanoate (chenodeoxycholate). As shown in Figure 59-4 biosynthesis of bile salts entails modification of cholesterol by hydroxylation of the sterol nucleus, saturation of the nucleus and epimerization of the 3β-hydroxyl group, and oxidation and shortening of the hydrocarbon side-chain by three carbons.[44,45] It is now appreciated that there are at least two distinct pathways for biosynthesis of primary bile salts. These two pathways involve complex enzymatic cascades. Details of these enzymatic pathways, regulation of bile salt biosynthesis, and enterohepatic cycling are the subject of a number of comprehensive reviews.[36,44-50] The following section summarizes salient features and recent advances in cloning and characterization of the key enzymes of bile salt synthesis.

The "neutral" or "classical" pathway of bile salt synthesis is initiated and rate-limited by cholesterol 7α-hydroxylase (CYP 7A1), a unique cytochrome P450 monooxygenase[51-53] that is localized to the smooth endoplasmic reticulum of hepatocytes.[54,55] This enzyme hydroxylates the C-7 position of the steroid ring of cholesterol. A series of enzymatic modifications of the steroid nucleus then takes place within the endoplasmic reticulum and cytosol.[44] An important intermediate step is addition of a hydroxyl group at position C-12 of the steroid nucleus by sterol 12α-hydroxylase, a cytochrome P450 enzyme (CYP 8B1)[56,57] in the smooth endoplasmic reticulum. The "neutral" pathway produces both cholate and chenodeoxycholate. The late steps of bile salt synthesis via the "neutral" pathway take place in mitochondria and peroxisomes, where oxidation of the hydrocarbon side chain occurs.[58] The activity of CYP 8B1 determines ratio of cholate to chenodeoxycholate in bile.[44,47] Under physiologic conditions in humans the neutral pathway produces chenodeoxycholate and cholate in roughly equal proportions.[45]

The second enzymatic cascade for biosynthesis of primary bile salts is known as the "acidic" or "alternative" pathway. The term *acidic* is used because carboxylic acid intermediates are formed at early steps during biosynthesis. The "acidic" pathway is initiated by sterol 27-hydroxylase (CYP 27), a mitochondrial cytochrome P450 mono-oxygenase[59-62] that adds a hydroxyl group to the hydrocarbon side-chain of cholesterol. CYP 27 is highly expressed in liver and in a number of extrahepatic tissues.[45,59] This observation taken together with discovery of 27-hydroxycholesterol in human blood has led to the suggestion that a fraction of bile salt biosynthesis could begin in the periphery and go to completion in the liver.[59] At a later step a hydroxyl group is added to position C-7 of the steroid nucleus by oxysterol 7α-hydroxylase (CYP 7B), another cytochrome P450 enzyme.[63] The "acidic" pathway produces principally chenodeoxycholic acid and only small amounts of cholic acid.[45]

The quantitative contributions of the "neutral" and "acidic" pathways to overall synthesis of bile salts have been estimated. Experiments in humans after cholecys-

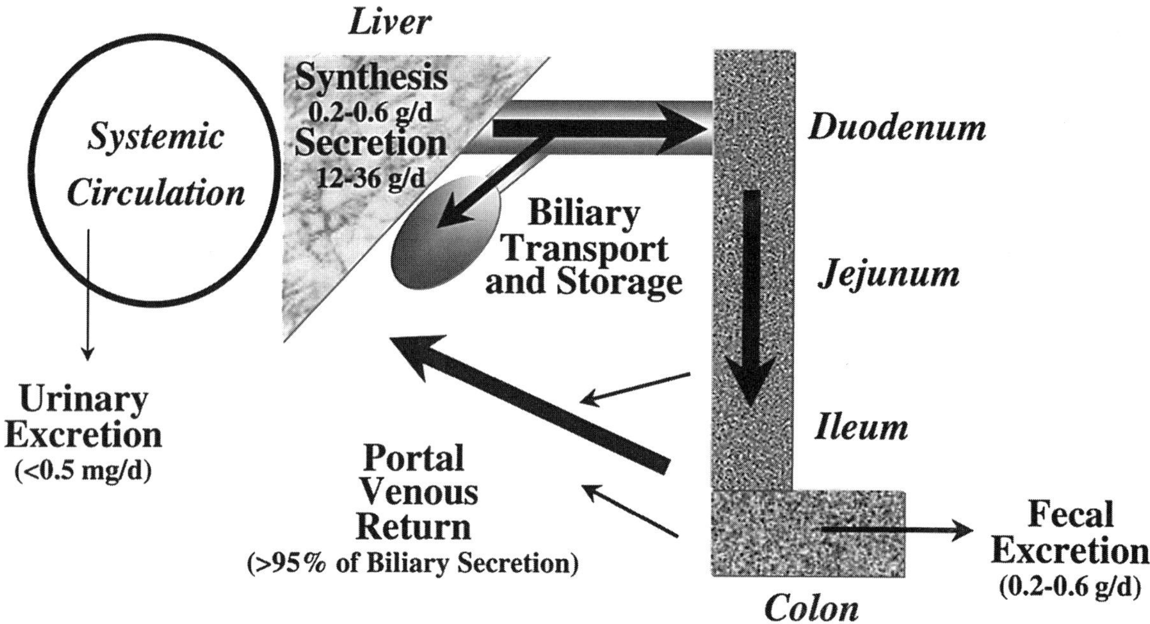

Figure 59-3 The enterohepatic circulation of bile salts. Typical values for hepatic synthesis and secretion and fecal and urinary losses are shown for healthy human beings. (Redrawn from Carey MC, Duane WC: Enterohepatic circulation. In Arias IM, Boyer JL, Fausto N, et al, eds: The Liver: Biology and Pathobiology. New York, Raven Press, Ltd., 1994:719.)

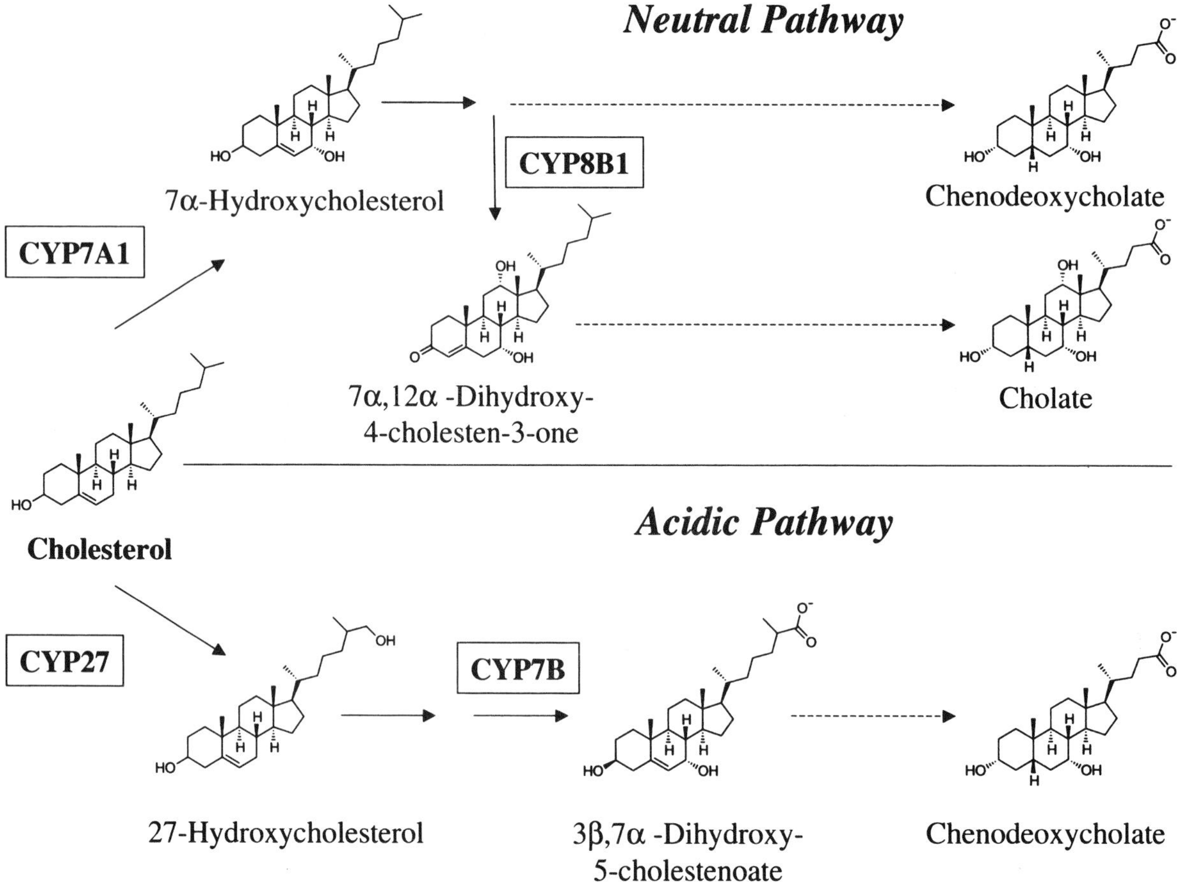

Figure 59-4 Two pathways for bile salt biosynthesis in the liver. The products of selected enzymes in the "neutral" and "acidic" pathways are displayed. *Solid arrows,* Single enzymatic steps; *dashed arrows,* two or more enzymatic reactions. (Modified from Carey MC, Duane WC: Enterohepatic circulation. In Arias IM, Boyer JL, Fausto N, et al: The Liver: Biology and Pathobiology, ed 3. New York, Raven Press, 1994:719.)

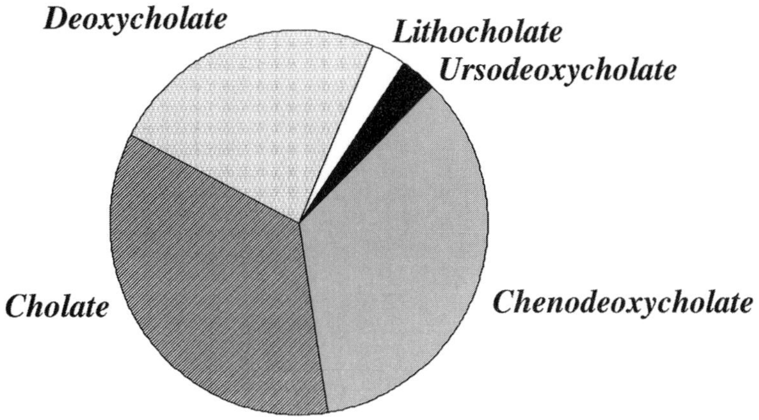

Figure 59-5 Composition of the bile salt pool in healthy human beings. *Cholate,* 3α,7α,12α-Trihydroxy-5β-cholanoate; *chenodeoxycholate,* 3α,7α-dihydroxy-5β-cholanoate; *deoxycholate,* 3α,12α-dihydroxy-5β-cholanoate; *ursodeoxycholate,* 3α, 7β-dihydroxy-5β-cholanoate; *lithocholate,* 3α-monohydroxy-5β-cholanoate.

tectomy suggest that the "neutral" pathway contributes the majority of bile salts synthesized in health.[64] The "acidic" pathway may become a more significant source of bile salts in chronic liver disease.[45] In rodents the contribution of the "acidic" pathway to bile salt synthesis may be as much as 50 percent.[65,66]

Conjugation of Bile Salts

At pH values that occur within the enterohepatic circulation, primary bile salts are only sparingly soluble in water.[67,68] When bile salts are conjugated in the liver by peptide linkage to either glycine or taurine,[48] solubility is increased markedly (i.e., pK_a values are greatly decreased) as is resistance to precipitation with physiologic calcium concentrations. Conjugation is accomplished in a two-step reaction.[69] The first step is catalyzed by bile acid–CoA synthetase, which promotes the formation of bile acid–CoA thioesters. The second step is catalyzed by bile acid CoA:amino acid N-acyltransferase.[48,70] In humans glycine conjugates predominate in a molar ratio of approximately 2:1 compared with taurine conjugates.[36] The extent to which taurine is used depends principally on dietary availability.[48] Conjugation of bile salts in the liver is a highly efficient process. Virtually all biliary bile salts are conjugated.[36]

Intestinal Modifications of Bile Salts

Within the enterohepatic circulation, primary bile salts are exposed to bacterial flora of the intestine, particularly in the cecum. The intestinal microflora can transform bile salts to a variety of metabolites.[71-73] During each cycle approximately 10 percent to 20 percent of bile salts are deconjugated (i.e., have their glycine or taurine removed from their side chains).[36] Hydrolysis of the amide bond of conjugated bile salts is mediated by a variety of bacterial species within the intestine.[72] After removal of the amino acid moiety, bile salts then may undergo 7α-dehydroxylation. Quantitatively, 7α-dehydroxylation of the primary bile salts represents the most common bacterial transformation.[72] Removal of the α-hydroxyl group from C-7 of cholate and chenodeoxycholate results in formation of the secondary bile salts deoxycholate and lithocholate, respectively. These are the principal bile salts present in human feces. The biochemistry and molecular genetics of the enzymatic machinery that removes the hydroxyl group from the C-7 position of unconjugated bile salts[72] have been described in *Clostridium* species.[74,75] Bacterial metabolism of bile salts also may cause epimerization (i.e., reorientation) of hydroxyl groups with respect to the steroid nucleus.[71] In this manner the primary bile salt chenodeoxycholate is converted to the tertiary bile salt ursodeoxycholate.

These common and other less common bacterial degradation products are absorbed passively to varying extents within the colon and returned to the liver via the portal circulation. After being taken up by the liver, secondary and tertiary bile salts are efficiently reconjugated with glycine or taurine and secreted into bile. Secondary and tertiary bile salts thereby join the enterohepatic circulation and contribute importantly to the heterogeneity of molecular species of bile salts within the bile salt pool (Figure 59-5). An important exception is lithocholate, which is highly insoluble even after conjugation. Its water solubility is increased by hepatic ester sulfation at C-3 of the steroid nucleus.[69,76] Sulfated lithocholate is poorly reabsorbed in the intestine, resulting in loss of most lithocholates in the feces.[36] Overall, secondary and tertiary bile salts contribute approximately 25 percent to the bile salt pool in healthy individuals.

Physical Chemistry of Bile Salts

Bile salts are highly soluble, detergent-like molecules. Their physical chemical properties have been the subject of several decades of study (for reviews, see refs. 67, 68, 77). As illustrated in Figure 59-6, bile salts are amphiphilic (i.e., possess both hydrophilic and hydrophobic surfaces). Their high aqueous solubility is due to their capacity to self-associate into micelles when a critical micellar concentration

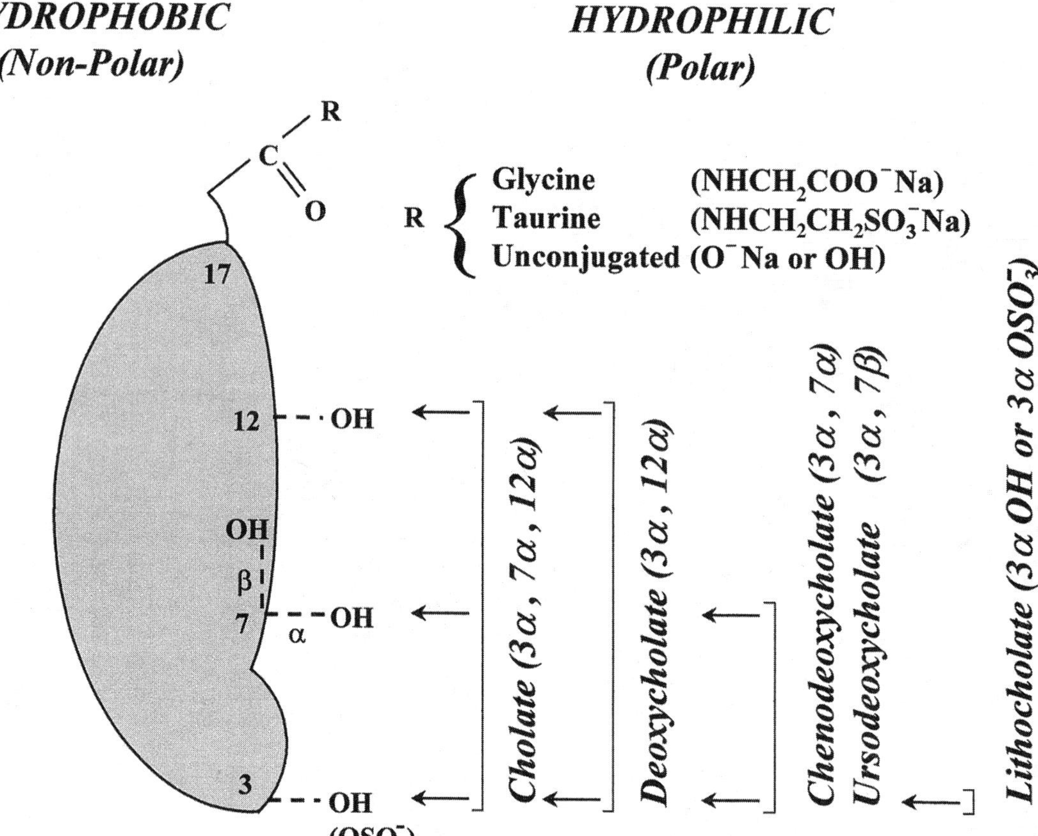

Figure 59-6 Amphipathic structures of the common human bile salts. In the liver the side chain (R) is conjugated to glycine or taurine. In the intestine the amino acid may be removed by bacteria to yield an unconjugated bile salt. Because of their relatively high pK_a values, unconjugated bile salts may exist in the dissociated (O^-Na) or undissociated (OH) form. (Modified from Carey MC, Duane WC: Enterohepatic circulation. In Arias IM, Boyer JL, Fausto N, et al, eds: The Liver: Biology and Pathobiology. New York, Raven Press, Ltd., 1994:719.)

(CMC) is exceeded. The CMC is a characteristic of species of bile salt, the ionic strength and composition, and the types and concentrations of other lipids present in solution. Aggregates formed when pure bile salts exceed their CMC values are known as simple micelles. CMC values for common bile salts under physiologic conditions are in the range of 1 to 20 mM.[48] Although not known with precision, hepatocellular concentrations of bile salt are submicellar and in the range of 100 to 200 μM.[78] Bile salt concentrations within the bile canaliculus are believed to be severalfold higher than hepatocellular concentrations[78] and likely exceed CMC values.[79] Because bile is concentrated within the biliary tree, bile salt concentrations further exceed their CMCs. Thus bile salts form simple micelles in bile. More importantly, micelles of bile salts solubilize other types of lipids to form mixed micelles (see the section on Aggregation of Lipids in Bile).

The potency of bile salts as detergents depends critically upon the distribution and orientation of hydroxyl groups around the steroid nucleus of the molecule. For example, 3α,7α-dihydroxy-5β-cholanoate (chenodeoxycholate) and 3α,7β-dihydroxy-5β-cholanoate (ursodeoxycholate) differ in structure by the spatial orientation of only a single hydroxyl group (see Figure 59-6). However, orientation of the C-7 hydroxyl group in the alpha orientation markedly expands the hydrophobic surface of the steroid nucleus. This explains why chenodeoxycholate is a potent detergent, whereas ursodeoxycholate is not.

The relative potency of a particular molecular species of bile salt as a detergent is commonly referred to as its hydrophobicity. Bile salt hydrophobicity can be quantified in the laboratory by high-performance liquid chromatography[80-82] and used to predict the biologic effects of individual bile salts. High-performance liquid chromatography is also used to determine the hydrophobicity of a mixture of bile salt species,[83] such as are present in human biles.

The physical chemical properties of bile salts also depend upon the nature and ionization state of functional groups on the side chain (see Figure 59-6).[48] Protonation of the side chain renders unconjugated bile salts only sparingly soluble in water.[67] Although protonation of unconjugated bile salts occurs in the intestine after deconjugation by bacterial flora, bile salts within the enterohepatic circulation of healthy individuals are otherwise conjugated. For an individual molecular species of bile salt, the glycine conjugate is more hydrophobic than the taurine conjugate.[80-83]

Transport of Bile Salts Within the Enterohepatic Circulation

Enterohepatic cycling of bile salts is primarily the consequence of specific transport proteins present in the liver and in the ileum, with contributions from gallbladder and intestinal motility. Applications of both classical biochemical approaches and newer molecular biologic technologies over the past decade have yielded remarkable progress in the identification and characterization of proteins that transport bile salts and the genes that encode them. In many cases these efforts also have revealed the molecular bases for inherited cholestatic syndromes.

Sinusoidal Bile Salt Transport. Bile salts returning from the intestine to the liver in the portal circulation are taken up with high (80 percent) first-pass clearance rates into the liver. Hepatocytes do not have the capacity to store bile salts, and these molecules are efficiently transported across the liver cell and re-secreted into bile. The remaining 20 percent of bile salts are cleared rapidly from the systemic circulation upon returning to the liver.

Three sinusoidal membrane transport proteins have been identified in rats that appear to contribute to the efficient clearance of bile salts from portal blood. These are sodium taurocholate co-transporting polypeptide (Ntcp),[84] organic anion-transporting polypeptide-1 (oatp-1),[85] and microsomal epoxide hydrolase.[86] Human homolog of these proteins have been identified.[87] Although the function of each protein as a bile salt transporter has been demonstrated in cell culture, the relative contributions of each to hepatocellular uptake of bile salts from the portal circulation remain uncertain.

In addition to proteins that promote uptake of bile salts from sinusoidal blood, proteins capable of exporting bile salts reside on the sinusoidal membrane.[87] These are members of the family of multi-drug resistance-associated proteins (MRP) family within the adenosine triphosphate (ATP)-binding cassette (ABC) superfamily of proteins.[88] ABCC1 (i.e., MRP1) and ABCC3 (i.e., MRP3) normally are present at low levels.[89,90] ABCC3 is up-regulated in Dubin-Johnson syndrome[89,91] and during cholestasis.[92] ABCC1 is up-regulated in endotoxemia-induced cholestasis.[93] Because ABCC1 and ABCC3 are ATP-dependent proteins capable of transporting di- and mono-anionic bile salts, respectively, these transporters may facilitate renal elimination of bile salts under cholestatic conditions in which down-regulation of canalicular transporters prevents biliary excretion.[87]

Transhepatocellular Bile Salt Transport. The mechanisms by which bile salts are transported from the sinusoidal to the canalicular membrane are not well understood. A vesicle-mediated pathway has been postulated, but this is not supported by current data.[94-96] In rat and human liver cytosol, bile salts bind to members of an aldo-keto reductase gene family (e.g., 3α-hydroxysteroid dehydrogenase in rat), to liver fatty acid binding protein, and to glutathione-*S*-transferases.[96,97] Although this supports the concept that cytosolic binding proteins are responsible for intracellular transport, functional data supporting intracellular bile salt transport by these proteins have not been presented.[96,97]

Canalicular Bile Salt Transport. Secretion of bile salts across the canalicular membrane is the rate-limiting step in the enterohepatic circulation of bile salts. ABCB11 (also referred to as the bile salt export pump or Sister-P-glycoprotein) represents the major canalicular bile salt transporting protein of mammalian liver and functions to extrude bile salts across the canalicular membrane against a concentration gradient.[98] It is also a member of the ABC superfamily.[88] Targeted disruption of the ABCB11 gene in mice decreases secretion of bile salts and causes non-progressive, intrahepatic cholestasis.[99] Naturally occurring mutations in ABCB11 in humans are associated with type 2 progressive familial intrahepatic cholestasis (PFIC2).[100,101] A second canalicular transporter ABCC2 (i.e., MRP2—formerly referred to as canalicular multi-specific organic anion transporter), which is mutated in Dubin-Johnson syndrome,[102,103] functions to secrete a wide variety of organic anions into bile, including bilirubin glucuronides, glutathione conjugates, and 3-sulfate and 3-glucuronide di-anionic bile salts.[87,104,105] The activity of ABCC2 represents a route for elimination of the hydrophobic and cytotoxic bile salt lithocholate, which is ester sulfated by the liver before secretion into bile.[36]

Bile Salt Transport Within the Biliary Tree and Intestine. After secretion from hepatocytes into bile ducts, bile salts are stored in the gallbladder and propelled into the biliary tree upon appropriate hormonal stimulus. It has become clear in recent years that the bile ducts are active with respect to bile salt transport. To explain the hypercholeretic effects of certain bile salts,[106] cholehepatic cycling from bile ducts to the hepatic sinusoid via the periductular capillary plexus was postulated.[48,107] It was shown subsequently that cholangiocytes express the sodium-dependent bile salt transporter on their apical membrane that is found in the ileum (see the following section).[108] Cholangiocytes express on the basolateral membrane, both an alternatively spliced form of the apical sodium-dependent bile salt transporter[109] and ABCC3.[90] Therefore the presence of apical and basolateral transporters provides a route for reabsorption of bile salts within the bile ducts.[87]

Intestinal Transport and Absorption of Bile Salts. Within the lumen of the small intestine, bile salt transit depends principally upon motility. Reabsorption of bile salts from intestine into portal circulation occurs by both passive and active mechanisms. Active transport of conjugated bile salts is localized to the ileum. Sodium-coupled absorption of bile salts occurs via an apical sodium-dependent transporter (also referred to as IBAT and formally named SLC10A2).[110-112] After uptake and during cytosolic transport, ileal bile salts appear to remain bound to an ileal bile acid–binding protein (I-BABP, also referred to as ileal lipid-binding protein).[96,113-115] ABCC3 may function as a bile salt transporter in the basolateral membrane of the ileocyte.[87] In addition to the ileum, bile salt reabsorption may occur proximally where organic anion transporting polypeptide-3 is expressed on the apical membrane of rat jejunal enterocytes. This protein may mediate uptake by an anion exchange-driven mechanism.[116] Passive reabsorption of unconjugated bile salts also occurs throughout the gastrointestinal tract.[36] This latter process is driven principally by protonation of the poorly soluble unconjugated bile salts within the intestinal lumen, which permits passive movement across membranes.

Transport of Bile Salts in Portal Blood. After reabsorption and transport across enterocytes, bile salts are returned to the liver in the portal circulation. Concentrations of bile salts in portal blood are approximately 20 μM, or roughly six times that of peripheral blood.[36,117] After a meal the concentration of bile salts in portal vein can increase by tenfold.[36] A fraction of bile salts in portal blood binds reversibly to albumin and to HDL in plasma. This fraction is transported with unbound bile salts to the hepatic sinusoids.[36]

Transport of Bile Salts in the Kidney. Urinary losses of bile salts are negligible in health but may increase dramatically in cholestatic conditions.[36,48] In cholestasis hepatic sulfation of bile salts is increased,[48] and sulfated bile salts are transported into blood across the sinusoidal membrane (see previous discussion). Although the kidney expresses transport proteins (e.g., apical sodium-dependent bile salt transporter and organic anion-transporting polypeptide-3) that apparently function to reclaim filtered bile salts, sulfated bile salts are not substrates for these transporters and are therefore eliminated in the urine.[87]

Regulation of the Enterohepatic Circulation of Bile Salts

When the enterohepatic circulation is intact, synthesis of bile salt from cholesterol precisely matches fecal losses. The relatively small loss on a percentage basis (less than 5 percent) amounts to 200 to 600 mg/day. However, this is a significant amount of cholesterol, accounting for about half the daily loss of cholesterol from the body. Bile salts returning from intestine to liver suppress bile salt synthesis. Removal of feedback inhibition by interruption of the enterohepatic circulation increases bile salt synthesis rates by up to tenfold.[36]

Short-term Regulation of Bile Salt Transport in Liver. The hepatocyte is regularly exposed to rapid fluctuations of bile salt concentrations. Because bile salt concentrations in portal blood vary widely between the fasted and fed states,[36] the liver responds in the short term by increasing hepatocellular bile salt transport over a time frame that is too rapid to be controlled by transcriptional mechanisms. The cellular mechanism of this response most likely involves rapid repositioning of bile salt transporters from storage vesicles within the cell to the plasma membrane to increase transport capacity.[118,119] This is presumably mediated by signal transduction mechanisms that regulate amounts of NTCP[120] and OATP-1[121] in the sinusoidal membrane and the amount of ABCB11 in the canalicular membrane.[119,122,123]

Hormonal Regulation of Bile Salt Synthesis. It is well appreciated that bile salt synthesis is under hormonal control. In hepatocytes insulin down-regulates CYP 7A1[124,125] and CYP 27.[125] Thyroid hormone and glucocorticoids synergistically up-regulate CYP 7A1 messenger ribonucleic acid (mRNA) and transcriptional activity, whereas the gene is down-regulated by insulin and glucagon.[45] Regulation of cholesterol CYP 7A1 by glucocorticoids may explain in part the diurnal variations in bile salt synthetic rates.[45] Detailed transcriptional mechanisms by which hormones regulate bile salt synthesis are complex and not completely understood.[47]

Transcriptional Control of Bile Salt Metabolism. Our understanding of bile salt homeostasis, including mechanisms by which bile salts regulate their own synthesis, has been revolutionized by the discovery that nuclear hormone receptors are transcriptional regulators of key enzymes in sterol metabolism. Nuclear hormone receptors are a superfamily of cellular receptors that regulate gene transcription.[126] In general, these proteins are activated upon binding small hydrophobic molecules (e.g., bile salts and steroid hormones). Two nuclear hormone receptors, the liver X receptor alpha (LXRα) and the farnesoid X receptor (FXR), are of particular importance in the transcriptional control of the enterohepatic circulation.[127] LXRα binds to oxidized cholesterol molecules known as oxysterols,[128] whereas FXR binds hydrophobic bile salts.[129-131] To influence gene transcription, each of these nuclear hormone receptors must bind to deoxyribonucleic acid (DNA) as a heterodimeric complex with the retinoid X receptor (RXR) and its ligand, 9-*cis* retinoic acid.[132]

The mechanisms by which LXRα and FXR control metabolism of cholesterol and bile salt have been studied principally in rodents and are summarized schematically in Figure 59-7. When the animal is challenged with a diet containing excess cholesterol, oxysterols accumulate in liver and intestine, where LXRα is expressed. Oxysterol binding to LXRα results in a marked increase in transcription of the CYP 7A1 gene in liver. This leads to catabolism of cholesterol to form bile salts.[133] Activation of LXRα by oxysterols in the intestine leads to a different physiologic response. There is increased expression of the Tangier disease gene product ABCA1 and the sitosterolemia gene products ABCG5 and ABCG8. These reduce cholesterol absorption apparently by pumping it from enterocytes back into the intestinal lumen.[134-136] In addition to these functions in the liver and intestine, LXRα increases expression of genes in liver and other tissues that promote reverse cholesterol transport.[134,137,138] In contrast to rodents, however, humans do not respond to dietary cholesterol by up-regulating CYP 7A1. This may be explained by a different nucleotide sequence in the human and rodent CYP 7A1 gene promoters that eliminates binding of LXRα in the human.[139,140]

As is also shown in Figure 59-7, FXR regulates a number of key genes that participate in maintaining bile salt homeostasis. In the liver FXR promotes down-regulation of Ntcp and CYP 7A1 but up-regulation of ABCB11.[141,142] Activation of FXR occurs as a result of binding to hydrophobic bile salts, which may explain why hydrophobic and not hydrophilic bile salts are potent inhibitors of

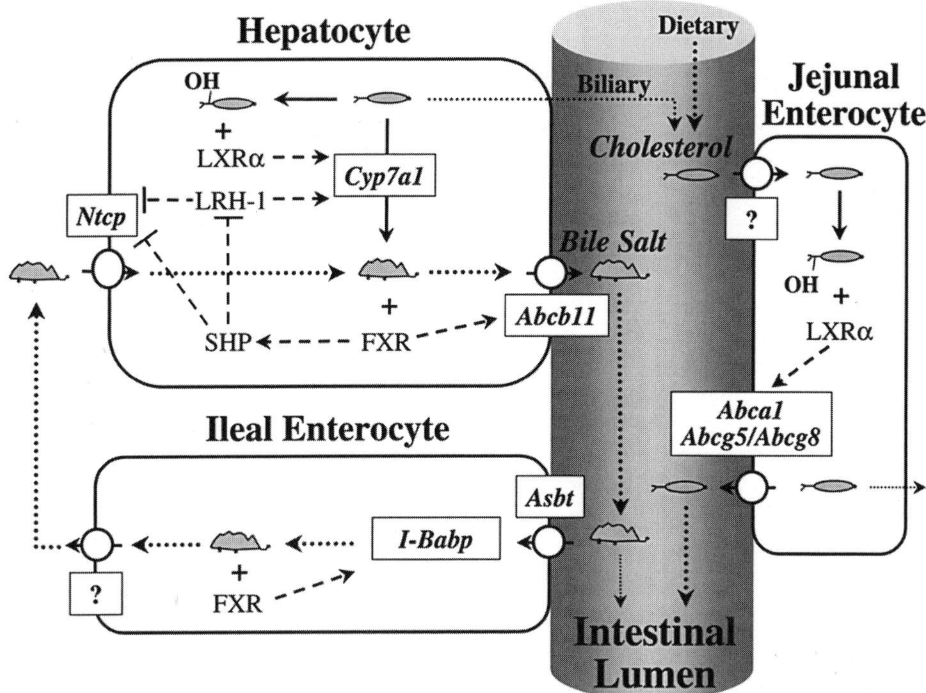

Figure 59-7 Nuclear hormone control of sterol metabolism within the enterohepatic circulation. Bile salt and cholesterol molecules are represented schematically, with the -OH group indicating oxidation of cholesterol to form an oxysterol. Solid arrows indicate metabolic pathways. A (+) indicates binding of a bile salt or oxysterol molecule to a nuclear hormone receptor. Dotted arrows point to genes that are up-regulated by nuclear hormone receptors, whereas dashed lines ending in solid bars denote genes that are down-regulated. Question marks indicate unidentified genes. Circles bisected by arrows indicate that gene products are membrane transport proteins. Dotted arrows signify transport pathways. Relative magnitudes of bile salt and cholesterol fluxes through transport pathways are represented qualitatively using dot sizes.

bile salt synthesis in vivo.[143] Up-regulation of ABCB11 is a direct result of binding by FXR and RXR to the gene promoter.[144] However, mechanistic studies show that FXR down-regulates gene expression of CYP 7A1 by an indirect mechanism.[145,146] A heterodimer of FXR and RXR promotes the transcription of a nuclear hormone receptor known as small heterodimer partner (SHP).[145] SHP binds and inactivates a DNA-binding protein called liver receptor homolog-1 (LRH-1), which is required for gene transcription of CYP 7A1.[145] Bile salts may also promote SHP transcription by activation of the c-Jun-N-terminal kinase/c-Jun pathway.[147] In addition, bile salt-mediated SHP activation leads to down-regulation of Ntcp in the liver.[148] FXR in the intestine promotes the expression of I-BABP[142] by binding to the gene promoter.[129,149] Although not known with certainty, I-BABP is believed to participate in transcellular transport of bile salts across ileal enterocytes.[97] Up-regulation of I-BABP by FXR therefore would provide a mechanism for enhancing bile salt absorption in response to increases in intestinal concentration of bile salts.

LXRα and FXR provide integrated mechanisms for the organism to respond to increases in cholesterol and bile salt levels (see Figure 59-7). When excess cholesterol is present, LXRα inhibits absorption, increases return of cholesterol to the liver from peripheral tissues, and promotes catabolism to bile salts. In contrast, elevations in hepatocellular bile salt concentrations provoke an adaptive response that is designed presumably to reduce bile salt-induced hepatotoxicity. FXR activation inhibits uptake of bile salt across the sinusoidal membrane, down-regulates of synthesis and enhances secretion into bile. By contrast, FXR in the intestine promotes conservation of bile salts by increasing absorption efficiency and thereby decreasing fecal losses.

Besides LXRα and FXR, other nuclear hormone receptors and transcription factors control metabolism of bile salts. Binding of lithocholate to the pregnane X receptor (PXR) in liver cells inhibits transcription of CYP 7A1 and induces expression of cytochrome P450 3A (CYP 3A).[150,151] In this manner, PXR provides an integrated response to the cholestatic effects of lithocholate. PXR decreases synthesis of endogenous bile salts to reduce hepatocellular bile salt concentrations, and it promotes hydroxylation of lithocholate to form more soluble species of bile salt.[150,151] The peroxisome proliferator-activated receptor alpha (PPARα) down-regulates CYP 7A1[152,153] and may alter bile salt composition by regulating

CYP 8B1.[154] Members of the hepatocyte nuclear factor (HNF) gene family also regulate several aspects of bile salt metabolism. These transcription factors bind to gene promoter regions and regulate transcription of CYP 7A1[155,156] and Ntcp.[157] In mice homozygous disruption of HNF-1α,[158] HNF-4α,[159] and HNF-3β[160] leads to multiple defects in bile salt metabolism.

Biliary Secretion of Lipids

Biliary secretion of bile salts promotes secretion of cholesterol and phospholipids into bile. In humans and laboratory animals[161,162] secretion rates of cholesterol and phospholipids into bile are curvilinear functions of bile salt secretion rates (Figure 59-8). An important consequence is that biliary lipid compositions vary as functions of bile salt secretion rate. As bile secretion rates decrease, bile becomes relatively more enriched with cholesterol.

Origins of Biliary Lipids

Bile Salts. Because bile salts are highly conserved within the enterohepatic circulation, synthesis of new bile salts within hepatocytes contributes only a small fraction (less than 5 percent) to biliary secretion of bile salts.[36] This contribution rises under conditions in which the enterohepatic circulation is partially or completely interrupted by surgery, disease states, or drugs (e.g., bile salt-binding resins). Complete interruption of the enterohepatic circulation results in up-regulation of bile salt synthesis sufficient to restore bile salt secretion rates to approximately 25 percent of their native values.[163]

Phospholipids. About 11 g of phospholipids are secreted into human bile per day.[164] Although these biliary phospholipids are derived from liver cell membranes, their compositions differ markedly. Hepatocyte membranes contain appreciable quantities of phosphatidylcholines (i.e., lecithins), phosphatidylethanolamines, phosphatidylinositols, phosphatidylserines, and sphingomyelins. In contrast, phosphatidylcholines make up more than 95 percent of biliary phospholipids in humans and most other species,[15,165] with phosphatidylethanolamines and sphingomyelins comprising the remainder. The main source of phosphatidylcholine molecules destined for secretion into bile is hepatic synthesis.[166,167] However, a fraction of biliary phosphatidylcholines may also originate in the phospholipid coat of HDL particles.[168]

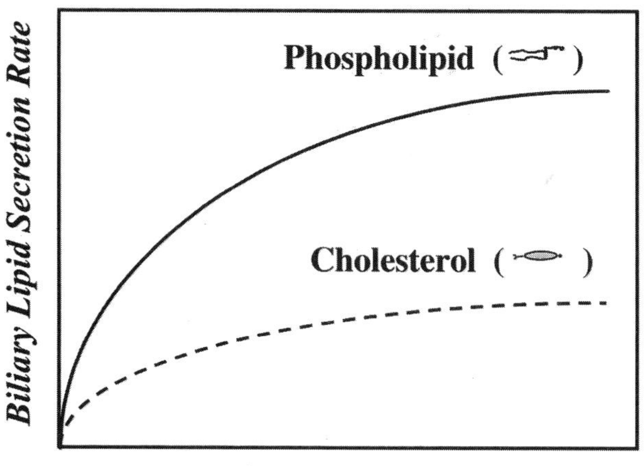

Figure 59-8 Schematic representation of quantitative relationships between secretion rates of phospholipid and cholesterol into bile and biliary bile salt secretion rates. (Redrawn from Cohen DE: Hepatocellular transport and secretion of biliary lipids. Curr Opin Lipidol 235:111, 1999.)

Cholesterol. Plasma lipoproteins are the principal source of cholesterol in bile. Consistent with their central role in reverse cholesterol transport, HDL particles appear to be the main lipoprotein source of cholesterol that is targeted for biliary secretion.[42,43,169,170] An appreciable fraction of cholesterol in bile also may be derived from the diet via apolipoprotein E-dependent delivery of chylomicron remnants to the liver.[171-173] Newly synthesized cholesterol in liver consists of only approximately 5 percent of biliary cholesterol.[174]

Mechanisms of Biliary Lipid Secretion

The principal driving forces for biliary lipid secretion appear to be two ATP-dependent membrane transporters situated in the canalicular membrane of the hepatocyte. As discussed previously, bile salts are extruded into bile by ABCB11. At the same time, phosphatidylcholines are translocated or "flipped" from the endoplasmic (inner) to ectoplasmic (outer) leaflet of the membrane bilayer by ABCB4 (formerly known as MDR3), a P-glycoprotein member of the multi-drug resistance gene family.[175] Indeed, biliary phospholipid secretion is eliminated in mice by disrupting the ABCB4 gene,[176] and mutations of this gene in humans are the molecular defect underlying type 3 progressive familial intrahepatic cholestasis (PFIC3).[177,178]

Although many mechanistic details remain uncertain, biliary lipid secretion appears to be initiated after extrusion of bile salts from the hepatocyte and translocation of phosphatidylcholines to the surface of the canalicular membrane (Figure 59-9). Detergent-like bile salt molecules within the canalicular space interact with canalicular membrane.[179] In general, the ectoplasmic leaflet of the canalicular membrane is cholesterol- and sphingomyelin-rich[180,181] and is relatively resistant to penetration by bile salts. However, the action of ABCB4 forms phosphatidylcholine-rich microdomains within the outer membrane leaflet.[182] Bile salts may partition preferentially into these areas to destabilize the membrane[175,182] and release phosphatidylcholine-rich vesicles.[183,184] A number of diverse observations indicate that bile salts promote vesicular secretion of biliary cholesterol and phosphatidylcholines. Biliary secretion of organic anions in laboratory animals does not influence bile salt secretion, but does inhibit secretion of phospholipid and cholesterol into bile.[185-188] This occurs because organic anions bind bile salts within bile canaliculi and prevent interactions with the canalicular membrane.[179,189,190] Additionally, physical evidence supports bile salt–stimulated secretion of vesicles. Unilamellar vesicles (diameter approximately 150 to 500 Å) have been demonstrated in hepatic biles freshly collected from laboratory animals.[191-193] When cultured under specified conditions, rat hepatocytes form couplets with isolated "bile canaliculi" at interfaces between adjoining cells.[194] Using laser light-scattering techniques, vesicle formation has been observed within these "bile canaliculi" after exposure to bile salts.[79] Finally, rapid fixation techniques have provided direct morphologic evidence for vesicle formation at the outer surface of the canalicular membrane.[182,195]

The mechanisms by which cholesterol is incorporated into biliary vesicles are less well understood. Cholesterol contents of vesicles may be determined simply by the degree to which cholesterol partitions into phosphatidylcholine-rich microdomains in the canalicular membrane. Another possibility is that bile salts may regulate partitioning of cholesterol into nascent vesicles. Because of the high affinity of sphingomyelin for cholesterol,[196] microdomains form in membranes with sufficient amounts of cholesterol and sphingomyelin (e.g., the canalicular membrane). Because bile salts reduce the affinity of cholesterol for sphingomyelin,[197] they could induce migration of cholesterol into phosphatidylcholine-rich microdomains (see Figure 59-9).

It is also possible that efflux of biliary cholesterol from the canalicular membrane is protein-mediated. ABCA1[198] and SR-BI[31] are two plasma membrane proteins that promote cellular efflux of cholesterol. The subcellular distribution of ABCA1 in liver is not yet known, but its significance for bile formation has been examined in genetically modified mice. Overexpression of ABCA1 in liver and macrophages increases the cholesterol content of gallbladder bile.[198] However, biliary lipid secretion is unaffected in ABCA1 knockout mice.[199,200] SR-BI is localized in both sinusoidal and canalicular membranes of the hepatocyte.[201,202] In transgenic and knockout mice biliary secretion of cholesterol varies in proportion to hepatic expression of SR-BI.[203-206] Additional data are required, however, to distinguish between canalicular regulation of biliary cholesterol secretion by SRT-BI and the established contribution of SR-BI to sinusoidal uptake of HDL cholesterol that is destined for secretion into bile.[207,208]

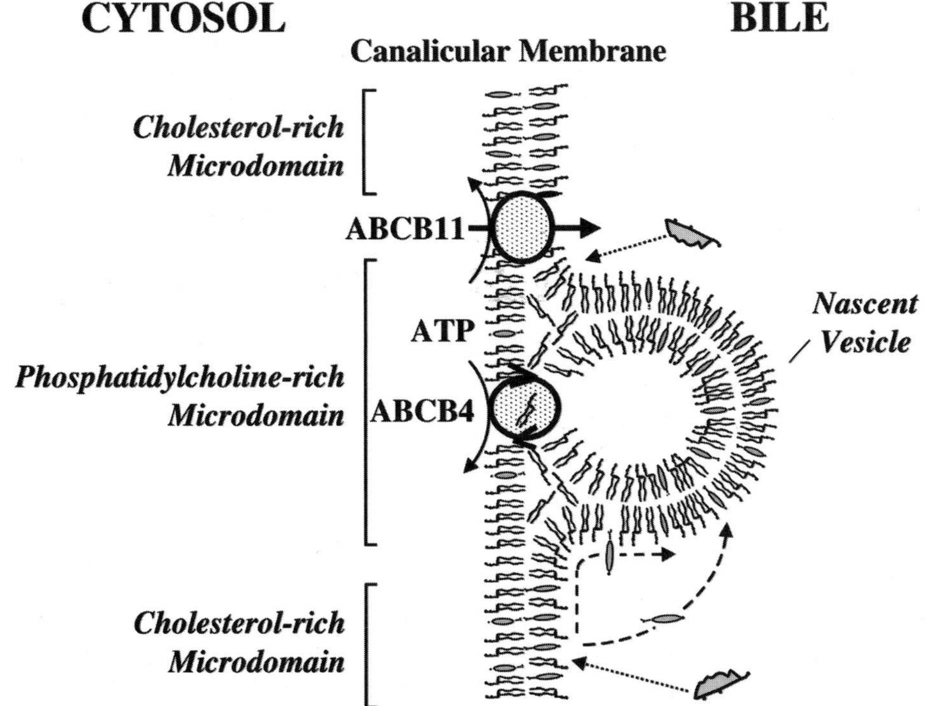

Figure 59-9 Diagrammatic representation of biliary vesicle formation. Bile salts are pumped into bile by ABCB11, and phosphatidylcholines are "flipped" by ABCB4 from endoplasmic (inner) to ectoplasmic (outer) leaflet of the membrane bilayer. As indicated by the dotted arrows, biliary bile salts interact with phosphatidylcholine-rich and cholesterol-rich microdomains in the canalicular membrane. Physical-chemical interactions of bile salts with phosphatidylcholine-rich microdomains promote formation of nascent vesicles. Bile salt interactions with cholesterol-rich microdomains reduce affinity of cholesterol for sphingomyelin, which is also enriched in these microdomains. Transfer of cholesterol to nascent vesicles *(dashed arrows)* occurs either by lateral diffusion within the ectoplasmic leaflet of the canalicular membrane or by transfer directly through the aqueous phase. (Redrawn from Cohen DE: Hepatocellular transport and secretion of biliary lipids. Curr Opin Lipidol 235:111, 1999.)

Trafficking of Biliary Lipids Within the Hepatocyte

Because membrane lipids are removed from the canalicular membrane for secretion into bile, they must be resupplied at the same rate. Despite years of study, hepatocellular mechanisms responsible for trafficking of biliary cholesterol and phospholipids to the canalicular membrane remain poorly understood. Transport of cholesterol and phosphatidylcholines to the canalicular membrane in the form of vesicles has been proposed,[209,210] but convincing evidence is lacking. Movement of insoluble membrane lipids to the canalicular membrane could occur via lipid transfer proteins that are enriched in liver cytosol. Sterol carrier protein 2 (SCP2) is a small (13 kD) protein that promotes transfer of cholesterol between membranes.[211,212] Evidence in humans[213] and in animal models[214-217] suggests that SCP2 is important for hepatocellular trafficking of biliary cholesterol. Phosphatidylcholine transfer protein (PC-TP) is a 25-kD cytosolic lipid transfer protein that is highly expressed in liver. It promotes intermembrane exchange and net transfer of phosphatidylcholines.[218] The observation that biliary phospholipids are highly enriched (more than 95 percent) in phosphatidylcholines has drawn attention to the possibility that PC-TP in liver might function to deliver phosphatidylcholines to the canalicular membrane.[219,220] In humans[11] hepatic expression of PC-TP appears to vary in proportion to secretion rates of biliary phosphatidylcholines. However, the presence of phosphatidylcholines in biles of mice after homozygous disruption of the gene encoding PC-TP[221] argues against a central role in biliary phosphatidylcholine secretion. Possibly biliary phosphatidylcholines are synthesized in situ within the canalicular membrane. But the only evidence for this mechanism is the presence in canalicular membrane of phosphatidylethanolamine-n-methyltransferase, which catalyzes conversion of phosphatidylethanolamine to phosphatidylcholine.[167]

Most cholesterol and some phosphatidylcholines in bile are derived from HDL. However, mechanisms by which HDL lipids are processed for biliary secretion are not well-understood. But, whereas HDL particles contain both unesterified and esterified cholesterol, all biliary cholesterol is unesterified.[15] It appears, therefore, that biliary cholesterol originates from either unesterified[170,222,223] or esterified[223] cholesterol in HDL. This implies that hydrolysis of HDL-derived cholesteryl esters in liver precedes secretion into bile. However, little is known about the process. Unesterified cholesterol delivered from HDL may remain confined to the plasma membrane before its biliary secretion, apparently without entering the hepatocyte.[222]

Gallbladder Physiology

The gallbladder stores bile during interdigestive periods and delivers it to the duodenum after ingestion of food. Normal gallbladder functions include absorption of solutes and water, secretion of mucin glycoproteins, and mechanical filling and emptying. As will be discussed later, abnormalities in each of these functions contributes to the pathogenesis of cholesterol and pigment gallstones.

Absorption

The gallbladder concentrates bile sixfold to tenfold and sequesters up to 60 percent of the bile salt pool during fasting.[224] This is accomplished by passive movement of water out of the gallbladder in response to vectorial transport of sodium chloride (NaCl), which does not change the tonicity of bile.[225] Based upon studies in a variety of animal models (reviewed in refs. 226, 227) that are consistent with observations in cultured human gallbladder epithelial cells,[228] key mechanistic concepts have emerged: (1) The driving force for movement of NaCl out of bile is by extrusion of sodium from gallbladder epithelial cells by an Na^+-K^+ adenosinetriphosphatase (ATPase) on the basolateral plasma membrane. (2) NaCl moves from bile across the apical membrane into gallbladder epithelium by "double exchange," a process in which Na^+ and Cl^- are exchanged for H^+ and HCO_3^-, respectively. (3) Protons that acidify bile come from Na^+-H^+ exchange. The protein responsible for this function in humans is NHE-3, a family member of the Na^+-H^+ exchange proteins.[229]

The gallbladder absorbs a variety of molecules in addition to NaCl. Earlier experiments in the guinea pig indicated that the gallbladder removes bile salts,[230] cholesterol,[231] and phospholipids[232] from bile. More recent studies utilizing the isolated perfused human gallbladder[233] have demonstrated greater absorption of biliary cholesterol and phospholipids compared with bile salts. The effect of this unequal uptake of lipids was to decrease cholesterol saturation in bile. Calcium is absorbed by the gallbladder, which may prevent precipitation of calcium salts.[234] The gallbladder also absorbs bilirubin, organic anions,[230,235] and albumin.[236] However, the physiologic significance associated with removal of these compounds from bile is not known.

Secretion

In addition to H^+ ions that enter bile during the course of NaCl absorption, the gallbladder secretes mucus. The principal protein components of mucus are called mucous glycoproteins or mucins. Mucins are high molecular weight glycoproteins (10^6 to 10^7 daltons) that are carbohydrate-rich. The major gallbladder mucin is a product of *MUC5B*, the same gene that encodes tracheobronchial mucin.[237] Radial orientation of oligosaccharide side chains around a peptide backbone results in a "bottle brush" configuration of the mucin molecule, which forms a gel at concentrations exceeding 20 to 40 mg/ml.[238] Mucin glycoproteins also contain hydrophobic binding domains that bind biliary lipids and bilirubin.[239,240]

Mucins are secreted into bile by exocytosis[241] by a mechanism that may require activity of the cystic fibrosis gene product, CFTR, in mucous granules within gallbladder epithelial cells.[242] Regulation of mucin secretion is complex. Potential physiologic stimuli include arachidonic acid, prostaglandins, vasoactive intestinal peptide, epinephrine, isoproterenol, extracellular ATP, oxygen radicals, and hydrophobic bile salts.[243-247] Hydrophobic bile salts stimulate mucin secretion independently of their detergent effects on membranes.[248] They are transported into the cell and activate Ca^{2+}/calmodulin-dependent protein kinase II.[249]

Filling and Emptying

Motility of the gallbladder is precisely regulated during fasting and after a meal. The sphincter of Oddi is principally responsible for controlling the flow of bile into the gallbladder versus the duodenum. Elevated tone of the sphincter of Oddi directs bile flow into the gallbladder. The process, referred to as receptive relaxation,[250] allows filling to occur without elevations in intraluminal pressure.[251] The gallbladder wall relaxes to avoid progressive increases in intraluminal pressure. In humans, bile is diverted into the gallbladder for storage during an overnight fast[252] to fill to a capacity of 17 to 25 ml.[253]

Gallbladder emptying occurs during fasting and in postprandial states. In the fasting state, emptying is coordinated with the migrating motor complex. Gallbladder contractions are timed to coincide with duodenal contractions, so that bile flows into the duodenum just before the burst phase of the migrating motor complex.[250,254,255] By stimulating intrinsic cholinergic neurons, motilin controls these events[256] in which gallbladder volume decreases by as much as 30 percent to 35 percent and is then rapidly refilled.[250] Cyclical emptying and refilling of the gallbladder in conjunction with the migrating motor complex occurs approximately every 120 minutes during fasting. This function helps to maintain the enterohepatic circulation of bile salts.[250]

In response to a meal, gallbladder volume is reduced by up to 75 percent.[257] Depending upon the composition of the meal, a minimum gallbladder volume is achieved in 0.5 to 4 hours[258] in two distinct phases. The cephalic phase occurs in response to sham feeding. Vagal stimulation causes contractions that evacuate approximately 30 percent of the gallbladder contents.[259,260] The intestinal phase is the component of gallbladder emptying that occurs in response to food in the intestine. It is mediated principally by cholecystokinin (CCK). In both phases, bile flows into the duodenum as the result of simultaneous gallbladder contraction and relaxation of the sphincter of Oddi.[261] Gallbladder motility is also influenced by a variety of gastrointestinal and neuropeptides (summarized in refs. 250, 258), the pathophysiologic significance of which is uncertain.

Aggregation of Lipids in Bile

Cholesterol and phosphatidylcholines are insoluble in water and must be packaged together with bile salts for transport in bile. Experimental evidence that bile salts function as natural detergents dates to the mid-twentieth century.[262,263] However, comprehensive analyses of model biles (i.e., laboratory-made mixtures of purified bile salts, phosphatidylcholines, and cholesterol) in the 1960s[264,265] were required to describe the aggregative behavior of biliary lipids in water at equilibrium. These studies provided the foundation for detailed characterizations of micelles and vesicles, which are the two main types of macromolecular aggregates in bile. It was discovered that micelles could be composed of either bile salts plus cholesterol (i.e., simple micelles) or of bile salts, phosphatidylcholines, and cholesterol (i.e., mixed micelles).[266-269] Biliary vesicles were shown to be spherical membrane bilayers that contained principally phosphatidylcholines and cholesterol with only traces of bile salts.[270,271] Vesicles are unilamellar (i.e., a single bilayer that encircles an aqueous core) or multi-lamellar (i.e., contain multiple concentric spherical bilayers). The precise compositions and proportions of micelles and vesicles are determined principally by the concentrations of biliary lipids,[20,272] which vary considerably within the bile ducts and gallbladder.

Micelles

Model biles containing high concentrations of bile salts compared with phosphatidylcholines and cholesterol are optically clear because they contain small micellar aggregates.[264,265,273] Micelles were first proposed to be shaped like disks, with phospholipid-cholesterol bilayers surrounded on their perimeters by bile salt molecules.[266] These particles were characterized in physiologically relevant model biles[269,270] and in native biles.[274] Mixed micelles range in size from 20 to 120 Å in radius and co-exist with simple micelles (10 to 20 Å in radius) of bile salt–cholesterol.[269,275,276] A refined molecular model of mixed micelles proposed that bile salts were incorporated into the phosphatidylcholine-cholesterol bilayers in addition to surrounding the perimeters.[269] This model now appears to be a valid description of small micelles (smaller than 50 Å in radius), but evidence[276-280] indicates that larger mixed micelles assume "worm-like" structures.[279]

Vesicles

Vesicles in bile have one of two distinct origins. Those formed at the canalicular membrane are unilamellar and rich in phosphatidylcholines compared with cholesterol (i.e., contain one cholesterol molecule per three phosphatidylcholine molecules). Because of increasing bile salt concentrations in the biliary tree, these vesicles rapidly undergo structural rearrangements and are therefore detectable only in bile specimens analyzed immediately after collection.[191-193]

A second type of vesicle forms spontaneously in bile when the capacity of mixed and simple micelles to solubilize cholesterol is exceeded.[78] These unilamellar or multi-lamellar vesicles are cholesterol-rich, with cholesterol contents reaching as high as two cholesterol molecules per phosphatidylcholine molecule. The identification of cholesterol-rich vesicles in bile was important historically because it led to a paradigm shift with respect to understanding the pathogenesis of cholesterol gallstones.

Early concepts of biliary lipid aggregation were based strictly on the equilibrium phase diagram (Figure 59-10).[264,265] It was believed that cholesterol in human

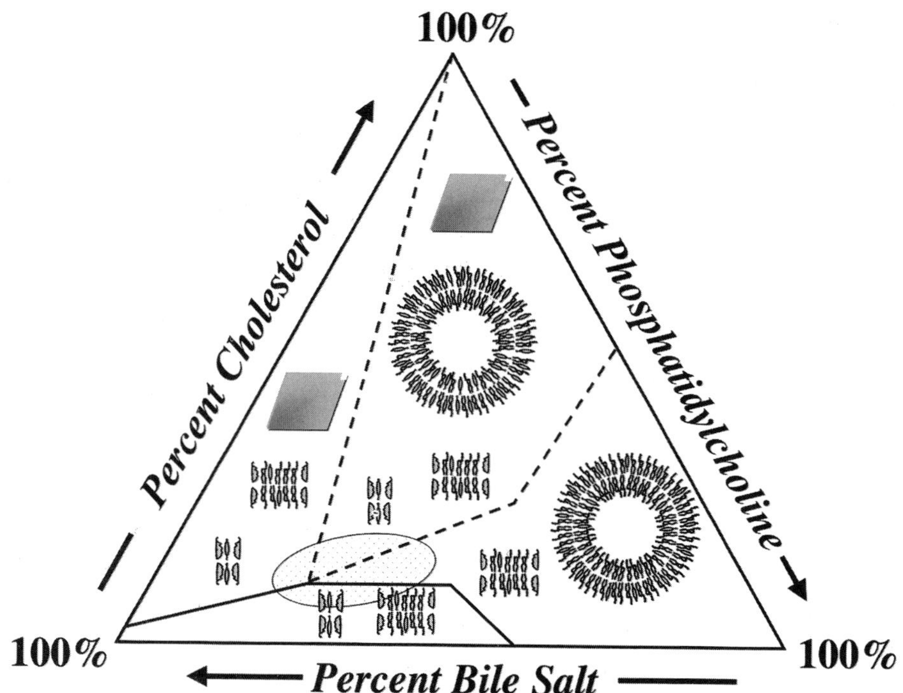

Figure 59-10 Schematic representation of the equilibrium phase diagram for human gallbladder bile. The solid line indicates the boundary of the micellar zone. Cholesterol in biles with compositions that fall within the micellar zone is solubilized in simple and mixed micelles. Bile compositions that fall outside the micellar zone are divided into three regions separated by the dashed lines. In the region on the left, simple and mixed micelles co-exist with cholesterol monohydrate crystals. In the center region, simple and mixed micelles co-exist with vesicles and cholesterol monohydrate crystals. Vesicles in this region are relatively enriched with cholesterol. In the region on the right, mixed micelles co-exist with vesicles that are relatively enriched with phosphatidylcholines.[20] The shaded region indicates the range of compositions of human biles. Biles from cholesterol gallstone patients and normal individuals that are supersaturated with cholesterol plot above the micellar zone.

gallbladder bile was solubilized in micelles and that cholesterol crystallized to form gallstones when its concentration exceeded the limit of solubility in micelles.[281] But gallbladder biles from many healthy humans were supersaturated with cholesterol (i.e., cholesterol concentrations exceeded what could be accommodated by micellar particles).[282] Moreover, dilute hepatic biles, in which cholesterol stones never formed, could be supersaturated with cholesterol in a high proportion of people.[40,283] Subsequently, cholesterol-rich vesicles were shown to encompass the particle responsible for solubilizing biliary cholesterol in excess of what could be solubilized in mixed micelles.[270,284] The discovery of biliary vesicles reconciled earlier reports of non-micellar particles in biles that lacked cholesterol crystals or gallstones.[285-287] Cholesterol-rich vesicles were shown to co-exist with mixed micelles and simple micelles.[270,275] Consistent with the absence of cholesterol crystallization in hepatic biles, cholesterol-rich vesicles proved to be remarkably stable in dilute biles. As will be discussed later, destabilization of cholesterol-rich vesicles in gallbladder constitutes an important step in the pathogenesis of cholesterol gallstones.

Co-existence and Interconversion of Micelles and Vesicles in Bile

Although bile is rarely at equilibrium, the physical states assumed by biliary lipids at equilibrium[68,288] (see Figure 59-10) have provided the underpinnings for describing biliary lipid aggregation in vivo. Because bile is concentrated within the biliary tree, bile salt concentrations approach their CMC values. When this occurs, bile salts begin to modify the structure of phospholipid-rich vesicles that are secreted into bile.[289] These interactions mark the start of a complex series of molecular rearrangements that ultimately form simple and mixed micelles.[289] In human bile supersaturated with cholesterol, there appear to be two pathways for forming cholesterol-rich vesicles from phospholipid-rich vesicles that are assembled at the canalicular membrane.[78,166] Figure 59-11 depicts the most likely mechanism for formation of cholesterol-rich vesicles. Because bile salts solubilize phospholipids more efficiently than cholesterol, cholesterol-rich vesicles may form when bile salts preferentially extract phospholipid molecules directly from phospholipid-rich vesicles.[289] Another possibility that has been demonstrated in model systems is rapid dissolution of phospholipid-rich vesicles by bile salts. This creates unstable mixed micelles with

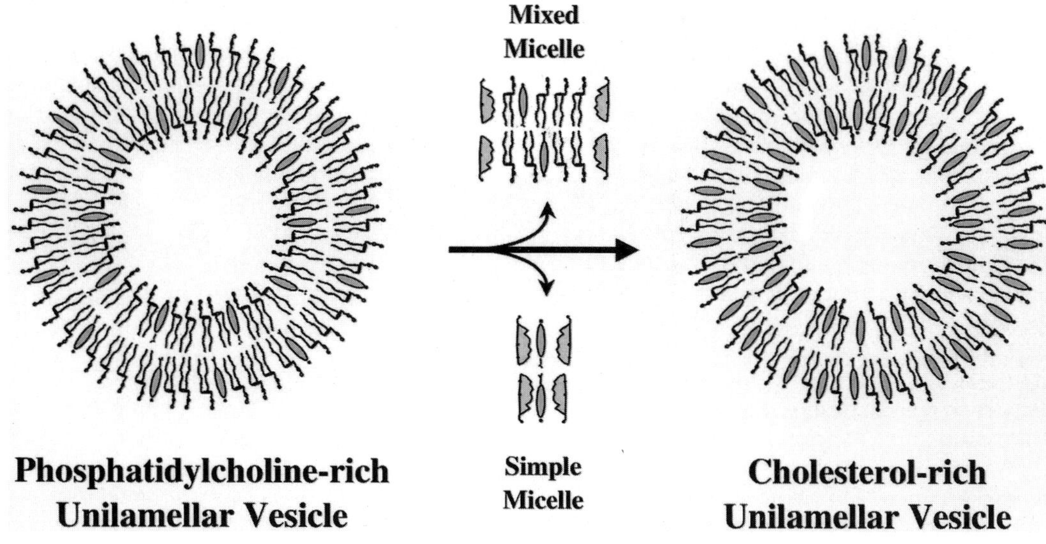

Figure 59-11 Formation of cholesterol-rich unilamellar vesicles from phosphatidylcholine-rich vesicles in bile.

excess cholesterol. Cholesterol-rich vesicles arise by structural rearrangements of these unstable micellar particles.[276,289]

PATHOGENESIS OF CHOLESTEROL GALLSTONES

Metabolic Abnormalities Associated with Cholesterol Gallstone Formation

Hypersecretion of biliary cholesterol is the primary metabolic abnormality responsible for initiating cholelithiasis.[14,166,290] However, the gallbladder and intestine also conspire as part of a "vicious cycle"[290,291] that creates physical-chemical instabilities in bile and culminates in formation of cholesterol gallstones.

Liver

Formation of cholesterol gallstones is the final consequence of excess secretion of cholesterol from the liver into bile.[40,292] Biliary secretion rates of bile salts are normal in patients with cholesterol gallstones.[36,166] In these individuals, however, bile salts promote biliary secretion of vesicles that contain approximately 33 percent more cholesterol molecules per phospholipid molecule than vesicles in control subjects.[14,293] This is commonly referred to as hypersecretion of biliary cholesterol. Despite intensive study of hepatic cholesterol metabolism in patients with gallstones,[290] the metabolic basis for hypersecretion of biliary cholesterol remains poorly understood.

Gallbladder

Hypomotility. Gallbladder hypomotility is an abnormality principally associated with the formation of cholesterol (but not pigment) gallstones. Both filling and emptying of the gallbladder are affected in patients with hypomotility.[294,295] Contractile abnormalities are observed in the postprandial state and during fasting.[296]

Gallbladder motor function is measured in vivo by a variety of techniques.[295,297] These techniques have revealed that moderately increased fasting gallbladder volumes and markedly increased residual volumes result in decreased ejection fractions of gallbladder bile in cholesterol gallstone patients.[298-300] A recent study has demonstrated that patients with black pigment stones have normal fasting gallbladder volumes but delayed emptying and residual volumes that are elevated to a more modest degree compared with cholesterol gallstone patients.[300] Studies in vitro comparing gallbladder function in cholesterol gallstone patients versus controls have demonstrated abnormalities in binding of agonists to plasma membrane receptors, alterations in contraction of isolated smooth muscle cells, and decreased contractility of isolated smooth muscle strips and whole gallbladder preparations.[301] In particular, there is impairment of signal transduction in response to binding of agonists (e.g., CCK).[302-304] Defects in contractility associated with cholesterol gallstones are reversible and are attributable primarily to excess accumulation of biliary cholesterol in membranes of gallbladder smooth muscle cells.[305,306] This mechanism appears to explain why gallbladder emptying is impaired before gallstone formation in animal models[307] at a time when bile is merely supersaturated with cholesterol. Similar effects of cholesterol on plasma membranes may cause diminished relaxation of the gallbladder, which is associated with cholesterol gallstone disease.[304,308]

Hypersecretion of Mucins. Mucus is an integral component of cholesterol and pigment gallstones, suggesting an important role for mucins in stone formation.[309] In a number of animal models of cholelithiasis, mucin accumulation occurs before development of stones. A detailed study in the cholesterol-fed prairie dog showed that a fivefold increase in mucin secretion coincided with supersaturation of bile with cholesterol and occurred before crystallization of cholesterol and gallstone formation.[310] The early appearance of mucins during the course of diet-induced cholelithiasis has been observed in other animal models[309] and in humans.[311,312] A pathogenic role for mucin was strongly suggested by prevention of cholelithiasis by aspirin in the prairie dog, apparently by selective inhibition of prostaglandin-induced mucin formation.[313] Concentrations of gallbladder mucin were lower in humans taking nonsteroidal anti-inflammatory drugs (NSAIDs)[314]; aspirin administration has been shown to prevent gallstone formation during rapid weight loss.[315] However, the influence of aspirin and NSAIDs on experimentally induced cholelithiasis in animals has been inconsistent[316-318] and epidemiologic data do not support an inverse relationship between NSAID use and gallstone disease.[319,320] Therefore other biliary constituents (e.g., lithogenic bile, hydrophobic bile salts, bacterial lipopolysaccharides) may contribute to promoting hypersecretion of mucins during the early phases of cholelithiasis.[321] In humans a critical consequence of mucin hypersecretion is the formation of biliary sludge,[311,322,323] which is discussed in the section on Formation and Growth.

Lipid Absorption. In contrast to normal subjects in whom differential absorption of bile salts, cholesterol, and phospholipid by the gallbladder reduces cholesterol saturation of bile,[233] the gallbladder epithelium of individuals with cholesterol gallstones loses the capacity for selective absorption of biliary cholesterol and phospholipids.[324] Impaired lipid absorption may contribute to gallstone formation by sustaining cholesterol supersaturation of bile during storage.[324] Because the concentrating function of the gallbladder is retained, the total concentration of lipids in bile increases. This has an important effect on the equilibrium phase diagram for the biliary lipids (see Figure 59-10). In more dilute hepatic biles the dashed phase boundaries are positions much further to the left.[325,326] Therefore even though hepatic biles are supersaturated with cholesterol, cholesterol crystallization does not occur because the bile compositions fall within the two phase region in which mixed micelles co-exist at equilibrium with vesicles.

Intestine

Increased proportions of deoxycholate are commonly found in biles of patients with cholesterol gallstone disease.[81,293,327] Deoxycholate is a hydrophobic bile salt that increases biliary cholesterol secretion[193,327,328] and suppresses synthesis of primary bile salts.[45,329] Deoxycholate also may contribute critically to cholesterol crystallization. The intestine, which is the source of deoxycholate in bile, thereby may contribute to the pathogenesis of cholesterol gallstones.[327]

Experimental evidence supports multiple mechanisms for increased formation of deoxycholate in the intestine. Motor dysfunction of the gallbladder associated with cholesterol gallstone disease may increase deoxycholate formation. This occurs because bile salts, which cycle more frequently between the liver and intestine in patients with gallstones, are exposed to intestinal microflora for longer periods of time.[290] Similarly, prolonged intestinal transit times in patients with cholesterol gallstones increase biliary deoxycholate content.[330-332] In addition to increase time of exposure of bile salts to bacteria, deoxycholate is elevated in cholesterol gallstone patients because of increased overall 7α-dehydroxylation activity of the intestinal microflora.[332,333] Finally, the bioavailability of deoxycholate is higher in patients with cholesterol gallstones because of the longer transit times in large bowel and higher values of pH in distal colon.[332]

Physical-chemical Events Leading to Cholesterol Gallstone Formation

As described previously, earlier studies have established that biles from patients with cholesterol gallstones and from controls are often supersaturated with cholesterol[334] and that the degree of cholesterol supersaturation is not a reliable predictor of gallstones. Useful discriminatory data have been provided by microscopic analyses, which reveal more rapid crystallization of cholesterol in biles of patients with gallstones compared with control biles of similar lipid composition.[335-337] The time required to observe cholesterol crystals forming in biles by light microscopy, under standardized conditions, was referred to initially as "nucleation time."[335] This measurement provided a reliable means of distinguishing biles from cholesterol gallstone patients and controls. Moreover, differences in nucleation times suggested that human biles might contain factors that control gallstone formation by inhibiting or accelerating the appearance of cholesterol crystals.[338,339]

Whereas the concept of nucleation time has remained useful, the terminology has been revised because it provided an inaccurate physical-chemical description of the measurement. Nucleation refers specifically to the very earliest events of crystallization in which cholesterol molecules cluster irreversibly to form a critical nucleus.[340] This critical nucleus of cholesterol molecules must then grow to become observable. Appreciating that nucleation and crystal growth are both essential components of what was originally referred to as "nucleation time,"[341] "crystal observation time" is now properly used to describe the period of time required to detect crystals by classical microscopic techniques.

Cholesterol Nucleation

The precise molecular mechanisms of nucleation remain incompletely understood, but we now understand many of the conditions associated with this process. Based upon video imaging techniques, it was first suggested that cholesterol-rich unilamellar vesicles aggregated before cholesterol nucleation[342,343] to form multi-lamellar vesicles.[270,344] The likelihood that vesicles represent the principal source of cholesterol for nucleation is supported by biochemical analyses[345,346] and high-resolution cryoelectron microscopy.[276]

Recent detailed analyses of cholesterol crystallization in model[290,347] and native[325] biles suggest that there are two distinct mechanisms for cholesterol nucleation.[290] These are illustrated in Figure 59-12. In biles with relatively high concentrations of phosphatidylcholines, aggregation and fusion of cholesterol-rich vesicles results in multi-lamellar vesicles that give rise to crystals of cholesterol monohydrate,[348] which are the "building blocks" of cholesterol gallstones. At lower concentrations of phosphatidylcholines, vesicles may become unstable and essentially implode. Crystals formed by this mechanism are composed principally of anhydrous cholesterol.[290] Eventually, these anhydrous crystals become hydrated to form cholesterol monohydrate.[349,350]

Crystal Growth

Growth of cholesterol crystals is an event distinct from nucleation.[340] In practice, however, the precise moment of nucleation cannot be distinguished clearly from growth of cholesterol crystals in a complex fluid such as bile.[351] Notwithstanding this limitation, combined measurements of nucleation and crystal growth (i.e., crystal observation time) have been standardized, quantified, and automated.[352-355] These have proven useful in the search for factors that influence cholesterol crystallization in human bile.

Factors that Affect Cholesterol Crystallization in Bile

More rapid crystallization of cholesterol in biles of patients with gallstones[335] implied that lithogenic bile contained components that accelerated crystallization (i.e., pronucleating agents) or that normal biles contained components that inhibited crystallization (i.e., anti-nucleating agents). Bile contains both accelerators and inhibitors of crystallization.

Mucin was the first biliary protein shown to accelerate cholesterol crystallization.[313,356] Subsequently, it was demonstrated that a number of glycoproteins that bind reversibly to concanavalin A-Sepharose also accelerate cholesterol crystallization.[357] These include aminopeptidase N,[358-360] immunoglobulins,[361] α1-acid glycoprotein,[362] phospholipase C,[363] fibronectin,[364] and haptoglobin.[365] Other accelerators of cholesterol crystallization include the amphipathic anionic polypeptide fraction/calcium-binding protein,[366] albumin-lipid complexes,[367] and group II phospholipase A2.[368] Non-protein components of bile also accelerate cholesterol crystallization. A low-density particle composed principally of lipids is a potent promoter of crystallization.[357] Calcium bound to micelles and vesicles in bile[369] may accelerate cholesterol nucleation by promoting fusion of cholesterol-rich vesicles.[370] The precipitation of calcium salts in biles that are supersaturated with calcium salts and cholesterol leads to rapid crystallization of cholesterol, an effect that is enhanced by the presence of mucins.[371] Rapidity of cholesterol crystal formation also varies in proportion to the deoxycholate content of bile.[372] This effect is due presumably to the influence of this hydrophobic bile salt on the equilibrium phase relationships

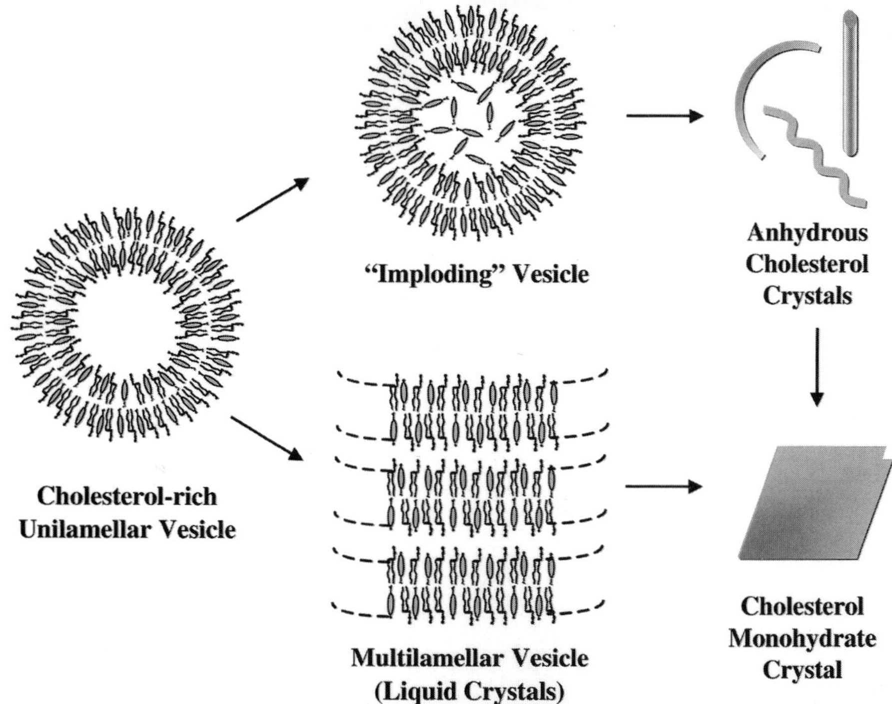

Figure 59-12 Two pathways for crystallization of cholesterol in bile. Cholesterol contained in cholesterol-rich unilamellar vesicles may "implode" into the core. Under these conditions anhydrous cholesterol crystals of varied morphology are formed initially. In the aqueous environment of bile, anhydrous cholesterol crystals eventually reorganize to form cholesterol monohydrate crystals. The other pathway begins with aggregation of cholesterol-rich unilamellar vesicles to form multi-lamellar vesicles, which give rise directly to cholesterol monohydrate crystals. (Redrawn from Carey MC: Formation and growth of cholesterol gallstones: the new synthesis. In Fromm H, Leuschner U, eds: Bile Acids—Cholestasis—Gallstones. Dordrecht, The Netherlands, Kluwer, 1996:147.)

of biliary lipids.[325] Finally, recent studies have shown that the degree of cholesterol supersaturation of bile per se may be a determinant of rapid crystallization of cholesterol.[373,374]

Although fewer in number than promoters, several inhibitors of cholesterol crystallization have been identified. These include apolipoproteins AI and AII,[375-377] a 120-kD glycoprotein,[378] a 15-kD protein,[379] and secretory immunoglobulin A and its heavy and light chains.[380,381]

Notwithstanding evidence supporting the significance of various pro- and anti-nucleating proteins for gallstone formation, the possibility has been raised that some of their effects are either non-specific[382] or unphysiologic.[373,383-386] As technologies improve for the study of cholesterol nucleation and crystal growth in bile,[348] the contributions of promoters and inhibitors of cholesterol crystallization to gallstone formation should become more clear.

Formation and Growth of Cholesterol Gallstones

Cholesterol gallstones consist of radially or horizontally oriented cholesterol crystals imbedded within an organic matrix.[387-389] This implies that crystal formation in bile is followed by assembly into larger structures. Many aspects of the process by which gallstones are assembled remain poorly understood. For example, it is not clear why cholesterol stones in a gallbladder may be small (1 to 15 mm) and numerous (more than 10,000), large (6 to 10 cm) and solitary, and how mucins, biliary proteins, bile pigments, and inorganic salts are deposited in cholesterol stones.[290]

Biliary sludge is a critical co-factor for formation of cholesterol gallstones. Sludge was originally described as an ultrasonographic finding.[390] Subsequent analysis revealed that sludge is a sediment consisting of cholesterol monohydrate crystals or bilirubinate granules trapped in a mucus gel.[311] Formation of sludge is a key precursor of cholelithiasis because it provides a viscous, gel-like microenvironment for assembly of stones (Figure 59-13).[322] Nevertheless, biliary sludge progresses to gallstone formation in only 5 percent to 15 percent of patients over a 3-year period.[323] When an etiology is transient (e.g., pregnancy, total parenteral nutrition), sludge frequently resolves upon removing its cause.[323]

In contrast to the relatively rapid processes of nucleation and growth of cholesterol crystals, organization of crystals into cholesterol gallstones occurs over periods that range from weeks to years (see Figure 59-13).[290,322,389] The presence of calcium salts and pigments within the center of most cholesterol stones suggests a requirement for a central nidus, about which cholesterol crystals assemble.[370,391,392] Assembly of a nidus and subsequent stone growth appear to be controlled by mucins, other biliary proteins,[393] and the cholesterol saturation of bile and the characteristics of any preexisting stones.[388] Growth of stones is most likely a discontinuous process[388] that is punctuated by deposition of rings of calcium bilirubinate and calcium carbonate.[8,9]

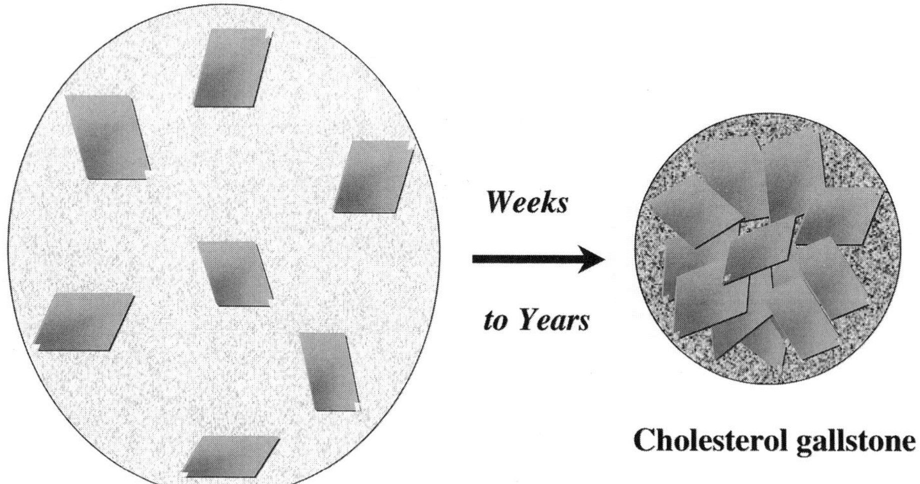

Figure 59-13 Growth of macroscopic cholesterol gallstones after cholesterol crystal formation. Cholesterol monohydrate crystals become trapped in the gallbladder within a mucin gel or sludge. Over weeks to years, crystals aggregate to form cholesterol gallstones. (Redrawn from Carey MC: Formation and growth of cholesterol gallstones: the new synthesis. In Fromm H, Leuschner U, eds: Bile Acids—Cholestasis—Gallstones. Dordrecht, The Netherlands, Kluwer, 1996:147.)

Role of Bacteria

Studies based on bacteriologic and morphologic analysis of bile and gallstones have strongly discounted the importance of infection in the pathogenesis of cholesterol and black pigment stones.[394-396] However, recent studies using molecular biologic analysis have demonstrated the presence of bacterial ribosomal RNA in cholesterol and pigment gallstones.[397-399] An exception in these studies was stones containing the highest cholesterol contents (more than 90 percent), which rarely contained bacterial RNA. By nucleotide sequencing, *Propionibacterium, Escherichia coli,* and *Pseudomonas* species were identified most frequently in gallstones. Whether transient infection with these organisms is pathogenic remains speculative. Nevertheless, transient, self-terminating infection or colonization of gallstones with bacteria at low concentrations may contribute to cholesterol gallstone formation.[321,397] Alternatively, the presence of bacteria in this setting may reflect secondary colonization that occurs after stone formation.

PATHOGENESIS OF PIGMENT GALLSTONES

Black Pigment Gallstones

The initiating event in formation of black pigment stones occurs when unconjugated bilirubin precipitates as calcium bilirubinate.[400] Under normal circumstances, unconjugated bilirubin is not secreted into bile.[14] Because of the presence of endogenous β-glucuronidase in bile,[401] however, unconjugated bilirubin is formed in small amounts (approximately 1 percent of bile pigments).[402] Unlike soluble bilirubin conjugates (e.g., bilirubin diglucuronide), unconjugated bilirubin and calcium bilirubinate are sparingly soluble and are bound only to limited extents to aggregates of biliary lipid.[14,400] Under conditions that increase bilirubin secretion into bile (see the section on Black Pigment Gallstones on p. 1732), the activity of endogenous β-glucuronidase leads to higher levels of unconjugated bilirubin. Moreover, increased biliary secretion of bilirubin inhibits secretion of cholesterol and phospholipid into bile at the level of the canalicular membrane.[179,185] Because mixed micelles and vesicles in bile solubilize unconjugated bilirubin and bind calcium,[369,403] a deficiency of mixed micelles[402] and vesicles[404] favors precipitation of calcium bilirubinate.[400] Defective acidification,[370,402] leading to more alkaline bile, may cause calcium to precipitate with carbonate and phosphate and become incorporated into pigment stones.[402] Whereas gallbladder contractility may be reduced modestly in the setting of pigment stones,[300,405] hypersecretion of mucin does occur.[406,407] Polymerization of bilirubin pigment and aggregation with calcium carbonate and calcium phosphate crystals within a mucin gel lead to mature black pigment stones.[400,402]

Brown Pigment Gallstones

Brown pigment stones form under conditions distinctly different from those for black pigment stones. Stasis within the bile duct leading to chronic infection sets the stage for forming brown pigment stones.[395,402,408] Bacteria are components of these stones and are uniformly cultured from bile.[12,409] Anaerobic organisms liberate β-glucuronidase,[410] phospholipase A1,[411] and conjugated bile salt hydrolase.[14,412] The respective degradation products produced by these enzymes include unconjugated bilirubin, free fatty acids, and unconjugated bile salts—all of which are sparingly soluble and precipitate as calcium salts.[14,413] Enzymatic degradation of bile salts and phospholipids that solubilize cholesterol leads to precipitation of cholesterol, which constitutes 10 percent to 40 percent of brown pigment stones.[14] An increase in mucin content of hepatic bile[414] appears to serve as a gel in which brown pigment stones develop.[402]

ETIOLOGIC FACTORS FOR GALLSTONE DISEASE

Pathophysiologic States

Several conditions and disease states are associated with increased risk of gallstone disease.This section highlights some common and uncommon risk factors for cholesterol, black pigment gallstones, and brown pigment gallstones.

Cholesterol Gallstones

Obesity, Weight Fluctuations, and Weight Loss. A strong association between obesity and cholesterol gallstone disease is well established.[6,415,416] The frequency of gallstones varies in proportion to body mass index[319,417] and distribution of body fat (e.g., waist-to-hip ratio).[416,418] The pathogenesis of cholesterol gallstones in obesity appears to be linked primarily to increased production and turnover of cholesterol,[419,420] leading to hypersecretion of cholesterol into bile.[39,421-423] Whether obesity is associated with impaired gallbladder function remains unclear.[424]

The incidence of gallstones is particularly high in obese individuals who lose weight rapidly[315,415,425,426] or experience frequent fluctuations in weight.[427] Measurements of bile composition after rapid weight loss show increases in cholesterol saturation, arachidonic acid, prostaglandin E2, calcium, and mucin,[312,403] with concomitant decreases in cholesterol crystal observation time.[312] Biliary sludge is an important co-factor in formation of gallstones in association with rapid weight loss.[323]

Leptin is a circulating hormone produced in adipocytes that promotes satiety, energy metabolism, and weight loss.[428] Plasma leptin levels are elevated in most obese individuals[429] and are highly correlated with the frequency of gallstone disease in Mexican Americans.[430] Recent studies in genetically obese animals[431,432] and humans[433] suggest that leptin may be important in obesity-related cholelithiasis through regulation of biliary lipid secretion.

Hyperlipidemia. Whereas most studies have failed to demonstrate a relationship between serum cholesterol and cholelithiasis, hypertriglyceridemia is a consistent finding in gallstone disease.[416] Biliary cholesterol saturation is increased in the setting of elevated plasma triglycerides[434,435] and may be the result of altered metabolism of bile salt.[436,437] Plasma levels of HDL cholesterol correlate inversely with prevalence of gallstones[416] and cholesterol saturation of bile.[435] Despite well-established correlations between elevated plasma triglycerides, low HDL cholesterol, and obesity, a preponderance of evidence suggests that high plasma triglycerides and low HDL are independent risk factors for cholelithiasis.[6,416]

Pregnancy. The prevalence of gallstones increases as a function of the number of full-term pregnancies.[319,416,438-440] Pregnancy is associated with increased saturation of bile by cholesterol[441] and impaired gallbladder function.[442] These effects are mediated respectively by estrogen and progesterone[6] and are compounded by prolonged intestinal transit times[443] that favor formation of deoxycholate.[327] This combination of factors during pregnancy contributes to the high incidence (approximately 30 percent) of biliary sludge. The sludge resolves spontaneously in most individuals but leads to cholesterol gallstones in approximately 2 percent to 5 percent of cases.[291,323,444]

Intestinal Hypomotility. Intestinal hypomotility appears be an independent risk factor for cholesterol gallstones,[445,446] as evidenced by prolonged transit times in patients otherwise at relatively low risk for cholesterol cholelithiasis.[447,448] This concept is supported by the uniform presence of cholesterol gallstones in individuals with somatostatinoma syndrome,[449] which can be attributed in part to prolonged intestinal transit.[6] As described previously, current concepts of cholethiasis suggest that increased formation of deoxycholate is the primary metabolic consequence of delayed intestinal transit.

Spinal Cord Injury. Patients with spinal cord injury are at very high risk for developing gallstones.[450,451] The type of gallstones present in these patients is not known, but they are likely to be cholesterol gallstones. The pathogenesis appears to be multi-factorial and secondary to weight loss and intestinal hypomotility.[291,452] The incidence of biliary sludge is increased in these patients,[453] but gallbladder emptying appears to be unaffected by spinal cord injury.[453,454]

Black Pigment Gallstones

Ileal Disease. Patients with compromised ileal function are at increased risk for pigment gallstones.[14] Increased incidences of gallstones are observed after ileal bypass surgery for treatment of obesity or hyperlipidemia[455,456] or after resection of diseased ileum.[457] Ileal resection in laboratory animals induces pigment stones,[458,459] apparently because malabsorption of bile salt promotes enterohepatic cycling and increased biliary secretion of bilirubin.[460] Crohn's disease of the ileum is associated with a high incidence of gallstones,[461-463] most of which are pigment stones.[14,463] Increased concentrations of bilirubin in the bile of these patients[464] appear to be explained by bile salt-induced enterohepatic cycling of bilirubin at the level of the colon.[465]

Chronic Hemolysis. Hemolysis is associated with pigment gallstones whether hemolysis is induced by heart-lung bypass,[466] sickle cell or other hemolytic anemias,[12,467,468] or malaria.[12]

Cirrhosis. Pigment gallstones occur with increased frequency in cirrhosis,[469] which is accompanied by hemolysis and increased production and biliary secretion of bilirubin.[470] Increased concentrations of bilirubin in bile are accompanied in these patients by decreased concentrations of bile salts.[36] Precipitation of calcium bilirubinate is a consequence of increased concentrations of biliary calcium coupled with decreased concentrations of lipid aggregates that solubilize bilirubin.[402,471]

Aging. Numerous studies have documented increased formation of gallstones as a function of age in most populations.[6] Biliary cholesterol saturation increases in the elderly.[472,473] This may be due primarily to increased biliary secretion of cholesterol,[472,473] which occurs in the absence[473] or presence of decreased synthesis of bile salts.[472,474] Nevertheless, the increased prevalence of gallstones with aging is due to the black pigment stones. The incidence of cholesterol gallstones peaks in mid-life. This is followed by a rise in the incidence of pigment stones that occurs later in life.[475,476]

Gilbert's Syndrome. In contrast to normal biles in which bilirubin diglucuronide is the predominant conjugate of bilirubin,[16] biles of patients with Gilbert's syndrome have elevated concentrations of bilirubin monoglucuronide.[477] This apparently predisposes to pigment stone formation because β-glucuronidase-mediated formation of unconjugated bilirubin is a single-step hydrolysis of bilirubin monoglucuronide rather than the slower two-step process in normal individuals.[402]

Brown Pigment Gallstones

Risk factors for brown pigment gallstones in bile ducts include conditions that predispose to biliary stasis and infection (e.g., foreign bodies such as sutures,[478] sphincterotomy,[479] parasites or ova from *Ascaris lumbricoides* and *Clonorchis senensis*[6]). Brown pigment stones also occur with increased frequency in patients with juxtapapillary duodenal diverticula, a condition associated with increased activity of bacterial β-glucuronidase in bile.[480]

Environmental Factors

Dietary

Diet represents an important co-factor in the pathogenesis of cholesterol and possibly pigment gallstones. The individual contributions of dietary components (i.e., total calories, cholesterol, fat, protein, carbohydrates, and alcohol) to the risk of gallstone disease have been reviewed recently.[6,482] These analyses emphasize the contributions to cholithiasis of chronic overnutrition, particularly with respect to increases in refined carbohydrates and low intake of fiber.

Pharmacologic

Therapy with a number of common medications predisposes to cholesterol gallstones. Hypolipidemic fibrates that activate PPARα are associated with up-regulation of HMG-CoA reductase, down-regulation of CYP 7A1, and increased secretion of biliary cholesterol.[482] Of the various fibrate drugs available, however, only clofibrate has been associated with an actual increase in the incidence of gallstones.[483]

Estrogens promote hypersecretion of biliary cholesterol; progesterone decreases gallbladder contractility.[291] However, currently prescribed anovulatory preparations of estrogen and progesterone do not appear to increase appreciably the risk of cholesterol gallstones (reviewed in ref. 6). In contrast, high-dose estrogen for management of metastatic prostate cancer does promote gallstone formation.[484]

The somatostatin analog octreotide, when used chronically for therapy for acromegaly or secretory diarrhea, is associated with an elevated risk of cholesterol gallstones.[446,485] This is likely the result of a combination of gallbladder stasis and intestinal hypomotility, which leads to enrichment of the bile salt pool with deoxycholate.[446]

Ceftriaxone is secreted into bile as a divalent anion and can precipitate as a calcium salt.[486] This leads to sludge composed mainly of calcium-ceftriaxone complexes.[323] Whereas sludge resolves after discontinuation of therapy in most patients, ceftriaxone gallstones can develop.[323] Finally, the immunosuppressant drugs Cyclosporin A and FK506 result in hyposecretion of bile salts because of a multiplicity of metabolic effects[6] and contribute to an increased risk of cholesterol gallstones in patients with organ transplants.[487-489]

Genetics

Human Genetics

Data for variations in prevalences of gallstones among geographically and ethnically diverse populations—as well as family and twin studies—strongly support a genetic component to susceptibility to gallstones (reviewed in ref. 6). An attractive theory asserts that *LITH* genes, which encode gallstone susceptibility, are "thrifty" genes that evolved under selective evolutionary pressure encountered by humans during epic migrations.[6,490-492] Whereas the identity of thrifty genes is currently unknown, other specific human genes have been associated with increased susceptibility to gallstones. The apolipoprotein E4 genotype is a risk factor for cholesterol gallstone disease.[493] The cholesterol content of gallstones may be increased by the apolipoprotein E4 allele.[494] However, an independent study failed to confirm this finding.[495] A recent study has demonstrated that mutations in *ABCB4* (*MDR3*) are associated with a peculiar form of gallstone disease that is characterized by intrahepatic sludge, cholesterol gallstones in the gallbladder, and mild chronic cholestasis.[496] Rapid advances in techniques for genetic analyses and the availability of the nucleotide sequence of the human genome will likely lead to identification and characterization of *LITH* genes in the coming years.

Mouse Genetics

Inbred mice represent a powerful model for the study of genetic diseases.[497] Current technologies permit rapid localization of both specific genes and phenotypic traits to precise locations on mouse chromosomes. Using observations that certain inbred strains of mice form gallstones when challenged with a high-fat and high-cholesterol lithogenic diet whereas other strains are resistant,[498,499] gallstone susceptibility in mice has been linked to two or more *Lith* genes.[499,500] *Lith1* is the major gallstone gene in mice[499] and is located in a narrowly restricted region of DNA on chromosome 2.[499,501] Independent experiments have assigned *Abcb11* (*Bsep*) to the same region,[501] suggesting that *Abcb11* may be identical to *Lith1*. A current "gallstone map" catalogs all known genetic loci that confer gallstone susceptibility in mice—as well as candidate genes.[502] A detailed understanding of gallstone genetics in mice will likely facilitate the search for *LITH* genes in humans.

ACKNOWLEDGMENTS

This chapter is dedicated to the author's father, Murray L. Cohen, MD, on the occasion of his 75th birthday.

This work was supported in part by Grant Nos. DK56626 and DK48873 from the National Institutes of Health. Support from the Alexandrine and Alexander L. Sinsheimer Fund (D.E.C.) is gratefully acknowledged. The author thanks Dr. Martin C. Carey for critical review of the manuscript.

References

1. Everhart JE, Khare M, Hill M, et al: Prevalence and ethnic differences in gallbladder disease in the United States. Gastroenterology 117:632, 1999.
2. Sandler RS, Everhart JE, Donowitz M, et al: The burden of selected digestive diseases in the United States. Gastroenterology: in press, 2002.
3. Fromm H: Medical management of gallstones. In Zakim D, Boyer TD, eds: Hepatology: A Textbook of Liver Disease, ed 4. 2002: in press.
4. Park YH, Igimi H, Carey MC: The "mirroring" of gallstones: description of a novel silvering method to determine the surface area of an irregular object. In vitro demonstration that multiple gallstones from the same gallbladder dissolve in unsaturated "bile" at the same rate. Gastroenterology 83:1071, 1982.
5. Cetta F, Lombardo F, Malet PF: Black pigment gallstones with cholesterol gallstones in the same gallbladder. 13 cases in a surgical series of 1226 patients with gallbladder stones. Dig Dis Sci 40:534, 1995.
6. Paigen B, Carey MC: Gallstones. In King RA, Rotter JI, Motulsky AG, eds: The Genetic Basis of Common Diseases, ed 2. London, Oxford, 2002:298-335.
7. Malet PF, Williamson CE, Trotman BW, et al: Composition of pigmented centers of cholesterol gallstones. Hepatology 6:477, 1986.

8. Taylor DR, Crowther RS, Cozart JC, et al: Calcium carbonate in cholesterol gallstones: polymorphism, distribution, and hypotheses about pathogenesis. Hepatology 22:488, 1995.
9. Malet PF, Weston NE, Trotman BW, et al: Cyclic deposition of calcium salts during growth of cholesterol gallstones. Scan Electron Microscop 775, 1985.
10. Ohta T, Nagakawa T, Takeda T, et al: Histological evaluation of the intrahepatic biliary tree in intrahepatic cholesterol stones, including immunohistochemical staining against apolipoprotein A-1. Hepatology 17:531, 1993.
11. Shoda J, Oda K, Suzuki H, et al: Etiologic significance of defects in cholesterol, phospholipid, and bile acid metabolism in the liver of patients with intrahepatic calculi. Hepatology 33:1194, 2001.
12. Trotman BW: Pigment gallstone disease. Gastroenterol Clin North Am 20:111, 1991.
13. Trotman BW, Soloway RD: Pigment gallstone disease: summary of the National Institutes of Health—international workshop. Hepatology 2:879, 1982.
14. Carey MC: Pathogenesis of gallstones. Am J Surg 165:410, 1993.
15. Hay DW, Carey MC: Chemical species of lipids in bile. Hepatology 12:6S, 1990.
16. Roy Chowdhury J, Jansen P: Bilirubin Metabolism and Its Disorders. In Zakim D, Boyer TD, eds: Hepatology: A Textbook of Liver Disease, ed 4. Philadelphia, Saunders, 2002:233-270.
17. Reuben A: Biliary proteins. Hepatology 4:46S, 1984.
18. LaRusso NF: Proteins in bile: how they get there and what they do. Am J Physiol 247:G199, 1984.
19. Albers CJEM, Huizenga JR, Krom RAF, et al: Composition of human hepatic bile. Ann Clin Biochem 22:129, 1985.
20. Carey MC, Small DM: The physical chemistry of cholesterol solubility in bile. Relationship to gallstone formation and dissolution in man. J Clin Invest 61:998, 1978.
21. Müller M: Bile Formation. In Zakim D, Boyer TD, eds: Hepatology: A Textbook of Liver Disease, ed 4. 2002:271-290.
22. Anderson RG: The caveolae membrane system. Annu Rev Biochem 67:199, 1998.
23. Smart EJ, Graf GA, McNiven MA, et al: Caveolins, liquid-ordered domains, and signal transduction. Mol Cell Biol 19:7289, 1999.
24. Gylling H, Miettinen TA: Cholesterol absorption and synthesis related to low density lipoprotein metabolism during varying cholesterol intake in men with different apoE phenotypes. J Lipid Res 33:1361, 1992.
25. Grundy SM, Ahrens EH: Measurements of cholesterol turnover, synthesis, and absorption in man, carried out by isotope kinetic and sterol balance methods. J Lipid Res 10:91, 1969.
26. Miettinen TA, Kesaniemi YA: Cholesterol absorption: regulation of cholesterol synthesis and elimination and within-population variations of serum cholesterol levels. Am J Clin Nutr 49:629, 1989.
27. Sehayek E, Nath C, Heinemann T, et al: U-shape relationship between change in dietary cholesterol absorption and plasma lipoprotein responsiveness and evidence for extreme interindividual variation in dietary cholesterol absorption in humans. J Lipid Res 39:2415, 1998.
28. Bosner MS, Lange LG, Stenson WF, et al: Percent cholesterol absorption in normal women and men quantified with dual stable isotopic tracers and negative ion mass spectrometry. J Lipid Res 40:302, 1999.
29. Vlahcevic ZR, Hylemon PB, Chiang JYL: Hepatic cholesterol metabolism. In Arias IM, Boyer JL, Fausto N, et al, eds: The Liver: Biology and Pathobiology. New York, Raven Press, Ltd., 1994:379.
30. Glomset JA: The plasma lecithins:cholesterol acyltransferase reaction. J Lipid Res 9:155, 1968.
31. Rothblat GH, de la Llera-Moya M, Atger V, et al: Cell cholesterol efflux: integration of new and old observations provides new insights. J Lipid Res 40:781, 1999.
32. Tall AR, Jiang X, Luo Y, et al: 1999 George Lyman Duff memorial lecture: lipid transfer proteins, HDL metabolism, and atherogenesis. Arterioscler Thromb Vasc Biol 20:1185, 2000.
33. Brown MS, Goldstein JL: A receptor-mediated pathway for cholesterol homeostasis. Science 232:34, 1986.
34. Ghosh S, Mallonee DH, Hylemon PB, et al: Molecular cloning and expression of rat hepatic neutral cholesteryl ester hydrolase. Biochim Biophys Acta 1259:305, 1995.
35. Buhman KF, Accad M, Farese RV: Mammalian acyl-CoA:cholesterol acyltransferases. Biochim Biophys Acta 1529:142, 2000.
36. Carey MC, Duane WC: Enterohepatic circulation. In Arias IM, Boyer JL, Fausto N, Jakoby WB, et al, eds: The Liver: Biology and Pathobiology. New York, Raven Press, Ltd., 1994:719.
37. Grundy SM, Metzger AL: A physiological method for estimation of hepatic secretion of biliary lipids in man. Gastroenterology 62:1200, 1972.
38. Grundy SM: Absorption and metabolism of dietary cholesterol. Annu Rev Nutr 3:71, 1983.
39. Reuben A, Maton PN, Murphy GM, et al: Bile lipid secretion in obese and non-obese individuals with and without gallstones. Clin Sci 69:71, 1985.
40. Northfield TC, Hofmann AF: Biliary lipid output during three meals and an overnight fast. I. Relationship to bile acid pool size and cholesterol saturation of bile in gallstone and control subjects. Gut 16:1, 1975.
41. Wilson MD, Rudel LL: Review of cholesterol absorption with emphasis on dietary and biliary cholesterol. J Lipid Res 35:943, 1994.
42. Hillebrant CG, Nyberg G, Einarsson K, et al: The effect of plasma low density lipoprotein apheresis on the hepatic secretion of biliary lipids in humans. Gut 41:700, 1997.
43. Carey MC: Homing-in on the origin of biliary steroids. Gut 41:721, 1997.
44. Bjorkhem I: Mechanism of bile acid biosynthesis in mammalian liver. In Danielsson H, Sjövall J, eds: Steroids and Bile Acids. Amsterdam, Elsevier, 1985:231.
45. Vlahcevic ZR, Pandak WM, Stravitz RT: Regulation of bile acid biosynthesis. Gastroenterol Clin North Am 28:1, 1999.
46. Russell DW, Setchell KD: Bile acid biosynthesis. Biochemistry 31:4737, 1992.
47. Chiang JYL: Regulation of bile acid synthesis. Front Biosci 3:D176, 1998.
48. Hofmann AF: Bile acids. In Arias IM, Boyer JL, Fausto N, et al, eds: The Liver: Biology and Pathobiology. New York, Raven Press, Ltd., 1994:677.
49. Vlahcevic ZR, Heuman DM, Hylemon PB: Physiology and pathophysiology of enterohepatic circulation of bile acids. In Zakim D, Boyer TD, eds: Hepatology: A Textbook of Liver Disease, ed 3. Philadelphia, W.B. Saunders, 1996:376.
50. Hofmann AF: Enterhepatic circulation of bile acids. In Schultz SG, Forte JG, Rauner BB, eds: Handbook of Physiology—The Gastrointestinal System III. Bethesda, MD, American Physiological Society, 1989:567.
51. Jelinek DF, Andersson S, Slaughter CA, et al: Cloning and regulation of cholesterol 7 alpha-hydroxylase, the rate-limiting enzyme in bile acid biosynthesis. J Biol Chem 265:8190, 1990.
52. Li YC, Wang DP, Chiang JY: Regulation of cholesterol 7 alpha-hydroxylase in the liver. Cloning, sequencing, and regulation of cholesterol 7 alpha-hydroxylase mRNA. J Biol Chem 265:12012, 1990.
53. Noshiro M, Nishimoto M, Morohashi K, et al: Molecular cloning of cDNA for cholesterol 7 alpha-hydroxylase from rat liver microsomes. Nucleotide sequence and expression. FEBS Lett 257:97, 1989.
54. Myant NB, Mitropoulos KA: Cholesterol 7 alpha-hydroxylase. J Lipid Res 18:135, 1977.
55. Shefer S, Hauser S, Bekersky I, et al: Biochemical site of regulation of bile acid biosynthesis in the rat. J Lipid Res 11:404, 1970.
56. Ishida H, Noshiro M, Okuda K, et al: Purification and characterization of 7 alpha-hydroxy-4-cholesten-3-one 12 alpha-hydroxylase. J Biol Chem 267:21319, 1992.
57. Eggertsen G, Olin M, Andersson U, et al: Molecular cloning and expression of rabbit sterol 12alpha-hydroxylase. J Biol Chem 271:32269, 1996.
58. Bjorkhem I: Mechanism of degradation of the steroid side chain in the formation of bile acids. J Lipid Res 33:455, 1992.
59. Javitt NB: Bile acid synthesis from cholesterol: regulatory and auxiliary pathways. FASEB J 8:1308, 1994.
60. Cali JJ, Russell DW: Characterization of human sterol 27-hydroxylase. A mitochondrial cytochrome P-450 that catalyzes multiple oxidation reaction in bile acid biosynthesis. J Biol Chem 266:7774, 1991.
61. Andersson S, Davis DL, Dahlback H, et al: Cloning, structure, and expression of the mitochondrial cytochrome P-450 sterol 26-hydroxylase, a bile acid biosynthetic enzyme. J Biol Chem 264:8222, 1989.

62. Usui E, Noshiro M, Okuda K: Molecular cloning of cDNA for vitamin D3 25-hydroxylase from rat liver mitochondria. FEBS Lett 262:135, 1990.
63. Schwarz M, Lund EG, Lathe R, et al: Identification and characterization of a mouse oxysterol 7alpha-hydroxylase cDNA. J Biol Chem 272:23995, 1997.
64. Swell L, Gustafsson J, Schwartz CC, et al: An in vivo evaluation of the quantitative significance of several potential pathways to cholic and chenodeoxycholic acids from cholesterol in man. J Lipid Res 21:455, 1980.
65. Princen HM, Meijer P, Wolthers BG, et al: Cyclosporin A blocks bile acid synthesis in cultured hepatocytes by specific inhibition of chenodeoxycholic acid synthesis. Biochem J 275:501, 1991.
66. Vlahcevic ZR, Stravitz RT, Heuman DM, et al: Quantitative estimations of the contribution of different bile acid pathways to total bile acid synthesis in the rat. Gastroenterology 113:1949, 1997.
67. Carey MC: Physical-chemical properties of bile acids and their salts. In Danielsson H, Sjövall J, eds: New Comprehensive Biochemistry. Amsterdam, Elsevier, 1985:345.
68. Cabral DJ, Small DM: The physical chemistry of bile. In Schultz SG, Forte JG, Rauner BB, eds: Handbook of Physiology—The Gastrointestinal System III. Bethesda, MD, American Physiological Society, 1989:621.
69. Elliot WH: Metabolism of bile acids in liver and extrahepatic tissues. In Danielsson H, Sjövall J, eds: Sterols and Bile Acids. Amsterdam, Elsevier, 1985:303.
70. Falany CN, Johnson MR, Barnes S, et al: Glycine and taurine conjugation of bile acids by a single enzyme. Molecular cloning and expression of human liver bile acid CoA:amino acid N-acyltransferase. J Biol Chem 269:19375, 1994.
71. Hylemon PB: Metabolism of bile acids in intestinal microflora. In Danielsson H, Sjövall J, eds: Sterols and Bile Acids. Amsterdam, Elsevier, 1985:331.
72. Hylemon PB: Biochemistry and genetics of intestinal bile salt metabolism. In Paumgartner G, Stiehl A, Gerok W, eds: Bile Acids as Therapeutic Agents. Dordrecht, Kluwer Academic Publishers, 1991:1.
73. Hylemon PB, Harder J: Biotransformation of monoterpenes, bile acids, and other isoprenoids in anaerobic ecosystems. FEMS Microbiol Rev 22:475, 1998.
74. Wells JE, Hylemon PB: Identification and characterization of a bile acid 7alpha-dehydroxylation operon in *Clostridium* sp. strain TO-931, a highly active 7alpha-dehydroxylating strain isolated from human feces. Appl Environ Microbiol 66:1107, 2000.
75. Kitahara M, Takamine F, Imamura T, et al: Assignment of Eubacterium sp. VPI 12708 and related strains with high bile acid 7alpha-dehydroxylating activity to *Clostridium scindens* and proposal of *Clostridium hylemonae* sp. nov., isolated from human faeces. Int J Syst Evol Microbiol 50:971, 2000.
76. Palmer RH: The formation of bile acid sulfates: a new pathway of bile acid metabolism in humans. Proc Natl Acad Sci U S A 58:1047, 1967.
77. Hofmann AF, Roda A: Physicochemical properties of bile acids and their relationship to biological properties: an overview of the problem. J Lipid Res 25:1477, 1984.
78. Cohen DE, Carey MC: Physical chemistry of lipids during bile formation. Hepatology 12:143S, 1990.
79. Möckel GM, Gorti S, Tandon RK, et al: Microscope laser light-scattering spectroscopy of vesicles within canaliculi of rat hepatocyte couplets. Am J Physiol 269:G73, 1995.
80. Armstrong MJ, Carey MC: The hydrophobic-hydrophilic balance of bile salts. Inverse correlation between reverse-phase high performance liquid chromatographic mobilities and micellar cholesterol-solubilizing capacities. J Lipid Res 23:70, 1982.
81. Rossi SS, Converse JL, Hofmann AF: High pressure liquid chromatographic analysis of conjugated bile acids in human bile: Simultaneous resolution of sulfated and unsulfated lithocholyl amidases and the common conjugated bile acids. J Lipid Res 28:589, 1987.
82. Cohen DE, Leonard MR: Immobilized artificial membrane chromatography: a rapid and accurate HPLC method for predicting bile salt-membrane interactions. J Lipid Res 36:2251, 1995.
83. Heuman DM: Quantitative estimation of the hydrophilic-hydrophobic balance of mixed bile salt solutions. J Lipid Res 30:719, 1989.
84. Hagenbuch B, Stieger B, Foguet M, et al: Functional expression cloning and characterization of the hepatocyte Na+/bile acid cotransport system. Proc Natl Acad Sci U S A 88:10629, 1991.
85. Jacquemin E, Hagenbuch B, Stieger B, et al: Expression cloning of a rat liver Na(+)-independent organic anion transporter. Proc Natl Acad Sci U S A 91:133, 1994.
86. von Dippe P, Amoui M, Stellwagen RH, et al: The functional expression of sodium-dependent bile acid transport in Madin-Darby canine kidney cells transfected with the cDNA for microsomal epoxide hydrolase. J Biol Chem 271:18176, 1996.
87. St-Pierre MV, Kullak-Ublick GA, Hagenbuch B, et al: Transport of bile acids in hepatic and non-hepatic tissues. J Exp Biol 204:1673, 2001.
88. Dean M, Rzhetsky A, Allikmets R: The human ATP-binding cassette (ABC) transporter superfamily. Genome Res 11:1156, 2001.
89. Konig J, Rost D, Cui Y, et al: Characterization of the human multidrug resistance protein isoform MRP3 localized to the basolateral hepatocyte membrane. Hepatology 29:1156, 1999.
90. Kool M, van der Linden M, de Haas M, et al: MRP3, an organic anion transporter able to transport anti-cancer drugs. Proc Natl Acad Sci U S A 96:6914, 1999.
91. Ogawa K, Suzuki H, Hirohashi T, et al: Characterization of inducible nature of MRP3 in rat liver. Am J Physiol 278:G438, 2000.
92. Soroka CJ, Lee JM, Azzaroli F, et al: Cellular localization and up-regulation of multidrug resistance-associated protein 3 in hepatocytes and cholangiocytes during obstructive cholestasis in rat liver. Hepatology 33:783, 2001.
93. Vos TA, Hooiveld GJ, Koning H, et al: Up-regulation of the multidrug resistance genes, Mrp1 and Mdr1b, and down-regulation of the organic anion transporter, Mrp2, and the bile salt transporter, Spgp, in endotoxemic rat liver. Hepatology 28:1637, 1998.
94. Crawford JM: Role of vesicle-mediated transport pathways in hepatocellular bile secretion. Semin Liver Dis 16:169, 1996.
95. El-Seaidy AZ, Mills CO, Elias E, et al: Lack of evidence for vesicle trafficking of fluorescent bile salts in rat hepatocyte couplets. Am J Physiol 272:G298, 1997.
96. Agellon LB, Torchia EC: Intracellular transport of bile acids. Biochim Biophys Acta 1486:198, 2000.
97. Bahar RJ, Stolz A: Bile acid transport. Gastroenterol Clin North Am 28:27, 1999.
98. Gerloff T, Stieger B, Hagenbuch B, et al: The sister-P-glycoprotein represents the canalicular bile salt export pump of mammalian liver. J Biol Chem 273:10046, 1998.
99. Wang R, Salem M, Yousef IM, et al: Targeted inactivation of sister of P-glycoprotein gene (spgp) in mice results in nonprogressive but persistent intrahepatic cholestasis. Proc Natl Acad Sci U S A 98:2011, 2001.
100. Strautnieks SS, Bull LN, Knisely AS, et al: A gene encoding a liver-specific ABC transporter is mutated in progressive familial intrahepatic cholestasis. Nat Genet 20:233, 1998.
101. Jansen PL, Strautnieks SS, Jacquemin E, et al: Hepatocanalicular bile salt export pump deficiency in patients with progressive familial intrahepatic cholestasis. Gastroenterology 117:1370, 1999.
102. Paulusma CC, Bosma PJ, Zaman GJR, et al: Congenital jaundice in rats with a mutation in a multidrug resistance-associated protein gene. Science 271:1126, 1996.
103. Paulusma CC, Kool M, Bosma PJ, et al: A mutation in the human canalicular multispecific organic anion transporter gene causes the Dubin-Johnson syndrome. Hepatology 25:1539, 1997.
104. Oude Elferink RP, Ottenhoff R, Radominska A, et al: Inhibition of glutathione-conjugate secretion from isolated hepatocytes by dipolar bile acids and other organic anions. Biochem J 274:281, 1991.
105. Akita H, Suzuki H, Ito K, et al: Characterization of bile acid transport mediated by multidrug resistance associated protein 2 and bile salt export pump. Biochim Biophys Acta 1511:7, 2001.
106. Yoon YB, Hagey LR, Hofmann AF, et al: Effect of side-chain shortening on the physiologic properties of bile acids: hepatic transport and effect on biliary secretion of 23-nor-ursodeoxycholate in rodents. Gastroenterology 90:837, 1986.
107. Hofmann AF: Current concepts of biliary secretion. Dig Dis Sci 34:16S, 1989.
108. Lazaridis KN, Pham L, Tietz P, et al: Rat cholangiocytes absorb bile acids at their apical domain via the ileal sodium-dependent bile acid transporter. J Clin Invest 100:2714, 1997.
109. Lazaridis KN, Tietz P, Wu T, et al: Alternative splicing of the rat sodium/bile acid transporter changes its cellular localization and transport properties. Proc Natl Acad Sci U S A 97:11092, 2000.

110. Wong MH, Oelkers P, Craddock AL, et al: Expression cloning and characterization of the hamster ileal sodium-dependent bile acid transporter. J Biol Chem 269:1304, 1994.
111. Wong MH, Oelkers P, Dawson PA: Identification of a mutation in the ileal sodium-dependent bile acid transporter gene that abolishes transport activity. J Biol Chem 270:27228, 1995.
112. Shneider BL, Dawson PA, Christie DM, et al: Cloning and molecular characterization of the ontogeny of a rat ileal sodium-dependent bile acid transporter. J Clin Invest 95:745, 1995.
113. Kramer W, Girbig F, Gutjahr U, et al: Intestinal bile acid absorption. Na(+)-dependent bile acid transport activity in rabbit small intestine correlates with the coexpression of an integral 93-kDa and a peripheral 14-kDa bile acid-binding membrane protein along the duodenum-ileum axis. J Biol Chem 268:18035, 1993.
114. Oelkers P, Dawson PA: Cloning and chromosomal localization of the human ileal lipid-binding protein. Biochim Biophys Acta 1257:199, 1995.
115. Gong YZ, Everett ET, Schwartz DA, et al: Molecular cloning, tissue distribution, and expression of a 14-kDa bile acid-binding protein from rat ileal cytosol. Proc Natl Acad Sci U S A 91:4741, 1994.
116. Walters HC, Craddock AL, Fusegawa H, et al: Expression, transport properties, and chromosomal location of organic anion transporter subtype 3. Am J Physiol 279:G1188, 2000.
117. Ahlberg J, Angelin B, Bjorkhem I, et al: Individual bile acids in portal venous and systemic blood serum of fasting man. Gastroenterology 73:1377, 1977.
118. Gatmaitan ZC, Nies AT, Arias IM: Regulation and translocation of ATP-dependent apical membrane proteins in rat liver. Am J Physiol 272:G1041, 1997.
119. Kipp H, Pichetshote N, Arias IM: Transporters on demand: intrahepatic pools of canalicular ATP binding cassette transporters in rat liver. J Biol Chem 276:7218, 2001.
120. Webster CR, Anwer MS: Role of the PI3K/PKB signaling pathway in cAMP-mediated translocation of rat liver Ntcp. Am J Physiol 277:G1165, 1999.
121. Glavy JS, Wu SM, Wang PJ, et al: Down-regulation by extracellular ATP of rat hepatocyte organic anion transport is mediated by serine phosphorylation of oatp1. J Biol Chem 275:1479, 2000.
122. Misra S, Ujházy P, Gatmaitan Z, et al: The role of phosphoinositide 3-kinase in taurocholate-induced trafficking of ATP-dependent canalicular transporters in rat liver. J Biol Chem 273:26638, 1998.
123. Misra S, Ujházy P, Varticovski L, et al: Phosphoinositide 3-kinase lipid products regulate ATP-dependent transport by sister of P-glycoprotein and multidrug resistance associated protein 2 in bile canalicular membrane vesicles. Proc Natl Acad Sci U S A 96:5814, 1999.
124. Wang DP, Stroup D, Marrapodi M, et al: Transcriptional regulation of the human cholesterol 7 alpha-hydroxylase gene (CYP7A) in HepG2 cells. J Lipid Res 37:1831, 1996.
125. Twisk J, Hoekman MF, Lehmann EM, et al: Insulin suppresses bile acid synthesis in cultured rat hepatocytes by down-regulation of cholesterol 7 alpha-hydroxylase and sterol 27-hydroxylase gene transcription. Hepatology 21:501, 1995.
126. Nuclear Receptors Nomenclature Committee: A unified nomenclature system for the nuclear receptor superfamily. Cell 97:161, 1999.
127. Repa JJ, Mangelsdorf DJ: The role of orphan nuclear receptors in the regulation of cholesterol homeostasis. Annu Rev Cell Dev Biol 16:459, 2000.
128. Janowski BA, Willy PJ, Devi TR, et al: An oxysterol signalling pathway mediated by the nuclear receptor LXR alpha. Nature 383:728, 1996.
129. Makishima M, Okamoto AY, Repa JJ, et al: Identification of a nuclear receptor for bile acids. Science 284:1362, 1999.
130. Parks DJ, Blanchard SG, Bledsoe RK, et al: Bile acids: natural ligands for an orphan nuclear receptor. Science 284:1365, 1999.
131. Wang H, Chen J, Hollister K, et al: Endogenous bile acids are ligands for the nuclear receptor FXR/BAR. Mol Cell 3:543, 1999.
132. Repa JJ, Mangelsdorf DJ: Nuclear receptor regulation of cholesterol and bile acid metabolism. Curr Opin Biotechnol 10:557, 1999.
133. Peet DJ, Turley SD, Ma W, et al: Cholesterol and bile acid metabolism are impaired in mice lacking the nuclear oxysterol receptor LXR alpha. Cell 93:693, 1998.
134. Repa JJ, Turley SD, Lobaccaro JA, et al: Regulation of absorption and ABC1-mediated efflux of cholesterol by RXR heterodimers. Science 289:1524, 2000.
135. Berge KE, Tian H, Graf GA, et al: Accumulation of dietary cholesterol in sitosterolemia caused by mutations in adjacent ABC transporters. Science 290:1709, 2000.
136. Schmitz G, Langmann T, Heimerl S: Role of ABCG1 and other ABCG family members in lipid metabolism. J Lipid Res 42:1513, 2001.
137. Luo Y, Tall AR: Sterol upregulation of human CETP expression in vitro and in transgenic mice by an LXR element. J Clin Invest 105:513, 2000.
138. Laffitte BA, Repa JJ, Joseph SB, et al: LXRs control lipid-inducible expression of the apolipoprotein E gene in macrophages and adipocytes. Proc Natl Acad Sci U S A 98:507, 2001.
139. Cheema SK, Agellon LB: The murine and human cholesterol 7alpha-hydroxylase gene promoters are differentially responsive to regulation by fatty acids mediated via peroxisome proliferator-activated receptor alpha. J Biol Chem 275:12530, 2000.
140. Chiang JY, Kimmel R, Stroup D: Regulation of cholesterol 7alpha-hydroxylase gene (CYP7A1) transcription by the liver orphan receptor (LXRalpha). Gene 262:257, 2001.
141. Chawla A, Saez E, Evans RM: Don't know much "bile-ology." Cell 103:1, 2000.
142. Sinal CJ, Tohkin M, Miyata M, et al: Targeted disruption of the nuclear receptor FXR/BAR impairs bile acid and lipid homeostasis. Cell 102:731, 2000.
143. Heuman DM, Hylemon PB, Vlahcevic ZR: Regulation of bile acid synthesis. III. Correlation between biliary bile salt hydrophobicity index and the activities of enzymes regulating cholesterol and bile acid synthesis in the rat. J Lipid Res 30:1161, 1989.
144. Ananthanarayanan M, Balasubramanian NV, Makishima M, et al: Human bile salt export pump (BSEP) promoter is transactivated by the farnesoid X receptor/bile acid receptor (FXR/BAR). J Biol Chem 276:28857, 2001.
145. Lu TT, Makishima M, Repa JJ, et al: Molecular basis for feedback regulation of bile acid synthesis by nuclear receptors. Mol Cell 6:507, 2000.
146. Chiang JY, Kimmel R, Weinberger C, et al: Farnesoid X receptor responds to bile acids and represses cholesterol 7alpha-hydroxylase gene (CYP7A1) transcription. J Biol Chem 275:10918, 2000.
147. Gupta S, Stravitz RT, Dent P, et al: Down-regulation of cholesterol 7alpha-hydroxylase (CYP7A1) gene expression by bile acids in primary rat hepatocytes is mediated by the c-jun n-terminal kinase pathway. J Biol Chem 276:15816, 2001.
148. Denson LA, Sturm E, Echevarria W, et al: The orphan nuclear receptor, shp, mediates bile acid-induced inhibition of the rat bile acid transporter, ntcp. Gastroenterology 121:140, 2001.
149. Grober J, Zaghini I, Fujii H, et al: Identification of a bile acid-responsive element in the human ileal bile acid-binding protein gene. Involvement of the farnesoid X receptor/9-cis-retinoic acid receptor heterodimer. J Biol Chem 274:29749, 1999.
150. Staudinger JL, Goodwin B, Jones SA, et al: The nuclear receptor PXR is a lithocholic acid sensor that protects against liver toxicity. Proc Natl Acad Sci USA 98:3369, 2001.
151. Xie W, Radominska-Pandya A, Shi Y, et al: An essential role for nuclear receptors SXR/PXR in detoxification of cholestatic bile acids. Proc Natl Acad Sci U S A 98:3375, 2001.
152. Marrapodi M, Chiang JY: Peroxisome proliferator-activated receptor alpha (PPARalpha) and agonist inhibit cholesterol 7alpha-hydroxylase gene (CYP7A1) transcription. J Lipid Res 41:514, 2000.
153. Patel DD, Knight BL, Soutar AK, et al: The effect of peroxisome-proliferator-activated receptor-alpha on the activity of the cholesterol 7 alpha-hydroxylase gene. Biochem J 351 Pt 3:747, 2000.
154. Hunt MC, Yang YZ, Eggertsen G, et al: The peroxisome proliferator-activated receptor alpha (PPARalpha) regulates bile acid biosynthesis. J Biol Chem 275:28947, 2000.
155. Chen J, Cooper AD, Levy-Wilson B: Hepatocyte nuclear factor 1 binds to and transactivates the human but not the rat CYP7A1 promoter. Biochem Biophys Res Commun 260:829, 1999.
156. Stroup D, Chiang JY: HNF4 and COUP-TFII interact to modulate transcription of the cholesterol 7alpha-hydroxylase gene (CYP7A1). J Lipid Res 41:1, 2000.

157. Trauner M, Arrese M, Lee H, et al: Endotoxin downregulates rat hepatic ntcp gene expression via decreased activity of critical transcription factors. J Clin Invest 101:2092, 1998.
158. Shih DQ, Bussen M, Sehayek E, et al: Hepatocyte nuclear factor-1alpha is an essential regulator of bile acid and plasma cholesterol metabolism. Nat Genet 27:375, 2001.
159. Hayhurst GP, Lee YH, Lambert G, et al: Hepatocyte nuclear factor 4alpha (nuclear receptor 2A1) is essential for maintenance of hepatic gene expression and lipid homeostasis. Mol Cell Biol 21:1393, 2001.
160. Rausa FM, Tan Y, Zhou H, et al: Elevated levels of hepatocyte nuclear factor 3beta in mouse hepatocytes influence expression of genes involved in bile acid and glucose homeostasis. Mol Cell Biol 20:8264, 2000.
161. Mazer NA, Carey MC: Mathematical model of biliary lipid secretion: a quantitative analysis of physiological and biochemical data from man and other species. J Lipid Res 25:932, 1984.
162. Cohen DE: Hepatocellular transport and secretion of biliary lipids. Curr Opin Lipidol 235:111, 1999.
163. Campbell CB, Burgess P, Roberts SA, et al: The use of rhesus monkeys to study biliary secretion with an intact enterohepatic circulation. Aust N Z J Med 2:49, 1972.
164. Cohen DE: Hepatocellular transport and secretion of biliary phospholipids. Semin Liver Dis 16:191, 1996.
165. Alvaro D, Cantafora A, Attili AF, et al: Relationships between bile salts hydrophilicity and phospholipid composition in bile of various animal species. Comp Biochem Physiol 83B:551, 1986.
166. Carey MC, LaMont JT: Cholesterol gallstone formation. 1. Physical-chemistry of bile and biliary lipid secretion. Prog Liver Dis 10:136, 1992.
167. Verma A, Ahmed HA, Davis T, et al: Demonstration and partial characterisation of phospholipid methyltransferase activity in bile canalicular membrane from hamster liver. J Hepatol 31:852, 1999.
168. Portal I, Thierry C, Sbarra V, et al: Importance of high-density lipoprotein-phosphatidylcholine in secretion of phospholipid and cholesterol into bile. Am J Physiol 264:G1052, 1993.
169. Schwartz CC, Halloran LG, Vlahcevic ZR, et al: Preferential utilization of free cholesterol from high-density lipoproteins for biliary cholesterol secretion in man. Science 200:62, 1978.
170. Robins SJ, Fasulo JM: High density lipoproteins, but not other lipoproteins, provide a vehicle for sterol transport to bile. J Clin Invest 99:380, 1997.
171. Cooper AD: Metabolic basis of cholesterol gallstone disease. Gastroenterol Clin North Am 20:21, 1991.
172. Amigo L, Quinones V, Mardones P, et al: Impaired biliary cholesterol secretion and decreased gallstone formation in apolipoprotein E-deficient mice fed a high-cholesterol diet. Gastroenterology 118:772, 2000.
173. Sehayek E, Shefer S, Nguyen LB, et al: Apolipoprotein E regulates dietary cholesterol absorption and biliary cholesterol excretion: Studies in C57BL/6 apolipoprotein E knockout mice. Proc Natl Acad Sci U S A 97:3433, 2000.
174. Empen K, Lange K, Stange EF, et al: Newly synthesized cholesterol in human bile and plasma: Quantitation by mass isotopomer distribution analysis. Am J Physiol 272:G367, 1997.
175. Elferink RP, Groen AK: The mechanism of biliary lipid secretion and its defects. Gastroenterol Clin North Am 28:59, 1999.
176. Smit JJM, Schinkel AH, Oude Elferink RPJ, et al: Homozygous disruption of the murine *mdr2* P-glycoprotein gene leads to a complete absence of phospholipid from bile and to liver disease. Cell 75:451, 1993.
177. de Vree JM, Jacquemin E, Sturm E, et al: Mutations in the *MDR3* gene cause progressive familial intrahepatic cholestasis. Proc Natl Acad Sci U S A 95:282, 1998.
178. Jacquemin E, De Vree JM, Cresteil D, et al: The wide spectrum of multidrug resistance 3 deficiency: from neonatal cholestasis to cirrhosis of adulthood. Gastroenterology 120:1448, 2001.
179. Verkade HJ, Vonk RJ, Kuipers F: New insights into the mechanism of bile acid-induced biliary lipid secretion. Hepatology 21:1174, 1995.
180. Kremmer T, Wisher MH, Evans WH: The lipid composition of plasma membrane subfractions originating from the three major functional domains of the rat hepatocyte cell surface. Biochim Biophys Acta 455:655, 1976.
181. Higgins J, Evans WH: Transverse organization of phospholipids across the bilayer of plasma-membrane subfractions of rat hepatocytes. Biochem J 174:563, 1978.
182. Crawford AR, Smith AJ, Hatch VC, et al: Hepatic secretion of phospholipid vesicles in the mouse critically depends on mdr2 or MDR3 P-glycoprotein expression. Visualization by electron microscopy. J Clin Invest 100:2562, 1997.
183. Yousef IM, Fisher MM: In vitro effect of free bile acids on the bile canalicular membrane phospholipids in the rat. Can J Biochem 54:1040, 1976.
184. Gerloff T, Meier PJ, Stieger B: Taurocholate induces preferential release of phosphatidylcholine from rat liver canalicular vesicles. Liver 18:306, 1998.
185. Apstein MD: Inhibition of biliary phospholipid and cholesterol secretion by bilirubin in the Sprague-Dawley and Gunn rat. Gastroenterology 87:637, 1984.
186. Verkade HJ, Wolbers MJ, Havinga R, et al: The uncoupling of biliary lipid from bile acid secretion by organic anions in the rat. Gastroenterology 99:1485, 1990.
187. Apstein MD, Russo AR: Ampicillin inhibits biliary cholesterol secretion. Dig Dis Sci 30:253, 1985.
188. Yamashita G, Tazuma S, Kajiyama G: Effects of organic anions on biliary lipid secretion in rats. Biochem J 286:193, 1992.
189. Yamashita G, Tazuma S, Horikawa K, et al: Partial characterization of mechanism(s) by which sulphobromophthalein reduces biliary lipid secretion. Biochem J 291:173, 1993.
190. Verkade HJ, Havinga R, Gerding A, et al: Mechanism of bile acid-induced biliary lipid secretion in the rat: Effect of conjugated bilirubin. Am J Physiol 264:G462, 1993.
191. Cohen DE, Angelico M, Carey MC: Quasielastic light scattering evidence for vesicular secretion of biliary lipids. Am J Physiol 257:G1, 1989.
192. Ulloa N, Garrido J, Nervi F: Ultracentrifugal isolation of vesicular carriers of biliary cholesterol in native human and rat bile. Hepatology 7:235, 1987.
193. Cohen DE, Leighton LS, Carey MC: Bile salt hydrophobicity controls biliary vesicle secretion rates and transformations in native bile. Am J Physiol 263:G386, 1992.
194. Weinman SA, Graf J, Boyer JL: Voltage-driven, taurocholate-dependent secretion in isolated hepatocyte couplets. Am J Physiol 19:G826, 1989.
195. Crawford JM, Möckel G-M, Crawford AR, et al: Imaging biliary lipid secretion in the rat: ultrastructural evidence for vesiculation of the hepatocyte canalicular membrane. J Lipid Res 36:2147, 1995.
196. Brown DA, London E: Structure and origin of ordered lipid domains in biological membranes. J Membr Biol 164:103, 1998.
197. van Erpecum KJ, Carey MC: Influence of bile salts on molecular interactions between sphingomyelin and cholesterol: relevance to bile formation and stability. Biochim Biophys Acta 1345:269, 1997.
198. Vaisman BL, Lambert G, Amar M, et al: ABCA1 overexpression leads to hyperalphalipoproteinemia and increased biliary cholesterol excretion in transgenic mice. J Clin Invest 108:303, 2001.
199. Groen AK, Bloks VW, Bandsma RH, et al: Hepatobiliary cholesterol transport is not impaired in Abca1-null mice lacking HDL. J Clin Invest 108:843, 2001.
200. Drobnik W, Lindenthal B, Lieser B, et al: ATP-binding cassette transporter A1 (ABCA1) affects total body sterol metabolism. Gastroenterology 120:1203, 2001.
201. Ikemoto M, Arai H, Feng D, et al: Identification of a PDZ-domain-containing protein that interacts with the scavenger receptor class B type I. Proc Natl Acad Sci USA 97:6538, 2000.
202. Silver DL, Nan W, Xiao X, et al: HDL particle uptake mediated by SR-BI results in selective sorting of HDL cholesterol from protein and polarized cholesterol secretion. J Biol Chem 276:25287, 2001.
203. Kozarsky KF, Donahee MH, Rigotti A, et al: Overexpression of the HDL receptor SR-BI alters plasma HDL and bile cholesterol levels. Nature 387:414, 1997.
204. Wang N, Arai T, Ji Y, et al: Liver-specific overexpression of scavenger receptor BI decreases levels of very low density lipoprotein ApoB, low density lipoprotein ApoB, and high density lipoprotein in transgenic mice. J Biol Chem 273:32920, 1998.
205. Sehayek E, Ono JG, Shefer S, et al: Biliary cholesterol excretion: a novel mechanism that regulates dietary cholesterol absorption. Proc Natl Acad Sci USA 95:10194, 1998.

206. Mardones P, Quinones V, Amigo L, et al: Hepatic cholesterol and bile acid metabolism and intestinal cholesterol absorption in scavenger receptor class B type I-deficient mice. J Lipid Res 42:170, 2001.
207. Rigotti A, Trigatti BL, Penman M, et al: A targeted mutation in the murine gene encoding the high density lipoprotein (HDL) receptor scavenger receptor class B type I reveals its key role in HDL metabolism. Proc Natl Acad Sci U S A 94:12610, 1997.
208. Varban ML, Rinninger F, Wang N, et al: Targeted mutation reveals a central role for SR-BI in hepatic selective uptake of high density lipoprotein cholesterol. Proc Natl Acad Sci U S A 95:4619, 1998.
209. Marzola MP, Rigotti A, Nervi F: Secretion of biliary lipids from the hepatocyte. Hepatology 12:134S, 1990.
210. Ahmed HA, Jazrawi RP, Goggin PM, et al: Intrahepatic biliary cholesterol and phospholipid transport in humans: effect of obesity and cholesterol cholelithiasis. J Lipid Res 36:2562, 1995.
211. Wirtz KWA: Phospholipid transfer proteins revisited. Biochem J 324:353, 1997.
212. Schroeder F, Frolov A, Schoer JK, et al: Intracellular sterol binding proteins: cholesterol transport and membrane domains. In Chang TY, Freeman DE, eds: Intracellular Cholesterol Trafficking. Boston, Kluwer Press, 1998:211.
213. Ito T, Kawata S, Imai Y, et al: Hepatic cholesterol metabolism in patients with cholesterol gallstones: enhanced intracellular transport of cholesterol. Gastroenterology 110:1619, 1996.
214. Puglielli L, Rigotti A, Amigo L, et al: Modulation of intrahepatic cholesterol trafficking: evidence by *in vivo* antisense treatment for the involvement of sterol carrier protein-2 in newly synthesized cholesterol transport into rat bile. Biochem J 317:681, 1996.
215. Fuchs M, Lammert F, Wang DQH, et al: Sterol carrier protein 2 participates in hypersecretion of biliary cholesterol during gallstone formation in genetically gallstone-susceptible mice. Biochem J 336:33, 1998.
216. Zanlungo S, Amigo L, Mendoza H, et al: Sterol carrier protein 2 gene transfer changes lipid metabolism and enterohepatic sterol circulation in mice. Gastroenterology 119:1708, 2000.
217. Fuchs M, Hafer A, Munch C, et al: Disruption of the sterol carrier protein 2 gene in mice impairs biliary lipid and hepatic cholesterol metabolism. J Biol Chem 276:48058, 2001.
218. Wirtz KWA: Phospholipid transfer proteins. Annu Rev Biochem 60:73, 1991.
219. Cohen DE, Leonard MR, Carey MC: In vitro evidence that phospholipid secretion into bile may be coordinated intracellularly by the combined actions of bile salts and the specific phosphatidylcholine transfer protein of liver. Biochemistry 33:9975, 1994.
220. LaMorte WW, Booker ML, Kay S: Determinants of the selection of phosphatidylcholine molecular species for secretion into bile. Hepatology 28:631, 1998.
221. van Heivoort A, de Brouwer A, Ottenhoff R, et al: Mice without phosphatidylcholine transfer protein have no defects in the secretion of phosphatidylcholine into bile or into lung airspaces. Proc Natl Acad Sci U S A 96:11501, 1999.
222. Robins SJ, Fasulo JM: Delineation of a novel hepatic route for the selective transfer of unesterified sterols from high-density lipoproteins to bile: studies using the perfused rat liver. Hepatology 29:1541, 1999.
223. Ji Y, Wang N, Ramakrishnan R, et al: Hepatic scavenger receptor BI promotes rapid clearance of high density lipoprotein free cholesterol and its transport into bile. J Biol Chem 274:33398, 1999.
224. Holzbach RT: Effects of gallbladder function on human bile: composition and structural changes. Hepatology 4:57S, 1984.
225. Dietschy JM: Recent developments in solute and water transport across the gall bladder epithelium. Gastroenterology 50:692, 1966.
226. Cremaschi D, Porta C: Sodium salt neutral entry at the apical membrane of the gallbladder epithelium: comparing different species. Comp Biochem Physiol 103A:619, 1992.
227. Reuss L: Ion transport across gallbladder epithelium. Physiol Rev 69:503, 1989.
228. Purdum PP, Ulissi A, Hylemon PB, et al: Cultured human gallbladder epithelium: methods and partial characterization of a carcinoma-derived model. J Lab Clin Med 68:345, 1993.
229. Silviani V, Gastaldi M, Planells R, et al: NHE-3 isoform of the Na+/H+ exchanger in human gallbladder. Localization of specific mRNA by in situ hybridization. J Hepatol 26:1281, 1997.
230. Ostrow JD: Absorption by the gallbladder of bile salts, sulfobromophthalein, and iodipamide. J Lab Clin Med 74:482, 1969.
231. Neiderhiser DH, Harmon CK, Roth HP: Absorption of cholesterol by the gallbladder. J Lipid Res 17:117, 1976.
232. Neiderhiser DH, Morningstar WA, Roth HP: Absorption of lecithin and lysolecithin by the gallbladder. J Lab Clin Med 82:891, 1973.
233. Ginanni Corradini S, Ripani C, Della Guardia P, et al: The human gallbladder increases cholesterol solubility in bile by differential lipid absorption: a study using a new in vitro model of isolated intra-arterially perfused gallbladder. Hepatology 28:314, 1998.
234. Rege RV, Nahrwold DL, Moore EW: Absorption of biliary calcium from the canine gallbladder: protection against the formation of calcium-containing gallstones. J Lab Clin Med 110:381, 1987.
235. Ostrow JD: Absorption of organic compounds by the injured gallbladder. J Lab Clin Med 78:255, 1971.
236. Toth JL, Harvey PR, Upadyha GA, et al: Albumin absorption and protein secretion by the gallbladder in man and in the pig. Hepatology 12:729, 1990.
237. Keates AC, Nunes DP, Afdhal NH, et al: Molecular cloning of a major human gall bladder mucin: complete C-terminal sequence and genomic organization of MUC5B. Biochem J 324:295, 1997.
238. LaMont JT, Smith BF, Moore JR: Role of gallbladder mucin in pathophysiology of gallstones. Hepatology 4:51S, 1984.
239. Smith BF, LaMont JT: Hydrophobic binding properties of bovine gallbladder mucin. J Biol Chem 259:12170, 1984.
240. Nunes DP, Afdhal NH, Offner GD: A recombinant bovine gallbladder mucin polypeptide binds biliary lipids and accelerates cholesterol crystal appearance time. Gastroenterology 116:936, 1999.
241. Wahlin T, Bloom GD, Carlsoo B: Histochemical observations with the light and the electron microscope on the mucosubstances of the normal mouse gallbladder epithelial cells. Histochemistry 42:119, 1974.
242. Kuver R, Klinkspoor JH, Osborne WR, et al: Mucous granule exocytosis and CFTR expression in gallbladder epithelium. Glycobiology 10:149, 2000.
243. Hale WB, Turner B, LaMont JT: Oxygen radicals stimulate guinea pig gallbladder glycoprotein secretion in vitro. Am J Physiol 253:G627, 1987.
244. Kuver R, Savard C, Oda D, et al: PGE generates intracellular cAMP and accelerates mucin secretion by cultured dog gallbladder epithelial cells. Am J Physiol 267:G998, 1994.
245. LaMont JT, Turner BS, DiBenedetto D, et al: Arachidonic acid stimulates mucin secretion in prairie dog gallbladder. Am J Physiol 245:G92, 1983.
246. Dray-Charier N, Paul A, Combettes L, et al: Regulation of mucin secretion in human gallbladder epithelial cells: predominant role of calcium and protein kinase C. Gastroenterology 112:978, 1997.
247. Klinkspoor JH, Kuver R, Savard CE, et al: Model bile and bile salts accelerate mucin secretion by cultured dog gallbladder epithelial cells. Gastroenterology 109:264, 1995.
248. Klinkspoor JH, Yoshida T, Lee SP: Bile salts stimulate mucin secretion by cultured dog gallbladder epithelial cells independent of their detergent effect. Biochem J 332:257, 1998.
249. Chignard N, Mergey M, Veissiere D, et al: Bile acid transport and regulating functions in the human biliary epithelium. Hepatology 33:496, 2001.
250. Shaffer EA: Review article: control of gall-bladder motor function. Aliment Pharmacol Ther 14(suppl 2):2, 2000.
251. Cole MJ, Shaffer EA, Scott RB: Gallbladder pressure, compliance, and hysteresis during cyclic volume change. Can J Physiol Pharmacol 65:2124, 1987.
252. Shaffer EA, McOrmond P, Duggan H: Quantitative cholescintigraphy: assessment of gallbladder filling and emptying and duodenogastric reflux. Gastroenterology 79:899, 1980.
253. Everson GT, Braverman DZ, Johnson ML, et al: A critical evaluation of real-time ultrasonography for the study of gallbladder volume and contraction. Gastroenterology 79:40, 1980.
254. Marzio L, Neri M, Capone F, et al: Gallbladder contraction and its relationship to interdigestive duodenal motor activity in normal human subjects. Dig Dis Sci 33:540, 1988.
255. Qvist N, Oster-Jorgensen E, Rasmussen L, et al: The relationship between gallbladder dynamics and the migrating motor complex in fasting healthy subjects. Scand J Gastroenterol 23:562, 1988.
256. Luiking YC, Peeters TL, Stolk MF, et al: Motilin induces gall bladder emptying and antral contractions in the fasted state in humans. Gut 42:830, 1998.

257. Fisher RS, Stelzer F, Rock E, et al: Abnormal gallbladder emptying in patients with gallstones. Dig Dis Sci 27:1019, 1982.
258. O'Donnell LJ, Fairclough PD: Gall stones and gall bladder motility. Gut 34:440, 1993.
259. Hopman WP, Jansen JB, Rosenbusch G, et al: Cephalic stimulation of gallbladder contraction in humans: role of cholecystokinin and the cholinergic system. Digestion 38:197, 1987.
260. Witteman BJ, Jebbink MC, Hopman WP, et al: Gallbladder responses to modified sham feeding: effects of the composition of a meal. J Hepatol 19:465, 1993.
261. Grider JR: Role of cholecystokinin in the regulation of gastrointestinal motility. J Nutr 124:1334S, 1994.
262. Hartley GS: The Colloid State. II. Aqueous Solutions of Paraffin-Chain Salts. A Study in Micelle Formation. Paris, Herman & Co., 1936.
263. Isaksson B: On the dissolving power of lecithin and bile salts for cholesterol in human bladder bile. Acta Soc Med Upsal 59:296, 1954.
264. Small DM, Bourgès M, Dervichian DG: Ternary and quaternary aqueous systems containing bile salt, lecithin, and cholesterol. Nature 211:816, 1966.
265. Bourgès MC, Small DM, Dervichian DG: Biophysics of lipid association. III. The quaternary systems lecithin-bile salt- cholesterol-water. Biochim Biophys Acta 144:189, 1967.
266. Small DM: Physico-chemical studies of cholesterol gallstone formation. Gastroenterology 52:607, 1967.
267. Carey MC, Small DM: The characteristics of mixed micellar solutions with particular reference to bile. Am J Med 49:590, 1970.
268. Mazer NA, Carey MC, Kwasnick RF, et al: Quasielastic light scattering studies of aqueous biliary lipid systems. Size, shape, and thermodynamics of bile salt micelles. Biochemistry 18:3064, 1979.
269. Mazer NA, Benedek GB, Carey MC: Quasielastic light-scattering studies of aqueous biliary lipid systems. Mixed micelle formation in bile salt-lecithin solutions. Biochemistry 19:601, 1980.
270. Mazer NA, Carey MC: Quasielastic light scattering studies of aqueous biliary lipid systems. Cholesterol solubilization and precipitation in model bile solutions. Biochemistry 22:426, 1983.
271. Somjen GJ, Gilat T: A non-micellar mode of cholesterol transport in human bile. FEBS Letters 156:265, 1983.
272. Carey MC: Critical tables for calculating the cholesterol saturation of native bile. J Lipid Res 19:945, 1978.
273. Small DM, Bourgès MC, Dervichian DG: The biophysics of lipidic associations. I. The ternary systems: lecithin-bile salt-water. Biochim Biophys Acta 125:563, 1966.
274. Mazer NA, Schurtenberger P, Carey MC, et al: Quasielastic light scattering studies of native hepatic bile from the dog: comparison with aggregative behavior of model biliary lipid systems. Biochemistry 23:1994, 1984.
275. Cohen DE, Carey MC: Rapid (1 hour) high-performance gel filtration chromatography resolves coexisting simple micelles, mixed micelles and vesicles in bile. J Lipid Res 31:2103, 1990.
276. Gantz DL, Wang DQ, Carey MC, et al: Cryoelectron microscopy of a nucleating model bile in vitreous ice: formation of primordial vesicles. Biophys J 76:1436, 1999.
277. Hjelm RP, Thiyagurajan P, Alkan H: A small-angle neutron scattering study of the effects of dilution on particle morphology in mixtures of glycocholate and lecithin. J Appl Cryst 21:858, 1988.
278. Chamberlin R, Thurston G, Benedek G, et al: Light scattering evidence for "worm-like" mixed detergent-diacylphosphatidylcholine (PC) micelles. Materials Research Society Fall Meeting, Boston, MA, 1989:697.
279. Cohen DE, Thurston GM, Chamberlin RA, et al: Laser light scattering evidence for a common wormlike growth structure of mixed micelles in bile salt- and straight-chain detergent-phosphatidylcholine aqueous systems: relevance to the micellar structure of bile. Biochemistry 37:14798, 1998.
280. Walter A, Vinson PK, Kaplun A, et al: Intermediate structures in the cholate-phosphatidylcholine vesicle-micelle transition. Biophys J 60:1315, 1991.
281. Admirand WH, Small DM: The physic-chemical basis of cholesterol gallstone formation in man. J Clin Invest 47:1045, 1968.
282. Holzbach RT, Marsh M, Olszewski M, et al: Cholesterol solubility in bile. Evidence that supersaturated bile is frequent in healthy man. J Clin Invest 52:1467, 1973.
283. McDougall RM, Walker K, Thurston OG: Prolonged secretion of lithogenic bile after cholecystectomy. Ann Surg 182:150, 1975.
284. Sömjen GJ, Gilat T: A non-micellar mode of cholesterol transport in human bile. FEBS Lett 156:265, 1983.
285. El Kodsi B, Cooperband SR, Bouchier IAD: Variations in the ultracentrifugal characteristics of human gallbladder and hepatic bile with diseases of the biliary tree. J Lab Clin Med 72:592, 1968.
286. Lairon D, Lafont H, Hauton J-C: Lack of mixed micelles bile salt-lecithin-cholesterol in bile and presence of a lipoproteic complex. Biochimie 54:529, 1972.
287. Stevens RD: An electron spin resonance study of cholestane spin label in aqueous mixtures of biliary lipids. J Lipid Res 18:417, 1977.
288. Small DM: General discussion III. Evening session, December 7, 1983. Hepatology 4:180S, 1984.
289. Cohen DE, Angelico M, Carey MC: Structural alterations in lecithin-cholesterol vesicles following interactions with monomeric and micellar bile salts: physical-chemical basis for subselection of biliary lecithin species and aggregative states of biliary lipids during bile formation. J Lipid Res 31:55, 1990.
290. Carey MC: Formation and growth of cholesterol gallstones: the new synthesis. In Fromm H, Leuschner U, eds: Bile Acids - Cholestasis - Gallstones. Dordrecht, The Netherlands, Kluwer, 1996:147.
291. Donovan JM: Physical and metabolic factors in gallstone pathogenesis. Gastroenterol Clin North Am 28:75, 1999.
292. LaMont JT, Carey MC: Cholesterol gallstone formation. 2. Pathobiology and pathomechanics. Prog Liver Dis 10:165, 1992.
293. Hofmann AF, Grundy SM, Lachin JM, et al: Pretreatment biliary lipid composition in white patients with radiolucent gallstones in the National Cooperative Gallstone Study. Gastroenterology 83:738, 1982.
294. Pellegrini CA, Ryan T, Broderick W, et al: Gallbladder filling and emptying during cholesterol gallstone formation in the prairie dog. A cholescintigraphic study. Gastroenterology 90:143, 1986.
295. Jazrawi RP, Pazzi P, Petroni ML, et al: Postprandial gallbladder motor function: refilling and turnover of bile in health and in cholelithiasis. Gastroenterology 109:582, 1995.
296. van Erpecum KJ, Venneman NG, Portincasa P, et al: Review article: agents affecting gall-bladder motility—role in treatment and prevention of gallstones. Aliment Pharmacol Ther 14(suppl 2):66, 2000.
297. Jazrawi RP: Review article: measurement of gall-bladder motor function in health and disease. Aliment Pharmacol Ther 14(suppl 2):27, 2000.
298. Everson GT: Gallbladder function in gallstone disease. Gastroenterol Clin North Am 20:85, 1991.
299. Pauletzki J, Paumgartner G: Review article: defects in gall-bladder motor function—role in gallstone formation and recurrence. Aliment Pharmacol Ther 14(suppl 2):32, 2000.
300. Portincasa P, Di Ciaula A, Vendemiale G, et al: Gallbladder motility and cholesterol crystallization in bile from patients with pigment and cholesterol gallstones. Eur J Clin Invest 30:317, 2000.
301. Portincasa P, Minerva F, Moschetta A, et al: Review article: in vitro studies of gall-bladder smooth muscle function. Relevance in cholesterol gallstone disease. Aliment Pharmacol Ther 14 Suppl 2:19, 2000.
302. Yu P, Chen Q, Harnett KM, et al: Direct G protein activation reverses impaired CCK signaling in human gallbladders with cholesterol stones. Am J Physiol 269:G659, 1995.
303. Behar J, Rhim BY, Thompson W, et al: Inositol trisphosphate restores impaired human gallbladder motility associated with cholesterol stones. Gastroenterology 104:563, 1993.
304. Xiao ZL, Chen Q, Amaral J, et al: Defect of receptor-G protein coupling in human gallbladder with cholesterol stones. Am J Physiol Gastrointest Liver Physiol 278:G251, 2000.
305. Xu QW, Shaffer EA: The potential site of impaired gallbladder contractility in an animal model of cholesterol gallstone disease. Gastroenterology 110:251, 1996.
306. Chen Q, Amaral J, Biancani P, et al: Excess membrane cholesterol alters human gallbladder muscle contractility and membrane fluidity. Gastroenterology 116:678, 1999.
307. Doty JE, Pitt HA, Kuchenbecker SL, et al: Impaired gallbladder emptying before gallstone formation in the prairie dog. Gastroenterology 85:168, 1983.

308. Chen Q, Amaral J, Oh S, et al: Gallbladder relaxation in patients with pigment and cholesterol stones. Gastroenterology 113:930, 1997.
309. Smith BF, LaMont JT: Gallbladder mucin and gallstone formation. In Cohen S, Soloway RD, eds: Gallstones. New York, Churchill Livingstone, 1984:101.
310. Lee SP, LaMont T, Carey MC: Role of gallbladder mucus hypersecretion in the evolution of cholesterol gallstones. Studies in the prairie dog. J Clin Invest 67:1712, 1981.
311. Lee SP, Nicholls JF: Nature and composition of biliary sludge. Gastroenterology 90:677, 1986.
312. Marks JW, Bonorris GG, Albers G, et al: The sequence of biliary events preceding the formation of gallstones in humans. Gastroenterology 103:566, 1992.
313. Lee SP, Carey MC, LaMont JT: Aspirin prevention of cholesterol gallstone formation in prairie dogs. Science 211:1429, 1981.
314. Sterling RK, Shiffman ML, Sugerman HJ, et al: Effect of NSAIDs on gallbladder bile composition. Dig Dis Sci 40:2220, 1995.
315. Broomfield PH, Chopra R, Sheinbaum RC, et al: Effects of ursodeoxycholic acid and aspirin on the formation of lithogenic bile and gallstones during loss of weight. N Engl J Med 319:1567, 1988.
316. O'Leary DP, LaMorte WW, Scott TE, et al: Inhibition of prostaglandin synthesis fails to prevent gallbladder mucin hypersecretion in the cholesterol-fed prairie dog. Gastroenterology 101:812, 1991.
317. MacPherson BR, Pemsingh RS: Ground squirrel model for cholelithiasis: role of epithelial glycoproteins. Microsc Res Tech 39:39, 1997.
318. Cohen BI, Mosbach EH, Ayyad N, et al: Aspirin does not inhibit cholesterol cholelithiasis in two established animal models. Gastroenterology 101:1109, 1991.
319. Attili AF, Capocaccia R, Carulli N, et al: Factors associated with gallstone disease in the MICOL experience. Multicenter Italian Study on Epidemiology of Cholelithiasis. Hepatology 26:809, 1997.
320. Kurata JH, Marks J, Abbey D: One gram of aspirin per day does not reduce risk of hospitalization for gallstone disease. Dig Dis Sci 36:1110, 1991.
321. Ko CW, Lee SP: Gallstone formation. Local factors. Gastroenterol Clin North Am 28:99, 1999.
322. Carey MC, Cahalane MJ: Whither biliary sludge? Gastroenterology 95:508, 1988.
323. Ko CW, Sekijima JH, Lee SP: Biliary sludge. Ann Intern Med 130:301, 1999.
324. Corradini SG, Elisei W, Giovannelli L, et al: Impaired human gallbladder lipid absorption in cholesterol gallstone disease and its effect on cholesterol solubility in bile. Gastroenterology 118:912, 2000.
325. Wang DQ-H, Carey MC: Complete mapping of crystallization pathways during cholesterol precipitation from model bile: influence of physical-chemical variables of pathophysiologic relevance and identification of a stable liquid crystalline state in cold, dilute and hydrophilic bile salt-containing systems. J Lipid Res 37:606, 1996.
326. Wang DQ, Carey MC: Characterization of crystallization pathways during cholesterol precipitation from human gallbladder biles: identical pathways to corresponding model biles with three predominating sequences. J Lipid Res 37:2539, 1996.
327. Marcus SN, Heaton KW: Deoxycholic acid and the pathogenesis of gall stones. Gut 29:522, 1988.
328. Carulli N, Loria P, Bertolotti M, et al: Effects of acute changes of bile acid pool composition on biliary lipid secretion. J Clin Invest 74:614, 1984.
329. Einarsson C, Hillebrant CG, Axelson M: Effects of treatment with deoxycholic acid and chenodeoxycholic acid on the hepatic synthesis of cholesterol and bile acids in healthy subjects. Hepatology 33:1189, 2001.
330. Marcus SN, Heaton KW: Intestinal transit, deoxycholic acid and the cholesterol saturation of bile—three inter-related factors. Gut 27:550, 1986.
331. Hussaini SH, Pereira SP, Veysey MJ, et al: Roles of gall bladder emptying and intestinal transit in the pathogenesis of octreotide induced gall bladder stones. Gut 38:775, 1996.
332. Thomas LA, Veysey MJ, Bathgate T, et al: Mechanism for the transit-induced increase in colonic deoxycholic acid formation in cholesterol cholelithiasis. Gastroenterology 119:806, 2000.
333. Berr F, Kullak-Ublick GA, Paumgartner G, et al: 7 alpha-dehydroxylating bacteria enhance deoxycholic acid input and cholesterol saturation of bile in patients with gallstones. Gastroenterology 111:1611, 1996.
334. Holzbach RT: Current concepts of cholesterol transport and crystal formation in human bile. Hepatology 12:26S, 1990.
335. Holan KR, Holzbach RT, Hermann RE, et al: Nucleation time: a key factor in the pathogenesis of cholesterol gallstone disease. Gastroenterology 77:611, 1979.
336. Sedaghat A, Grundy SM: Cholesterol crystals and the formation of cholesterol gallstones. N Engl J Med 302:1274, 1980.
337. Gollish SH, Burnstein MJ, Ilson RG, et al: Nucleation of cholesterol monohydrate crystals from hepatic and gall-bladder bile of patients with cholesterol gall stones. Gut 24:836, 1983.
338. Holzbach RT: Recent progress in understanding cholesterol crystal nucleation as a precursor to human gallstone formation. Hepatology 6:1403, 1986.
339. Jirsa M, Groen AK: Role of biliary proteins and non-protein factors in kinetics of cholesterol crystallisation and gallstone growth. Front Biosci 6:E154, 2001.
340. Small DM: Cholesterol nucleation and growth in gallstone formation. N Engl J Med 302:1305, 1980.
341. Holzbach RT: Nucleation of cholesterol crystals in native bile. Hepatology 12:155S, 1990.
342. Kibe A, Dudley MA, Halpern Z, et al: Factors affecting cholesterol monohydrate crystal nucleation time in model systems of supersaturated bile. J Lipid Res 26:1102, 1985.
343. Halpern Z, Dudley MA, Kibe A, et al: Rapid vesicle formation and aggregation in abnormal human biles. A time-lapse video enhanced microscopy study. Gastroenterology 90:875, 1986.
344. Olsewski MF, Holzbach RT, Saupe A, et al: Liquid crystals in human bile. Nature (Lond) 242:336, 1973.
345. Lee SP, Park HZ, Madani H, et al: Partial characterization of a nonmicellar system of cholesterol solubilization in bile. Am J Physiol 252:G374, 1987.
346. Konikoff FM, Cohen DE, Carey MC: Phospholipid molecular species influence crystal habits and transition sequences of metastable intermediates during cholesterol crystallization from bile salt-rich model bile. J Lipid Res 35:60, 1994.
347. Konikoff FM, Chung DS, Donovan JM, et al: Filamentous, helical, and tubular microstructures during cholesterol crystallization from bile. Evidence that cholesterol does not nucleate classic monohydrate plates. J Clin Invest 90:1155, 1992.
348. Konikoff FM, Danino D, Weihs D, et al: Microstructural evolution of lipid aggregates in nucleating model and human biles visualized by cryogenic transmission electron microscopy. Hepatology 31:261, 2000.
349. Konikoff FM, Laufer H, Messer G, et al: Monitoring cholesterol crystallization from lithogenic model bile by time-lapse density gradient ultracentrifugation. J Hepatol 26:703, 1997.
350. Chung DS, Benedek GB, Konikoff FM, et al: Elastic free energy of anisotropic helical ribbons as metastable intermediates in the crystallization of cholesterol. Proc Natl Acad Sci U S A 90:11341, 1993.
351. Holzbach RT, Busch N: Nucleation and growth of cholesterol crystals. Kinetic determinants in supersaturated native bile. Gastroenterol Clin North Am 20:67, 1991.
352. Busch N, Tokumo H, Holzbach RT: A sensitive method for determination of cholesterol growth using model solutions of supersaturated bile. J Lipid Res 31:1903, 1990.
353. Ginanni Corradini S, Cantafora A, Capocaccia L, et al: Development and validation of a quantitative assay for cholesterol crystal growth in human gallbladder bile. Biochim Biophys Acta 1214:63, 1994.
354. Somjen GJ, Ringel Y, Konikoff FM, et al: A new method for the rapid measurement of cholesterol crystallization in model biles using a spectrophotometric microplate reader. J Lipid Res 38:1048, 1997.
355. Harvey PR, Upadhya GA: A rapid, simple high capacity cholesterol crystal growth assay. J Lipid Res 36:2054, 1995.
356. Levy PF, Smith BF, LaMont JT: Human gallbladder mucin accelerates nucleation of cholesterol in artificial bile. Gastroenterology 87:270, 1984.
357. de Bruijn MA, Mok KS, Nibbering CP, et al: Characterization of the cholesterol crystallization-promoting low-density particle isolated from human bile. Gastroenterology 110:1936, 1996.
358. Groen AK, Noordam C, Drapers JA, et al: Isolation of a potent cholesterol nucleation-promoting activity from human gallbladder bile: role in the pathogenesis of gallstone disease. Hepatology 11:525, 1990.

359. Nunez L, Amigo L, Rigotti A, et al: Cholesterol crystallization-promoting activity of aminopeptidase-N isolated from the vesicular carrier of biliary lipids. FEBS Lett 329:84, 1993.
360. Offner GD, Gong D, Afdhal NH: Identification of a 130-kilodalton human biliary concanavalin A binding protein as aminopeptidase N. Gastroenterology 106:755, 1994.
361. Harvey PR, Upadhya GA, Strasberg SM: Immunoglobulins as nucleating proteins in the gallbladder bile of patients with cholesterol gallstones. J Biol Chem 266:13996, 1991.
362. Abei M, Nuutinen H, Kawczak P, et al: Identification of human biliary alpha 1-acid glycoprotein as a cholesterol crystallization promoter. Gastroenterology 106:231, 1994.
363. Pattinson NR: Identification of a phosphatidylcholine active phospholipase C in human gallbladder bile. Biochem Biophys Res Commun 150:890, 1988.
364. Chijiiwa K, Koga A, Yamasaki T, et al: Fibronectin: a possible factor promoting cholesterol monohydrate crystallization in bile. Biochim Biophys Acta 1086:44, 1991.
365. Yamashita G, Ginanni Corradini S, Secknus R, et al: Biliary haptoglobin, a potent promoter of cholesterol crystallization at physiological concentrations. J Lipid Res 36:1325, 1995.
366. Ostrow JD: Properties of APF/CBP in bile and gallstones. Hepatology 16:1493, 1992.
367. Mala I, Zikova J, Spundova M, et al: Lipid-protein complexes as cholesterol pronucleating agents in human bile. Int J Biochem Cell Biol 30:251, 1998.
368. Shoda J, Ueda T, Ikegami T, et al: Increased biliary group II phospholipase A2 and altered gallbladder bile in patients with multiple cholesterol stones. Gastroenterology 112:2036, 1997.
369. Donovan JM, Leonard MR, Batta AK, et al: Calcium affinity for biliary lipid aggregates in model biles: complementary importance of bile salts and lecithin. Gastroenterology 107:831, 1994.
370. Moore EW: Biliary calcium and gallstone formation. Hepatology 12:206S, 1990.
371. van den Berg AA, van Buul JD, Tytgat GN, et al: Mucins and calcium phosphate precipitates additively stimulate cholesterol crystallization. J Lipid Res 39:1744, 1998.
372. Hussaini SH, Pereira SP, Murphy GM, et al: Deoxycholic acid influences cholesterol solubilization and microcrystal nucleation time in gallbladder bile. Hepatology 22:1735, 1995.
373. Miquel JF, Nunez L, Amigo L, et al: Cholesterol saturation, not proteins or cholecystitis, is critical for crystal formation in human gallbladder bile. Gastroenterology 114:1016, 1998.
374. Chijiiwa K, Hirota I, Noshiro H: High vesicular cholesterol and protein in bile are associated with formation of cholesterol but not pigment gallstones. Dig Dis Sci 38:161, 1993.
375. Kibe A, Holzbach RT, LaRusso NF, et al: Inhibition of cholesterol crystal formation by apolipoproteins in supersaturated model bile. Science 225:514, 1984.
376. Tao S, Tazuma S, Kajiyama G: Apolipoprotein A-I stabilizes phospholipid lamellae and thus prolongs nucleation time in model bile systems: an ultrastructural study. Biochim Biophys Acta 1166:25, 1993.
377. Secknus R, Darby GH, Chernosky A, et al: Apolipoprotein A-I in bile inhibits cholesterol crystallization and modifies transcellular lipid transfer through cultured human gall-bladder epithelial cells. J Gastroenterol Hepatol 14:446, 1999.
378. Ohya T, Schwarzendrube J, Busch N, et al: Isolation of a human biliary glycoprotein inhibitor of cholesterol crystallization. Gastroenterology 104:527, 1993.
379. Secknus R, Yamashita G, Ginanni Corradini S, et al: Purification and characterization of a novel human 15 kd cholesterol crystallization inhibitor protein in bile. J Lab Clin Med 127:169, 1996.
380. Busch N, Lammert F, Marschall HU, et al: A new subgroup of lectin-bound biliary proteins binds to cholesterol crystals, modifies crystal morphology, and inhibits cholesterol crystallization. J Clin Invest 96:3009, 1995.
381. Busch N, Lammert F, Matern S: Biliary secretory immunoglobulin A is a major constituent of the new group of cholesterol crystal-binding proteins. Gastroenterology 115:129, 1998.
382. Ahmed HA, Petroni ML, Abu-Hamdiyyah M, et al: Hydrophobic/hydrophilic balance of proteins: a major determinant of cholesterol crystal formation in model bile. J Lipid Res 35:211, 1994.
383. Wang DQ, Cohen DE, Lammert F, et al: No pathophysiologic relationship of soluble biliary proteins to cholesterol crystallization in human bile. J Lipid Res 40:415, 1999.
384. Abei M, Schwarzendrube J, Nuutinen H, et al: Cholesterol crystallization-promoters in human bile: comparative potencies of immunoglobulins, alpha 1-acid glycoprotein, phospholipase C, and aminopeptidase N1. J Lipid Res 34:1141, 1993.
385. Miquel JF, Von Ritter C, Del Pozo R, et al: Fibronectin in human gallbladder bile: cholesterol pronucleating and/or mucin "link" protein? Am J Physiol 267:G393, 1994.
386. de Bruijn MA, Mok KS, Out T, et al: Immunoglobulins and alpha 1-acid glycoprotein do not contribute to the cholesterol crystallization-promoting effect of concanavalin A-binding biliary protein. Hepatology 20:626, 1994.
387. Osuga T, Mitamura K, Miyagawa S, et al: A scanning electron microscopic study of gallstone development in man. Lab Invest 31:696, 1974.
388. van Den Berg AA, van Buul JD, Ostrow JD, et al: Measurement of cholesterol gallstone growth in vitro. J Lipid Res 41:189, 2000.
389. Wolpers C, Hofmann AF: Solitary versus multiple cholesterol gallbladder stones. Mechanisms of formation and growth. Clin Investig 71:423, 1993.
390. Conrad MR, Janes JO, Dietchy J: Significance of low level echoes within the gallbladder. AJR Am J Roentgenol 132:967, 1979.
391. Kaufman HS, Magnuson TH, Pitt HA, et al: The distribution of calcium salt precipitates in the core, periphery and shell of cholesterol, black pigment and brown pigment gallstones. Hepatology 19:1124, 1994.
392. Wosiewitz U: Scanning electron microscopy in gallstone research. Scan Electron Microscop 419, 1983.
393. de la Porte PL, Domingo N, van Wijland M, et al: Distinct immunolocalization of mucin and other biliary proteins in human cholesterol gallstones. J Hepatol 25:339, 1996.
394. Cetta F: The role of bacteria in pigment gallstone disease. Ann Surg 213:315, 1991.
395. Kaufman HS, Magnuson TH, Lillemoe KD, et al: The role of bacteria in gallbladder and common duct stone formation. Ann Surg 209:584, 1989.
396. Wetter LA, Hamadeh RM, Griffiss JM, et al: Differences in outer membrane characteristics between gallstone-associated bacteria and normal bacterial flora. Lancet 343:444, 1994.
397. Swidsinski A, Khilkin M, Pahlig H, et al: Time dependent changes in the concentration and type of bacterial sequences found in cholesterol gallstones. Hepatology 27:662, 1998.
398. Swidsinski A, Ludwig W, Pahlig H, et al: Molecular genetic evidence of bacterial colonization of cholesterol gallstones. Gastroenterology 108:860, 1995.
399. Lee DK, Tarr PI, Haigh WG, et al: Bacterial DNA in mixed cholesterol gallstones. Am J Gastroenterol 94:3502, 1999.
400. Ostrow JD: The etiology of pigment gallstones. Hepatology 4:215S, 1984.
401. Ho KJ, Hsu SC, Chen JS, et al: Human biliary beta-glucuronidase: correlation of its activity with deconjugation of bilirubin in the bile. Eur J Clin Invest 16:361, 1986.
402. Cahalane MJ, Neubrand MW, Carey MC: Physical-chemical pathogenesis of pigment gallstones. Semin Liver Dis 8:317, 1988.
403. Shiffman ML, Sugerman HJ, Kellum JM, et al: Changes in gallbladder bile composition following gallstone formation and weight reduction. Gastroenterology 103:214, 1992.
404. Schriever CE, Jungst D: Association between cholesterol-phospholipid vesicles and cholesterol crystals in human gallbladder bile. Hepatology 9:541, 1989.
405. Behar J, Lee KY, Thompson WR, et al: Gallbladder contraction in patients with pigment and cholesterol stones. Gastroenterology 97:1479, 1989.
406. Malet PF, Deng SQ, Soloway RD: Gallbladder mucin and cholesterol and pigment gallstone formation in hamsters. Scand J Gastroenterol 24:1055, 1989.
407. LaMont JT, Ventola AS, Trotman BW, et al: Mucin glycoprotein content of human pigment gallstones. Hepatology 3:377, 1983.
408. Cetta FM: Bile infection documented as initial event in the pathogenesis of brown pigment biliary stones. Hepatology 6:482, 1986.
409. Leung JW, Sung JY, Costerton JW: Bacteriological and electron microscopy examination of brown pigment stones. J Clin Microbiol 27:915, 1989.
410. Maki T: Pathogenesis of calcium bilirubinate gallstone: role of *E. coli,* beta-glucuronidase and coagulation by inorganic ions, polyelectrolytes and agitation. Ann Surg 164:90, 1966.

411. Nakano T, Yanagisawa J, Nakayama F: Phospholipase activity in human bile. Hepatology 8:1560, 1988.
412. Akiyoshi T, Nakayama F: Bile acid composition in brown pigment stones. Dig Dis Sci 35:27, 1990.
413. Ostrow JD: Brown pigment gallstones: the role of bacterial hydrolases and another missed opportunity. Hepatology 13:607, 1991.
414. Yamasaki T, Nakayama F, Tamura S, et al: Characterization of mucin in the hepatic bile of patients with intrahepatic pigment stones. J Gastroenterol Hepatol 7:36, 1992.
415. Everhart JE: Contributions of obesity and weight loss to gallstone disease. Ann Intern Med 119:1029, 1993.
416. Diehl AK: Epidemiology and natural history of gallstone disease. In Cooper AD, eds: Gastroenterology Clinics of North America. Philadelphia, W.B. Saunders, 1991:1.
417. Field AE, Coakley EH, Must A, et al: Impact of overweight on the risk of developing common chronic diseases during a 10-year period. Arch Intern Med 161:1581, 2001.
418. Kodama H, Kono S, Todoroki I, et al: Gallstone disease risk in relation to body mass index and waist-to-hip ratio in Japanese men. Int J Obes Relat Metab Disord 23:211, 1999.
419. Miettinen TA: Cholesterol production in obesity. Circulation 44:842, 1971.
420. Nestel PJ, Schreibman PH, Ahrens EH Jr: Cholesterol metabolism in human obesity. J Clin Invest 52:2389, 1973.
421. Shaffer EA, Small DM: Biliary lipid secretion in cholesterol gallstone disease. The effect of cholecystectomy and obesity. J Clin Invest 59:828, 1977.
422. Mabee TM, Meyer P, DenBesten L, et al: The mechanism of increased gallstone formation in obese human subjects. Surgery 79:460, 1976.
423. Bennion LJ, Grundy SM: Effects of obesity and caloric intake on biliary lipid metabolism in man. J Clin Invest 56:996, 1975.
424. Petroni ML: Review article: gall-bladder motor function in obesity. Aliment Pharmacol Ther 14(suppl 2):48, 2000.
425. Liddle RA, Goldstein RB, Saxton J: Gallstone formation during weight-reduction dieting. Arch Intern Med 149:1750, 1989.
426. Shiffman ML, Sugerman HJ, Kellum JM, et al: Gallstone formation after rapid weight loss: a prospective study in patients undergoing gastric bypass surgery for treatment of morbid obesity. Am J Gastroenterol 86:1000, 1991.
427. Syngal S, Coakley EH, Willett WC, et al: Long-term weight patterns and risk for cholecystectomy in women. Ann Intern Med 130:471, 1999.
428. Friedman JM, Halaas JL: Leptin and the regulation of body weight in mammals. Nature 395:763, 1998.
429. Considine RV, Sinha MK, Heiman ML, et al: Serum immunoreactive-leptin concentrations in normal-weight and obese humans. N Engl J Med 334:292, 1996.
430. Duggirala R, Mitchell BD, Blangero J, et al: Genetic determinants of variation in gallbladder disease in the Mexican-American population. Genet Epidemiol 16:191, 1999.
431. VanPatten S, Ranginani N, Shefer S, et al: Impaired biliary lipid secretion in obese Zucker rats: leptin promotes hepatic cholesterol clearance. Am J Physiol 281:G393, 2001.
432. Bouchard G, Carver T, Tovbina M, et al: Genetic factors underlying obesity, but not obesity per se, determine cholesterol gallstone formation in inbred mice. Hepatology 32:391A, 2000 (abstract).
433. Mendez-Sanchez N, Gonzalez V, Suarez JA, et al: Plasma leptin levels modulate cholesterol secretion in patients losing weight. Gastroenterology 116:A1245, 1999 (abstract).
434. Ahlberg J, Angelin B, Einarsson K, et al: Biliary lipid composition in normo- and hyperlipoproteinemia. Gastroenterology 79:90, 1980.
435. Thornton JR, Heaton KW, Macfarlane DG: A relation between high-density-lipoprotein cholesterol and bile cholesterol saturation. BMJ 283:1352, 1981.
436. Duane WC: Abnormal bile acid absorption in familial hypertriglyceridemia. J Lipid Res 36:96, 1995.
437. Angelin B, Hershon KS, Brunzell JD: Bile acid metabolism in hereditary forms of hypertriglyceridemia: evidence for an increased synthesis rate in monogenic familial hypertriglyceridemia. Proc Natl Acad Sci U S A 84:5434, 1987.
438. Scragg RK, McMichael AJ, Seamark RF: Oral contraceptives, pregnancy, and endogenous oestrogen in gall stone disease—a case-control study. BMJ 288:1795, 1984.
439. Barbara L, Sama C, Morselli Labate AM, et al: A population study on the prevalence of gallstone disease: the Sirmione Study. Hepatology 7:913, 1987.
440. Prevalence of gallstone disease in an Italian adult female population. Rome Group for the Epidemiology and Prevention of Cholelithiasis (GREPCO). Am J Epidemiol 119:796, 1984.
441. Kern F, Jr., Everson GT, DeMark B, et al: Biliary lipids, bile acids, and gallbladder function in the human female. Effects of pregnancy and the ovulatory cycle. J Clin Invest 68:1229, 1981.
442. Everson GT, McKinley C, Lawson M, et al: Gallbladder function in the human female: effect of the ovulatory cycle, pregnancy, and contraceptive steroids. Gastroenterology 82:711, 1982.
443. Gilat T, Konikoff F: Pregnancy and the biliary tract. Can J Gastroenterol 14(suppl D):55D, 2000.
444. Maringhini A, Ciambra M, Baccelliere P, et al: Biliary sludge and gallstones in pregnancy: incidence, risk factors, and natural history. Ann Intern Med 119:116, 1993.
445. Heaton KW: Review article: epidemiology of gall-bladder disease—role of intestinal transit. Aliment Pharmacol Ther 14 Suppl 2:9, 2000.
446. Dowling RH: Review: pathogenesis of gallstones. Aliment Pharmacol Ther 14(suppl 2):39, 2000.
447. Heaton KW, Emmett PM, Symes CL, et al: An explanation for gallstones in normal-weight women: slow intestinal transit. Lancet 341:8, 1993.
448. Spathis A, Heaton KW, Emmett PM, et al: Gallstones in a community free of obesity but prone to slow intestinal transit. Eur J Gastroenterol Hepatol 9:201, 1997.
449. Krejs GJ, Orci L, Conlon JM, et al: Somatostatinoma syndrome. Biochemical, morphologic and clinical features. N Engl J Med 301:285, 1979.
450. Apstein MD, Dalecki-Chipperfield K: Spinal cord injury is a risk factor for gallstone disease. Gastroenterology 92:966, 1987.
451. Moonka R, Stiens SA, Resnick WJ, et al: The prevalence and natural history of gallstones in spinal cord injured patients. J Am Coll Surg 189:274, 1999.
452. Lynch AC, Antony A, Dobbs BR, et al: Bowel dysfunction following spinal cord injury. Spinal Cord 39:193, 2001.
453. Tandon RK, Jain RK, Garg PK: Increased incidence of biliary sludge and normal gall bladder contractility in patients with high spinal cord injury. Gut 41:682, 1997.
454. Ketover SR, Ansel HJ, Goldish G, et al: Gallstones in chronic spinal cord injury: is impaired gallbladder emptying a risk factor? Arch Phys Med Rehabil 77:1136, 1996.
455. Buchwald H, Varco RL, Matts JP, et al: Effect of partial ileal bypass surgery on mortality and morbidity from coronary heart disease in patients with hypercholesterolemia. Report of the Program on the Surgical Control of the Hyperlipidemias (POSCH). N Engl J Med 323:946, 1990.
456. Sorensen TI, Ingemann Jensen L, Klein HC, et al: Risk of gallstone formation after jejunoileal bypass increases more with a 1:3 than with a 3:1 jejunoileal ratio. Scand J Gastroenterol 15:979, 1980.
457. Davies BW, Abel G, Puntis JW, et al: Limited ileal resection in infancy: the long-term consequences. J Pediatr Surg 34:583, 1999.
458. Pitt HA, Lewinski MA, Muller EL, et al: Ileal resection-induced gallstones: altered bilirubin or cholesterol metabolism? Surgery 96:154, 1984.
459. Bickerstaff KI, Moossa AR: Effects of resection or bypass of the distal ileum on the lithogenicity of bile. Am J Surg 145:34, 1983.
460. Brink MA, Mendez-Sanchez N, Carey MC: Bilirubin cycles enterohepatically after ileal resection in the rat. Gastroenterology 110:1945, 1996.
461. Andersson H, Bosaeus I, Fasth S, et al: Cholelithiasis and urolithiasis in Crohn's disease. Scand J Gastroenterol 22:253, 1987.
462. Whorwell PJ, Hawkins R, Dewbury K, et al: Ultrasound survey of gallstones and other hepatobiliary disorders in patients with Crohn's disease. Dig Dis Sci 29:930, 1984.
463. Lapidus A, Bangstad M, Astrom M, et al: The prevalence of gallstone disease in a defined cohort of patients with Crohn's disease. Am J Gastroenterol 94:1261, 1999.
464. Lapidus A, Einarsson C: Bile composition in patients with ileal resection due to Crohn's disease. Inflamm Bowel Dis 4:89, 1998.
465. Brink MA, Slors JF, Keulemans YC, et al: Enterohepatic cycling of bilirubin: a putative mechanism for pigment gallstone formation in ileal Crohn's disease. Gastroenterology 116:1420, 1999.

466. Azemoto R, Tsuchiya Y, Ai T, et al: Does gallstone formation after open cardiac surgery result only from latent hemolysis by replaced valves? Am J Gastroenterol 91:2185, 1996.
467. Rescorla FJ, Grosfeld JL: Cholecystitis and cholelithiasis in children. Semin Pediatr Surg 1:98, 1992.
468. Walker TM, Hambleton IR, Serjeant GR: Gallstones in sickle cell disease: observations from The Jamaican Cohort study. J Pediatr 136:80, 2000.
469. Bouchier IA: Postmortem study of the frequency of gallstones in patients with cirrhosis of the liver. Gut 10:705, 1969.
470. Raedsch R, Stiehl A, Gundert-Remy U, et al: Hepatic secretion of bilirubin and biliary lipids in patients with alcoholic cirrhosis of the liver. Digestion 26:80, 1983.
471. Ostrow JD: Unconjugated bilirubin and cholesterol gallstone formation. Hepatology 12:219S, 1990.
472. Einarsson K, Nilsell K, Leijd B, et al: Influence of age on secretion of cholesterol and synthesis of bile acids by the liver. N Engl J Med 313:277, 1985.
473. Valdivieso V, Palma R, Wunkhaus R, et al: Effect of aging on biliary lipid composition and bile acid metabolism in normal Chilean women. Gastroenterology 74:871, 1978.
474. Bertolotti M, Abate N, Bertolotti S, et al: Effect of aging on cholesterol 7 alpha-hydroxylation in humans. J Lipid Res 34:1001, 1993.
475. Trotman BW, Soloway RD: Pigment vs cholesterol cholelithiasis: clinical and epidemiological aspects. Am J Dig Dis 20:735, 1975.
476. Nagase M, Tanimura H, Setoyama M, et al: Present features of gallstones in Japan. A collective review of 2,144 cases. Am J Surg 135:788, 1978.
477. Fevery J, Verwilghen R, Tan TG, et al: Glucuronidation of bilirubin and the occurrence of pigment gallstones in patients with chronic haemolytic diseases. Eur J Clin Invest 10:219, 1980.
478. Cetta F, Baldi C, Lombardo F, et al: Migration of metallic clips used during laparoscopic cholecystectomy and formation of gallstones around them: surgical implications from a prospective study. J Laparoendosc Adv Surg Tech A 7:37, 1997.
479. Cetta F: Do surgical and endoscopic sphincterotomy prevent or facilitate recurrent common duct stone formation? Arch Surg 128:329, 1993.
480. Skar V, Skar AG, Bratlie J, et al: Beta-glucuronidase activity in the bile of gallstone patients both with and without duodenal diverticula. Scand J Gastroenterol 24:205, 1989.
481. Tseng M, Everhart JE, Sandler RS: Dietary intake and gallbladder disease: a review. Public Health Nutr 2:161, 1999.
482. Stahlberg D, Reihner E, Rudling M, et al: Influence of bezafibrate on hepatic cholesterol metabolism in gallstone patients: reduced activity of cholesterol 7 alpha-hydroxylase. Hepatology 21:1025, 1995.
483. Gallbladder disease as a side effect of drugs influencing lipid metabolism. Experience in the Coronary Drug Project. N Engl J Med 296:1185, 1977.
484. Henriksson P, Einarsson K, Eriksson A, et al: Estrogen-induced gallstone formation in males. Relation to changes in serum and biliary lipids during hormonal treatment of prostatic carcinoma. J Clin Invest 84:811, 1989.
485. Daughaday WH: Octreotide is effective in acromegaly but often results in cholelithiasis. Ann Intern Med 112:159, 1990.
486. Shiffman ML, Keith FB, Moore EW: Pathogenesis of ceftriaxone-associated biliary sludge. In vitro studies of calcium-ceftriaxone binding and solubility. Gastroenterology 99:1772, 1990.
487. Menegaux F, Dorent R, Tabbi D, et al: Biliary surgery after heart transplantation. Am J Surg 175:320, 1998.
488. Steck TB, Costanzo-Nordin MR, Keshavarzian A: Prevalence and management of cholelithiasis in heart transplant patients. J Heart Lung Transplant 10:1029, 1991.
489. Lord RV, Ho S, Coleman MJ, et al: Cholecystectomy in cardiothoracic organ transplant recipients. Arch Surg 133:73, 1998.
490. Weiss KM, Ferrell RE, Hanis CL, et al: Genetics and epidemiology of gallbladder disease in New World native peoples. Am J Hum Genet 36:1259, 1984.
491. Lowenfels AB: Gallstones and glaciers: the stone that came in from the cold. Lancet 1:1385, 1988.
492. Neel JV: The "thrifty genotype" in 1998. Nutr Rev 57:S2, 1999.
493. Bertomeu A, Ros E, Zambon D, et al: Apolipoprotein E polymorphism and gallstones. Gastroenterology 111:1603, 1996.
494. Juvonen T, Kervinen K, Kairaluoma MI, et al: Gallstone cholesterol content is related to apolipoprotein E polymorphism. Gastroenterology 104:1806, 1993.
495. Van Erpecum KJ, Van Berge-henegouwen GP, Eckhardt ER, et al: Cholesterol crystallization in human gallbladder bile: relation to gallstone number, bile composition, and apolipoprotein E4 isoform. Hepatology 27:1508, 1998.
496. Rosmorduc O, Hermelin B, Poupon R: MDR3 gene defect in adults with symptomatic intrahepatic and gallbladder cholesterol cholelithiasis. Gastroenterology 120:1459, 2001.
497. Paigen K: A miracle enough: the power of mice. Nat Med 1:215, 1995.
498. Alexander M, Portman OW: Different susceptibilities to the formation of cholesterol gallstones in mice. Hepatology 7:257, 1987.
499. Khanuja B, Cheah YC, Hunt M, et al: *Lith1,* a major gene affecting cholesterol gallstone formation among inbred strains of mice. Proc Natl Acad Sci U S A 92:7729, 1995.
500. Paigen B, Schork NJ, Svenson KL, et al: Quantitative trait loci mapping for cholesterol gallstones in AKR/J and C57L/J strains of mice. Physiol Genomics 4:59, 2000.
501. Bouchard G, Nelson HM, Lammert F, et al: High-resolution maps of the murine Chromosome 2 region containing the cholesterol gallstone locus, Lith1. Mamm Genome 10:1070, 1999.
502. Lammert F, Carey MC, Paigen B: Chromosomal organization of candidate genes involved in cholesterol gallstone formation: a murine gallstone map. Gastroenterology 120:221, 2001.

CHAPTER

60

The Medical Management of Gallstones

Veronica A. Arteaga, MD, BS, and Hans Fromm, MD

As a common medical condition that is increasing worldwide, gallstone disease presents a significant burden for the public health system. About 10 percent to 15 percent of the population in the United States and Western Europe has gallstones.[1-3] Gallstones seem to be even more common in Latin America.[2] About 90 percent of the gallstones are composed predominantly of cholesterol. The remaining 10 percent are pigment stones, which are made up mainly of calcium bilirubinate. The growing prevalence of cholelithiasis appears to be related mainly to the propagation of cholesterol gallstones resulting from the spreading influence of the so-called Western lifestyle.[3] Overeating and sedentary behavior with the consequent development of obesity and diabetes mellitus promote disturbances in cholesterol metabolism. Bile becomes supersaturated in cholesterol, with gallstones frequently forming. Our understanding of the metabolic disturbances underlying the pathogenesis of cholesterol gallstones and the recognition of its epidemiologic link to lifestyle provide opportunities for gallstone prevention. Therefore the discussion of gallstone management will consider preventive measures, in addition to the more traditional methods of gallstone management.

PATHOGENESIS AND RISK FACTORS OF GALLSTONES

Cholesterol Gallstones

Cholesterol gallstones form on the basis of cholesterol-supersaturated bile.[4] The pathophysiologic chain of events leading to cholesterol cholelithiasis is thought to be initiated by a decrease in propulsive intestinal motility, possibly because of an increased deposition of dietary cholesterol in small intestinal smooth muscle membrane.[5,6] It is interesting to note that this pathogenic mechanism of decreased smooth muscle contractility appears to be identical to that underlying the development of decreased gallbladder emptying.[7] Decreased intestinal transit leads to prolonged exposure of bile acids to bacteria, with increased dehydroxylation of the trihydroxy bile acid cholic acid to its more hydrophobic dihydroxy metabolite, deoxycholic acid. Because of its hydrophobicity, deoxycholic acid stimulates the hepatic secretion of cholesterol mainly by facilitating its solubilization in the canalicular membrane. Deoxycholic acid also increases the proportion of arachidonate-rich species of phosphatidyl choline in bile. As a result, more mucin, which has strong nucleating properties, is secreted by the gallbladder mucosa. The increase of cholesterol in gallbladder bile in the form of both a supersaturated solution and crystals sets the stage for deposition of cholesterol in gallbladder smooth muscle membranes with the consequent impairment of gallbladder contractility. In addition to gallbladder mucin and decreased gallbladder emptying, cholesterol crystallization and gallstone growth are facilitated by the secretion of a number of pronucleating proteins, such as apoprotein A1 and A2, aminopeptidase N, phospholipase A2 and C, haptoglobin, and immunoglobulins.

The main risk of cholesterol gallstones relates to an increase in the biliary secretion of cholesterol.[4] Risk factors include obesity, rapid weight loss, hypertriglyceridemia, low high-density lipoprotein levels, increasing age, the presence of the apo E4 isoform, and parity. Another important risk factor that is also based primarily on the presence of increased cholesterol secretion is genetic predisposition in certain ethnic groups, such as Native Americans and Northern Europeans, and in patients with a family history of gallstones.[8-11] The power of gallstone (lith) genes is also evidenced by recent studies in inbred mice, which are characterized by a very high incidence of cholesterol gallstones.[12] Under certain conditions nutritional changes, which are associated with diminished stimulation of gallbladder contraction, present major risks for cholesterol gallstone formation. Examples are both parenteral nutrition and rapid-weight-loss diets that contain less than 10 g of fat per day.[13]

Pigment Stones

Pigment stones form when calcium bilirubinate precipitates in bile because of an increased presence of unconjugated bilirubin, which is less soluble than is its conjugated moiety. Risk factors are hemolysis, cirrhosis of the liver, inflammatory bowel disease, and ileal resection. The increased risk of pigment stones in the latter two conditions appears to be related to an increased intestinal absorption of unconjugated bilirubin.

Acalculous Gallbladder Disease

Although this review concerns the management of gallstones, a few words should be said about acalculous gallbladder disease. The reason for directing attention to this entity relates to the problem of managing patients with symptoms indistinguishable from those of biliary pain in whom no gallstones can be found. The pain may be caused by passage of the gallstone through the bile ducts, by microlithiasis, or by a recently defined muscle defect in the gallbladder.[14-17] Recent studies by Amaral and colleagues suggest that acalculous gallbladder disease may be related to a dysfunction of the contractile apparatus of the gallbladder. The contraction induced by cholecystokinin was markedly reduced both in vivo and in vitro. This contractility defect could not be corrected by G-protein activators or with the second messenger 1,2-dioctanoyl-sn-glycerol. The clinical significance of these findings remains uncertain, although patients with this disorder have been reported to experience relief of pain after cholecystectomy.[18] How decreased motility of an acalculous gallbladder could cause biliary pain is not clear. Therefore further studies are needed, and it appears premature to endorse the recommendation made by surgeons to subject patients to cholecystectomy if their gallbladder ejection fraction is less than 35 percent.[18]

CLINICAL PRESENTATION

Symptoms

Most gallstones cause no symptoms or complications. In 70 percent to 80 percent of patients cholelithiasis is asymptomatic (i.e., biliary pain, the only symptom characteristic for active gallstone disease, is absent).[19] Therefore a careful history from the patient is essential for distinguishing biliary pain from nonspecific symptoms. Although often referred to as biliary colic, biliary pain is not colicky. Rather it presents as a steady, severe pain in the epigastrium or right upper abdomen that lasts at least 30 minutes, typically with a crescendo-plateau-decrescendo sequence of intensity and with radiation into the right scapula. The pain often awakens the patient at night and is frequently associated with nausea and vomiting.

Complications

The main complications of gallstones are acute cholecystitis, common bile duct stones, acute pancreatitis, and ascending cholangitis. The diagnosis of acute cholecystitis is based largely on clinical symptoms and signs, a careful physical examination, and certain laboratory findings. Murphy's sign, a distinct tenderness on inspiration in the area of the gallbladder, is probably the most reliable finding pointing toward an acute inflammation of the gallbladder. Although ultrasonographic changes, such as increased thickness of the gallbladder wall or pericholecystic fluid collection, are consistent with the diagnosis of acute cholecystitis, they are not diagnostic per se. Similar caution should be used in the interpretation of nucleotide imaging studies of the gallbladder, such as a cholecystokinin scintigram (HIDA) scan. Although a normal study does not rule out acute gallbladder disease, an abnormal finding (i.e., no appearance of the nucleotide in the gallbladder) is diagnostically useful only in conjunction with the described typical symptoms and signs. Acute cholecystitis with or without the additional complication of common bile duct obstruction has to be suspected if biliary pain develops in association with fever, leucocytosis with a left shift, and a transient rise in alanine aminotransferase, aspartate aminotransferase, and γ-glutamyl transpeptidase (GGT). These enzyme abnormalities may be followed by alkaline phosphatase (AP) and bilirubin elevations.

Very high serum amylase and lipase values may also be present, and they are indicative of acute pancreatitis, which can be serious, often requiring endoscopic retrograde cholangiopancreatography (ERCP) and, if a stone is found in the bile duct, endoscopic sphincterotomy and stone extraction. In a small percentage of cases choledocholithiasis can evolve into ascending cholangitis, which characteristically presents with rigors, fever, and jaundice.

With few exceptions, complications of gallstones are preceded by repeated episodes of biliary pain.[20] Exceptions are elderly patients or patients immunocompromised by conditions—such as poorly controlled diabetes mellitus or chronic renal insufficiency—in whom biliary complications can develop without pain or typical findings on physical examination. In these cases liver test abnormalities, usually consisting of bilirubin, AP, GGT, and transaminase elevations, prompt the appropriate diagnostic studies (i.e., ultrasonography, computed tomography [CT] scan, magnetic resonance imaging, or ERCP). Unfortunately, cholecystectomies are too often performed unnecessarily for symptoms not related to gallstones, such as abdominal discomfort resulting from irritable bowel syndrome or dyspepsia, which is easily distinguishable from biliary pain.

MANAGEMENT

Expectant Management and Preventive Measures

The annual risk of patients with asymptomatic cholelithiasis to develop biliary pain is 1 percent to 4 percent. In the majority of cases significant symptoms or complications from the gallstones never develop. No treatment, therefore, represents an important management strategy for asymptomatic gallstone carriers.[20,21] The risk of symptomatic gallstones may be decreased by physical activity and by increased coffee consumption.[22,23] Recent studies also suggest that long-term treatment with ursodeoxycholic acid (UDCA) may markedly decrease the recurrence of biliary pain, the development of complications, and the consequent need for cholecystectomy.[24]

Cholecystectomy

Cholecystectomy is the main treatment for symptomatic gallstones. The question is whether surgery should be considered after the first episode of biliary pain or after the second attack. The life expectancy has been estimated to be virtually the same with either management strategy. Even if surgery would be delayed until a complication occurs, the life expectancy would not decrease by more than 23 to 25 days in comparison to operative treatment immediately after the first episode of biliary pain. The strategy of waiting with surgery until the second episode of biliary pain appears particularly appropriate for middle-aged or older patients because in approximately 30 percent biliary symptoms do not recur in 10 years.[25] Age of the patient is a factor that needs to be weighed carefully in the decision between surgical and medical therapy of symptomatic gallstones. The cumulative death rate for a 30-year-old patient undergoing immediate cholecystectomy has been estimated to be 0.11 percent. Elderly patients, specifically those 65 years or older, are at increased risk from surgical treatment. The cumulative lifetime risk of mortality from gallstones is 2.3 percent. The experience of the surgeon influences the risk of cholecystectomy. Intraoperative complications are both more common and more serious in laparoscopic than in open cholecystectomy. For example, the incidence of bile duct injury in laparoscopic cholecystectomy, which, on average, is around 0.25 percent, has been reported to be as high as 0.95 percent.[26]

Oral Bile Acid Dissolution Therapy

Medical management plays a major role in gallstone patients who have biliary pain for the first time, who are at increased risk from surgery, or who do not want to have surgery. The choice of medical treatment is based on selection criteria related to the patient's condition and gallstone features, to the familiarity of the treating physician with the different therapeutic options, and to the availability of the treatment method that appears most promising.

Oral dissolution therapy with UDCA can be very effective in selected patients with small, non-calcified gallstones.[21,27-29] UDCA is therapeutically attractive for at least two reasons. First, it is extraordinarily safe (i.e., virtually free of significant side effects). Second, as has already been referred to, UDCA appears to markedly decrease the incidence of both gallstone complications and recurrent biliary pain, effects that are independent of its cholelitholytic action. Patients considered for UDCA dissolution treatment should have uncomplicated gallstone disease with infrequent episodes of biliary pain. Gallstone calcifications can be excluded with a plain roentgenogram of the abdomen, although a CT scan is substantially more sensitive. However, a CT scan may not be cost-effective because minor calcifications not detected by conventional radiography do not preclude gallstone dissolution.[30] UDCA is taken twice per day with meals at a total dose of 8 to 10 mg/kg/day. The best treatment results, complete dissolution in up to 90 percent of patients, are obtained in gallstones not exceeding 5 mm in diameter. The success rate decreases with increasing stone size. Gallstones that are larger than 1 cm rarely dissolve. If stones dissolve, they do so at an average rate of 1 mm per month. A drawback of UDCA therapy is that gallstones recur in about 30 percent of patients who had single stones versus approximately 50 percent of those with multiple stones. Most recurrences are seen during the first years after dissolution at an annual rate of about 10 percent. Fortunately, most stone recurrences are asymptomatic. Although it decreases gallstone recurrence, maintenance treatment with UDCA is not considered cost-effective.

Extracorporeal Shock-wave Lithotripsy

Extracorporeal shock-wave lithotripsy (ESWL), which is being used mainly in Europe and Asia, may soon also become available in the United States. Medstone, a US-based company, has recently received approval by the Food and Drug Administration (FDA) for ESWL treatment of gallstones under the provision that a treatment study be carried out according to an FDA-approved protocol. This study is currently in progress. Similar to oral bile acid dissolution therapy, ESWL is indicated in selected patients with uncomplicated symptomatic gallstones.[31] The gallstones have to be non-calcified. The highest success rate is achieved in single stones with a size of up to 2 cm. Although patients receive adjuvant therapy with UDCA at a dose of 8 to 10 mg/kg/day to promote the dissolution of the stone fragments, studies have shown that stones that are broken up to very small fragments often clear the gallbladder spontaneously. Optimal fragmentation of the gallstones to particles not larger than 1 to 2 mm considerably improves the success of ESWL. With observation of the described optimal selection criteria, about 80 percent of the patients become stone-free within 12 months. The rate of complications, such as acute pancreatitis and common bile duct obstruction by gallstone fragments, is extremely low.

Topical Dissolution Therapy

Gallstones can be topically dissolved using either methyl-tert butyl ether (MTBE) or ethyl propionate. The solvent is infused into the gallbladder through a pigtail catheter, which can be placed either endoscopically or transhepatically. Although the success rate can be high in properly selected patients with non-calcified gallstones, the treatment is experimental and rarely used. In addition to the special precautions required, because of the fire hazard and risk of other side effects caused by the volatility of MTBE, the topical dissolution procedure is labor intensive, unless a specially designed pump and computerized delivery system, currently under study, are used.[32] Although ethyl propionate is considered to be safer than MTBE, the experience with this compound in human studies is limited.

GALLSTONE RECURRENCE

A drawback of all medical methods that achieve clearance of the gallbladder of gallstones is that gallstones recur in about 30 percent of patients who had single stones versus approximately 50 percent of those with multiple stones.[33] Most recurrences are seen during the first years after successful treatment at an annual rate of about 10 percent. If gallstones recur after UDCA therapy, most of them do so without biliary pain. However, the incidence of symptomatic recurrences appears to be higher after ESWL. This may be due to the possibility that patients selected for ESWL were more symptomatic than those chosen for UDCA therapy. Although decreasing gallstone recurrence, maintenance treatment with UDCA is not considered cost-effective.

MICROLITHIASIS

Microlithiasis constitutes a clinically very important stage of gallstone disease. It occurs either in the form of biliary crystals that can be detected only by microscopic examination of a bile sample or as sonographically evident sludge in the gallbladder.[14-16] Although probably involved in the pathogenesis of biliary pain and complications in gallstone disease, in general, biliary microcrystals have been shown to be the cause of so-called idiopathic acute pancreatitis in about 70 percent of the cases. Gallbladder sludge is often found in hospitalized patients in association with prolonged fasting and parenteral nutrition. As with typical cholelithiasis, these crystals can be birefringent cholesterol monohydrate crystals, birefringent calcium carbonate microspheroliths, or calcium bilirubinate granules. The management of microlithiasis-related acute pancreatitis is controversial. Although removal of the gallbladder as the locus of crystal formation is likely to be curative, expectant management or ursodiol treatment may be reasonable alternatives in view of insufficient data regarding the recurrence rate of microlithiasis-induced acute pancreatitis. The latter is likely to vary in different patient populations and associated disease conditions.

SUMMARY

Gallstones are not only very prevalent in most parts of the world, but also a significant burden for the public health system. Considerable progress has been made both in the understanding of the pathogenesis of gallstones and in their management. Although cholecystectomy is standard therapy for symptomatic gallstones, medical treatment alternatives are appropriate in selected patients who either do not want surgery or are at increased risk from cholecystectomy. Gallstone patients are often subjected unnecessarily to cholecystectomy for gastrointestinal symptoms not related to gallstones. Most gallstones are asymptomatic. If symptoms are absent or non-specific, cholelithiasis should be managed expectantly. Selected patients with non-calcified, small gallstones may benefit from oral dissolution therapy with ursodiol. ESWL, which may soon be available in the United States, is particularly successful in 5- to 20-mm solitary, non-calcified gallbladder stones. The role of potentially effective methods of topical dissolution therapy in the management of gallstones requires further study. Biliary microlithiasis represents a clinically very important stage of gallstone disease. Its management as the most common cause of so-called idiopathic acute pancreatitis is controversial and in need of further investigation.

References

1. Sama C, Morselli Labate AM, et al: Epidemiology and natural history of gallstone disease. Semin Liver Dis 10:149-158, 1990.
2. Diehl AK: Epidemiology and natural history of gallstone disease. Gastroenterol Clin North Am 20:1-19, 1991.
3. Everhart JE, Khare M, Hill M, Maurer KR: Prevalence and ethnic differences in gallbladder disease in the United States. Gastroenterology 117:632-639, 1999.
4. Apstein MD, Carey MC: Pathogenesis of cholesterol gallstones: a parsimonious hypothesis. Eur J Invest 26:343-352, 1996.
5. Xu Q, Scott RB, Tan DTM, Shaffer EA: Slow intestinal transit: a motor disorder contributing to cholesterol gallstone formation in the ground squirrel. Hepatology 23:1664-1672, 1996.
6. Van Erpecum KJ, Van Berge-Henegouwen GP: Gallstones: an intestinal disease? Gut 44:435-438, 1999.
7. Chen Q, Amaral J, Biancani P, Behar J: Excess membrane cholesterol alters human gallbladder muscle contractility and membrane fluidity. Gastroenterology 116:678-685, 1999.
8. Sampliner RE, Bennett PH, Comess LJ, et al: Gallbladder disease in Pima Indians. Demonstration of high prevalence and early onset by cholecystography. N Engl J Med 283:1358-1364, 1970.
9. Van der Linden W, Simonsen N: The familial occurrence of gallstone disease. Incidence in parents of young patients. Hum Hered 23:123-127, 1973.
10. Gilat T, Feldman C, Halpern Z, et al: An increased familial frequency of gallstones. Gastroenterology 84:242-246, 1983.
11. Jorgensen T: Gallstones in a Danish population: familial occurrence and social factors. J Biosoc Sci 20:11-120, 1988.
12. Wang DQ-H, Paigen B, Carey MC: Phenotypic characterization of Lith genes that determine susceptibility to cholesterol cholelithiasis in inbred mice: physical chemistry of gallbladder bile. J Lipid Res 38:1395-1411, 1997.
13. Festi D, Colecchia A, Orsini M, et al: Gallbladder motility and gallstone formation in obese patients following very low calorie diets. Use it (fat) to lose it (well). Int J Obes Relat Metab Disord 22:592-600, 1998.
14. Ros E, Navarro S, Bru C, et al: Occult microlithiasis in idiopathic acute pancreatitis: prevention of relapses by cholecystectomy or ursodeoxycholic acid therapy. Gastroenterology 101:1701-1709, 1991.
15. Lee SP, Nicholls JF, Park HZ: Biliary sludge as a cause of acute pancreatitis. N Engl J Med 326:589-593, 1992.
16. Ko CW, Sekijima JH, Lee SP: Biliary sludge. Ann Intern Med 130:301-311, 1999.
17. Amaral J, Xiao Z-L, Chen Q, et al: Gallbladder muscle dysfunction in patients with chronic acalculous disease. Gastroenterology 120:506-511, 2001.
18. Mulholland MW: Progress in understanding of acalculous gallbladder disease. Gastroenterology 120:570-572, 2001.
19. Ricci G, the GREPCO Group (Rome Group for the Epidemiology and Prevention of Cholelithiasis): The GREPO research programmes: aims and prevalence data. In Cappocaccia L, Ricci G, Angelico F, et al, eds: Epidemiology and Prevention of Gallstone Disease. Lancaster, England, MTP Press, 1984:9.
20. Ransohoff DF, Gracie WA: Treatment of gallstones. Ann Intern Med 119:606-619, 1993.
21. Howard DE, Fromm H: Overview of non-surgical therapy of gallstones. Gastroenterol Clin North Am 28(1):133-144, 1999.
22. Leitzmann MF, Rimm EB, Willett WC, et al: Recreational physical activity and the risk of cholecystectomy in women. N Engl J Med 341:777-784, 1999.
23. Leitzmann MF, Willett WC, Rimm EB, et al: A prospective study of coffee consumption and the risk of symptomatic gallstone disease in men. JAMA 281:2106-2112, 1999.
24. Tomida S, Abei M, Yamaguchi T, et al: Long-term ursodeoxycholic acid therapy is associated with reduced risk of biliary pain and acute cholecystitis in patients with gallbladder stones: a cohort analysis. Hepatology 30:6-13, 1999.
25. Ransohoff D: Management of patients with symptomatic gallstones: a quantitative analysis. Am J Med 88:154-160, 1990.
26. Targarona EM, Marco C, Balague C, et al: How, when, and why bile duct injury occurs: a comparison between open and laparoscopic cholecystectomy. Surg Endosc 12:322, 1998.
27. Fromm H, Roat JW, Gonzalez V, et al: Comparative efficacy and side effects of ursodeoxycholic and chenodeoxycholic acids in dissolving gallstones: a double blind controlled study. Gastroenterology 85:1257-1264, 1983.
28. Fromm H: Gallstone dissolution therapy. Current status and future prospects. Gastroenterology 91:1560-1567, 1986.

29. Levenson DE, Fromm H: Management of gallbladder disease. In Zakim D, Boyer TD, eds: Hepatology. A Textbook of Liver Disease. Philadelphia, WB Saunders Co., 1996:1877-1897.
30. Sarva RP, Farivar S, Fromm H, Poller W: Study of the sensitivity and specificity of computerized tomography in the detection of calcified gallstones which appear radiolucent by conventional roentgenography. Gastrointest Radiol 6:165-167, 1981.
31. Mulagha E, Fromm H: Extracorporeal shock wave lithotripsy of gallstones revisited: current status and future promises. J Gastroent Hepatol 15:239-243, 2000.
32. Zakko S, Hofmann AF: Microprocessor-assisted solvent-transfer system for gallstone dissolution. In vitro and in vivo validation. Gastroenterology 99:1807-1813, 1990.
33. Fromm H, Malavolti M: Gallstone recurrence after medical therapy. Viewpoints Dig Dis 24(1):1-7, 1992.

CHAPTER

61

Non-surgical Treatment of Biliary Tract Diseases

Michael J. Levy, MD, and Steve Goldschmid, MD

PROCEDURAL-RELATED ASPECTS

Introduction

Since the first endoscopic retrograde cholangiopancreatography (ERCP) in 1968,[1] endoscopic techniques have assumed an expanding role in the diagnosis and treatment of biliary tract diseases. Safe and effective endoscopic techniques now exist to diagnose and treat biliary tract disorders. Because endoscopy is less invasive than percutaneous or surgical approaches, endoscopy is often the preferred method for evaluating and treating patients with biliary tract disease. However, optimal patient care can only be achieved through an interdisciplinary approach that bases management decisions not only on the clinical scenario but also on available expertise. Although a multi-disciplinary approach is ideal, in this chapter we will focus on the role of endoscopic techniques in the management of biliary disorders.

Complications

Complications occurring during or soon after ERCP include pancreatitis, bleeding, retroduodenal perforation, stone and basket impaction, medication reaction, cardiopulmonary insult, and, rarely, death.[2-8] Late complications include acute cholecystitis, cholangitis, papillary stenosis, retained bile duct stones, and the predisposition to new stone formation.[2-8] Most investigators have found that the complication rate, especially pancreatitis, is higher for therapeutic, as opposed to diagnostic, procedures.[5,9] Others have found that the level of intervention does not alter the complication rate.[10,11] The overall complication rate is approximately 5 percent to 10 percent, with lower rates noted for the more highly skilled endoscopist.[3-7,12-14]

Anatomic and disease-related factors may hinder the ability to technically perform an ERCP. Altered duodenal anatomy (e.g., neoplastic invasion, duodenal stricture, Billroth II, Roux-en-Y) may limit access to the papilla.[15,16] Selective cannulation of the bile duct is not always possible and may result from a periampullary diverticula, ampullary neoplasm, or papillary stenosis.[17] The inability to perform an adequate sphincterotomy may also affect the success of ERCP. The presence of a short intraduodenal sphincter segment or procedure-induced bleeding often limits the ability to perform a sphincterotomy of adequate length. For patients with choledocholithiasis, morphologic characteristics of the stone or stones also influence the success of ERCP. It is often more difficult to remove large stones (larger than 1-2 cm), hard stones, square stones, multiple stones, intrahepatic stones, cystic duct stones, or stones proximal to a biliary stricture or tumor. The presence of refractory coagulopathy may limit the therapeutic options of ERCP and may represent an absolute contraindication to the procedure. Adequate sedation is necessary, and in those patients for whom conscious sedation cannot be administered safely, general anesthesia is necessary.

INDICATIONS

Choledocholithiasis

General

Before the development of endoscopic sphincterotomy (ES) in 1974,[18,19] surgical laparotomy and bile duct exploration were required to manage patients with bile duct stones (Figure 61-1). Initially, the use of ES for choledocholithiasis was restricted to elderly patients after cholecystectomy. Now, advances in equipment, increased numbers of skilled endoscopists, and the trend to laparoscopic cholecystectomy have resulted in a broadening of the indications for ES in patients with choledocholithiasis (Table 61-1). Endoscopic therapy is associated with a lower morbidity and mortality rate compared to percutaneous transhepatic[20-24] or surgical[20,25-27] approaches and is therefore considered the technique of choice.[20,27] Endoscopic management of bile duct stones is indicated for patients with a gallbladder in situ who have a high operative risk as a result of their age or underlying health. ES and stone retrieval is also indicated before laparoscopic cholecystectomy, and in the setting of cholangitis, severe or non-resolving gallstone pancreatitis, or for patients who decline surgery. Endoscopy is now regarded as the technique of choice for patients with choledocholithiasis after cholecystectomy.

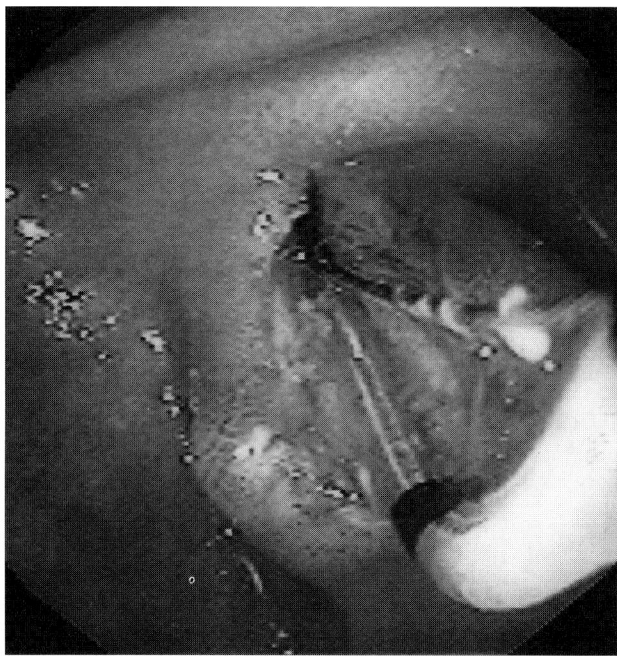

Figure 61-1 Endoscopic sphincterotomy.

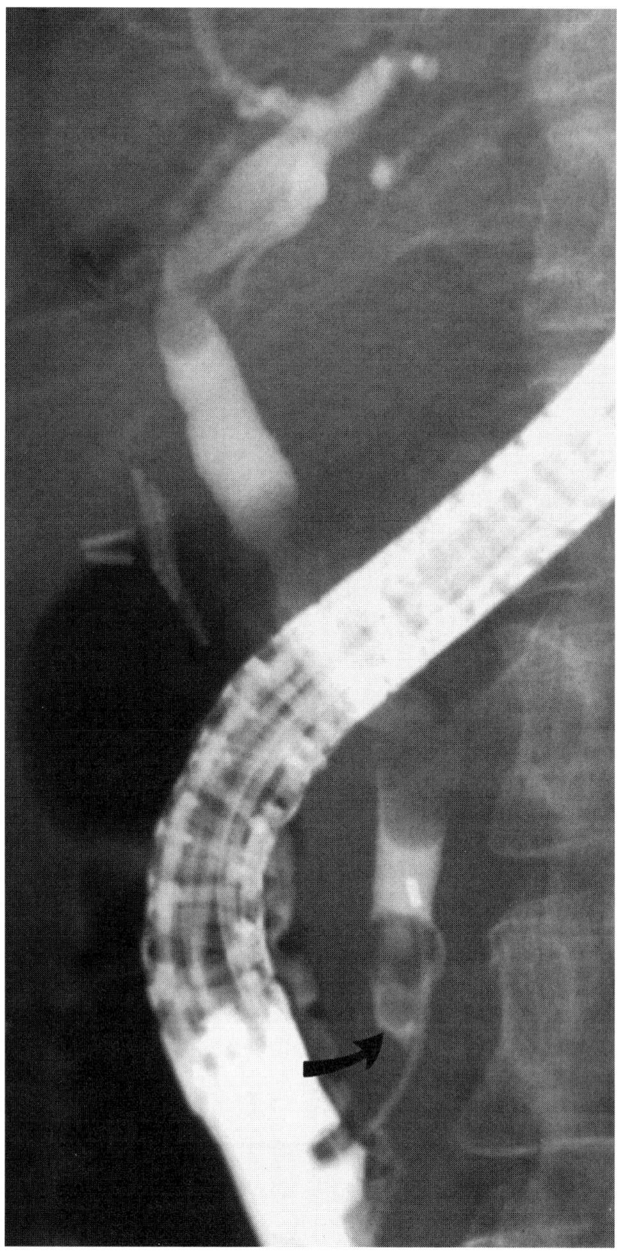

Figure 61-2 Balloon extraction of a small common bile duct stone *(curved arrow)* performed without the need for a prior sphincterotomy.

TABLE 61-1
Indications for Endoscopic Sphincterotomy for Choledocholithiasis

Gallbladder Present
High operative risk (relative to alternative or no therapy)
Elderly
Co-morbid illness
Before laparoscopic cholecystectomy
Acute cholangitis
Acute gallstone pancreatitis (severe or non-resolving)
Patient preference (non-operative management of gall bladder stones)
Gallbladder Absent (Postcholecystectomy)
T tube absent
T tube present
Immature T tube tract
Failed T tube extraction

Stone Extraction

When performed by experienced endoscopists, selective bile duct cannulation is possible in >95 percent of patients.[7,28,29] After cannulation, the bile duct can be cleared of stones in approximately 90-95 percent of patients, with an overall success rate of about 80-100 percent.[29-36] The use of special cannulas or papillotomes may be required to assist cannulation.[28,37-40] Precut papillotomy is seldom required.

The presence of choledocholithiasis is confirmed by endoscopic cholangiography, after which an endoscopic sphincterotomy is performed to aid in stone removal. The length of the sphincterotomy is based on the size of the stone and the length of the intramural bile duct, both determined at endoscopy. Because of the short-term and uncertain long-term risks of papillary sphincterotomy, some prefer to remove small stones (smaller than 5 mm) without performing a sphincterotomy. These tiny stones may be removed with the aid of a wire basket or balloon without the need for sphincter ablation (Figure 61-2).

Balloon papillary dilation with an 8- to 10-mm hydrostatic balloon may also obviate the need of ES for stones up to 10 mm in diameter. Some have found the short-term risk of balloon dilation and ES to be similar.[41] Because of the potential long-term risk of ES, these physicians favor balloon dilation for retrieval of small

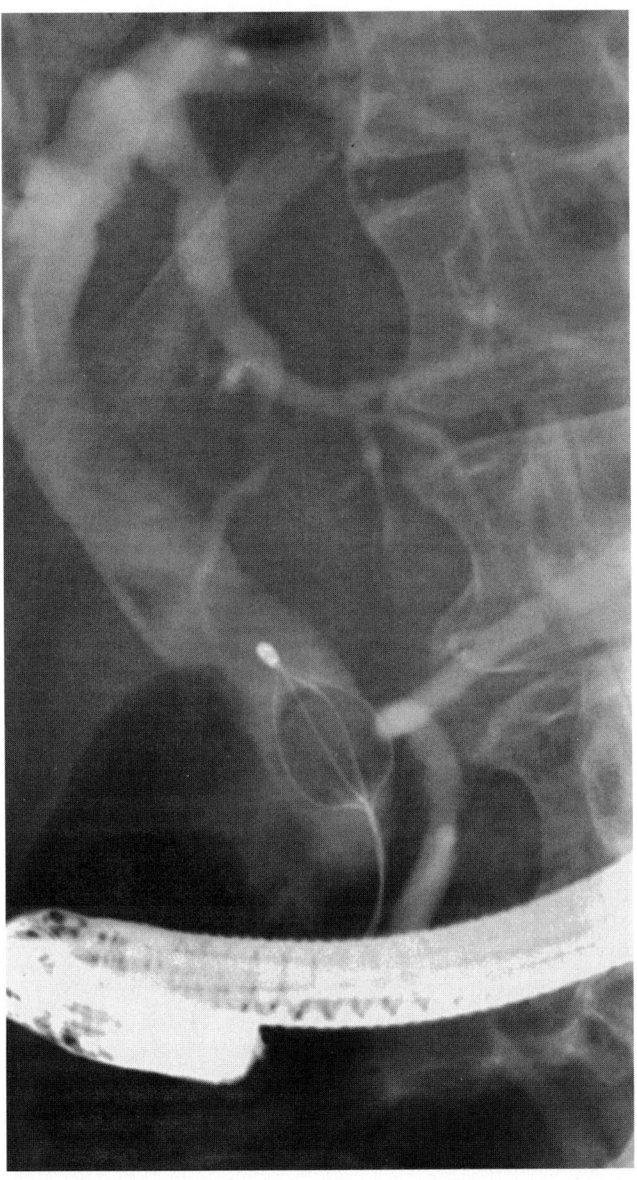

Figure 61-3 Extraction of a common bile duct stone with the aid of a basket.

stones.[41] Others have found the short-term complication rate and procedure time to be significantly greater for balloon dilation.[42] In most centers balloon dilation is seldom performed except in a select population in whom the potential risks of ES are too great, for example, patients with refractory coagulopathy.[43,44]

After ES or balloon dilation, stones are removed with the aid of either a balloon catheter or wire basket (Figure 61-3). Of note, balloon catheters differ from balloon dilators and are used to sweep stones from a duct and do not serve to dilate the sphincter. Balloon catheters are especially effective in removing stones smaller than 10 mm within a non-dilated duct. A wire basket may be favored for stones larger than 10 mm, small stones in a dilated duct, intrahepatic stones, and stones proximal to a downstream bile duct stricture. However, the stone and basket may become impacted as the result of a large stone size relative to the distal bile duct or papilla.

Retained Stones

When standard techniques such as balloon catheters or wire baskets fail to clear the bile ducts, then lithotripsy techniques[45-52] or chemical dissolution therapy[53,54] may be used to facilitate stone removal. The various techniques for lithotripsy include mechanical,[45,46] electrohydraulic,[47,48] laser,[49,50] and extracorporeal shockwave lithotripsy.[51,52] When an experienced endoscopist uses such measures, the success rate for crushing and removing refractory stones is similar to that of standard stones and approaches 80 percent to 95 percent.[30-34,45,46,55]

Mechanical lithotripsy is the most widely used form of lithotripsy because of its ease, safety, efficacy, and low cost. This technique involves passing a "crushing basket," which is located within a metal sheath, through the scope and into the bile duct at the time of ERCP. This piece of equipment consists of an internal wire basket surrounded by a plastic sheath and an outer metal sheath. After capture of the stone, longitudinal force is applied via a crank handle until either the stone is crushed against the metal sheath or the wire basket itself breaks. Rarely does this technique fail to remove a stone as a result of insufficient force, but instead failure usually results from an inability to engage the stone. Another type of mechanical lithotripter is available to remove impacted standard wire baskets and is an essential piece of equipment for all endoscopy centers. When a standard basket becomes impacted within the duct or papilla, the basket handle is cut off and the endoscope is removed. A metal sheath is advanced over the cut standard basket wires and then the metal sheath is back-loaded as the endoscope is reinserted. Use of the crank handle allows stone crushing and removal of the impacted basket.

Acute complications develop in approximately 8 percent to 10 percent of patients after endoscopic sphincterotomy, including acute pancreatitis (1 percent-6 percent), hemorrhage (2 percent-3 percent), cholangitis (1 percent-3 percent), and retroduodenal perforation (less than 1 percent).[4,8,30,56,57] The reported 30-day mortality rate is 3 percent to 16 percent[58] with death occurring in 0.1 percent to 1.0 percent of patients.* Delayed complications are reported in 10 percent to 15 percent of patients after endoscopic sphincterotomy[61,62] and occur at a rate similar to that for surgical bile duct exploration and biliary drainage.[63-65] These late complications include recurrent stone formation and cholangitis (despite a widely patent sphincterotomy) and ampullary stenosis, but can usually be managed endoscopically.

It is imperative to establish biliary drainage in the 5 percent of patients for whom stone extraction fails or is incomplete to prevent distal stone impaction and acute cholangitis.[66] This is accomplished by endoscopic placement of either a nasobiliary stent or an internal biliary stent.[66-73] Endoscopic or surgical efforts for stone removal are undertaken at a later date when the patient's clinical status permits. Nasobiliary tubes allow one to obtain a cholangiogram without having to repeat an ERCP but are poorly tolerated and may unintentionally become dislodged. Internal stents are generally favored[66] because

*References 4, 8, 30, 31, 56, 59, 60.

of greater patient satisfaction. In addition, the presence of internal stents may serve to mechanically fragment existing stones and aid subsequent removal.[74,75] The addition of an oral dissolution agent may serve to soften stones and therefore further decrease stone caliber and facilitate removal.[76] The drawback of internal stents is the risk of occlusion or distal migration that may lead to ductal obstruction, cholangitis, and the need for repeat endoscopy.

An alternative approach in poor surgical candidates and the very elderly is simply to perform a sphincterotomy to allow biliary drainage with permanent stent placement that prevents stone impaction.[76-78] With this approach approximately 11 percent to 15 percent of patients will develop late complications, most commonly cholangitis.* However, more recent reports have noted the risks of this approach to be far greater, with complications developing in about 40 percent and biliary-related death occurring in roughly 15 percent of patients.[73,80] Therefore the decision to offer this form of therapy should be made with care.

Precholecystectomy (Gallbladder Present)

The need and optimal timing of preoperative endoscopic clearance of bile duct stones in patients with choledocholithiasis and cholelithiasis is unclear. Clinical, laboratory, and radiologic parameters are poorly predictive of the presence of choledocholithiasis. Even when these parameters suggest their presence, the majority of preoperative ERCPs fail to detect bile duct stones.[29,81] However, bile duct stones should still be suspected in people with an elevated bilirubin or when imaging studies demonstrate a dilated biliary system.[82] Minimally elevated liver enzymes and mild gallstone pancreatitis are poorly predictive of choledocholithiasis.[82] Two prospective randomized trials determined that endoscopy before open cholecystectomy offered no advantage.[83,84] Another prospective randomized trial[85] and other retrospective trials[86,87] in patients undergoing laparoscopic cholecystectomy came to the same conclusion. Decisions regarding the need and timing of ERCP with respect to laparoscopic cholecystectomy should be based on the probability of stones and the skill and experience of the endoscopist and surgeon. This should help increase the number of positive or therapeutic ERCPs, avoid unnecessary ERCPs, and decrease the number of undiagnosed bile duct stones.

Initial experience suggests that routine ERCP is not indicated before laparoscopic cholecystectomy in people with a low likelihood of choledocholithiasis.[85,88] On the other hand, patients who are likely to have bile duct stones most likely benefit from ERCP and stone removal.[36,89] When the presence of bile duct stones is less certain, minimally invasive studies such as endoscopic ultrasound (EUS) and magnetic resonance cholangiography (MRCP) are useful to assess the presence and to help guide therapy.[90-92] Studies have found EUS to be of comparable or greater accuracy than ERCP for diagnosing choledocholithiasis (Figure 61-4).[93,94] Although EUS is of value in establishing the diagnosis, it does not allow therapeutic intervention—ERCP is still required in appropriately selected patients. It may be even more important to perform MRCP or EUS on patients with a history of post-ERCP pancreatitis, after a failed ERCP, for patients with acute pancreatitis, and during pregnancy. When uncertainty remains as to the presence of bile duct stones, the choice and timing of procedures must be based on the availability and skill of the endoscopist and surgeon. The feasibility of combined laparoscopic cholecystectomy and intraoperative ERCP in patients with suspected cholelithiasis and choledocholithiasis has been demonstrated. This approach allows a one-stage procedure with avoidance of preoperative ERCP and eliminates the need for repeat surgery after a failed ERCP. However, logistic issues will likely diminish the enthusiasm for this approach, especially in centers with extensive endoscopic and surgical expertise.

In centers with available expertise we recommend that ERCP be performed postoperatively when attempted surgical stone removal is unsuccessful. This allows attempted surgical clearance that would obviate the need for endoscopy. Bile duct stones are removed at the time of open cholecystectomy via bile duct exploration or at the time of laparoscopic cholecystectomy via percutaneous approaches. Delaying endoscopy until after surgery is only suggested for centers that have a high success rate for selective bile duct cannulation and stone clearance because failure necessitates repeat surgery and bile duct exploration. Postoperative ERCP is also the procedure of choice for evaluating symptoms or lab results that suggest laparoscopic cholecystectomy-induced injury. Preoperative ERCP is recommended when there is a high likelihood of bile duct stones, cholangitis is sus-

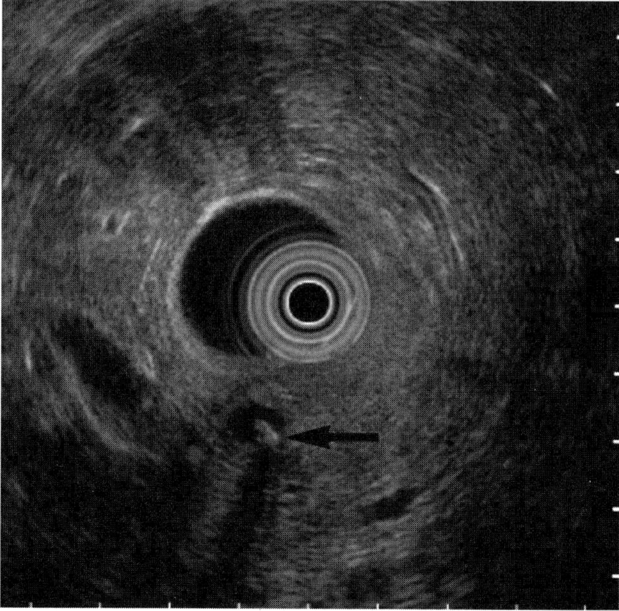

Figure 61-4 Endoscopic ultrasound detection of a distal common bile duct stone *(arrow)*. (Courtesy of Dr. Maurits J. Wiersema.)

*References 68, 69, 71, 74, 75, 79.

pected, severe gallstone pancreatitis is present, or the diagnosis is in question.

Elective cholecystectomy is indicated in good operative candidates of almost any age because the risks of future gallbladder-related symptoms and complications outweigh the operative risks. The use of ES and stone clearance may obviate the need for cholecystectomy in the very elderly or in those with significant co-morbid illness. With this approach gallbladder-related symptoms or complications requiring further therapy develop in 10 percent of patients over 5 to 10 years, with most occurring within the first year. This rate is similar to that in patients with asymptomatic cholelithiasis.[67] Therefore people with choledocholithiasis who are poor operative candidates or have an anticipated shortened life span may be best served by endoscopic stone removal that leaves the gallbladder intact, unless their clinical course mandates further intervention.

Postcholecystectomy

Bile duct stones are identified in about 2 percent to 5 percent of patients during or after laparoscopic cholecystectomy.[95] For most patients stone removal is achieved by the means previously described. Stones may also be detected during T-tube cholangiography after cholecystectomy. For patients with a T tube in place, other therapeutic options are available. Stones smaller than 5 mm that do not pass spontaneously may be removed by simple maneuvers such as T-tube flushing, which increases biliary hydrostatic pressure. Larger stones typically require additional measures to clear the duct. Most favor endoscopic approaches for stone removal because of the lower morbidity and mortality compared to surgical approaches and because there is no need to delay ERCP while awaiting T-tube maturation. Endoscopic stone clearance is successful in more than 90 percent of cases, with a morbidity of about 5 percent.[96-99] Percutaneous approaches through a T tube include hydraulic irrigation in conjunction with glucagon or nitrate administration to induce sphincter relaxation,[100] infusion of solvents or cholesterol,[100] choledochoscopy with lithotripsy, and stone extraction through a mature track.[101,102]

Acute Cholangitis

Acute cholangitis most often results from choledocholithiasis and bile duct obstruction, which leads to bile stasis and bacterial infection (Figure 61-5).[103] The organisms most commonly implicated include *Escherichia coli, Klebsiella* spp., *Enterobacter* spp., *Enterococcus* spp., and *Streptococcus* spp.[104] Cholangitis less frequently occurs as a result of malignant biliary obstruction, sump syndrome, choledochal cyst, papillary stenosis, or benign postoperative strictures. Regardless of the underlying pathology, bacteria and their toxins may reflux into the bloodstream as a result of the elevated intraductal pressure, leading to systemic manifestations of bacteremia or even sepsis.[103,105]

Most patients respond to initial conservative management of intravenous fluids and antibiotics, which should be administered soon after diagnosis, followed later by elective endoscopic or surgical biliary decompression.[26] The timing and extent of therapy must be tailored to the underlying pathology and the patient's clinical status. Urgent endoscopy is indicated when initial conservative measures fail and in the setting of severe cholangitis, as suggested by hypotension, shock, or confusion.[27,106] When therapy is delayed in this subgroup of patients, death is almost certain.[24] Regardless of the underlying pathology, the goal of therapy is to achieve biliary drainage and decompression. An endoscopic technique is favored because of its efficacy and safety compared with other approaches.[20-27,107] Percutaneous and surgical options are available when endoscopic approaches fail or are unavailable. Internal stents or nasobiliary tubes may be inserted to allow patient stabilization, when necessary.

Acute Gallstone Pancreatitis

Gallstones account for approximately half of all cases of acute pancreatitis.[108,109] Approximately 8 percent of all patients with cholelithiasis develop pancreatitis.[110] Gallstones are believed to lead to pancreatitis by transiently obstructing the ampulla of Vater.[111] This theory is supported by the fact that bile duct stones are found in 62 percent to 75 percent of patients when surgery is performed within 48 hours of admission. Many of these stones are impacted at the ampulla of Vater.[108] Although most patients fully recover after an attack of gallstone pancreatitis, some develop significant morbidity.[112] The reported mortality of about 10 percent to 20 percent is at least twice that of alcoholic pancreatitis.[112] The mortality rate is even higher (13 percent-50 percent) for patients developing concurrent cholangitis.[113,114]

Surgery was once the favored therapy for severe gallstone pancreatitis because of concern over the safety of

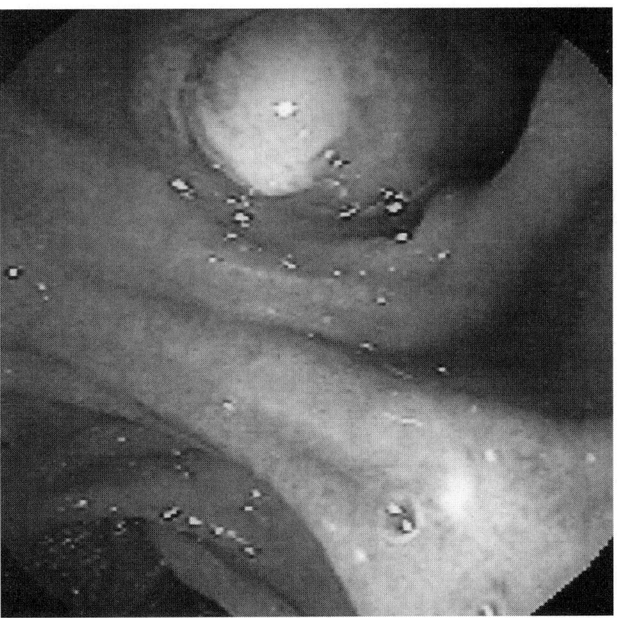

Figure 61-5 Pus and a stone extruding from the papilla in a patient with suppurative cholangitis secondary to choledocholithiasis.

ERCP and possible effects of ERCP on the course of pancreatitis. A prospective, randomized surgical study reported a mortality of 48 percent in patients who underwent early operative intervention for severe disease.[115] This significant mortality rate encouraged a shift in the focus of treatment to a safer, non-surgical approach for removing bile duct stones.

Initial trials involving ERCP and endoscopic sphincterotomy for gallstone pancreatitis reported dramatic clinical and biochemical improvements in the majority of patients.[116,117] These studies did little to change practices, however, partly because of their methodologic flaws. In these early studies, the disease severity, timing of sphincterotomy, and definition of complications varied widely, and therefore limited the conclusions that could be drawn. More recent studies, although having some design variations, have served to more clearly define the role of ERCP and sphincterotomy in this patient population.

In 1988 Neoptolemos and colleagues performed the first prospective randomized trial comparing urgent ERCP (within 72 hours of hospitalization) with sphincterotomy and stone removal to conservative therapy in patients with acute gallstone pancreatitis.[118] They not only established the safety of this approach but also noted a decrease in morbidity (24 percent versus 61 percent) and shortened hospital stay (median 9.5 days versus 17 days) in the subset of patients with severe pancreatitis. However, early endoscopy did not improve mortality. Fan and colleagues conducted a similar prospective randomized study in 1993.[119] They found that ERCP with sphincterotomy (within 24 hours of admission) was superior to conventional therapy in severely ill patients with gallstone pancreatitis and cholangitis. They noted a reduction in morbidity (16 percent versus 32 percent) from biliary sepsis, irrespective of disease severity, but failed to detect a statistically significant difference in overall survival.

Fölsch and colleagues, in a multi-center prospective trial in 1997, found no benefit to ERCP in acute biliary pancreatitis.[120] This study, however, excluded patients with biliary obstruction, jaundice, and cholangitis—those most likely to benefit from such therapy. The findings of this study should not discourage the use of ERCP and stone removal in acute pancreatitis but instead serve to remind us of those patients most likely to benefit from such intervention. ERCP should be reserved for patients with severe acute biliary pancreatitis with an elevated or rising bilirubin or when cholangitis is suspected. If stone extraction fails, appropriate measures should be taken to ensure adequate biliary drainage and to prevent recurrent stone impaction or worsening biliary sepsis. Although ERCP is of benefit in this select group of patients, one should note that no study has demonstrated a positive influence on the course of biliary pancreatitis itself or on survival.

Bile Duct Leak (Fistula)

Bile duct leaks most commonly occur as a result of cholecystectomy and are more frequently seen in the era of laparoscopic cholecystectomy (Figure 61-6).[121-123] They may also occur after bile duct exploration, a local infection, penetrating trauma, or in the setting of prolonged biliary tract disease. Most patients with a bile duct leak present within a week of surgery[124,125] and may complain of abdominal pain, tenderness, fever, nausea, vomiting, jaundice, and rarely, a palpable mass or ascites.[124]

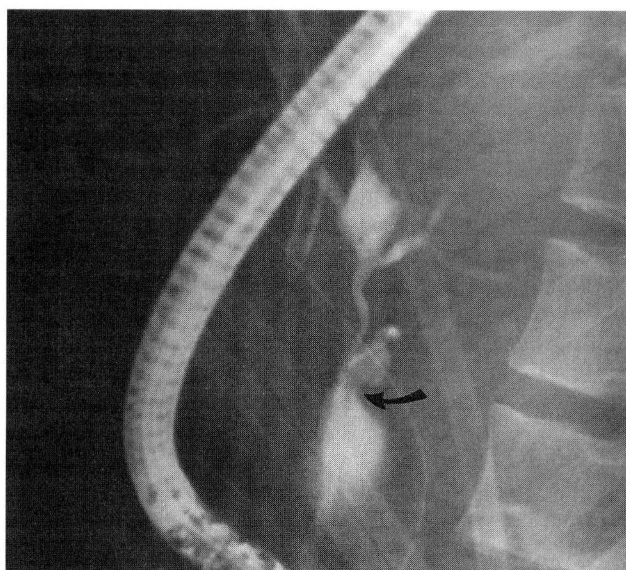

Figure 61-6 Bile duct leak *(curved arrow)* at cystic duct following laparoscopic cholecystectomy.

Biliary leaks most often develop after misapplication or spontaneous dislodgement of clips to the cystic duct stump during laparoscopic cholecystectomy.[126] Ischemia, cautery-induced injury, disruption of the duct of Luschka in the gallbladder bed, trauma during cholangiography, and loss of integrity of the bile duct anastomotic site may induce fistula formation.[127-132] Fistulas may also develop at the time of T-tube removal after liver transplantation. The presence of choledocholithiasis or a biliary stricture (benign or malignant) may predispose to fistula formation and delay healing because of the resulting elevation in intraductal pressure.[131,133] Immunosuppressed patients, those with infected bile peritonitis, and those with large leaks or hilar leaks are at risk for delayed or failed healing.

A low threshold should be maintained for the diagnosis in postcholecystectomy patients who do not recover rapidly from surgery. Laboratory values vary and are of little use in establishing or excluding the diagnosis. Transabdominal ultrasound and computed tomography may detect a biloma, and an HIDA scan may demonstrate the leak. However, ERCP is the most sensitive test to establish the diagnosis, with detection rates of 98 percent to 100 percent.[124,131,133]

Although surgical intervention was once the therapy of choice, today most leaks are treated by endoscopic techniques with healing rates of 90 percent to 100 percent.[131,133] The goal of endoscopy is to decrease the intraductal pressure by temporarily or permanently ablating the papilla. This creates a low-resistance pathway for the flow of bile into the duodenum, as opposed to the peritoneum, and allows healing of the disrupted duct. This may be accomplished endoscopically by performing a sphincterotomy, or by placement of an internal transpapillary stent or nasobiliary tube, with most favoring the use of internal transpapillary stents.[123-126,133-141] Although a few reports have found greater results with the use of larger stents[131] or stents that traverse the leak site,[131,133] most have found that the stent caliber and length do not affect the efficacy.[123-126,134-141] This is most likely because healing results simply from removing the transpapillary pressure gradient. In fact, healing rates do not appear to vary with respect to the choice of endoscopic therapy offered.[131,133] Resolution typically occurs within 7 days of therapeutic intervention.[142]

Although definitive data are lacking, there are specific situations that may require the use of additional or different therapy. A nasobiliary tube may be favored in patients with an ileus because of their elevated intraduodenal pressure. In this situation the use of an internal stent would not lead to a decrease in the pressure gradient between the bile duct and duodenum. The presence of a stone or stricture (benign or malignant) may require a sphincterotomy with or without long-term stenting. Most favor insertion of large-caliber stents that traverse the fistula site for patients with large bile duct leaks. Patients with a large biloma, especially those that are infected, often require percutaneous drainage. Surgery is required for completely transected ducts or when the placement of clips across the bile duct prohibits endoscopic techniques.

Benign Biliary Stricture

General

Benign biliary strictures typically occur as a result of surgery-induced injury. Non-surgical causes of benign biliary strictures include Mirizzi's syndrome, long-standing choledocholithiasis, primary sclerosing cholangitis, and chronic pancreatitis. Although termed "benign," these strictures are of concern given the potential consequences, including cholangitis and secondary biliary cirrhosis. Benign biliary strictures, regardless of etiology, respond well soon after stenting, with relief of cholangitis and jaundice. The long-term efficacy is good for postoperative strictures but often unsatisfactory for others, such as those secondary to chronic pancreatitis.

Postoperative

Surgical trauma may occur at the time of laparoscopic or open cholecystectomy, bile duct exploration, or at the site of the biliary anastomosis after liver transplantation. Benign bile duct strictures may also develop after hepatic, pancreatic, or gastric surgery. The frequency with which these strictures occur has increased as the use of laparoscopic cholecystectomy has broadened. Stricture formation is usually induced by ischemic, thermal, or inflammatory injury. Patients typically present within a few months of surgery; however, more delayed presentation may be seen. The cholangiogram usually reveals a smoothly tapered stricture with proximal ductal dilation.

Endoscopic therapy is generally favored because of its relative ease and safety compared to surgery. In most cases balloon dilation is performed with 4- to 10-mm balloons. Long-term stent therapy is another option. Increasing numbers and diameters of stents are inserted over a few months to a year. The number and caliber of stents, and duration of stenting, are based on the appearance of the stricture as compared to the adjacent distal duct at follow-up exam. At 5 years postendoscopic therapy, approximately 25 percent of patients will have developed cholestasis with or without cholangitis, necessitating surgical intervention.[143-145] Surgery is also indicated for strictures refractory to endoscopic therapy and extremely "tight" or long (more than 2 cm) strictures.[146]

Chronic Pancreatitis

A distal bile duct stricture develops in approximately one third of patients with chronic pancreatitis and may be manifest by any combination of pain, cholestasis, jaundice, or cholangitis. Endoscopic biliary stent placement is favored by some and does offer good short-term relief of cholestasis.[147] Stent therapy may suffice in a subgroup of patients with chronic pancreatitis who experience biliary obstruction—not as a result of chronic scarring but because of inflammation resulting from an acute exacerbation of pancreatitis. Stenting also has a diagnostic role in helping to determine whether a patient is experiencing pain as a result of the biliary obstruction or as a result of chronic pancreatitis itself.[148] In these patients the use of stents may help predict those who are likely to have a good response to surgical biliary decompression.

The majority of patients, however, require either prolonged stent therapy with multiple stent exchanges or surgical intervention.[147] Therefore in patients with chronic pancreatitis–induced bile duct strictures and complications of obstruction, stent placement should be considered a temporizing measure or simply used as a diagnostic tool. Chronic stent therapy may be considered in poor operative candidates. In general, surgical decompression is regarded as the only effective long-term therapy.

Primary Sclerosing Cholangitis

The frequency with which primary sclerosing cholangitis (PSC) is diagnosed continues to rise as the use of screening liver chemistries and ERCP increases. This disease represents a chronic progressive cholestatic disorder of uncertain etiology.[149-151] Patients develop intrahepatic or extrahepatic biliary strictures as a part of their disease process.[149-151] Over time biliary cirrhosis, liver failure, and portal hypertension commonly develop.[149-151]

The diagnosis is based on the presence of cholestatic liver chemistries, a compatible cholangiogram, liver biopsy, and the absence of other disorders that are associated with secondary sclerosing cholangitis.[152] Although the bile duct may appear normal in "small duct PSC,"[153] the cholangiogram is generally considered the gold standard for establishing the diagnosis of PSC. Most centers prefer to obtain a cholangiogram via an endoscopic approach. The disadvantages of using the percutaneous route is the potential difficulty of cannulating a small fibrotic intrahepatic bile duct, the inability to obtain a pancreatogram, and relative morbidity compared to endoscopy. Cholangiography most commonly demonstrates diffuse multifocal strictures within intrahepatic and/or extrahepatic bile ducts (Figure 61-7).[150,151,154,155] The biliary system may appear beaded because of the presence of normal or dilated segments between the strictures. Bile duct pseudodiverticulae, mural irregularity, and stones are commonly seen as well. Concomitant or isolated cystic duct or pancreatic duct involvement may exist in a minority of patients.

The presence of a dominant stricture, stones, or debris may be associated with a more rapid decline in a patient's clinical condition and warrants therapeutic intervention. A dominant stricture or stone may lead to an elevation in intraductal pressure and hasten the decline in liver function. Therapy to relieve obstruction usually results in an improvement in clinical status, and often, partial reversal of liver damage, slowed disease progression, and a delayed need for liver transplantation.[153,156-158] Patients with worsening lab results, jaundice, pruritus, cholangitis, a dominant stricture, or bile duct stone should be considered for endoscopic intervention. For many patients endoscopic therapy may be definitive and should be considered the first line of therapy. Liver transplantation may be required to manage refractory strictures.[152,153,159]

Endoscopic options for dominant strictures include catheter dilation, balloon dilation, and insertion of internal stents or nasobiliary tubes.[152,153,157-159] Bile duct stones and debris are removed with the aid of a balloon catheter or wire basket with or without a prior endoscopic sphincterotomy. Most physicians favor performing an ES during the first ERCP in patients with PSC because the papilla often becomes involved in the fibrotic process. An ES facilitates passage of brushes and biopsy equipment into the papilla and is useful because multiple ERCPs are often required in these patients. However, an ES may add to the already increased risk of cholangitis that occurs after an ERCP in patients with PSC by allowing reflux of bacteria and food into the bile duct. The increased risk of cholangitis, particularly after stent placement, necessitates the prophylactic administration of antibiotics before ERCP, which should be continued for 3 to 7 days after the procedure.

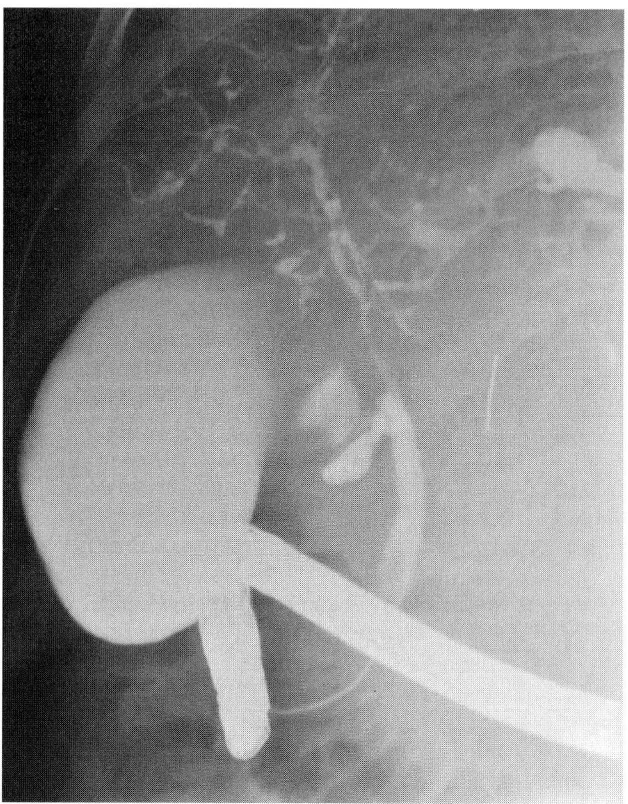

Figure 61-7 Cholangiographic features of primary sclerosing cholangitis.

It is often difficult to traverse these strictures because of the severity of the stenosis and the presence of pseudodiverticula. As a result, the risk of perforation or creation of a false passage is increased in these patients. Fortunately, these complications typically resolve without clinical consequence. Most respond to antibiotics with repeat ERCP in a few days if the initial exam was unsuccessful. After a guidewire is in place, catheter (4-10 Fr) or balloon (4-6 mm) dilation is performed. Although not always possible, the goal is to dilate the stricture to the diameter of the adjacent duct. Severe strictures often require serial dilations. Some favor the use of biliary stents in place of dilation for strictures associated with PSC.[158,160] However, others argue against the placement of internal stents in this patient population because of the risk of cholangitis, except in those patients with an inadequate response to balloon dilation.[153]

Consideration should be given to the presence of cholangiocarcinoma, which develops in up to 15 percent of patients with PSC.[150] Risk factors and potential clues include the presence of ulcerative colitis, cirrhosis, rapidly worsening liver chemistries, or a decline in clinical status. Comparison of the current cholangiogram with prior exams is important because it may help to identify changes such as a recalcitrant stricture, marked proximal ductal dilation, or a polypoid lesion, each of which may signify the presence of cholangiocarcinoma.[150]

Malignant Bile Duct Stricture

Malignant bile duct obstruction may result from a neoplasm arising from the bile duct, ampulla, liver, or pancreas. When the evaluation reveals a potentially resectable lesion, surgery should be offered to good operative candidates. Options for palliative therapy include endoscopic, radiologic, surgical, or medical interventions.

Endoscopic stenting of malignant biliary strictures effectively palliates more than 80 percent of patients and has an overall morbidity of 0 percent to 36 percent, with significant morbidity occurring in less than 10 percent of patients.[161-172] Endoscopic stent insertion compares favorably to percutaneous[163,164,166,167,171] and surgical[164,166,169,172] techniques for the palliation of malignant bile duct obstruction and is the preferred approach. Although stent occlusion can be expected to develop, the 6-month average life expectancy of these patients[161,162] lessens the importance of this occurrence. Before inserting a plastic or metal stent, antibiotics should be given and any significant coagulopathy corrected.[170] After guidewire placement and stricture dilation, the stent is inserted so that the proximal tip clears the tumor by 2 to 3 cm. Although at times difficult, traversal of malignant strictures is facilitated by the use of special coated wires and steerable guidewires and sphincterotomes. In general, an initial sphincterotomy is unnecessary except when papillary stenosis is present or to facilitate insertion of more than one stent.

In patients with hilar tumors the need to drain both the right and left intrahepatic bile ducts is debated.[170] Some favor the placement of a unilateral stent, citing the fact that such therapy usually allows resolution of the cholestasis and jaundice.[173] Others believe that bilateral stenting is necessary because of the increased risk of cholangitis and mortality seen with unilateral stenting (Figure 61-8).[165] We favor placement of bilateral stents when technically feasible, especially when contrast has been injected proximal to a stricture. This can be accomplished by initially placing two wires, one into each intrahepatic bile duct, followed by stent insertion. A single stent is placed if bilateral insertion is not possible. Patients are then closely followed. At the first sign of cholestasis or cholangitis, endoscopic or percutaneous biliary decompression of the contralateral side is performed. If the endoscopic approach fails, then percutaneous or a combined endoscopic and percutaneous approach should be considered. Surgical drainage is generally reserved for patients failing less-invasive maneuvers or those with concomitant outlet obstruction.

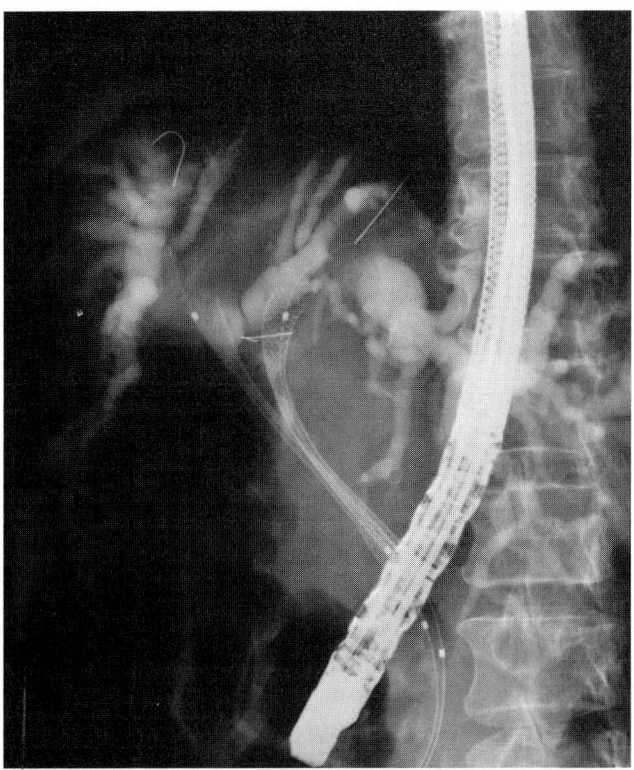

Figure 61-8 Bilateral placement of metal stents in a patient with a Klatskin tumor. (Courtesy of Dr. Christopher J. Gostout.)

Plastic Stents

Plastic bile duct stents are successfully placed in approximately 90 percent to 95 percent of patients, with a lower success rate for hilar tumors.[161-169,174,175] More than 80 percent of patients experience relief of jaundice and pruritus, with most reporting an improved quality of life.[161-169,174,176,177]

Plastic biliary stents (10 Fr) remain patent for an average of 3 to 6 months, but occlusion has been noted within a few days to as late as a year after placement.[174,178-185] Stent occlusion is strongly suggested by the recurrence of jaundice, pruritus, or fever. The presence of fatigue, low-grade temperature, and minimally elevated liver tests may also suggest stent occlusion. Certain characteristics of the stent (small caliber, long stent), bile composition (low mucin level, presence of bacteria), or the tumor itself (long, proximal tumor) influence stent occlusion. Except for stent diameter, attempts to modify these variables have minimally affected stent patency.[174,179-182,186-188] The stent diameter has been shown to correlate with duration of patency. Larger stents (10 Fr) should be placed instead of smaller stents whenever possible.[180,181] The benefit of larger stents may result from improved flow and diminished opportunity for sludge deposition. However, studies have not demonstrated any added benefit from inserting plastic stents larger than 10 Fr.

Stents must be exchanged after they occlude to avoid complications. Snares, forceps, and special stent extractors are available for stent retrieval.[184] The optimum timing of stent exchange is unclear. Because of expected stent occlusion that occurs over time and its associated morbidity, some prefer planned elective stent exchange every 3 to 4 months.[161-163] However, others have not found any benefit to this approach and instead prefer to base the timing of stent exchange on the presence of objective parameters of occlusion.[189,190] With this approach nearly 50 percent of patients die without ever requiring a stent exchange.[188] Regardless of the approach, close follow-up is necessary, with a low index of suspicion for stent occlusion and the need for exchange.

Metal Stents

The problem of plastic stent occlusion encouraged the development of expandable metal stents. Because of their much greater diameter, metal stents offer a more prolonged patency. Because of the relative permanency of these stents they are generally placed only in patients that clearly will not undergo surgical resection. There are several types of metal stents, including the Gianturco Z stent (Wilson-Cook), the Strecker stent (Boston Scientific Corporation), and the Wallstent (Schneider, Inc.), for which the most experience exists.[191-202] These stents are available in various lengths and diameters, with the choice of stent size based on the appearance of the malignant stricture. They are inserted over a guidewire and often may be placed with a "diagnostic" endoscope because of their small caliber before deployment. Covered metal stents have been developed to inhibit tumor ingrowth but can make initial placement more difficult.[203]

Using metal stents instead of plastic stents leads to a shorter hospitalization, less frequent cholangitis, prolonged patency, and a decreased need for reintervention.[199,200,204,205] The total cost for using metal stents is lower than plastic stents, despite the greater cost of the metal stent itself. This cost advantage is due to the decreased need for repeat intervention. The cost advantage for metal stents is only realized in those patients in whom a relatively prolonged survival is expected.[206] The use of plastic stents in these patients would likely necessitate another endoscopy and stent exchange. The need for a second endoscopy increases the total cost of plastic stent therapy beyond that for metal stent therapy. Two studies determined that patients expected to live longer than 3 to 4 months should be considered for metal stent therapy.[200,206] Another subgroup of patients who should be considered for metal stent therapy is that which have experienced rapid and repeated plastic stent occlusion.

Sphincter of Oddi Dysfunction

The sphincter of Oddi is a 5- to 15-mm-long fibromuscular sheath that encircles the terminal common bile duct, pancreatic duct, and common channel. This sphincter regulates the flow of bile and pancreatic juice into the duodenum, inhibits reflux of duodenal contents into the common bile duct and pancreatic duct, and promotes gallbladder filling with bile. Sphincter of Oddi dysfunction (SOD) causes diminished transsphincteric flow of bile or pancreatic juice because of organic obstruction (stenosis) or functional obstruction (dysmotility). The diagnosis is typically suspected in young patients with biliary-like abdominal pain after cholecystectomy in the absence of other pathology such as a bile duct stone, stricture, or malignancy.

Patients with SOD are classified as having either biliary-type or pancreatic-type disease (Table 61-2).[207-209]

TABLE 61-2

Sphincter of Oddi Dysfunction (Geenen and Hogan Classification)

Biliary type	Pancreatic type
Type I	**Type I**
Biliary-type pain	Pancreatic-type pain
LFT elevated	Amylase/lipase elevation
CBD dilation	PD dilation
Delayed drainage	Delayed drainage
Type II	**Type II**
Biliary-type pain	Pancreatic-type pain
One or two of above criteria	One or two of above criteria
Type III	**Type III**
Biliary-type pain only	Pancreatic-type pain only

LFT, Liver function tests; *CBD,* common bile duct; *PD,* pancreatic duct.

Subclassifying patients (types I, II, or III) helps to predict the underlying pathology. Type I disease usually results from stenosis alone; type III disease is typically a consequence of dysmotility alone.[207-209] Stenosis, dyskinesia, or an element of both is nearly evenly seen in patients with type II disease. Subclassifying also helps us predict the likelihood of pain relief after therapy, with the highest response rate occurring in patients with type I disease.

Sphincter of Oddi manometry (SOM) is the gold standard for diagnosing SOD. SOM employs a water-perfused catheter system that is inserted endoscopically into the common bile duct or pancreatic duct to measure the sphincter pressure. The diagnosis is established by finding a hypertensive sphincter of Oddi pressure (more than 40 mm Hg) during manometry.[207] Because of the risk of pancreatitis, SOM is reserved for patients with clinically significant or disabling symptoms. SOM is only performed if sphincter ablation is planned after confirming the diagnosis. This procedure is unnecessary in type I disease because of the almost absolute prevalence of SOD in this subset of patients, and empiric therapy without confirmatory SOM is reasonable.[210] Patients with type III disease often experience abdominal pain not as a result of sphincter dysmotility but from another functional or organic problem. In this group (type III) the decision to proceed with SOM must be carefully made given the inherent risks of the procedure. SOM is most likely to benefit patients with type II disease and it is important to establish the diagnosis of SOD by manometry before offering therapy.

Endoscopic sphincterotomy is effective and generally regarded as the therapy of choice for SOD.[211,212] Infrasphincteric botulinum toxin[213] or nitric oxide[214] injection and balloon dilation[215] are no longer performed because they have a limited efficacy and frequent, often severe, complications. The complication rate of endoscopic sphincterotomy, when performed for SOD, is greater than for other indications,[4,216] especially when the bile duct is not dilated.[4,217] Pancreatitis develops in up to 25 percent of patients, with 1 percent to 3 percent developing severe pancreatitis. The risk of sphincterotomy is potentially ameliorated by placement of a pancreatic duct stent.[218] Surgical sphincteroplasty is more invasive and should only be performed when endoscopic sphincterotomy fails.

Sump Syndrome

Patients who undergo a side-to-side choledochoduodenostomy may develop sump syndrome, which is manifested by cholangitis, pain, or pancreatitis. Symptoms result from filling of the bypassed segment of the bile duct with food, stones, or debris and eventually occluding the anastomotic orifice. Stenosis of the surgical anastomotic site is typically present. An endoscopic sphincterotomy is nearly always curative for these patients.[219,220] When an endoscopic sphincterotomy is contraindicated, one can simply remove the food, stone, or debris via the choledochoduodenostomy, but at a high risk of recurrence.

SUMMARY

Many disorders previously treated by surgical means can now be treated endoscopically, most often, with decreased cost, morbidity, and mortality. We stress, however, that optimal care is achieved through an interdisciplinary approach that bases management decisions on the clinical scenario and available expertise. We expect this field to expand as safer and more effective techniques are developed to treat the host of abnormalities related to the pancreatic and biliary ducts.

References

1. McCune WS, Shorb PE, Moscovitz H: Endoscopic cannulation of the ampulla of vater: a preliminary report. Ann Surg 167(5): 752-756, 1968.
2. Dunham F, Bourgeois N, Gelin M, et al: Retroperitoneal perforations following endoscopic sphincterotomy; clinical course and management. Endoscopy 14(3):92-96, 1982.
3. Escourrou J, Cordova JA, Lazorthes F, et al: Early and late complications after endoscopic sphincterotomy and biliary lithiasis with and without the gallbladder 'in situ.' Gut 25(6):598-602, 1984.
4. Freeman ML, Nelson DB, Sherman S, et al: Complications of endoscopic sphincterotomy. N Engl J Med 335:909-918, 1996.
5. Loperfido S, Angelini G, Benedetti G, et al: Major early complications from diagnostic and therapeutic ERCP: a prospective multicenter study. Gastrointest Endosc 48(1):1-10, 1998.
6. Leese T, Neoptolemos JP, Carr-Locke DL: Successes, failures, early complications and their management following endoscopic sphincterotomy: results in 394 consecutive patients from a single centre. Br J Surg 72(3):215-219, 1985.
7. Vaira D, D'Anna L, Ainley C, et al: Endoscopic sphincterotomy in 1000 consecutive patients. Lancet 2(8660):431-434, 1989.
8. Thornton J, Axon A: Towards safer endoscopic retrograde cholangiopancreatography. Gut 34(6):721-724, 1993.
9. Catalano MF, Geenen JE, Schmalz MJ, et al: ERCP induced acute pancreatitis: risk assessment based on diagnostic and specific therapeutic cases. Gastrointest Endosc 43:376A, 1996.
10. Cavallini G, Tittobello A, Frulloni L, et al: Gabexate for the prevention of pancreatic damage related to endoscopic retrograde cholangiopancreatography. N Engl J Med 335(13):919-923, 1996.
11. Vandervoort J, Tham TCK, Wong RCK, et al: Prospective study of post-ERCP complications following diagnostic and therapeutic ERCP. Gastrointest Endosc 43:401A, 1996.
12. Cotton PB, Lehman G, Vennes J, et al: Endoscopic sphincterotomy complications and their management: an attempt at consensus. Gastrointest Endosc 37:383-393, 1991.
13. Shemesh E, Klein E, Czerniak A, et al: Endoscopic sphincterotomy in patients with gallbladder in situ; the influence of periampullary duodenal diverticula. Surgery 107(2):163-166, 1990.
14. Worthley CS, Toouli J: Gallbladder non-filling: an indication for cholecystectomy after endoscopic sphincterotomy. Br J Surg 75(8):796-798, 1988.
15. Katon RM, Bilbao MK, Parent JA, et al: Endoscopic retrograde cholangiopancreatography in patients with gastrectomy and gastrojejunostomy (Billroth II). A case for the forward look. Gastrointest Endosc 21(4):164-165, 1975.
16. Goldschmiedt M, Marcon N, Kandel P, et al: A review of 160 endoscopic retrograde cholangiopancreatographies (ERCP): inpatients with Billroth II anastomosis. Gastrointest Endosc 37:247A, 1991.
17. Lobo DN, Balfour TW, Iftikhar SY: Periampullary diverticula: consensus of failed ERCP. Ann Roy Coll Surg Engl 80(5):326-331, 1998.
18. Siegel JH, Ben-Zvi JS, Pullano WE: Mechanical lithotripsy of common duct stones. Gastrointest Endosc 36:351-356, 1990.
19. Shaw MJ, Mackie RD, Moore JP, et al: Results of a multicenter trial using a mechanical lithotripter for the treatment of large bile duct stones. Am J Gastroenterol 88:730-733, 1993.
20. Boey JH, Way LW: Acute cholangitis. Ann Surg 191(3):264-270, 1980.
21. Gould RJ, Vogelzang RL, Neiman HL, et al: Percutaneous biliary drainage as an initial therapy of the biliary tract. Surg Gynecol Obstet 160(6):523-527, 1985.
22. Kadir S, Baassiri A, Barth KH, et al: Percutaneous biliary drainage in the management of biliary sepsis. AJR 138(1):25-29, 1982.
23. Pessa ME, Hawkins IF, Vogel SB: The treatment of acute cholangitis. Percutaneous transhepatic biliary drainage before definitive therapy. Ann Surg 205(4):389-392, 1987.
24. Fitzgibbons RJ, Ryberg AA, Ulualp KM, et al: An alternative technique for treatment of choledocholithiasis found at laparoscopic cholecystectomy. Arch Surg 130(6):638-642, 1995.
25. Leese T, Neoptolemos JP, Baker AR, et al: Management of acute cholangitis and the impact of endoscopic sphincterotomy. Br J Surg 73(12):988-992, 1986.
26. Leung JW, Chung SC, Sung JJ, et al: Urgent endoscopic drainage for acute suppurative cholangitis. Lancet 1(8650):1307-1309, 1989.
27. Lai EC, Mok FP, Tan ES, et al: Endoscopic biliary drainage for severe acute cholangitis. N Engl J Med 326(24):1582-1586, 1992.
28. Rossos PG, Kortan P, Haber G: Selective common bile duct cannulation can be simplified by the use of a standard papillotome. Gastrointest Endosc 39:67-69, 1993.
29. Chan AC, Chung SC, Wyman A, et al: Selective use of preoperative endoscopic retrograde cholangiopancreatography in laparoscopic cholecystectomy. Gastrointest Endosc 43(3):212-215, 1996.
30. Leese T, Neoptolemos JP, Carr-Locke DL: Successes, failures, early complications and their management following endoscopic sphincterotomy: results in 394 consecutive patients from a single centre. Br J Surg 72:215-219, 1985.
31. Cotton PB, Vallon AG: British experience with duodenoscopic sphincterotomy for removal of bile duct stones. Br J Surg 68:373-375, 1981.
32. Foutch PG: Endoscopic management of large common duct stones. Am J Gastroenterol 86(11):1561-1565, 1991.
33. Sherman S, Hawes RH, Lehman GA: Management of bile duct stones. Semin Liv Dis 10(3):205-221, 1990.
34. Cotton PB: Endoscopic management of bile duct stones (apples and oranges). Gut 25(6):587-597, 1984.
35. Kalimi R, Cosgrove JM, Marini C, et al: Combined intraoperative laparoscopic cholecystectomy and endoscopic retrograde cholangiopancreatography: lessons from 29 cases. Surg Endosc 14(3):232-234, 2000.
36. Huynh CH, Van de Stadt J, Deviere J, et al: Preoperative endoscopic retrograde cholangiopancreatography: therapeutic impact in a general population of patients needing a cholecystectomy. Hepatogastroenterology 43(12):1484-1491, 1996.
37. Shakoor T, Geenen JE: Pre-cut papillotomy. Gastrointest Endosc 38:623-627, 1992.
38. Cotton PB: Precut papillotomy—a risky technique for experts only. Gastroenterology 35(6):578-579, 1989.
39. Huibregtse K, Katon RM, Tytgat GN: Precut papillotomy via fine-needle knife papillotomy: a safe and effective technique. Gastrointest Endosc 32(6):403-405, 1986.
40. Weisberg MF, Miller GL, McCarthy JH: Needle knife papillotomy: a valuable yet dangerous technique. Gastrointest Endosc 37:267A, 1991.
41. Bergman JJGHM, Rauws EAJ, Fockens P, et al: Randomised trial of endoscopic balloon dilation versus endoscopic sphincterotomy for removal of bile duct stones. Lancet 349(9059):1124-1129, 1997.
42. DiSario JA, Freeman ML, Bjorkman DJ, et al: Endoscopic balloon dilation compared to sphincterotomy (EDES) for extraction of bile duct stones: preliminary results. Gastrointest Endosc 45:129A, 1997.
43. Prat F, Tennenbaum R, Ponsot P, et al: Endoscopic sphincterotomy in patients with liver cirrhosis. Gastrointest Endosc 43(2 Pt 1):127-131, 1996.
44. Kawabe T, Komatsu Y, Tada M, et al: Endoscopic papillary balloon dilation in cirrhotic patients: removal of common bile duct stones without sphincterotomy. Endoscopy 28(8):694-698, 1996.
45. Siegel JH, Ben-Zvi JS, Pullano WE: Mechanical lithotripsy of common duct stones. Gastrointest Endosc 36:351-356, 1990.
46. Shaw MJ, Mackie RD, Moore JP, et al: Results of a multicenter trial using a mechanical lithotripter for the treatment of large bile duct stones. Am J Gastroenterol 88:730-733, 1993.
47. Hixson LJ, Fennerty MB, Jaffee PE, et al: Peroral cholangioscopy with intracorporeal electrohydraulic lithotripsy for choledocholithiasis. Am J Gastroenterol 87:296-299, 1992.
48. Leung JW, Chung SS: Electrohydraulic lithotripsy with peroral choledochoscopy. BMJ 299:595-598, 1989.

49. Cotton PB, Kozarek RA, Schapiro RH, et al: Endoscopic laser lithotripsy of large bile duct stones. Gastroenterology 99:1128-1133, 1990.
50. Birkett DH: Biliary laser lithotripsy. Surg Clin North Am 72:641-654, 1992.
51. Ponchon T, Martin X, Barkun A, et al: Extracorporeal lithotripsy of bile duct stones using ultrasonography for stone localization. Gastroenterology 98:726-732, 1990.
52. Sauerbruch T, Stern M: Fragmentation of bile duct stones by extracorporeal shock waves. A new approach to biliary calculi after failure of routine endoscopic measures. Gastroenterology 96(1):146-152, 1989.
53. Palmer KR, Hofmann AF: Intraductal mono-octanoin for the direct dissolution of bile duct stones: experience in 343 patients. Gut 27(2):196-202, 1986.
54. Neoptolemos JP, Hall C, O'Connor HJ, et al: Methyl-tert-butyl-ether for treating bile duct stones: the British experience. Br J Surg 77(1):32-35, 1990.
55. Lee JG, Leung JW: Endoscopic management of difficult common bile duct stones. Gastrointest Endosc Clin North Am 6(1):43-55, 1996.
56. Cotton PB, Geenen JE, Sherman S, et al: Endoscopic sphincterotomy for stones by experts is safe, even in younger patients with normal ducts. Ann Surg 227(2):201-204, 1998.
57. Sherman S, Ruffolo TA, Hawes RH, et al: Complications of endoscopic sphincterotomy. A prospective series with emphasis on the increased risk associated with sphincter of Oddi dysfunction and non-dilated bile ducts. Gastroenterology 101:1068-1075, 1991.
58. Siegel JH: Endoscopic papillotomy in the treatment of biliary tract disease: 258 procedures and results. Dig Dis Sci 26:1057-1064, 1981.
59. Dowsett JF, Vaira D, Hatfield RW, et al: Endoscopic biliary therapy using the combined percutaneous and endoscopic technique. Gastroenterology 96:1180-1186, 1989.
60. Cotton PB, Vallon AG: British experience with duodenoscopic sphincterotomy for removal of bile duct stones. Br J Surg 68:373-375, 1981.
61. Hawes RH, Cotton PB, Vallon AG: Follow-up 6 to 11 years after duodenoscopic sphincterotomy for stones in patients with prior cholecystectomy. Gastroenterology 98:1008-1012, 1990.
62. Ikeda S, Tanaka M, Matsumoto S, et al: Endoscopic sphincterotomy: long-term results in 408 patients with complete follow-up. Endoscopy 20:13-17, 1988.
63. Baker AR, Neoptolemos JP, Leese T, et al: Long term follow-up of patients with side to side choledochoduodenostomy and transduodenal sphincteroplasty. Ann Roy Coll Surg 69:253-257, 1987.
64. Cranley B, Logan H: Exploration of the common bile duct—the relevance of the clinical picture and the importance of preoperative cholangiography. Br J Surg 67(12):869-872, 1980.
65. Sheridan WG, Williams HO, Lewis MH: Morbidity and mortality of common bile duct exploration. Br J Surg 74(12):1095-1099, 1987.
66. Leung JWC, Cotton PB: Endoscopic nasobiliary catheter drainage in biliary and pancreatic disease. Am J Gastroenterol 86(4):389-394, 1991.
67. Gracie WA, Ransohoff DF: The natural history of silent gallstones: the innocent gallstone is not a myth. N Engl J Med 307(13):798-800, 1982.
68. Cairns SR, Dias L, Cotton PB, et al: Additional endoscopic procedures instead of urgent surgery for retained common bile duct stones. Gut 30(4):535-540, 1989.
69. Soomers AJ, Nagengast FM, Yap SH: Endoscopic placement of biliary endoprostheses in patients with endoscopically unextractable common bile duct stones. A long-term follow-up study of 26 patients. Endoscopy 22(1):24-26, 1990.
70. Peters R, MacMathuna P, Lombard M, et al: Management of common bile duct stones with a biliary endoprosthesis. Report on 40 cases. Gut 33(10):1412-1415, 1992.
71. Navicharem P, Rhodes M, Flook, D, et al: Endoscopic retrograde cholangiopancreatography (ERCP) and stent placement in the management of large common bile duct stones. Aust NZ J Surg 64(12):840-842, 1994.
72. Maxton DG, Tweedle DE, Martin DF: Retained common bile duct stones after endoscopic sphincterotomy: temporary and long-term treatment with biliary stenting. Gut 36(3):446-449, 1995.
73. Bergman JJ, Rauws EA, Tijssen JG, et al: Biliary endoprosthesis in elderly patients with endoscopically irretrievable common bile duct stones: report on 117 patients. Gastrointest Endosc 42(3):195-201, 1995.
74. Kubota Y, Takaoka M, Fujimura K, et al: Endoscopic endoprosthesis for large stones in the common bile duct. Intern Med 33(10):597-601, 1994.
75. Maxton DG, Tweedle DE, Martin DF: Stenting for choledocholithiasis: temporizing or therapeutic? Am J Gastroenterol 91(3): 615-616, 1996.
76. Johnson GK, Geenen JE, Venu RP, et al: Treatment of non-extractable common bile duct stones with combination ursodeoxycholic acid plus endoprostheses. Gastrointest Endosc 39(4):528-531, 1993.
77. Cotton PB, Forbes A, Leung JW, et al: Endoscopic stenting for long-term treatment of large bile duct stones: 2- to 5-year follow-up. Gastrointest Endosc 33(6):411-412, 1987.
78. Foutch PG, Harlan J, Sanowski RA: Endoscopic placement of biliary stents for treatment of high risk geriatric patients with common duct stones. Am J Gastroenterol 84(5):527-529, 1989.
79. Dowsett JF, Vaira D, Polydorou A, et al: Interventional endoscopy in the pancreatobiliary tree. Am J Gastroenterol 83(12):1328-1336, 1988.
80. Chopra KB, Peters RA, O'Toole PA, et al: Randomised study of endoscopic biliary endoprosthesis versus duct clearance for bile duct stones in high-risk patients. Lancet 348(9030):791-793, 1996.
81. Tham TC, Lichtenstein DR, Vandervoort J, et al: Role of endoscopic retrograde cholangiopancreatography for suspected choledocholithiasis in patients undergoing laparoscopic cholecystectomy. Gastrointest Endosc 47(1):50-56, 1998.
82. Rijna H, Kemps WG, Eijsbouts Q, et al: Preoperative ERCP approach to common bile duct stones: results of a selective policy. Dig Surg 17(3):229-233, 2000.
83. Neoptolemos JP, Carr-Locke DL, Fossard DP: Prospective randomised study of preoperative endoscopic sphincterotomy versus surgery alone for common bile duct stones. Br Med J Clin Res Ed 294(6570):470-474, 1987.
84. Stiegmann GV, Goff JS, Mansour A, et al: Precholecystectomy endoscopic cholangiography and stone removal is not superior to cholecystectomy, cholangiography, and common duct exploration. Am J Surg 163(2):227-230, 1992.
85. Chang L, Lo S, Stabile BE: Preoperative versus postoperative endoscopic retrograde cholangiopancreatography in mild to moderate gallstone pancreatitis: a prospective randomized trial. Ann Surg 231(1):82-87, 2000.
86. Himal HS: Preoperative endoscopic retrograde cholangiopancreatography (ERCP) is not necessary in mild pancreatitis. Surg Endosc 13(8):782-783, 1999.
87. Geron N, Reshef R, Shiller M, et al: The role of endoscopic retrograde cholangiopancreatography in the laparoscopic era. Surg Endosc 13(5):452-456, 1999.
88. Neuhaus H, Feussner H, Ungeheuer A, et al: Prospective evaluation of the use of endoscopic retrograde cholangiography prior to laparoscopic cholecystectomy. Endoscopy 24(9):745-749, 1992.
89. Esber EJ, Sherman S: The interface of endoscopic retrograde cholangiopancreatography and laparoscopic cholecystectomy. Gastrointest Endosc Clin North Am 6(1):57-80, 1996.
90. Anouyal P, Anouyal G, Levy P, et al: Diagnosis of choledocholithiasis by endoscopic ultrasound. Gastroenterology 106:106(4):1062-1067, 1994.
91. Guidbaud L, Bret PM, Reinhold C, et al: Diagnosis of choledocholithiasis: value of MR cholangiography. Am J Roentgenol 163(4):847-850, 1994.
92. Stockberger SM, Wass JL, Sherman S, et al: Intravenous cholangiography with helical CT: comparison to endoscopic retrograde cholangiopancreatography. Radiology 192(3):675-680, 1994.
93. Chak A, Hawes RH, Cooper GS, et al: Prospective assessment of the utility of EUS in the evaluation of gallstone pancreatitis. Gastrointest Endosc 49(5):599-604, 1999.
94. Sahai AV, Mauldin PD, Marsi V, et al: Bile duct stones and laparoscopic cholecystectomy: a decision analysis to assess the roles of intraoperative cholangiography, EUS, and ERCP. Gastrointest Endosc 49(3 Pt 1):334-343, 1999.
95. Bickerstaff KI, Berry AR, Chapman RW, et al: Early postoperative endoscopic sphincterotomy for retained biliary stones. Ann Roy Coll Surg Engl 70(6):350-351, 1988.

96. Hammarstrom LE, Stridbeck H, Ihse I: Long-term follow-up after endoscopic treatment of bile duct calculi in cholecystectomized patients. World J Surg 20(3):272-276, 1996.
97. O'Doherty DP, Neoptolemos JP, Carr-Locke DL: Endoscopic sphincterotomy for retained common bile duct stones in patients with T-tube in-situ in the early postoperative period. Br J Surg 73(6):454-456, 1986.
98. Bickerstaff KI, Berry AR, Chapman RW, et al: Early postoperative endoscopic sphincterotomy for retained biliary stones. Ann Roy Coll Surg Engl 70(6):350-351, 1988.
99. Cranley B, Logan H: Exploration of the common bile duct—the relevance of the clinical picture and the importance of preoperative cholangiography. Br J Surg 67(12):869-872, 1980.
100. Tritapepe R, di Padova C, di Padova F: Non-invasive treatment for retained common bile duct stones in patients with T tube in-situ: saline washout after intravenous ceruletide. Br J Surg 75(2):144-146, 1988.
101. Nussinson E, Cairns SR, Vaira D, et al: A 10 year single centre experience of percutaneous and endoscopic extraction of bile duct stones with T tube in-situ. Gut 32(9):1040-1043, 1991.
102. Soehendra N, Kempeneers I, Eichfuss HP, et al: Early postoperative endoscopy after biliary tract surgery. Endoscopy 13(3):113-117, 1981.
103. Connors PJ, Carr-Locke DL: Endoscopic retrograde cholangiopancreatography findings and endoscopic sphincterotomy for cholangitis and pancreatitis. Gastrointest Endosc Clin North Am 1:27-50, 1991.
104. Leung JW, Ling TK, Chan RC, et al: Antibiotics, biliary sepsis, and bile duct stones. Gastrointest Endosc 40(6):716-721, 1994.
105. Csendes A, Sepulveda A, Buriles P, et al: Common bile duct pressure in patients with common bile duct stones with or without acute suppurative cholangitis. Arch Surg 123(6):697-699, 1988.
106. Welch JP, Donaldson GA: The urgency of diagnosis and surgical treatment of acute suppurative cholangitis. Am J Surg 131(5):527-532, 1976.
107. Siegel JH, Rodriguez R, Choen SA, et al: Endoscopic management of cholangitis: critical review of an alternative technique and report of a large series. Am J Gastroenterol 89(8):1142-1146, 1994.
108. Acosta JM, Pellegrini CA, Skinner DB: Etiology and pathogenesis of acute biliary pancreatitis. Surgery 88(1):118-125, 1980.
109. Houssin D, Castaing D, Lemoine J, Bismuth H: Microlithiasis of the gallbladder. Surg Gynecol Obstet 157(1):20-24, 1983.
110. Armstrong CP, Taylor TV, Jeacock J, Lucas S: The biliary tract in patients with acute gallstone pancreatitis. Br J Surg 72:551-555, 1985.
111. Opie EL: The etiology of acute hemorrhagic pancreatitis. Bull Johns Hopkins Hosp 12:182, 1901.
112. Trapnell JE, Duncan EH: Patterns of incidence in acute pancreatitis. BMJ 2(5964):179-183, 1975.
113. Lawson DW, Daggett WM, Civetta JM, et al: Surgical treatment of acute necrotizing pancreatitis. Ann Surg 172(4):605-617, 1970.
114. Imrie CW, Whyte AS: A prospective study of acute pancreatitis. Br J Surg 62(6):490-494, 1975.
115. Kelly TR, Wagner DS: Gallstone pancreatitis: a prospective randomized trial of the timing of surgery. Surgery 104(4):600-605, 1988.
116. Safrany L, Cotton PB: A preliminary report: urgent duodenoscopic sphincterotomy for acute gallstone pancreatitis. Surgery 89(4):424-428, 1981.
117. Rosseland AR, Solhaug JH: Early or delayed endoscopic papillotomy (EPT) in gallstone pancreatitis. Ann Surg 199(2):165-167, 1984.
118. Neoptolemos JP, Carr-Locke DL, London NJ, et al: Controlled trial of urgent endoscopic retrograde cholangiopancreatography and endoscopic sphincterotomy versus conservative treatment for acute pancreatitis due to gallstones. Lancet 2(8618):979-983, 1988.
119. Fan ST, Lai EC, Mok FP, et al: Early treatment of acute biliary pancreatitis by endoscopic papillotomy. N Engl J Med 328(4):228-232, 1993.
120. Fölsch UR, Nitsche R, Ludtke R, et al: Early ERCP and papillotomy compared with conservative treatment for acute biliary pancreatitis. The German Study Group on Acute Biliary Pancreatitis. N Engl J Med 336(4):237-242, 1997.
121. Southern Surgeons Club: A prospective analysis of 1518 laparoscopic cholecystectomies. N Engl J Med 324(16):1073-1078, 1991.
122. Gouma DJ, Go PM: Bile duct injury during laparoscopic and conventional cholecystectomy. J Am Coll Surg 178(3):229-233, 1994.
123. Bergman JJ, van den Brink GR, Rauws EA, et al: Treatment of bile duct lesions after laparoscopic cholecystectomy. Gut 38(1):141-147, 1996.
124. Barkun AN, Rezieg M, Mehta SN, et al: Postcholecystectomy biliary leaks in the laparoscopic era: risk factors, presentation, and management. McGill Gallstone Treatment Group. Gastrointest Endosc 45(3):277-282, 1997.
125. Woods MS, Shellito JL, Santoscoy GS, et al: Cystic duct leaks in laparoscopic cholecystectomy. Am J Surg 168(6):560-563, 1994.
126. Kozarek RA, Traverso LW: Endoscopic stent placement for cystic duct leak after laparoscopic cholecystectomy. Gastrointest Endosc 37(1):71-73, 1991.
127. Traverso LW, Kozarek RA, Ball TJ, et al: Endoscopic retrograde cholangiopancreatography after laparoscopic cholecystectomy. Am J Surg 165(5):581-586, 1993.
128. Ferguson CM, Rattner DW, Warshaw AL: Bile duct injury in laparoscopic cholecystectomy. Surg Lap Endosc Percut Tech 2(1):1-7, 1992.
129. Brooks DC, Becker JM, Connors PJ, Carr-Locke DL: Management of bile leaks following laparoscopic cholecystectomy. Surg Endosc 7(4):292-295, 1993.
130. Frakes JT, Bradley SJ: Endoscopic stent placement for biliary leak from an accessory duct of Luschka after laparoscopic cholecystectomy. Gastrointest Endosc 39(1):90-92, 1993.
131. Foutch PG, Harlan JR, Hoefer M: Endoscopic therapy for patients with a post-operative biliary leak. Gastrointest Endosc 39(3):416-421, 1993.
132. Mergener K, Strobel JC, Suhocki P, et al: The role of ERCP in diagnosis and management of accessory bile duct leaks after cholecystectomy. Gastrointest Endosc 50(4):527-531, 1999.
133. Davids PH, Rauws EA, Tytgat GN, Huibregtse K: Postoperative bile leakage: endoscopic management. Gut 33(8):1118-1122, 1992.
134. Esber EJ, Sherman S: The interface of endoscopic retrograde cholangiopancreatography and laparoscopic cholecystectomy. Gastrointest Endosc Clin North Am 6(1):57-80, 1996.
135. Binmoeller K, Katon RM, Shneidman R: Endoscopic management of postoperative biliary leaks: review of 77 cases and report of two cases with biloma formation. Am J Gastroenterol 86(2):227-231, 1991.
136. Bjorkman DJ, Carr-Locke DL, Lichtenstein DR, et al: Postsurgical bile leaks: endoscopic obliteration of the transpapillary pressure gradient is enough. Am J Gastroenterol 90(12):2128-2133, 1995.
137. Peters JH, Ollila D, Nichols KE, et al: Diagnosis and management of bile leaks following laparoscopic cholecystectomy. Surg Endosc 4(3):163-170, 1994.
138. Brandabur JJ, Kozarek RA: Endoscopic repair of bile leaks after laparoscopic cholecystectomy. Semin Ultrasound CT MR 14(5):375-381, 1993.
139. Raijman I, Catalano MF, Hirsch GS, et al: Endoscopic treatment of biliary leakage after laparoscopic cholecystectomy. Endoscopy 26(9):741-744, 1994.
140. Barton JR, Russell RC, Hatfield AR: Management of bile leaks after laparoscopic cholecystectomy. Br J Surg 82(7):980-984, 1995.
141. Bjorkman DJ, Carr-Locke DL, Lichtenstein DR, et al: Postsurgical bile leaks: endoscopic obliteration of the transpapillary pressure gradient is enough. Am J Gastroenterol 90(12):2128-2133, 1995.
142. Sherman S, Shaked A, Cryer HM, et al: Endoscopic management of biliary fistulas complicating liver transplantation and other hepatobiliary operations. Ann Surg 218(2):167-175, 1993.
143. Davids PH, Rauws EA, Coene PP, et al: Endoscopic stenting for postoperative biliary strictures. Gastrointest Endosc 38(1):12-18, 1992.
144. Berkelhammer C, Kortan P, Haber GB: Endoscopic biliary prosthesis as treatment for benign postoperative bile duct strictures. Gastrointest Endosc 35(2):95-101, 1989.
145. Geenen DJ, Geenen JE, Hogan WJ, et al: Endoscopic therapy for benign bile duct strictures. Gastrointest Endosc 35(5):367-371, 1989.
146. Davis P, et al: Benign postoperative biliary strictures: endoscopic management and long-term follow-up. Gastrointest Endosc 37:267A, 1991.
147. Deviere J, Devaere S, Baize M: Endoscopic biliary drainage in chronic pancreatitis. Gastrointest Endosc 36(2):96-100, 1990.
148. Meier P, et al: Nonoperative biliary drainage differentiates chronic pancreatitis (CP) from biliary pain in CP patients with benign bile duct strictures. Gastrointest Endosc 37:250A, 1991.

149. LaRusso NF, Wiesner RH, Ludwig J, MacCarthy RL: Primary sclerosing cholangitis. N Engl J Med 310(14):899-903, 1984.
150. Lee YM, Kaplan MM: Primary sclerosing cholangitis. N Engl J Med 14(332):924-933, 1995.
151. Wiesner RH: Current concepts in primary sclerosing cholangitis. Mayo Clin Proc 69(10):969-982, 1994.
152. Gaing AA, Geders JM, Cohen SA, et al: Endoscopic management of primary sclerosing cholangitis: review, and report of an open series. Am J Gastroenterol 88(12):2000-2008, 1993.
153. Johnson GK, Geenen JE, Venu RP, et al: Endoscopic treatment of biliary duct strictures in sclerosing cholangitis: a larger series and recommendations for treatment. Gastrointest Endosc 37(1):38-43, 1991.
154. MacCarty RL, LaRusso NF, Wiesner RH, Ludwig J: Primary sclerosing cholangitis: findings of cholangiography and pancreatography. Radiology 149(1):39-44, 1983.
155. Majoie CB, Huibregtse K, Reeders JW: Primary sclerosing cholangitis. Abdom Imaging 22(2):194-198, 1997.
156. Cotton PB, Nickl N: Endoscopic and radiologic approaches to therapy in primary sclerosing cholangitis. Semin Liver Dis 11(1):40-48, 1991.
157. Lee JG, Schutz SM, England RE, et al: Endoscopic therapy of sclerosing cholangitis. Hepatology 21(3):661-667, 1995.
158. van Milligen de Wit AW, van Bracht J, Rauws EA, et al: Endoscopic stent therapy for dominant extrahepatic bile duct strictures in primary sclerosing cholangitis. Gastrointest Endosc 44(3):293-299, 1996.
159. Siegel JH, Guelrud M: Endoscopic cholangiopancreatoplasty: hydrostatic balloon dilation in the bile duct and pancreas. Gastrointest Endosc 29(2):99-103, 1983.
160. van Milligen de Wit AW, Rauws EA, van Bracht J, et al: Short-term endoscopic stent therapy for dominant extrahepatic bile duct strictures in primary sclerosing cholangitis. Gastrointest Endosc 41:419A, 1995.
161. Huibregtse K, Katon RM, Coene PP, et al: Endoscopic palliative treatment in pancreatic cancer. Gastrointest Endosc 32(5):334-338, 1986.
162. Siegel JH, Snady H: The significance of endoscopically placed prostheses in the management of biliary obstruction due to carcinoma of the pancreas: results of nonoperative decompression in 277 patients. Am J Gastroenterol 81(8):634-641, 1986.
163. Brandabur JJ, Kozarek RA, Ball TJ, et al: Nonoperative versus operative treatment of obstructive jaundice in pancreatic cancer: cost and survival analysis. Am J Gastroenterol 83(10):1132-1139, 1988.
164. Shepherd HA, Royle G, Ross AP, et al: Endoscopic biliary endoprosthesis in the palliation of malignant obstruction of the distal common bile duct: a randomised trial. Br J Surg 75(12):1166-1168, 1988.
165. Deviere J, Baize M, de Toeuf J, et al: Long-term follow-up of patients with hilar malignant stricture treated by endoscopic internal biliary drainage. Gastrointest Endosc 34(2):95-101, 1988.
166. Andersen JR, Sorensen SM, Kruse A, et al: Randomised trial of endoscopic endoprosthesis versus operative bypass in malignant obstructive jaundice. Gut 30(8):1132-1135, 1989.
167. Dowsett JF, Russell RCG, Hatfield ARW, et al: Malignant obstructive jaundice: what is the best management? A prospective randomised trial of surgery vs endoscopic stenting. Gut 30:128, 1989.
168. Cullingford GL, Srinivasan R, Carr-Locke DL: Endoscopic endoprosthesis for malignant biliary obstruction. Gut 30:1458A, 1989.
169. Boender J, Nix GA, Schutte HE, et al: Malignant common bile duct obstruction: factors influencing the success rate of endoscopic drainage. Endoscopy 22(6):259-262, 1990.
170. Kozarek RA: Endoscopy in the management of malignant obstructive jaundice. Gastrointest Endosc Clin North Am 6(1):153-176, 1996.
171. Wagner HJ, Knyrim K, Vakil N, Klose KJ: Plastic endoprostheses versus metal stents in the palliative treatment of malignant hilar biliary obstruction. A prospective and randomized trial. Endoscopy 25(3):213-218, 1993.
172. Speer AG, Cotton PB, Russell RC, et al: Randomised trial of endoscopic versus percutaneous stent insertion in malignant obstructive jaundice. Lancet 2(8550):57-62, 1987.
173. Polydorou AA, Cairns SR, Dowsett JF, et al: Palliation of proximal malignant biliary obstruction by endoscopic endoprosthesis insertion. Gut 32(6):685-689, 1991.
174. Cheung KL, Lai EC: Endoscopic stenting for malignant biliary obstruction. Arch Surg 130(2):204-207, 1995.
175. Liu CL, Lo CM, Lai EC, Fan ST: Endoscopic retrograde cholangiopancreatography and endoscopic endoprosthesis insertion in patients with Klatskin tumors. Arch Surg 133(3):293-296, 1998.
176. Ballinger AB, McHugh M, Catnach SM, et al: Symptom relief and quality of life after stenting for malignant bile duct obstruction. Gut 35(4):467-470, 1994.
177. Sherman S, Lehman G, Earle D, et al: Endoscopic palliation of malignant bile duct obstruction: improvement in quality of life. Gastrointest Endosc 43:321A, 1996.
178. Kadakia SC, Starnes E: Comparison of 10 French gauge stent with 11.5 French gauge stent in patients with biliary tract diseases. Gastrointest Endosc 38(4):454-459, 1992.
179. Leung JW, Ling TK, Kung JL, Vallance-Owen J: The role of bacteria in the blockage of biliary stents. Gastrointest Endosc 34(1):19-22, 1988.
180. Speer AG, Cotton PB, Rhode J, et al: Biliary stent blockage with bacterial biofilm. Ann Intern Med 108(4):546-553, 1988.
181. Speer AG, Cotton PB, MacRae KD: Endoscopic management of malignant biliary obstruction: stents of 10 French gauge are preferable to stents of 8 French gauge. Gastrointest Endosc 34(5):412-417, 1988.
182. Seitz U, Vadeyar H, Soehendra N: Prolonged patency with a new-design Teflon biliary prosthesis. Endoscopy 26(5):478-482, 1994.
183. Frakes JT, Johanson JF, Stake JJ: Optimal timing for stent replacement in malignant biliary tract obstruction. Gastrointest Endosc 39(2):164-167, 1993.
184. Soehendra N, Maydeo A, Eckmann B, et al: A new technique for replacing an obstructed biliary endoprosthesis. Endoscopy 22(6):271-272, 1990.
185. Pereira-Lima JC, Jakobs R, Maier M, et al: Endoscopic biliary stenting for the palliation of pancreatic cancer: results, survival predictive factors, and comparison of 10-French with 11.5-French gauge stents. Am J Gastro (10):2179-2184, 1996.
186. Hurwich DB, Poterucha JJ, Nixon DE, et al: Preventing biliary stent occlusion. Gastrointest Endosc 38:263, 1992.
187. Leung JWC, Banez VP: Clogging of biliary stents: mechanisms and possible solutions. Dig Endosc 2:97-104, 1990.
188. Sherman S, Lehman G, Earle D, et al: Multicenter randomized trial of 10-French versus 11.5 French plastic stents for malignant bile duct obstruction. Gastrointest Endosc 43:396A, 1996.
189. Coene PPLO, Tytgat G, Obertop H, et al: Prophylactic versus symptomatic exchange of biliary stents. Gastrointest Endosc 41:394, 1995.
190. Tarnasky PR, Miller C, Mauldin P, et al: Comparison of prophylactic versus indicated stent exchange for malignant obstructive jaundice using computer modeling. Gastrointest Endosc 43:399A, 1996.
191. Lammer J: Biliary endoprosthesis. Plastic versus metal stents. Radiol Clin North Am 28(6):1211-1222, 1990.
192. Kozarek RA, Ball TJ, Patterson DJ: Metallic self-expanding stent application in the upper gastrointestinal tract: caveats and concerns. Gastrointest Endosc 38(1):1-6, 1992.
193. Jackson JE, Roddie ME, Cherry N, et al: The management of occluded metallic self-expandable biliary endoprostheses. Am J Roentgenol 157(2):291-292, 1991.
194. Shim CS, Lee MS, Kim JH, Cho SW: Endoscopic application of Gianturco-Rosch biliary Z-stent. Endoscopy 24(5):436-439, 1992.
195. Kawase Y, Takemura T, Hashimoto T: Endoscopic implantation of expandable metal Z stents for malignant biliary strictures. Gastrointest Endosc 39(1):65-67, 1993.
196. Neuhaus H, Hagenmuller F, Classen M: Self-expanding biliary stents, preliminary clinical experience. Endoscopy 21(5):225-228, 1989.
197. Huibregtse K, Carr-Locke DL, Cremer M, et al: Biliary stent occlusion–a problem solved with self-expanding metal stents? European Wallstent Study Group. Endoscopy 24(5):391-394, 1992.
198. Cotton PB: Metallic mesh stents—is the expanse worth the expense? Endoscopy 24(5):421-423, 1992.
199. Carr-Locke DL, Ball TJ, Connors PJ, et al: Multicenter randomized trial of Wallstent biliary endoprosthesis versus plastic stents. Gastrointest Endosc 39:310, 1993.
200. Davids PH, Groen AK, Rauws EA, et al: Randomised trial of self-expanding metal stents versus polyethylene stents for distal ma-

lignant biliary obstruction. Lancet 340(8834-8835):1488-1492, 1992.
201. Cremer M, Deviere J, Sugai B, Baize M: Expandable biliary metal stents for malignancies: endoscopic insertion and diathermic cleaning for tumor ingrowth. Gastrointest Endosc 36(5):451-457, 1990.
202. Dertinger S, Ell C, Fleig WE, et al: Long-term results using self-expanding metal stents for malignant biliary obstruction. Gastroenterology 102:310A, 1992.
203. Sievert CE, Silvis SE, Vennes JA, et al: Comparison of covered vs uncovered wire stents in the canine biliary tract. Gastrointest Endosc 38:262A, 1992.
204. Knyrim K, Wagner HJ, Pausch J, Vakil N: A prospective, randomized, controlled trial of metal stents for malignant obstruction of the common bile duct. Endoscopy 25(3):207-212, 1993.
205. Wagner HJ, Knyrim K, Vakil N, Klose KJ: Plastic endoprostheses versus metal stents in the palliative treatment of malignant hilar biliary obstruction. A prospective and randomized trial. Endoscopy 25(3):213-218, 1993.
206. Yeoh KG, Zimmerman MJ, Cunningham JT, et al: Comparative costs of metal versus plastic biliary stent strategies for malignant obstructive jaundice by decision analysis. Gastrointest Endosc 49(4 Pt 1):466-471, 1999.
207. Hogan WJ, Geenen JE, Dodds WJ: Dysmotility disturbances of the biliary tract: classification, diagnosis, and treatment. Semin Liver Dis 7(4):302-310, 1987.
208. Geenen JE, Hogan WJ, Dodds WJ, et al: Intraluminal pressure recording from the sphincter of Oddi. Gastroenterology 78(2):317-324, 1980.
209. Hogan WJ, Geenen JE: Biliary dyskinesia. Endoscopy 20(suppl 1):179-183, 1988.
210. Hogan WJ, Sherman S, Pasricha P, Carr-Locke D: Sphincter of Oddi manometry. Gastrointest Endosc 45(3):342-348, 1997.
211. Geenen JE, Hogan WJ, Dodds WJ, et al: The efficacy of endoscopic sphincterotomy after cholecystectomy in patients with sphincter-of-Oddi dysfunction. N Engl J Med 320(2):82-87, 1989.
212. Neoptolemos JP, Bailey IS, Carr-Locke DL: Sphincter of Oddi dysfunction: results of treatment by endoscopic sphincterotomy. Br J Surg 75(5):454-459, 1988.
213. Wehrmann T, Seifert H, Seipp M, et al: Endoscopic injection of botulinum toxin for biliary sphincter of Oddi dysfunction. Endoscopy 30(8):702-707, 1998.
214. Slivka A, Chuttani R, Carr-Locke DL, et al: Inhibition of sphincter of Oddi function by the nitric oxide carrier S-nitroso-N-acetylcysteine in rabbits and humans. J Clin Invest 94(5):1792-1798, 1994.
215. Kozarek RA: Balloon dilation of the sphincter of Oddi. Endoscopy 20(suppl 1):207-210, 1988.
216. Masci E, Toti A, Mariani S, et al: Complications of diagnostic and therapeutic ERCP: a prospective multicenter study. Am J Gastroenterol 96:417-423, 2001.
217. Neoptolemos JP, Bailey IS, Carr-Locke DL: Sphincter of Oddi dysfunction: results of treatment by endoscopic sphincterotomy. Br J Surg 75(5):454-459, 1988.
218. Tarnasky PR, Palesch YY, Cunningham JT, et al: Pancreatic stenting prevents pancreatitis after biliary sphincterotomy in patients with sphincter of Oddi dysfunction. Gastroenterology 115(6):1518-1524, 1998.
219. Baker AR, Neoptolemos JP, Carr-Locke DL, Fossard DP: Sump syndrome following choledochoduodenostomy and its endoscopic treatment. Br J Surg 72(6):433-436, 1985.
220. Marbet UA, Stalder GA, Faust H, et al: Endoscopic sphincterotomy and surgical approaches in the treatment of the 'sump syndrome.' Gut 28(2):142-145, 1987.

Index

Page references followed by "f" indicate figures, "t" indicate tables, and "b" indicate boxes

D

F

G

U